PRACTICAL MANAGEMENT OF PAIN

PRACTICAL MANAGEMENT OF PAIN

Fifth Edition

Honorio T. Benzon, MD
Professor of Anesthesiology
Associate Chair for Academic Affairs and Promotions
Northwestern University Feinberg School of Medicine
Chicago, Illinois

James P. Rathmell, MD
Professor of Anesthesia
Harvard Medical School
Vice Chair and Chief, Division of Pain Medicine
Department of Anesthesia, Critical Care, and Pain Medicine
Massachusetts General Hospital
Boston, Massachusetts

Christopher L. Wu, MD
Professor of Anesthesiology and Critical Care Medicine
Johns Hopkins School of Medicine
Baltimore, Maryland

Dennis C. Turk, PhD
John and Emma Bonica Professor of Anesthesiology and Pain Research
University of Washington School of Medicine
Director, Center for Pain Research on Impact, Measurement, and Effectiveness (C-PRIME)
Seattle, Washington

Charles E. Argoff, MD
Professor of Neurology
Director, Comprehensive Pain Management Center
Albany Medical College
Albany, New York

Robert W. Hurley, MD, PhD
Professor of Anesthesiology
Chief, Division of Pain Medicine
Medical Director, University of Florida Pain and Spine Center
University of Florida College of Medicine
Gainesville, Florida

ELSEVIER
MOSBY

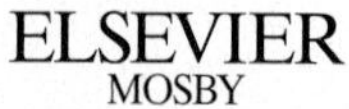

ELSEVIER
MOSBY

1600 John F. Kennedy Blvd.
Ste 1800
Philadelphia, PA 19103-2899

PRACTICAL MANAGEMENT OF PAIN ISBN: 978-0-323-08340-9

Notices

Knowledge and best practice in this field are constantly changing. As new research and experience broaden our understanding, changes in research methods, professional practices, or medical treatment may become necessary.

Practitioners and researchers must always rely on their own experience and knowledge in evaluating and using any information, methods, compounds, or experiments described herein. In using such information or methods they should be mindful of their own safety and the safety of others, including parties for whom they have a professional responsibility.

With respect to any drug or pharmaceutical products identified, readers are advised to check the most current information provided (i) on procedures featured or (ii) by the manufacturer of each product to be administered, to verify the recommended dose or formula, the method and duration of administration, and contraindications. It is the responsibility of practitioners, relying on their own experience and knowledge of their patients, to make diagnoses, to determine dosages and the best treatment for each individual patient, and to take all appropriate safety precautions.

To the fullest extent of the law, neither the Publisher nor the authors, contributors, or editors, assume any liability for any injury and/or damage to persons or property as a matter of products liability, negligence or otherwise, or from any use or operation of any methods, products, instructions, or ideas contained in the material herein.

Library of Congress Cataloging-in-Publication Data

Practical management of pain / [edited by] Honorio T. Benzon ... [et al.]. – 5th ed.
p. ; cm.
Rev. ed. of: Raj's practical management of pain / [edited by] Honorio T. Benzon ... [et al.].
4th ed. 2008.
Includes bibliographical references and index.
ISBN 978-0-323-08340-9 (hardcover : alk. paper)
I. Benzon, Honorio T. II. Raj's practical management of pain.
[DNLM: 1. Pain Management. WL 704.6]
RB127
616'.0472–dc23 2013014564

Publishing Manager: Michael Houston
Senior Content Development Specialist: Joan Ryan
Publishing Services Manager: Patricia Tannian
Senior Project Manager: Sharon Corell
Senior Designer: Ellen Zanolle

Printed in China

Last digit is the print number: 9 8 7 6 5 4 3 2 1

To my family–Juliet, Hazel, Paul, Annalisa, Jonathan, Hubert, and Nathalie.
To those who helped me succeed–Ed Brunner, Ben Covino, Gerry Ostheimer, Dave Brown, Jim Rathmell, Admir Hadzic, and Tim Deer.
To my co-editors, your expertise is invaluable and your hard work is very much appreciated.

Honorio T. Benzon, MD

To Nori Benzon, who once again led this project with patience, persistence, and kindness; it is a privilege and pleasure to work with you always.
To Warren Zapol and Jeanine Wiener-Kronish, who have served as critical supporters and guides.
To my wife and children—Bobbi, Lauren, James, and Cara—thank you.

James P. Rathmell, MD

To my parents, Shy-Hsien and Tsai-Lien Wu and Chi-Jen and Sue-Yuan Lee, my wife, Lucia, and my children, Emily and Alex.

Christopher L. Wu, MD

To my many students, collaborators, and colleagues who have contributed to my understanding of the plight of "normal" people who find themselves in unimaginable circumstances. They have truly enriched the journey. And to Lorraine M. Turk, more than a wife, a partner, and my best friend, for her consistent and unyielding patience, tolerance, sacrifices, and understanding throughout our marriage.

Dennis C. Turk, PhD

To my wife and best friend, Pat, for your constant understanding and incessant patience throughout our relationship.
To our children, David, Melanie and Emily. Your support of my professional activities is so appreciated, and I look forward to your continued development of those interests and activities that you are truly passionate about.
To Nori Benzon for asking me to be a part of this amazing project and for his determination and diligence in assuring its completion.
To Robert Y. Moore, MD, PhD, Roscoe Brady, MD, John Halperin, MD, and Michael Gruenthal, MD, PhD, for your encouragement and counsel throughout my career.

Charles E. Argoff, MD

To my wife, Meredith, and my two children, Gibson and Alexandra, who make me smile every time they enter my thoughts.
To Nori Benzon, MD, Steve Cohen, MD, Chris Wu, MD, and Donna Hammond, PhD, who are mentors and friends. I feel nothing but gratitude for their support and guidance over the years.
To Nori and all of the co-editors, it has been an honor and privilege to work on this project.

Robert W. Hurley, MD, PhD

Contributors

Bernard M. Abrams, MD
Clinical Professor
Department of Neurology
University of Missouri-Kansas City
Village of Loch Lloyd, Missouri

Meredith C.B. Adams, MD
Assistant Professor
Departments of Anesthesiology, Psychiatry, and Neurology
University of Florida
Gainesville, Florida

Ashley Agerson, MD
Assistant Professor
Department of Anesthesia
Northwestern University Feinberg School of Medicine
Chicago, Illinois

Dustin Anderson, MD
Resident, Department of Anesthesiology
The University of Florida College of Medicine
Gainesville, Florida

Magdalena Anitescu, MD, PhD
Associate Professor
Director, Pain Management Fellowship Program
Department of Anesthesia and Critical Care
University of Chicago Medical Center
Chicago, Illinois

A. Vania Apkarian, PhD
Professor
Department of Physiology
Northwestern University Feinberg School of Medicine
Chicago, Illinois

Charles E. Argoff, MD
Professor of Neurology
Director, Comprehensive Pain Management Center
Albany Medical College
Albany, New York

Juan Francisco Asenjo, MD
Associate Professor
Department of Anesthesia and Alan Edwards McGill Pain Center
Director, Regional Anesthesia and Spine Perioperative Fellowships
McGill University Health Center
Montreal, Quebec, Canada

John A. Bailey, MD
Medical Director
Pain Care Physicians of Charleston, LLC
Charleston, South Carolina

Stephen J. Bekanich, MD
Associate Professor of Medicine
Medical Director, Palliative Care Services
University of Miami Miller School of Medicine
Miami, Florida

Benoy Benny, MD
Associate Professor
Director, Spine and Sports Medicine
Department of Physical Medicine and Rehabilitation
Baylor College of Medicine
Houston, Texas

Honorio T. Benzon, MD
Professor of Anesthesiology
Associate Chair for Academic Affairs and Promotions
Northwestern University Feinberg School of Medicine
Chicago, Illinois

Klaus Bielefeldt, MD
Associate Professor of Medicine
Division of Gastroenterology
Department of Internal Medicine
Center for Pain Research
University of Pittsburgh School of Medicine
Pittsburgh, Pennsylvania

Brian Birmingham, MD
Assistant Professor
Department of Anesthesiology
Rush Medical College
Associate Clinical Director
Department of Anesthesiology
Rush University Medical Center
Chicago, Illinois

Michael M. Bottros, MD
Assistant Professor of Anesthesiology and Pain Medicine
Washington University School of Medicine
St. Louis, Missouri

Randall P. Brewer, MD
River Cities Interventional Pain Specialists
Willis-Knighton Health System
Shreveport, Louisiana

Jason C. Brookman, MD
Assistant Professor
Department of Anesthesiology and Critical Care
Division of Regional Anesthesia and Acute Pain
Johns Hopkins School of Medicine
Baltimore, Maryland

David L. Brown, MD
Chairman
Anesthesiology Institute
Cleveland Clinic
Cleveland, Ohio

Chad M. Brummett, MD
Assistant Professor
Director, Pain Research
Department of Anesthesiology
Division of Pain Medicine
University of Michigan Health System
Ann Arbor, Michigan

Kim J. Burchiel, MD
Department of Neurological Surgery
Oregon Health & Science University
Portland, Oregon

Allen W. Burton, MD
Houston Pain Associates
Houston, Texas

Asokumar Buvanendran, MD, MBBS
Professor
Department of Anesthesiology
Director of Orthopedic Anesthesia
Rush University Medical Center
Chicago, Illinois

Alex Cahana, MD
Professor
Department of Anesthesiology and Pain Medicine
Center for Pain Relief
University of Washington Medical Center
Seattle, Washington

Kenneth D. Candido, MD
Chairman and Professor
Department of Anesthesiology
University of Illinois College of Medicine
Advocate, Illinois Masonic Medical Center
Chicago, Illinois

James Celestin, MD
Harvard Vanguard Medical Associates
Boston, Massachusetts

Kwai-Tung Chan, MD
Baylor College of Medicine
Houston, Texas

Ronil V. Chandra, MBBS
Department of Neuro-interventional Radiology
Massachusetts General Hospital
Boston, Massachusetts

Kailash Chandwani, MD
Institute for Pain Diagnostics and Care
Ohio Valley General Hospital
Pittsburgh, Pennsylvania

Delia Chiaramonte, MD
Clinical Assistant Professor
Director of Education
Center for Integrative Medicine
University of Maryland School of Medicine
Baltimore, Maryland

Roger Chou, MD
Associate Professor
Department of Medical Informatics and Clinical Epidemiology
Scientific Director
Oregon Evidence-Based Practice Center
Oregon Health and Science University
Portland, Oregon

Daniel Clauw, MD
Professor
Department of Anesthesiology and Medicine (Rheumatology)
University of Michigan
Ann Arbor, Michigan

Steven P. Cohen, MD
Professor, Walter Reed National Military Medical Center
Bethesda, Maryland
Professor, Division of Pain Management
Department of Anesthesiology and Critical Care Medicine
Johns Hopkins School of Medicine
Baltimore, Maryland

David Copenhaver, MD, MPH
Director of Cancer Pain Management
Assistant Professor of Anesthesiology and Pain Medicine
University of California, Davis,
School of Medicine
Lawrence J. Ellison Ambulatory Care Center
Sacramento, California

Megan H. Cortazzo, MD
University of Pittsburgh Physicians
Department of Physical Medicine and Rehabilitation
Rehab Medicine Center
Pittsburgh, Pennsylvania

Edward C. Covington, MD
Director, Chronic Pain Rehabilitation
Cleveland Clinic
Cleveland, Ohio

Nessa Coyle, RN, PhD
Pain and Palliative Care Service
Department of Medicine
Memorial Sloan-Kettering Cancer Center
New York, New York

Chris D'Adamo, PhD
Assistant Professor
Department of Family and Community Medicine
Department of Epidemiology and Public Health
Assistant Director of Medical Education
University of Maryland School of Medicine
Center for Integrative Medicine
Baltimore, Maryland

Carlton Dampier, MD, CPI
Professor of Pediatrics
Emory University School of Medicine
Co-Director, Pediatric Program, and Director, Ethics and Regulatory Program, Atlanta
Clinical and Translational Science Institute
Aflac Cancer and Blood Disorders Center
Atlanta, Georgia

Miles Day, MD
Professor
Department of Anesthesiology and Pain Medicine
Medical Director, The Pain Center at Grace Clinic
Texas Tech University HSC
Lubbock, Texas

Oscar de Leon-Casasola, MD
Professor of Anesthesiology and Medicine
Vice-Chair for Clinical Affairs
Department of Anesthesiology
University of Buffalo School of Medicine
Chief, Pain Medicine and Professor of Oncology
Roswell Park Cancer Institute
Buffalo, New York

Andrew Dubin, MD
Associate Professor
Department of Physical Medicine and Rehabilitation
Albany Medical College
Albany, New York

Michael A. Erdek, MD
Program Director
Division of Pain Medicine
Johns Hopkins School of Medicine
Baltimore, Maryland

Vania E. Fernandez, MD
Attending Physician, Miami VA Medical Center
Assistant Professor of Clinical Anesthesiology
Clinical Director, UMH Chronic Pain Service
Assistant Program Director, Pain Management Fellowship
University of Miami Miller School of Medicine
Miami, Florida

Perry G. Fine, MD
Professor of Anesthesiology
Pain Research Center
School of Medicine
University of Utah
Salt Lake City, Utah

Scott M. Fishman, MD
Professor and Vice Chair
Department of Anesthesiology and Pain Medicine
Chief, Division of Pain Medicine
University of California, Davis
School of Medicine
Lawrence J. Ellison Ambulatory Care Center
Sacramento, California

Julie S. Franklin, MD
Director, Pain Service
White River Junction, Vermont

Timothy Furnish, MD
Assistant Clinical Professor
Division of Pain Medicine
Department of Anesthesiology
University of California, San Diego Medical Center
San Diego, California

Vicente Garcia Tomas, MD
Assistant Professor of Anesthesiology and Critical Care Medicine
The Johns Hopkins Hospital
Baltimore, Maryland

Robert J. Gatchel, PhD
Nancy P. and John G. Penson Endowed Professor of Clinical Health Psychology
Professor and Chairman
Department of Psychology
College of Science
The University of Texas at Arlington
Arlington, Texas

G.F. Gebhart, PhD
Director, Center for Pain Research
Departments of Anesthesiology and Neurobiology
University of Pittsburgh School of Medicine
Pittsburgh, Pennsylvania

Myra Glajchen, DSW
Assistant Professor
The Saul R. Korey Department of Neurology and the Department of Anesthesiology
Albert Einstein College of Medicine
Bronx, New York
Director, Institute for Education and Training in Pain and Palliative Care
Co-Director, Fellowship Training Programs
Department of Pain Medicine and Palliative Care
Beth Israel Medical Center
New York, New York

Michael Gofeld, MD
Assistant Professor
University of Toronto
Pain Management Program, Palliative Care Initiative
Sunnybrook Health Sciences Centre
Toronto, Ontario, Canada

Rachael Gooberman-Hill, PhD
Senior Research Fellow
Musculoskeletal Health Unit
School of Clinical Sciences
University of Bristol
Bristol Implant Research Centre
Southmead Hospital
Westbury-on-Trym
Bristol, United Kingdom

Andrew H. Gordon, MD
Resident, Department of Physical Medicine and Rehabilitation
Johns Hopkins School of Medicine
Baltimore, Maryland

Martin Grabois, MD
Professor and Chairman
Department of Physical Medicine and Rehabilitation
Baylor College of Medicine
Houston, Texas

Carmen R. Green, MD, MPH
Professor, Health Management and Policy
Professor, Anesthesiology
Professor, Obstetrics and Gynecology
Department of Anesthesiology
University of Michigan
Ann Arbor, Michigan

Anil Gupta, MD, PhD
Associate Professor
Department of Anesthesiology and Intensive Care
Institution for Medicine and Health
University Hospital
Örebro, Sweden

Admir Hadzic, MD, PhD
Professor of Clinical Anesthesiology
College of Physicians and Surgeons
Columbia University
St. Lukes-Roosevelt Hospital
New York, New York

Robbie Haggard, MS, LPC-S
Social Science Research Associate
University of Texas at Arlington
Arlington, Texas

Marie N. Hanna, MD
Associate Professor
Department of Anesthesia and Critical Care Medicine
Director, Regional Anesthesia and Acute Pain Management
The Johns Hopkins University
Baltimore, Maryland

R. Norman Harden, MD
Addison Chair in Pain Studies
Director, Center for Pain Studies
Rehabilitation Institute of Chicago
Associate Professor
Department of Physical Medicine and Rehabilitation
Northwestern University
Chicago, Illinois

Simon Haroutiunian, MD
Danish Pain Research Center
Aarhus University Hospital
Aarhus, Denmark

Richard L. Harvey, MD
Medical Director, Center for Stroke Rehabilitation
The Rehabilitation Institute of Chicago
Chicago, Illinois

Alicia Heapy, PhD
Assistant Professor of Psychiatry
Yale School of Medicine
New Haven, Connecticut

Omar H. Henriquez, MD
Anesthesiology Resident
Department of Anesthesiology
University of Florida
Gainesville, Florida

Joshua A. Hirsch, MD
Chief, Minimally Invasive Spine Surgery
Department of Radiology
Massachusetts General Hospital
Boston, Massachusetts

Marc A. Huntoon, MD
Professor, Department of Anesthesiology
Chief, Division of Pain Medicine
Vanderbilt University
VUMC Interventional Pain Center
Nashville, Tennessee

Robert W. Hurley, MD, PhD
Professor of Anesthesiology
Chief, Division of Pain Medicine
Medical Director, University of Florida Pain and Spine Center
University of Florida College of Medicine
Gainesville, Florida

Mohammed Issa, MD
Clinical Fellow in Anaesthesia
Brigham and Women's Hospital
Boston, Massachusetts

Kenneth C. Jackson, II, PharmD
Associate Dean, Professor
School of Pharmacy
Pacific University
Hillsboro, Oregon

Benjamin W. Johnson, Jr., MD, MBA
Department of Anesthesiology
Vanderbilt University
Nashville, Tennessee

Leonardo Kapural, MD, PhD
Professor, Department of Anesthesiology
Wake Forest University School of Medicine
Medical Director
Carolinas Pain Institute
Wake Forest University Health Sciences Chronic Pain Center
Winston-Salem, North Carolina

Robert D. Kerns, PhD
National Program Director for Pain Management
Veterans Health Administration Director
VA Connecticut Healthcare System
Professor of Psychiatry, Neurology, and Psychology, Yale University
Pain Research, Informatics, Medical Comorbities, Education (PRIME) Center
West Haven, Connecticut

Farooq Khan, MD
OSF Saint Elizabeth Medical Center
Ottawa, Illinois

Amy J. Kirsling, MPA
Northwestern University School of Medicine
Department of Physical Medicine and Rehabilitation
Chicago, Illinois

Kanupriya Kumar, MD
Assistant Professor of Anesthesiology and Critical Care Medicine
Department of Anesthesiology and Critical Care Medicine
Johns Hopkins School of Medicine
Baltimore, Maryland

Kwesi Kwofie, MD
Regional Anesthesia Fellow
Department of Anesthesiology
St. Luke's-Roosevelt Hospital Center
New York, New York

Irfan Lalani, MD, PA
Interventional Pain, Neurodiagnostics and Rehabilitation
Methodist Sugar Land Hospital
Sugar Land, Texas

Jennifer M. Lee, MD
Resident, Department of Anesthesiology and Pain Medicine
University of Washington
Seattle, Washington

Thabele M. Leslie-Mazwi, MD
Department of Interventional Neuroradiology
Massachusetts General Hospital
Boston, Massachusetts

Yuan-Chi Lin, MD, MPH
Associate Professor of Anaesthesia and Pediatrics
Harvard Medical School
Director, Medical Acupuncture Service
Senior Associate in Anesthesia and Pain Medicine
Boston Children's Hospital
Boston, Massachusetts

Matthew J.P. LoDico, MD
Fellow in Pain Medicine
Department of Anesthesiology
University at Buffalo School of Medicine
Buffalo, New York

Khalid Malik, MD
Associate Professor
Anesthesiology, Pain, and Critical Care Medicine
Northwestern University Feinberg School of Medicine
Chicago, Illinois

Asha Manohar, MD
Assistant Professor of Anesthesiology and Critical Care Medicine
The Johns Hopkins Hospital
Baltimore, Maryland

Edward R. Mariano, MD, MAS
Associate Professor of Anesthesiology
Stanford University School of Medicine
Stanford, California

Timothy P. Maus, MD
Department of Radiology
Mayo Clinic
Rochester, Minnesota

Gary McCleane, MD
Consultant in Pain Management
Rampark Pain Centre
Northern Ireland, United Kingdom

Brian E. McGeeney, MD, MPH
Assistant Professor of Neurology
Boston University School of Medicine
Boston, Massachusetts

Noshir R. Mehta, DMD, MDS, MS
Professor and Associate Dean, International Relations
Chairman, Department of General Dentistry
Director, Craniofacial Pain Center
Tufts University School of Dental Medicine
Boston, Massachusetts

Sonal Mehta, MD
Assistant Professor of Medicine
Division of Geriatrics and Gerontology
Weill Cornell Medical College
New York, New York

Douglas G. Merrill, MD, MBA
Professor of Anesthesiology
Dartmouth Medical School
Director, The Center for Perioperative Services
Medical Director, Outpatient Surgery
Dartmouth-Hitchcock Medical Center
Lebanon, New Jersey

Harold Merskey, MD
Professor Emeritus
Department of Psychiatry
University of Western Ontario
London, Ontario, Canada

James R. Miner, MD
Emergency Medicine
Hennepin County Medical Center
Minneapolis, Minnesota

Brian Morrison, DC
Morrison Chiropractic
Ellicott City, Maryland

Geeta Nagpal, MD
Assistant Professor of Anesthesiology
Northwestern University Feinberg School of Medicine
Chicago, Illinois

Patrick Narchi, MD
Anesthesia Department
Soyaux Centre Clinical
Soyaux, France

Joseph M. Neal, MD
Department of Anesthesiology
Virginia Mason Medical Center
Clinical Professor of Anesthesiology
University of Washington
Seattle, Washington

Barry Nicholls, MD
Taunton and Somerset NHS Foundation Trust
Musgrove Park Hospital
Taunton, Somerset
United Kingdom

Lone Nikolajsen, MD, PhD
Danish Pain Research Center
Aarhus University Hospital
Aarhus, Denmark

Jean-Pierre P. Ouanes, DO
Assistant Professor
Department of Anesthesiology and Critical Care Medicine
Johns Hopkins School of Medicine
Baltimore, Maryland

Xavier Paqueron, MD, PhD
Anesthesia Department
Soyaux Centre Clinical
Soyaux, France

Sagar S. Parikh, MD
Department of Medicine
Saint Peter's University Hospital
New Brunswick, New Jersey

Winston C.V. Parris, MD
University Hospital and Medical Center
Tamarac, Florida

Meenal Patil, MD
Assistant Professor of Clinical Anesthesiology
Division of Pain Medicine
Vanderbilt University
VUMC Interventional Pain Center
Nashville, Tennessee

Frederick M. Perkins, MD
Chief, Anesthesia
VA Medical Center
White River Junction, Vermont

David A. Provenzano, MD
Executive Director
Institute for Pain Diagnostics and Care
Ohio Valley General Hospital
McKees Rocks, Pennsylvania

James D. Rabinov, MD
Department of Radiology
Massachusetts General Hospital
Boston, Massachusetts

Mohammed Ranavaya, MD
Professor of Occupational and Environmental Medicine
Marshall University School of Medicine
Huntington, West Virginia

Ahmed M. Raslan, MD
Assistant Professor
Department of Neurological Surgery
Oregon Health and Science University
Portland, Oregon

James P. Rathmell, MD
Professor of Anesthesiology
Harvard Medical School
Vice Chair and Chief, Division of Pain Medicine
Department of Anesthesia, Critical Care, and Pain Medicine
Massachusetts General Hospital
Boston, Massachusetts

M. Cary Reid, MD, PhD
Associate Professor of Medicine
Division of Geriatrics and Gerontology
Weill Cornell Medical College
New York, New York

W. Evan Rivers, DO
Assistant Professor of Neurosurgery
University of New Mexico School of Medicine
Albuquerque, New Mexico

Robert D. Rondinelli, MD, PhD
Medical Director, Rehabilitation Services
Iowa Health System
Des Moines, Iowa

Marta J. Rozanski, MD
Research Fellow in Anaesthesia
Massachusetts General Hospital
Boston, Massachusetts

Francis V. Salinas, MD
Department of Anesthesiology
Virginia Mason Medical Center
Seattle, Washington

Emine Aysu Salviz, MD
Resident
Department of Anesthesiology
Columbia University College of Physicians and Surgeons
New York, New York

Amod Sawardekar, MD
Assistant Professor of Anesthesiology
Northwestern University's Feinberg School of Medicine
Ann and Robert H. Lurie Children's Hospital of Chicago
Chicago, Illinois

Pat Schofield, PhD
Professor of Nursing
School of Health and Social Care
University of Greenwich
London, United Kingdom

Steven J. Scrivani, DDS, DMedSc
Clinical Professor
The Craniofacial Pain and Headache Center
Tufts University School of Dental Medicine
Adjunct, Department of Public Health and Community Medicine
Pain Research, Education and Policy Program
Tufts University School of Medicine
Boston, Massachusetts
Research Associate
Pain and Analgesia Imaging and Neuroscience Group
Brain Imaging Center
McLean Hospital
Belmont, Massachusetts

Elizabeth Seng, MS
Graduate Student
Clinical Health Psychology
Ohio University
Athens, Ohio

Ravi Shah, MD
Assistant Professor of Anesthesiology
Northwestern University Feinberg School of Medicine
Attending Physician
Lurie Children's Hospital
Chicago, Illinois

Hariharan Shankar, MD
Associate Professor
Department of Anesthesiology
Medical College of Wisconsin
Program Director, Pain Medicine Fellowship Program
Director, Pain Clinic
Department of Anesthesiology
Clement Zablocki VA Medical Center
Milwaukee, Wisconsin

Vandana Sharma, MD
Fellow in Pain Medicine
Department of Anesthesiology
Buffalo, New York

Uma Shastri, MD
Regional Anesthesia Fellow
New York School of Regional Anesthesia
Department of Anesthesiology
St. Luke's-Roosevelt Hospital Center
New York, New York

Stephen D. Silberstein, MD
Professor of Neurology
Jefferson Headache Center
Philadelphia, Pennsylvania

François Singelyn, MD, PhD
Anesthesia Department
Soyaux Centre Clinical
Soyaux, France

Howard S. Smith, MD
Albany Medical Center
The Neurosciences Institute
Albany, New York

Melanie B. Smith, PA-C
River Cities Interventional Pain Specialists
Shreveport, Louisiana

Egilius L.H. Spierings, MD, PhD, CPI
Associate Clinical Professor
Consulting Neurologist
Craniofacial Pain and Headache Center
Tufts University School of Dental Medicine
Boston, Massachusetts
Director and Principal Investigator
MedVadis Research Corporation
Watertown, Massachusetts

Jeanette S. Springer, MD
Danish Pain Research Center
Aarhus University Hospital
Aarhus, Denmark

Steven P. Stanos, DO
Medical Director
Chronic Pain Care Center
Rehabilitation Institute of Chicago
Northwestern University Fienberg School of Medicine
Department of Physical Medicine and Rehabilitation
Chicago, Illinois

Carrie Stewart, BSc
Centre of Academic Primary Care
University of Aberdeen
Aberdeen, United Kingdom

Santhanam Suresh, MD
Chairman
Department of Pediatric Anesthesiology
Director, Pain Management Team
Professor of Anesthesiology and Pediatrics
Northwestern University Feinberg School of Medicine
Lurie Children's Hospital of Chicago
Chicago, Illinois

David Tauben, MD
Departments of Internal Medicine and Anesthesiology and Pain Medicine
Director, Center for Pain Relief
University of Washington
Seattle, Washington

Gregory W. Terman, MD, PhD
Professor and Director of Pain Medicine Research
Department of Anesthesiology and Pain Medicine
Professor, Graduate Program in Neurobiology and Behavior
University of Washington
Seattle, Washington

Brian R. Theodore, PhD
Acting Instructor
Department of Anesthesiology and Pain Medicine
University of Washington
Seattle, Washington

Katrina M. Thomas, MD
Northwestern University School of Medicine
Department of Physical Medicine and Rehabilitation
Chicago, Illinois

Knox H. Todd, MD, MPH
Chair, Department of Emergency Medicine
MD Anderson Cancer Center
Houston, Texas

Vincente Garcia Tomas, MD
Instructor
Department of Anesthesiology and Critical Care Medicine
Johns Hopkins School of Medicine
Baltimore, Maryland

Dennis C. Turk, PhD
John and Emma Bonica Professor of Anesthesiology and Pain Research
University of Washington School of Medicine
Director, Center for Pain Research on Impact, Measurement, and Effectiveness (C-PRIME)
Seattle, Washington

Mark D. Tyburski, MD
Department of Physical Medicine and Rehabilitation
The Permanente Medical Group
Roseville Medical Center
Roseville, California

Meredith G. van der Velden, MD
Instructor in Anaesthesia
Children's Hospital
Boston, Massachusetts

Maarten van Eerd, MD
Department of Anesthesiology and Pain Management
University Medical Centre Maastricht
Maastricht, The Netherlands

Maarten van Kleef, MD, PhD
Department of Anesthesiology and Pain Management
Maastricht University Medical Centre
Maastricht, The Netherlands

Jan Van Zundert, MD, PhD
Department of Anesthesiology and Multidisciplinary Pain Centre
Ziekenhuis Oost-Limburg
Campus André Dumont
Genk, Belgium

Renata Variakojis, MD
President
The Center for Pain Treatment
Palos Heights, Illinois

Jeanine A. Verbunt, MD, PhD
Adelante Center of Expertise in Rehabilitation and Audiology
Maastricht University
Hoensbroek, The Netherlands

Thomas R. Vetter, MD, MPH
Maurice S. Albin Professor of Anesthesiology
Vice Chair and Director of Division of Pain Medicine
Medical Director, UAB Preoperative Assessment, Consultation and Treatment Clinic
Quality and Safety Officer, UAB Hospital Highlands
Associate Professor of Pediatrics
Associate Professor of Health Policy and Organization
University of Alabama at Birmingham
Birmingham, Alabama

David B. Waisel, MD
Associate Professor of Anaesthesia
Harvard Medical School
Program Director
Pediatric Anesthesiology Fellowship
Children's Hospital
Boston, Massachusetts

Howard J. Waldman, DO
Mid-America Physiatrists
Leawood, Kansas

Mark S. Wallace, MD
Professor of Clinical Anesthesiology
Chief, Division of Pain Medicine
Department of Anesthesiology
University of California, San Diego
La Jolla, California

Ajay D. Wasan, MD, Msc
Assistant Professor
Harvard Medical School
Brigham and Women's Hospital
Pain Management Center
Chestnut Hill, Massachusetts

Karin N. Westlund, PhD
Professor, Department of Physiology
University of Kentucky
Lexington, Kentucky

Harriët M. Wittink, PhD, MS, PT
Research Group Lifestyle and Health
Faculty of Health Care
Utrecht University of Applied Sciences
Utrecht, The Netherlands

Christopher L. Wu, MD
Professor of Anesthesiology and Critical Care Medicine
Johns Hopkins School of Medicine
Baltimore, Maryland

Daquan Xu, MD, MBBS
The New York School of Regional Anesthesia
New York, New York

Tony L. Yaksh, PhD
Professor of Anesthesiology and Pharmacology
University of California, San Diego
School of Medicine
San Diego, California

Robert P. Yezierski, PhD
Director of Education
Pain Research and Intervention Center of Excellence
Professor of Orthodontics, Neuroscience, and Anesthesiology
University of Florida
Gainesville, Florida

Albert J. Yoo, MD
Department of Radiology
Massachusetts General Hospital
Boston, Massachusetts

Preface

This, the fifth edition of the *Practical Management of Pain,* provides cutting-edge developments in pain medicine and reflects maturity of this medical specialty as it has progressed since earlier editions. As in the previous edition, the Editors represent the specialties of anesthesiology, psychology, and neurology that, together with physical medicine and rehabilitation and psychiatry, provide the core of pain medicine. In addition, we recruited Robert Hurley, MD, PhD, to join us as an editor. Rob brings an added perspective to the book. He is knowledgeable in the pharmacological management of acute and chronic pain, performs interventional techniques, and has conducted basic science pain research.

The current edition retains the format of the previous volume. It includes sections on general considerations, basic aspects, evaluation and assessment, clinical conditions, pharmacologic, psychological, and physical medicine treatments, nerve block techniques, interventional techniques, and pain management in special situations. The topics represent the multidisciplinary nature of pain medicine. Similar to the previous edition, the fifth includes an international group of authors, recognizing the scientific contributions of experts from around the world. We have expanded the number of chapters from 72 to 83 with the new chapters covering ultrasound-guided techniques in regional anesthesiology and pain management procedures. In addition to the suggested reading list, there is an extensive set of references in supplementary materials accompanying the published volume.

This volume is intended for the diverse range of pain clinicians looking for applications in their daily practice, pain researchers seeking extensive background on relevant topics, fellows reviewing for the pain medicine boards, and residents who want a complete discussion of the breadth of the field. Each chapter provides practical applications of the various and diverse acute and chronic pain syndromes. Throughout the volume there are distillations of research on all relevant aspects of pain medicine, including current knowledge of mechanisms involved and strategies for assessing and treating patients with chronic pain.

A project of this magnitude could not come to fruition without the efforts and assistance of a large number of people, and the result is truly a team effort. The contributors took time out of their busy academic, clinical, and administrative responsibilities to prepare their chapters. The editors spent an enormous amount of time finalizing the book. Our publishing team at Elsevier, led by Publishing Manager Michael Houston, Senior Content Developmental Specialist Joan Ryan, and Senior Project Manager Sharon Corell, did an excellent job of developing the book and keeping it on track. On a personal note, it is a delight to work with Michael Houston again as he was Dr. Benzon's executive publisher in the first book that he edited, *Essentials of Pain Medicine.* We hope that you will agree that our collective efforts have resulted in an up-to-date, practical, and comprehensive volume worthy of your attention.

The Editors

Contents

PRACTICAL MANAGEMENT OF PAIN

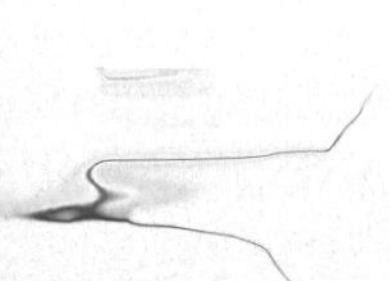

PART 1

GENERAL CONSIDERATIONS

HONORIO T. BENZON, EDITOR

PART OUTLINE

1 The History of Pain Medicine

Winston C.V. Parris | Benjamin W. Johnson, Jr.

History is a distillation of rumor.

THOMAS CARLYLE (1795-1881)

Management of pain, like management of disease, is as old as the human race. In the view of Christians, the fall of Adam and Eve in the Garden of Eden produced for man (and woman) a long life of suffering disease and pain. This one act allegedly set the stage for several disease concepts, including the experience of pain in labor and delivery; the concept that hard work is painful; the notion that blood, sweat, and tears are needed to produce fruit; the introduction of pain and disease to human existence; establishment of the fact that hell and its fires are painful; and the expectation that heaven is pure, delightful, spiritually pleasing, and of course, pain free. In these concepts, pain is viewed as a negative experience and one that is associated with disease, morbidity, and the dying process. Many diseases, including infections, plagues, metabolic disorders (e.g., diabetes mellitus), endocrine disorders, hypertension, and cancer, of course, afflict humankind spontaneously and usually cause significant pain without any wrongdoing, negligence, or irresponsibility on the part of the afflicted person.

As we consider the historical perspective, humans have deliberately and knowingly inflicted on one another many experiences associated with pain—from the earliest wars to the more recent irrational shooting incidents in the Arkansas and Oregon public school systems, from the scourging of Jesus to contemporary strife in the Middle East, the Rwandan genocide, the Irish "religious" fratricide, and the conflicts in Bosnia and the Balkans. All wars, including the great wars, World War I and World War II, the American Civil War, the Korean War, and the Vietnam War, have been associated with untold pain, suffering, and death.

Although we as human beings have not learned from these painful episodes and continue to inflict pain on others, the advances and increasing sophistication of the 21st century have brought about new concepts of disease and the painful states that diseases produce. The social illnesses—venereal diseases; the pulmonary, cardiovascular, and neoplastic consequences of smoking; the trauma associated with automobile accidents; the pathology caused by drug abuse and misuse; and the proliferation of viral illnesses (e.g., acquired immunodeficiency syndrome)—have all contributed further pain and suffering to our lot. Therefore, any review of history and politics, economics, and the social interrelationships of the world is inevitably a review of the history of pain. This chapter focuses on some of the major historical events that have influenced pain, its development, and its management and highlights the important phases that have led to the current conceptualization of pain and its treatment as an independent specialty in modern medicine.

PAIN AND RELIGION

The early concept of pain as a form of punishment from supreme spiritual beings for sin and evil activity is as old as the human race.[1] In the book of *Genesis*, God told Eve that following her fall from grace she would endure pain during childbirth: "I will greatly multiply your pain in childbearing; in pain you shall bring forth children, yet your desire shall be for your husband and he shall rule over you" (Genesis 3:16). This condemnation led early Christians to accept pain as a normal consequence of Eve's action and to view this consequence as being directly transferred to them. Thus any attempt to decrease the pain associated with labor and delivery was treated by early Christians with disdain and disapproval. It was not until 1847, when Queen Victoria was administered chloroform by James Simpson[2] for the delivery of her eighth child, Prince Leopold, that contemporary Christians and in particular Protestants accepted the notion that it was not heretical to promote painless childbirth as part of the obstetric process.

From the Old Testament, Job has been praised for his endurance of pain and suffering. Yet Job's friends wondered whether these tribulations were an indication that he had committed some great sin for which God was punishing him (Job 5:17). Nonetheless, Job was considered a faithful servant by God and was not guilty of any wrongdoing. In fact, he was described as a man who was "blameless and upright" and one who feared God and turned away from evil.[3]

In the 5th century, St. Augustine wrote that "all diseases of Christians are to be ascribed to demons; chiefly do they torment the fresh baptized, yea, even the guiltless newborn infant," thus implying that not even innocent infants escape the work of demons. Today, major typhoons, hurricanes, fires, earthquakes, volcanoes, tsunamis, floods, and droughts destroy hundreds and at times thousands of innocent, defenseless people. One ponders the rationale of such pain and suffering endured by otherwise good people while seemingly ruthless and evil persons apparently triumph and prosper in an atmosphere of luxury and comfort.

This paradox can be discouraging at times but is usually upheld by firm Christian belief. In the 1st century, many people who belonged to the Catholic Church were rebuked and suffered ruthless persecution, including death, because of their belief in Jesus as the Messiah. Some who were subsequently described as martyrs endured their suffering in the belief that they did it for the love of Christ, and they felt that their suffering identified them with Christ's suffering on the cross during his crucifixion.[4] This may be the earliest example of the value of psychotherapy as an important modality in managing pain. Thus, many present-day cancer patients with strong Christian beliefs view their pain and suffering as part of their journey toward eternal salvation. This concept has led to several scientifically conducted and government-sponsored studies evaluating intercessory prayer as an effective modality for controlling cancer pain.

To fully appreciate the historical significance of pain, it is important to reflect on the origins of the "pain patient." The word *pain* comes from the Latin word *poena*, which means "punishment." The word *patient* is derived from the Latin word *patior*, meaning "to endure suffering or pain." Thus, it is not too outrageous to appreciate that in ancient days persons who experienced pain were interpreted to have received punishment in the form of suffering that was either dispensed by the gods or offered up to appease the gods for transgressions.[5]

As spinal and epidural modes of anesthesia have developed and the techniques have been refined so that mortality and morbidity from them are negligible, childbirth and delivery are increasingly considered relatively painless in most developed societies. Unfortunately, in many countries neither the personnel nor the technology for obstetric regional analgesia is available, and resources to provide such personnel and technology are inadequate, thus making childbirth a primitively painful and at times disastrous event. The history of anesthesia is full of instances wherein attempts to relieve pain were initially met with resistance and sometimes violence. In the mid-19th century, Crawford Long from the state of Georgia in the United States attempted to develop and provide anesthesia, but contemporary Christians of that state considered him a heretic for his scholarly activity. As a result, he literally had to flee for his life from Georgia to Texas. Although surgical anesthesia was well developed by the late 19th century, religious controversy over its use required Pope Pius XII to give his approval before anesthesia could be used extensively for surgical procedures.[6] Pope Pius XII wrote, "The patient, desirous of avoiding or relieving pain, may without any disquietude of conscience, use the means discovered by science which in themselves are not immoral."

PAIN AND THE ANCIENT CULTURES

Disease, pain, and death have always been considered undesirable. The principles on which medicine was founded were based on measures to overcome human suffering from disease. Thus pain was usually thought of as either emanating from an injury or originating from the dysfunction of an internal organ or system. Traditionally, pain after physical injury (e.g., a gunshot wound or spear injury) was not considered problematic since as soon as the offending injurious agent was removed or once the consequences of the offending injury were corrected, the patient either recovered rapidly or, on occasion, died.[7] On the other hand, pain from disease (e.g., the pain of an inflamed gallbladder or ruptured appendix) was regarded with more mystique, and treatment was usually tinged with superstitious tradition. The tribal concept of pain came from the belief that it resulted from an "intrusion" from outside the body. These "intruders" were thought to be evil spirits sent by the gods as a form of punishment. It was in this setting that the role of medicine men and shamans flourished because these were the persons assigned to treat the pain syndromes associated with internal disease. Since it was thought that spirits entered the body by different avenues, the rational approach to therapy was aimed at blocking the particular pathway chosen by the spirit.

In Egypt, the left nostril was considered the specific site where disease entered. This belief was confirmed by the Papyri of Ebers and Berlin,[8] which stated that the treatment of headache involved expulsion of the offending spirit by sneezing, sweating, vomiting, urination, and even trephination. In New Guinea it was believed that evil spirits entered via a spear or an arrow, which then produced spontaneous pain.[7] Thus it was common for the shaman to occasionally purge the evil spirit from a painful offending wound and neutralize it with his special powers or special medicines. Egyptians treated some forms of pain by placing an electric fish from the Nile over the wounds to control the pain.[9] The resulting electrical stimulation that produced relief of pain actually works by a mechanism similar to transcutaneous electrical nerve stimulation (TENS), which is frequently used today to treat pain.

The Papyrus of Ebers, an ancient Egyptian manuscript, contains a wide variety of pharmacologic information and describes many techniques and recipes, some of which still have validity.[8] This papyrus describes the use of opium for the treatment of pain in children. Other concoctions for treating pediatric pain have included wearing amulets filled with a dead man's tooth (Omnibonus Ferraruis, 1577) as treatment of teething pain. Although early documents specifically address the management of pain in children, it is unfortunate that even today treatment of pediatric pain is far from optimal. This glaring deficiency was highlighted in 1977 by Eland, who demonstrated that in a population of children 4 to 8 years of age, only 50% received analgesics for postoperative pain.[3] The results are even more unsatisfactory for the treatment of chronic pain and cancer pain in children. It is unfortunate that the observations of earlier scholars have been ignored. Two erroneous assumptions—that children are less sensitive to pain and that the central nervous system is relatively undeveloped in neonates—are partially responsible for this deficiency.

Early Native Americans believed that pain was experienced in the heart, whereas the Chinese identified multiple points in the body where pain might originate or might be self-perpetuating.[10] Consequently, attempts were made to drain the body of these "pain points" by inserting needles, a concept that may have given birth to the principles of acupuncture therapy, which is well over 2000 years old.[11]

The ancient Greeks were the first to consider pain to be a sensory function that might be derived from peripheral stimulation.[12] In particular, Aristotle believed that pain was a central sensation arising from some form of stimulation of the flesh, whereas Plato hypothesized that the brain was the destination of all peripheral stimulation.[1] Aristotle advanced the notion that the heart was the originating source or processing center for pain. He based his hypothesis on the concept that an excess of vital heat was conducted by the blood to the heart, where pain was modulated and perceived.

Because of his great reputation, many Greek philosophers followed Aristotle and embraced the notion that the heart was the center for pain processing.[13] Another Greek philosopher, Stratton, and other distinguished Egyptians, including Herophilus and Eistratus, disagreed with Aristotle and proposed the concept that the brain was the site of pain perception as suggested by Plato. Their theories were reinforced by actual anatomic studies showing the connections of the peripheral and central nervous systems.[14]

Nevertheless, controversies between the opposing theories of the brain and the heart as the center for pain continued, and it was not until 400 years later that the Roman philosopher Galen rejuvenated the works of the Egyptians Herophilus and Eistratus and greatly re-emphasized the model of the central nervous system. Although Galen's work was compelling, he received little recognition for it until the 20th century.

Toward the period of the Roman Empire, steady progress was made in understanding pain as a sensation similar to other sensations in the body. Developments in anatomy and, to a lesser extent, in physiology helped establish that the brain, not the heart, was the center for the processing of pain.[15] While these advances were taking place, simultaneous advances were occurring in the development of therapeutic modalities, including the use of drugs (e.g., opium), as well as heat, cold, massage, trephination, and exercise, to treat painful illnesses. These developments brought about establishment of the principles of surgery for treating disease. Electricity was first used by the Greeks of that era as they exploited the power of the electrogenic torpedo fish (*Scribonius longus*) to treat the pain of arthritis and headache. Electrostatic generators were used in the late Middle Ages, as was the Leyden jar; these developments resulted in the re-emergence of electrotherapy as a modality for managing medical problems, including pain. There was a relative standstill in the development of electrotherapy as a medical modality until the electric battery was invented in the 19th century. Several attempts were then made to revive its use as an effective medical modality, but these concepts did not catch on and were largely used only by charlatans and obscure scientists and practitioners. Throughout the Middle Ages and the Renaissance, debate on the origin and processing center of pain raged. Fortunes fluctuated between proponents of the brain theory and proponents of the heart theory, depending on which theory was favored.

Heart theory proponents appeared to prosper when William Harvey, recognized for his discovery of the circulation, supported the heart as the focus for pain sensation. Descartes disagreed vehemently with the Harvey hypothesis, and his description of pain conducted from peripheral damage through nerves to the brain led to the first plausible pain theory, that is, the *specificity theory*.[16] It is interesting to note that the specificity theory followed Descartes' description by some 2 centuries. Several other theories followed the specificity theory and contributed to the foundation for understanding pain and pain mechanisms.

PAIN AND PAIN THEORIES

The specificity theory, originally proposed by Descartes, was formally revised by Schiff based on animal research. The fundamental tenet of the theory was that each sensory modality, including pain, was transmitted along an independent pathway. By examining the effect of incisions in the spinal cord, Schiff[16] demonstrated that touch and pain were independent sensations. Furthermore, he demonstrated that sectioning of the spinal cord deferentially resulted in the loss of one modality without affecting the other. Further work along the same lines by Bliz,[17] Goldscheider,[18] and von Frey[19] contributed to the concept that separate and distinct receptors exist for the modalities of pain, touch, warmth, and cold.

During the 18th and 19th centuries, new inventions, new theories, and new thinking emerged. This period was known as the Scientific Revolution, and several important inventions took place, including discovery of the analgesic properties of nitrous oxide, followed by the discovery of local anesthetic agents (e.g., cocaine). The study of anatomy was also developing rapidly as an important branch of science and medicine; most notable was discovery of the anatomic division of the spinal cord into sensory (dorsal) and motor (ventral) divisions. In 1840 Mueller proposed that based on anatomic studies, there was a straight-through system of specific nerve energies in which specific energy from a given sensation was transmitted along sensory nerves to the brain.[20] Mueller's theories led Darwin to propose the intensive theory of pain,[21] which maintained that the sensation of pain was not a separate modality but instead resulted from a sensory overload of sufficient intensity for any modality. This theory was modified by Erb[22] and then expanded by Goldscheider[18] to encompass the roles of both stimulus intensity and central summation of stimuli. Although the intensive theory was persuasive, the controversy continued, with the result that by the mid-20th century, the specificity theory was universally accepted as the more plausible theory of pain.

With this official, though not unanimous blessing of the contemporary scientific community, strategies for pain therapy began to focus on identifying and interrupting pain pathways. This tendency was both a blessing and a curse. It was a blessing in that it led many researchers to explore surgical techniques that might interrupt pain pathways and consequently relieve pain, but it was a curse in that it biased the medical community for more than half a century into believing that pain pathways and their interruption were the total answer to the pain puzzle. This trend was begun in the late 19th century by Letievant, who first described specific neurectomy techniques for treating neuralgic pain.[23] Afterward, various surgical interventions for chronic pain were developed and used, including rhizotomy, cordotomy, leukotomy, tractotomy, myelotomy, and several other operative procedures designed to interrupt the central nervous system and consequently reduce pain.[24] Most of these techniques were abysmal failures that not only did not relieve pain but also on occasion produced much more pain than was previously present. A major consequence lingers today—the notion that pain can be "fixed" by a surgical procedure or other modality.

PAIN AND DISEASE

The cardinal features of disease as recognized by early philosophers included calor, rubor, tumor, and dolor; the English translation is heat, redness, swelling, and pain. One of the important highlights in the history of pain medicine was the realization that even though heat, redness, and swelling may disappear, pain can continue long after and be unresponsive on occasion to different therapeutic modalities. When pain continues long after the natural pathogenic course of disease has ended, a chronic pain syndrome develops with characteristic clinical features, including depression, dependency, disability, disuse, drug misuse, drug abuse, and of course, "doctor shopping." John Dryden once wrote, "For all the happiness mankind can gain is not in pleasure, but in rest from pain." Thus many fatal nonpainful diseases are not as feared as relatively trivial painful ones.

Throughout the ages, physicians and healers have focused their attention on managing pain. Thus in managing cancer, an important measure of successful treatment is the success with which any associated pain is managed. Although many technological advances have been made in medicine, it is only within the past 10 to 20 years that significant strides have been made in dealing with chronic pain as a disease entity per se—one requiring specialized study, specialized evaluation, and specialized therapeutic interventions. As better techniques and more effective methods for evaluation and treatment of pain, especially chronic pain, are developed, management of pain will be considered more complete and an important supplement to the great strides made in other areas of chronic disease management.

PAIN IN THE 20TH CENTURY

General anesthesia was formally discovered by William Morton in 1846; in 1847, Simpson used chloroform to provide anesthesia for the labor pains of Queen Victoria during the delivery of her eighth child, Prince Leopold.[9] This action helped legitimize the practice of pain relief during childbirth. Heretofore, even the concept of analgesia for the relief of labor pain was considered heretical and unchristian. Around the same time the hollow needle and the syringe were invented. Many local anesthetic agents were also discovered in this era. In 1888, Corning described the use of a local anesthetic, cocaine, for the treatment of nerve pain. Techniques for local and regional anesthesia for both surgery and pain disorders proliferated rapidly.

In 1907, Schlosser reported significant relief of neuralgic pain for long periods with injection of alcohol into damaged and painful nerves. Reports of similar treatment came from the management of pain resulting from tuberculous and neoplastic invasion.[25] In 1926 and 1928, Swetlow and White, respectively, reported on the use of alcohol injections into thoracic sympathetic ganglia to treat chronic angina. In 1931, Dogliotti described the injection of alcohol into the cervical subarachnoid space to treat pain associated with cancer.[26]

One consequence of war has been the development of new techniques and procedures to manage injuries. In World War I (1914-1918), numerous injuries were associated with trauma (e.g., dismemberment, peripheral vascular insufficiency, and frostbite). In World War II (1939-1946), not only peripheral vascular injuries but also phantom limb phenomena, causalgia, and many sympathetically mediated pain syndromes occurred. Leriche developed the technique of sympathetic neural blockade with procaine to treat the causalgic injuries of war.[27] John Bonica, himself an army surgeon during World War II, recognized the gross inadequacy of managing war injuries and other painful states of veterans with the existing unidisciplinary approaches.[28] This led him to propose the concept of multidisciplinary, multimodal management of chronic pain, including behavioral evaluation and treatment. Bonica also highlighted the fact that pain of all kinds was being undertreated; his work has borne fruit in that he is universally considered the "father of pain," and he was the catalyst for the formation of many established national and international pain organizations. The clinic that he developed at the University of Washington in Seattle remains a model for the multidisciplinary management of chronic pain. As a result of his work, the American Pain Society (APS) and the International Association for the Study of Pain (IASP) have been formed, are still active, and continue to lead in pain research and pain management. Bonica's lasting legacy is his historic volume *The Management of Pain*, first published in 1953.

Anesthesiology as a specialty developed but was still associated with significant mortality and morbidity. Anesthesiology departments were considered divisions of surgery and did not reach full autonomy until after World War II. As a result of the morbidity associated with general anesthesia and because several new local anesthetics were being discovered, regional anesthesia and its associated techniques began to flourish in the United States. Bonica also played a major role in advancing the use of epidural anesthesia to manage the pain associated with labor and delivery. Regional anesthesia suffered a significant setback in the United Kingdom with the negative publicity surrounding the 1954 cases of Wooley and Roe, in whom serious and irreversible neurologic damage occurred after spinal anesthesia. It took 3 more decades to fully overcome that setback and to see regional anesthesia widely accepted as safe and effective in the United Kingdom. Several persons contributed significantly to the development of regional anesthesia, including Corning, Quincke-August Bier, Pitkin, Etherington-Wilson, Barker, and Adriani.

As recent society has developed and science has prospered, the general public has come to consider pain to be unsatisfactory and unacceptable. Consequently, demands have been made that resulted in the development of labor and delivery anesthesia services, acute pain services, and more recently, chronic pain clinics. Bonica's vision was not only the development of these clinics but also the founding and maintenance of national and international pain organizations to promote research and scientific understanding of pain medicine. As a result, a tremendous amount of research continues, almost quadrupling each year.

An outstanding contribution in the field of research was the development and publication of the *gate control theory* by Melzack and Wall in 1965.[29] This theory, built on the preexisting and prevalent specificity and intensive theories, provided a sound scientific basis for understanding pain mechanisms and for developing other concepts on which sound hypotheses could be developed. The gate control theory emphasizes the importance of both of ascending and descending modulation systems and laid down a solid framework for the management of different pain syndromes. The gate control theory almost single-handedly legitimized pain as a scientific discipline and led not only to many other research endeavors building on the theory but also to the maturity of pain medicine as a science.[30] As a consequence, the APS, the American Academy of Pain Medicine (AAPM), the American Society of Regional Anesthesia and Pain Medicine, the IASP, and the World Institute of Pain (WIP) flourish today as serious and responsible organizations that deal with various aspects of pain medicine, including education, science, certification, and credentialing of members of the specialty of pain medicine.

PAIN AND THE IMPACT OF PSYCHOLOGY

The history of pain medicine would be incomplete without acknowledging the noteworthy contributions of psychologists. Their influential research and clinical activities have been an integral part of a revolution in conceptualization of the pain experience.[31] For example, in the early 20th century the role of the cerebral cortex in the perception of pain was controversial because of a lack of understanding of the neuroanatomic pathways and the neurophysiologic mechanisms involved in pain perception.[32,33] This controversy largely ended with introduction of the gate control theory by Wall and Melzack in 1965.[29] The gate control theory has stood the test of time in that subsequent research using modern brain-imaging techniques such as positron emission tomography, functional magnetic resonance imaging, and single-photon emission computed tomography has also described the activation of multiple cortical and subcortical sites of activity in the brain during pain perception. Further elaboration of the psychological aspects of the pain experience includes the three psychological dimensions of pain: sensory-discriminative, motivational-affective, and cognitive-evaluative.[34]

Psychological researchers have greatly advanced the field of pain medicine by reconceptualizing both the etiology of the pain experience and the treatment strategy. Early pain researchers conceptualized the pain experience as a product of either somatic pathology or psychological factors. However, psychological researchers have convincingly challenged this misconception by presenting research that illustrates the complex interaction between biomedical and psychosocial factors.[35-37]

This biopsychosocial approach to the pain experience encourages the realization that pain is a complex perceptual experience modulated by a wide range of biopsychosocial factors, including emotions, social and environmental contexts, and cultural background, as well as beliefs, attitudes, and expectations. As the acutely painful experience transitions into a chronic phenomenon, these biopsychosocial abnormalities develop permanency. Thus, chronic pain affects all facets of a person's functional universe, at great expense to the individual and society. Consequently, logic dictates that this multimodal etiology of pain requires a multimodal therapeutic strategy for optimal cost-effective treatment outcomes.[38,39]

Additional contributions from the field of psychology include therapeutic behavioral modification techniques for the management of pain. Such techniques as cognitive behavioral intervention, guided imagery, biofeedback, and autogenic training are the direct result of using the concepts presented in the gate control theory. In addition, neuromodulatory therapeutic modalities such as TENS, peripheral nerve stimulation, spinal cord stimulation, and deep brain stimulation are also logical offspring of the concepts presented in the gate control theory.

Evaluation of candidates for interventional medical procedures is another valuable historical contribution from the field of psychology. Not only is the psychologist's expertise in the identification of appropriate patients valuable for the success of therapeutic procedural interventions for the management of pain, but the psychologist's expertise is also helpful in identifying patients who are not appropriate candidates for procedural interventions. Thus, psychologists have contributed positively toward the cost-effectiveness and utility of diagnostic and therapeutic pain medicine.

PAIN AND PAIN INSTITUTIONS

THE INTERNATIONAL ASSOCIATION FOR THE STUDY OF PAIN

The IASP is the largest multidisciplinary international association in the field of pain. Founded in 1973 by John J. Bonica, MD, the IASP is a nonprofit professional organization dedicated to furthering research on pain and improving the care of patients experiencing pain. Membership is open to scientists, physicians, dentists, psychologists, nurses, physical therapists, and other health professionals actively engaged in pain and to those who have special interest in the diagnosis and treatment of pain. The IASP has members in more than 100 national chapters.

The goals and objectives of the IASP are to foster and encourage research on pain mechanisms and pain syndromes and to help improve the management of patients with acute and chronic pain by bringing together scientists, physicians, and other health professionals of various disciplines and backgrounds who have interest in pain research and management. Goals of the IASP also include mandates to promote education and training in the field of pain, as well as to promote and facilitate the dissemination of new information in the field of pain. One of the instruments of dissemination is sponsorship of the journal *Pain*. In addition, the IASP promotes and sponsors a highly successful triennial world congress, as well as other meetings. The IASP encourages the development of national chapters for national implementation of the international mission of the IASP. In addition, the IASP encourages the adoption of a uniform classification, nomenclature, and definition of pain and pain syndromes. Development of a uniform records system in regard to information related to pain mechanisms, syndromes, and management is also a stated goal of the IASP, and education of the general public on the results and implications of current pain research is another mission of the IASP.

The IASP has partnered with the World Health Organization in providing guidelines for assessment and management of chronic pain, especially in developing countries. Cancer pain awareness and its management have been noteworthy contributions of the IASP.

Special interest groups (SIGs) within the IASP have successfully promoted research, understanding, education, and enhanced pain management of the particular special interest. Areas of interest include pain in children, neuropathic pain, herbal medicine, and cancer pain, among others. The IASP also promotes and administers Chronic Pain Fellowship programs for deserving candidates all over the world.

THE AMERICAN PAIN SOCIETY

Spurred by burgeoning public interest in pain management and research, as well as by formation of the Eastern and Western USA Chapters of the IASP, the APS was formed in 1977 as a result of a meeting of the Ad Hoc Advisory Committee on the Formation of a National Pain Organization. The need for a national organization of pain professionals was realized as growth of the IASP continued. The APS became the first national chapter of the IASP and has constituent regional and state chapters. The APS has its own journal, *The Journal of Pain*, and holds national meetings. Its main function is to carry out the mission of the IASP on a national level.

COMMISSION ON THE ACCREDITATION OF REHABILITATION FACILITIES

As pain clinics developed, it became clear that there was a need for credentialing, not only of pain centers and pain clinics but also of pain clinicians. In 1983, the Commission on Accreditation of Rehabilitation Facilities (CARF) was the first to offer a system of accreditation for pain clinics and pain treatment centers. The CARF model was based on the rehabilitation system, and it quickly became clear that the orientation of the CARF would be physical and psychosocial rehabilitation of patients suffering pain, in contrast to modality treatment to reduce pain sensation. CARF standards mandated that multidisciplinary pain management programs offer medical, psychological, and physical therapy modalities for the management of pain. Pain clinicians were not accredited by CARF, and it quickly became apparent that one could have an accredited pain center without having accredited pain clinicians. The CARF model gained modest acceptance among insurance carriers and third-party payers, primarily because of its emphasis on accountability and program evaluation. Its major goals included such objective measures as increased physical function, reduced intake of medication, and return-to-work issues.

THE AMERICAN ACADEMY OF PAIN MEDICINE

As CARF gained prominence, many pain clinicians realized that neither CARF nor the APS completely met their practice and professional needs. Furthermore, it became obvious that there was a major deficiency in evaluating the competence of pain physicians in that there were no uniform standards for training and credentialing of these pain clinicians. Thus in 1983, at a meeting of the APS in Washington, DC, a group of physicians (of whom chapter author Winston Parris was privileged to be a member) formed the American Academy of Algology (the term *algology* is derived from the words *algos* [Greek for "pain"] and *logos* [Greek for "study"]). The name was changed 2 years later to the AAPM, a name that is more acceptable in mainstream medicine.

This academy was formed to meet the needs and aspirations of pain physicians in the United States. Its major focus was to address the specific concerns of pain physicians and to enhance, authenticate, develop, and lead to the credentialing of pain medicine specialists. As a medical specialty society, the academy is involved in education, training, advocacy, and research in the specialty of pain medicine. The practice of pain medicine is multidisciplinary in approach and incorporates modalities from various specialties to ensure comprehensive evaluation and treatment of patients with pain. The AAPM represents the diverse scope of the field through membership from a variety of origins, including such specialties as anesthesiology, internal medicine, neurology, neurologic surgery, orthopedic surgery, physiatry, and psychiatry. Goals of the AAPM include the promotion of quality care of both patients experiencing pain as a symptom of a disease and patients with the primary condition of pain through research, education, and advocacy, as well as advancement of the specialty of pain medicine.

As we enter the managed care era, it is clear that issues such as reimbursement, contract negotiations, fee scheduling, practice management, mergers, acquisitions, and other business-related matters are becoming increasingly important to pain practitioners. The political and business arms of the AAPM are becoming instrumental in helping guide physicians through the murky waters of managed care and pain medicine.

In an attempt to provide creditable credentialing in pain medicine, the AAPM sponsored the American College of Pain Medicine (ACPM), which organized, developed, and administered the first credentialing examination in 1992. Successful candidates received the Fellowship of the American College of Pain Medicine. In the process of attempting to receive recognition of the American Board of Medical Specialties (ABMS), the name was changed on the recommendation of the ABMS to the American Board of Pain Medicine (ABPM).

Since the development of AAPM, most of the organization's goals have been met:

1. Successful lobbying for a seat for pain medicine in the House of Delegates of the American Medical Association.
2. Successful establishment of a credentialing body, the ABPM (formerly the ACPM), which offers annual credentialing examinations for eligible physicians. Among the many criteria, the minimum criterion is that candidates be ABMS-certified in their primary specialty.
3. Establishment of *The Clinical Journal of Pain*, which initially served as the official journal of the AAPM and has now been replaced by the journal *Pain Medicine.*

Additional goals include an attempt to establish uniform practice parameters and outcome measures for different pain modalities.

THE AMERICAN BOARD OF PAIN MEDICINE

The ABPM is the examination division of the AAPM and serves the public by improving the quality of pain medicine through certification of pain specialists. It evaluates candidates who voluntarily appear for examination after a credentialing process and certifies them as *Diplomates in Pain Medicine* if they successfully pass the examination process.

This mission serves the public by helping ensure that physicians passing the examination have an approved level of expertise and currency of knowledge in pain medicine. More than 2000 physicians have become diplomates of the ABPM.

THE AMERICAN SOCIETY OF REGIONAL ANESTHESIA AND PAIN MEDICINE

The American Society of Regional Anesthesia (ASRA) is the preeminent society on regional anesthesia. The society is based in the United States; other societies on regional anesthesia are based in Europe, Asia, and Latin America. Cognizant of the fact that anesthesiologists account for the majority of pain medicine practitioners and interventional pain physicians and perform translational and clinical research, the ASRA started another annual meeting dealing exclusively with pain medicine. The annual meeting of the ASRA that deals with regional anesthesia is held in the spring, whereas its annual meeting on pain medicine is held in the fall. To better fulfill its mission, the ASRA has changed its name to the American Society of Regional Anesthesia and Pain Medicine and the name of their highly cited journal, *Regional Anesthesia,* to *Regional Anesthesia and Pain Medicine.* This journal is the official publication of the American, European, Asian and Oceanic, and Latin American Societies of Regional Anesthesia.

THE AMERICAN SOCIETY OF INTERVENTIONAL PAIN PHYSICIANS

The American Society of Interventional Pain Physicians (ASIPP) is a national organization that represents the interests of interventional pain physicians in the United States. The society was founded in 1998 by Dr. Laxmaiah Manchikanti and associates for the purpose of improving the delivery of interventional pain management services to patients across the United States, whether in hospitals, ambulatory surgical centers, or medical offices. The ASIPP has an active political action committee that has been instrumental in achieving numerous legislative victories benefiting its constituents and their patients. Goals of the ASIPP include the preservation of insurance coverage, coverage for interventional pain procedures, advancement of patient safety, advancement of cost-effectiveness, and establishment of accountability in the performance of interventional procedures. Also included in the goals of the ASIPP are the pursuit of excellence in education in interventional pain management, improvement of practice management, enhancement of regulatory compliance, and elimination of fraud and abuse. The ASIPP journal is indexed and called *Pain Physician.*

THE AMERICAN ACADEMY OF HOSPICE AND PALLIATIVE MEDICINE

The American Academy of Hospice and Palliative Medicine (AAHPM) was founded in 1988 to advance the specialty of hospice medicine in the United States. Goals of the AAHPM include providing education and clinical practice standards, fostering research, facilitating personal and professional development, and sponsoring public policy advocacy for the terminally ill and their families. The academy's philosophy includes the belief that the proper role of the physician is to help the sick, even when cure is not possible. In addition, the AAHPM aims to help patients achieve an appropriate and easy passage to death as one of the most important and rewarding services that a physician can provide. The academy endorses the philosophy that the medical profession should attend to all the needs of the dying patient and family and should encourage and promote patient autonomy.

THE AMERICAN ACADEMY OF OROFACIAL PAIN

The American Academy of Orofacial Pain (AAOP) is an organization of health care professionals dedicated to the alleviation of pain and suffering through education, research, and patient care in the field of orofacial pain and associated disorders. Goals of the AAOP include the establishment of acceptable criteria for the diagnosis and treatment of orofacial pain and temporomandibular disorders, sponsorship of annual meetings and a medical journal, and encouragement of the study of orofacial pain and temporomandibular disorders at undergraduate and postgraduate levels of dental education.

THE AMERICAN ACADEMY OF PAIN MANAGEMENT

The American Academy of Pain Management (AAP Management), founded in 1988, is an inclusive interdisciplinary organization serving clinicians who treat people with pain through advocacy and education and by setting standards of care. AAP Management is open to a diverse group of pain clinicians and emphasizes inclusivity of all health care specialties. The organization boasts a large, diverse membership and an online University of Integrated Studies that offers graduate-level online courses for health practitioners. In addition, various levels of pain credentialing are available, depending on the level of education of the student or practitioner.

AMERICAN SOCIETY FOR PAIN MANAGEMENT NURSING

Founded in 1990, the American Society for Pain Management Nursing (ASPMN) is an organization of professional nurses dedicated to promoting and providing optimal care of individuals with pain through education, standards, advocacy, and research. Their goals include providing access to specialized care for patients experiencing pain, providing education of the public regarding self-advocacy for their pain needs, and providing a network for nurses working in the pain management field. This society also sponsors educational conferences and is formulating a means of adding compensational value to the specialty of pain management nursing. The ASPMN has published a number of scholarly position papers regarding best-practice nursing standards for such situations as male infant circumcision, procedural analgesia and sedation, patients who are unable to self-report pain complaints, and others.

THE NATIONAL HEADACHE FOUNDATION

Founded in 1970, the National Headache Foundation (NHF) works to create an environment in which headaches are viewed as a legitimate health problem. Goals of the NHF include promotion of research into the causes and treatment of headache and education of the public regarding the legitimacy of headache as a biologic disease.

THE WORLD INSTITUTE OF PAIN

The WIP is an international organization that aims to promote the best practice of pain medicine throughout the world. Its goals are to educate and train personnel of member pain centers by the use of local hands-on training international seminars and exchange of clinicians. Updating member pain centers with state-of-the-art pain information via newsletters, scientific seminars, and journal and book publications is an additional goal. One of the most important goals of the WIP is to develop an international examination process for testing and certifying qualified interventional pain physicians. After showing proficiency in both general pain knowledge and safe performance of interventional procedures, successful candidates are awarded the designation of *Fellow of Interventional Pain Practice* (FIPP). The journal of the WIP, *Pain Practice,* is indexed and has a very respectable initial impact factor.

THE WORLD SOCIETY OF PAIN CLINICIANS

The World Society of Pain Clinicians (WSPC) is an international organization whose goals are to bring together clinicians with a common interest in the treatment of pain. Additional goals are to stimulate education and learning in the field of pain and to encourage dissemination of information on pain throughout the world. The WSPC also endorses and encourages auditing and scientific research on all aspects of pain, especially treatment. The WSPC sponsors a biannual international congress on the clinical aspects of pain and has its own journal, *Pain Clinic.*

THE INTERNATIONAL SPINE INTERVENTION SOCIETY

The International Spine Intervention Society (ISIS) is a society of physicians interested in the development, implementation, and standardization of percutaneous techniques for precision diagnosis of spinal pain. The organization sponsors forums for exchange of ideas, encourages research undertaking, and holds public lectures. The mission of the ISIS includes consolidation of developments in diagnostic needle procedures, identification and resolution of controversies, public dissemination of developments, and recommendation of standards of practice based on scientific data.

THE INTERNATIONAL NEUROMODULATION SOCIETY

Founded in 1989, the International Neuromodulation Society (INS) is a multidisciplinary international society that promotes therapeutic neuromodulation at a clinical and scientific level. The primary means of exchanging knowledge consist of regular scientific meetings and the journal *Neuromodulation.* The first national chapter of the INS was the American Neuromodulation Society.

AMERICAN PAIN FOUNDATION

Founded in 1997 by three past presidents of the APS, the American Pain Foundation (APF) was an independent, nonprofit, grassroots organization serving people with pain through information, advocacy, and support. Its goals included serving as an information clearinghouse for people with pain, promoting recognition of pain as a critical health issue, and advocating for changes in professional training regulatory policies and health care delivery systems to ensure that people with pain have access to proper medical care. The APF was the first pain organization specifically formed to serve the interests of people with diverse disorders associated with the presence of significant pain. Regrettably, the organization was dissolved in early 2012 because of financial difficulties.

THE NATIONAL PAIN FOUNDATION

Founded in 1998, the National Pain Foundation (NPF) seeks to advance the recovery of persons in pain through education, information, and support. The NPF empowers patients by helping them become actively involved in the design of their treatment plan. The organization's website has interactive features that encourage patients to identify the information that they need to manage their pain in the most understandable way. The NPF strives to fill the gap in the understanding, awareness, and accessibility of pain treatment options.

PAIN AND THE HOSPICE MOVEMENT

Hospice is a medieval term representing a welcome place of rest for pilgrims to the Holy Land. The concept of hospice dates back to the reign of Emperor Julian the Apostate, when Fabiola, a Roman matron, created a place for sick and healthy travelers and cared for the dying.[40] Hospitals in general were regarded as Christian institutions, and in medieval times most hospitals were used as hospices and vice versa.[41]

During the 11th century, several hospices were based in and operated by monasteries. The 17th century Catholic priest St. Vincent DePaul founded the Sisters of Charity in Paris as a home for the poor, the sick, and the dying. St. Vincent DePaul's work for the poor and the sick created a significant impact not only on the Catholic Church but also on other contemporary religions. The Protestant pastor Fliedner was so influenced that he founded Kaiserwerth 100 years later. Nuns from the Sisters of Charity and Kaiserwerth accompanied Florence Nightingale to Crimea to care for wounded soldiers and other citizens who were either sick or dying.[42]

In 1902, the Irish Sisters of Charity founded St. Joseph's Hospice, which was staffed by Cecily Saunders 50 years later. Dr. Saunders was the first full-time hospice medical officer, and she was regarded as the founder and medical director of St. Christopher's Hospice in England. She was initially trained as a nurse and served in World War II. After becoming injured, she received training as a medical social worker. She subsequently developed a keen interest in terminal cancer patients and underwent training in medical school to become a physician. She emphasized the importance of taking patients at their word during pain assessment and of scheduling the dosing of opioids on a time-contingent basis as compared with an as-needed dosing schedule. She also advocated the need for frequent pain assessment to effectively manage cancer patients' pain. In addition, she sought to convince the medical community that it was totally unnecessary and inhumane for cancer patients to die in pain.[43] For all her efforts and leadership, she is regarded as the "mother of palliative care" and was knighted for her contributions to the hospice movement and care of dying cancer patients. Dame Saunders' views and works are widely taught in medical and nursing schools today and form the basis of palliative care.

PAIN AND THE FUTURE

Pain medicine has come a long way. A review of the history of pain demonstrates that until the time of Bonica, pain management was considered to be unimodal and unidisciplinary and was largely managed haphazardly and without any clear structural organization. Today, new drugs, innovative techniques, and creative procedures have expanded the scope of pain medicine. In addition, new research is contributing daily to modern concepts of pain and its management; these concepts are having positive effects on the development of pain medicine. Evidence-based guidelines on neuropathic pain by distinguished groups such as the IASP NeuroP SIG, European Federation of Neurological Sciences, and Canadian Pain Society have been published.

The contributions of the IASP, WIP, WSPC, APS, AAPM, ASRA, and the many other international, national, regional, state, and local organizations devoted to pain and pain management are all having a significant impact on the dissemination of knowledge, promotion of research, and realization of networking on local, national, and international levels. Pain practitioners and investigators are no longer isolated, and a flurry of published manuscripts and textbooks now cover a wide array of topics on pain medicine. Credentialing is well on its way, and two credible organizations are responsible for credentialing pain physicians in the United States. They include the diploma offered by the ABPM and the Certificate of Added Qualification by the American Board of Anesthesiology. Diplomas are offered by examination. In addition, the WIP offers a FIPP certification by examination.

With the recent trend of adverse changes in the global economy, including changes in medical economics, such as the realities created by managed care and the different health maintenance organizations, pain medicine has had to redirect its strategies for effective delivery and fair reimbursement for services rendered. These developments have also spawned new health care provider relationships and payment models for more cost-effective delivery of pain evaluation and treatment services. Many pain-oriented SIGs are dealing with these issues, and it is clear that the scientific community concerned with pain must develop reliable and reproducible outcome measures to maintain high quality, credibility, integrity, and competence in the management of chronic pain.

To this end, training of pain specialists is being given serious consideration, and a matching program for pain medicine fellowship positions is on the horizon. It is likely that in addition to the current 1-year pain medicine fellowships, attempts will be made to establish residencies in pain medicine. It is clear that in addition to offering these postgraduate measures, administrators of medical schools must re-evaluate their educational programs and make their curricula more inclusive of pain medicine. With such changes taking place, the future of pain medicine looks bright as a result of major contributions at all levels by dedicated and committed pain clinicians and researchers.

KEY POINTS

- The word *pain* comes from the Latin word *poena*, which means "punishment." The word *patient* is derived from the Latin word *patior*, meaning "to endure suffering or pain."
- The history of anesthesia is full of instances in which attempts to relieve pain were initially met with resistance and at times violence.
- Developments made in anatomy and physiology helped establish that the brain, not the heart, was the center for processing pain.
- The tenet of the specificity theory, proposed by Descartes and revised by Schiff, was that each sensory modality, including pain, was transmitted along an independent pathway.
- The use of chloroform to provide anesthesia for the labor pains of Queen Victoria helped legitimize the practice of pain relief during childbirth.
- The clinic that Bonica developed at the University of Washington in Seattle remains a model for the multidisciplinary management of chronic pain.
- Regional anesthesia suffered a significant setback with the negative publicity surrounding the 1954 cases of Wooley and Roe, in whom serious and irreversible neurologic damage occurred after spinal anesthesia. It took 3 decades to overcome this setback and establish regional anesthesia as safe and effective.
- An outstanding contribution in the field of research was development and publication of the *gate control theory* by Melzack and Wall in 1965.
- Psychological researchers have greatly advanced the field of pain medicine by reconceptualizing both the etiology of the pain experience and the treatment strategy.
- Several organizations advance the science and practice of pain medicine, including the International Association for the Study of Pain (IASP), American Pain Society (APS), American Society of Regional Anesthesia and Pain Medicine, American Academy of Pain Medicine (AAPM), World Institute of Pain (WIP), International Spine Intervention Society (ISIS), National Headache Foundation (NHF), and the American Society of Interventional Pain Physicians (ASIPP).
- Pain medicine practitioners are certified by the American Board of Anesthesiology and the American Board of Pain Medicine (ABPM).
- Changes in the pain medicine fellowship program related to the length of training and a matching program are being considered.

SUGGESTED READINGS

Abram SE. Advances in chronic pain management since gate control. *Reg Anesth.* 1993;18:66.

Campbell L. History of the hospice movement. *Cancer Nurs.* 1986;9:333.

Fordyce WE. Behavioral factors in pain. *Neurosurg Clin N Am.* 1991;2:749.

Melzack R, Wall PD. Pain mechanisms: a new theory. *Science.* 1965;150:971.

Raj PP. Pain relief: fact or fancy? *Reg Anesth.* 1990;15:157.

Saunders C. The last stages of life. *Am J Nurs.* 1965;65:70.

Turk DC. Clinical effectiveness and cost-effectiveness of treatments for patients with chronic pain. *Clin J Pain.* 2002;18:355.

Turk DC, Okifuji A. Psychological factors in chronic pain: evolution and revolution. *J Consult Clin Psychol.* 2002;70:678.

Unruh AM. Voices from the past: ancient views of pain in childhood. *Clin J Pain.* 1992;8:247.

Warfield C. A history of pain relief. *Hosp Pract.* 1988;7:121.

The references for this chapter can be found at www.expertconsult.com.

2

Taxonomy and Classification of Chronic Pain Syndromes

Harold Merskey

DEFINING PAIN

The first task of the authors of any taxonomy is to know what they are talking about. Sometimes knowledge is taken for granted. A taxonomy of pain needs some understanding of the term itself. We all assume that we know the meaning of the word pain—and indeed we do. Nevertheless, for a long time there was no unanimity about how to define pain. There is still no absolute unanimity, but a consensus appears to have formed in favor of the definition of pain offered by the International Association for the Study of Pain (IASP) in 1979[1] and subsequently published in the *Classification of Chronic Pain* produced by the IASP.[2] The definition of pain—"an unpleasant sensory and emotional experience associated with actual or potential tissue damage or described in terms of such damage"—was based on an earlier one[3] that had achieved some recognition; it was intended to deal with the situation that although pain was normally understood to be the consequence of physically damaging stimulation or a disorder in the body, many patients appeared to have pain but did not have overt tissue damage.

Morris[4] observed that the key to the IASP definition is to dissolve any necessary connection between pain and tissue damage. It depends on use of the word *pain* regardless of whether physical change is apparent. It is important to recognize that pain is always a subjective psychological state. At the same time, the note on this definition emphasized that pain "most often has a proximate physical cause."[3] The IASP definition has been adopted fairly broadly and helps minimize the idea that there is some sort of pain that patients imagine and that is not the same as the pain of "real injury or disease." In the personal opinion of this writer, much pain that is primarily organic in origin has an organic basis that is incompletely explained. Sometimes this happens for reasons of mere convenience; that is, every-day transient pain is not usually investigated, nor does it need to be. At other times it may happen because of difficulties in diagnosis, even with chronic severe disorders. The lack of physical proof should never be taken on its own as a sufficient indicator of a psychological cause of pain.

THE NATURE OF CLASSIFICATION

Taxonomy means the arrangement of rules. *Taxonomy* as a term is derived from two Greek words—*tasso* and *nomia*—meaning "arrangement" and "rules." In other words, it deals with the principles of classification and not with the content of classifications. It is about how to set up a classification and not about the detail of what goes into it. It ordinarily applies to the science of classification of living organisms. Classifications are also produced for nonliving organisms and material that was never alive.

There are two types of classification, natural and artificial. A *natural* classification deals with the material of physics and biology and anything else in the natural world, such as types of stars or forms of animals—in other words, the material world. An *artificial* classification deals with arrangement of the products of human activity, for example, a telephone directory.

In an artificial classification there is no necessary connection between the basis on which the classification is produced and the inherent nature of the subject matter. Thus, the list of names in a telephone directory by alphabetical order is arbitrary but works extremely well.[5]

An ideal classification should not only be comprehensive but should also locate each item within it in a place of its own without overlap. The periodic table in chemistry is a wonderful example of scientific beauty and a perfect or almost perfect classification wherein every element belongs in its own place relative to the other elements. In biology, a superior form of classification is a phylogenetic one based on evolutionary relationships.

Medical classifications are established on a very different basis. In the International Statistical Classification of Diseases and Diagnostic Guidelines, 10th Revision (ICD-10),[6] the classification is arranged by causal agents, such as infectious diseases or neoplasms; by systems of the body, such as cardiovascular or musculoskeletal; by symptom pattern and type of symptoms, as in psychiatric illnesses; and even by whether the condition or event is related to the artificial intervention of an operation. Illnesses or categories may be grouped by time of occurrence, such as congenital or perinatal disorders, and at the basic level are grouped as symptoms, signs, and abnormal clinical and laboratory findings.

In the ICD-10 there is code 080 for delivery in an uneventful case, including spontaneous breech delivery. Major groups are subdivided by system (e.g., neurology), by symptom pattern (e.g., epilepsy or migraine), by the presence of hereditary or degenerative disease (e.g., Huntington's disease and hereditary ataxia), by location of the disorder (e.g., extrapyramidal disorders), by anatomic and physiologic characteristics (e.g., extrapyramidal and movement disorders, such as Parkinson's disease and dystonia), by location (e.g., polyneuropathies), and by infectious and chemical causes. With these approaches, categories overlap repeatedly. Pain is found in the group of symptoms, signs, and clinical and laboratory findings as "R52—pain not elsewhere classified." This particular code excludes some 19 others that reflect pain in different parts of the body and excludes "psychogenic" pain (code F45.4) and renal colic (N33). Thus, pain occurs at various levels of diagnosis and categorization in the ICD-10.

The overlap found in medicine is inevitable. There must always be some provision for conditions that are not well described and will overlap with others that are well described. The purposes of medicine require attention to the many different aspects of disease that enter into the classifications. That should be apparent from the examples cited.

WHICH TYPES OF PAIN NEED CLASSIFICATION

From the point of view of a pain practitioner, only some types of pain need classification, and indeed it would be inappropriate to classify all types of pain in a chronic pain classification. A large proportion of the pain that human beings and other creatures experience in the world is brief and transitory. As a rule, it is accompanied by overt damage that needs its own appropriate treatment or it passes quickly. Pain is the most common symptom in the whole of medicine. Therefore, any attempt to classify all types of pain would inevitably lead to an overall classification of medicine that would have a particular focus that is unnecessary for most medical cases. Illnesses with pain that have needed a special classification are those in which pain is a significant persistent problem. This conclusion still leaves a large field for a classification of pain but saves the pain specialist from having to write the classification for all the rest of medicine as well.

Among specific systems of classification, the ICD-10 is used worldwide for the purpose of documenting mortality and morbidity.[6] In the United States, a slightly modified version of the previous international system of classification, namely, ICD-9CM, is used. (CM stands for Clinical Modification.) This modification was promoted by the U.S. government to provide the additional data required by clinicians, researchers, epidemiologists, medical record librarians, and administrators of inpatient and outpatient community programs. In the United States, ICD-9CM is published by the Department of Health and Human Services, Public Health Services, Health Care Financing Administration.

The international ICD-10 system comprises a table of names and numerical codes for these names. The ICD-10 consists of three volumes. Volume I is a tabular list that contains the report of the International Conference for the 10th Revision, the classification itself at three- and four-character levels, a classification of the morphology of neoplasms, a special tabulation list for mortality and morbidity, definitions, and the nomenclature regulations. Volume II includes an instruction manual, and Volume III is an alphabetical index. The latter also includes expanded instructions on use of the index.

In the United States, ICD-9CM coding has particular importance because of the 1988 Medical Catastrophic Coverage Act, which although later repealed, required the use of ICD-9 codes on "Medicare Part B" claims. This requirement continued with ICD-9CM, and to date, ICD-9CM has not been replaced in the United States. Pain specialists in the United States may believe that the ICD-9CM classification does not cover their requirements for appropriate billing of work done and may prefer a pain-based classification.

Of course, classifications have a number of purposes besides billing. The primary one is to exchange standardized information so that "stroke," "cholecystitis," and "depressive disorder," for example, have the same meanings to different colleagues. Meanings should be the same both within the same country and throughout the world. This should facilitate statistical comparisons of the occurrence and management of disease and serve as a basic tool for scientific progress by establishing standards of diagnosis and description that can be compared between workers within countries and internationally.

Such classification can help provide an understanding of disorders, but it does so only by giving shape to the advances of investigators, whether alone, in working groups, or in national and international organizations. Classifications also serve as a means of recognizing work done and providing standards for payment. This is one of the reasons for their relative popularity with both medical professionals and administrators.

Classifications, of necessity, cannot provide "absolute truth." Thus even when a classification recognizes a disorder as a "condition," a "disorder," or a "disease," it is not the classification that provides the knowledge that justifies these various titles but rather the existing level of scientific knowledge. To the extent that a classification identifies current scientific knowledge and claims it to be acceptable, it may establish unity, but classifications as a rule only follow scientific knowledge.

This also means that just as classifications take material as they find it, they are not expected to provide perfect decisions or standards by which we can state that something is "a disease," a "disorder," a "syndrome," or merely a "symptom." The one word of these four for which the meaning is not in dispute is *symptom*, the patient's statement of a complaint. All four words involve or have involved some dispute regarding whether they reflect the true nature of the phenomena with which physicians deal. Physicians become concerned about whether they recognize something as a disease or "only a syndrome" or "just a symptom." It is not the function of a classification to determine the answers to such questions. In fact, it can be extraordinarily hard to determine what constitutes a syndrome and whether diseases should have a fixed standard.[7]

THE INTERNATIONAL ASSOCIATION FOR THE STUDY OF PAIN CLASSIFICATION

The IASP classification focuses on chronic pain. A small number of pain syndromes that are not necessarily chronic were included for comparative purposes because they might be relevant to pain specialists (e.g., acute herpes zoster, burns with spasm, pancreatitis, prolapsed intervertebral disk) or because the acute version frequently becomes chronic. The classification is based on five axes. The first axis is anatomic localization, which was chosen for both historical and practical reasons. The historical reasons are that there was previously difficulty in establishing a chronic pain classification based on etiology and that there was too much argument or potential argument about causes. It was also recognized that in essence pain is referred to parts of the body and it is always a somatic symptom, whatever its cause. In addition, location provides a useful means of distinction between different conditions. Accordingly, the IASP classification presents a list of relatively generalized syndromes followed by regional ones. Relatively generalized syndromes include peripheral neuropathy, stump pain, phantom pain, complex regional pain syndrome, central pain, syringomyelia, polymyalgia rheumatica, fibromyalgia, rheumatoid arthritis, and so forth. Pain of psychological origin is also included. Relatively localized syndromes are subdivided according to whether they affect the head and neck, limbs, thorax, or abdomen or whether they have a spinal or radicular distribution or origin.

The IASP classification set out to provide categories and codes for all the relevant conditions. Not all pain is continuously chronic. Some pain that is severe *and* chronic remits between episodes (e.g., migraine and cluster headache), but these types of pain are also included under the rubric of chronic pain. Some chronic pain consists of pain that persists past what has usually been considered to be the normal time needed for healing. However, this is not always the case, and the decision of what constitutes the normal time for healing is much argued. Indeed, it is now understood—but not so well understood in 1986 when the first edition of the classification was published—that pathophysiologic processes may well maintain pain long after the normal expectation of pain from injury has ended. I personally question whether we should even mention the normal time needed for healing when discussing chronic pain.

Be that as it may, the IASP Taxonomy Committee recognized that some pain persists despite no apparent explanation, other pain persists with an explanation (e.g., the pain of osteoarthritis), and still other pain, which is not always continuous, can recur. Patients with these types of pain, by virtue of their intractability, were considered proper subjects for a classification of chronic pain.

MULTIPLE AXES

An anatomic classification alone is not sufficient. Some effort has to be made, even if it is tentative, to describe the nature of the pain and different types of pain, to note the system in which it occurs, to set up a system that indicates which disturbance seems to be most responsible for the pain, to describe the features of the pain even though they might vary within diagnoses, and to attribute cause when possible. Accordingly, the classification of chronic pain specifies five axes for describing pain.

The first axis is the anatomic axis, and the second axis is the system most related to the cause of the pain (besides the nervous system, which is always involved in pain). The systems identified were (1) the central, peripheral, and autonomic nervous systems and special senses; (2) psychological and social function of the nervous system (which was given a separate coding); (3) respiratory and vascular systems; (4) the musculoskeletal system and connective tissue; (5) cutaneous and subcutaneous tissue and associated glands (e.g., breast, apocrine), the gastrointestinal system, the genitourinary system, and other organs or viscera (e.g., thyroid, lymphatic); and (6) unknown systems. A code was also allowed wherein more than one system was found to contribute to the pain.

The third axis describes the temporal characteristics of the pain and its pattern of occurrence. A code was allowed for instances in which temporal patterns were not recorded but distinctions were made as follows: single episode, continuous or nearly continuous, nonfluctuating or fluctuating, recurring irregularly, paroxysmal (e.g., tic douloureux), occurring regularly (e.g., premenstrual pain), sustained with superimposed paroxysms and other combinations, and none of the above.

The fourth axis accepts statements of intensity, and the fifth axis identifies etiology. Causes can include genetic or congenital disorders; operations; burns; infections; inflammation; neoplasms; toxic, metabolic, degenerative, mechanical, or functional (including psychophysiologic) causes; or those resulting from ideas (e.g., conversion hysteria or depressive hallucination—both of which are either hard to show or particularly rare).

The actual system has served well as a guide for making a diagnosis and establishing priorities in making a diagnosis. It has served poorly as a means of exchanging information on certain cases of different sorts. Thus, I do not think that I have seen any example of a study in which pain was selected solely on the basis that it had a particular pattern on the third axis, such as *continuous* or *nearly continuous.* These features have of course been found and reported frequently in studies in which the patients were selected on the basis of other criteria (e.g., the anatomic location or the etiologic diagnosis, to take the first and the fifth axes). The system does, however, provide fairly well for individual codes to be given if they are required for a specific study of a group, mainly relying on the anatomic, systemic, and diagnostic axes (e.g., I, II, and V). The third axis (i.e., the temporal characteristics) serves well only for identifying continuous or discontinuous pain, which is often merely a feature of the diagnosis and not a feature of the selection of cases or the exchange of information. The fourth axis has also contributed relatively little in its present shape, with intensity frequently being recorded separately from the diagnosis.

The codes can serve as a means of identifying unique patterns. Each of the five axes provides a place in the code for a condition. However, Vervest and Schimmer[8] showed that not all the codes are unique, and allowance for this is made by adding the letters a, b, c, and so forth to the five-number code when necessary.

Chronic pain was defined as pain that had been present for more than 6 months. It was thought that although many types of pain become persistent and chronic at 3 months, a 6-month division did not present difficulties in practice, was fairly characteristic, and served as a good entry to the population treated by pain specialists. The term *chronic pain* was not intended—and still is not intended—to mean a particular syndrome or pattern, and the notion of "chronic pain syndrome," which tends to mix the physical and psychological consequences of pain, was not accepted by the Taxonomy Committee of the IASP. In its deliberations the committee proceeded to adopt an anatomic classification as the starting point for its classification of chronic pain on a model originally developed by John Bonica.[9]

PARTICULAR DIAGNOSES

The provision of categories is particularly useful when existing knowledge of painful syndromes is weak. For example, the understanding of reflex sympathetic dystrophy, whose name was changed on the advice of a special subcommittee to *complex regional pain syndrome* (CRPS) type 1, has served as a means for identifying criteria that would provide either a clinical means for agreement between different investigators or a special sample for research purposes. In this case, the first step taken in conjunction with the classification system was to define CRPS type 1 merely by its clinical phenomena and not by its theoretical relationship to the sympathetic nervous system. The second step, taken more recently,[10] proposed changes in the diagnostic criteria that provided both clinical diagnostic criteria for general use and more stringent research diagnostic criteria for specific research investigations. This seems to be a satisfactory solution to the problem of how many people may claim the label and what sort of cases should be concomitantly studied to establish convincing evidence of the research findings. Other examples in which the classification has been useful include pioneering the spread of understanding about relatively new syndromes (e.g., the syndrome of painful legs and moving toes [see Merskey and Spear[3]] or the syndrome of paroxysmal hemicrania). In these cases, the classification has given an appropriate place to syndromes that have not yet entered the general lexicon although they are described in the literature.

PSYCHIATRIC ASPECTS OF CHRONIC PAIN

The psychiatric aspects of chronic pain may be coded in two ways. The first recognizes that patients seen in clinical practice often have some degree of emotional difficulty in association with chronic pain. In such cases the psychological changes are most often anxiety or depression and may be attributed to the persistence of pain causing distress, loss of employment, altered marital relationships, decline in self-image, and so forth, as well as independent events that cause depression or anxiety (e.g., bereavement or illness in a close relative). In these circumstances it is important to describe the psychological status of patients, to understand why they are troubled, and to provide appropriate treatments, which first of all may consist of better analgesia but in addition may include antidepressant medication and social support. Whenever psychological help is requested, it should include assistance with emotional difficulties, whether it be supportive or cognitive therapy. Behavioral therapy usually has only a very limited role in managing the secondary effects of pain, but assistance in adjustment to pain can be of great importance and can involve rehabilitation experts.

The second option in regard to psychiatry and pain would be to see the psychological illness as a cause of the pain. This is thought to be much less common as a sustained cause of pain than was originally suggested. Headache from emotional problems and precordial pain from anxiety are fairly typical examples of situations in which some pain, but less often chronic pain, may be due to depression or anxiety disorders. In such cases, psychiatric methods of care are appropriate after physical examination. However, these situations hardly ever account for the great majority of patients with chronic pain and emotional disturbance. One explanation that was formerly favored suggests that the pain solves a problem, but this explanation seems to be less and less realistic as time goes by, and psychiatry has failed to prove by systematic methods that sustained pain results from a chronic emotional disorder. We provided psychological categories notwithstanding; thus, the IASP system laid down the following categories: pain of psychological origin: muscle tension; delusional hallucinatory; hysterical conversion or hypochondriacal; and associated with depression. It appears that these categories are not used much. Factitious illness and malingering were not included as disorders as they were thought appropriate to describe as part of the psychiatric condition.

INTERNATIONAL PSYCHIATRIC CLASSIFICATIONS

The classification of mental and behavioral disorders recommended by the World Health Organization[11] is a part of the overall international classification. Categories have been established with an eye to agreement with the layout of the *Diagnostic and Statistical Manual of Mental Disorders, Fourth Edition* (*DSM-IV*), of the American Psychiatric Association (APA),[12] which is well known in many countries. The ICD-10 classification of mental and behavioral disorders preserves categories parallel to those used in DSM-IV, although the descriptions are often different. However, the ICD-10 classification does not use the "checklist approach" but rather gives a general description and the major criteria required. The APA DSM-IV and DSM-IV TR (in which the explanatory text changed but not the codes) retain the same criteria as each other.

With respect to pain, the options in both systems are as follows: First, any particular diagnosis such as schizophrenia or depression of some sort may be made and indicated as a cause of the patient's pain in cases in which it is understood that the diagnosis applies and pain may be accepted as resulting from such conditions. Then, the ICD-10 classification provides a category of Pain Disorder, Somatoform Persistent (F45.44). This category in essence corresponds to what the DSM-IV now calls Persistent Somatoform Pain Disorder. In the ICD-10 classification, the predominant complaint is persistent, severe, and distressing pain that cannot be explained fully by a physiologic process or a physical disorder. It is presumed to be of psychological origin, but pain occurring during the course of a depressive disorder or schizophrenia is not included. Pain that is due to known or inferred psychophysiologic mechanisms such as muscle tension pain or migraine but is still believed to have a psychogenic cause is coded under Psychological or Behavioral Factors Associated with Disorders or Diseases Classified Elsewhere (e.g., muscle tension pain or migraine). In ICD-10, the most common problem is to differentiate this disorder from the histrionic elaboration of organically caused pain. Thus, this category is essentially meant to deal with pain that serves an unconscious motive. For a number of practical reasons this is an extremely difficult proposition to prove clinically.

Under DSM-IV the criteria are similarly stringent but the diagnosis is made much more frequently, both in the United States and in Canada. According to the description of chronic pain disorder in DSM-IV, the word *somatoform* was dropped from the title. Pain disorder is the predominant focus of the clinical manifestation, and it must cause significant stress or impairment in social, occupational, or other important areas of functioning. Psychological factors must be judged to have an important role in the onset, severity, exacerbation, or maintenance of the pain, and the symptom or deficit must not be intentionally produced. This condition is not to be diagnosed if the pain is better accounted for by a mood, anxiety, or psychotic disorder or if it meets the criteria for dyspareunia.

These criteria have the effect of limiting the condition to one that is not associated with significant depression or anxiety or that results from a physical illness. Within DSM-IV, two versions of pain disorder were allowed. One is "pain disorder associated with psychological factors," wherein the necessary criteria are met as above but psychological illness is not present. The other is "pain disorder associated with both psychological factors and a general medical condition." In this case the same rules apply as for pain disorder on its own, but it is thought that a physical condition may be present but not sufficient to account for a large part of the syndrome. It is stated as follows: "Both psychological factors and a general medical condition are judged to have important roles in the onset, severity, exacerbation, or maintenance of the pain." The associated general medical condition or anatomic site of the pain is coded separately.

In my observation, many diagnosticians who are sincerely interested in the patient's welfare welcome this category as a means of diagnosing a distressing psychological state for which they do not see an adequate physiologic or general medical explanation. In my view, however, this is not the way it should be used. It would only logically be justifiable with respect to the criteria for cognate diagnoses if it could be demonstrated that there was some psychological cause that was unconsciously producing the symptom at the same time as producing anxiety or depression—in other words, what used to be called *hysteria*. For reasons discussed elsewhere,[13] the diagnosis of pain as "a conversion disorder" can rarely be made adequately. Persons with doubts should try to imagine whether they could produce, by thinking about it, a physical symptom such as paralysis that they would maintain consciously and whether they could produce a state of feeling of chronic pain in themselves by reflecting on it and then ask how is it possible that pain could be produced unconsciously if it cannot even be produced consciously? Overall then, psychological diagnoses as causes of pain are not favored by this writer except in very limited situations. Occasionally, patients with classic depressive illness suffer from severe headaches that go away when the depression is better. Occasionally, patients with post-herpetic neuralgia have much worse pain when they become depressed and much less pain when the depression is treated, but this situation is relatively rare and does not reflect the bulk of either general medical, neurologic, or psychiatric practice.

The diagnosis of chronic pain related to psychiatry is, at present, a controversial issue with respect to DSM-V, which has the category Pain Disorder. The current proposal of the APA is that there will be substantial changes in the pain disorder criteria involving both Pain Disorder and other so-called "Somatoform Disorders." It appears that the "Somatic Symptom Disorder Work Group" is proposing radical changes in this category and will (or may) rename the Somatoform Disorders section as "Somatic Symptom Disorders," eliminate four existing DSM-IV categories (Somatization Disorder, Hypochondriasis, Pain Disorder, and Undifferentiated Somatoform Disorder), replace these discrete categories and their criteria with a single new category ("[Complex] Somatoform Symptom Disorder"), and apply new criteria.

To receive a diagnosis of complex somatic symptom disorder, patients must complain of at least one somatic symptom that is distressing or disruptive of their daily lives. Also, patients must have at least one of the following from the E type criteria: "emotional/cognitive/behavioural disturbances: high levels of health anxiety, disproportionate and persistent concerns about the medical seriousness of the 'symptoms,' and an excessive amount of time and energy devoted to the symptoms and health concerns. Finally, the symptoms and later concerns must have lasted for at least six months." There are some further qualifications, and the development of the system has been vigorously criticized by Dr. Allen Frances, the principal architect and editor in chief of DSM-IV, which has been widely used and officially adopted by various bodies.

The diagnosis of "Pain Disorder" in DSM-IV was not entirely satisfactory in this author's view, and reasons have been given for not using it. Nonetheless (for reasons connected with funding the diagnosis on insurance claims from either side of the fence), many expert witnesses have tended to rely on the DSM-IV diagnoses. Some have also relied on the DSM-IV grading systems with respect to functional abilities. Others, like myself, who have treated pain—entirely—as a physical disorder for medicolegal purposes have made use of whichever version of the American Medical Association Guides to the Evaluation of Impairment was relevant in their particular jurisdiction. For psychiatric purposes in evaluating the disability caused by pain, one can reasonably apply the criteria for disability of the Somatoform Disorders Scale as published in DSM-IV by reference to the Global Assessment of Functioning scale. In jurisdictions outside the United States the same scale can also reasonably be used for both physical and psychological illness. Thus, rather than the questionable diagnosis of "Pain Disorder," the Global Assessment of Functioning scale may be used independent of the diagnosis simply on the basis of what the patient can and cannot do—without necessarily applying a psychiatric diagnosis.

In my experience to date, similar situations have been interpreted in the medicolegal situation more often to the benefit of the defense than to the benefit of the injured party in compensation disputes. However, on a fair presentation it should work equally well for both sides of the argument and better than any arbitrary scaling unrelated to the life experience of the individual.

CONCLUSION

Classification is required in medical practice to identify like phenomena observed by practitioners. There is no absolute rule of what a syndrome or classification should be. The basis for the use of different classification systems is outlined in this chapter.

SUGGESTED READINGS

American Psychiatric Association. *Diagnostic and Statistical Manual of Mental Disorders* (DSM-IV). 4th ed. Washington, DC: American Psychiatric Association; 1994.

Bonica JJ. *The Management of Pain.* Philadelphia: Lea & Febiger; 1953.

Galbraith DI, Wilson DG. *Biological Science: Principles and Patterns of Life.* Toronto: Holt, Reinhart & Winston; 1966.

Harden RN, Bruehl SP. Diagnostic criteria: the statistical derivation of the four criterion factors. In: Stanton-Hicks M, Harden RN, eds. *CRPS Current Diagnosis and Therapy.* Seattle: IASP Press; 2005:45-58.

Lindblom U, Merskey H, Mumford JM, et al. Pain terms: a current list with definitions and notes on usage. *Pain.* 1979;3(suppl):S215-S221.

Merskey H. Pain disorder, hysteria, or somatization [commentary]? *Pain Res Manage.* 2004;9:67-71.

Merskey H. Variable meanings for the definition of disease. *J Med Philos.* 1986;11:215-232.

Merskey H, Bogduk N, eds. *Classification of Chronic Pain: Descriptions of Chronic Pain Syndromes and Definitions of Pain Terms.* 2nd ed. Seattle: International Association for the Study of Pain; 1994.

Merskey H, Spear FG. *Pain: Psychological and Psychiatric Aspects.* London: Bailliere, Tindall & Cassell; 1967.

Morris D. The challenges of pain and suffering. In: Jensen TS, Wilson PR, Rice SC, eds. *Chronic Pain.* London: Arnold; 2003:1-13.

Vervest A, Schimmer G. Taxonomy of pain of the IASP [letter]. *Pain.* 1988;34:318-321.

World Health Organization. *The ICD-10 Classification of Mental and Behavioural Disorders: Clinical Descriptions and Diagnostic Guidelines.* Geneva: World Health Organization; 1992.

World Health Organization. *International Statistical Classification of Diseases and Related Problems, 10th Revision (ICD-10).* Geneva: World Health Organization; 1992.

The references for this chapter can be found at www.expertconsult.com.

3

Organizing an Inpatient Acute Pain Service

Jennifer M. Lee | Alex Cahana | Gregory W. Terman

THE RATIONALE

An estimated 48 million inpatient surgical procedures are performed annually in the United States (National Center for Health Statistics, National Hospital Discharge Survey: 2009, cdcinfo@cdc.gov). Although it is to be expected that surgical treatment results in some degree of patient discomfort, acute postsurgical pain has been widely undertreated. In one survey, 80% of patients reported experiencing moderate to extreme pain after surgery.[1] Ineffective postoperative pain management is associated with economic and medical implications, including extended lengths of treatment, readmissions, and patient dissatisfaction with medical care.[2,3]

Consequently, in 2001 the American Pain Society (APS) declared the start of a "Decade of Pain Control and Research" and urged health professionals to treat pain as "the fifth vital sign." Thereafter, a flood of practice guidelines emerged in the literature in an attempt to emphasize and provide instructions for realization of this proposal. Nonetheless, a decade later, the parent organization of the APS, the International Association for the Study of Pain (IASP), designated 2011 the *Global Year Against Acute Pain.* This campaign sought to highlight "the persistent problem of acute pain…the most commonly experienced pain (e.g., surgery, childbirth, trauma)…treatable with currently available medications and techniques [but with] a large gap between evidence and practice—resulting in widespread under-treatment" (http://www.iasp-pain.org/Content/NavigationMenu/GlobalYearAgainstPain/GlobalYearAgainstAcutePain/default.htm).

It turns out that achieving satisfactory acute pain management is quite challenging. It is often difficult to estimate what a patient's postoperative analgesic requirements will be.

The following factors, for example, may influence postoperative opioid requirements:

- Preoperative pain sensitivity[4]
- Coexisting medical conditions and associated multiple drug administration
- Presurgical opioid tolerance or a history of drug abuse
- Psychological factors, including catastrophizing and anxiety[5,6]
- Age[7]
- Type of surgery[8]

Great care must be applied to consider all the aforementioned characteristics when deriving an analgesic plan for managing an individual's response to a surgical insult.

The sequelae associated with surgical procedures result from various components of the stress response and include cardiopulmonary, infectious, and thromboembolic complications; cerebral dysfunction; nausea and gastrointestinal paresis; fatigue; and prolonged convalescence. Throughout the process of organizing an acute pain program, it is helpful to keep the following statements in mind:

- The postoperative pain management regimen should be designed with attention to providing patient comfort and also inhibiting nociceptive impulses sufficient to allow a patient to participate fully in active rehabilitation when appropriate.
- A time-, energy-, and cost-effective acute pain program should optimally provide multimodal and multidisciplinary interventions, including systemic and regional pharmacological treatments, stress reduction, transcutaneous electrical nerve stimulation, music therapy, and acupuncture.[9-11]
- Surgical stress responses are inhibited mostly by the neuraxial administration of local anesthetics; the administration of other agents—systemically, neuraxially, or perineurally—appears to contribute little additional reduction of the endocrine (metabolic and catabolic) stress response following operative procedures.[12,13]
- Parenteral opioids exaggerate the perioperative immune system depression already triggered by the neuroendocrine response to surgery, although the clinical relevance of this observation is controversial.[14] Opioids administered into the epidural space have minor suppressive effects on surgically induced proinflammatory cytokines.[15]
- Effective analgesia can reduce postoperative morbidity. As an example, thoracic epidural analgesia has been shown to improve postoperative spirometry and reduce pulmonary infections and atelectasis.[16,17] In many settings the routine and "gold standard" of care involves such facilitation of the patient's recovery of pulmonary function.

The experience of a skilled anesthesiologist easily lends itself to providing leadership within an acute pain service. Anesthesiologists are proficient in the use of systemic and regional analgesic techniques, including peripheral and neuraxial blockade. They also often have an understanding of the surgical techniques and consequent insults that they impose. Additionally, anesthesiologists are well equipped with leadership skills for working within a multidisciplinary team; these are also vital skills within the operating theater. Nonetheless, an anesthesiologist-based team is not the only service model.

Nurse-based, anesthesiologist-supervised inpatient acute pain services have also been demonstrated to provide safe and effective postoperative pain management.[18,19] Regardless of the service model, nursing involvement in an acute pain service is essential. Bedside nurses' impression of a patient's analgesic needs and recovery is an invaluable element in the decision-making process for any given patient, and because it is the nurse who will ultimately be delivering the care, it is vital that the nurse understand the analgesic plan and goals.

Detailed practice guidelines and protocols can help streamline the ordering and implementation of patient care. Well-established protocols have been shown to reduce errors in realms outside pain management[20] and decrease the cost associated with prescribing choices.[21] At the University of Washington Medical Center, for example, we have instituted multiple protocols, including order sets for patient-controlled analgesia (PCA), continuous and patient-administered epidural analgesia, ketamine infusions, and continuous perineural catheter infusions (Figs. 3.1 to 3.4; we have recently switched to electronic order sets mirroring these past paper protocols). The PCA and epidural analgesia protocols must include titration and bolus instructions to treat breakthrough or incident pain. The order sets should also include routine and specific monitoring orders, as well as treatment options for common or dangerous side

PAIN SERVICE: Parenteral (IV/SQ) Patient Controlled Analgesia (PCA) Orders Page 1 of 2

1. Discontinue current opioids and/or benzodiazepines except:

____

____

2. Call pain service regarding any new orders for opioids or benzodiazepines not ordered by the pain service.
3. Call pain service for orders to manage nausea/vomiting, itching, anxiety, or inability to sleep if PRN medications ordered below (see #7 and #8) are not effective.
4. **PCA Orders: Standard Concentration (standard) OR ☐ Non Standard Concentration**

DRUG: *(check one)*	☐ MORPHINE	☐ HYDROMORPHONE	☐ FENTANYL	☐ MEPERIDINE	☐ OTHER ________
Standard Concentration	5 mg/mL	1 mg/mL	50 mcg/mL	10 mg/mL	Concentration ________
PCA Dose	______mg	______mg	10 mcg (standard) or ______mcg	10 mg (standard) or ______mg	______mg/mcg
PCA Lockout	6 minutes	6 minutes	6 minutes	6 minutes	6 minutes
4 Hour Limit	30 mg (standard) or ☐ ______mg or ☐ turn off	6 mg (standard) or ☐ ______mg or ☐ turn off	300 mcg (standard) or ☐ ______mcg or ☐ turn off	150 mg (standard)	________ or ☐ turn off
Volume (25 mL IV bag is standard)	25 mL IV bag ☐ 100 mL IV bag	25 mL IV bag ☐ 100 mL IV bag	25 mL IV bag ☐ 100 mL IV bag	25 mL IV bag	25 mL IV bag ☐ 100 mL IV bag

OPTIONAL CLINICIAN BOLUS DOSES AT START OF THERAPY &/OR FOR INCIDENT/BREAKTHROUGH PAIN

2X the current PCA dose every 5 minutes up to a maximum of 5 doses (standard) **or**

☐ ______**mg/mcg** (circle one) **every 5 minutes up to a maximum of 5 doses.**

- Limit clinician bolus doses to every 4 hour interval. *(If needed more often than every 4 hours, call Pain Service.)*
- Series of clinician bolus doses should be given from pump *(except in PACU)* and completed within one hour.
- **Monitor and document SpO2, respiratory rate, sedation score, and pain score every 15 min x 4.**

☐ **USE IV PCA optional clinician bolus dose orders to treat incident/breakthrough pain** if patient has **both** neuraxial route *(epidural or intrathecal)* pain management **AND** IV PCA pain management.

CONTINUOUS INFUSION MODE : **None (standard)**

☐ Start continuous infusion at the time(s) and dose(s) below.

☐ 0600 – 2200 hours daily AND/OR ☐2200 – 0600 hours nightly OR ☐ Continuous

______mg/mcg/hr (circle one) ______mg/mcg/hr (circle one) ______mg/mcg/hr (circle one)

RN Independent Double Check:

Check patient identifiers, drug, drug concentration, pump settings, and PCA connection to compatible IV line. Check with PCA initiation, change in drug, change in concentration.

Initiated by:______________________ Date:__________ Time:__________

Verified by:______________________ Date:__________ Time:__________

PROVIDER SIGNATURE	PRINT NAME	☐ ACUTE PAIN SVC ☐ CHRONIC PAIN SVC	NPI	DATE	TIME

PT.NO

NAME

DOB

UW Medicine Health System
Harborview Medical Center – UW Medical Center
Northwest Hospital & Medical Center – University of Washington Physicians
Seattle, Washington

PAIN SERVICE IV PCA ORDERS
PAGE 1 OF 2

U0840

WHITE - MEDICAL RECORD

UH0840 REV NOV 10

A

Figure 3.1 A and B, University of Washington Medical Center parenteral (intravenous/subcutaneous) patient-controlled analgesia standardized order set. Courtesy of University of Washington Medical Center, Seattle, Washington.

PAIN SERVICE: Parenteral (IV/SQ) Patient Controlled Analgesia (PCA) Orders Page 2 of 2

5. **MONITORING & DOCUMENTATION:**

STANDARD MONITORING:
Respiratory rate, pain score, and sedation score – every 2 hours for 8 hours,
Then, respiratory rate, pain score, and sedation score every 4 hours while patient is on PCA.

CHECK BOX if Special Monitoring is required:

☐ SPECIAL MONITORING:

For first 12 hours, monitor SpO2 via continuous pulse oximetry, respiratory rate, sedation score and pain score every 1 hour. Administer oxygen per MD order to keep SpO2 > 92%.

☐ If patient has **both** neuraxial route *(epidural or intrathecal)* pain management **AND** IV PCA route pain management, **USE neuraxial monitoring orders to monitor the patient.**

DOCUMENTATION:
Clear pump and document the total dose delivered every 8 hours (e.g.. 0600, 1400, 2200) in the clinical record.

6. **TREATMENT OF SIDE EFFECTS:**

A. **Call Pain Service for sedation score = 2, RR < 8/ minute, or pCO2 > 50 mmHg or Sp02 <92%**

B. SEDATION SCORE = 3 and/or RR < 8/minute:
Administer **Naloxone** 0.08 mg IV STAT every 2 minutes PRN. (See Naloxone Kit instructions).
Call Pain Service.

C NAUSEA/VOMITING:
Metoclopramide 10 mg IV every 6 hours PRN.

IF NOT EFFECTIVE, GIVE: **Ondansetron** 4 mg IV every 8 hours PRN X 24 hours.
Call pain service if Ondansetron is ineffective and/or continued unrelieved nausea/vomiting.

In addition, if age < 60 years, **Transdermal Scopolamine** patch to either mastoid area PRN.
Change scopolamine patch every 72 hours.

D. ITCHING:
Diphenhydramine 25 mg IV every 6 hours PRN severe itching.
IF NOT EFFECTIVE, discontinue Diphenhydramine AND GIVE:
Nalbuphine 2.5 – 5 mg IV every 4 hours PRN.

E. URINARY RETENTION:
If patient unable to void or symptoms of urinary retention, check bladder volume with Bladder Scan.
If volume > 400 mL & unable to void, "in and out" bladder catheter, PRN.

7. If age < 60 years, **Zolpidem** 5 mg PO at bedtime PRN for sleep. Call Pain Service if not effective.

8. **FOR INADEQUATE PAIN RELIEF OR OTHER PROBLEMS RELATED TO PCA:**
Call Pain Service physician at pager 986-3334.

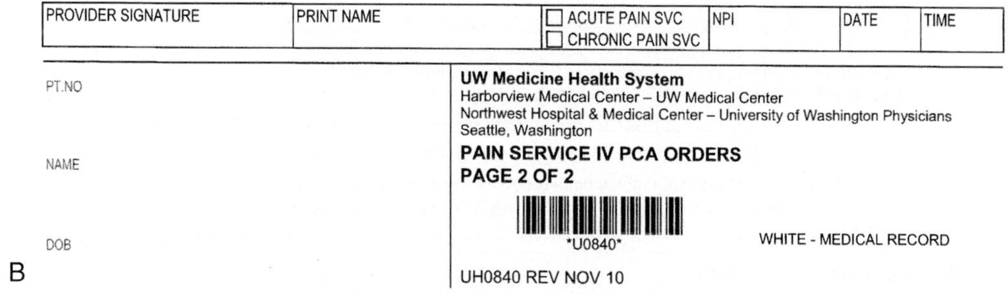

PROVIDER SIGNATURE	PRINT NAME	☐ ACUTE PAIN SVC ☐ CHRONIC PAIN SVC	NPI	DATE	TIME

PT.NO

NAME

DOB

UW Medicine Health System
Harborview Medical Center – UW Medical Center
Northwest Hospital & Medical Center – University of Washington Physicians
Seattle, Washington

PAIN SERVICE IV PCA ORDERS
PAGE 2 OF 2

U0840

WHITE - MEDICAL RECORD

UH0840 REV NOV 10

B

Figure 3.1, cont'd.

effects (e.g., antiemetics or antipruritics and opioid receptor antagonists to reverse respiratory depression). Ketamine and perineural anesthetics are most frequently ordered as adjuncts to other analgesic therapies (e.g., PCA). Recovery room, intensive care unit, and medical/surgical floor nurses must be trained to be familiar with the order set parameters. In most cases, nurses are able to assess the patient and implement changes that successfully achieve adequate analgesia with minimal side effects autonomously.

An emerging area of concern for any anesthesiology-based pain service is the increasing complexity of invasive pain management techniques in an era of ever-increasing numbers of anticoagulants given as treatment or prophylaxis for an ever-increasing number of medical and surgical indications (including, for example, treatment of cardiac arrhythmias or valve disease and deep vein thrombosis prophylaxis). To aid in treating such patients with the least risk, the University of Washington Medical Center has designed institutional guidelines (based on national guidelines such as those of the American Society of Regional Anesthesia, for instance) for the management of indwelling neuraxial and peripheral nerve catheters in patients treated concomitantly with anticoagulants (Table 3.1). The document was designed to address placement, maintenance, and removal of the catheter in several common anticoagulation scenarios. The intention of such guidelines is to distill the existing scientific evidence and opinion into a format that is easily accessible and simple to apply to patient care.

PERSONAL INVENTORY

It is important to recognize at the outset that establishing a pain service is a major endeavor. Planning, design, and implementation of a successful service will require substantial human and material resources.

If the need and desire for an acute pain service exist within a hospital facility, one must first elicit the support of the department chairperson. Although multiple design models for an acute pain management service are possible, most will require that an anesthesiologist be made available for some level of participation in the service. Unless resources allow an anesthesiologist to be easily released from operating room obligations, the staffing conflict will present a certain challenge. An agreeable arrangement of service responsibilities must allow the anesthesiologist to be available to provide safe and consistent care to whomever he or she is responsible.

PAIN SERVICE EPIDURAL INFUSION ORDERS
Page 1 of 2

1. Discontinue current opioids and/or benzodiazepines except: ________________________
2. Epidural Catheter: ***(check one)***
   ☐ Thoracic placement ☐ Lumbar placement ☐ Other:________________
3. Infusion: ***(check one)***
   ☐ **Continuous + Patient Controlled Epidural Analgesia (PCEA)**
   Continuous rate: 6 mL **(standard)** ________mL/hr *(Maximum infusion rate is 14 mL/hr)*
   PCEA dose: 2 mL **(standard)** **or** ☐ ________mL
   PCEA dose lockout: 10 min **(standard)** **or** ☐ ________min
   OR
   ☐ **Continuous Infusion ONLY**
   Continuous rate = ________mL/hr
4. Drug(s): ***(check one)***
   ☐ FENTANYL 2 mcg/mL + BUPIVACAINE 1/16% (0.625 mg/mL)
   ☐ FENTANYL 2 mcg/mL + BUPIVACAINE 1/10% (1 mg/mL)
   ☐ FENTANYL 2 mcg/mL + BUPIVACAINE 1/8% (1.25 mg/mL)
   ☐ BUPIVACAINE 1/16% (0.625mg/mL)
   ☐ BUPIVACAINE 1/10% (1 mg/mL)
   ☐ BUPIVACAINE 1/8% (1.25 mg/mL)
   ☐ BUPIVACAINE ________% (________/mg/mL)
   ☐ Opioid (specify) ________________mcg/mL or mg/mL + BUPIVACAINE ________% (________mg/mL)
5. VOLUME OF EPIDURAL SOLUTION = 250 mL in normal saline **(standard)**
6. BREAKTHROUGH PAIN MANAGEMENT ***(check one)***
   A. ☐ **Continuous + Patient Controlled Epidural Analgesia (PCEA) (check box)**
   Give clinician bolus equal to ☐ continuous hourly infusion rate or ☐ ______mL into epidural catheter
   and increase continuous hourly rate by 2 mL/hrs every 2 hours PRN
   MAXIMUM RECOMENDED INFUSION RATE is 14 mL/hr.
   B. ☐ **Continuous Infusion only (NO PCEA – no patient controlled settings): (check box)**
   ☐ **Fentanyl** 50 mcg (1 mL) into epidural catheter every 2 hours PRN. *(check box)*
   ☐ Use IV PCA clinician bolus dose orders to treat incident/breakthrough pain if patient has **both** epidural pain management **AND** IV PCA pain management. (check box)
   C. ☐ Other:________________________

RN Independent Double Check:
Check patient identifiers, drug, drug concentration, pump settings, and PCA connection to compatible IV line. Check with PCA initiation, change in drug, and change in concentration.
Initiated by:________________ Date:____________ Time:________
Verified by: :________________ **Date:**____________ **Time:**________

PROVIDER SIGNATURE	PRINT NAME	☐ ACUTE PAIN SVC ☐ CHRONIC PAIN SVC	NPI	DATE	TIME

PT.NO

NAME

DOB

UW Medicine Health System
Harborview Medical Center – UW Medical Center
Northwest Hospital & Medical Center – University of Washington Physicians
Seattle, Washington
PAIN SERVICE EPIDURAL INFUSION ORDERS
PAGE 1 OF 2

U0949

WHITE - MEDICAL RECORD

UH0949 REV NOV 10

A

Figure 3.2 A and B, University of Washington Medical Center epidural infusion standardized order set. Courtesy of University of Washington Medical Center, Seattle, Washington.

PAIN SERVICE EPIDURAL INFUSION ORDERS
Page 2 of 2

MONITORING: Includes epidural continuous infusion and epidural continuous infusion with Patient Controlled Epidural Analgesia (PCEA).

7. **First 24 hours:** Respiratory rate & sedation scale every 1 hour. **Respiratory Effort:** RN assess for changes in the pattern and quality of ventilation (rate, depth, regularity, and effort to breathe).
8. **First 24 hours:** Assess pulse oximetry reading while on room air every 2 hours. If patient is on oxygen, remove oxygen for 5 minutes and assess pulse oximetry reading every 2 hours. Notify Pain Service with changes in respiratory assessment and if SP02 <92% on room air when oxygen removed.
9. BP/Pulse from start of infusion every 30 min x 3 hours: then every 2 hours x 24 hours; then every 4 hours. **Postural BP/P prior to first ambulation.**
10. After 24 hours: Respiratory rate & sedation scale every 4 hours during epidural use.
11. Pain assessment every 4 hours and PRN.
12. Lower extremity motor function assessment every 4 hours. (e.g. bilateral straight leg lifts).
13. After epidural catheter discontinued, check: Respiratory rate, sedation scale, and lower extremity motor function assessment every 4 hours x 12 hours.

BREAKTHROUGH PAIN DOSE MONITORING:

14. Blood pressure, pulse, respiratory rate, sedation scale, and pain assessment rechecked every 15 minutes x 1 hour after each clinician bolus dose and/or with each continuous rate increase.
15. See "notify pain service" section below (See A thru F) related to breakthrough pain monitoring.

---

16. Maintain IV access (drip or peripheral lock with flushes) until 12 hours after epidural analgesia continuous infusion discontinued.
17. **No other opioid or central nervous system depressant medications except those ordered by the pain service.**
18. **TREATMENTS OF SIDE EFFECTS:**
    a) SEDATION SCALE = 3 plus RR < 8/minute: **Naloxone** 0.08 mg IV every 2 minutes PRN (See Naloxone Kit instructions.)
    b) NAUSEA/VOMITING: **Metoclopramide** 10 mg IV every 6 hours PRN
    In addition, if age < 60 years, **Transdermal Scopolamine** patch to either mastoid area.
    Change scopolamine patch every 72 hours PRN
    If ineffective, give: **Ondansetron** 4 mg IV every 8 hours PRN x 24 hours.
    c) ITCHING: **Diphenhydramine** 25 mg IV every 6 hours PRN
    If ineffective, discontinue and give: **Nalbuphine** 2.5 – 5 mg IV every 4 hours PRN
    d) URINARY RETENTION: **Urinary catheters are not routinely required with thoracic epidural catheter placement**. If no urinary catheter and patient is unable to void - check bladder volume with bladder scan. If volume > 400 mL, "in & out" bladder catheter PRN
19. FOR SLEEP: and if age < 60 years, **Zolpidem** 5 mg PO every bedtime PRN

NOTIFY PAIN SERVICE (PAGER 986-3334) FOR ANY OF THE FOLLOWING

A. RR < 8/min. or pCO2 > 50 mm Hg.
B. Sedation scale = 2 or pattern of progressive sedation.
C. BP < ______mm Hg and/or P < ______/min.
D. Inability to ambulate independently.
E. Inadequate analgesia or other problems related to epidural.
F. Temperature > 38.5°C.
G. New orders for pharmacologic anticoagulation or antiplatelet therapy.

PROVIDER SIGNATURE	PRINT NAME	☐ ACUTE PAIN SVC ☐ CHRONIC PAIN SVC	NPI	DATE	TIME

PT.NO

NAME

DOB

UW Medicine
Harborview Medical Center – UW Medical Center
University of Washington Physicians
Seattle, Washington

PAIN SERVICE EPIDURAL INFUSION ORDERS
PAGE 2 OF 2

U0949

WHITE - MEDICAL RECORD

UH0949 REV NOV 10

B

Figure 3.2, cont'd.

Once the intradepartmental issues of resource allocation have been discussed with the chairperson, the proposal to begin an acute pain service should be brought to the medical director and team. Commitment of the medical director to the project will be necessary for provision of resources in the form of personnel and money.

Finally, appropriate leadership for the acute pain service must be selected. Operating the service will require a diverse constellation of skills. The individual must have knowledge of the mechanisms of acute postsurgical pain and the methods of treatment, including opioid and nonopioid analgesia, epidural placement and maintenance, peripheral nerve catheter placement and maintenance, and ketamine and other adjuvant drug therapies—as well as treatments of the side effects from these therapies. An anesthesiologist is often the best fit since he or she has experience with these therapies. Of course, as mentioned previously, a number of nonpharmacological therapies (e.g., physical and alternative or complementary medicine therapies) also have a role in acute pain management, and leaders of any acute pain service must likewise be aware of these therapeutic strategies.

PAIN SERVICE: Pain Management Ketamine Continuous Infusion Orders

1. Prescription:

Drug:	Ketamine – Non Anesthetic Dosing
Concentration:	1mg/mL Send in 250mL normal saline bag
Route:	IV infusion
Infusion Rate: DO NOT TITRATE, DO NOT BOLUS	________mg/hour (For Postoperative patients: Do not exceed 8mg/hour infusion rate on medical surgical and oncology floors)
Infusion Device:	Standard pain infusion pump Drug is to be secured in locked box with the pump.

2. Change Ketamine bag every 24 hours (related to stability in IVF bag).
   Order next bag in sufficient time to avoid disruption of continuous ketamine infusion.
3. Monitoring and Documentation:

   Ketamine drip initiation: Blood pressure (BP), respiratory rate (RR), pain score, sedation score every 30 minutes for one hour and then every two hours for 8 hours. After 8 hours, monitor RR, pain score, and sedation score every 4 hours while on infusion.
   Ask the patient if they are having hallucinations or unpleasant, disturbing dreams every 8 hours. Document in the clinical record.

   NOTE: Anticipate decreasing opioid requirement/use.

   Infusion rate increases: BP, RR, pain score, sedation score every 30 minutes for one hour, then every two hours for 4 hours and then every 4 hours.

   Check box if special monitoring is required:
   ☐ if patient has **both** neuraxial route (epidural or intrathecal) pain management and Ketamine infusion, **USE neuraxial (epidural or intrathecal) monitoring orders** for RR, pain score and sedation score. BP every 30 minutes for one hour and then every two hours for 8 hours and then every 4 hours.
4. **Call Pain Service pager 986-3334 if**:

   Systolic BP if > or < 30 mm Hg from pre-infusion baseline parameters Baseline BP = ________
   Sedation score > 2 and/or RR < 8 breaths/minute
   Patient reports hallucinations (auditory or visual); feeling dissociated; or reports of unpleasant, disturbing dreams.
   Inadequate pain management
5. Call Pain Service regarding any new orders for opioids or benzodiazepines not ordered by the Pain Service.
6. Patient also has pain service pain management orders for:
   ☐ PCA
   ☐ Neuraxial analgesia (Epidural or Intrathecal)
   ☐ Other: ________

PHYSICIAN/MID LEVEL SIGNATURE	PRINT NAME	PAGER	UPIN/NPI	DATE	TIME

PT.NO

NAME

DOB

UW Medicine
Harborview Medical Center – UW Medical Center
University of Washington Physicians
Seattle, Washington
KETAMINE CONTINUOUS INFUSION ORDERS

U2694

UH2694 REV MAY 09

WHITE - MEDICAL RECORD
CANARY - PHARMACY
PINK - NURSING

PHYSICIAN ORDER — YELLOW

Figure 3.3 University of Washington Medical Center intravenous ketamine infusion standardized order set. Courtesy of University of Washington Medical Center, Seattle, Washington.

In addition to expertise in analgesic therapies, the success and stability of any new acute pain service will require that the service director also possess certain nonclinical skills, including strong leadership, organizational, and administrative abilities. Clinical success demands the integration of multiple clinical disciplines, such as nursing, medicine, pharmacy, and others. These diverse professionals need to operate independently and in collaboration. Additionally, the leader will need to understand the place of the acute pain service within the structure of the hospital organization. The service should be structured so it is made both efficient and valuable to the hospital and its surgical services. Selection of a qualified director of an acute pain service is vital to its success.

ASSESSMENT OF NEED

Once the challenge of organizing an acute pain service is accepted, assessment of need is mandatory. This might be accomplished by surveying the patient population, nurses, types of specialty services, procedures commonly performed, and the people performing these procedures. Furthermore, the Joint Commission on Accreditation of

DIAGNOSIS	CONDITION

Peripheral Nerve/Wound Infusion Pump Physician Orders

1. Type of catheter:

   ☐ Peripheral nerve catheter

   ☐ Surgical wound catheter

2. Initiate peripheral nerve/wound infusion pump.

   Type of Pump: ☐ Disposable Pain Pump (i.e. Stryker PainPump2 BlockAid) ☐ other:____________________

3. Anesthetic to be used in the peripheral nerve/wound infusion pump:

   Initial Pump Fill:

   ☐ Ropivacaine 0.2% 400 mL volume (prepared in OR pharmacy)

   ☐ Ropivacaine 0.5% 400 mL volume (prepared in OR pharmacy)

   ☐ Bupivacaine 0.25% 400 mL volume (prepared in OR pharmacy)

   ☐ other: ______________________________ (prepared in the OR pharmacy)

4. Peripheral nerve/wound pump settings:

   Continuous Flow Rate (mL/hr): ☐ 2 mL/hr ☐ 4 mL/hr ☐ 6 mL/hr ☐ Other: __________

   NOTE: Maximum recommended volume continuous infusion rate for local anesthetic concentrations ≥ 0.5% is 10 mL/hour.

   Patient controlled anesthetic Bolus Dose (mL): ☐ 1 mL ☐ 2 mL ☐ other__________

   Lockout Time (min.): ☐ 60 minutes ☐ 120 minutes ☐ other__________

5. **CHECK BOX** if neurovascular checks are needed for this patient.

   ☐ Assess and document neurovascular check

   of ______________________________ every 4 hours.

6. Monitor pump screen every 4 hours for warning symbols or messages on display screen.
7. Document total volume of local anesthetic infused every 8 hours.
8. If signs and symptoms of infection, unusual/excessive drainage from the insertion site, catheter pump leaks, signs/symptoms of local anesthetic toxicity, or inadequate analgesia, contact physician/service above that placed peripheral nerve/wound pump.
9. Pump Refill Orders:

   ☐ Ropivacaine 0.2% 400 mL volume. Send in IV bag. (prepared in inpatient pharmacy)

   ☐ Ropivacaine 0.5% 400 mL volume. Send in IV bag (prepared in inpatient pharmacy)

   ☐ Bupivacaine 0.25% 400 mL volume. Send in IV bag. (prepared in inpatient pharmacy)

   ☐ other:____________________ Send in IV bag. (prepared in inpatient pharmacy)

10. Other:______________________________

PHYSICIAN SIGNATURE	PRINT NAME	PAGER	NPI/UPIN	DATE	TIME

PT.NO

NAME

DOB

UW Medicine
Harborview Medical Center – UW Medical Center
University of Washington Physicians
Seattle, Washington

PERIPH NERVE/WOUND INFUS PUMP ORDS

U2245

UH2245 REV JUL 07

WHITE - MEDICAL RECORD
CANARY - PHARMACY
PINK - NURSING

Figure 3.4 University of Washington Medical Center peripheral nerve/wound infusion standardized order set. Courtesy of University of Washington Medical Center, Seattle, Washington.

Healthcare Organizations (JCAHO) has set forth standards declaring the patient's right to adequate pain assessment and treatment and has explicitly acknowledged that pain is a coexisting condition with a number of diseases and injuries that requires explicit attention. It is on this basis that the mission statement of the service should be defined.

Those constructing the service might also consider whether they wish to distinguish or separate different types of pain management challenges or manage them as a conglomerate. As an example, the University of Washington Inpatient Pain Services is divided into three factions: acute pain, chronic/cancer pain, and interventional pain. The service was separated into these groups to preserve continuity of care and more practically manage the high volume of patients. Admittedly, the boundaries between these categories are artificial and may overlap. As an example, consider a patient with acute postsurgical pain superimposed on chronic cancer pain or a patient who has recently undergone placement of an implanted epidural neuromodulating device for treating chronic pain.

Whatever the organization, an acute postoperative pain management service is likely to require 24-hour,

Table 3.1 University of Washington Medical Center Anticoagulation Guidelines for Neuraxial or Peripheral Nerve Procedures

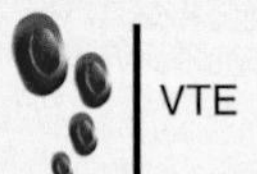

VTE

University of Washington Medical Center (UWMC)

ANTICOAGULATION GUIDELINES FOR NEURAXIAL OR PERIPHERAL NERVE PROCEDURES

Guidelines to prevent spinal hematoma following epidural/intrathecal/spinal procedures and perineural hematoma following peripheral nerve procedures

ATTENTION: When can you safely do neuraxial/peripheral nerve procedures or give anticoagulants?
Neuraxial routes include epidural and intrathecal infusions, implanted intrathecal pumps, and spinal injections.
Peripheral routes include all peripheral nerve and plexus infusions.

NOTE: Bloody tap/procedure? Anesthesia to call pain service

MEDICATION	PRIOR TO NEURAXIAL/NERVE PROCEDURE Minimum time between last dose of anticoagulant and spinal injection OR neuraxial/nerve catheter placement	WHILE NEURAXIAL/NERVE CATHETER IN PLACE Restrictions on use of anticoagulants while neuraxial/nerve catheters are in place and prior to their removal	AFTER NEURAXIAL/NERVE PROCEDURE Minimum time between neuraxial/nerve catheter removal OR spinal nerve injection and next anticoagulant dose
Anticoagulants for VTE prophylaxis			
Heparin unfractionated, 5000 unit q8h or q12h	May be given; no time restrictions for catheter placement/removal or spinal injections Do NOT call pain service		
Heparin unfractionated, 7500 units SQ q8h	8 hr	CONTRAINDICATED while catheter in place May NOT be given unless approved by pain service attending	2 hr
Dalteparin (Fragmin), 5000 u/day SQ	12 hr (longer in renal impairment)	May be given BUT: • Must wait 8 hr after catheter PLACEMENT before giving dose • Must wait 12 hr after last dose before REMOVING catheter	2 hr
Enoxaparin (Lovenox), 40 mg/day SQ			
Enoxaparin (Lovenox), 30 mg SQ q12h or 40 mg SQ q12h	12 hr (longer in renal impairment)	CONTRAINDICATED while catheter in place. May NOT be given unless approved by pain service attending	2 hr
Fondaparinux (Arixtra), < 2.5 mg SQ qday	48 hr (longer in renal impairment)		
Rivaroxaban (Xarelto), 10 mg PO	24 hr (longer in renal impairment)	May be given BUT contact pain service regarding dose timing • Must wait 8 hr after catheter PLACEMENT before giving dose • Must wait 24 hr after last dose before REMOVING catheter	6 hr (per manufacturer recommendations)
Agents used for full systemic anticoagulation			
Dabigatran (Pradaxa)	72 hr (longer in renal impairment)	CONTRAINDICATED while catheter in place. May NOT be given unless approved by pain service attending	2 hr
Dalteparin (Fragmin), 200 U/kg/day SQ or 100 U/kg SQ q12h	24 hr (longer in renal impairment)		
Enoxaparin (Lovenox), 1.5 mg/kg/day SQ or 1 mg/kg SQ q12h	24 hr (longer in renal impairment)		
Fondaparinux (Arixtra), 5-10 mg/day SQ	72 hr (longer in renal impairment)		
Heparin unfractionated, IV continuous infusion or >5000 units SQ bid or tid	When aPTT <40 sec		
Rivaroxaban (Xarelto), 15-20 mg PO day	24 hr (longer in renal impairment)		6 hr (per manufacturer recommendations)
Warfarin (Coumadin)	When INR <1.5		2 hr

aPTT, activated partial thromboplastin time; INR, international normalized ratio; IV, intravenous; PO, orally; SQ, subcutaneously; VTE, venous thromboembolism.

Courtesy of University of Washington Medical Center, Seattle, Washington.

Table 3.2 Options for Acute Pain Treatment Based on Available Resources

Analgesic Technique	Personnel*	Knowledge	Skills†	Equipment‡	Comment§
Basic anxiety reduction	Any				1, 8, 9
PO/PR nonopioids	A, B	Dose, range, side effects	M, N		1, 8, 9
PO/PR opioids	A, B	Dose, range, side effects	M, N		1, 8, 9
SC/IM opioids	A, B, G	Dose, range, side effects	M, N, O, R	T	1, 8, 9
IV opioids	A, B, G	Dose, range, side effects, loading titration	M, N, O, P, R	T, U, W, X, Y	1, 8, 9
Local anesthetic infiltration	B	Anatomy, dose, range, side effects	M, R, S, T		4, 7
Opioid PCA	A, C or E, G	Dose, range, side effects, PCA principles	M, N, P	U, V, X, Y	8, 9
Ketamine	C	Dose, range, side effects	M, N, P, R	U, W, X, Y	4
Nitrous oxide	B	Dose, range, side effects, administration	M, N, R	Delivery system	4, 8
TENS	A, B	Anatomy	M	Units, accessories	Adjunctive therapy
Intraspinal opioids	A, C, E	Dose, range, side effects	M, N, P, Q, R	T, U, W, X, Z	1, 2, 8, 9
Plexus blocks	A, C	Dose, range, side effects, anatomy	M, N, P, Q, R, S	T, W, X, Y	2
Neuraxial block	A, C	Dose, range, side effects, anatomy	M, N, P, Q, R, S	T, U, W, X, Y, Z	1, 2, 3, 5, 6, 7, 8
Interpleural	A, C, D, E	Dose, range, side effects, anatomy	M, N, P, Q, R, S	T, U, W, X, Y, Z	1, 3, 7
Cryoanalgesia	E, D	Anatomy		Delivery system	1, 3, 7
Psychological support	A, B, C, D, E, F	Coping strategies	Relaxation, breathing exercises	All the above	Time-consuming, adjunct
Acute pain service	A, C, D, E, F, G	All of the above	M, N, O, P, Q, R, S, leadership		Policies, procedures, education, quality assurance

**Personnel*: A, nurse; B, physician; C, anesthesiologist; D, surgeon; E, pain specialist; F, psychologist; G, pharmacist.

†*Skills*: M, evaluate effects; N, monitor; O, injection technique; P, start IV line; Q, block technique; R, support ventilation; S, treat convulsion.

‡*Equipment*: T, needles, syringes; U, IV equipment; W, PPV equipment; X, oxygen; Y, suction; Z, epidural catheters.

§*Comments*: 1, dose regularly; 2, continuous infusion; 3, tachyphylaxis; 4, aspiration; 5, possible hypotension; 6, possible high block; 7, possible convulsion; 8, hypoventilation; 9, antagonist available.

IM, intramuscular; IV, intravenous; PCA, patient-controlled analgesia; PO, by mouth; PPV, positive pressure ventilation; PR, by rectum; SC, subcutaneous; TENS, transcutaneous electrical nerve stimulation.

7-day-a-week call coverage, with appropriately available medical supervision. Immediate availability is important with regard to patient safety and patient satisfaction. Inadequacy of pain relief has been highlighted as a quality-of-care measure and a focus of patients' concern. In a questionnaire survey, 57% of patients identified pain after surgery as their primary fear.[1] The competitive health care environment mandates that hospitals share a focus on the issues that are most important to patients. Favorable reports of patient satisfaction may attract patients to partake of services in a given hospital facility and also encourage patient loyalty with return for future medical services. Furthermore, immediate postoperative patient satisfaction with care is a predictor of long-term, positively self-perceived health status according to one multicenter prospective cohort study.[22] Indeed, data from the Hospital Consumer Assessment of Healthcare Providers and Systems (HCAHPS) are likely to put hospital pain management, as well as patient satisfaction with that management, front and center not only with regard to comparisons between hospitals but ultimately for reimbursement of hospital services.

DEFINITION OF THE SERVICE

Once the mission statement has been formulated in response to the perceived institutional and community needs, it is necessary to define the resources that will be required. The resources and modalities that an acute pain service may use are diverse and depend on the patient population, the skills of the personnel, and the service's therapeutic approach. Ideally, a scientific approach to the selection of treatment modalities that specifically evaluates the efficacy and cost-effectiveness of each therapy is used. Ultimately, the resources required to implement and operate an acute pain service will represent a synthesis of characteristics of the patient population, evidence-based selection of therapeutic modalities, and consistency with the service's mission.

The feasibility of various treatment plans based on the availability of resources has been defined by the IASP task force on the management of acute pain (Table 3.2). Again, individualized treatment of patients should ideally be chosen from a rational, evidence-based selection list, also outlined by

Table 3.3 Evidence-Based Guides for the Treatment of Acute Pain

Group	Guidelines	Website
Prospect	Procedure-specific postoperative pain management	www.postoppain.org/frameset.htm
European Society of Regional Anaesthesia and Pain Therapy	Postoperative pain management, good clinical practice	www.esraeurope.org/PostoperativePain Management.pdf
Arbeitsgemeinschaft der Wissenschaftlichen Medizinischen Fachgesellschaften (AWMF) (Association of the Scientific Medical Societies in Germany), Deutsche Interdisziplinäre Vereinigung für Schmerztherapie (DIVS) (German Interdisciplinary Association for Pain Therapy, Germany)	Behandlung akuter perioperativer und posttraumatischer Schmerzen (Guidelines on acute perioperative and post-traumatic pain [in German])	www.uni-duesseldorf.de/awmf/II/
Association of Paediatric Anaesthetists, United Kingdom	Good practice in postoperative and procedural pain (2008)	www.britishpainsociety.org/book_apa_part I.pdf www.britishpainsociety.org/book_apa_part2.pdf
Society for Anaesthesiology, Analgesia, Reanimation and Intensive Care (SIAARTI), Italy	Postoperative pain treatment, SIAARTI recommendations 2010, short version (2010)	www.minervamedica.it/en/journals/minerva-anesthesiological/article.php?cod=R02Y2010N08A0657
American Academy of Pediatrics Committee on Fetus and Newborn, American Academy of Pediatrics Section on Surgery, Canadian Paediatric Society Fetus and Newborn Committee	Prevention and management of pain in the neonate, an update (2010)	http://aappolicy.aappublications.org/cgi/content/abstract/pediatrics:118/5/2231
American Society of Anesthesiologists	Practice guidelines for acute pain management in the perioperative setting	www2.asahq.org/publications/pc-115-4-practive-guidelines-for-acute-pain-management-in-the-perioperative-setting.aspx

the IASP task force on management of acute pain (Table 3.3). Such ideal care allows maximal improvement of patients' outcome with the most cost-effectiveness possible. To achieve this aim, resources in the form of medications, equipment, and personnel must be anticipated and negotiated with the institution's administrative, business, and clinical departments when one is designing the structure of the service.

After the resources are defined, it is imperative to assess the safety of the proposed plan. The principles of therapy to be implemented in the practice of pain medicine should allow one to do the following:

1. Evaluate the source and severity of the pain.
2. Understand the relationship between pain and other components of suffering (e.g., a poor prognosis creating reactive depression or anxiety).
3. Achieve and maintain adequate analgesia and incorporate it into the acute rehabilitation scheme.
4. Refine therapy based on individual needs.

After the available resources are settled, the type of service that can be organized can be determined. A *single-modality service* allows the provision of analgesia with intravenous opioid systems to all inpatients and provision of regional analgesia in selected instances. This model can be nurse based with physician supervision and offers a limited, yet cost-effective, method to treat postoperative patients. A *multimodal service* includes diverse health care professionals from a variety of domains. Extracting and integrating the relevant expertise from multiple health care disciplines often allow individualized and optimized pain management. Disciplines commonly used include psychology, pharmacy, physical therapy, and nutrition. The comprehensive approach of a multidisciplinary pain service functions in a consultative capacity for inpatients with complicated pain issues. Examples include patients with chronic pain suffering from acute exacerbations and postsurgical patients with severe opiate tolerance following long-term opioid treatment.[23] This model has been most frequently used in the context of inpatient palliative care consultation at the end of life, but it may have utility in the acute care arena as well.

Ongoing quality assurance evaluation can be managed on a service, departmental, or institutional level but should be transparent to participants and provide an opportunity for feedback and improvement for trainees, faculty, and the service itself.

FINANCING AND THE BUSINESS PLAN

The next step in the process of organizing an inpatient acute pain service is to construct the business plan. This is often the most difficult phase since the financial and business skills needed may not be innate to clinical anesthesiologists and are rarely covered in their training. Furthermore, the value analysis of this type of service is not entirely monetary.

It should be emphasized that although the cost of delivering care may be considerable, calculation of the cost analysis is a more complicated determination. The ideal measurement of utility regarding pain management is controversial. Researchers have examined outcome measures, including hospital stay, hospital readmissions, quality of life, and productivity.[24] However, regardless of the cost analysis, there is a cultural expectation and ethical imperative supporting the philosophy that appropriate treatment of pain is independently valuable. The JCAHO has emphasized this sentiment in their statement that appropriate pain management is "good medicine" and that "excuses for inadequate pain control will no longer be accepted because poor pain control is unethical, clinically unsound, and economically wasteful."[25]

With that acknowledgement, the purpose of an acute pain service business plan is to describe the inner workings of the proposed service, including its organizational strategy, marketing plan, tentative schedule for implementation, and overall cost. This must occur before the first cent is spent on the project. The business plan has two components. The first arm of the plan is a narrative that includes the mission statement, its structure, and the responsibilities of the service. Here, the job descriptions of involved personnel are outlined, facility requirements are listed, and the marketing plan is presented. This document should clarify the role, responsibilities, duties, and expectations of various personnel key to a successfully operating service. Guidelines and manuals for nurses and house staff are key to this first portion of the business plan.

The second portion of the business plan is prepared as a spreadsheet that outlines the finances of the business endeavor, and these estimates must be as accurate as possible. Estimates of fixed and variable incomes, the start-up capital necessary until revenue produces profit, and a month-by-month expenditure estimate for at least the first year must be among the data provided in this document. The plan should also consider the acquisition cost of analgesic medications and other pharmacy costs.

Macario and McCoy reviewed the records of 298 patients who underwent hip or knee replacement surgery and found that pharmacy cost accounted for only 3% of the total hospital cost but that postoperative analgesia cost represented 31% of the total pharmacy cost.[26] Other cost drivers include human resources in the form of pharmacists and nurses, as well as equipment, including PCA and epidural pumps. Medication errors are another rarely considered factor that increases the cost of postoperative analgesia. Adverse drug events, for example, have been shown to result in extending hospital stay by 4.6 days at a cost of $5857 per patient.[27] Finally, this second section of the business plan ought to include a discussion of anticipated challenges to reimbursement either within or outside the institution.

For instance, it is necessary to examine the insurance characteristics of the patient population that the acute pain program will serve. Based on the payer mix or the percentage of the population that is served by health maintenance (HMO), preferred provider (PPO), and medical care (MCO) organizations, it may be necessary to arrange plans for preauthorization of acute pain services with the administrators of local health plans. To prepare for this step in the business plan, it is ideal to have an estimate of the anticipated monthly patient load and the minimum number of patients that will be required to support service expenses. If there is a risk that the number of postsurgical patients using the acute pain services will not suffice, expansion to include nonsurgical or cancer patients with pain may be considered. When assessing these sources, one must be sure that reimbursement will adequately cover the expense of the additional time, energy, and personnel required to deliver and document daily care.

In construction of the business plan, total revenue minus total cost will produce a *predicted* financial position. This calculation begins with estimation of the approximate charge per patient for each therapeutic modality that is to be used. With this revenue in mind, the cost of providing the service and the various therapeutic modalities can be determined. Ideally, the financial design of the acute pain service should include elements promoting flexibility as the patient load waxes and wanes. This is best accomplished by shifting fixed cost (e.g., permanent employees) to variable cost (e.g. temporary employees) as much as possible. Remember that the result of this calculation will fluctuate over time. Financial solvency of the service will be most protected by hoping for the best while planning for the worst-case scenario.

BILLING AND COLLECTION

A well-organized structure for billing and collection for services is imperative to ensure the solvency of any medical organization. Knowledgeable personnel, the necessary hardware, and efficient software for data collection are necessities if the service's business plan includes an internal billing and collection group. As medical coding and billing accelerate in complexity and specialty, many organizations have elected to employ outside billing and collection services that operate on a percentage-based contract.

It is crucial to be aware of current Centers for Medicare and Medicaid Services (CMS) guidelines for documentation and billing and to remain informed about modifications as they occur. Accurate documentation of services will facilitate correct and timely reimbursement, as well as represent what was actually done in the medical record. Furthermore, accurate documentation will make clear what was *not* done both to other health care professionals and to third party payers—thereby avoiding time-consuming changes in documentation, fines, and even criminal charges if discrepancies between CMS guidelines and physician billing are judged to be fraudulent. (Example reference guides regarding chart notation and CMS-required documentation can be found in Appendexes A through F.)

MARKETING PLAN

Once design and planning of the up-and-coming acute pain service have been completed, a marketing plan will be important to promoting its utilization. Potential referring providers and patients will need to be introduced to the concept and to the benefits that the service has to offer.

Although conventional medical education often leaves physicians naïve to the business and marketing dimensions of medicine as an industry, help can be garnered from the hospital's public relations office or from a private marketing firm. Implementation of the marketing plan is another cost that must be considered in the service's budget.

The marketing strategy must be designed with care. It should present a consistent image of the mission and services offered by the budding acute pain service in a light that emphasizes the added value to patient care. The marketing strategy may also delicately make a case for the potential cost and convenience advantages of using the new service. Methods for circulating such information may include announcements and brochures, professionally prepared stationary, logo, newsletters, and websites.

Internal education is another vital part of marketing an acute pain service. Frequent positive interactions between the acute pain service and other departments and their personnel (e.g., presentations at interdepartmental case conferences) are crucial for increasing the visibility of the service and expanding its referral base. In an academic institution, this might also include the involvement of nonanesthesiology residents in the service. When residents rotating from other specialties participate, particularly from the surgical department, they can learn about the treatment modalities offered and the advantages that they provide. Finally, the importance of education and involvement of nursing colleagues cannot be overestimated since they are often in a position to suggest that a patient be referred to the acute pain service.

It is also important that the acute pain service remain attentive and responsive to changes in patient care needs. Recently, for example, some acute pain services have found utility in providing formal or informal perioperative pain clinic services as well. Such clinics can be helpful in preoperatively identifying and planning for patients who are likely to have difficult pain management problems postoperatively (e.g., patients with chronic pain or opiate tolerance), thus improving perceived service efficacy and efficiency. Moreover, a perioperative pain clinic can help surgeons wean their difficult postoperative pain patients from a complicated analgesic regimen or transition them back to their chronic pain therapies. Such outpatient services can help market more classic acute pain inpatient services to surgical colleagues, as well as provide better (and perhaps safer) continuity of care.

Finally, the marketing plan of an acute pain service should align itself with the JCAHO and its standards and expectations. Implementation and compliance with these standards should serve to propel an acute pain service toward success since both aim to make pain a top priority.

CONCLUSION

Although health care providers acknowledge that providing analgesia to acute postsurgical patients is important, this task is often easier said than done. Challenges to meeting this aim include opioid tolerance, acute-on-chronic pain scenarios, and the great variety of surgical procedures and techniques. An acute inpatient pain service can often offer insight and experience when dealing with these complex clinical issues. However, the design, planning, and implementation of an acute inpatient pain service must be performed with great care and intention. Only with thoughtful construction will a successful service emerge that is able to meet and exceed the needs of the hospital, its surgical services, and the patients whom they serve.

KEY POINTS

- Acute, postoperative pain remains widely undertreated even though it is a primary concern of patients anticipating planned surgery.
- An optimal postoperative pain management program will integrate multimodal and multidisciplinary interventions.
- Several systems for organizing an inpatient acute pain service have been described, although most use a partnership between nursing and anesthesiology.
- Detailed practice guidelines, protocols, and order sets can streamline and simplify care.
- Enlisting the support of hospital administration and defining resources are a vital first step in organizing an inpatient acute pain service.
- Treatments provided by the pain service should be individualized and evidence based.
- The business plan of the service must include a cost analysis, although deliverance of pain relief is inherently valuable beyond a calculable measure.
- The business plan should be flexibly constructed by shifting fixed cost to variable cost whenever possible.
- Accuracy in documentation and billing is crucial to facilitate timely and correct reimbursement.
- A marketing plan introduces potential referring providers to the concept and benefits that the service presents.

SUGGESTED READINGS

Bardiau FM, Taviaux NF, Albert A, et al. An intervention study to enhance postoperative pain management. *Anesth Analg.* 2003;96:179-185.

Chrubasik S, Chrubasik J, Grote U, et al. Practicability of the multimodal postoperative approach. *Reg Anesth.* 1996;21:43.

Donihi AC, DiNardo MM, DeVita MA, et al. Use of a standardized protocol to decrease medication errors and adverse events related to sliding scale insulin. *Qual Saf Health Care.* 2006;15:89-91.

Hahnenkamp K, Herroeder S, Hollmann MW. Regional anaesthesia, local anaesthetics and the surgical stress response. *Best Pract Res Clin Anaesthesiol.* 2004;18:509-527.

Hebl JR, Dilger JA, Byer DE, et al. A pre-emptive multimodal pathway featuring peripheral nerve block improves perioperative outcomes after major orthopedic surgery. *Reg Anesth Pain Med.* 2008;33:510-517.

Ip HY, Abrishami A, Peng PW, et al. Predictors of postoperative pain and analgesic consumption: a qualitative systemic review. *Anesthesiology.* 2009;111:657-677.

Philips DM. JCAHO pain management standards are unveiled. Joint Commission on Accreditation of Healthcare Organizations. *JAMA.* 2000;284:428-429.

Practice guidelines for acute pain management in the postoperative setting: a report by the American Society of Anesthesiologists Task Force on Pain Management, Acute Pain Section. *Anesthesiology.* 1995;82:1071-1081.

Shapiro A, Zohar E, Kantor M, et al. Establishing a nurse-based, anesthesiologist-supervised inpatient acute pain service: experience of 4,617 patients. *J Clin Anesth.* 2004;16:415-420.

Stadler M, Schlander M, Braeckman M, et al. A cost-utility and cost-effectiveness analysis of an acute pain service. *J Clin Anesth.* 2005;16:159-167.

Warfield CA. Acute pain management: programs in US hospitals and experiences and attitudes among US adults. *Anesthesiology.* 1995;83:1090-1094.

The references for this chapter can be found at www.expertconsult.com.

Appendix 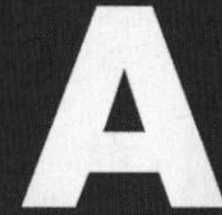

HPI (history of present illness): Characterize HPI by considering either the status of chronic conditions or the number of elements recorded. ☐ 1 condition ☐ 2 conditions ☐ 3 conditions or ☐ Location ☐ Severity ☐ Timing ☐ Modifying factors ☐ Quality ☐ Duration ☐ Context ☐ Associated signs and symptoms	☐ Status of 1-2 chronic conditions	☐ Status of 1-2 chronic conditions	☐ Status of 3 chronic conditions	☐ Status of 3 chronic conditions
	☐ Brief (1-3)	☐ Brief (1-3)	☐ Extended (4 or more)	☐ Extended (4 or more)
ROS (review of symptoms) ☐ Constitutional (wt loss, etc.) ☐ Ears, nose, mouth, throat ☐ GI ☐ GU ☐ Integumentary (skin, breast) ☐ Endo ☐ Me/lymph ☐ Eyes ☐ Cardiovasc ☐ Musculo ☐ Resp ☐ Neuro ☐ Psych ☐ All/immuno ☐ Psych	☐ N/A	☐ Pertinent to problem (1 system)	☐ Extended (Pert and others) (2-9 systems)	☐ Complete (Pert and all others) (10 systems)
PFSH (past, family, social history) ☐ Past history (the patient's past experiences with illnesses, operations, injuries, and treatments) ☐ Family history (a review of medical events in the patient's family, including diseases that may be hereditary or place the patient at risk) ☐ Social history (an age-appropriate review of past and current activities)	☐ N/A	☐ N/A	☐ Pertinent (1 history area)	☐ *Complete (2 or 3 history areas)
*Complete PFSH: 2 history areas: (a) established patients—office (outpatient) care, domicilliary care, home care; (b) emergency department; (c) subsequent nursing facility care; and, (d) subsequent hospital care	Problem focused	Exp. problem focused	Detailed	Comprehensive
3 history areas: (a) new patients—office (outpatient) care, domicilliary care, home care; (b) consultations; (c) initial hospital care; (d) hospital observation; and (e) initial nursing facility care	Final history requires all 3 components above met or exceeded			

B Appendix

Examination CPT Examination Description	1995 Guideline Requirements	1997 Guideline Requirements	CPT Type of Examination
Limited to affected body area or organ system	One body area or organ system	1-5 bulleted elements	Problem-focused examination
Affected body area or organ system and other symptomatic or related organ systems	2-7 body areas and/or organ systems	6-11 bulleted elements	Expanded problem-focused examination
Extended examination of affected body area or organ system and other symptomatic or related organ systems	2-7 body areas and/or organ systems	12-17 bulleted elements for 2 or more systems	Detailed examination
General multisystem	8 or more body areas and/or organ systems	18 or more bulleted elements for 9 or more systems	Comprehensive examination
Complete single-organ system examination	Not defined	See requirements for individual single-system examinations	

CPT, Current Procedural Terminology.

Appendix C

Data Reviewed or Ordered		Point Value
Order and/or review medically reasonable and necessary clinical laboratory procedures. Note: Count laboratory panels as one procedure.	1-3 procedures	1
	≥4 procedures	2
Order and/or review medically reasonable and necessary diagnostic imaging studies in radiology section of CPT.	1-3 procedures	1
	≥4 procedures	2
Order and/or review medically reasonable and necessary diagnostic procedures in medical section of CPT.	1-3 procedures	1
	≥4 procedures	2
Discuss tests results with performing physician.		1
Discuss case with other physician(s) involved in patient's care or consult another physician (i.e., true consultation meaning seeking opinion or advice of another physician regarding the patient's care). This does not include referring patient to another physician for future care.		1
Order and/or review old records. Record type and source must be noted. Review of old records must be reasonable and necessary based on the nature of the patient's condition. Practice or facility protocol–driven record ordering does not require physician work and thus should not be considered when coding E/M services. Perfunctory notation of old record ordering/review solely for coding purposes is inappropriate and counting such is not permitted.	Order/review without summary	1
	Order/review and summarize	2
Independent visualization and interpretation of an image, ECG or laboratory specimen not reported for separate payment. Note: Each visualization and interpretation is allowed 1 point.		1
Review of significant physiologic monitoring or testing data not reported for separate payment (e.g., prolonged or serial cardiac monitoring data not qualifying for payment as rhythm ECGs).		1
	Total points	

CPT, Current Procedural Terminology; ECG, electrocardiogram; E/M, evaluation and management.

D Appendix

Risk for Complications and/or Morbidity or Mortality			
Level of Risk	**Presenting Problem(s)**	**Diagnostic Procedure(s) Ordered**	**Management Options Selected**
Minimal	• One self-limited or minor problem, e.g., cold, insect bite, tinea corporis	• Laboratory test requiring venipuncture • Chest x-rays • ECG/EEG • Urinalysis • Ultrasound, e.g., echocardiography • KOH preparation	• Rest • Gargles • Elastic bandages • Superficial dressings
Low	• Two or more self-limited or minor problems • One stable chronic illness, e.g., well-controlled hypertension or non-insulin–dependent diabetes, cataract, BPH • Acute uncomplicated illness or injury, e.g., cystitis, allergic rhinitis, simple sprain	• Psychological test not under stress, e.g., pulmonary function tests • Noncardiovascular imaging studies with contrast, e.g., barium enema • Superficial needle biopsies • Clinical laboratory tests requiring arterial puncture • Skin biopsies	• Over-the-counter drugs • Minor surgery with no identified risk factors • Physical therapy • Occupational therapy • IV fluids without additives
Moderate	• One or more chronic illnesses with mild exacerbation, progression, or side effects of treatment • Two or more stable chronic illnesses • Undiagnosed new problem with uncertain prognosis, e.g., lump in the breast • Acute illness with systemic symptoms, e.g., pyelonephritis, pneumonitis, colitis • Acute complicated injury, e.g., head injury with brief loss of consciousness	• Physiologic tests under stress, e.g., cardiac stress test, fetal contraction stress test • Diagnostic endoscopy with no identified risk factors • Dee needle or incisional biopsy • Cardiovascular imaging studies with contrast and no identified risk factors, e.g., arteriogram, cardiac catheter • Obtain fluid from body cavity, e.g., lumbar procedure, thoracentesis, culdocentesis	• Minor surgery with identified risk factors • Elective major surgery (open, percutaneous, or endoscopic) with no identified risk factors • Prescription drug management • Therapeutic nuclear medicine • IV fluids with additives • Closed treatment of fracture or dislocation without manipulation
High	• One or more chronic illnesses with severe exacerbation, progression, or side effects of treatment • Acute or chronic illnesses or injuries that may pose a threat to life or bodily function, e.g., multiple trauma, acute MI, pulmonary embolus, severe respiratory distress, progressive severe rheumatoid arthritis, psychiatric illness with potential threat to self or others, peritonitis, acute renal failure • An abrupt change in neurologic status, e.g., seizure, TIA, weakness, or sensory loss	• Cardiovascular imaging studies with contrast • Cardiac electrophysiologic tests • Diagnostic endoscopy with identified risk • Diskography	• Elective major surgery (open, percutaneous, or endoscopic) with no identified risk factors • Emergency major surgery (open, percutaneous, or endoscopic) • Parenteral controlled substances • Drug therapy requiring intensive monitoring for toxicity • Decision not to resuscitate or to de-escalate care because of poor prognosis

BPH, benign prostatic hyperplasia; ECG, electrocardiogram; EEG, electroencephalogram; IV, intravenous; MI, myocardial infarction; TIA, transient ischemic attack.

Appendix E

Final Assignment of Medical Decision-Making Type				
A. Number of diagnoses or management options	1 Point—minimal	2 Points—limited	3 Points—multiple	≥4 Points—extensive
B. Amount and complexity of data reviewed/ordered	≤1 Point—none/minimal	2 Points—limited	3 Points—multiple	≥4 Points—extensive
C. Risk	Minimal	Low	Moderate	High
Type of medical decision making	Straightforward	Low complexity	Moderate complexity	High complexity
Final medical decision making requires 2 of 3 components above met or exceeded.				

F

Appendix

Inpatient

	Initial Hospital/Observation			Subsequent Inpatient/Follow-up		
	Requires 3 components within shaded area			Requires 2 components within shaded area		
History	D or C	C	C	PF interval	EPF interval	D interval
Examination	D or C	C	C	PF	EPF	D
Complexity of medical decision	SF/L	M	H	SF/L	M	H
Average time (minutes) (observation care has no average time)	30 Init hosp (99221) Observ care (99218)	50 Init hosp (99222) Observ care (99219)	70 Init hosp (99223) Observ care (99220)	15 Subsequent (99231)	25 Subsequent (99232)	35 Subsequent (99233)
Level	I	II	III	I	II	III

C, comprehensive; D, detailed; EPF, expanded problem-focused; H, high; L, low; M, moderate.

4 Measurement-Based Stepped Care Approach to Interdisciplinary Chronic Pain Management

David Tauben | Brian R. Theodore

INTRODUCTION

Chronic pain is an urgent public health concern that significantly impairs the physical, psychological, and social functioning of those experiencing it and their significant others.[1,2] The Institute of Medicine (IOM) recently estimated that more than 110 million adults, over one third of the population of the United States, experience some form of chronic pain,[2] with the symptom of pain being the most common reason for people to consult a primary care physician.[3] Despite the magnitude of this problem, pain management is severely under-represented in the content of medical education and is delivered by many providers who feel unprepared to manage it.[2,4,5] Consequently, treatment of pain is highly variable and often unstructured, with important decisions being based primarily on clinician intuition, personal bias, and the severe time constraints present in hurried practices.[6]

It is estimated that chronic pain costs between $565 and $635 billion per year in health care and reduced productivity; these costs have increased fivefold in the past decade and will probably increase with the aging population.[2] However, these increases in health care expenditures have not translated into improvements in clinical outcomes.[7,8] In addition, the National Center for Health Statistics noted that 40% of people reporting chronic pain indicate moderate to severe degradation in their functioning,[9] thereby contributing to the high direct and indirect costs of chronic pain. Poor provider self-reported pain care competency reduces clinician productivity and increases practice dissatisfaction in those managing chronic pain. Most importantly, these costs do not reflect the incalculable impact of pain on the lives of patients and their significant others.

Given that chronic pain is a complex biopsychosocial disorder, successful management of it requires a systematic multidimensional approach to assessment and strategically targeted interdisciplinary therapies. Care of complex chronic illness requires defined processes for rapid identification of problems and "stepped" systems that reliably direct services to intensified treatment strategies for challenging patients who have a limited or poor response to initial treatments. This chapter discusses a patient-centered approach to the care of chronic pain and how outcomes are improved when an interspecialty collaborative model is followed.

STEPPED CARE

The *stepped care* model entails a well-established primary care response to the management of chronic disease that systematically adjusts medical treatment when patients are not responding to initial interventions.[10] Wagner and colleagues cited five components of stepped care[11]:

1. Use of explicit plans and protocols
2. Reorganization of the practice to meet the needs of patients who require more time, a broad array of resources, and closer follow-up
3. Systematic attention to the information and behavioral change needs of patients
4. Ready access to necessary expertise
5. Supportive information systems

Von Korff and Tiemans subsequently described a model involving the stepwise introduction of targeted interventions to improve the care of patients with chronic illness; this model provides a framework for achieving cost-effective care based on patients' observed response to treatment.[12]

STEPPED CARE IN PAIN

The World Health Organization (WHO) cancer pain analgesic ladder is a historic example of a stepped care model, though with a sharply delineated focus on relief of the intensity of cancer pain alone (Fig. 4.1).

This is undoubtedly a useful and effective model for relieving acute and progressive pain from cancer and for palliative and end-of-life care of pain when reducing the intensity of pain becomes the primary and often sole goal of treatment, even, when necessary, at the expense of function. The WHO ladder continues to be useful even though it does not include pain's other domains of biopsychosocial distress. Care of chronic *noncancer* pain focuses its outcome on *function—not primarily comfort—*in patients not at the end of life and thus needs to incorporate other of pain's domains beyond reported pain intensity.

John Loeser from the University of Washington has depicted the individual's experience of chronic pain as a concentric series of domains and specifically differentiated the painful nociceptive experience from the enveloping experience of suffering and maladaptive behavior that

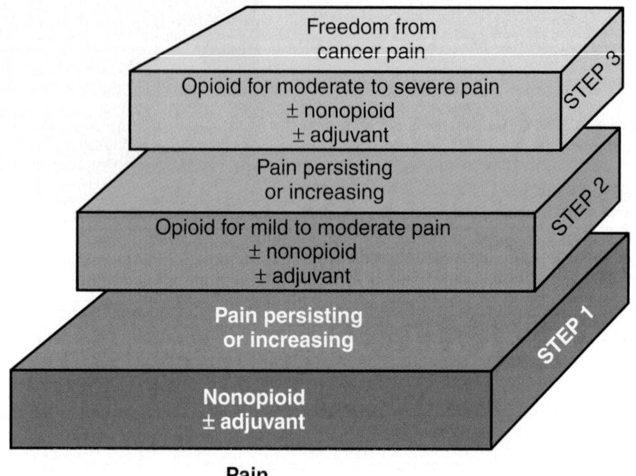

Figure 4.1 World Health Organization cancer pain treatment ladder. (Redrawn from www.cancerpain.org.uk/module2b.htm.)

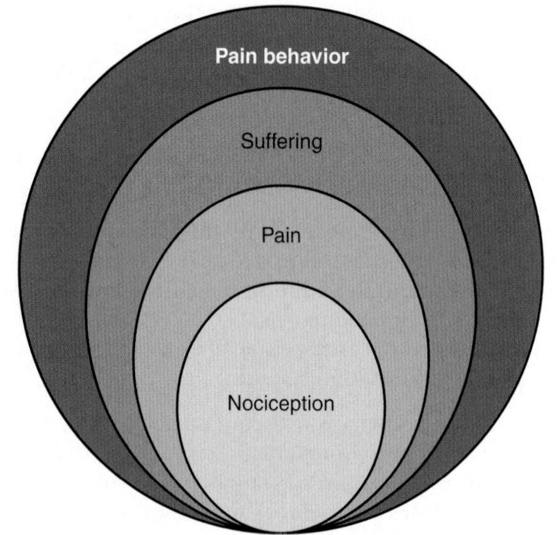

Figure 4.2 The Loeser model of pain. (Redrawn from Loeser JD. Perspectives on pain. In: Turner P, ed. *Clinical Pharmacology and Therapeutics*. London: Macmillan; 1980:313-316.)

patients with chronic pain often demonstrate.[13] A search for the elusive nociceptive pain generator that can be numbed, burned, or otherwise removed will undoubtedly result in exclusion of care for complex pain disorders, which often require systematic multidimensional assessment of pain. Loeser's "onion" (Fig. 4.2) is a multilayered rather than a multistepped care model, and although he does not delineate algorithmic plans, protocols, and measures in detail, it still anticipates a stepped approach to the care of pain in patients with chronic illness.

Von Korff and Moore proposed a stepped care approach specifically for the primary care management of chronic back pain in which interventions are sequenced "so that the intensity, complexity, and costs of care are guided by each patient's observed outcome."[14] Otis and coauthors also published a convincing case-based rationale for the stepwise integration of coordinated mental health services into progressively more treatment-resistant pain care coordinated within a primary care practice setting.[15]

COLLABORATIVE CARE APPROACH

The most robust demonstration of the effectiveness of collaborative care has been described in the management of depression.[16] Unützer and Park described a model of "measurement-based care, treatment to target, and stepped care in which treatments are systematically adjusted and 'stepped up' if patients are not improving as expected."[17] This approach has demonstrated improved patient satisfaction and health outcomes.[18-20]

COLLABORATIVE CARE OF PAIN

Dobscha and others described a model and the preliminary outcomes of collaborative care for chronic musculoskeletal pain in primary care practice.[21,22] A clustered randomized trial that evaluated collaborative care for chronic pain in five primary care settings within a single Veterans Administration medical center demonstrated greater improvement in pain-related disability, and in patients with baseline depression, greater improvement in the severity of depression was achieved in those receiving the intervention than in patients receiving treatment as usual. The study intervention followed the stepped care approach and included patient assessment, monitoring of symptoms, a two-session program for education of clinicians, education and activation, feedback and recommendations to clinicians, and facilitation of specialty care. Outcome measures used in this study were the Roland-Morris Disability Questionnaire and the Patient Health Questionnaire 9-item (PHQ-9) depression inventory.

EXISTING GUIDELINES

Multiple guidelines and algorithms have been published for specific painful disorders, including back pain, headache, and other chronic pain conditions commonly encountered in both specialty and primary care clinical practice.[23,24] Many guidelines exist for opioid management[25-28]; however, there are limited published and widely accepted clinical practice guidelines for comprehensive measurement-based, stepped care for chronic pain beyond efforts by the Department of Veterans Affairs to streamline the treatment of pain within its health care setting.[29] This gap persists despite published evidence that such a stepped care approach leads to better overall outcomes. The following sections summarize various studies in the published literature that have evaluated the stepped care approach, as well as efforts made to date that hold promise for more standardized and widely accepted clinical practice guidelines.

PAIN CARE PROGRESSION MODEL

Dubois and colleagues proposed a pyramidal model for implementing a "population-based stepped-care approach to chronic pain" (Fig. 4.3).[30] Their future model for management of pain in the U.S. Veterans Health Administration medical system calls for increased levels of expertise based on a patient's level of complexity. Although it does recognize that specific degrees of expertise are necessary for effective

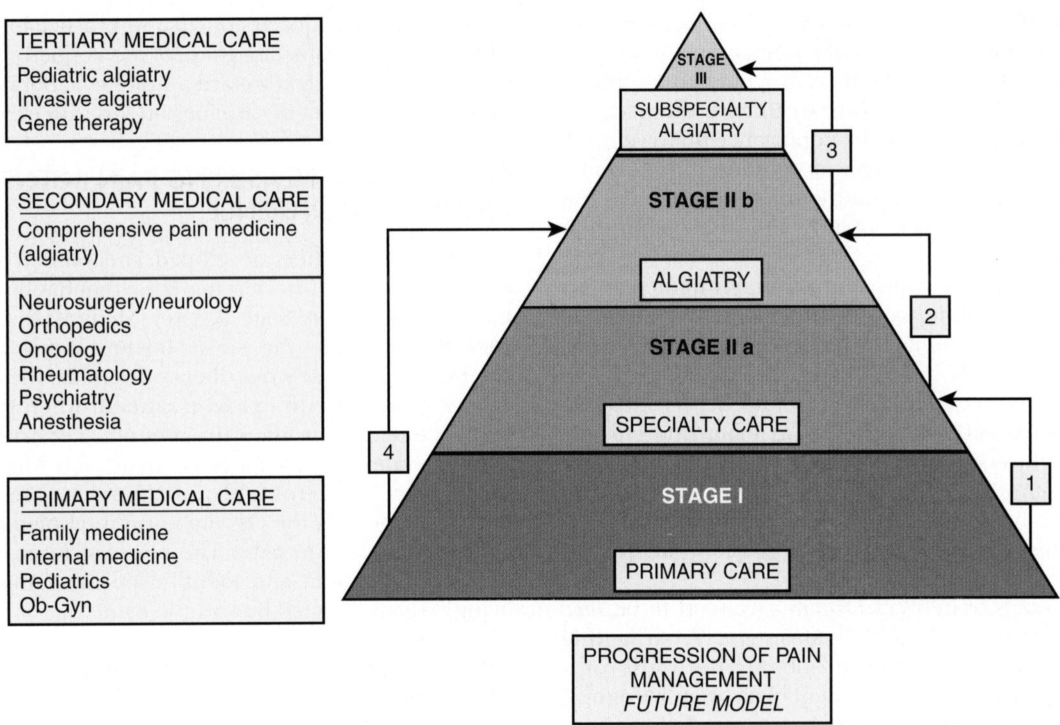

Figure 4.3 Progression of the pain management stepped care pyramid. Ob-Gyn, obstetrics and gynecology. (Redrawn from Dubois MY, Gallagher RM, Lippe PM. Pain medicine position paper. *Pain Med*. 2009;10:987.)

treatment outcomes, being essentially a stepped model extending up through the continuum of primary to tertiary pain care, it does not anchor these levels with measurement-based benchmarks that systematize the assessment to determine who progresses and to which type of physician or other health care professional. A proposed linkage of stepped care with a measurement-based approach is described below.

MEASUREMENT-BASED STEPPED CARE: THE PAIN TREATMENT DOMAINS

Because chronic pain is a multidimensional disorder, achieving the best outcomes requires attention to more domains than just self-reported pain intensity. The "fifth vital sign," which is useful for the care of acute pain, is an insufficient assessment measure for achieving the best outcomes in patients with chronic pain.[31,32] Measurement-based care directed toward *physical and emotional function, quality of sleep, risk for chemical dependency, adherence to treatment, patient satisfaction,* and *self-reported quality of life* is well recognized and in fact involves critical patient response domains that, when followed over time, permit useful assessment of outcomes.[31] Adjusting pain treatment on the basis of immediate clinical outcomes follows the fundamental tenet of "stepped care."[14] Just as a random blood sugar measurement is not a sufficient measure of care in a diabetic patient, chronic pain in a complex chronic illness such as diabetes requires measurement and tracking of many biobehavioral and comorbid health outcomes over time. By systematizing standard metrics, measurement-based care is expected to improve assessment and facilitate adjustments in treatment to match the response of individual patients to care; improved quality and consistency of measurement will enhance the quality of care and the patient's satisfaction with it, increase the health of the population, and probably reduce the per capita cost of care, the so-called *triple aim* of the Institute for Health Improvement.[33]

A collaborative care chronic illness process for chronic pain would need assessment measures for the specific chronic pain domains frequently encountered in patients with complex chronic pain. This model would require formulating an individualized stepped care plan that matches a patient's unique combination of active co-occurring disorders with the interspecialty domains of chronic pain. Measurement-based stepped care would systematically identify multidimensional signs and symptoms of poor physical, emotional, and sleep function and longitudinally track treatment outcomes across these specific domains. Structured multidimensional pain measurement and consistent tracking of treatment outcomes are needed to reliably and routinely prompt modifications in any care provided.

At the University of Washington, chronic pain is currently being measured with a number of specific evidence-based public domain tools. These measures are recorded in an electronic database, which can individually report the patient's status at each visit, starting with the initial identification of chronic noncancer pain (advised to begin at day 90 of opioid therapy) and at all subsequent pain treatment follow-up visits. Different tracking versions are in place that range from pain specialty consultation to primary care practice. Unique modules are being developed for specialties commonly encountering challenges in pain management, such as orthopedics, physical medicine and rehabilitation, rheumatology, and neurology.

PROBLEM OF NONCOLLABORATIVE PAIN CARE

Many challenges confront chronic pain care as a result of gaps in policy, treatments, attitudes, education, and research, as detailed in the 2011 report *Relieving Pain in America* by the IOM.[2] Not only does the IOM fundamentally identify pain management as a moral imperative, but it also outlines the importance of comprehensive treatment, the need for interdisciplinary approaches, the importance of prevention, wider use of existing knowledge, recognition of the conundrum of opioid use, collaborative roles for patients and clinicians, and the value of a public health– and community-based approach.

Pain care also suffers from the frustratingly limited ability of most current chronic pain treatments, either interventional or noninterventional, to reduce the *intensity of pain*, with efficacy typically being less than 30%.[34] These therapeutic limitations redirect attention to what else beyond pain intensity predicts success or failure in managing chronic illness. Stepped care is such a structured process for assessing and reducing the adverse impact of chronic pain on additional life measures—less of "how much does it hurt?" and more about physical function, mood, quality of life, and access to systematic care.

Current models of delivery of pain care tend to be *noncollaborative*, fragmented, and inconsistent. A struggling primary care provider unable to identify the cause of a patient's disabling, severe persistent pain may recognize that the patient is doing poorly despite escalating doses of opioids without improvement in pain or function and with high levels of patient distress and problems in adherence and compliance. Referral to a wide range of specialists should follow, but to which specialist, triggered by what measures, and with what goal? Figure 4.4 illustrates the status quo in today's common treatment approach to chronic pain. Common issues, questions, and potential problems that arise from such an inadequate model of care include the following:

- How and when does the primary care provider determine which specialist to refer to?
- How likely is it that the recommendations will be coordinated with other members of the care team?
- Are all specialists in agreement about what to measure to meet the diagnosis and treatment goals?
- Can all agree on which care guideline to use?
- How does the patient make sense of all this advice and move forward into a meaningful treatment plan?
- Who is measuring compliance and adherence to whatever treatment plan is chosen?
- Are records shared?

Given the inadequacies of current practice in the management of chronic pain, discussion of the stepped care approach provides some context toward a more collaborative and integrated management of care for patients with chronic pain.

STEPS 1 AND 2: MEASURING PAIN INTENSITY AND PAIN INTERFERENCE

Von Korff and others developed and validated a two-item pain intensity and interference scale that has been endorsed by the Washington State Agency Medical Diretors Group (AMDG) guideline (Fig. 4.5).[25] It is specifically intended for use by primary care prescribers of opioids, with the goal of assessing response to opioid treatment when given for the management of chronic pain of noncancer origin.

Other validated but more detailed tools to measure how much pain interferes with function have been used for decades, especially the Oswestry and the Roland-Morris Disability Questionnaires.[35-37] These measures provide a more detailed assessment and identify specific activities of daily living directly affected by chronic pain.

STEP 3: ASSESSMENT OF MOOD AND RISK FACTORS

SCREENING FOR DEPRESSION AND ANXIETY

Given the biopsychosocial impact of chronic pain, it is imperative that the impact of chronic pain on mood be measured

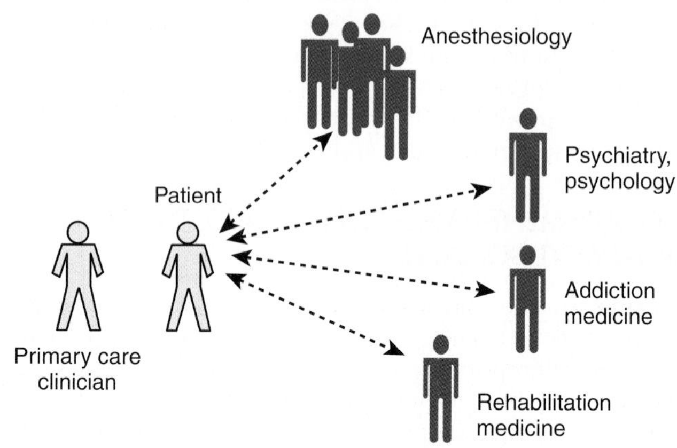

Figure 4.4 A current noncollaborative model of pain care. (From University of Washington Division of Pain Medicine/TelePain; original figure courtesy of Kent Unruh.)

Pain intensity and interference

In the last month, on average, how would you rate your pain? Use a scale from 0 to 10, where 0 is "no pain" and 10 is "pain as bad as could be." [*That is, your usual pain at times you were in pain.*]

No Pain **As bad as pain could be**

0	1	2	3	4	5	6	7	8	9	10

In the last month, how much has pain interfered with your daily activities? Use a scale from 0 to 10, where 0 is "no interference" and 10 is "unable to carry on any activities."

No interference						**Unable to carry on any activities**				
0	1	2	3	4	5	6	7	8	9	10

Figure 4.5 Two-question pain intensity and interference measure. (From Agency Medical Directors' Group. Interagency guideline on opioid dosing for chronic non-cancer pain: an educational aid to improve care and safety with opioid therapy. 2010 update. Available at www.agencymeddirectors.wa.gov/Files/OpioidGdline.pdf.)

consistently. Many studies have documented the utility of specific measures to assess and address depression, in particular, the PHQ-9 (Fig. 4.6).[38,39] Pain with co-occurring psychological disorders managed in 14 rural primary care practices demonstrated improved outcomes when longitudinally measured with the Medical Outcomes Study Short-Form 36-Item (SF-36) survey and the Functional Interference Estimate at baseline, 6 months, and 12 months.[40]

Measuring the mood of chronic pain patients at every clinical encounter is as reasonable as measuring blood pressure and weight in addition to pulse when evaluating cardiac status. Direct observation has shown that the time needed for patients to complete the nine-item PHQ-9 paper form is just 15 to 30 seconds (personal observations by D.T.). Clinicians may also adopt a shorter version for assessment of mood in place of the PHQ-9. For example, the PHQ-4 is a validated shortened combination of two measures from the PHQ-9 depression questionnaire and two measures from the Generalized Anxiety Disorder 7-item scale (GAD-7) anxiety questionnaire (Fig. 4-7).[41] In addition, the publicly available item banks of the Patient-Reported Outcomes Measurement Information System (PROMIS) developed by the National Institutes of Health include well-developed mood and other pain-related affective disorder assessments that deploy computer adaptive testing technology to provide the shortest selection of questionnaire items needed to reliably assess the domains of interest.[42] Other tools to measure mood are also widely available, and although the diversity of instruments will stimulate research in psychometrics, the use of diverse questionnaires in clinical effectiveness research inhibits direct comparisons between outcomes from different study populations. Therefore, a move toward the selection of standard measures holds much promise in the development and continuing advancement of the PROMIS item banks.

RISKS ASSOCIATED WITH CHRONIC OPIOID THERAPY

Opioid dose–prescribing limits have been proposed in response to the dramatic increase in accidental overdoses of prescription opioids and deaths in most regions of the United States. The initial opioid dose limit proposed by the 2010 Washington State AMDG of 120 mg morphine equivalent dose (MED), beyond which specialty consultation is advised when pain and function are not improved or risk for poor mood, high distress, or substance abuse is present, was based on a consensus of Washington State clinicians from both community and academic practices.[25] There is now growing evidence-based support for safety limits with escalating opioid doses for chronic noncancer pain (Fig. 4.8). Elevated risk also extends to fractures from accidental falls,[43] sleep disordered breathing,[44] endocrinologic disturbances,[45-48] and immune dysfunction.[49] Limited support for benefit and increasingly evident risk for escalating opioid doses in chronic pain management differentiate the *comfort*-directed goals for palliative and end-of-life pain from the *function*-directed goals for chronic noncancer pain.[50-53]

SUBSTANCE USE DISORDERS AND PAIN

The value of a stepped care model when managing alcoholism has been reported by Sobell and Sobell,[54] and many tools to assess and refer primary care patients for treatment of alcoholism are well described and have been proved effective. Measurement-based tools to assess for alcoholism include the long-familiar CAGE (*c*ut down, *a*nnoyed by criticism, *g*uilty about drinking, *e*ye-opener drinks), the Alcohol Use Disorder Identification Test (AUDIT), the brief Michigan Alcoholism Screening Test (bMAST), and others.[55-58]

With estimates of co-occurring addiction and pain ranging from 18% to 30% and the well-established increased

PHQ-9 Scoring Tally Sheet	Not at all	Several days	More than half the days	Nearly every day
	0	1	2	3
Little interest or pleasure in doing things				
Feeling down, depressed, or hopeless				
Trouble falling or staying asleep or sleeping too much				
Feeling tired or having little energy				
Poor appetite or overeating				
Feeling bad about yourself, feeling that you are a failure, or feeling that you have let yourself or your family down				
Trouble concentrating on things such as reading the newspaper or watching television				
Moving or speaking so slowly that other people could have noticed or being so fidgety or restless that you have been moving around a lot more than usual				
Thinking that you would be better off dead or that you want to hurt yourself in some way				
Totals				

Figure 4.6 Patient Health Questionnaire 9-item (PHQ-9) depressive symptom screener. (From Kroenke K, Spitzer RL, Williams JB. The PHQ-9: validity of a brief depression severity measure. *J Gen Intern Med.* 2001;16:606-613.)

Over the past 2 weeks have you been bothered by these problems?	Not at all	Several days	More days than not	Nearly every day
Feeling nervous, anxious, or on edge	0	1	2	3
Not being able to stop or control worrying	0	1	2	3
Feeling down, depressed, or hopeless	0	1	2	3
Little interest or pleasure in doing things	0	1	2	3

Figure 4.7 Patient Health Questionnaire 4-item depression and anxiety screener. (From Löwe B, Wahl I, Rose M, et al. A 4-item measure of depression and anxiety: validation and standardization of the Patient Health Questionnaire-4 (PHQ-4) in the general population. *J Affect Disord*. 2010;122:86-95.)

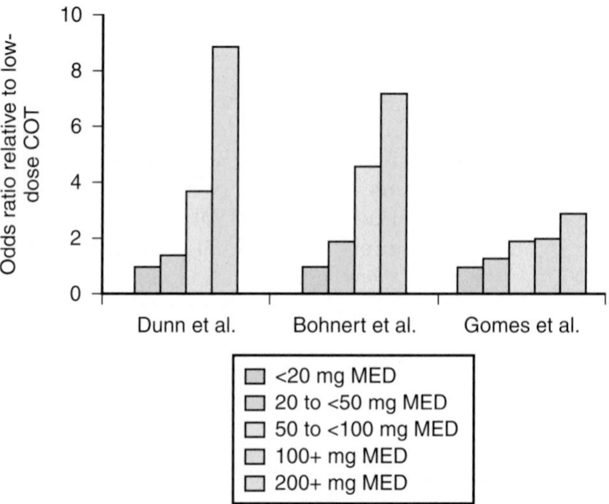

Figure 4.8 Morphine equivalent dose (MED) relative risks: recent data. COT, chronic opioid therapy. (Courtesy of Von Korff M. Presentation to the Food and Drug Administration in June 2012. Data reported from Dunn KM, Saunders KW, Rutter CM, et al. Opioid prescriptions for chronic pain and overdose: a cohort study. *Ann Intern Med*. 2010;152:85-92; Bohnert AS, Valenstein M, Bair MJ, et al. Association between opioid prescribing patterns and opioid overdose–related deaths. *JAMA*. 2011;305:1315-1321; and Gomes T, Mamdani MM, Dhalla IA, et al. Opioid dose and drug-related mortality in patients with nonmalignant pain. *Arch Intern Med*. 2011;171:686-691.)

complexity of care for pain patients with active or remote substance abuse disorders, it is of vital importance to pay careful attention to assessment and outcomes when prescribing opioids and other at-risk drugs such as benzodiazepines and other sedatives.[59-63] Based on a 1-year evaluation of function in primary care patients with musculoskeletal pain and a substance abuse disorder, Morasco and associates proposed stepped-up interventions in pain patients with chemical dependency problems: "Chronic non-cancer pain patients with a history of a substance use disorder (SUD) report poorer pain-related functioning and are less likely to experience clinically significant improvements from usual pain treatment. Providers should assess for SUD status and provide more intensive interventions for these patients."[64]

Evidence that the use of opioids for pain is a risk factor for the development of substance use disorder patterns of behavior is robust.[65-68] Furthermore, measurement of opioid misuse may be needed not only at the outset of chronic opioid therapy (COT) but also throughout treatment.[69] Fleming and coworkers reported a ninefold increase in the likelihood of a substance abuse disorder when four or more types of aberrant drug behavior occurred (in particular, self oversedation, report of feeling intoxicated, early refill requests, self-directed dose increase) in more than 900 chronic pain patients seen in a primary care practice, with no cases of abuse being diagnosed when no aberrancies occurred.[70] The challenge of uncovering or inducing frank addiction and less clear-cut addictive behavior to the many scheduled drugs used for the treatment of chronic pain complicates the management of patients who, as a result of medically prescribed and despite compliant use of long-term high-dose opioids, may proceed to develop *complex persistent opioid dependency*, a syndrome becoming evident to clinicians struggling to wean chronic pain patients off long-term high doses of opioids.[71] Drug-dependent behavior and urine drug-monitoring aberrancies occur along a spectrum, including in many highly functioning patients, mostly those managed with long-acting and high-dose COT,[72-74] many of whom may not meet addiction diagnoses by clinical or *Diagnostic and Statistical Manual of Mental Disorders, Fourth Edition* (*DSM-IV*), criteria (and pending DSM-V criteria).

ADVERSE SELECTION

There is a growing evidence base to support the high risk for psychiatric and substance use diagnoses in patients receiving the highest doses of opioids for chronic pain. The 2006 Trends and Risks of Opioid Use for Pain (TROUP) study found opioid use to be higher in individuals with mental health and substance use disorders, and in individuals with chronic pain, those with mental health and substance use disorders were more likely to receive opioids than those without these diagnoses.[75] A misuse score was generated on the basis of days of short-acting opioids supplied, days of long-acting opioids supplied, number of opioid pharmacies, and number of opioid prescribers. The authors concluded that patients with chronic pain and mental health or substance use disorders are more distressed and more complicated to care for than patients who have only chronic pain. High prescriptive use of sedatives and opioids was found particularly in young depressed women receiving higher-dose COT for multiple pain problems.[76] The authors noted that this "potent combination of risk factors since younger age, higher daily opioid doses, and depression have all been shown to be independently associated with worse opioid-related outcomes and, in the case of depression, higher rates of long-term COT use." Since patients at the highest risk are being prescribed the highest opioid doses, so-called adverse selection,[77] systematic measurement-based assessment of mental health will add critical structure and pain care consistency when making clinical decisions regarding the most appropriate opioid dose for patients at the highest risk.

STEP 4: MEASURING CHRONIC OPIOID TREATMENT RISKS

Several widely used opioid risk scales can be used by clinicians to determine the safety of prescribing opioids long-term. As reviewed by Chou and colleagues,[78] these scales include the Opioid Risk Tool (ORT); the Screener to Predict Opioid Misuse Among Chronic Pain Patients (SOAPP-R); the Current Opioid Misuse Measure (COMM); and the Diagnosis, Intractability, Risk, and Efficacy (DIRE) Score. Each tool offers advantages and disadvantages, although the length and total number of questions needed are a crucial determinant of applicability in the workflow of community and academic primary care practices. All are validated instruments, so selection of the optimal tool depends on clinician preference and the logistics of administration (i.e., self-report vs. clinician administered). Regardless, some measure of opioid risk must be recorded before committing to opioids for COT, and the degree of risk can also be used to systematically determine the frequency of urine drug monitoring or the frequency of accessing state prescription drug–monitoring programs, which are available in nearly all states in the United States.

The use of urine drug toxicology to monitor adherence to pain medication treatment has been extensively reviewed by Christo and colleagues.[79] The results of urine drug toxicology are often complicated by false positives and negatives, incomplete knowledge of the expected metabolism of opiates, variable testing thresholds in different laboratories and available commercial products, and cross-reactivity of enzyme-linked dipstick assays; additional training and support by laboratory experts are often needed when unexpected results are seen in clinical practice.[80] A clinically useful algorithm for urine testing based on risk assessment is available in Appendix D of the Washington State AMDG guidelines.[25]

STEP 5: CALCULATING OPIOID DOSE EQUIVALENCY

Because high opioid doses increase risk, they need be consistently reviewed on an ongoing basis. Many different formulas are available to convert different opioids into a comparable "equianalgesic" value, typically called the "morphine equivalent dose."[81] To consistently record the opioid dose according to a standard equianalgesic formula, the Washington State AMDG has published a web-based calculator that is a recommended conversion tool to determine the opioid dose and hence risk. This can be accessed at the URL www.agencymeddirectors.wa.gov/opioiddosing.asp.

STEP 6: MEASURING THE EFFECT OF PAIN ON SLEEP

Pain nearly always disrupts sleep, and disordered sleep or sleep deprivation increases pain intensity.[82] Managing sleep disturbances is thus a valuable first-line approach to the care of patients with acute, chronic, or palliative pain conditions. Additionally, either isolated or combined obstructive and

1. *S*noring
   Do you *s*nore loudly (louder than talking or loud enough to be heard through closed doors)?
   Yes No
2. *T*ired
   Do you often feel *t*ired, fatigued, or sleepy during the daytime?
   Yes No
3. *O*bserved
   Has anyone *o*bserved you stop breathing during your sleep?
   Yes No
4. Blood *p*ressure
   Do you have or are you being treated for high blood *p*ressure?
   Yes No
5. *B*MI
   *B*MI higher than 35 kg/m^2?
   Yes No
6. *A*ge
   *A*ge older than 50 years?
   Yes No
7. *N*eck circumference
   *N*eck circumference greater than 40 cm?
   Yes No
8. *G*ender
   *G*ender male?
   Yes No

High risk for OSA: answering yes to three or more items
Low risk for OSA: answering yes to less than three items

Figure 4.9 STOP-Bang sleep apnea screening tool. BMI, body mass index; OSA, obstructive sleep apnea. (From Chung F, Yegneswarian B, Liao P, et al. STOP questionnaire: a tool to screen patients for obstructive sleep apnea. *Anesthesiology*. 2008;108:812-821.)

central sleep apnea increases in frequency with the dose of opioid.[44,83] A variety of tools are available, including the STOP-Bang sleep apnea screening tool (Fig. 4.9).[84]

LONGITUDINAL MULTIDIMENSIONAL PAIN TRACKING

The use of evidence-based multidimensional longitudinal data for clinical decision making has only recently been introduced into pain treatment protocols. A number of proprietary systems that combine extensive public domain questionnaires are available, and some are linked to large registry data banks, which offers the potential to improve research on the effectiveness of specialty-based pain treatments in real-time clinical practice.[85,86] Less lengthy paper-based and electronic systems have been designed for primary care. One example is *PainTracker*, developed by Mark Sullivan and his group at the University of Washington. It is designed to record and graphically present several pain treatment–related domains in a format that is easily reviewed and implemented in day-to-day clinical decision making for patients taking opioids for chronic noncancer pain. Limited to 17 questions, it records pain intensity, interference of pain with function, mood, sleep, opioid risk, and treatment compliance, and it is presented graphically alongside concurrent opioid MED dosing (Fig. 4.10).

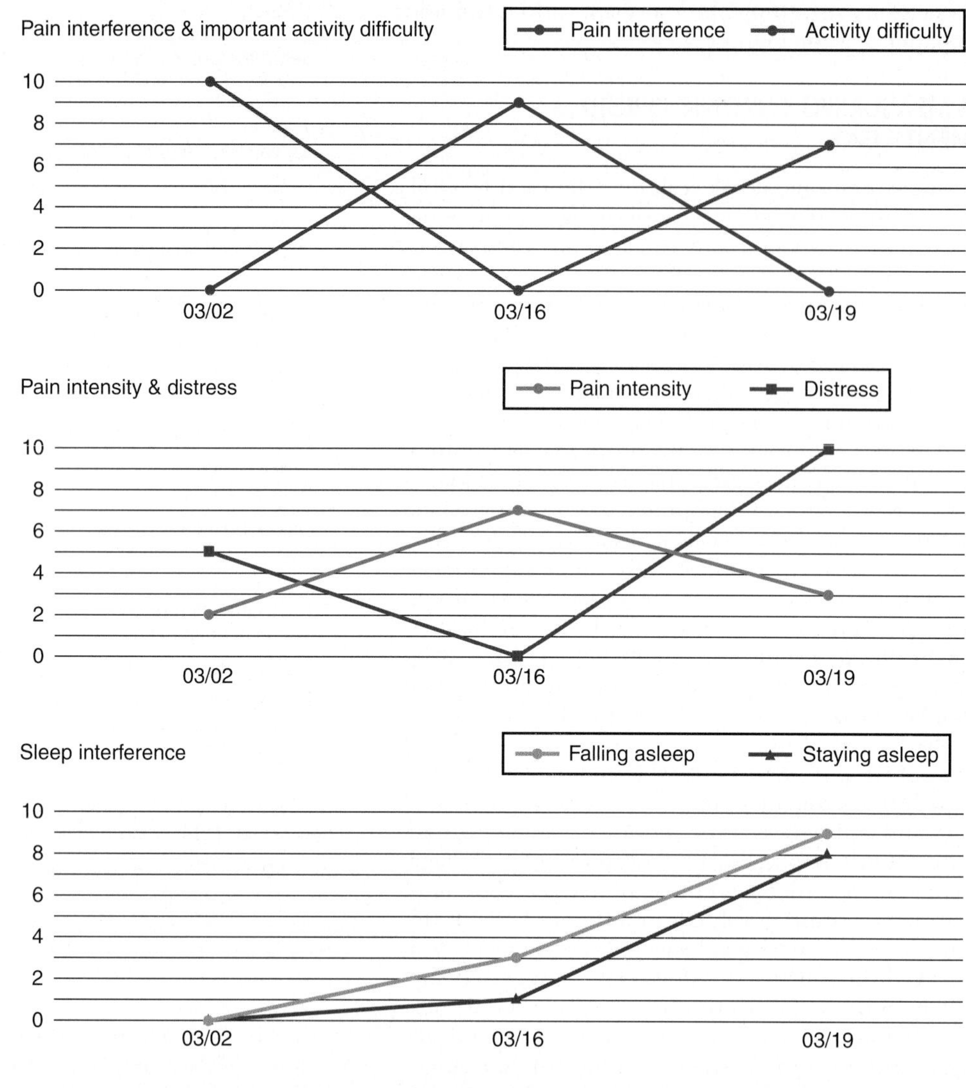

	03/02	03/16	03/19
Pain sites ***Bold* indicates worst**	Head, neck, chest, stomach	Head, neck, chest, stomach, back, arm, hand, buttocks, genital/urinary, leg, knee, foot	
Morphine equivalents, mg/day	**191**	**2605**	**1600**
Exceed Rx, days/mo	1–2	1–2	
ORT	8	0	26
Nonopioid pain meds	Kids' vitamins, daily vitamins	Vitamin D	

Figure 4.10 University of Washington PainTracker report. ORT, Opioid Risk Tool. (Courtesy of the University of Washington, Seattle.)

ACCESS TO EXPERT PAIN CARE

Limited access to pain specialists contributes to problems in pain care. In the United States, fewer than 3500 physicians were board-certified in pain care between 2000 and 2009. This shortage in expertise leaves more than 33,000 people with chronic pain for every specialist, and 80% of people experiencing severe pain are never referred to a specialized pain program or clinic.[2] Solving this problem calls for a new approach to pain management, at least in the United States, if not globally. Opioid-based management of chronic pain also represents an ongoing U.S. public health problem. Pain medications are inherently dangerous, with five of the top six fatal drug outcomes in the United States attributed to this category of drug.[87]

INNOVATIVE MODELS OF PAIN CARE

Because improved access to pain specialty care remains a major problem, is it possible to fix the problem by simply increasing the supply of highly trained pain specialists? This does not follow the progressive care model proposed earlier[25-30] since it

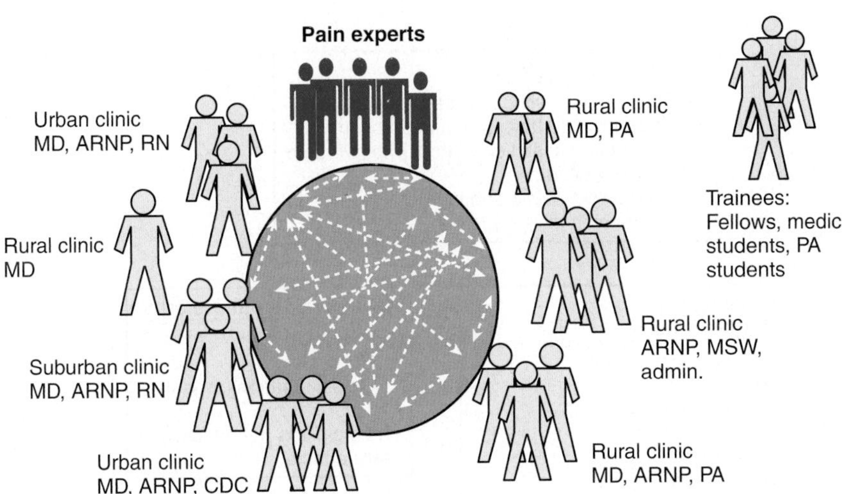

Figure 4.11 Telehealth Knowledge Network for Pain Care. ARNP, advance registered nurse practitioner; CDC, chemical dependency counselor; MD, doctor of medicine; MSW, medical social worker; PA, physician assistant; RN, registered nurse. (From the University of Washington Division of Pain Medicine/TelePain; original figure courtesy of Kent Unruh.)

increases the number of pain specialists without the called-for increase in collaborative and coordinated care. An alternative is to identify and train "pain champions" from the existing pool of primary care providers. This would allow more proficient *nonspecialty* pain clinicians to be embedded in the community clinic setting, where nearly all pain is treated.[88] This "stepped-up" clinician proficiency could add process support and technical information for a robust measurement-based stepped care approach. This kind of postgraduate educational program is now being piloted at the University of Washington and is called *Pain Champions: A Look Over the Expert's Shoulder* (available at depts.washington.edu/anesth/education/forms/pain/UW-Pain-Champions-Overview.pdf).

Another solution is to deploy multidisciplinary expertise through a telehealth platform. These experts would promote measurement-based care strategies, train providers on how and which tools to use, and assist in the interpretation of poorly performing patients based on objective measures that can be tracked over time. A model of pain care delivery following a provider-to-provider educational consultation has been developed at the University of New Mexico and was further advanced for chronic pain and addiction consultation at the University of Washington (Fig. 4.11). This "Extension for Community Healthcare Outcomes" (ECHO)[89] is designed to be an interactive learning environment, or "knowledge network." Consistent with the measurement-based stepped care approach to improve pain care outcomes, using defined measurements to assess multidimensional domains and following them over time would be expected to improve provider and patient satisfaction and clinical outcomes and reduce cost. Studies are now under way to determine how large and durable these effects will be in areas of provider knowledge, competency, and patient multidimensional outcomes.

MEASUREMENT-BASED STEPPED CARE APPROACH TO CHRONIC PAIN MANAGEMENT

Figure 4.12 illustrates the process and components in the systematic measurements specific to the multidisciplinary domains of chronic pain management. This then allows clinicians to quickly identify specific problem areas either at the outset of care or as pain treatment progresses. This structured approach to chronic pain care, in which treatments are systematically "stepped up" when patients are not improving as expected, follows the core principles outlined in currently effective processes of complex disease management. Attending to crucial functional and psychosocial measurements beyond *pain intensity* alone will facilitate consistent and rapid referral to an appropriate specialist. For instance, when a patient shows a high degree of limitation in *physical function*, rehabilitation medicine with physical and occupational therapy will be consistently considered. Vocational counseling can be added when pain interferes with or prevents return to work after an unexpectedly prolonged time until recovery from an injury. Evidence of a serious *behavioral health* problem will quickly prompt referral to a psychiatrist or clinical psychologist. Poor *treatment adherence* can trigger referral to a nurse care coordinator, social worker, or both. *Sleep disorders* can be addressed readily and treatments attempted by the treating clinician, and when tracking shows the sleep difficulty to be refractory to primary efforts, timely referral to a sleep specialist can determine whether central or obstructive sleep apnea is a factor and, if indicated, the need to step up to more expert cognitive behavioral therapies for insomnia.

When a systematic process is in place to assess and monitor for evidence of risk for a *substance use disorder*, there can be a consistent increase in the intensity of monitoring for adherence, such as more frequent urine drug monitoring or access to state prescription drug–monitoring programs. With systematically recorded evidence of noncompliance with a controlled substance (i.e., need for early refills, unexpected urine drug results, lost or stolen prescriptions), referral to an addiction specialist, specialized counseling, or both will be routinely triggered.

When the pain persists without a diagnosis and treatments result in no improvement in pain relief and function, especially when opioid dose escalation has occurred, timely referral to a pain specialist is indicated. This stepped care incorporates specific benchmarks to consistently and collaboratively guide the progression of pain care. Structured and systematic measurement-based care has demonstrated improved patient outcomes and satisfaction and reduces cost by treating according to prespecified care plans. Integration and coordination of mental health and primary care have

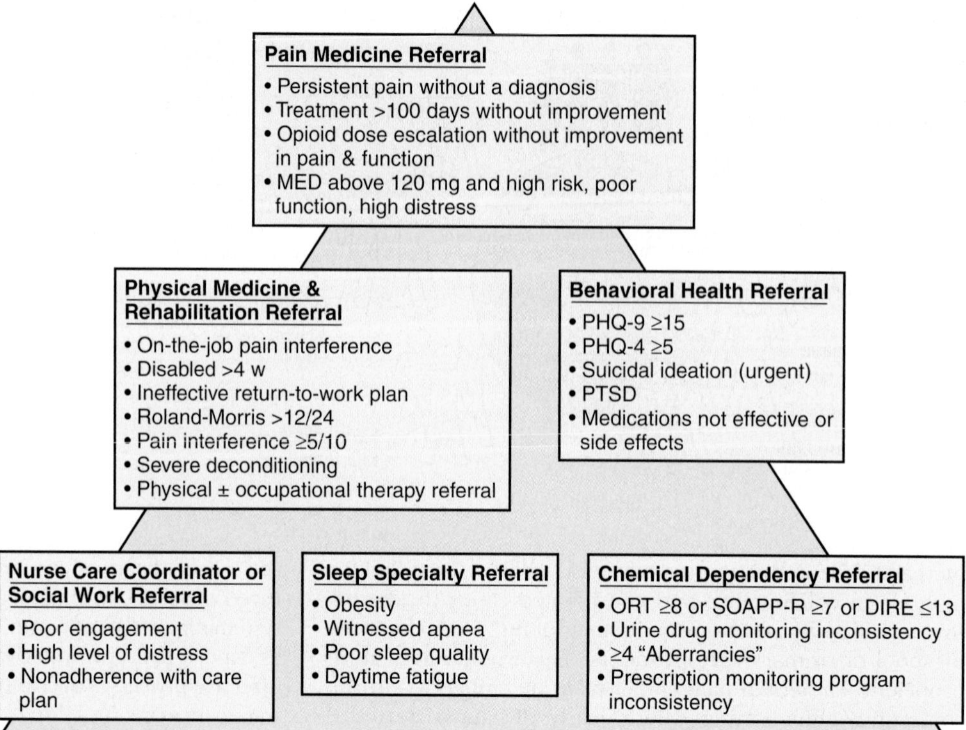

Figure 4.12 Conceptual model of the measurement-based stepped care approach to chronic pain management. DIRE, Diagnosis, Intractability, Risk, and Efficacy score; MED, morphine equivalent dose; ORT, Opioid Risk Tool; PHQ-9, Patient Health Questionnaire 9-item depression inventory; PTSD, post-traumatic stress disorder; SOAPP-R, Screener to Predict Opioid Misuse Among Chronic Pain Patients. (From Tauben D. University of Washington, Seattle Division of Pain Medicine.)

been shown to enhance patient and provider satisfaction,[90] improve patient outcomes,[91] and decrease health care costs.[92]

CONCLUSION

Pain is more than nociception, and chronic pain always requires a multidimensional approach to care. Stepped care is a well-established approach to chronic illness, with increased levels of treatment intensity being added when improvement is not observed in response to earlier interventions. Measuring the multidimensional disturbances that occur when pain progresses from a symptom of a disease to a disease itself increases the pain care provider's ability to consistently identify and diagnose pain complaints and impairments related to the often accompanying biopsychosocial difficulties, including physical deconditioning unrelated to or as a sequela of the initial injury or disease, co-occurring and newly developing behavioral health disorders, abnormal sleep function, and risks relevant to the frequent occurrence of chemical dependency in this population. Finally, measurement-based care identifies the correct next step up the referral pathway for pain patients who are not doing well and prompts early referral to a specialist in pain medicine before the problem becomes intractable.

SUGGESTED READINGS

Agency Medical Directors Groups. Interagency guideline on opioid dosing for chronic non-cancer pain: an educational aid to improve care and safety with opioid therapy. 2010 update. Cited March 7, 2012. Available at www.agencymeddirectors.wa.gov/Files/OpioidGdline.pdf.

Ballantyne JC, Shin NS. Efficacy of opioids for chronic pain: a review of the evidence. *Clin J Pain.* 2008;24:469-478.

Chelminski PR, Ives TJ, Felix KM, et al. A primary care, multi-disciplinary disease management program for opioid-treated patients with chronic non-cancer pain and a high burden of psychiatric comorbidity. *BMC Health Serv Res.* 2005;5:3.

Committee on Advancing Pain Research, Care, and Education. *Relieving Pain in America: A Blueprint for Transforming Prevention, Care, Education, and Research.* Washington, DC: Institute of Medicine; 2011.

Dobscha SK, Corson K, Perrin NA, et al. Collaborative care for chronic pain in primary care. *JAMA.* 2009;301:1242-1252.

Dubois MY, Gallagher RM, Lippe PM. Pain medicine position paper. *Pain Med.* 2009;10:987.

Dworkin RH, Turk DC, Farrar JT, et al. Core outcome measures for chronic pain clinical trials: IMMPACT recommendations. *Pain.* 2005;113:9-19.

Lippe PM, Brock C, David J, et al. The First National Pain Medicine Summit—final summary report. *Pain Med.* 2010;11:1447-1468.

Mezei L, Murinson BB, for the Johns Hopkins Pain Curriculum Development Team. Pain education in North American medical schools. *J Pain.* 2011;12:1199-1208.

Sullivan MD. Who gets high-dose opioid therapy for chronic non-cancer pain? *Pain.* 2010;151:567-568.

Sweeny K, Bodenheimer T, Wagner EH, et al. Improving primary care for patients with chronic illness: the chronic care model, part 2. *JAMA.* 2002;288:1909-1914.

Turk DC, Wilson HD, Cahana A. Treatment of chronic non-cancer pain. *Lancet.* 2011;377:2226-2235.

Unützer J, Park M. Strategies to improve the management of depression in primary care. *Prim Care Clin Office Pract.* 2012;39:415-431.

Upshur CC, Luckmann RS, Savageau JA. Primary care provider concerns about management of chronic pain in community clinic populations. *J Gen Intern Med.* 2006;21:652-655.

Von Korff M, Moore JC. Stepped care for back pain: activating approaches for primary care. *Ann Intern Med.* 2001;134:911-917.

The references for this chapter can be found at www.expertconsult.com.

5 The Health-Care Policy of Pain Management

Thomas R. Vetter

INTRODUCTION

Chronic pain is a major cause of suffering, disability, lost productivity, and diminished quality of life across the entire life course.[1,2] Cross-sectional studies have revealed that upward of 55% of adults experience chronic pain.[3-6] Likewise, up to 45% of children experience at least one episode of chronic pain,[7-10] with an attendant similar adverse effect on their daily activities and quality of life.[11-13] Many pediatric patients with chronic pain eventually experience similar recurrent pain as adults.[14,15]

In its 2011 report *Relieving Pain in America: A Blueprint for Transforming Prevention, Care, Education, and Research*, the Institute of Medicine (IOM) estimated that more than 116 million Americans struggle with chronic pain—greater than the combined prevalence of heart disease, cancer, and diabetes—which results in associated medical cost and lost productivity of US $635 billion annually.[16,17] Even in a country such as Canada, with its more constrained, universal health insurance, the recently estimated (and escalating) yearly expenditure of Can $3500 per chronic pain sufferer translates into annual direct system costs of greater than Can $400 million.[18] Acute pain also has major adverse effects on individual health and well-being, as well as a major impact on the health care delivery system.[19-21] Furthermore, inadequate treatment of acute postoperative and traumatic pain in adults and children can lead to particularly severe and unremitting chronic pain.[22-26]

Based on focus groups of key stakeholders, six major themes have been identified by the Pain Action Initiative: A National Strategy (PAINS) regarding chronic pain, all of which speak to its interconnected ethical, economic, and health care policy elements (Box 5.1).[27] Pain management thus has a myriad of implications on major health care policy, several of which are discussed here. Health care policy per se is a very broad and continually evolving topic for which more comprehensive resources are available.[28-30]

THE ROLE OF ECONOMIC EVALUATION IN FORMULATING CHRONIC PAIN MANAGEMENT POLICY

The individual and societal costs of pain are multifaceted and extensive, and it is essential that informed policy makers and practitioners be fully aware of them (Box 5.2).[18,31] Of note, the acute and chronic pain-related cost borne by the individual, such as uninsured treatments, informal care, and intangibles related to loss of quality of life, is unquestionably substantial but difficult to estimate, and consequently it is often underappreciated.[18,31]

As discussed in the current accompanying chapter on clinical trial design (Chapter 80), appraisal of a new or existing treatment involves three aspects: *efficacy*, *effectiveness*, and *efficiency*.[32-35] Even though randomized controlled trials can rigorously assess the *efficacy* of a pain treatment, their findings often lack external validity (generalizability to other settings). This weakness underscores the need for more naturalistic observational studies of treatment *effectiveness* in real-world practice (e.g., as part of multidrug, multimodal pain therapy, in more demographically and clinically diverse patients, and for much longer periods).

There are simply not enough financial resources in the health care systems around the world—even in the most developed countries—to fund all technically feasible and potentially beneficial health care interventions.[36] Given such inevitably constrained health care resources, difficult choices have to be made, and a formal economic evaluation offers a systematic and transparent process for informing such choices. Specifically, the comparative *efficiency* (incremental cost per clinical outcome) of a pain intervention can be determined. However, there is a great need for more robust, longitudinal cost-effectiveness studies on assessment and treatment of chronic pain.[35,37,38]

Health care economic evaluation methods have matured considerably in the last 25 years, with a plethora of published resources.[36,39-44] Nonetheless, despite widespread promotion to this audience, many physicians, health services researchers, and policy makers remain reluctant to apply economic evaluation methods in their clinical decision making and clinical trials.[45] Much of this gap has been attributed to physicians and their inherent tendency to think more in terms of clinical effectiveness and advocacy at the individual patient level rather than about cost-effectiveness (efficiency) at the population or health policy level.[45] This resistance to collecting, analyzing, and incorporating health economic data in the presently well-established era of both evidence-based medicine and demand for value in health care is particularly notable.[45,46]

THE EQUITY OF CHRONIC PAIN: HOW CAN SCIENCE GUIDE HEALTH POLICY?

In addition to assessing the efficacy, effectiveness, and efficiency of a new or existing pain assessment or treatment modality, a fourth key health policy element is *equity* of

Box 5.1 Current Major Themes in Chronic Pain Management

- Reducing disparities in access to pain care in the young, elderly, and lower socioeconomic groups
- Defining quality of care in pain management
- Need to train qualified providers and offer training programs in pain medicine
- Need for evidence-based public policy regarding opioid use and diversion
- Need to raise awareness about chronic pain as a disease to prevent stigmatization and discrimination
- Promotion of multimodal therapies for pain care as a way of diverting attention from opioid abuse problem

From McGee SJ, Kaylor BD, Emmott H, et al. Defining chronic pain ethics. *Pain Med.* 2011;12:1376-1384.

Box 5.2 The Multifaceted and Extensive Individual and Societal Costs of Pain

- Cost of interventions and therapies for treating pain and securing pain relief (e.g., cost of drugs and staff)
- Cost that is incurred as a result of ineffective interventions being provided (e.g., cost of additional primary care consultations)
- Cost to health service and to patients and their families because of lack of appropriate facilities within a locality (e.g., cost of accessing alternative therapies)
- Cost resulting from inappropriate self-medication and treatment by patients (e.g., cost of treating overdoses)
- Cost of treating and preventing adverse events that arise as a result of prescribing decisions (e.g., cost of gastrointestinal bleeding)
- Cost of disability claims resulting from people's inability to work
- Cost to the economy of reductions in productivity and absenteeism
- Cost of providing social care and support to people suffering with pain (e.g., cost of home care and respite care)
- Cost of informal care provided by families (e.g., loss of earnings)
- Cost of intangibles associated with deterioration in the quality of life of patients and their families

Data from Phillips CJ. The real cost of pain management. *Anaesthesia.* 2001;56:1031-1033.

patient access to comparable health care—including pain management.[18,31] Pioneered by John Bonica and Wilbert Fordyce more than 50 years ago, a multidisciplinary pain treatment program has been advocated as the optimal way to manage chronic pain.[47,48] This long-standing recognition of the merit of multidisciplinary pain treatment clinics, combined with an increasing prevalence of chronic pain, has led to a growth in demand, clinic waiting list size and time, and international concerns over limited pain treatment resources—all prompting the question of how can science guide health policy regarding chronic pain.[49]

Given its national health insurance program ("universal coverage" framed by the Canada Health Act of 1984), Canada presents a unique opportunity to examine the health policy and economics of pain management in a developed country. An initial survey of Canadian multidisciplinary pain treatment facilities (MPTFs) conducted by the STOP-PAIN Research Group found the median wait time for a first appointment in public MPTFs to be 6 months, approximately 12 times longer than the wait time for nonpublic MPTFs. The existing capacity of MPTFs in all of Canada could meet only 20% of the demand.[50] The authors and others concluded that current Canadian MPTFs are unable to meet the clinical needs of adult patients with chronic pain in terms of both regional accessibility and reasonable wait time for patients' first appointment.[50,51] The STOP-PAIN Research Group reported similarly inadequate access, with variable and prolonged wait times for pediatric patients suffering from chronic pain.[52]

Two subsequent STOP-PAIN studies focused on the biopsychosocial and economic burden of adult patients on Canadian MPTF wait lists.[49] In STOP-PAIN-1, patients on MPTF wait lists experienced severe pain (61%), marked limitations in activity (66%), significant depression (50%), and frequent suicide ideation (35%).[53] These biopsychosocial findings from STOP-PAIN-1 are similar to those from large concurrent samples of pain treatment clinic patients in Australia and Germany.[54,55] In STOP-PAIN-2, the median monthly cost was Can $1462 per study participant on an MPTF wait list, 95% of which was due to lost productivity (wages) and personal out-of-pocket expenses.[56]

An extensive systematic review of the literature and a survey of International Association for the Study of Pain (IASP) chapter presidents and other key stakeholders identified no established benchmarks or guidelines for acceptable wait times for the treatment of chronic pain.[57] However, another systematic literature review indicated that patients with chronic pain experience a significant deterioration in health-related quality of life and psychological well-being from the time of referral to treatment.[58] This consistent pattern of evidence underscores the need to improve access to appropriate care for patients with chronic pain—an escalating public health problem with major human and economic cost.[58]

PAIN MANAGEMENT AS A GLOBAL PUBLIC HEALTH PRIORITY AND HUMAN RIGHT

The World Health Organization (WHO) has estimated that more than 80% of the world's population is inadequately treated for moderate to severe pain and that 5 billion people live in countries with minimal to no appropriate access to controlled analgesics.[59] Given this enormous worldwide burden, pain should ostensibly represent a major global public health concern.[60,61] Yet pain management has been relatively neglected by national governmental agencies and international nongovernmental organizations.[62-68] Acute, chronic, and cancer pain collectively represents the often unreported and hence silent dimension of many of the worldwide causes of both adult and pediatric morbidity and mortality.[64] Although acute pain may reasonably be considered a symptom of disease, illness, or injury, chronic and

Box 5.3 IASP Declaration of Montreal

Article 1. The right of all people to have access to pain management without discrimination
Article 2. The right of people in pain to acknowledgment of their pain and to be informed about how it can be assessed and managed
Article 3. The right of all people with pain to have access to appropriate assessment and treatment of the pain by adequately trained health care professionals

From International Association for the Study of Pain. *Declaration of Montreal: Declaration That Access to Pain Management Is a Fundamental Human Right*. Seattle: IASP; 2010.

Box 5.4 Barriers to Access to Pain Treatment Globally

1. Failure of governments to put functioning drug supply systems in place
2. Failure to enact policies on pain treatment and palliative care
3. Poor training of health care workers
4. Existence of unnecessarily restrictive drug control regulations and practices
5. Fear among health care workers of legal sanctions for legitimate medical practice
6. Unnecessarily high cost of pain treatment

From Lohman D, Schleifer R, Amon JJ. Access to pain treatment as a human right. *BMC Med.* 2010;8:8.

recurrent pain is a specific health care problem—a disease in its own right.[61,69] It has been persuasively posited that this pervasive view of chronic pain as a symptom of disease rather than a disease state in itself has contributed to the paucity of public health and health policy attention (and funding) that chronic pain has received.[27,60]

Consequently, the WHO, IASP, and European Federation of the IASP chapters jointly declared in 2004 that such widespread, inadequately treated chronic pain must not be tolerated and, furthermore, that relief of pain should be a universal human right.[62-64,70] In 2010 the IASP issued the *Declaration of Montreal: Declaration That Access to Pain Management Is a Fundamental Human Right* (Box 5.3), which, in addition to emphasizing that chronic pain is a disease entity, reaffirmed the basic human right to access effective pain management and the obligation of governments and health care institutions to establish laws, policies, and systems that help promote—not inhibit—access to pain management.[69,71]

The two ultimate aims of this ongoing global pain initiative are to inform policy makers about the personal burden and economic cost of chronic pain and to educate physicians and allied health care professionals about assessment and management of pain to promote higher standards of care worldwide.[63,69] Similar attention has focused on effective palliative care being a universal, international human right.[67,72-74] Finally, denial of adequate pain treatment, when used as a form of punishment or torture, is a grossly egregious human rights violation.[75]

INCREASING WORLDWIDE ACCESS TO ANALGESICS

Even though simple, cost-effective treatments exist, a major gap exists between our increasingly sophisticated understanding of the pathophysiology of pain and its continued widespread inadequate management.[64,65] Despite international human rights laws, calls for the reform of laws and policies inhibiting access to pain treatment worldwide, and the attendant obligation of sovereign states to provide their citizens access to pain relief medicine, obstacles still commonly exist in providing pain treatment and palliative care (Box 5.4).[76,77] Of the 42 million grams of morphine consumed legally worldwide in 2010, 78% went to six countries—Australia, Canada, France, Germany, the United Kingdom, and the United States (Fig. 5.1*A*).[78,79] As a result, access to even basic treatment, such as oral analgesics, including opioids (e.g., morphine), for cancer pain and antiepileptic and antidepressant drugs for neuropathic pain, is widely variable and commonly deficient (Fig. 5.1*A* and *B*).[77,79-84]

Pain is a universal, multicultural experience that affects all people regardless of demographics or geography; however, inadequate treatment and the adverse effects of pain are not equally distributed worldwide.[60] This gap is most apparent and problematic in the poorest and most socially dysfunctional developing nations in Africa and Asia, which are contending with widespread poverty, oppression and violence, and sometimes war and its aftermath (Fig. 5.2).[64,65,79] However, a similar disparity in pain treatment exists in Europe between the European Union member countries and the former Iron Curtain Eastern European and Balkan countries.[80,85,86] Many cancer patients in Eastern Europe do not receive adequate relief of pain because of excessive regulatory restrictions on the availability and accessibility of opioids.[87] According to a Human Rights Watch report, the Ukraine is one of several Eastern European and Central Asian countries that consume only enough opioids in total to treat less than 30% of their citizens with terminal cancer and human immunodeficiency virus (HIV) infection or acquired immunodeficiency syndrome (AIDS).[66] Pain medicine and palliative care practitioners thus need to advocate for reform of governmental policy to overcome impediments to patient access to opioids.[79,88] For example, a 4-year project in which health care professionals collaborated with governmental officials culminated in the Romanian Parliament passing new, more progressive legislation on the medical use of opioids and psychotropic substances, with an ensuing nationwide practitioner educational program.[89]

THE NEED FOR A MORE COMPREHENSIVE AND ORGANIZED APPROACH TO PRESCRIBING OPIOIDS CHRONICALLY

Although many in the world suffer needlessly, prescribing of opioids for chronic non–cancer-related pain has paradoxically escalated in the United States recently; yet such use has outpaced the growth of scientific evidence on the benefits

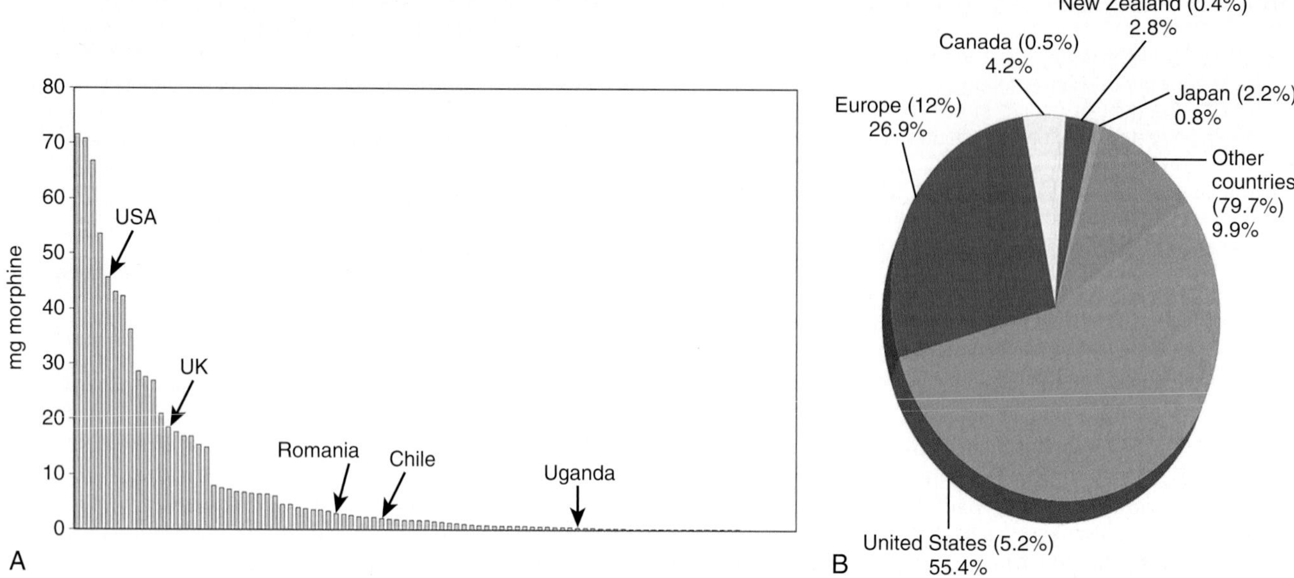

Figure 5.1 **A,** Global per capita consumption of morphine.[79] **B,** Maldistribution of regional legal opioid consumption versus population and morphine distribution of consumption, 2010. *Note*: Percentages in parentheses refer to share of the world population (i.e., total population of all reporting countries). (From International Narcotics Control Board. Available at http://www.incb.org/.)

and harm of these medications.[90,91] Critical research gaps exist on use of opioids for chronic non–cancer-related pain, and the need for a stronger evidence base is hence urgent.[90,91] Nevertheless, a recent multidisciplinary expert panel commissioned by the American Pain Society and the American Academy of Pain Medicine concluded that based on a systematic review of the available, albeit limited evidence, chronic opioid therapy can be an effective treatment in carefully selected and monitored patients with chronic non–cancer-related pain.[92]

Even in countries such as the United States with its ample, if not perhaps overabundant supply of opioids, there are inconsistent prescribing patterns and thus frequently unequal and inadequate access to opioids. As with many other elements of the U.S. health care system, there are racial, socioeconomic, and age disparities in pain assessment and opioid prescribing patterns, with minorities, the poor, and the elderly less likely to have access to needed controlled substances.[93-97] In many large U.S. medical centers, such marginalized patients with a legitimate need for opioids are customarily passed around from clinic to clinic. These patients thus out of necessity frequently visit emergency departments, where assessment and treatment of pain are widely variable and inadequate and where racial disparities in opioid prescribing also exist.[98-102] An innovative pharmacy- and primary care–based chronic opioid management program (an "Opioid Renewal Clinic") for such high-risk patients has been implemented successfully at the Philadelphia Veterans Affairs Medical Center.[103-105] To be more widely applied, this comprehensive practice model requires close collaboration between primary care physicians and pain medicine specialists.[106] However, there appears to be little support for such a labor-intensive, comparatively low-margin program among nongovernmental health care administrators and interventional pain practitioners.

ADDRESSING PAIN IN THE ESPECIALLY VULNERABLE PEDIATRIC AND GERIATRIC POPULATIONS

Given their respective potential and historically major societal contributions, it can be cogently argued that equitable and compassionate health care of children and the elderly is a hallmark of a just, higher-order society.[107-109] It is thus quite problematic that the especially vulnerable pediatric and geriatric populations remain quite prone to inadequate pain management—even in developed countries.

There is abundant published guidance on the assessment and treatment of pediatric pain, as well as robust data on its widespread prevalence and adverse effects.[110-113] Thus, inadequate pediatric management can no longer be attributed to a lack of evidence-based medicine but rather to an inability to apply what is known in everyday practices.[114] Clinicians, educators, administrators, and policy makers have an individual and collective responsibility to decrease pain and suffering in children and adolescents by narrowing the gap between current clinical practice and the existing research evidence and ethics supporting optimal patient care.[114-117] In developed countries, including the United States, Canada, and the United Kingdom, there is a need for increased training, resources, and reimbursement for primary care physicians and pain clinicians who seek to manage pediatric chronic pain via an often indicated biopsychosocial approach.[17,52,118,119] This need is especially great in smaller communities and rural settings, which are typically quite distant from formal pediatric pain medicine programs.[17,52] However, the situation is even more dire throughout the developing world (in low- and middle-income countries), where access to even basic pain treatment services is largely unavailable to the vast majority of children and adolescents who suffer pain from diseases (e.g., HIV/AIDS, cancer, sickle

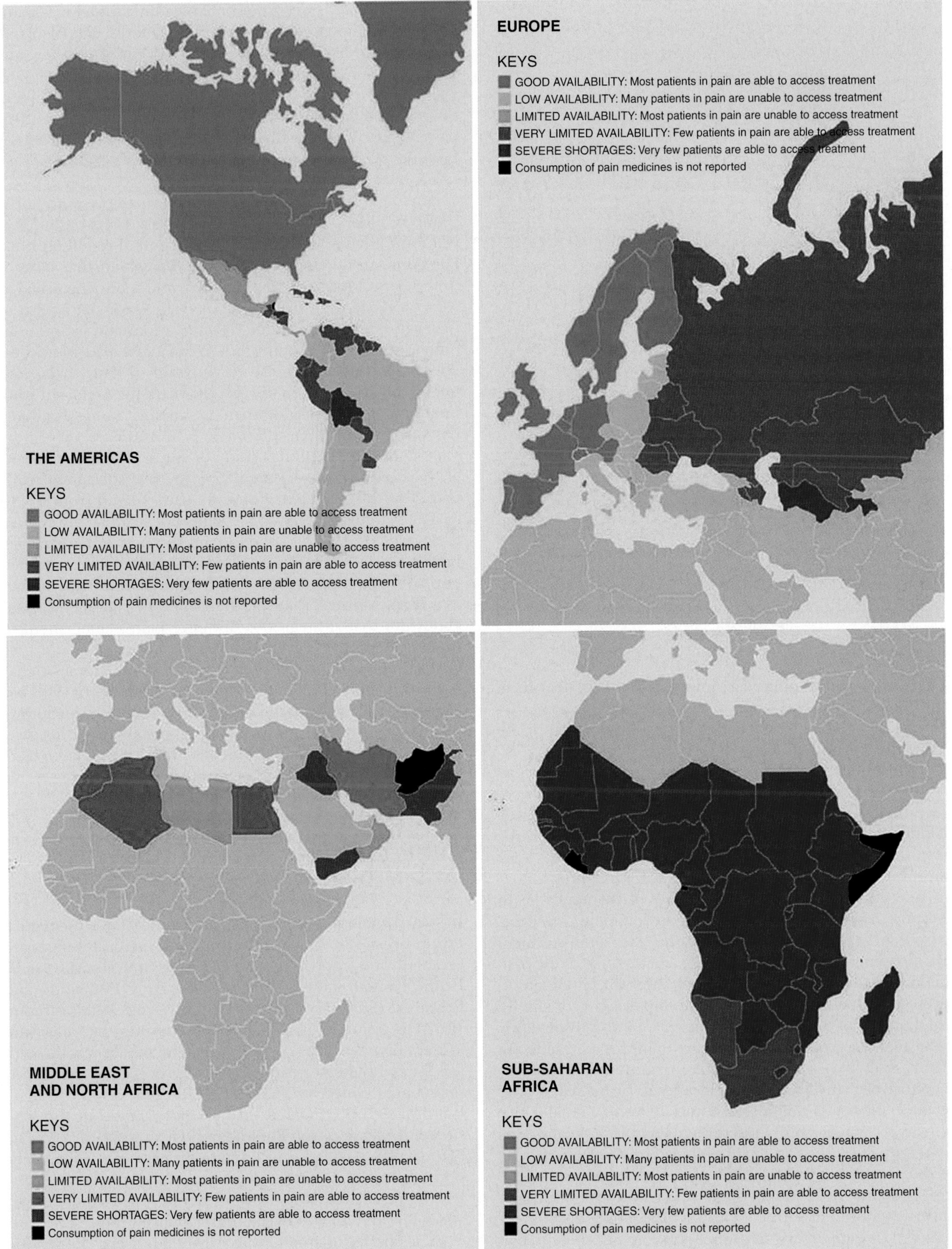

Figure 5.2 Regional access to pain treatment. (From Human Rights Watch. *Global State of Pain Treatment*. New York: Human Rights Watch; 2011:1-23. Reprinted with permission.)

Continued

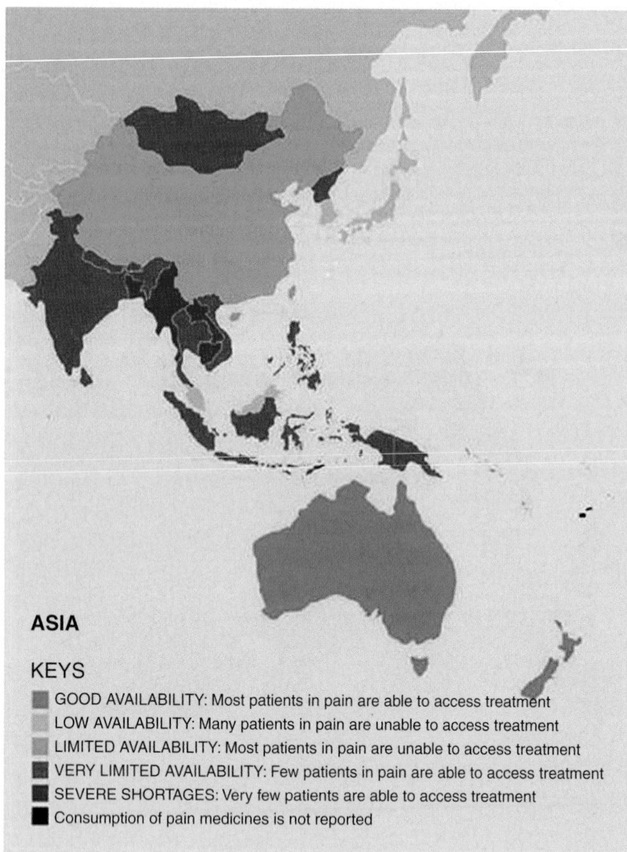

Figure 5.2, cont'd

cell disease) and trauma (e.g., injury, burns, war, terrorism, land mines).[68,120] The scope of this collective pediatric suffering and a global plan of action have been detailed by the WHO and a group of invested clinicians.[120,121]

At the other end of the age spectrum, assessment and treatment of geriatric pain have also been well described.[122-128] Nevertheless, chronic pain affects an estimated 25% to 50% of elderly people living in the community. Geriatric chronic pain management remains similarly suboptimal, with improvement needed in screening, clinical evaluation, follow-up, and attention to potential toxicities of therapy.[129-132] In 2009 the American Geriatric Society recommend low-dose, low-potency opioids (e.g., hydrocodone) over a nonsteroidal anti-inflammatory drug (NSAID; [e.g., ibuprofen]) as the first-line drug of choice for all elderly patients with moderate to severe pain, pain-related functional impairment, or diminished quality of life because of pain.[133,134] Two subsequently published, large-scale, retrospective analyses of Medicare claims data have questioned these recommendations. In a cohort of arthritis patients (mean age of 80 years, 85% female), the use of opioids was associated with a greater risk for cardiovascular events, safety events requiring hospitalization, and all-cause mortality than was the use of NSAIDs.[135] In the same database of patients, the risk for fractures of the hip, pelvis, wrist, or humerus was lower with propoxyphene and tramadol than with codeine, hydrocodone, and oxycodone.[136] Despite the use of propensity score matching to balance the potentially confounding covariates identified, these authors did not consider the potential dose-response gradient or account for key confounders, such as over-the-counter analgesic use and gastrointestinal bleeding, functional status and falls, and tobacco exposure and cardiovascular events.[137] The National Institutes of Health Pain Consortium recently sponsored an "Expert Panel Discussion on the Pharmacological Management of Chronic Pain in Older Adults" to identify research gaps and strategies to address them. This 2010 panel focused specifically on the use of opioids and NSAIDs because of these continued uncertainties regarding their risks versus benefits.[138,139]

Nursing home residents are a particularly vulnerable group of elders. The Centers for Disease Control and Prevention estimated that there are currently 1.5 million nursing home residents in the United States and that 43% of Americans older than 65 years will enter a nursing home at some point in their lives, with an average 835-day length of time since initial admission.[140] Pain is a common symptom in older residents of nursing homes and can lead to adverse effects such as a decrease in activities of daily living and quality of life.[141] Over the last 20 years the reported multinational prevalence of pain in nursing home residents has varied from 3.7% to 79.5%.[142] Moreover, a very large-scale U.S. cross-sectional study of nursing home residents 65 years and older revealed 17% to have substantial daily pain, but this prevalence of daily pain ranged from 0% to 54.7% by individual facility.[143] Thus not surprisingly, regulatory agencies, health care policy makers and administrators, health services researchers, and clinicians have identified improving pain assessment and treatment in nursing homes as a high priority. However, there has been little consensus about the best strategies to optimize pain management in nursing homes.[144] Given the unique population and care environment, clinical leadership in nursing homes needs not only proficient pain assessment and treatment skills but also working knowledge of organizational change, including quality improvement, team building, collaborative decision making, and system-level problem solving.[144,145] Of note, failure to provide adequate pain control in the nursing home setting has been legally interpreted as elder abuse.[64,146]

THE REGULATORY PROCESS FOR DRUGS AND MEDICAL DEVICES

It is worthwhile to compare, contrast, and critique the regulatory processes by which new drugs and medical devices are reviewed and approved for marketing and clinical use.[147] In the United States, the Center for Drug Evaluation and Research (CDER) of the Food and Drug Administration (FDA) is primarily responsible for assessing the safety and efficacy of a new drug. As a new drug makes its way through this federal regulatory and approval process, a series of four phases are defined by the FDA CDER (Table 5.1).[148,149] Medical devices are regulated in the United States by the FDA Center for Devices and Radiological Health (CDRH).[150] The FDA CDRH classifies a new medical device according to its perceived risk by using a three-tiered system (class I, II, or III), with escalating supporting evidence required for efficacy and safety and for postmarket surveillance (Table 5.2).[150]

In a similar manner, the Australian Drug Evaluation Committee makes recommendations to the national Therapeutic Goods Administration.[151] As in the United States, after a drug is initially approved, marketed, and distributed

Table 5.1 Food and Drug Administration and Center for Drug Evaluation and Research New Drug Review and Approval Process

Phase	Goal	Subject Enrollment	Typical Time Period
Preclinical Investigational new drug application	Preclinical (animal) data to justify testing of the drug in humans	Not applicable	1 yr
Phase I	Basic safety profile and pharmacokinetics of the drug	50-100 human subjects	1-3 yr
Phase II	Drug dosage, broad efficacy, and additional safety	100-500 human subjects	2 yr
Phase III	Confirmation of the safety and effectiveness of the drug, its dosages, and drug interactions in a broader population	1000-4000 human subjects	3-4 yr
Phase IV	New or expanded use (indication) for patient population and long-term risks vs. benefits	2000-5000 patients	2-5 yr

Data from Novo Nordisk (Bagsvaerd, Denmark). *From Idea to Patient*. 2010; and Overview of device regulation. 2009. Available at http://www.fda.gov/MedicalDevices/DeviceRegulationandGuidance/Overview/default.htm. Accessed April 3, 2012.

Table 5.2 Food and Drug Administration and Center for Devices and Radiological Health New Medical Device Risk Classification

Risk Classification	FDA Level of Evidence and Regulatory Requirements	Examples
Class I: lowest risk	None General controls: prohibitions against adulteration and misbranding, requirements for establishing registration and device listing, adverse event reporting, and good manufacturing practices	Elastic bandages, examination gloves, and handheld surgical instruments
Class II: low risk	Manufacturer must provide data to demonstrate that a new class II device is "substantially equivalent" to a legally marketed device Special controls: may require performance standards, design controls, and postmarket surveillance programs	Epidural and spinal needles Acupuncture needles Totally implanted spinal cord stimulators Powered wheelchairs Infusion pumps Surgical drapes
Class III: high risk	Clinical data demonstrating reasonable assurance that the device is safe and effective in the target population Full premarket approval required	Implantable infusion pumps, including for intrathecal and epidural medications Heart valves, pacemakers, implantable defibrillators, and coronary stents

Data from Overview of device regulation. 2009. Available at http://www.fda.gov/MedicalDevices/DeviceRegulationandGuidance/Overview/default.htm. Accessed April 3, 2012.

in Australia, it is considered eligible for phase IV trials in which new or expanded uses or populations (or both) can be approved and long-term risk versus benefits explored. In the European Union, either a state (i.e., country) level or a more centralized process is followed for drug approval. In the more centralized process, the Committee for Human Medicinal Products evaluates and makes recommendations to the European Medicines Agency (EMA), which grants community marketing authorization.[152,153] In the United Kingdom, after a drug is approved and licensed by the EMA, it undergoes further review for clinical indications and cost-effectiveness by the National Institute for Health and Clinical Excellence (NICE) in England and Wales or the Scottish Medicines Consortium in Scotland, which must approve its use by the respective branch of the National Health Service.[154-156]

In China, under the auspices of the State Food and Drug Administration, the Center for Drug Evaluation oversees approval of new drugs for marketing, with the new drug approval and registration process predicated on suitable clinical study data.[157] In India, the Central Drugs Standard Control Organization undertakes the data review process and makes recommendations to the Drugs Controller General. Drugs previously approved in the United States, Great Britain, Switzerland, Australia, Canada, Germany, South Africa, Japan, or the European Union (category A) are eligible for fast tracking in India, whereas in the absence of such a previous national approval, a similar multiphase process (category B) is followed.[158]

Given this very similar drug regulatory structure and process, one might expect a similar level of evidence required (i.e., threshold) and time line for approval; however, such is not the case.[147] In the United States the threshold for regulatory approval of a pharmaceutical is much lower than in Canada, the United Kingdom, and the European Union. Under the current Code of Federal Regulations, new drug approval by the U.S. FDA is typically based on demonstration of efficacy in only two or more randomized clinical trials, often in comparison to placebo—not the currently approved competing generic drug.[159] Given the perceived continued progress of medical science, governmental marketing approval of a new drug implies to clinicians and the general public that the new product represents an advance over older treatments. However, these current FDA standards for approval fail to assess whether newly approved drugs are less efficacious or less well tolerated than existing, often lower-cost alternatives. This raises the possibility that patients may be harmed by receiving a newly approved, typically more expensive, yet less efficacious treatment instead of a less costly alternative with well-established effectiveness and safety.[159] Aggressive pharmaceutical industry marketing to clinicians, as well as directly to consumers in the United States, increases the likelihood of this scenario.

In contrast, health care systems in several developed countries (e.g., Australia, Canada, and Britain) are applying comparative effectiveness research methods to allow decision makers (patients, clinicians, purchasers, politicians, and policy makers) to make informed decisions on specific health practices.[160] Such countries are now specifically using cost-effectiveness analysis—a form of comparative effectiveness research—to make drug approval decisions and to determine what medications will be reimbursed from the finitely available collective funding.[161] Such a cost-effectiveness analysis involves a head-to-head comparison of the cost and outcomes of the proposed proprietary drug versus an existing (if available, generic) drug.[162] A similar approach is used for so-called "me too" drugs.[161] NICE makes such decisions in the British National Health Service.[156,163,164] The cost-effectiveness–based approval process used by NICE has not been without controversy—with some clinicians and patients deriding it as being tantamount to overt rationing of health care and restricting access to potentially vital therapies.[165] Supporters of the NICE system argue that markedly higher patient co-payments for such drugs in the United States amount to barriers to access and covert rationing.[166,167]

Some have contended that the introduction of a new medical device into clinical practice is typically and unnecessarily delayed between 1 and 3 years in the United States when compared with the European Union.[168] This is especially so with class III high-risk devices, which to receive approval for marketing in the United States, the manufacturer must demonstrate the device to be reasonably safe and effective, typically with a prospective, randomized controlled clinical trial.[168] To receive approval to market the same device in the European Union, the manufacturer must demonstrate only that it is safe and that it performs in a manner consistent with the manufacturer's intended use.[168] Nevertheless, in recent years, well-publicized device recalls and lawsuits in the United States have led to concern that the FDA does not require sufficiently well-designed and valid supporting studies and does not keep unsafe devices off the market.[169,170] A recent study observed that of 78 class III ("high risk") cardiovascular devices that were approved through the FDA full premarket approval (PMA) process between 2000 and 2007, only 27% of the devices had been subjected to a single randomized trial and only 5% had undergone two or more blinded randomized studies.[171] The failure of certain medical devices such as implantable defibrillators—despite full PMA by the FDA—could pose deadly risks.[169] Of the 113 medical devices recalled from 2005 through 2009 by the FDA for life-threatening or very serious hazards, 78% were originally approved for marketing under the less stringent Section 510(k) FDA process or were considered so low risk that they were exempt from review.[172]

MEDICAL REVERSAL: WHY WE MUST RAISE THE BAR BEFORE ADOPTING NEW MEDICATIONS AND TECHNOLOGIES

In medicine, therapies, diagnostic tests, and screening modalities decline over time in clinical popularity for two reasons. The first reason is the occurrence of *replacement*—when an existing practice is supplanted by one that works better.[173] An example of replacement is the use of low-molecular-weight heparin (e.g., dalteparin) instead of unfractionated heparin or warfarin for the treatment and secondary prevention of deep vein thrombosis in cancer patients.[174] The second reason is the occurrence of *reversal*—when an existing practice falls out of favor not by being surpassed by another but when it is shown to have failed to achieve its intended goal or to result in harm that outweighs its benefits.[173] Although such medical reversals should be rare given the widely promulgated guidelines for study design and reporting of findings and the well-established tenets of evidence-based medicine, they are ubiquitous.[173] A recent study reviewed all 212 "original articles" published during 1 year in the *New England Journal of Medicine* and found that 16 (13%) of the 124 dealing with medical practice constituted reversal of existing practice,[175] thus confirming a previously observed reversal rate of 16% in highly cited original clinical research studies.[176] One of the most publicized examples involved rofecoxib (Vioxx). Its manufacturer, Merck, withdrew the drug in September 2004 because of an excess risk for myocardial infarction and stroke—after more than 80 million patients had taken the drug. This represents the largest prescription drug withdrawal (medical reversal) in history.[177]

Although replacement represents a logical progression in medical care, reversal reveals frequent missteps.[173] Specifically, medical reversal occurs primarily when a new clinical trial that is superior to its published predecessors by virtue of more robust design, controls, sample size, or primary end points contradicts current clinical practice.[173,175] For example, since first described in the mid to late 1990s, vertebroplasty quickly achieved widespread use such that in 2004 the procedure was performed more than 27,000 times in the United States—despite a lack of strong evidence in support of its efficacy.[178-180] To the contrary, two eventual well-designed randomized controlled trials conclusively demonstrated that vertebroplasty was no better than placebo (sham) in treating the pain and pain-related disability associated with osteoporotic compression fractures.[181-183] Unfortunately, the available evidence in support of conservative therapy (bed rest, analgesic medication, physiotherapy, and bracing) for osteoporotic compression fractures is also not strong.[184]

Medical reversal is problematic for three reasons: (1) it implies that mistakes or patient harm occurred with the previous but now abandoned, ineffective practice; (2) removing a once-common practice can be difficult, and continued adherence despite the contradicted claim furthers malfeasance; and (3) it undermines trust in the medical system.[173] Therefore, raising the bar for adoption of new medical practices has been proposed. The "common sense" approach that a new treatment will or should work can no longer justify

Box 5.5 Underlying Principles of the Institute of Medicine's *Relieving Pain in America: A Blueprint for Transforming Prevention, Care, Education, and Research*

A moral imperative. Effective pain management is a moral imperative, a professional responsibility, and the duty of people in the healing professions.

Chronic pain can be a disease in itself. Chronic pain has a distinct pathology that causes changes throughout the nervous system that often worsen over time. It has significant psychological and cognitive correlates and can constitute a serious, separate disease entity.

Value of comprehensive treatment. Pain results from a combination of biologic, psychological, and social factors and often requires comprehensive approaches to prevention and management.

Need for interdisciplinary approaches. Given chronic pain's diverse effects, interdisciplinary assessment and treatment may produce the best results for people with the most severe and persistent pain problems.

Importance of prevention. Chronic pain has such a severe impact on all aspects of the lives of its sufferers that every effort should be made to achieve both primary prevention (e.g., during surgery for a broken hip) and secondary prevention (of transition from the acute to the chronic state) through early intervention.

Wider use of existing knowledge. Although there is much more to be learned about pain and its treatment, even the existing knowledge is not always used effectively, and thus substantial numbers of people suffer unnecessarily.

The conundrum of opioids. The committee recognizes the serious problem of diversion and abuse of opioid drugs, as well as questions about their usefulness long-term, but believes that when opioids are used as prescribed and appropriately monitored, they can be safe and effective, especially for acute, postoperative, and procedural pain, as well as for patients near the end of life who desire more pain relief.

Roles for patients and clinicians. The effectiveness of pain treatments depends greatly on the strength of the clinician-patient relationship; pain treatment is never about the clinician's intervention alone but about the clinician and patient (and family) working together.

Value of a public health– and community-based approach. Many features of the problem of pain lend themselves to public health approaches—concern about the large number of people affected, disparities in occurrence and treatment, and the goal of prevention cited above. Public health education can help counter the myths, misunderstandings, stereotypes, and stigma that hinder better care.

From Institute of Medicine, Committee on Advancing Pain Research, Care, and Education. *Relieving Pain in America: A Blueprint for Transforming Prevention, Care, Education, and Research*. Washington, DC: National Academies Press; 2011.

its adoption.[173] Instead, rigorous efficacy and effectiveness studies need to be done before new modalities and technologies are adopted.

CONCLUSION

Given the widespread and substantial human and financial impact of pain, the economics and health policy of pain management are inextricably linked. As noted earlier, all health care systems—across the entire socioeconomic spectrum—are confronting the same fundamental health economic and health policy problem: how best to allocate finite resources to satisfy infinite health care demands.[185] Ultimately, as observed by a leading health care economist, "In a world of budget constraints there are no easy solutions."[186] Yet clear guidance and recommendations are readily at hand. Cited at the outset of this discussion, it is fitting to conclude by revisiting the 2011 IOM report *Relieving Pain in America: A Blueprint for Transforming Prevention, Care, Education, and Research.* It offers a set of underlying principles (Box 5.5) and a series of 16 salient recommendations, provides a time line for implementing them, and designates the groups responsible for doing so.[17,187] Though focused on the U.S. health care system, these IOM findings are universally applicable and an urgent call to action.

SUGGESTED READINGS

Barr DA. *Introduction to U.S. Health Policy: The Organization, Financing, and Delivery of Health Care in America.* 3rd ed. Baltimore: Johns Hopkins University; 2011.

Bodenheimer T, Grumbach K. *Understanding Health Policy: A Clinical Approach.* 6th ed. New York: McGraw-Hill; 2012.

Brennan F, Carr DB, Cousins MJ. Pain management: a fundamental human right. *Anesth Analg.* 2007;105:205-221.

Gilron I, Johnson A. Economics of chronic pain: how can science guide health policy? *Can J Anaesth.* 2010;57:530-538.

Gupta A, Mehdi A, Duwell M, et al. Evidence-based review of the pharmacoeconomics related to the management of chronic nonmalignant pain. *J Pain Palliat Care Pharmacother.* 2010;24:152-156.

Human Rights Watch. *Global State of Pain Treatment.* New York: Human Rights Watch; 2011:1-128.

Institute of Medicine, Committee on Advancing Pain Research, Care, and Education. *Relieving Pain in America: A Blueprint for Transforming Prevention, Care, Education, and Research.* Washington, DC: National Academies Press; 2011.

Phillips CJ, Schopflocher D. The economics of chronic pain. In: Rashiq S, Schopflocher D, Taenzer P, et al, eds. *Chronic Pain: A Health Policy Perspective.* Weinheim, Germany: Wiley-VCH Verlag; 2008:41-50.

Prasad V, Cifu A. Medical reversal: why we must raise the bar before adopting new technologies. *Yale J Biol Med.* 2011;84:471-478.

Robinson RL, Vetter TR. Healthcare economic evaluation of chronic pain: measuring the economic, social and personal impact of chronic pain and its management. In: Moore RJ, ed. *Biobehavioral Approaches to Pain.* New York: Springer; 2009:219-258.

Schopflocher D, Harstall C. The descriptive epidemiology of chronic pain. In: Rashiq S, Schopflocher D, Taenzer P, et al, eds. *Chronic Pain: A Health Policy Perspective.* Weinheim, Germany: Wiley-VCH Verlag; 2008:29-40.

Sultz HA, Young KM. *Health Care USA: Understanding Its Organization and Delivery.* Sudbury, Mass: Jones & Bartlett; 2011.

World Health Organization. *The Framework for the Access to Controlled Medications Programme.* Geneva: WHO; 2007.

The references for this chapter can be found at www.expertconsult.com.

6 Quality Assessment and Improvement and Patient Safety in the Pain Clinic

Vania E. Fernandez | Marta J. Rozanski | James P. Rathmell | Douglas G. Merrill

This chapter covers both quality assessment and improvement systems and patient safety issues. These are in some cases distinct and in others inextricably interrelated. They are each debated on national and international levels, and both are fundamental elements of the daily practice of pain medicine. The first section considers quality assessment and improvement programs and some practical steps to take to create a "QA/QI" program in a pain practice. The second section discusses the patient safety movement, both on a national scale and in terms of how each pain practitioner can expect to be involved.

SECTION 6.1 QUALITY ASSESSMENT AND IMPROVEMENT IN THE PAIN CLINIC

A significant factor in the deficits of our nation's health is the broader social dysfunction of the nation: the inequities of education, income, employment, social support, and opportunity that still exist in this country.[1] Nonetheless, we are cognizant that our health care system is also severely troubled. In the ensuing two sections we discuss the topics of quality and patient safety separately. These sections review the practical efforts that pain physicians can make to address these issues at the level that they can control: in the pain clinic.

WHAT IS "QUALITY" IN HEALTH CARE: DO WE HAVE IT?

Quality as an issue in health care is a relatively recent phenomenon. Starr's massive and Pulitzer Prize–winning 1982 review of health care policy and its relationship to society has no entry in its index for the word "quality" (or "value" or "outcome" for that matter).[2] Health care quality has been defined in many ways over the past several years. Since providers are not the only parties interested in defining and determining quality, many opinions are available on what constitutes health care quality.[3]

Lohr created a definition that the National Academy of Sciences' Institute of Medicine (IOM) has included in its discussion of quality[4]: "Quality is the degree to which health services for individuals and populations increase the likelihood of desired health outcomes and are consistent with current professional knowledge." This definition, with its emphasis on targeting known "desired" goals of health and its link to evidence-based medicine, is attractive to most physicians. As Donabedian wrote in his landmark paper on quality assessment in medicine in 1966[5]: "As such, the definition of quality may be almost anything anyone wishes it to be, although it is, ordinarily, a reflection of values and goals current in the medical care system and in the larger society of which it is a part."

A recommended addition to the "medical" definition that was offered by Lohr is one that recognizes the importance of process (delivery of an intervention), as well as the structures that support that care in determining the actual outcome of the care.[5] This three-legged stool provides opportunity for measurement (and improvement) of more than just report cards, which leads to a more comprehensive definition of health care quality if we add what is suggested by Bowers and Kiefe[6]: "quality being the extent to which structure and process maximize the likelihood of good outcomes."

Again, the emphasis is on the "likelihood" of good outcomes because high-quality care and outcomes are not necessarily directly linked. As Chassin and Galvin stated, the vagaries of the human condition mean that good-quality medical care can be followed by a poor outcome and excellent outcomes can occur despite poor care.[7]

QUALITY VERSUS VARIATION IN HEALTH CARE: MISUSE, OVERUSE, UNDERUSE, OR NONE OF THE ABOVE?

Another important definition of quality in health care is the absence of misuse, underuse, or overuse of therapy. These three embodiments of poor quality, originally cited by Donabedian in the 1960s, remain a common reference in discussions of health care quality.[5,8] The process of avoiding or eliminating these three problems is inherent in the standards of evidence-based medicine and in the effort to assess and eliminate unwarranted variation in care patterns. It is important to recognize that variation may be good or bad, or neither. It may indicate significant overuse or underuse of a therapy and thereby signal that either the science of the therapy is poor or it is being applied haphazardly.

However, before practice data can truly be defined as "variation," it must be assayed for any underlying reasons for diverse practices (including dissimilarities in supply and demand because of geographic economics and climate, for instance). Only if these factors are similar can any variation detected be linked to quality, rather than just being *associated* with confounding factors unrelated to quality. For instance, an increased number of obstetricians in an area may be associated with a higher birth rate in that area, but physician supply does not cause pregnancy (or birth).[9]

An important example of misinterpretation of variation is found in the influential monograph "The Care of Patients with Severe Chronic Illness: A Report on the Medicare Program by the Dartmouth Atlas."[10] Here the authors counted the number of physician visits by Medicare beneficiaries with various chronic medical conditions—filtered by hospital and by geographic region—and determined that the geographic regions where there are fewer physician visits are the same locations where the Medicare beneficiaries have higher levels of patient satisfaction and quality of care. From this they extrapolated to the conclusion that we have a surplus of physicians. One example cited is the contrast between the Mayo Clinic, where there are fewer physician visits, and nonintegrated health care systems in New York City and Los Angeles.

In reality, variation in health care practitioner visits may be associated with a diversity of genetic, cultural, and social situations. These three geographic areas are markedly different in their genetic, social, and cultural homogeneity, as well as in the percentage of older adults who live below the poverty level. They vary with regard to availability of nonphysician providers and thus access to preventive care. These three areas are also quite different in their rate of uninsured, so it is unimaginable that health care would be comparable between New York City or Los Angeles and Minnesota.[11]

This study's conclusion is a reminder of the critical importance of risk adjustment for dissimilitude in population types when analyzing variation in clinical processes or outcomes. The value in finding variation in care is to provide a signal that there may be "best practices" that can be emulated, but best practices can be determined only if patient and disease characteristics are similar.[12] Not all variation is misuse, overuse, or underuse.

THE SEVEN PILLARS OF QUALITY

In 1990, Donabedian enumerated seven attributes, or "pillars," of health care quality[13]:

1. Efficacy—the ability of care to actually improve health
2. Effectiveness—how well care achieves improvement in health in the circumstances of "everyday practice"
3. Efficiency—the cost of any given improvement in health
4. Optimality—the point at which incremental increases in care begin to diminish in their return on investment, such that health may be improved, but in a less efficient manner
5. Acceptability of care to patients—accessibility, the practitioner-patient relationship, amenities of care, patient valuation of care outcomes, patient estimation of care's economic worth
6. Legitimacy—consideration of the value of care by others than the patient receiving that care, the aspect of societal valuation as mentioned above
7. Equity—the balance between what individuals and what society consider appropriate distribution of care and resources

Donabedian continued, "quality cannot be judged by technical terms, by health care practitioners alone; that the preferences of individual patients and society at large have to be taken into account as well."

This last lesson should be kept in mind when choosing any single definition of "quality" as most appropriate.

WHAT FORCES PROPEL THE MODERN QUALITY MOVEMENT?

The concern about quality in health care became more intense in the latter 1980s as the systems of quality research and management that grew out of the business and manufacturing world were first applied to health care.[14] Despite the improved outcomes with increased economy achieved by the application of these methods in some health care organizations, quality science did not widely penetrate the national health care delivery system.

In 1998, the IOM published its first large report detailing the problems in the quality of U.S. health care: "The Urgent Need to Improve Health Care Quality."[7] This was followed in 1999 by *To Err Is Human: Building a Safer Health System. Report from the Committee on Quality of Health Care in America*, which focused on patient safety and claimed that between 40,000 and 98,000 patients die annually in hospitals because of defects in the quality of their care.[15] In addition, that report stated that 5.4% of patients suffered perioperative complications, almost 50% of which were due to caregiver error.

In addition to concerns about safety, five forces are driving the resurgence of concern about quality[16]:

1. Cost—health care expenditures have grown well past the trillion dollar mark, and it is now the perception of many in business, government, and the public that more than one third of that sum, or almost $400 billion annually, is a waste of money.[17] Correct or not, this impression is a huge motivator for the modern concern about quality—and value—among those who are paying the bills for health care. This concern extends to pain medicine because it is a high dollar item: in 1998, $26.3 billion was expended on the care of back pain alone.[18] Furthermore, it has been shown that low back pain episodes are associated with increased expenditure for other health conditions.[19]
2. Variation in the application of care—geographic variation exists in cost and care, often without linkage between more care and better quality. This situation is a red flag for those who evaluate quality and who believe that variation represents an absence of evidence of value (see Figs. 6.1 and 6.2).[20]

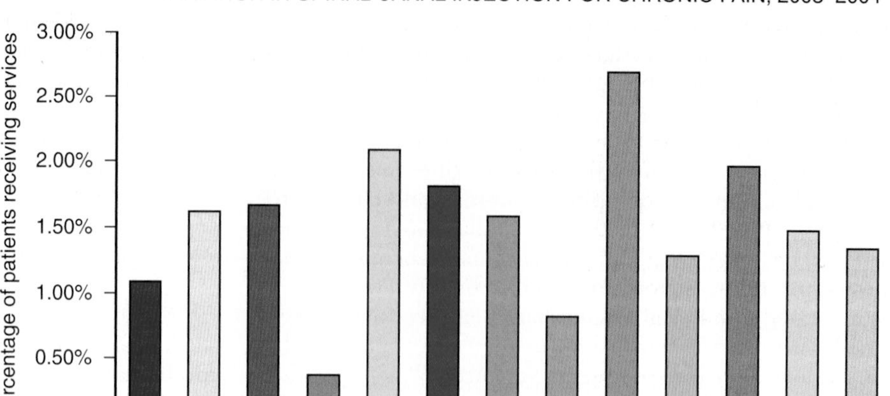

Figure 6.1 Variation in the rate of spinal canal injections for chronic pain, 2003 to 2004. This chart shows the remarkable variation in spinal canal injections recorded by the Medicare carrier Noridian in the 11 states that it served in 2003 and part of 2004. (From Friedly J, et al. Geographic variation in epidural steroid injection use in Medicare patients. *J Bone Joint Surg Am.* 2008;90:1730-1737.)

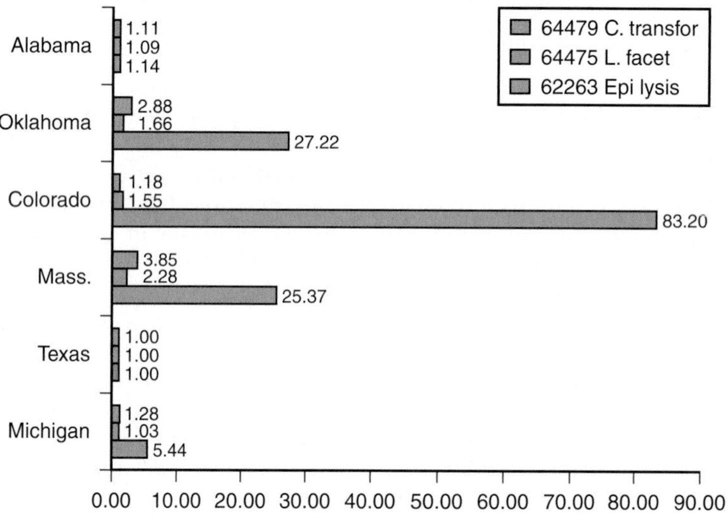

Figure 6.2 Inverse probability of receiving an injection anywhere but Texas. This graph shows the Centers for Medicare and Medicaid Services data for six states with regard to three injections: cervical transforaminal epidural steroids; lumbar facet injection, single level; and epidural lysis of adhesions. The variation in care is most notable in that all bars to the right portray a diminished incidence of the use of these procedures, with Texas serving as the baseline. Epidural neurolysis shows the most variation, with more than 80 times less use in Colorado per capita than in Texas. Such variation in care has been shown to be associated with a deficit in the quality of evidence for appropriate indications and is noted by health care policy experts as an indication of overuse. (From Merrill DG. Hoffman's glasses: evidence-based medicine and the search for quality in the literature of interventional pain medicine. *Reg Anesth Pain Med*. 2003;28:547-560.)

3. The increase in for-profit health care delivery systems, specialty ("boutique") hospitals, and office-based surgery is a concern for some health care policy makers, who view these as potential drivers of increased cost. In addition, there is a fear that such practice modes "skim" the most profitable segment of income from traditional hospitals, thereby leaving the larger nonprofit and public entities at risk for financial ruin. This same argument was used against ambulatory surgery centers when they were first introduced in the 1970s and is the impetus behind the Certificate of Need requirements that the American Hospital Association was able to lobby for in many states.[21] Furthermore, there is a potential conflict of interest when the providers are stakeholders in these health care entities.[22]
4. The increase in medical malpractice litigation, seen by some as an indicator of poor quality, is viewed by others as a driving force of the defensive overutilization of services that leads to increased spending and exposure of the patient to unnecessary risk.
5. The expanding role of government and industry in scrutinizing health care and regulating its practice is due in part to the importance of these groups as the largest purchasers/consumers of health care, coupled with the business sector's internal history of quality innovation.

PATIENT SAFETY AND THE "CULTURE OF SAFETY"

There is reasonable debate on whether a specific patient may be safe and whether a specific error contributes to real morbidity.[23,24] However, the public, legislators, and payers are convinced that both patient safety and human error are significant problems in today's health care delivery system.[25,26] The health care industry is now urged to create a "culture of safety" at all levels of practice, which will put in place processes that will eliminate or decrease the impact of human error.[27]

The majority of error committed in health care is due to system defects rather than individual mishaps, as was pointed out in the IOM's *Crossing the Quality Chasm: A New Health System for the 21st Century*. This book also presented a framework for improving health care quality with six specific targets for improvement[28]:

1. Safety
2. Effectiveness
3. Efficiency
4. Timeliness of care
5. Patient-centered care
6. Equitable care

This anxiety about safety has led the Centers for Medicare and Medicaid Services (CMS) to make contracts with Quality Improvement Organizations (QIOs) and spend in excess of $200 million per year on them, despite evidence that QIOs do not make a difference in the quality of care.[29] Congress appropriated more than $300 million to the Agency for Health Care Research and Quality (AHRQ) in the 5 years that followed the publication of *To Err is Human*, yet there is still much on the IOM list that has not been addressed.[30]

Among these larger forces of business, government, and society, a lesson sometimes lost is that the individual practitioner *can* improve the quality of health care. If practitioners identify outcomes that are desired, use the tenets of evidence-based medicine to find "best practices," and measure both their delivery of these therapies (process) and the results of these therapies (outcomes), it is more likely that quality will improve.[31] Adherence to evidence-based "best practice" begins with the individual practitioner and is associated with significant improvement in patient outcomes, including mortality.[32]

CONTINUOUS QUALITY IMPROVEMENT OR TOTAL QUALITY MANAGEMENT DEFINED

Continuous quality improvement (CQI) or total quality management (TQM) is a seven-step process that consists of the identification of desired knowledge, design of appropriate measures to obtain the necessary assessments, measurement, investigation of the measurements to find trends and best practices, return of that information to those who can effect change, implementation of change in practice to increase the incidence of best practice, and then remeasurement to assess the program of change. It is an outgrowth of the "total quality control" movement that spread from the business sector to health care in the 1980s.[33] Its origins may be traced to Walter Shewart's work in the 1920s, including the "plan-do-study-act" cycle that was further amplified by Deming in the 1970s.[14] In medicine, CQI has been valuable in creating significant improvement in practice patterns, even among multiple practitioners in multiple sites across geographically large distances.[34]

HEALTH CARE QUALITY AND BUSINESS

The health care quality movement has attracted significant attention from the business community, the group that often pays the bill. Indeed, there is a widespread belief that business management tools can provide the solutions to the health care quality problem.[35] Recognition of this potential industry crossover is the reason that the business community, so oddly placed as our nation's primary provider of health care insurance, has created powerful organizations, such as the Leapfrog Group (www.leapfroggroup.org/home), the Bridges to Excellence program (www.hci.org), and, in league with insurers, the Integrated Health Care Association (www.iha.org). Each of these organizations aims to push health care providers to embrace specific goals and types of behavior that are likely to improve patient safety and outcome.[36] These organizations have recommended financial incentives (pay for performance [P4P]), public disclosure of hospital safety rankings ("report cards"), and institutional changes in quality methodology and behavior, including the use of electronic health records (EHRs) and computerized physician order entry (CPOE). They have spawned interest in these programs within CMS and pushed along initiation of the CMS P4P programs that are growing in parallel with those being created by private payers.[37]

QUALITY ASSESSMENT AND QUALITY IMPROVEMENT: RISK ADJUSTMENT AND REPORT CARDS

Success in quality improvement as a result of employer-based initiatives has been mixed. This is in part due to the choice of quality initiatives with insufficient evidence of validity, as occurred when Leapfrog pushed for high-risk surgical procedures to be limited only to hospitals whose volume had already reached a chosen minimum level.[38] In addition, participation has been voluntary and the financial incentives have been either paltry, easily gained, or both. Some revision of the Leapfrog criteria occurred with late recognition of the importance of risk adjustment.[36]

One challenge is that the correlation between process measures (those most easily measured) and outcome measures (more difficult to measure) remains controversial in the most basic and oft-studied clinical circumstances (e.g., outcome of treatment of myocardial infarction by hospital).[39] This critical aspect of the application of quality science must be certain before any real value can be attached to public reporting of hospital (or physician) performance. Moreover, evidence is growing that even when accurate, report cards alone do not induce improved performance.[35,40,41]

APPLICATION OF CONTINUOUS QUALITY IMPROVEMENT AND TOTAL QUALITY MANAGEMENT: NATIONAL SURGICAL QUALITY IMPROVEMENT PROGRAM

There is a known means of improving quality of care: the simple act of measuring controllable clinical outcomes in a way in which they can be systematically analyzed and the information provided to the caregivers, with guidance on opportunities for change.[42-44] Using specific measures to guide improvement initiatives is the key to success of the application of quality science. By contrast, monitoring of broadly defined outcome measures (such as mortality in hospital report cards) fails to effectively improve care because their causative factors are so diverse and are often independent of the practice of the caregivers under observation. The failures of a "shotgun" approach to measurement are exacerbated by a lack of risk adjustment.[45]

The Department of Veterans Affairs (VA) National Surgical Quality Improvement Program (NSQIP) was created by surgeons in the VA system and in 1991 began to collect data to allow assessment of surgical outcomes and quality in the many hospitals in the system.[46] Nurses hired specifically to work on the study collected the data. It included variables (e.g., preoperative serum albumin levels) to allow risk stratification of patients. Three important principles have been elucidated:

1. It is an absolute requirement that all evaluations of health care quality be amended by stratification of patient risk factors (risk adjustment). Not doing so introduces an error rate as high as 60% when comparing the unadjusted quality of programs.
2. Provider volume does *not* necessarily correlate with outcome. This finding disputes the Leapfrog tenet that outcomes are improved by directing surgical procedures only to hospitals with "sufficient" volumes. Instead, there is no clearly "safer volume," but what is important is the quality of the program.[42] This exemplifies the error of choosing "obvious" quality goals before gathering adequate data.
3. Regular provision to surgeons of the results of their institutions' outcomes allows identification of "best practice" and is an effective means of improving quality of care. This approach improved patient outcome measures such as mortality and length of stay by as much as 45%.

The VA system experience has further shown that there are aspects of the Leapfrog and 100,000 Life Initiatives that are of value: the use of EHRs, CPOE, financial incentives for compliance of providers with designated performance goals, and routine comprehensive quality measurement has led to improved quality and delivery of warranted care.[46]

However, there are still barriers to comprehensive CQI programs: physician-specific outcome monitoring is unlikely to be accurate because any single doctor treats too few patients for accurate statistical evaluation, in most settings there is still a lack of extant evidence-based benchmarks, and technical barriers still prevent accurate collection of data.[47] In addition, the lack of good data on the appropriate management of patients with multisystem disease means that a physician who holds back from treating one disease with guideline-specific treatments because of concern about disease-disease or disease-drug interactions would be "punished" if scrutinized under the current quality assessment and improvement paradigm.[48] This illustrates the difficulty of attributing specific patient outcomes to "causative" individual provider actions.

Iezzoni, a pioneer in the science of risk adjustment, noted that outcomes in health care cannot be simplistically linked directly to care but are actually part of an equation that she terms an "algebra of effectiveness." This "algebra" is determined by three factors: the patient's condition and inherent risk, the effectiveness of the treatment provided, and an unaccountable or uncontrollable set of random variables.[49] The NSQIP has proved that collection of risk-adjusted data regarding surgery site outcomes, rather than physician-specific outcomes measurement, is a successful strategy for improving outcomes. Notably, the NSQIP data collection and analysis that were facility specific were accurate enough that it prevented the planned closure of several "poorly" performing sites once risk adjustment for patient comorbidity was invoked.[42] At this point in time, concentration on evaluation of facilities rather than individual physicians is the only appropriate CQI approach in view of the current limitations of technology and evidence-based medicine.

QUALITY IMPROVEMENT IN PAIN MEDICINE

Community pain practice quality is improved if a cohesive program of measurement, identification of best practice, education, and reassessment is applied.[50,51] CQI programs may improve the quality of therapy simply by inducing a more extensive review of a patient's history. For instance, inquiry about patient risk adjustors may lead to the recognition of mental health issues that could significantly affect the outcomes of any pain treatment plan.[52] The use of baseline measures can both direct care and provide an understanding of the probable potential for meaningful improvement in function and pain scores by identifying risk factors for long-term treatment failure.[53,54] Verhoef and colleagues made the point that the best set of outcome measures for a pain practice will include some open-ended questions and also to let patients take on part of the role of setting goals for their own therapy.[55] In this way, patients can be expected to be additionally motivated to reach these goals.

An active CQI program will also allow practitioners to evaluate the effects of the introduction of new therapies or treatment algorithms into their practices and either prove or disprove their value.[56] CQI provides a means to achieve accreditation for facilities and may even influence which quality measurements are adopted by regulatory agencies as sources of "grading" quality of care.[57] Finally, the use of a clinical database for monitoring patient outcomes also provides a sense of participation in the process for the staff members whose work is being assessed, a key factor in their acceptance of and enthusiasm for the benefits of CQI.[58]

The most significant hurdle in CQI for pain medicine is a lack of apparent benchmarks or national "best practices" that providers can emulate. Using the literature to establish benchmarks is prone to error because of the significant positive bias in the reporting of success of techniques. Overall, the evidence is not clear which, if any, interventions improve many chronic pain states.[59]

Analysis of practice patterns by either partners or an unassociated local group of pain physicians is potentially an excellent source of evidence in situations in which there is a lack of randomized controlled trials in the peer-reviewed literature. Assessment programs that are under the mantle of "peer review" statutes will allow participating physicians rapid and open means of sharing their own best practices with one another in an attempt to increase the quality of the community's pain care. Such evaluation may be accomplished with very short questionnaires. Patient interest in and compliance with such assessments are usually avid.[60]

Pain medicine practitioners can find a useful template for CQI programs that can be used in their own practices in Patel and colleagues' description of such programs in mental health[61]:

Quality improvement programs are practice and system strategies that support efficiency, appropriate care, and acceptable outcome. Comprehensive approaches that support client and provider education; encourage consumers to take a more active role in their recovery; and make use of support structures, such as case management to coordinate care have been shown to improve quality, in terms of both processes and outcomes of care.

CONSTRUCTING A CONTINUOUS QUALITY IMPROVEMENT PROGRAM FOR A PAIN PRACTICE

There are several steps in creating a CQI program for pain:

1. Identify the practitioners (physicians, nurses, therapists) who will be involved.
2. Gather these caregivers together to align their information goals and to craft a set of measures toward which all can agree that the program should be directed. A good starting point is the list put forth by the IOM[28]:
   a. Care should be *safe.*
   b. Care should be *effective* and based on proven *evidence and science.*
   c. Care should be *efficient* and *cost-effective with no waste.*
   d. Care should be *timely,* with no waiting or delays.
   e. Care should be *patient centered*–respect patient preference and give the patient control.
   f. Care should be *equitable* with no unequal treatment.
3. The most effective CQI program will start with the participants deciding what they personally believe are the most interesting (initial) questions to be answered. For instance, four or five separate practices in a delivery area might decide to evaluate the outcomes of referral to physical and behavioral therapists in the area or the value of a particular invasive pain technique.
4. Pick outcome measures that will allow accurate assessment of the problem. Weinstein and Deyo recommended separation of assessment into four domains: patient health status, cost, patient expectation, and clinical status.[62] Within these areas, indicators are chosen that answer the questions most important to the practitioners. Indicators are of three types[63]:
   a. *Structure measures* assess the characteristics of the practice or a facility, such as staff-to-patient ratios or patterns of diagnosis. Such information may alert the practitioner to unforeseen aspects of practice that are causing quality issues. For instance, a growth in the number of return visits of patients with complex regional pain syndrome who demonstrate increased dysfunction after an initial period of improvement could alert the care teams to an unrealized issue of reimbursement denials for the prolonged physical and behavioral therapy required in the care of this syndrome.
   b. *Process measures* assess how care is provided in the practice. For instance, the compliance audits regarding documentation by practitioners and therapists that support evaluation and management coding fit into this category. The disadvantage of process measures is primarily in determining a link with outcome, because these measures must be considered surrogates for outcome in the many situations in which direct measurement of the outcomes is impeded by difficulty in risk adjustment or other barriers. Another problem is that process measures are frequently used since they are relatively easy to measure, but they may have little connection to true clinical outcomes. An example is how long it takes for a patient to be roomed after arrival. Finally, quality assessment is best if it considers a continuum of care, but process measures tend to evaluate only small pieces of care.[64]
   c. *Clinical outcome measures* are those on which most practitioners focus, although an effective CQI program will monitor all three types. An example of clinical outcome measures is the use of repeated patient health status testing to determine health status longitudinally after interventions. In most practices, it would be expected that some sort of evaluation of patients in this regard would be collated and sorted by diagnosis, demographics, and intervention. This is a critical step in monitoring for overuse or underuse of medical therapies.
5. The measures chosen should have the following characteristics[65,66]:
   a. *Relevance.* They should relate directly to the goals of the group, and it should be true that the interventions on the group have an effect on them.
   b. *Timeliness.* The measures should be collected in a timely manner so that they can be related as closely as possible to the interventions that the practitioners wish to assess.
   c. *Reliability.* The measures should be accurate and consistent no matter when or who is assessing and recording them.
   d. *Validity.* A valid measure is sensitive to changes that the practitioner can effect.
   e. *Precision.* The measures should be clearly defined and leave little potential for individual or erroneous interpretation.
   f. *Cost-effectiveness.* A CQI program costs money, and the measures should be significant enough to your patients and your practice that they are worth the time and money expended on the process of collection and analysis.

g. *Provider control.* The variable measured must be one that the provider or organization can actually control or it is not worth measuring. For instance, measuring patient self-reported pain levels 1 year after an intervention for a chronic pain condition is unlikely to reflect a process that the provider can control because of the impact of the intervening health care and patient activity over the course of 1 year.
h. *Clear meaning.* The measure must be one that is easily understood by all concerned.

6. Terminology—once the practitioners have chosen the outcome measures, the terms must be adjusted to be in congruence with standard nomenclature. The accepted standard is a somewhat moving target, but SNOMED-CT (Systemized Nomenclature of Medicine—Clinical Terms) is produced by the College of American Pathologists (CAP) and has been designated by the National Institutes of Health (NIH) and the National Library of Medicine (NLM) for use in electronic transfer of medical information in the United States. Thus all practitioners should make sure that their own terms are "cross-walked" to SNOMED terms so that they report data that are standardized by accreditation and certification bodies and by payers in the years to come. This crosswalk process may be done in one of (at least) four ways:
   a. One can download all of SNOMED at the NLM site, which has licensed SNOMED for use by any entity within the United States. This site is www.nlm.nih.gov/research/umls, but the data sets are raw and most practitioners would need help manipulating them.
   b. The CAP has a complete version for sale at www.ihtsdo.org/snomed-ct, although the price may vary depending on the nature of the entity requesting it.
   c. Apelon (www.apelon.com) has two products that will take care of the translation process. One is Mycroft, which is a translator that is free via Web browser and allows the user to find the crossmatch in SNOMED for any other term. This requires a fair amount of time and may not be useful if there are a lot of terms to look up. The other option is Termworks, a translator that will automatically translate a body of terms (in a spreadsheet format). However, this product is obtained by subscription, which, as of this writing, costs $1000 per month or $10,000 per year. Another product (TermManager) allows you to upload your terms to their server, and the translation is done at that level for a subscription fee of $100 per month per user. Though expensive, in the case of a large volume of terms this may be a good way to cut down on the hunting time that would otherwise be necessary for translation of terms.
7. *Risk adjustment* must be included in the design of the monitoring system for the measurements to have any utility in identifying high quality and best practice.[67,68] In the past, newly minted measures of quality have been introduced without attention to risk or to scientific investigation to ascertain that they were valid estimators of outcome.[69] As the NSQIP proved, without accounting for the severity of patient morbidity, "significant correlation" between care processes and clinical outcomes may prove spurious when such comorbidities are later considered.[42] Risk adjustment is a young and still potentially confounding science, and many of its controversies are yet unsolved.[70,71]

The vagaries of risk adjustment require that practitioners use tools of measurement that are already validated. For instance, it is true to say that age and diabetes are significant comorbid conditions that should be considered when determining the probable outcome after surgery, but their relative importance can vary depending on which surgical procedure is under consideration, who is determining the severity of the comorbid condition, whether administrative or clinical determinants are used to determine the presence of disease and its severity, or which administrative coding tool is used to identify the condition.[72,73] If a pain practitioner or group decides to create a completely new measure, careful attention to risk adjustment theory and its evaluation in the literature or appropriate texts is recommended.[74] Nonetheless, it is possible for small groups of clinical experts to choose risk adjustment indices with validity if the process is done with bias controls and if there is involvement of biostatisticians and epidemiologists.[75]

Risk adjustment in chronic pain practice poses very significant challenges in view of the wide diversity in the types of adjustors that are operant in the widely varied population known as "chronic pain patients." The variegated nature of patients with multiple comorbid conditions ranging from physical disabilities, economic and social burdens, and mental health disorders makes it difficult to allocate risk "cohorts."[76] Risk adjustment in pain treatment outcome *research* is also a new science, and more rigorous studies than yet exist in the literature are needed before clarity and certainty exist in this area.

SPECIFIC OUTCOME TOOLS AND MEASURES FOR YOUR PRACTICE

Box 6.1 lists some measures and tools that might be considered for a pain CQI program. They have been used in scientific studies to measure some of the variables that would be valuable to a pain program. The reader is cautioned, however, that a great deal of variation exists in the versions of some of these instruments published in the literature.[77]

Many organizations are still attempting to codify and make uniform the "dictionary" of terms that are used in quality databases. An excellent source of guidance in this endeavor is a document from the American Society of Anesthesiologists (ASA) titled "Guiding Principles for Management of Performance Measures by the American Society of Anesthesiologists," available on the ASA website www.asahq.org. Several organizations are involved in the effort to codify terminology in addition to the ASA, including the Anesthesia Patient Safety Foundation (APSF) and its Data Dictionary Taskforce, and international groups such as the World Health Organization (WHO). The number of societies, the importance of the task, and the lack of certainty in the area mean that any database will be mutable over the next decade. The benefit of such malleability of design, which will always cost money, is that the practitioners who use it will be better assured that they will be in compliance with the requirements of accreditation agencies (e.g., The Joint Commission [TJC], Accreditation Association for Ambulatory Health Care [AAAHC], and others), which will also be set and amended in the years to come. A review of the challenges and some tools for measuring outcomes specific to

Box 6.1 Examples of Data Measures and Quality Assessment Tools Adaptable for Quality Assessment and Improvement Programs in Pain Practices

Basic Patient Information

Some of this information will be gleaned from the patient chart and some will require further questioning by staff.

Demographics

- Gender
- Age
- Ethnicity
- Residential zip code
- Referred? Y/N
- Live alone? Y/N
- Care for self without help? Y/N
- Other caregivers/providers (list)

Disability and Litigation

Litigation active? Y/N
Legally disabled? Y/N
—percentage?
Working? Y/N

Mental Health

DSM-IV codes assigned
Psychiatric hospitalization DRGs
Annual psychiatric hospitalization days

Patient Expectations

Expected degree of return of function
Expected job status after treatment
Expected changes in medication after treatment
Expected decrease in pain level after treatment

Costs

Direct Health Care Costs

Physician visits
Emergency department and hospitalization costs
Physical therapist fees
Physical therapy modalities
Occupational therapy
Vocational rehabilitation therapy
Behavioral health therapy
Laboratory studies
Imaging costs
Professional home care
Stimulator or pump and implantation fees
Analgesic and behavioral medications
Alternative therapy costs

Indirect Health Care Costs

Litigation fees
Lost wages
Cost of housekeeping
Cost of other home care
Travel cost for care
Time expended by family, others in care

Tools

Be aware that multiple versions may exist in the literature for some of these tools. When available, the most definitive source is listed below.

Overall Quality-of-Life Status

SF-12 or SF-36 measures: www.qualitymetric.com
U.S. National Health Interview Survey (U.S. NHIS)
Spitzer's Quality of Life Uniscale—a one-question set that records patient self-assessment of the past week in terms of quality of life[78]
Spitzer's QOL Index—five items[78]

Pain- and Function-Specific Questionnaires

TOPS (Treatment Outcomes in Pain Survey)[79]
PIQ-6 (Pain Impact Questionnaire): www.qualitymetric.com
PIQ-R (Revised Chronic and Acute Pain Impact): www.qualitymetric.com
ASA9: http://old.asahq.org/Newsletters/1997/08_97/Outcomes_0897.html
Fibromyalgia Impact Questionnaire[80]
Roland-Morris Back Pain[81]
Patient Specific Functional Scale[82]
Quebec Back Pain Questionnaire
Waddell Disability Index
West-Haven-Yale Multidimensional Pain Inventory (MPI)

Condition-Specific Measures

These are somewhat more specialized tools that may work in pain assessment programs.
Pain Disability Questionnaire[83]
Patient Specific Index/Patient Specific Functional Scale
Problem Elicitation Technique
Patient Generated Index
Canadian Occupational Performance Measure
Schedule for the Evaluation of Individual Quality of Life
Measure Yourself Medical Outcome Profile
Juvenile Arthritis Quality of Life Questionnaire

Risk Adjustment

Functional Comorbidity Index[84]

Patient Satisfaction

Picker Patient Experience Questionnaire[85]—this is a superb assessment of how your practice measures up to the patient's expectations. It would be worth assessing at intermittent, fixed intervals to watch for trends and administrative areas that could be improved.

Measures Used in Health Quality and Function Studies

Utility measures—patient assessment of the value of the overall health state
Euroqol (EQ-5D)[86]—highly recommended as a short and insightful look at your patient's attitudes
Health Utility Index[87]
Generic measures—these measures quantify the patient's self-assessment of overall health
Sickness Impact Profile[88]—progenitor of the Roland-Morris questionnaire
Nottingham Health Profile[89]
SF-12, SF-36: www.qualitymetric.com

Work and Function

Work Limitations Questionnaire
Oswestry Disability Index
Simple Shoulder Test
Neck Disability Index
Short Musculoskeletal Functional Assessment

Continued

Box 6.1 Examples of Data Measures and Quality Assessment Tools Adaptable for Quality Assessment and Improvement Programs in Pain Practices (Continued)

Pain

Visual analog scale (VAS) or Pain Intensity Difference (PID)—there are many confounding factors in the measurement of pain intensity; also, there are validity concerns regarding the importance of change over time (studies indicate that 2 points may be a valid cutoff for clinically significant improvement).[90]

Von Korff's Pain Scale[91]

Graded Chronic Pain Scale[92]

Neuropathic Pain Specific tools[93]

Neuropathic Pain Scale

Neuropathic Pain Symptom Inventory

Leeds Assessment of Neuropathic Symptoms and Signs (LANSS)

Neuropathic Pain Questionnaire (NPQ)[94]

Neuropathic Pain Screening Tool (NPST)

Neuropathic Pain Diagnostic Questionnaire (DN4)

Neuropathic Pain Screening Tool (NPST)

Palliative Care

Patient Needs Assessment Tool (PNAT)[95]

DRG, diagnosis-related group; DSM-IV, *Diagnostic and Statistical Manual of Mental Disorders, Fourth Edition*; QOL, quality of life; SF-36, Medical Outcomes Study Short-Form 36-Item Survey.

assessing outcomes in back pain therapy has recently been published.[96]

An excellent review is one by Resnik and Dobrykowski that involves outcome measurement in patients with low back pain.[97] The entire December 15, 2000, issue of *Spine* is highly recommended reading because it contains in-depth reviews of several of the back pain measurement tools.[98] Obviously, not all the measures listed will be applicable to every pain practice, and the practitioner is urged to review the references in Box 6.1 for information on how best to use the various measures.

One important issue is the significance of any change observed in the various measures over time in each patient. Some of the tools recommended were developed primarily to look at patient cohorts rather than an individual patient. This area of research is still emerging, and readers are encouraged to monitor the literature closely to assure them that their use of the tools is valid.[90]

THE TOOLS

The Brief Pain Inventory is adaptable to computer use, although it has not been validated for all pain conditions.[99] Another valuable tool is a modification of the Medical Outcomes Study Short-Form 36-Item (SF-36) survey, the Low-Back SF-36PF$_{18}$.[100] This instrument is also amenable to computer use and includes aspects of the SF-36 and the Oswestry and Quebec back pain questionnaires. A newer instrument that may lend itself to prediction of outcomes is the Pain Disability Questionnaire (PDQ), which is a short list of 15 questions that uses a continuum line for responses, similar to the visual analog scales for rating pain that most chronic pain patients have seen.[83] It may also be used on a computer. TOPS (Treatment Outcomes of Pain Survey) is a valuable tool that includes the SF-36 and additional questions that are specific to pain medicine.[79] It has the added value of having been validated in clinical practice and as a research tool.

Over the next several years, advancement in the nomenclature of clinical outcomes monitoring will occur and lead to more specific definitions of the vocabulary of pain quality databases. This will improve the comparability of data across databases and tools, further refine the science of pain management, and increase the probability that we will be able to fix national benchmarks of quality and best practices.

A RISK ADJUSTMENT TOOL FOR PAIN PRACTICE CONTINUOUS QUALITY IMPROVEMENT

As mentioned, it is important within a pain practice to calibrate expectations of improvement in a given patient by factoring in comorbid conditions and any evident functional disabilities and including other confounding conditions, such as ongoing litigation. One new index that allows for this is the Functional Comorbidity Index.[84]

WHICH TOOL TO USE AND HOW?

Gathering data is best managed in part by using patient surveys before and after provision of services, with timing appropriate to the nature of the patient's condition and the expected effective duration of the intervention. Several very good reviews of the relative merits of these measurement tools advocate well for certain tools in certain patients or for certain conditions.[87,101,102]

Brevity and speed of both information entry (either by the patient or staff) and data analysis are salutatory aspects of an outcome measurement system, and these aspects should be considered when determining which instruments will be used. The use of both a short general health assessment and a specific pain evaluation tool is probably the most basic approach. Using computerized surveys (e.g., in the waiting room) improves data integrity by decreasing omitted responses and improving internal consistency.[103] They should be used instead of written surveys whenever possible.

WHAT IS THE VALUE OF CONTINUOUS QUALITY IMPROVEMENT TO A PAIN PRACTICE?

A QA/QI program can help a pain practice in several ways:

1. *Accreditation* of a pain practice facility is discussed in the section on safety. However, accreditation bodies are very interested in the nature of any CQI programs. Thus an added benefit of such a program, in addition to improved care for patients, is the approbation of accreditors.
2. *Payment for quality* is the newest impetus for providers and facilities to participate in quality improvement programs.

P4P is the general term used to describe reimbursement programs that tie some portion of provider income to either process or outcome achievements. P4P will also effect changes in patient referral patterns as the information gathered on provider performance is made available to payers, employers, and patients.[104] Therefore, investment in a CQI program will have potential benefits in terms of patient census and reimbursement rates in the coming years.

3. *Benchmarking providers* in an objective and appropriate manner is another value of a well-crafted CQI program. By evaluating practice patterns of providers at a single site or at many sites, benchmarks can be identified that allow all physicians and staff members to assess their own performances against other practitioners and thus elucidate "best practices." Allowing practitioners to see their own process outcome data and compare it with others working in the same facility has improved efficiency with no alteration in patient satisfaction.[105]

WHAT WILL A QUALITY ASSURANCE AND IMPROVEMENT PROGRAM COST?

PERSONNEL

A busy practice will require between 0.5 and 1.0 full-time employees to manage data input. This staff person, if not completely occupied by this work, might also serve as the Health Insurance Portability and Accountability Act (HIPAA) compliance officer and oversee all policies regarding the quality initiatives of the practice. Though relatively expensive, a registered nurse is of great value in this role.

TECHNOLOGY

It would be convenient if each practice location were to have access to an EHR to allow automated capture of accurate data to provide evidence of quality. We may be some years away from an EHR in every procedure room and are even further away from an accurate EHR in every procedure room. Sadly, investment in changes in infrastructure that might bolster improved quality is often squelched by the nature of reimbursement in our current medical system.[106]

In the meantime, therefore, it is appropriate to concentrate on inexpensive and already available means of capturing such data and transmitting it to practitioners.[107] Probably the most efficacious single-site approach is to use a computer relational database (e.g., Microsoft Access) to capture information gathered by more traditional methods, such as chart assessment by clerks and patient interviews by nurses. Such databases have been valuable in determining areas of potential cost savings, improvement in efficiency, and potential error and shortfalls in quality.[105]

If the practitioner is not a skilled programmer, it is reasonable to hire one and build his or her own database with modes of risk adjustment and automated capture of demographic and laboratory data. They can be built with a graphic user interface (GUI) that is intuitive for even the most non–technology-savvy staff member and that will allow patients to directly interface with waiting room kiosks. This can all be done with about 60 hours of programming (Fig. 6.3).

Physicians and staff will spend somewhat less time helping with design and testing.[108] Licensing for the software and for use of the American Medical Association Current Procedural Terminology codes will be needed, and the purchase of additional computer monitors or kiosks may also be necessary, depending on the current configuration of technology at the clinic. In all, an investment of $15,000 would create a superb single-office product with automated reporting and measures very specific to the goals and practice patterns of the pain clinic whose practitioners created it.

THE FUTURE IS NOW FOR QUALITY ASSESSMENT IN PAIN MANAGEMENT

In 2011 the IOM issued a comprehensive report that underscores the need for an extensive transformation in all aspects of our treatment of pain in America.[109] One of the resultant findings of its work was the lack of existing data on which to support our current practice and advance our evolving field. This influential review calls for a bird's eye view of pain management, expanded from the practitioner-patient relationship to the care of patients on a societal level.

While we are still striving to implement CQI in individual pain management practices, as detailed earlier, the Stanford Pain Registry has taken this a step further by aggregating data in the form of a National Pain Registry.[110] This effort exemplifies the broader view that is required to improve patient care and facilitate the discovery of novel solutions for pain management. The registry is currently shared by numerous pain centers and will eventually be open to clinics nationwide. Such metadata systems already exist in primitive form online as both not-for-profit and profitable entities that collect quality assessment data on behalf of providers. The practice generally has access to its individual data and analysis, but the business essentially "owns" the collective database. This information can then be subjected to countless analyses. Thus, it is not only used by providers to assess and improve the quality of care in their private clinic but can also be pooled for research purposes. Comparative effectiveness between distant practices and longitudinal data analysis are examples of the many uses of Web-based data collection programs such as these.

Still further, the vision is coming full circle by reintroducing the patient as part of the transformation in pain management called for by the IOM. Patients are already participating in daily sampling of data, such as pain scores or accelerometry activity, via Android cell phones that remotely report to the provider and by extension to the registry.[111,112] This information will allow the provider to track a patient's progress, evaluate ongoing treatment, and gather data that can later contribute to evidence-based practice and document accountable care.

CONCLUSIONS ABOUT QUALITY IMPROVEMENT IN PAIN PRACTICE

This chapter separates patient safety and quality improvement as independent sections. However, both must be considered when reviewing strategies to improve either

PAIN EVENT MRN: 1235467 Patient: DOE, JANE DOB: 1/28/1958 Close

Patient Information | Questions | Pain Event | First Call Back | Second Call Back

Date of Service: 2/12/2004

ARRIVAL: (24 hr) Arrival Time: 14:00

Pain Rating:

PATIENT CARE TEAM:

Staff Anes:

PACU RN:

FLUROSCOPY USED? Yes No

DISCHARGE: (24 hr) D/C Time:

Pain Rating at D/C:

Disposition: Home

A. Activity level:
Before this visit with the doctor, would you say that this pain has caused significant interference with your activities of daily life?
Completely unable to do my usual activity.

B. Work status:
Cannot work, temporary disability due to this problem.

C. Your health status:
How would you rate your overall health now compared to 4 weeks ago?
Much worse now compared to then.

D. Quality of Life
How have things been going for you during the past 4 weeks?
Pretty bad.

A

PAIN EVENT MRN: 1235467 Patient: DOE, JANE DOB: 1/28/1958 Close

Patient Information | Questions | Pain Event | First Call Back | Second Call Back

Date of Service: 2/12/2004

ARRIVAL: (24 hr) Arrival Time: 14:00

Pain Rating:

PATIENT CARE TEAM:

Staff Anes:

PACU RN:

FLUROSCOPY USED? Yes No

DISCHARGE: (24 hr) D/C Time:

Pain Rating at D/C:

Disposition: Home

Diagnosis

Order	Dx	Description
1	723.4	Cervical Radiculitis
2	722.0	Disc displacement

Adverse Rxn

Order	Rxn

Procedures

Order	CPT	Desc
1	62310	ESI cervical or thoracic inject
2	99242	Consult, Level 2, expanded prob focus (routine) 30 min

Plan

Order	Plan_Description
1	Return as needed for possible repeat injection
2	Water Walking

B

PAIN EVENT MRN: 1235467 Patient: DOE, JANE DOB: 1/28/1958 Close

Patient Information | Questions | Pain Event | First Call Back | Second Call Back

FIRST Call Back Information

Call Back Date:

Pain Rating:

Satisfaction Level:

Overall, patient comments were:

Comments / Notes

A. Activity level:
Before this visit with the doctor, would you say that this pain has caused significant interference with your activities of daily life?

B. Work status:

C. Your health status:
How would you rate your overall health now compared to 4 weeks ago?

D. Quality of Life
How have things been going for you during the past 4 weeks?

E. Did this procedure seem to help you and was it worthwhile?

F. "If you were ever told in the future that this procedure might be of help to you, would you agree to have it done again?"

C

Figure 6.3 A, Pain clinic database: initial questions screen. This image shows a typical interface for recording the answers to an initial set of screening questions regarding the pain problem and quality of health as described by a patient on a visit to a pain clinic. Using the Microsoft Access Relational Database or similar technology, this user-friendly graphic interface allows clerical personnel to record the events and answers in a relational database that can then be used to monitor individual and collective patient outcomes for quality management in a pain practice. **B,** Pain clinic database: procedures screen. This image shows a typical interface for prompting and recording the events that typically occur on the day of a pain service, which allows the information to be placed into a relational database for quality management purposes. **C,** Pain clinic database: first callback screen. This image shows a typical interface for prompting and recording the questions and answers for phone calls to a pain patient, which allows the information to be placed into a relational database for quality management purposes. (Microsoft Access is a registered trademark of Microsoft Corporation.)

of them.[113] The following are necessary to improve pain CQI programs:

1. CQI programs should be used at each individual clinic to discover which processes and structures beget the best clinical outcomes.
2. The data for each clinic should be linked to all the others to create national quality benchmarks that will provide a means of identifying and duplicating best practices.
3. Innovations in care systems should be welcomed, but only in settings that allow their study in comparison to the best practices that already exist.
4. Evidence-based approaches to pain medicine must be improved. Practitioners must be scrupulous in evaluating procedures and therapies with rigorous doubt and eliminate those that do not prove valuable in comparison to alternatives that may be more banal and less lucrative.
5. Access to high-quality multidisciplinary care, including mental health care, which may often be expensive and long term, must be a priority of our specialty so that we can advocate for it to payers, health care policy makers, and legislators, who too frequently ignore the benefits of such care.[61]

Finally, pain medicine—and health care in general—needs more robust federal support for inexpensive methods to engender clinical measurement of outcomes, risk adjustment, and clinician feedback if quality improvement is to occur rapidly. Computerized systems should be made available to primary and ambulatory care facilities to allow the identification of national benchmarks of care. Only in this way can we rapidly discover best practices and decrease the waste inherent in the current care model, where individual clinicians often practice in the dark with regard to evidence and the effects of their own interventions.

SECTION 6.2 PATIENT SAFETY

TO ERR IS HUMAN AND PREVENTION OF HARM

The publication *To Err Is Human: Building a Safer Health System. Report from the Committee on Quality of Health Care in America* in 1999 was the Institute of Medicine's (IOM) public alarm about patient safety and error in the health care delivery system.[1] The authors estimated—based among others on the Harvard Medical Practice Study of 1991—that the iatrogenic injury rate was nearly 4% in U.S. hospitalized patients. They concluded that more than half of these injuries were due to errors in medical care and that two thirds of all iatrogenic injuries could be prevented.[2] Similar results were presented in a systematic review of eight studies conducted in the United States, Canada, Australia, and the United Kingdom that encompassed nearly 75,000 in-hospital patients: 9.2% encountered adverse events and the authors concluded that 43.5% of such events could be classified as preventable.[3] However, the rate of induced harm can be as high as 25%.[4] The doctor's fear of punishment for making errors, as well as the difficulty of detecting errors, makes these estimates disputable.[5] Despite other triggered controversies,[6-8] all these reports expanded the conversation considerably and focused the attention of practitioners, payers, patients, and governments on these preventable errors. Patient safety is, based on the World Health Organization (WHO) definition, "the absence of preventable harm to a patient during the process of health care."[9] Patient safety, with its fundamentals of collecting and analyzing events, as well as prevention of adverse events in a confidential environment, has become an indispensable discipline and element of health care quality.[10,11]

A significant hurdle in the effort to improve safety is that there are insufficient data to assess health care safety or even definitively identify uniformly valid indicators of safety in health care.[12] Therefore, which solutions, which information, and which technology will be of value in improving patient safety are still disputable.[13]

To improve patient safety, the IOM motivated hospitals, as well as professional societies, and recommended the creation of centers and organizations for focusing on patient safety. As an effect of the efforts of the IOM, the government was one of the first to support research on safety.[14] As a further consequence, the Patient Safety and Quality Improvement Act signed into law in 2005 also encouraged the development of a Patient Safety Organization (PSO) and defined the role of PSOs. The act called for a confidential culture of patient safety and for the establishment of a Network of Patient Safety Database (NPSD) to provide an interactive evidence-based management resource.[15]

Based on different facets of patient safety and with varied scopes, an increasing number of agencies and organizations have emerged:

1. The Agency for Healthcare Research and Quality (AHRQ) has the federal lead in patient safety; it supports research of causes and the development of new strategies in patient safety, as well as their integration into the health care industry. This center coordinates the PSOs and distributes knowledge about effective practices. The AHRQ offers the Patient Safety Network (PSNet), a Web-based resource of news on patient safety,[15] and the Web M&M, a morbidity and mortality round on the Web.[16]
2. The National Quality Forum helps improve the quality of U.S. health care by building, endorsing, and promoting national consensus about priorities, measurements, and their education.[17]
3. The Joint Commission (TJC: Joint Commission on Accreditation of Healthcare Organizations), advised by a panel of safety experts, has published its national patient safety goals since 2002. These goals are provided as clear, actionable statements, such as "use at least two patient identifiers when providing care, treatment, or services" or "mark the procedure site," along with the rationale behind these goals, as well as the elements of

performance.[18] The main topics are to identify patients correctly, improve staff communication, use medications safely, prevent infection, identify patient safety risk factors, and prevent mistakes in surgery.

4. Another PSO is the National Patient Safety Foundation (NPSF), an independent not-for-profit organization that works on improving patient safety by providing knowledge and developing, as well as enhancing, the culture of safety.[19] Lucian Leape, a contributor to *To Err is Human*, was one of the founders of the NPSF.[20]
5. Large businesses, understanding the fundamental issue as being poor quality in the face of high prices, organized themselves via the Leapfrog Group and created programs for change while also pushing for new regulation and legislation to improve safety.[21] The goal of the Leapfrog Group, a voluntary program, is to reward the safety efforts of health care providers and thereby trigger big leaps in health care safety. They aim to reduce preventable medical mistakes, improve the quality and affordability of health care, and encourage health care providers to publish their quality and outcomes and reward them for improving quality. This group focuses on four leaps: computerized physician order entry (CPOE), evidence-based hospital referral, intensive care unit physician staffing, and a Leapfrog safe practices score that assesses a hospital's progress.[22] These measures are variable in their evidentiary support for improving quality, and they are all potentially expensive.[23] Nonetheless, Leapfrog and its proponents quickly declared that the most important next step was and is urging of the public to push for health care professionals to adopt these goals.[24] The Leapfrog Group and its tenets have also imbued the discussion of patient safety in our health care system with an economic and political imperative that makes further objective evaluation of the true nature of health care's safety more difficult, even as new solutions are recommended.
6. The Institute for Healthcare Improvement (IHI), another independent not-for-profit organization founded in 1991, initiated the 100,000 Lives Campaign (2004 to 2006), which was designed to save lives by introducing six safety guidelines into health care.[25] The institute added another six guidelines and launched the 5 Million Lives Campaign in 2006 (Box 6.2).[26] How many lives could actually have been saved is not clear, but the effect was tremendous: more than 4000 hospitals in the United States enrolled in this project committed to somehow integrate these 12 goals into their clinical routines.[27]
7. Patient safety is not just a problem in industrialized countries, it is also a global problem. Similar to these 12 goals, in 2004 the WHO launched the World Alliance for Patient Safety in all member states to improve safety in

Box 6.2 Goals of the 100,000 and the 5 Million Lives Campaign

1. *Deploy rapid response teams or medical emergency teams.* Small interdisciplinary medical teams are dispatched to the bedside in anticipation of significant medical deterioration that could lead to cardiopulmonary arrest.
2. *Deliver reliable evidence-based care for acute myocardial infarction.* Use the guidelines of the American College of Cardiology and American Heart Association to lessen the impact of or prevent myocardial infarction.
3. *Prevent adverse drug events through medication reconciliation.* Medication reconciliation is the process of reviewing the patient's medication orders before and after any change in caregiver or in the site of care to monitor for any discrepancies in ordered versus administered medication.
4. *Prevent central line infections.* Five components of care were identified by the Centers for Disease Control and Prevention (CDC) that if used, will diminish the risk for infection: hand hygiene, maximal barrier protection (including gowns and gloves), chlorhexidine skin antisepsis, optimal site selection (subclavian vein in adults), and daily review of the indications for the catheter and removal as quickly as possible.
5. *Prevent surgical site infections.* The CDC recommended four practices to decrease surgical site infections: evidence-based medicine–guided use of prophylactic antibiotics, as little hair removal via shaving the site as possible, perioperative glucose control (in the intensive care unit after major cardiac surgery), and maintenance of perioperative normothermia after colorectal surgery.
6. *Prevent ventilator-assisted pneumonia.* Four practices were recommended: elevation of the head of the bed to between 30 and 45 degrees, daily "sedation vacation" with daily assessment for possible extubation, prophylaxis for peptic ulcer disease, and prophylaxis for deep vein thrombosis.
7. *Prevent pressure ulcers by reliably using science-based guidelines for prevention of this serious and common complication.* Strategies to prevent pressure ulcers are turning of patients, basic skin care, proper nutrition, and hydration.
8. *Reduce methicillin-resistant* Staphylococcus aureus *(MRSA) infection through basic changes in infection control processes throughout the hospital.* Hand, especially with infected patients, contact precautions for infected and colonized patients and adequate cleaning and decontamination of the equipment and facility are the key factors to reduce MRSA infections.
9. *Prevent harm from high-alert medications starting with a focus on anticoagulants, sedatives, narcotics, and insulin.* Use standardized medication orders or protocols, visual reminders, and double checks.
10. *Reduce surgical complications by reliably implementing the changes in care recommended by the Surgical Care Improvement Project.*
11. *Deliver reliable, evidence-based care for congestive heart failure to reduce readmission.* Clear discharge instructions and prevention of infection need to be provided to reduce readmission.
12. *Get boards on board by defining and spreading new and leveraged processes for hospital boards of directors so that they can become far more effective in accelerating the improvement of care.*

From Berwick DM, Calkins DR, McCannon CJ, et al. The 100,000 Lives Campaign: setting a goal and a deadline for improving health care quality. *JAMA.* 2006;295:324-327; and McCannon CJ, Hackbarth AD, Griffin FA. Miles to go: an introduction to the 5 Million Lives Campaign. *Jt Comm J Qual Patient Saf.* 2007;33:477-484.

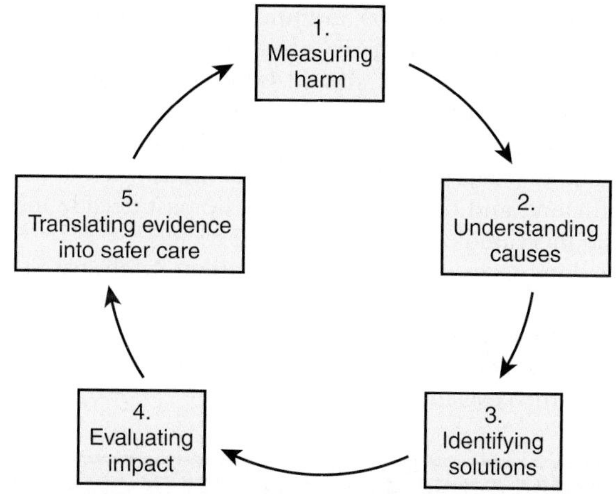

Figure 6.4 The circle of patient safety. This figure shows how patient safety can be explored most effectively. It consists of five steps. The aim is to analyze reasons for errors and to reduce preventable harm in daily practice.

health care. Prevention of health care–associated infections, hand hygiene, surgical safety, and patient engagement were the targeted issues that were to be addressed by implementing guidelines and establishing a uniform classification of patient safety concepts with an emphasis on prevention, detection, and reduction of risk.[28]

UNDERSTANDING THE COMPONENTS OF PATIENT SAFETY

The health care system has become very complex. There is no single reason why an adverse event happens; rather, it is a combination of individual errors and errors in the system. Caregivers can be inattentive or careless, and errors are seen as a moral issue or a consequence.[29] We are then faced with active failures, which are mistakes, procedural violations, or bearish behavior directly causing adverse events.[30] From another point of view, workers can be seen as being able to fail, and errors consequently occur as a result of conditions that are the source of the error and are a consequence rather than a cause.[31] Hence the system can provoke an environment in which such errors arise because of organizational decisions, also called latent conditions. These conditions may be undetected for a long time before leading to a problem when combined with active failures.[29] In creating safer processes it is best to focus on system changes rather than on scrutiny of individual practitioner errors because system errors are most causative of adverse events.[31,32]

It is necessary to conduct research to determine which solutions are effective in making patient treatment safer. The analysis and the aim to reduce preventable harm led to the key areas presented in Figure 6.4, adapted from the WHO.[33] As a first step the harm must be clearly defined, measured, and collected in a database. It can then be analyzed. Based on these thoughts, a treatment strategy can be evolved, proved, and integrated into daily practice to improve patient safety. However, this circle is effective only in a confidential environment in which the providers involved do not fear punishment, which causes under-reporting.[34]

Standardized and reliable definitions are needed to accurately measure harm and to evaluate the effect on patient safety. First, a medical error has to be distinguished from an adverse event. Medical errors are "the failure to complete a planned action as intended or the use of a wrong plan to achieve an aim."[35] Drug errors are the most common medical errors.[1,36] Most often they are not directly linked to the patient's medical condition; however, they have the potential of being harmful.[37] An adverse event is a harmful injury resulting from a treatment and is not caused by the underlying medical problem.[38] These events can be lethal, life-threatening, and disabling; prolong hospital stay; and require additional monitoring. They can be further classified as preventable or nonpreventable.[39]

There is a retrospective (reactive) and a prospective (proactive) way to measure and improve safety.[11,40] The retrospective way consists of a "root cause analysis" (RCA), error-reporting systems, morbidity and mortality conferences, or malpractice claims. These methods seek to answer the question of what went wrong and why. We use these techniques widely to understand the causes of harm and to improve safety. They increase the awareness of fault processes and are more likely to detect latent errors and adverse events[41] but bear the risk of spending resources on interventions that have little chance of diminishing harm.[42] A group of anesthesiologists from Seattle and Boston, for example, investigated conditions and patterns in malpractice claims after interventional pain treatment at the level of the cervical spine. They found that injuries leading to malpractice claims were most often caused by direct needle trauma to the spinal cord, these injuries were often severe, and they appeared more frequently in unresponsive patients.[43]

Failure Modes and Effects Analysis (FMEA) is a proactive assessment tool. It helps anticipate and prevent adverse events based on knowledge from past failures by aiming to foresee potential failures. It involves a care team that meets on a regular basis, a serious challenge in our health care system. The advice can be scarce.[44] Another prospective tool is based on Patient Safety Indicators (PSIs), developed by the AHRQ and revised by the University of California at San Francisco–Stanford University Evidence-based Practice Center (UCSF-Stanford EPC). They identify hospitalizations with potentially preventable patient safety events based on standardized algorithms, which are available for free.[45,46] They demonstrated that the specificity was high (99.1%), sensitivity was moderate (19% to 56%), and positive predictive value was 22% to 74% for the original PSI definition when compared with the NSQIP adverse events.[46]

In 1974, Jick introduced a prospective concept based on trigger events.[47] Trigger tools such as the Global Trigger Tool (GTT) identify patient safety events during hospitalization. Clearly defined events (e.g., ordering of specific drugs such as antidotes, or the presence of abnormal laboratory values) serve as a trigger to activate further investigation of the case.[48] This tool seems to be more reliable than other methods in detecting possible events. Whereas a combination of AHRQ PSIs and provider-reported events found 4% of adverse events, the GTT found 27% of adverse events.[49] The potential reported adverse events have a low association with documented harm, differ across organizations, and raise concern about using these patient safety measures for public reporting and comparison of organizational performance.[49]

Box 6.3 Pronovost's Four Points for Translation of Evidence into Practice

- Summarize evidence into checklists; identify (maximum of seven) interventions with the greatest benefit and convert them into behavior.
- Identify and reduce barriers to compliance with the checklist; "walk" through the process and observe the staff performing the intervention to recognize deficiencies, potential gains, and losses with the implementation.
- Measure and provide feedback. Be encouraging; develop and pilot-test measures that evaluate the process or the outcome and provide feedback.
- Ensure that all patients receive the interventions; recognize work, improve culture, and monitor performance.

From Pronovost PJ, Holtzmueller CG, Ennen CS, et al. Overview of progress in patient safety. *Am J Obstet Gynecol*. 2011;204:5-10.

Patient safety research developed and helped identify many solutions. There is ample evidence for the benefit of specific patient safety practices: use of prophylaxis to prevent venous thromboembolism in patients at risk, use of perioperative β-blockers to prevent perioperative morbidity and mortality, use of maximum sterile barriers while placing central intravenous catheters to prevent infections, use of antibiotic prophylaxis in surgical patients to prevent surgical site infections, asking patients to recall and restate what they have been told during the informed consent process, continuous aspiration of subglottic secretions to prevent ventilator-associated pneumonia, use of pressure-relieving bedding material to prevent pressure ulcers, use of real-time ultrasound guidance during central line insertion to prevent complications, patient self-managed outpatient anticoagulation, provision of nutrition with a particular emphasis on early enteral nutrition in critically ill and surgical patients, and use of antibiotic-impregnated central venous catheters to prevent catheter-related infections.[50]

The next step is the translation of evidence, research, or clinical guidelines into daily practice. Major difficulties can arise, but there are many different models on how to proceed. However, it is not yet clear which models are most effective and efficient.[51] Pronovost and colleagues described one practically oriented method consisting of four key elements in an approach to integrate evidence into practice.[52] This strategy has been used successfully to reduce bloodstream infection associated with central lines.[52,53] Box 6.3 shows Pronovost's four points for translation of evidence into practice.[54]

SUCCESS?

The IHI declared victory on June 14, 2006, by stating that the 100,000 Lives Campaign had saved more than 122,000 lives.[55] However, support for this contention is a retrospective calculation of a statistical probability of how many lives "would have been lost" had the statistical analysis of 2004 been applied, versus the number of lives that were actually lost between January 2005 and June 2006.[56] Those who were skeptical of the mathematics used to calculate the original numbers of lives at risk should be just as skeptical of the methodology used to verify this success.

Safety in medicine is a very complex problem, and progress is slow.[4,14,57] Progress may remain unknown[58] or at least insufficient, and the main effect in the past decade instead was an increased overall sensitivity of society.[59]

For long-term improvement in patient safety, we need a benevolent culture of safety in which health care providers can obtain an adequate education, including education on all available sources and technologies with an understanding that the costs must be monitored.

CULTURE OF SAFETY AND SAFETY CLIMATE

The IOM proposed to not only build centers and organizations but also create a culture of safety. A safety culture is crucial for improvements in safety.[60,61] The concept of a patient safety culture originated from the experience in hazardous industries. It depends on attitudes, beliefs, behaviors, perceptions, values, and practices shared by employees.[62] However, the safety culture differs considerably between hospitals and persons.[63] Finding the commonalities may be imperative to any type of safety improvement program.[64]

There is a difference between a culture of safety and a safety climate.[65] A safety climate is a quantitative description or a way of measuring safety culture by taking a closer look at adverse events (outcomes measures), analyzing adherence to practices (process measures), or calibrating health care teams' attitudes about issues relevant to safety.[66-68] Nevertheless, culture and climate are positively related: a higher level of group culture correlates with higher safety climates, whereas hierarchic structures lead to lesser safety climates.[69]

It has been suggested that engaged senior leaders are important to an organization's successful development of a culture of safety.[70,71] Improved leadership in which boards and medical staff share responsibility and focus on improvement strategies together may offer great potential.[72] Teamwork and collaboration such as open communication[71] have been defined as a second important behavior to support a culture of safety, especially if the increasing complexity of patients today is taken into account.[73] Evidence-based medicine (EBM) with standardized processes leads to high reliability and, together with patient-centered medicine, has an important influence on patient safety culture.[74,75] James Rogers[76] underlined that a culture of safety can be built up through social engineering. A just culture in which providing safety-related information in a blame-free environment is rewarded and in which people have the will and the knowledge to learn from mistakes (learning culture) is essential to develop a culture of safety.[77]

EDUCATION

In the past decade, education has altered significantly as a result of safety issues.[78] One of the most important amendments was the work hour restriction. Because operator fatigue has been recognized as a potential source of error in many industries, the U.S. Congress and the IOM asked for limitations on work hours to improve patient safety. However, this led to many disputes about the feasibility of education and the competency of residents. Practitioners who have completed their training tend to work longer hours with less rest than is considered appropriate in almost any other work setting. This should be particularly concerning for pain practices that use interventional therapies. All aspects of cognition are adversely affected by fatigue, although there is insufficient evidence to pinpoint a specific amount of rest as being "enough" in medicine. In general, practitioners tend to ignore or discount the potential impact of fatigue on their own error rate.[79] Each practitioner is encouraged to create and follow personal and practice-wide policies regarding continuous time spent on clinical activity.[80] Besides the work hour limitations, many professional societies have also adapted their curricula to focus on safety. The American College of Surgeons has already integrated six core competencies defined by the Accreditation Council for Graduate Medical Education (ACGME) and the American Board of Medical Specialties (ABMS), including listings of patient safety topics, teaching and learning strategies, and assessment methods. Guidelines for implementation and dissemination are also provided; the curriculum content underscores the need to create an organizational culture of safety and focuses on both individuals and systems.[63] Individual residency programs may prioritize the content of the curriculum according to their specific needs.[81]

Education is tightly linked with the introduction of new technologies. There are different ways to adopt new techniques and technologies into clinical use. Peyton's four-step approach (1, trainer demonstrates; 2, talk the trainee through; 3, trainee talks the trainer through; and 4, trainee does) was shown to be superior to standard instructions; faster performance when learned skills were performed for the first time was seen.[82] For physicians and other health care professionals at all levels, simulation tools in which mistakes can be made without harming the patient provide a good alternative to real patients. Simulation-based education is expensive, but it is cost-effective if used properly and has been proved to increase patient safety.[83] Simulation-based training complements medical education in patient care settings[84] but does not replace educational activities based on actual patient care experiences.[85] How effective the use of simulation is depends on informed use, providing feedback, engaging trainees in deliberate practice, integrating simulation into an overall curriculum, and instruction and competence of the faculty in its use.[85] Bohmer and Edmondson pointed out that learning is essential to improve health care and to prevent becoming outdated. Individual learning success is linked directly to the experience of the learner. However, they could show that the slopes of learning curves for a distinct complex surgical procedure were significantly different in two groups despite equal levels of experience. They highlighted the usefulness of organizational learning consisting of managed reflection, interpretation, and repetition as a team.[86,87]

Checklists have also become part of the education process. They help confirm the completion of crucial steps and appear to be particularly useful in improving performance during emergencies, as seen in the aviation industry. The WHO introduced the Surgical Safety Checklist in 2008 after preliminary research demonstrated that half of major surgical complications are preventable.[88] Haynes and colleagues showed that implementation of the checklist lowered the rate of death from 1.5% to 0.8% and the rate of inpatient complications from 11% to 7%.[66] The American Society of Regional Anesthesia and Pain Medicine (ASRA) showed in a randomized simulation study that checklists not only improve medical management of systemic toxicity secondary to local anesthesia but also augment nontechnical performance.[89]

Other important sources aimed at providing evidence to improve patient safety and clinical outcomes are guidelines and practice advisories, such as those published and steadily updated for regional anesthesia and pain medicine.[90,91] Based on the current literature, expert opinion, and clinical data, these systematically formulated advisories aim to improve patient safety by reducing the incidence and severity of adverse outcomes in daily practice.[92] These recommendations usually focus on clinical topics for which treatment is as yet unclear.[93] The recommendations may be adapted and changed to fit individual institutional and provider needs.[92] Consensus statements based on opinions today may be rewritten and changed when overruled by new scientific facts, and readers and writers are encouraged to continuously re-evaluate these recommendations.[94,95]

TECHNOLOGY

Information technology can reduce error and the negative impact of error by providing critical information at the point of care, improving the speed of response once an error has occurred, and tracking the occurrence of errors to allow monitoring for trends and feedback to providers.[96] Even though an investment, today's practitioners cannot afford to not have electronic health records, with which they can easily track and document the course of their patients' care.[97] It appears increasingly desirable to have a nationwide, Internet-based monitoring program, such as a prescription drug–monitoring program, to not only avoid multiple prescriptions for opioids but also improve patient safety and distribute important information about the health of patients.[98] An example of the promise of improvement in safety through innovative technology is in patient identification. Correct patient identification and elimination of wrong-site surgery have been identified by the IOM and TJC as a significant opportunity for improved safety.[99] The use of a bar code system can virtually eliminate the potential for patient misidentification and can also diminish medication errors. Unfortunately, high cost and slow speed of the systems have led to their adoption by only a few U.S. hospitals.[100,101]

The use of technology has facilitated many steps in patient care. Calculation of medication doses, exchange of patient data between geographically or temporally separated practitioners, providing references such as guidelines for care, and monitoring of patient outcomes, adverse events, and practice patterns can all help improve patient safety.[96] Not only is the technology itself crucial, but the organization also plays a part. Systems that support clinicians with access to guidelines and monitoring of medication errors have improved the quality of care and decreased error.[102]

IMAGING TECHNOLOGIES

Besides the administrative technologies, more and more medical technologies are emerging into the field of health care. Imaging modalities in interventional pain medicine help identify relevant structures accurately, which intuitively appears to ensure safer interventional therapy in pain medicine. Ultrasound techniques, fluoroscopy, and computed tomography are being used. Indirect methods such as nerve stimulation can help identify nerves and increase the likelihood of success of neural blockade; however, they have limited sensitivity.[103] There are also direct methods to differentiate the properties of the target from those of the surrounding tissue. The safe use of ultrasound techniques for performing nerve blocks has increased in past years,[104] although this has not been proved to increase safety to date.[105] Ultrasound is likely to substitute for the use of fluoroscopy in specific techniques, such as stellate ganglion blockade.[106] Ultrasound can demonstrate the location of not only an intercostal nerve but also the pleura; pneumothorax can also be readily identified, which contributes to safer procedures.[107] Fluoroscopic guidance, with or without radiographic contrast enhancement, helps ensure intravascular catheter location or detection of intravascular needle perforation, and it can be used to prevent unintentional intravascular or subarachnoid injection of local anesthetics or steroids.[106] New techniques, such as the use of an "optical" spinal needle that provides spectrophotometric information from the tip of the needle, can safely identify the epidural space and may be complementary to fluoroscopic imaging of the epidural space.[108] Brynolf and associates have shown that detection of nerves with optical reflectance spectroscopy is complementary to ultrasound and might replace nerve stimulation. It might also lower vascular complications while detecting intra-arterial placement of the tip of the needle.[109] Although imaging guidance has become routine in pain medicine, there is still insufficient evidence to prove that it increases the safety of procedures.[106]

BARRIERS: COST AND STANDARDIZATION

At this point it is not certain whether the investment in technology will be worth the cost. Cost is a primary reason that health care providers have not quickly adopted technology as a means of improving care.[110] As a measure of federal and state governments' belief in the IOM report on patient safety and the potential role of technology, several bills have been introduced and passed that subsidize the cost of introduction of technology at hospitals and offices.[96] Other concerns that are holding back the widespread adoption of technology in practice include variations in software design standards that would allow different systems in different practices to directly transfer data, particularly among older "legacy" databases. In view of the cost of implementation of new systems, including education of staff and acquisition costs for software and hardware, the inability of a new system to "read" the data already on hand in the practice is a significant disincentive.

With increasing health care costs in the United States, it is essential to reduce these costs.[111] Comparative effectiveness research (CER) offers a mean to identify feasible targets in health care. It was introduced by the Patient-Centered Outcome Research Institute, which was established by the Affordable Care Act. It helps in making informed health decisions by advancing the quality and relevance of evidence concerning the manner in which diseases can effectively and appropriately be prevented, diagnosed, treated, monitored, and managed through research, synthesis of evidence, and EBM while helping cut costs.[112] The 2009 American Recovery and Reinvestment Act allocated about $1 billion toward CER, and the 2010 Patient Protection and Affordable Care Act established a national center to support CER.[113] EBM and CER have been introduced as cost-cutting and rationing measures; however, EBM principles have to be implemented in a proper manner.[111,114,115] It is important that improvement strategies be developed locally to target specific problems.[116] Although EBM is linked to the best scientific knowledge available, it should not be disregarded that the most important improvement goal is the outcome for the patient in the real world, and direct assessment of outcomes in practice should be a basic element integrated into our routine evaluation.[117]

NEXT STEPS FOR THE PAIN PRACTITIONER

Practitioners should work to discern practical ways to improve patient safety and the most efficient and economical means of practicing in congruence with the regulations and legislation now evolving from the public safety campaign. Whatever safety improvement programs are chosen, they should be repeatedly evaluated for efficacy and abandoned if they are not efficient and effective.

"Mistake-proofing" care will require minimizing variation in its delivery, monitoring every patient's course of care for error and adverse outcomes, and making care delivery systems within the clinic as simple as possible to avoid the complexities that lead to variation and error.[118] Such efforts have been effective in other industries, including aviation, nuclear power, and the military. Clinicians may believe that medical care is not amenable to the safety-monitoring systems of other industries, yet emulation of highly reliable organizations (HROs) within these other industries does lead to improvements in safety in health care.[119,120] HROs succeed by making their systems as simple as possible, amenable to as little disruption as possible, and easy to understand.[121] They combine these three characteristics with high priority on safety at the highest levels of the organization—including willingness to spend money and person-power.[122]

Box 6.4 lists specific targets that the pain practitioner can focus on to improve patient safety. It is critical to document these efforts and their results to be sure that resources are not wasted and also to portray the diligence of the practice at times when payers and regulators inquire about safety efforts.

TREATMENT OUTCOME DATABASES: RECORDING ADVERSE EVENTS

Practitioners will best ensure their patients' safety by recording their outcomes and all adverse events in a database. There are many ways to measure outcomes, which is

Box 6.4 Interventions That May Improve Patient Safety in the Pain Clinic

Facility Procedures and Structure

- Routinely and repetitively conduct drills for emergency situations by assigning specific roles to personnel in the case of patient medical emergencies, facility emergencies (e.g., power outage, fire, earthquake, severe weather), and selected adverse events in patient care.
- If relocating or creating a new facility, locate it as near a hospital as possible. Arrange to create a legal transfer agreement with that hospital.
- Furnish the facility with in-wall piped oxygen and suction, as well as adequate lighting and space to allow full access to patients by sufficient personnel in the case of an emergency.
- Consider accreditation by the AAAHC, TJC, CARF, or another agency. If accreditation is not possible, consider annual inspection by one of these agencies for evaluation of your facility and practice regarding safety.
- Daily cleaning should include bactericidal cleansing of all surfaces contacted by staff, patients, or family members of patients in all parts of the facility.
- Place hand cleanser dispensers in multiple locations readily available to all clinical and nonclinical staff.
- Drawers and supply cabinets should be clearly organized and standardized in their organization between rooms.

Medication Management

- Use and enforce contracts for opioids and controlled substances.
- Monitor and document patient response and the frequency of renewals for opioids and sedatives.
- All medications used at the facility should be labeled (including an outdate once opened) and carefully read aloud before being drawn up and before administration.
- All syringes should be labeled in a standard manner regarding label color, font, size, and information on outdate.
- The facility should be regularly inventoried (weekly or monthly) for outdated medications and other supplies.
- Use medication reconciliation techniques to confirm doses and the frequency of all medications when there is a transition in caregiver, location, or date.
- Use computer technology to monitor for potential adverse drug events.
- Contract with a clinical pharmacist for consultation services as needed.
- Use protocols for monitoring the prescription of any medication that may lead to significant morbidity with continued use, such as NSAIDs, opioids, tricyclic antidepressants, and so on. These protocols should include timely and repetitive monitoring for known risks via either laboratory or electrocardiographic studies or mandated office visits.
- Communicate prescriptions of all medications to all practitioners providing care to your patient.
- Any adverse drug events should be reported immediately and recorded in a database that is regularly reviewed for trend analysis. The patient should be notified about the adverse event. The patient's other caregivers outside the practice should be notified about the adverse drug event.
- Prompt attention by staff should be focused on open discussion and adjustment of protocols and policies by the end of the day to avoid any repetition of errors that occurred either with or without an adverse drug event.

Technology

- Track the outcomes of all care. Use relational database technology to allow evaluation of outcomes for trends, both positive and negative. Do not make this a punitive system, but provide information on outcomes to staff regularly to invite input on changes in the system that may avert negative events.
- Consider the use of an electronic medical record.
- Use technology to allow the integration of clinical and laboratory systems to ensure that all critical information is available at the point of care.
- Use a computerized physician order entry system that also includes transmittal of outpatient prescriptions direct to a pharmacy.
- Use a computer system to track patients' medications that has automated alerts regarding potential drug interactions and anticoagulant use.
- Use technology to provide practitioners with all necessary reference material for decision support (e.g., medication dose, cross-reaction, and toxicity information).
- Use technology to ensure accurate matching of patient identity, medication history, and current medications at each point of care. Consider the use of a bar code system.
- Create or obtain audiovisual (e.g., DVD) material about procedures and medications to allow patients to review them before obtaining informed consent for procedures or before beginning a new medication.

Staff

- Establish a pattern of regular use of hand cleansing by all personnel.
- Create and enforce protocols for handoff of patients between practitioners.
- Create and enforce protocols for two-person patient identification interaction.
- Use standard teams with assigned roles for medical and invasive procedures.
- Involve all staff in discussions of quality and safety issues and invite open and nonpunitive review of adverse events and trends with freedom of each staff member to contribute ideas for improvement of the system.
- Create a plan in advance to respond to adverse events, including honest discussions with patients and family, as well as support for the staff involved.
- Do not allow employees to work beyond the limits of their education and training.
- Monitor, track, and report all practitioner work hours and do not allow them to extend beyond 80 hours per week or for more than 16 consecutive hours.
- Maintain sufficient staffing to ensure adequate care for sedated or recovering patients. These staff levels should be equivalent to or more intensive than the local standard of care as used in hospitals in the area.

Procedures

- Use full barrier protection during invasive procedures.
- Administer appropriate prophylactic antibiotics.
- Use imaging technology when appropriate during invasive procedures.
- Use the minimum necessary contrast material.
- Develop and enforce the use of standard protocols for medical and invasive procedures, including sterile preparation and critical medication checks, such as anticoagulants.
- Use guidelines, checklists, or both.
- Develop and enforce protocols to ensure that invasive procedures are carried out at the correct site, including marking of the patient's body area before preparation and a pause for

Continued

Box 6.4 Interventions That May Improve Patient Safety in the Pain Clinic (Continued)

verbal confirmation among all staff present of patient identification and procedural intent.
- Follow state and other applicable regulations regarding radiation safety.
- Avoid patient sedation beyond loss of the ability to discern and communicate paresthesia or other changes in sensation during neuraxial or perineural procedures.
- Refer procedures that you rarely or never perform to higher-volume practitioners or facilities. Monitor the outcomes of these patients.
- Provide both written and audiovisual informed consent material and give patients time to review them, as well as to ask questions, before obtaining informed consent for procedures.
- Use supplemental oxygen and monitor oximetry whenever sedation is used.
- Use supplemental oxygen and monitor oximetry whenever the prone position is used.
- Mandate and enforce that all patients have a driver before beginning either sedation or any procedure.
- Obtain written agreement from patients that they will not drive for 8 hours following a neuraxial procedure, sedation, or any procedure that could impair their motor skills.

Extrafacility Considerations

- Maintain close interaction with any provider also involved in your patient's care.
- Provide information about prescriptions of all controlled substance that you have begun, as well as any other medication or treatment interventions that you have made.
- Make direct phone contact with written confirmation regarding significant changes in condition or the treatment plan.
- Create a transfer agreement with a hospital to prepare for a patient emergency.
- Participate in exchange of regular peer review of procedures and standards with other practitioners who have no economic stake in your practice or facility.

AAAHC, Accreditation Association for Ambulatory Health Care; CARF, Commission on Accreditation of Rehabilitation Facilities; NSAID, nonsteroidal anti-inflammatory drug; TJC, The Joint Commission.

important to adequately reflect the quality provided. The Medical Outcomes Study Short-Form 36-Item (SF-36) Survey and the more comprehensive Treatment Outcome in Pain Survey (S-TOPS) are used, among others.[123,124] Such an outcomes database or registry is vital for practitioners to discover their own best practices and to monitor for any trends that would reveal a lack of efficacy of therapeutic interventions. With this said, the routine use of standardized outcomes measures in pain practice is more the exception than the rule at this point; there is no agreement on what measures best reflect relevant change in the well-being of individual patients. Simple recording of adverse events, without affixing blame, can provide opportunities for solo physicians and large groups to spot trends in which certain care patterns are associated with significant rates of error or even injury.[125] Regardless of whether such adverse events are ever reported outside the practice, their scrutiny by practitioners "in house" can improve care.[126,127] Box 6.5 lists some of the adverse events that might be might be monitored in a pain medicine practice.

SOME PRACTICAL TIPS TO IMPROVE PATIENT SAFETY

In the environment of national safety initiatives that emphasize significant investment in information technology, some of the simpler steps in improving patient safety may be overlooked. For an office that engages in interventional therapy, there are parallels to the safety features needed in offices that perform any kind of surgery. Recently, Bridenbaugh[128] offered recommendations regarding safer office care that include: improved office emergency equipment that is routinely updated and maintained by biotechnical personnel; training and certification of personnel in delivery of medications and resuscitative techniques; use of written practice policies and procedures that are routinely reviewed with the staff, including emergency procedures; use of monitoring that conforms to the same levels as would be expected in an accredited ambulatory surgical center or hospital; guidelines for sedation and anesthesia that conform to those of the American Society of Anesthesiologists; and compliance with any local or state standards of office safety and quality standards. One cheap but creative use of technology to improve patient safety at home is the simple handheld camera phone. This may serve as a means to monitor patient wound status, a technique that could be of value to a pain practice in which patients with invasive catheters are cared for at home.[129]

PATIENT SAFETY AND THE IMPAIRED DRIVER: CHRONIC PAIN AND ANALGESICS

A controversial topic is the role that a physician plays in determination of the ability of patients to drive an automobile. Most state regulations require health care practitioners to report any patients who have a medical or surgical impairment that would make them unsafe if they have not voluntarily given up driving. This is a significant concern for practitioners whose practice has a large percentage of older patients, many of whom may have vision or hearing impairments that warrant concern about safety while driving a car.[130]

Additional concerns for the pain practitioner are patients who are taking opioid medications or who undergo procedures that may impair their motor skills or mentation. The real risk of driving in the setting of long-term use of opioids is unclear, but impairment is probably present in some patients.[131,132] It is also significant to consider that both opioid use and peripheral neuropathy are risk factors for impaired driving.[133] Some evidence exists that middle-aged drivers with chronic pain, with or without treatment, are involved more often in serious accidents than are drivers who do not report

Box 6.5 A List of Potential Adverse Events to Be Monitored in a Pain Practice Safety Program

Procedural Events

Procedure on the wrong body part or location
Procedure performed on the wrong patient
Wrong procedure performed
Unintended retention of a foreign object in a patient
Product or device events
  Contamination
  Function other than intended
Intravascular air embolism
Infection following a procedure
Unexpected death following a procedure
Unexpected hospitalization within 24 hours of a procedure
Unintentionally compromised nerve function following any procedure
Lack of consent or incongruous consent
Allergic reaction
Anaphylaxis
Abortion of a procedure—anxiety
Abortion of a procedure—other
Burn
CV—angina
CV—arrest
CV—congestive heart failure
CV—dysrhythmia
CV—electrocardiographic changes
CV—hypertension
CV—hypotension
CV—infarction
Death
Dehiscence of wound
Dizziness
Electrolyte abnormality
Failure to follow up or communicate laboratory, pathology, or radiology test results
Fainting
Fall
Fever—not malignant hyperthermia
Headache
Hemorrhage
Increased pain
Itching
IV site pain
IV site infection
Malignant hyperthermia
Neurologic change
No home care
No instructions given
No ride available
Physician delay
Patient delay
Respiratory arrest/apnea
Respiratory asthma
Respiratory pneumothorax
Respiratory pulmonary edema
Return to the operating room
Sepsis
Signed out against medical advice
Somnolence
Transient neurologic syndrome
Urinary retention
Viscus perforation

Non-procedural Care-Related Adverse Events

Serious adverse event secondary to a medication prescription
Any medication prescription error requiring follow-up by a pharmacist or physician
Serious injury to a patient or other person secondary to misuse of a device or medication
Nerve injury, fall, or skin breakdown in an anesthetized body part following treatment
Hypoglycemia
Allergic reaction to medication or other treatment
Patient fall while on site at the facility for treatment
Patient fall while taking medication that may impair balance or mentation
Patient involvement in a motor vehicle accident subsequent or consequent to treatment
Any staff or patient injury while on site at the facility for treatment
Patient misidentification
Release of any patient to an inappropriate or incorrect caregiver
HIPAA privacy or security rule violation
Incomplete medication list documentation
Incomplete allergy list documentation
Incomplete problem list documentation
Incomplete or incorrect "other provider" list
Inability to access health records at the point of care

CV, cardiovascular; HIPAA, Health Insurance Portability and Accountability Act; IV, intravenous.

pain.[134] Recently, a study raised the possibility that just the presence of chronic pain of any severity is a risk for impaired driving skills when tested on a controlled course.[135]

PATIENTS UNDERGOING INJECTION THERAPY: SHOULD THEY HAVE A DRIVER?

Literature searches do not reveal a controlled study that provides the answer to this question. Many practitioners require all patients undergoing interventional therapy to have a driver for the following reasons:

1. Frequently, the patient's original diagnosis entails some degree of neural dysfunction and therefore driving capability is probably already impaired.
2. Pain, which may actually increase during the initial treatment period, can cause mental distraction and muscle spasm, which could impair driver focus and function.
3. The activity of driving will very frequently exacerbate muscle spasm and is often among the activities that patients complain worsens their pain, so driving is on the list of activities that we ask our patients not to do any more than absolutely necessary during the days that treatment is in progress.
4. Theoretically, even procedures that do not intentionally block neural transmission (e.g., an epidural steroid injection with only steroid and normal saline) may cause a diminished motor response because of either volumetric compression on nerve tissue or increased pain after the injection.

5. We ask our patients to engage in therapeutic activities the day of their procedure, including the use of massage, bath, and relaxation therapy. The efficacy of these measures is opposed by the stress associated with the activity of driving.
6. In our practice, we have found that patients who are required to procure a driver for their return home are less likely to return to work immediately after the procedure or to ignore postprocedure instructions.
7. Finally, with no definitive study in the literature showing that driving after injection therapy is safe and with plausible theoretical reasons to consider that such patients might be more prone to accidents, it is a reasonable and prudent precaution.

WHAT TO DO WHEN AN ADVERSE EVENT DOES OCCUR

The intent of this section is to promote the use of methods to diminish the likelihood of error and avoid adverse events. Nonetheless, adverse events will happen. How should the practitioner respond? Most often the initial impulse will be to deny the event, to "cover up" any role that error played in the outcome, and to—at all costs—not implicate any practitioner as being culpable when communicating with the affected patient.

However, recent work by the APSF has emphasized the importance of open and frank communication, with open answers to even difficult questions, with the patient and family involved.[136] An attitude of learning and correcting error rather than blaming the practitioners involved, combined with complete honesty about the events that occurred, is recommended.[137] Above all, a strategy for dealing with patient injury should be worked out in advance among all the practice participants. The APSF has placed an "adverse event protocol" on its website at www.apsf.org that is oriented toward an anesthetic adverse event (see the drop-down list under "resource center" and click on "clinical safety tools"). It would provide guidance in the pain clinic as well.

The practice's adverse event plan should also include discussions with malpractice carriers and practice management attorneys in advance of any events. Having a plan—and confidence in it—is the best approach to management of any breaches in patient safety. Such events should always be examined closely to find the system flaws that led to any errors.

ACCREDITATION

It is strongly recommended that all practitioners invite an independent agency to inspect their practice annually and provide advice about improving the quality and safety of care delivered there, even if formal accreditation does not ensue. Options include state health departments, as well as either TJC (http://www.jointcommission.org/accreditation/ambulatory_healthcare.aspx) or the AAAHC (http://www.aaahc.org/en/accreditation/). Both will certify multiple- and single-specialty ambulatory surgical centers, as well as physician practices and offices that practice pain medicine. If the program in question is a multidisciplinary program, another accrediting organization to consider is the Commission on Accreditation of Rehabilitation Facilities (http://www.carf.org/home/), which is willing to accredit what it terms "interdisciplinary pain rehabilitation programs."

Certainly, full accreditation or even just a letter from an inspector describing a practice's positive and negative attributes—assuming that the former outweigh the latter—can be valuable in contracting with third-party payers as a means of proving a salutatory commitment to patient safety and practice quality. Such accreditation has been used successfully to decrease liability insurance for a facility and malpractice insurance for both a facility and the physicians who are part of its practice or ownership group. It is also probably true that such documentation would be of value in the event of any later tort action concerning a patient's safety.

CONCLUSIONS

Mistakes are a fact of life. It's the response to the error that counts. The only real mistake is the one from which we learn nothing.

JOHN POWELL

SUMMARY

- The quality movement in health care is less than 3 decades old and is still evolving. However, it is being rapidly driven by alarm among the public, payers, regulators, and the business community spurred by widespread evidence of unsafe care.
- The various stakeholders in health care define quality in different ways, and physicians must consider these alternative attitudes as they work to improve and prove the value of their practices.
- At each clinic a "culture of safety" must be established by creating new systems that will decrease the impact of human error on patient outcomes.
- Many of the current reforms aimed at improved safety and higher quality are based on as yet unproven theories and may well fall out of favor in the coming years.
- One certain way in which to improve quality is the measurement of practice to determine "best practice." This should be done by all practitioners and all facilities and involves monitoring measures of structure, process, and clinical outcomes.
- Use continuous quality improvement (also known as total quality management) techniques to increase the number of practitioners who can replicate the best practices.
- Combining a practice that includes a comprehensive care approach and behavioral and vocational therapies with computer-based continuous quality improvement strategies will improve the quality of care in pain medicine.

SUGGESTED READINGS

Section 6.1

Donabedian A. Evaluating the quality of medical care. *Milbank Q.* 1966;44:166-203.

Donabedian A. The seven pillars of quality. *Arch Pathol Lab Med.* 1990;114:1115-1118.

Donabedian A. *An Introduction to Quality Assurance in Health Care.* Oxford: Oxford University Press; 2002:45–58.

Farrar JT, Portenoy RK, Berlin JA, et al. Defining the clinically important difference in pain outcome measures. *Pain.* 2000;88:287-294.

Grotle M, Brox JI, Vollestad NK. Functional status and disability questionnaires: what do they assess? A systematic review of back-specific outcome questionnaires. *Spine.* 2004;30:130-140.

Iezzoni L. *Risk Adjustment for Measuring Health Care Outcomes.* 3rd ed. Ann Arbor, Mich: Health Administration Press; 2004.

Institute of Medicine. *Crossing the Quality Chasm: A New Health System for the 21st Century.* Washington, DC: National Academies Press; 2001.

Section 6.2

Berwick DM, Calkins DR, McCannon CJ, et al. The 100,000 Lives Campaign: setting a goal and a deadline for improving health care quality. *JAMA.* 2006;295:324-327.

Bridenbaugh PO. Office-based anesthesia: requirements for patient safety. *Anesth Prog.* 2005;52:86-90.

Goeschel CA, Wachter RM, Pronovost PJ. Responsibility for quality improvement and patient safety: hospital board and medical staff leadership challenges. *Chest.* 2010;138:171-178.

Kohn LT, Corrigan JM, Donaldson MS, eds. *To Err Is Human: Building a Safer Health System. Report from the Committee on Quality of Health Care in America.* Washington, DC: National Academy Press; 1999.

Leape LL, Brennan TA, Laird N, et al. The nature of adverse events in hospitalized patients: results of the Harvard Medical Practice Study II. *N Engl J Med.* 1991;324:377-384.

Leape LL, Berwick DM. Five years after To Err Is Human: what have we learned? *JAMA.* 2005;293:2384-2390.

McCannon CJ, Hackbarth AD, Griffin FA. Miles to go: an introduction to the 5 Million Lives Campaign. *Jt Comm J Qual Patient Saf.* 2007;33:477-484.

Singer SJ, Falwell A, Gaba DM, et al. Identifying organizational cultures that promote patient safety. *Health Care Manage Rev.* 2009;34:300-311.

The references for this chapter can be found at www.expertconsult.com.

7 Education, Training, and Certification in Pain Medicine

James P. Rathmell | David L. Brown

THE EVOLUTION OF PAIN MEDICINE AS A SUBSPECIALTY

As knowledge expands and the need for detailed skills arises, specialization ensues. This is a natural progression, and it has become impossible for any physician to become an expert in every field. There has long been discomfort with specialization despite unflagging progression in this direction. The urge to both specialize and remain unspecialized dates back to the earliest recorded history in medicine. The first specializations were between barber-surgeons and internists, and a rivalry of sorts remains to this day. Writing about Ambrose Paré, the 16th century physician who elevated the role of barber-surgeons to that of other physicians, the present-day surgeon and historian Sherwin Nuland reflected on the ongoing distinction between internist and surgeon[1]:

Surgery is an exercise in the use of the intellect. Heckling internists, with tongues barely in check, would prefer that surgical specialists be viewed merely as dexterous craftsman who carry out the routing errands assigned to them by their more cerebrally endowed medical overseers. I attribute this teasing raillery to a kind of good-natured fraternal envy, not so much of our celebrity status, but rather of the visibility of the cures we surgeons achieve and the particular personal gratification we have while doing it.

In the United States, anesthesiology has progressed toward further specialization, first with the establishment of critical care, then pain management (now pain medicine), and more recently pediatric anesthesiology and cardiothoracic anesthesiology. The addition of pain medicine as a subspecialty of anesthesiology is just one recent example of the growth of medical specialties. With specialization comes a conscious effort to focus practice so that one becomes intricately familiar with a more limited realm. The obvious result is loss of the skills and knowledge needed to practice in the broader parent specialty. In pain medicine, many now view this as a full-time vocation. The scientific meetings and journals that keep pain medicine specialists up-to-date have little overlap with those that are designed to serve anesthesiologists practicing in the operating room. The only common thread between the technical skills needed in the pain clinic and those required for anesthesiology in the operating room is expertise in neural blockade. The pain medicine practitioner must acquire a vastly different skill set from those practicing anesthesiology, including expanding their skills as diagnosticians.

Much has been written about the origins of pain medicine as a distinct discipline, and anesthesiologists have played a primary role since the start.[2] It really started with the introduction of effective general anesthetics in the mid-19th century, when surgical pain could be separated from surgery. Almost 100 years later, the late John Bonica, an anesthesiologist and recognized father of the specialty that we now call pain medicine, developed his career by promoting multidisciplinary pain care and formal training of specialists. From his life's work we now have extensive ongoing efforts to recognize and treat pain effectively, to train subspecialists, and to conduct basic and clinical research to further our understanding of pain and its treatment. The International Association for the Study of Pain, founded in 1974, its U.S. chapter the American Pain Society, and the journal *Pain* are legacies left by Dr. Bonica for our patients.

Accredited fellowship training in pain medicine is a relatively recent development. Before 1992, training was frequently obtained in academic anesthesiology departments, including those of Bonica, Bridenbaugh, Carron, Haugen, Moore, Raj, Winnie, and others, and subsequently in programs run by their trainees. These unaccredited programs advanced the specialty, widened interest in pain medicine as a career, and propagated pain care in smaller and smaller communities across the country. Outside the United States, this type of informal training remains the rule for those seeking expertise in pain medicine. In the United States, the American Board of Anesthesiology (ABA) developed interest in certifying pain medicine specialists following their training. Through the leadership of Dr. William Owens in his roles in both the ABA and the Accreditation Council on Graduate Medical Education (ACGME) and through his representations of the subspecialty to the American Board of Medical Specialties, formal training programs were accredited and physicians were certified. Drs. Stephen Abram and John Rowlingson were both key members of the group that assisted Dr. Owens in moving the new subspecialty forward.

The first programs were accredited by the ACGME in 1992. The number of ACGME-accredited programs and trainees in accredited programs has grown steadily over the past decade, and there are now just more than 100 training programs that turn out about 300 new pain specialists each year. Working in parallel with ACGME, the ABA developed a subspecialty certification examination in pain medicine, first named the "Certificate of Added Qualifications in Pain Management" and now titled "Subspecialty Certification in Pain Medicine." The first examination was given in 1993. The number of candidates taking the examination has grown steadily since the initial examination.

Dr. Bonica's original push to develop multidisciplinary pain care recently evolved into collaboration between four specialties that agreed to a single and unified set of program requirements for all ACGME-accredited pain fellowships, regardless of the sponsoring specialty. The ACGME Residency Review Committees for Anesthesiology, Neurology, Physical Medicine, and Rehabilitation and Psychiatry agreed on these requirements in late 2005, and the ACGME board approved their implementation for 2007.[3] These requirements have standardized pain fellowship training programs. After introduction of the new training requirements in 2007, a number of programs closed because of unwillingness to adopt a multidisciplinary approach, and thus only the more comprehensive programs were left to continue the training of physician pain specialists (Fig. 7.1). Programs have begun to produce more comprehensive and multidisciplinary focused physicians from a wider range of primary disciplines (Figs. 7.2 and 7.3). Other groups are also encouraging a more comprehensive approach to pain care, with the linked American Academy of Pain Medicine and the American Board of Pain Medicine likewise devoting energy to a multidisciplinary approach. There remain a number of experienced pain specialists who believe that eventually the ACGME-accredited fellowships will be extended to 2 years to cover an expanding knowledge base. Equally important in evolution of the discipline is the creation of academic physicians within the fellowships who undertake research programs to add new knowledge to guide clinical practice in this area of medicine.

Pain and its consequences draw on resources from all medical disciplines. Dr. Bonica's experiences during World War II suggested that each medical specialist had unique expertise to bring to patients suffering pain—hence his consistent and effective promotion of a multidisciplinary process for pain care. Also thanks largely to Dr. Bonica, anesthesiology has led the development of formal training programs. Indeed, the majority of currently accredited programs reside within academic anesthesiology departments, and most program directors are anesthesiologists. Specialists from other disciplines have also focused their clinical and research efforts on pain. The most obvious example is neurology, from which the majority of clinical treatment and research on headache has arisen. The field of physical medicine and rehabilitation has also had a focus and expertise on functional restoration, and physiatrists lead many chronic pain rehabilitation programs. Moreover, psychiatrists and psychologists have of course been closely involved when pain, depression, and substance abuse overlap. During the last decade, specialists from these other disciplines have been seeking subspecialty training in pain medicine with increasing regularity.

The range of practitioners declaring themselves pain medicine specialists is extraordinary, from clinics that provide largely or solely cognitive-behavioral approaches to chronic pain through functional restoration programs all the way to the type of clinic that offers nothing more than injections of various sorts. "Interventional pain medicine" is a phrase that has been coined for techniques that involve minimally invasive treatments and minor surgery as part of their application, including neural blockade and implantable analgesic devices. Despite the paucity of scientific evidence to guide pain practitioners, particularly evidence to support the use of many interventional modalities, many techniques appear to have efficacy based on limited observational data and have been adopted into widespread use. As practitioners, we are left to choose among the treatment modalities

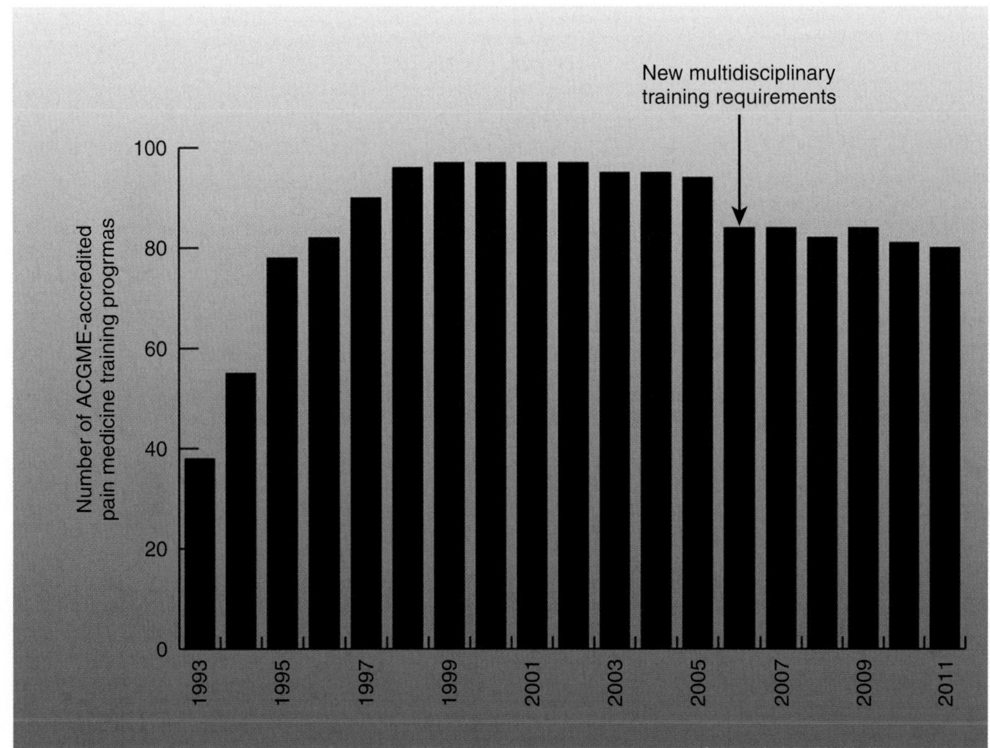

Figure 7.1 Trends in the number of pain medicine fellowship training programs accredited by the Accreditation Council for Graduate Medical Education (ACGME) since the first programs were established in 1992. (Data courtesy of the American Board of Anesthesiology, October 2011.)

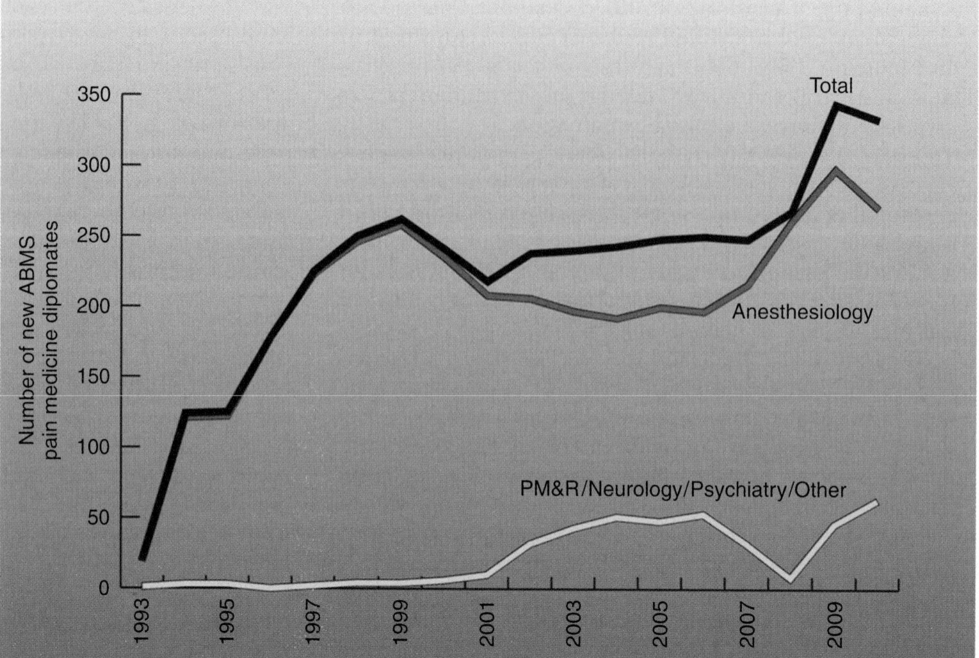

Figure 7.2 Trends in the number of new subspecialty board-certified diplomates in pain medicine recognized by the American Board of Medical Specialties (ABMS) and their primary discipline of ABMS board certification. PM&R, physical medicine and rehabilitation. (Data courtesy of the American Board of Anesthesiology, October 2011.)

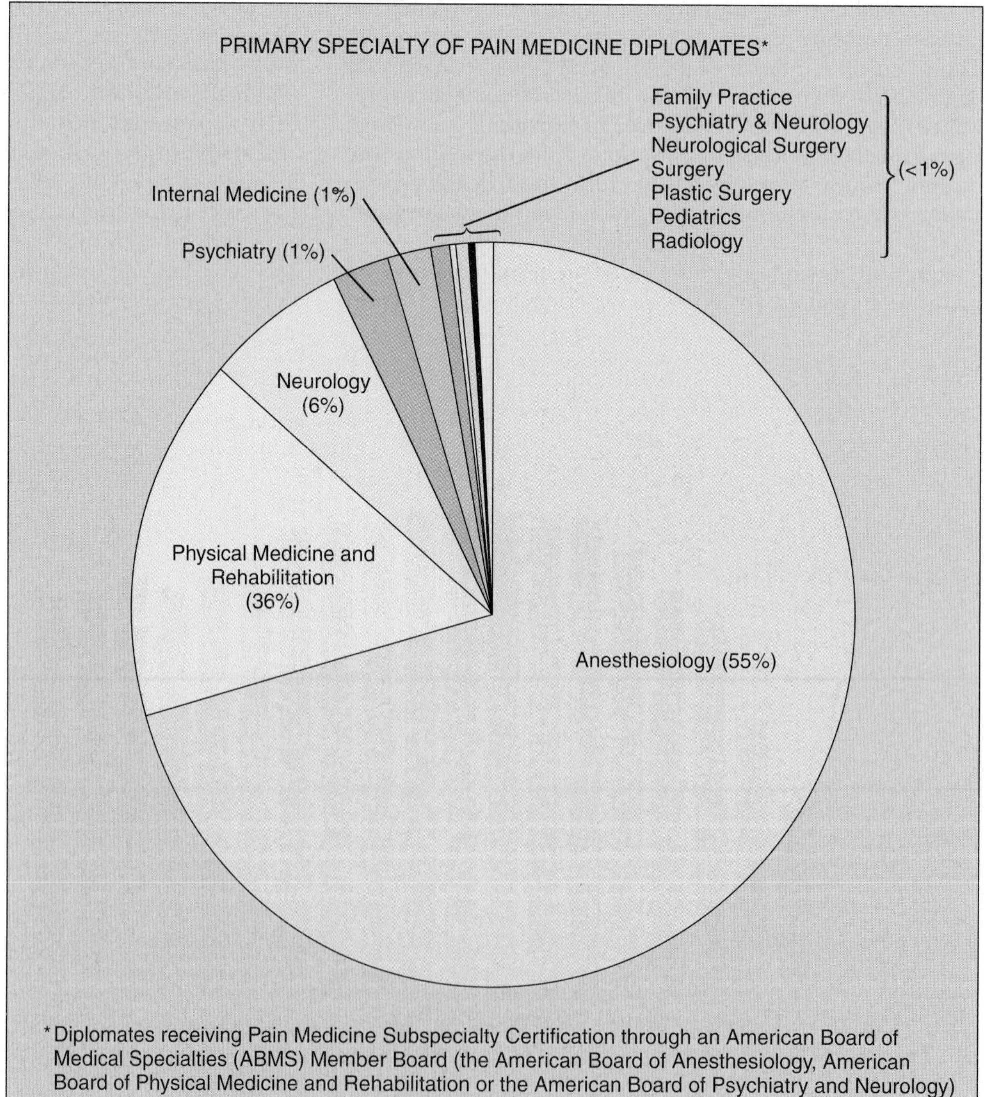

Figure 7.3 Primary specialty of board certification of diplomates receiving subspecialty certification in pain medicine through a member board of the American Board of Medical Specialties (ABMS; member boards offering pain medicine subspecialty certification include the American Board of Anesthesiology [ABA], the American Board of Physical Medicine and Rehabilitation [ABPMR], and the American Board of Psychiatry and Neurology [ABPN]). (All data provided by the ABA, ABPMR, and ABPN, July 2010.)

available, often with only anecdotal and personal experience to guide us in treating a group of desperate patients with intractable pain who are willing to accept almost any treatment, even though it remains unproven. There is no single practice pattern that pain specialists can point to as being the correct way to treat patients with chronic pain. Training programs vary widely in the scope of what they train practitioners to do. The best pain medicine practitioners strike a reasonable balance between interventional and noninterventional management. This practice pattern is sustainable, and those adopting a balanced style of practice will be able to adapt to the evolving scientific evidence that appears in support of pain treatment, regardless of the type of treatment. A balance between treatment modalities also allows practitioners to switch from one mode to another or to incorporate multiple treatment approaches simultaneously. Use of these interventional modalities is just a small part of the armamentarium of a skilled pain practitioner.

TRAINING AND CREDENTIALING IN INTERVENTIONAL PAIN MEDICINE

In our rapidly changing world of modern health care, new technologies are appearing at a dizzying rate. Many of these new treatments require physicians to acquire detailed new knowledge and technical skills. The introduction of new techniques typically extends from centers in the public or private sector, where the ideas are conceived and tested in a limited realm among innovators. From there, anecdote can often take over, and many techniques in pain medicine have blossomed into widespread use with nothing more than word of mouth to propagate their use. The use of pulsed radiofrequency treatment of pain is one such example in which clinical application has preceded detailed clinical testing.[4]

In the United States and Europe, industry often leads innovation by testing and initiating the introduction of new devices. When the innovation appears to have merit in limited trials, many devices are introduced to the market with approval through the Food and Drug Administration's 510K "substantially similar device" process with little or no data regarding efficacy. Once on the market, the means by which practitioners decide to adopt new technologies, the speed of progression of these new techniques, and—of great importance—the means by which practitioners gain enough expertise to introduce new techniques into their own practice are all highly variable and seemingly without any rational or consistent approach.

Interventional pain medicine is evolving as a distinct discipline that requires detailed new knowledge and expertise. Familiarity with radiographic anatomy for performing image-guided injections and the minor surgical skills needed to implant devices such as spinal cord stimulators and drug delivery systems are just a few of the techniques that practitioners must master. As we set out to introduce new interventional techniques into our own pain practices, we must be sure that we have been properly trained to perform these techniques in a manner that ensures safety and success.

Adequate exposure to these newer treatment alternatives during the fellowship training period is necessary to ensure appropriate application and optimize patient outcomes. Although we do not have scientific data that define the average minimum level of experience that will be necessary to achieve competence, especially for complex procedures associated with significant risk, logic dictates that that trainees should be exposed to a minimum number of these procedures during a fellowship. The ACGME has established requirements for the average minimum number of epidural, spinal, and peripheral nerve blocks necessary for the accreditation of anesthesiology residency programs. Other medical subspecialties also require a minimum number of specified procedures to achieve and maintain competence: subspecialty training in gastroenterology has a requirement for performing a minimum of 100 esophagogastroduodenoscopy and 100 colonoscopy procedures with polyp removal[5] during formal training, and subspecialty training in cardiovascular disease requires 100 cardiac catheterization procedures to demonstrate minimum proficiency.[6] Indeed, the ACGME's Residency Review Committee for Anesthesiology has accepted revised Program Requirements for Pain Medicine Training Programs that specify the minimum exposure of trainees to various procedures, including image-guided injection techniques for the cervical and lumbar spine; sympathetic blockade; neurolytic block, including radiofrequency treatment of pain; spinal cord stimulation; and placement of permanent spinal drug delivery systems. For techniques that are now widely accepted as a core element of pain practice, we must ensure that our trainees gain enough experience to conduct these procedures independently. One key element of the ACGME deliberations about unified pain training is to acknowledge that not all pain fellows will have experience in the wide variety of interventional techniques. Rather, it is hoped that these fellows will gain an understanding of all available options for patients with pain and yet demonstrate and have competence documented in only techniques for which formal training is made available during fellowship training.

It is difficult to define the techniques that are core for a pain practitioner, but it does seem that detailed knowledge of the radiographic anatomy of the spine and the minor surgical expertise required to implant spinal cord stimulators and permanent spinal drug delivery systems are among the skills that most practicing pain physicians would expect a new graduate from a pain fellowship program to have. New techniques are appearing at a staggering rate, and we cannot rely on pain fellowship programs to provide all the technical training that is needed. Stronger standards for minimum training following fellowship programs are also urgently needed. Some pain practitioners believe that too many of their colleagues find it perfectly acceptable to attend a brief weekend course and then introduce a highly technical new treatment into practice without additional study, training, or oversight.[7] Practitioners themselves must take the lead in obtaining adequate training *before* proceeding with any new and unfamiliar technique. A weekend workshop is just a start, often a good start—the best workshops will give practitioners a detailed understanding of anatomy, pathophysiology of disease related to use of the new technique, patient selection, conduct of the procedure, outcomes, and avoidance, management, and recognition of complications. Box 7.1 is a suggested method for practitioners to introduce a new technique into clinical practice.[8]

Box 7.1 Suggested Training and Experience When Introducing a New Technique into Clinical Practice

1. *Study the new technique* and the published literature and gain detailed knowledge of all aspects of the technique.
2. *Attend a workshop*, preferably a hands-on cadaver-based workshop that allows introduction of the technique in as realistic a setting as can be assembled.
3. *Plan* adequate time for your initial procedures.
4. *Get help* at the bedside during the initial performance of new procedures—perhaps another experienced practitioner at your institution or an invited expert to assist or team up with a colleague in a related discipline.
5. *Inform your patients* that you are introducing a new technique and include this discussion as part of the informed consent process.
6. *Examine your outcomes* carefully in the initial stages of using any new technique and compare them with those of your colleagues and the published literature.

Reprinted with permission from Lubenow TR, Rathmell JP. Let's take a rational approach to technical training in pain medicine. *Am Soc Anesth Newsl.* 2005;69:6-8.

FUTURE DIRECTIONS

The field of evidence-based medicine has emerged as a new paradigm to guide practicing physicians. This field aims to educate practitioners on how to frame specific questions based on the clinical problems that they encounter every day. They then venture to the published scientific literature with focused questions on prevention, treatment, and diagnosis of a specific clinical condition. Many evidence-based medicine centers offer concise and periodically updated summaries on specific clinical conditions. The idea is to get the best information available to practicing clinicians. They describe the best available evidence, and if there is no good evidence, they say so. In pain medicine we are faced with an expanding array of treatment options that strike us as logical developments that *should* provide pain relief for our patients. However, there is a dearth of clinical evidence to guide rational choice and application of the majority of these emerging treatments. So how are we to decide when to apply them?

Nearly a decade ago, Merrill[9] presented an analysis of the state of evidence guiding the use of interventional treatments in the field of pain medicine. He pointed out the frequent flaws in existing studies (largely the lack of valid comparators, such as no treatment) and concluded that "the practice of invasive pain medicine teeters at a particularly critical juncture…crippled by a lack of vigorous self-evaluation of its role in the treatment of chronic pain." Merrill went on to detail the means by which we, as scientists and clinicians, can proceed to build a better body of evidence for the treatments that we are using. However, the field of pain medicine is young and early in development, and randomized clinical trials are still lacking for many treatments.

New treatments evolve slowly. Application of the scientific method in clinical medicine begins with observation, perhaps a chance observation that a certain drug typically used for another purpose provides analgesia to a given patient. If the drug is readily available, a clinician may choose to try treatment of other patients with similar conditions. If academically minded, the clinician may choose to report the limited success in a case series. Case series are a valuable beginning, the very beginning of emerging new ideas. If the problem is uniform and prevalent enough, the new treatment may gain the attention of investigators willing to assemble a randomized clinical trial. All too often, sound treatments are never tested because of lack of interest or funding. Those that are tested tend to be under patent, and the manufacturer proceeds with large trials understandably in the hope of financial return in the event that the treatment proves useful. Patients who are suffering from severe and intractable pain are desperate and can easily be convinced that desperate measures, however new or unproven, are warranted.

How then are we to proceed? Our patients are begging for us to try anything that offers a glimmer of hope in reducing their pain, and we as scientists embrace the rigor of the scientific method and want desperately to do what is best for our patients. We have treatment after treatment that makes logical sense and shows early promise in case series and observational studies, but few data that support an evidence-based approach to practice. Using acute low back pain with sciatica as an example, a number of evidence-based reports have emerged to guide clinicians.[10] The only modalities that are rated as "beneficial" or "likely to be beneficial" are advice to stay active and use of nonsteroidal anti-inflammatory drugs, behavioral therapy, and multidisciplinary treatment programs. Opioid analgesics, acupuncture, back schools, epidural steroid injections, and spinal manipulation were all judged to be of "unknown effectiveness." Yet in actual clinical practice in the United States, a short course of an opioid analgesic plus early intervention with epidural steroid injections is common. To complicate matters, the use of fluoroscopic guidance to direct injections to the affected level via an interlaminar or transforaminal approach has gained widespread acceptance, but with only uncontrolled case series to guide us as clinicians. Those with persistent pain and contained disk herniations now have a dizzying array of treatment options, including laser diskectomy, thermal disk decompression, and vacuum disk extraction, all using Food and Drug Administration–approved devices with only uncontrolled observational studies that suggest effectiveness.[11] The new devices are intellectually appealing and minimally invasive, yet only open surgical diskectomy has proved superior to conservative management in patients with persistent sciatica secondary to intervertebral disk prolapse.[12]

The evidence-based medicine movement gives little guidance to practitioners whose tools are still under development. They simply remind us that no evidence regarding many of our techniques exists. Without declaring a moratorium on all interventional pain techniques, Merrill[9] offers the individual practitioner advice: monitor your own outcomes with valid measures, be more reflective and systematic in studying your own outcomes and patterns of care, and provide this information to your patients as part of the decision-making process. As pain practitioners we have an expanding range of treatment options available to us, few with convincing evidence of efficacy superior to that of alternative treatments.

We must evaluate each patient and use the limited evidence available to us today to guide compassionate and rational, if not evidence-based, use of therapy for our desperate patients.

The urgent need for expanded clinical research in pain medicine, coupled with recent efforts to improve multidisciplinary training, are straining the ability of training programs to adequately provide the needed education and research experience for pain medicine fellows in the course of a 1-year fellowship. The ACGME and ABA are currently working to further restructure pain medicine training to accomplish these goals (for a recent review see Rathmell[13]). The idea is to provide more comprehensive and multidisciplinary training and to require meaningful research experience during fellowship training. With this approach we will create a more homogeneous group of pain medicine specialists who emerge with similar knowledge and skills, regardless of the parent discipline in which they trained. This will move us toward improving the consistency and quality of care of patients with acute, chronic, and cancer-related pain.

KEY POINTS

- The first multidisciplinary pain clinic was established by the late Dr. John Bonica. The International Association for the Study of Pain, founded in 1974, its U.S. chapter the American Pain Society (APS), and the journal *Pain* are his legacies.
- The initial accredited pain medicine fellowship programs were based on anesthesiology programs. The ACGME Residency Review Committees for Anesthesiology, Neurology, Physical Medicine, and Rehabilitation and Psychiatry agreed on standard multidisciplinary requirements in late 2005, and the ACGME board approved their implementation for 2007. A number of programs closed and the more comprehensive programs continued the training of physician pain specialists (see Fig. 7.1). These programs have begun to produce more comprehensive and multidisciplinary focused physicians from a wider range of primary disciplines.
- The ACGME has established requirements for the average minimum number of epidural, spinal, and peripheral nerve blocks necessary for accreditation of anesthesiology residency programs, similar to other subspecialties. The anesthesiology revised Program Requirements for Pain Medicine Training Programs specify the minimum exposure of trainees to various techniques, including image-guided injection techniques on the cervical and lumbar spine; sympathetic blockade; neurolytic block, including radiofrequency treatment of pain; spinal cord stimulation; and placement of permanent spinal drug delivery systems.

KEY POINTS—cont'd

- Detailed knowledge of the radiographic anatomy of the spine and the minor surgical expertise required to implant spinal cord stimulators and permanent spinal drug delivery systems are among the skills that a new graduate from a pain medicine fellowship program is expected to have.
- The ABA, together with the ACGME, developed a subspecialty certification examination in pain medicine, first named the "Certificate of Added Qualifications in Pain Management" and now titled "Subspecialty Certification in Pain Medicine." The first examination was given in 1993, and the number of candidates taking the examination has steadily grown.
- Many devices have been introduced to the market with approval through the Food and Drug Administration's 510K "substantially similar device" process with little or no data regarding efficacy. The means by which practitioners decide to adopt new technologies, the speed of progression of these new techniques, and the means by which practitioners gain enough expertise to introduce new techniques into their own practices are all highly variable. Rational steps in incorporating a new interventional technique into someone's practice are outlined in Box 7.1.
- Efforts to provide multidisciplinary training and the need for clinical research are straining the ability of training programs to provide the education and research experience for pain medicine fellows in the course of a 1-year fellowship. The ACGME and ABA are currently working to further restructure pain medicine training to accomplish these goals.

SUGGESTED READINGS

Lubenow TR, Rathmell JP. Let's take a rational approach to technical training in pain medicine. *Am Soc Anesth Newsl.* 2005;69:6-8.

Merrill DG. Hoffman's glasses: evidence-based medicine and the search for quality in the literature of interventional pain medicine. *Reg Anesth Pain Med.* 2003;28:547-560.

Program Requirements for Fellowship Education in Pain Medicine. Available at http//www.acgme.org/acWebsite/downloads/RRC_progReq/sh_multiPainPR707_TCC.pdf.

Rathmell JP. The injectionists. *Reg Anesth Pain Med.* 2004;29:305-306.

Rathmell JP. American Society of Regional Anesthesia and Pain Medicine 2011 John J. Bonica award lecture: the evolution of the field of pain medicine. *Reg Anesth Pain Med.* 2012;37:652-656.

Rathmell JP, Brown DL. The evolution of training in pain medicine in the United States. *American Society of Anesthesiologists Newsletter.* November 2002.

The references for this chapter can be found at www.expertconsult.com.

PART 2

BASIC CONSIDERATIONS

ROBERT W. HURLEY, EDITOR

PART OUTLINE

8 Pain Pathways: Peripheral, Spinal, Ascending, and Descending Pathways

Karin N. Westlund

INTRODUCTION

The neural circuits that are responsible for pain and the reactions to pain[1] can be termed the *pain system*[2-4] or, perhaps more appropriately, the *pain systems*. The pain systems include (1) peripheral neurons with a set of peripheral receptive elements, the nociceptors; (2) numerous central neuronal relay pathways; and (3) sets of integrative neurons that impose excitatory or inhibitory influences on nociceptive information at numerous levels of the neuraxis.

The initial reception of input perceived to be painful occurs on the peripheral terminations of nociceptors transducing noxious mechanical, temperature, and chemical stimuli. Nociceptors transmit information about internal or external stimuli that are noxious, distressing, or damaging to second-order neurons located in the spinal cord or brainstem level innervated (i.e., the lumbar spinal cord for leg input, the thoracic spinal cord for stomach lining input, and the trigeminal spinal nucleus for face input). Nociceptive signals are then transmitted by projection neurons of the pain system to integration sites in the brainstem. A primary integration site for sensory information is the thalamus, but numerous other brainstem and higher brain structures are participants in the integrative neuronal circuits responding to pain.

A variety of coordinated pain reactions are generated, including protective somatic and autonomic reflexes, endocrine actions, emotional responses, learning and memory about the event, and cortical awareness of pain. In addition to pain transmission and pain reactions, the brain centers that receive nociceptive information also provide either negative or positive feedback that reduces or accentuates pain and pain reactions. Negative feedback to the spinal cord circuitry is mediated by descending pathways that are often called the "endogenous analgesia system." The mechanism and pathways responsible for accentuation of pain and pain reactions, referred to as central sensitization or facilitation, can involve increased responsiveness at all levels of the pain system, including the peripheral nociceptors, spinal cord, brainstem, and higher centers. The net effect of the positive and negative alterations in circuitry leads to the perceptual experience of "pain."

NOCICEPTORS

PERIPHERAL RECEPTIVE ELEMENTS

The initial reception of noxious input perceived to be painful occurs at the specialized endings of primary afferent sensory neurons known as nociceptors. Reception of noxious input occurs in functionally specialized free nerve endings of the skin, muscle,[5] joints,[6,7] viscera,[8,9] and dura[10] (Fig. 8.1). Nociceptive endings are also located in the fascia and adventitia of blood vessels.[11] Glutamate receptors, as well as μ- and δ-opiates, substance P (SP), somatostatin, and vanilloid receptors, have been identified immunohistochemically on the peripheral endings of cutaneous nerve fibers.[12-16] Nociceptor subtypes respond best to either mechanical (mechanical nociceptors), mechanical and thermal (mechanothermal nociceptors), or mechanical, thermal, and chemical stimuli (polymodal nociceptors).[17,18] Common types of cutaneous nociceptors are Aδ mechanoreceptors and C polymodal nociceptors, which relay the transduced information about potentially harmful input via Aδ and C fibers, respectively.[19,20]

PERIPHERAL NERVES

The axons that relay information about noxious input from the skin and other tissues to the central nervous system (CNS) fall characteristically into the range of small, unmyelinated axonal fibers with conduction velocities lower than 2.5 m/sec for C fiber (or group IV) nociceptors[21] (Fig. 8.2) and small fibers wrapped in a thin layer of myelin produced by Schwann cells with a conduction velocity of 4 to 30 m/sec in the case of Aδ fibers (or group III).[22] Primary afferent C fibers are more numerous than myelinated primary afferents in peripheral nerves. For example, in dorsal roots, the ratio of C fibers to A fibers is about 2.5:1,[23] and in joint nerves (after sympathetic postganglionic axons are removed by sympathectomy), the ratio of C to A fibers is 2.3:1.[24]

The peripheral nerves carry both sensory and motor axons. Regardless of whether they innervate cutaneous, deep, vascular, or visceral tissue, the primary afferent (incoming) fibers carrying sensory information separate from the motor nerve axons near the spinal cord and become the dorsal root that enters the spinal cord on the dorsal surface (Fig. 8.3). Motor commands are sent out to the periphery through the ventral root by large, rapidly conducting somatic efferent nerve fibers and by small, slowly conducting autonomic motor fibers. Whereas the motor neurons are located in the ventral horn of the spinal cord or intermediate regions in the case of autonomic motor neurons, the sensory afferent fibers have their cell bodies in the dorsal root ganglia (DRGs) (or cranial nerve ganglia) located outside the spinal cord or brainstem.

Noxious mechanical, temperature, and chemical (nociceptive) information is first relayed across a synapse located in the dorsal horn of the spinal cord before transmission to brainstem sites (including the ventral posterolateral [VPL] nucleus of the thalamus) (see Figs. 8.1 and 8.3). Cutaneous and visceral nociceptive input is provided to spinal

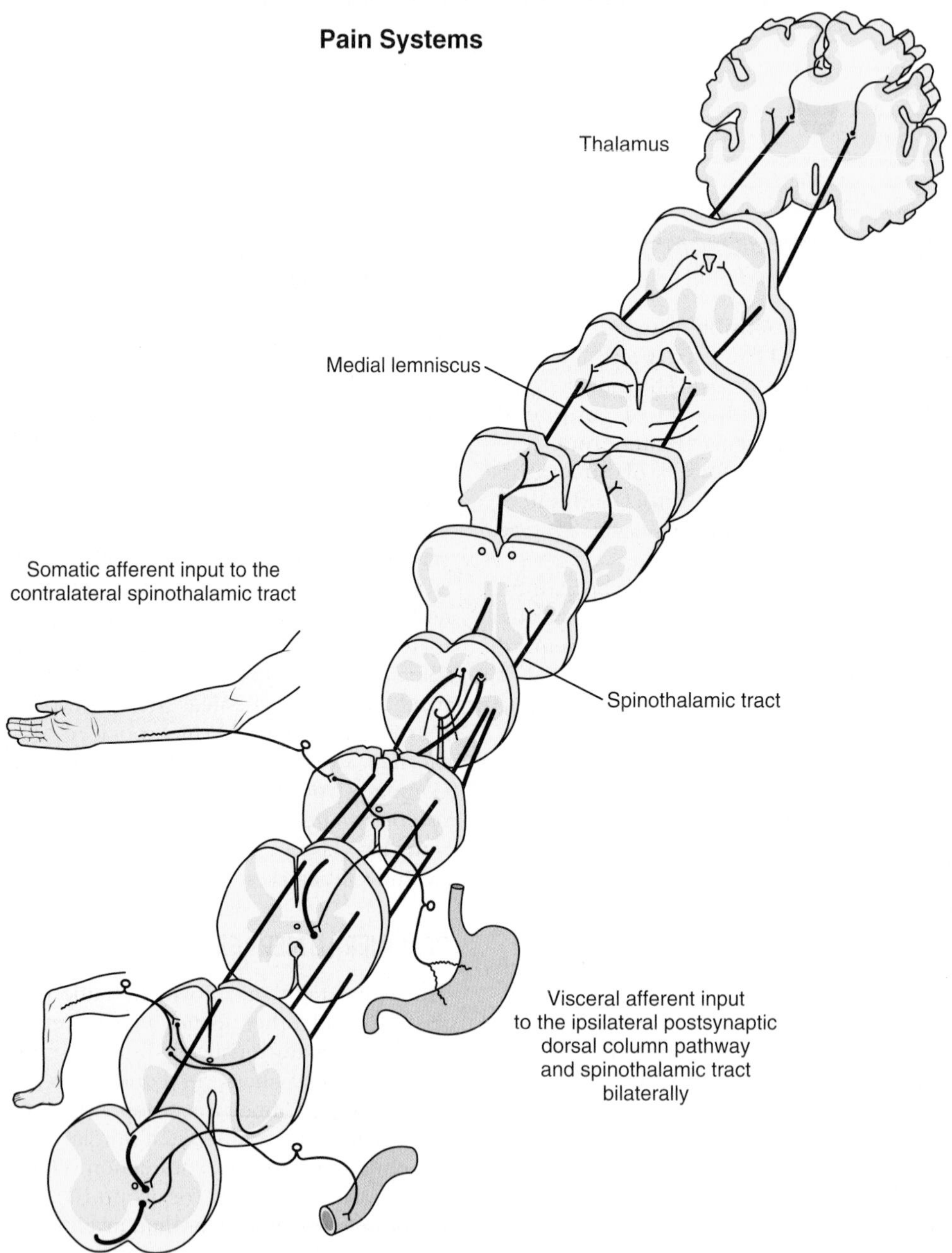

Figure 8.1 The pain systems convey input from somatic structures, as well as from viscera and other deep tissues, via peripheral nerves. Afferent nerve fibers carrying nociceptive information have free nerve endings in peripheral tissue and terminate in the superficial spinal cord dorsal horn. Information about pain is relayed through at least one synapse to cells in the spinal cord dorsal horn. Two parallel ascending pathways provide the information to integration centers in the thalamus, which provide the information to cortical regions. Input primarily from somatic structures is relayed to spinothalamic tract cells whose axons cross the midline and ascend in the lateral and ventrolateral spinal white matter as the spinothalamic tract. As the spinothalamic tract courses through the brainstem, collateral fibers innervate a variety of brainstem centers involved in providing responses to nociceptive input on its path to the thalamus. Nociceptive input arising from visceral structures is relayed by postsynaptic dorsal column cells whose axons course in the dorsal columns. After a synaptic relay in the dorsal column nuclei and crossing to the opposite side of the brainstem, the medial lemniscus carries nociceptive information to the thalamus. Both these routes are somatotopically arranged throughout their length.

neurons in different spinal regions, has different ascending spinal projection pathways, and has different brainstem terminations.

In contrast, incoming cutaneous non-noxious input important for discerning fine, discriminative touch, pressure, and position in space is transmitted by large, myelinated peripheral nerve fibers directly through the dorsal column of the spinal cord. The first synapse of these large, uncrossed ascending primary afferent fibers is in the dorsal column nuclei of the medulla. From there, cutaneous sensory information is transmitted as the decussated medial lemniscal pathway to the contralateral VPL nucleus of the thalamus, the primary sensory integrative relay of the sensory system. Similar information is relayed to the brainstem through several tracts whose cells of origin are within the spinal cord, including the tactile component of the postsynaptic dorsal column pathway, the spinocervical tract, and the proprioceptive pathway that projects to nucleus Z in the medulla.[19]

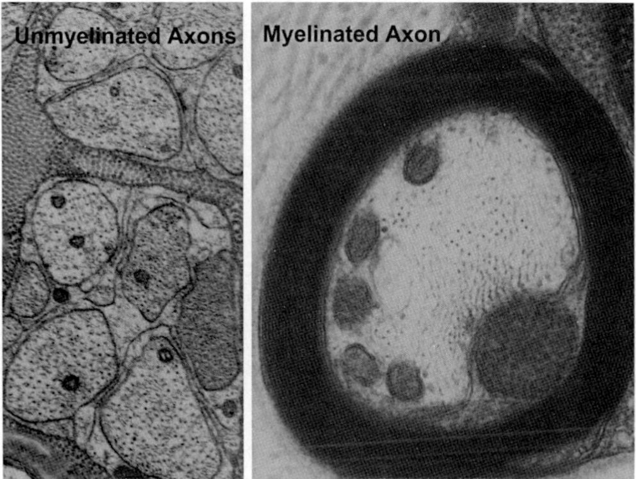

Figure 8.2 Peripheral nerves conveying information about pain are either small, slowly conducting fibers found unmyelinated in bundles or medium-sized axons with thin myelin, which provides a higher conduction velocity.

Primary afferent fibers providing input to autonomic regions of the spinal cord from visceral structures and the vasculature travel along with the sympathetic efferent nerves. They pass directly through the sympathetic trunk, however, to join other afferent fibers entering the dorsal horn of the spinal cord (see Fig. 8.3).

As in most central neuronal circuits, glutamate is the primary neurotransmitter substance in primary afferent nociceptors. Its action is modulated by neuropeptides co-released at their terminal endings and by activation molecules. Calcitonin gene–related peptide (CGRP), SP, neurokinin A, galanin, and somatostatin are just a few examples of the many neuropeptides that provide neurogenic modulation and inflammation peripherally.[25,26] Afferent nerve endings

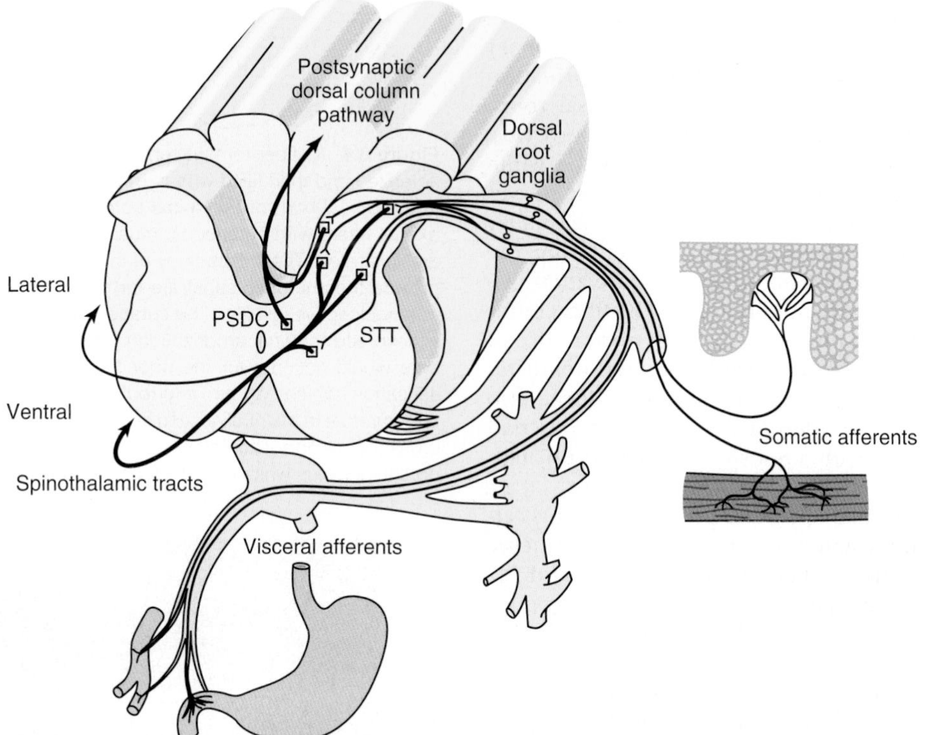

Figure 8.3 Nociceptive afferent nerve fibers have receptive free nerve endings in the dermal papillae of skin, in muscle, in the vasculature, and in visceral structures. Nerves carrying nociceptive information travel with other somatic and autonomic motor axons, even passing through the autonomic ganglia, but have their cell bodies in the dorsal root ganglia located in the spinal vertebral column. The central axonal projection of afferent nerve fibers then passes through the dorsal root to innervate the spinal cord dorsal horn. Nociceptive information is relayed across at least one synapse in the dorsal horn to alert cells with projections to higher centers. The spinothalamic tract (STT) cells in the superficial dorsal horn send an axonal projection across the midline to travel in the lateral SST. SST cells in the deep dorsal horn send axons across the midline to ascend in the ventral white matter. SST cells bring information about both somatic and visceral pain to the thalamic levels. Postsynaptic dorsal column (PSDC) cells relay information about visceral pain through the ipsilateral dorsal column.

are also activated by inflammatory mediators, such as tumor necrosis factor-α, interleukin-1 (IL-1), and IL-6.[27-29] Other activators include the small molecules adenosine, adenosine triphosphate, nitric oxide, and other reactive oxygen species.[30-33] All these substances have been identified at terminal sites, in DRGs, and in the dorsal horn.

CELL BODIES IN DORSAL ROOT GANGLIA

The large, medium, and small neuronal cell bodies of the primary afferent nerve fibers lie just outside the spinal column clustered in DRGs, with many of the small and medium DRG cells belonging to the nociceptors.[34] The pseudounipolar DRG neurons extend their axons peripherally as primary afferent fibers and centrally as dorsal roots. The modulatory neuropeptides produced in DRGs are transported quickly to terminal endings in the periphery and the spinal cord and thus may not necessarily be evident in the cell body without experimental manipulations. The small satellite glia, the other component of DRGs, provide support but are also capable of exerting modulatory influence on the neurons that promote peripheral sensitization.

SPINAL CORD TERMINATIONS

The primary afferent fiber type and its site of termination centrally are relevant to its function. The afferent fibers enter the gray matter of the spinal cord through the dorsal root entry zone and primarily innervate regions of the spinal cord within the same or adjacent spinal segments matching that spinal nerve. In general, large myelinated primary afferent fibers carrying discriminative sensory information (tactile, pressure, vibratory sense) enter the dorsal roots, traverse the top of the dorsal horn of the spinal cord (Lissauer's tract), and turn to ascend uncrossed as the white matter dorsal column. The large sensory afferent nerves provide only collateral input to the dorsal horn. The smaller myelinated and unmyelinated axonal fibers entering the dorsal root carry information about temperature and nociceptive input perceived as pain in humans. The fibers enter Lissauer's tract and then innervate the gray matter core of the spinal cord, where neuronal cell bodies and dendrites receive their arborized synaptic endings (Fig. 8.4; see also Fig. 8.3). However, these afferent fibers may also ascend rostrally or descend caudally a few spinal segments through Lissauer's tract.

Two populations of small-diameter primary afferents carrying pain-related information to the dorsal horn are classified as (1) peptidergic, containing CGRP and SP, and (2) nonpeptidergic, containing no peptides but expressing purinoceptors for ATP (P2X3) and binding isolectin B4 (IB4).

Since the sole source of CGRP in the dorsal horn of the spinal cord is from primary afferents, this peptide serves as a convenient marker for primary afferent peptidergic terminal endings in the spinal cord (Fig. 8.5).[35-37] CGRP fibers extend extensive fiber terminations up and down the superficial spinal cord dorsal horn through numerous spinal levels on entering at a particular spinal segment and can even cross the midline in small numbers.[35] Numerous other neuropeptides have been localized in the dorsal horn.[26] Visceral afferents are rich in vasoactive intestinal polypeptide (VIP), bombesin, CGRP, and SP[20,25] and would account for some of

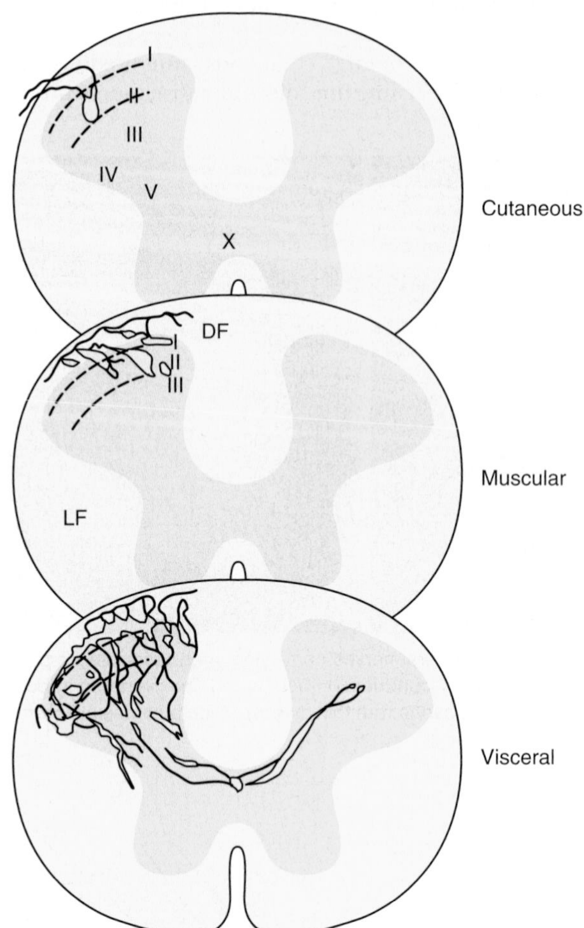

Figure 8.4 C-fiber terminal endings have been physiologically characterized and then filled with dye to reveal their terminal arborizations in the dorsal horn of the spinal cord. Examples of terminal arbors of axonal fibers with cutaneous, muscular, and visceral receptive fields are illustrated. The morphology of the cutaneous axonal ending would provide the anatomic substrate for precise point-to-point localization of a nociceptive insult on the cutaneous surface. Likewise, the diffuse widespread terminal arborization pattern of visceral afferent nerve fibers would account for the poor localization of visceral nociceptive sensation, which can be "referred" to other structures. Most visceral structures lie in the midline, and some of the visceral fibers shown even cross the midline. The Roman numerals indicate Rexed's laminae. DF, dorsal funiculus white mater; LF, lateral funiculus white matter.

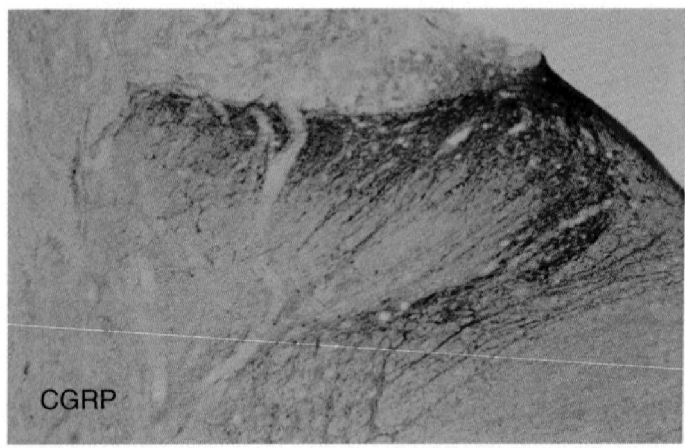

Figure 8.5 Calcitonin gene–related peptide (CGRP) is a good marker of the population of primary afferent nerve terminals innervating the dorsal horn.

the population of these peptides in the dorsal horn. Other neurotransmitters and neuromodulators are discussed more thoroughly in a subsequent chapter.

Nociceptive primary afferent endings contain small, round, clear glutamate containing vesicles[37] for synaptic transmission and relay of nociceptive information. Other large, glomerular-type afferent endings typically contain large, densely cored vesicles containing peptides (Fig. 8.6). CGRP receptors have been localized on postsynaptic membranes opposite glomerular, elongated, and dome-shaped synaptic endings in the superficial dorsal horn.[38] The spinal cord–specific modulatory effects of specific neuropeptides such as SP, CGRP, VIP, and cholecystokinin (CCK)[39-41] contribute to enhanced nociception. In high activation states, increased release of glutamate and increased activation of dorsal horn neurons by glutamate, small-molecule activators, and cytokines occurs as in other sites of neural integration. In the spinal cord this generates enhanced nociception, referred to as central sensitization.

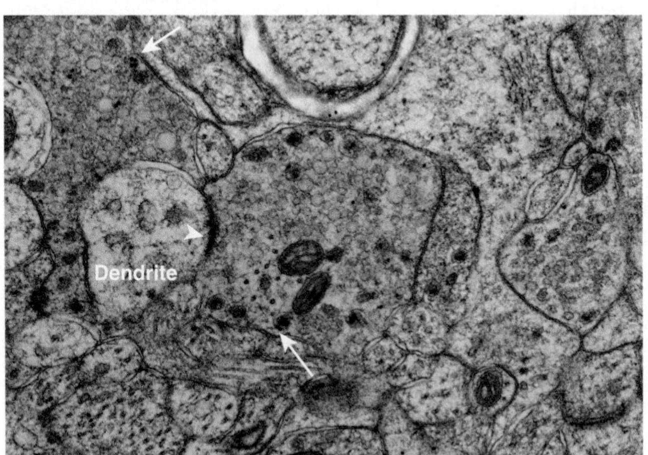

Figure 8.6 Many afferent nerve terminals in the spinal cord dorsal horn terminate in irregular, scalloped endings filled with both clear and dense core vesicles containing neurotransmitter substances. The scalloped endings (colored yellow) are formed as the endings contact numerous small dendrites of spinal neurons, such as the one shown containing the arrowhead. The arrowhead is directed toward a synaptic contact. Several of the dense core vesicles illustrated (arrows) in the terminal endings contain dense gold particles indicating immunolocalization of calcitonin gene–related peptide.

SPINAL CORD AND SPINAL TRIGEMINAL NUCLEUS

SPINAL CORD DORSAL HORN

The noxious input relayed by primary afferent fibers is received by neurons in the dorsal horn of the spinal cord. The dorsal horn contains both local interneurons and the projection neurons that provide the information to higher processing centers in the brain. Signals from nociceptors are relayed across at least one synapse before arriving at higher brain regions, in contrast to the input for non-noxious sensation, which is relayed directly to dorsal column nuclei in the brainstem (see Figs. 8.1 and 8.3).

The gray matter at the core of the spinal cord is a matrix of synaptic terminations and cells that form the first tier of processing and integration of sensory information. The gray matter has been subdivided topographically into 10 laminae by Rexed[42] based on histologic appearance as a result of the distribution of neuronal cells and axons (Fig. 8.7; see also Fig 8.4 and Paxinos[43]). The gray matter of the dorsal horn includes laminae I to VI. Some cells in deeper laminae (VII and X) also relay nociceptive information to the brainstem.

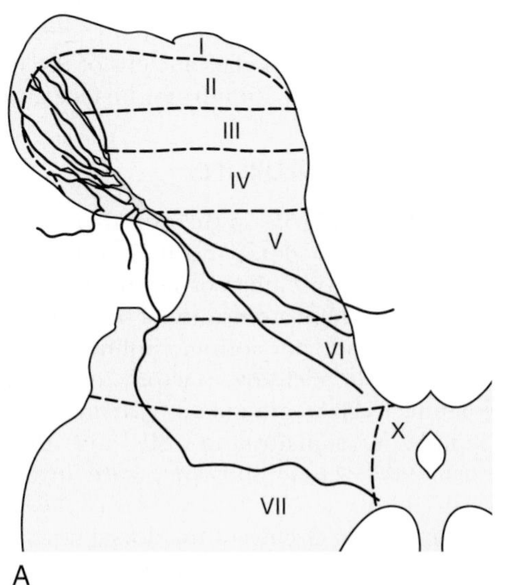

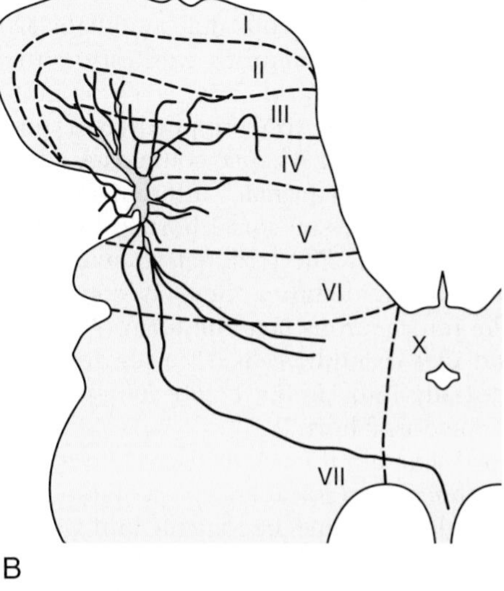

Figure 8.7 Spinal cord cells that were physiologically characterized were filled with a stainable dye and reconstructed over many spinal cord slices to provide details of their dendritic arborization. The cell in **A** was characterized as a high-threshold cell since it responded to intense stimulation in the digit of the hind limb. The cell body is situated in lamina IV, and its dendrites extend into all laminae. Dendrites extend almost a millimeter in the rostrocaudal direction. Its axon bifurcates to cross the midline ventrally in lamina X, as well as passing into the dorsal column. The cell in **B** was characterized as a "wide-dynamic range cell" responding to a broader range of cutaneous input. The cell body is situated in lamina V, and its dendrites extend radially in all directions, including 1.2 mm in the rostrocaudal direction. The axon is seen crossing the midline in lamina X. The dashed lines and Roman numerals indicate Rexed's laminae.

Laminae VII to IX and lamina X are involved in somatic and autonomic motor function, respectively.

The white matter encasing the gray matter is composed of ascending and descending fiber bundles traveling longitudinally and connecting the spinal cord and the brain. Many of the axons are ensheathed in myelin formed by oligodendroglia. These myelin-producing glial cells are unique to the CNS. Other glial cells in the CNS include astrocytes and microglia.

Most of the primary afferent endings carrying nociceptive information heavily innervate the superficial dorsal horn of the spinal cord (laminae I and II) (see Figs. 8.4 and 8.5). Somatic nociceptor C-fiber afferent endings are distributed rather focally in the spinal cord, mainly to laminae I and II in the same and adjacent segments, whereas visceral C-fiber afferents can extend for more than five segments before they terminate widely distributed in laminae I, II, V, and X ipsilaterally, as well as in laminae V and X contralaterally[44-46] (see Fig. 8.4). Cutaneous Aδ mechanical nociceptors terminate in the ipsilateral laminae I and V, and they may also have endings in lamina X and the contralateral dorsal horn.[47] Noxious cutaneous input is relayed by lamina I, IV, and V projection neurons as the crossed spinothalamic tract (STT) pathway traveling in the lateral and ventrolateral white matter en route to the VPL and posterior thalamus.[2,48-52]

In addition to afferent endings, fiber terminations of the descending pathways and local interneurons also heavily innervate the superficial dorsal horn, thus adding to the dense crescent of terminal endings observed when stained immunocytochemically for many neurotransmitters and receptors.

The outer marginal layer, or lamina I, contains nets of spiny dendrites of cells that are longitudinally arranged along the length of the cord. Many of the cells are interneurons, but there are also lamina I cells that send axonal projection to the brainstem, thalamus, and hypothalamus (for review see Willis and Westlund[53]).

Lamina II, or the substantia gelatinosa, contains both excitatory and inhibitory interneurons that modulate projection neurons. Lamina II interneurons synthesize either inhibitory or excitatory neurotransmitters, such as glutamate and γ-aminobutyric acid (GABA), respectively. Typical of lamina II are large glomerular synaptic complexes, sometimes referred to as scalloped primary afferent endings, that contact multiple dendrites of dorsal horn cells simultaneously[19,54-57] (see Fig. 8.6). The terminals contain large dense-core vesicles, which identifies them as containing neuropeptides. The interneurons take the form of stalked (limiting) cells and islet (central) cells,[58-60] with dendrites extending both dorsally into lamina I and ventrally into deeper laminae of the dorsal horn.

Laminae III and IV contain interneurons and large projection neurons of the spinocervical and postsynaptic dorsal column pathways that relay mechanotactile and visceral nociceptive information, respectively. The deeper laminae IV to VI contain interneurons and nociceptive projection neurons that distribute nociceptive input to the brainstem, thalamus, and hypothalamus. The projections of these cells form the spinoreticular, spinothalamic, and spinohypothalamic tracts. The dendrites of the interneurons and projection neurons in deeper laminae are oriented radially and flattened and resemble slabs stacked in the spinal cord. The dendrites of identified STT cells can extend through all laminae dorsolaterally and may extend over several millimeters in the rostrocaudal direction.[61,62]

The central region of the spinal cord is a visceral nociceptive and autonomic processing area, including lamina X and adjacent parts of laminae III, IV, V, VII, and VIII. This region contains second-order projection neurons that transmit information about visceral and somatic pain in the body core, in addition to interneurons and neurons with autonomic-related functions. These cells are "silent" neurons and thus have been studied significantly less than other spinal cord neurons. In fact, the early intermediate gene product c-Fos in cells in the deeper laminae only appears after noxious visceral and prolonged pain states.[63] The visceral nociceptive projection cells are postsynaptic dorsal column, spinoreticular (ventromedial and ventrolateral medulla, raphe, locus coeruleus, periaqueductal gray [PAG]), spinoparabrachial, spinoamygdalar, spinothalamic (parafascicular and central lateral), and spinohypothalamic projection neurons.[64-70] These are the cells of origin of the medial pain pathways that ascend to higher brain levels through routes separate and parallel to those of the lateral pain pathway originating from lamina I, IV, and V STT neurons.[71-77] Their axonal projections and relay neurons innervate the brainstem core and the medial and intralaminar thalamus rather than the ventrobasal thalamus en route to the limbic and insular cortices (anterior cingulate and medial frontal cortices). The nociceptive information delivered ultimately has an impact on motivational, affective, and illness responses.

Incoming sensory information received from the head, neck, and dura arrives via afferent fibers from the trigeminal nerve. The terminal distribution in the dorsal horn of the spinal trigeminal nucleus in the caudal medulla is in a position equivalent to the spinal cord dorsal horn and appears very similar when stained for peptides. Glutamate and glutaminase have been found in spinal trigeminal neurons.[78] The projection neurons of the spinal trigeminal nucleus terminate in the ventromedial nucleus of the thalamus and relay nociceptive information from the face and dura.

SPINAL INTERNEURONS

Most of the neurons in the dorsal horn are interneurons.[79] Neurons in the dorsal horn have been found to contain any of a large number of neuroactive substances that are presumably neurotransmitters or modulators. These substances include adenosine, choline acetyltransferase, CCK, corticotropin-releasing factor, dynorphin, enkephalin, galanin, GABA, glutamate, glycine, neurotensin, neuropeptide Y, somatostatin, SP, and thyrotropin-releasing hormone.[20] These substances are involved in excitatory or inhibitory modulation of nociceptive processing by the interneuronal circuits of the dorsal horn.

Inhibition of spinal transmission, by non-noxious mechanical stimulation, for example, can occur through activation of either the segmental or supraspinal circuitries. Events that can inhibit nociceptive transmission can occur by reducing release of neurotransmitters from nociceptor terminals at the dorsal horn. Even though physiologists have conveniently explained "surround"-type inhibition of dorsal horn synaptic transmission in terms of dorsal horn axo-axonic synaptic transmission, only a few anatomic figures of this type have been described for the dorsal horn.[60,80,81] Rather, the anatomic arrangement of synapses for the gate theory of pain proposed by Melzack and Wall[82] is probably mediated through axodendritic arrangements of CGRP primary afferent terminals innervating the dendrites of GABA interneurons in lamina II and reciprocal interactions. Fine myelinated and unmyelinated CGRP-labeled afferent fibers are observed synapsing with GABAergic dendritic profiles.[81] GABA interneurons are primarily the islet cells,[59] which are also found in laminae I and III and have been stained for another inhibitory amino acid, glycine.[48] GABA interneurons are uniquely qualified to provide the "presynaptic" inhibition of nociceptive input either through contacts provided by their dendrites back onto CGRP primary afferent endings, through dendro-axonal contacts back onto primary afferent endings, or onto other dorsal horn neurons. Other inhibitory neurons in the dorsal horn contain dynorphin and glycine. Likewise, an interposed excitatory interneuron, such as one containing glutamate, would provide an excitatory boost to spinal nociceptive processing. Interestingly, neurons in lamina II, the substantia gelatinosa, do not respond to release of SP since they lack neurokinin 1 (NK1 or SP) receptors.[83] SP terminal endings are located on nociceptive projection cells in both lamina I and the deep dorsal horn, including lamina I cells with NK1 receptors that rapidly internalize the receptors on nociceptive stimulation.[84,85]

In the case of intense or prolonged nociceptive stimulation, the same anatomic arrangement of the dorsal horn circuitry providing "presynaptic inhibition" by GABA interneurons can override the inhibition and result in sensitization.[86,87] Prolonged membrane hyperpolarization evokes a secondary role of $GABA_B$ receptors that changes their role from inhibition to excitation by altering the membrane conductance of central primary afferent terminals. This results in diminished presynaptic inhibition and depolarization of the afferent nerve terminal endings themselves, which generates an action potential that travels back out the afferent nerve toward the periphery. These "dorsal root reflexes" release neurotransmitters such as glutamate and peptides from the axonal terminals into the damaged tissue and allow increased release of transmitter at the central terminals in the dorsal horn. This sets up a reverberating positive feedback loop that amplifies nociceptive input and results in both peripheral and central sensitization, which can promote the establishment of chronic pain.

Thus, nociceptive information entering the spinal cord dorsal horn is modulated by both excitatory and inhibitory influences at the periphery and at the level of the spinal cord before being relayed by projection neurons to higher centers. Modulation occurs not only through influences of the primary afferent nerve on the local interneuronal circuitry but also through the input provided to projection neurons by descending input from the brainstem. This modulatory input probably also involves the spinal interneuronal circuitry.

PROJECTION NEURONS

Several types of projection neurons in lamina I have been described by Lima and Coimbra that send their axon rostrally to the brainstem.[88-91] These cell types include fusiform (spindle-shaped), multipolar, flattened, and pyramidal neurons. Different subsets of these cells project their axons to the nucleus of the solitary tract; to the dorsal and lateral reticular nuclei in the medulla, pons, and midbrain; and to the thalamus. Neurons of the same morphologic types express SP, enkephalin, dynorphin, or GABA,[92] although some of the cells may have been interneurons. Three morphologic types of lamina I STT cells have been described in cats and monkeys: fusiform, pyramidal, and multipolar.[93,94] Evidence has been provided that the fusiform and multipolar STT cells are nociceptive whereas the pyramidal STT cells are thermoreceptive.[95] Consistent with this finding, most fusiform and multipolar lamina I STT neurons express NK1 receptors and most pyramidal STT cells do not.[83,96]

The projection cells that are found in deeper laminae of the dorsal horn are typically large, multipolar neurons with extensive dendritic arborization. The dendrites of deep projection cells tend to arborize radially in the spinal cord dorsal horn, in contrast to lamina I projection cells, whose dendrites are longitudinally distributed along the dorsal surface of the spinal cord gray matter such that in the coronal plane they are barely visible. A radial dendrite arrangement provides for the integration of convergent input encoded by STT cells in the deeper laminae, as opposed to the superficial projection neurons, which are situated to have ready access to specific incoming nociceptive and thermal input directly via the afferent nerve fibers. Some STT cells in deeper laminae do have dendrites that extend dorsally into laminae I and II (see Fig. 8.7). These STT cells receive direct synaptic connections from the terminals of nociceptors ending in the superficial dorsal horn and are particularly responsive to "high-threshold" input.[52,97,98] Other STT cells identified as "wide–dynamic range" cells respond to a variety of mechanical, thermal, and nociceptive input. They have dendrites that extend chiefly in the ventral direction and receive convergent input from afferents supplying both deep somatic and visceral structures.

The SST and interneuronal cells in the dorsal horn have been shown to express the early intermediate gene activation marker c-Fos in many pain models.

It is reported that brief nociceptive stimulation causes activation of c-Fos in laminae I, IV, and V whereas sustained nociceptive stimulation is needed to activate c-Fos in laminae III, V, VII, and X, as in models of joint and visceral inflammation.[63] The STT neurons contain glutamate,[99] and some also contain peptides such as SP, enkephalin, dynorphin, or VIP.[100,101] Lamina X STT cells have been shown to contain CCK, bombesin, galanin, or any combination of these substances.[102,103] Synapses found on the cell bodies of STT neurons in deep layers of the dorsal horn have been shown to contain glutamate, GABA, glycine, SP, CGRP, vasopressin, norepinephrine, or serotonin,[62,84,103-109] thus indicating that these STT cells are affected by both excitatory and inhibitory events associated with nociceptive processing. The dorsally directed dendrites of many deep dorsal horn neurons contain NK1 (SP) receptors,[83] and these are internalized following the presumably painful stimulation occurring during inflammation.[110] Ultrastructural studies have revealed postsynaptic localization of the glutamate receptor subunits *N*-methyl-D-aspartate (NMDA) R1, α-amino-3-hydroxy-5-methyl-4-isoxazolepropionate (AMPA)

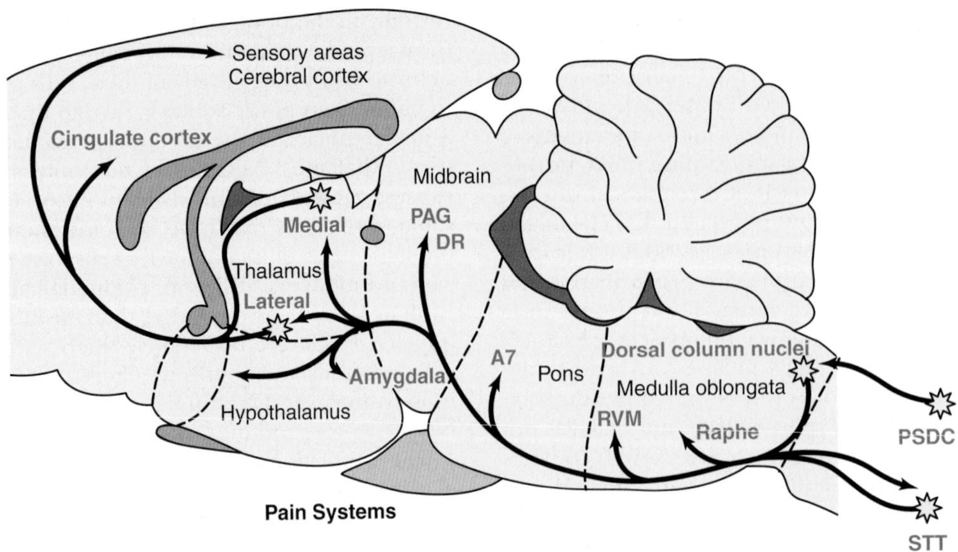

Figure 8.8 Pain systems include the spinothalamic tract and the postsynaptic dorsal column pathways. These parallel pain systems ascending from the spinal cord converge to course through the brainstem as the spinothalamic tract and the medial lemniscus. Although the primary termination site for sensory integration is the thalamus, abundant collateral terminations are provided to integration sites throughout the brainstem. The ventral posterolateral nucleus of the thalamus is the principal somatosensory relay for information provided to the sensory areas of the cerebral cortex for localization of pain sensation. The medial and intermediate portions of the thalamus project to the anterior cingulate and frontal cortex, respectively, and provide input relevant to the affective responses to pain. Autonomic adjustments occur in response to the input provided to the hypothalamus. A7, noradrenergic cell group; DR, dorsal raphe; PAG, periaqueductal gray; PSDC, postsynaptic dorsal column cell; RVM, rostral ventromedial medulla; STT, spinothalamic tract cell.

GluR1 and GluR2/3, and metabotropic mGluR1 and mGluR2/3 associated with terminals in contact with identified STT neurons.[111,112] NMDA R1 and AMPA GluR2/3 receptors were also localized presynaptically on terminals contacting STT neurons.

CENTRAL ASCENDING PATHWAYS

Nociceptive transmission neurons in the spinal cord send axonal fiber projections to the many sensory-processing regions in the brain, including the dorsal column nuclei, dorsal and ventral medullary reticular formation, dorsolateral pontine locus coeruleus/parabrachial region, midbrain PAG, medial and lateral thalamus, anterior pretectal nucleus, hypothalamus, and amygdala (Fig. 8.8; see also Fig. 8.1). Anterograde tract tracing studies demonstrate the second-order ascending pathways crossing to the opposite side as they project through the spinal cord white matter to the brainstem as the spinoreticular, spinoparabrachial, spinoamygdalar, and spinohypothalamic tracts.[67,69,70] These tracts terminate bilaterally on reaching several specific brainstem levels. Nonoverlapping but parallel medial and lateral pain pathways are described.[67,69-77] The lateral pain pathway, the STT, transmits site-specific (discriminative) information about the location, quality, and intensity of noxious input to the lateral thalamus and then to the primary (SI) and secondary (SII) somatosensory cortices. The medial pain system transmits nociceptive information to the midline brainstem, hypothalamus, amygdala, and medial and intralaminar thalamus, which interact with limbic structures, including the anterior cingulate cortex, to activate affective, motivational, and autonomic responses to pain. Medial pain pathways include the spinoamygdalar, spinohypothalamic, medial spinothalamic, and spinoreticular pathways and connections to the anterior cingulate and prefrontal and insular limbic cortices.

SPINOTHALAMIC TRACT

STT neurons are the primary relay cells providing nociceptive input from the spinal cord to the thalamus, a major integration site for sensory information. Tactile information from the same body region converges on the same thalamic neurons. This point-to-point reception of information in the lateral thalamus provides somatotopic encoding for specific localization of the input onto the cortical representation of the specific body region.[112] This provides the ability to precisely locate the origin of the nociceptive input. The STT cells receiving noxious cutaneous and temperature input are largely situated in lamina I and the lateral half of the neck of the dorsal horn in laminae IV and V.[48,49,51,52] Other STT neurons are scattered throughout the deep dorsal horn and intermediate region (including lamina X[113]) and even in lamina VII of the ventral horn. Many of the STT cells in deeper laminae receive both cutaneous and visceral nociceptive information.[114]

The axons of STT cells cross the midline of the spinal cord in the anterior white commissure ventral to the central canal[52] (see Figs. 8.1, 8.3, and 8.7) and ascend primarily in the contralateral (opposite) white matter in the lateral and ventro(antero)lateral funiculi.[115] The axons of STT cells terminate laterally in the posterior ventrobasal thalamic complex (VPL, ventral posterior inferior) or medially in the medial and intralaminar thalamus (subparafascicular, centrolateral [CL], and other nuclei of the thalamus). Lamina I STT neurons send their axonal projections in the middle of the lateral funiculus to terminate in the posterior part of the ventral medial nucleus of the thalamus, as well as in the ventral posterior and medial dorsal nuclei.[116] Early electrophysiologic studies reported parallel processing of nociceptive input in the cortex arising from the ventrobasal thalamus to sensory (SI, SII), cingulate, and insular cortices, including input from the VPL and CL, and tooth pulp input from the ventromedial nuclei of the thalamus.[117-119] Clear visualization of activation in cortical sites is now available with functional magnetic resonance imaging (fMRI)[120] and is reviewed in a later chapter.

POSTSYNAPTIC DORSAL COLUMN PATHWAY

The spinal cord dorsal column contains ascending axons of the postsynaptic dorsal column neurons, in addition to the first-order ascending axons of primary afferent neurons relaying touch, pressure, and vibratory sensation. These second-order projection neurons are responsive to noxious visceral input. The cell bodies of many of these cells are located in laminae III and IV[121] but have also been reported in lamina X.[65,67] The postsynaptic dorsal column cell neurons may respond to noxious visceral stimulation. These cells send a direct projection uncrossed to the dorsal column nuclei in the dorsal medulla. Sacral lamina X neurons have axons traveling near the dorsal column midline septum and, from the thoracic spinal level axons, travel along the intermediate septum of the dorsal column and then travel with the crossed third-order medial lemniscal fibers to the thalamus. Cells in the sacral spinal levels terminate in the gracile nucleus, and cells in the thoracic spinal levels terminate in both the gracile and cuneate nuclei. Postsynaptic dorsal column neurons in lamina X transmit visceral nociceptive information to the thalamus and converge on some of the same thalamic cells receiving nociceptive information from the skin and other somatic structures[66,68,122,123] (see Figs. 8.1 and 8.7).

SPINORETICULAR PATHWAYS

Many projection axons from the spinal cord also provide direct and collateral innervation to brainstem regions involved in pain-related activities, including descending modulation of pain, autonomic responsiveness, alerting response, escape response, and limbic and cortical activation. Collectively, these neurons are referred to as the spinoreticular system (see Figs. 8.1 and 8.8). These integrative regions modulate and balance excitatory and inhibitory neuronal influences on nociception through reciprocal higher brain connectivity, which ultimately determines the pain state.[53,76]

A dorsal spinomedullary pathway arises from cells in laminae I, IV, and X and terminates bilaterally in the subnucleus reticularis dorsalis (SRD) of the dorsal medullary reticular formation, which is located just ventral to the cuneate and solitary nuclei of the dorsal medulla.[124] This nucleus is a brainstem site active in balancing descending inhibition and facilitation of nociceptive processes. The diffuse noxious inhibitory controls (DNICs) inhibiting wide–dynamic range neurons in the spinal cord competing with afferent input are dependent on a supraspinal loop through the SRD and a descending pathway.[125,126] Projections from this region innervate the contralateral somatosensory, motor, limbic, and insular cortices and the PAG, pons, cerebellum, trigeminal, and other brainstem nuclei[127] Connections to the anterior cingulate gyrus participate in descending facilitatory modulation of pain.[128]

Major ascending axonal projections relaying information about pain pass laterally through the brainstem but have collateral terminations in the reticular formation of the ventrolateral medulla,[90,129,130] the rostral ventromedial medulla (RVM) (nucleus gigantocellularis pars alpha and nucleus raphe magnus [NRM]). The midline raphe nuclei contain serotonergic and nonserotonergic neurons with descending projections to the spinal cord.[131] The direct spinal projection pathway also traverses brainstem regions containing catecholaminergic neurons, including the C1, A1, A2, A5, A6, and A7 regions of both the pons and medulla.[132] The catecholaminergic neurons of the brainstem are involved in diverse functions, including modulation of pain, stress responses, arousal, and learning. The connectivity described between the ventromedial medulla and the catecholamine cells of the pons[133,134] and the anterior cingulate gyrus,[128] as well as between brainstem catecholaminergic cells and the thalamus[74] and anterior cingulate cortex,[75] assists in coordination of descending and facilitatory influences on pain perception and affective and stress responses.

Many of the spinal axonal projections terminate in the parabrachial region. Small injections of retrograde tracer into the parabrachial nucleus confirm that this nucleus receives projections primarily from lamina I nociceptive neurons[135] and directly projects to the PAG, amygdala, and ventrobasal thalamus.[136,137] Involvement in visceral nociceptive processing is reported for the parabrachial nucleus.[138]

Ascending pathways relaying nociceptive information also terminate in the PAG and midline midbrain reticular formation.[106,132,139-142] The PAG and the raphe magnus are major sources of input driving the descending inhibition and facilitation that are known to affect the perception of pain. Direct neuronal projections from the central region of the spinal cord to the midline brainstem nuclei, including the rostral ventromedial nucleus of the medulla and the midbrain PAG and raphe magnus, have been described as well.[67]

Another termination site innervated directly by ascending pathways from the spinal cord and from the dorsal column nuclei is the anterior pretectal nucleus.[143] The anterior pretectal nucleus is thought to be an important source of descending inhibition of nociceptive pathways. Evidence suggests that it sends axons to catecholaminergic neurons of the parabrachial region.[144]

SPINOHYPOTHALAMIC, LIMBIC, AND CORTICAL CONNECTIONS

Pain is often accompanied by motivational-affective responses, including suffering, anxiety, increased attention and arousal, increased heart rate and blood pressure, and changes in endocrine and autonomic responses. The neural structures that relay these changes are likely to be parallel to those relaying information localizing the source of the noxious input on the body map. An interesting hypothesis is that the medial and lateral pain pathways provide affective and epicritic (discriminative) pain sensation, respectively. The ventrolateral STT clearly provides information for specific discrimination of pain and temperature, somatotopic localization, and the quality and intensity coding of cutaneous pain. Some of the pathways in unique positions to assume a role in affective pain awareness would include the spinoamygdalar pathway, spinal pathways relaying visceral pain through the postsynaptic medial dorsal column route, and ventromedial projections to midline structures, including the RVM, PAG, hypothalamus, and CL and medial thalamus.[67] Interestingly, some thalamic cells in the CL nucleus are activated only by noxious visceral stimulation.[145] CL and medial thalamic projections to the anterior cingulate and frontal cortices, respectively, have been described.[146] The thalamic connections to the somatosensory (SI, SII) cortices have not been well studied.

Spinohypothalamic and spinoamygdalar pathways have been described that may be involved in autonomic and affective responses to pain.[147-149] The ascending axonal projections of these pathways arise primarily from spinal cord laminae I and X, as well as from the lateral reticulated region of the spinal cord. Synapses are made in the lateral hypothalamus and the central nucleus of the amygdala. Both these regions are also involved in antinociceptive actions, as well as in autonomic and affective responses to nociceptive input through connections with the medial thalamus and other parts of the limbic system.

The ascending axonal projections of these pathways arise primarily from spinal cord lamina I and from deep spinal laminae (VII, VIII, and X). Spinal projections to the ventrolateral medulla are conveniently located to relay to the paraventricular nucleus of the hypothalamus,[150] amygdala,[151] and medial preoptic region.[152] A direct route to the medial thalamus, amygdala, and spinal-parabrachial-amygdalar pathways[153,154] is clearly involved. A spinal-reticular-thalamic-cortical pathway was originally proposed as a projection to the forebrain that relays information about painful input, presumably for subjective interpretation based on known anatomic projections of the reticular formation to higher brain centers.[155] Relays to insular cortical structures have also been described.

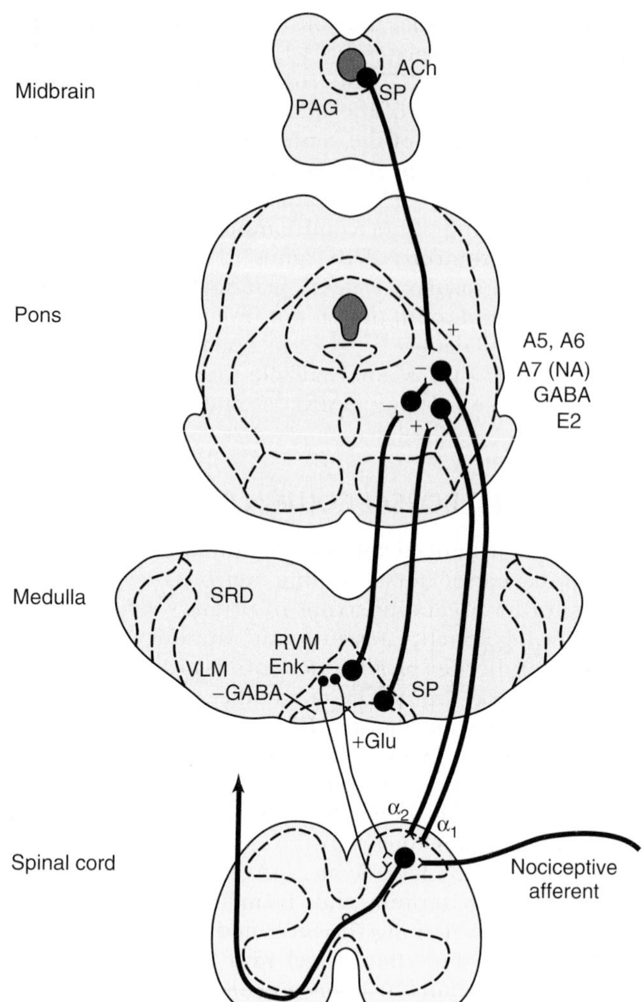

Figure 8.9 Multiple integration sites in the brainstem receive nociceptive input from the ascending pain systems. Complex brainstem circuitry provides both descending inhibitory and excitatory alterations of nociceptive responses at the level of the spinal cord. Cells are situated side by side in the rostral ventromedial medulla (RVM) that impose either excitatory or inhibitory influence. Cells in the RVM are both serotonergic (5-hydroxytryptamine) and nonserotonergic. They provide both a direct descending pathway to the spinal cord and a major input to the dorsolateral pons. The A5 to A7 noradrenergic (NA) cell groups in the dorsolateral pons provide major inhibitory feedback to the spinal cord. The periaqueductal gray (PAG) and the anterior pretectal nuclei provide inhibitory input to the spinal cord through connections with descending pathways from the dorsolateral pons. Specific neurotransmitters within brainstem regions are noted, as are specific receptors having an impact on nociception in the spinal cord dorsal horn. ACh, acetylcholine; E2, estrogen receptor 2; Enk, enkephalin; GABA, γ-aminobutyric acid; Glu, glutamate; SRD, subnucleus reticularis dorsalis; SP, substance P; VLM, ventrolateral medulla.

DESCENDING PATHWAYS MODULATING PAIN

Descending inhibition of spinal nociceptive processes was initially described in behavioral experiments in which electrical stimulation of the PAG resulted in antinociception.[156] The antinociception was proposed, based on behavioral, electrophysiologic, and morphologic studies, to occur through a PAG relay to the RVM and then to the spinal cord[157-166] (also see reviews[139,167-169]). Subsequent findings suggest that the process is mediated through more complicated circuitry (Fig. 8.9). It is now known that both inhibitory and excitatory influences on spinal cord nociceptive processing occur after the activation of recurrent loops through the brainstem by ascending pathways from the spinal cord. Extensive behavioral and electrophysiologic studies have found that bulbospinal facilitatory projections and in particular those descending from the RVM promote tactile and thermal hyperesthesia.[170-173] The RVM is responsible for the maintenance, although not the initiation, of neuropathic central[174-176] and visceral pain.[177,178] The RVM is composed of the midline raphe system and the adjacent ventral reticular formation. The raphe-spinal pathway is largely, but not entirely serotonergic.[131,179,180] The component that originates from the NRM descending in the dorsolateral funiculus is primarily associated with inhibitory control, and a ventrolateral descending pathway is typically thought to exert facilitatory control of nociceptive responses. Excitatory SP and inhibitory enkephalinergic connections between the NRM and noradrenergic neurons of the dorsolateral pons are a major component of the descending control system that promotes both facilitatory and inhibitory influences modulating pain.[133,181] An additional supraspinal loop from the dorsal horn to the dorsal reticular nucleus and back to the dorsal horn also mediates both descending inhibition and facilitation.

Descending noradrenergic input to the spinal cord from the dorsolateral pons has been shown to limit responses to acute noxious stimulation[137]; however, elimination of the A6 locus coeruleus nucleus provides facilitation in the case of long-term nociceptive activation.[182] The largest percentage of spinally projecting noradrenergic neurons has been identified in the locus coeruleus, subcoeruleus, parabrachial, and Kölliker-Fuse nuclei.[183-185] The noradrenergic A5 cell group in the ventrolateral pons/medulla and the adrenergic neurons of the ventrolateral medulla also send axonal projections to influence nociception in the spinal cord and thalamus as well.[74,186]

The PAG in the midbrain makes descending connections not only with the RVM[187] but also with the noradrenergic system of the dorsolateral pons.[188] A net inhibition of spinal nociceptive processing is initiated from the PAG through glutamate and SP input to these brainstem regions with major descending axonal projections. The cholinergic neuronal system is another major reticular system of the midbrain and other portions of the brainstem that provides descending influence on nociception. The cholinergic mechanisms can reduce nociception, as well as potentiate opiate analgesia.[189,190] These analgesic actions may be mediated through presynaptic terminations of laminae III to V cholinergic interneurons, which are reported to synapse directly onto primary sensory endings.[191]

The anterior pretectal nucleus has also been associated with inhibition of nociceptive somatosensory function.[143] The anterior pretectal region evokes antinociceptive responses in the tail flick, formalin, and paw pressure tests. However, this region has minor direct input from laminae I and X in the spinal cord, and direct innervation of the spinal cord by the anterior pretectal nucleus has not been reported. Indications are that these effects are mediated through anatomic connectivity with the dorsolateral pontine pathways.

Many hypothalamic nuclei, including those in the lateral hypothalamus, have descending connections with the PAG.[192-194] The hypothalamic input to the PAG is topographic, with particular hypothalamic nuclei linked with particular regions of the PAG. Hypothalamic axons form the largest input to the PAG.[194]

Several forebrain areas with descending projections have an influence on nociception, including the central nucleus of the amygdala, the SI cortex, and many parts of the limbic cortex.[192,195] Limbic regions include the anterior cingulate gyrus, the infralimbic and prelimbic cortices medially, the precentral medial cortex, and laterally the anterior and posterior insular cortices and the perirhinal cortex.

A simplified schema of the supraspinal circuitry of the descending control systems imposing facilitatory and inhibitory modulation of nociceptive processing is shown in Figure 8.9. Current evidence has shown that descending modulation from higher centers involves the circuitry of the dorsolateral pons to the medial and intralaminar thalamic nuclei.[74] Nociceptive insults, such as nerve damage or tissue inflammation, increase the tone of both modulatory events and shift the balance toward facilitation. Even though increased activation of pain systems and increased descending facilitation predominate during pain states, descending inhibitory systems continue to dampen the increasing nociceptive activation. Conversely, "stress-induced analgesia" would imply a shift in balance favoring activation of the descending inhibitory pathway. In truth, it is the sum of the effects of this complex polysynaptic circuitry that establishes the level of pain intensity perceived.

CENTERS FOR HIGHER PROCESSING OF NOCICEPTION

Specific discriminative input in response to noxious somatic stimulation is received in the VPL nucleus of the thalamus. The midline and intralaminar thalamic CL and parafascicular nuclei receive nondiscriminative visceral nociceptive input. The ventromedial nuclei of the thalamus receive face and tooth pulp input. Early electrophysiologic studies reported parallel processing of nociceptive input from the ventrobasal thalamus to the sensory (SI, SII), cingulate, and insular cortices.[117-119]

Confirmation in humans of the activation of cortical sites reported in animal studies became available with the advent of positron emission tomography and fMRI.[196-206] The studies confirmed brain activation in response to painful input in the human thalamus, SI and SII somatosensory cortices, anterior cingulate gyrus, insula, prefrontal cortex, lentiform nucleus, and cerebellum. The improved resolution of fMRI has made it possible to determine changes imposed by pharmacologic agents on the higher processing of pain, as has been shown for a pancreatitis model persisting 1 week in rats[207] (see Fig. 8.8). The VPL thalamus and SI and SII cortices are known to be somatosensory-processing regions, and evidence from imaging studies is consistent with a sensory-discriminative role of these structures. The anterior cingulate cortex is presumably involved in interpretation of the emotional significance of the painful input by the limbic system,[201] whereas the lentiform nucleus and cerebellum may be involved in the learning of reflexive motor responsiveness to painful input that is necessary to protect the individual. The insula, cerebellum, and frontal cortex may contribute to memory and learning of events related to painful stimuli, such as avoidance behavior based on previous experience.[204] A more detailed discussion of the clinical correlation of these topics is available in other chapters.

KEY POINTS

- Nociceptive nerve endings transduce information about internal and external mechanical, thermal, and chemical stimuli that are noxious, distressing, or damaging. Sensory nerves transmit the information centrally.
- Pain is communicated from nerve endings to the spinal cord, relayed across a synapse in the spinal cord, and then transmitted to brainstem integration sites.
- Spinal cord and spinal trigeminal dorsal horn interneurons provide state-dependent signal modification that either amplifies or inhibits the pain signal before relay of the information to brainstem integration sites.
- Central ascending spinothalamic pathways carry discriminative pain-related information coded for location, intensity, and quality of the noxious input. Axons of lamina I spinothalamic tract neurons cross the midline and ascend in the lateral spinal cord white matter on the opposite side. Spinothalamic tract neurons in deeper laminae send their axons through the ventrolateral spinal white matter on the opposite side and through the ventrolateral brainstem to the primary integrative site for discriminatory sensory information in the ventral posterolateral nucleus of the thalamus.
- Discriminative information about pain is relayed by neurons of the ventral posterolateral thalamus primarily to the primary and secondary somatosensory cortices with connectivity to the motor cortex to plan and execute appropriate escape responses.
- Collateral axons of the ascending spinothalamic tract or direct innervation of other integrative brainstem sites includes the lateral medullary and pontine reticular formation, parabrachial nuclei, periaqueductal gray, hypothalamus, and amygdala. Termination sites suggest that the lateral pain-related pathways have an impact on autonomic regulation, limbic activation, and emotional response, along with the spinoamygdalar pathway.
- Phylogenetically older axonal pathways carrying visceral pain and mechanotactile information from deep tissues arise from neurons in laminae III, VII, VIII, and X. These axons ascend in the dorsal column to innervate the caudal dorsal column nuclei in the midline of the caudal medulla or travel in the ventral white matter midline to innervate the ventral and medial brainstem sites, periaqueductal gray, hypothalamus, amygdala, substantia innominata, nucleus basalis of Meynert, globus pallidus, insular cortex, and medial and intralaminar thalamus. The termination sites suggest that the medial pain-related pathways have an impact on autonomic responses, limbic activation, fear-motivated avoidance, and emotional response, along with the spinoamygdalar and spinoparabrachial pathways.
- Descending input to the spinal cord modulates the primary sensory information to either facilitate or inhibit the sensory signal.
- Descending pathways to the spinal cord that modulate pain include axons originating in the pontine locus coeruleus and medullary reticular formation. These centers are influenced by input from higher brain centers, as well as by incoming spinal sensory transmission.

KEY POINTS—cont'd

- Centers for higher processing have complex integrative connectivity among the cortical, limbic, medial thalamic, hypothalamic, and brainstem sites that has an impact on the awareness of pain, motivational responses to pain, and regulation of autonomic, emotional, and motor responses to pain.
- Functional magnetic resonance imaging provides better information about pain processing in higher brain centers.

SUGGESTED READINGS

Carlton SM, Lamotte CC, Honda CN, et al. Ultrastructural analysis of axosomatic contacts on functionally identified primate spinothalamic tract neurons. *J Comp Neurol.* 1989;281:555-566.

Cliffer KD, Burstein R, Giesler GJ. Distributions of spinothalamic, spinohypothalamic, and spinotelencephalic fibers revealed by anterograde transport of PHA-L in rats. *J Neurosci.* 1991;11:852-868.

Keay KA, Feil K, Gordon BD, et al. Spinal afferents to functionally distinct periaqueductal gray columns in the rat: an anterograde and retrograde tracing study. *J Comp Neurol.* 1997;385:207-229.

Mayer DJ, Wolfe TL, Akil H, et al. Analgesia from electrical stimulation in the brain stem of the rat. *Science.* 1971;174:1351-1354.

Meller ST, Dennis BJ. Afferent projections to the periaqueductal gray in the rabbit. *Neuroscience.* 1986;19:927-964.

Newman HM, Stevens RT, Apkarian AV. Direct spinal projections to limbic and striatal areas: anterograde transport studies from the upper cervical spinal cord and the cervical enlargement in squirrel monkey and rat. *J Comp Neurol.* 1996;365:640-658.

Oliveras JL, Redjemi F, Guilbaud G, et al. Analgesia induced by electrical stimulation of the inferior centralis nucleus of the raphe in the cat. *Pain.* 1975;1:139-145.

Oliveras JL, Woda A, Guilbaud G, et al. Inhibition of the jaw opening reflex by electrical stimulation of the periaqueductal gray matter in the awake, unrestrained cat. *Brain Res.* 1974;72:328-331.

Rees H, Roberts MHT. The anterior pretectal nucleus: a proposed role in sensory processing. *Pain.* 1993;53:121-135.

Ren Y, Lu Y, Yang H, et al. Central lateral thalamic neurons receive noxious visceral mechanical and chemical input in rats. *J Neurophysiol.* 2009;102:244-258.

Reynolds DV. Surgery in the rat during electrical analgesia induced by focal brain stimulation. *Science.* 1969;164:444-445.

Saper CB, Levisohn D. Afferent connections of the median preoptic nucleus in the rat: anatomical evidence for a cardiovascular integrative mechanism in the anteroventral third ventricle. *Brain Res.* 1983;288:21-31.

Sawchenko PE, Swanson LW. The organization of noradrenergic pathways from the brainstem to the paraventricular and supraoptic nuclei in the rat. *Brain Res.* 1982;257:275-325.

Silverman DHS, Munakata JA, Ennes H, et al. Regional cerebral activity in normal and pathological perception of visceral pain. *Gastroenterology.* 1997;112:64-72.

Vera-Portocarrero LP, Xie J, Kowal J, et al. Descending facilitation from the rostral ventromedial medulla maintains visceral pain in rats with experimental pancreatitis. *Gastroenterology.* 2006;130:2155-2164.

Vera-Portocarrero LP, Zhang ET, Ossipov MH, et al. Descending facilitation from the rostral ventromedial medulla maintains nerve injury–induced central sensitization. *Neuroscience.* 2006;140:1311-1320.

Wang CC, Shyu BC. Differential projections from the mediodorsal and centrolateral thalamic nuclei to the frontal cortex in rats. *Brain Res.* 2004;995:226-235.

Zhuo M, Gebhart GF. Facilitation and attenuation of a visceral nociceptive reflex from the rostroventral medulla in the rat. *Gastroenterology.* 2002;122:1007-1019.

The references for this chapter can be found at www.expertconsult.com.

9

A Review of Pain-Processing Pharmacology

Tony L. Yaksh

In the early 1900s, Sir Charles Sherrington designated high-intensity stimuli that signaled a potential injury to the body as being *nociceptive* in character. The application of such stimuli to the body produces a syndrome that includes withdrawal of the affected body part, signs of autonomic activation, and a complex set of behavioral responses that in intact animals include agitation and vocalization. In humans, an unconditioned high-intensity stimulus evokes discrete sensations that have the assigned attribute of being *painful* (e.g., the sensation initiated by picking up a very hot cup of coffee). The reported sensation is referred to the site of stimulation, and the magnitude of the report or response varies with the intensity of the stimulus. Termination of the stimulus before injury results in cessation of the sensation. Accordingly, *nociception* is a descriptor that refers to the physiologic response generated by such high-intensity, potentially tissue-injuring stimuli, whereas *pain* represents the interpretation of that event as a sensation with highly aversive properties. Such stimuli have powerful motivating effects that can support the generation of escape behavior when cued by innocuous stimuli that have previously been paired with a nociceptive stimulus. Thus, a strong shock evokes the nociceptive state (e.g., hypertension). A light paired with that shock would soon become conditionally associated with the shock such that in a short time, it alone can initiate the same profile of nociception.

Should the stimulus be of sufficient magnitude to result in local injury (tissue disruption, plasma extravasation), a pain sensation will persist after removal of the stimulus, and the injury will be accompanied by increased sensitivity to subsequent stimuli applied to the injury site (primary hyperalgesia) and enhanced sensitivity to stimuli applied at sites adjacent to the injury site (e.g., secondary hyperalgesia). Again, as mentioned, these states of enhanced sensation indicate that the non–tissue-injuring stimulus now acquires an aversive property (e.g., warm water on a sunburn).

As an overview, these effects of a high-intensity, tissue-injuring stimulus reflect an initial activation of the primary afferents that project to the dorsal horn of the spinal cord, from which transmitters are released that activate a complex dorsal horn circuitry. Under normal circumstances these spinal neurons respond maximally to input arising from the root projecting to the spinal segments in which the cell lies. However, even though these afferents primarily activate these homosegmental neurons, they also send collaterals rostrally and caudally up to several spinal segments away, where they make synaptic contact with neurons in adjacent segments (heterosegmental). These distal neurons are less efficiently activated than the homosegmental cells (and may not be activated sufficiently to generate an action potential), but together these homosegmental and heterosegmental cells form the real or potential dimension of the dermatome of that spinal segment. As will be shown later, if the *excitability* of these higher-order spinal heterosegmental neurons is increased, cells that were not activated by a given input now become depolarized, and the size of the dermatome of a given segment will be increased. These dorsal horn neurons then project by long tracts in the ventrolateral quadrant either (1) directly to diencephalic sites (e.g., thalamus, hypothalamus) or (2) indirectly through an intermediate synapse on neurons in the medulla, pons, or mesencephalon, which then project to a variety of diencephalic and limbic forebrain sites. The anatomic details of these pathways have previously been discussed (see Chapter 8).

In general, the processes leading to a pain state secondary to a high-intensity peripheral stimulus reflect the frequency of traffic that appears in these spinofugal pathways. Activity in the spinofugal systems is primarily dependent on the intensity of the afferent stimulus, but as will be made evident, a variety of systems serve to increase the gain of the spinal input-output function and to depress this gain. In the first case, we would anticipate that there would be an increased pain sensation associated with any given stimulus, whereas in the second case, the pain sensation produced by a given stimulus would be diminished. This dynamic property of the input-output systems represents an important characteristic of systems that process nociceptive stimuli. In the following sections we wish to consider the transmitter pharmacology that defines these synaptic linkages.

PRIMARY AFFERENT SIGNALING

ACUTE STIMULATION

The systems underlying this acute psychophysical experience begin with the primary sensory neuron, the afferent fiber. It possesses several intrinsic attributes:

1. In the absence of a stimulus, most primary afferents show little if any ongoing activity.
2. Activity in these afferents is initiated by a variety of physical or chemical stimuli, which respectively activate specific populations of primary afferents.
3. The nature of the sensory information encoded by a given primary afferent is dependent on the properties of the transduction channels or receptors that are expressed on the terminals of that sensory axon.

4. The frequency of firing in these afferents generated by a particular stimulus varies in a monotonic fashion with the intensity of the stimulus (e.g., temperature for a thermal-sensitive afferent). Thus, the specific population of primary afferents activated and the frequency of discharge encode the intensity of the message.
5. Sensory afferents are morphologically described as Aβ, which are large, myelinated, fast-conducting axons that are typically activated by low-intensity mechanical stimuli; Aδ, smaller, myelinated, fast-conducting afferents with subpopulations that preferentially respond to thermal or mechanical, low- or high-threshold stimuli; and C, small, unmyelinated, very slowly conducting afferents that are activated by high-intensity thermal or mechanical stimuli (or both). A myelinated afferent axon typically displays specialized terminals that are particularly sensitive to mechanical distortion, which leads to a local increase in sodium current that depolarizes the axon. Unmyelinated afferent axons typically show "free nerve endings"; that is, they display no evident morphologic specialization. However, these terminals express a variety of specific transducer channels that are sensitive to specific stimuli and serve to increasingly depolarize the afferent terminal as stimulus intensity rises. When activated by the appropriate stimulus, these channels in turn activate voltage-sensitive sodium (Na_v) channels that pass Na^+ and initiate action potentials. As indicated in Figure 9.1, some of these channels that transduce a physical stimulus may also be activated by a variety of chemicals. In this case, these chemicals produce a sensation that reflects the physical stimulus that is transduced by that channel (e.g., the transient receptor potential vanilloid-1 [TRPV1] receptor is activated by capsaicin, which produces a painful burning sensation, whereas menthol activates the TRPM8 cold receptor and initiates the sensation of a low temperature).

TISSUE-INJURING STIMULI

High-intensity stimuli may result in local tissue injury. Such injury will lead to cellular disruption, injury to local vascular integrity and subsequent plasma extravasation, and migration of inflammatory cells such as macrophages and neutrophils. These events give rise to the release of a variety of active factors (Box 9.1). These products act through eponymous receptors that are present on the terminals of many unmyelinated axons. Activation of these receptors serves to initiate two events: (1) depolarization of the terminal leading to discharge of the afferent, with the frequency of activation being dependent on concentration, and (2) activation of intraterminal processes (phosphorylation of local membrane channels), which sensitizes the terminal such that the degree of depolarization for a given stimulus is enhanced. Such effects yield "spontaneous afferent activity" and an enhanced response to a second stimulus applied to the site of injury. These changes in the milieu of the peripheral terminal occur secondary to tissue damage and the accompanying extravasation of plasma as a result of increased permeability of the capillary wall (see Box 9.1). These events are responsible for the "triple response": reddening at the site of the stimulus (reflecting local arterial dilation), local edema (increased capillary permeability), and a regional reduction in the magnitude of the stimulus required to elicit a pain response (i.e., hyperalgesia).

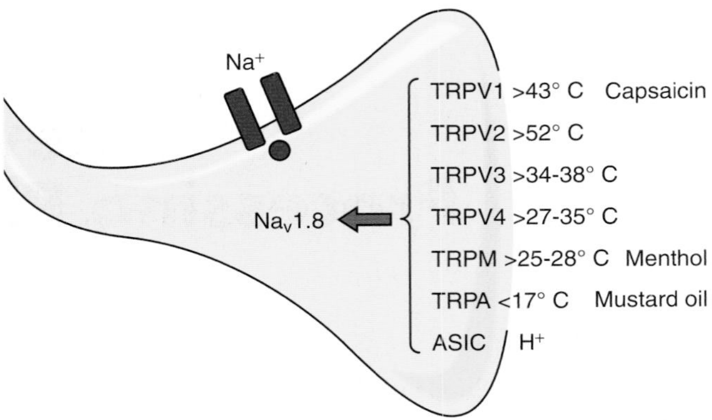

Figure 9.1 Transducer channels on a small afferent terminal. Optimal stimulus intensities for activating channels and various chemicals that also activate these channels are indicated. Different terminals express different combinations of channels, which would define the response properties of that afferent. Channel activation leads to activation of voltage-sensitive sodium (Na_v) channels. The $Na_v1.8$ subtype of channels is frequently present only in unmyelinated axons (C fibers). ASIC, acid-sensing ion channel; TRP, transient receptor potential.

NERVE INJURY AS A STIMULUS

Following nerve injury arising from a variety of insults, the organisms will frequently display the development of a variety of highly aversive "spontaneous" sensations over time. These sensations are believed to arise in part from afferent traffic. Sensory axons typically display little spontaneous activity in the absence of a stimulus. This is particularly true for small, high-threshold afferents. However, after a chemical, immune, or mechanical injury to the nerve, afferent axons exhibit (1) an initial burst of afferent firing, (2) electrical silence for an interval of hours to days, and (3) the appearance over hours to days of "spontaneous " bursting activity in both myelinated and unmyelinated axons. This ongoing activity reflects the initial dying back of the injured axon (retrograde chromatolysis) and then initiation of sprouting. Collections of these sprouts form neuromas. Recording from the afferent axon indicates that the ongoing activity originates after an interval of days to weeks from the lesioned site (neuroma) and from the dorsal root ganglion (DRG) of the injured nerve.

Several lines of evidence support the assertion that the ectopic activity in the afferent arising from the neuroma or the DRG of the injured axon is in part responsible for the observed pain behavior: (1) the onset of ectopic activity in the neuroma or DRG and the onset of pain behavior have parallel time courses, (2) pain behavior can be blocked by the application of tetrodotoxin (TTX) or local anesthetic to the neuroma or DRG, (3) dorsal rhizotomy will transiently reverse the pain behavior, and (4) irritants applied to DRG will initiate activity and yield pain behavior. A number of changes occur that can lead to prominent alterations in ongoing afferent activity.

ALTERED CHANNEL EXPRESSION

A variety of channels in the sensory afferent can modulate excitability. Two major classes are the sodium channel, which carries the primary current for axonal depolarization, and a number of potassium channels. Activation of such potassium channels can reduce axon excitability. Clearly, upregulation of sodium channels or downregulation of potassium channels would have the net effect of increasing axon excitability.

Box 9.1 Agents Released by Tissue Injury That Depolarize and Sensitize Small Primary Afferent Terminals

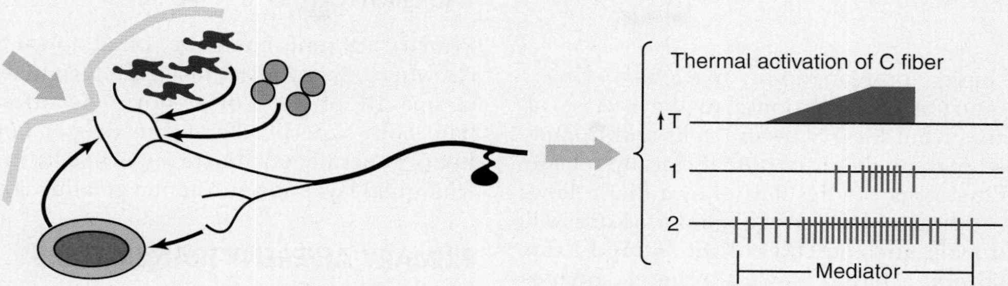

The mediators listed below are released by injury from macrophages, mast cells, and blood vessels. These mediators evoke spontaneous activity in otherwise silent C fibers and lower the threshold for activation in response to a ramped thermal stimulus (right: 1 vs. 2).

1. **Amines.** Histamine (mast cells, basophils, and platelets) and serotonin (mast cells and platelets) are released by a variety of stimuli, including mechanical trauma, heat, radiation, and certain products of tissue damage.
2. **Kinin.** Bradykinin is synthesized by a cascade triggered via activation of factor XII by agents such as kallikrein and trypsin and by physical trauma. It acts through specific bradykinin receptors (B1/B2).
3. **Lipidic acids.** Tissue injury activates a variety of widely distributed phospholipases that free arachidonic acid (AA). AA is a substrate for a large family of enzymes, such as cyclooxygenase, to synthesize lipid mediators, including prostaglandin E_2, prostacyclin, and thromboxane A_2, all of which can facilitate the excitability of C fibers through specific membrane receptors (EP-r, IPR, Tx-R, respectively).
4. **Cytokines.** Cytokines such as tumor necrosis factor-α and interleukins such as IL-1β are released by inflammatory cells (macrophages) and sensitize C fibers through eponymous binding sites.
5. **Proteinases.** Thrombin or trypsin is released from inflammatory cells and activates specific receptors (proteinase-activated receptors).
6. **Neurotrophic factors.** Nerve growth factor (NGF) will activate primary afferent terminals by binding to TrkA tyrosine kinase. NGF is released from fibroblasts and mast cells by injury and inflammation.
7. **[H]/[K].** Elevated H^+ (low pH) and high K^+ are found in injured tissue. A variety of channels present on C fibers (e.g., transient receptor potential vanilloid-1 [TRPV1]/acid-sensing ion channels [ASICs]) are activated by H^+. Acid pH potentiates terminal activation by noxious heat and other chemical mediators.
8. **Primary afferent peptides.** Calcitonin gene–related peptide and substance P are found in and released from the peripheral terminals of C fibers. These peptides produce vasodilation, plasma extravasation, and degranulation of mast cells through their respective receptors. This leads to local reddening and swelling in skin innervated by the stimulated sensory nerve.

Sodium Channels

A large increase in the expression of sodium channels in neuromas and DRGs occurs after nerve injury. Several sodium channel variants exist in primary afferent neurons, including subtypes designated as $Na_v1.6$, $Na_v1.7$, $Na_v1.8$, and $Na_v1.9$. Those designated as being resistant to the sodium channel blocker TTX, $Na_v1.8$ and $Na_v1.9$, are found primarily in small DRG cells (C fibers). These channels mediate slowly activating and slowly inactivating sodium currents. The importance of some of these variants in nerve injury pain states is suggested by knock-down studies wherein reduction of, for example, $Na_v1.8$ has no effect on baseline pain thresholds but reverses nerve injury–evoked pain states in animal models. In humans and animal models, systemic lidocaine at plasma concentrations that block ectopic activity has the ability to attenuate the hyperpathic state observed after nerve injury, thus confirming the importance of sodium channels in the post–nerve injury pain state. In humans, mutations in one sodium channel ($Na_v1.7$) can cause *extremely painful conditions.* Conversely loss-of-function mutations lead to a *prominent insensitivity* to pain generated by tissue-injuring stimuli. Conversely, other mutations can result in a "gain of function," and this is correlated with syndromes such as erythromelalgia, which is characterized by severe episodic pain.

Potassium Channels

Following nerve injury, potassium currents have been shown to be reduced, thus suggesting downregulation of these channels. Potassium channel blockers increase ectopic firing after peripheral nerve injury.

CHANGES IN THE CHEMICAL SENSITIVITY OF NEUROMAS AND DORSAL ROOT GANGLIA

Sprouted terminals of an injured axon display sensitivity to a number of humoral factors, including prostanoids, catecholamines, and cytokines such as tumor necrosis factor (TNF). Several examples of how this sensitivity is related to the appearance of ongoing activity will be noted.

Cytokines

After nerve injury, release of a variety of cytokines, particularly TNF, is noted from various local inflammatory cells. These cytokines directly activate the nerve and neuroma through eponymous receptors that become expressed in the membrane after the nerve injury. The mechanisms of the TNF interaction are multiple and complicated. Acutely, TNF decreases potassium conductance in neurons, whereas longer-term effects may be initiated through activation of a variety of kinases (mitogen-activated protein kinases

[MAPKs]). Behaviorally, application of TNF to the nerve results in hyperalgesia, and systemic delivery of TNF-binding protein reduces free TNF and decreases pain behavior in animals with neuropathic pain.

Catecholamines

Following nerve injury, postganglionic *sympathetic efferents* sprout into the injury site. In response to the release of nerve growth factors from local Schwann cells and inflammatory cells, these postganglionic terminals locally release catecholamines. Physiologic studies have shown that following nerve injury, stimulation of postganglionic axons will excite the injured axon and the DRG of the injured axon and that such activation is blocked by α-adrenergic antagonism. After nerve injury, upregulation of the expression of α_1-adrenergic receptors has been demonstrated. Accordingly, increased catecholamine concentrations in the vicinity of the DRG or the injured neuroma can translate into enhanced activity.

Prostaglandin Receptors

Prostanoids are released by inflammatory cells secondary to tissue injury. They can enhance the opening of TTX-insensitive sodium channels by acting through eponymous receptors on the afferent terminal. TTX-insensitive channels are typically found on small unmyelinated axons, which emphasizes the association of these observations with axons carrying information having "nociceptive" content.

These events are believed to contribute to the development of "spontaneous" afferent traffic after peripheral nerve injury.

THE FIRST-ORDER SYNAPSE

Primary afferents enter the spinal dorsal horn. As reviewed elsewhere, large afferents (Aβ) terminate deep to Rexed lamina III of the dorsal horn. Aδ afferent fibers terminate both superficially and in deeper laminae, whereas C fibers generally terminate superficially in laminae I and II (marginal layer and substantia gelatinosa).

PRIMARY AFFERENT TRANSMITTERS

It has classically been appreciated that primary afferent input results in a postsynaptic excitatory event, thus emphasizing that primary afferent transmitters are uniformly excitatory. As a general statement, it appears that the principal primary afferent neurotransmitter evoking acute excitation is glutamate. It is contained in the synaptic vesicles of most spinal afferent terminals, and its synthetic enzymes have been identified in virtually every primary afferent DRG cell body, regardless of size or state of myelination. These acute effects are mediated by the α-amino-3-hydroxy-5-methyl-4-isoxazolepropionate (AMPA)-type glutamate ionophore present on the second-order neuron. This receptor produces a robust, but short-lasting depolarization of the postsynaptic membrane by increasing sodium conductance (Table 9.1).

Table 9.1 Summary of Primary Afferent Transmitter Organization

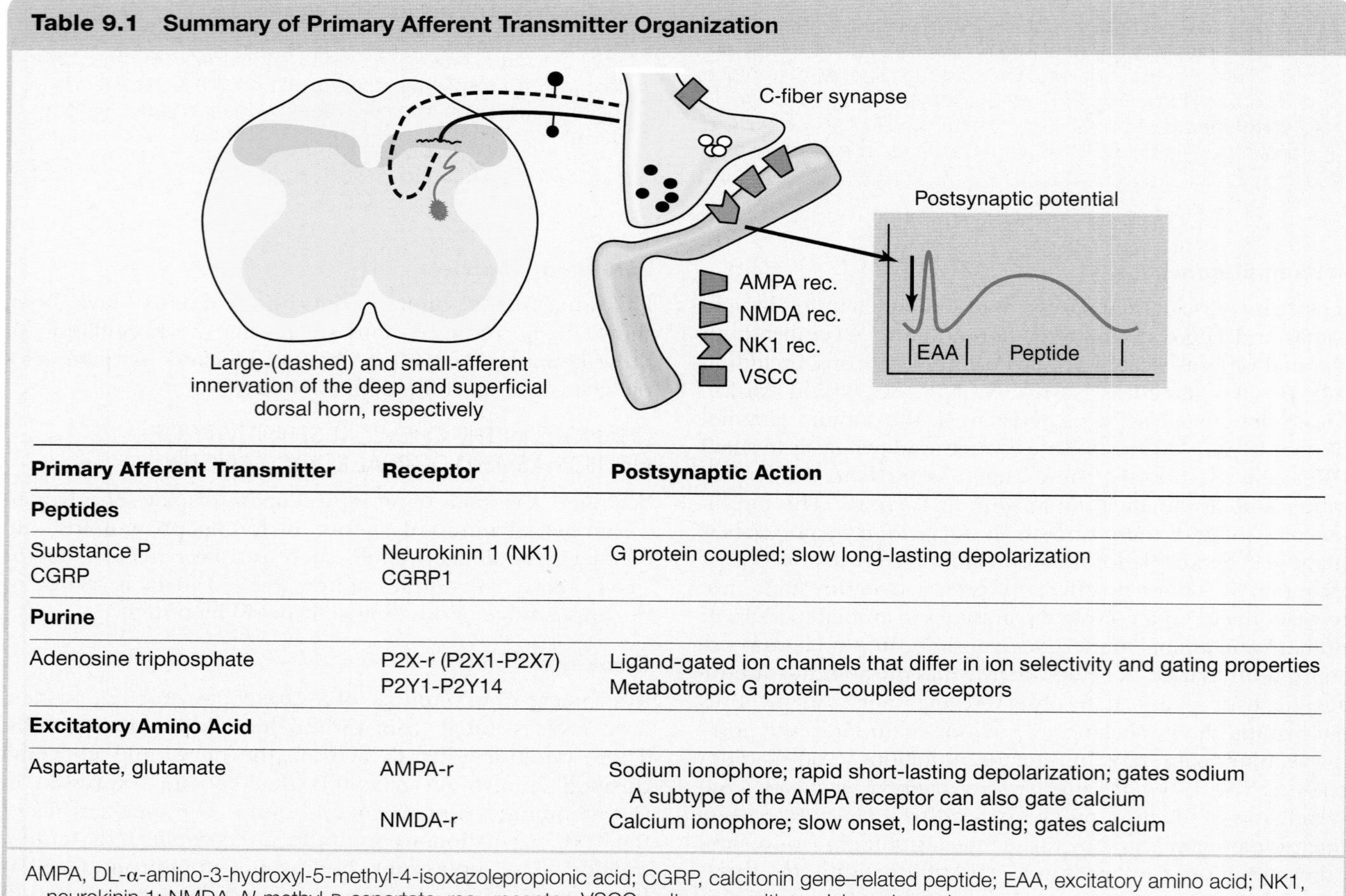

Primary Afferent Transmitter	Receptor	Postsynaptic Action
Peptides		
Substance P CGRP	Neurokinin 1 (NK1) CGRP1	G protein coupled; slow long-lasting depolarization
Purine		
Adenosine triphosphate	P2X-r (P2X1-P2X7) P2Y1-P2Y14	Ligand-gated ion channels that differ in ion selectivity and gating properties Metabotropic G protein–coupled receptors
Excitatory Amino Acid		
Aspartate, glutamate	AMPA-r	Sodium ionophore; rapid short-lasting depolarization; gates sodium A subtype of the AMPA receptor can also gate calcium
	NMDA-r	Calcium ionophore; slow onset, long-lasting; gates calcium

AMPA, DL-α-amino-3-hydroxyl-5-methyl-4-isoxazolepropionic acid; CGRP, calcitonin gene–related peptide; EAA, excitatory amino acid; NK1, neurokinin 1; NMDA, *N*-methyl-D-aspartate; rec., receptor; VSCC, voltage-sensitive calcium channel.

In addition to glutamate, populations of primary afferents may contain and release a number of neuropeptides, notably substance P (SP) and calcitonin gene–related peptide (CGRP), and even certain growth factors such as brain-derived neurotrophic factor. Given the complexity of the coding, it is likely that nociceptive information is processed by a variety of transmitters. The transmitters in these small high-threshold afferents display several general properties:

1. Consistent with their location in small afferent terminals, high levels of peptides are present in laminae I and II, and these levels are reduced by rhizotomy or ganglionectomy or by treatment with the small afferent neurotoxin capsaicin. The sensitivity of these afferent to capsaicin indicates that one important characteristic of many (but not all C fibers) is expression of the TRPV1 (capsaicin) receptor. A second population of C fibers that do not express TRPV1 typically express a second marker (isolectin B4 [IB4]). These IB4-positive afferents characteristically project to the deeper layers of the dorsal horn and do not express neuropeptides.
2. Glutamate and many peptides are co-contained and co-released (e.g., glutamate, SP, and CGRP in the same C-fiber terminal).
3. Release is dependent on the opening of voltage-sensitive calcium channels, and the magnitude of release is proportional to stimulus frequency.
4. Iontophoretic application of glutamate and the peptides found in primary afferents onto the dorsal horn will produce postsynaptic excitation. Amino acids produce a rapid, short-lasting depolarization, whereas the peptides produce a delayed and long-lasting discharge (see Table 9.1).

REGULATION OF DORSAL HORN EXCITABILITY

As noted in the introduction, the intensity of the painful stimulus is encoded in the projection to higher centers by the frequency of the output function. Accordingly, factors that enhance the excitability of spinal afferent terminals (leading to increased release of transmitter) or the excitability of the dorsal horn projection neuron will increase the apparent magnitude of a given stimulus, whereas factors that diminish the excitability of the primary afferent or the projection neuron will lead to a reduction in the apparent stimulus intensity. In the following section we will consider substrates that respectively enhance and diminish the response of the dorsal horn to a given stimulus.

FACILITATION OF DORSAL HORN EXCITABILITY

Persistent small (C fiber), but not large (A fiber) afferent activation of lamina I (marginal cell) and lamina V (wide dynamic range [WDR]), as occurs with tissue injury and inflammation, has been shown to (1) enhance the response to subsequent dorsal horn input and (2) increase the receptive field of the activated neurons. Thus, the conditioning afferent input increases the receptive field size of the neurons such that afferent input from dermatomal areas that previously did not activate the given neuron now evokes a prominent response. Moreover, low-threshold tactile stimulation also becomes increasingly effective in driving these neurons. This phenomenon, first described by Lorne Mendell and Patrick Wall in the mid-1960s, is broadly referred to as "wind-up." These physiologic effects reflect events that are referred to as *central* or, more specifically, *spinal sensitization* and are believed to underlie the psychophysical correlates of tissue injury wherein tissue injury leads to hyperalgesia and secondary hyperpathia (e.g., increased sensitivity to stimuli applied outside the area of injury). The relevance of this small-afferent–evoked facilitation in humans has been emphasized by psychophysical studies in human subjects. Here, local activation of C fibers by the intradermal injection of capsaicin leads to an initial pain report followed for an extended period by a surrounding region showing enhanced mechanical and thermal sensitivity. This effect is blocked by a transient local anesthetic block of the nerves innervating the capsaicin-injected area. These observations emphasize that ongoing small-afferent input can initiate central sensitization of pain processing.

Based on the above commentary, a decrease in C-fiber–evoked excitation in the dorsal horn produced by a reduction in the release of small-afferent transmitter or block of the postsynaptic receptor (e.g., AMPA for glutamate) will diminish the magnitude of the afferent drive and, accordingly, diminish the facilitated processing evoked by protracted small-afferent input. The facilitated state, however, reflects more than the repetitive activation of a simple excitatory system.

GLUTAMATE RECEPTORS AND SPINAL FACILITATION

The first real demonstration of the unique pharmacology of the facilitated state was achieved by showing that spinal wind-up was prevented by the spinal delivery of antagonists of the *N*-methyl-D-aspartate (NMDA) receptor, a glutamate ionophore composed of a number of subunits that is potently excitatory. When activated, it passes large amounts of Ca^{2+} and Na^+ current. An important observation is that NMDA antagonists have no effect on acute evoked activity but reduce the wind-up induced by repetitive C-fiber stimulation. Correspondingly, behavioral studies have revealed that such drugs have no effect on behavior evoked by an acute noxious stimulus (e.g., acute thermal escape) but do reduce the hyperalgesia observed after tissue injury and inflammation.

The absence of an effect of NMDA antagonism on acute afferent-evoked activation or the pain state reflects an important property of this receptor. At resting membrane potential the NMDA receptor displays a block of the channel by Mg^{2+}. Occupancy of the NMDA receptor by glutamate will not activate the ionophore in the presence of Mg^{2+}. With ongoing depolarization of the membrane (as produced during repetitive stimulation) secondary to the activation of AMPA and SP receptors, the Mg^{2+} block is removed. If several allosteric binding sites on the NMDA ionophore are occupied (glycine/polyamine sites), glutamate may now activate the NMDA channel and permit passage of Ca^{2+} and Na^+ current. This opening thus serves to further depolarize the membrane and, importantly, to increase intracellular Ca^{2+}, which serves to initiate downstream components of the excitatory and facilitatory cascade (see below).

It has become increasingly apparent that although AMPA mediates an acute depolarization reflecting an increase in Na^+ influx, in the presence of repetitive stimulation, Ca^{2+} permeability develops in the AMPA channels (e.g., calcium-permeable AMPA channels with a distinct antagonist pharmacology).

Downstream Cascades

Primary afferent C fibers release peptides (e.g., SP, CGRP), purines (adenosine triphosphate [ATP]), and excitatory amino acid (glutamate) products. These peptides and excitatory amino acids induce excitation in second-order neurons. As noted for glutamate, direct monosynaptic excitation is mediated by AMPA receptors (i.e., acute primary afferent excitation of WDR neurons is not mediated by the NMDA or neurokinin 1 [NK1] receptor). This initial activation leads to enablement of the NMDA ionophore (and the generation of Ca^{2+}-permeable AMPA channels), which in turn initiates a number of complex cascades that reflect processes that serve to "sensitize" the postsynaptic dorsal horn neuron. Several primary examples of such facilitatory cascades initiated by repetitive small-afferent input are presented in the following text.

Local Neuronal Circuits

NMDA Receptors. The best example of a cascade initiated by small-afferent input is activation of the NMDA receptor. As noted above, with ongoing membrane depolarization, the NMDA ionophore loses its Mg^{2+} block, which allows the large increase in intracellular Ca^{2+}.

AMPA Receptors. Although the AMPA receptor is largely considered to be an acutely activated ionophore that allows the primary passage of sodium, there are structural variants on the AMPA receptor that allow it to pass calcium. These "calcium-permeable" AMPA receptors are believed to participate along with the NMDA receptor in various aspects of spinal facilitation.

Neurokinin 1 Receptors. NK1 receptors are G protein–coupled receptors that are activated by the SP released from small primary afferents. Activation of this receptor leads to prolonged depolarization and mobilization of intracellular calcium. Spinal delivery of agents that block the NK1 site for SP can diminish wind-up and significantly reduce the second-phase response to intradermal formalin injection.

Prostaglandin Cascade. The increase in intracellular calcium serves to promote the transmigration of a variety of phospholipases to the membrane, where they then serve to cleave arachidonic acid. Arachidonic acid serves as a substrate for cyclooxygenase (COX) to produce a number of prostanoids. All these enzymes have been found to be constitutively expressed in spinal neurons and non-neuronal cells. This cascade leads to the release of a number of prostaglandins that act on a number of eponymous receptors that are located *presynaptically* on the primary afferent terminal and *postsynaptically* on second-order neurons. The presynaptic effect has been shown to enhance the opening of voltage-sensitive calcium channels, which serves to mediate vesicular mobilization and release of transmitter. A postsynaptic action that attenuates the activation of *inhibitory* glycine receptors has been demonstrated. This leads to loss of the regulatory inhibition that otherwise limits postsynaptic activation. In turn, this results in an enhanced response of the second-order (projection) neuron to a given afferent input (Fig. 9.2).

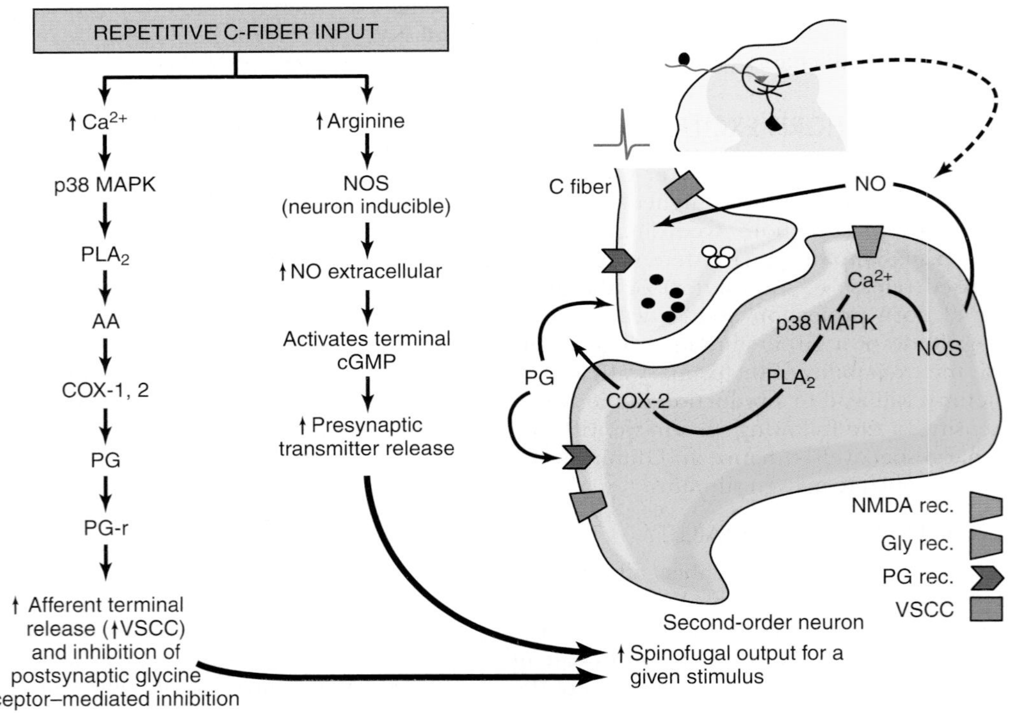

Figure 9.2 Small-afferent input activates second-order neurons and thereby leads to increased intracellular calcium, which initiates several intracellular cascades. (1) Activation of phospholipase A_2 (PLA_2) increases free arachidonic acid (AA). This serves as a substrate for cyclooxygenase (COX-1 and COX-2), which leads to the release of a number of prostaglandins (PG) that act on a variety of eponymous prostanoid receptors that are located presynaptically on the primary afferent terminal and postsynaptically on the higher-order neurons. See text for further comment. (2) Activation of nitric oxide synthase (NOS) in the presence of arginine leads to release of nitric oxide (NO), which diffuses to enhance the release of transmitter (e.g., glutamate). These events can serve to increase terminal release and increase postsynaptic excitability. cGMP, cyclic guanine monophosphate; Gly, glycine; NMDA, *N*-methyl-D-aspartate; p38 MAPK, p38 mitogen-activated protein kinase; rec., receptor; VSCC, voltage-sensitive calcium channel.

Nitric Oxide Synthase. Small-afferent input also leads to the activation of nitric oxide synthase (NOS). Both neuronal NOS and inducible NOS are present in neurons and other cells. In the presence of arginine, nitric oxide forms and diffuses to act presynaptically (retrograde transmission) through cyclic guanosine monophosphate to enhance release of transmitter (e.g., glutamate). These events can serve to increase terminal release and increase postsynaptic excitation (see Fig. 9.2).

Phosphorylation. As reviewed, small-afferent input serves to increase intracellular Ca^{2+} in second-order neurons. This leads to the activation of a number of protein kinases such as PKC and PKA or MAPK (Fig. 9.3). There are many isoforms of these kinases. All serve to phosphorylate consensus sites on various proteins. PKC has been shown to phosphorylate amino acids sites on NMDA and AMPA receptors. This phosphorylation tends to lower the threshold for activation, which leads to greater membrane permeability. In the case of the NMDA ionophore, it serves to lower the threshold for removal of the Mg^{2+} block that otherwise prevents channel activation. p38 MAPK, when activated, phosphorylates phospholipase A_2, thereby leading to its activation (see Fig. 9.2), and it activates various transcription factors, such as the nuclear factor NF-κB, which serves to increase the synthesis of various proteins, such as COX, and a variety of channels (Na_v, Ca_v), receptors (TRPV1), and transcription factors (activation transcription factor 3 [ATF-3]).

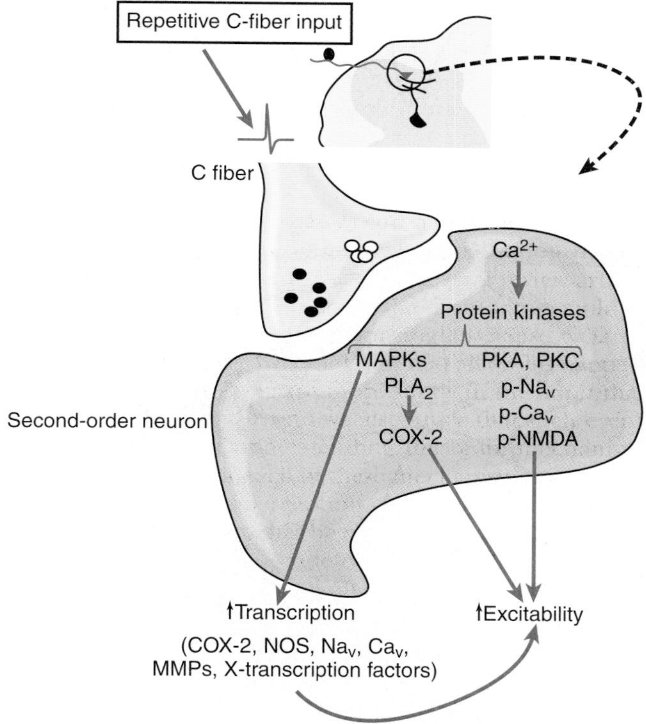

Figure 9.3 Small-afferent input serves to increase intracellular calcium in second-order neurons, which activates a number of protein kinases such as PKC and PKA or mitogen-activated protein kinases (MAPKs), which serve to phosphorylate various proteins. Specifically, in this schema, PKC and the NMDA and AMPA receptors are phosphorylated, which leads to lower activation thresholds. When activated, p38 MAPK phosphorylates PLA_2, which results in its activation (see Fig. 9.2) and serves to activate various transcription factors (e.g., nuclear factor κB) that increase the synthesis of various proteins (e.g., COX) and a variety of channels (Na_v, Ca_v), receptors (transient receptor potential vanilloid 1 [TRPV1]), and transcription factors (activation transcription factor 3 [ATF-3]). AMPA, DL-α-amino-3-hydroxyl-5-methyl-4-isoxazole propionic acid; COX, cyclooxygenase; MMP, matrix metalloproteinase; NMDA, *N*-methyl-D-aspartate; NOS, nitric oxide synthase; PLA_2, phospholipase A_2; rec., receptor; VSCC, voltage-sensitive calcium channel.

Bulbospinal Pathways. Of particular interest has been the growing appreciation that small-afferent input can initiate facilitated activation through spinobulbospinal linkages (Fig. 9.4). Thus, it has been shown that C fibers make synaptic contact with superficial dorsal horn neurons (lamina I neurons). These neurons project into the brainstem and make synaptic contact with medullary midline raphe spinal neurons that are serotonergic. These cells in turn project into the spinal dorsal horn and make synaptic contact with a number of neuronal populations but, importantly, those with cell bodies in the deep dorsal horn (lamina V). The serotonergic projections act through excitatory $5\text{-}HT_3$ receptors to enhance the firing of these lamina V neurons. As stated, these cells are noted for their ability to display a facilitated state called "wind-up." Block of this bulbospinal linkage or the use of $5\text{-}HT_3$ inhibitors has been reported to reduce this facilitated state.

Non-neuronal Cells

The central nervous system has a wide variety of non-neuronal cells. Among these are astrocytes and microglia. These astrocytes, microglia, and neurons form a complex network in which each can influence the excitability of the others (Fig. 9.5).

Transmitter Mediators of Non-neuronal Cell Activation. Primary afferents and intrinsic neuron transmitters (glutamate, ATP, SP) can overflow from the synaptic cleft to these adjacent non-neuronal cells and lead to their activation. Activation of neurons can result in the release of chemokines such as fractalkine. Astrocytes may communicate with microglia by the release of a number of products, including glutamate/cytokines and "S-100" protein. These products have eponymous receptors, which can lead to changes in the biology of astrocytes and microglia and result in the extracellular movement of a variety of neuroactive products, such as free radicals, cytokines (interleukin-1β [IL-1β] and TNF), and a host of lipid mediators, including arachidonic acid, platelet-activating factor, prostaglandins, and leukotrienes. Astrocytes have the well-known ability to regulate extracellular glutamate through an active uptake system. Conversely, during certain activation or stress, these intracellular glutamate stores can be released and result in significant increases in the extracellular glutamate concentration.

Gap Junctions. Astrocytes may communicate over a distance by the spread of excitation through local nonsynaptic contacts referred to as "gap" junctions. These junctions represent specialized proteins (hexagonal multimers made up of connexin macromolecules) that serve to link the adjacent membranes of two cells. Through such linkages, local excitation in one astrocyte can lead to increased Ca^{2+} reversal

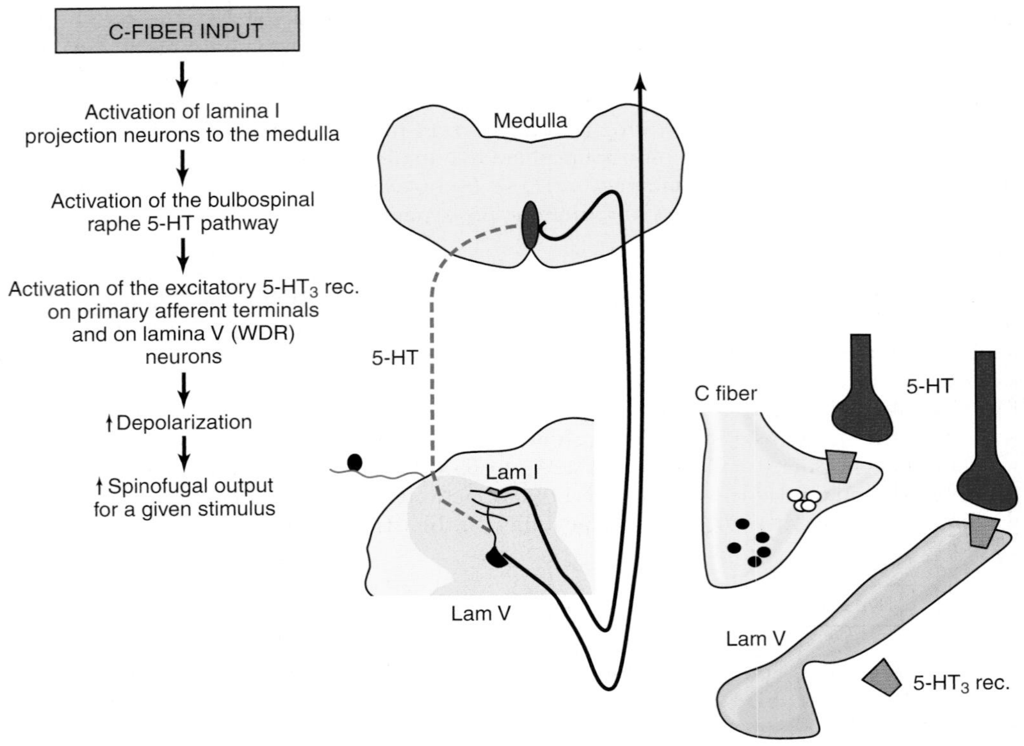

C-FIBER INPUT

Activation of lamina I projection neurons to the medulla

Activation of the bulbospinal raphe 5-HT pathway

Activation of the excitatory 5-HT_3 rec. on primary afferent terminals and on lamina V (WDR) neurons

↑Depolarization

↑Spinofugal output for a given stimulus

Medulla

5-HT

Lam I

Lam V

C fiber

5-HT

Lam V

5-HT_3 rec.

Figure 9.4 Small-afferent–evoked activation of lamina I neurons that project into the medullary raphe nuclei and serve to excite bulbospinal serotonin (5-hydroxytryptamine [5-HT]) pathways that activate excitatory 5-HT_3 receptors on lamina V neurons. This projection serves to facilitate the firing of these lamina V projection neurons and may underlie the phenomenon of "wind-up." rec., receptor; WDR, wide dynamic range.

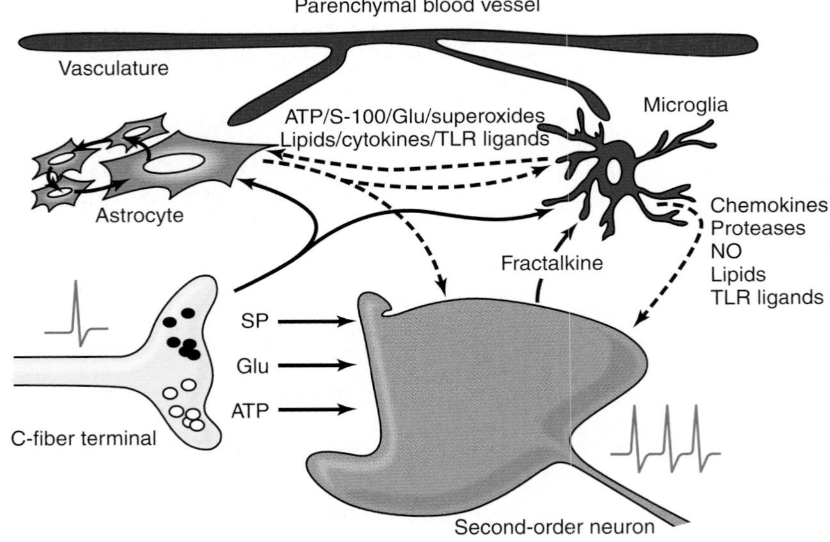

Figure 9.5 Schematic showing the complex assemblage in the dorsal horn with respect to astrocytes, microglia, and neurons. Products released from neurons can activate the release of a variety of active products from astrocytes and microglia. Astrocytes can activate other astrocytes through gap junctions, as well as activate microglia, and can induce the excitability of neurons by releasing a variety of active factors. As indicated, postsynaptic neuronal activation can lead to the release of chemokines such as fractalkine, which can act on eponymous receptors on microglia. See text for further details. ATP, adenosine triphosphate; Glu, glutamate; NO, nitric oxide; SP, substance P; TLR, toll-like receptor.

of a glutamate transporter and increased extracellular ATP, which can depolarize local neuronal processes and produce local cerebrovascular constriction. Though classically limited to astrocytes, it is currently evident that such linkages may also occur between astrocytes and neurons and microglia. The gap junction thus represents a mechanism whereby a syncytium of excitability can be created.

Circulating Factors. Finally, after tissue injury and inflammation, circulating cytokines (such as IL-1β/TNF-α) can activate perivascular astrocytes and microglia. As noted, microglia are in fact brain-resident macrophages. Such mechanisms provide an important linkage for the somatic sensations associated with systemic infection (e.g., such as in the course of a common cold or the "flu").

The relevance of the non-neuronal cell population to the facilitation process in pain processing after peripheral injury is supported by a variety of observations. First, peripheral injury and inflammation will lead to the acute and chronic activation of microglia and astrocytes. Thus, p38 MAPK-β is present in microglia and shows activation in minutes after a peripherally injuring stimulus. Over longer periods, other markers of microglia (OX42) and astrocytes (glial fibrillary acidic protein [GFAP]) show a significant increase in expression. Drugs such as minocycline (a second-generation tetracycline) and pentoxifylline have been reported to block microglia activation and diminish hyperalgesic states. Similar metabolic inhibitors that block astrocyte activation (fluorocitrate) can likewise diminish hyperalgesia after nerve and tissue injury. These agents, though not clinically implemented, suggest important directions in drug therapy development.

Innate Immune Systems. It has become increasingly appreciated that components of the innate immune response systems may also play a role in the development of ongoing pain after injury. One component is the toll-like receptors (TLRs). The TLRs recognize molecules derived from damage and infectious products and are expressed in cells involved in immune function (e.g., macrophages, neutrophils). They are also found in spinal cord neurons, glial cells, and DRGs. Several TLRs have been implicated in pain processing through the use of mutant mice. These receptors signal via a complex series of downstream cascades that can lead to signaling mediated by a wide variety of cytokines. As an example, in DRG neurons, consistent with expression of TLR message, TLR4 agonists increase intracellular calcium and thereby lead to release of neurotransmitters. Importantly, it has been increasingly appreciated that many ligands, such as tenascin C, which can activate various TLRs, are generated in neuraxial tissue after peripheral injury and inflammation.

IMPORTANCE OF FACILITATORY SYSTEMS TO INJURY-EVOKED PAIN

The preceding section reviewed a number of systems that serve to increase the gain of the spinal transmission system. This facilitation serves two interrelated functions. First, it explains in part the mechanisms whereby a peripheral injury that leads to repetitive small-afferent input can result in a potent hyperalgesic state (i.e., the response to any subsequent afferent stimulus is enhanced). Second, as was noted, following local injury there is frequently the development of enlarged receptive fields that extend beyond the territory of original injury. As discussed earlier, the dermatome for any given root is represented in part by spinal collaterals of afferents that project to neurons in adjacent segments. When these cells undergo facilitation, the input from distal dermatomes becomes sufficient to drive activity in these cells. Accordingly, the receptive field of that cell now incorporates this distal body surface. Given this perspective, it is not surprising that agents targeted at these facilitatory mechanisms can have profound effects on injury-induced pain states. Agents such as COX inhibitors are an important example for emphasizing the role of the facilitated state in the pain experience. COX inhibitors act to diminish hyperesthesia secondary to tissue injury. This reaction reflects the important role of prostaglandins released not only in the periphery but also in the spinal cord, where they can act to facilitate the release of C-fiber transmitters such as SP. Current evidence suggests that both COX-1 and COX-2 are important constitutive enzymes in the spinal systems. However, spinal COX-2 inhibitors appear to be particularly important in regulating injury-induced spinal facilitation. Nonetheless, work also points to other facilitatory mechanisms that may likewise be useful targets in the development of future agents. The potency of NOS inhibitors on behavior suggests the importance of spinal release of nitric oxide in facilitatory processes leading to hyperalgesia. Agents that inhibit microglial and astrocyte activation can also diminish hyperalgesic states. These agents, though not clinically useful or defined as safe after spinal delivery, suggest important directions in drug therapy development.

As a final *caveat* to this discussion of neuraxial facilitation, it is important to note that central facilitation studies examining the effects of repetitive C-fiber stimulation on dorsal horn neurons (described earlier) are carried out in animals that are under 1 MAC (minimum alveolar concentration) anesthesia (typically isoflurane or halothane). It has indeed been demonstrated that behavioral models of facilitation wherein the injury is induced under the effect of a systemic anesthetic (barbiturate, volatile agent, etc.) show that the hyperalgesic state may be initiated despite the fact that the injury is produced under anesthesia. The relevance of this observation to the performance of surgery on patients "anesthetized" with volatile anesthetics or with barbiturates alone is clear. Though preventing the ascending pain message, these anesthetics surprisingly do not appear to block the facilitatory processes that are initiated by small-afferent input, probably at the level of transmitter release at the first spinal synapse. This lack of effect of anesthetic on primary afferent release is believed to represent the basis of the consideration for the concept of "preemptive analgesics" via such therapeutic approaches as regional anesthesia.

PHARMACOLOGY OF SPINAL INHIBITION

Second-order dorsal horn neurons (WDR neurons) receive excitatory input from large afferents, as well as from excitatory interneurons. This input is typically mediated by glutamate. The output from the spinal dorsal horn evoked by such excitation is subject to upregulation of excitability, but it has long been appreciated that these cells are also subject to mechanisms that downregulate local excitability. In the following sections we will consider the pharmacology of such processes.

LOCAL INHIBITORY CIRCUITS

This section considers systems that are local to the dorsal horn and regulate local excitability.

INHIBITORY AMINO ACIDS

Based on the effects of various inhibitory amino acid antagonists, it appears that the excitatory effect of primary afferents, both small and large but particularly large (Aβ) ones, are subject to potent inhibition that is expressed by inhibitory γ-aminobutyric acid (GABA) and glycine receptors, which are both presynaptic on the primary afferent and postsynaptic on the second-order neuron. This relationship is indicated in Figure 9.6. Release of GABA and glycine from local interneurons will act on $GABA_A/GABA_B$ receptors and glycine receptors, respectively. The $GABA_A$ receptor and glycine receptors are ionophores that when activated, serve to increase Cl^- conductance. Based on resting transmembrane Cl^- gradients, such an increase in permeability leads to modest membrane hyperpolarization and an increase in shunting current. These effects reduce the ability of an excitatory

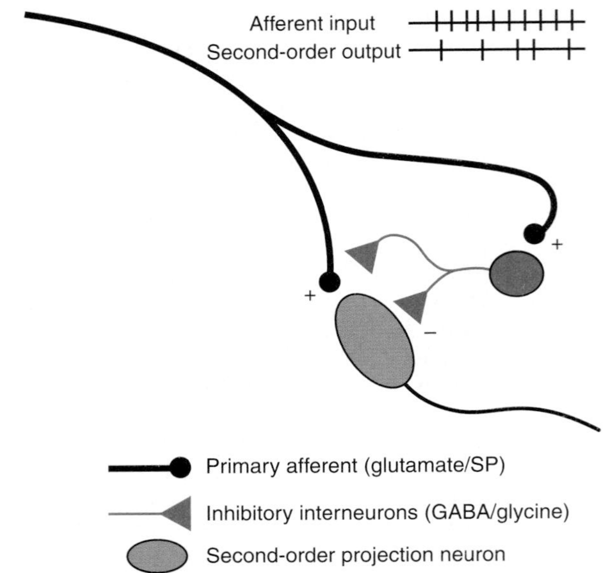

Figure 9.6 Schematic showing presynaptic and postsynaptic regulation by glycine/γ-aminobutyric acid (GABA) interneurons of Aβ afferents input onto a second-order dorsal horn neuron. As indicated, the afferent input activated the second-order projection neurons and inhibitory interneurons. The delay in GABA/glycine release results in delayed inhibition of the second-order neurons. This results in a sculpting of second-order neuron output. In the absence of such inhibition, the afferent input yields a pronounced increase in second-order neuron outflow. SP, substance P.

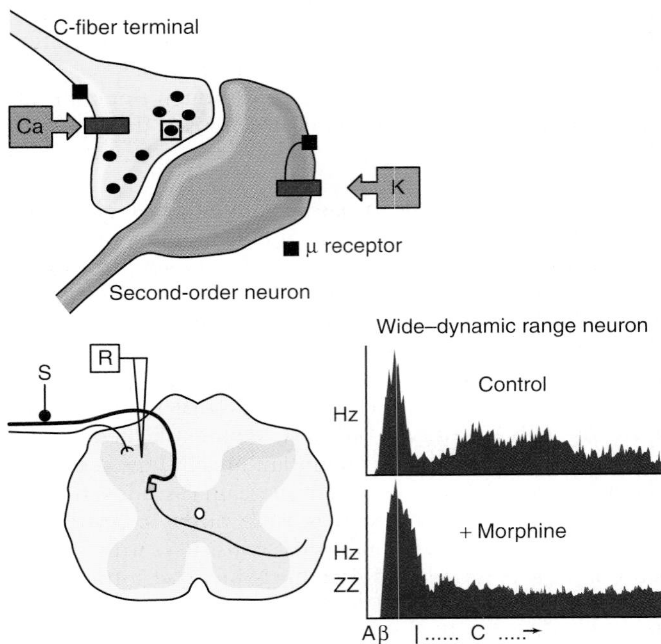

Figure 9.7 Opiate receptors are located presynaptically and postsynaptically on small primary afferents terminating in the substantia gelatinosa. A local action of opiates in the spinal cord will selectively depress the discharge of spinal dorsal horn neurons activated by small (high threshold, delayed) but not large (low threshold, short latency) afferents. C, C-fiber; R, recording electrode; S, stimulating electrode.

input to depolarize the cell. $GABA_B$ receptors are G protein–coupled receptors that are also inhibitory. The relevance of this ongoing inhibitory organization to ongoing sensation is substantiated by the fact that local application of $GABA_A$ (bicuculline) or glycine (strychnine) receptor inhibitors will lead to powerful augmentation of the discharge of dorsal horn neurons evoked by large (Aβ)-afferent input.

OPIOIDS

The potent analgesic effect of opiates reveals the efficient role played by opiate receptors in regulating pain transmission. Systematic study has shown that opiate receptors that regulate the pain response are located both at the spinal level and in several brain loci.

Spinal Opiate Action

Intrathecal delivery of opiate agonists will potently inhibit the injury-evoked discharge of superficial and deep dorsal horn neurons induced by small high-threshold afferents (C fiber). The deep dorsal horn neurons also receive input from low-threshold large (Aβ) afferents, but this evoked component is not typically blocked by opiates. These effects are mediated by an action on opioid receptors (typically characterized as μ-opioid based on agonist and antagonist pharmacology). Localization of these μ receptors has revealed them to be largely on C-fiber primary afferents that terminate in the superficial dorsal horn and on the dendrites and cell bodies of deeper dorsal horn neurons (Fig. 9.7).

Intrathecal administration will reliably attenuate the response of the animal to a variety of unconditioned somatic and visceral stimuli that would otherwise evoke organized escape behavior in all species. Confirmation of the presynaptic action is provided by the observation that opiates reduce the release of primary afferent peptide transmitters, such as the SP contained in small afferents. The presynaptic action corresponds to the ability of opiates to prevent the opening of voltage-sensitive Ca^{2+} channels, thereby preventing mobilization and release of transmitter. A postsynaptic action is demonstrated by the ability of opiates to block the excitation of dorsal horn neurons evoked by glutamate, a process reflecting direct activation of the dorsal horn. The activation of potassium channels leading to membrane hyperpolarization is consistent with direct postsynaptic inhibition.

Supraspinal Opiate Action

Direct injection of opiates into the brain has shown that opioid receptors that modulate pain behavior are found in several restricted brain regions, including the amygdala and the midline medulla, but the best characterized of these supraspinal sites so identified is the mesencephalic periaqueductal gray (PAG). Microinjection of opiates into this region will block the nociceptive response in a naloxone-reversible fashion. Several mechanisms exist whereby opiates acting in the PAG may alter nociceptive transmission:

1. Activation of bulbospinal projection. In the PAG, opiate receptors are presynaptic on GABAergic terminals that inhibit projection to the medulla. Morphine acts to block the release of GABA, which terminates the inhibitory control over PAG outflow. The PAG has excitatory projections into the medulla, which then activates bulbospinal noradrenergic and serotonergic pathways. The noradrenergic projection acts through spinal α_2-receptors to reduce dorsal horn excitation.

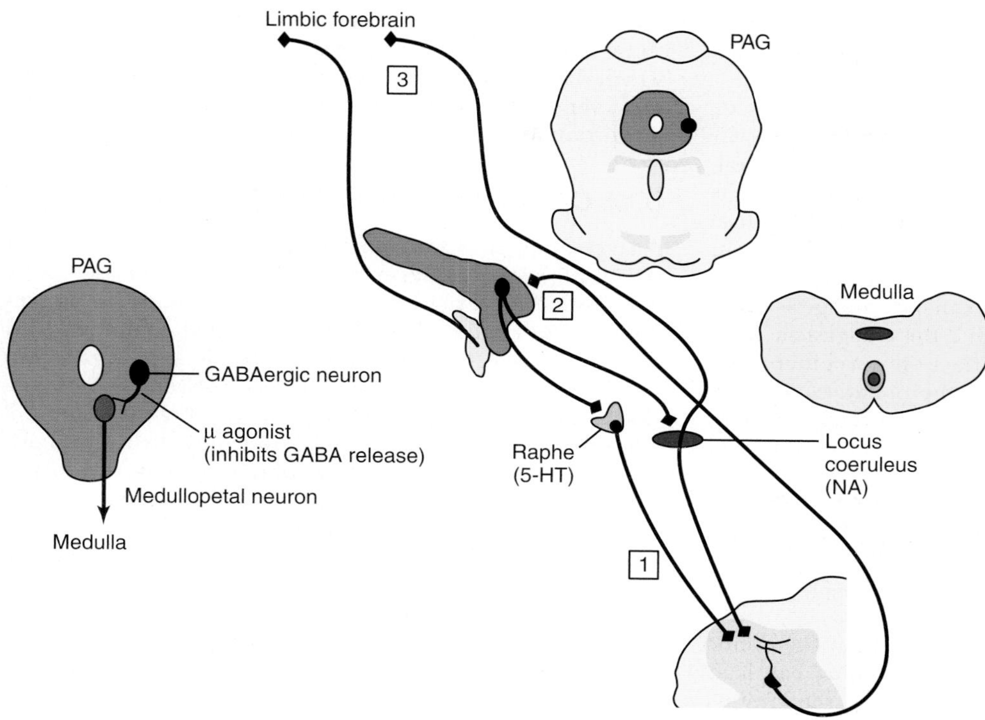

Figure 9.8 Schematic of organization of opiate action within the periaqueductal gray (PAG) whereby μ-opiate actions block the release of γ-aminobutyric acid (GABA) from tonically active systems that otherwise regulate projections to the medulla and lead to activation of PAG outflow. (1) Excitatory outflow from the PAG activates bulbospinal projections that release serotonin (5-hydroxytryptamine [5-HT]) or noradrenaline (NA), or both, at the spinal level. (2). Preterminal opiate binding within the PAG on the ascending spinofugal projection. (3) Outflow from the PAG increases excitability of the dorsal raphe and locus coeruleus, from which ascending serotonergic and noradrenergic projections originate and project to the limbic forebrain.

2. Opiate binding within the PAG. Such binding may be preterminal on the ascending spinofugal projection. This preterminal action would inhibit input into the medullary core and mesencephalic core.
3. Outflow from the PAG. PAG outflow can increase excitability of the dorsal raphe and locus coeruleus/lateral tegmental nuclei from which ascending serotonergic and noradrenergic projections, respectively, originate and project to limbic forebrain. These projections are thought to modulate emotionality (see later).

These three mechanisms are summarized in Figure 9.8.

Endogenous Opiates

Opiate receptors are presumed to be targeted by endogenous compounds released from local interneurons. A number of such functionally qualified families of agents have been identified according to the family of prohormones from which they are derived: proenkephalin (enkephalins), prodynorphins (dynorphins), and pro-opiomelanocortins (β-endorphin). Other endogenous opioids have also been described, such as the endomorphins. These are all peptides that have been shown to have significant affinity for one or more of the several identified opioid receptors. Enkephalins have been found in dorsal horn interneurons and in bulbospinal pathways. Such interneuronal systems are present throughout the brain. β-Endorphin is present in long projection pathways that largely originate in the hypothalamus. Even though opiate receptors can regulate spinal nociceptive processing, there is surprisingly limited data to suggest that the endogenous systems have a robust effect on pain processing. Naloxone, an opioid antagonist, has modest effects on ongoing pain processing. Enkephalins are rapidly metabolized by a variety of peptidases, and changes in the pain threshold in animal models have been shown to alter pain thresholds in a number of experimental pain states.

BULBOSPINAL PROJECTION SYSTEMS

A number of transmitters are known to be contained in and released from bulbospinal projecting pathways; however, those best characterized are the monoamines norepinephrine and serotonin.

Bulbospinal Norepinephrine

Norepinephrine projections to the spinal cord arise from lateral medullary sites and the locus coeruleus, whereas norepinephrine projections to the forebrain arise from the locus coeruleus (see Fig. 9.8). The rostral projections are believed to play the primary role in altering the affective components of behavior. The caudal adrenergic projections play a principal role in regulating spinal nociceptive processing through an action on spinal dorsal horn α_2-adrenergic receptors that are located presynaptic and postsynaptic to the primary afferent. Spinal delivery of α_2-adrenoceptor agonists such as clonidine and dexmedetomidine produces significant analgesia. This spinal action of an α_2-agonist is mediated by a mechanism similar to that used by spinal opiates, but the receptor is distinct: (1) α_2 binding is presynaptic on C fibers and postsynaptic on dorsal horn neurons, (2) α_2-receptors can depress the release of C-fiber transmitters, and (3) α_2-agonists can hyperpolarize dorsal horn neurons through a G_i-coupled potassium channel.

Bulbospinal Serotonin

Serotonin (5-hydroxytryptamine [5-HT]) arises from the nucleus raphe magnus, which projects spinally, and from the raphe dorsalis, which provides the principal source of forebrain 5-HT. As reviewed earlier, spinipetal 5-HT projections can have multiple effects, including excitation and inhibition. These complex effects suggest that under certain conditions, increasing spinal 5-HT tone may *facilitate* nociceptive processing.

Altering Terminal Monoamine Concentrations

Importantly, agents that regulate the extracellular concentrations of these monoamines can have pronounced effects on emotional tone and nociceptive transmission. Because extracellular levels depend not only on release but also on their reuptake, agents that block the reuptake transporter, such as the tricyclic antidepressants, can have analgesic properties. Current evidence suggests that the analgesic actions are largely mediated through an effect on norepinephrine and not serotonin. This difference in their relative contributions to analgesic efficacy may reflect the several opposing effects that are associated with the action of serotonin.

PHARMACOLOGY OF FACILITATORY STATES THAT OCCUR SECONDARY TO NERVE INJURY

From the preceding sections it was evident that the events that take place following peripheral tissue injury can lead to potent facilitation of neuraxial processing that results in large part from the persistent small-afferent traffic that occurs with injury and inflammation. These changes reflect events that occur in the injured nerve (as reviewed in a preceding section): alteration of protein expression leading to upregulation of some proteins and downregulation of others. The increased spontaneous activity arising from neuromas and DRGs provides a tentative explanation for the ongoing dysesthesias that are associated with a variety of nerve injury conditions. The prominent finding that low-threshold tactile stimulation acquires an aversive component appears to present a more complex set of events. Current thinking is that it is mediated by low-threshold mechanosensitive (Aβ) afferents. The precise mechanism of this involvement of low-threshold afferents in initiation of pain is not known, although several possibilities have been considered credible.

CROSSTALK BETWEEN LARGE AND SMALL AFFERENTS

Following nerve injury, "crosstalk" mediated by ephaptic contacts may develop between afferents in DRGs and neuromas. Here, depolarizing currents in one axon would generate a depolarizing voltage in an adjacent quiescent axon. In this manner, a large low-threshold afferent would drive activity in an adjacent high-threshold afferent.

LARGE-AFFERENT SPROUTING

As reviewed previously, large myelinated (Aβ) afferents project into the spinal Rexed lamina III and deeper. Small afferents (C fibers) tend to project into spinal laminae I and II, a region populated by neurons responding to this high-threshold input. Following peripheral nerve injury, it has been argued that the central terminals of myelinated afferents (A fibers) sprout into lamina II of the spinal cord. With this synaptic reorganization, stimulation of low-threshold mechanoreceptors (Aβ fibers) could produce excitation of these neurons and be perceived as painful. The degree to which this sprouting occurs is a point of current discussion, and even though it does appear to occur, it is considerably less prominent than originally reported.

LOSS OF INTRINSIC INHIBITORY CONTROL

A large number of small interneurons lie in the superficial dorsal horn; these interneurons contain and release GABA and glycine. As reviewed earlier, these terminals are presynaptic to the large central afferent terminal complexes and form reciprocal synapses, and GABAergic axosomatic connections have been identified on second-order and projection neurons (see Fig. 9.6). Accordingly, these transmitters exert powerful inhibitory control over the activity of Aβ primary afferent terminals and second-order neurons in the spinal dorsal horn. As discussed earlier, the importance of this local inhibitory circuitry is indicated by the observation that intrathecal delivery of a $GABA_A$ (bicuculline) receptor or glycine (strychnine) receptor antagonist evokes a powerful tactile allodynia. Such observations led to the hypothesis that nerve injury may induce a loss of GABAergic/glycinergic neurons. Although some data do support a loss of such neurons, this loss appears to be minimal. Recent observations now suggest a second alternative. After nerve injury, spinal neurons are altered in such a fashion that $GABA_A$ and glycine receptor activation becomes excitatory. As noted previously, these receptors are chloride ionophores. When these ionophores are activated, chloride moves according to its transmembrane gradient. The transmembrane gradient is maintained by transporters that export chloride. After nerve injury the activity of the chloride transporter is reduced, which leads to an increase in intracellular chloride, and increasing membrane Cl^- conductance, as occurs with $GABA_A$ receptor activation, now results in membrane depolarization. Thus, paradoxically, afferent input that activates $GABA_A$/glycine channels may actually serve to facilitate membrane depolarization and lead to a much enhanced response to the Aβ drive.

ENHANCED EXCITATORY DRIVE

GLUTAMATE RELEASE

Spinal glutamate release plays an important role in post–nerve injury pain states. There is a significant enhancement in resting spinal glutamate secretion after nerve injury. Such release is in accord with (1) increased spontaneous activity in the primary afferent and (2) loss of the intrinsic inhibition that may serve to modulate resting glutamate secretion (see below). The significance of this release is emphasized by several observations: (1) Intrathecally delivered glutamate will evoke a powerful tactile allodynia and thermal hyperalgesia through the activation of spinal NMDA and non-NMDA receptors. (2) Spinal delivery of NMDA antagonists has been shown to attenuate the hyperpathic states arising in animal models of nerve injury. NMDA receptor activation mediates an important facilitation in neuronal excitability. In addition, the NMDA receptor is a calcium ionophore, which when activated, leads to prominent increases in intracellular calcium. The increase in intracellular Ca^{2+} initiates a cascade of events that includes the activation of a variety of enzymes (kinases), some of which phosphorylate membrane proteins (e.g., calcium channels and the NMDA receptors) and others such as the MAPKs serve to mediate intracellular signaling, thereby leading to the altered expression of a variety of proteins and peptides (e.g., COX and dynorphin). A number of factors have been shown to enhance release of glutamate. Two examples will be discussed further.

Spinal Dynorphin

Nerve injury leads to a prominent increase in spinal dynorphin expression. Intrathecal delivery of dynorphin can initiate the concurrent release of spinal glutamate and a potent tactile allodynia; NMDA antagonists reverse the latter effect. Even though dynorphin is an endogenous opioid peptide, these effects appear to be independent of any action on an opiate receptor.

Altered Channel Expression

As reviewed previously, nerve injury leads to the upregulation of a variety of sodium channels and downregulation of potassium channels. This altered expression is referred to as the *neonatal phenotype*. This assertion belies the enormous changes in channel expression that are associated with nerve injury. As an example, it has been shown that after nerve injury there is a significant increase in expression of the $\alpha_2\delta$ subunit. This subunit is found in the structures of several members of the voltage-sensitive calcium channel family. At the spinal level, this binding site is densely present in the substantia gelatinosa of the superficial dorsal horn and in the DRG. The relevance of this increased expression is suggested by the potent anti-allodynic effects associated with the actions of the agent gabapentin. This molecule appears to exert its effects by highly selective binding to the $\alpha_2\delta$ subunit. N-type voltage-sensitive calcium channels also show an increase in expression, and spinal delivery of N-type calcium channel blockers such as ziconotide also produces potent anti-allodynic effects.

NON-NEURONAL CELLS AND NERVE INJURY

As reviewed in preceding sections, astrocytes and microglia have been shown to play a powerful constitutive role in increasing synaptic excitability through the release of a variety of active factors (see Fig. 9.5). After nerve injury, significant activation of spinal microglia and astrocytes takes place in the spinal segments receiving input from the injured nerves. Work with TLRs suggests that products released centrally by nerve injury can activate these cells through the constitutively expressed TLRs. This activation is manifested by morphologic changes in these cells, as well as by increased expression of cellular markers for microglia (e.g., OX42/p38 MAPK) and astrocytes (GFAP). Of particular interest is that in the presence of pathology such as bone cancer, extravagant activation of these non-neuronal cells has been shown. Although the origin of this activation is not clear, increased afferent traffic and release of excitatory transmitters, as well as products that appear to be increased secondary to nerve injury, such as growth factors, appear to be involved. This activation of intracellular transcription factors serves to increase the spinal expression of COX, NOS, glutamate transporters, and proteinases and to downregulate other systems such as the chloride transporters discussed in the preceding section. Such biochemical components have previously been shown to play an important role in the facilitated state.

In addition to the role played by glia, there is also the appreciation that after injury, a variety of cell surface markers are expressed in the DRG that promote the migration of macrophages and neutrophils into the DRG. These cells are believed to contribute to the inflammatory milieu.

OVERVIEW

In summary, the post–tissue injury pain state reflects sensitization of the peripheral terminal in response to the local release of a variety of factors that initiate spontaneous activity and sensitization of the peripheral terminal. There is also a potent central (spinal) sensitization that leads to enhanced responsiveness of dorsal horn neurons that receive ongoing small-afferent traffic. This condition results in an enhanced response to input from the injured receptive field and enlargement of the peripheral fields, which can now activate these neurons through originally ineffective subliminal input. The augmentation reflects not only the local synaptic circuitry (glutamate/SP) but also spinobulbospinal linkages (5-HT) and by-products released from local non-neuronal cells. The afferent activation and sensitization are subject to regulation by a variety of systems, including those that regulate release of transmitter from the primary afferent and activation of the second-order or projection neuron.

Regarding the events that occur after nerve injury, it is evident that there are two principal elements, those that account for the spontaneous pain and those that lead to an alteration in the encoding of normally innocuous low-threshold mechanical stimuli. The spontaneous activity is probably a reflection of the complex events that arise from channel expression and the inflammatory factors that appear after nerve injury and lead to ectopic activity. The alterations related to the facilitated response represent evident changes in dorsal horn function. The net effect appears to be enhanced excitability secondary to the increased expression of excitatory elements and reduced inhibitory contribution. The increased excitation probably arises from a number of sources, including the activation of non-neuronal cells.

Finally, peripheral nerve injury, such as that caused by compression or trauma and chemotherapy, leads to a persistent pain state. In contrast, local tissue injury or inflammation results in hyperpathic states, with the time course paralleling the onset and resolution of the injury state. However, as reported in humans, the pain state originating from prolonged inflammation may persist even when the inflammatory state resolves (loss of neutrophils/macrophages and cytokines). Comparable pain states have been identified in preclinical models. Recognition of this propensity of an acute injury to transition to a persistent or chronic pain condition raises important issues about the convergence of mechanisms that underlie the inflammatory and nerve injury conditions. For example, it is noteworthy that trophic and persistent changes in the DRG have been identified after long intervals (days to weeks) in animal models. In this case, transcription factors (e.g., ATF-3) are activated that show little tendency to reverse even over extended intervals. This suggests the possibility that in populations of patients and in certain preclinical models, peripheral inflammation may lead to persistent changes in afferent neuraxial coupling. In studies involving TLR mutants, these changes in persistent pain and upregulation of transcription factors have been prevented. Other persistent changes will probably also be identified.

KEY POINTS

- Aβ afferents, which are large, myelinated, fast-conducting axons, are typically activated by low-intensity mechanical stimuli. Aδ fibers, smaller, myelinated, fast-conducting afferents, have subpopulations that preferentially respond to thermal or mechanical, low- or high-threshold stimuli. C fibers, small unmyelinated, very slowly conducting afferents, are activated by high-intensity thermal or mechanical stimuli (or both).
- With tissue injury, ongoing activity is initiated by changes in the local milieu that evoke activity and sensitize the peripheral terminal. With ongoing small afferent input, there is a spinal sensitization that reflects acute increases in neuronal responsiveness mediated by NMDA receptors and longer term events reflecting activation of kinases, generation of pro-inflammatory intermediaries, and yet more persistent events mediated by transcriptional activation.
- After a chemical, immune, or mechanical injury to the nerve, afferent axons display (1) an initial burst of afferent firing, (2) electrical silence for an interval of hours to days, and (3) the appearance of "spontaneous" bursting activity in both myelinated and unmyelinated axons over hours to days. This ongoing activity reflects the initial dying back of the injured axon (retrograde chromatolysis) and then initiation of sprouting.
- Bulbospinal serotonergic projections act through excitatory 5-HT_3 receptors to enhance the firing of these lamina V neurons. These cells are noted for their ability to display a facilitated state called "wind-up." Blockade of this bulbospinal linkage or the use of 5-HT_3 inhibitors has been reported to reduce this facilitated state.
- It has been demonstrated that behavioral models of facilitation wherein the injury is carried out under a systemic anesthetic (barbiturate, volatile agent, etc.) show that the hyperalgesic state may be initiated despite the fact that the injury is inflicted under the influence of an anesthetic.

KEY POINTS—cont'd

- Though preventing the ascending pain message, anesthetics surprisingly do not appear to block the facilitatory processes that are initiated by small-afferent input, probably at the level of transmitter release at the first spinal synapse.
- Prostaglandins act on a number of eponymous receptors that are located *presynaptically* on the primary afferent terminal and *postsynaptically* on second-order neurons.
- Following peripheral nerve injury, ongoing pain appears to represent ectopic activity in the neuroma and the DRG, a phenomena reflecting upregulation of sodium channels and the expression of receptors activated by changes in the local milieu. The enhanced response to low threshold stimulation may reflect loss of intrinsic GABA and glycinergic inhibition and activation of non-neuronal cells.

SUGGESTED READINGS

Bardin L. The complex role of serotonin and 5-HT receptors in chronic pain. *Behav Pharmacol.* 2011;22:390-404.

Bohlen CJ, Julius D. Receptor-targeting mechanisms of pain-causing toxins: how? *Toxicon.* 2012;60:254-264.

Chiang CY, Sessle BJ, Dostrovsky JO. Role of astrocytes in pain. *Neurochem Res.* 2012;37:2419-2431.

Christianson CA, Dumlao DS, Stokes JA, et al. Spinal TLR4 mediates the transition to a persistent mechanical hypersensitivity after the resolution of inflammation in serum-transferred arthritis. *Pain.* 2011;152:2881-2891.

Old EA, Malcangio M. Chemokine mediated neuron-glia communication and aberrant signalling in neuropathic pain states. *Curr Opin Pharmacol.* 2012;12:67-73.

Sorkin LS, Yaksh TL. Central pharmacology of nociceptive transmission. In: Koltzenburg M, McMahon SB, eds. *Wall and Melzack's Textbook of Pain.* 6th ed. St. Louis: Elsevier; 2012:371-414.

Todd AJ. Chapter 6 Anatomy and neurochemistry of the dorsal horn. *Handb Clin Neurol.* 2006;81:61-76.

Todd AJ. Neuronal circuitry for pain processing in the dorsal horn. *Nat Rev Neurosci.* 2010;11:823-836.

Trang T, Beggs S, Salter MW. Brain-derived neurotrophic factor from microglia: a molecular substrate for neuropathic pain. *Neuron Glia Biol.* 2011;7:99-108.

Willis Jr WD. The somatosensory system, with emphasis on structures important for pain. *Brain Res Rev.* 2007;55:297-313.

Wood JN. Ion channels in analgesia research. *Handb Exp Pharmacol.* 2007;177:329-358.

Xu Q, Yaksh TL. A brief comparison of the pathophysiology of inflammatory versus neuropathic pain. *Curr Opin Anaesthesiol.* 2011;24:400-407.

The comments in this chapter related to the pharmacology of the substrates activated after tissue injury and nerve injury must be considered as a broad overview. More detailed considerations and citations can be found in a several detailed reviews and texts listed above.

Pain and Brain Changes

10

A.Vania Apkarian

Change, alternatively referred to as reorganization or plasticity, is a fundamental property of the brain that enables it to adapt and thus enhance survival of the organism. It has been documented and studied across all the scales of the brain. The smallest unit of neural processing is the individual channel and its related receptor. Its efficacy can be modulated by various mechanisms, for example, changes in the availability or concentration of various chemicals within the intracellular or extracellular environment. Such a change can lead to an increase either in local resting membrane potential or, when it influences the excitability of the neuron, in an increased or decreased rate of firing. A change in either resting membrane potential or individual neuronal firing rate can in turn modulate individual synapse strength, which can be demonstrated experimentally as phenomena called long-term potentiation and long-term depression. Cumulative changes across these microscopic scales would in turn lead to reorganization of whole territories of the cortex, in which one functional specialization may be abandoned and replaced by another. Several review articles highlight the recent excitement in the topic across multiple brain functional systems, from the single synapse to large-scale reorganization.[1-6] We now know that all of this happens in the human brain, perhaps more subtly in the adult than in the developing brain, and we also know that such events are fundamental for understanding the brain mechanisms of pain. We will revisit each of these mechanisms specifically in the context of pain perception.

Regarding pain, there has been a fundamental shift in our concept of the functional role of the brain. Until about 15 years ago, most basic research on pain involved charting the "telephone lines" and the "code" for these lines. Basically, most work in the field was an attempt to establish pain as a sensory modality with its unique pathways and presentation within the peripheral nervous system (PNS) and central nervous system (CNS). Chapter 8, which discusses the anatomy of pain systems, nicely demonstrates this knowledge and shows the distinct PNS and CNS components that participate in coding pain. This work has been highly successful in showing that unique receptors in the skin are involved in responding to mechanical, thermal, and chemical noxious stimuli. This information is transmitted through specialized myelinated and unmyelinated fibers to the spinal cord, where the nociceptive input converges on specific populations of cells, which in turn transmit the signal cephalad through multiple ascending pathways to give rise to the perception of pain. Descending modulatory pathways converge back on nociceptive neurons in the spinal cord and control their level of excitability based on environmental conditions. This is the "telephone line" view of pain perception, also known as the specificity theory of pain, which some researchers criticized for years as being too limited and simplistic in scope.[7-9] Its basic underlying assumption is a unidirectional flow of information from the environment to the cortex through specific pathways, disruption of any parts of which would break the telephone lines of communication and relieve the pain. Within this viewpoint there is little space to accommodate some of the most debilitating clinical pain conditions, namely, chronic pain, and in fact even the existence of these conditions was highly controversial for large portions of the past century. There remain hard-core scientists who still adhere to this notion[10]; however, the brunt of scientific evidence generated recently shows that the plasticity of the brain and peripheral nerves is a fundamental component of pain, especially for clinical pain in general and even more specifically for chronic pain. Recent studies have repeatedly uncovered the fact that disruption of any of the PNS or CNS components of the network underlying pain perception results, in most cases, in exacerbation of pain behavior rather than its diminution and that the specific site and extent of injury result in mimicking, at least in part, various clinical pain conditions. Plasticity of the PNS and CNS seems to be a universal consequence of persistent pain, the details of which depend on the type and extent of injury giving rise to the persistent pain. Accordingly, Woolf and Salter[11] concluded, "All living organisms need to be able to react to noxious stimuli, and a major evolutionary drive for the development of a plastic nervous system might have been the acquisition of the capacity to detect and remember pain." This suggests the possibility that the ability of the brain to change was driven by its need to adapt to coping with pain rather than the other way around.

ACUTE NOCICEPTION IN CONTRAST TO PERSISTENT PAIN

Activation of the nociceptive system in the absence of changes in the PNS or CNS is supposed to happen only when short-lasting stimuli (on the scale of a few seconds and not persisting for more than minutes) are applied that can evoke pain but do not cause inflammation or injury. Under such restricted conditions, one expects to observe a primarily neuroelectric response in which, depending on the stimulus, nerve endings of unmyelinated and small myelinated nociceptors are excited and, in turn, activate second-order spinal cord cells that project to multiple supraspinal sites. The best known and best characterized of these is the spinothalamic pathway, which has all the characteristics necessary for coding stimulus properties such as its location, intensity, and modality. The spinothalamic pathway has also been classically attributed with conveying the emotional properties of noxious stimuli,[12] although recent brain-imaging studies are beginning to question this notion, at least in humans.[13,14] As soon as noxious stimuli increase in duration or intensity, they are accompanied by inflammation or injury, which in turn results in a long list of PNS and CNS changes.

DEFINITIONS OF GENERAL PAIN TYPES

- **Nociceptive pain** refers to normal, acute pain perception evoked by short-lasting noxious stimuli in intact tissue in the absence of peripheral or central sensitization.
- **Inflammatory pain** refers to pain following tissue injury but with no neural injury. Some group this under nociceptive, others under pathophysiologic pain. There is ample evidence of peripheral and central reorganization in such conditions; thus, it cannot be regarded as normal pain.
- **Neuropathic pain** refers to pain after neural injury. It is generally accepted as a pathophysiologic state accompanied by peripheral and central reorganization.

DEFINITIONS OF ABNORMAL PAIN

- **Allodynia** is the perception of pain from a stimulus that in a healthy organism is not painful.
- **Hyperalgesia** is an enhanced perception of pain from a stimulus that does evoke pain in a healthy organism but to a lesser extent.
- **Primary sensitization** is an enhanced sensation and related enhanced neuronal transmission within and around the site of injury, which suggests that the effect is a consequence of reorganization of neuronal signaling directly from the injury.
- **Secondary sensitization** is an enhanced sensation and neural transmission at body sites removed from the site of injury. It is usually attributed to changes in neuronal properties in the spinal cord where the end product of various changes leads to increased excitability of neurons involved in transmitting nociceptive input cephalad. The process is assumed to be a result of reorganization of the spinal cord nociceptive circuitry.
- **Supraspinal sensitization** is the term used to distinguish between spinal and supraspinal changes in nociceptive coding. Such processes are assumed to change the cortical elements involved in pain perception. These in turn would modulate the spinal cord processing of afferent nociceptive input through descending modulatory pathways.

INFLAMMATION AND CHANGES IN RESPONSE IN FREE NERVE ENDINGS

Free nerve endings terminating in the skin and viscera are the machinery for signaling local mechanical, thermal, and chemical changes,[15,16] as well as for modulating this local environment (Fig. 10.1). Thus, even at the level of the afferent receptor, nociceptive afferents are involved in two-way communication. Moreover, these receptors undergo changes in their response properties that affect the trafficking of chemicals, as well as the sensitivity to local events. Free nerve endings possess a long list of receptors (proteins that span the lipid bilayer membrane that separates the extracellular and intracellular spaces) specialized for detecting the presence of specific chemicals or stimuli (Fig. 10.2) that act as agonists and, by binding to the receptor, either activate intracellular second-messenger events or directly open the channel. To provide inflow of Na^+ ions, for example, the VR1 cation channel is activated at around 43° C and is also sensitive to capsaicin and acidity.[17,18] This process initiates a current, which then generates an action potential that by propagating centrally into the spinal cord may in turn activate second-order neurons that transmit this information farther centrally. Injury or inflammation results in local release of the "inflammatory soup," which includes peptides (bradykinin), neurotransmitters (serotonin), and neurotrophins (nerve growth factor). These factors interact with

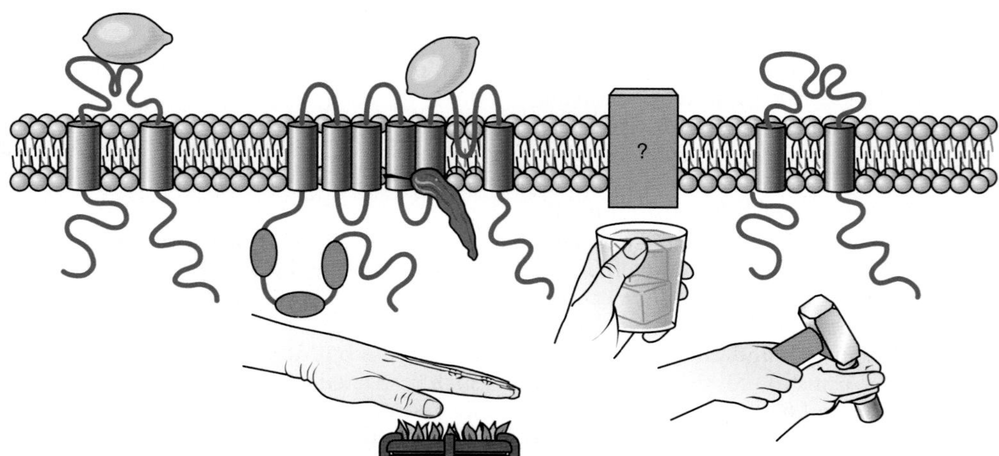

Figure 10.1 Nociceptors use a variety of signal transduction mechanisms to transmit local mechanical, thermal, and chemical events. Changes in local pH can be detected directly by a variety of types of receptors, whereas other receptors may be more specialized for mechanical deformation. The receptor for detecting cold pain remains controversial, although a number of candidates have recently been identified. Transient receptor potential vanilloid-1 (TRPV1) responds to noxious heat, as well as to acidity and capsaicin, the pungent ingredient in chili pepper, and these three dimensions interact and enhance responses from each other. The large majority of free nerve endings in the skin are called polymodal nociceptors because they contain multiple receptors and thus respond to various combinations of mechanical, heat, cold, and chemical stimuli. (Adapted from Julius D, Basbaum AI. Molecular mechanisms of nociception. *Nature*. 2001;413:203-210, with permission.)

cell surface receptors (see Fig. 10.2) to activate the nociceptor. Besides transmitting the information centrally, this process also initiates neurogenic inflammation by locally releasing various neurotransmitters such as substance P and calcitonin gene–related peptide (CGRP). Release of these substances by terminals on the free endings of nociceptors induces local vasodilation and plasma extravasation, as well as activation of non-neuronal cells such as mast cells and neutrophils, all of which contribute to the inflammatory soup (Fig. 10.3) and further sensitize these peripheral nociceptors by binding to their respective receptors, thus enhancing intracellular processes.[11,19]

NEUROPATHIC PAIN AND PERIPHERAL CHANGES

Neuropathic pain is distinct from nociceptive and inflammatory pain conditions in that the injury is itself neuronal whereas inflammatory injuries are caused by disease of non-neural tissue. Osteoarthritis is the prime example of a persistent (or chronic) non-neuropathic condition, whereas clinical conditions such as post-herpetic neuralgia (PHN) and diabetic neuropathy are classic examples of neuropathic pain following metabolic disease or infection. When the neuropathic pain is of central origin (e.g., after autoimmune disease, stroke, trauma, or cancer), it has been proposed that it occurs only if the central insult directly involves the nociceptive pathways.[20] The opposite does not seem to be true. That is, an injury to the nociceptive system does not imply the necessity of having pain. A partial lesion of a peripheral nerve commonly induces neuropathic pain.[21] However, severing of dorsal roots seems to have little chance of creating lasting pain.[22] Generally, neuropathic pain conditions are associated with abnormal neuronal activity at the site of the injury, as well as with central sensitization.[23] Thus, neuropathic pain is generally viewed as paradoxical because it involves severing portions of the nociceptive system and thereby usually causing various types of sensory deficits, which rather than decreasing pain transmission results in long sustained increased pain because of reorganization of the peripheral and central neural elements participating in pain perception.

When neuropathic pain is a consequence of injury to the PNS, the extent to which it depends on peripheral as opposed to central sensitization continues to be debated, with strong evidence provided for both views. The mechanisms underlying such conditions have been studied extensively, and peripheral and central changes have been well characterized, primarily because of a number of animal models that have been advanced over the past 15 years. In contrast, pain induced by central neural injury remains less well characterized and is best studied following spinal cord injury (SCI).[24] Neuropathic as well as inflammatory pain conditions are commonly accompanied by tactile allodynia, heat or cold hyperalgesia, and spontaneous pain. The extent of the contribution of each of these abnormalities to specific clinical conditions varies with the type of clinical

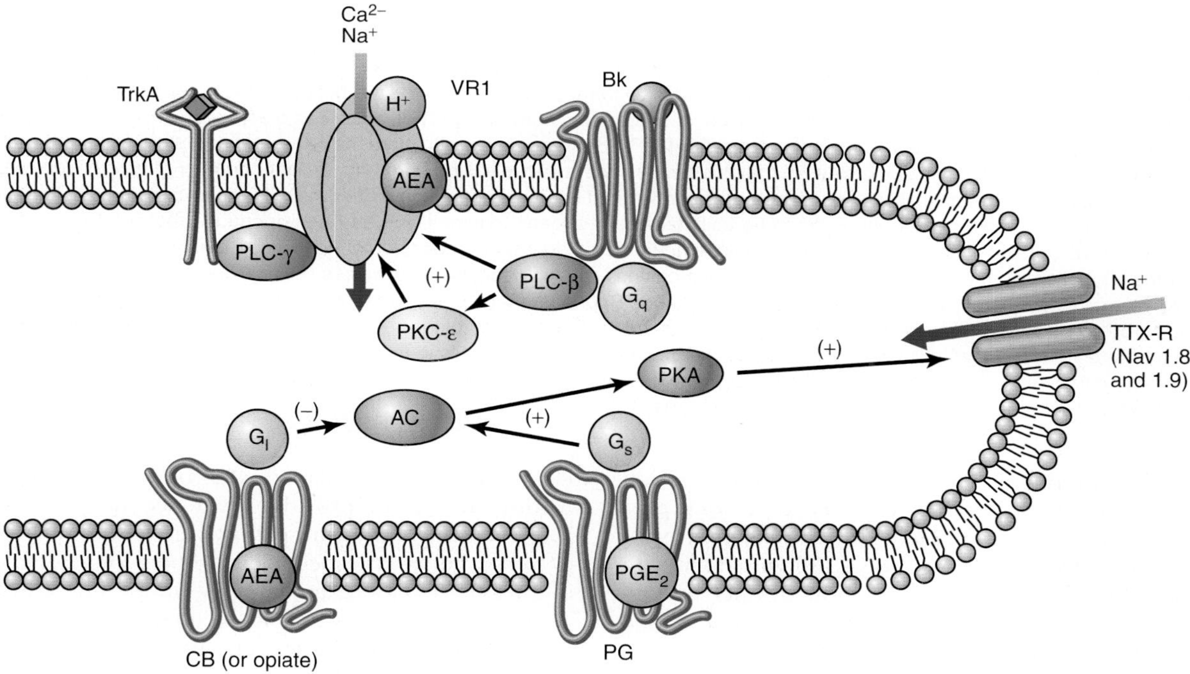

Figure 10.2 A variety of receptors spanning the nociceptive free nerve ending interact intracellularly to either enhance or diminish excitability as a function of the extracellular milieu. If the nociceptor's environment changes as a result of inflammation or injury, its excitability is altered. The effect of such changes on the vanilloid receptor (VR1) and voltage-gated sodium channels (Nav 1.8 and 1.9) is illustrated. An extracellular increase in the concentration of bradykinin (Bk) and nerve growth factor, acting through its own receptor (TrkA), shifts the excitability of VR1 to heat and acidity through intracellular pathways. Similarly, inflammatory products such as prostaglandin (PG) increase the excitability of sodium channels through intracellular messengers, whereas cannabinoids (CB) or opioids counteract this effect. AC, adenylate cyclase; AEA, arachidonyl ethanol amide; PGE2, prostaglandin E2; PKA, protein kinase A; PKC, protein kinase C; PLC, phospholipase C; TTX, tetrodotoxin. (Adapted from Julius D, Basbaum AI. Molecular mechanisms of nociception. *Nature*. 2001;413:203-210, with permission.)

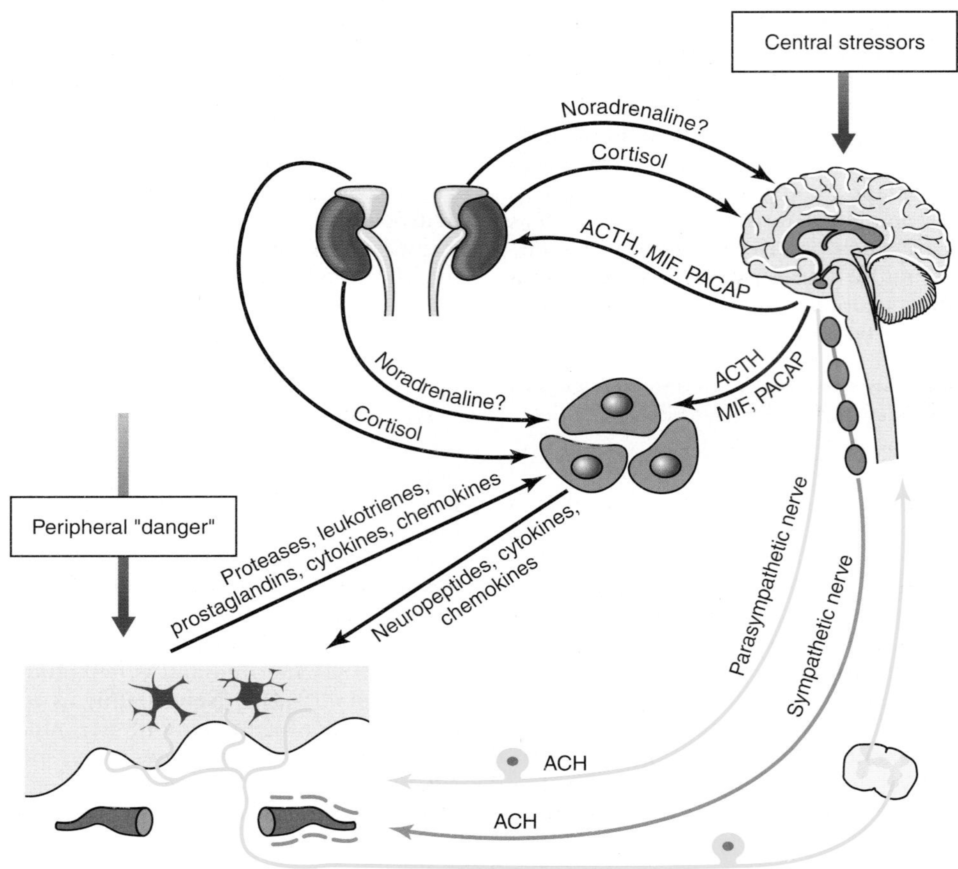

Figure 10.3 The inflammatory response at the skin is more complex than presented in text. This figure illustrates the main components that influence local inflammatory responses in the skin. The skin is regarded as a neuroimmunoendocrine organ and is associated with the peripheral nervous system, central nervous system, and autonomic nervous system. Stressors activate the hypothalamus/hypophysis in the central nervous system, thereby releasing neuromediators such as adrenocorticotropic hormone (ACTH), as well as macrophage migration inhibitory factor (MIF) and pituitary adenylate cyclase–activating polypeptide (PACAP). They may either stimulate the release of norepinephrine and cortisol from the adrenal glands or directly stimulate leukocytes in the blood via corticotropin-releasing hormone, melanocortin, or pituitary adenylate cyclase receptors and thereby modulate the immune responses during inflammation. Norepinephrine and cortisol affect several immune cells, including lymphocytes, granulocytes, and macrophages. Immune cells release cytokines, chemokines, and neuropeptides that modulate inflammatory responses in the skin. On stimulation, sensory nerves release neuromediators that modulate cutaneous inflammation and pain. Skin inflammation affects the activation of immune cells via cytokines, chemokines, prostaglandins, leukotrienes, nitric oxide, and melanocyte-stimulating hormone, which may have a proinflammatory effect (e.g., substance P) or an anti-inflammatory effect (e.g., calcitonin gene–related peptide), as well as PACAP by upregulating or downregulating inflammatory mediators such as cytokines. Autonomic nerves in the skin, mainly sympathetic cholinergic and rarely parasympathetic cholinergic nerves (ACH), innervate several cells in the skin, thereby maintaining skin homeostasis and regulating inflammation as well as host defense. (From Roosterman D, Goerge T, Schneider SW, et al. Neuronal control of skin function: the skin as a neuroimmunoendocrine organ. *Physiol Rev*. 2006;86:1309-1379.)

condition; for example, PHN is associated with a very high incidence of tactile allodynia, whereas chronic back pain (CBP) is dominated by spontaneous pain. Consistent with this clinical picture, animal models of inflammatory pain that persists for different durations show distinct peripheral and central reorganization. Similarly, different animal models of neuropathic pain, in which the differences sometimes seem trivial (for example, different approaches used to induce partial sciatic nerve injury), also show various differences in reorganization.

In intact healthy organisms, nociceptive input is transmitted through Aδ and C nociceptors. However, there is now very good evidence that following central sensitization caused by inflammation or neuropathic injury, peripheral input to the CNS through non-nociceptive, thickly myelinated Aβ touch afferents may evoke pain.[25,26] The latter is clear evidence that the functional roles of afferent fibers can be disturbed, again providing evidence that notions regarding specificity of the pain pathway are tenuous.

Nerve injury provides a new source of afferent activity as a result of ectopic discharges from the injured axons, in contrast to normal tissue, in which electrogenesis is limited to excitation of free nerve endings through transduction of noxious stimuli.[27] When an axon is severed, its proximal stump seals off and forms a terminal swelling, or end-bulb. In adults, axotomized cells survive and begin to regenerate from the proximal cut end. Many of these cells grow back and reinnervate peripheral target tissue. When growth is blocked, as commonly occurs with most injury conditions, the terminal end-bulbs persist, turn back on themselves, and form a tangled mass termed a neuroma. There is good evidence that neuromas generate spontaneous ectopic activity that directly contributes to the perception of spontaneous pain. Neuromas are also sensitive to mechanical and chemical stimuli; their activity is exacerbated by temperature. Both A fibers and C fibers show ectopic activity, although the latter persist longer after injury, and sympathetic-sensory coupling may occur at the neuroma through noradrenergic sensitization.[27] Overall, these changes, which are a consequence of damage to peripheral nerves, are triggered by metabolic and functional responses of the sensory cell that render it hyperexcitable, thereby contributing to the positive sensory symptoms of neuropathic pain, as well as triggering and maintaining central sensitization. Nerve injury induces alterations at multiple sites along the neural axis. Abnormalities occur in the injured and uninjured afferents, accompanied by central sensitization at the spinal cord level coupled with cell death. Additionally, there are changes in the descending control system, and immune responses in the periphery and the spinal cord are observed. As described later, such changes are also accompanied by reorganization of the cortical-subcortical circuitry involved in pain perception, in which immune responses as well as signs of cell death have also been observed. Generally, the literature on central sensitization simply refers to the fact that spinal cord transmission of nociceptive information is enhanced. Here, I argue that there is a specific cortical-subcortical reorganization that accompanies neuropathic pain and perhaps persistent inflammatory pain states as well. I label the latter "supraspinal sensitization."

The following is a summary of the evidence regarding the roles of various sources of afferent input in neuropathic pain. (1) Systemic administration of a selective CB2 cannabinoid receptor agonist reverses the mechanical and thermal hyperalgesia–related behavior in an animal model of peripheral neuropathy.[28] Because CB2 is expressed only in the periphery, the result is strong evidence of the role of peripheral afferents. (2) Similarly, reducing the efficacy of specific sodium channel subtypes in the periphery can decrease signs of mechanical hyperalgesia.[29] (3) In addition to the hyperexcitable injured afferents, there is also good evidence that neuropathic pain can develop in the absence of activity from the injured nerve.[30] (4) Spontaneous activity develops in uninjured, unmyelinated nociceptive afferents that innervate the same territory as the injured afferents, similar spontaneous activity develops following inflammatory injury, and in both the rate of this activity relates to spontaneous pain as assessed by the frequency of lifting the injured limb.[31] (5) There is also evidence for sensitization of intact afferents that develop adrenergic sensitivity[32] and increased responsiveness to thermal and mechanical stimuli.[33] (6) Messenger RNA for a variety of receptors is upregulated in the cell bodies of dorsal root ganglion (DRG) neurons of both injured and uninjured afferents, which are regulated by trophic factors transported from the site of injury to these cell bodies.[23] These processes contribute to changes in sensitivity to heat, cold, and mechanical stimuli in intact and injured afferents, as well as their responses to various modulatory input.

CENTRAL SENSITIZATION FOLLOWING INFLAMMATORY, NEUROPATHIC, OR CANCER PAIN

Glutamate is the dominant excitatory neurotransmitter in all nociceptors, and all primary nociceptors terminate and make synaptic contact with second-order neurons in the dorsal horn gray matter of the spinal cord. Unlike the rest of the CNS, nociceptive afferents also contain a long list of neuropeptides that are co-released from afferents and can modulate neurotransmission at longer distances than just at the synapse. Substance P is a peptide neurotransmitter that binds preferentially to the neurokinin-1 (NK1) receptor in the spinal cord. Changes in NK1 receptor expression and internalization can be used to identify the spatial and temporal effects of peripheral nociceptive input on individual spinal cord neurons (Fig. 10.4). In animal models of both inflammatory and neuropathic injury there is ample evidence that second-order synaptic transmission becomes sensitized, though with distinct properties for each general type of injury.[23] Moreover, newer evidence shows that in animal models of cancer pain there is yet another set of distinct cellular and molecular signs of reorganization regarding the state of second-order neurons within the spinal cord.[34]

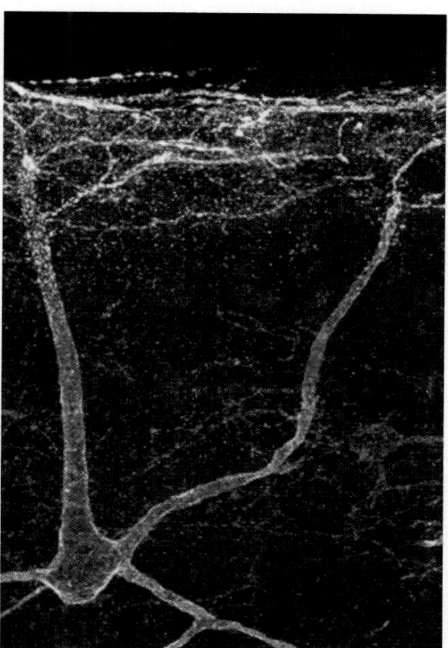

Figure 10.4 Internalization of the neurokinin-1 (NK1) receptor, a receptor that preferentially binds to substance P released from afferent terminals in the spinal cord. The cell body is located in layers 3 and 4 of the dorsal horn, whereas its dendrites extend to layer 1. The highest concentration of NK1 receptors is in layer 1, and a noxious stimulus induces internalization of these receptors from the cell surface into intracellular compartments. Changes in the location of expression and concentration of NK1 have been used to chart central sensitization processes. (Adapted from Hunt SP, Mantyh PW. The molecular dynamics of pain control. *Nat Rev Neurosci*. 2001;2:83-91, with permission.)

Inflammatory pain involves the sensitization of both primary afferent and spinal cord neurons. The neurochemical changes that contribute to inflammatory pain have been examined via expression and internalization of the NK1 receptor in the spinal cord (see Fig. 10.4) in acute, short-term, and long-term inflammatory pain states.[35] With acute inflammatory pain there is ongoing release of substance P as measured by NK1 internalization in layer 1 neurons (neurons located at the marginal zone; these neurons send supraspinal projections to a variety of targets). Although there is no tonic release of substance P with short-term inflammatory pain, 3 hours after injury, both noxious and non-noxious somatosensory stimulation induces NK1 internalization in neurons located in layers 1, 3, and 4. This is significant because neurons in layers 3 and 4 are classically responsive only to innocuous stimuli and in intact, healthy organisms do not show NK1 internalization. In longer-term inflammatory pain models (3 weeks after the initial injury), the same pattern of substance P release and NK1 activation occurs as in short-term inflammation, with the addition of significant upregulation of NK1 in layer 1 neurons. These changes suggest that there are unique neurochemical signatures for acute, short-term, and long-term inflammatory pain, and given that NK1 internalization is associated with potentiation of glutamatergic neurotransmission, it is clear that the longer that inflammatory conditions persist, the more spinal cord circuitry is recruited and associated with the behavior.

With inflammation there is significant upregulation of substance P and other neuropeptides, such as CGRP, in the dorsal horn, whereas these same primary afferent neurotransmitters are downregulated with neuropathic pain. In contrast, in a bone cancer pain model, no change in these peptidergic neurotransmitters takes place. Likewise, galanin and neuropeptide Y are markedly upregulated in sensory neurons with neuropathic pain, but no change is observed in these neurotransmitters with cancer pain. Even more marked are the different neurochemical changes induced by each pain state in the spinal cord. Whereas inflammation induces an increase in substance P and CGRP in layers 1 and 2 of the spinal cord, nerve injury induces downregulation of these same markers in this area of the spinal cord with an additional upregulation of galanin and neuropeptide Y. In contrast, with cancer pain, the concentrations of these molecules or markers are not significantly changed. However, the greatest change observed in the spinal cord in response to metastatic bone cancer pain is the activation of astrocytes. These results imply that with inflammatory, neuropathic, or cancer pain, a unique and highly distinct set of neurochemical changes occur in the spinal cord and DRG.[36]

Central sensitization occurs following inflammation or neuropathic injury and involves homosynaptic and heterosynaptic mechanisms.[11,23] Homosynaptic mechanisms involve changes in the response properties of second-order neurons with direct afferent input from the site of injury, whereas heterosynaptic mechanisms underlie the spread of hyperexcitability to neurons with input from intact afferents. The latter accounts for the mechanisms of allodynia. In this case, nociceptive input alters synaptic efficacy such that Aβ mechanoreceptors acquire the capacity to activate second-order nociceptors. Additionally, uninjured nociceptors can acquire spontaneous activity after neuropathic injury, and this leads to enhanced excitability of the spinal cord nociceptors supplied by this input. Sensitization, both homosynaptic and heterosynaptic, involves the increased release of excitatory neurotransmitters, such as glutamate and substance P, or enhanced synaptic efficacy, all of which result in a reduction in the threshold for activation, increased responsiveness as measured by the number of action potentials generated for a given stimulus, and expansion of the receptive fields of dorsal horn neurons.[11] There is a long list of mechanisms that can contribute to different extents to this outcome, including (1) presynaptic changes, (2) postsynaptic changes, (3) interneuron changes, (4) changes in descending modulation, (5) immune and microglial mechanisms, and (6) cell death. Convincing evidence along all these lines is outlined only briefly here.

1. Regarding presynaptic effects, the best evidence is for opioid receptors, which are downregulated with neuropathic pain and upregulated with inflammatory pain. Because opioid receptors control presynaptic and postsynaptic neural transmission from nociceptive afferents, these changes in expression result in modulation of central nociceptive transmission by both mechanisms.[11,37]
2. There is ample evidence for involvement of postsynaptic mechanisms in central sensitization. Primarily, release of substance P and other peptides opens the *N*-methyl-D-aspartate (NMDA) glutamate-gated channel, thereby leading to increased calcium entry, which in turn may also potentiate glutamate transmission through α-amino-3-hydroxy-5-methyl-4-isoxazolepropionate (AMPA) receptors.[38]
3. Inhibitory γ-aminobutyric acid (GABAergic) interneurons control the overall excitability of neuronal transmission throughout the CNS and play an important role in governing the sensitivity of dorsal horn–projecting neurons. The reduced expression of inhibitory receptors observed following nerve injury[35] decreases the inhibitory control on afferent input. Also, nerve injury is accompanied by downregulation of the potassium chloride (KCl) transporter, which reverses the effects of GABA release in that opening of the Cl channel now leads to excitation rather than inhibition.[39]
4. Descending modulatory pathways seem to reorganize with neuropathic pain and play a critical role in associated behavior. The rostral ventromedial (RVM) medulla receives input from the periaqueductal gray (PAG), which in turn receives convergent input from cortical, basal ganglia, and amygdala input. The RVM medulla projects to the spinal cord and has excitatory and inhibitory innervations within the dorsal horn. Many of the RVM cells express opioid receptors, ablation of which either before or after induction of neuropathic behavior eliminates hyperalgesic behavior.[29] This evidence is important from two viewpoints: first, the descending modulation must be substantially reorganized with neuropathic pain, and second, the supraspinal, including cortical, input interacts with the spinal cord processing of nociceptive afferent input and plays an important role in hyperalgesic behavior. Again, this provides the view that pain behavior is the integrated output of ascending and descending signals throughout the CNS and casts grave doubt on the unidirectional, dedicated telephone line model of pain perception.
5. Involvement of the immune system in peripheral inflammation is well established (see Fig. 10.3). There is now also good evidence for its role in neuropathic conditions.[40] Peripheral nerve damage evokes a cascade of peripheral immune responses that lead to macrophage infiltration and increased expression of proinflammatory cytokines.[23] Knockout of the proinflammatory interleukin-1 (IL-1) receptor along with overexpression

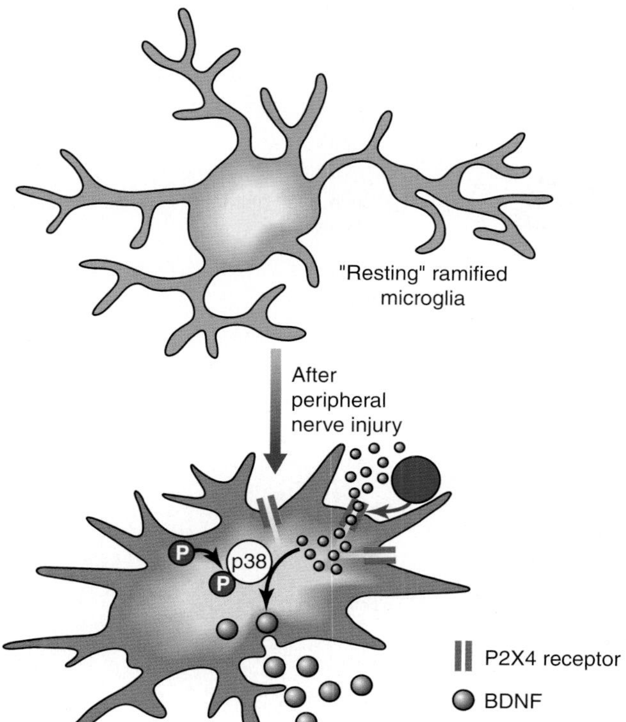

Figure 10.5 Numerous changes in spinal microglia take place after peripheral nerve injury and result in the phenomenon of activation, which leads to enhancement of central sensitization and mechanical allodynia. A critical factor in relation to neuropathic pain is upregulation of expression of the P2X4 receptor. Influx of calcium into microglia through P2X4 receptors results in an intracellular cascade involving phosphorylation (P), the result of which is the release of brain-derived neurotrophic factor (BDNF). BDNF then acts on neurons in the dorsal horn to drive the spinal hyperexcitability underlying neuropathic pain. (From Trang T, Beggs S, Salter MW. Purinoceptors in microglia and neuropathic pain. *Pflugers Arch*. 2006;452:645-652, with permission.)

of the IL-1 receptor antagonist decreases hyperalgesia and results in reduced spontaneous activity as recorded from dorsal root fibers.[41] Thus, peripheral IL-1 clearly participates in neuropathic pain. There is recent evidence that central immune mechanisms, mediated through activation of microglia, are also essential in neuropathic pain (Fig. 10.5).[42]

6. Cell death has now been repeatedly documented to occur in the spinal cord following peripheral nerve injury.[43,44] It seems to have a limited time course, underlies apoptosis, and affects primarily GABAergic inhibitory interneurons (Fig. 10.6).

This summary of peripheral and spinal cord changes with persistent pain of various types highlights the main components involved. It also ignores or skims over much of the detail. In fact, the literature on the subject is vast and growing rapidly. Here I have attempted to identify cellular, molecular, and structural changes that accompany persistent or chronic pain. This overview also sets the stage so that one can examine the literature regarding human brain activity with respect to pain and its relationship to the expected equivalences between supraspinal sensitization and peripheral and central sensitization.

NOCICEPTIVE SUPRASPINAL PROJECTIONS AND CORTICAL-SUBCORTICAL PAIN CIRCUITRY

There is a long list of pathways that convey nociceptive information from the spinal cord to higher brain centers (see Chapter 8). These pathways can generally be subdivided into two groupings: pathways accessing the cortex through the thalamus, which is the spinothalamic pathway, and pathways that access the cortex more indirectly through synapses at the brainstem, amygdala, and basal ganglia, as well as direct projections from the spinal cord to the prefrontal cortex. The relative size of these projections and the response properties of spinal cord neurons that participate in the different pathways have been studied relatively well in mammals, but such information is mostly lacking in humans. It is quite possible that some of these pathways may be preferentially enhanced in humans as compared with other mammals. The spinothalamic pathway has been studied most extensively, and the supraspinal circuitry regarding pain is usually cast within the anatomic framework of this pathway while ignoring the contribution of the others.

Conscious perception of external stimuli requires encoding by sensory organs, processing within the respective sensory system, and activation of the appropriate sensory cortical areas. Based on a small case series of infratentorial and supratentorial brain lesions in 1911, Head and Holmes[45] postulated that the sensation of pain is an exception to this rule and that its conscious perception occurs in the "essential organ of the thalamus." Despite evidence to the contrary from clinical reports,[46,47] single-unit recordings in animals,[48,49] and neuroanatomic tracings,[50] it was maintained for a long time that the cortical representation of pain was a negligible one.

This situation changed when modern neuroimaging techniques (positron emission tomography [PET] and functional magnetic resonance imaging [fMRI]) demonstrated systematic changes in metabolism and perfusion in a large number of cortical areas following the application of painful stimuli.[51-54] These findings were supported by invasive and noninvasive electrophysiologic studies in humans using magnetoencephalography (MEG), electroencephalography (EEG), and subdural and depth recordings. Meanwhile, it has been recognized that painful stimuli activate a vast network of cortical (and subcortical) areas, including the primary and secondary somatosensory (SI, SII) cortices, insula, posterior parietal cortex, anterior and midcingulate cortex, and parts of the prefrontal cortex (Fig. 10.7). These areas are now presumed to be involved in the generation of pain perception, as well as in the descending control of pain.[14,55,56] A recent meta-analysis examined the incidence of statistically significant activity across all brain-imaging studies of pain in healthy subjects over the past 15 years and indicated that in 68 studies the incidence of activity across these regions was 55% to 94%, with the lowest incidence seen for the prefrontal cortex (55%) and the highest for the insula (94%).[14] Hence the nociceptive system converges with other systems for generation of the conscious percept of pain. In this sense the nociceptive system is not different from, for example, the visual system. However, to what extent any cortical regions can be considered nociceptive specific is still an open question.

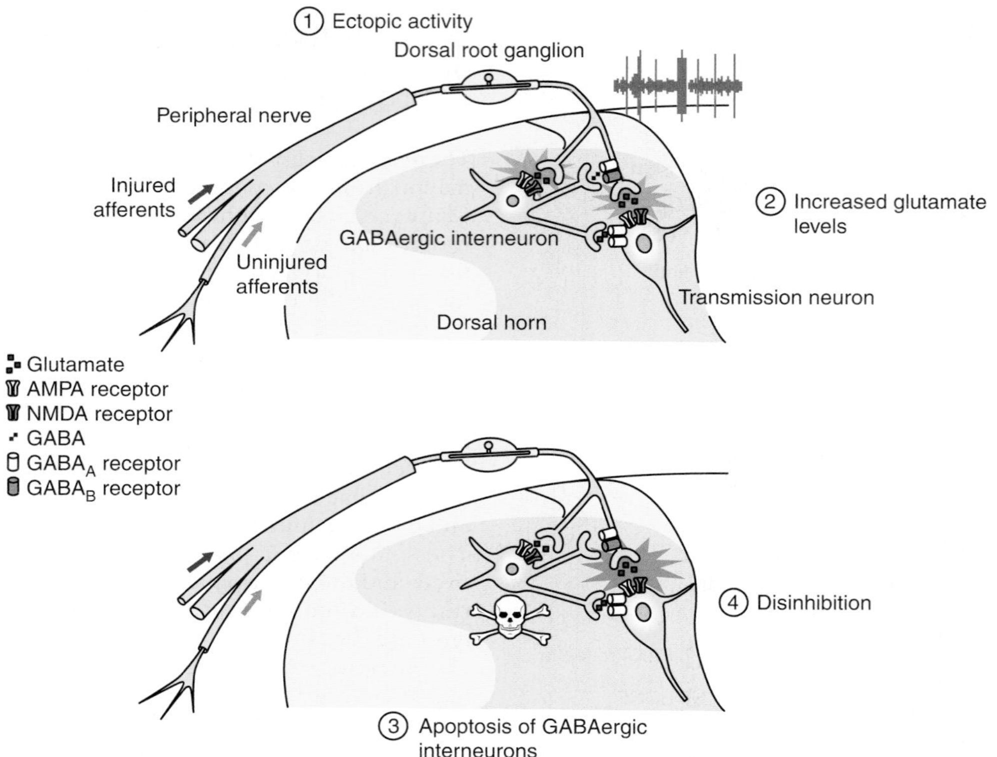

Figure 10.6 Mechanisms of neurodegeneration in the spinal cord following peripheral nerve injury. (1) Abnormal ectopic activity from injured and neighboring uninjured primary afferents generates increased extracellular glutamate levels in the dorsal horn. (2) Excess activation of *N*-methyl-D-aspartate (NMDA), glutamate, and α-amino-3-hydroxy-5-methyl-4-isoxazolepropionic acid (AMPA) receptors leads to a rising influx of Ca^{2+} into dorsal horn neurons, which over time exhausts the buffering capacity of mitochondria. (3) Apoptosis is induced in γ-aminobutyric acid (GABAergic) interneurons. (4) As a result, the GABA-mediated presynaptic and postsynaptic inhibition of sensory transmission is diminished, and input from nociceptive and non-nociceptive afferents is conveyed without adequate control. The response to noxious stimulation becomes exaggerated (producing hyperalgesia), and normally innocuous stimuli begin to produce pain (allodynia). (From Apkarian AV, Scholz J. Shared mechanisms between chronic pain and neurodegenerative disease. *Drug Disc Today Dis Mech*. 2006;3:319-326, with permission.)

Over the past 15 years or so, activation of the cortical and subcortical areas (including the thalamus, basal ganglia, amygdala, and brainstem) by pain in healthy subjects has been examined in terms of the specific dimensions of pain that can be mapped within this network, as well as its modifications with various cognitive and pharmacologic manipulations. Traditionally, pain perception has been conceived to consist of sensory-discriminative, affective-motivational, and cognitive-evaluative dimensions.[57] The sensory-discriminative dimension includes intensity discrimination, pain quality, stimulus localization, and timing discrimination; this dimension is traditionally thought to involve the lateral thalamic nuclei and the SI and SII cortices. The affective-motivational dimension includes perception of the negative hedonic quality of pain, autonomic nervous system manifestations of emotions, and motivated behavioral responses; this dimension is traditionally thought to involve the medial thalamic nuclei and the limbic anterior and medial cingulate cortices (ACC and MCC, respectively). The insula has an intermediate position in this concept and receives input from the lateral thalamus but projects into the limbic system. The cognitive-evaluative dimension includes interaction with previous experience, cognitive influence on perceived pain intensity, and an overall evaluation of its salience; this dimension is traditionally thought to involve the prefrontal cortex. However, numerous neuroimaging studies have assessed various experimental paradigms derived from several psychological concepts that do not easily fit into the traditional three dimensions of pain. Therefore, I discuss the evidence for involvement of cortical areas in specific functions instead of the dimensions of pain.

LOCATION AND QUALITY OF PHASIC PAIN

Neuroimaging studies have examined brain regions activated by many types of painful stimulation, including noxious heat and cold, muscle stimulation, topical and intradermal capsaicin, colonic distention, rectal distention, gastric distention, esophageal distention, ischemia, cutaneous electric shock, ascorbic acid, laser heat, and the illusion of pain evoked by combinations of innocuous temperatures.[14,58] Despite the differences in sensation, emotion, and behavioral responses provoked by these different types of pain, individuals can easily identify each as being painful. Thus, there appears to be a common construct of "pain" with an underlying network of brain activity in the areas described. Nevertheless, despite the similarities in pain experiences and similarities in neural activation patterns, each pain experience is unique. Subjects can usually differentiate noxious heat from noxious cold and from noxious pressure. Given that there is ubiquitous convergence of information from cutaneous, visceral, and muscle tissue

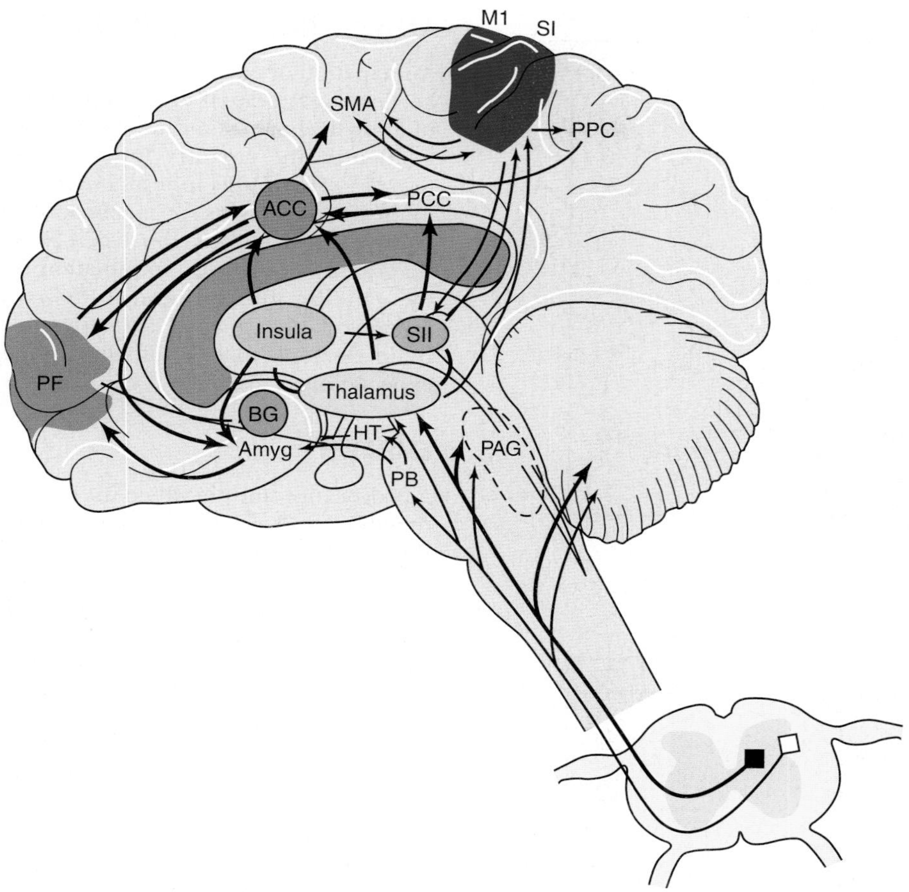

Figure 10.7 Cartoon of the main cortical-subcortical brain regions implicated in pain. Multiple ascending pathways are shown transmitting nociceptive information cephalad. The spinothalamic pathway with connectivity between the thalamus, primary and secondary somatosensory cortices (SI, SII), insula, and anterior cingulate cortex (ACC) is supposed to provide both sensory and affective information to the cortex. However, nociceptive information flowing through pathways outside the spinothalamic tract accesses the cortex through limbic and prefrontal pathways and may be more important in the hedonic and emotional aspects of pain. The cartoon is misleading in that it emphasizes unidirectional flow of nociceptive information. As emphasized throughout the chapter, there is now very good evidence that the cortical-subcortical circuitry projects through the periaqueductal gray (PAG), parabrachial nucleus (PB), basal ganglia (BG), and rostral ventromedial medulla (RVM) back to the spinal cord and affects afferent excitability. HT, hypothalamus; PF, prefrontal cortex; PCC, posterior cingulate cortex; PPC, posterior parietal cortex; SMA, supplementary motor area. (From Apkarian AV, Bushnell MC, Treede RD, et al. Human brain mechanisms of pain perception and regulation in health and disease. *Eur J Pain*. 2005;9:463-484, with permission.)

throughout the afferent nociceptive system,[59] differentiation of types of pain must be achieved by feature extraction via interactions between neurons in the cortical-subcortical circuitry (Fig. 10.8). Although this has not yet been demonstrated, somatotopic organization for noxious stimuli has been shown in human brain imaging, at least for the SI and SII cortices and the basal ganglia, and electrophysiologically in nonhuman primates in the thalamus. Thus these regions can all play a part in localization of pain. Strigo and colleagues[60] directly compared the brain activation produced by esophageal distention and by cutaneous heat on the chest that were matched for pain intensity. They found that the two qualitatively different pain types produced different primary loci of activation within the insula, SI cortex, and motor and prefrontal cortices. Such local differences in response within the "nociceptive network" might subserve our ability to distinguish visceral and cutaneous pain, as well as the differential emotional, autonomic, and motor responses associated with these different sensations.

REPRESENTATION IN THE TIME DOMAIN

The dual pain sensation elicited by a single brief painful stimulus is caused by the different conduction times in nociceptive A and C fibers (about 1-sec difference) and is reflected in two sequential brain activations on EEG and MEG recordings from the SI and SII cortices and the MCC.[61-64] Intracranial recordings[65,66] show that the earliest pain-induced brain activity originates in the vicinity of the SII cortex. These observations support the suggestion derived from anatomic studies that the SII region and adjacent insula are primary receiving areas for nociceptive input to the brain.[67,68]

ATTENTION AND DISTRACTION EFFECTS

Early human brain-imaging studies examining the effects of attention and distraction showed modulation of pain-evoked activity in a number of cortical regions, including

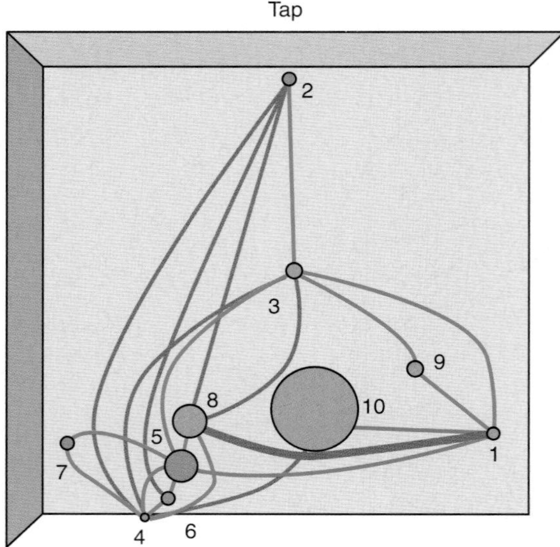

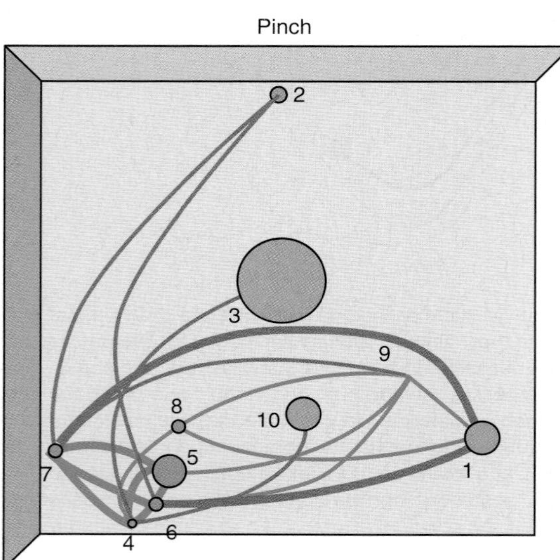

Figure 10.8 Changes in connectivity and firing rate in a group of 10 neurons recorded within the lateral thalamus in an anesthetized monkey in response to either tapping or pinching the skin. The 10 neurons are numbered, and their mean firing rate is indicated by the size of each circle; the strength of positive and negative functional connections is indicated by the colored connections (red and green lines of different thickness). The data demonstrate that functional connectivity between neighboring neurons in the thalamus shifts with the type of stimulus applied to the skin. (From Apkarian AV, Shi T, Bruggemann J, et al. Segregation of nociceptive and non-nociceptive networks in the squirrel monkey somatosensory thalamus. *J Neurophysiol*. 2000;84: 484-494, with permission.)

the sensory and limbic structures, as well as the prefrontal areas.[69-71] Other studies extended these notions by showing that during distraction there is a functional interaction between the pregenual ACC and the frontal cortex that exerts a top-down modulation on the PAG and thalamus to reduce activity in cortical sensory regions and correspondingly decrease the perception of pain.[72-74]

ANTICIPATION AND EXPECTATION

Anticipation or expectation of pain can activate many of the cortical areas related to perception of pain in the absence of a physical pain stimulus.[75-78] Two studies have attempted to identify the circuitry for modulation of pain expectation.[79,80] The results indicated that the expectation of pain intensity is necessary for maximal activation of the afferent pain circuitry and maximal perceived pain intensity, thus suggesting that cortical modulation by expectancy changes the gain for afferent input to the cortex. Generally, there remains a strong need for systematic studies to identify brain elements that modulate pain responses as a result of expectation.

EMPATHY

A provocative study in which the authors defined empathy as the ability to have an experience of another's pain opened the field regarding the interaction between pain and empathy. Using this definition and comparing brain activity when experiencing pain or knowing that a loved one, present in the same room, was experiencing the same pain, the authors showed that many cortical regions were similarly activated for both conditions.[81] These results were interpreted as evidence that the affective component of pain is active in both empathy and pain, and they thus concluded that empathy for pain involves the affective component but not the sensory component of pain. The study induced a flurry of activity in attempting to understand the relationship between empathy and pain. Multiple groups have replicated the main finding and proposed different underlying mechanisms.[82-84] Even though these results are internally consistent, their interpretation remains problematic. Simple introspection casts doubt on the notion that empathy means actually experiencing another person's pain. Instead, what is called empathy may be assessment of the magnitude of negative emotion that the other person may be experiencing, that is, a cognitive function of interpersonal communication. According to this concept, empathy may be conceived of as a psychological process involving cognitive-evaluative and affective mechanisms that allows us to understand the personal experience of another person. A study in patients with congenital insensitivity to pain[85] reported a deficit in rating pain-inducing events, but normal inference of pain from facial expressions ("empathy"), thus indicating that empathy for pain does not require an intact pain percept.

MOOD AND EMOTIONAL STATES

Studies show that experimental procedures that improve mood generally reduce pain whereas those that have a negative effect on mood increase pain. One study showed that looking at fearful faces increases the level of anxiety and discomfort, which also resulted in enhanced esophageal stimulation and evoked activity in limbic regions such as the ACC and insula.[86]

PLACEBO

Placebo is a potent modulator of pain; it affects all clinical studies of pain pharmacology. Placebo effects have also been seen in depression and Parkinson's disease, and recent brain-imaging studies have shown robust involvement of the brain and subcortical reward circuitry in these conditions.[87] The first neurochemical evidence for opioid involvement in placebo was demonstrated about 35 years ago by showing that placebo analgesia can be blocked by naloxone.[88] Consistent with this notion, changes in endogenous opioid release have been shown to be involved in placebo-induced analgesia, in which the prefrontal cortex (medial and lateral), as well as the insula and ventral striatum, seem to be involved, and in high placebo responders, increased opioid release in the ventral striatum is positively correlated with pain ratings.[89] Results generally consistent with this brain response pattern have been demonstrated by a number of other groups[80,90,91]; the medial prefrontal/rostral ACC responses to placebo seem to recruit the PAG and amygdala,[92] and involvement of the PAG in placebo-induced analgesia is experimentally observed as well, which links opioid descending modulation with prefrontal cortical control of placebo analgesia. The correspondence between placebo analgesia and reward was studied directly, and the results showed a strong correspondence between the brain regions involved in each.[93]

PHARMACOLOGIC MODULATION OF PAIN

OPIOIDS

The literature is vast regarding opioid descending modulation through the PAG and its effects on inhibitory interneurons in the spinal cord. The presence of large concentrations of opioid receptors at the cortical and subcortical levels has also been known for decades, yet little effort has been devoted to understanding the role of the latter in pain. Recent studies of opioid responses in the brain have used two approaches: examination of metabolic function in response to pharmacologic agents and direct measurement of receptors. The effect of the μ-opioid agonist fentanyl on brain responses to painful stimuli has been explored, and it was found that most cortical responses to pain are reduced or eliminated, thus confirming the analgesic effects of the opioid.[94,95] Changes in the endogenous opioid system are studied with a selective μ-opioid radiotracer, which shows activation of opioid neurotransmission in the ACC, prefrontal cortex, insular cortex, and subcortical areas during tonic muscle pain.[96-98]

DOPAMINE

Dopamine is best known for its role in motor, motivation, and pleasure control; accumulating evidence suggests that dopamine, primarily acting at the level of the subcortical basal ganglia, may also be involved in pain modulation. Human brain-imaging studies have documented increased pain sensitivity associated with lower levels of endogenous dopamine,[99-101] and sustained experimental pain has been shown to result in the release of dopamine in the basal ganglia.[101] Moreover, abnormal levels of dopamine in the basal ganglia have been associated with chronic pain in burning mouth syndrome, atypical facial pain,[102-104] and perhaps fibromyalgia.[105]

ESTROGEN

Women far outnumber men in susceptibility to many autoimmune disorders, fibromyalgia, and chronic pain. Differences in physiologic responses to stress may be an important risk factor for these disorders inasmuch as physiologic responses to stress seem to differ according to sex, phase of the menstrual cycle, menopausal status, and pregnancy status.[106] Some studies have documented that the threshold for and tolerance of pain is lower in women.[107,108]

The association of sex hormones with pain perception and pain memory was studied by Zubieta and colleagues.[97] Their studies showed that more μ-opioid receptors were available in the presence of high estrogen levels and that women reported less pain in response to acute painful stimuli than when their estrogen levels were low. Moreover, estrogen-associated variations in the activity of μ-opioid neurotransmission correlated with individual ratings of the sensory and affective perceptions of pain and the subsequent recall of that experience. These data demonstrate a significant role of estrogen in modulating endogenous opioid neurotransmission and the associated psychophysical responses to an acute pain stressor in humans.

OVERVIEW OF THE ROLE OF THE CORTEX IN ACUTE PAIN PERCEPTION

The preceding section describes the contribution of modern imaging studies to our understanding of the involvement of the cortex in pain perception. Cortical activity has been demonstrated to possess the properties necessary for involvement in pain perception, such as somatotopic representation of painful stimuli, correlation with stimulus intensity, modulation with attention, modulation with expectation and other psychological variables, and distinct brain regions showing differential activity for the sensory and affective dimensions of pain, as well as attenuation of responses with analgesic drugs. Thus human brain-imaging studies have asserted the role of the cortex in acute pain.

However, because imaging studies identify brain responses in a correlative manner, they may all reflect secondary processes. Perception of pain automatically directs attention to the source of the pain and results in autonomic responses, motor reflexes to escape from the pain, and other emotional and cognitive responses that are undoubtedly at least partially mediated through cortical processes. Therefore, the role of the cortex in pain perception, in contrast to its activity as a consequence of these secondary responses, remains unclear and needs to be properly addressed in future studies.[109] In fact, unpublished data from the author's laboratory suggest that a large proportion of the brain network activated by acute pain may be responses that are commonly involved in estimation of general magnitude for any sensory modality and, as a result, are not specific for nociception, thus suggesting that the majority of cortical activity for acute pain is instead sensory, cognitive, emotional, and attentional responses to nociceptive input. Therefore, the extent to which any given cortical region is necessary for acute pain needs further studies using multiple technological approaches. For most parts of the nociceptive cortical network, as illustrated earlier, it is likely that they participate only partly in pain perception (by providing certain feature extraction functions) and also participate in other functions in different contexts.

CLINICAL PAIN

It should be emphasized that although the subjective phenomenon of being in pain can be considered an emergent phenomenon of cortical activity,[56] there is currently no measure of brain activity that would objectively show whether a person is in pain. Therefore, neither electrical studies (EEG or MEG) nor imaging with fMRI or PET can be used to verify the presence of ongoing spontaneous pain in an individual. Neither fMRI nor PET allows clinical assessment of nociceptive pathways in individual cases because thus far no activation paradigm has been developed that would reliably induce a particular cortical activation pattern in each and every healthy subject. Consequently, negative findings with these techniques are inconclusive.

For the study of pathologic nociceptive processing at the group level, however, fMRI and PET techniques are extremely powerful. These techniques have broadened our understanding of the pathophysiology of conditions involving decreased pain perception, such as afferent pathway lesions or borderline personality disorder, as well as conditions involving increased pain perception, such as neuropathic pain or fibromyalgia.[110-114] Nevertheless, there are also large gaps in our current knowledge regarding general clinical pain states. For example, we have yet to begin to understand how the duration of pain in simple clinical states affects the brain's processing of pain. Do patients suffering from tooth pain for 24 hours versus others suffering for a week have similar or distinct brain responses? Clearly, animal data on spinal cord processing of inflammatory pain suggest that the two conditions should engage and excite a greater number of projection neurons, but clinical data are missing. Similarly, we have little knowledge on inflammatory clinical pain states in general. However, chronic pain conditions have been studied more extensively, which is appropriate because these are the conditions that we understand the least and this knowledge may translate into new avenues for therapy.

CHRONIC PAIN

STUDYING BRAIN ACTIVITY IN CHRONIC PAIN WITH NONSPECIFIC PAINFUL STIMULI

Chronic pain might result from cortical processing of chronic nociceptive input according to the same mechanisms as for acute pain, or there might be specific changes in the cortical processing of nociceptive input in patients with chronic pain. Such changes could then be either a causal factor for or a consequence of the chronicity of the pain condition. The primary expectation from animal model studies of persistent pain, whether inflammatory or neuropathic, is enhanced excitability of spinal cord nociceptive neurons, which would translate into generally larger cortical activity throughout the brain regions activated by acute pain. This is exactly what has not been observed for a long list of chronic pain conditions. Pointing to an important disconnect between the animal models and human studies, it is unclear whether the mismatch is a result of inadequate animal models or inappropriate explanation of the results seen in animal models.

A recent meta-analysis has in fact shown that across some 100 studies one can establish statistically significant differences in the incidence of different brain areas activated by experimental painful stimuli between acute and chronic pain conditions: the prefrontal cortex shows stronger activation in patients with chronic pain, whereas other nociceptive cortical areas and the thalamus show a weaker response.[14] A simple interpretation of these findings is that nociceptive signal processing of experimental painful stimuli in chronic pain patients involves a reduced sensory-discriminative component and an increased affective-motivational or cognitive-evaluative component. This interpretation is also consistent with the stronger affective component of clinical pain than of experimental pain.[115] However, there are further implications: Is the result a consequence of some trivial confounding factors, or does it signify changes in the physiology of pain? One could construct a long list of confounders that may underlie the observation, from shifts in attention to coping mechanisms to the effects of drug use to heightened anxiety and depression.

The standard approach for studying brain activity in subjects with acute pain is to induce pain with a mechanical or thermal stimulus and determine the brain regions modulated with the stimulus period and even with the various intensities used. Therefore, it is natural to carry the same technology to the clinical arena and apply it to patients with chronic pain. An example is one study that attempted to identify brain activity in patients with chronic regional pain syndrome (CRPS) via fMRI.[116] The design of the study was to examine brain activity when thermal stimuli were applied to the body part where CRPS pain was present and compare brain responses to this stimulus in CRPS and healthy subjects. Moreover, because the pain in CRPS patients with sympathetically maintained pain may be modulated by a sympathetic block, it was reasoned that one could decrease the patients' ongoing pain and then re-examine brain activity responses to the same stimulus. The study was done in a small group of patients, and this by itself is an important weakness, endemic throughout clinical pain brain-imaging studies. The main observation was that thermal stimuli in patients with CRPS evoked more prefrontal cortical activity than usually seen in healthy subjects, and this was reversed (became more similar in pattern to normal subjects' brain activity in response to thermal stimuli) following sympathetic blocks. The introduction of sympathetic blocks necessitated use of the same procedure in healthy subjects as well, and its effects were minimal. The study also observed that when a placebo block resulted in decreased pain perception, the cortical response pattern changed similarly to that of an effective block. These results show that brain activity with thermal stimuli may be distinct between CRPS and healthy subjects, but they raised a number of unanswered questions, many of which challenge the validity of the approach. For example, the simple assumption that sympathetic blocks were only or mainly affecting the CRPS pain without interfering with afferent sensory transmission was unclear. The analysis was based on the idea that spontaneous pain per se would not affect subjects' ability to assess stimulus pain, which may not be true, and that contrasting the effects of sympathetic blocks in CRPS and healthy subjects is valid.

CLINICAL PAIN CONDITIONS STUDIED BY STIMULATION AND THE ROLE OF THE CORTEX

A direct approach to studying clinical pain states is to provoke them and examine brain activity. This is feasible with the use of drugs that induce headache and cardiac pain. As a result, there is a growing literature in both fields. There is also now good evidence that migraine with aura is accompanied by decreased blood flow and reduced activity in the occipital cortex and that migraine with or without aura is associated with increased cortical thickness in the visual cortical regions involved in motion detection.[117]

MIGRAINE

Migraine attacks are characterized by unilateral severe headache often accompanied by nausea, phonophobia, and photophobia. Activation of the trigeminovascular system is thought to be responsible for the pain itself, and cortical spreading depression (CSD) seems to underlie the aura symptoms. This view has been greatly advanced and substantiated by brain-imaging studies. fMRI studies show the typical cerebrovascular changes of CSD in the cortex of migraineurs while experiencing a visual aura.[118] The subsequent decrease in fMRI signal is temporally correlated with the scotoma that follows the scintillations. These changes in fMRI signal develop first in the extrastriate cortex, contralateral to the visual changes. It then slowly migrates toward more anterior regions of the visual cortex, which represent the peripheral visual fields, in agreement with progressive movement of the scintillations and scotoma from the center of vision toward the periphery. A recent study that analyzed visually triggered attacks showed hyperemia in the occipital cortex independent of whether the headache was preceded by visual symptoms.[119] An alternative view considers migraine aura and headache as being parallel rather than sequential processes and proposes that the primary cause of migraine headache is an episodic dysfunction in brainstem nuclei involved in the central control of nociception.[120]

CLUSTER HEADACHE

The pathophysiology of cluster headache is thought to involve multiple brain regions. Brain-imaging studies imply that the associated, excruciatingly severe unilateral pain is probably mediated by activation of the first (ophthalmic) division of the trigeminal nerve whereas the autonomic symptoms are caused by activation of cranial parasympathetic outflow from the seventh cranial nerve.

Using PET in patients with cluster headaches, significant activations ascribable to the acute cluster headaches were observed in the ipsilateral hypothalamic gray matter and in multiple cortical areas, including the cingulate and prefrontal cortices. When compared with the headache-free state, only hypothalamic activity was distinct.[121] This highly significant activation was observed in patients only while they were experiencing an acute cluster headache attack. Newer magnetic resonance spectroscopy (MRS) results further substantiate this idea by showing reduced metabolites within the hypothalamus of patients with cluster headache in contrast to healthy or migraine headache controls.[122] These data suggest that although primary headaches such as migraine and cluster headache may share a common pain pathway (the trigeminovascular innervation) and activate similar cortical regions, the underlying pathogenesis may be quite different.

CARDIAC PAIN

Cardiac pain and its variants have been studied by brain imaging and the use of various drugs that induce these symptoms.[123-125] Overall, these studies imply that differences between different cardiac pain conditions are a result of central processing. Syndrome X, for example, is interpreted as a cortical pain syndrome, a "top-down" process, in contrast to the "bottom-up" generation of a pain percept caused by myocardial ischemia in coronary artery disease.

IRRITABLE BOWEL SYNDROME

Irritable bowel syndrome (IBS) is a disorder of abdominal pain or discomfort associated with bowel dysfunction. Hypersensitivity to visceral but not somatic stimuli has been demonstrated in IBS. A number of groups have examined brain activity in this condition, mainly by monitoring responses to painful and nonpainful rectal distention, as well as responses to the anticipation of painful distention. Two studies are interesting in that both show a significant positive correlation between cingulate cortex activity and subjective ratings of rectal distention pain in normal subjects, and in both studies this relationship completely disappeared in IBS patients.[126,127]

More recent studies show a hint of sensitization in IBS patients inasmuch as the use of subliminal and supraliminal rectal distention seems to indicate small differences between IBS and healthy controls in the total cortical volume activated or in regional activity as a function of distention volume.[128,129] A study of IBS versus healthy subjects examined thermal and visceral hyperalgesia and related brain activity.[130] This seems to be the only study in which, besides pain intensity and unpleasantness measures, the authors also documented fear and anxiety and showed that all are rated higher by patients with IBS undergoing both heat and rectal distention and that, not surprisingly, these increased sensations and emotions give rise to larger cortical activations in IBS patients. The latter is most likely a reflection of a mismatch in perceptual magnitude between the groups and says little regarding abnormalities in cortical activity in IBS patients. Such mismatches, at least for fear and anxiety, are most likely common in the majority of IBS studies. One assumes that the simple introduction of a rectal balloon in IBS patients would result in increased anxiety, which undoubtedly affects cortical activity in response to visceral and somatic pain, yet its specific contribution has remained unexplored.

In an elegant study, perception-related ratings were used during rectal distention to evoke either the urge to defecate or pain, and brain activity related to the ratings was compared in IBS patients and healthy subjects.[131] The approach is similar to the technique used for mapping brain activity in response to spontaneous pain in patients with CBP and PHN.[132,133] The results showed large differences between the two groups contrasted, with far more extensive brain activation in the healthy subjects. The results are complicated by the fact that the authors did not take into consideration the influence of spontaneous pain. Still, this is perhaps one of the best-controlled IBS studies and indicates distinct cortical areas involved in the urge and pain perceptions in each group.

SPONTANEOUS PAIN AS A CONFOUNDER IN ASSESSING BRAIN ACTIVITY

A person who has lived for years with pain must have developed some coping mechanisms that aid in pursuing everyday life interests. How does this affect the brain? Can one consider the brain of a patient in chronic pain as being a brain signaling pain together with a brain undertaking other tasks as in healthy subjects? Or does the presence of ongoing pain interact with and affect other processes as well? There is now direct evidence of the modulation that ongoing pain imposes on brain activity in general.

A recent study reported brain activity in patients with spontaneous pain and PHN before and after topical lidocaine treatment.[133] The PHN patients were imaged with fMRI before treatment, after 6 hours, and then again after 2 weeks' treatment with lidocaine. Behaviorally and based on questionnaires, most participants showed a modest but significant decrease in their ongoing pain. The patients were scanned while they were either rating their pain or rating a visual bar that varied in time in a pattern that mimicked their ratings of pain. Thus, the latter is a control task that captures the motor and cognitive parts of the task, but of course it does not reflect the pain. Brain activity with both tasks increased from the first to the third session. This observation is similar to earlier reports in which a decrease in clinical pain in many instances resulted in increased brain activity. In this case, however, the internal control was also changing in a manner parallel to the pain condition, thus hinting that the effects of decreased pain were modulating more than just the pain-related circuitry.

To identify the role of spontaneous pain on brain activity in general, a correlation analysis was performed for both tasks with mean spontaneous pain. The result showed that brain activity for both tasks was influenced by the level of spontaneous pain, which implies that pain intensity in general influences task performance. This is in line with previous studies showing that ongoing pain may interfere with cognitive function.[134] The finding indicates that the intensity of spontaneous pain affects brain activity for any task that the subject attempts to perform, with some aspects being enhanced and others inhibited. Therefore, the decreased brain activity reported for pain tasks in many clinical pain conditions is most likely a reflection of the presence of the spontaneous pain and is not specific to the task being investigated. The fact that pain intensity seems to modulate brain activity in general has another powerful consequence. It suggests that by simply studying brain activity in tasks unrelated to pain, one should be able to identify the presence of pain and study its effects on sensory, cognitive, motor, and attentional processing, an exciting prospect that remains to be pursued.

FUNCTIONAL MAGNETIC RESONANCE IMAGING OF SPONTANEOUS PAIN

Spontaneous pain is highly prevalent in clinical pain conditions and is usually the primary drive for patients to seek medical care. Thus, understanding its related brain circuitry is scientifically as well as therapeutically imperative. Cortical responses to standard mechanical or thermal stimulation are of limited value for understanding these clinical pain conditions. Spontaneous pain fluctuates unpredictably on the time scale of seconds to minutes, and these fluctuations have characteristic properties that differentiate between different chronic pain conditions such as PHN and CBP.[135] This variability can also be observed in fMRI signals when such patients rate their spontaneous pain. Therefore, this technique was applied to study brain activity in patients with CBP and PHN[132,133] with respect to their subjective report of fluctuations of spontaneous pain.

The combination of relating brain activity to spontaneous pain and correcting for confounders by subtracting the brain activity for visual bar lengths provides a robust approach with which clinical pain may be studied directly. Note that in this case the brain activity is related to exactly the event about which the patient complains. With this approach it was shown in CBP patients[132] that the brain regions activated when the pain was increasing corresponded to the brain regions activated with acute pain in normal subjects. In contrast, at times when the pain was high and sustained, brain activity was limited mainly to the medial prefrontal cortex, a region not usually activated with acute pain (Fig. 10.9). The resultant brain activity was strongly correlated with the patients' reported pain intensity at the time of the scan, specifically with medial prefrontal activity. Also, the duration or chronicity of the pain was captured in the insular activity, a region activated only during increases in spontaneous pain. Thus, two fundamental properties of CBP—its intensity and duration—were directly reflected in the brain activity identified in these patients (Fig. 10.10). By applying a painful thermal stimulus in the same patients (as well as in healthy subjects), the same study showed that brain regions reflecting the intensity of the stimulus were not related to that reflecting the intensity of the spontaneous pain. In turn, the brain region that reflected spontaneous pain intensity was activated only for the latter and did not reflect painful thermal stimulus intensity. Therefore, at least in the patient group studied, spontaneous pain involved a different brain activity pattern than acute pain did.

NEUROPATHIC PAIN

An MRS study showed that level of *N*-acetylaspartate (NAA), a neuronal marker, was decreased in the thalamus of patients with chronic neuropathic pain after SCI but not in patients with SCI and no pain.[136] Thus, neurochemical brain imaging provides evidence for the occurrence of long-term changes in the brain chemistry and morphology of patients with chronic neuropathic pain. Thalamic activity in neuropathic patients was also reported to increase after pain relief[137] and to be significantly negatively correlated with the duration of the condition in patients with CRPS.[138] Thus, the reduced activation of the thalamus may also be an altered functional state rather than an irreversible degeneration. Patients with neuropathic pain in addition show reduced availability of opioid receptor binding sites.[139] This reduction was symmetrical in those with peripheral neuropathic pain, which suggests possible release of endogenous opioids, but lateralized to the hemisphere contralateral to

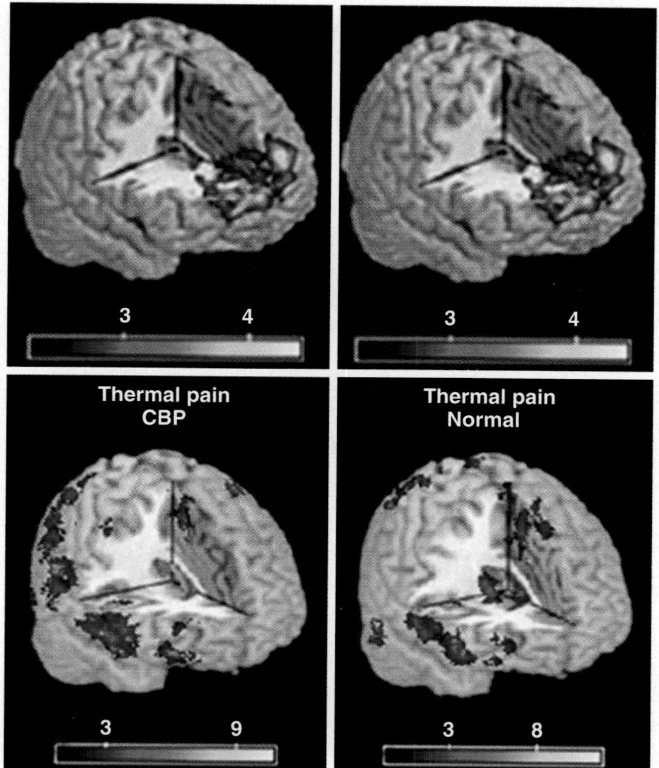

Figure 10.9 Brain activity with spontaneous pain in patients with chronic back pain (CBP). **Top left panel**: Brain activity in patients with CBP specifically for spontaneous pain periods when it is rated as high intensity. Activity is limited to the medial prefrontal cortex, a brain region involved in emotional assessment, especially in relation to self. In contrast, when the pain is transitioning from low to high, brain activity is very different (**top right panel**). **Lower left panel**: Brain activity for thermal painful stimuli applied to the back in patients with CBP at a location where the back pain was indicated to be most intense. **Lower right panel**: Brain activity in response to thermal painful stimuli applied to approximately the same back area in healthy subjects. Note that there is no difference between the two activity patterns, which shows that thermal pain responses are not different between patients with CBP and healthy subjects. Moreover, the brain activity shown in the lower panels is similar to that shown in top right panel. Therefore, the increases in spontaneous pain are most likely mediated through a nociceptive signal that invades the cortex, which is in turn sustained in the prefrontal cortex. (From Baliki MN, Chialvo DR, Geha PY, et al. Chronic pain and the emotional brain: specific brain activity associated with spontaneous fluctuations of intensity of chronic back pain. *J Neurosci*. 2006;26:12165-12173, with permission.)

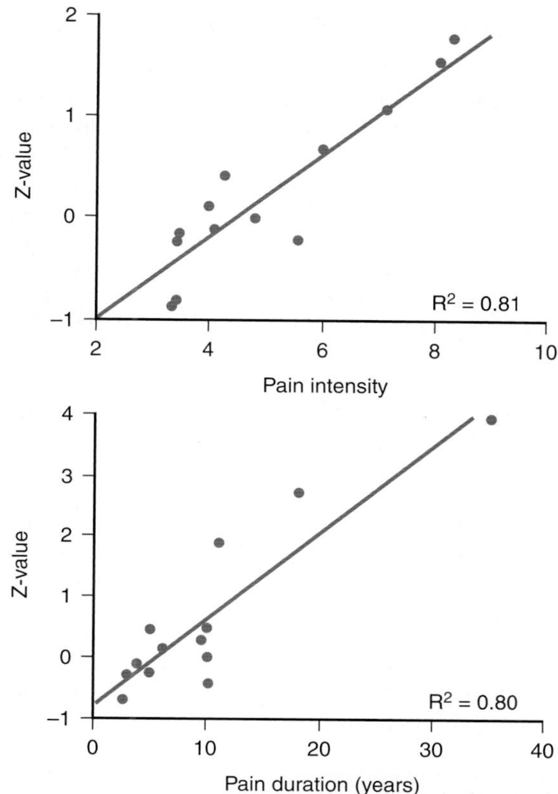

Figure 10.10 Brain activity in patients with chronic back pain reflects pain intensity and pain duration. The **top panel** shows that activity in the medial prefrontal cortex, for time periods when spontaneous pain was rated to be of high intensity, very strongly correlates with the intensity of pain that patients with chronic back pain report at the time of scanning. Each point on the graph represents an individual participant's pain, whereas the Z-value is the intensity of brain activity extracted from the medial prefrontal cortex in each individual. The **lower panel** shows the relationship between the number of years that each patient has had pain and activity in the insula when the spontaneous pain was increasing. Again, there is a very strong correlation between brain activity and pain duration in this case. These results demonstrate that by simply looking at brain activity at these two sites, one can predict, at the individual level, pain intensity and pain duration with very high confidence.

the pain in patients with central pain, consistent with a loss of receptors.[140]

Differences in brain activity between healthy subjects and patients in activation paradigms are difficult to interpret because they do not distinguish between brain activity specifically related to the clinical condition and abnormalities in sensory processing secondarily associated with the clinical state. Particularly in neuropathic pain, the accompanying sensory deficit may be reflected in the imaging results and not the pain. Reduced relevance of the acute stimulus in subjects who are already in pain may also account for much of the decreased regional brain activity in those with neuropathic pain. To overcome such nonspecific differences in brain activity, one needs to compare brain activity in response to stimuli for which perceptual evaluation has been equated between patients and healthy subjects.

A number of studies[76,116,133,137] have looked at the regions of the brain modulated by relief of chronic neuropathic pain. The brain regions modulated by these procedures were quite disparate. This heterogeneity is not surprising because the pattern of brain activity may be specific to each neuropathic pain condition. The most recent study[133] illustrates how such therapeutic procedures can be used to functionally subdivide brain responses to areas related to acute changes as a result of therapy and those that respond with longer-term treatment: regions involved in sensory coding such as the thalamus seem to be associated with the former, whereas areas involved in emotions and hedonics, such as the ventral striatum and amygdala, seem to respond to the longer-term treatment.

LOW BACK PAIN AND FIBROMYALGIA

As mentioned, the brain activity in healthy subjects and patients with increased pain sensitivity should be compared in such a way that the perceived intensity has been matched across the two groups. A recent study used such a design and showed generally heightened brain activity in response to painful mechanical stimuli of equivalent perceptual intensity in both patients with fibromyalgia and patients with CBP versus healthy subjects.[111,141] Morphometric and neurochemical brain-imaging studies provide evidence for the occurrence of long-term changes in the brain chemistry and morphology of patients with chronic pain. The level of NAA, a neuronal marker, was decreased in the medial and lateral prefrontal cortex of patients with CBP in comparison to an age- and gender-matched control group.[142] A morphometric study of patients with CBP also showed a decrease in gray matter density in the dorsolateral prefrontal cortex and thalamus when compared with matched controls.[109] Furthermore, these long-term chemical and morphologic changes are significantly correlated with different characteristics of pain such as pain duration,[13] pain intensity,[13,136,143-145] and sensory-affective components.[145] The morphometric and neurochemical studies imply an active role of the CNS in chronic pain and suggest that supraspinal reorganization may be critical for chronic pain.

EVIDENCE FOR SUPRASPINAL NEURODEGENERATION IN CHRONIC PAIN

Neurodegeneration in the spinal cord, which changes the topography as well as the gain for transmission of nociceptive signal, probably provokes parallel reorganizations in the supraspinal pathways. Human brain-imaging studies are beginning to address this question in relation to specific chronic pain conditions.

THALAMIC ACTIVITY IN CHRONIC PAIN

In contrast to experimentally induced pain in normal subjects, chronic clinical pain conditions are consistently associated with decreased baseline activity or decreased stimulus-related activity in the thalamus.[14] Interpretation of these results, though, is hampered by inadequate controls. The most elegant study on the topic thus far has been a single-photon emission computed tomography (SPECT) blood flow experiment,[138] which showed a strong relationship between the time of onset of CRPS and thalamic activity, thus suggesting that thalamic activity undergoes adaptive changes in the course of CRPS and indicating a transition from an acute to a chronic state. Unfortunately, there are no biologic markers for pain that would define standard time lines for the transition from acute to chronic pain. This ambiguity complicates interpreting the thalamic adaptive changes seen in CRPS. Early hyperperfusion in the thalamus might be a consequence of central sensitization or spinal disinhibition as a result of apoptosis of interneurons. Increased polysynaptic excitation after the removal of GABAergic inhibitory control may prompt a vicious circle that causes the degeneration of more dorsal horn neurons, including nociceptive transmission neurons, which would explain the long-term thalamic hypoperfusion.

Regional brain activation with experimental pain in humans is usually interpreted in relation to the spinothalamic pathway. The decreased thalamic signaling in chronic pain poses a puzzling dilemma from this viewpoint and suggests that nociceptive pathways outside this projection may be more important in chronic pain. Given the changes in thalamic activity seen with CRPS,[138] one possible explanation is early activation of the spinothalamic pathway, which at longer periods becomes hypoactive and is compensated by enhanced activity in other nociceptive pathways, such as the spinal-parabrachial-amygdala, spinal–basal ganglia, spinal-prefrontal, and spinal-hypothalamic pathways.

DECREASED METABOLISM IN THE THALAMUS AND CORTEX

In most human neurodegenerative conditions, such as Alzheimer's disease (AD) or Parkinson's disease, proton MRS shows decreased levels of brain metabolites, primarily NAA, either in absolute terms or in relation to internal markers such as creatine, phosphocreatine, inositol, or choline. Because NAA is found mainly in neuronal cell bodies, it has become accepted as a parameter for neuronal density and a tool with which neurodegeneration can be studied noninvasively. Recent studies indicate that NAA levels discriminate between patients with amyotrophic lateral sclerosis and healthy controls with 71% sensitivity and 93% specificity and predict survival outcomes in this population.[146,147] In AD, higher parietal lobe NAA levels are reported to be predictive of a positive treatment outcome, and lower levels correlate with AD progression as strongly as the rate of ventricular expansion does.[148,149]

With chronic pain, NAA decreases in the dorsolateral prefrontal cortex (DLPFC) of patients with CBP.[142] The concentration of NAA in the DLPFC correlated with pain intensity, as well as with the affective dimensions of back pain. In contrast, NAA in the orbitofrontal cortex was not associated with particular pain descriptors but correlated with state and trait anxiety parameters.[143] The association of decreased thalamic NAA levels and pain intensity has also been observed in patients with central pain after SCI[136] and in patients with CRPS or PHN.[150] Decreased concentrations of metabolites such as glucose or inositol have been found in the cerebrospinal fluid of patients with back pain caused by disk herniation or spinal stenosis.[151]

REDUCTION OF CEREBRAL GRAY MATTER

Given the baseline activity pattern and metabolic changes in the brain that have been found in functional imaging studies, one would expect a decrease in neocortical gray matter volume and regional gray matter density in the thalamus and DLPFC. Such changes were in fact the main observation of the first morphometric study in which the morphology of CBP patients was contrasted with that of sex- and age-matched healthy control subjects (Fig. 10.11).[13] Total neocortical gray matter volume was negatively correlated with the duration of chronic pain. Every year of living with the condition decreased cortical volume by an additional 1.5 cm^3 beyond the decrease in volume attributable to normal

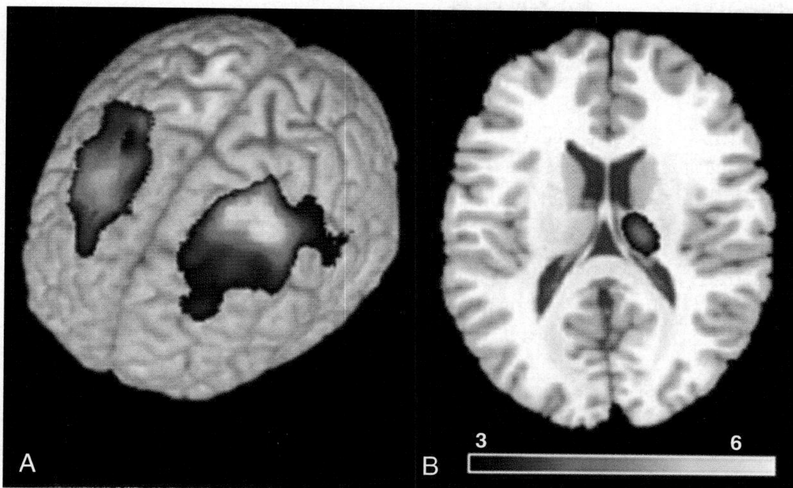

Figure 10.11 Brain regions that show reduced regional gray matter in patients with chronic back pain in matched healthy control subjects. The regional atrophy is shown in increasing brightness; a brighter color indicates increased confidence that the region has reduced gray matter in the patient group. The main brain regions are the bilateral dorsolateral prefrontal cortex (**A**) and the unilateral thalamus (**B**). The results suggest that such patients undergo a continued decrease in regional gray matter as long as they are living with their chronic pain. (Adapted from Apkarian AV, Sosa Y, Sonty S, et al. Chronic back pain is associated with decreased prefrontal and thalamic gray matter density. *J Neurosci*. 2004;24:10410-10415, with permission.)

aging. The specificity of the outcome is corroborated by the fact that the magnitude of DLPFC gray matter changes in patients with spinal nerve root injury differed from that in patients with non-neuropathic back pain. Furthermore, gray matter variability correlated with the sensory and affective dimensions of back pain. A recent independent study replicated most of these results.[152] Specific changes in regional gray matter density have also been found in patients with tension headache[152] and recently in those with fibromyalgia.[153] Details of the morphologic changes may be specific to particular chronic pain states, thus potentially providing biologic parameters that allow differentiation of chronic pain conditions.

The results imply that chronic pain is accompanied by cerebral atrophy. Yet the mechanisms underlying this atrophy remain to be elucidated. Cortical neurodegeneration may occur secondary to spinal cord neurodegeneration or reflect stress impinging on neurons that are trying to cope with increased afferent input. Genetic factors may render subjects vulnerable to chronic pain either because they have genetically determined lower gray matter density in brain regions such as the DLPFC or because neurons in brain regions at risk for chronic pain–related degeneration are more susceptible to stress, such as increased excitatory input. The brain atrophy in patients with chronic pain may be caused by an irreversible loss of neurons or by changes in volume, which could recover when the chronic pain is treated properly. The extent of reversibility of the brain atrophy in those with chronic pain is a crucial issue, and its relationship to successful therapy deserves to be investigated.

INCREASED AMYGDALA EXCITABILITY IN PERSISTENT PAIN

As part of the limbic system, the amygdala plays a key role in attaching emotional significance to sensory stimuli, emotional learning and memory, and affective states and disorders.[154] The amygdala also mediates conditioned and environmentally and morphine-induced analgesia, thus suggesting coupling to descending inhibition.[155] The amygdala is one of the higher brain centers with direct links to brainstem centers that are important for pain inhibition and facilitation.[156] Only recently, however, was a systematic analysis of pain processing and pain modulation in the amygdala performed.[157] In these studies an arthritis model was used to show pain-related sensitization and synaptic plasticity of amygdala neurons and, as a consequence, increased nocifensive and affective pain behavior.[158]

Neuroimaging pain studies using PET and fMRI have produced mixed results regarding pain-related amygdala function in humans. Some studies identified pain-related changes in signal in the human amygdala. The experimental conditions included the application of brief noxious heat stimuli to the skin of humans,[159-161] noxious rectal distention in patients with IBS,[162,163] and mechanical allodynia in neuropathic pain patients.[164] In these studies both activation and deactivation were measured. Importantly, a significant number of neuroimaging pain studies were unable to detect any changes in signal in the amygdala in response to painful stimuli or in certain pain states.[157] Evidence from recent studies suggests a correlation between activity in the amygdala and spontaneous pain in patients with CBP[132] or neuropathic pain,[133] with an absence of activity in the amygdala in response to acute thermal pain in patients with CBP and in healthy control subjects.[132] The latter, consistent with the results of animal studies, suggests that amygdala activity is increased in those with chronic pain, at least in proportion to spontaneous pain.

CYTOKINES IN THE BRAIN AND THALAMUS

The role of proinflammatory cytokines has been extensively studied in the periphery, spinal cord, and hypothalamus following peripheral inflammation. Recent results indicate that mice with a deficiency in the IL-1 gene have reduced responses to inflammatory and neuropathic injury. The authors concluded that IL-1 modulates both the generation and maintenance of inflammatory and neuropathic pain.[165] Another study in rats with neuropathic pain indicated increased endogenous levels of the proinflammatory cytokine IL-1β only in the animals in which there were clear behavioral signs of the presence of pain.[166] The latter is proposed as a marker for brain regions undergoing synaptic plasticity because changes in neuronal activity can result in cytokine induction in the brain and in long-term potentiation of synaptic activity in the hippocampus.[167]

ROLE OF THE CORTEX IN CHRONIC PAIN PERCEPTION

Despite a plethora of data, there remain a host of uncertainties about their significance. Overall, clinical brain-imaging studies indicate reduced transmission of information through the thalamus to the cortex and increased activity in the prefrontal cortex, coupled with regional atrophy. The number of studies remains small, and hence our confidence in the reproducibility of these changes remains minimal. Still, the observations regarding changes in cortical and thalamic activity in subjects with chronic pain are in general consistent with the notion that chronic pain conditions preferentially engage brain areas involved in cognition and emotion with decreased activity in regions involved in the sensory evaluation of nociceptive input.

Evidence has been presented that brain activity, chemistry, and morphology may be reorganized in chronic pain conditions. Does this evidence imply that there is supraspinal reorganization above and beyond what is established in the periphery and spinal cord? That is, even if we establish a brain pattern of activity for some chronic pain condition, does this reflect some unique contribution of the brain to this state or is it simply a reflection of lower-level reorganization? The answer is not straightforward. However, only by answering such questions will brain imaging be able to provide new information on the myriad mechanisms described for peripheral and spinal cord reorganization with chronic pain. Overall, this evidence provides signs regarding supraspinal sensitization and the long list of changes that may underlie this phenomenon, a process in which the primary or critical parameters that control these changes remain essentially unknown.

CONCLUSION

This chapter outlines the peripheral and central events that accompany pain with an emphasis on the cellular, molecular, anatomic, and physiologic changes that accompany various types of pain conditions. The review also attempts to highlight the gaps that continue to become apparent as the field moves forward and unravels the large number of factors that shift in relation to pain. The gap between animal models of pain and human clinical conditions should be apparent. Yet in many cases there seems to be growing evidence from studies involving both groups that similar and parallel changes accompany persistent pain. The animal studies provide convincing evidence of changes in receptor properties in both the periphery and the spinal cord, as well as changes in excitability and neurodegeneration, especially in the spinal cord. Human studies, however, provide better evidence of topographic changes in pain encoding between acute and chronic pain states, especially the finding that distinct portions of the cortex may be involved in each. The accumulating evidence for cortical neurodegeneration poses new questions regarding the driving forces for chronic pain, namely, are the latter a consequence or predisposing events for such conditions? More important, the chapter indicates that pain perception cannot be viewed as unidirectional transmission of information from the periphery to the cortex but rather that pain is caused by an interaction between ascending and descending pathways that reorganize the system at all levels.

Images of brain activation by painful stimuli leave the impression that at least half of the brain participates in processing nociceptive information. At other times, many of the same areas participate in visual, motor, emotional, cognitive, or other signal processing. In that sense our current understanding of the nociceptive network in the brain is consistent with the current understanding of how the brain uses distributed processing for its many functions. It is not clear, however, to what extent any part of the cerebral cortex is specific for nociception. The best candidate region for such a function lies in the parasylvian cortex, in the vicinity of the SI and SII cortices and portions of the ACC. In chronic pain, nociceptive processing in the cerebral cortex is partly preserved and partly altered, in particular with respect to prefrontal cortex functions. This reorganization may be a neuroplastic response to the chronicity of pain, it may reflect activation of antinociceptive processes, or it may even represent a factor predisposing to the development of chronic pain.

KEY POINTS

- Free nerve endings terminating in the skin and viscera are the machinery for signaling local mechanical, thermal, and chemical changes, as well as for modulating this local environment.
- The VR1 cation channel is activated at around 43° C and is also sensitive to capsaicin and acidity.
- Neuropathic pain is generally viewed as paradoxical because it involves severing portions of the nociceptive system and thereby usually causing various types of sensory deficits, which rather than decreasing pain transmission results in long sustained increased pain as a result of reorganization of the peripheral and central neural elements participating in pain perception.
- In intact healthy organisms, nociceptive input is transmitted through Aδ and C nociceptors. However, there is now very good evidence that following central sensitization caused by inflammation or neuropathic injury, peripheral input to the central nervous system through non-nociceptive, thickly myelinated, Aβ touch afferents may evoke pain.
- Neuromas generate spontaneous ectopic activity that directly contributes to the perception of spontaneous pain. Neuromas are also sensitive to mechanical and chemical stimuli; their activity is exacerbated by temperature. Both A and C fibers show ectopic activity, although the latter persists longer after injury, and sympathetic-sensory coupling may occur at the neuroma through noradrenergic sensitization.
- The sensory-discriminative dimension includes discrimination of intensity, pain quality, stimulus localization, and timing; this dimension is traditionally thought to involve lateral thalamic nuclei and the primary and secondary somatosensory cortices.
- The affective-motivational dimension includes perception of the negative hedonic quality of pain, autonomic nervous system manifestations of emotions,

KEY POINTS—cont'd

and motivated behavioral responses; this dimension is traditionally thought to involve medial thalamic nuclei and the limbic anterior and medial cingulate cortices.

- The cognitive-evaluative dimension includes interaction with previous experience, cognitive influence on perceived pain intensity, and an overall evaluation of its salience; this dimension is traditionally thought to involve the prefrontal cortex.

SUGGESTED READINGS

Apkarian AV, Stea RA, Manglos SH, et al. Persistent pain inhibits contralateral somatosensory cortical activity in humans. *Neurosci Lett.* 1992;140:141-147.

Bushnell MC, Duncan GH, Hofbauer RK, et al. Pain perception: is there a role for primary somatosensory cortex? *Proc Natl Acad Sci U S A.* 1999;96:7705-7709.

Caterina MJ, Schumacher MA, Tominaga M, et al. The capsaicin receptor: a heat-activated ion channel in the pain pathway. *Nature.* 1997;389:816-824.

Craig AD. Pain mechanisms: labeled lines versus convergence in central processing. *Annu Rev Neurosci.* 2003;26:1-30.

Devor M. Centralization, central sensitization and neuropathic pain. Focus on "sciatic chronic constriction injury produces cell-type–specific changes in the electrophysiological properties of rat substantia gelatinosa neurons." *J Neurophysiol.* 2006;96:522-523.

Gracely RH, Petzke F, Wolf JM, et al. Functional magnetic resonance imaging evidence of augmented pain processing in fibromyalgia. *Arthritis Rheum.* 2002;46:1333-1343.

Julius D, Basbaum AI. Molecular mechanisms of nociception. *Nature.* 2001;413:203-210.

Tominaga M, Caterina MJ, Malmberg AB, et al. The cloned capsaicin receptor integrates multiple pain-producing stimuli. *Neuron.* 1998;21:531-543.

Verne GN, Himes NC, Robinson ME, et al. Central representation of visceral and cutaneous hypersensitivity in the irritable bowel syndrome. *Pain.* 2003;103:99-110.

Willis WD, Westlund KN. Neuroanatomy of the pain system and of the pathways that modulate pain. *J Clin Neurophysiol.* 1997;14:2-31.

Woolf CJ, Salter MW. Neuronal plasticity: increasing the gain in pain. *Science.* 2000;288:1765-1769.

The references for this chapter can be found at www.expertconsult.com.

11 An Introduction to Pharmacogenetics in Pain Management: Knowledge of How Pharmacogenomics May Affect Clinical Care

Charles E. Argoff

CASE 11.1

A 58-year-old Asian male with no significant past medical history presents with acute herpes zoster in the left T4 dermatome. Presenting signs and symptoms include severe localized pain and tactile allodynia associated with a vesicular eruption. Even after the rash resolves, 3 months later he continues to complain of severe burning pain in addition to allodynia and hyperalgesia in the left T4 dermatomal region, suggesting that he has developed postherpetic neuralgia (PHN). Ten milligrams of nortriptyline, a tricyclic antidepressant (TCA), is prescribed with a plan to titrate up to a higher dose to achieve effective pain relief if the initial 10-mg dose is not helpful enough. Unfortunately, he is unable to tolerate the initial dose because he quickly develops intolerable adverse effects (sedation, orthostatic hypotension, and dry mouth) shortly after he begins taking it.[1] Tramadol and then hydrocodone/acetaminophen are prescribed but these are also poorly tolerated. He is then prescribed gabapentin at an initial dose of 300 mg taken at night, which is titrated over several weeks to an effective analgesic dose for PHN: 1800 mg/day in three divided doses. Although the burning pain is lessened, it is still not sufficiently controlled and the patient returns for further treatment. From the time of presentation for treatment, it has taken over 6 weeks for him achieve any notable degree of pain reduction.

This patient was treated according to available evidence-based, current guidelines,[1-3] yet he did not obtain adequate analgesic benefit from the prescribed medications. Clinicians recognize that individual variations in responses to pain itself, as well as in the response to pharmacotherapies for pain relief, are routinely observed; however, advances in pharmacogenomics may allow us to better understand why patients may have variable responses to various analgesic therapies and may soon allow an opportunity for clinicians to identify the most appropriate pharmacotherapies for a patient *before* prescribing and hence improve patient-specific outcomes. The knowledge and use of relevant pharmacogenomic information may indeed help a clinician to truly individualize a patient's care, an example of personalized health care.

In this example, the patient's treatment responses require a careful evaluation of possible reasons for them. Variability in patient response, including intolerable adverse effects, can be due to nonadherence with the prescribed medication or medication schedule, a drug interaction inhibiting the medication's effectiveness, mechanisms of pain generation that fail to respond to the prescribed medication's mechanism of action, or a combination of these. It is also possible that the patient's genetic background has affected his ability to clinically respond to or metabolize the prescribed medications, and this is where the emerging field of pharmacogenomics becomes important to recognize. This patient example illustrates the variable analgesic response and adverse event profile when analgesics are prescribed. As noted, clinicians are only too well aware how often individuals may not obtain the expected therapeutic benefit from analgesic medications.[4] The response rates in well-designed studies of various analgesic therapies are approximately 50% to 60%; this "treatment success" rate is similar to trials of therapies used to treat congestive heart failure and epilepsy.[5-7] Many key areas of medicine are similarly affected by poor responder rates in clinical trials of diverse drug types. Knowledge of relevant pharmacogenomic factors that may influence the effect of a prescribed analgesic should allow clinicians to improve analgesic treatment outcomes.

THE IMPACT OF PHARMACOGENOMIC RESEARCH ON CLINICAL MEDICINE

Pharmacogenomics is the study of the impact of genetics on pharmacotherapeutic responses and tolerability, in an effort to improve drug safety and efficacy through genetically guided, individually tailored treatments.[4] As noted previously, the same drug can be associated with different clinical responses among a group of individuals. This is because each individual's unique genetics provides the genetic blueprint for the generation of singular protein expression profiles, which subsequently leads to functional variations observed as clinical responses. Indeed, taking into account such genetic predisposition and receptor subtype expression has the potential to result in a more satisfactory reduction in symptoms or resolution of disease. This approach is certainly at the core of so-called personalized medicine. When the clinician is aware of a patient's genetic predisposition and receptor subtype expression, this knowledge may lead to more individually focused prescribing with improved efficacy and safety for the patient.[4]

Ongoing research on the genetic determinants of various diseases have been derived from the Human Genome Project, including The SNP Consortium (TSC).[8] Single nucleotide polymorphisms (SNPs; pronounced "snips") are the most important contributors to the observed regular variation in the genetic code, which lead to the human population's diversity of appearance and, at a deeper level, to our diversity in physiology. SNPs are defined as deoxyribonucleic acid (DNA) sequence variations resulting from a single nucleotide (adenine [A], thymine [T], cytosine [C], or guanine [G]) change in the genome sequence. As an example, the most commonly observed change is when a C is replaced by a T, as in when the sequence ACGGCTAA is changed to ATGGCTAA.[8] Overall there are approximately 9 million to 10 million common SNPs.[9] In many cases, this minimal change amid a background of the approximately 3.3 billion base pairs of DNA contained in one somatic cell does not lead to any significant observable change in an individual. Many of these DNA changes do not translate into differences at the protein level. However, there are SNPs that in fact do lead to phenotypic differences, and some single base pair changes do affect a noticeable, clinically relevant change in phenotype. Unique SNPs have been identified that lead to lower activity of various enzymes, red hair color and fair skin, and a lack of or diminished expression of one of the red blood cell antigens.[10,11]

The most commonly observed DNA sequences of a gene are called "wild-type," and the less common alleles are "variants" if they are prevalent in more than 1% of the population. The even less prevalent alleles have another name; DNA sequences in genes found in less than 1% of the population are called "mutations."[12] For example, within pain management, an autosomal dominantly inherited peripheral neuropathy, hereditary sensory, and autonomic neuropathy (HSAN) type I confers insensitivity to pain mediated through the progressive degeneration of the dorsal root ganglia (DRG) and motor neurons as the result of mutations within a specific location in chromosome 9.[13,14] Individuals with this genetic background cannot sense pain, making them particularly prone to painless but potentially severe injuries, with detrimental complications, such as chronic skin ulcers and distal amputations. Additional types of changes to our DNA can occur, such as deletions and insertions, which also can result in catastrophic consequences. Large population studies have analyzed hundreds of thousands of SNPs in an attempt to establish the genetic linkages to a diversity of diseases.[12] The Wellcome Trust Consortium published a particularly important study in the June 2007 issue of *Nature*. The authors assessed the genetic influence on seven major diseases by comparing the SNPs of 14,000 patients (2000 with each disease to those of 3000 healthy patients).[15] Genomic hot spots (regions of DNA connected to biologic functions/diseases) were linked to a susceptibility to developing bipolar disorder, Crohn's disease, coronary artery disease, diabetes (both type 1 and type 2), hypertension, and rheumatoid arthritis.[15] Key terms used in pharmacogenomics can be viewed in Table 11.1.

Table 11.1 Key Pharmacogenetic Terminology

Term	Definition
Genome	The entire collection of genetic information (or genes) that an organism possesses
Genotype	The genetic constitution of an individual, either overall or at a specific gene
Heterozygous	The presence of two different alleles (one on the maternal chromosome and one on the paternal chromosome) at a gene location
Homozygous	The presence of two identical alleles at a gene location
Isoform	A variant in the amino acid sequence of a protein
Messenger RNA	An RNA-containing single-strand copy of a gene that migrates out of the cell nucleus to the ribosome, where it is translated into a protein
Mutation	A rare variant in a gene, occurring in less than 1% of a population
Pedigree	A diagram depicting heritable traits across two or more generations of a family
Phenotype	The observable characteristics of a cell or organism, usually resulting from the product coded by a gene (genotype)
Polymorphism	The existence of two or more variants of a gene in a population, with at least 1% frequency of the less common variant
Prodrug	A medication that is inactive until it is converted enzymatically to its active metabolite
Single-nucleotide polymorphism (SNP)	A single base-pair change in a DNA sequence compared with the "common" or "wild-type" sequence
Variant allele	The allele at a particular SNP that is the least frequent in a population
Wild-type allele	The allele at a particular SNP that is most frequent in a population, also called "common" allele

From Attia J, Ioannidis JP, Thakkinstian A, et al. How to use an article about genetic association, A: background concepts. *JAMA.* 2009;301:74-81.

The integration of genetic information into clinical practice has far-reaching implications. For example, the clinical integration of genetic information has been increasingly used in oncology to guide treatment. Other areas of medicine are also beginning to tailor pharmacotherapies based on an individual's genetic information, and certain biomarkers are now known that can help to guide treatment in many areas of medicine including pain management. Pharmacogenomic testing has benefited patients and clinical medicine in general by improving the ability to stratify the risks of various treatments for individual patients by identifying groups of patients with a higher potential for poor efficacy or for treatment side effects (Table 11.2).[16] The beneficial effects of utilizing information derived from pharmacogenomics in the future of clinical medicine may lead to improved success rates, decreased side effect burdens, and reduced health care costs.[16]

Table 11.2 Metabolizer Status by Racial/Ethnic Group

Gene or Enzyme	Examples of Drugs Metabolized by This Enzyme	Phenotype and Frequency by Groups	Clinical Effect
CYP1A2	Anticonvulsants: phenytoin, carbamazepine substrates Antidepressants: clomipramine, fluoxetine, fluvoxamine, imipramine, maprotiline, nortriptyline Muscle relaxant: cyclobenzaprine NSAIDs: acetaminophen, naproxen	PM: Caucasian, 12%	Weak metabolism of enzyme
CYP2C9	Warfarin substrates Phenytoin Angiotensin II blockers: irbesartan, losartan NSAIDs: celecoxib, diclofenac, ibuprofen, meloxicam, naproxen Oral antidiabetics: glipizide, tolbutamide	PM: Caucasian, 2%-6%	Weak metabolism of enzyme
CYP2C19	Anticonvulsants: diazepam, phenytoin substrates Proton pump inhibitors: omeprazole, pantoprazole	PM: Caucasian, 2%-6%; Chinese,15%-17%; Japanese, 18%-23%	Weak metabolism of enzyme
CYP2D6	Analgesics: codeine, dextromethorphan, oxycodone, tramadol substrates Antiarrhythmic drugs: ajmaline, flecainide, mexiletine, propafenone Antiemetics: metoclopramide Antipsychotics + SSRIs: fluoxetine, haloperidol, paroxetine β-blockers: metoprolol, propranolol, timolol 5-HT3 antagonists: ondansetron, tropisetron TCAs: amitriptyline, clomipramine, desipramine, imipramine	PM: Caucasian, 3%-10%; Chinese/Japanese/ African American, <2% UR: Ethiopian, 20%; Hispanic, 7%; Scandinavian, 1.5%	Weak metabolism of enzyme Enhanced metabolism of enzyme substrates

5-HT_3, serotonin; NSAIDs, nonsteroidal anti-inflammatory drugs; PM, poor metabolizer; SSRIs, selective serotonin reuptake inhibitors; TCAs, tricyclic antidepressants; UR, ultra-rapid.

Adapted from Fishbain DA, Fishbain D, Lewis J, et al. Genetic testing for enzymes of drug metabolism: does it have clinical utility for pain medicine at the present time? A structured review. *Pain Med.* 2004;5:81-93; and Stamer UM, Stuber F. Genetic factors in pain and its treatment. *Curr Opin Anaesthesiol.* 2007;20:478-484.

THE IMPACT OF PHARMACOGENOMIC RESEARCH ON PAIN MEDICINE

Individuals have differential responses to pain and different likelihoods for developing chronic pain.[17] In 2006, Tegeder and colleagues reported that GTP cyclohydrolase (GCH1), the rate-limiting enzyme for tetrahydrobiopterin (BH4) synthesis, is a key modulator of peripheral neuropathic and inflammatory pain, tracing the predisposition for high pain tolerance to this enzyme cofactor, which is upregulated in primary sensory neurons of the dorsal root ganglion following nerve injury.[18] This cofactor modulates both inflammatory and neuropathic pain. These investigators identified a "pain protective" polymorphism in 15% of the population within the gene that encodes for this essential cofactor involved in this specific pain pathway, which yields reduced pain sensitivity.[19] Individuals with this "pain protective" genotype could potentially confound analgesic trial results, unless they were identified and randomized. Polymorphisms in other genes have also been linked to pain sensitivity.[20]

Genetic predisposition also affects an individual's susceptibility to specific complications of common disease states such as diabetes-associated nephropathy. A genome-wide scan identified two novel candidate genetic loci associated with diabetic nephropathy, implicating new pathways in the pathogenesis of this debilitating complication of diabetes.[21] Pharmacogenomic research has the potential to lead to great strides in the optimization of analgesics as well. Genetic variance can impact the therapeutic response of specific pain medications or predispose an individual to adverse effects. Differences in clinical response to pain medications, in terms of efficacy, toxicity, pharmacokinetics, metabolism, and drug transport, have been linked in part to genetic variations.[4] In 2004, Fishbain and colleagues concluded that "genomic testing for enzymes of drug metabolism has significant potential for improving the efficacy of drug treatment and reducing adverse drug reactions," notably for the pain therapies: tricyclic antidepressants, anti-inflammatory drugs, and opioids, among others.[4]

TRICYCLIC ANTIDEPRESSANTS

Consider the patient example, in which the TCA administered to the patient presenting with PHN led to intolerable adverse effects. TCAs are metabolized in the liver by the cytochrome P450 (CYP450) system, which is responsible for the breakdown of 40% to 50% of all commonly prescribed medications.[22] CYP450 is the most intensely studied gene family, and polymorphisms within this class of enzymes can lead to reduced or accelerated metabolism of their substrates, including specific medications.[23] As such, two individuals having the same weight and given the same drug dosage can have more than a 1000-fold difference in their plasma drug levels.[4] This can be extremely important to recognize from a clinical viewpoint. In studies, individuals have been grouped by their phenotype: poor metabolizers, who have two nonfunctional enzyme alleles; intermediate metabolizers, who have at least one reduced functional allele of an enzyme; extensive metabolizers, who have at least one functional allele; and ultra-rapid metabolizers, who have multiple copies of a functional allele or an allele with a promoter mutation that confers increased transcription of that gene.[22] Extensive metabolizers obtain the expected therapeutic benefit from standard doses of a drug, whereas individuals who are poor metabolizers are at risk of poor efficacy or adverse effects if given a prodrug that is incompletely metabolized due to genetic differences in their liver enzyme systems. On the other hand, ultra-rapid metabolizers can be prone to adverse effects because of higher than expected drug concentrations from enhanced metabolism. The plasma drug concentrations in individuals given the same dose of antidepressants have been found to vary—primarily based on the polymorphisms present in the CYP2D6 enzyme (as well as CYP1A2, CYP2C19, and CYP3A4/5).[24,25] Relevant to the patient presented at the beginning of this chapter, individuals who are poor metabolizers of TCAs (approximately 7% of the Caucasian population) tend to accumulate drug concentrations outside of the narrow therapeutic range of the drug classes, leading to adverse TCA effects at lower than expected doses.[22,24] In contrast, patients who are CYP2D6 ultra-rapid metabolizers may require higher doses to achieve analgesia.[22,24,25] Potentially, the patient presented is a CYP2D6 poor metabolizer.

The value of genotyping before prescribing antidepressants was considered in a large population-based study of 1198 elderly Dutch patients. Perhaps not surprisingly, poor metabolizers of TCA's more than extensive metabolizers required either lower maintenance doses or discontinuation of TCAs altogether.[26] Although research does not provide clear evidence to support the routine clinical use of liver enzyme genotyping before analgesic treatment, an increasing number of commercial entities have developed the capabilities to perform these assays and thus they are now available for the clinician to consider using.[4] Clinically, the recognition that an individual patient could be a poor metabolizer, with or without confirmatory testing, can assist the prescriber to consider medication changes (dose adjustment or frank discontinuation) when poor efficacy or adverse events are observed.

NONSTEROIDAL ANTI-INFLAMMATORY DRUGS (NSAIDs)

Pharmacogenomic research in pain management has identified wide interindividual variation in the analgesic efficacy of both nonspecific NSAIDs and selective inhibitors of cyclooxygenase-2 (COX-2) due to SNPs within the COX genes.[26] A SNP in the promoter for the gene encoding COX-2 (the -1195G to A change) has a prevalence of greater than 10% and has been associated with mild asthmatic reactions.[27] Indeed, another functional effect of the increased expression of COX-2 potentially mediated by several SNPs is the enhanced susceptibility to hypersensitivity in response to standard doses of aspirin and other NSAIDs that inhibit COX-2, otherwise known as aspirin-intolerant asthma (AIA).[28] Additionally, a large genotyping study has determined that individuals with specific variants of the COX-1 and COX-2 genes have an increased risk of cardiovascular disease when taking aspirin.[29] Other studies have investigated an association between genotypes of the cytochrome P450 enzyme CYP2C9 and taking NSAIDs metabolized by that enzyme. An increased risk of developing gastroduodenal bleeding was noted in patients with this co-occurrence.[30-32]

OPIOID ANALGESICS

SNPs

In properly selected patients, opioids can be effective treatments for acute moderate to severe pain, as well as chronic moderate to severe pain.[33] Similar to tricyclic antidepressants, most opioids are metabolized by the CYP450 enzyme class (Table 11.3).[22] Hence, SNPs in CYP450s can have an impact on clinical analgesic and adverse effect responses.

In particular, codeine has been associated with variable individual clinical responses. Codeine itself is a prodrug: a medication that is inactive until it is enzymatically converted to its active metabolite. Codeine must be converted to morphine via CYP2D6 to provide analgesia.[34] In addition to codeine, CYP2D6 poor metabolizers may experience suboptimal analgesic efficacy when prescribed "routine" doses of tramadol. This is because the analgesic benefit attributed to its opioid-related mechanism of action requires that tramadol first be metabolized via a CYP2D6-based mechanism to an active metabolite.[34] The metabolism of many currently available opioids can be affected by SNPs with the CYP450 system; however, three opioid analgesic medications are not metabolized through this system at prescribed doses: hydromorphone, morphine, and oxymorphone.[34,35] Therefore, if it has been identified, perhaps by noting poor analgesic efficacy or intolerable adverse effects (or even possibly actual pharmacogenetic testing) that an individual has a SNP that alters the enzymatic activity of one or more of the CYP450 isoenzymes, an opioid analgesic (if otherwise appropriate for that patient) might be considered that is not metabolized through this mechanism in order to increase the likelihood of a successful treatment outcome.

The current clinical value of pharmacogenomic research illustrates that pharmacogenomic data may play a role in risk stratification and may help guide prescribers in their decision making. Relevant to the patient presented previously, 41% to 51% of individuals of Asian origin express an unstable CYP2D6 enzyme, whereas 12% to 21% of Caucasian people express an inactive CYP2D6 enzyme.[36] However, in clear contrast, 10% to 29% of people of Ethiopian or Saudi Arabian descent have heightened CYP2D6 activity.[36] When considered for the purposes of clinical decision making, this pharmacogenomic information can provide clues about how a specific patient may respond to codeine and

Table 11.3 Enzymes Involved in Opioid Metabolism

Class	Drug	Metabolism
Opium alkaloids	Codeine	10% CYP3A4 (to norcodeine); 5% CYP2D6 (to morphine); 80% UGT2B7
	Hydrocodone	CYP2D6 (to hydromorphone) and CYP3A4 (to norhydrocodone); other minor non-CYP oxidative enzymes
	Morphine	UGTs (GYP-metabolized products)
	Oxycodone	Hepatic glucuronide by UGT1A3 and UGT2B7
		CYP2D6 (to oxymorphone) and CYP3A4 (to noroxycodone); GYP-metabolized product(s) by UGTs
Semisynthetic derivatives	Dihydrocodeine	5%-10% CYP2D6 (to dihydromorphine) and CYP3A4 (to nordihydrocodeine); 85% UGT2B7
	Hydromorphone	Hepatic glucuronide conjugation via UGT1A3, UGT2B7; dihydromorphinone ketone reductase
	Oxymorphone	UGT1A3 and UGT2B7,with UGT2B7 being the predominant enzyme
Phenylheptylamine	Methadone	N-demethylation by CYP3A4
Oripavine derivatives	Buprenorphine	CYP3A4 (65%), CYP2C8 (30%), CYP3A5, CYP3A7,CYP2C9, CYP2C19, and CYP2C18; GYP-metabolized product(s) further cleared by UGTs
Phenylpiperidines	Fentanyl	N-dealkylation by CYP3A4
	Meperidine	CYP3A4, CYP286, and CYP2C19
	Remifentanil	Nonspecific blood and tissue esterases to remifentanil acid
	Sufentanil	N-dealkylation by CYP3A4
Diphenylpropylamine derivatives	Loperamide	N-demethylation by CYP2B6, CYP2C8, CYP2D6, and CYP3A4
	Propoxyphene	N-demethylation by CYP3A4
Others	Naloxone	Conjugation with glucuronic acid via UGTs, mainly UGT2B7
	Naltrexone	Aldo-keto reductase (dihydrodiol dehydrogenase); glucuronidation via UGTs
	Tramadol	O-demethylation by CYP2D6; N-demethylation by CYP286 and CYP3A4

CYP, cytochrome P450; UGT, uridine diphosphate glycosyltransferase.
From Kadiev E, Patel V, Rad P, et al. Role of pharmacogenetics in variable response to drugs: focus on opioids. *Expert Opin Drug Metab Toxicol.* 2008;4:77-91.

other opioids metabolized by CYP2D6 and, thereby, offer prescribing guidance (see Table 11.3). The patient presented earlier may be genetically predisposed to low CYP2D6 activity, and his inherent enzymatic capacity may be not be sufficient to obtain analgesia from the prodrug codeine as well as other opioids such as hydrocodone (hydrocodone is metabolized to hydromorphone through a CYP450-dependent process).[37] Pharmacogenomic information may provide the connection between the opioid prescribed and the lack of expected clinical response or the presence of unexpected adverse effects. Opioid responsiveness is widely recognized as a highly individualized phenomenon that depends on many factors, including pain etiology, prior exposure to opioids and opioid tolerance level, and other psychophysiologic determinants. Consequently, pharmacogenomics can have a significant impact on the clinical response to opioid therapy.[38]

Genetic determinants beyond metabolic enzymes (such as the CYP450 family) also affect an individual's responses to opioid analgesics. These include drug transporters and drug targets such as the μ-opioid receptor gene OPRM1. A common polymorphism of OPRM1 is the substitution of a single nucleotide at position 118 with an adenine substitution by a guanine. The reported allelic frequencies for this are estimated at 10% to 30% among Caucasians, lower among African Americans, and higher among Asians.[39] There is great interest in this polymorphism because it has been associated with pharmacologic and physiologic consequences affecting not only experimental pain models but also neuraxial opioid use for labor analgesia, postoperative analgesia, and cancer-related pain.[39] The different combination of these SNPs within genes that code for the targets of opioid analgesics (e.g., OPRM1) may result in different clinical effects and thus knowledge of these for a specific patient could one day allow for improved outcomes for opioid prescribing. In addition to the CYP450 family of enzymes, the μ-receptor gene (OPRM1, p.118A/G), and the catechol-O-methyltransferase (COMT Val158Met), several types of the adenosine triphosphate (ATP)–binding cassette and subfamily B member 1 gene (ABCB1) have been extensively studied.[39] At the same time it has been determined that interaction of several polymorphisms likely influence the pharmacokinetics and pharmacodynamics of medications—for example, inherited differences—in drug targets (receptors), as well as drug metabolism and drug transport.[39] Recognizing that morphine and most clinically used opioids act via the μ-opioid receptor, the concept of μ-receptor multiplicity has been studied with the recognition that different splice variants of the MOR-1 gene exist with the potential to clinically affect the benefits or lack thereof of morphine as well as other opioid analgesics.[40] This kind of information will likely affect the manner in which clinicians prescribe opioids in the future.

ALTERNATIVE SPLICING

Although most studies concerning opioid-response variability have focused on SNPs, other investigators are examining cellular mechanisms that may contribute to the interindividual variable response to opioid analgesics. Evidence has identified multiple μ-opioid receptor subtypes, often referred to as "splice variants," with distinct properties that influence the pharmacodynamics of individual opioids.[41] To understand this source of diversity, consider a brief review of the central tenets of molecular biology.[12] Genetic material, DNA, is transcribed into ribonucleic acid (RNA) and then translated into proteins, with cellular structural, enzymatic, and receptor functions. SNPs are sources of variation in the DNA, while diversity is also introduced during the transcription of RNA, during which alternative splice variants are produced. This idea was proposed in the 1980s by Nobel Prize winner Walter Gilbert and has since been well characterized and is recognized as the major source of proteome diversity enabling the complexity of human traits.[23]

Alternative splice variants of the μ-opioid receptor have been identified and have been correlated with the clinical phenomenon of incomplete cross-tolerance by which tolerance to one opioid does not translate to tolerance to other opioids.[40] In addition, although most clinically used opioids are selective for the μ-opioid receptor, their ability to activate the receptor can vary, leading to widely different efficacies and side effect profiles between individual patients. In fact, the minimal effective analgesic concentration for morphine can vary among patients by as much as 10-fold.[42] Further response variation within an individual is related to gene expression patterns changing over time and even diverging across organ systems and tissues, based on an individual's state of health and the degree or type of physiologic or emotional stress present.

As previously mentioned, clinically significant response variation in both the efficacy and adverse events of opioids as well as other analgesics has been noted for many years.[43] Chronic opioid therapy treatment guidelines developed by the American Pain Society and the American Academy of Pain Medicine recommended considering "opioid rotation" (e.g., switching from one opioid to another) if the initially prescribed opioid is neither well tolerated nor clinically effective after a reasonable trial.[44] Grilo and colleagues completed a study of 67 patients with difficult-to-treat rheumatologic pain, in which most patients rotated from morphine to either transdermal fentanyl or hydromorphone.[45] Those patients who underwent opioid rotation experienced a mean reduction of 30 mm on a visual analogue scale, indicating a clinically meaningful reduction in pain intensity.[46] In a study of opioids for the treatment of chronic noncancer pain, Quang-Cantagrel and colleagues reported that the first long-acting opioid prescribed was effective for 36% of patients. However, the initially prescribed opioid had to be discontinued because of adverse effects in 30% or ineffectiveness in 34% of those studied. Eventually, a clinical response was obtained by changing to a second (31% responded), third (40% of the remainder responded), fourth (56% of the remainder responded), and fifth (14% of the remainder responded) opioid.[47] These data, however, do not indicate that eventually a patient will respond to a particular opioid and thus it is important to note that the failure of one opioid does not predict the patient's response to another opioid analgesic.[48] The concept of opioid rotation is based not only on empirical clinical observations but also on the pharmacogenetic considerations discussed earlier. Safe and effective opioid rotation requires specific clinical knowledge; if opioid rotation is believed to be an appropriate approach to managing the care of an individual patient, guidelines are available for the calculation of equianalgesic dosing and other important steps in this process.[49]

FUTURE OUTLOOK AND CONCLUSIONS

Advances in pharmacogenomics will optimistically allow clinicians to more precisely individualize optimal pharmacologic care for their patients with acute and chronic pain. Commercial pharmacogenomic testing is currently available; however, it is not yet clear how practical and helpful this is in a real-world setting. The potential benefits of such testing are attractive enough given the potential for more effective and safer management of patients with acute and chronic pain to warrant further study to improve their clinical applicability.

KEY POINTS

- Pharmacogenomics is the study of the impact of genetics on pharmacotherapeutic responses and tolerability, in an effort to improve drug safety and efficacy through genetically guided, individually tailored treatments.
- Advances in pharmacogenomics may begin to allow us to better understand why patients may have variable responses to various analgesic therapies and may soon allow an opportunity for clinicians to identify the most appropriate pharmacotherapies for a patient *before* prescribing.
- Single nucleotide polymorphisms (SNPs; pronounced "snips") are the most important contributors to the observed regular variation in the genetic code, which lead to the human population's diversity of appearance, and at a deeper level, to our diversity in physiology.
- Genetic variance can impact the therapeutic response of specific pain medications or predispose an individual to adverse effects.
- Extensive metabolizers obtain the expected therapeutic benefit from standard doses of a drug, while individuals who are poor metabolizers are at risk of poor efficacy and/or adverse effects if given a prodrug that is incompletely metabolized due to genetic differences in their liver enzyme systems.

SUGGESTED READINGS

Attia J, Ioannidis JP, Thakkinstian A, et al. How to use an article about genetic association, A: background concepts. *JAMA*. 2009;301:74-81.

Fishbain DA, Fishbain D, Lewis J, et al. Genetic testing for enzymes of drug metabolism: does it have clinical utility for pain medicine at the present time? A structured review. *Pain Med.* 2004;5:81-93.

Frazer KA, Ballinger DG, Cox DR, et al. A second generation human haplotype map of over 3.1 million SNPs. *Nature.* 2007;449:851-861.

Hosford DA, Lai EH, Riley JH, et al. Pharmacogenetics to predict drug-related adverse events. *Toxicol Pathol.* 2004;32(suppl 1):9-12.

Mogil JS, Ritchie J, Smith SB, et al. Melanocortin-1 receptor gene variants affect pain and mu-opioid analgesia in mice and humans. *J Med Genet.* 2005;42:583-587.

The references for this chapter can be found at www.expertconsult.com.

12

Psychosocial Aspects of Chronic Pain

Dennis C. Turk

When a patient seeks treatment from a health care provider because of a symptom such as pain, the initial focus is on the patient's medical history and the underlying pathology—a hunt to identify the broken body part, which is treated to eliminate the symptom. In chronic diseases there may be no cure currently available and the best that can be accomplished is alleviation of the symptoms. However, it is important to maintain a longituidinal perspective that a patient with symptoms has a learning history that existed before the onset of the symptoms, as well as contextual factors that are present throughout the course of the medical condition. Both will have important influence on how symptoms are experienced and how the patient adapts to the symptoms and responds to treatment.

Chronic pain, like many chronic diseases, is a demoralizing state that confronts individuals not only with the distress created by the symptoms but also with many other ongoing difficulties that compromise all aspects of their lives. Living with chronic disease requires considerable emotional resilience because it depletes people's emotional reserves. Individuals with chronic pain have a continuing quest for relief that often remains elusive; this can lead to feelings of demoralization, helplessness, hopelessness, and outright depression.

It is also important to keep in mind that most people do not live in isolation but within a social context. Thus, chronic symptoms tax not only the individual but also the capacity of significant others who provide instrumental and emotional support. Health care providers share patients' and significant others' feelings of frustration as reports of symptoms continue despite providers' best efforts and at times in the absence of pathologic signs that can account for the symptoms reported.

In chronic pain syndromes (e.g., osteoarthritis, fibromyalgia, diabetic painful neuropathy), the pain does not appear to have any obvious useful function. Pain that is chronic can significantly compromise quality of life and, if unremitting, may actually produce physical harm by suppressing the body's immune system.[1] Historically, a number of models have been postulated to explain chronic pain. Several are outlined below.

BIOMEDICAL MODEL OF CHRONIC PAIN

The traditional biomedical model of pain—which dates back to the ancient Greeks and was inculcated into medical thinking and practice by Descartes in the 17th century—assumes that people's reports of pain result from a specific disease state represented by disordered anatomy and physiology. The diagnosis is confirmed by data from objective tests showing physical damage and impairment, and medical interventions are specifically directed toward correcting the organic dysfunction or organic source of pathology.

Health care providers often undertake Herculean efforts (frequently at great expense to the patient or third-party payer) in an attempt to establish the specific link between objective indications of tissue damage and the reported severity of pain. The expectation is that once the physical cause has been identified, appropriate treatment will follow. Treatment will then focus on eliminating or blocking the putative cause or causes of the pain by chemical (e.g., oral medication, regional anesthesia, implantable drug delivery systems), surgical (e.g., laminectomy, spinal fusion), or electrical (e.g., spinal cord stimulation, transcutaneous electrical nerve stimulation) manipulation of the pain pathway.

There are several perplexing features of chronic pain that do not fit neatly within the traditional biomedical model, specifically, its suggestion of an isomorphic relationship between pathology and symptoms. For example, pain may be reported even in the absence of an identified pathologic process. It is estimated that one third to one half of all visits to primary care physicians are prompted by symptoms for which no biomedical causes can be detected.[2] In up to 86% of cases, the cause of back pain is unknown despite the performance of sophisticated imaging.[3]

Conversely, significant pathology is noted in up to 35% of *asymptomatic* people with imaging studies such as computed tomography and magnetic resonance imaging.[4-6] Yet these individuals do not appear to experience any pain. Thus, some report severe pain with *no* identifiable pathology, and those with demonstrable pathology may *not complain* of or even experience any pain.

People differ markedly in how frequently they report physical symptoms, in their propensity to visit physicians when experiencing identical symptoms, and, as noted, in their response to the same treatments.[7,8] There are large numbers of people with chronic pain problems who do not seek medical attention. For example, in a survey of nurses, Linton and Buer[9] found that the majority reported moderate to severe pain "often or always," but they indicated that they had not missed a single day of work because of pain. Similarly, Hicks and colleagues[10] observed that almost half of a community-dwelling sample of older people reported considerable back pain, yet the majority did not seek any medical care.

Often the nature of patients' responses to treatment has little to do with their objective physical condition.[11]

For example, White and associates[12] noted that less than a third of people with clinically significant symptoms consult a physician. Conversely, 30% to 50% of patients who seek treatment in primary care do not have specific diagnosable disorders,[13] and in up to 80% of people reporting back pain[3] and the majority of people with chronic headache, no physical basis for the pain can be identified.

There are several potential explanations, not the least of which is the availability of health insurance to cover the costs. As often happens in medicine, when biologic explanations for symptoms are unknown, inadequate, or inconsistent, psychogenic explanations are posed as alternatives.

PSYCHOGENIC MODEL OF CHRONIC PAIN

The psychogenic view is the reverse side of the coin of the biomedical model. In this case, if a patient's report of pain occurs in the absence of objective physical pathology or is disproportionate to the pathology, the pain reports are attributed to a psychological etiology and thus are "psychogenic." It may be treated as a psychiatric diagnosis within the fourth edition of the American Psychiatric Association's *Diagnostic and Statistical Manual of Mental Disorders, Revised*[14]: pain disorder associated with psychological factors or even a pain disorder associated with psychological factors *and* a general medical condition.

Although the notion of psychogenic pain is ubiquitous, empirical evidence supporting it is scarce. A substantial number of patients with chronic pain do not exhibit significant psychopathology. Moreover, studies suggest that in the majority of cases, the emotional distress observed in these patients occurs in response to the persistence of pain and not as a causal agent[15,16] and may resolve once the pain is adequately treated.[17]

SECONDARY-GAIN MODEL OF CHRONIC PAIN

The secondary-gain (motivational) model is an alternative to the psychogenic model. From this perspective, reports of pain in the absence of or in excess of the physical pathology are attributed to the desire of the patient to obtain some benefit, such as attention, time off from undesirable activities, or financial compensation—*secondary gains*. In contrast to the psychogenic model, in the secondary-gain view the assumption is that the patient is *consciously* attempting to acquire a desirable outcome. Simply put, the complaint of pain in the absence of a pathologic process is regarded as fraudulent.[18]

BEHAVIORAL CONCEPTUALIZATIONS

Pain is an unavoidable part of human life. No learning is required to activate nociceptive receptors. However, pain is a potent and salient experience. Beyond mere reflexive actions, people must learn to avoid, modify, or cope with noxious stimulation. There are three major principles of behavioral learning that can help us understand the acquisition of adaptive as well as dysfunctional behavior associated with pain.

CLASSIC (RESPONDENT) CONDITIONING

In his classic experiment, Pavlov discovered that a dog could be taught, or "conditioned," to salivate at the sound of a bell by pairing the sound with food presented to a hungry dog. Salivation of dogs in response to food is a natural response; however, by preceding the feeding with the sound of a bell, Pavlov's dogs learned to associate the sound of the bell with imminent feeding. Once this association was learned, or "conditioned," the dogs were found to salivate at the mere sound of the bell *even in the absence of food.*

The influence of classic conditioning can be observed in pain patients. Consider physical therapy, a mainstay of treatment for chronic pain patients, where treatment may evoke a conditioned fear response. For example, a patient who experienced increased pain following physical therapy may become conditioned and experience a negative emotional response to the presence of the physical therapist, to the treatment room, and to any contextual cues associated with the nociceptive stimulus. The negative emotional reaction may lead to tensing of muscles, which in turn may exacerbate the pain and thereby further strengthen the association between the presence of the physical therapist and pain.

Once a pain problem persists, fear of motor activities may become increasingly conditioned and result in avoidance of activity in the anticipation of avoidance of pain. Avoidance of pain is a powerful rationale for reduction of activity, where the muscle soreness associated with exercise functions as a justification for further avoidance. Consequently, although it may be useful to reduce movement in the acute stage of pain, limitation of activities can be maintained not only by the pain but also by an *anticipatory* fear that has been acquired through the mechanism of classic conditioning. Thus, cognitive processes may interact with pure conditioning. It is the anticipation that motivates a conscious decision to avoid specific behavior or stimuli.

With chronic pain, many activities that were initially neutral or even pleasurable may now elicit or exacerbate pain. As a consequence, they are experienced as aversive and actively avoided. Over time, a greater number of stimuli (e.g., activities) may be expected to elicit or exacerbate pain and will be avoided. This process is referred to as *stimulus generalization*. Thus, the anticipatory fear of pain and restriction of activity—and not just the actual nociception—may contribute to disability. Anticipatory fear can also elicit physiologic reactivity, which may aggravate the pain. As a result, conditioning may directly increase nociceptive stimulation and subsequently the perception of pain.

The conviction by patients that they should remain inactive is difficult to modify as long as avoidance of activity succeeds in preventing aggravation of the pain. By contrast, repeatedly engaging in behavior—*exposure*—that produces progressively less pain than was predicted (corrective feedback) will be followed by a reduction in anticipatory fear and anxiety associated with the activity.[19] Such transformations add support to the importance of a quota-based physical exercise program, with patients gradually and progressively increasing their activity levels despite fear of injury and discomfort associated with the use of deconditioned muscles.[20]

This exposure, in the absence of anticipated pain, provides the *corrective feedback* that should be positively reinforcing and increase the likelihood of continuing previously avoided activities.

OPERANT CONDITIONING—CONTINGENCIES OF REINFORCEMENT

The effect of environmental factors in shaping the experience of people with pain was acknowledged long ago.[21] However, a new era in thinking about pain began with Fordyce's extension of *operant conditioning* to chronic pain.[22] The main focus of operant learning is modifying the frequency of a given behavior—increasing desirable behavior and extinction of maladaptive behavior. The fundamental principle is that if the consequence of a given behavior is rewarding, its occurrence increases, whereas if the consequence is aversive, the likelihood of its occurrence decreases.

When a person is exposed to a stimulus that causes tissue damage, the immediate behavioral response is withdrawal in an attempt to escape from noxious sensations. Such reflexive behavior is adaptive and appropriate. Behavior associated with pain, such as limping and moaning, is called *pain behavior*. Pain behavior includes overt expressions of pain, distress, and suffering. A critical defining feature of overt behavior is that it is observable and thus has a communicative function. If behavior is observable, it is capable of evoking responses, and it is the consequences following the behavior that are particularly important because they can serve to maintain or diminish the likelihood of the behavior recurring. According to Fordyce,[22] pain behavior can become subjected to the principles of operant conditioning. Such behavior may be positively reinforced directly, such as by attention from a family member, acquaintance, or health care provider. The principles of learning suggest that behavior that is positively reinforced will occur more frequently. Pain behavior may also be maintained by escaping the noxious stimulation with the use of drugs or rest or by avoiding undesirable activities. In addition, *well behavior* (e.g., activity, working) may not be positively reinforced, and the more rewarding pain behavior may therefore be maintained.

The following example illustrates the role of operant conditioning. When back pain flares up, the individual may lie down and hold her back. Her husband may observe her behavior and respond by offering to rub her back. This response may positively reward the woman, and her pain behavior (i.e., lying down) may be repeated even in the absence of severe pain. In other words, her pain behavior is being maintained by the learned consequences. The woman's pain behavior may be negatively reinforced if she is permitted to avoid undesirable activities. For example, her husband may suggest that they cancel their evening plans with his brother, an activity that she preferred to avoid in the past. In this situation, her husband provided extra attention, comfort, and the opportunity to avoid an undesirable social obligation.

Table 12.1 presents examples of basic operant principles in chronic pain. The operant learning paradigm does not explain the etiology of pain or initiation of the behavior but rather focuses primarily on maintenance of pain behavior and deficiency of well behavior. Adjustment of reinforcement principles will likely modify the probability of recurrence of pain behavior and well behavior.

Table 12.1 Operant Principles of Reinforcement

Principle	Consequence	Probability of the Behavior Recurring
Positive reinforcement	Reward the behavior	More likely
Negative reinforcement	Prevent or withdraw aversive results	More likely
Punishment	Punish the behavior	Less likely
Neglect	Prevent or withdraw positive results	Less likely

It is important to not make the mistake of viewing pain behavior as being synonymous with *malingering*. Malingering involves the patient *consciously* and *purposely* faking a symptom such as pain for some gain, usually financial (secondary gain). In the case of pain behavior, there is no suggestion of conscious deception but rather the unintended performance of pain behavior resulting from environmental reinforcement contingencies. Contrary to the beliefs of many third-party payers, there is little support for the contention that outright faking of pain for financial gain is prevalent.[23]

SOCIAL-LEARNING PROCESSES

From the social-learning perspective, pain behavior may be acquired through *observational learning* and *modeling* processes. That is, people can acquire behavioral responses that were not previously in their repertoire by the observation of others, particularly those whom they view as similar to themselves.

Children develop attitudes about health and health care and the perception and interpretation of symptoms and physiologic processes from their parents and the social environment. They learn appropriate and inappropriate responses to injury and disease and thus may be more or less likely to ignore or over-respond to the symptoms that they experience as a result of behavior modeled in childhood. The culturally acquired perception and interpretation of symptoms determine how people deal with disease states. The observation of others in pain is an event that captivates attention. Such attention may have survival value, may help avoid experiencing more pain, and may help learn what to do about acute pain.

From the earliest years, infants, toddlers, and young children are exposed to numerous painful episodes from bumps and falls. Thus they have plenty of opportunity to observe the reactions that they receive.[24] Children of parents with chronic pain may make more pain-related responses during stressful times than would children with healthy parents. These children tend to exhibit greater illness behavior (e.g., complaints, days absent from school, visits to the school nurse) than do children of healthy parents.[25] *Models* can influence the expression, localization, and methods of coping with pain.[26] Physiologic responses may even be conditioned during observation of others in pain.[27] Expectancies and actual behavioral responses to nociceptive stimulation are based, at least partially, on prior experience either directly or from the observation of others. This may contribute to the marked variability in response to objectively similar degrees of physical pathology observed.

The biomedical, psychogenic, secondary-gain, and behavioral views are unidimensional. Reports of pain are ascribed to *either* physical *or* psychological factors. Rather than being categorical, either somatogenic or psychogenic, both physical and psychological components may interact to create and influence the perception and experience of pain.

Any physical abnormalities that are identified may be moderated by coexisting psychosocial influences. The complexity of pain is especially evident when it persists over time, during which a range of psychological, social, and economic factors interact with the physical pathology to modulate patients' reports of pain and the impact of pain on their lives. In the case of chronic pain, health care providers need to not only search for the physical source of the pain through examination and diagnostic tests but also examine the patient's mood, fears, expectancies, coping efforts, and resources; the responses of significant others; and the impact of pain on the patient's life.

Persons experiencing pain, particularly chronic pain, have a continuing quest for relief that remains elusive, which can lead to feelings of frustration, demoralization, and depression, thus compromising the quality of all aspects of their lives. People with chronic pain are confronted with not only the stress of pain but also a cascade of ongoing problems (e.g., financial, interpersonal). Moreover, the experience of "medical limbo" (i.e., the presence of a painful condition that eludes diagnosis and carries the implication of either psychiatric causation or malingering on the one hand or an undiagnosed potentially disabling condition on the other) is itself a source of significant stress and can result in psychological distress.

Biomedical factors, in the majority of cases, appear to instigate the initial report of pain. Over time, however, psychosocial and behavioral factors may serve to maintain and exacerbate the level of pain, influence adjustment, and contribute to excessive disability. Following from this view, pain that persists over time should not be viewed as being solely physical or solely psychological; the experience of pain is maintained by an interdependent set of biomedical, psychosocial, and behavioral factors.[28,29]

People with chronic pain frequently terminate active efforts to manage the pain and instead turn to passive coping strategies, such as inactivity, medication, or alcohol, to reduce the pain and emotional distress. They also absolve themselves of personal responsibility for managing their pain and as a substitute rely on family and health care providers. The thinking of chronic pain patients has been shown to contribute to the exacerbation, attenuation, and maintenance of pain, pain behavior, affective distress, adjustment to chronic pain, health care seeking, response to treatment, and disability.[30-33]

The important role of the behavioral and environmental contingencies of reinforcement in chronic pain has already been described. However, another set of psychological factors—affective and cognitive factors—play equally important roles.

AFFECTIVE FACTORS

Pain is ultimately a subjective, private experience, but it is invariably described in terms of sensory and affective properties. As defined by the International Association for the Study of Pain, "[Pain] is unquestionably a sensation in a part or parts of the body but it is also always unpleasant and therefore also an emotional experience."[34] The central and interactive roles of sensory information and the affective state are supported by an overwhelming amount of evidence.[35] The affective components of pain include many different emotions, but they are primarily negative emotions. Depression and anxiety have received the greatest amount of attention in chronic pain patients; however, anger has recently attracted considerable interest as an important emotion in chronic pain patients.

In addition to affect being one of the three interconnected components of pain, pain and emotions interact in a number of ways. Emotional distress may predispose people to experience pain, be a precipitant of symptoms, be a modulating factor that amplifies or inhibits the perception of pain severity, be a consequence of persistent pain, or be a perpetuating factor. Moreover, these potential roles are not mutually exclusive, and any number of them may be involved in a particular circumstance and interact with cognitive appraisal. For example, the literature is replete with studies demonstrating that the current mood state modulates reports of pain, as well as tolerance of acute pain.[36] Levels of anxiety have been shown to influence not only the severity of pain but also complications following surgery and the number of days of hospitalization required.[37,38] The level of depression has been observed to be closely tied to chronic pain.[39]

Although we provide an overview of research on the predominant emotions—anxiety, depression, and anger—associated with pain individually, it is important to acknowledge that these emotions are not as distinct when it comes to the experience of pain. They interact and augment each other over time.

ANXIETY

It is common for patients with symptoms of pain to be anxious and worried, especially when the symptoms are unexplained, as is often the case with chronic pain syndromes. For example, in a large-scale, multicenter study of patients with fibromyalgia syndrome, between 44% and 51% acknowledged that they were anxious.[40] People with persistent pain may be anxious about the meaning of their symptoms and their future—will their pain increase, will their physical capacity diminish, or will their symptoms result in progressive disability wherein they ultimately need a wheelchair or are bedridden? In addition to these sources of fear, those with persistent pain may be worried that, on the one hand, people will not believe that they are suffering and, on the other, they may be told that they are beyond help and will "just have to learn to live with it." Fear and anxiety also relate to activities that people with pain anticipate will increase their pain or exacerbate whatever physical factors might be contributing to the pain. These fears may contribute to avoidance and motivate inactivity and, ultimately, greater disability.[41] Continual vigilance and monitoring for noxious stimulation and the belief that it signifies progression of disease may render even low-intensity aversive sensations less bearable. In addition, such fears will contribute to increased muscle tension and physiologic arousal, which may exacerbate and maintain the pain.[42,43]

The threat of intense pain captures attention in such a way that individuals have difficulty disengaging from it. The experience of pain may initiate a set of extremely negative thoughts, as noted previously, and arouse fear—fear of inciting more pain and injury or fear of their future impact.[44] Fear and anticipation of pain are cognitive-perceptual processes that are not driven exclusively by the actual sensory experience of pain and can exert a significant impact on the level of function and pain tolerance. People are motivated to avoid and escape from unpleasant consequences; they learn that avoidance of situations and activities in which they have experienced acute episodes of pain will reduce the likelihood of re-experiencing pain or causing further physical damage. They may become hypervigilant to their environment as a way of preventing the occurrence of pain.

Investigators[19,45] have suggested that fear of pain, driven by the anticipation of pain and not by the sensory experience of pain itself, produces strong negative reinforcement for the persistence of avoidance behavior and the putative functional disability in pain patients. Avoidance behavior is reinforced in the short term through a reduction of the suffering associated with noxious stimulation.[46] Avoidance, however, can be a maladaptive response if it persists and leads to increased fear, limited activity, and other physical and psychological consequences that contribute to disability and persistence of the pain.

Studies have demonstrated that fear of movement and fear of injury or reinjury are better predictors of functional limitation than biomedical parameters or even the severity and duration of the pain are.[47,48] For example, Crombez and colleagues[47] showed that pain-related fear was the best predictor of behavioral performance in trunk extension, flexion, and weight-lifting tasks, even after the effects of pain intensity are statistically controlled. Moreover, Vlaeyen and associates[49] found that fear of movement and injury or reinjury was the best predictor of self-reported disability in chronic back pain patients and that the physiologic sensory perception of pain and biomedical findings did not add any predictive value. The importance of fear of activity appears to generalize to daily activities, as well as the to clinical experimental context. Approximately two thirds of people with chronic low back pain avoid back-straining activities because of fear of injury.[47] For example, fear avoidance beliefs about the physical demands of a job are strongly related to disability and work lost during the previous year, even more so than the severity of pain or other pain variables.[49,50] Interestingly, a reduction in pain-related anxiety predicts improvement in functioning, affective distress, pain, and pain-related interference with activity.[51] Clearly, fear, pain-related anxiety, and concerns about avoidance of harm all play important roles in chronic pain and need to be assessed and addressed during treatment.

Pain-related fear and concerns about avoidance of harm both appear to exacerbate symptoms.[19] Anxiety is an affective state that is greatly influenced by appraisal processes; to cite the stoic philosopher Epictetus, "There is nothing either bad or good but thinking makes it so." Thus, there is a reciprocal relationship between the affective state and cognitive-interpretive processes. Thinking affects mood, and mood influences appraisals and, ultimately, the experience of pain.

DEPRESSION

Clinical data suggest that 40% to 50% of chronic pain patients experience significant depression.[39] Epidemiologic studies provide abundant evidence confirming a strong association between chronic pain and depression but do not address whether chronic pain causes depression or depression causes chronic pain. Prospective studies of patients with chronic musculoskeletal pain have suggested that chronic pain can cause depression,[52] that depression can cause chronic pain,[53] and that they exist in a mutually reinforcing relationship.[28,29]

One fact often raised to support the idea that pain causes depression is that the current depressive episode often began after onset of the pain problem. The majority of studies appear to support this contention.[54] However, several studies have documented that many patients with chronic pain, especially disabled patients seen in pain clinics, have often had previous episodes of depression that predated their pain problem by years.[55] It is important to acknowledge that studies based on patients treated at pain treatment facilities may be biased in that patients treated at these facilities have been shown to have exceedingly high levels of depression, which may have prompted referral,[56] and they may not be representative of all individuals with persistent pain. One important prospective study[32] demonstrated that levels of depression predicted the development of low back pain 3 years following the initial assessment. Patients with depression were 2.3 times more likely to report back pain than were those who did not report depression. Depression was a much stronger predictor of incident back pain than any clinical or anatomic risk factors. This has led some investigators to propose that there may exist a common trait of susceptibility to dysphoric physical symptoms (including pain) and to negative psychological symptoms (including anxiety and depression). They concluded that "pain and psychological illness should be viewed as having reciprocal psychological and behavioral effects involving both processes of illness expression and adaptation."[57] Once chronic pain has been diagnosed, it no longer matters which is the cause and which is the consequence—pain or depression. Both need to be treated.

It is not surprising that a large number of chronic pain patients are depressed. It is interesting to ponder the converse. Given the nature of the symptom and the problems created by chronic pain, why is it that all such patients are *not* depressed? Turk and colleagues[16,58] examined this question and determined that patients' appraisal of the effects of the pain on their lives and their ability to exert any control over the pain and their lives mediated the link between pain and depression. That is, patients who believed that they could continue to function despite their pain and who believed that they could maintain control despite their pain did not become depressed.

ANGER

Anger has been widely observed in people with chronic pain.[59] Pilowsky and Spence[60] reported "bottled-up anger" in 53% of chronic pain patients. Kerns and coworkers[61] noted that internalization of angry feelings was strongly related to measures of pain intensity, perceived interference, and the reported frequency of pain behavior. Summers and colleagues[62] examined patients with spinal cord injuries and found that anger and hostility were powerful predictors of pain severity. Moreover, even though chronic pain patients in psychotherapy might present an image of themselves as being even tempered, 88% of the patients treated acknowledged their feelings of anger when explicitly sought.[63]

Frustrations related to the persistence of symptoms, limited information on etiology, and repeated treatment failures, along with anger toward employers, insurers, the health care system, family members, and themselves, all contribute to the general dysphoric mood of these patients. The effects of anger and frustration on exacerbation of pain and acceptance of treatment have not received much attention, but it would be reasonable to expect that the presence of anger may serve as a complicating factor that increases autonomic arousal and blocks motivation and acceptance of treatments oriented toward rehabilitation and management of the disability rather than cure, which are often the only treatments available for chronic pain.[64]

When a person with pain is angry, there are a range of possible targets (e.g., employer, insurance company, health care providers). Fernandez and Turk[64] proposed that the specificity of targets toward which patients direct angry feelings may be important in understanding the relationship between pain and anger. There may be some targets of anger that are more relevant to the chronic pain experience than others.

Okifuji and colleagues[65] found that 60% of patients expressed anger toward health care providers, 39% toward significant others, 30% toward insurance companies, 26% toward employers, and 20% toward attorneys. The target of anger most commonly acknowledged, however, was oneself (endorsed by approximately 70% of the sample). Overall, correlations between anger and pain severity have been shown to be statistically significant and range from .17 to .35.[61,66] Okifuji and coauthors[65] reported that anger was significantly correlated with pain intensity ($r = .30$ to .35). They also reported that anger was significantly correlated with disability ($r = .26$) and was highly associated with depression ($r = .52$).

The precise mechanisms by which anger and frustration exacerbate pain are not known. One reasonable possibility is that anger exacerbates pain by increasing physiologic arousal.[67] For example, Burns and coauthors[66] reported the results of a study in which it was demonstrated that anger-induced stress produces increased muscle tension, which in turn predicts greater severity of pain in chronic back pain patients. It was found that this effect was specific to anger; a measure of depression that was significantly correlated with pain was not associated with increased muscle reactivity.

A negative mood in chronic pain patients is likely to affect treatment motivation and adherence to treatment recommendations. For example, patients who are anxious may fear engaging in what they perceive as demanding activities, patients who are depressed and feel helpless may have little initiative to comply, and patients who are angry with the health care system are not likely to be motivated to respond to recommendations from yet another health care professional.

COGNITIVE FACTORS

Persistent pain beliefs, appraisals, and expectations about pain, the ability to cope, social supports, the disorder, the medicolegal system, the health care system, and employers are all important because they may facilitate or disrupt an individual's sense of control. These factors also influence patients' investment in treatment, acceptance of responsibility, perceptions of disability, adherence to treatment recommendations, support from significant others, expectancies regarding treatment, and acceptance of the treatment rationale.

Cognitive interpretations also affect how patients relate symptoms to others, including health care providers. Overt communication of pain, suffering, and distress will elicit responses that may reinforce pain behavior and impressions about the seriousness, severity, and uncontrollability of the pain. That is, reports of pain may induce physicians to prescribe more potent medications, order additional diagnostic tests, and in some cases perform surgery.[68] Family members may express sympathy, excuse the patient from responsibilities, and encourage passivity, thereby fostering further physical deconditioning. The cognitive-behavioral perspective integrates the emphasis of operant conditioning on external reinforcement and the respondent view of conditioned avoidance within the framework of information processing.

People with persistent pain often have negative expectations about their own ability and responsibility to exert any control over their pain. Moreover, they often view themselves as helpless. Such negative, maladaptive appraisals about their condition, situation, and personal efficacy in controlling their pain and problems associated with the pain reinforce their experience of demoralization, inactivity, and overreaction to nociceptive stimulation. These cognitive appraisals are posited as having an effect on behavior that leads to reduced effort, reduced perseverance in the face of difficulty, decreased activity, and increased psychological distress.

Pain and emotions interact in a number of ways, which in turn may interact with cognitive appraisal of the pain state. Research has consistently demonstrated that patients' attitudes, beliefs, and expectancies about their plight, themselves, their coping resources, and the health care system affect reports of pain, activity, disability, and response to treatment.

BELIEFS ABOUT PAIN

People respond to medical conditions in part based on their subjective ideas about illness and their symptoms. Health care providers working with chronic pain patients are aware that patients with similar pain histories and reports of pain may differ greatly in their beliefs about their pain. Behavior and emotions are influenced by interpretation of events and expectations rather than solely by objective characteristics of the event itself. Thus pain, when interpreted as signifying ongoing tissue damage or a progressive disease, is likely to produce considerably more distress and behavioral dysfunction than if it is viewed as being the result of a stable problem that is expected to improve.

People build fairly elaborate views of their physical state, and these views or representations provide the basis for action plans and coping. Beliefs about the meaning of pain and individuals' ability to function despite discomfort are important aspects of expectations about pain. For example, a cognitive representation that you have a very serious, debilitating condition, that disability is a necessary aspect of pain, that activity is dangerous, and that pain is an acceptable excuse for neglecting responsibilities will probably result in maladaptive responses.

Chronic pain patients often demonstrate poor behavioral persistence in exercise tasks. Their performance on these tasks may be independent of physical exertion or actual self-reports of pain but rather be related to *previous* pain reports or anticipation and fear of injury, reinjury, or exacerbation of their pain.[19] These people appear to have a negative view of their ability and expect increased pain if they perform physical exercises. Thus, the rationale for their avoidance of exercise was not the presence of pain but their *learned expectation* of heightened pain and the accompanying physical arousal that might exacerbate the pain and reinforce their beliefs regarding the pervasiveness of their disability. When people experience pain and have a negative perception of their capability for physical performance, a vicious circle is formed, with failure to perform activities reinforcing the perception of helplessness and incapacity. Once again we can see how behavioral (conditioning) factors interact with cognitive processes.

Certain beliefs may lead to maladaptive coping, increased distress, and greater disability. People who believe that their pain will persist may be passive in their coping and fail to make use of strategies to cope with pain. People who consider their pain to be an unexplainable mystery may negatively evaluate their own ability to control or decrease pain and are less likely to rate their coping strategies as effective in controlling and decreasing pain.[69] People's beliefs, appraisals, and expectancies regarding the consequences of an event *and their ability* to cope and adapt to their symptoms and changed life circumstances are hypothesized to function in two ways. There may be a direct influence on physiologic arousal and mood and an indirect one through their effects on coping efforts.[70,71]

Once beliefs and expectancies are formed, they become stable and are very difficult to modify. As noted, individuals with persistent pain tend to avoid experiences that could invalidate their beliefs and guide their behavior in accordance with these beliefs, even in situations in which these beliefs are no longer valid. Consequently, as noted previously, they do not obtain corrective feedback.

It is essential for people with chronic pain to develop adaptive beliefs about the relationships among impairment, pain, distress, and disability and to de-emphasize the role of experienced pain in their regulation of functioning. In fact, results from numerous treatment outcome studies have shown that changes in pain level do not parallel changes in other variables of interest, including activity level, medication use, return to work, rated ability to cope with pain, and pursuit of further treatment. If health care providers hope to achieve better outcomes and to reduce their frustration from patients' lack of compliance with their advice, they need to learn about and to address patients' concerns within this therapeutic context.

SELF-EFFICACY

Self-efficacy is a personal expectation that is particularly important in patients with chronic pain. A self-efficacy expectation is specifically defined as a personal conviction that you can successfully execute a course of action (perform the required behavior) to produce a desired outcome in a given situation. Given sufficient motivation to engage in a behavior, it is a person's self-efficacy beliefs that determine the choice of activities that the person will initiate, the amount of effort that will be expended, and how long the individual will persist in the face of obstacles and aversive experiences. Efficacy judgments are based on four sources of information regarding capabilities, listed in descending order of effects: (1) past performance at the task or similar tasks, (2) the performance accomplishments of others who are perceived to be similar, (3) verbal persuasion about capabilities, and (4) perception of the state of physiologic arousal.

In chronic pain patients, self-efficacy positively affects physical and psychological functioning.[72,73] Self-efficacy is also an important mediator of therapeutic change.

Prospective studies in patients who underwent orthopedic surgery have demonstrated that high self-efficacy before the start of rehabilitation and larger increases over the course of rehabilitation speed recovery and predict better long-term outcomes.[74-76] Improvements in self-efficacy after self-management and cognitive-behavioral interventions have been shown to be associated with improvements in pain, functional status, and psychological adjustment.[77,78]

The experience of performance mastery can be created by encouraging patients to undertake subtasks that are initially attainable but become increasingly difficult and subsequently approach the desired level of performance.[20] In a quota-based physical therapy system, the initial goal is set below the initial performance to increase mastery of performance. It is important to remember that coping behavior is influenced by a person's beliefs that the demands of a situation do not exceed the person's coping resources. For example, Council and colleagues[79] asked patients to rate their self-efficacy, as well as their expectancy of pain related to performance during movement tasks. Patients' performance levels were highly related to their expectations of self-efficacy, which in turn appeared to be determined by their expectancy regarding levels of pain that would be experienced.

CATASTROPHIC THINKING

Pain catastrophizing can be defined as an exaggerated negative orientation toward actual or anticipated pain experiences. There has been much debate about the specific nature of catastrophizing as a psychological construct.[80,81] However, current conceptualizations most often describe it in terms of appraisal or as a set of maladaptive beliefs.[82,83]

It appears to be a particularly potent way of thinking that greatly influences pain and disability. Evidence for the role of pain catastrophizing in chronic pain adjustment is overwhelming and has been summarized in several review articles and studies.[77,80]

Prospective studies have indicated that catastrophizing might be predictive of the inception of chronic musculoskeletal pain in the general population[84,85] and of more intense pain and slower recovery after surgical intervention.[86-88] Several investigators have demonstrated the therapeutic efficacy of reducing catastrophizing.[89,90]

COPING

Self-regulation of pain and its effects depends on the individual's specific ways of dealing with pain, adjusting to pain, and reducing or minimizing the pain and distress caused by pain—in other words, the individual's coping strategies.[91] Coping is assumed to be implemented by spontaneously used purposeful and intentional acts, and it can be assessed in terms of overt and covert behavior. Overt behavioral coping strategies include rest, medication, and the use of relaxation. Covert coping strategies include various means of distracting yourself from pain, reassuring yourself that the pain will diminish, seeking information, and problem solving. Coping strategies act to alter both the perception of the intensity of the pain and one's ability to manage or tolerate the pain and continue everyday activities.

Studies have found active coping strategies (efforts to function despite pain or to distract oneself from pain, such as being active and ignoring the pain) to be associated with adaptive functioning and passive coping strategies (depending on others for help in pain control and restriction of activities) to be related to greater pain and depression.[92] However, beyond this, there is no evidence to support the greater effectiveness of any individual active coping strategy over any other.[93] It seems more likely that different strategies will be more effective than others for some people at some times but not necessarily for all people all of the time.

A number of studies have demonstrated that if patients are instructed in the use of adaptive coping strategies, their rating of intensity of pain decreases and their tolerance of pain increases.[92] The most important factor in poor coping appears to be the presence of catastrophic thinking, not the nature of specific adaptive coping strategies.[80]

Given our discussion of the psychological factors that play a role in pain, we can now consider how these factors can be integrated within a multidimensional model of pain. Pain is a complex subjective phenomenon that consists of a range of factors, each of which contributes to the interpretation of nociception as pain. Thus, each person uniquely experiences pain. A significant factor contributing to the current situation relates to diagnostic uncertainty. The diagnosis of pain is not an exact science. A major problem in understanding pain is that it is a subjective (internal) state. There is no *pain thermometer* that can accurately measure the amount of pain that a person feels or should be experiencing.

BIOPSYCHOSOCIAL MODEL

In contrast to the biomedical model's emphasis on disease, the biopsychosocial model focuses on illness, which is the result of a complex interaction of biologic, psychological, and social variables. From this perspective, diversity in expression of illness (which includes its severity, duration, and consequences for the individual) is accounted for by the interrelationships among biologic changes, psychological status, and social and cultural contexts; all these variables shape the person's perception and response to illness.

The biopsychosocial way of thinking about the different responses of people to symptoms and the presence of chronic conditions is based on an understanding of the dynamic nature of these conditions. That is, by definition, chronic syndromes extend over time. Therefore, these conditions need to be viewed longitudinally as ongoing, multifactorial processes in which there is a dynamic and reciprocal interplay among biologic, psychological, and social factors that shapes the experience and responses of patients. Biologic factors may initiate, maintain, and modulate physical perturbations; psychological variables influence appraisal and the perception of internal physiologic signs; and social factors shape patients' behavioral responses to the perceptions of their physical perturbations.

At the same time, psychological factors may influence biology by affecting hormone production,[94] brain structure and processes,[95,96] and the autonomic nervous system.[97,98] Behavioral responses may also affect biologic contributors, such as when a person avoids engaging in certain activities to reduce the symptoms. Although avoidance may initially reduce the symptoms, in the long run it will lead to further physical deconditioning, which can exacerbate nociceptive stimulation.

The picture is not complete unless we consider the direct effects of disease factors and treatment on cognitive and behavioral factors. Biologic influences and medications (e.g., steroids, opioids) may affect the ability to concentrate, cause fatigue, and modulate peoples' interpretation of their state, as well as their ability to engage in certain activities.

At different points during the evolution of a disease or impairment, the relative weighting of physical, psychological, and social factors may change. For example, during the acute phase of a disease, biologic factors may predominate, but over time, psychological and social factors may assume a disproportionate role in accounting for the symptoms and disability. Moreover, there is considerable variability in the behavioral and psychological manifestations of dysfunction, both across persons with comparable symptoms and within the same person over time.[99]

To understand the variable responses of people to chronic conditions, it is essential that biologic, psychological, and social factors all be considered. Moreover, a longitudinal perspective is essential. A cross-sectional approach will permit consideration of these factors only at a specific point in time, and chronic conditions continually evolve. What is observed at any one point in time is a person's adaptation to interacting biologic, personal, and environmental factors. In sum, the hallmarks of the biopsychosocial perspective are (1) integrated action, (2) reciprocal determinism, and (3) development and evolution. No single factor in isolation—pathophysiologic, psychological, or social—will adequately explain chronic pain status. This can be contrasted with the traditional biomedical model, whose emphasis on the somatogenic-psychogenic dichotomy is too narrow in scope to accommodate the complexity of chronic pain.

From an integrative biopsychosocial perspective, pain is viewed as a subjective perception that results from the transduction, transmission, and modulation of sensory input filtered through a person's genetic composition and previous learning history and modulated further by the person's current physiologic state, idiosyncratic appraisals, expectations, present mood state, and sociocultural environment.

CONCLUDING COMMENTS

It is abundantly clear that pain is not a monolithic entity. No isomorphic relationship exists among tissue damage, nociception, and pain report. The variability in patients' responses to nociceptive stimuli and treatment is somewhat more understandable when we consider that pain is a personal experience influenced by attention, the meaning of the situation, and previous learning history, as well as by physical pathology. In the majority of cases, biomedical factors appear to instigate the initial report of pain. Over time, however, secondary problems associated with deconditioning may exacerbate and serve to maintain the problem. Inactivity leads to an increased focus on and preoccupation with the body and pain, and these cognitive-attentional changes increase the likelihood of misinterpretation of symptoms, overemphasis on symptoms, and the patient's self-perception as disabled. Reduction of activity, anger, fear of reinjury, pain, loss of compensation, and an environment that perhaps unwittingly supports the *pain patient role* can impede alleviation of pain, successful rehabilitation, reduction of disability, and improvement in adjustment.

Pain that persists over time should not be viewed as either solely physical or solely psychological. Rather, the experience of pain is a complex amalgam maintained by an interdependent set of biomedical, psychosocial, and behavioral factors whose relationships are not static but evolve and change over time. The various interacting factors that affect a person with chronic pain suggest that the phenomenon is quite complex and requires a biopsychosocial perspective.

From the biopsychosocial perspective, each of these factors contributes to the experience of pain and the response to treatment. The interaction among the various factors is what produces the subjective experience of pain. There is a synergistic relationship whereby psychological and socio-enviromental factors can modulate nociceptive stimulation and the response to treatment. In turn, nociceptive stimulation can influence patients' appraisal of their situation and the treatment, their mood states, and the ways that they interact with significant others, including medical practitioners. An integrative, biopsychosocial model of chronic pain needs to incorporate the mutual interrelationships among physical, psychological, and social factors and the changes that occur in these relationships over time.[28,29] A model and treatment approach that focuses on only one of these three core sets of factors will inevitably be incomplete.

The current state of knowledge suggests that pain must be viewed as a complex biopsychosocial phenomenon that incorporates physical, psychosocial, and behavioral factors. Failure to incorporate each of these factors will lead to incomplete understanding and unsuccessful treatment of people who experience and live with chronic pain.

KEY POINTS

- Focusing exclusively on the symptoms, anatomy, and physiology of patients with chronic pain is inadequate because a range of individual variables, prior experiences and learning history, and social context all influence reporting of symptoms, adaptation, disability, and response to treatments.
- To understand patients with chronic pain, a longitudinal perspective must be taken.
- Chronic pain is not exclusively somatogenic or psychogenic, but rather both somatic and psychosocial factors interact and are synergistic.
- All people, not just those experiencing chronic pain, are influenced by their attitudes, beliefs, and expectations.
- People with chronic pain avoid activities (e.g., exercise) that they fear will either exacerbate their pain or increase the possibility of further physical pathology and increase behavior (e.g., reclining) that they believe will prevent the occurrence of pain or injury.
- Responses from significant others (e.g., family, health care providers) that are positive (e.g., attention, sympathy) will increase the likelihood of more adaptive behaviors.
- People learn, even without their awareness, what to expect and how to respond by observation of others, especially those whom they perceive as being similar to themselves.
- Anxiety, depression, and anger are prevalent in people with chronic pain, and these emotional states influence the perception of nociception, adaptation, and response to treatment.
- People with persistent pain often have negative expectations about their ability and responsibility to exert any control over their pain and view themselves as helpless, all of which contributes to a general state of demoralization.
- A self-efficacy expectation, or a personal conviction that you can successfully execute a course of action (perform the required behavior) to produce a desired outcome in a given situation, is particularly important in patients with chronic pain because it is a person's self-efficacy beliefs that determine the choice of activities that the person will initiate, the amount of effort that will be expended, and how long the individual will persist in the face of obstacles and aversive experiences.
- Pain catastrophizing, an exaggerated negative orientation toward actual or anticipated pain experiences, appears to be a particularly potent way of thinking that greatly influences pain and disability.
- In contrast to the biomedical model's emphasis on disease, the biopsychosocial model focuses on illness, which is the result of a complex interaction of biologic, psychological, and social variables.
- Pain that persists over time should not be viewed as being either solely physical or solely psychological; rather, the experience of pain is a complex amalgam maintained by an interdependent set of biomedical, psychosocial, and behavioral factors whose relationships are not static but evolve and change over time.

SUGGESTED READINGS

Burns JW, Kubilus A, Bruehl S, et al. Do changes in cognitive factors influence outcome following multidisciplinary treatment for chronic pain? A cross-lagged panel analysis. *J Consult Clin Psychol.* 2003;71:81-91.

Burns JW, Wiegner S, Derleth M, et al. Linking symptom-specific physiological reactivity to pain severity in chronic low back pain patients: a test of mediation and moderation models. *Health Psychol.* 1996;16:319-326.

Carragee EJ, Alamin TF, Miller JL, et al. Discographic, MRI and psychosocial determinants of low back pain disability and remission: a prospective study in subjects with benign persistent back pain. *Spine J.* 2005;5:24-35.

Flor H, Turk DC. *Chronic Pain: An Integrated Biobehavioral Approach.* Seattle: IASP Press; 2011.

Fordyce WE. *Behavioral Methods in Chronic Pain and Illness.* St. Louis: Mosby; 1976.

Gatchel RJ, Peng YB, Peters ML, et al. The biopsychosocial approach to chronic pain: scientific advances and future directions. *Psychol Bull.* 2007;133:581-624.

Jarvik JG, Hollingworth W, Heagerty PJ, et al. Three-year incidence of low back pain in an initially asymptomatic cohort. Clinical and imaging risk factors. *Spine.* 2005;30:1541-1548.

Jensen MP, Turner JA, Romano JM. Changes in beliefs, catastrophizing, and coping are associated with improvements in multidisciplinary pain treatment. *J Consult Clin Psychol.* 2011;69:655-662.

Leeuw M, Goossens ME, Linton SJ, et al. The fear-avoidance model of musculoskeletal pain: current state of scientific evidence. *J Behav Med.* 2007;30:77-94.

Sullivan MJL, Thorn B, Haythornthwaite JA, et al. Theoretical perspectives on the relation between catastrophizing and pain. *Clin J Pain.* 2001;15:52-64.

Turk DC, Okifuji A. What factors affect physicians' decisions to prescribe opioids for chronic non-cancer pain patients? *Clin J Pain.* 1997;13:330-336.

Turk DC, Swanson KS, Wilson HD. The biopsychosocial model of pain and pain management. In: Ebert M, Kerns RD, eds. *Behavioral and Pharmacological Pain Management.* New York: Cambridge University Press; 2011:16-43.

Vlaeyen JW, Kole-Snijders AM, Boeren RB, et al. Fear of movement/(re)injury in chronic low back pain and its relation to behavioral performance. *Pain.* 1995;62:363-372.

Woby SR, Watson PJ, Roach NK, et al. Coping strategy use: does it predict adjustment to chronic back pain after controlling for catastrophic thinking and self-efficacy for pain control? *J Rehabil Med.* 2005;37:100-107.

The references for this chapter can be found at www.expertconsult.com.

PART 3

EVALUATION AND ASSESSMENT

CHARLES E. ARGOFF | JAMES P. RATHMELL, EDITORS

PART OUTLINE

13

History and Physical Examination of the Pain Patient

Andrew Dubin | Irfan Lalani | Charles E. Argoff

Physical examination serves to further explore and confirm the findings from the clinical history. Objective data obtained from the examination are essential to accurately diagnose the etiology of the pain. This chapter provides an overview of a structured approach to the physical examination of a pain patient, along with the anatomic and physiologic basis of the physical findings.

The key components of the physical examination include a general physical examination, a detailed neurologic examination, a detailed musculoskeletal examination, and an examination for cutaneous or trophic findings. The musculoskeletal examination includes inspection, palpation, percussion, auscultation, and provocative maneuvers.

GENERAL PHYSICAL EXAMINATION

Vital signs, including temperature, heart rate, respiratory rate, blood pressure, and weight, should be noted at each visit. This information is useful in forming an impression of the overall health and comorbid conditions of the patient.

A few moments should be spent in observing and documenting the general appearance and gait of the patient. Whenever possible, the examining physician should make every effort to bring the patient back to the examining room from the waiting room. This allows the physician the opportunity for examination as the patient transitions from sitting to standing and ambulates to the examining room. This observation time allows an "unofficial" examination that may reveal inconsistencies not noted on the "official formal" examination.

Attributes include how the patient dresses and personal hygiene. Pain behavior, posture, and anatomic abnormalities such as contractures, amputation, and asymmetries should also be noted. Maladaptive postural dynamics play an important role in generating myofascial pain. Excessive lumbar lordosis places strain on the lumbar extensor muscles and results in low back pain. Similarly, forward flexion of the cervical spine with drooping of the shoulders strains the cervical paraspinous and scapular muscles and thereby causes neck and upper back pain.

Evaluation of gait includes assessment of stride length, base, arm swing, and stability. An unsteady, wide-based ataxic gait can be seen in patients with cerebellar and proprioceptive disorders. In patients with hip and lower extremity pain, the stance phase is reduced in the affected limb, along with a shortened swing phase on the uninvolved side, which results in an antalgic gait pattern. A waddling gait can be seen in patients with weakness of the hip girdle muscles or bilateral degenerative hip joint disease. A multitude of gait deviations can occur in patients with footdrop, including vaulting, steppage gate, circumduction, and persistent abduction of the affected limb.[1]

NEUROLOGIC EXAMINATION

The following are components of the neurologic examination:

1. Mental status examination
2. Cranial nerve testing
3. Motor strength examination
4. Deep tendon reflexes
5. Sensation
6. Coordination
7. Special tests

MENTAL STATUS EXAMINATION

A reasonable assessment of mental status can often be made as part of history taking and inquiry into activities of daily living and function. A basic mental status examination includes assessment of the level of consciousness; orientation to person, place, time, and situation; registration and short-term memory; attention and concentration; and assessment of language for aphasia. The Folstein Mini-Mental Status Examination is a useful screening tool for detecting cognitive deficits and dementia.

Assessment of mood, affect, suicidal and homicidal ideation, and neurovegetative symptoms such as sleep, appetite, and energy level should be inquired about routinely. This helps uncover comorbid psychiatric conditions (e.g., depression, anxiety, and psychosis), which can have a profound impact on the treatment of pain patients.

CRANIAL NERVE TESTING

The cranial nerve examination localizes pathology primarily at the level of the brainstem. Central pain conditions associated with brainstem pathology (e.g., strokes, tumors, demyelinating disease, and vascular malformations) can be associated with cranial nerve deficits.[1]

CRANIAL NERVE I

OLFACTORY NERVE

Test one nostril at a time. Odors such as coffee, mint, or cloves can be used. Noxious odors such as ammonia should be avoided because they activate trigeminal nerve receptors in the nasal passages.

The most common cause of smell dysfunction is nasal and sinus pathology. Dementia, neurodegenerative conditions, and basal frontal tumors can also result in smell dysfunction.

CRANIAL NERVE II

OPTIC NERVE

Visual acuity is determined with a Snellen chart. Visual fields are tested by the confrontation method at the bedside. More formal visual field testing with perimetry can be requested if indicated. Pupillary reaction to light and accommodation tests the optic and ophthalmic nerves. Funduscopic examination is done to evaluate the optic disc and retina. Papilledema and enlargement of the blind spot can be seen in conditions associated with elevated intracranial pressure, including idiopathic intracranial hypertension, which is a relatively common cause of intractable headache.

CRANIAL NERVES III, IV, AND VI

OPHTHALMIC, TROCHLEAR, AND ABDUCENS NERVES

These nerves control eye movement and can be tested by asking the patient to track a moving object in the eight positions of cardinal gaze. Eyelid elevation and pupillary constriction are controlled by the third cranial nerve and are evaluated by assessing the direct, consensual, and accommodation reflexes. Sympathetic fibers innervate the pupillary dilator muscles. Horner's syndrome can be detected in several clinical conditions, including after stellate ganglion blockade. This syndrome includes ipsilateral ptosis, miosis, and anhidrosis. However, the mechanism of these changes involves sympatholysis and is independent of cranial nerve function.

CRANIAL NERVE V

TRIGEMINAL NERVE

This nerve supplies sensory input to the face, mouth, tongue, and scalp up to the vertex. The mandibular division of the trigeminal nerve also supplies the muscles of mastication (i.e., temporalis, masseter, medial, and lateral pterygoid muscles).

Sensation along the ophthalmic, maxillary, and mandibular divisions of the trigeminal nerve can be tested with temperature, pinprick, and light touch. The trigeminal nerve also provides the afferent limb of the corneal blink reflex.

Peripheral lesions of the trigeminal nerve result in ipsilateral loss of facial sensation with weakness and atrophy of the ipsilateral jaw muscles.

CRANIAL NERVE VII

FACIAL NERVE

The facial nerve innervates the muscles of facial expression, the submandibular and lacrimal glands, and taste in the anterior two thirds of the tongue. Testing is usually limited to checking facial motor function (e.g., forehead wrinkling, eye closure, smile, pursing lips, and corneal blink). Supranuclear lesions of the seventh nerve typically spare the forehead, whereas nuclear and infranuclear lesions do not.

Sensory testing of the facial nerve is not routinely performed but can be accomplished by applying sweet, sour, and salt stimuli to the ipsilateral half of the anterior two thirds of the tongue.

CRANIAL NERVE VIII

VESTIBULOCOCHLEAR NERVE

The vestibulocochlear nerve mediates hearing and balance. Hearing can be assessed with a 512-Hz tuning fork. The Rinne and Weber tests are commonly used to assess for sensorineural and conductive deafness.

In the Weber test, the base of a gently vibrating tuning fork is placed on the midforehead or the vertex. The patient is asked which ear hears the sound better. Normally, the sound is heard equally in both ears. With unilateral sensorineural hearing loss, sound is heard better in the unaffected ear. With unilateral conductive hearing loss, sound is heard better in the affected ear.

The Rinne test is conducted by placing the base of a gently vibrating tuning fork on the mastoid bone behind the ear. When the patient can no longer hear the sound, the fork is quickly moved next to the patient's ear. In patients with sensorineural deafness and normal hearing, air conduction is better than bone conduction. With conductive deafness, bone conduction is better than air conduction.

Nystagmus noted on eye movement testing may be a sign of vestibular dysfunction. In patients with complaints of episodic vertigo, the Dix-Hallpike maneuver is useful for making the diagnosis of benign paroxysmal positional vertigo.

CRANIAL NERVE IX

GLOSSOPHARYNGEAL NERVE

The glossopharyngeal nerve subserves taste in the posterior third of the tongue and sensation in the pharynx. It provides the afferent limb of the gag reflex.

CRANIAL NERVE X

VAGUS NERVE

The vagus nerve innervates the pharyngeal and laryngeal muscles and forms the efferent limb of the gag reflex. Symptoms of vagus nerve lesions include dysarthria and dysphagia.

CRANIAL NERVE XI

ACCESSORY NERVE

The cranial segment of the accessory nerve supplies the muscles of the larynx, whereas the spinal segment innervates the trapezius and sternocleidomastoid muscles. These muscles are tested by ipsilateral shoulder shrug and contralateral head turn maneuvers.

CRANIAL NERVE XII

HYPOGLOSSAL NERVE

The hypoglossal nerve provides motor supply to the tongue. Testing is performed by tongue protrusion and pushing the tongue against the cheek on either side. Lesions of the hypoglossal nerve produce ipsilateral deviation on tongue protrusion.

MOTOR STRENGTH EXAMINATION

Manual muscle testing is performed by asking the patient to place each muscle in its position of maximal mechanical advantage. Muscle strength is commonly assessed with the Medical Research Council scale (Table 13.1). Grades 1 to 3 are relatively objective and less prone to interobserver variation. Grade 1 implies a palpable contraction but with no associated movement noted. Grade 2 implies an ability to move the limb with gravity eliminated (this may require special postioning to assess). A grade 3 finding on motor examination is consistent with the ability to move against gravity but an inability to move against further resistance. The gastrocnemius muscle presents unique challenges when performing a manual muscle test. In the case of the gastrocnemius, a grade 3 muscle is able to perform one toe raise with the patient standing and lightly holding onto something for balance. A grade 4 muscle is able to perform 5 toe raises, and a grade 5 gastrocnemius is capable of performing 10 toe raises. Grades 4 and 5 are difficult to standardize among different examiners. Factors such as a patient's body habitus, age, and expected functional status, as well as examiner strength, contribute to the difficulty of grading muscle strength above grade 3.[2]

The screening muscle strength examination should correspond to a template that evaluates sequential nerve roots and peripheral nerves. Tables 13.2 and 13.3 provide a summary of the commonly tested muscles along with their corresponding nerve root and peripheral nerve innervation.[3]

Table 13.1 Medical Research Council Grading of Muscle Strength

Grade 0	No movement
Grade 1	Flicker of movement
Grade 2	Movement only with gravity eliminated
Grade 3	Full range of movement against gravity
Grade 4	Full range of movement against some resistance
Grade 5	Full power against resistance

The muscle strength examination depends significantly on patients' comprehension and effort. Suboptimal or volitional lack of effort may be apparent as "give-way weakness," with the patient applying intermittent resistance to the examiner interspersed with moments of nearly complete cessation of effort. Weakness as a result of radiculopathy, focal compressive peripheral neuropathy, diffuse peripheral neuropathy, or myopathy should fit specific patterns. A nonphysiologic pattern should raise suspicion for potential psychogenic weakness. The Hoover test is useful to detect psychogenic weakness of the lower extremities. The patient is examined while lying supine in bed and is asked to elevate the paretic leg. The examiner's hand should be placed underneath the contralateral heel. A positive Hoover test result occurs if the patient fails to exert downward force on the examiner's hand. The Hoover sign is based on the crossed extensor reflex mediated by interneurons in the spinal cord. This reflex was first described by Sherrington and can be demonstrated in decorticate animals.[1]

REFLEX TESTING

The deep tendon reflexes are mediated by a monosynaptic arc. The afferent limb is provided by sensory fibers, which innervate muscle spindles. These fibers project centrally toward the spinal cord and synapse with alpha motor neurons in the ventral horn. The alpha motor neurons comprise the efferent limb of the reflex arc. It is important to note that normal individuals can have diminished deep tendon reflexes. The Jendrassik maneuver can be used to elicit deep tendon reflexes in this situation. The patient is asked to interlock the fingers of both hands and pull them apart. Jaw clenching can also be used to achieve a similar effect. Lesions of the afferent or efferent limb of this arc can cause diminished or absent deep tendon reflexes. This includes conditions such as peripheral neuropathy and radiculopathy. However, patients with small-fiber neuropathy have preserved deep tendon reflexes because the neural deficit spares large myelinated Ia fibers.

Deep tendon reflexes are best examined with a Queen Square or Troemner hammer while the patient is seated

Table 13.2 Upper Extremity Muscles: Innervation and Action

Muscle	Action	Nerve Root	Nerve
Infraspinatus	Shoulder external rotation	C5-6	Suprascapular
Deltoid	Shoulder abduction, extension, and flexion	C5-6	Axillary
Biceps	Forearm flexion and supination	C5-6	Musculocutaneous
Triceps	Forearm extension	C7-8	Radial
Brachioradialis	Forearm flexion in the midprone position	C6	Radial
Extensor carpi radialis longus and brevis	Wrist extension	C6-7	Radial
Flexor carpi ulnaris	Wrist flexion with ulnar deviation	C8-T1	Ulnar
Flexor digitorum profundus	Flexion at the distal interphalangeal joints	C7-8	Anterior interosseus branch of the median nerve
Abductor pollicis brevis	Abduction of the thumb	C8	Median
Adductor pollicis longus	Abduction of the thumb	C8-T1	Ulnar

comfortably in the upright position. Table 13.4 explains the grading of deep tendon reflexes. Table 13.5 reviews the important deep tendon reflexes and their corresponding nerve root level.

Upper motor neuron lesions cause hyperreflexia. The Babinski and Hoffman signs may be present in patients with upper motor neuron dysfunction. A subtly positive Hoffman response can be seen in young women, as well as in people taking selective serotonin reuptake inhibitor antidepressants, and in these scenarios may not represent pathology. The Babinski sign is elicited by stroking the lateral aspect of the sole of the foot with a blunt object (e.g., a disposable wooden spatula). A positive sign is indicated by extension of the great toe (Fig. 13.1). Care should be taken to not stimulate the more medial aspect of the sole, which will evoke a withdrawal response. Hoffman's sign is elicited by briskly flicking the dorsal or volar aspect of the distal phalanx of the middle finger. Reflex flexion of the index finger and thumb constitutes a positive response.[4]

Table 13.3 Lower Extremity Muscles: Innervation and Action

Muscle	Action	Nerve Root	Nerve
Iliopsoas	Hip flexion	L2-4	Femoral
Adductor longus and brevis	Hip adduction	L2-4	Obturator
Gluteus maximus	Hip extension	L5-S2	Inferior gluteal
Gluteus medius and minimus	Hip abduction	L5-S2	Superior gluteal
Quadriceps femoris	Knee extension	L2-4	Femoral
Hamstrings (i.e., semitendinosus, semimembranosus, and biceps femoris)	Knee flexion	L5-S1	Sciatic
Tibialis anterior	Foot dorsiflexion	L4-5	Deep peroneal
Extensor hallucis longus	Extension of the big toe	L5	Deep peroneal
Peroneus longus	Foot eversion	L5	Superficial peroneal
Gastrocnemius/soleus	Foot plantar flexion	S1-2	Tibial
Tibialis posterior	Foot inversion and plantar flexion	L5-S1	Tibial

Table 13.4 Grading of Deep Tendon Reflexes

Grade 0	Absent
Grade 1+	Hypoactive
Grade 2+	Normal
Grade 3+	Spread of reflex contraction to muscles innervated by the adjacent root level
Grade 4+	Sustained clonus

Table 13.5 Nerve Root Innervation of the Deep Tendon Reflexes

Muscle Tendon	Nerve Root Level
Biceps	C5-6
Brachioradialis	C6
Triceps	C7-8
Quadriceps femoris	L3-4
Gastrocnemius/Achilles tendon	S1-2

SENSATION

Sensory examination should include the modalities of temperature, pinprick, proprioception, and vibration. Pinprick and temperature are mediated by Aδ and C small fibers and are transmitted in the spinal cord by the lateral spinothalamic tract. Proprioception and vibration are mediated by Aβ large fibers and are carried by the dorsal columns in the spinal cord.

Pinprick testing can be performed with a clean disposable safety pin. A distal-to-proximal pattern of testing is useful in evaluating patients with length-dependent peripheral neuropathy. In patients with nerve root pathology, testing in a dermatomal pattern is recommended (Fig. 13.2). Temperature sensation can be assessed rapidly by using the cold metal portion of a tuning fork and warm water in a test tube. The format for testing is identical to that for pinprick testing.

Proprioception is assessed at individual synovial joints. The most sensitive test for proprioception involves the interphalangeal joint of the big toe. The toe is grasped at its lateral margins between the thumb and index finger of the examiner's hand. The big toe is then abducted from the remaining toes and moved superiorly and inferiorly in increments of 5 degrees while the patient's eyes are closed. The patient is then asked to identify whether the toe is being moved up or down. If proprioception is impaired at the toe, the same test can be repeated at the ankle, knee, and distal interphalangeal joint of the index finger.

Vibration sense is usually examined by placing a vibrating 128-Hz tuning fork over a distal bony prominence. The dorsal surface of the interphalangeal joint of the big toe, medial malleolus, tibial tuberosity, and patella are the relevant lower extremity landmarks. The distal phalanx of the index finger, distal end of the radius, and olecranon process of the ulna are the important sites for testing vibration in the upper extremity. Recently, the Rydel-Seiffer 64-Hz quantitative tuning fork has been shown to have better correlation than the traditional 128-Hz tuning fork with sural nerve sensory nerve action potential and ankle reflex results.[5]

COORDINATION

Cerebellar function can be divided into midline/vermal and hemispheric functions. The vermis controls axial coordination and balance, whereas the hemispheres coordinate the limbs. Vermian function is assessed by observation of gait and standing balance. Hemispheric function is assessed with the finger-to-nose and heel-to-shin tests. Other tests include rapidly alternating movements (e.g., sequential hand pronation and supination) and examination for motor tone, which is reduced in patients with cerebellar disease. Chronic alcohol abuse and long-term use of medications such as phenytoin can cause acquired cerebellar degeneration.[4]

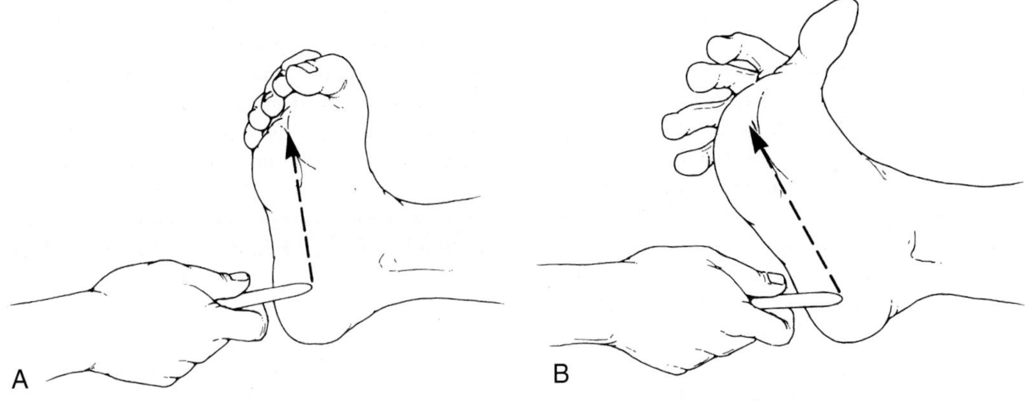

Figure 13.1 Babinski test. **A,** Normal. **B,** Abnormal.

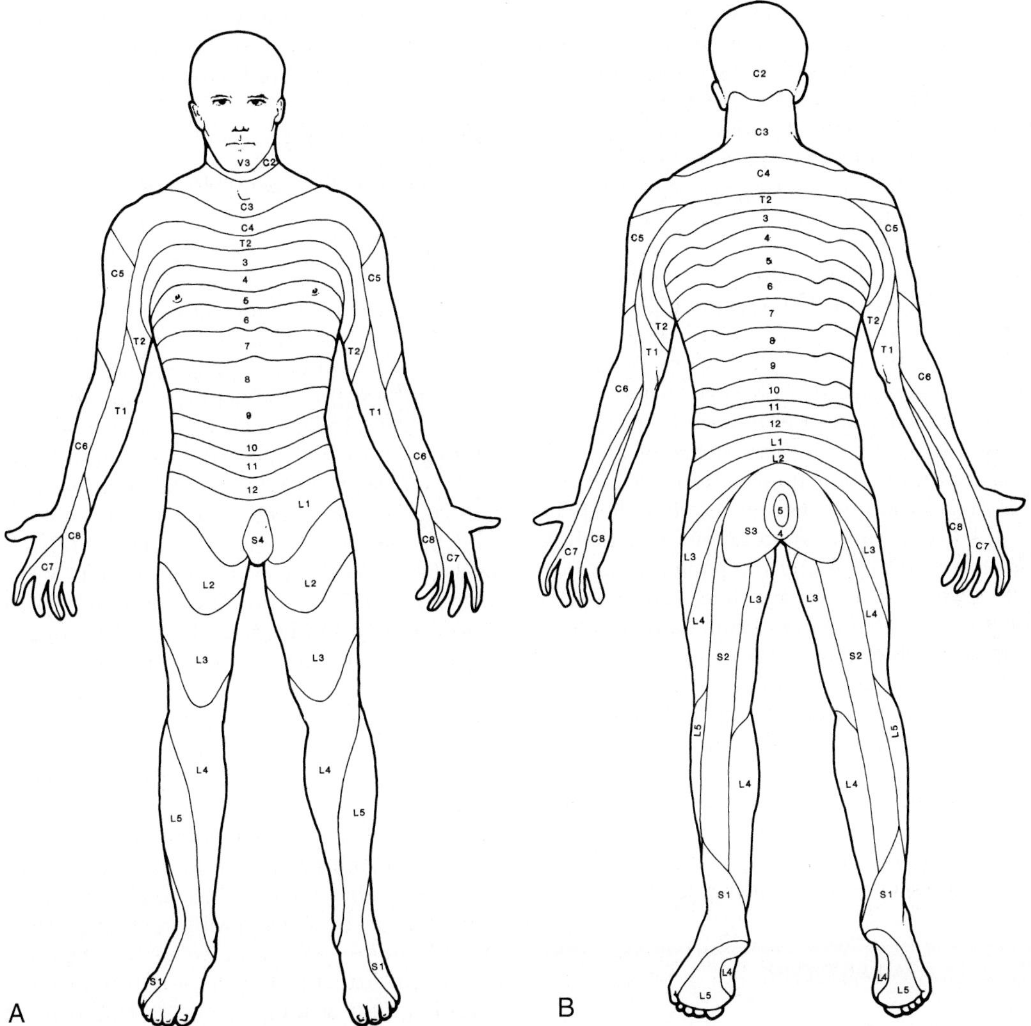

Figure 13.2 Anterior (**A**) and posterior (**B**) dermatomes of the body. (From Baker AB, Baker LH. *Clinical Neurology*. Vol 1. New York: Harper & Row; 1983.)

MUSCULOSKELETAL EXAMINATION

The musculoskeletal examination serves to evaluate the integrated functioning of bones, joints, supporting ligaments, and muscular tissue. Information from the examination can be used to localize possible sources of pain in various structures, including the skin, subcutaneous tissue, tendons, joints, ligaments, and periosteum. The format of the musculoskeletal examination follows the steps of inspection, palpation, range of motion, and special tests. The components tested are the spine (cervical, thoracic, lumbar) and the extremities with their respective joints.

SPINAL EXAMINATION

Inspection of the cervical and thoracolumbar spine provides information on posture and alignment. Abnormal kyphosis, lordosis, or scoliosis should be noted. Palpation of the spinous processes can reveal localized tenderness, which is seen in patients with conditions such as vertebral compression fractures, epidural tumor, or abscess. A step-off (i.e., a sudden change in prominence of the spinous processes) is also indicative of a vertebral compression fracture with resultant loss of height. Tenderness in the paraspinous regions can be seen in patients with facet arthropathy and myofascial pain syndrome. Normal range of motion of the cervical spine is 60 degrees of forward flexion, 75 degrees of extension, 45 degrees of lateral flexion, and 80 degrees of lateral rotation. Range-of-motion testing should be performed with the patient in both the supine and sitting positions. Improvement in range of motion in the supine position suggests that muscle spasm is responsible for restricting cervical mobility. However, there is no positional improvement in cervical range of motion with cervical arthropathy. Normal thoracolumbar spine range of motion is 90 degrees of forward flexion, 30 degrees of back extension, 25 degrees of lateral flexion, and 60 degrees of lateral rotation. Pain that is provoked by back extension and lateral rotation is suggestive of facet arthropathy in that these maneuvers result in zygapophyseal joint loading. Pain that is provoked by forward flexion is consistent with a discogenic or vertebral body source of pain because flexion causes axial loading. Lumbar discogenic pain is often restricted to the axial spine and is associated with intolerance of the sitting position and pain provoked by coughing, sneezing, and Valsalva maneuvers. A positive abduction tension release sign is highly specific in determining whether the shoulder pain is secondary to C5-6 root compression or shoulder pathology. The test is performed by asking the patient to abduct the affected arm such that the forearm is placed in a resting position on top of the patient's head. With shoulder pathology, attempts to achieve this position will cause pain. In patients with C5-6 root compression, this test position will commonly result in a marked reduction in pain in the shoulder and medial scapular (rhomboid) region. The Spurling maneuver is highly specific for confirming the diagnosis of cervical radiculopathy. The patient is asked to perform simultaneous lateral flexion and extension of the neck toward the symptomatic side. Provocation of ipsilateral neck and arm pain constitutes a positive Spurling sign.[6,7]

MYOFASCIAL EXAMINATION

Myofascial pain is manifested by the presence of tender palpable bands of muscle called *trigger points*. Active myofascial trigger points are associated with complaints of spontaneous pain and restricted range of motion. Latent trigger points are tender and palpable on direct examination, but they do not produce spontaneous pain.

Myofascial examination should start with assessment of posture and joint function to determine any underlying cause of the regional myofascial pain. Myofascial trigger points can be identified by gentle palpation in the direction of muscle fibers. Trigger points can be felt as a ropelike region of nodularity. Trigger points also are exquisitely tender, and palpation produces local as well as referred pain. The referral pain pattern may mimic a radicular or peripheral nerve distribution. Commonly affected muscles include the trapezius, gluteus, and cervical and lumbar paraspinous musculature, but many others may be affected as well.[8]

EXAMINATION OF THE EXTREMITIES

Inspection and, when indicated, measurement of the extremities may reveal discrepancies in limb length, deformities, and alterations in muscle bulk. Range of motion can be demonstrated by asking the patient to perform specific tasks such as raising the hands above the head. The lower extremities can be assessed during evaluation of gait. The pattern of gait abnormality can direct the clinician to the underlying cause of dysfunction, such as footdrop, leg length discrepancy, or hip or knee pain.[6,7,9,10]

UPPER EXTREMITY

SHOULDER JOINT EXAMINATION

Inspection should evaluate for symmetry, bulk of the deltoid muscles, and posture. Palpation of the shoulder joint should include the sternoclavicular joint, clavicle, acromioclavicular joint, glenohumeral joint, and the scapular spine and scapulothoracic articulation. Normal range of motion for the shoulder joint is 180 degrees of flexion and extension in the sagittal plane, 180 degrees of abduction and adduction in the frontal plane, 90 degrees of external rotation, and 40 degrees of internal rotation. Common causes of shoulder pain include glenohumeral arthritis, acromioclavicular arthritis, subacromial or subdeltoid bursitis, supraspinatus and bicipital tendonitis, and rotator cuff tendonitis, tears, and labral lesions, commonly noted as SLAP (superior labrum anterior to posterior) lesions. A variety of special tests are used to diagnose these conditions. The tests most commonly used in clinical practice are described below.

Pain on shoulder abduction and elevation is seen with impingement syndrome. The etiology involves entrapment of soft tissue between the humeral head and the coracoacromial arch. Subacromial bursitis, supraspinatus tendinitis, and partial or complete tears of the rotator cuff tendons can be present at the same time. In case of a complete tear, the patient will be unable to abduct the arm if it is tested to isolate supraspinatus function. Horizontal abduction in the plane of the scapula with the thumb turned down—the tipped can test—is a sensitive test for rotator cuff pathology. Untreated tears of the rotator cuff tendons result in disuse atrophy of the scapular muscles. The drop arm test is used to diagnose complete rotator cuff tears. The patient's arm is passively abducted to 90 degrees and then released. Failure to maintain shoulder abduction suggests a complete rotator cuff tear. The diagnosis can be investigated further with magnetic resonance imaging.

Adhesive Capsulitis

Frozen shoulder, or adhesive capsulitis, is characterized by diminished range of motion at the scapulothoracic and glenohumeral joints. There is progressive fibrosis of the shoulder joint capsule, which disrupts normal shoulder mobility and scapulothoracic rhythm. Normally, the shoulder joint can be abducted to 180 degrees. Scapulothoracic motion begins at 90 degrees of shoulder abduction, and there is a 2:1 ratio of glenohumeral to scapulothoracic motion. Adhesive capsulitis results in gradual loss of range of motion, with little to no shoulder movement present in advanced cases.

ELBOW JOINT

Inspection of the elbow joint includes assessment of humeral and radial-ulnar symmetry. The carrying angle between the arm and forearm is measured with the patient standing and the arms at the side and facing anteriorly. The normal carrying angle is 10 to 15 degrees of valgus for men and up to 18 degrees for women. Readily palpable landmarks of the elbow joint include the olecranon process and the medial and lateral epicondyles. Normal range of motion at the elbow starting from the anatomic position is 0 degrees of extension to 150 degrees of flexion at the humeroulnar joint and 170 degrees of pronation and supination at the radioulnar joint.

Lateral Epicondylitis

Overuse of the forearm extensor muscles results in inflammation of the common extensor tendon insertion at the lateral epicondyle. Patients report constant elbow pain that is worse with wrist movement. Bedside testing is performed by asking the patient to extend the wrist and resist forcible wrist flexion. Pain over the lateral epicondyle confirms the diagnosis of lateral epicondylitis. In severe cases, passive flexion of the wrist may also replicate pain in the extensor mass.

Medial Epicondylitis

This condition is similar to lateral epicondylitis and results from overuse of the forearm flexor muscles. Pain is experienced over the medial epicondyle and can be reproduced by forcibly extending the patient's flexed wrist.

WRIST JOINT

Inspection plus palpation of the wrist joint is used to evaluate joint symmetry. Range of motion is 60 degrees of extension, 70 degrees of flexion, 20 degrees of abduction, and 30 degrees of adduction. The most common clinically encountered specific wrist joint pain disorder is carpal tunnel syndrome. This entity is a result of entrapment of the median nerve at the wrist, which causes symptoms of wrist pain with associated numbness and weakness of the hand. A diagnosis of carpal tunnel syndrome is supported by the presence of the Tinel and Phalen signs. In the Tinel sign, percussion of the proximal volar wrist crease produces paresthesias in the thumb and index and middle fingers of the symptomatic hand. To elicit the Phalen sign, the patient is asked to forcibly flex both wrists against one another for 1 minute. Reproduction of sensory dysesthesias in a median nerve distribution is consistent with a positive Phalen test. Caution must be used when interpreting the results of these tests because neither test has a high degree of specificity or sensitivity. The "gold standard" test for evaluation of suspected carpal tunnel syndrome is formal electrodiagnostic testing.

EVALUATION OF THE DIGITS

The digits are inspected to evaluate for symmetry and the presence of any deformities. Heberden's nodes at the distal interphalangeal joints and Bouchard's nodes at the proximal interphalangeal joints can be seen in patients with osteoarthritis. Range of motion can be assessed by asking patients to open and close their fist. Normal range of motion in the sagittal plane is 90 degrees at the metacarpophalangeal joints, 120 degrees at the proximal interphalangeal joints, and 70 degrees at the distal interphalangeal joints. The first metacarpophalangeal joint has 50 degrees of motion in abduction, 50 degrees in adduction, and 35 degrees in opposition.

EVALUATION OF THE HIP JOINT

Inspection of the hip joint should pay attention to symmetry, muscle bulk, and surgical scars. Normal range of motion at the hip is 100 degrees of flexion, 30 degrees of extension, 20 degrees of adduction, and 40 degrees of abduction. With the hip joint in a flexed position, range of motion is 45 degrees for internal rotation and 40 degrees for external rotation. Hip pain may result from pathology of the acetabulum, femoral neck or head, periosteum, or joint capsule. It may also result from abnormalities in a surrounding structure such as the bursae or may be referred from the lumbar spine or sacroiliac joint. Hip joint pathology classically results in referral of pain to the groin and anteromedial or lateral aspect of the thigh over the greater trochanter region. However, referral of pain from knee pathology can also cause anteromedial thigh pain. Additionally, lateral thigh pain can be seen as a "typically atypical" referral pain pattern of an L5 radiculopathy, with pain involving the L5-innervated gluteal muscles.

As one can see, pain referral patterns alone are often insufficient to diagnose the etiology of hip pain, and an appropriate imaging evaluation is helpful in this regard.

TROCHANTERIC BURSITIS

Patients report a deep, dull, aching pain with radiation to the lateral hip region. The pain is worse at night. Inflammation primarily involves the trochanteric bursa, which lies between the gluteus maximus and gluteus medius tendons. The diagnosis is supported by tenderness with palpation over the greater trochanter and pain on hip extension and resisted hip abduction.

PATRICK'S TEST

Patrick's test evaluates hip and sacroiliac joint pathology. With the patient in the supine position, the examiner passively flexes, abducts, and externally rotates the hip. Pain in the groin suggests hip joint pathology, whereas sacroiliac pain indicates dysfunction of the sacroiliac joint (Fig. 13.3).

STRAIGHT-LEG RAISE TEST

With the patient in the supine position, the examiner passively elevates one leg by holding it at the ankle. The hip is flexed to an angle of 70 to 90 degrees with the knee extended (Fig. 13.4). A positive straight-leg raise test produces pain starting at the hip with radiation down to the ankle. Pain that remains localized to the posterior thigh region is caused by tension on the hamstrings. A crossed straight-leg raise sign is present if testing of the uninvolved leg produces contralateral symptoms. Both the straight and crossed straight-leg raise tests place the lumbosacral nerve roots under tension, and a positive test is suggestive of lumbosacral radiculopathy. Straight-leg testing can also be performed with the

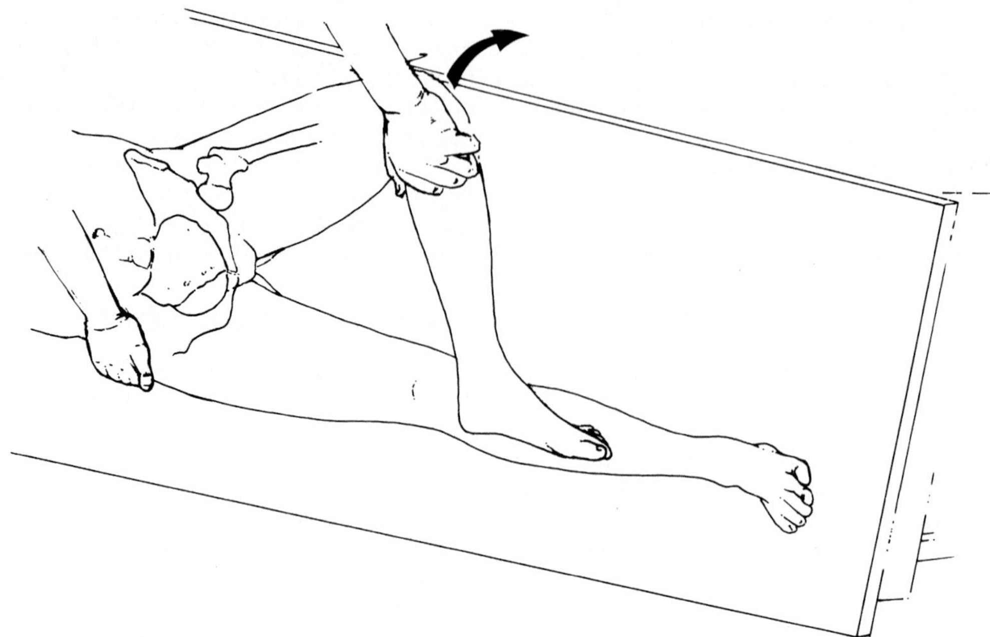

Figure 13.3 The Patrick or flexicon abduction external (FABER) test.

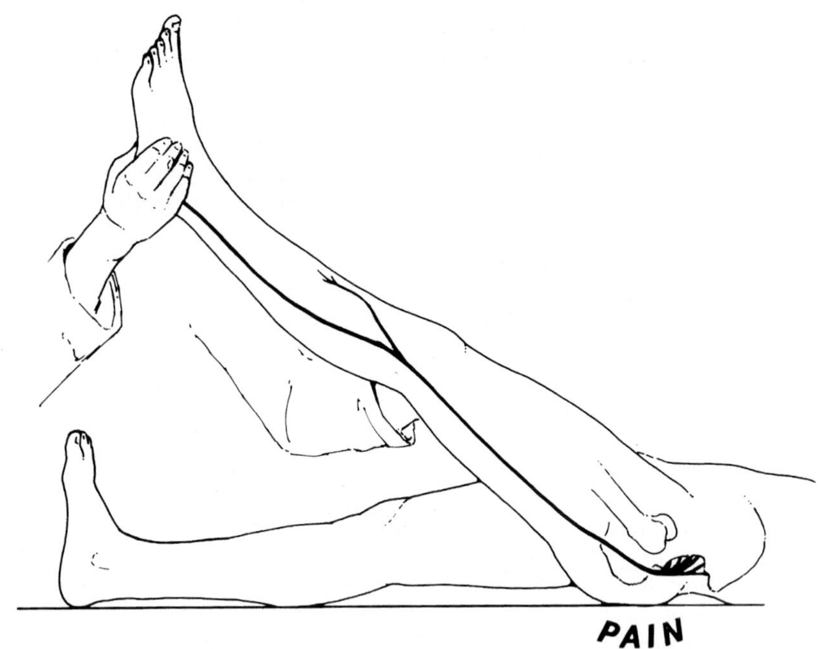

Figure 13.4 Straight-leg raise test (Lasègue's sign).

patient in the seated position. In this setting the patient is asked to extend the knee. This stretches the lumbosacral roots as the hip is flexed to 90 degrees when the patient is seated. If augmentation is needed, the patient can be asked to dorsiflex the foot, or the examiner can passively dorsiflex the patient's foot if needed.

EVALUATION OF THE KNEE

Inspection should assess symmetry, position of the patella, surgical scars, and the bulk of the surrounding musculature, including the quadriceps femoris muscle. Particular attention should be placed on inspection of the vastus medialis because this muscle atrophies rapidly when patients have chronic knee pain and reflex inhibition of quadriceps function. Varus deformity of the knee is a result of medial compartment loss, whereas valgus deformity is caused by lateral compartment loss. Bilateral genu valgum (knock-knees), genu varum (bowed legs), or genu recurvatum (back knees) should be noted as well. Palpation should include the surrounding bursae (i.e., the pes anserinus and prepatellar bursae) because these are common sources of pain. Normal range of motion at the knee joint is 150 degrees in the sagittal plane.

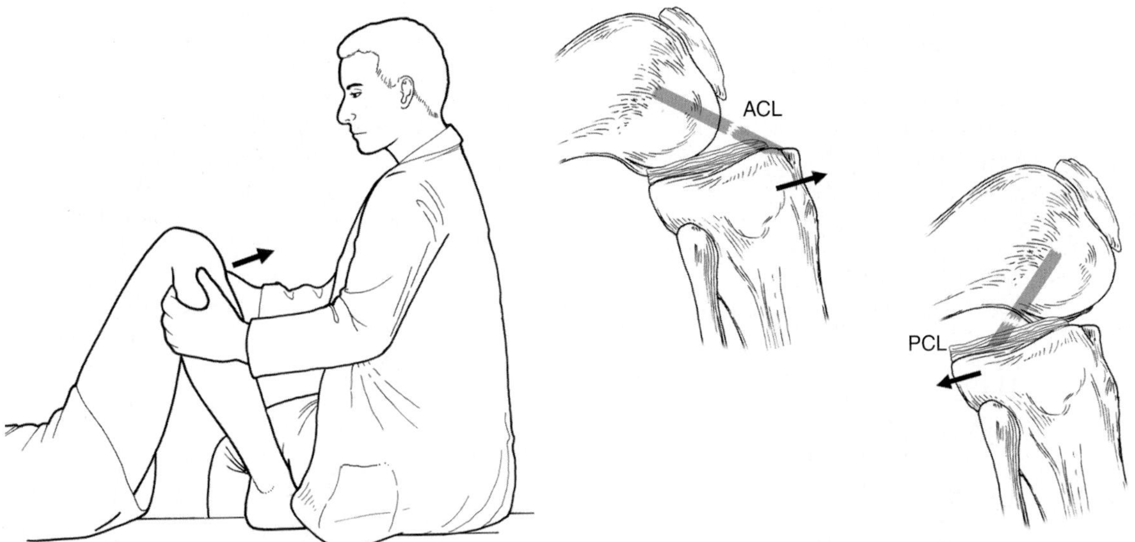

Figure 13.5 Drawer sign test for the cruciate ligaments. The standard drawer sign test for the cruciate ligaments immobilizes the foot and stresses the lower part of the leg on the femur. Pulling the leg forward tests the anterior cruciate ligament (ACL), whereas posterior pressure tests the posterior cruciate ligament (PCL). (Redrawn from Calliet R. *Knee Pain and Disability*. 3rd ed. Philadelphia: FA Davis; 1992:1-69.)

SPECIAL TESTS

Drawer Sign

With the patient's knee in the flexed position and the foot anchored to stabilize the lower part of the leg, the examiner draws the tibia anteriorly. Movement of the tibia in the forward direction constitutes a positive anterior drawer sign and suggests a tear of the anterior cruciate ligament. Similarly, if the tibia moves posteriorly when pulled backward, this is a positive posterior drawer sign and is caused by a torn posterior cruciate ligament (Fig. 13.5).

Patellar Femoral Grinding Test

Knee pain on rising to a standing position or while climbing stairs can occur with chondromalacia patellae. With the patient's knee extended, the examiner exerts downward pressure on the patella into the femoral groove. Patients with chondromalacia patellae will complain of pain with this maneuver.

Apley's Compression or Grinding Test

This test is used to evaluate for medial and lateral meniscal tears. With the patient in the prone position, the knee is flexed to 90 degrees, downward force is applied to the heel, and the tibia is rotated medially and laterally against the femur (Fig. 13.6). Pain provoked in the medial or lateral aspect of the knee indicates a tear in the respective collateral ligament.

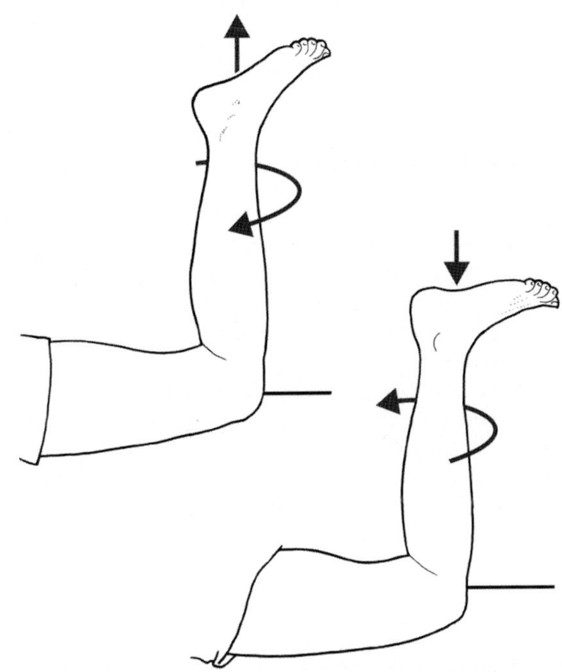

Figure 13.6 Examination of ligament injury, including the meniscus (Apley's test). The Apley test checks the integrity of the knee ligamentous structures and the menisci. It is performed in two aspects. *Left,* With the patient prone and the knee flexed to a right angle, downward pressure is applied to the lower part of the leg. The leg is then rotated to test the menisci. This maneuver compresses the menisci between the femoral condyles and the tibial plateau, as in the McMurray test. With the lower part of the leg internally rotated, the medial meniscus is tested. Grating, crepitation, limitation, and pain imply meniscal damage. From the same position, the leg is elevated *(right),* which places traction on the ligaments. Excessive motion, deduced by comparison to the contralateral side, indicates laxity or injury to the knee ligaments and capsule. (Redrawn from Calliet R. *Knee Pain and Disability*. 3rd ed. Philadelphia: FA Davis; 1992:1-69.)

EVALUATION OF THE ANKLE

Inspection should include evaluation of bony landmarks, symmetry, and edema. Normal range of motion of the ankle is 20 degrees of dorsiflexion and 40 degrees of plantar flexion through the tibiotalar joint. The 30 degrees of inversion and 15 degrees of eversion noted at the ankle are a result of subtalar motion, not tibiotalar motion.

Pain and excessive motion on pulling the ankle joint anteriorly indicate a tear in the anterior talofibular ligament, whereas similar findings on forced inversion occur with tears of the calcaneofibular ligament. The posterior

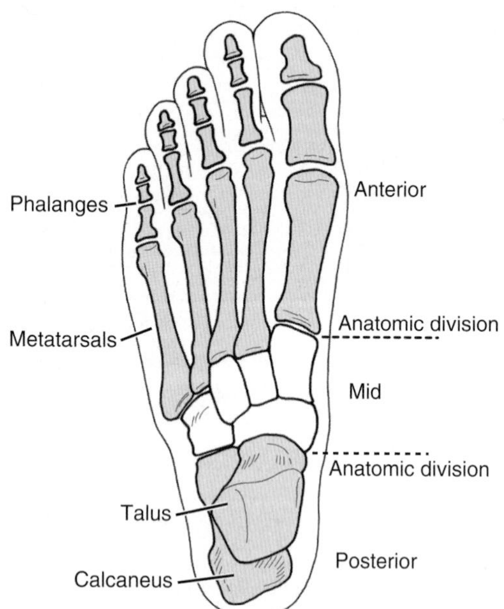

Figure 13.7 Anatomy of the foot with functional segmentation. (Redrawn from Abrams B, Glaser L. Painful conditions of the foot and ankle: evaluation and treatment. *Pain Diagn*. 1997;7:351-363.)

talofibular ligament is usually damaged only in patients with a significant history of preceding trauma.

EVALUATION OF THE FOOT

Functional assessment of the foot is targeted toward its anterior, middle, and posterior segments. The anterior segment consists of the 5 metatarsal and 14 phalangeal bones; the middle segment includes the navicular, cuboid, and 3 cuneiform bones; and the posterior segment includes the talus and calcaneus (Fig. 13.7).

The posterior segment of the foot transmits body weight to the ground. The middle segment provides flexibility and the ability to adapt gait to uneven surfaces. The anterior segment acts as a fulcrum to provide forward thrust during ambulation. The impact of the foot against the ground is cushioned by its longitudinal and transverse arches.

Foot pain is a common symptom in patients (Fig. 13.8). The more common pain syndromes that are diagnosed by physical examination are described in the following sections.

TARSAL TUNNEL SYNDROME

In tarsal tunnel syndrome, the posterior tibial nerve is entrapped beneath the lancinate ligament, posterior to the medial malleolus. Patients complain of pain and paresthesias affecting the toes and sole of the foot. Physical examination may demonstrate atrophy of the intrinsic foot muscles and hypoesthesia of the sole of the foot. Percussion posterior to the medial malleolus can provoke paresthesia in the ipsilateral sole and toes in patients with tarsal tunnel syndrome.

MORTON'S NEUROMA

Morton's neuroma is characterized by pain between the metatarsal bones, usually between the third and fourth toes and less commonly between the second and third toes. The pain is reproducible on palpation of the space between the metatarsal heads. The etiology of Morton's neuroma is not well understood, but it probably represents a form of interdigital neuritis. Interestingly, surgically resected specimens in patients with Morton's neuroma do not show any significant changes in nerve histology when compared with control tissue obtained from cadavers.

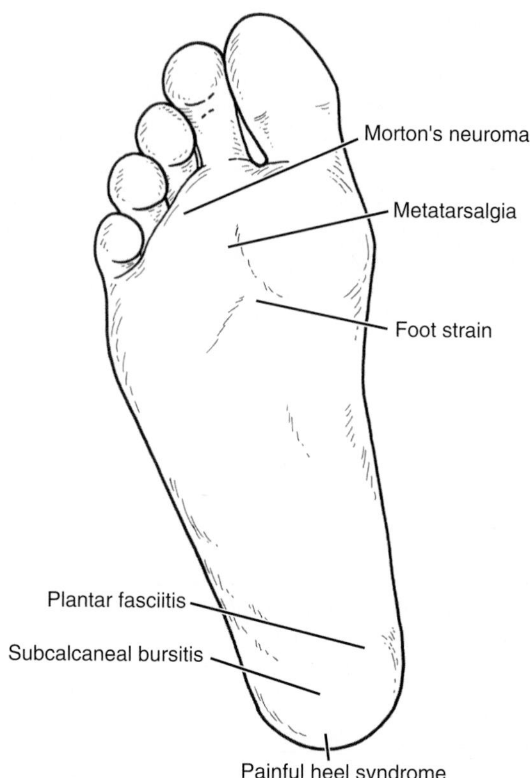

Figure 13.8 Location of common painful conditions involving the plantar surface of the foot. (Redrawn from Abrams B, Glaser L. Painful conditions of the foot and ankle: evaluation and treatment. *Pain Diagn*. 1997;7:351-363.)

METATARSALGIA

Pain in patients with metatarsalgia occurs on weight bearing and is localized to the plantar aspect of the metatarsal heads. The pain occurs maximally over the first metatarsal head and can be reproduced by direct palpation. With foot inversion, weight is shifted to the heads of the second and third metatarsal bones, and repetitive stress can result in pain over these sites as well. Patients may walk with a characteristic antalgic gait, with the foot being held in the inverted position. This can serve as a useful clue to the diagnosis.

FOOT STRAIN

Foot strain affects the middle segment of the foot. Repetitive patterns of overuse result in elongation of the longitudinal arch and alterations in the normal alignment of the talus and calcaneus. Elongation of the longitudinal arch produces excessive strain on the plantar fascia, medial collateral ligament, and talocalcaneal ligament. Physical findings include flattening and pain on compression of the longitudinal arch.

PLANTAR FASCIITIS

Plantar fasciitis is manifested as plantar foot pain on weight bearing. Patients often have a history of prolonged standing in footwear lacking arch support or on hard surfaces.

Inflammation develops at the point of attachment of the plantar fascia to the calcaneus. Calcaneal bone spurs can develop from chronic straining of the plantar fascia. Clinically, tenderness on palpation can be elicited over the anterior portion of the calcaneus with radiation into the plantar fascia. A common finding is pain the first thing in the morning. Patients will frequently note severe plantar foot pain with weight bearing on arising and temporary improvement with weight bearing or after the morning shower.

PAINFUL HEEL SYNDROME

Painful heel syndrome is a result of degenerative changes in the weight-bearing aspect of the calcaneus and occurs primarily in morbidly obese individuals or those who stand or walk excessively. Pain is often worse in the morning on waking up or after prolonged rest. Examination is significant for tenderness on palpation over the posterior portion of the plantar aspect of the calcaneus.

TESTS FOR A NONORGANIC ETIOLOGY OF PAIN

WADDELL'S SIGNS

Waddell's tests were intended to evaluate patients with low back pain for functional overlay. There are five signs in total, and the presence of any three of these five signs in a patient was considered suggestive of a nonorganic pain etiology.[11]

1. Tenderness to palpation
   Widespread skin tenderness with light touch
   Tenderness on deep palpation that is not restricted to a single anatomic area
2. Simulation
   Low back pain provoked by axial loading pressure on the skull of a standing patient or rotation of the shoulders and pelvis in the same plane resulting in increased low back pain
3. Distraction
   For example, a patient with a positive response to the straight-leg raise test in the supine position but no pain on the same test repeated in the sitting position
4. Regional disturbance in function
   Weakness involving multiple muscle groups in a nonmyotomal distribution with "give-way" effort
   Sensory loss in a segmental pattern (e.g., glove-stocking rather than a dermatomal distribution) observed in a patient in whom polyneuropathy is not an appropriate diagnosis
5. Overreaction
   Disproportionate facial or verbal behavior (e.g., moaning and grimacing on light touch, posturing, and withdrawing from the examiner)

However, there are several limitations of Waddell's signs. Widespread superficial tenderness is commonly found in patients with fibromyalgia, and tenderness on deep palpation is part of myofascial pain syndrome. Sensory loss in a glove-stocking distribution is present with peripheral polyneuropathy. Moreover, studies have not found a consistent relationship between the presence of Waddell's signs and subscale scores on the Minnesota Multiphasic Personality Inventory. In fact, recent data suggest that Waddell's signs cannot accurately distinguish between organic and nonorganic causes of pain.[12]

The physical examination may be helpful in elucidating the cause of a patient's pain complaints; however, when used alone it has limitations, and the results of physical examination need to be considered in the context of the patient's history, as well as in the context of the results of diagnostic studies.

The references for this chapter can be found at www.expertconsult.com.

14 Electromyography and Evoked Potentials

Bernard M. Abrams | Howard J. Waldman

Electrodiagnosis is a broad term that includes multiple electrodiagnostic techniques, including needle electrode examination (NEE); motor and sensory nerve conduction studies (NCSs), including late responses; and evoked potentials (EPs). Electrodiagnostic techniques such as electromyography (EMG) and EPs are very useful adjuncts to physical examination of patients in pain. Conditions in which EMG or EPs may be of use include painful peripheral neuropathies, entrapment neuropathies, traumatic nerve injuries, radicular and multiradicular problems, lumbar spinal stenosis, arachnoiditis, and painful myopathies.

In recent years there has been increased reliance on anatomic measures such as intradermal nerve biopsy for small-fiber neuropathy and magnetic resonance imaging (MRI) for larger neural structures. This "anatomic" approach fails to recognize the differences and respective advantages and shortcomings of physiologic versus anatomic testing and, above all, fails to recognize the inherent nature of pain, a subjective experience that can only be *correlated* with the clinical picture.

The problems inherent in applying electrodiagnostic techniques to the diagnosis and management of pain are no different from those encountered in history taking, physical examination, radiologic evaluation, and therapeutic diagnostic testing (e.g., nerve blocks). Pain is a subjective experience, often without an objective "litmus test," and final diagnosis of the etiology and presumptive treatment of a pain syndrome is a *clinical* one that can be *supported* only by relevant data, including findings on EMG.

Electrodiagnostic techniques can be applied virtually without complications to large portions of the body and hence the nervous system to gain an overall understanding of the distribution of abnormalities, if present, or relative normalcy if not. The distribution of abnormalities correlates strongly with the etiology of a disease process causing pain. Questions that can be posed and answered through the use of electrodiagnostic techniques include the following:

- Is a disease of nerves present?
- If so, is it a mononeuropathy, polyneuropathy, or mononeuritis multiplex?
- Does the distribution of abnormalities suggest involvement at the nerve root, plexus, or nerve level?
- If there is a disease process involving a single (or multiple) nerve such as injury or compression, is it improving, worsening, or static?
- Is the nerve involved motor, sensory, or mixed?
- Is the process one of nerve, muscle, or both?
- Are small fibers selectively involved or is this mainly a large-fiber disorder, or are both involved?
- Is there autonomic as well as somatic involvement?
- Are more proximal structures rather than distal ones involved?
- Is the central nervous system involved?

These are the types of inquiries that add substantially to diagnostic information about the etiology, severity, and prognosis of painful disorders. Although many painful disorders do not affect either the peripheral or central nervous system, electrodiagnostic testing can often add reassuring negative results to the diagnostic picture.

Electrodiagnosis is an extremely useful investigative technique for evaluating patients with pain because it satisfies two fundamental steps in the assessment of a neuropathic painful syndrome before any attempt at therapy: (1) rigorously establishing the presence or absence of a peripheral nervous system lesion and (2) determining the relevance of an established peripheral neuropathic lesion to the subjective clinical complaint. In addition, with the advent of new treatments, including enzyme replacement and potential insertion of genetic material into cells, early diagnosis and the ability to monitor treatment outcomes objectively become of great importance. Recent enzyme replacement therapy for Pompe's disease is an example of the potential diagnostic, therapeutic, and prognostic importance of electrodiagnosis.[1]

The parent organization of electrodiagnosis is the American Association of Neuromuscular and Electrodiagnostic Medicine (AANEM), which has promulgated a *Recommended Policy for Electrodiagnostic Medicine Position Statement.*[2] This document seeks to lay out the scope of electrodiagnosis by using consensus expert opinion to ensure adequate examination while attempting to conserve scarce resources by listing the indications for testing and the maximum number of studies per diagnosis in 90% of cases. Since there has been some abuse of the number of studies done on patients and since many pain specialists are not familiar with the techniques of electrodiagnosis, this may serve as an important source of information on the appropriate measures to be used when these diagnostic methods are being considered.

ELECTROMYOGRAPHY

EMG is a method of testing both the physiologic state and the anatomic integrity of lower motor neuron structures (anterior horn cells, nerve roots, plexuses, peripheral nerves, neuromuscular junction, and muscles), their sensory components, and some spinal and brainstem reflex pathways.[3] The term *electromyography* previously caused considerable confusion because strictly speaking, it was needle electrode evaluation (NEE) of muscle function but often was expanded to include nerve conduction velocity (NCV) or NCSs and other tests. However, its common usage has come to mean needle EMG, determination of NCV, and less frequently, testing such as the *H-reflex* and *F-response*, cranial nerve reflexes (e.g., the blink reflex), and studies of the neuromuscular junction. The all-inclusive term *EMG* is used here in an effort to avoid confusion among tests.

Longmire[4] pointed out the puzzling dichotomy regarding pain and electrodiagnostic testing in the medical literature. In standard textbooks on electrodiagnostic testing,[4-9] little or no reference is made to painful syndromes and their diagnosis despite their excellent discussion of physiology, technique, and clinical correlation. On the other hand, a perusal of pain textbooks[3,10,11] reveals cogent attempts to correlate neurophysiologic studies with pain management. The reason for the paucity of references appears to be at least in part the attitudes of pain specialists themselves, who point out that "large caliber afferent fibers are physiologically unrelated to pain, a submodality mediated by small caliber fibers. Additionally, the test is unable to explore the bases for positive sensory phenomena, generated by dysfunction even of large caliber afferent channels."[12]

ELECTRICAL TESTING OF NERVES AND MUSCLES

BRIEF HISTORY

As early as 1791, Galvani found that electricity was produced by muscular contractions.[13] The first experimental work with EMG was performed by Lord Adrian in 1925. In 1928, Proebster first described the presence of "spontaneous irregular action potentials in denervated muscle."[13] In its progression to clinical application, EMG made a major step forward with use of the cathode ray oscilloscope by Erlanger and Gasser, as well as the concentric needle electrode and loudspeaker.[14] Vast numbers of nerve injuries in World War II and later conflicts added further impetus to the study of nerve and muscle by electrodiagnostic technique.

THE ELECTRODIAGNOSTIC METHOD

Electrical diagnostic measurement systems have only four basic components[4]:

1. Electrodes
2. Stimulator
3. High-gain differential amplifier
4. Recording display or central processing device

The EMG apparatus amplifies and displays biologic information derived from either surface or needle electrodes. Electrical information may be recorded from muscles, nerves, or other nervous system structures and is displayed on an oscilloscope. In addition to the visual display on the oscilloscope, a permanent recording may be made, audio amplification may allow it to be heard over a loudspeaker, and analog-digital analysis of signals may be used. Nerves are electrically stimulated to measure conduction.

For NCSs, skin surface electrodes are generally used for recording compound muscle or nerve action potentials. Rarely, needle electrodes are used. For needle EMG, needle electrodes are used with a strong trend toward disposable needles. For sensory testing, ring electrodes are used for measurement (Fig. 14.1). Modern EMG equipment is manufactured by numerous companies and is generally standardized to allow reliable and reproducible testing by different laboratories,[10] but normative data, including data for special populations such as geriatric, pediatric, diabetic, and even active workers, may differ among laboratories and require standardization by each laboratory.[8,15-17]

NEE is an invasive procedure but complications are rare; however, patients should be apprised of them. The most common is transient muscle soreness. Aseptic precautions should be observed. Precautions for testing include extra care with patients who are taking warfarin or other anticoagulants or who have hemophilia or other blood dyscrasias, but since most muscles tested are superficial, they can easily be compressed and the bleeding abated. Severe thrombocytopenia is a relative contraindication and should be considered carefully. Patients positive for human immunodeficiency virus (HIV) represent a transmission risk, but the use of disposable needles (which should be universal) should protect against this hazard. One should carefully consider persons who have a cardiac pacemaker or transcutaneous stimulator when doing stimulation for NCSs.[3] Certain muscles, such as the rhomboids and abdominals, which are sometimes interrogated by NEE in pain patients, and the diaphragm (almost never), carry a risk for pneumothorax and infectious peritonitis, respectively. Beyond placing a needle through an infected site, there are probably no absolute but only relative contraindications to EMG. Extremely anxious patients and some children occasionally require

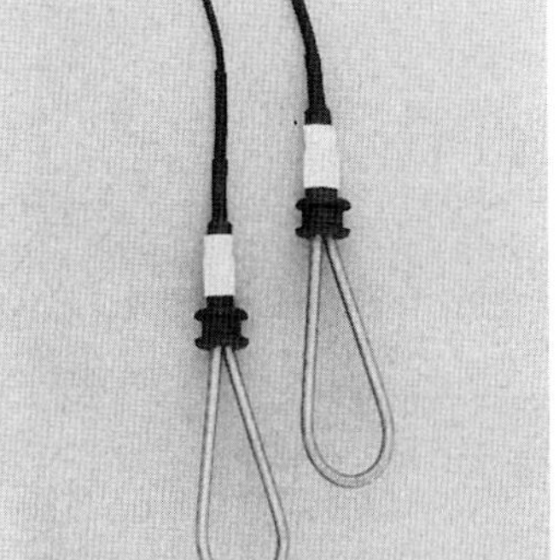

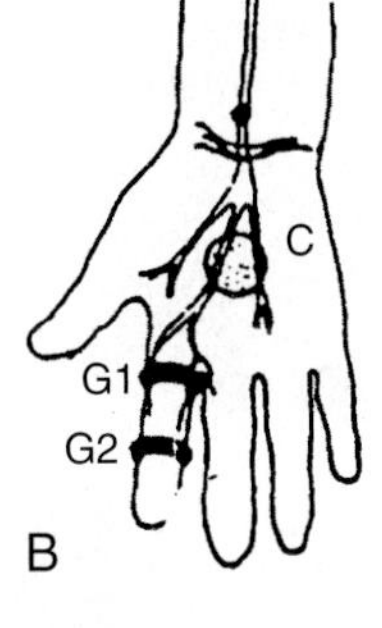

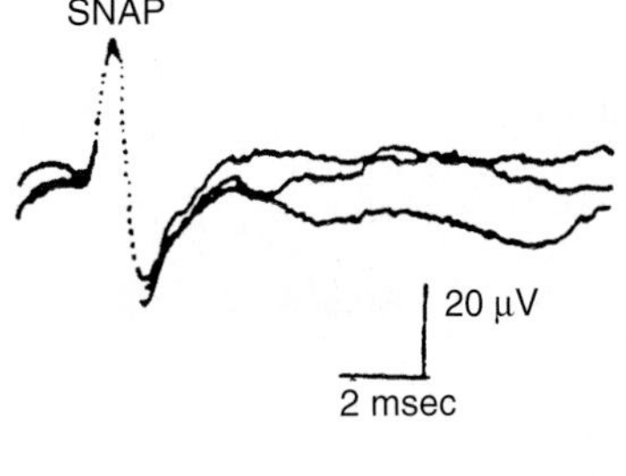

Figure 14.1 **A,** Commonly used ring electrodes for measurement of median and ulnar sensory nerve conduction studies. **B,** Placement of electrodes for median sensory nerve conduction studies and sensory nerve action potentials (SNAPs) obtained on stimulation of the median nerve at the wrist. C, ground electrode; G1, recording electrode; G2, reference electrode. (**A,** Courtesy of Oxford Instruments Medical, Inc., Hawthorne, NY.)

some sedation. Aftereffects are negligible, with rare bruising, although occasionally a highly disturbed, suggestible, or litigious patient may complain vehemently of increased pain or disability. To the contrary, patients may occasionally report a salutary effect on their condition![18]

PHYSIOLOGY

PHYSIOLOGIC MECHANISMS IN THE PRODUCTION OF MUSCLE POTENTIALS

When an impulse arrives at the region of the junction between a nerve and muscle, at the nerve terminal, a depolarization takes place and triggers the opening of voltage-gated calcium channels, which in turn triggers the release of acetylcholine in the synaptic cleft between the axon terminal and the neuromuscular junction. Acetylcholine activates nicotinic receptors, which are ligand-gated sodium channels that activate the tubule system of the muscle. The stimulus is transmitted along the fiber by an excitable membrane that surrounds the muscle fiber. The action potential results from breakdown of the surface membrane potential, which is associated with critical changes in ionic permeability. In a resting muscle fiber, the potential difference across the surface membrane is 90 mV, with negative inside and positive outside. During excitation, the resting potential temporarily reverses to 40 mV, negative outside. This action potential travels along the muscle fiber at velocities ranging from 3.5 to 5 m/sec in different fibers.[19]

In recording extracellularly, as with EMG, the electrode picks up the action potential as it is conducted through the medium that surrounds the active fiber. The impedance of the external medium is small in comparison to the impedance of the fiber interior, and hence the voltage of the extracellularly recorded potentials is maximally only 2% to 10% of the intracellularly recorded potential changes. The functional unit (Fig. 14.2) in reflex or voluntary activity is the *motor unit*; a motor unit is the group of muscle fibers innervated by a single anterior horn cell.

Conduction along the fine intramuscular branches of the anterior horn cell axon occurs so rapidly that all muscle fibers in a motor unit are activated nearly simultaneously. The number of muscle fibers per motor unit varies considerably from muscle to muscle; for example, in the gastrocnemius the motor unit consists of about 1600 muscle fibers, whereas in the small muscles of the eye there are only 5 to 10 fibers. The motor units in various muscles cover different areas of the muscle's cross section (e.g., brachial biceps, 55 mm; rectus femoris, anterior tibial, and opponens pollicis, 8 to 9 mm). The distribution of fibers is such that fibers from several different motor units are intermingled, which is why four to six motor units can be identified by EMG from the same intramuscular recording point. In normal muscle, these single motor unit potentials can be differentiated only during weak voluntary effort.[15,20]

The potentials from different motor units are recognized by their frequency of discharge, which varies for each motor unit (some are more or less excitable). Moreover, the various potentials often differ in appearance because of the differential distance of the recording electrode from the individual fibers of the activated motor units and the differential distribution of the motor end plates in the several units within "range" of a concentric or single needle electrode in one position in the muscle. An upward deflection on the oscilloscope is considered electrically negative, and a downward deflection is considered electrically positive. In the immediate vicinity of a potential there is an upward, or negative, deflection.

PHYSIOLOGY OF NERVE CONDUCTION

The cell membrane (axolemma) of a nerve axon separates the intracellular axoplasm from the extracellular fluid.[8] The unequal distribution of ions between these fluids produces a difference in potential across the cell membrane. This resting potential is about 70 mV and is negative on the inside with respect to the outside of the cell membrane. When a nerve fiber is stimulated, it causes a change in the membrane potential; a rapid but brief flow of sodium ions occurs through ionic channels inward across the cell membrane and gives rise to an action potential.

The way in which an action potential is conducted along an axon depends on whether the axon is myelinated or unmyelinated.[21] In a *myelinated* fiber, the action potential is regenerated only at the nodes of Ranvier, so the resulting action potentials "jump" from node to node, thereby resulting in saltatory conduction. The velocity of nerve conduction depends on the diameter of the myelinated fiber. Small myelinated fibers may conduct as slowly as 12 m/sec,

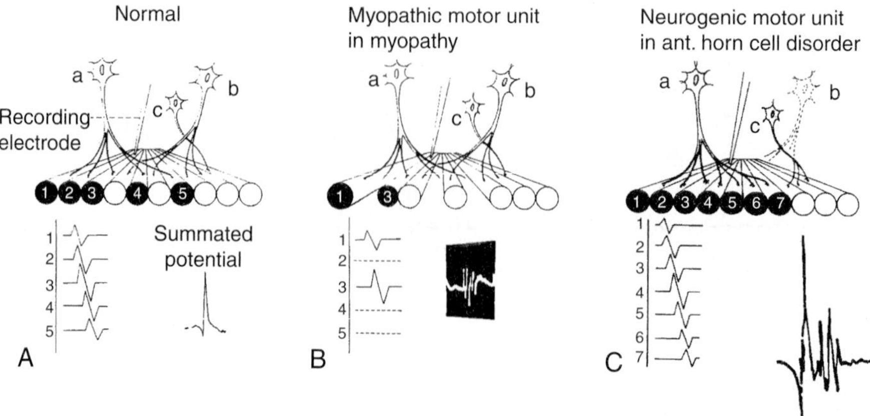

Figure 14.2 A, Schematic illustration of three normal motor units, "a," "b," and "c." *Note:* Muscle fibers of different motor units are normally intermingled. Below the motor units are action potentials of five individual muscle fibers of a motor unit and its summated motor unit potential. **B,** Myopathic changes in motor unit "a." Of the original five muscle fibers, three have undergone degeneration, thus reducing the size of the motor unit. **C,** Neurogenic transformation of motor unit "a." Anterior horn cell "b" is shown undergoing degeneration, and its two muscle fibers are not innervated by axons of anterior horn cell "a," thus leading to an increase in the territory and size of motor unit "a."

whereas large motor and sensory fibers conduct at a rate of 50 to 70 m/sec in humans. In an *unmyelinated* fiber in humans, the conduction rate is about 2 m/sec.

Several factors affect conduction velocity other than whether the axon is myelinated:

- Temperature of the limb (low temperatures decrease conduction velocity)[22]
- Age of the patient (infants have slow conduction velocities and older adults have increasingly slowed conduction velocities)
- Height of an individual (increased height may increase the internodal distances of the nodes of Ranvier)[8]

BASIC ELECTROMYOGRAPHY EXAMINATION

EMG must be combined with clinical examination of the patient by the electromyographer. This includes grading of muscle strength. It is of prime importance for the electromyographer to personally correlate the clinical data and that obtained by EMG. Each examination must be planned individually. There is no "cookbook" formula to follow. Because the EMG examination is an extension of the clinical examination, the patient must be evaluated fully and the problem tentatively assigned to the portion of the anterior horn cell system that seems most likely to be involved. The electromyographer determines the segment or segments of the peripheral nervous system suspected to be involved, and the examination is planned to either substantiate or invalidate the presumptive clinical diagnoses.

CONDUCTING THE EXAMINATION

Needle examination of a patient is designed to determine the following:

1. Integrity of a muscle and its nerve supply
2. Location of any abnormality
3. Any abnormalities of the muscle itself

The electrodes may be monopolar or concentric (Fig. 14.3). The examination proceeds through the following steps (Fig. 14.4):

1. Determination of activity of the muscle in the relaxed state[9,15]
2. Evaluation of any insertional activity that arises
3. Assessment of the activity seen on weak voluntary effort
4. Determination of the pattern seen on maximum voluntary effort, which is known as the *interference pattern* (there is interference in discerning individual muscle action potentials from the resting baseline)

NEEDLE FINDINGS IN NORMAL MUSCLE

INSERTIONAL ACTIVITY

When the needle is inserted into a normal muscle, it evokes a brief burst of electrical activity that lasts no more than 2 to 3 msec, a little longer than the actual movement of the needle.[10] This activity is described as insertional activity and is generally 50 to 250 mV in amplitude (see Fig. 14.4*A*). These insertional potentials are believed to represent discharges from muscle fibers produced by injury, mechanical stimulation, or irritation of the muscle fibers.

SPONTANEOUS ACTIVITY (ACTIVITY AT REST)

When the needle is stationary and the muscle is relaxed, there is no electrical activity present in normal muscle except when the needle is in the area of the end plate. Two types of end-plate "noise" are normal (see Fig. 14.4*C*): (1) low-amplitude and undulating, which probably represents extracellularly recorded miniature end-plate potentials, and (2) high-amplitude intermittent spike discharges, which probably represent discharges of single muscle fibers excited by intramuscular nerve terminals irritated by the needle. Any other spontaneous activity at rest is abnormal.

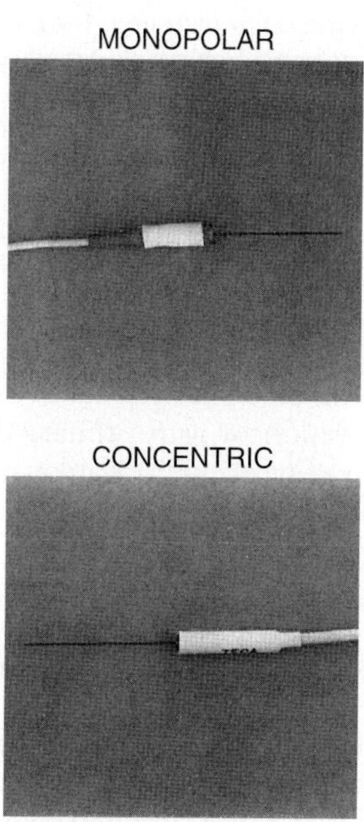

Figure 14.3 Commonly used monopolar and concentric needle electrodes. (Courtesy of Oxford Instruments Medical, Inc., Hawthorne, NY.)

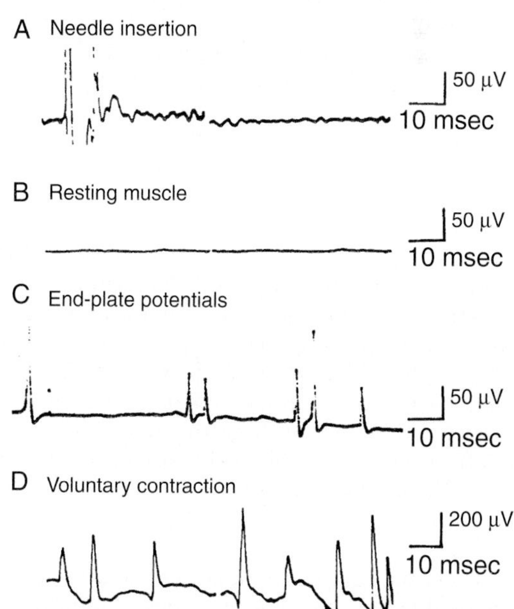

Figure 14.4 **A,** Trace showing normal insertional activity. **B,** No spontaneous activity in a normal muscle at rest. **C,** Spontaneous end-plate potentials. **D,** Normal biphasic and triphasic motor unit potentials during weak voluntary contraction.

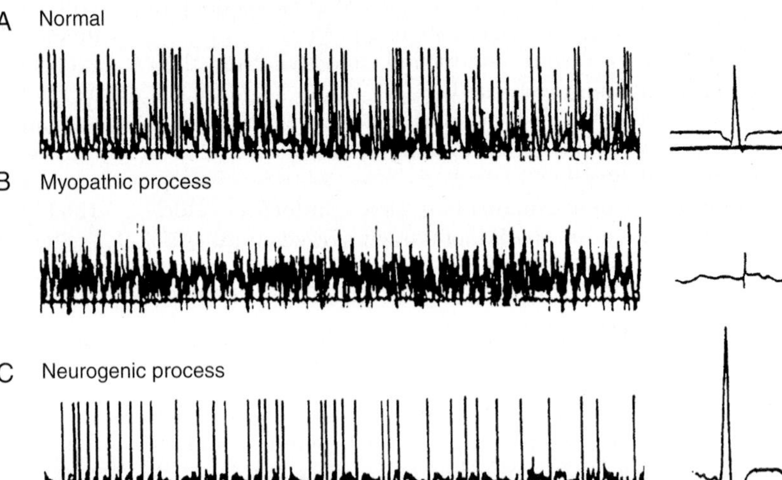

Figure 14.5 **A,** Full interference pattern on maximum effort in a normal muscle. **B,** Full interference pattern in a myopathic muscle on submaximal effort. The number of spikes is greater (each spike represents a motor unit) because of an increase in the firing rate of motor units with early recruitment. **C,** Reduced interference pattern in a denervated muscle on maximal effort resulting from loss of motor units. *Note:* The decreased number of spikes is evident by an increased gap between spikes.

An increased duration of insertional activity may be seen with loss of innervation or with primary disease of muscle fiber.[10] Reduction may occur in patients with myopathies or more advanced degeneration in which muscle tissue has been replaced by fat or fibrous connective tissue.[23]

VOLUNTARY ACTIVITY

Voluntary activity of the muscle is analyzed after the muscle is studied at rest (see Fig. 14.4*D*). Electrical activity (termed a *motor unit action potential*) is noted. As mentioned previously in the discussion on physiology, a motor unit refers to the number of muscle fibers supplied by one motor neuron and its axon. This number varies from muscle to muscle and may be as few as 10 to more than 1000 muscle fibers. When a motor neuron discharges, it activates all the muscle fibers of the motor unit.

The force of contraction determines the number of motor units brought into play.[15,18] This begins with a single motor unit that fires and can be identified on the screen by its distinctive morphology. As effort is increased, other motor units come into play, which can still be individually discerned and have their own individual morphology and audio representation on the loudspeaker. As the contraction increases, the firing rate of each individual motor unit action potential increases, and the action potential is subsequently joined by other motor unit action potentials, whose firing rates also increase. This phenomenon is known as *recruitment* (Fig. 14.5). In normal muscles, the strength of a voluntary muscle contraction is directly related to the number of individual motor units that have been recruited and their firing rate.[20,24] Analysis of motor units includes (1) waveform, (2) amplitude, and (3) interference patterns.

Waveform

Most units are biphasic or triphasic. The number of phases is determined by the "baseline crossings." Motor units that cross the baseline or have more than five phases are called *polyphasic motor units.* Though occasionally seen in healthy muscle, they do not exceed 15% of the total number of motor units. In some muscles, polyphasic motor units are more prevalent. Polyphasic potentials are a measure of fiber synchrony.

Amplitude

The amplitude depends on the number of fibers in the motor unit and the type of EMG needle used. Monopolar needles are associated with higher-amplitude potentials than bipolar or coaxial needles are. Normal amplitude ranges from 1 to 5 mV. Because the motor unit is the sum of the action potentials of each muscle fiber of the unit, a large motor unit has a larger amplitude; conversely, a smaller motor unit has a smaller amplitude.

Interference Patterns

With maximum voluntary effort, a large number of motor units are brought into play and their firing rate increases. They tend to "interfere" with each other and are not recognized further as individual units. This gives rise to a situation called an *interference pattern* (see Fig. 14.5). A normal muscle has a "full" interference pattern.

NEEDLE FINDINGS IN ABNORMAL MUSCLE

Various abnormalities may occur that indicate the presence of total denervation—neurogenic paresis, peripheral type, or neurogenic paresis, anterior horn cell type. In addition, myogenic paresis may be detected. Generally, on the basis of abnormal findings and with a well-determined examination, the presence of a radiculopathy, generalized neuropathy, focal neuropathy or mononeuropathy, or plexopathy can be determined. The following are needle abnormalities in abnormal muscle:

1. Insertional activity (decreased or increased)
2. Spontaneous activity (fibrillations, positive sharp waves, or fasciculations) (Fig. 14.6)
3. Abnormalities in voluntary motor unit activity, especially recruitment (see Fig. 14.5)
4. Abnormal motor unit morphology (e.g., excessive or extreme polyphasia)

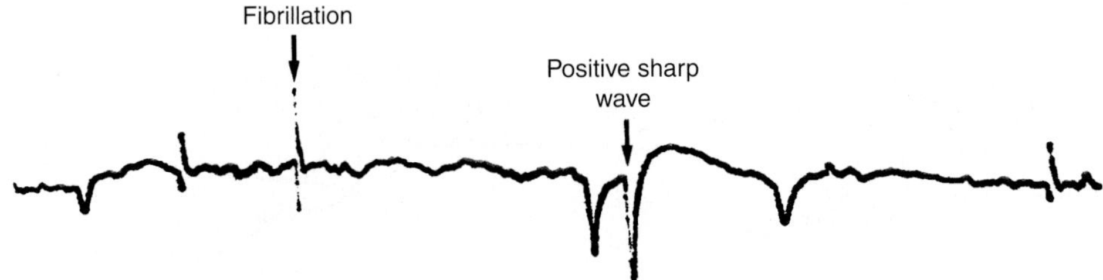

Figure 14.6 Positive sharp wave and fibrillation potentials recorded from a denervated muscle.

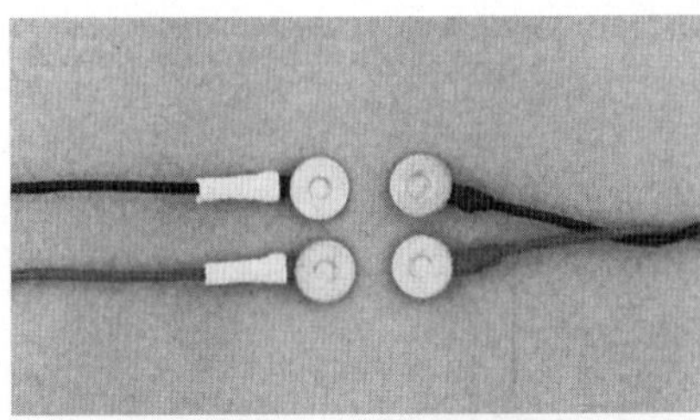

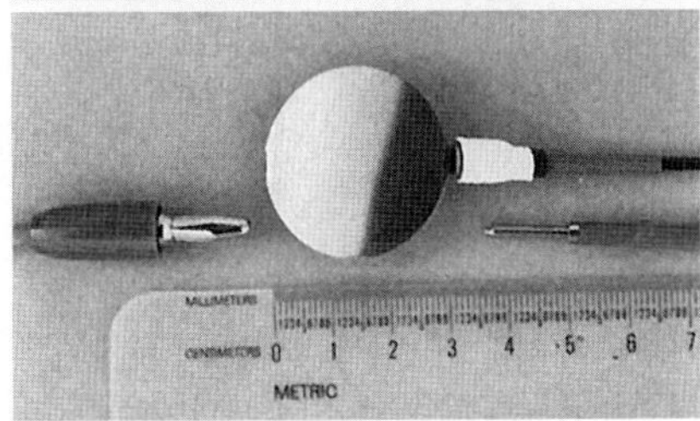

Figure 14.7 Disk surface electrodes and a ground electrode are used for measurement of motor nerve conduction velocity. (Courtesy of Oxford Instruments Medical, Inc., Hawthorne, NY.)

Nerve conduction studies are of value in the following cases:

1. Determining whether a disease of nerve is present
2. Determining the distribution of a neuropathy (e.g., mononeuritis, polyneuropathy, mononeuritis multiplex; this may be a valuable point in the differential diagnosis of the cause of a neuropathy)
3. Determining at what point in a nerve a conduction block is present and locating an entrapment site
4. Studying the progress of disease of a peripheral nerve (e.g., Is it getting better? Worse? Staying the same?)
5. Seeing whether reinnervation of a previously sectioned nerve has taken place
6. Establishing in a disease of the myoneural junction (e.g., myasthenia gravis) the fact that conduction along the nerve is adequate or normal

There are a few important limitations to the use of NEE in muscle disease. Some disorders may not result in abnormal findings on EMG, including certain congenital conditions and endocrine disorders such as steroid myopathy and polymyalgia rheumatica, an important cause of muscle pain and weakness in the elderly. EMG affects primarily type I fibers during minimal voluntary effort before the interference pattern makes discernment of individual motor units difficult.[18]

Conduction velocity studies are carried out by inserting a needle electrode into a muscle innervated by the nerve under study or by the use of surface electrodes over that muscle (Fig. 14.7). For example, the first dorsal interosseous muscle may be examined to determine the function of the ulnar nerve (Fig. 14.8). The nerve is stimulated at the elbow in the case of the ulnar nerve, and the latency of the response is determined. The response is generally a spike-like large motor unit action potential. The ulnar nerve is then stimulated in the wrist or the axillary region, or both. The difference in latencies between the two points of stimulation and the distance between the two points of stimulation provide the basis for calculation of conduction velocity. Conduction velocity is determined by the following formula:

$$\text{MCV (m/sec)} = \text{DMM}/(\text{PML} - \text{DML})$$

where DMM is the distance between the two stimulus points in millimeters, PML is proximal motor latency (in milliseconds), DML is distal motor latency (in milliseconds), and MCV is motor conduction velocity in meters per second.[3]

Textbooks of stimulation points and pickup points are readily available.[7,8] Normal values are usually established for each nerve in individual laboratories, but normal values for commonly tested sensory and motor nerves are generally available (Table 14.1). Median nerve stimulation is comparable to ulnar nerve stimulation (Fig. 14.9).

F WAVE

DEFINITION

Motor conduction velocity along the whole axon, including the proximal portions, can be studied by eliciting the F-wave response, a small, late muscle response that occurs as a result of backfiring of anterior horn cells.[25-27] F waves may be obtained from almost any mixed nerve that can be stimulated, but the median, ulnar, peroneal, and posterior tibial nerves are the most commonly used (Fig. 14.10). If the standard distal motor conduction velocities are normal but the F-wave value is prolonged, slowing must be occurring somewhere more proximal to the distal normal segment. (The method used to determine F-wave latency varies from laboratory to laboratory; the F-wave value with each successive shock stimulus shows a variability of several milliseconds, with some examiners averaging 10, 30, or 50 responses and some taking the shortest of 10, 20, or more responses.) Limb temperature and arm or leg length may also be important to know. Comparison with the opposite limb may be most helpful if that limb is asymptomatic.

PITFALLS AND COMMENTS

In addition to the variability in F waves and how they are obtained in different laboratories, many electromyographers overuse (or at least overperform) the F-wave study when proximal slowing in a nerve or nerve root is not even in the differential diagnosis. The most accepted use of the study is for suspected early *Guillain-Barré syndrome,* when results of the usual studies are still normal—typically in the

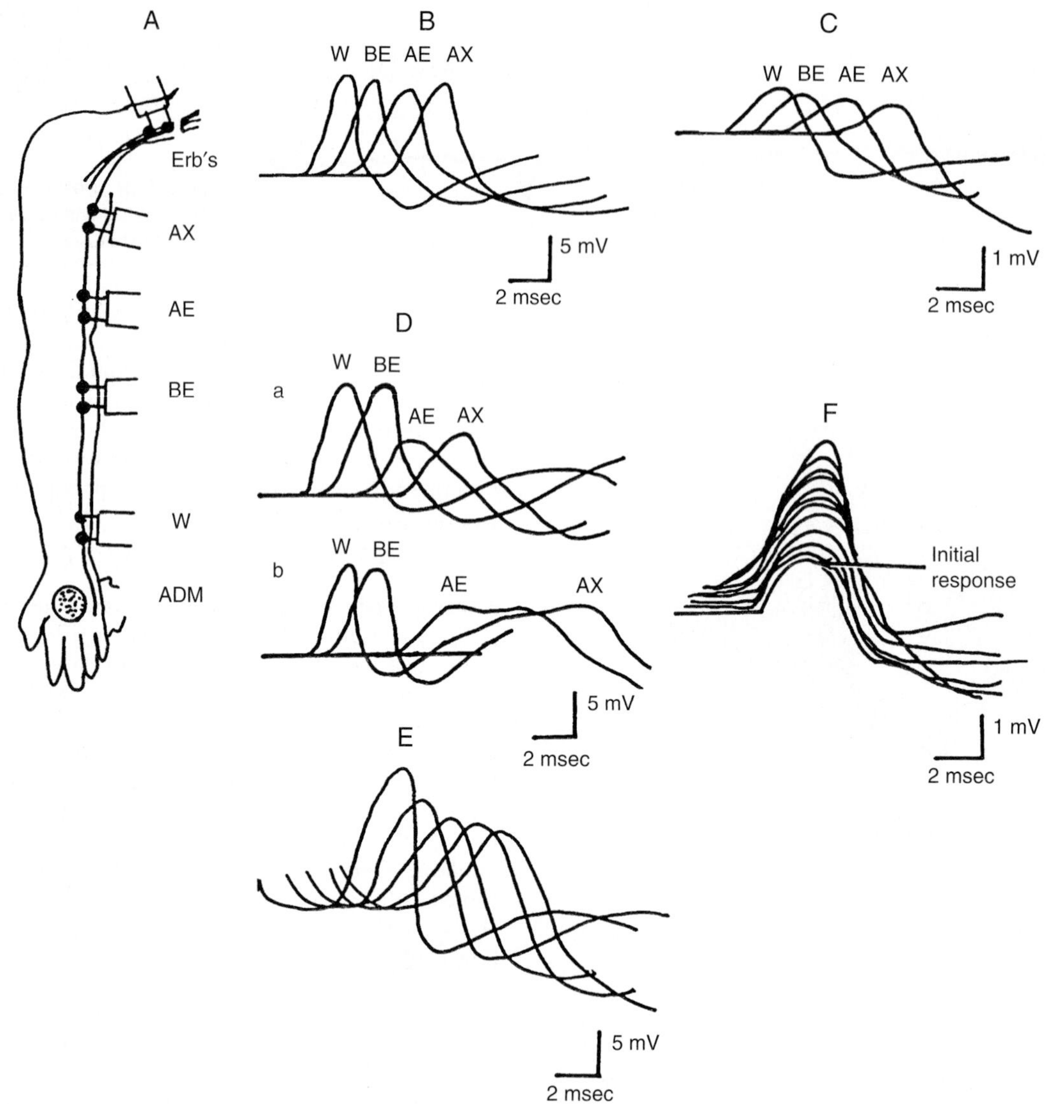

Figure 14.8 **A,** Commonly used site of stimulation of the ulnar nerve at the wrist, below the elbow, above the elbow, and at the axilla. The ulnar nerve can also be stimulated at Erb's point in the supraclavicular fossa. **B,** Normal-amplitude compound motor action potentials (CMAPs) recorded from the abductor digiti minimi manus (ADM) following stimulation of the ulnar nerve at these various sites. **C,** Low-amplitude CMAPs in a patient with axonal neuropathy. All CMAPs are of the same amplitude but are much smaller than normal. **D,** Decremental response (a) and decremental and dispersed response (b) on stimulation above the elbow and at the axilla and normal response on stimulation below the elbow and wrist. **E,** Repetitive nerve stimulation of the ulnar nerve at the wrist in a patient with myasthenia gravis. Note the initial normal response and subsequent decremental response at the slow rate (3 pulses/sec). **F,** Repetitive nerve stimulation in Lambert-Eaton syndrome. With a rapid rate (20 to 50 pulses/sec), a marked incremental response occurs. Note the very low initial response and the twofold to fourfold increase following the rapid rate of stimulation. AE, above the elbow; AX, axilla; BE, below the elbow; W, wrist.

first 10 days of the illness. It is highly controversial in the evaluation of radiculopathies.[28,29]

HOFFMAN REFLEX (H-REFLEX)

DEFINITION

The H-reflex is obtained by electrostimulation of the posterior tibial nerve in the popliteal space at a slow rate with a long duration and submaximal electrical shock; it is recorded with surface electrodes over the gastrocnemius-soleus (Fig. 14.11). The impulse travels up the sensory fibers to the spinal cord, synapses with the alpha motor neuron, and returns down the motor fibers to the calf muscle. H-reflex latencies are therefore long, in the range of 40 to 45 msec. They are carried mostly in the S1 nerve root distribution and cannot be recorded consistently from other muscles. To determine a delay or an asymmetry, one should always study the opposite leg for comparison.[30-33]

PITFALLS AND COMMENTS

The H-reflex is somewhat more useful than the F wave, but the main reason for the study is to evaluate patients with suspected S1 radiculopathy whose history or findings on physical examination are suggestive but the EMG is normal.[34] Usually, when an absent H-reflex is noted, which suggests a problem with S1 nerve root conduction, an absent or depressed ankle reflex has already been noted on the physical examination, so the study is, for many, redundant. Pitfalls occur when the opposite leg is not studied to show

Table 14.1 Normal Values for Commonly Tested Sensory and Motor Nerves

Nerves	Amplitude (Avg.)	Distal Latency in msec (Avg.)*	Conduction Velocity in m/sec (Avg.)
Median (sensory)	10-85 μV (20)	2.0-3.7 (3.2)	
Ulnar (sensory)	5-70 μV (15)	1.6-3.2 (2.8)	
Radial (sensory)	10-60 μV (18)	1.7-2.8 (2.4)	
Median (motor)	5-25 mV (8)	2.0-4.0 (3.3)	48-69 (54)
Ulnar (motor)	5.5-20 mV (8)	1.6-3.1 (2.6)	50-69 (55)
Sural (sensory)	3-38 mV (8)	2.3-4.6 (4.1)	41-61 (46)
Peroneal (motor)	2.5-18 mV (4)	2.3-6.0 (4.1)	41-58 (45)
Posterior tibial (motor)	4-38 mV (11)	2.1-6.0 (4.3)	

*Distal latencies are based on standard distance: 13 cm for the median (S), 11 cm for the ulnar (S), 10 cm for the radial (S), 14 cm for the sural (S), 4 to 6 cm for the median (M) and ulnar (M), 6 to 8 cm for the peroneal (M), and 8 to 12 cm for the posterior tibial (M) nerves.

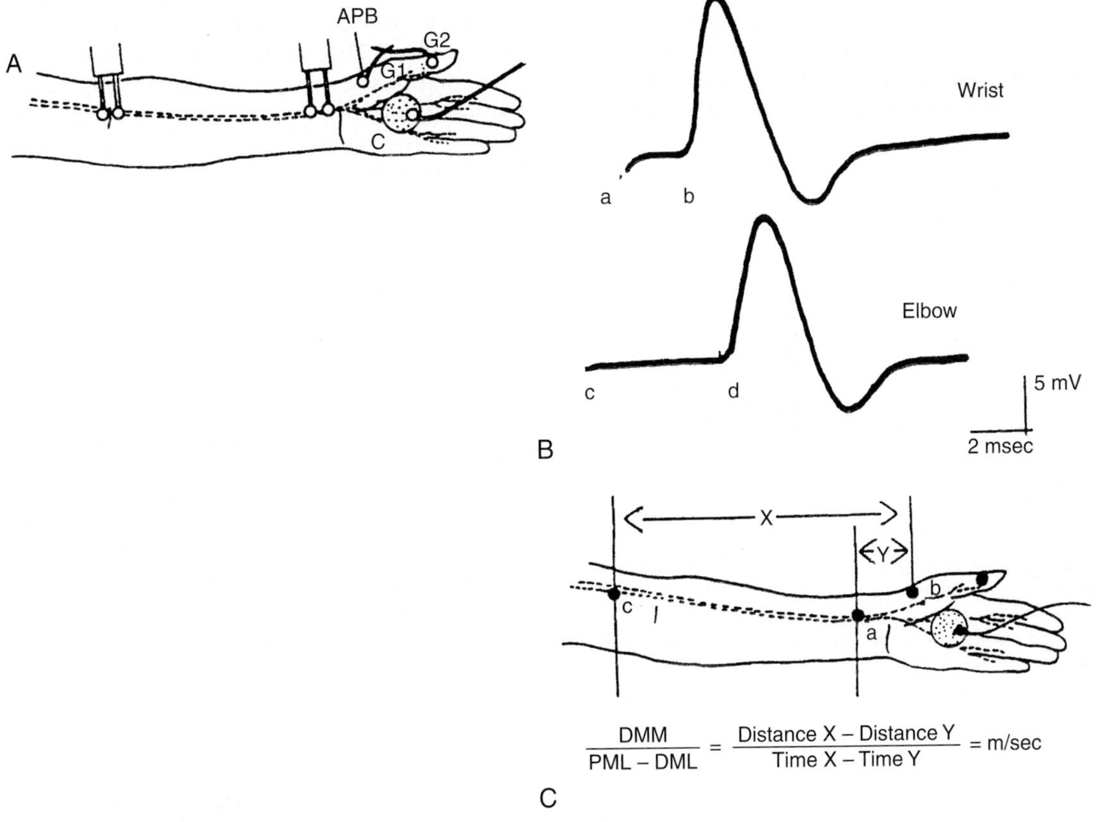

Figure 14.9 **A,** Site of stimulation of the median nerve at the wrist and the elbow. **B,** Thenar abductor pollicis brevis (APB) compound motor action potentials obtained following stimulation of the median nerve at the wrist and elbow. a-b, motor latency at the wrist; c-d, motor latency at the elbow. **C,** Distance and latency measurements for the median nerve and the method used to calculate motor conduction velocity in the segment of the median nerve between the wrist and elbow. PML, proximal motor latency; DML, distal motor latency; DMM, distance in millimeters.

a normal H-reflex as a contrast. If the H-reflex is absent bilaterally, it may reflect more generalized disease, such as peripheral neuropathy. Older patients often do not have good H-reflexes as a normal finding. In addition, a unilaterally absent H-reflex with normal findings on needle EMG does not indicate when the injury occurred; the findings may have been the result of a previous injury.

QUANTITATIVE SENSORY TESTING (PSEUDOMOTOR AXON REFLEX TEST)

Quantitative sensory testing takes various forms, including the quantitative somatosensory thermotest using a controlled ramp of ascending or descending temperature through a Peltier device.[35] Measurement of the threshold for cold sensation reflects the function of small-caliber Aδ myelinated afferents. The threshold for warm sensation reflects the function of warm-specific small unmyelinated afferent channels. Cold pain and heat pain thresholds test the function of unmyelinated C-fiber, polymodal nociceptors, and, to a lesser extent, Aδ-fiber nociceptors. Certain abnormal patterns are characteristic of dysfunction of small-caliber peripheral nerve afferents.[36] To obtain maximal information from a quantitative somatosensory thermotest, it is necessary to test for cold, pain, and heat sensations, which is mandatory in the evaluation of painful syndromes.[37] Quantitative sensory testing performed at different sites along an extremity in patients with polyneuropathy yields useful information about staging of the pathologic process along the extremity.

The quantitative pseudomotor axon reflex test (QSART) is a quantitative thermoregulatory sweat test. It has been used to detect postganglionic pseudomotor failure in neuropathies[38,39] and preganglionic neuropathies with presumed trans-synaptic degeneration.[40] In patients with distal small-fiber neuropathy, it is the most sensitive diagnostic test.[41] Various commercial devices have been used to differentiate axonal from demyelinating polyneuropathy.[42]

CLINICAL CORRELATIONS OF ELECTROMYOGRAPHIC TESTING

Clinical correlations can be based on a careful history, clinical examination, and electrodiagnostic studies. Electrodiagnostic studies are best for distinguishing neuropathy from myopathy and determining whether a neuropathy is generalized axonal, demyelinating, mixed, or focal, thus giving important clues about the cause. Furthermore, nerve trauma can be monitored serially to determine recovery. In many instances, a diagnosis of plexopathy or radiculopathy can be made.

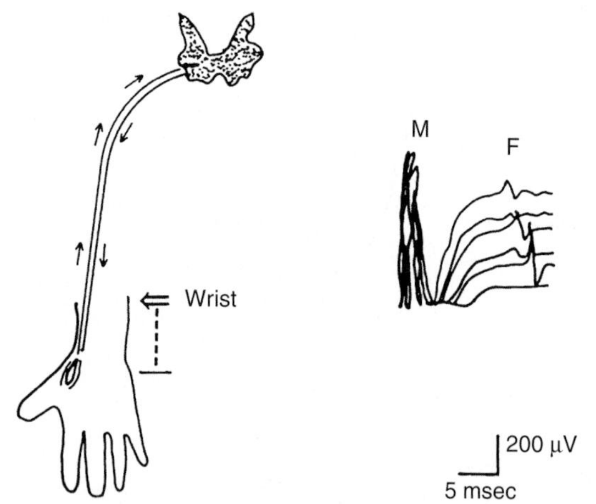

Figure 14.10 Consecutive tracings showing M responses and F waves recorded from the abductor pollicis brevis after stimulation of the median nerve at the wrist.

NERVE TRAUMA

Often after an injury, such as a laceration, the nerve is completely severed. At rest, denervation potentials are recorded in the muscles supplied by that nerve in the form of positive sharp waves or fibrillation potentials, and on EMG, no motor unit action potentials are seen. Sometimes, however, an injury is incomplete and the type of nerve lesion is uncertain.

Neurapraxia

Neurapraxia is the mildest form of nerve injury. It consists of loss of conduction without associated changes in axonal structure. This form of conduction block often occurs with compressive or ischemic nerve injuries, such as a mild entrapment syndrome or compression (e.g., "Saturday night palsy"). In neurapraxic injuries, focal demyelination occurs. Serial nerve conduction determinations along the course of the nerve enable one to locate the site of the conduction block. The prognosis for complete recovery is generally good, and healing occurs within days or weeks, barring further injury.

Axonotmesis

In axonotmesis, a more severe form of nerve injury, the axon is disrupted in its myelin sheath. The neural tube, which consists of the endoperineurium and epineurium, remains intact. The nerve undergoes wallerian degeneration, with fragmentation of the axon distal to the site of injury. Motor and sensory paralysis occurs along with associated atrophy of the muscles supplied and loss of reflexes. After about 4 to 5 days, the distal segments of the nerve become inexcitable. In 1 to 2 weeks, positive sharp waves are seen; fibrillations in the involved musculature occur in 2 to 3 weeks. The intact neural tube forms a lattice for the regenerating axon, and the prognosis for recovery is generally good.

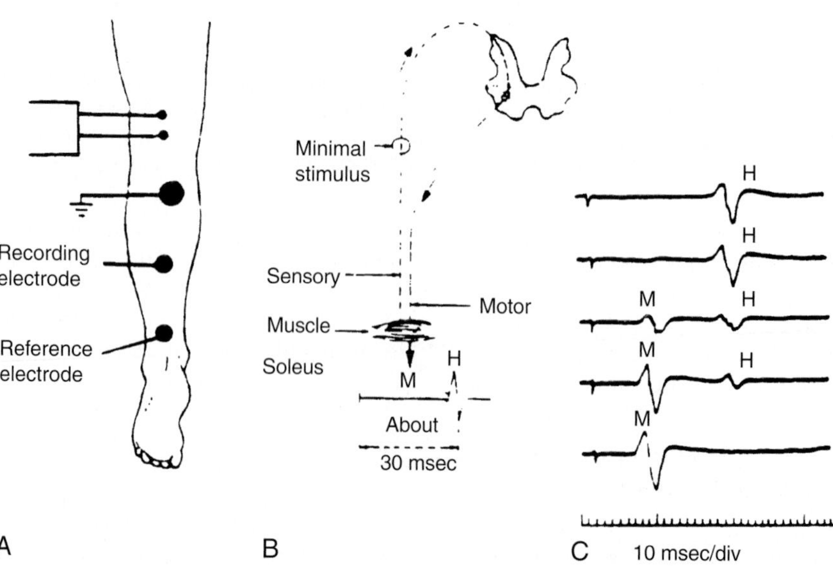

Figure 14.11 **A,** Placement of recording electrodes and site of stimulation of the posterior tibial nerve for recording of the Hoffman (H) reflex from the soleus muscle. **B,** H-reflex pathways. An electrical impulse generated on stimulation of the tibial nerve travels along the sensory axon (afferent) within the spinal cord and along the motor axon (efferent). **C,** Motor response (M) and H-reflex (H). Five consecutive traces are shown. Starting from the top, each trace is obtained with increasing stimulus intensity. With minimal stimulus only, the H response is obtained. As the intensity of the stimulus is increased, the M response begins to appear and the H response begins to decrease until it finally becomes unobtainable.

Neurotmesis

Neurotmesis is the most severe form of nerve injury and consists of severe disruption or transection of the nerve. Nerve regeneration and recovery are often incomplete, and surgical reanastomosis may be required. Neuromas may form and are commonly associated with pain. Only serial determinations over time can determine the difference between axonotmesis and neurotmesis.

NONTRAUMATIC NEUROPATHIES

In a patient with a nontraumatic neuropathy, segmental demyelination is generally associated with slowing of NCV and temporal dispersion of evoked responses. With axonal degeneration, however, a reduction in the evoked response amplitudes with mild or minimal slowing of NCV is typical. EMG provides early information regarding reinnervation before clinical recovery is evident. The earliest positive evidence of reinnervation is the appearance during voluntary effort of motor unit potentials that are of low amplitude in the beginning but are highly polyphasic ("nascent") units. They may be present several weeks before clinical evidence of functional recovery is apparent.

POLYNEUROPATHY

EMG and evaluation of nerve conduction are useful in diagnosing polyneuropathy and in determining whether the pathologic process is axonal and demyelinating. A diagnosis of polyneuropathy is made when abnormal nerve conduction and EMG findings are bilateral and symmetrical.

Generalized peripheral neuropathies frequently associated with pain are noted in Box 14.1.[43-48] The following electrodiagnostic findings are characteristic of axonal neuropathy:

1. Abnormally low or absent sensory nerve action potentials and compound muscle action potential amplitudes
2. Normal distal latencies
3. Near-normal motor and sensory conduction velocities

If a disease process affects the large-diameter axons, some slowing of conduction occurs; the velocity is seldom reduced by more than 20% to 30% of normal. However, fibrillations and positive sharp waves are present in muscles innervated by the affected nerves and are generally worse distally. The feet are more involved than the hand muscles, and the leg muscles are involved more than the arm muscles. Motor unit potentials are decreased in number with deficient recruitment and an incomplete interference pattern. Some motor units have increased amplitude and duration.

In contrast, diffuse demyelinating neuropathy is characterized by a reduction in conduction velocity, usually more than 40% of the normal range. Distal latencies are also prolonged. The sensory nerve action potentials and compound muscle action potentials usually exhibit low amplitudes and temporal dispersion. Needle EMG shows no fibrillations or positive sharp waves unless secondary axonal degeneration is present. In a pure demyelinating neuropathy, there is no denervation of muscle fibers. Motor units are decreased in number; the decreased recruitment is attributable to conduction block in some fibers. Usually, no significant change in the duration, amplitude, or morphology of motor units occurs, but the number of polyphasic potentials may be increased if the terminal axons have become demyelinated.

Once it has been determined by EMG whether a neuropathy is primarily axonal or demyelinating, one can then consider clinically which neuropathies are diffusely axonal and which are demyelinating. Subacute and chronic diffuse axonal types include most toxic and nutritional neuropathies, uremia, diabetes, hypothyroidism, HIV infection, Lyme disease, paraneoplastic disease, dysproteinemia, and amyloidosis.

Demyelinating polyneuropathies include hereditary motor and sensory neuropathy types I and III, Refsum's disease, multifocal leukodystrophy, and Krabbe's disease. *Acute* nonuniform demyelinating diseases include Guillain-Barré syndrome, diphtheria, and acute arsenic intoxication, whereas *chronic* versions include inflammatory demyelinating peripheral neuropathy, idiopathic disease, and neuropathies accompanying HIV disease, as well as various paraproteinemias, dysproteinemias, and osteosclerotic myeloma.[49]

Box 14.1 Generalized Peripheral Neuropathies with Emphasis on Painful Conditions

- Diabetes mellitus
- Polyneuropathy associated with insulinoma
- Polyneuropathy associated with nutritional deficiency
- Alcohol-nutritional deficiency polyneuropathy
- Vasculitis-associated neuropathy
- Amyloidosis
- Cancer and chemotherapeutic-related neuropathies
- Sjögren's syndrome
- Pompe's disease
- Toxic substances (arsenic and thallium)
- HIV-related distal symmetrical polyneuropathy
- Fabry's disease
- Guillain-Barré syndrome (acute inflammatory demyelinating polyneuropathy)
- Cryptogenic sensory or sensorimotor neuropathy
- Polyneuropathy secondary to neoplasm, including paraneoplastic syndromes such as acute sensory neuropathy or sensorimotor neuropathy associated with carcinoma

HIV, human immunodeficiency virus.

MONONEUROPATHIES AND ENTRAPMENT NEUROPATHIES

With an entrapment neuropathy, the most commonly involved nerves are the median, ulnar, radial, common peroneal, and tibial. Entities such as trauma, vasculitis, diabetes mellitus, leprosy, and sarcoidosis can affect any nerve in the body. Electrophysiologic studies are of great assistance in localizing the lesion in the individual nerve and in differentiating mononeuropathy from diffuse polyneuropathy, plexopathy, and radiculopathy.

MEDIAN NERVE

The median nerve is most commonly entrapped at the wrist as it passes through the carpal tunnel, but it may also be injured at the elbow where it passes between the two heads of the pronator teres or, less frequently, is compressed by a dense band of connective tissue (the ligament of Struthers immediately above the elbow) (see Fig. 14.9).[50,51] The median nerve is derived from the C6 through T1 nerve roots (lateral and medial cords of the brachial plexus). The diagnosis of carpal tunnel syndrome is made by demonstrating localized slowing of sensory and motor conduction across the wrist as evidenced by prolonged sensory and motor distal latencies.[3] In addition, with late changes there may be denervation in the form of fibrillations, positive sharp waves, and reduced motor units with polyphasia in the hand muscles innervated by the median nerve. The need for reference values for special populations, including diabetics and active workers, has been emphasized in a recent AANEM monograph.[17]

A recent review has emphasized that carpal tunnel syndrome may represent a focal intracanal condition such as pregnancy, lipoma, an arterial condition, and the hereditary neuropathy of amyloidosis.[17]

Pronator Teres and Anterior Interosseous Syndromes. The pronator teres and anterior interosseous syndromes consist of proximal compression or entrapment neuropathies of the median nerve. Patients with pronator teres syndrome may also have normal distal latency but no evidence of denervation in the median-innervated hand and forearm muscles except for the pronator teres.[51] The anterior interosseous nerve is a motor branch of the median nerve, with its origin just distal to the pronator teres.[51]

Ulnar Nerve

The ulnar nerve is derived from the C8 and T1 cervical nerve roots (medial cord of the brachial plexus). It is usually injured at the elbow but occasionally at the wrist in the canal of Guyon or deep in the palm (silver beater's palsy). EMG helps differentiate C8 and T1 radiculopathies from plexopathy or more distal ulnar nerve palsy (see Fig. 14.8).[52,53] When the lesion is in the wrist at the canal of Guyon, usually both sensory and motor fibers are involved and the amplitude of the sensory nerve action potential and muscle action potential is reduced. Distal sensory and motor latency across the wrist is prolonged, and there is no focal slowing of motor NCV or decrement in compound muscle action potential across the elbow. With a lesion in the deep palmar branch, no sensory abnormality occurs and all the changes are in the motor distribution distal to the lesion.[54] When the abnormality is at the elbow, there may be localized slowing of NCV across the elbow, often as much as 25% to 40% below normal. Normal values may depend on the method used (arm straight vs. arm bent). The sensory potential may be affected, as may EMG findings in the ulnar hand muscles.

Radial Nerve

The radial nerve is a continuation of the posterior cord of the brachial plexus and receives fibers from the C5 to C8 cervical roots. It is usually involved at the spiral groove of the humerus, often secondary to a humeral fracture. With a lesion at the spiral groove, the triceps muscle is noted to be spared on EMG, but all the extensor muscles of the forearm are involved. An isolated superficial radial nerve palsy sometimes occurs at the wrist, with the only abnormality being in the radial sensory nerve action potential.

Posterior Interosseous Syndrome. The posterior interosseous nerve syndrome (sometimes known as *complicated lateral epicondylitis*) is caused by entrapment of this branch of the radial nerve at the arcade of Fröhse between the two heads of the supinator. EMG shows involvement of the extensor carpi ulnaris, extensor digitorum longus, extensor pollicis longus, and extensor indicis with sparing of the more proximal supinator and extensor carpi radialis longus and brevis.[55] Sensation is unaffected.

Common Peroneal Nerve

The common peroneal nerve is derived from the L4 through S1 roots but primarily from L5. It may be compressed at the head of the fibula. Peroneal NCSs show reduced compound action potentials, as recorded from the extensor digitorum brevis on stimulation above the fibular head, and normal compound action potentials below the fibular head and at the ankle.

Posterior Tibial Nerve at the Ankle

The posterior tibial nerve is derived from the L4 through S3 roots and may be compressed in the tarsal tunnel. NCSs show prolongation of the distal motor and sensory latency of the tibial nerve.[56-58] There may be EMG changes in the appropriate foot muscles. This syndrome is relatively uncommon.

Sciatic Nerve

The sciatic nerve arises from the L4, L5, S1, S2, and S3 nerve roots. A controversial syndrome is entrapment by the piriformis muscle as it passes through the greater sciatic notch. A lesion of the sciatic nerve is defined and localized by detailed needle examination of muscle in the lower limb.[59]

Other Uncommon Neuropathies

There are numerous potential mononeuropathies, including those involving the long thoracic nerve, dorsal scapular nerve, suprascapular nerve, musculocutaneous nerves, and axillary nerves in the shoulder girdle and upper extremity, as well as those in the pelvic girdle, including the femoral, obturator, saphenous, lateral femoral cutaneous, genitofemoral, ilioinguinal, and superior and inferior gluteal nerves. Needle EMG reveals denervation changes in muscle innervated by individual nerves. NCSs are rarely useful in their evaluation.[60]

RADICULOPATHIES

Radiculopathies are diseases of the nerve roots and must be differentiated from plexopathies, as well as from complex individual nerve root lesions. Roots are commonly involved by compression, especially in the cervical and lumbar region, but they may also be involved in diseases such as diabetes mellitus, herpes zoster, carcinomatous infiltration, and lymphomatous infiltration of nerves, as well as by rare sarcoidosis and infectious processes. Determination of motor and sensory nerve conduction is rarely useful because the lesion in a radiculopathy is proximal to the dorsal root ganglion and motor conduction studies are usually normal, although they may be reduced in amplitude if the lesion is severe enough to cause axonal loss. The H-reflex is absent or latency-delayed when the S1 root is involved. Typically, nerve root lesions are identified by abnormal needle examination results in the appropriate paraspinal and limb muscles.[57] Because most limb muscles are supplied by more than one nerve root (Tables 14.2 and 14.3), a normal study does not exclude the diagnosis of radiculopathy; however, when the findings on EMG are abnormal, they provide objective evidence of functional impairment in the nerve root and localize the lesion to one or more roots in addition to revealing the severity of involvement.[3,61-63]

Table 14.2 Segmental Innervation of Commonly Tested Muscles in the Upper Extremity

Muscle	Spinal Segment	Nerve Supply
Cervical paraspinal	C2 to C8	Corresponding cervical root
Trapezius	C2, C3, C4	Spinal accessory
Supraspinatus	C5, C6	Subscapular
Infraspinatus	C5	Subscapular
Deltoid (circumflex)	C5, C6	Axillary
Biceps brachii	C5, C6	Musculocutaneous
Brachioradialis	C6, C7	Radial
Flexor carpi radialis	C6, C7, C8	Median
Pronator teres	C6, C7	Median
Triceps brachii	C7, C8	Radial
Extensor digitorum communis	C7, C8	Radial
Extensor indicis	C7, C8	Radial
Flexor carpi ulnaris	C8, T1	Ulnar
Abductor pollicis brevis	C8, T1	Median
First dorsal interosseus	C8, T1	Ulnar
Abductor digiti minimi manus	C8, T1	Ulnar

Table 14.3 Segmental Innervation of Commonly Tested Muscles in the Lower Extremity

Muscle	Spinal Segment	Nerve Supply
Lumbosacral paraspinal	L1 to S1	Corresponding roots
Iliacus	L2, L3, L4	Femoral
Adductors of the thigh	L2, L3, L4	Obturator
Quadriceps femoris	L2, L3, L4	Femoral
Tibialis anterior	L4, L5	Deep peroneal
Gluteus medius	L4, L5, S1	Superior gluteal
Gluteus maximus	L5, S1	Inferior gluteal
Peroneus longus	L5, S1	Superficial peroneal
Biceps femoris—long head	L5, S1	Sciatic
Biceps femoris—short head	L5, S1	Sciatic
Flexor digitorum longus	L5, S1	Posterior tibial
Tibialis posterior	L5, S1	Posterior tibial
Extensor digitorum brevis	L5, S1	Deep peroneal
Gastrocnemius—lateral	L5, S1	Posterior tibial
Gastrocnemius—medial	S1, S2	Posterior tibial
Abductor hallucis	S1, S2	Posterior tibial
Abductor digiti quinti	S1, S2	Posterior tibial
Tensor fasciae latae	L5, S1	Superior gluteal

PLEXOPATHIES

In plexopathies, motor NCSs are useful in excluding a peripheral nerve lesion; otherwise, the findings are normal except that the amplitudes of compound muscle action potentials may be reduced. Sensory NCSs are usually helpful in excluding other causes. Again, needle examination is most helpful, but it requires knowledge of which muscles are supplied by which portions of the plexus.

ANTERIOR HORN CELL DISEASE

Disorders of the anterior horn cell do not generally cause pain except for acute poliomyelitis (acute febrile stage). When diseases such as amyotrophic lateral sclerosis cause pain, the etiology is usually multifactorial (spasticity, musculoskeletal, positioning) and not usually discernible with EMG.

DISORDERS OF THE CENTRAL NERVOUS SYSTEM

Findings on EMG are almost always normal in diseases of the central nervous system.

PRIMARY MUSCLE DISORDERS

One of the clearest applications of EMG is for differentiating myopathies from neuropathic processes.[64-68] The differentiation in EMG studies between myopathy and neuropathy should be obvious by needle examination. In myopathy, the potentials are reduced in amplitude and may be very polyphasic, recruit paradoxically (i.e., more potentials seen on the screen than would be expected for the corresponding amount of effort), and are accompanied by marked signs of irritability. In polymyositis and metabolic muscle disorders, sensory nerve conduction is always normal. The compound muscle action potential amplitude may be low, but otherwise motor conduction results are normal. EMG findings are commonly normal in myofascial pain syndromes and fibromyalgia, but in polymyositis and metabolic muscle disorders (e.g., glycogen and lipid storage disease), muscle pain, cramps, and weakness can occur. Box 14.2[64-66] lists the painful myopathies.

Unusual diseases characterized by muscle cramping, including stiff man syndrome (Moersch-Woltman syndrome), simply show muscle contraction and spasms. Conditions with continuous muscle fiber activity (Isaacs-Mertens syndrome) show continuous, low-amplitude, fibrillation-type potentials.[64-66]

USEFULNESS AND LIMITATIONS OF ELECTROMYOGRAPHY

EMG and NCSs are useful in localizing neuromuscular disease sites and in providing information about the nature of the process (demyelinating, axonal, primary muscular, radicular) but cannot give the cause (diabetes, Guillain-Barré syndrome, myositis, tumor, ruptured disk). Figure 14.12 presents a summary of EMG findings in various conditions. In addition, a normal result does not mean that the patient does not have pain. Electrodiagnostic studies in the EMG laboratory, as usually performed, measure only activity related to the motor nerve fibers, the larger sensory nerve

Box 14.2 Painful Myopathies[64-66]

Dermatomyositis
Polymyositis
Corticosteroid myopathies
Amyloid myopathies
Thyroid myopathies
Alcoholic myopathy
HIV myopathy
Critical care myopathy
Drugs reported to cause myopathy
- Alcohol
- ε-Aminocaproic acid*
- Amiodarone*
- Anesthetic: intravenous propofol
- Carbimazole
- Chloroquine*
- Cholesterol-lowering agents* (all have been implicated)
- Cimetidine
- Clozapine
- Colchicine*
- Corticosteroids*
- Cyclosporine
- Emetine
- Fluoroquinolone antibiotics: ofloxacin, levofloxacin
- Gene therapy: direct insertion of transgenes into the muscle (Dalakas 2009)
- Germanium
- Glycyrrhizin* (licorice)
- Gold salts
- Growth hormone
- Hydroxychloroquine
- Interferon alpha-2b
- Ipecac
- Labetalol
- Omeprazole
- Perhexiline
- D-Penicillamine
- Phenylbutazone
- Phenytoin
- Propylthiouracil
- Pyrazinamide
- Retinoids
  - Etretinate
  - Isotretinoin
  - Tretinoin
- Sulfonamide
- Tranilast
- Vincristine
- Zidovudine*

*Well documented. The rest are based on isolated case reports, and a causal relationship has not been established.

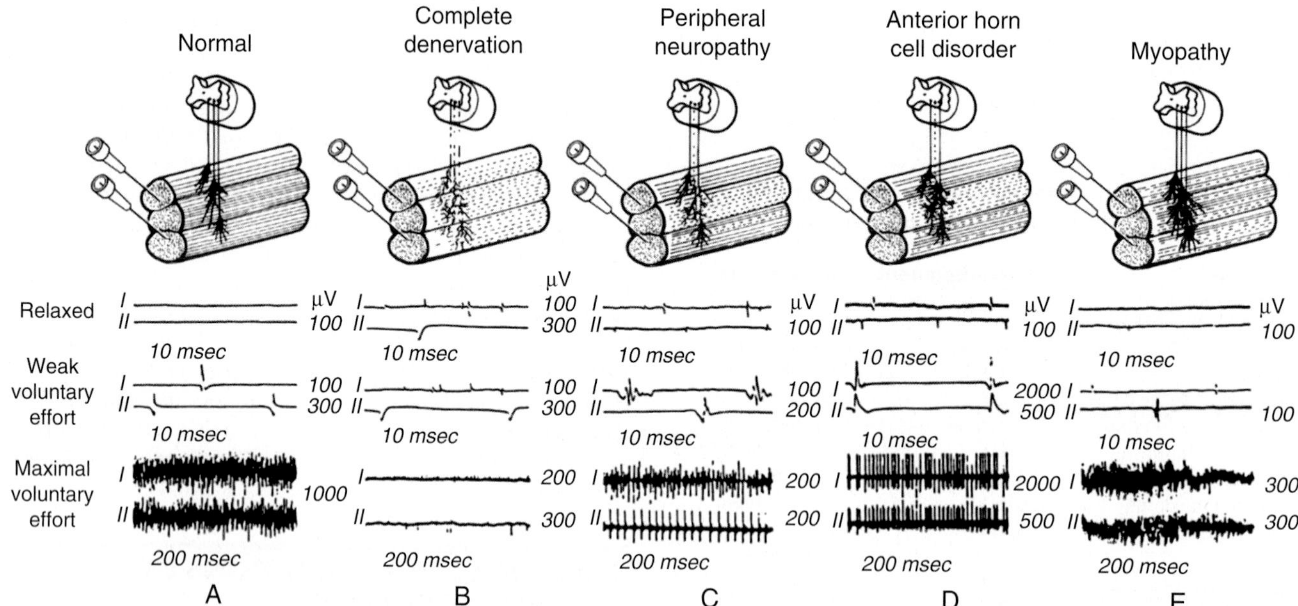

Figure 14.12 Summary of electromyographic findings in various conditions. Diagrams show electromyograms from normal muscle and from muscles with paresis of neurogenic and myogenic origin with a schematic presentation of the muscle fibers from three motor units (affected fibers are dotted). Two recording electrodes, I and II, and the corresponding recordings I and II are shown. Up is negative. **A,** Normal. *At rest*: no action potentials. *Weak voluntary effort*: single motor unit potentials. *Maximal voluntary effort*: interference pattern, no synchronization. **B,** Total denervation with diffuse atrophy of muscle fibers. *At rest*: diphasic and positive denervation potentials. *Voluntary effort*: no motor unit potentials. **C,** Peripheral neurogenic paresis with patchy loss of muscle fibers. *At rest*: denervation potentials. *Voluntary effort*: often with increased action potential duration, polyphasic potentials. The pattern of single motor unit potentials or a mixed pattern during maximal voluntary effort is shown. There is no synchronization between the various leads. **D,** Neurogenic paresis in diseases of the anterior horn cells with patchy loss of muscle fibers. *At rest*: denervation potentials. *Voluntary effort*: increased action potential duration and voltage, polyphasic potentials. Single motor unit potentials with maximal voluntary effort are shown, often synchronous in different leads. **E,** Myogenic paresis with diffuse atrophy of muscle fibers. *At rest*: spontaneous discharges of short duration (in severe cases). *Voluntary effort*: diminished action potential duration, diminished action potential voltage, polyphasic potentials. An interference pattern occurs with maximal effort; a short duration of the single spike potentials is often seen. (From Buchthal F. *An Introduction to Electromyography*. Copenhagen: Scandinavian University Books; 1957:40.)

fibers, and the muscles. Sympathetic and small unmyelinated nerve fiber functions are not evaluated except by quantitative sensory testing.

The timing of EMG in relation to injury or the onset of symptoms may be very important. Early after nerve injury (0 to 14 days), EMG may show only electrical silence, which is not helpful. If any motor units are seen at that time, the nerve to that muscle is at least partially intact. Fibrillation potentials appear only after 2 to 3 weeks. If reinnervation is occurring, small, very polyphasic recovery or "nascent" units will be noted. Serial studies after nerve injury are more helpful than a single study.

EVOKED POTENTIALS

EPs are electrical responses of the nervous system to external sensory stimuli. It has been known for decades that these responses are present; however, their clinical usefulness did not become possible until the development of computerized averaging and advanced signal processing in the late 1960s.[61] Since then, the importance of EPs in diagnosing diseases of the peripheral and central nervous system has undergone exponential growth.

The utility of EPs is based on their ability to provide objective and reproducible data concerning the status of the sensory nervous system. EP testing can demonstrate abnormalities in the sensory system when clinical signs and symptoms are ambiguous. In addition, evidence of clinically unsuspected lesions may be provided when the history and findings on physical examination are normal. EP testing may help delineate the anatomic distribution of nervous system lesions and help monitor their progression or regression; such testing may be used to demonstrate the integrity of nervous system pathways placed at risk during surgery.[61,62]

GENERAL PRINCIPLES

EP responses have very low amplitude (0.1 to 20 mV); consequently, they are obscured by random noise consisting primarily of spontaneous electroencephalographic activity, muscle artifact, and environmental interference. Extraction of the EP response is accomplished by signal averaging. This process summates the "time-locked" EP response, which occurs at the same interval after the stimuli and minimizes unwanted noise.

Although EPs can be elicited by a wide variety of stimuli, the most commonly used stimuli are visual, auditory, and somatosensory.[67-69] This gives rise to the *visual evoked potential* (VEP) test, the *brainstem auditory evoked potential* (BAEP) test, and the *somatosensory evoked potential* (SEP) test. In each of these tests the EP response consists of a sequence of upward and downward deflections (e.g., peaks and waves). The characteristics to be evaluated are the presence or absence, polarity, configuration, amplitude, latency, and interval between individual peaks (*interpeak latency* [IPL]).

Standardized nomenclature for identification of individual peaks or waves has not been universally established,[70,71] although some general principles for labeling have been agreed on.[72,73] Peaks or waves, or both, may be identified by their polarity and the latency at which they occur. For example, the positive peak occurring at 100 msec in the VEP is commonly designated *P100*. Labeling may also be based on the anatomic site at which the response is recorded (e.g., Erb's point), or the deflections may simply be numbered in sequence (e.g., waves I through V in the BAEP).

Normal values for the components of the EP response are affected by numerous factors, including the technique and equipment used by different laboratories. Therefore, each laboratory generally establishes its own normal values by using 2.5 or 3 SD from the mean to determine the limits of normality. Normal values are also influenced by subject factors, including gender, age, body size, and temperature. Clinical interpretation of the EP requires consideration of these factors.[67,74,75]

EQUIPMENT

Most laboratories use commercially available EP equipment that should meet the standards established by the American Association of Electrodiagnostic Medicine and the American Electroencephalographic Society.[72,73,76] In simplest terms, the EP is recorded by attaching electrodes to the patient over specific areas on the extremities, spine, and scalp, depending on the type of test being performed. After the electrodes are attached to record the EP signals, repetitive stimuli timed with the recording process are presented to the patient. The EP signal is collected by the recording electrodes and amplified, filtered, averaged, and displayed for evaluation, printing, and storage. Careful application of the recording electrodes is critical to obtain an EP response of good quality.[70] The electrode site must be cleaned, and the electrode must be attached with a medium that conducts electricity. Standard metal electroencephalographic cup electrodes are commonly used, although other types of electrodes, including needles, may be used.

Placement of electrodes on the scalp is standardized according to the International 10-20 System.[77] This system refers to placement of electrodes either 10% or 20% of the total distance between prominent landmarks on the skull (Fig. 14.13). The specific configuration of electrode placement for a given test is referred to as the *montage*.

SPECIFIC TESTS OF EVOKED POTENTIALS

The three tests of EPs that are used most often measure the visual, brainstem auditory, and somatosensory pathways.

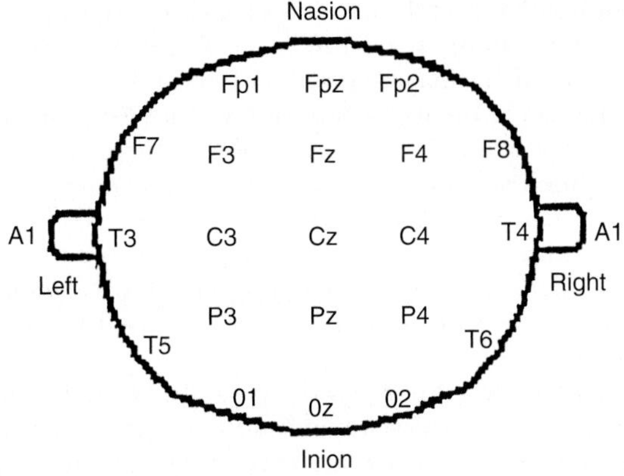

Figure 14.13 The International 10-20 System of electrode placement uses 10% or 20% increments between bony skull landmarks to determine individual electrode locations.

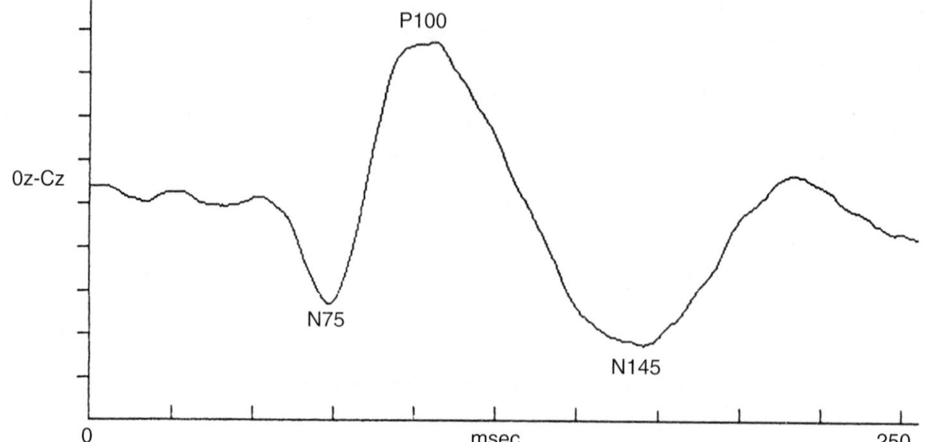

Figure 14.14 Normal visual evoked potential response from one eye to a pattern shift stimulation recorded from the midocciput. The typical response consists of three peaks designated N75, P100, and N145.

Testing of cognitive function and transcranial[72] magnetic stimulation to determine central motor conduction may also be performed. In patients with pain, SEP testing generally offers the greatest clinical utility and is therefore discussed here in the greatest detail.

VISUAL EVOKED POTENTIALS

VEPs are used to evaluate pathologic conditions affecting the visual pathways. VEPs are generated primarily in the visual cortex and may be affected by abnormalities anywhere along the visual pathway from the cornea to the occipital cortex.[70,78,79] Because the anterior visual pathway from the cornea to the retina may be evaluated directly by ophthalmologic examination, the VEP is used mainly to assess the optic pathway posterior to the retina.

The most common stimulus used to elicit the VEP is a reversing checkerboard pattern, typically transmitted through a video monitor and producing checks that alternate from black to white and vice versa. This is referred to as a *pattern-reversal* VEP. Flashes of light may also be used to produce VEPs, but they result in greater variability in response and are less sensitive to abnormalities in the pathway than pattern-reversal testing is.[79]

Flash-elicited VEPs are used primarily when an individual cannot cooperate with pattern-reversal testing and gross determination of visual pathway integrity is required (e.g., in infants or comatose patients and during general anesthesia).[68,74] A flash stimulus is also used to produce the electroretinogram, a specialized type of VEP that reflects the function of the retina and distal portion of the optic nerve.

During performance of pattern-reversal VEPs, each eye is tested separately to localize the lesion to the affected side. Because the visual pathways cross at the optic chiasm, evaluation of chiasmal and retrochiasmal pathology requires that the individual temporal and nasal portions of the visual fields of each eye be tested. This is referred to as *partial-field stimulation*, whereas *full-field stimulation* is used to evaluate prechiasmal lesions.[74]

For pattern-reversal VEPs, the patient is seated comfortably in front of the video monitor producing the alternating checkerboard pattern. The distance of the patient from the monitor and the size of the checks are adjusted to produce a visual angle of 10 to 20 degrees. This stimulates the central part of the retina, which is responsible for the greatest proportion of the VEP response.[67,79] If the patient wears eyeglasses, they should be worn during the test because decreased visual acuity will alter the results. Recording electrodes are placed on the scalp, typically over the midline occiput, vertex, and forehead (Oz, Cz, and Fpz, respectively, in the International 10-20 System). Additional electrodes are placed lateral to the midline occipital electrode if partial-field stimulation is performed. The eye not being tested is patched, and the patient is instructed to gaze at the center of the monitor screen. The checkerboard pattern reverses one to two times per second, and 100 reversals (trials) are generally required to produce a clearly defined response. The test is repeated under identical conditions to demonstrate reproducibility of the response.

The VEP response consists of three peaks (Fig. 14.14). The primary peak of interest is positive with a latency of approximately 100 msec and is referred to as the *P100*. The remaining two peaks are negative and occur at latencies of about 75 and 145 msec, respectively. They are more variable than the P100 and are of less clinical usefulness. Normal values vary among laboratories, although the upper limits of normal generally range from 117 to 120 msec, with differences in latency between eyes no greater than 6 to 7 msec for the P100 response.

Clinical Utility

VEPs are used for the evaluation of many conditions affecting the visual system. In clinical settings, the VEP is used primarily for the diagnosis of multiple sclerosis. Numerous studies have shown that a high percentage of patients with multiple sclerosis exhibit VEP abnormalities, most commonly a prolongation of P100 latency.[67,80-82] As in conventional NCSs, conditions producing demyelination elicit an increase in response latency, whereas axonal loss produces a reduction in response amplitude (Fig. 14.15). Of patients undergoing VEP testing for evaluation of multiple sclerosis, 63% have abnormal results. Abnormality rates of at least 85% have been reported in patients known definitely to have multiple sclerosis.[67] Additionally, abnormalities have been found to persist for years after a single episode of optic neuritis, even if the individual remains free of symptoms.[78] The addition of BAEP and SEP testing improves the diagnostic yield over that of VEP alone.[74,83,84]

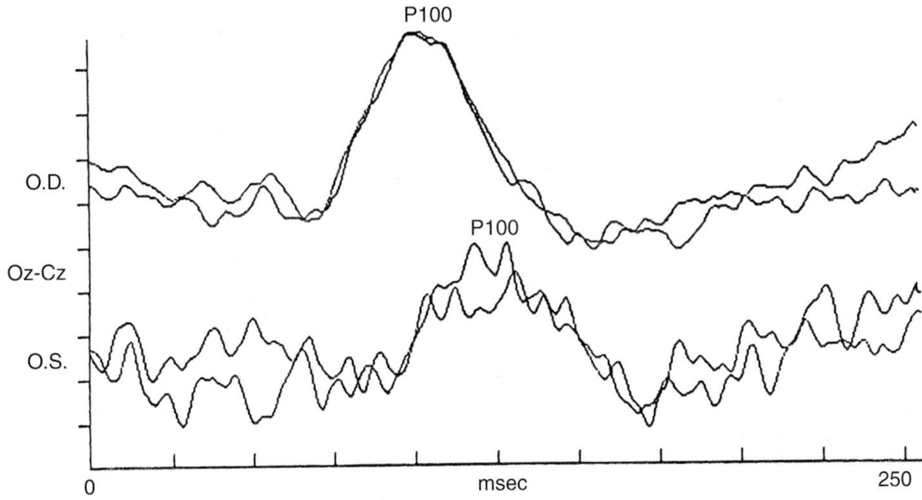

Figure 14.15 Abnormal visual evoked potential response from a patient with multiple sclerosis demonstrating prolonged latency and reduced amplitude of the left eye (O.S.) P100 response. The response from the right eye (O.D.) is normal.

VEP abnormalities have been reported in patients with migraine headaches, with some researchers claiming the ability to classify the type of migraine.[85-88] Abnormalities may be more common if the VEP is performed soon after the migraine attack.[86] Flash-elicited VEPs may reveal a higher frequency of abnormality than seen with pattern-reversal testing. Nevertheless, the use of VEPs for the diagnosis of migraine headache remains controversial.[87]

Diseases of the eye, such as cataracts, glaucoma, and diminished visual acuity, may produce VEP abnormalities, most frequently a decrease in P100 amplitude. Because a direct correlation exists between visual acuity and VEP amplitude, VEP testing may be used to determine visual acuity.[74,89] This is done primarily in patients who are unable to undergo conventional refraction, such as infants and patients with severe mental retardation.

Diseases affecting the anterior visual pathways, such as tumors and ischemia, may produce VEP abnormalities.[90,91] Tumors and infarctions in the posterior optic pathways may also produce VEP abnormalities, especially with partial-field stimulation. Unfortunately, "masking" effects from the normal side in patients with unilateral retrochiasmal lesions may result in normal VEPs. At present, the use of VEPs for diagnosis of retrochiasmal disease remains complicated and contentious.[67,70,74,89] Diseases associated with VEP abnormalities are listed in Box 14.3.

Monitoring visual pathway integrity during surgical procedures that jeopardize the visual system has become increasingly widespread. Various techniques involving the use of strobe lights, light-emitting diode goggles, and fiberoptic contact lenses have been developed to stimulate the optic system in anesthetized patients.[92] In addition to providing information concerning pathway integrity, VEPs can help identify optic nerve elements that may be embedded in tumors, thereby reducing the risk for accidentally disrupting these structures.[68,93]

Box 14.3 Diseases Associated with Abnormalities in Visual Evoked Potentials

Multiple sclerosis
Optic pathway tumors
Spinocerebellar degeneration
Charcot-Marie-Tooth disease
Pernicious anemia
Retinopathy
Optic neuropathy
Glaucoma
Refraction errors

AUDITORY EVOKED POTENTIALS

Just as visual stimuli are used to produce VEPs for evaluation of the visual pathway, auditory stimuli may be used to assess the auditory pathway. The auditory pathway extends from the middle ear structures through the eighth cranial nerve and brainstem and into the auditory cortex. The *auditory evoked potential* (AEP) is produced by presenting auditory stimuli to each ear, which results in a sequence of waveforms that bear a close relationship to these auditory pathway structures and allows relatively specific localization of pathology in the auditory pathway, particularly in the eighth cranial nerve and brainstem.

Although the AEPs parallel hearing, they do not test hearing per se; rather, they reflect a synchronous neural discharge in the auditory system.[93] Thus an individual may have a normal behavioral audiogram and a grossly abnormal AEP or, conversely, a normal AEP and central auditory deafness.

Brainstem Auditory Evoked Potential

The BAEP is one of several tests included under the general heading of "auditory evoked potentials" that are differentiated by recording techniques and latency of responses. Of these tests, the BAEP is most used clinically. The BAEP is also referred to as the *auditory brainstem response* (ABR) and the *brainstem auditory evoked response* (BAER).

Method. Recording the BAEP response is accomplished by presenting an auditory stimulus to each ear individually and recording the response from electrodes placed on the scalp and on or near each ear. Typically, a montage of four electrodes is used on the forehead, vertex, and each earlobe (Fpz, Cz, A1/A2, respectively). The auditory stimulus

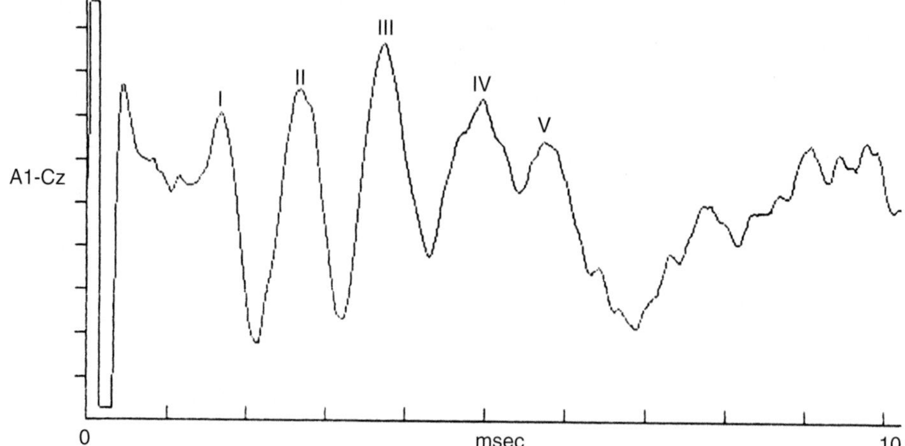

Figure 14.16 Normal brainstem auditory evoked potential response recorded from the left ear to click stimuli demonstrating the five principal peaks. The peaks are labeled with Roman numerals I through V.

used most frequently consists of a brief (100-msec) electrical pulse referred to as a "click." Usually, these clicks are presented to the patient through standard audiologic earphones or insert earphones that fit into the ear canal. Clicks are presented normally at an intensity of 65 to 70 dB above the normal hearing level and at a rate of 10 to 50 clicks/sec. Averaging of 1000 to 2000 stimuli is usually necessary to produce a well-defined BAEP response.

The typical response consists of a series of seven positive waves numbered by Roman numerals I through VII (Fig. 14.16). For the purpose of clinical evaluation, the first five waves are used because waves VI and VII are not present consistently. The BAEP waveform normally occurs within the first 10 msec following presentation of the stimulus; the latency of each wave and the IPL among waves I, III, and V are measured (IPL, or interpeak latency, refers to the latency between each individual wave). Generally, the amplitude of the BAEP response varies too much to be clinically useful, but the ratio of amplitudes between waves I and V may be abnormal in patients with demyelinating disease.[88]

Normal values for the waves and IPLs vary among laboratories, but average normal values are presented in Table 14.4. Many factors may affect the absolute latencies of the BAEP waves (e.g., peripheral hearing loss). IPLs offer a more reliable measure of pathology in the auditory pathway since they frequently remain constant despite changes in the absolute latencies of the waves themselves. Several technical factors, such as varying the stimulus rate or intensity, alter the BAEP. These factors must be considered when the results obtained are evaluated.

Because clinical use of the BAEP relies on the relationship between individual BAEP waves and the anatomic structures that produce them, identification of individual generator sources of BAEPs has been researched extensively. Some controversy remains,[67,68,74,94] particularly concerning waves IV and V, which appear to have multiple generator sources: wave I is thought to be produced by the auditory portion of the eighth cranial nerve; wave II by the eighth cranial nerve and the cochlear nucleus; wave III by the lower pons (probably in the superior olivary complex); and waves IV and V in the upper pons and lower midbrain, possibly in the lateral lemniscus or inferior colliculus.

The status of the patient does not usually affect the ability to obtain a BAEP response. This response may even be obtained from patients who are under general anesthesia or are comatose.[68,95] Mild to moderate peripheral hearing loss may alter absolute wave latencies, although IPLs are not generally changed significantly, thus allowing interpretation of the BAEP. Marked hearing loss, however, may make interpretation of the BAEP extremely difficult or impossible because of degradation of the response. If possible, behavioral audiometry should be performed before BAEP testing to allow more accurate interpretation of the results.[67,93]

Table 14.4 Normative Parameters for Brainstem Auditory Evoked Potentials*

Wave	Normal Value (msec)	Standard Deviation (msec)
I	1.7	0.2
II	2.8	0.2
III	3.8	0.2
IV	5.1	0.2
V	5.6	0.2
I-III	2.1	0.4
III-V	1.9	0.4
I-V	3.9	0.4

Wave V/I amplitude ratio >1.0; wave V interaural latency difference = 0.4 msec.

*Normative values from Waldman HJ, Leawood, KS.

Clinical Utility. BAEPs are useful in evaluating various disease states affecting the auditory pathways. In addition to their VEP abnormalities, patients with multiple sclerosis may demonstrate abnormal BAEPs.[93,94,96] Reported rates of abnormality range from 32% to 72%.

The most common BAEP abnormalities are increased IPLs and a decreased wave V–to–wave I amplitude ratio. Although the BAEP has been found to be useful in evaluating patients with multiple sclerosis, most studies have found it the least sensitive diagnostically when compared with the VEP and SEP.[84,97,98] BAEPs are extremely useful in the diagnosis of acoustic neuromas and other tumors of the cerebellopontine angle. BAEP abnormality rates greater than 90% have been noted in most studies. In addition, the

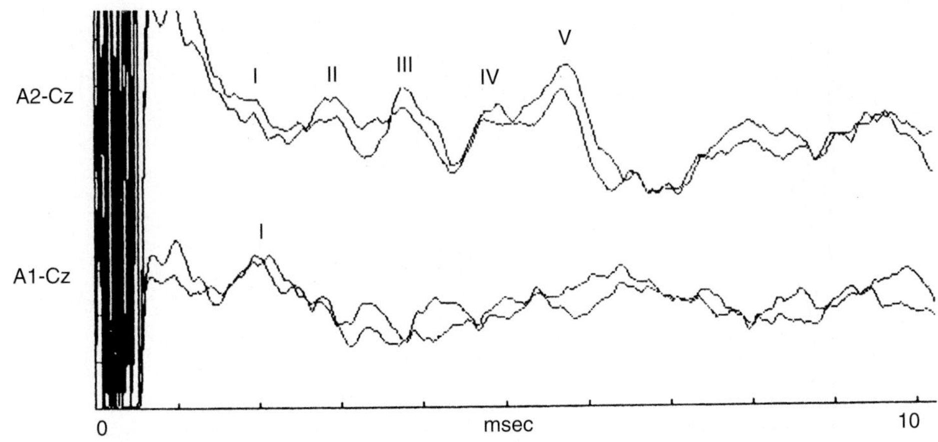

Figure 14.17 Abnormal brainstem auditory evoked potential response from a patient with a left acoustic neuroma. The left trace (A1-Cz) demonstrates only the presence of wave I with an absence of subsequent waves.

BAEP was superior to routine audiometry and computed tomography in early detection of these lesions. An increase in wave I–to–wave III IPL is the most common BAEP abnormality (Fig. 14.17).[99-101]

Brainstem tumors and strokes frequently produce abnormalities in the BAEP if the areas involved lie in the auditory pathway. Prolongation of interpeak or absolute latencies, or both, and absence of waves may be seen, depending on the anatomic site of the lesion.[74,78,97]

The BAEP aids in evaluation of comatose and head-injured patients. Coma produced by toxic or metabolic causes does not generally produce BAEP abnormalities, whereas BAEPs are frequently abnormal in patients with coma secondary to structural brainstem lesions. In patients with head injuries, BAEPs have been predictors of outcome: more severe BAEP abnormalities indicate a poorer prognosis.[102,103] AEP abnormalities have also been described in patients with minimal head injuries, such as postconcussive syndrome.[104] Many other disorders have been associated with BAEP abnormalities,[67,74,105] including degenerative disorders such as Friedreich's ataxia, vertebrobasilar transient ischemic attacks, basilar migraine, and spasmodic torticollis.[106,107]

As with VEPs and the visual pathway, BAEPs may be used to monitor integrity of the auditory pathway during surgical procedures. Operative monitoring of BAEPs has been used most frequently during resection of acoustic neuromas and tumors of the cerebellopontine angle.[68] The primary use of BAEPs has been to determine hearing sensitivity in patients who are unable to undergo behavioral audiometry (e.g., infants). Estimates of hearing sensitivity are usually obtained by progressively decreasing the intensity of the auditory stimulus until no discernible BAEP response is obtained. Because click stimuli are broadband with a frequency range between 1000 and 4000 Hz, filtered clicks and tone bursts with narrower frequency spectra have been used to obtain better frequency specificity of hearing.[94,108,109]

Other Auditory Evoked Potentials

Although the BAEP is the most commonly used AEP, other AEPs have been developed to expand clinical utility. The electrocochleogram begins within the first 3 msec after the presentation of auditory stimuli and reflects electrical activity of the cochlear hair cells and the auditory nerve. This measurement has been used clinically to evaluate patients with Meniere's disease, to monitor damage caused by ototoxic drugs, and to evaluate sensorineural hearing loss.[110]

The 40-Hz, middle-latency, and long-latency AEPs occur later in latency than does the BAEP. They are thought to be generated primarily by structures above the brainstem and therefore may be useful in evaluating more central auditory disorders, as well as in determining hearing sensitivity. These responses are less reliable and more commonly affected by the patient's state than the BAEP is.[94,111]

SOMATOSENSORY EVOKED POTENTIALS

SEPs are responses evoked by stimulation of sensory nerves. Allowing assessment of somatosensory pathway function, SEPs have been obtained by stimulating sensory and mixed nerves in the upper and lower extremities, dermatomal sensory areas of the skin, and cranial nerves. Recording of the SEP response depends on stimulation of large, fast-conducting sensory fibers in the peripheral nerve. From the peripheral nerve, the SEP pathway enters the spinal cord through the dorsal root ganglion and ascends in the ipsilateral dorsal columns. The pathway crosses at the medial lemniscus, travels to the contralateral ventroposterolateral nucleus of the thalamus, and then proceeds to the primary sensory cortex.

The correlation between SEPs and disorders affecting joint and position sense is generally accepted. SEPs are usually normal in patients with abnormalities affecting only pain and temperature sensation.[67,70] Cortical evoked potentials have been recorded following noxious stimuli, although these pain-related potentials currently offer limited clinical usefulness.[74] Recent studies have suggested that some individuals with altered pain-temperature sensation may have abnormalities in pain-related EPs. Some disagree on whether this reflects abnormalities in spinothalamic function or whether these potentials are related to the cognitive processing of pain.[112-119]

Method

Numerous methods have been described to record SEPs, with attempts at standardization occurring only recently.[120-122] Consequently, recording technique, waveform nomenclature, and normal values may vary between investigators.[70,71] Certain general principles, however, apply to most studies. The stimulus of choice for the SEP is electrical and consists of a square wave pulse delivered to the patient by surface or,

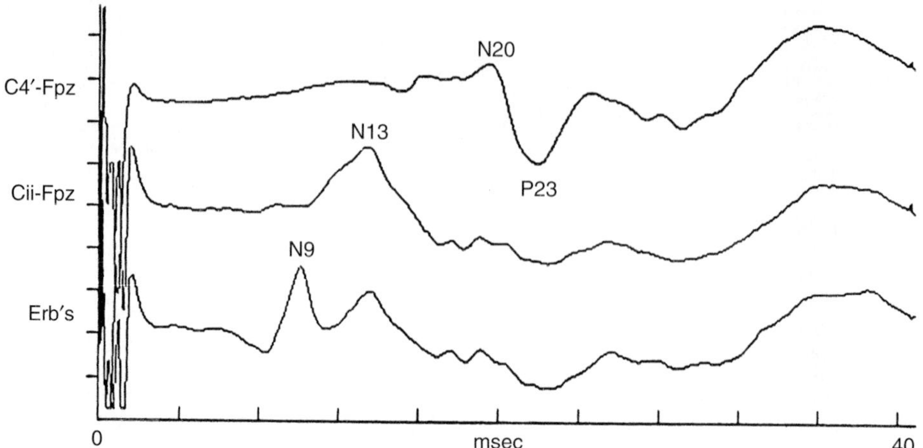

Figure 14.18 Normal upper extremity somatosensory evoked potential response from stimulation of the left median nerve. Responses were recorded from Erb's point (N9), the second cervical vertebra (N13), and the cortex (N20-P23).

less commonly, by needle electrodes. Stimulus duration is usually 100 to 200 msec at a rate of three to seven stimuli per second. Stimulus intensity is adjusted to the point of producing an observable muscle twitch for mixed nerves or 2.5 to 3 times the sensory threshold for sensory nerve stimulation. When applied properly, the stimulus is not generally painful.

Unilateral stimulation is used routinely to permit lateralization of abnormalities, with bilateral stimulation often being reserved for intraoperative monitoring.[68] The site of stimulation depends on the nerve being studied. Typically, distal sites overlying the nerve are used (e.g., median nerve stimulation at the wrist).

The ascending SEP response is recorded by placing pairs of recording electrodes at different locations along the somatosensory pathway being studied. Placement of these recording electrodes depends on whether the nerve being evaluated is located in the upper or lower extremity and on the specific nerve being tested.

Upper Extremity Somatosensory Evoked Potential

Sites for recording electrodes to study nerves in the upper extremity generally include Erb's point in the supraclavicular fossa, the cervical spine (typically over the C2 or C5 spinous process), and the contralateral scalp overlying the area of the primary sensory cortex (corresponding to C3 or C4 of the International 10-20 System). Also, a reference electrode is placed on the forehead (Fz) and a ground electrode is placed proximal to the stimulation site. A noncephalic reference electrode may also be used to allow better visualization of subcortical potentials.

The median nerve has been the most extensively studied upper extremity nerve and is prototypical of an upper extremity SEP.[120,121] When the median nerve is stimulated at the wrist, the expected responses are recorded at each electrode site (Fig. 14.18):

1. At Erb's point, a negative peak with a latency of about 9 msec (designated N9)
2. From the cervical spine, a negative peak at about 13 msec (designated N13)
3. From the scalp, a negative peak at about 20 msec (designated N20), followed by a positive peak at around 23 msec (designated P23)

The sources of these responses remain controversial, although N9 may be generated by fibers in the brachial plexus.[122] N13 is thought to be generated by the dorsal column nuclei and N20 by thalamocortical radiations and possibly the primary sensory cortex. Occasionally, a negative peak of approximately 11-msec latency (N11) precedes the N13 response and is believed to reflect activity in the posterior columns and the dorsal root entry zone of the spinal cord.[67,74,123]

Lower Extremity Somatosensory Evoked Potential

Recording the SEP from nerves situated in the lower extremity generally includes placement of recording electrodes on the lumbar spine over the L3 spinous process, on the lower thoracic spine at T12, and on the scalp over the primary sensory cortex (Cz). In studies of the extremity, SEP responses are difficult to record above the thoracic spine; thus cervical spine recording sites are not usually included.

As in upper extremity SEPs, a reference electrode and ground electrode are necessary. Like the median nerve in the upper extremity, the tibial nerve provides a characteristic SEP of the lower extremity.[121,124] When the tibial nerve is stimulated at the ankle, the responses expected include the following (Fig. 14.19):

1. A negative peak with an approximate latency of 19 msec recorded at L3 (designated L3S)
2. At T11, a negative peak at about 21 msec (designated T11S)
3. At the scalp, a positive peak at approximately 37 msec (designated P37), followed by a negative peak with a latency of about 45 msec (designated N45)

The L3S response is thought to reflect activity in the nerve roots of the cauda equina. The T11S response is thought to be generated by the dorsal fibers of the spinal cord, and the scalp potentials are considered reflections of thalamocortical activity.[67,121,123]

In general, cortical responses can be obtained easily, with as few as 100 to 200 stimuli being required. Lumbar and thoracic spinal responses are difficult to acquire and may not be recordable in obese or uncooperative patients without the use of sedation. Frequently, 1000 to 2000 stimuli are required to obtain clearly defined responses.

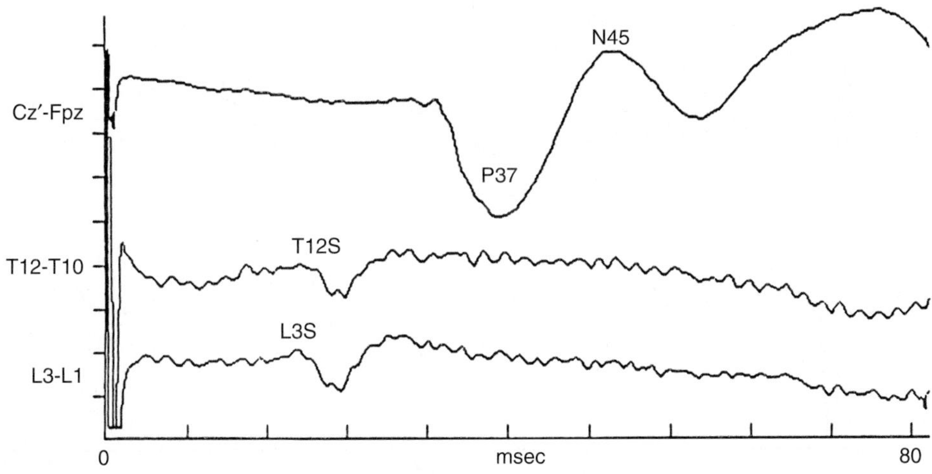

Figure 14.19 Normal lower extremity somatosensory evoked potential response from stimulation of the left posterior tibial nerve. Responses were recorded from the 3rd lumbar vertebra (L3S), the 12th thoracic vertebra (T12S), and the cortex (P37-N45).

Interpretation

Interpretation of SEPs depends on the presence or absence of expected waves and, when present, their absolute latencies and IPLs. Latencies beyond 2.5 to 3 SD from the mean are deemed abnormal. If the SEP is considered a wave traveling from the stimulation site at the peripheral nerve and ascending proximally through the various recording sites on its way to the cortex, it can be seen that a lesion along the ascending somatosensory pathway will result in normal responses distal to the lesion and abnormal responses proximally. Thus, if the brachial plexus response (N9) is normal and the cervical spine potential (N13) is delayed or absent, a lesion is located central to the brachial plexus but below the lower medulla in the cervical root or cord. Similarly, if the brachial plexus potential (N9) is absent or prolonged, a lesion distal to the plexus in the peripheral nerve is likely.

Because diseases of the peripheral nerves that cause slowing of conduction velocity (e.g., demyelinating neuropathies) prolong the latency of all peaks proximal to the nerve, IPLs are useful to confirm normal conduction through the central nervous system despite peripheral nerve abnormalities.[119] Conduction through the central nervous system is referred to as central conduction time and is measured from N13 to N20 in the upper extremity and from L3S to P37 in the lower extremity. Besides peripheral nerve disease, decreased body temperature and increased limb length result in prolongation of absolute peak latencies, thus making determination of central conduction time critical.[67,74,113]

Clinical Uses of Somatosensory Evoked Potentials

Peripheral Nerve Disease. The occurrence of central nervous system amplification of the peripheral nerve volley permits cortical SEPs to be recorded when sensory nerve responses are not recordable by conventional techniques.[113,116,117] Therefore, in cases of severe peripheral nerve disease in which conventional determination of nerve conduction is impossible, NCV may be calculated by stimulating a peripheral nerve at two sites and subtracting the latencies of the corresponding scalp-recorded SEPs. Similarly, conduction can be determined in cases of peripheral nerve entrapment in which conventional nerve conduction responses are difficult or impossible to obtain, as in the case of entrapment of the lateral femoral cutaneous nerve (meralgia paresthetica).[116]

Radiculopathy. Much has been published on the use of SEPs in the diagnosis of radiculopathy.[116,118-138] These studies have shown that SEPs recorded from nerves derived from several nerve roots (e.g., median and peroneal nerves) have limited value in diagnosing radiculopathies because abnormalities in a single involved root would be "overshadowed" by contributions from uninvolved roots supplying that nerve. To circumvent this problem, techniques to derive SEPs from single nerve roots have been investigated. This has been accomplished by stimulation of an area of skin derived from a single dermatome (e.g., the great and first toe web space innervated by the L5 nerve root).[129-132] Another method has involved stimulation of segmentally innervated cutaneous sensory nerves (e.g., using the sural nerve to evaluate the S1 nerve root) (Fig. 14.20).[133]

Results from these "segmentally specific" techniques have ranged from excellent to "essentially useless," with reported abnormality rates in radiculopathy ranging from 7% to 92%.[134-137] Some of the controversy stems from differences in the diagnostic criteria used to determine abnormality. Because any slowing of NCV from a focal lesion of an individual nerve root would be "diluted" by normal conduction along the remainder of the nerve, abnormalities in latency are found less often than a reduction in amplitude. Since amplitude varies even among normal individuals, reduction of amplitude as an indication of abnormality is less reliable than abnormalities in latency.[83,123,128]

Abnormalities in latency were observed in some individuals, and the diagnostic yield was improved when latency and amplitude values were compared with those of an opposite uninvolved extremity that was used as a control. Reports of using spinal rather than cortical SEPs after segmental sensory stimulation suggest a more reliable method for diagnosis of radiculopathies.[138]

Despite the controversy, some consensus exists regarding the usefulness of SEPs in diagnosing radiculopathies. They are purportedly useful for radiculopathies in which sensory symptoms predominate and diagnosis by other techniques such as EMG is difficult.[126,129,133,139] Nevertheless, EMG

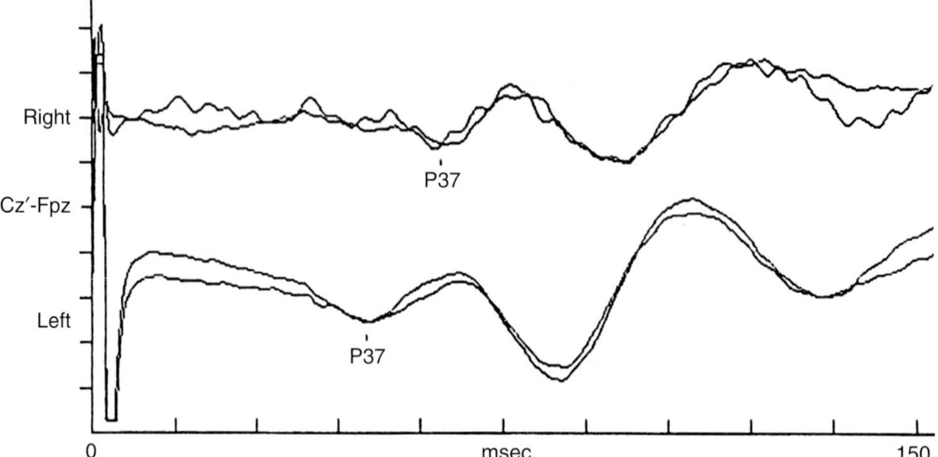

Figure 14.20 Abnormal cortically recorded somatosensory evoked potential response from stimulation of the right sural nerve in a patient with a right lumbar radiculopathy. The P37 response demonstrates prolonged latency and reduced amplitude in comparison to the normal left-sided response.

remains the "gold standard" for the electrodiagnostic evaluation of radiculopathies.

Thoracic Outlet Syndrome. Although ulnar nerve SEPs are controversial, they have been used in an attempt to identify thoracic outlet syndrome. In patients with suspected thoracic outlet syndrome who demonstrated no objective signs of neurologic involvement (e.g., weakness of the hand muscle, numbness, and abnormal findings on EMG), ulnar nerve SEPs were generally normal.[140]

In neurogenic thoracic outlet syndrome, SEP abnormalities included prolonged, attenuated, or absent N9 or N13 peaks, or both, and an increased N9-to-N13 IPL. Normal findings on SEP studies of the median nerve in the involved extremity and side-to-side comparisons were also used to confirm the diagnosis. In cases treated surgically, postoperative improvement in ulnar SEPs was reported.[141-144]

Brachial Plexopathy. Studies have shown that SEPs may provide useful information for the management of patients with brachial plexopathies.[125,126] The ability to record SEPs helps confirm axonal continuity and may help determine whether lesions are preganglionic or postganglionic. As in the case of radiculopathy, segmentally specific testing rather than stimulation of multisegmented nerves provides more specific and accurate information.[145,146]

SEPs are limited in that they test the sensory portions of nerves, which allows only inference concerning motor function. Furthermore, when multiple lesions are present, SEP abnormalities may reflect just the most distal lesions. Therefore, in a patient with a postganglionic lesion, a preganglionic lesion involving the same nerve fibers may go undetected.

Lumbar Spinal Stenosis and Cervical Spondylosis. SEPs have been useful in the diagnosis of lumbar and cervical spinal stenosis, with dermatomal SEPs reported to be superior to EMG in diagnosing central and lateral recess lumbar stenosis.[144,147,148] SEP abnormalities have improved after surgical decompression of these lesions.[149] In central spondylosis, SEP abnormalities correlated well with the presence of myelopathy but not with radiculopathy alone.[150]

Spinal Cord Lesions. SEPs are frequently abnormal in patients with spinal cord lesions affecting the posterior columns. Intramedullary and extramedullary tumors, traumatic spinal cord injury, and vascular lesions may produce these abnormalities. Complete spinal cord lesions generally abolish all recordable SEP responses above the lesion. Partial lesions may or may not produce SEP abnormalities, depending on the extent of posterior column involvement.[151-154] In traumatic spinal cord injury, good correlation between SEP results and the severity of spinal cord injury has been noted. The prognosis for recovery is better when the SEPs are normal in the early post-traumatic period.[155,156]

Trigeminal Nerve Lesions. SEPs recorded from the trigeminal nerve are reported to be abnormal in approximately 41% of patients with idiopathic and multiple sclerosis–related trigeminal neuralgia. In patients undergoing retrogasserian injection of glycerol, alteration in SEP waveforms correlated well with successful treatment as measured by pain relief. Trigeminal SEPs have been used successfully in the diagnosis of parasellar and cerebellopontine angle tumors affecting the trigeminal nerve, even if the involvement was subclinical. In addition, information concerning the site of the lesion along the trigeminal pathway can be obtained.[154,157-159]

Lesions of the Brainstem and Cerebral Hemisphere. Tumor, infarct, and hemorrhage involving the somatosensory pathway of the brainstem and cerebrum generally produce SEP abnormalities.[73,81,160] SEPs may be particularly useful in patients with thalamic pain, in whom abnormalities in N20 and P23 have been reported following median nerve stimulation. Thalamic lesions involving areas other than the ventroposterolateral nucleus are usually associated with normal SEPs.[154,161] Lesions involving the thalamocortical radiations or the sensory cortex may produce a normal N20 and an abnormal P23 response unless retrograde degeneration of the thalamic nuclei has occurred, which results in abnormalities in both responses.[74,155]

Median nerve SEPs have demonstrated prognostic value in patients with right hemiplegia. Abnormalities in N20 and P23 correlate with a poorer prognosis for functional recovery.[161] In cases of traumatic head injury and coma, SEPs have proved valuable in localizing lesions and as a predictor of both favorable and unfavorable outcomes.[102,103,162]

Multiple Sclerosis. SEPs are used frequently in conjunction with VEPs and AEPs to evaluate patients with suspected multiple sclerosis. The incidence of SEP abnormalities is higher in patients with sensory symptoms. Furthermore, SEP abnormalities are more frequent in the lower extremities.[84,83,155] The sensitivity of SEPs in the diagnosis of multiple sclerosis has been comparable to that of VEP testing. Some studies have demonstrated SEPs to be equal to or better than MRI for diagnosis of this disease.[127,163] SEP abnormalities include prolongation of latencies and attenuation or absence of responses.

Monitoring during Surgery. SEPs have been used to monitor the integrity of the somatosensory pathway and cerebral status during various vascular and neurosurgical procedures, most notably carotid endarterectomy and scoliosis surgery. The use of SEP surgical monitoring has become routine in many communities, and its applications continue to expand.[68,164,165]

Other Uses. SEP abnormalities have been found in various degenerative, hereditary, and metabolic disorders. Abnormal SEPs have been reported with Friedreich's and other cerebellar ataxias, Huntington's chorea, motor neuron disorders, Guillain-Barré syndrome, Charcot-Marie-Tooth disease, vitamin B_{12} deficiency, diabetes, and hyperthyroidism.[67,74,113,166,167] SEPs have been used in conjunction with electroencephalography to determine brain death.[152,168] Pudendal nerve SEPs have been applied in the evaluation of bladder and sexual dysfunction.[169-171]

MOTOR EVOKED POTENTIALS

Because of the inability of conventional NCSs to evaluate anatomically deep structures (e.g., cortical structures, lumbosacral plexus), alternative techniques were sought. EPs allowed evaluation of the sensory portions of anatomically deep structures, but the motor portions of these structures remained inaccessible. It had long been known that a high-voltage, short-duration electrical pulse could stimulate these remote structures, but the technique was painful and, in some cases, required direct electrical stimulation (e.g., via needle insertion or during surgical exposure of the structure).[79,172] It had also been known that a magnetic field was able to induce flow of electric current in neuronal structures, but it was not until the 1980s that a practical technique was developed. Essentially an extension of conventional NCSs, motor EPs allow assessment of the motor pathways in peripheral neuronal structures. Unlike conventional NCSs, assessment of the central motor conduction pathways may also be performed. Stimulation may be electrical or magnetic, although magnetic stimulation is the most commonly used form because it is relatively painless.

Motor EPs have found their greatest usefulness in determining central conduction through the motor structures of the brain and spinal cord. By recording from distant sites (e.g., muscles in the extremities), one can determine motor conduction throughout the entire motor pathway. This test is performed in a manner similar to that for SEPs, with the exception that the stimulus is applied centrally and recorded peripherally.[79,113,172,173]

Clinical Utility

Motor EPs have found wide clinical utility in the diagnosis of disorders that affect the central or peripheral motor pathways. Abnormalities in motor EPs have been described in patients with multiple sclerosis, Parkinson's disease, cerebrovascular accident, myelopathy in the cervical and lumbar spines, plexus lesions, and motor neuron disorders.[113,172-176] Cortical hyperexcitability has been demonstrated in migraine patients with transcranial magnetic stimulation.[177] Motor EPs are also finding a role in intraoperative monitoring of neuronal structures placed at surgical risk.[113,172,173]

EVENT-RELATED POTENTIALS

Unlike the previously discussed EPs, which are recorded from simple sensory or motor stimuli, event-related potentials record cortical activity evoked by a stimulus with cognitive significance. Various techniques have been developed to assess the temporal aspects of cognitive processing. The most common technique uses the presentation of randomly occurring infrequent stimuli interspersed among more frequently occurring stimuli of a different type (i.e., an infrequent deep tone occurring randomly among more frequently occurring high-pitched tones). The subject is instructed to attend only to (or to count) the infrequent stimuli, which results in an evoked waveform with a latency of approximately 300 msec and positive polarity. This waveform is referred to as the *P300 response.* Prolongation of the P300 response is associated with disorders that impair cognition, such as dementia, neurodegenerative disorders, schizophrenia, and autism.[67,74,178-180] It has also been used as a predictor of early outcome after emergence from traumatic coma.[181]

CONCLUSION

In conclusion, electrodiagnostic techniques such as EMG and EP testing remain useful techniques for the diagnosis of central and peripheral neuropathies. Even though they have been found helpful in diagnosing some disorders of the central nervous system,[10] they are much more useful in disorders of the nerve roots, plexus lesions, neuropathies, and disorders of the peripheral nerves and less frequently fo painful myopathies. Neuromuscular junction disorders, amyotrophic lateral sclerosis, and other anterior horn cell disorders, except poliomyelitis in its acute stage, rarely produce pain.

Clinical use of electrodiagnostic techniques has expanded rapidly because of improvements in equipment and increased standardization of techniques. Recent advances in magnetic stimulation are allowing evaluation of central motor pathways and deep peripheral nerves that was not possible previously with SEPs and conventional nerve conduction techniques. Advancements in quantitative electroencephalographic and topographic brain mapping are being applied to EPs and promise additional information beyond that provided currently by EP testing alone.

Although electrodiagnostic techniques may find, confirm, and localize a nerve or muscle disease process, the relevance of the electrodiagnostic finding to the patient's pain symptomatology must be determined by the referring physician and the electromyographer, who should work together to assess all available history, physical examination findings, other laboratory tests, and imaging findings before finalizing the diagnosis and establishing a treatment plan.

KEY POINTS

- Electromyography (EMG) and evoked potentials (EPs) are physiologic tests, and their relationship to anatomy must be inferred.
- Little has been written about the use of EMG and EPs in relation to pain, largely because pain is mostly carried by C fibers and Aδ fibers and these are poorly represented in EMG in comparison to larger fibers.
- EMG and EPs need to be correlated with the clinical picture to arrive at a proper diagnosis and may be considered an extension of the clinical examination.
- EMG and nerve conduction studies (NCSs) may differentiate between neuropathic and myopathic conditions and determine whether single nerves, multiple nerves or plexuses, or nerve roots are involved.
- From the distribution of pathology on EMG and NCSs, an anatomic distribution can be inferred and the differential diagnosis of painful conditions narrowed.
- Needle EMG determines the state of a given muscle (i.e., normal, neuropathic, or myopathic). Needle examination of multiple muscles determines the pattern of involvement, if present, and gives an anatomic diagnosis of a painful condition.
- NCSs may indicate normal conduction, conduction block, or slowed conduction and may differentiate among entrapment neuropathies, axonal neuropathies, and demyelinating neuropathies and hence narrow the differential diagnosis of a painful condition affecting the nerves primarily.
- There are few significant side effects with EMG, NCSs, or EPs and very few absolute contraindications to their performance.
- The needle portion of the EMG is performed at rest, with minimal voluntary effort, and with maximum voluntary effort.

KEY POINTS—cont'd

- Spontaneous activity at rest is usually abnormal, and a gradual increase in voluntary effort may help in discerning the nature and distribution of abnormalities.
- Special tests may indicate the presence of pathology in the peripheral portion of cranial nerves.
- Quantitative sensory testing gives information about the physiologic state of smaller fibers concerned with pain transmission.
- There are various painful neuropathies and myopathies, and EMG and NCSs may provide an objective measure of their presence.
- The H-reflex may be of use in lumbar radiculopathies.
- EPs are derived from the electroencephalogram by averaging. Visual EPs may be useful in determining the presence of optic neuritis, and sensory EPs may be useful in neuropathies producing slow conduction velocities.

SUGGESTED READINGS

American Electroencephalography Society. Clinical evoked potential guidelines. *J Clin Neurophysiol.* 1984;1:6-52.

Barohn RJ. Approach to peripheral neuropathy and neuronopathy. *Semin Neurol.* 1998;18:7-18.

Longmire D. Tutorial 10: electrodiagnostic studies in the assessment of painful disorders. *Pain Dig.* 1993;3:116-122.

Lynch MC, Cohen JA. A primer on electrophysiologic studies in myopathy. *Rheum Dis Clin North Am.* 2011;37:253-268.

AAEM Education and Marketing Department Recommended Policy for Electrodiagnostic Medicine Position Statement. Available at www.aaem.com. Accessed March 7, 2012.

Sandoval AEG. Electrodiagnostics for low back pain. *Phys Med Rehabil Clin N Am.* 2010;21:767-776.

Sivak M, Ochoa J, Fernandez JM. Positive manifestations of nerve fiber dysfunction: clinical, electrophysiologic, and pathologic correlates. In: Brown WF, Bolton CF, eds. *Clinical Electromyography.* 2nd ed. Boston: Butterworth-Heinemann; 1993:119-137.

Verdugo RJ, Ochoa JL. Quantitative somatosensory thermotest: a key method for functional evaluation of small caliber afferent channels. *Brain.* 1992;115:893-913.

Waldman HJ. Neurophysiologic testing in the evaluation of the patient in pain. In: Waldman SD, Winnie AP, eds. *Interventional Pain Management. Dannemiller Memorial Educational Foundation.* Philadelphia: Saunders; 1996:104-118.

Werner RA, Andary M. Electrodiagnostic evaluation of carpal tunnel syndrome. *Muscle Nerve.* 2011;44:597-607.

The references for this chapter can be found at www.expertconsult.com.

Radiologic Assessment of the Patient with Spine Pain

15

Timothy P. Maus

Imaging is a significant, but not independent, component of the multifaceted evaluation of the patient with spine or limb pain. Imaging must be interpreted in concert with the history, physical exam, electrodiagnostic evaluation, and responses to image-guided anesthetic or provocative procedures. It does not stand alone, but can only be understood in its proper context: the individual patient's unique syndrome of pain or neurologic dysfunction.

Pain of spinal origin is extremely common; low back pain is the second most common cause of symptomatic office visits in the United States.[1,2] There is a nearly 75% lifetime prevalence of back pain in the United States,[3] and one third of U.S. adults report back pain in the previous 3 months.[1] Advanced imaging is applied to this complaint with ever-increasing frequency; the number of lumbar magnetic resonance imaging (MRI) scans among Medicare beneficiaries rose fourfold from 1994 to 2005.[4] Over 40% of patients with acute low back pain underwent immediate imaging in a private insurance claims database study.[5] In another Medicare-based study of low back pain patients without red flags for systemic disease, nearly 30% underwent imaging (radiography or advanced imaging) within 28 days.[6] In a study in an emergency department environment, the use of advanced imaging (computed tomography [CT] or MRI) for low back pain tripled from 2002 to 2006.[7] Approximately one third of Medicare low back pain patients who undergo outpatient MRI studies have not received any prior conservative therapy.[8]

Despite this intensity of imaging and the downstream effects of increasing minimally invasive interventions and surgical procedures that flow from them, there is no evidence that patient outcomes are improving. Measures of physical functioning, work/school limitations, and mental health in U.S. adults with back or neck complaints were similar or worse in 2005 than in 1997.[9] A regional study (North Carolina) demonstrated that the proportion of adults with chronic low back pain causing activity impairment rose from 3.9% in 1992 to 10.2% in 2006.[10] A review article by Chou, Deyo, and Jarvik examined the evidence for our inefficient utilization of imaging in the back pain patient, underlying causal forces and mechanisms for initiating improvements.[11] The purpose of this chapter is to foster the rational decision making they advocate in the use of spine imaging, based on evidence, as we in the pain management community seek to improve patient outcomes.

THE GOAL OF IMAGING

The primary goal of imaging in the patient with spine or limb pain is to identify patients who are suffering from an undiagnosed systemic process causal of the pain/dysfunction syndrome. This is an uncommon phenomenon. An analysis by Jarvik and Deyo[12] suggests that 95% of low back pain is due to benign processes. In patients presenting to a primary care setting with low back pain, only 0.7% suffer from undiagnosed metastatic neoplasm. Spine infection, including pyogenic and granulomatous diskitis, epidural abscess, or viral processes, is present in only 0.01% of subjects. Noninfectious inflammatory spondyloarthropathies, such as ankylosing spondylitis, account for 0.3% of presentations. Osteoporotic compression fractures are the most common systemic pathologic process to present as back pain, accounting for 4% of patients.[12] Imaging seeks to identify the approximately 5% of patients with back or limb pain who have undiagnosed systemic disease as the etiology of their pain. A related imaging goal is to characterize and assist in therapy planning in the very small percentage of patients who have neural compressive disease resulting in radiculopathy or radicular pain syndromes that fail conservative therapy and require surgical or minimally invasive intervention.

SPECIFICITY: ASYMPTOMATIC IMAGING FINDINGS

The low prevalence of systemic disease as a cause of back pain implies that most imaging studies primarily describe what are often, and inappropriately, termed "degenerative" phenomena. These may include anterior and lateral vertebral body osteophytes, loss of T2 signal in the intervertebral disk, and structural changes of facet arthrosis. Degeneration is a pejorative term implying disease; these changes have no relationship to pain syndromes and correlate only with age. They are best referred to as age or age-related change. These age changes are typically relatively uniform across the spine, although the lowest lumbar segments are over-represented. Evidence for the lack of specificity of such imaging findings for spine pain syndromes is evident in cadaver studies, imaging studies in asymptomatic populations, and population studies.

Nathan[13] described the presence of anterior and lateral osteophytes in 100% of cadavers at the age of 40, whereas posterior osteophytes are present only in a minority of cadavers at 80 years of age. Hult[14] studied adults with spine radiographs and showed that by age 50 years, 87% will have radiographic evidence of disk age-related change (narrowing of the disk space, marginal sclerosis with osteophytes, vacuum phenomena). In a second study including a cohort of asymptomatic workers, Hult[15] noted radiographic evidence of disk

Table 15.1 Imaging Abnormalities in Asymptomatic Subjects

Test	Author (reference), Date	Patients (N)	Age Range (mean)	Disk Herniation	Disk Bulge	Disk Degeneration	Central Canal Stenosis	Annular Fissure
X-ray	Hult (15) 1954	1200	40-44 55-59			56% 95%		
X-ray	Hellstrom (20) 1990	143	14-25			20%		
Myelogram	Hitselberger (16) 1968	300	(51)	31%				
CT	Wiesel (17) 1984	51	(40)	20%			3.4%	
MRI	Weinreb (21) 1989	86	(28)	9%	44%			
MRI	Boden (18) 1990	53	< 60 ≥ 60	22% 36%	54% 79%	46% 93%	1% 21%	
MRI	Jensen (22) 1994	98	(42)	28%	52%		7%	
MRI	Boos (23) 1995	46	(36)	76%	51%	85%		
MRI	Stadnik (24) 1998	36	(42)	33%	81%	56%		56%
MRI	Weishaupt (25) 1998	60	(35)	60%	28%	72%		20%
MRI	Jarvik (19) 2001	148	(54)	38%	64%	91%	10%	38%

From Maus T. Imaging the back pain patient. *Phys Med Rehabil Clin N Am.* 2010; 21:725-766, Table 3.

"disease" in 56% of those aged 40 to 44 years, which rose to 95% in subjects 50 to 59 years old. With the evolution of more sophisticated spine imaging techniques, this lack of specificity of degenerative findings has not improved. Hitselberger and Witten[16] studied plain myelography of asymptomatic volunteers and noted that 24% showed abnormalities that would have been considered significant in a clinical context of back or leg pain. A study of lumbar spine CT in asymptomatic volunteers by Wiesel and colleagues[17] showed that in patients older than 40 years, 50% had "significant" abnormalities. Similarly, Boden and colleagues[18] evaluated MRI of the lumbar spine in asymptomatic volunteers; in patients older than 60 years, 57% had abnormalities that would have been considered significant in an appropriate clinical setting. Jarvik and colleagues[19] studied a large patient population with MRI. This study noted that only extrusions, moderate to severe central canal stenosis, and direct visualization of neural compression were likely to be significant and would separate patients with pain from asymptomatic volunteers. Disk protrusions, zygapophysial joint (z-joint or facet joint) arthrosis, and anterolisthesis or retrolisthesis were virtually always asymptomatic findings. Imaging studies of asymptomatic volunteers are compiled in Table 15.1.[20-25]

A study by Kanayama[26] in 200 healthy adults (mean age 40, with no current complaint or therapy for back pain nor any history of lumbar surgery) segregated lumbar MRI findings by segmental level (Table 15.2). Asymptomatic T2 signal loss and disk herniations were most common at the L4 and L5 segmental levels; this series also had a high prevalence of asymptomatic high intensity zones (HZ) (24% at L4 and L5). More recent studies have addressed the prevalence of disk "degenerative" imaging findings (T2 signal loss, loss of disk space height) in younger populations, primarily in Scandinavian countries; these are MRI population-based studies without regard to symptomatology. Kjaer and colleagues,[27] studying children age 13 years, found a 21% prevalence of disk "degeneration." In a study of adolescents, Salminen and colleagues[28] found a 31% prevalence of disk "degeneration" in 15-year-olds, which rose to 42% in 18-year-olds. Takatalo and colleagues[29] evaluated 558 young adults aged 20 to 22 years. Using the 5-point Pfirrmann classification of disk degeneration, they noted disk degeneration of grade 3 or higher in 47% of these young adults. There was a higher prevalence in males (54%) than in females (42%). Multilevel degeneration was identified in 17%.

As in the lumbar region, age changes in the cervical and thoracic spine are common, asymptomatic, and increase in prevalence with age. Matsumoto studied nearly 500 asymptomatic patients with MRI; he noted a loss of T2 signal within cervical disks in 12% to 17% of patients in their twenties, but in 86% to 89% of patients older than 60 years of age.[30] Asymptomatic cervical cord compression was observed in 7.6% of patients, largely over the age of 50. Similarly, Boden studied 63 asymptomatic subjects with MRI and noted cervical disk "degeneration" in 25% of those younger than 40, and in excess of 60% of patients older than 40 years of age.[31] Asymptomatic subjects older than 40 years of age had a 5% rate of disk herniations and a 20% rate of foraminal stenosis. Teresi studied 100 asymptomatic subjects with MRI and noted asymptomatic cervical cord compression in 7% and either disk protrusion or annular bulge in 57% of subjects older than 64 years of age.[32] In the thoracic spine, Wood studied 90 asymptomatic patients with MRI.[33] In this population, 73% of the patients had positive thoracic imaging findings, 37% had disk herniations, 53% demonstrated disk bulges, and asymptomatic cord deformity was present in 29%.

Table 15.2 Segmental Distribution of Asymptomatic Lumbar Age-Related Change

Segment	Disk Herniation	Nuclear T2 Signal Loss	Modic Change	HIZ
L1	0.5%	7%	1%	0%
L2	3.5%	12%	3%	4%
L3	16.5%	15.5%	4%	5%
L4	25%	49.5%	11%	23.5%
L5	35%	53%	10%	24%

Data abstracted from Kanayama M, Togawa D, Takahashi C, et al. Cross-sectional magnetic resonance imaging study of lumbar disk degeneration in 200 healthy individuals. *J Neurosurg Spine.* 2009;11:501-507.

The evidence is deep and overwhelming. The structural spine imaging findings most commonly referred to as "degenerative changes" or "degenerative disk disease," including anterior and lateral osteophytes, loss of T2 signal in the disk, loss of disk space height, disk bulges and protrusions, and facet arthrosis, are ubiquitous and unassociated with pain syndromes; their only association is with age. They can only be avoided by a youthful death. They are not a disease state and are best referred to as normal age change or age-related change.

A consequence of this high prevalence of asymptomatic age-related changes is that the imager must know the nature of the pain syndrome if he or she is to properly focus on findings significant to the unique patient under consideration. There must be concordance of the imaging finding and the pain syndrome it is postulated to elicit. Imaging cannot prove causation, hence the need for anesthetic and provocative procedures. Communication regarding the nature of the pain syndrome is essential, whether this occurs through a robust electronic medical record, an intake document at the imaging site, or direct interaction of the imager with the patient.

SENSITIVITY: PHYSIOLOGIC IMAGING

There is also a major sensitivity fault associated with spine imaging. The majority of patient symptoms referable to the spine occur in axially loaded positions, either sitting or standing. A substantial portion of radiographs and most advanced imaging (CT and MRI) are obtained in a recumbent position, removing the effects of axial load and physiologic posture. This may fail to reveal the lesion responsible for the index pain.

There is ample evidence of the effect of axial load and physiologic posture on the biomechanical and structural characteristics of the spine, derived from biomechanical, cadaver, and imaging studies. Lumbar intradiskal pressures are higher when sitting or standing than when in a recumbent position.[34] The cadaver study of Inufusa demonstrated a reduction in the cross-sectional area of the lumbar central canal and lateral recesses in extension, with an increase in flexion.[35] Lumbar neural foraminal cross section is also diminished in extension and increased in flexion. Fujiwara noted a reduction in cadaveric lumbar neural foraminal area with side bending or rotation toward the index foramen; an increase in area was observed with side bending or rotation away from the foramen.[36] Studying normal volunteers, Schmid observed a 40-mm^2 reduction in the cross-sectional area of the dural sac at the L3-L4 level with movement from flexion to extension.[37] The lumbar neural foraminal cross-sectional area was reduced by 23% in moving from an upright neutral to an upright extended position. Danielson[38] noted a significant decrease in the dural sac cross-sectional area with axial loading in 56% of subjects, most commonly at L4-L5; this was more common with increasing age. Dynamic reduction in dural sac area with loading was less frequent in normal volunteers than in a population of patients with neurogenic intermittent claudication. Hansson and colleagues identified the ligamentum flavum as the most important structure resulting in dynamic reduction in the lumbar central canal area under physiologic loading.[39] Physiologic posture (lumbar lordosis) is likely more important than axial load.[40] Multiple studies in patients with upright imaging have demonstrated the enlargement of lumbar disk bulges or protrusions with axial load, which may be further exacerbated with extension.[41,42] Synovial cysts, which may be provocative of radicular pain syndromes or contribute to neurogenic intermittent claudication, may be undetectable on recumbent imaging when synovial fluid remains in the facet joint space. Upon the assumption of axial load and apposition of the facet articular surfaces, the fluid is forced from the joint space into the cyst, where it may act as a neural compressive lesion.

The cervical spine similarly exhibits dynamic physiologic change with posture and load. Cadaveric studies have demonstrated increased disk bulging and buckling of the ligamentum flavum in cervical spine extension; the ligamentum flavum effect was most significant.[43] MRI studies of patients[44,45] noted an increase in central canal stenosis with both extension and flexion of the cervical spine relative to neutral posture; the decrease was most marked in extension. Cervical neural foramina diminish in cross section, width, and height in extension and increase in all these parameters in flexion.[46]

In summary, physiologic extension and axial load reduce the area of all lumbar spine compartments; these are increased in flexion. The cervical central canal is diminished in areas in extension more so than in flexion; it is maximal in the neutral position. Cervical foramina increase in all dimensions in flexion and diminish in extension. These dynamic changes constitute the greatest sensitivity fault in imaging: conventional supine imaging may fail to reveal a lesion that is causal of the patient's symptoms when that lesion is only expressed in physiologic postures.

Several methods have been devised to overcome this sensitivity fault. Radiographs should always be obtained upright; this allows assessment of sagittal and coronal balance in a physiologic posture. Flexion-extension radiographs may detect instability not observed on neutral upright views, but the yield of diagnostic information is very low. In studies in both the lumbar and cervical spine segments, less than 1% of flexion-extension radiographic studies provided information over that noted on static upright radiographs.[47,48] The cost and radiation exposure is best deferred to a presurgical setting, not during an initial evaluation of the back or neck pain patient.

Advanced imaging can be performed with axial loading devices on conventional CT or MRI scanners. These devices can improve the sensitivity to the detection of clinically significant central canal compromise.[49] The 2011 North American Spine Society's evidence-based guidelines on evaluation and treatment of spinal stenosis suggest axially loaded imaging in the setting of suspected neurogenic intermittent claudication and stenosis unconfirmed by conventional imaging, with a canal diameter of less than 110 mm.[22,50] Willén and colleagues demonstrated that surgical results of cases of occult lumbar spinal stenosis detected only by axially loaded MRI were comparable to those of stenosis observed in unloaded MRI examinations.[51]

MRI scanning in an upright position—sometimes referred to as dynamic, positional, or kinetic MRI—is now commercially available and widely marketed. The practical challenge is that currently available systems are of low field strength (0.6T), with an unavoidable reduction in image quality. This reduction in image quality can have important consequences for clinical image interpretation. If current low field strength dynamic systems were applied selectively to cases where conventional imaging failed to demonstrate a correlative lesion causal of the patient's pain, the patient would likely benefit. All too often, however, the cost of these systems results in their routine use, or even promotion as the best available imaging tool for all spine conditions. This practice could harm patients, as diminished image quality reduces sensitivity to the detection of sinister lesions, which is the primary goal of imaging the back pain patient (Fig. 15.1).

VALIDITY

Spine imaging must be undertaken with a full understanding of the specificity and sensitivity faults inherent in its use. The ultimate question, of course, is one of validity: Does performing an imaging study of the spine segment in question result in improved patient outcomes through a more timely and accurate diagnosis of the process causing the patient's pain? This is well studied, particularly in the application of imaging to the acute presentation of back pain. Chou and colleagues performed a meta-analysis of the six randomized controlled trials (n = 1804) examining the role of imaging in the acute presentation of back or limb pain with no clinical features suggesting systemic disease.[52] They identified no benefit in pain, function, quality or life, or patient-rated improvement in patients undergoing imaging (radiographs, CT, or MRI) at presentation versus those undergoing clinically directed conservative care. Although routine imaging might have been expected to provide reassurance, imaged patients did not have better psychological outcomes.

Carragee and colleagues elegantly demonstrated the lack of utility of imaging in the acute setting in a 5-year prospective observational study.[53] A cohort of asymptomatic subjects deemed to be at risk for back pain resulting from labor-intensive vocations underwent lumbar spine MRI. This patient cohort was followed periodically over the subsequent 5 years; a subset of these subjects presented to a medical care provider with acute back or leg pain during this 5-year period and a second lumbar MRI was obtained. Less than 5% of the MRI scans obtained at the time of acute presentation with back or leg pain showed clinically relevant new findings; virtually all of the "positive findings" noted on the images at the time of presentation with back/leg pain had been present on the baseline studies obtained when the patient was asymptomatic. Only direct evidence of neural compression in patients with a corresponding radicular pain syndrome was considered to be useful imaging information. Of particular note, psychosocial factors, not the morphology seen on imaging, were the best predictors of the degree of functional disability caused by back or leg pain.[53]

A study by Modic,[54] also in the acute presentation of low back pain or radiculopathy, showed no relationship between the extent of disk herniations and presenting signs or symptom. The type, size, or location of a herniation at presentation, or change in size or type over time, did not correlate with clinical outcomes. MRI imaging characteristics did not have measurable value in planning conservative care. The study emphasized that the surgical decisions must be made on clinical grounds, given the inability of imaging to predict outcomes. The Modic study, like that of Carragee, demonstrated that psychosocial factors predict functional disability better than imaging parameters.[54]

Although the depth of evidence regarding the inability of imaging to improve outcomes in back and limb pain patients is most profound in the acute setting, it applies more broadly as well. Chou and colleagues[11] explored the seemingly counterintuitive finding that routine imaging does not lead to better outcomes in back or limb pain. This lack of utility can be attributed to the favorable natural history of back and limb pain, the low prevalence of sinister disease as causal of back pain, the weak correlation between imaging findings and symptoms (the specificity fault), and the minimal impact of imaging on clinical decision making. Given the demonstrable modest utility of imaging, the decision to undertake this path must be a carefully reasoned one.

IMAGING RISK/BENEFIT

The decision to proceed with any medical test or procedure should be preceded by a consideration of likely benefit weighed against risk or actual harms. Certainly there are benefits to be derived from imaging. Foremost, imaging may suggest the diagnosis of previously unsuspected systemic disease. In the patient with a radicular pain syndrome or radiculopathy that has not responded to conservative therapy, imaging may supply invaluable information that allows planning of minimally invasive or surgical procedures. Negative imaging should also have value in providing reassurance that there is no sinister disease present and in stopping further workup in appropriate circumstances. Finally, in patients with chronic pain syndromes, imaging may assist in the identification of the structural or inflammatory cause of such pain. Only when a specific pain generator is identified can a specific plan of therapeutic intervention, whether it be conservative or invasive, be developed.

There are direct harms and potential risks associated with imaging, which must be balanced against potential benefits. These include radiation dose, cost, the labeling effect, and

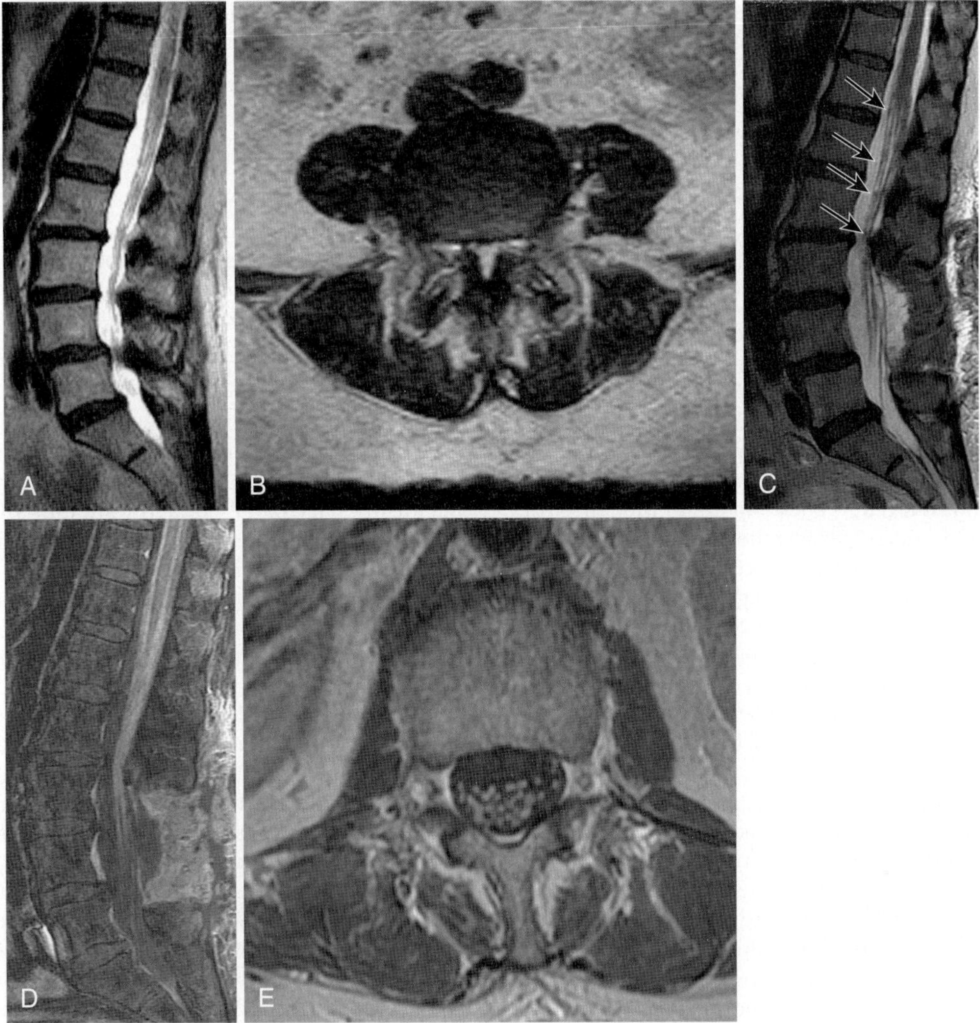

Figure 15.1 Diminished sensitivity of low field strength upright MRI to sinister lesions. A 74-year-old female presented with bilateral lower extremity weakness and pain with a low field strength upright MRI from another institution. Sagittal T2 image **(A)** and axial T2 image **(B)** at the L4 level show degenerative spondylolisthesis at L4 with central canal compromise. She underwent an L3-L5 decompression without change in symptoms. A 1.5 Tesla MRI performed 3 weeks postoperatively demonstrated nodularity *(arrows)* in the cauda equina on a T2 sagittal image **(C).** Gadolinium-enhanced fat-saturated T1 sagittal **(D)** and axial **(E)** images demonstrate diffuse leptomeningeal metastases from breast cancer. She died in 2 months. A high-quality preoperative MRI would have likely led to the diagnosis and avoided an unnecessary operation. (From Khalil JG, Nassr A, Maus TP. Physiologic imaging of the spine. *Radiol Clin North Am.* 2012;50:599-611.)

the downstream risk of provoking minimally invasive or surgical interventions of dubious efficacy.

Radiation dose in radiography, CT or CT/myelography, and nuclear medicine studies constitutes a direct patient harm. Radiation exposure from radiographs, CT, and nuclear medicine studies carries a cumulative risk of neoplasm induction. This risk becomes particularly problematic when serial studies are performed. The biologically effective absorbed radiation dose is measured by the Sievert (Sv); in North America, the average annual natural background exposure is approximately 3 mSv.[55] A frontal and lateral chest radiograph is often considered the common currency of radiation exposure, incurring a dose of approximately 0.1 mSv. A three-view lumbar spine radiographic series is then worth approximately 15 chest radiographs, or 1.5 mSv; cervical spine radiographs incur a dose 0.2 mSv. A dose of 6 mSv is typical for a lumbar spine CT scan, a value of 60 chest radiographs. Cervical spine CT incurs 2 mSv, or 20 chest radiographs. A technetium bone scan has a dose of 6.3 mSv. The cumulative radiation exposure creates real harm; the 2.2 million lumbar spine CT scans performed in the United States in 2007 were projected to result in 1200 future cancers.[56] Although less radiation intensive, lumbar radiography is performed much more frequently than CT and contributes nearly fivefold the cumulative radiation burden to the U.S. population.[57] The average annual radiation exposure from lumbar radiographs is 75 times that of chest radiography.[57] Radiation risks of spine imaging are made more acute by the necessary inclusion of radiosensitive tissues, the gonadal structures in the pelvis, and the thyroid in the neck.

Imaging studies of the spine are costly. In the United States, the medical imaging community incurs more than $100 billion of societal cost per year. The 2012 Medicare reimbursements[58] for lumbar spine imaging include radiographs: $41; noncontrast CT: $264; myelogram: $506; noncontrast MRI: $439; whole-body positron emission tomography (PET)/CT: $1183; bone scan with single-photon emission CT (SPECT): $261.[18] Nominal fees are typically 3 to 5 times the Medicare reimbursements. It is easy to appreciate how quickly imaging costs can accrue.

The labeling effect refers to the inevitable identification of age-related change, usually described as "degenerative change," or "degenerative disk disease" on imaging studies obtained in evaluation of back or limb pain. The patient may then perceive that he or she suffers from a degenerative spine condition; the term *degenerative* has only negative connotations. Fearing further damage to their "degenerative" spine, they may give up favorite activities and exercise, resulting in deconditioning and contributing to depression. These fear-avoidance behaviors can be a major impediment to recovery. In a study in which back pain patients were randomized to either receiving or being blinded to the results of their MRI imaging, those who were privy to the results (which were all benign) had a lesser sense of well-being.[54] A study of subacute or chronic back pain patients showed that those who underwent spine radiography reported more pain, had a diminished global health state, and consumed more follow-up care than those who were not imaged.[59] These findings emphasize the need for patient education regarding the insignificance of age-related imaging findings; imaging professionals should carefully choose descriptive language in imaging reports and avoid the use of pejorative terms such as "degenerative change."

Finally, and most ominously, imaging may precipitate interventions that have little evidence of efficacy and expose the patient to harm. Jarvik and colleagues[60] documented that obtaining advanced imaging (MRI) early in a patient's spine pain syndrome leads to increased surgical interventions despite equivalent pain and disability profiles, when compared with un-imaged patients. Likewise, Lurie and colleagues[61] examined the dramatic regional variation (12-fold) in the rate of surgical intervention for central canal stenosis. These investigators noted that the rate of surgical intervention correlated directly with the intensity of CT and MRI use. Webster and colleagues, evaluating subjects with acute job-related back pain, noted that undergoing an MRI in the first month of symptoms was associated with an eightfold increased risk for surgery and a fivefold risk for more medical care consumption than that noted for clinically matched, un-imaged subjects.[62] Many of the interventions directed toward spine pain, both surgical and minimally invasive, have only modest, if any, evidence basis.

IMAGING RECOMMENDATIONS

Imaging is performed to identify sinister disease as a cause of a patient's back or limb pain. Spine imaging has major specificity and sensitivity faults. The decision to initiate imaging must occur as a reasoned decision, weighting potential benefit against real harms and risk. The evidence is clear that there is no benefit to imaging in the acute presentation of back or limb pain in the absence of signs or symptoms of systemic disease. These principles are firmly based on evidence and have led to the imaging guidelines promulgated by several scientific societies.

These guidelines are not new. In 1994, the Agency for Health Care Policy and Research recommended against imaging patients with back pain within the first month of a pain syndrome in the absence of signs of systemic disease.[63] The American College of Radiology (ACR) consensus practice guidelines were restated in 2009.[64] Imaging is not indicated in the patient who presents with acute low back pain with or without radiculopathy except in the presence of "red flag" features including the following:

- Recent significant trauma, minor trauma in a patient older than 50 years
- Unexplained weight loss
- Unexplained fever
- Immunosuppression
- History of neoplasm
- Prolonged steroid use or osteoporosis
- Age greater than 70 years
- Known intravenous drug abuse
- Progressive neurologic deficit with intractable symptoms
- Duration longer than 6 weeks

A 2007 joint recommendation from the American College of Physicians (ACP) and the American Pain Society stated that imaging should not be obtained in patients with nonspecific low back pain.[65] Imaging should only be performed when severe or progressive neurologic deficits are present or when serious underlying systemic disease is suspected. Furthermore, patients with signs or symptoms of radiculopathy or spinal stenosis should be imaged only if they are candidates for surgical or minimally invasive intervention (e.g., epidural steroid injection). In a further elaboration on these guidelines, the ACP, in its initiative to promote high-value medical care, provided more specific imaging recommendations based on clinical scenarios (Table 15.3).[66]

There is evidence that of the small proportion of subjects with sinister disease as the cause of their back or limb pain, virtually all have risk factors that trigger imaging under these guidelines. A retrospective study of 963 patients presenting with acute low back pain noted that the 8 subjects with neoplasm all had clinical risk factors.[67] In a prospective study of 1170 acute low back pain patients without clinical risk factors, no cases of neoplasm were found.[68] No sinister disease was missed in the absence of clinical risk factors in a subsequent systematic review.[69]

Despite these well-supported, evidence-based guidelines, clinical practice in the United States remains greatly divergent from this ideal. By one estimate, between one third and two thirds of all advanced spine imaging is inappropriate when measured against existing guidelines.[4] Utilization of spine imaging is accelerating despite a complete lack of evidence of its effectiveness in improving the outcomes of back and limb pain patients. Chou and colleagues have enumerated causes of this overutilization: inappropriate patient expectations, direct and indirect financial incentives on the part of providers, defensive medicine, and provider time constraints.[11] These issues present great challenges to imaging professionals and those who utilize imaging to improve the clinical state of their patients. Solutions will undoubtedly be multifactorial, but education of the patient, the imaging professional, and imaging consumers would seem to be at the heart of the matter. It is hoped that the evidence presented here will assist in more rational decision making regarding imaging the spine pain patient (Box 15.1).

RADIOGRAPHS

With the failure of clinically directed conservative care, and having made a reasoned decision to initiate imaging of

Table 15.3 Suggestions for Imaging in Patients with Acute Low Back Pain

Imaging Action and Clinical Situation	Suggestions for Initial Imaging
Immediate Imaging	
Radiography plus erythrocyte sedimentation rate*	Major risk factors for cancer (new onset of low back pain with history of cancer, multiple risk factors for cancer, or strong clinical suspicion for cancer)
Magnetic resonance imaging	Risk factors for spinal infection (new onset of low back pain with fever and history of intravenous drug use or recent infection)
	Risk factors for or signs of the cauda equina syndrome (new urine retention, fecal incontinence, or saddle anesthesia)
	Severe neurologic deficits (progressive motor weakness or motor deficits at multiple neurologic levels)
Defer Imaging after a Trial of Therapy	
Radiography with or without erythrocyte sedimentation rate	Weaker risk factors for cancer (unexplained with weight loss or age > 50 years)
	Risk factors for or signs of ankylosing spondylitis (morning stiffness that improves with exercise, alternating buttock pain, awakening because of back pain during the second part of the night, or younger age (20 to 40 years)
	Risk factors for vertebral compression fracture (history of osteoporosis, use of corticosteroids, significant trauma, or older age [> 65 years for women or > 75 years for men])
Magnetic resonance imaging	Signs and symptoms of radiculopathy (back pain with leg pain in an L4, L5, or S1 nerve root distribution or positive result on straight leg raise or crossed straight leg raise test) in patients who are candidates for surgery or epidural steroid injection
	Risk factors for or symptoms of spinal stenosis (radiating leg pain, older age, or pseudoclaudication) in patients who are candidates for surgery
No imaging	No criteria for immediate imaging and back pain improved or resolved after a 1-month trial of therapy
	Previous spinal imaging with no change in clinical status

*Consider magnetic resonance imaging if the initial imaging result is negative but a high degree of clinical suspicion for cancer remains.
Adapted from Chou R, Qaseem A, Owens DK, et al. Diagnostic imaging for low back pain: advice for high-value health care from the American College of Physicians. *Ann Intern Med*. 2011;154:181-189, Table 4.)

the spine pain patient, imaging should begin with upright, weight-bearing radiographs of the appropriate spine segment. The ACR and the ACP are consistent in their recommendations that patients with “red flag” features of recent trauma, osteoporosis, age greater than 70 years, or clinically suspected inflammatory spondyloarthropathy should initially undergo radiographs; advanced imaging should be reserved for patients with progressive neurologic deficits or a strong clinical suspicion of infection or neoplasm.[64-66] Radiographs provide a modest sensitivity screen for sinister conditions, establish spine enumeration, and when performed in physiologic positions allow assessment of sagittal and coronal plane balance.

Spine enumeration is a critical but underappreciated role of radiographs. The typical spine morphology of 24 mobile, presacral spine segments (7 cervical, 12 rib-bearing thoracic, and 5 lumbar type vertebral bodies) is not uniformly present; deviation can result in confusion in establishing the origin of pain syndromes, or wrong segment minimally invasive or surgical interventions. It can be reasonably assumed in the human species that there are 7 cervical vertebrae. There is considerable variation in the number and distribution of thoracic and lumbar segments that may be difficult to appreciate on MRI alone; radiographs can establish this enumeration and serve as the foundation for subsequent advanced imaging description.

In a study by Carrino and colleagues using complete spine radiographs, 91.8% of subjects had 24 presacral vertebral segments: 4.8% had 23 and 3.4% had 25.[70] Akbar and colleagues, using full spine sagittal MRI localizer images,

Box 15.1 Spine Imaging Principles

- The primary role of imaging is the identification of undiagnosed systemic disease.
- Spine imaging has a significant specificity fault: a high prevalence of asymptomatic age-related “degenerative” findings.
- Significance of imaging findings depends on concordance: the imager must know the pain/dysfunction syndrome.
- Spine imaging may be insensitive to dynamic lesions.
- No imaging is indicated in the acute presentation of back or limb pain in the absence of “red flag” features.
- The decision to undertake imaging must be a reasoned harms and risk/benefit judgment.
- Imaging correlates poorly with clinical presentation and course.

identified 23 presacral segments in 3.3% of subjects and 25 in 3.3%; these anomalies of spine enumeration were not mentioned in the radiology report in nearly 70% of cases.[71] In Carrino’s study, if one considers both anomalous number and distribution (e.g., 13 rib-bearing vertebrae + 4 lumbar type vertebrae) of thoracolumbar spine segments, 10.9% of subjects have nonclassical anatomy.[70] For the spine interventionalist, this implies these situations are in the procedure room regularly; failure of recognition virtually guarantees wrong segment procedures.

Anomalous segmentation is predicted by the presence of transitional thoracolumbar or lumbosacral vertebral bodies,

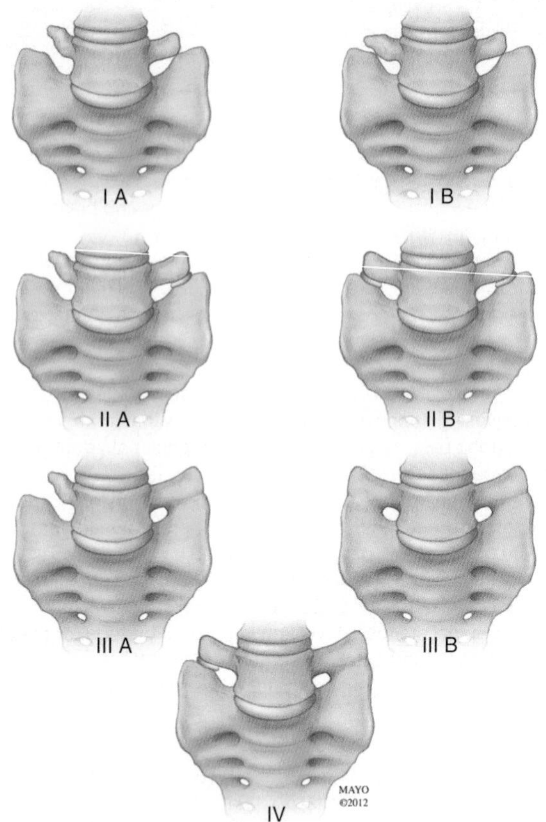

Figure 15.2 Castellvi classification of lumbosacral transitional segments.

which may be a source of confusion in their own right. Thoracolumbar transitional segments have hypoplastic ribs at the lowest rib-bearing segment; they were present in 4.1% of subjects in Carrino's study.[70] Lumbosacral transitional segments have characteristics of both the L5 lumbar body and the superior sacral segment; their described prevalence ranges from 4% to 30%.[72] The Castellvi classification (Fig. 15.2) describes the morphologic types, ranging from an expanded (height > 19 mm) dysplastic transverse process (type I), through a pseudoarticulation between the transverse process and sacral ala (type II), to osseous fusion between the transverse process and the sacrum (type III).[73] Type IV denotes the presence of a type II transition on one side and a type III on the other. Unilateral (a) and bilateral (b) subtypes are also described. On lateral radiographs or sagittal MRI images, a transitional segment can be suggested in the presence of a perceived narrow S1-S2 disk, which extends for the entire anterior-posterior (AP) width of the sacral body with parallel end plates and a squared upper sacral segment (Fig. 15. 3).[72] The presence of a transitional lumbosacral segment increased by sevenfold the likelihood of an anomalous number of presacral segments. In patients with radicular pain syndromes and lumbosacral transitional anatomy, the pain practitioner must also be aware of the possibility of an extraforaminal nerve entrapment between the enlarged transverse process and sacral ala.

Correlation of pain syndromes with imaging findings can be confounded in patients with transitional anatomy or anomalous segmentation. It is best to consider that, in general, radicular innervation patterns remain relatively constant when counted caudally from the skull base, but the skeletal anatomy may change about them. For example, the 26th nerve (8 cervical nerves, 12 thoracic, 5 lumbar, 1st sacral nerve) from the skull base most commonly innervates the medial head of the gastrocnemius and the soleus muscles, the basis of the S1 radicular pain pattern. In a patient with 25 presacral vertebral segments, this may exit under the pedicle of the lowest lumbar type vertebral body, creating confusion for the unwary practitioner (Fig. 15.4). There is also variation in typical innervation patterns in the presence of transitional anatomy, which may introduce further localization challenges. Only meticulous attention to spine enumeration, best provided by plain radiographs, sometimes supplemented by total spine MRI localizer images, will protect the spine pain patient and interventionalist from wrong segment invasive procedures (Box 15.2).

When radiographs are obtained, they should be upright, weight-bearing images. Only in a physiologic posture can one assess sagittal and coronal balance (Fig. 15.5). Upright radiographs demonstrate more thoracic kyphosis and lumbar lordosis than do recumbent images.[74] Weight-bearing images may also demonstrate instability, most commonly L4-L5 degenerative spondylolisthesis, which would be occult on recumbent films.[75] In spinal deformity patients, the exacerbation of spinal curves with weight bearing can be dramatic. Flexion-extension radiographs in the lumbar or cervical spine are not indicated as part of an initial imaging investigation. There is no role for oblique radiographs of the spine; in the lumbar region they double the gonadal dose and do not provide useful information that will affect clinical decision making.[75] Cervical spine oblique views similarly serve only to irradiate sensitive tissue (thyroid, lens of the eye) without clinical benefit.

ADVANCED IMAGING MODALITIES

When radiographs are not explanatory of an unremitting pain syndrome or suggest underlying systemic disease, advanced imaging (CT, MRI, nuclear medicine) may be obtained. CT has undergone a revolution since the early 2000s with the advancement of multidetector technology. A data set for the lumbar spine can now be obtained in a few seconds, eliminating motion artifact and dramatically improving patient tolerance. This data set can then be reconstructed in any plane without a loss of spatial resolution or additional radiation exposure. CT provides superior imaging of cortical and trabecular bone when compared with MRI. For this reason, CT may be necessary to characterize primary bone tumors of the spine. CT also provides reasonable contrast resolution and can identify root compressive lesions such as disk herniations or characterize central canal, lateral recess, and foraminal compromise in the majority of cases. CT cannot identify intrathecal pathology and is less sensitive than MRI in the detection of early inflammatory or infectious processes, neoplasm, or paraspinal soft tissue lesions. Radiation dose must always be considered when employing CT, particularly in young patients or in serial studies. One by-product of the rapid technological advance of CT is that the literature contains no comparative studies between MRI and the latest generation of multidetector CT scanners in the detection and characterization of disk herniations.

MRI has been the dominant spine imaging modality since the 1990s, despite modest technological advancement

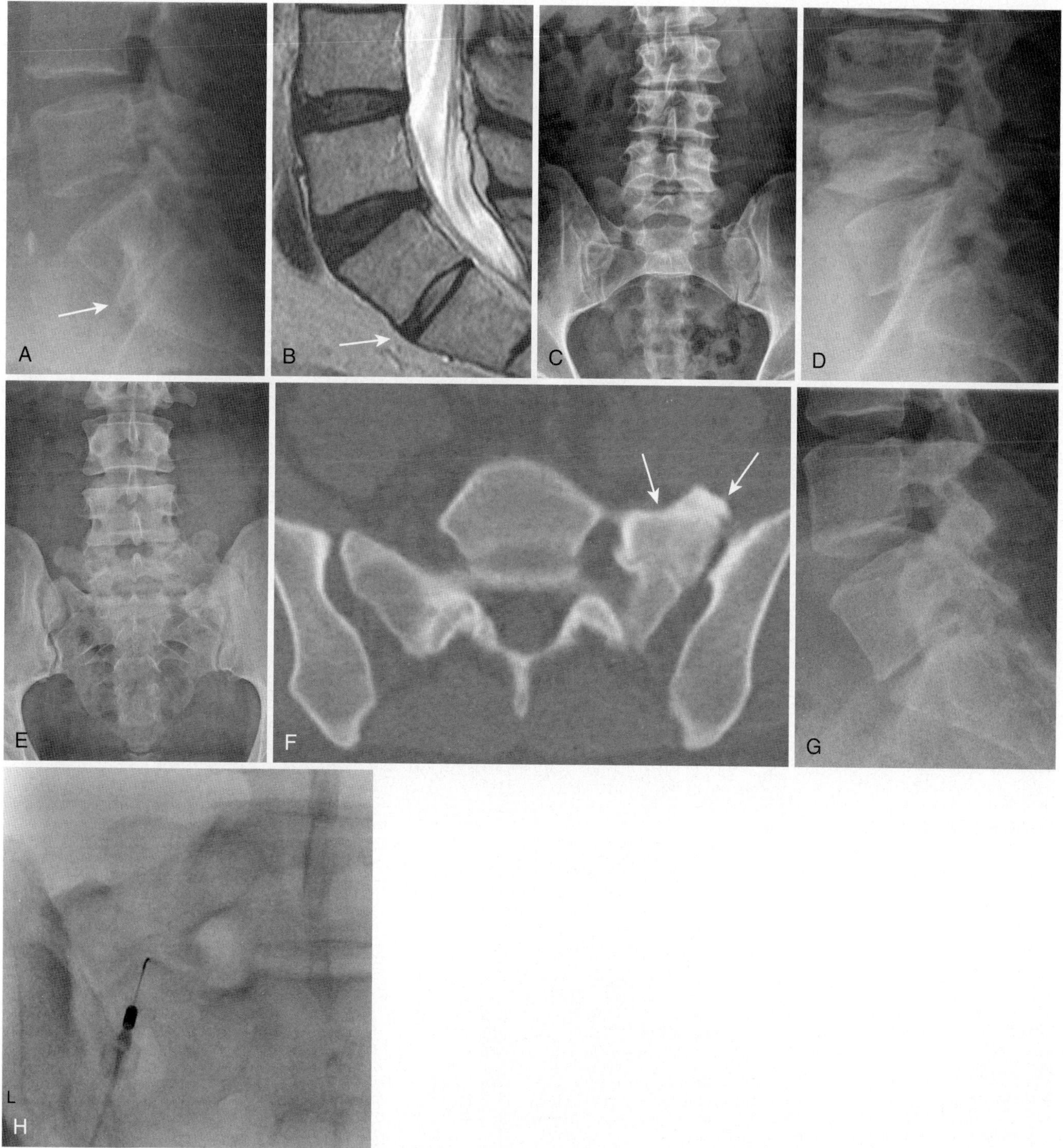

Figure 15.3 Transitional segments. Lateral radiograph **(A)** and sagittal T2 MRI image **(B)** demonstrate typical findings of a transitional segment interspace *(arrows):* a narrow disk space with parallel end plates and normal T2 signal intensity. Castellvi IIa transitional segment is demonstrated in frontal **(C)** and lateral **(D)** radiographs. Note right pseudoarticulation. In another patient, frontal radiograph **(E)** shows a left-sided pseudoarticulation, also seen on the axial CT image (*arrows* in **[F]**). Narrow, parallel end plates are visible in the transitional interspace on the lateral radiograph **(G)**. This patient had axial pain attributed to the pseudoarticulation; this was injected **(H)** with relief of the index pain.

in the realm of spine imaging in that time span. MRI has superior contrast resolution and thus the ability to distinguish between soft tissue types, allowing it to detect intrathecal pathology and identify subtle root compressive lesions. MRI has superior sensitivity in the detection of neoplasm and infection. With the use of gadolinium contrast, or heavily T2-weighted imaging sequences (short-tau inversion recovery [STIR] or fast spin echo T2 sequences with fat saturation), MRI can detect the physiologic parameters of edema, hyperemia, and inflammatory change. It has greater specificity than CT in characterizing the chronicity of fractures. With gadolinium enhancement, MRI can distinguish between recurrent disk herniation and scarring in the post-operative patient. MRI does not evaluate cortical bone well. Patient acceptance remains problematic because of prolonged imaging times and up to 10% examination failures caused by claustrophobia. Open magnets have improved patient acceptance, but at the cost of image quality. A small percentage of patients are MRI incompatible due to pacemakers, spinal cord stimulators, or other implanted devices. MRI remains costly. The sensitivity challenges imposed by recumbent MRI imaging were discussed earlier; the hope is that the engineering challenges of high field strength, weight-bearing MRI imaging will be met in the near future.

CT myelography retains a problem-solving role in the lumbar spine; it will substitute for MRI in the incompatible patient. CT myelography has superior spatial resolution when compared with MRI but lacks its soft tissue contrast resolution. It can provide an exquisite demonstration of root compressive lesions and central canal, lateral recess, and foraminal compromise. In the cervical spine, the superior spatial resolution of CT myelography and its ability to discriminate between bone and soft tissue compressive lesions give it a continuing role. CT myelography is minimally invasive, expensive, operator dependent to a degree, and also requires current CT technology to be maximally useful.

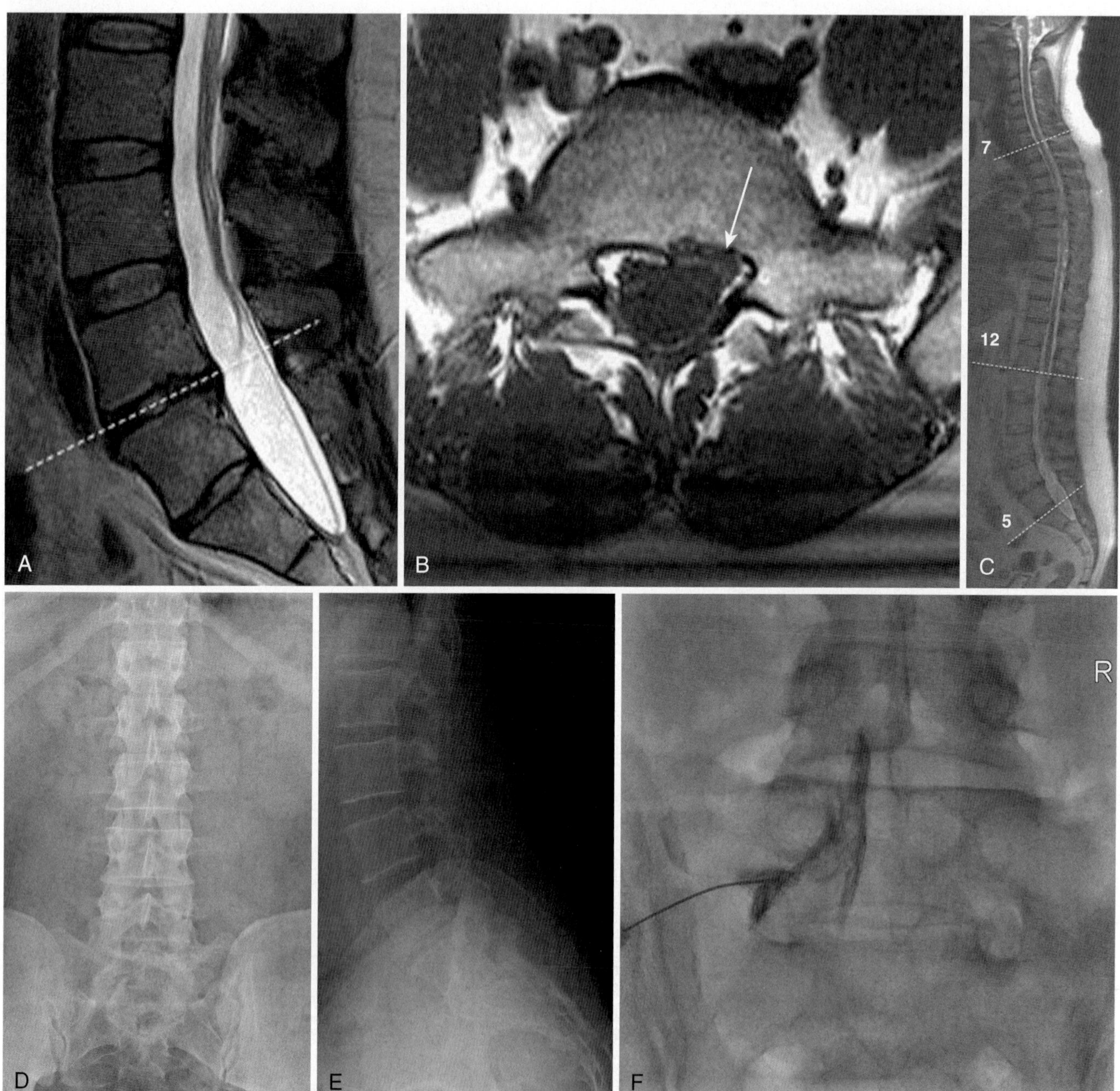

Figure 15.4 The importance of segmental enumeration. This 36-year-old male who has failed conservative care presents with a left-sided L5 radicular pain pattern involving the lateral thigh, lateral calf, and dorsum of the foot. His MRI (sagittal T2 **[A]** and axial T1 **[B]** at level of dotted line) shows a subtle disk extrusion in the left lateral recess (*arrow* in **[B]**) at the penultimate interspace. The lowest-most disk appears transitional. MRI scout **(C)** image demonstrates 24 presacral segments. Frontal and lateral radiographs (**D** and **E**) may suggest 5 lumbar vertebrae on cursory examination; careful counting at fluoroscopy noted 11 rib-bearing vertebrae. T12 has no ribs and L5 is transitional, Castellvi type 4. The transforaminal epidural steroid injection (**F** and **G**) was performed under the pedicle bearing the dysplastic left T5 transverse process and relieved the patient's pain.

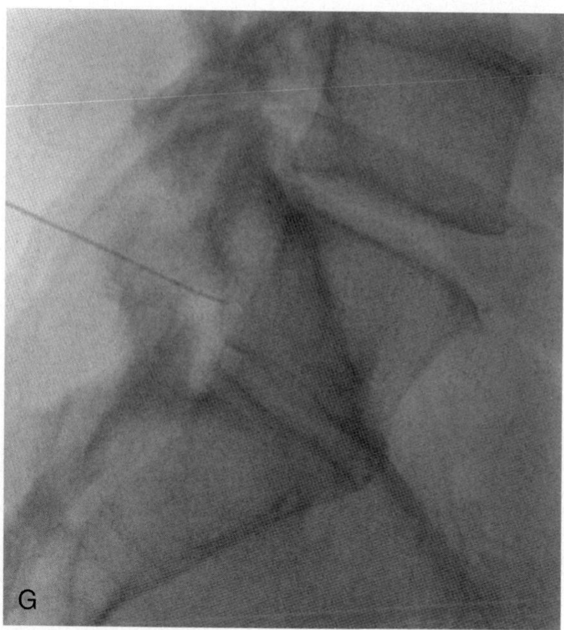

Figure 15.4, cont'd Note **(G)** the typical appearance of a transitional disk space. Careful enumeration of every case is the only way to avoid wrong segment interventions.

Box 15.2 Spine Enumeration

- Approximately 11% of subjects will have anomalies of number or distribution of thoracolumbar vertebral bodies.
- Anomalous segmentation is predicted by the presence of transitional thoracolumbar or lumbosacral vertebral bodies.
- Ideally, vertebral numbering should occur from the skull base caudally.
- Practically, the human cervical spine is homologous and can be assumed to have seven segments.
- T1 is marked by the first upward inclined transverse process.
- Meticulous enumeration on every case will prevent wrong segment procedures.

Cone-beam CT, weight-bearing myelography holds promise for assessing position-dependent pain syndromes, at least in part defeating the sensitivity fault of recumbent advanced imaging. In this technology, arising from rotational angiography roots, the C-arm rapidly rotates about the standing patient who has had contrast introduced into the thecal sac. A flat panel fluoroscopy detector gathers a data set that can be reconstructed in any plane. Soft tissue contrast does not approach that of true CT, and the longitudinal field of view is limited to the length of the flat panel detector. Despite these limitations, the high inherent contrast among intrathecal contrast, the soft tissue structures of the spinal column, and bone allows for a very good depiction of central canal, lateral recess, and foraminal compromise. This technology will only improve (Fig. 15.6).

Nuclear medicine studies are growing in importance in spine imaging. Technetium pyrophosphate bone scans detect increased blood flow and accelerated bone metabolic activity. With the addition of SPECT and SPECT/CT image fusion, significant additional spatial localization of hyperemia and increased metabolic activity are possible. This imaging is traditionally useful in assessing the burden of metastatic disease but can also be valuable in assessing non-neoplastic inflammatory states such as spondylolysis. SPECT/CT can potentially identify inflammatory synovitis in the facet and sacroiliac joints, which might guide interventions. However, validation studies of these techniques against accepted reference standards such as comparative blocks in the facet joints or intra-articular sacroiliac blocks have not yet been done. When MRI is not technically feasible, technetium bone scanning can be used to characterize the chronicity of vertebral fractures in selecting patients for bone augmentation. The technetium bone scan, in combination with gallium scan, offers sensitivity equal to MRI in the detection of spondylodiscitis. However, these techniques provide less anatomic information and MRI may ultimately be necessary to characterize the degree of central canal compromise that may influence surgical decision making. PET or PET/CT scans have an increasing role in assessing the burden of metastatic disease and in selecting lesions for percutaneous biopsy.

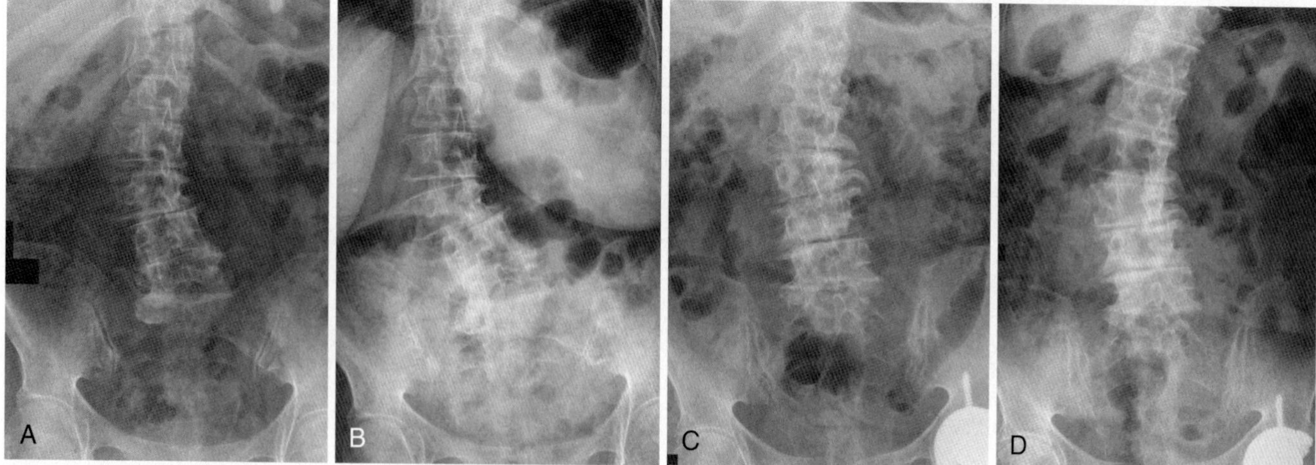

Figure 15.5 The effect of upright weight-bearing radiographs on balance and deformity. Recumbent radiograph **(A)** shows lumbar scoliosis with a rotatory component, which is significantly exacerbated in a subsequent upright radiograph **(B)**. In another patient, the recumbent radiograph **(C)** underestimates the true scoliotic curve seen on an upright radiograph **(D)**. Sagittal and coronal balance can only be assessed on upright, weight-bearing imaging.

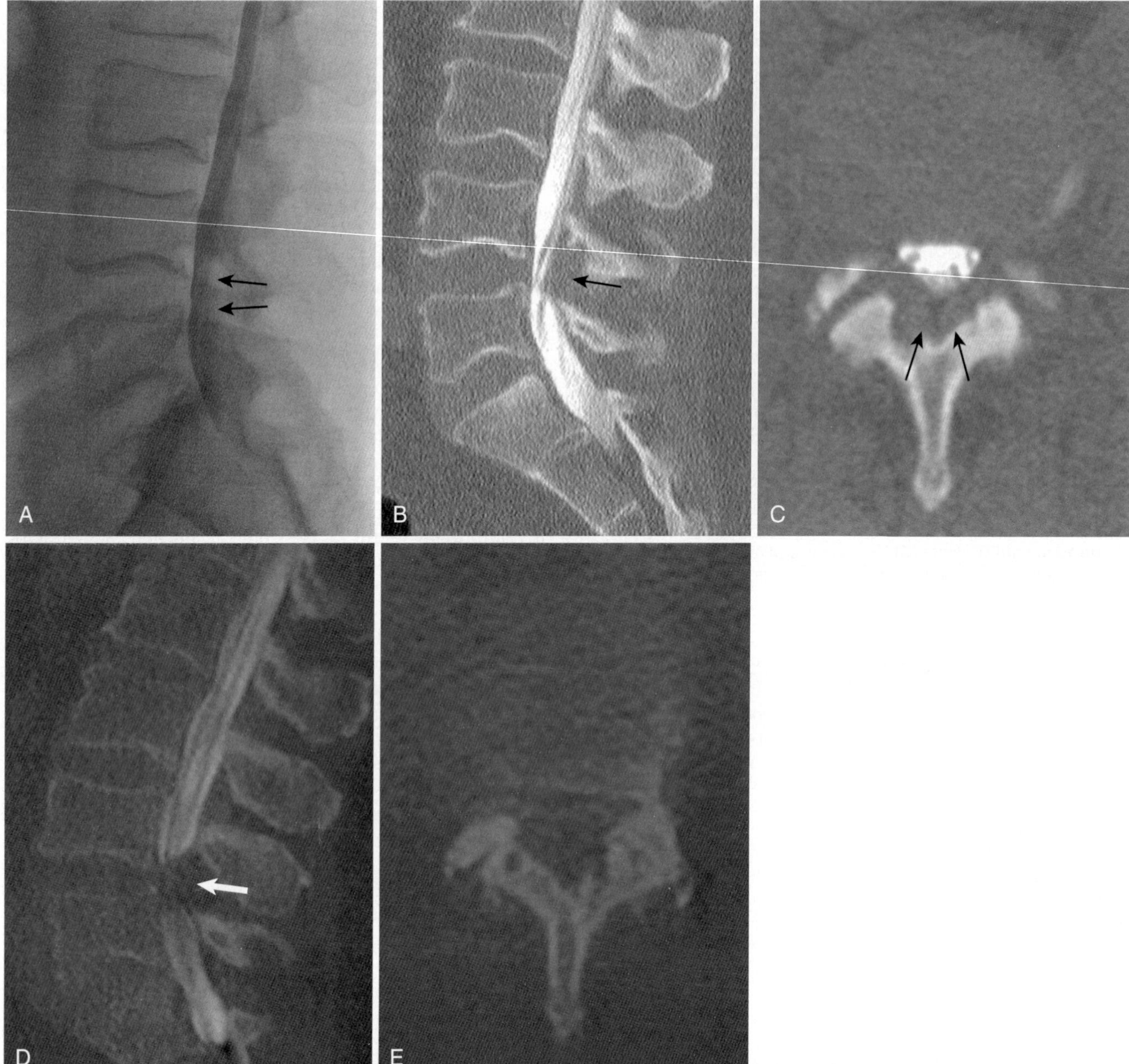

Figure 15.6 Ligamentum flavum redundancy (buckling) on upright myelography (cone beam CT). A 66-year-old man imaged for neurogenic intermittent claudication. Conventional myelogram in the lateral plane with the patient in the prone position **(A)** and postmyelogram sagittal **(B)** and axial CT at L4-5 interspace **(C)** with the patient in the prone position show minimal redundancy of the ligamentum flavum *(black arrows)* and mild central canal compromise at the L4-5 level. Cone beam CT myelography with the patient in an upright position demonstrates a marked increase in ligamentous buckling *(white arrow)* on the sagittal reconstruction **(D)** and complete effacement of the thecal sac on the axial reconstruction **(E)**. (Courtesy of Kent Thielen, MD, Mayo Clinic, Rochester, MN.)

IMAGING OF AXIAL PAIN GENERATORS

Axial pain that may have an imaging correlate derives primarily from stimulation of nociception of the spinal articulations: the intervertebral disk, the zygapophysial or facet joints, and the sacroiliac joint. More broadly, it may include pain originating from the muscular or ligamentous structures in the supporting architecture of the spine. Axial pain is clinically characterized as constant, dull, deep, poorly localized, and aching, located primarily in the paraspinous region with inconstant referral to the proximal extremities. This is in distinction to the neuropathic pain of radicular character, which is typically sharp, electric, lancinating, and experienced in a bandlike distribution into the more distal extremities. The prevalence of axial spine pain generators has been well described by Depalma (Table 15.4).[76,77] Intervertebral disk disruption (IDD) was the most common axial pain generator in this series, followed by the facet joint, the sacroiliac joint, and insufficiency fractures of the spine or pelvis. This work also emphasized the age dependence of these pain sources. Patients with diskogenic pain (IDD) were significantly

Table 15.4 Prevalence of Sources of Axial Low Back Pain, Age Correlation

Pain Source	Prevalence (%)	Mean Age (Std Dev)
Intervertebral disk disruption (IDD)	41.8	43.7 (10.3)
Facet joint	30.6	59.6 (13.1)
Sacroiliac joint	18.2	61.4 (17.7)
Vertebral insufficiency fracture	2.9	79 (11.8)
Pelvic insufficiency fracture	1.8	71.3 (11.7)
Baastrup's disease	1.8	75.3 (4.7)
Fusion hardware	2.9	59.6 (19.4)

Data from DePalma MJ, Ketchum JM, Saullo T. What is the source of chronic low back pain and does age play a role? *Pain Med.* 2011;12:224-233.

younger than patients with facet or sacroiliac joint pain. As age increased, the probability of IDD as a pain source decreased and the probability of facet or sacroiliac pain increased, up to approximately age 70.[76] A later multivariable analysis also showed a gender relationship, with IDD more prevalent in young men.[78] This echoes the earlier work of Schwarzer, who demonstrated that lumbar facet–mediated pain was uncommon in a population of young workers (~15%) but more highly prevalent in an aged population (~32%).[79,80]

IMAGING CORRELATES OF DISKOGENIC PAIN

The imaging diagnosis of diskogenic pain is made challenging by the lack of a pathoanatomic gold standard against which to assess imaging parameters. It is not possible to evaluate a disk, either at surgery or upon histologic examination, and deem it painful. The current most stringent reference standard for the diagnosis of diskogenic pain is manometrically controlled provocation diskography with normal control levels as documented in the practice guidelines of the International Spine Intervention Society (ISIS).[81]

It is important to observe, however, that examination of the same body of evidence regarding the validity of diskography as the reference standard has resulted in diametrically opposed recommendations regarding its use by different physician societies. The ISIS,[81] the North American Spine Society,[82] and the International Association for the Study of Pain[83] accept diskography as a useful diagnostic tool in back pain patients and recommend its use. The American Pain Society rejects diskography as a diagnostically useful test.[84] A comprehensive review of diskography in the journal of the American Society of Regional Anesthesia and Pain Medicine notes that whereas CT diskography is the gold standard for the assessment of structural disk alteration, there is no convincing evidence that the use of diskography as a selection tool improves surgical outcomes.[85] Any analysis of imaging findings in diskogenic pain patients thus remains based on a reference standard (provocation diskography) that is ultimately unproved against a pathoanatomic gold standard. This is further confounded by evolution of the criteria for a positive diskogram since the 1990s. For the purposes of this discussion, only concordant pain responses were considered to represent a positive diskogram. A significant concordant pain response without a specification of pain intensity or the use of manometry is defined as a Walsh criterion.[86] Inclusion of the requirement for a normal control disk elevates the criteria to that of the International Association for the Study of Pain (IASP).[83] None of the studies reviewed here meaningfully used manometric control or met the ISIS criteria for positive diskography.[81]

Although challenging, there is motivation to make the diagnosis of diskogenic pain via noninvasive imaging. Diskography has until recently been considered a minimally invasive and nondestructive test. There is now in vitro and in vivo evidence suggesting that disk puncture or diskography may contribute to disk dysfunction. Korecki and colleagues[87] noted that in a bovine disk model, single punctures with a 25-gauge needle resulted in biomechanical degradation of disk function with cyclic loading. Carragee and coworkers[88] demonstrated on 10-year follow-up MR imaging that asymptomatic subjects who had undergone investigational diskography showed more degenerative phenomena than did matched control subjects. Although the clinical significance of these observations remains uncertain, noninvasive diagnosis is desirable.

The specificity fault inherent in spine imaging was previously discussed: manifestations of disk "degeneration" are ubiquitous, usually asymptomatic, and primarily represent normal age change. In a population of symptomatic patients with suspected diskogenic pain, however, are there imaging findings that correlate with positive provocation diskography? The findings evaluated in the literature include (1) loss of disk space height, (2) generalized alterations in T2 signal within the disk, (3) alterations of disk contour, (4) Modic end plate marrow changes, and (5) the presence of high intensity zones (HIZ) or fissures within the posterior disk annulus. These imaging features are examined initially as independent variables with subsequent discussion of the more limited literature in which they are combined in a multivariate analysis. A significant portion of the presented data were drawn from a systematic review of imaging and clinical markers of axial pain generators in the lumbar spine performed by Hancock and colleagues.[89] Additional studies not included in that report or published subsequent to it have been added.[90] A common set of measures was compiled from the many studies: sensitivity, specificity, positive predictive value (PPV), negative predictive value (NPV), and likelihood ratios (LRs). When imaging features were quantified (T2 signal loss in the disk was reported as normal, moderate, or severe), a threshold was used. Original data were combined and recalculated to reflect setting a detection threshold as moderate (including moderate and severe cases) or severe only. Because the diagnosis of diskogenic pain may provoke therapeutic interventions (most of which carry risk and have unproved efficacy), emphasis was placed on those measurements that inform about false-positive results: specificity (true negatives/ true negatives + false positives) and PPV (true positives/true positives + false positives).

Table 15.5 T2 Signal Loss as a Predictor of Positive Provocation Diskography

Author (ref), Date	Diskogram Criteria	T2 Signal Criteria	Prevalence	Sensitivity	Specificity	PPV	NPV	+LR (CI)	–LR (CI)
Osti (95) 1992	Walsh	Moderate + Severe	47%	70%	64%	50%	80%	1.9 (1.3-2.7)	0.49 (0.3-0.8)
		Severe only	13%	23%	92%	60%	70%	2.8 (1.1-7)	0.83 (0.7-1)
Horton(96) 1992	Walsh	Moderate + Severe	69%	95%	43%	44%	94%	1.6 (1.2-2.2)	0.18 (0.04-0.9)
		Severe only	20%	37%	88%	58%	74%	2.8 (1.1-7.3)	0.72 (0.5-1)
Ito (91) 1998	Walsh	Moderate + Severe	63%	96%	46%	34%	97%	1.7 (1.4-2.2)	0.14 (0.03-0.6)
		Severe only	25%	70%	89%	64%	91%	5.7 (3-11)	0.36 (0.2-0.7)
Weishaupt (97) 2001	IASP	3-5 of 5-grade Pearce	65%	98%	59%	64%	98%	2.3 (1.8-3.1)	0.05 (0.01-0.3)
Lim (92) 2005	Walsh	4 and 5 of 5-grade Pearce	62%	88%	52%	50%	89%	1.8 (1.4-2.4)	0.25 (0.1-0.6)
Lei (98) 2008	IASP	3 and 4 of 4-point Woodward	57%	94%	77%	78%	94%	4 (2.5-6.4)	0.07 (0.02-0.2)
O'Neill (93) 2008	IASP	Moderate + Severe	62%	90%	67%	75%	86%	2.7 (2.2-3.3)	0.16 (0.1-0.2)
		Severe only	15%	24%	96%	87%	54%	6 (3-11.7)	0.79 (0.7-0.9)
Kang (94) 2009	IASP	3, 4, and 5 on Pfirrmann 5-point scale	70%	95%	39%	34%	96%	1.6 (1.3-1.8)	0.12 (0.03-0.5)

PPV, positive predictive value; NPV, negative predictive value; LR, likelihood ratio; IASP, International Association for the Study of Pain.
From Maus TP, Martin DP. Imaging for discogenic pain. In: Kapural L, Kim P, Deer T, eds. *Diagnosis, Management, and Treatment of Discogenic Pain.* Philadelphia: Elsevier/Saunders; 2012, p 38, Table 3-5.)

DISKOGENIC PAIN

LOSS OF DISK SPACE HEIGHT

The reports of Ito and colleagues,[91] Lim and colleagues[92] and O'Neill and colleagues[93] studied loss of disk space height as an imaging finding that may correlate with positive provocation diskography. The studies of Ito and colleagues and O'Neill and colleagues both suggest that in a population of symptomatic patients with axial pain considered diskogenic in nature, severe disk space narrowing, although an uncommon imaging finding (approximately 10%), is strongly predictive of a painful disk. Specificity of this finding was at least 97% in these studies with PPVs of 78% and 90%, respectively. Lim's study was less supportive. It is reasonable to conclude that in a patient with suspected diskogenic pain undergoing provocation diskography, severe loss of disk space height is a strong predictor of a positive diskogram.

NUCLEAR T2 SIGNAL LOSS

Studies addressing the correlation between MR imaging evidence of disk "degeneration," primarily nuclear T2 signal loss, and diskogenic pain reach back to the 1990s.[91-98] The challenges in this analysis are well illustrated in Table 15.5.[91-100] Although disk "degeneration" definitions are inconsistent, original data have been recalculated into threshold values to provide a reasonable basis of comparison. The changes in diskography criteria over time are also noted. Despite these shortcomings, conclusions can be reasonably drawn. The NPV of disks of normal nuclear signal is uniformly high and –LRs are highly informative; disks of normal nuclear signal are rarely painful. Severe, uniform loss of T2 signal, with or without loss of disk space height, is a finding of high specificity (88% to 96% in studies using a three-part classification system) with strongly informative +LR. Disks with severe T2 signal loss are rarely nonpainful. The utility of this finding is reduced by its low prevalence (it is found in 13% to 25% of disks undergoing diskography) and low sensitivity (23%, 24%, 37%, and 70% in the studies with a three-part classification system). Disks with intermediate signal loss may be painful but with less certainty (Fig. 15.7).

DISK CONTOUR ABNORMALITY

The studies of O'Neill and colleagues[92] and Kang and colleagues[93] included data correlating disk contour abnormalities and diskography. Both studies showed a statistically significant correlation of disk contour abnormality with positive provocation diskography. In O'Neill and colleagues' study, a disk bulge was the contour abnormality most predictive of a positive diskogram, with a +LR of 5.3.

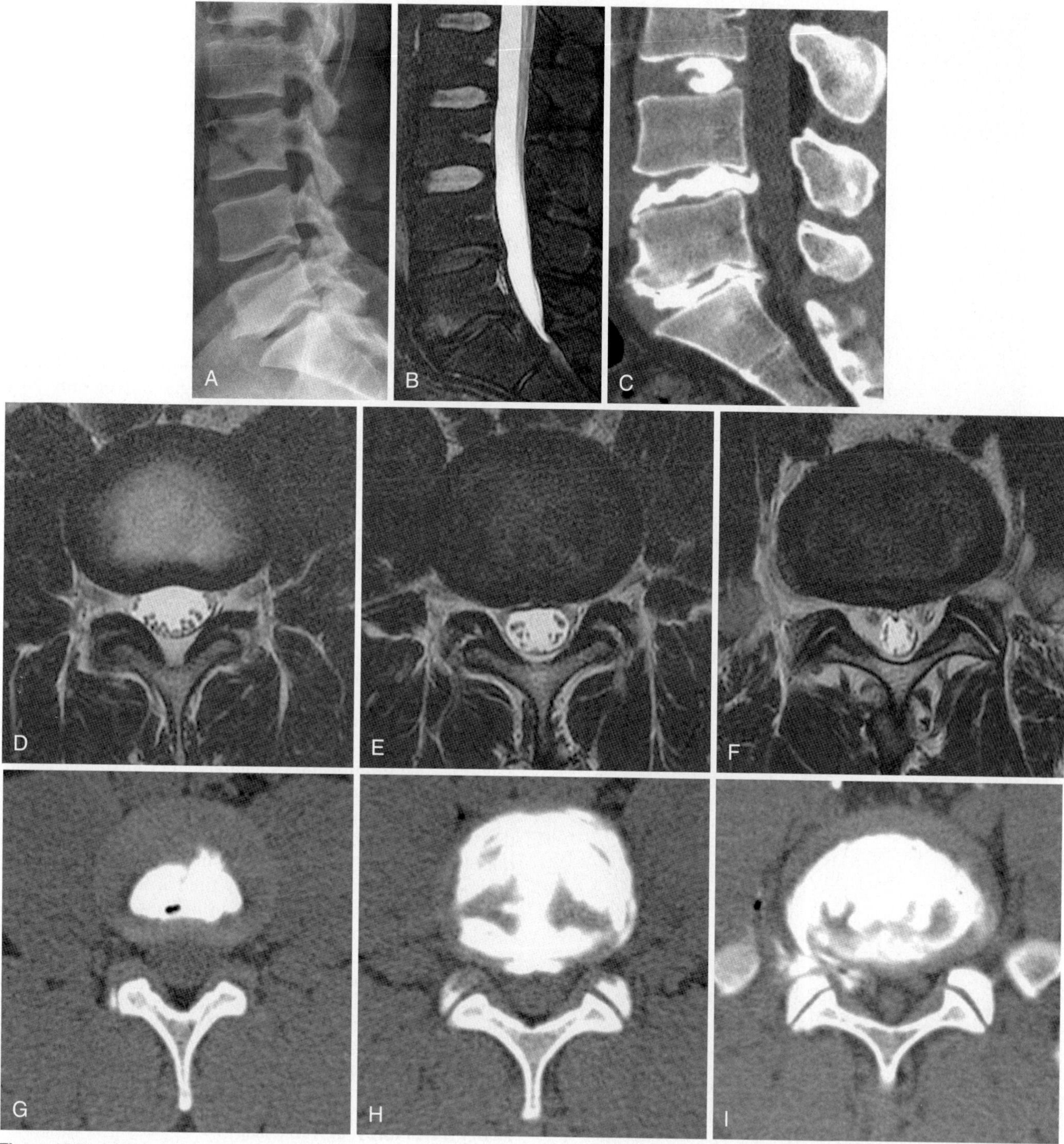

Figure 15.7 Disk height and nuclear T2 signal loss. Lateral radiograph **(A)** of a 50-year-old male with intractable axial pain. Note loss of height of lumbosacral disk, which contains gas. There is slight retrolisthesis of L4 on L5 and L5 on S1. Sagittal fat-saturated T2-weighted MRI **(B)** shows loss of T2 signal in the L4-5 and L5-S1 disks; normal upper lumbar disks. Axial T2-weighted images at L3-4 **(C)**, L4-5 **(D)**, and L5-S1 **(E)** demonstrate normal L3-4 disk, loss of T2 signal in L4-5 with a small central herniation, and a broad bulge at L5-S1. Sagittal CT diskogram **(F)** and axial images at L3-4 **(G)**, L4-5 (**H,** and L5-S1 **(I)** shows normal L3-4 disk, Grade IV annular disruption at L4-5 and L5-S1 with leak of contrast from the right posterolateral annulus at L5-S1. Patient had concordant axial pain at L4-5 and L5-S1 with a normal control disk at L3-4. (From Maus TP, Aprill CN. Lumbar discogenic pain, provocation diskography, and imaging correlates. *Radiol Clin North Am.* 2012;50:681-704.)

MODIC END PLATE CHANGES

The functional unity of the disk and the cartilaginous end plate is manifest in signal changes within the end plate and adjacent subchondral marrow that accompany nuclear matrix degradation. End plate marrow changes were originally classified by Modic in 1988 (Fig. 15.8).[101] Type I change represents ingrowth of vascularized granulation tissue into sub–end plate marrow; it exhibits a hypointense T1 and hyperintense T2 signal on MRI and may enhance with gadolinium. Type II change exhibits elevated T1 and T2

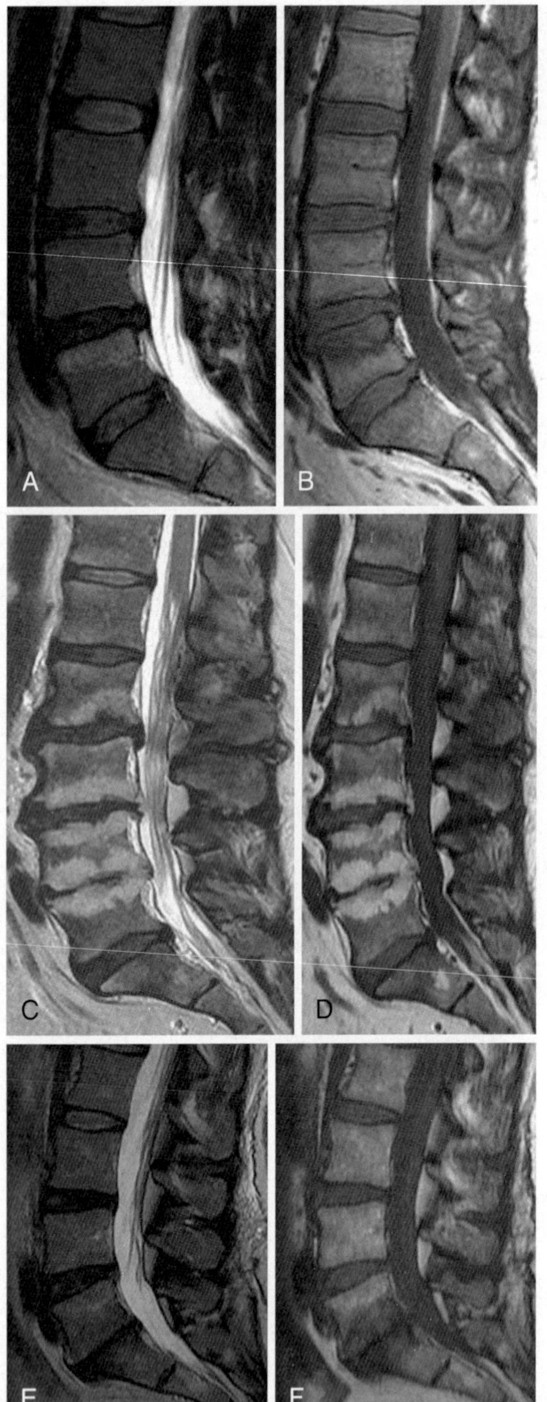

Figure 15.8 Modic end-plate changes. Modic I Sagittal T2 **(A)** and T1 **(B)** images demonstrate elevated T2 and diminished T1 signal involving the superior half of the L5 vertebral body. The histologic correlate of Modic I is vascularized granulation tissue. There are disk herniations at the L3-4 and L4-5 disks.

Modic II Sagittal T2 **(C)** and T1 **(D)** images reveal elevated T1 and T2 signal in the sub–end plate marrow involving L2-L5. The histologic correlate of Modic II is fatty infiltration.

Modic III Sagittal T2 **(E)** and T1 **(F)** images show diminished T2 and T1 signal in the sub–end plate marrow about the L5 interspace. The histologic correlate of Modic III is sclerotic bone.

signal and reflects fatty infiltration of sub–end plate marrow. Type III change is hypointense on T1 and T2; it correlates with bony sclerosis. Type I change is thought to represent an active inflammatory state, with type II more quiescent and type III post-inflammatory. Ohtori and colleagues[102] noted elevated levels of protein gene product 9.5–immunoreactive nerve fibers and TNF-α immunoreactive cells in the cartilaginous end plates of patients with Modic changes. The immunoreactive nerve ingrowth was noted exclusively in patients with diskogenic low back pain. TNF-α immunoreactive cells were more common in type I end plate changes.

Modic end plate changes do carry an association with low back pain, particularly type I change. Toyone and colleagues[103] found that 73% of patients with type I change had low back pain as opposed to 11% of type II patients. Likewise, Albert and Manniche[104] reported low back pain in 60% of patients with Modic changes but in only 20% of those without Modic changes. Type I change was more strongly associated with low back pain than type II change. Modic type I change may also be associated with segmental instability. Persistent type I change after fusion surgery raises concern for pseudarthrosis; patients with solid fusions more likely have either persistent type II change or resolution of all marrow abnormality.

The data in Table 15.6[91-94,97,98,105,106] describe Modic-type end plate changes as predictors of diskogenic pain. The studies discussed previously suggested that type I Modic change would be more strongly correlated with positive provocation diskography than type II; that conclusion is not borne out by the data, which suggest that either type I or type II Modic change correlates with positive diskography, although not uniformly. The studies of Braithwaite and colleagues,[105] Weishaupt and colleagues,[97] Lei and colleagues,[98] and O'Neill and colleagues[93] had few false-positive results (i.e., disks with adjacent type I or type II end plate changes that were nonpainful). The specificity, PPV, and +LRs in these studies were high. The usefulness of the MR imaging findings were only hampered by their infrequency. Other studies were less supportive but may be confounded by technical flaws. The compelling results presented by Weishaupt and colleagues[97] suggest a significant threshold for marrow change; with a threshold at 25% of vertebral body height, there were no false-positive results in this series. A reasonable conclusion is that Modic type I or II marrow change of this severity (25% of vertebral height) is an infrequent but highly specific finding, with a high PPV for diskogenic pain.

HIGH INTENSITY ZONE (HIZ)

In 1992, Aprill and Bogduk described the HIZ as an imaging marker of a painful disk at provocation diskography.[107] Their definition of the HIZ is a

high-intensity signal (bright white) located in the substance of the posterior annulus fibrosis, clearly dissociated from the signal of the nucleus pulposis in that it is surrounded superiorly, inferiorly, posteriorly and anteriorly by the low intensity (black) signal of the annulus fibrosis and is appreciably brighter than that of the nucleus pulposis. Page 362

This finding was identified on a midsagittal T2-weighted image; it may occur centrally in an otherwise normal

Table 15.6 End Plate (Modic) Change as a Predictor of Positive Provocation Diskography

Author (reference), Date	Diskogram Criteria	Modic Type	Prevalence per Disk	Sensitivity	Specificity	PPV	NPV	+LR	-LR
Braithwaite (105) 1998	Walsh	I + II	25% imaged 15% tested	24%	96%	91%	47%	6 (1.7-21.2)	0.80 (0.7-0.9)
		I	4% tested	5%	100%	100%	42%	7.4 (0.4-131)	0.95 (0.9-1)
		II	12% tested	18%	96%	89%	48%	4.4 (1.2-16.1)	0.86 (0.8-0.9)
Ito (91) 1998	Walsh	I + II + III	9%	23%	94%	56%	80%	4 (1.3-12.8)	0.82 (0.7-1)
Weishaupt (97) 2001	IASP	I	14%	29%	97%	88%	66%	9.9 (2.4-41.6)	0.73 (0.6-0.9)
		II	9%	19%	99%	90%	63%	12.75 (1.7-97.3)	0.83 (0.7-0.9)
		I + II	22%	48%	96%	88%	72%	10.86 (3.5-34.1)	0.55 (0.4-0.7)
		I + II Mod + Severe	16%	38%	100%	100%	69%	52.1 (3.2-844)	0.63 (0.5-0.8)
Kokkonen (106) 2002	Walsh	I	17%	19%	85%	41%	65%	1.25 (0.5-3)	0.96 (0.8-1.2
		II	19%	19%	80%	35%	64%	0.96 (0.4-2.2)	1 (0.8-1.2)
		I + II	36%	38%	65%	38%	65%	1.1 (0.6-1.8)	0.95 (0.7-1.3)
Lim (92) 2005	Walsh	I + II	14%	9%	83%	21%	62%	0.6 (0.2-1.7)	1.1 (0.9-1.3)
Lei (98) 2008	IASP	I + II	14%	32%	98%	94%	62%	19.25 (2.7-140)	0.69 (0.6-0.8)
O'Neill (93) 2008	IASP	I	4%	6%	99%	88%	49%	6.94 (1.6-29.9)	0.95 (0.9-1)
		II	4%	7%	99%	90%	50%	8.32 (1.9-35.5)	0.93 (0.9-1)
		I + II	8%	14%	98%	89%	51%	7.63 (2.8-21.2)	0.88 (0.8-0.9)
Kang (94) 2009	IASP	I + II	13%	14%	87%	26%	76%	1.08 (0.5-2.6)	0.99 (0.9-1.1)

PPV, positive predictive value; NPV, negative predictive value; LR, likelihood ratio; IASP, International Association for the Study of Pain.
From Maus TP, Martin DP. Imaging for discogenic pain. In: Kapural L, Kim P, Deer T, eds. *Diagnosis, Management, and Treatment of Discogenic Pain.* Philadelphia: Elsevier/Saunders; 2012.

annulus, in a bulging annulus, or be located superiorly or inferiorly behind the edge of the vertebral body in a severely bulging annulus. In a series of 500 consecutive patients, the per-patient prevalence was 29%; the per-disk prevalence of an HIZ was 6%. The majority of HIZs were present at the L4 and L5 disk levels, confirmed on later studies.

The relationship of the HIZ to pain production was evaluated in a subset of 41 patients, selected for the presence of an HIZ on prediskography MR imaging.[107] Diskography was performed with the requirement of a nonpainful control disk for a diagnosis of diskogenic pain. Pain responses were tabulated both as "exact" reproduction of pain as well as "similar" pain (Table 15.7). In all, 118 disks were tested in 41 patients; the per-disk prevalence of the HIZ was 34%, reflecting the selection bias. In detecting exact pain, the HIZ had a sensitivity of 82% and specificity of 89%, a 70% PPV, and a +LR of 7.3. When the diskographic criteria were relaxed to exact or similar pain, the specificity rose to 97% with a PPV of 95%; there were only two false-positive cases where a disk bearing an HIZ was nonpainful. The investigators postulated that the HIZ represents a complex grade 4 fissure where the nuclear material has been trapped within the lamellae of the annulus fibrosis and become inflamed, accounting for the T2 hyperintensity, brighter than that of the parent nucleus. They advanced the HIZ finding as pathognomonic of a symptomatic disk. The publication of these findings elicited considerable interest and many subsequent studies[91,93,94,97,98,108-113] attempting to verify or refute its conclusions.

Table 15.7 demonstrates informative +LR and high specificity in most of the studies. There are dissenting voices. Carragee and colleagues evaluated the correlation of the HIZ and painful disks at provocation diskography in both symptomatic and asymptomatic subjects. In symptomatic patients, 30% of disks had an HIZ; only 9% of disks in asymptomatic subjects contained an HIZ (significant, $P < 0.0001$).

Table 15.7 High Intensity Zone (HIZ) as a Predictor of Positive Provocation Diskography

Author (reference), Date	Diskogram Criteria	HIZ Criteria	Prevalence per Disk	Sensitivity	Specificity	PPV	NPV	+LR (CI)	−LR (CI)
Aprill (107) 1992	IASP Exact pain	Aprill	34%*	82%	89%	78%	91%	7.3 (3.9-13.7)	0.21 (0.1-0.4)
	Exact or similar pain	Aprill		63%	97%	95%	72%	18.4 (4.6-72.7)	0.38 (0.3-0.5)
Schellhas (108) 1996	IASP	Schellhas†	60%*	97%	83%	87%	97%	5.7 (3.5-9.3)	0.03 (0.01-0.11)
Ricketson (109) 1996	Walsh	Aprill	9%	12%	92%	57%	54%	1.5 (0.4-5.6)	0.96 (0.8-1.1)
Saifuddin (110) 1998	Walsh	Aprill	18%	27%	94%	89%	47%	4.8 (1.7-14.2)	0.77 (0.7-0.9)
Ito (91) 1998	Walsh	Aprill	20%	52%	89%	60%	87%	4.8 (2.3-10.2)	0.54 (0.4-0.8)
Smith (111) 1998	Walsh	Aprill	13%	27%	90%	40%	80%	2.6 (1.2-5.6)	0.82 (0.7-1)
Carragee (112) 2000	Walsh	Carragee‡	30%	45%	84%	73%	62%	2.8 (1.5-5.5)	0.7 (0.5-0.9)
Weishaupt (97) 2001	IASP	Aprill	20%	27%	85%	56%	62%	1.8 (0.8-3.7)	0.86 (0.7-1)
Peng (113) 2006	Walsh	Aprill	12%	NC	NC	100%	NC	NC	NC
Lei (98) 2008	Walsh	Aprill	19%	25%	87%	62%	57%	1.8 (0.8-4.1)	0.87 (0.7-1.1)
O'Neill (93) 2008	IASP	O'Neill§ 1+2+3 Intensity grades	28%	44%	89%	82%	60%	4.1 (2.7-6.1)	0.62 (0.5-0.7)
		2+3	16%	26%	95%	86%	54%	5.7 (3-10.9)	0.78 (0.7-0.8)
		3	9%	15%	98%	86%	52%	6.8 (2.7-17.1)	0.87 (0.8-0.9)
Kang (94) 2009	IASP	Aprill	26%	57%	84%	53%	86%	3.46 (2.2-5.5)	0.52 (0.4-0.7)

*Sensitivity and prevalence values are not meaningful due to this selection bias.
†Includes lesions with thin line of T2 hyperintensity within annulus or connecting nucleus to HIZ
‡Includes posterolateral lesions, HIZ signal intensity within 10% of CSF T2 signal
§Schellhas criteria plus posterolateral and lateral lesions
PPV, positive predictive value; NPV, negative predictive value; LR, likelihood ratio; IASP, International Association for the Study of Pain.
From Maus TP, Martin DP. Imaging for discogenic pain. In: Kapural L, Kim P, Deer T, eds. *Diagnosis, Management, and Treatment of Discogenic Pain.* Philadelphia: Elsevier Saunders; 2012:43, Table 3-7.

The statistics for the symptomatic group are presented in Table 15.7; an HIZ disk had an 84% specificity, a 73% PPV, and a +LR of 2.8 for diskogenic pain. These data are supportive of the HIZ as a useful marker for the painful disk. The investigators, however, point out that the presence of an HIZ disk was strongly predictive of a positive pain response at diskography in both the symptomatic (73%) and asymptomatic (69%) groups. The asymptomatic group had also been stratified by psychometric evaluation; in participants with either chronic pain or abnormal psychometric studies, all HIZ disks produced pain with pressurization. The investigators contend that the similar painful response rate of HIZ disks in symptomatic and asymptomatic subjects devalues the HIZ as a useful finding, because the total weight of diagnosis depends on concordance versus nonconcordance of pain response.

The study by O'Neill and associates[93] stratified HIZ lesions by relative signal intensity, and expanded the definition of the HIZ to include posterolateral and lateral lesions and those that demonstrated a connection to the nuclear compartment. Original data were recalculated to establish a three-part threshold of HIZ intensity: markedly intense cases, markedly and moderately intense cases, and a combination of all three. As the threshold tightened, the specificity and +LR rose; the PPV remained high for all three threshold levels. For only markedly hyperintense HIZs, the specificity was 98%, the PPV was 86%, and the +LR was 6.8. This would support Bogduk's comments that "low intensity zones may well occur in asymptomatic volunteers, but that when activated (ostensibly inflamed), these fissures become painful and assume a higher signal intensity" (Fig. 15.9) page 1260.[114]

MULTIVARIATE ANALYSIS

The studies of Kang[94] and O'Neill[93] included multivariate analyses. O'Neill and associates showed that the disk

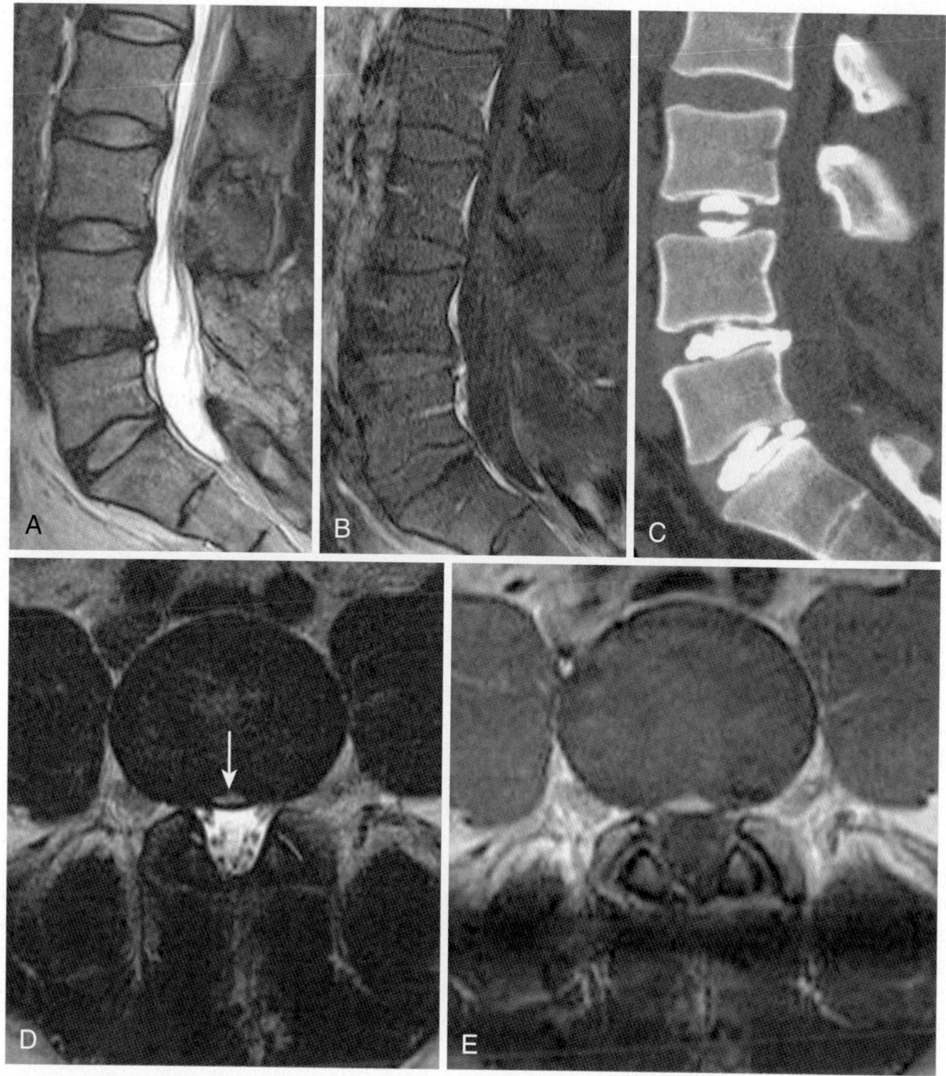

Figure 15.9 High Intensity Zone (HIZ). Middle-aged male has previously undergone L4-5 decompressive procedure, without diskectomy, for back and leg pain. Axial back pain was unrelieved. **A,** Sagittal T2-weighted MRI shows loss of T2 signal in the L4 disk with an HIZ in the posterior annulus. **D,** Axial T2 MRI image at L4-5 interspace demonstrates the HIZ *(arrow)* in the posterior annulus. **E,** Axial-enhanced T1 MRI image showing enhancement in the HIZ, also demonstrated in the sagittal fat-saturated T1 image **(B)**. Sagittal postdiskogram CT **(C)** demonstrates annular fissure at L4-5 leading to HIZ. Pressurization of the L4-5 disk produced concordant axial pain at < 20 pounds per square inch (PSI) above opening pressure. (From Maus TP, Aprill CN. Lumbar discogenic pain, provocation diskography, and imaging correlates. *Radiol Clin North Am.* 2012;50:681-704.)

structural findings—loss of disk height, loss of nuclear signal, and disk contour abnormalities—correlated strongly with each other; the inflammatory findings, HIZ, and end plate change did not, with the exception of HIZ and disk contour abnormality. The rank correlation of the MRI findings with a positive diskogram was as follows: signal abnormality > disk height > disk contour > HIZ > end plate change. Disk signal change alone was as accurate as other individual parameters or combinations thereof. This was most evident at the two extremes of the receiver operating characteristic (ROC) curve: when disk signal was normal, it was highly unlikely the disk was painful regardless of other findings, and when there was severe signal loss, the disk was highly likely to be painful. Other parameters become useful when disk signal was intermediate. Kang and colleagues[47] introduced a new MRI classification system combining the findings that were previously addressed as independent variables: class 1, normal or bulging disk without an HIZ; class 2, normal or bulging disk with an HIZ; class 3, disk protrusion without HIZ; class 4, disk protrusion with HIZ. Disk extrusions and sequestrations were excluded from the analysis. Logistic regression analysis showed that class 4, disk protrusion with HIZ, had the strongest correlation with concordant pain at diskography. This combination had a specificity of 87% and a PPV of 98%. This finding had a prevalence of 13% and a sensitivity of 45%.

IMAGING CORRELATES: CONCLUSION

Imaging identification of diskogenic pain is challenging for a variety of reasons. (1) There is no pathologic or surgical gold standard. (2) The existing standard of comparison, diskography, is ultimately unproven, subjective in its interpretation, and has evolved over time in its criteria for a positive test. None of the studies reviewed earlier use the most current and restrictive criteria, those of ISIS. (3) The

Box 15.3 Imaging Correlates of Diskogenic Pain (IDD)

- The disk structural markers—loss of disk space height, loss of nuclear T2 signal, and disk herniation—correlate strongly with one another; loss of nuclear signal is most significant.
- Severe nuclear signal loss or severe loss of disk space height strongly predicts a painful disk.
- Normal nuclear signal virtually excludes a painful disk.
- When nuclear signal is intermediate, the inflammatory markers of the high intensity zone and end plate marrow change come into play.
- A truly *high*-intensity zone is infrequent but strongly predicts a painful disk.
- When an HIZ is observed in combination with a disk protrusion, it strongly predicts a painful disk.
- Marrow end plate change of type I or type II involving greater than 25% of the vertebral body is uncommon, but it strongly predicts a painful disk.

imaging findings likely have threshold effects, where only a significant expression of the finding (intensity of an HIZ, extent of marrow change) is a useful predictor of diskogenic pain. Most studies do not account for this factor. (4) Imaging findings are likely technique dependent to an unknown degree, and imaging techniques are evolving.

From the tangle of data, useful information can emerge; the imaging correlates of diskogenic pain are summarized in Box 15.3. These imaging predictors of diskogenic pain, when applied to a select population of patients with axial back pain, in whom other pain generators have been excluded, could perhaps be used to initiate a proven therapy possessing a good safety profile. No such therapy exists. Diskography remains the reference standard for the diagnosis of diskogenic pain.

CERVICAL DISKOGENIC PAIN: IMAGING CORRELATES

This discussion has purposely focused on the lumbar spine. The lumbar spine segment is most commonly afflicted with diskogenic pain, and the literature regarding its pathogenesis and evaluation with imaging and provocation diskography, although challenging, is of greatest depth. The cervical intervertebral disk is structurally distinct from the lumbar disk. These is no posterior annulus, and the small nuclear compartment disappears early in life; the residual fibrocartilaginous plate normally develops fissures as mere age-related change.[81] There are no morphologic features at diskography that contribute to a diagnosis of diskogenic pain. Diagnosis is reliant entirely on the provocation of concordant pain, with the requirement of nonpainful control disks.

As in the lumbar segment, structural age changes (loss of T2 signal, loss of disk space height, contour abnormality) are ubiquitous on cervical MRI studies. The Matsumoto[30] study cited earlier examined 2480 cervical disks in asymptomatic subjects and noted loss of T2 signal in 17% of males and 12% of females between ages 20 to 30, and 89% of males and 86% of females over 60 years of age. In another study by Okada,[115] 89% of asymptomatic subjects (mean age 49) exhibited structural age changes on MRI; another group of patients (mean age 46) with symptomatic lumbar disk herniations but asymptomatic of neck pain showed cervical disk age-related change in 98%. There is a paucity of literature addressing the correlation of imaging findings with cervical diskography. An early study by Parfenchuck (1994) showed only a modest ability of MRI findings of T2 signal loss or disk contour abnormality to predict a positive cervical diskogram (sensitivity = 73%, specificity = 67%).[116] Schellhas' 1996 study suggested that MRI cannot reliably predict a positive cervical diskogram.[117] A more recent study by Zheng[118] again demonstrated only a modest predictive value of MRI using parameters of T2 signal loss and disk contour abnormality (sensitivity = 73%, specificity = 49%). The inflammatory disk parameters that proved to have such high specificity in the lumbar region are either unusual or little studied (Modic change) or have no anatomic existence (HIZ) in the cervical region. Occasionally foci of elevated T2 signal are observed in the posterior cervical disk, but in the absence of a posterior annulus, the anatomic correlate is unclear. Imaging identification of diskogenic pain in the cervical spine remains elusive. Cervical diskography remains the reference standard in diagnosis of cervical diskogenic pain.

The imaging investigation of diskogenic pain highlights a theme common to this chapter: physiologic parameters have greater significance in pain syndromes than purely structural alteration. To be ultimately valuable in the diagnosis of diskogenic pain, imaging must move beyond macroscopic descriptions of morphology to the realm of biochemical imaging, quantifying the change in nuclear constituents over time. In addition to characterizing biochemical nuclear matrix degradation, imaging will also need to more precisely identify inflammatory mediators in the disk and adjacent cartilaginous end plate. Perhaps then we will truly be capable of the noninvasive diagnosis of diskogenic pain.

IMAGING OF AXIAL PAIN GENERATORS

ZYGAPOPHYSIAL JOINT (Z JOINT, FACET JOINT)

The supporting structure of the posterior column of the spine includes the paired facet joints with their associated capsules, the ligamentum flavum, the intraspinous and supraspinous ligaments joining the spinous processes, and the intertransverse ligaments. The inferior articular process of the facet joint faces anteriorly and is convex in configuration; on axial images the inferior articular process is the more posterior component of the joint. The superior articular process (SAP) has a concave articular surface that faces posteriorly and medially; on axial images it appears as the anterior component of the joint. In an erect standing position, the lumbar facet joints bear approximately 16% of the compressive load; in a flexed sitting position they bear essentially no load. With loss of disk space height, the lumbar facet joints will bear proportionally more axial load. The fibrous joint capsule has been demonstrated to be richly innervated by nociceptors and proprioceptive fibers.[119] In a normal state, nociceptors such as those seen in the facet joint capsule have a high threshold and would not be expected to discharge unless loads are supraphysiologic. However, in the presence of pathologic joint inflammation, synovitis, chemical mediators may sensitize these nociceptors and supraphysiologic levels of stress may no longer be required to stimulate pain. Such inflammatory mediators (substance P, bradykinin, phospholipase A2) have been detected in the facet joint capsule.[120]

There is thus a pathoanatomic basis for facet joint-mediated pain, particularly in the presence of facet synovitis. The imaging challenge in identifying a potentially painful joint lies in the well demonstrated specificity fault, that imaging changes of morphologic facet arthrosis (subchondral sclerosis, erosions, or cyst formation, osteophytes, joint space narrowing, vacuum phenomena) are age related change and do not correlate with pain. The reference standard for facet pain is positive comparative dual medial branch blocks, as there are no reliable physical exam or historical features allowing a confident diagnosis of Z-joint pain.[81] Schwarzer and colleagues semi-quantitatively scored CT finding of structural facet arthrosis and found no relationship to Z-joint pain as determined by placebo controlled medial branch blocks.[121] More recently, Cohen and associates showed no association between MRI findings of structural facet arthrosis and pain relief with dual medial branch blocks and subsequent radiofrequency rhizotomy.[122] These structural changes become universal by the sixth or seventh decade of life; they do not represent active inflammatory disease causal of pain.[123]

Rather, imaging must look to identify physiologic, not structural, markers of active facet synovitis. Imaging techniques that may be applicable include the technetium pyrophosphate bone scan (including its technologic evolution SPECT and SPECT/CT) and the MRI physiologic imaging parameters of T2 hyperintensity and gadolinium enhancement. Technetium pyrophosphate bone scans detect hyperemia and accelerated bone turnover, which may be considered manifestations of active inflammation. Dolan and associates[124] compared the response to intra-articular facet joint injection guided by clinical exam versus positive SPECT studies; there was a significantly greater short term (1- to 3-month) clinical response in the SPECT-guided injections. A similar study by Holder and colleagues, using response to uncontrolled intra-articular injections as the reference standard, identified a 100% sensitivity and 71% specificity for SPECT scans in the detection of facet joint–mediated pain.[125] Pneumaticos and colleagues prospectively studied patients undergoing intra-articular injections in three groups: injections guided by positive SPECT scans, injections in patients with negative SPECT scan guided by clinical exam, and injections in patients without SPECT studies guided by clinical exam.[126] The patients whose injections were directed to SPECT-positive joints had significantly better clinical outcomes than the other two groups, as well as lower costs as fewer joints were injected. McDonald used SPECT/CT to identify joints for injection in 37 patients with clinical facet joint lumbar pain. The mean visual analog score (VAS) dropped from 7.2 to 2.8, with an average duration of benefit of 2.2 months; only 1 in 37 patients did not report benefit. The fused SPECT/CT images were useful in distinguishing the L4-5 and L5-S1 facet joints.[127]

There is no correlation between the degree of morphologic facet arthrosis and the intensity of SPECT activity.[124] Rather, the phase of active synovitis correlating with pain production may occur relatively early in the progressive development of structural changes of facet arthrosis. Kim and colleagues correlated MRI findings in the facet joints with SPECT; they noted that the MRI appearance of T2 hyperintensity in the synovium, intrasynovial fluid, and cartilage disruption best correlated with a positive SPECT, here used as a reference standard for active facet synovitis.[128] More extensive structural manifestations of facet arthrosis did not demonstrate the physiologic finding of SPECT activity. Cervionke and colleagues have demonstrated an indirect association of T2 hyperintensity within and about the facet joint with axial pain.[129] T2 hyperintensity in the adjacent pedicle has also been associated with axial pain of facet origin; this finding can also be seen in pedicle or pars stress fractures. T2 hyperintensity accompanying facet synovitis may also be seen in the surrounding multifidus muscle, occasionally sufficiently extensive as to raise concern for a sinister process. Gadolinium enhancement in and about the facet joint is also suggestive of facet synovitis. Ultimately, the physiologic parameters of edema, hyperemia and accelerated metabolic activity as detected by increased SPECT or SPECT/CT activity, and T2 hyperintensity and gadolinium enhancement on MRI must be evaluated as predictors of facet joint pain against the current reference standard, comparative medial branch blocks. Prevalence studies of these parameters in populations asymptomatic of back pain are also needed for researchers to understand the specificity of these imaging observations. Despite the lack of absolute validation, if the patient is going to undergo an MRI for evaluation of axial pain, a fat-saturated or short tau inversion recovery (STIR) sequence should be performed, as it represents the best chance of demonstrating physiologic findings (T2 hyperintensity), which may identify an axial pain generator (Fig. 15.10).

SPACE OF OKADA

A tissue pathway between same segment, contralateral facet joints was initially described in the cervical region by Dr. Kikuzo Okada in 1981; 80% of cervical facets demonstrated a communication between the joint capsules via a space situated dorsal to the ligamentum flavum in the axial plane and in the interlaminar space in the coronal plane.[130] This communication is frequently observed in intra-articular injections of cervical facet joints that are structurally normal on imaging or exhibit only modest evidence of synovitis or structural arthrosis. In the lumbar region, this communicating pathway is commonly observed only in the face of advanced facet arthrosis; it may also be observed in the presence of defects in the pars interarticularis. This lumbar retroligamentous pathway also commonly communicates with an adventitial bursa within the interspinous ligament (i.e., Baastrup's disease).[131]

This pathway may serve as a means of transmission of infection or, more commonly, noninfectious inflammatory change between multiple joints and tissue compartments.[131] In patients with lumbar axial pain and spondylolytic defects, this posterior element inflammatory complex may involve four facet joints, the bilateral pars defects, and the interspinous ligament. It may have a capacity of 4 to 6 cc of fluid in the author's experience. It is also a potential confounding space in interlaminar epidural steroid injections. This space may provide a false loss of resistance superficial to the dorsal epidural space; contrast injection may subsequently

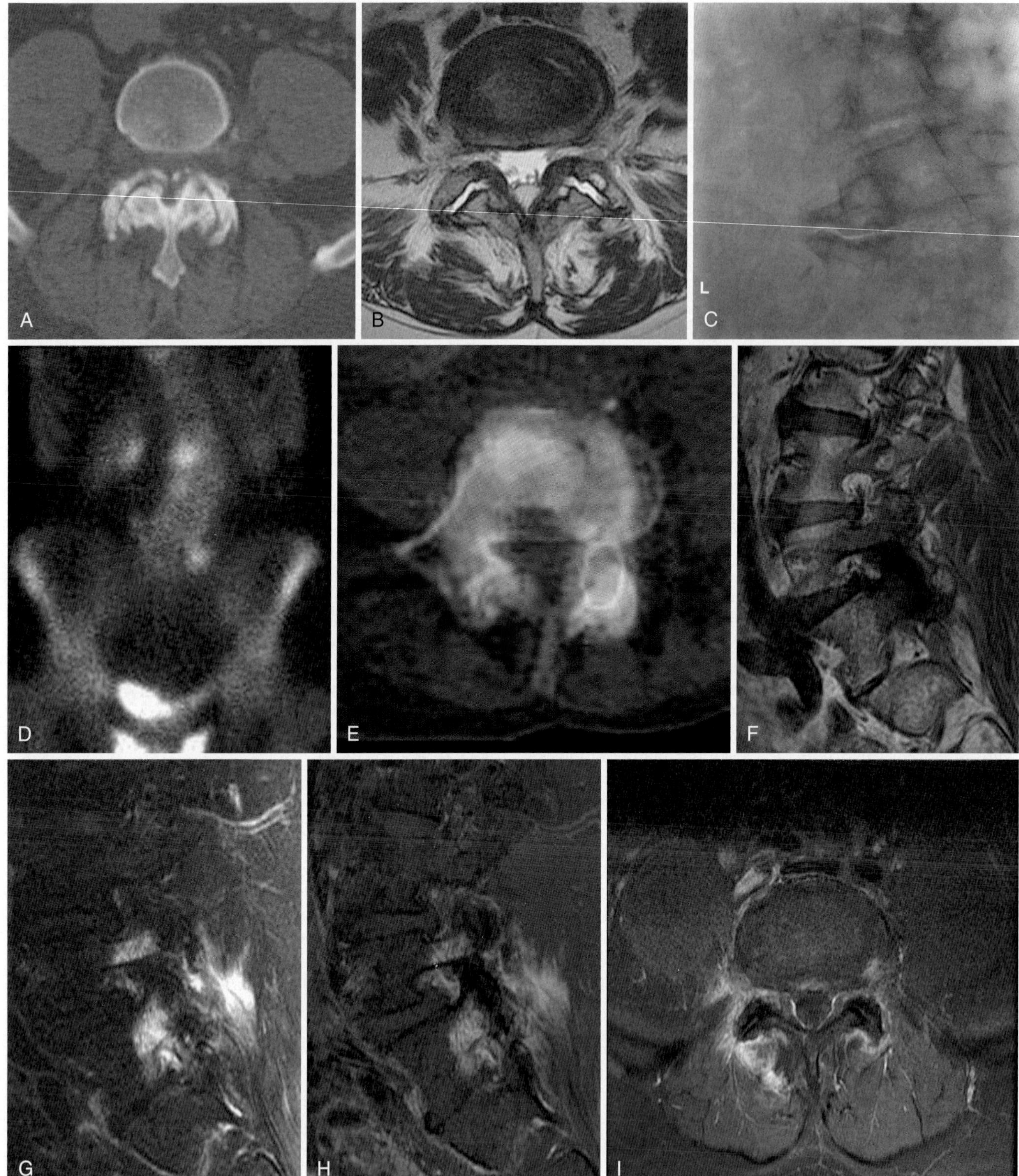

Figure 15.10 Imaging of facet arthrosis and synovitis. The changes of arthrosis (i.e., joint space narrowing, osteophytes, subchondral cysts, or sclerosis) as seen in the CT image **(A)** the T2 MRI image **(B)** or the radiographic image **(C)** do not correlate with pain. Planar bone scan image **(D)** of the same patient as **(C)** shows increased uptake near the lumbosacral junction on the left in this patient with left-sided axial pain. SPECT/CT image **(E)** provides better anatomic localization to the left L4-5 facet. In another patient with right-sided axial lumbar pain, T1 MRI image **(F)** shows low signal in right L5 pedicle, right L4-5 facet. Fat-saturated T2 sagittal image **(G)** demonstrates T2 hyperintensity in L4 and L5 pedicles, L4-5 facet, and adjacent soft tissues. Enhanced T1 sagittal **(H)** and axial **(I)** images also demonstrate the extensive inflammatory response in this patient with active synovitis. T2 hyperintensity or enhancement in pedicles can occur in facet synovitis or stress fractures of the pars or pedicle.

fill either facet joint at that segment level or the interspinous ligament (Fig. 15.11).

SACROILIAC JOINT

The sacroiliac joint is a large irregular synovial joint lined by thick hyaline cartilage on its sacral surface and thinner fibrocartilage on its iliac surface. The inferior and antero-superior aspects of the radiographically perceived joint are synovial; its superior and posterior aspect is ligamentous. The posterior surface of the joint is covered by thick interosseous and dorsal sacroiliac ligaments. There is minimal movement of the joint, except under the hormonal influences of pregnancy. This modest mobility is, however, vital to appropriate gait. The synovial portion of the joint is uniformly present in young adults, with a cartilage thickness

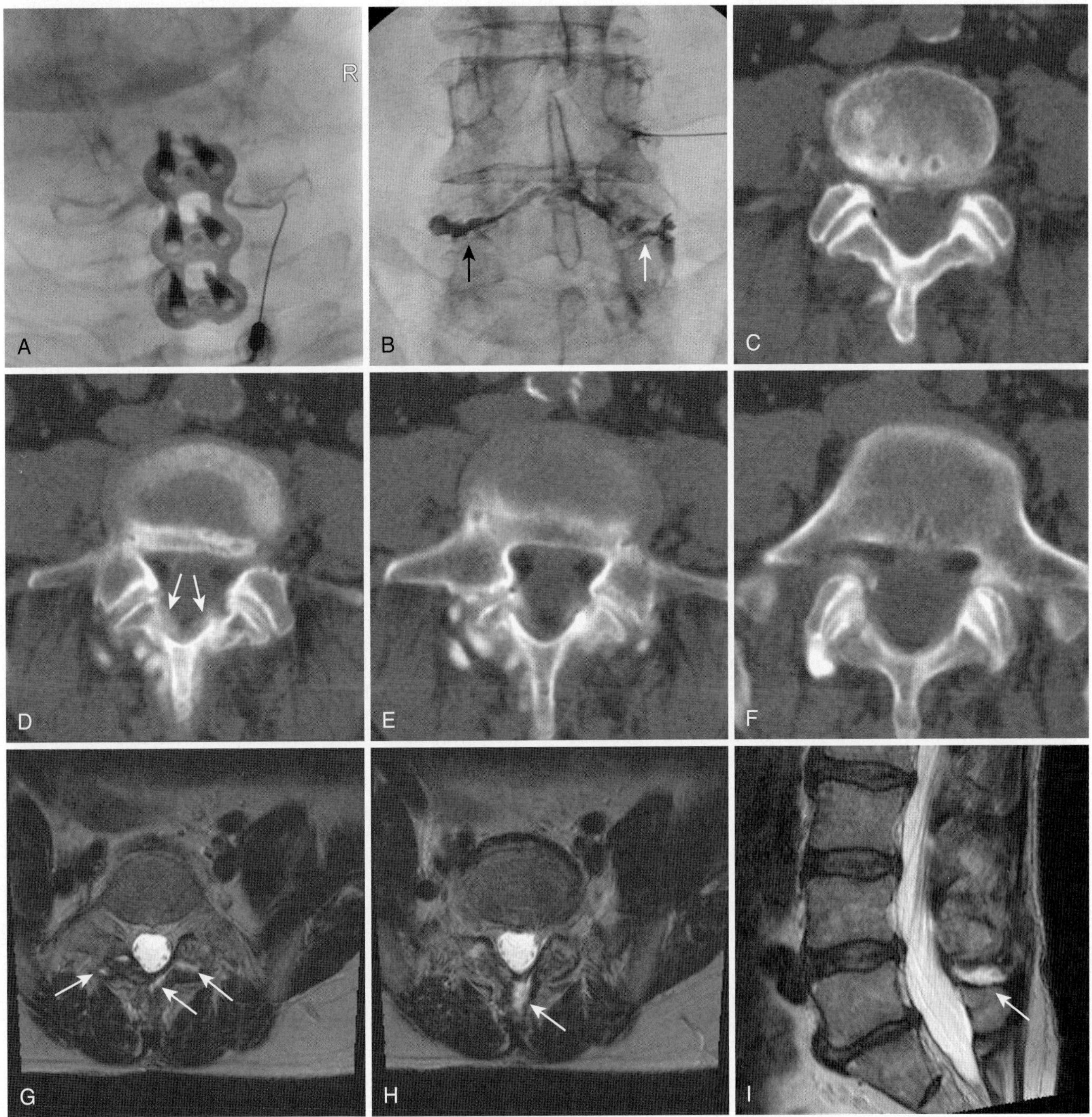

Figure 15.11 The Space of Okada. Frontal fluoroscopic image **(A)** demonstrates the space of Okada providing communication between the bilateral C6-7 facets via the right-sided injection. In another patient **(B),** an attempted right L4 transforaminal injection opacified the superior recess of the L4-5 facet, traversed an L5 pars defect *(white arrow)* to the right L5-S1 facet, and opacified the space of Okada to a left L5 pars defect *(black arrow)* and the left L4 and L5 facets. Subsequent CT **(C, D, E, F)** confirms opacification of all these structures. The space of Okada is marked by the *white arrows* in **(D)**. The space of Okada may contain a small amount of fluid, which appears as T2 hyperintensity (*white arrows,* **G, H, I**). Note continuity with interspinous ligament (*arrow* in **[H]** and **[I]**).

Continued

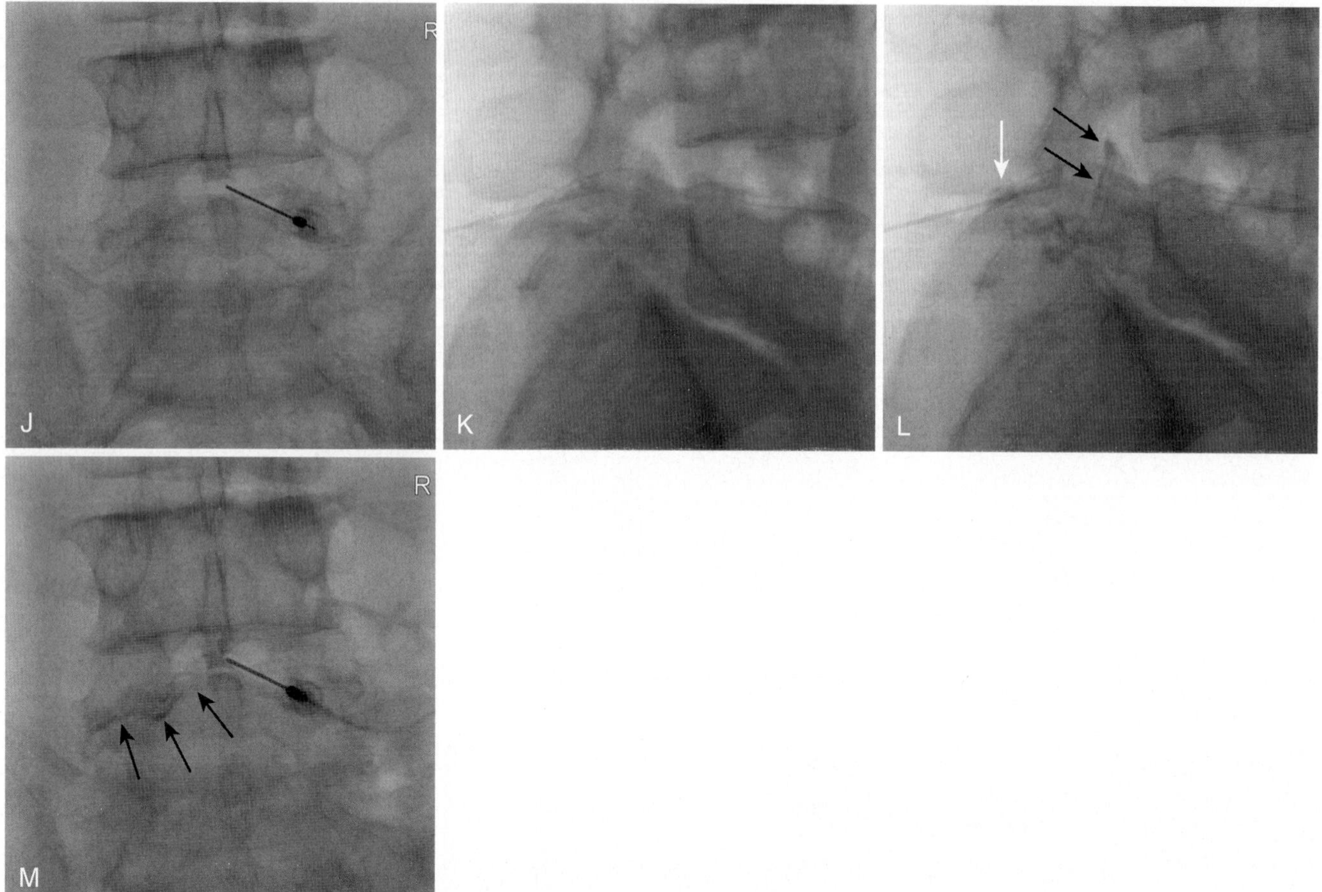

Figure 15.11 cont'd, In a final patient, an attempted interlaminar injection (needle placement images **J, K**) opacified the interspinous ligament (*white arrow* in **[L]**) and the left L4-5 facet (*black arrows* in **[L]**) via the space of Okada. This space (*black arrows* in **[M]**) is posterior to the ligamentum flavum; the needle was advanced ventrally into the epidural space without incident. (From Murthy NS, Maus TP, Aprill C. The retrodural space of Okada. *AJR Am J Roentgenol.* 2011;196:W784-W789.)

of 2 to 5 mm; the synovial space may be attenuated in older adults by fibrous adhesions, but fusion across the joint is not a normal change of aging. Potential communications between the synovial space and the dorsal sacral foramina, the L5 epiradicular sheath, and the ventrally situated lumbosacral plexus have been observed.[132] These could explain radicular pain associated with sacroiliac joint dysfunction. Although the surface area of the joint is large, its synovial space is of small volume, ranging from 1 to 2.5 cc.[133,134] Innervation of the sacroiliac joint is complex and remains controversial. Consensus suggests a dominant dorsal innervation from the L5 and S1-S4 dorsal rami.

Osteoarthrosis of the sacroiliac joints may be seen in pathologic specimens of young adults, but it is not generally appreciable radiographically until middle age. Changes of cartilage degeneration are more prominent on the iliac side of the joint. Beyond age 40, many subjects have detectable narrowing of the sacroiliac joint, especially in its inferior portion. This may be accompanied by subchondral sclerosis and osteophyte formation, most prominent anteriorly and inferiorly. A vacuum phenomenon may be seen. As in the facet joint, changes of osteoarthrosis are a normal aging phenomenon and are not predictive of pain.

Evaluation of imaging features predictive of sacroiliac joint pain is yet again confounded by the lack of a pathoanatomic gold standard. Medical history and physical exam provocative maneuvers are not capable of consistently identifying painful sacroiliac (SI) joints.[135] The reference standard for sacroiliac joint pain is relief of index pain with an intra-articular anesthetic block; this should ideally be either placebo controlled or a comparative block paradigm. Potential leakage from the joint capsule may complicate diagnostic specificity. Schwarzer[136] studied patients with chronic low back pain experienced below the lumbosacral junction. Using response to single blocks as the diagnostic criteria for sacroiliac pain yielded a prevalence of 30%. Requiring a positive block and a ventral capsular tear on postarthrographic CT yielded a prevalence of 21%; adding pain provocation with joint distension to the criteria lowered prevalence to 16%. The Maigne study using double blocks suggested a prevalence of 18.5%.[137] More recent work by DePalma[76] identified a prevalence of 18%; sacroiliac joint pain increased in prevalence with age up to approximately 70 years.

Structural changes of osteoarthrosis in the sacroiliac joint are poor predictors of pain. Elgafy and colleagues[138] scored CT features of arthrosis in SI joints and noted a sensitivity of 58% and a specificity of 69%. Physiologic imaging parameters suggesting the presence of hypervascularity, edema, or inflammation are more likely to predict pain. In the studies of Maigne[139] and Slipman,[140] technetium bone scans

Box 15.4 Zygapophysial (Facet) and Sacroiliac Joint Pain

- Structural arthrosis as seen by radiographs, CT, or MRI does not predict pain.
- Physiologic parameters of hyperemia, edema, and increased metabolic activity may predict pain.
- These physiologic parameters may be assessed by T2 hyperintensity (STIR or fat-saturated T2 images), gadolinium enhancement, or increased uptake on SPECT or SPECT/CT.
- There are no validation studies of physiologic parameters against accepted reference standards (dual, comparative blocks).
- There are no studies addressing specificity—that is, the prevalence of these findings in asymptomatic subjects.

achieved specificities of 89.5% and 100%, although with low sensitivity, for sacroiliac pain as referenced by uncontrolled intra-articular injections. The MRI physiologic parameters of T2 hyperintensity and gadolinium enhancement have been studied primarily in the context of inflammatory spondyloarthropathies. MRI evidence of active inflammation (sacroiliitis) is intrinsic to the diagnoses of spondyloarthropathies and correlates well with clinical disease activity and therapeutic response to disease modifying agents (TNFα inhibitors) (Box 15.4).

BAASTRUP'S DISEASE

Baastrup's disease, the apposition of the lumbar spinous processes resulting from hyperlordosis, segmental instability, or loss of disk space height, may degrade the interspinous ligament with formation of a pseudarthrosis or pseudobursa.[141] This may be a cause of focal midline lumbar pain. Such pseudobursa may have a synovial membrane and can communicate with facet joints or pars defects via the retroligamentous space of Okada.[130] The pseudobursa may extend anteriorly through a midline cleft in the ligamentum flavum and present on MRI or CT as a midline posterior epidural cyst, causing neural compression and contributing to radicular or claudicatory pain. It may be mistaken for a synovial cyst of facet origin but is distinguished by its midline posterior location, the relative absence of facet degeneration, and inflammatory change in the interspinous ligament.

Baastrup's disease may be identified on radiographs as contact between adjacent spinous processes with sclerosis, flattening, and enlargement. Not surprisingly, this structural change is commonly observed in asymptomatic individuals; in one study it was present in 81% of individuals greater than 80 years of age.[142] The authors also noted that "Baastrup's phenomenon" was observed in 41% of patients undergoing CT imaging for non-low-back pain indications.[142] MRI findings of edema, inflammation (T2 hyperintensity, gadolinium enhancement), or a cystic fluid collection in the interspinous ligament are more likely to represent symptomatic disease, although this has not been well validated against anesthetic blocks. DePalma's study suggested that Baastrup's disease accounted for approximately 2% of axial low back pain.[76] In an MRI study by Maes and associates, imaging evidence of Baastrup's disease was present in 8.2% of subjects, most commonly at the L4-5 segment; nearly half of the patients had multiple-level involvement.[143] Baastrup's disease may also be identified as hyperemia and increased metabolic activity on technetium pyrophosphate SPECT or SPECT/CT studies as well as Fluorodeoxyglucose (FDG)-PET/CT scans. Focal uptake in the spinous processes is most likely to be inflammatory and should not be misinterpreted as metastatic disease; the distinction should be obvious when correlated with the simultaneously obtained CT images, which will show typical structural changes of arthrosis.

BERTOLOTTI'S SYNDROME

Bertolotti's syndrome describes the controversial association of transitional lumbosacral segments with mechanical back pain. It does not imply a specific mechanism of pain production. Transitional lumbosacral segments occur in 4% to 30% of the general population.[72] In a large study of 4000 patients, Tini found no correlation between the presence of a transitional segment and low back pain.[144] The disk at the level of the transitional segment is often rudimentary, with little nuclear material; disk herniations seldom occur at this level.[72] Rather, stresses may be accentuated at the supra-adjacent disk level, where accelerated disk degeneration and an increased incidence of disk herniations have been reported.

Axial low back pain in the presence of an asymmetric transitional segment has also been attributed to abnormal unbalanced motion at this level, with the neoarticulation of the transverse process with the sacral ala or the contralateral facet as the specific pain generator. Jonsson reported 11 cases of mechanical pain attributed to the neoarticulation despite normal bone scans. Nine of 11 patients obtained pain relief with local anesthetic injection in the neoarticulation; a similar proportion of patients had improvement in pain with resection of the neoarticulation.[145] Physiologic imaging parameters (MRI T2 fat-saturated or STIR images, SPECT/CT) are more likely to be useful than structural changes, although no systematic studies have been performed. Brault reported a case of an adolescent athlete with focal mechanical pain consistently relieved by intra-articular injection of the facet contralateral to the neoarticulation. Interestingly, bone scan showed increased uptake at the neoarticulation, but not at the contralateral facet. Surgical resection of the neoarticulation resulted in complete relief of the contralateral pain at 1 year.[146] This may represent a case of pain generated by excessive facet capsular stresses caused by the asymmetric motion at this level, without detectable facet synovitis.

Transitional lumbosacral segments thus may be associated with axial pain, related to a neoarticulation, the contralateral facet at the level of an asymmetric neoarticulation, or IDD in the at-risk disk above a transitional segment. Radicular pain may be caused by a herniation in the adjacent segment disk or an extraforaminal entrapment at a neoarticulation. The presence of a transitional segment should always prompt meticulous attention to segmental enumeration, because of both its intrinsic capacity for confusion and the sevenfold increased likelihood of an anomalous number of mobile presacral segments (Fig. 15.12).[72]

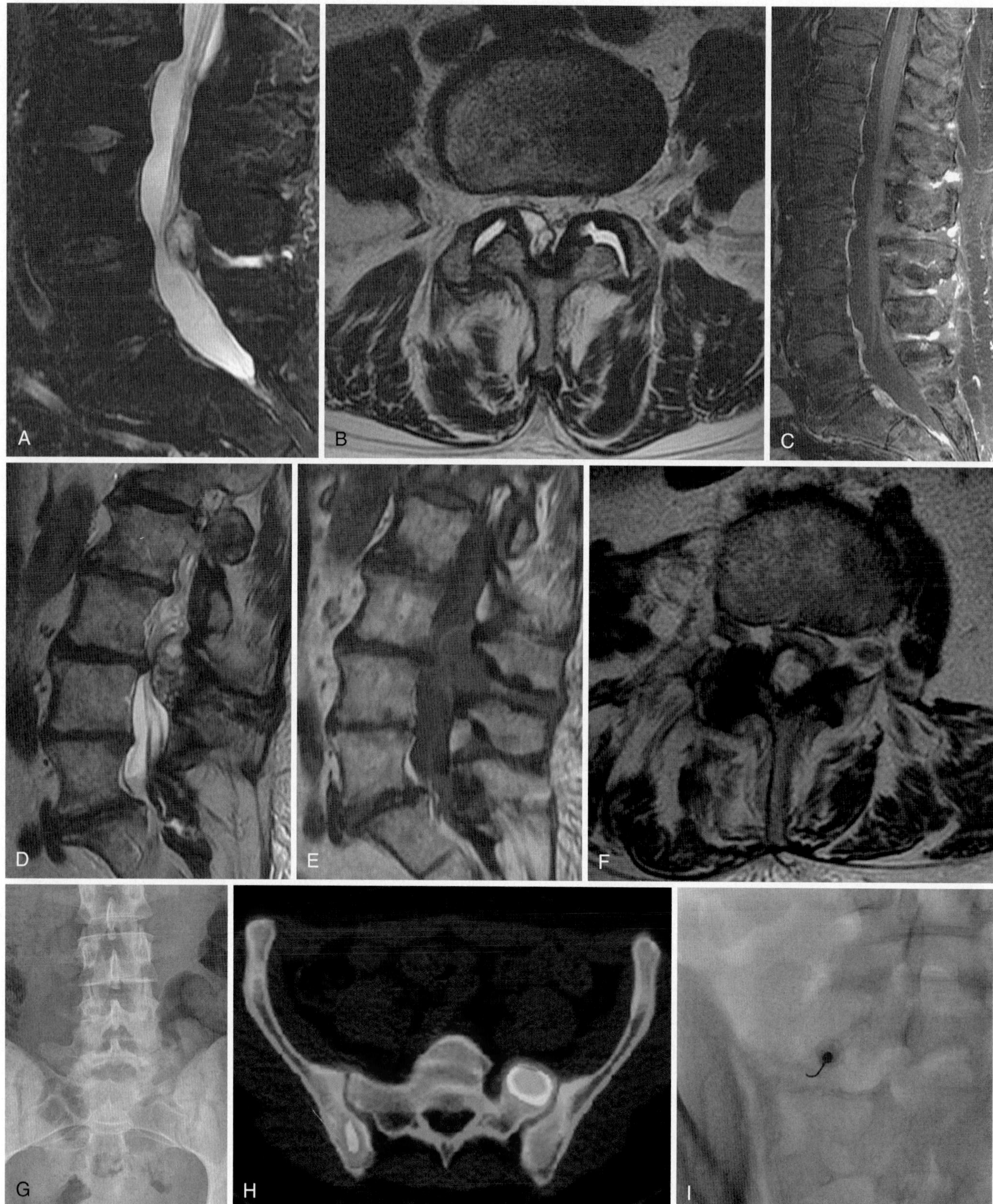

Figure 15.12 Baastrup's disease and Bertolotti's syndrome as posterior element pain generators. An elderly male presents with neurogenic intermittent claudication. T2 fat-saturated sagittal image **(A)** and axial T2 image at the L4-5 interspace **(B)** demonstrate that the compressive lesion is a right paramedian dorsal cyst in continuity with the interspinous pseudobursae of Baastrup's disease. There are also facet joint effusions. In another patient with axial pain **(C),** a fat-saturated, enhanced T1-weighted image shows inflammatory enhancement in the interspinous ligaments of T12-L4. Sagittal T2 **(D)** and T1 **(E)** images of another patient demonstrate a large complex midline dorsal cyst emerging from an interspinous pseudobursae at the L3-4 interspace (axial T2 image **[F]**). A 17-year-old female (frontal lumbar spine radiograph **[G]**) presented with intractable left lumbosacral junction region pain. Note left pseudoarticulation (Bertolotti's syndrome). SPECT/CT image **(H)** shows markedly increased uptake at the pseudoarticulation; pain was relieved with injection into this site (fluoro image **[I]**; note that the patient is prone).

COCCYDYNIA

The radiographic evaluation of the sacrococcygeal region in patients with coccydynia remains controversial. This largely female pain syndrome is probably multifactorial in origin with contributions by somatic and neuropathic pain.[147] A single lateral view of the coccyx to evaluate for destructive bony lesions is a reasonable screening study. Maigne has described a dynamic radiographic study to more fully evaluate the mobility of the coccyx.[148] This consists of a lateral radiograph with the patient standing for 10 minutes to visualize the coccyx without load, followed by a sitting lateral view, with the patient altering the pelvic position to that which stimulates the usual pain. Maigne and colleagues have studied coccygeal mobility and suggested that a normal coccyx may undergo from 5 to 25 degrees of angulation in moving from a standing to a sitting position. Flexion of the coccyx by more than 25 degrees with sitting as well as posterior subluxation of the coccyx with sitting and reduction with standing are considered pathologic and may be the anatomic basis of coccydynia.[148] Aggressive treatment decisions based on this evaluation are controversial. Advanced imaging has little role in this setting unless there is clinical suspicion of underlying systemic disease.

PSEUDARTHROSIS, POSTOPERATIVE AXIAL PAIN

Patients with posterior fusion instrumentation may develop pain related to pseudarthrosis, infection, implant fracture or loosening, or at the interface between the metal and the overlying soft tissue. Radiographs should be scrutinized for integrity of the implant construct, loosening of pedicle screws (which will manifest as a halo of lucency surrounding the screws), or imaging evidence of pseudarthrosis. Anesthetic injection about prominent hardware may be useful in identifying this as a pain generator.

Despite advances in surgical technique and fixation hardware, fusion remains an imperfect procedure. Pseudarthrosis is defined as the failure to achieve a solid bony fusion 1 year after attempted surgical fusion. It is manifested as persistent motion at the segment and absence of bony trabeculae bridging the vertebrae. Approximately 15% of lumbar spinal fusions result in pseudarthrosis; the range of successful reported technical and clinical outcomes spans 16% to 95%.[149] Rates of pseudarthrosis increased with the increasing number of fused levels and with risk factors including prior surgery, instability, deficient bone graft quality and quantity, and nicotine use (Fig. 15.13).

Detection of pseudarthrosis with imaging is of significance, as it is a cause of persistent or recurrent pain following surgery. The correlation is not exact; patients with radiographic pseudarthrosis may be pain free and patients with solid fusions by all imaging techniques may have persistent pain arising from other factors. The clinical questions, therefore, are twofold: Is a pseudarthrosis present, and, if so, is it the cause of persistent or recurrent pain? The ultimate gold standard for fusion is surgical exploration; even this is not foolproof, as patients who have had hardware removal after intra-operative evaluation of stability have subsequently gone on to develop progressive deformity.[150]

Weight-bearing radiographs are the primary tool in assessing stability and adequate fusion. In this setting, flexion-extension views likely add value. Radiographic evidence of instability includes translation of 3 mm or more at L1-L4 or 5 mm at L5-S1. Radiographic fusion may take 6 to 9 months, with ongoing remodeling for up to 2 years. Criteria for a radiographic solid interbody fusion are as follows:[151]

- No motion, or less than 3 degrees of intersegment position change on lateral flexion and extension views
- Lack of a lucent area around the implant
- Minimal loss of disk height
- No fracture of the implant, bone graft, or vertebrae
- No sclerotic change in the bone graft or adjacent vertebrae
- Visible osseous formation in or around the cage

CT will provide greater sensitivity in the detection of pseudarthrosis, which manifests as lucent fracture lines with adjacent sclerosis or fragmentation of the bone graft, and fracture or lucency about implants. Ideally, to verify solid fusion, one would like to be able to confirm the presence of continuous bony trabeculae across the site of fusion. In patients with intervertebral cage devices, bony trabeculae should be seen bridging the interspace through the cage and external to the cage.

Technetium bone scans with SPECT may be helpful. The fusion mass will be metabolically active for a prolonged period after surgery, and increased tracer uptake diffusely in the fusion mass is expected for several months. In normal healing, studies with serial bone scans have shown a steady decrease in tracer uptake after 3 months, with only minimal increased uptake at 1 year.[152] Increased uptake within the fusion mass beyond 1 year after surgery, or new increased uptake not present on prior studies, should raise concern for pseudarthrosis. On MRI, solid bone graft should exhibit signal characteristics of normal marrow. Focal zones of T1 hypointensity, T2 hyperintensity, and gadolinium enhancement may indicate a site of pseudarthrosis with ongoing motion and inflammation. This requires careful inspection.

With disk arthroplasty, postoperative evaluation can occur by radiography or CT; radiography is more conservative of cost and radiation for serial follow-up. The implant should be centered between the pedicles on AP images without penetration of the end plates. On lateral or sagittal images, the center of rotation should be in the posterior half of the disk space, but the implant should not extend beyond the posterior vertebral line.

The clinician and imager must also be aware of symptomatic adjacent segment disease as a cause of recurrent pain in the post fusion patient. Although controversial, this likely occurs at a rate of approximately 3% per year following lumbar fusion;[153] a similar rate has been associated with cervical fusion. The imaging findings will be those of diskogenic pain. Radiographic evidence of adjacent segment disease may or may not be clinically symptomatic.

Pseudarthrosis and adjacent segment disease are two primary causes of pain in the post-operative patient, sometimes labeled the “failed back.” Although conventionally considered a dread diagnosis, studies have shown that careful clinical evaluation, augmented by high-quality imaging and provocation and anesthetic interventions, can identify the specific cause of pain in the majority of cases. Waguespack and Slipman have each published large series of patients with so-called failed back syndrome.[154,155] A specific diagnosis identifying the pain generator was achieved in over

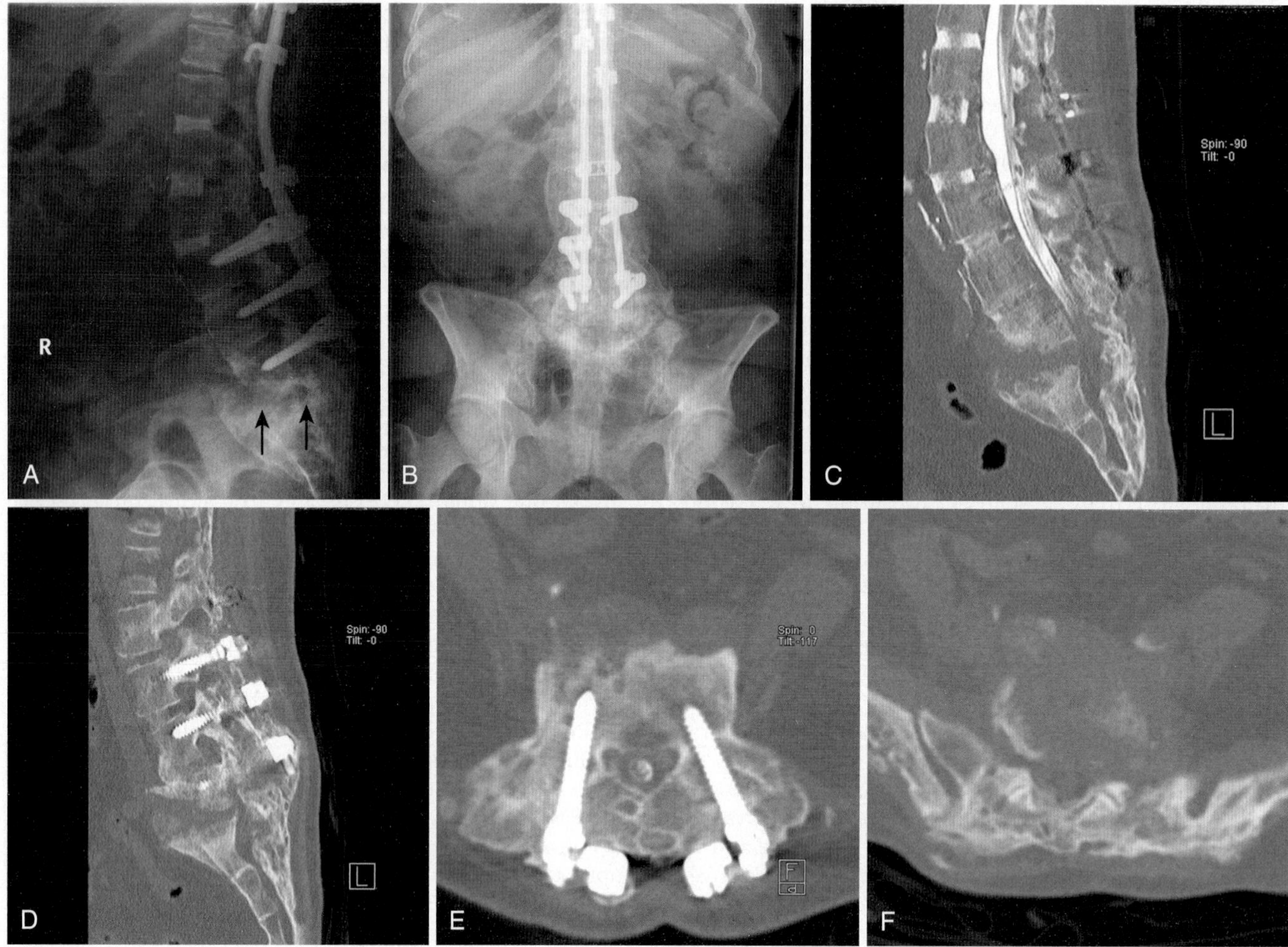

Figure 15.13 Pseudarthrosis on CT Myelography. This 71-year-old female is post multiple spine surgeries and has an instrumented fusion from the upper thoracic region to L5. She presents with bilateral leg pain in an L5 radicular distribution. Radiographs **(A, B)** show lucency with surrounding sclerosis at the L5 level. CT myelography sagittal reconstructions **(C, D)** reveal a pseudarthrosis at L5-S1 with Charcot or infectious features. Cultures were negative. Despite the instrumentation, the thecal sac is well demonstrated; it is patent at the L5 vertebral level **(E)** but obliterated at the L5-S1 disk level **(F)**. (From Thakkar RS, Malloy JP, Thakkar SC, et al. Imaging the postoperative spine. *Radiol Clin North Am.* 2012;50:731-747.)

90% of patients in both of these series. The most common diagnoses were foraminal stenosis (> 20%), diskogenic pain (20%), pseudarthroses (14%), neuropathic pain (10%), and recurrent disk herniation (7% to 12%), with lesser contributions from facet and SI joints. Each of these morphologic lesions has been individually addressed in preceding sections. The imaging challenge is to systematically evaluate each segmental level for these potential pain generators despite the confusion of the surgically altered anatomy.

IMAGING OF RADICULAR PAIN, RADICULOPATHY, AND MYELOPATHY

DISK HERNIATION

Radicular pain, or radiculopathy or myelopathy, has as its substrate neural compression and inflammation. Degradation of the nuclear matrix of the disk may occur in response to a variety of insults, including end plate infraction, genetically determined apoptotic chondrocyte cell death, diabetes mellitus, ochronosis, smoking, or infection. The nuclear compartment of the disk can no longer bear axial load, shifting its burden to the posterior annulus, which may undergo structural failure in the form of radial fissures, the anatomic basis of IDD. In addition to potentially causing axial pain, these fissures may allow herniation of nuclear material into the outer annular lamellae as a contained protrusion or breach the annulus and pass into the epidural space as an extrusion. The mechanical compression of neural tissue and an induced inflammatory response conspire to provoke radicular pain or radiculopathy.

Mixter and Barr initially described the disk herniation as the cause of sciatica in 1934; this observation, and the ability to relieve pain and neurologic dysfunction by surgical extirpation of the offending herniation, provided the basis for the first 70+ years of spine imaging. Myelography, CT, CT/myelography, and MRI were deemed useful in the patient with radicular pain or radiculopathy in the ability to first indirectly and later directly visualize the disk herniation and neural compression. The pathogenesis of radicular pain or radiculopathy is more complex than the simple compression of neural elements; an inflammatory response is also necessary to produce pain. The evidence supporting an inflammatory component in radicular pain was summarized by Mulleman and colleagues.[156,157] Neural compression in isolation produces nerve dysfunction, but not pain; exposure of compressed neural elements to the inflammatory response induced by disk nucleus pulposis results in radicular pain. This inflammatory response is mediated by phospholipase A2, interleukins 1 and 6, TNFα, and nitric oxide. The necessity of an induced inflammatory response for pain production provides a measure of understanding for the glaring specificity fault of disk herniation imaging: large disk herniations are often asymptomatic, and the severity of symptoms bears no relationship to herniation size.

The imaging description of disk herniations has historically been chaotic, with significant disparities among medical specialties and regionally. Clarity was restored by a lexicon of nomenclature produced as a cooperative venture between multiple spine societies in 2001.[158] In this construct, spondylosis deformans describes those changes thought to be due to normal aging. Degradation of the nuclear matrix may occur without structural failure of the annulus, hence there is preservation of disk space height and normal cartilaginous end plate and subchondral marrow. Anterior and lateral osteophytes are observed. MRI imaging shows loss of the normal intranuclear cleft and mild to moderately diminished T2 signal within the disk. Small concentric and transverse annular tears may be seen in spondylosis; radial tears are not considered a normal aging phenomenon. Small amounts of gas may be present within the disk that may be detected on plain films.

In this lexicon, pathologic discovertebral change is termed intervertebral osteochondrosis. This includes the changes of IDD, radial and large circumferential fissures extending to the outer annulus. They may be accompanied by the development of posterior osteophytes that encroach on the central canal. In addition to posterior osteophytes, plain film manifestations of intervertebral osteochondrosis include large amounts of gas within the interspace, loss of disk space height, and end plate irregularity. On T2-weighted MRI images, the disk is of markedly diminished signal intensity. Disk herniations are common.[158]

The inclusive term for displacement of disk material is *herniation.* A localized herniation is defined as involving less than 50% of the disk circumference; generalized disk displacement of more than 50% of the circumference is a bulging disk. Localized herniations are further subdivided: displacement of the disk over less than 25% of its circumference is called a focal herniation, and disk displacement between 25% and 50% is called a broad-based herniation. The distinction between protrusion and extrusion is one of shape (Fig. 15.14). In a protrusion, the width of displaced disk material, in any plane, does not exceed the width of its base against the normal ring apophysis. In an extrusion, the width of the displaced disk material exceeds its base in any plane. The presence of an extrusion shape suggests that there has been complete disruption of the outer annulus and disk material has entered the epidural space. *Sequestration* is the term for loss of continuity of a disk fragment with the parent disk from which it arose. Displacement of disk material away from the parent disk is termed *migration.* Migration can occur caudally or cranially. A herniated disk can further be classified as contained or uncontained. A contained disk herniation is one in which the outer annulus fibrosis is intact, whereas an uncontained herniation is one in which the annulus is completely disrupted. The shape definitions of protrusion and extrusion speak to this, but only by implication, not direct observation. CT or MRI can only rarely directly establish containment; post-CT diskography can make this distinction.

Description of displaced disk material (Fig. 15.15) in the axial plane is defined by zones: the central zone defined by the medial margins of the facets, the subarticular zone extending from the medial facet margin to the medial pedicle margin, the foraminal zone extending from the medial to lateral margins of the pedicle, and the extraforaminal zone peripheral to the lateral pedicle margin. A right-sided focal disk herniation may therefore be described as right central, right subarticular, right foraminal, or right extraforaminal. Similarly, the location in the sagittal plane (superior-inferior) is defined by levels in relationship to the vertebral end plate and pedicle margins. Extending from superior to inferior, the designations include the disk level, suprapedicular level, pedicle level, infrapedicular level, and the subsequent disk level. Although an element of subjectivity remains inherent in any usable system of terminology, careful adherence to these descriptors should allow a more coherent discussion of disk pathology.

Imaging of patients with radicular pain or radiculopathy should begin with upright radiographs of the involved spine segment. This will establish the enumeration, assess balance and stability, and act as a low-sensitivity screen for sinister disease. Advanced imaging may be needed in the setting of intractable radicular pain or progressive neurologic deficit. MRI has long been considered the primary imaging modality in the evaluation of disk herniations, but this has little basis in evidence. There are no studies comparing current generation CT with MRI technology in the detection and characterization of disk herniations. MRI remains the initial modality of choice largely because of its superior sensitivity and specificity in the detection of sinister disease causal of back or limb pain, which, it must be remembered, is the primary goal of imaging. CT myelography retains a problem-solving role in the lumbar region, but it plays a more prominent role in the cervical spine, where its ability to distinguish disk from bone may impact surgical planning.

IMAGING RELIABILITY

MRI has shown good reliability in the assessment of disk herniations. Lurie and colleagues[159] analyzed MRI studies of patients with disk herniations from the Spine Patient Outcomes Research Trial (SPORT) trial; interobserver reliability was high ($\kappa = 0.81$) for disk morphology when classified as normal/bulge, protrusion, and extrusion/sequestration. There was moderate inter-observer agreement for thecal sac ($\kappa = 0.54$) and nerve root compression ($\kappa = 0.47$). Pfirrmann and colleagues[160] proposed a grading system for nerve root compression. The authors divided the relationship of the herniated disk and the nerve root into four categories: no compromise, contact with the nerve root, deviation of the nerve root, and compression of the nerve root. The intra-observer ($\kappa = 0.62$ to 0.67) and intra-observer ($\kappa = 0.72$ to 0.77) reliability results were good. The correlation for a higher grade of nerve root involvement (compression) was better than for low-grade nerve root involvement.

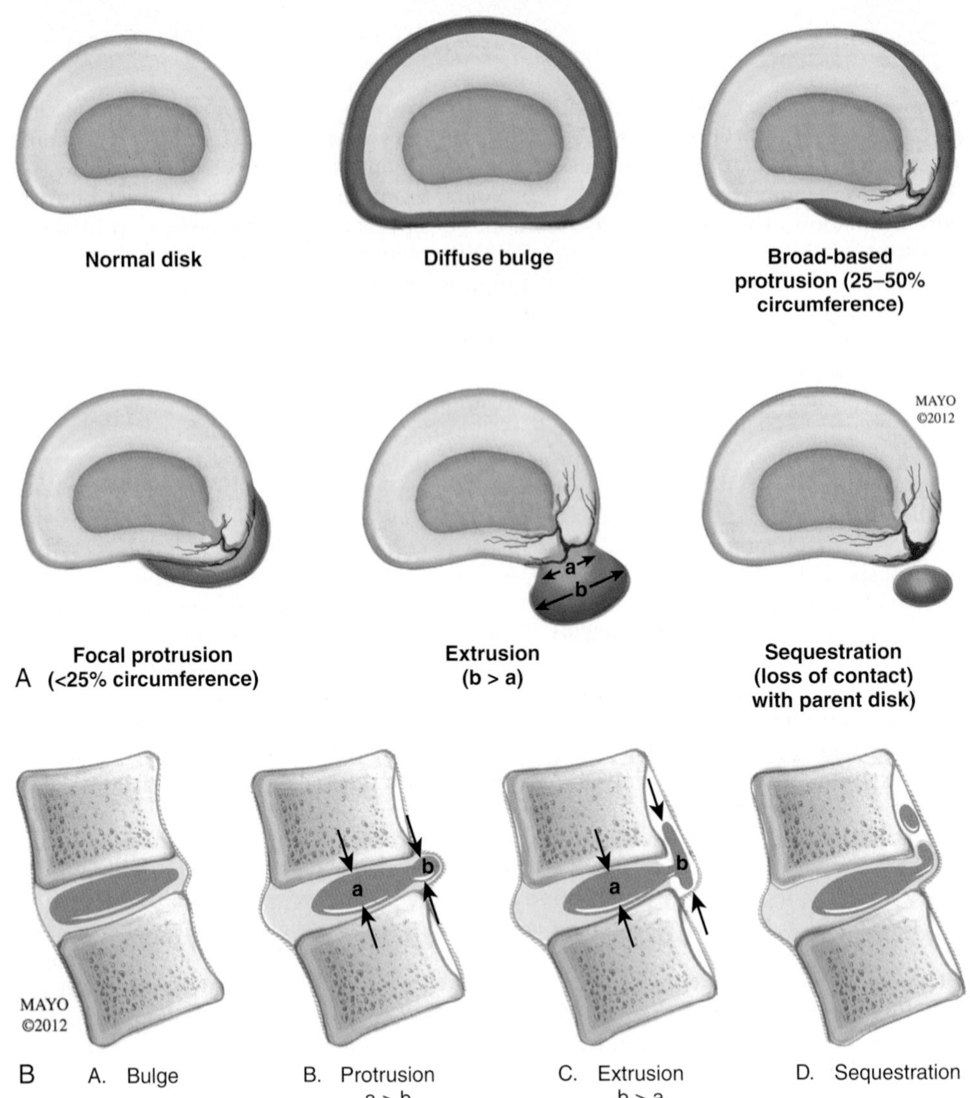

Figure 15.14 Disk herniation definitions. Disk herniation definitions are depicted in the axial **(A)** and sagittal **(B)** planes. Note that the normal L1-L4 disks, shown here, are not round, but an oblate structure whose dorsal margin is convex anteriorly. The L5 disk is normally oval in configuration, convex posteriorly. The definitions are elaborated in the accompanying text.

Central canal zone
Subarticular zone (lateral recess)
Foraminal zone
Extraforaminal zone (far lateral zone)
MAYO ©2012
A

Central canal zone
Subarticular zone
Foraminal zone
Extraforaminal zone
Suprapedicle level
Pedicle level
Infrapedicle level
Disk level
MAYO ©2012
B

Suprapedicle level
Pedicle level
Infrapedicle level
Disk level
MAYO ©2012
C

Figure 15.15 Zones and levels of disk displacement. In the axial plane **(A)** the location of displaced disk material is described by zones. Moving from the midline laterally, these zones are the right or left central zone, demarcated by the medial margins of the facet joints; the subarticular zone (lateral recess), bounded by the medial aspect of the facet joint and the medial aspect of the pedicle; the foraminal zone, bounded by the medial and lateral aspects of the pedicle; and the extraforaminal or far-lateral zone, peripheral to the lateral margin of the pedicle. These zones are also illustrated in the coronal plane **(B)**. The displacement of disk material in the cephalocaudal dimension is described by levels, as illustrated in **(B)** and **(C)**.

IMAGING OBSERVATIONS

MRI T2-weighted images can well display the interface between disk herniations and the thecal sac. The herniated material may be of low T2 signal intensity comparable to the parent disk that has undergone nuclear matrix degradation, but not uncommonly extruded disk material is of higher T2 signal than its parent disk. This may in part reflect inflammatory reaction surrounding extruded material; it can make detection of extruded material in the lateral recesses or foramina challenging on Fast Spine Echo, Turbo Spin Echo (FSE, TSE) T2-weighted images in which fat is also bright. Comparison with matched T1-weighted images will identify the now dark disk material against the bright fat in the lateral recess or foramina. Occasionally, disk herniations may be associated with a small amount of hemorrhage in the epidural space, which may manifest itself as an epidural process of high T1 and variable T2 signal intensity. This hemorrhage may be related to the pathogenesis of discal cysts, relatively rare cystic lesions in the epidural space, which may present with radicular pain and be the result of prior disk extrusion and hemorrhage with incomplete resorption.[161]

Ninety percent of lumbar disk herniations occur at the L4 or L5 interspace levels. The vector of disk displacement in most herniations is posterolateral. In the lumbar spine, the exiting nerve passes immediately inferior to the vertebral pedicle and exits the foramen above the interspace level. Therefore, most disk herniations do not affect the exiting nerve, but rather impinge on the traversing nerve, which exits under the next lower vertebral pedicle. For example, a posterolateral L4-L5 disk herniation results in an L5 radicular pain syndrome or radiculopathy. For a lumbar disk herniation to affect the like numbered nerve, it must be an extrusion with lateral and cephalad migration of disk material into the neural foramen. The greater spatial resolution of CT myelography may identify subtle lateral recess or foraminal lesions less well seen on MRI.

Contrast material is not typically used when MRI is undertaken to evaluate for causes of radicular pain or radiculopathy except in the presence of red flag features raising concern for infection of neoplasm, or prior surgery. Unenhanced imaging can primarily detect the mechanical compression of a nerve, not the inflammatory response, which is also necessary to provoke radicular pain. T2 hyperintensity on STIR or fat-saturated images may identify this reaction. If gadolinium is given, it is often observed that the soft tissue seen on unenhanced images, thought to be herniated disk material, is largely enhancing inflammatory/granulation tissue about a small disk fragment. When confronted by a patient with clinically evident radicular pain or radiculopathy and no evidence of a neural compressive lesion on standard imaging, an enhanced exam may reveal an inflammatory process associated with a disk whose annulus is incompetent.[162] This is described as chemical radiculitis. The neural compressive component of the lesion may only be present on imaging with axial load and physiologic positioning (Fig. 15.16).

POSTOPERATIVE IMAGING

Gadolinium-enhanced MRI does have a well-defined role in the evaluation of the postoperative patient. Plain films, CT, and CT myelography are relatively uninformative in the postoperative patient, as they cannot reliably distinguish recurrent disk herniation from epidural fibrosis/scar. Following diskectomy, extensive anatomic changes evolve over time, confounding imaging interpretation. Great caution must be used in interpreting MRI within 6 weeks of surgery.[163] In this time frame, MRI is most useful in the evaluation for hemorrhage, pseudomeningocele, or diskitis; evaluation for recurrent disk herniation is tenuous. The diagnosis of postoperative diskitis is also complicated by the normal linear enhancement that may be observed in the postoperative disk.[163] As postoperative tissue disruption and edema stabilize, MRI with gadolinium enhancement has been reported to be 96% to 100% accurate in distinguishing recurrent disk herniation from scar.[163] Scar or epidural fibrosis enhances rapidly and uniformly following gadolinium administration; disk material does not enhance for the first 20 to 30 minutes. Early post-gadolinium images in the postoperative patient will show recurrent disk herniation as a nonenhancing zone; enhancing epidural fibrosis may surround this. Extensive scar or epidural fibrosis is in itself a negative prognostic sign, associated with an increased incidence of postoperative radiculopathy.[164] In the postoperative setting, the thecal sac should be examined for evidence of arachnoiditis. In this condition, the roots of the cauda equina are either clumped together or adherent to the dural tube. The dural tube may even appear empty of roots, which are smoothly scarred to its wall. Roots may exhibit enhancement in this condition.

IMAGING NATURAL HISTORY

The imaging natural history of disk herniation is resolution.[165] Large disk herniations, extrusions, and sequestrations, which have entered the highly vascular epidural space, are most likely to undergo resorption mediated by macrophage produced metalloproteases.[166-168] This inflammatory response is integral to the profound pain these patients feel, but it will ultimately resorb the extruded disk material. If the inflammatory response can be attenuated by the targeted administration of corticosteroids, thus allowing the patient to remain functional, over time natural history will bear out with resolution of the herniated disk material and the radicular pain syndrome. Contained protrusions and bulges, with intact outer annulus shielding the herniation from the full fury of the immune system, tend not to change over time.

VALIDITY OF DISK HERNIATION IMAGING: CORRELATION WITH SYMPTOMS/SIGNS

The fundamental specificity fault of spine imaging is very evident in the imaging of disk herniations. Modic[54] demonstrated that there was no relationship between herniation type, size, or change over time and patient outcome. Most of the imaging findings observed on an imaging study obtained at presentation with radicular pain will have been present at a time when the patient was asymptomatic.[53] In another study by Masui, disk herniations treated conservatively were followed over 7 years.[169] Clinical outcomes were unrelated to the size of the herniation or age changes in the disk. To assign causality to a disk herniation, there must be concordance, a perfect match of the patient's pain or dysfunction syndrome, and the expected detriment caused by

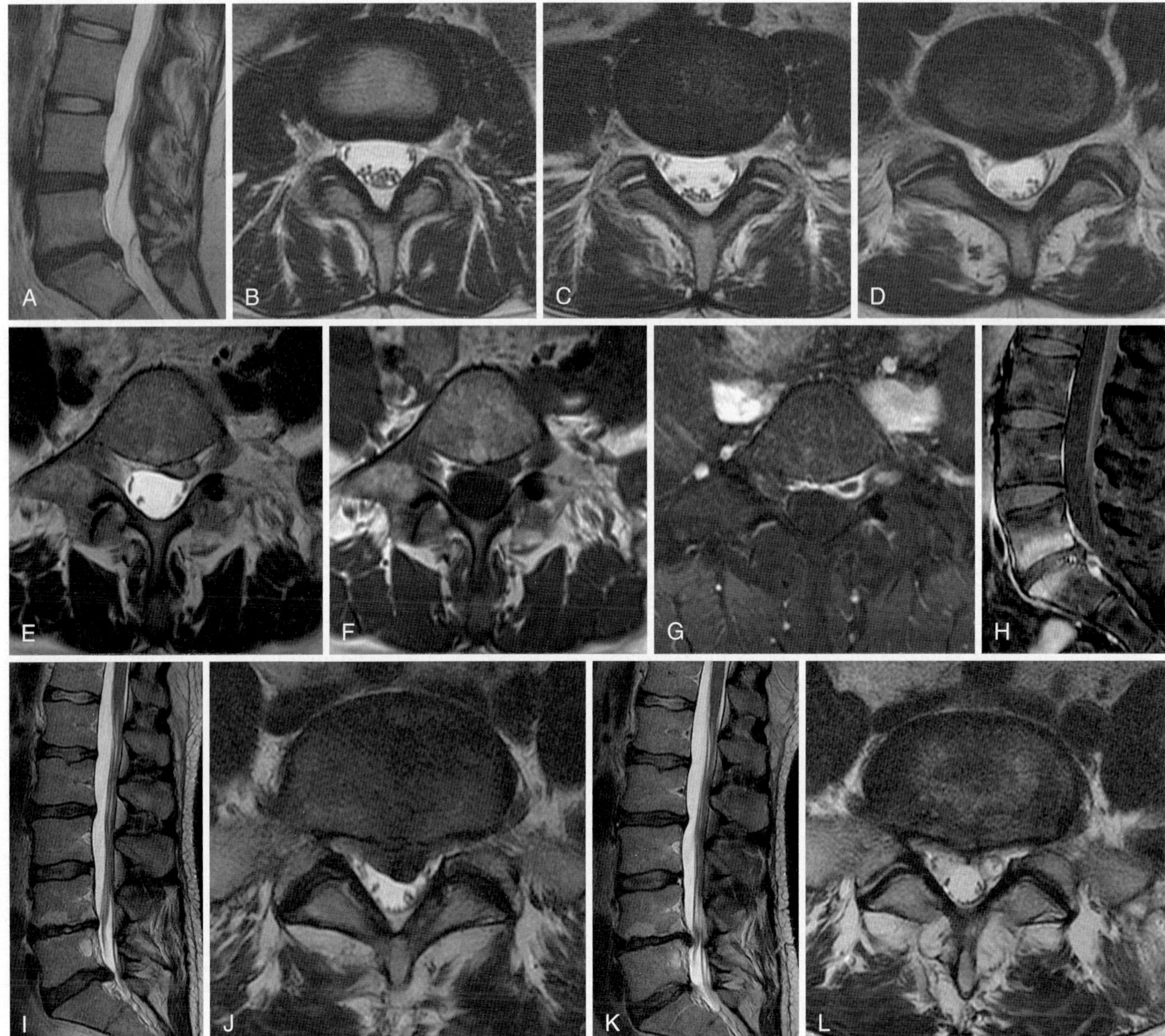

Figure 15.16 Disk herniations. Sagittal T2 MRI **(A)** and axial T2 images at L3-4 **(B)**, L4-5 **(C)**, and L5-S1 **(D)** disks demonstrate a normal L3-4 disk, a central protrusion at L4-5, and a right central extrusion with caudal migration at L5-S1. Axial T2 **(E)** and T1 **(F)** MRI images at the S1 end plate level demonstrate a left-sided sequestered disk fragment contacting the thecal sac. Fat-saturated T1 axial image **(G)** and sagittal image **(H)** show that much of the apparent disk herniation enhances and is inflammatory reaction about a small disk fragment. Enhancing Modic I change is present. Another patient with left S1 radicular pain due to an L5-S1 disk extrusion **(I, J)** was treated with a transforaminal epidural steroid injection with resolution of pain. He returned 4 years later with new L5 distribution pain and was reimaged **(K, L)**. Note that the L5-S1 extrusion has completely resolved; **([L]** is at the identical level as **[J])** and a new L4-5 extrusion has developed. The natural history of disk extrusion is resolution.

an observed herniation. The imager must know the nature of the pain syndrome to identify its likely cause among the distracters of asymptomatic findings. The sensitivity fault is also evident; disk herniations that do not appear to contact neural tissue on recumbent imaging may be compressive under axial load and physiologic posture. Willén and Danielson demonstrated that significant additional information was demonstrated in 14% of sciatica patients on images obtained under extension and axial load, including accentuation of disk herniations, increasing lateral recess or foraminal stenosis, and distension of synovial cysts that contributed to root compression (Box 15.5).[170]

RADICULAR PAIN

LATERAL RECESS, FORAMINAL STENOSIS

As the nerve root exits the common dural sac into its root sleeve, it leaves the central canal, passing caudally and laterally into the lateral recess or subarticular zone. Compromise of the lateral recess may be causal of radicular pain or radiculopathy. Lateral recess stenosis is primarily a product of facet joint arthrosis with overgrowth of the superior articular process. This encroaches on the posterior aspect of the lateral recess, impinging on the exiting nerve root. This is

Box 15.5 Disk Herniations and Radicular Pain

- Radicular pain requires both compression of neural tissue and an inflammatory response, likely mediated by TNFα.
- Standard imaging can only detect nerve root displacement or compression, which are necessary but insufficient to cause symptoms.
- This is in part the basis of the specificity fault: many disk herniations are asymptomatic.
- Assignment of causality of symptoms to a disk herniation requires concordance: there must be a key in lock match of the lesion and the syndrome of pain and neurologic dysfunction.
- The imager must know the nature of the radicular pain/radiculopathy syndrome to consider ascribing symptoms to a disk herniation.
- The natural history of disk herniations is resolution; larger herniations, extrusions, and sequestrations are more likely to resolve.
- There is no relationship between the size, type, or change in disk herniations over time and patient outcomes.
- Decisions regarding surgical intervention must be based on clinical grounds, not imaging appearance.

best demonstrated on axial MRI or CT myelographic images (Fig. 15.17). These images should be scrutinized to be certain that the nerve root in question is indeed entrapped within the lateral recess rather than simply displaced medially into the central canal. The minimum normal A-P dimensions of the lateral recess have been variably reported as 3 mm to 4 mm.[171] The lumbar level most commonly involved with lateral recess stenosis is the L4-5 interspace level.

As the exiting nerve root continues to progress caudally and laterally under its similarly numbered lumbar pedicle, it enters the foraminal zone. The intervertebral foramen is an inverted teardrop-shaped orifice; the exiting root is situated in the larger, superior aspect of the foramen. An annular bulge or lateral protrusion may intrude into the inferior portion of the neural foramen without causing neural compression. A disk extrusion with cranial migration of disk material into the foramen may compress the exiting root. Other degenerative phenomena causing foraminal stenosis include osteophytes arising from the posterior margin of the vertebral body or superior articular process, synovial cysts, or abnormalities of vertebral alignment, including the concavity of a scoliotic curve or spondylolisthesis resulting from spondylolysis or facet arthropathy. Foraminal stenosis is best demonstrated on sagittal MRI images (see Fig. 15.17). The low signal nerve root and accompanying small veins should always be surrounded by high-signal fat on T1- or T2-weighted sagittal MRI images. Axial MRI images may also demonstrate foraminal stenosis, although to less advantage.

SYNOVIAL CYSTS

Synovial cysts may accompany facet osteoarthrosis and may be a cause of radicular pain, neurogenic claudication, and may be associated with axial low back pain. Synovial cysts are thought to originate with a degenerative or traumatic defect in the fibrous facet joint capsule, with subsequent herniation of the synovial membrane through the defect. Expansion of the synovial outpouching, no longer constrained by the joint capsule, results in a cystic lesion, which may impinge on adjacent neural structures or simply serve as an imaging marker of capsular pathology. Synovial cysts may retain or potentially lose their communication with the facet joint. Ganglion cysts may have a similar gross appearance but histologically lack a synovial lining; they may be indistinguishable on imaging studies.

Although relatively unusual, synovial cysts are not rare: the series of Doyle and associates[172] demonstrated a prevalence of nearly 10% in a population of patients undergoing MRI for back or leg pain. In this series, anterior or intraspinal cysts, often arising from the superior recess, had a prevalence of 2.3%; posterior or extraspinal cysts were more common with a 7.3% prevalence. Synovial cysts are prevalent in an elderly population, with an average age of 63 in Metellus' study,[173] 61 in Apostolaki's[174] study population, and 66 years in the large surgical series of Lyons.[175] Reported male-to-female ratios are inconsistent, varying from a 1:1 ratio in the Lyons series to 1.2:1 in the Metellus series to 1:2 in the Apostolaki study; Doyle noted a female predominance in posterior cysts only. Synovial cysts are far more common in the lumbar region than in the thoracic or cervical spine. The literature has consistently shown that 60% to 70% of lumbar synovial cysts will be at L4/5 level, followed in relative order by L5/S1, L3/4, and L2/3. Anterior or intraspinal synovial cysts most commonly occur posterolateral to the thecal sac in close association to the facet joint. They may be embedded in the ligamentum flavum. Uncommonly, cysts may be located directly dorsal to the thecal sac, laterally within the neural foramen, or in a far lateral or extraforaminal site. Far lateral synovial cysts typically arise from the superior recess of the joint, which extends over the superior margin of the superior articular process; the communication with the joint will not be seen on an axial image but may be apparent on sagittal images.

Synovial cysts often arise from facet joints exhibiting significant arthrosis, with sclerosis, osteophytes, and increased joint fluid, although most joints with arthrosis do not produce cysts. Segmental hypermobility is postulated as an underlying cause of synovial cysts. This is supported by the strong association with the most mobile lumbar segment (L4/5) and the frequent (42% to 65%) association with degenerative spondylolisthesis.[174] Disk age-related changes are commonly present at the level of the cyst. Metellus[173] also noted that most cysts arise from joints with a predominant sagittal orientation; this orientation is also associated with segmental instability.

Synovial cysts may be detected by CT, CT myelography, or MRI; MRI is thought to be most sensitive (Fig. 15.18). Calcified cysts may rarely be seen on plain radiographs. Synovial cysts have great variation in their histology, with corresponding variety in their imaging appearance. Synovial cysts may be thin-walled collections of pure synovial fluid, or they may be complicated by varying degrees of chronic or acute hemorrhage and inflammation. Pure cysts have a high T2 signal, equal to or exceeding that of cerebrospinal fluid (CSF), with a thin, low-signal wall. With chronic hemorrhage, cyst contents may develop a high T1 signal (methemoglobin) and a variable T2 signal; the wall often enhances with gadolinium. In the presence of chronic inflammation and calcification,

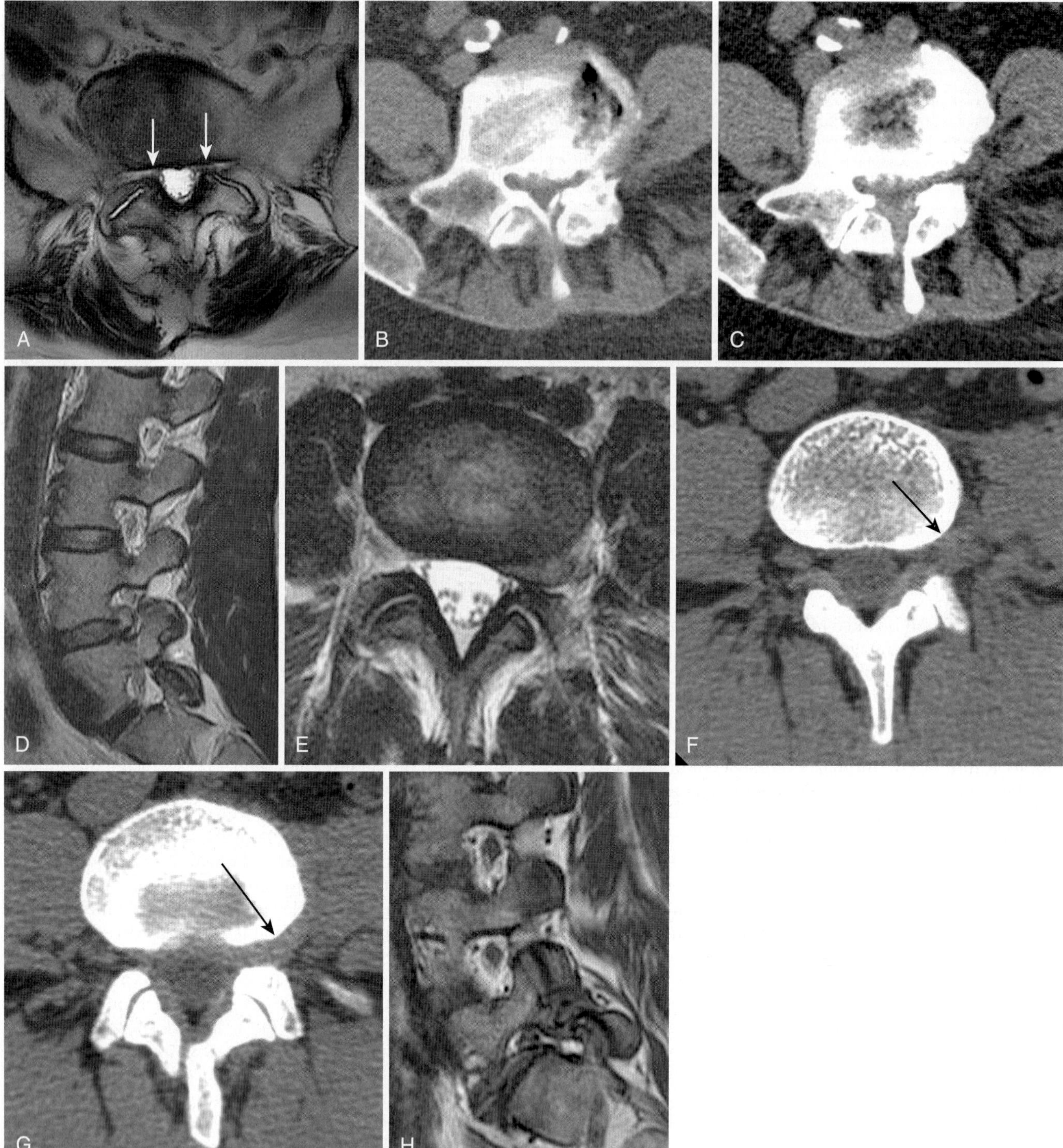

Figure 15.17 Subarticular zone (lateral recess) and foraminal compromise. Axial T2 MRI image **(A)** at the S1 superior end plate demonstrates a widely patent central canal, but severe bilateral subarticular zone stenosis *(arrows)* resulting from facet hypertrophy. Consecutive CT images **(B, C)** at the L5 pedicle level in another patient show severe central canal stenosis, but also severe subarticular zone stenosis primarily caused by end plate osteophytes. T2 sagittal and L4-5 disk axial images **(D, E)** in a patient with left anterior thigh pain reveal a left foraminal disk extrusion, displacing the dorsal root ganglion (DRG) superiorly and laterally. Axial CT images **(F, G)** in another patient with left L4 radicular pain also demonstrate a left L4 foraminal and extraforaminal extrusion *(arrows)* effacing the fat about the exiting L4 DRG and ventral ramus. A final patient with L5 spondylolysis **(H)** demonstrates the typical S-shaped foraminal stenosis at L5-S1 seen in this setting. Note normal foramina at L3-4 and L4-5 with abundant fat surrounding the DRG and small veins.

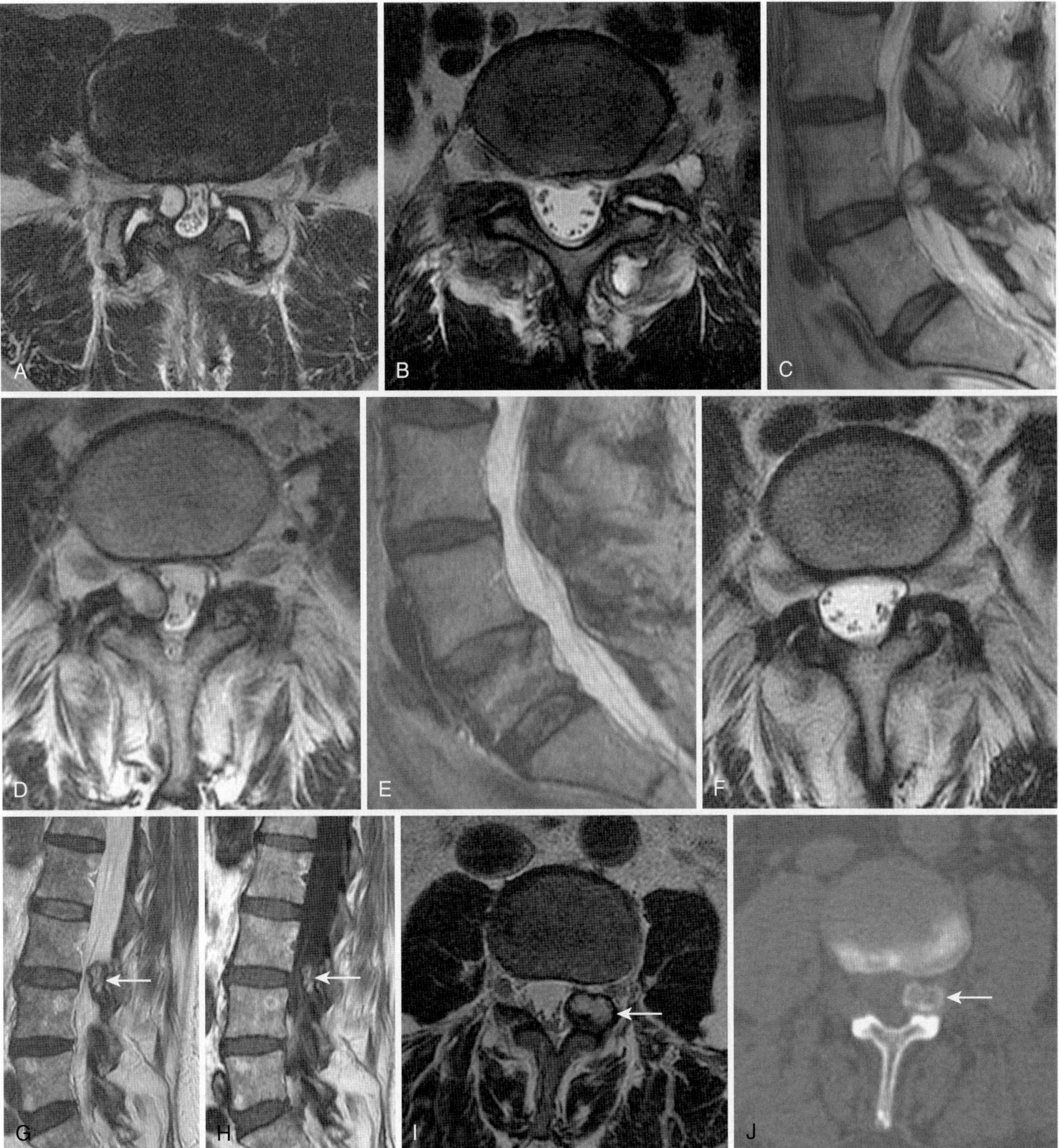

Figure 15.18 Synovial cysts. Typical bilateral L4 intraspinal synovial cysts **(A)** compress the thecal sac on a T2 axial image. A different patient **(B)** demonstrates a synovial cyst in the left L5-S1 neural foramen as well as a posterior extraspinal cyst. Another patient with right L5 radicular pain demonstrates an L4-5 synovial cyst on sagittal **(C)** and axial **(D)** T2 images. The patient underwent a right L5 transforaminal epidural steroid injection and an intra-articular injection of the facet joint/cyst. Her pain resolved. She presented 4 years later with axial pain. MRI T2 sagittal **(E)** and axial **(F)** show a new L5 compression fracture; the synovial cyst has resolved. A final patient demonstrates an irregular thick-walled cyst *(arrows)* arising from the left 3-4 facet **(G, H, I).** Note the T1 hyperintensity **(H).** CT **(J)** shows the cyst is calcified *(arrow).*

the wall may become quite thick, with a very low T1 and T2 signal. On CT, calcification is variably observed and cyst contents range from hypodense to slightly hyperdense relative to muscle. Changes of arthrosis in the adjacent facet joint are typical, including abnormal marrow signal (T2 hyperintensity, T1 hypointensity) in the articular processes and pedicle. A direct communication with the facet joint is not always demonstrable on either CT or MRI. Synovial cysts may not be evident on recumbent CT or MRI imaging, as the synovial fluid recedes into the joint space, collapsing the cyst; when the patient assumes axial load, the joint surfaces are opposed, driving the fluid into the cyst, which then exerts mass effect on neural elements. Not infrequently synovial cysts will fill when the joint is pressurized by intra-articular injection, despite no evidence of their existence on recumbent advanced imaging. The imaging differential diagnosis includes conjoined nerve root sleeves, sequestered disk fragments, cystic nerve sheath tumors, and degenerative cysts of other origins, such as pseudobursae in Baastrup's disease.

Anterior or intraspinal synovial cysts often present as lesions causing unilateral radicular pain or contributing to neurogenic claudication. Anterior synovial cysts may cause focal neural compression in the lateral recess, foramen, or extraforaminal space, or they may contribute to central canal stenosis. Posterior cysts do not cause neural compression but may be associated with axial pain and be an imaging sign of facet capsular disease. Synovial cysts may regress spontaneously. Radicular pain resulting from synovial cysts may be treated by an injection of corticosteroid into the facet joint bearing the cyst, with a transforaminal epidural steroid injection at the same procedural setting. This strategy successfully allowed 50% of patients to avoid surgical injection in a series by Sabers and colleagues.[176] Other nonoperative therapies have included aspiration, fenestration, or rupture of cysts under CT or fluoroscopic guidance. A large case series (n = 101) of percutaneous cyst rupture showed surgical sparing in about 50% of cases.[177] Surgical resection of synovial cysts generally has a favorable outcome, but it may require facetectomy, laminectomy, and possible fusion.

CERVICAL DISK HERNIATIONS

The cervical intervertebral disks differ structurally from the lumbar disk. The cervical disks are thicker anteriorly than posteriorly and have a less well defined nuclear/annular structure. There is no discrete annulus at the posterior disk margin. The cervical disks function less to disburse axial load. They undergo maturational change with age; intradiskal T2 signal loss is a poor predictor of axial pain. Cervical radicular pain or radiculopathy is less common than lumbar symptomatology. Cervical radicular pain is most commonly caused by foraminal compromise of multifactorial origin: uncovertebral joint and facet hypertrophy, loss of disk space height, and less frequently disk herniation. In a population-based study in Rochester, Minnesota, disk herniations were causal of only 22% of cervical radiculopathies.[178] The C6 and C7 nerves were most commonly affected. As in the lumbar region, the vector of herniation is usually posterolateral, but as the cervical nerves exit low in the foramen, a herniation will likely affect the exiting nerve, not the traversing nerve. The C6 nerve exits low in the C5-6 neural foramen; a herniation at this segment will most likely impinge on the C6 nerve.

The natural history of cervical disk herniations parallels the lumbar region. Cervical disk herniations may undergo spontaneous regression. As in the lumbar region, extrusions, migrated disk material, and laterally situated disk herniations are more likely to undergo spontaneous regression. As most lesions causing cervical radicular pain are not purely soft disk but are, at least in part, bony, overall regression of the root compressive lesion is less likely than in the lumbar region. MRI remains the primary advanced imaging modality, but CT myelography may play a larger role. It provides the best spatial resolution, critical in the narrow confines of the cervical region, and excels at discriminating bone from soft disk, which may alter the surgical approach (Fig. 15.19).

THORACIC DISK HERNIATIONS

Symptomatic thoracic disk herniations are rare; only 1% to 2% of all disk surgeries are performed in the thoracic segment.[179] The expected specificity fault applies; disk age-related changes are ubiquitous, and herniations are often asymptomatic. The majority of disk herniations occur in the mid and lower thoracic region. In the surgical series of Stillerman,[180] the T8 to T11 levels were most commonly affected. In this series, 76% of patients presented with pain, 61% with either motor or sensory dysfunction, and 24% with bladder dysfunction. Nearly two thirds of the disk herniations showed evidence of calcification on CT imaging. At surgery, 7% showed intradural extension. Thoracic disk herniations involving the conus can mimic lumbar radicular pain; MRI studies of the lumbar spine should always extend to the conus on the sagittal sequences.

Imaging of thoracic radicular pain should involve MRI or CT myelography. CT myelography has the greatest spatial resolution and may better demonstrate the presence of calcification within thoracic disks. MRI can detect signal abnormality within the cord, which may identify cord edema or venous hypertension, verifying the physiologic significance of a disk herniation. All imaging evaluation for thoracic disk disease must include careful enumeration of the segmental level involved. If a lesion that may require surgical or percutaneous intervention is detected, the imaging study should be extended to include sagittal images from the sacrum to the skull base. Communication between radiologist and surgeon or spine interventionalist is critical to avoid wrong segment interventions.

DEGENERATIVE SPONDYLOLISTHESIS

Spondylolisthesis refers to the abnormal anterior or posterior displacement of one vertebral body relative to another. Displacement caused by defects in the pars interarticularis (spondylolytic spondylolisthesis) will be discussed later. Degenerative anterolisthesis is the anterior displacement of a vertebral body relative to the body immediately caudal to it. The etiology of degenerative anterolisthesis is primarily facet joint arthrosis, often with a relative sagittal orientation of the facets. Disk structural failure is also necessary. Degenerative anterolisthesis may be present in 4% to 14% of elderly patients.[181] Anterolisthesis is most frequent at the L4 level, with less common occurrence at L5, followed by L3. It is significantly more common in women than in men.[181] Radiographic findings of degenerative anterolisthesis include the obvious displacement itself, joint space narrowing and sclerosis in the associated facets, and findings of intervertebral osteochondrosis, including a loss of disk space height, gas within the disk, and subchondral sclerosis.

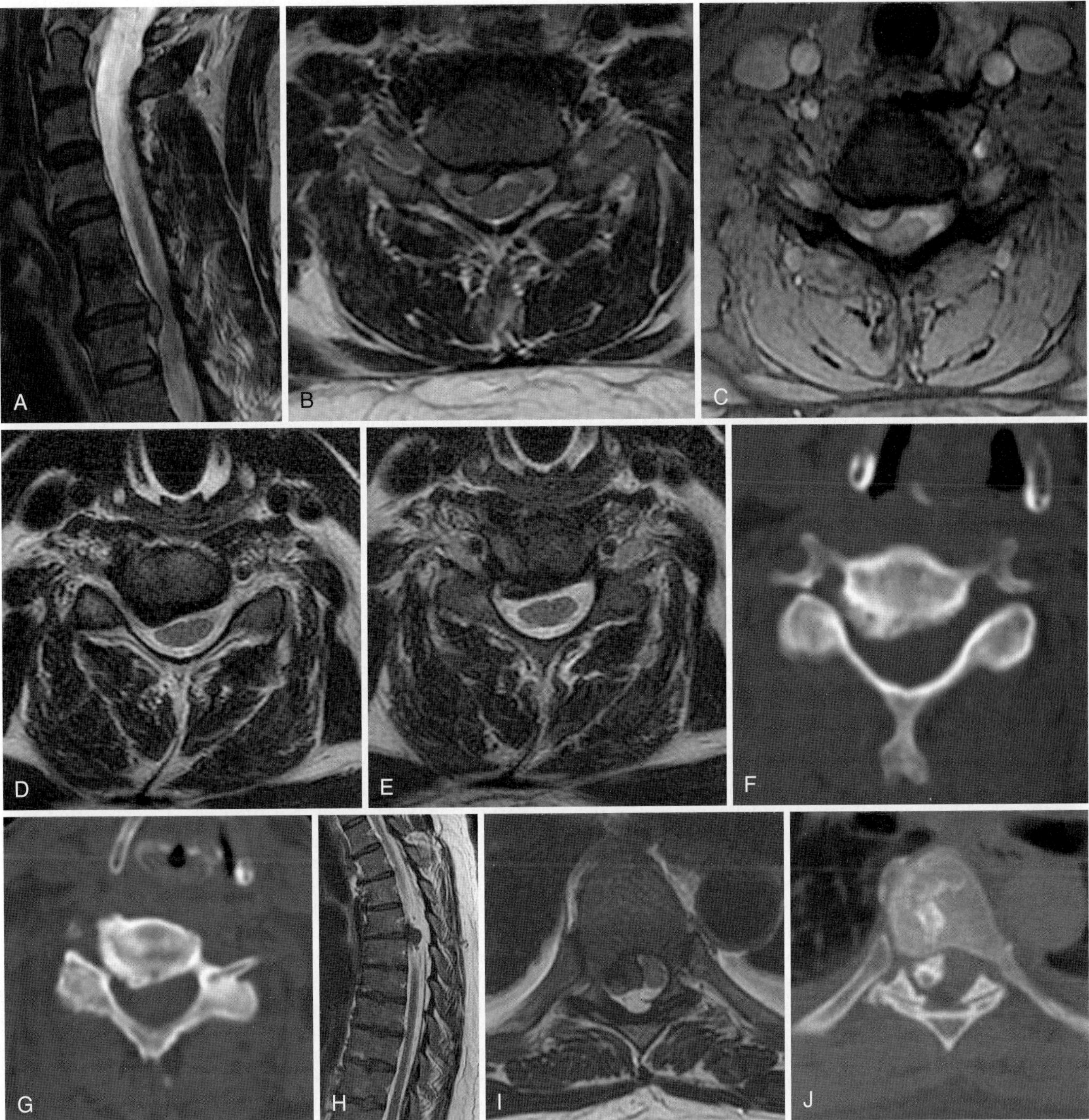

Figure 15.19 Cervical and thoracic disk herniations. A patient with prior C5-6 anterior cervical diskectomy and fusion presents with new right C7 distribution radicular pain. Sagittal T2 image **(A)** shows disk extrusion with caudal migration from the adjacent C6-7 segment. Note that the extruded material has higher T2 signal than parent disk, perhaps a reflection of the inflammatory response. Axial fast spine echo (FSE) T2 **(B)** and gradient echo **(C)** axial images at the C6-7 interspace well demonstrate the extrusion. In another patient with a right C6 radiculopathy axial FSE T2 images **(D, E)** at the C5-6 interspace suggest a disk-osteophyte complex and uncovertebral joint osteophytes compromise the right C5-6 foramen. The primary bony nature of the process is confirmed on CT images **(F, G).** In the cervical spine, compressive lesions are more likely to be osseous than soft disk alone. Thoracic disk extrusion in a 51-year-old woman with progressive thoracic myelopathy is shown in images **H, I,** and **J**. Sagittal T2 MR image **(H)** shows large T5-6 disk extrusion. Low T2 signal suggests calcification. The cord is displaced and compressed by the right-sided extrusion on T2-weighted axial MR image **(I)**. Axial CT image **(J)** demonstrates coarse calcification in the disk extrusion. Note the linear defect with marginal sclerosis in the end plate, a finding often accompanying disk herniations.

Degenerative retrolisthesis describes the posterior displacement of the index vertebral body relative to that below it; the primary causative process is intervertebral osteochondrosis. As there is a loss of disk space height, the oblique orientation of the facet results in the more superior vertebral body gliding posterior relative to its inferior counterpart. Degenerative retrolisthesis is most commonly seen at the L2 interspace level, with less common occurrence at L1, followed by L3. There is no significant gender difference.

Degenerative spondylolisthesis may be associated with axial low back pain. The Kauppila study showed that patients with degenerative spondylolisthesis had a higher prevalence of daily low back symptoms.[181] There was, however, no increased disability in spondylolisthesis patients relative to controls. In this study, the overall incidence of degenerative spondylolisthesis approached 20%. Degenerative spondylolisthesis carries with it the risk of neural element compromise with secondary central canal stenosis, lateral recess stenosis, or foraminal compromise.

SPINAL STENOSIS: LUMBAR NEUROGENIC INTERMITTENT CLAUDICATION (NIC)

Lumbar spinal stenosis is an imaging observation; it may give rise to the clinical syndrome of NIC. NIC is the most common cause of spine surgery in patients over 65 years of age.[182] The hallmark is the induction of gluteal and lower extremity pain with upright exercise or specific postural positions, and palliation by forward flexion, sitting, or recumbency. The most common symptoms in patients with lumbar spinal stenosis are back pain (prevalence of 95%), claudication (91%), leg pain (71%), weakness (33%), and voiding disturbances (12%).[183] There may be a paucity of physical findings, even in the presence of symptoms.

Despite its significance, few prevalence or natural history data are available for NIC. Kalichman and colleagues utilized data from the Framingham study to establish the prevalence of congenital and acquired lumbar central canal stenosis in a community population.[184] Using the anterior-posterior dimension of the central canal derived from CT studies (12 mm = relative stenosis, 10 mm = absolute stenosis), they noted congenital central canal narrowing of relative degree in 4.7% of the population and absolute stenosis in 2.6%. Acquired stenosis was identified in 22.5% (relative) and 7.3% (absolute) of individuals. Their review of the literature noted that the prevalence of acquired lumbar stenosis ranged from 1.7% to 13.1%. The prevalence of acquired stenosis (absolute) increased from 4% in patients younger than 40 years of age to 14.3% in patients older than 60. The North American Spine Society (NASS) 2011 evidence-based guidelines on the diagnosis and treatment of spinal stenosis suggest, in the absence of reliable evidence, that the natural history of patients with clinically mild to moderately symptomatic degenerative stenosis is favorable in one third to one half of patients.[185] In patients with mild to moderately symptomatic stenosis, rapid or catastrophic neurologic decline is a rare phenomenon.

PATHOPHYSIOLOGY

The pathogenesis of NIC in lumbar spinal stenosis has been a subject of investigation for half a century. Verbiest initially described mechanical compression of the nerve roots of the cauda equina as a cause of NIC in 1954.[186] Subsequent investigators have postulated that arterial and venous ischemia, perhaps exacerbated by restriction of CSF flow (which participates in nerve root nutrition), are contributors to the clinical syndrome. The current preponderance of evidence favors venous congestion secondary to mechanical compression. This hypothesis emphasizes the importance of multiple levels of compression and the physiologic effects of lumbar extension. Both of these observations have significant relevance to imaging.

The animal work of Takahashi and Olmarker demonstrated that two zones of modest compression in the cauda equina would dramatically reduce blood flow to the intervening nerve segment because of venous congestion; this venous congestion could precipitate neural dysfunction.[187,188] Kobayashi examined cauda equina histology after the application of a modest stenosis (30% of cross-sectional area) to the dural tube.[189] The cauda equina demonstrated congestion and dilatation of intraradicular veins and an inflammatory cellular infiltrate. There was disruption of the blood-nerve barrier, both at the site of the compression and also in more distant sites of Wallerian degeneration. The necrotic debris created by Wallerian degeneration stimulated macrophage activity generating inflammatory molecules such as interleukin-1 and TNFα. Macrophages stimulate cytotoxic activity by the release of nitric oxide and proteases. They are considered the chief effector cells causing an inflammatory neuritis that results in aberrant ectopic neural discharge and conduction disturbance leading to the pain and neural dysfunction of neurogenic intermittent claudication.[189]

Multiple sites of venous congestion are key to this model of NIC; it is supported by clinical studies. Sato demonstrated that patients with two-level central canal stenosis were significantly more likely to exhibit NIC than were patients with a single level of canal compromise. In two-level stenosis, the symptomatic expression most closely matched the radicular distribution of the more caudal of the two stenotic levels; in patients with compromise at the L3 and L4 disk levels, the pain pattern matched that of the traversing L5 roots.[190] Porter and Ward noted that the sites of compression may be either in the central canal or in the neural foramina.[191] In their cohort of 49 patients with NIC, 94% had either multilevel central canal stenosis or central canal plus neural foraminal stenosis. The work of Morishita emphasized the importance of the neural foramen as a potential zone of compression, particularly with dynamic changes in posture.[192] Even without demonstrable foraminal compromise by imaging in a neutral position, in lumbar extension intraforaminal pressures exceeded venous pressure and neural dysfunction was documented by electromyography (EMG). All levels of neural compromise, central, lateral recess, and foraminal, are potentially significant and must be detected by imaging.

CONGENITAL CENTRAL CANAL STENOSIS

A small proportion of patients with clinical NIC will have developmental narrowing of the lumbar central canal, with only modest spondylotic changes necessary to produce clinical symptoms. Singh and colleagues studied the morphologic characteristics of a cohort of surgically treated patients carrying the clinical diagnosis of congenital lumbar stenosis.[193] They noted that these patients had a significantly shorter pedicle length and, as a result, a smaller cross-sectional spinal canal area when compared with age- and sex-matched controls. The patients with a congenitally narrowed lumbar central canal typically exhibit these morphologic characteristics over several vertebral segments, maximal at the L3 level. This contrasts with purely acquired stenosis, which is often more focal, particularly at the L4 disk level. Congenital central canal stenosis patients tend to present at a younger age (40 to 50 years old) and with less spondylotic change than typical.

ACQUIRED SPINAL STENOSIS

The great majority of patients presenting with neurogenic intermittent claudication have acquired spondylotic change as their primary cause of central canal, lateral recess, or foraminal compromise. The changes that result in compromise of the central canal are rooted in the three-joint structure of the spine motion segment: the disk and the paired facet joints. In the anterior column, degradation of the disk nuclear matrix places excessive load on the posterior annulus, and annular failure results in posterior end plate osteophytes and disk herniation. These changes encroach on the ventral aspect of the central canal or lateral recesses. Loss of disk space height obligates narrowing of the neural foramina and contributes to increased facet load and ultimately arthrosis; facet capsular hypertrophy and superior articular process osteophytes compromise the lateral recesses. Synovial cysts, particularly at the L4 level, may contribute to central canal, lateral recess, or foraminal compromise. The reduced height of the segment and the loss of elasticity of the ligamentum flavum result in its buckling centrally as a dominant cause of the loss of cross-sectional area of the central canal. The ligamentum flavum may also thicken, although it is unclear if this represents true hypertrophy. These several anterior and posterior column phenomena conspire to narrow the central canal most commonly at the L4-5 disk level, followed by L3-4, L5-S1, and L1-2.[194]

There are a number of measurable parameters that could quantify the degree of stenosis depicted by radiography, myelography, CT, or MRI. Verbiest, in his early descriptions of the entity of spinal stenosis, suggested that a 10- to 12-mm anterior-posterior diameter of the dural sac on conventional myelography constituted relative stenosis, with a measurement of < 10 mm denoting absolute stenosis.[186] Steurer, in a 2011 review, surveyed the numerous measurements applied by various authors in the intervening decades in 25 unique studies and four systematic reviews.[171] The most common descriptors of central stenosis include the anterior-posterior (AP) dimension of the osseous canal or the dural sac and the cross-sectional area of the dural sac. A dural sac AP dimension of < 10 mm or a dural sac cross-sectional area of < 100 mm^2 constitutes stenosis. Descriptors of lateral recess (LR) or subarticular stenosis include the height and the lateral recess angle. Height is defined as the shortest distance between the most anterior point of the superior articular process (SAP) and the posterior vertebral body, and the LR angle is the angle formed by the posterior vertebral body and the pars interarticularis. LR stenosis is typically defined as height < 3 mm or angle < 30 degrees. Descriptors of foraminal stenosis most commonly used suggest a diameter of ≤ 2 to 3 mm as indicative of stenosis.

The multiplicity of quantitative parameters suggests that no single measurement has proven satisfactory. Indeed, the very notion of a readily quantifiable measure of stenosis may be flawed. There is a wide normal variation in central canal and dural tube diameters; an assessment of stenosis must address not simply diameter or cross-sectional area but the crowding or compression of neural tissue. The semiquantitative criteria advanced in 2001 by Fardon and Milette[158] simply defines reduction in expected area by less than one third as mild, by one third to two thirds as moderate, and by greater than two thirds as severe. This allows a subjective judgment of neural compression at the potential cost of reliability. Lurie and associates studied the reliability of the subjective grading of stenosis of the central canal, lateral recesses, and neural foramina and measurement of central canal and dural sac area aided by specific definitions and imaging examples of the criteria.[195] Stenosis was subjectively rated as none, mild, moderate, and severe using the Fardon and Milette definitions; nerve root compromise in the foramen was categorized as none, touching, displacing, or compressing. Inter-reader reliability in assessing the central canal was substantial, with a $\kappa = 0.73$. There was moderate to substantial reliability for foraminal stenosis and nerve root impingement (κ = 0.58. 0.51, respectively). Reliability for subarticular stenosis was only moderate at $\kappa = 0.49$. These results emphasize the importance of a clear definition of criteria for reliably grading stenosis by subjective scales.

Other imaging observations have been employed in an attempt to identify significant stenosis. The observation of nerve root redundancy as a qualitative marker of central canal compromise dates from the original description of the entity of spinal stenosis by Verbiest.[186] This is presumed to originate from mechanical entrapment of the root at the site of compression, with subsequent elongation of the nerve above this site under the tensile stress of physiologic flexion and extension motion. Some of these prominent structures may also represent dilated veins. Although frequently observed, this sign has been subjected to little study. Redundant nerve roots are present in 34% to 42% of surgical candidates with clinical NIC.[196] In a 2007 study by Min and colleagues, redundant nerve roots were more commonly observed in older patients, but there was no significant association with duration of symptoms, diameter of the spinal canal, preoperative symptom intensity or surgical outcomes.[196] There was a nonsignificant trend toward poorer surgical outcomes in patients with redundant roots.

A 2010 study by Barz described the "nerve root sedimentation sign" as a marker of symptomatic NIC.[197] In patients without central canal compromise, the roots of cauda equina lie in the dorsal aspect of the dural sac on supine MRI imaging. A positive sedimentation sign was defined as the absence of nerve root sedimentation to the dorsal dural sac on at least one axial MRI image at a level above or below the zone of compression; the two nerve roots leaving the dural sac at the next most caudal segment are exceptions. This retrospective study utilized a total of 200 patients: 100 patients with low back pain but without clinical NIC, and a dural cross-sectional area (DCSA) of > 120 mm^2 and a cohort of 100 patients with clinical NIC, a maximum walking distance of less than 200 m, and a DCSA of less than 80 mm^2 on at least one level. There was no correlation between the smallest DCSA and patient disability as measured by the Oswestry Disability Index (ODI). The sedimentation sign, however, was identified in 94 of the patients in the NIC cohort but in none of the low back pain group. It remains to be demonstrated that this sign provides additional specificity over a quantitative measurement of the DCSA.

Given the specificity challenges of purely anatomic imaging, the more physiologic parameter of gadolinium enhancement may have a role. This is not a new observation; in 1993, Jinkins observed abnormal intrathecal nerve root enhancement at the site of stenosis on enhanced MRI in patients with NIC.[198] He postulated that this represented a breakdown of the blood-nerve barrier at sites of nerve root injury with subsequent Wallerian degeneration. This has been elegantly confirmed in a canine model by the work of Kobayashi.[189] Histologic examination demonstrated congestion and dilatation of intra-radicular veins and an inflammatory cellular infiltrate at sites of gadolinium enhancement. Gadolinium enhancement may provide added specificity in the correlation of imaging and the clinical symptomatology of NIC; this remains to be proven in clinical studies (Fig. 15.20).

SPECIFICITY OF IMAGING FINDINGS

The ultimate challenge in establishing the utility of diagnostic imaging in the diagnosis of NIC is the lack of a gold standard against which to measure imaging parameters. Surgical findings may be subjective. Clinical outcomes are highly dependent on the technical success of the instituted surgical therapy and the outcome instruments used in any such measurement.

The specificity fault in imaging of central canal stenosis can be seen in studies of asymptomatic volunteers. Boden and associates noted significant central canal stenosis on MRI in 21% of asymptomatic subjects over the age of 60.[18] Jarvik and colleagues demonstrated that asymptomatic stenosis on MRI increases in prevalence with age: moderate to severe central canal stenosis was observed in 7% of subjects < 45; in 6% of subjects age 45 to 55; in 11% of subjects age 55 to 65, and in 21% of subjects over age 65.[19]

Against this background of asymptomatic central canal narrowing, numerous conflicting studies have attempted to establish a relationship between imaging quantitation of central canal or dural size and clinical expression of NIC. For example, Hamanishi and colleagues showed that a decrease in the DCSA to less than 100 mm^2 at more than two of three lumbar levels (L2-3, L3-4, L4-5) was highly associated with the presence of clinical NIC.[199] For each study showing such an association, several others refute it. Sirvanci examined patients undergoing decompressive surgery for NIC.[200] Morphologic stenosis was assessed by DCSA (> 100 mm^2: normal; 76 to 100 mm^2: moderately stenotic; < 76 mm^2: severely stenotic) and a 4-point grading of subarticular and foraminal stenosis. There was no correlation between any of the measured parameters in any spine compartment and patient disability as measured by the Oswestry Disability Index (ODI). This applied both to patients with multilevel central stenosis and to a subset with degenerative spondylolisthesis. The NASS guidelines[185] conclude that there is insufficient evidence to recommend for or against a correlation between clinical symptoms or function and the presence of anatomic narrowing of the spinal canal on cross-sectional imaging.

SENSITIVITY OF IMAGING FINDINGS

There is also a basic sensitivity flaw in advanced imaging. NIC is by definition intermittent; most patients with NIC report exacerbation of symptoms with extension and weight bearing. It is well known that the cross-sectional area of the central spinal canal, subarticular zone or lateral recess, and neural foramina is maximized with flexion positioning; the dimensions of these structures diminish with extension and axial load. Intradiskal pressures are significantly lower when one is in a recumbent position than when sitting or standing. A 2009 study by Hansson and associates identified the ligamentum flavum as the greatest dynamic contributor to central canal compromise with axial load and extension.[39] The average cross-sectional area of the central canal diminished by 23 mm^2 at the L3 disk level and 14 mm^2 at the L4 level under load. The ligamentum flavum was responsible for 50% of the reduction at the L3 level and 85% of the reduction at the L4 level. Madsen and associates attempted to distinguish between the effects of axial load and extension; their work suggested that lumbar spine extension is the dominant cause of reduction in DCSA in the standing patient.[40] Mechanisms circumventing this flaw include upright axial loading devices, the technologically immature upright MRI, and cone beam CT myelography (Box 15.6).

THORACIC SPINAL STENOSIS

Symptomatic central canal stenosis in the thoracic segment of the spine resulting from age-related change is far less common than in the cervical and lumbar regions, likely because of the added mechanical stability imparted by the rib cage. Systemic disease accounts for a correspondingly greater proportion of cases. Systemic processes leading to thoracic central canal compromise include achondroplasia, osteochondrodystrophy, Scheuermann's disease, diffuse idiopathic skeletal hyperostosis (DISH), and Paget's disease.

Compromise of the thoracic spinal canal may be manifest clinically as myelopathy, radiculopathy, or a mixed presentation. The segmental level of canal compromise is most commonly reported to be in the lower thoracic region. Thoracic spine mobility, particularly flexion-extension motion, is greatest near the thoracolumbar junction, likely the biomechanical underpinning to this distribution of age-related pathology. Posterior element age-related changes play a greater role in the genesis of thoracic central canal compromise. This takes the form primarily of unilateral or bilateral facet joint hypertrophy. Thoracic disk herniations or disk-osteophyte complexes may also contribute. Both the ventral and dorsal contributions to thoracic central canal compromise are clearly visible on CT, CT/myelography, and MRI.

Other causes of thoracic central canal stenosis include ossification of the thoracic ligamentum flavum (OLF), a well-recognized cause of thoracic stenosis in an Asian population, but rare among Caucasian subjects. Epidural lipomatosis is a rare cause of central canal compromise in the thoracic or lumbar spine. It may be idiopathic or secondary to endogenous or exogenous steroid excess. Obesity is a common factor in both groups. Excess epidural fat acts as a mass compressing the dural sac, most commonly from a dorsal vector in the thoracic region; it is more likely to be circumferential in the lumbar region.

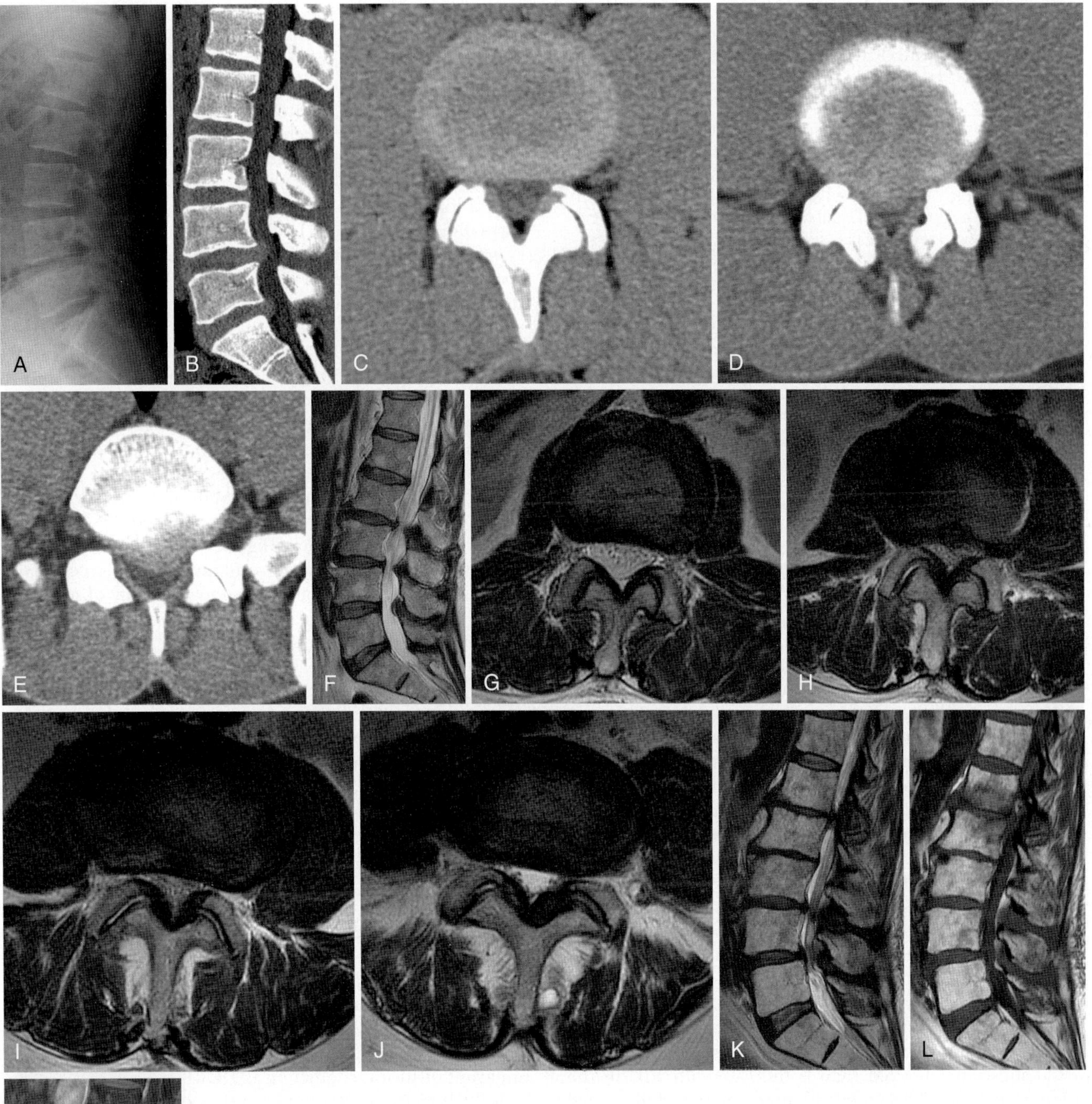

M

Figure 15.20 Central canal stenosis manifest as neurogenic intermittent claudication (NIC). A 24-year-old male presents with incapacitating leg pain with walking and recent voiding disturbance. Lateral radiograph **(A)** demonstrates short pedicles throughout the lumbar spine. Sagittal CT image **(B)** and axial images at L3-4 **(C)**, L4-5 **(D)**, and L5-S1 **(E)** demonstrate the developmentally narrow spinal canal with superimposed disk herniations at L4-5 and L5-S1. There is severe central canal compromise at L4-5 and L5-S1. The L3-4 disk has a broad bulge without canal compromise. A 62-year-old male has classic symptoms of NIC; a sagittal T2 MRI image **(F)** demonstrates mild loss of disk space height and annular bulges at L2-3 and L3-4; the dominant element constricting the spinal canal is the ligamentum flavum. Axial T2 images at L1-2 to L4-5 **(G, H, I, J**, respectively**)** confirm the severe central canal compromise at L2-3 and L3-4 primarily because of ligamentum flavum thickening. A 68-year-old male has severe NIC with a walking tolerance of 10 to 20 m. A T2 sagittal image **(K)** shows severe stenosis at L4-5 and an L1-2 herniation. T1 unenhanced **(L)** and fat-saturated, T1-enhanced **(M)** images show intrathecal enhancement at L4-5 consistent with breakdown of blood-nerve barrier and Wallerian degeneration. Note also enhancing Modic I change and disk herniation at L1-2.

Box 15.6 Lumbar Spinal Stenosis: Neurogenic Intermittent Claudication

- Decompression procedures for lumbar spinal stenosis are the most common spine surgery in the elderly.
- Neurogenic intermittent claudication (NIC) is a clinical syndrome; spinal stenosis is an anatomic observation.
- The best evidence of NIC pathophysiology suggests venous congestion from multiple sites of compression initiates an inflammatory reaction and Wallerian degeneration with blood-nerve barrier disruption and intra-radicular edema.
- Clinically, multiple sites of compression, at different segment levels or different spine compartments (central, lateral, foraminal) are necessary for NIC.
- Beware the specificity fault: The correlation between quantitative measures of central canal or dural sac size and patient symptoms or function is poor.
- Beware the sensitivity fault: Dynamic lesions, present only with extension and axial load, may make recumbent imaging insensitive.

CERVICAL STENOSIS: CERVICAL SPONDYLOTIC MYELOPATHY (CSM)

Cervical spondylotic myelopathy (CSM) is the most common cause of spinal cord dysfunction in patients over 55 years of age.[201] Stookey originally described cervical spondylotic myelopathy in 1928.[202] Although its pathophysiology remains incompletely understood, it is widely acknowledged to involve static factors causing stenosis of the cervical canal and dynamic factors causing repetitive cord injury.[201] These mechanical factors both directly injure neural tissue and initiate secondary ischemia, inflammation, and apoptosis. The histologic characteristics in the cord in CSM include cystic cavitation and gliosis of the central gray matter and demyelination of the medial portions of the white matter long tracks. There is Wallerian degeneration in the posterior columns and posterolateral tracts cephalad to the site of compression. Loss of anterior horn cells and corticospinal tract degeneration are visible at and caudal to the site of compression.

The developmentally narrow spinal canal is a more universal substrate for CSM than is the case with NIC in the lumbar region. The sagittal diameter of the adult spinal cord is nearly constant, measuring about 8 mm from C3-C7; the cervical cord enlargement occurs primarily in the transverse plane.[201] The normal cervical spinal canal sagittal diameter (posterior vertebral body to spinolaminar line) is 17 to 18 mm (C3-C7) in a Caucasian population; these subjects rarely develop sufficient age-related change to provoke CSM. Edwards and LaRocca observed that patients with developmentally narrowed midcervical sagittal diameters of < 10 mm were often myelopathic, patients with canals of 10 to 13 mm were at risk for CSM, canals of 13 to 17 mm were noted in patients with symptomatic spondylosis but rarely myelopathy, and subjects with canals > 17 mm were not prone to develop spondylosis.[203] Morishita studied the kinematics of subjects with congenitally narrowed canals; there is hypermobility in the lower cervical region, providing a biomechanical explanation for the significantly greater age-related change seen in this setting.[204] Hence, the individual with a congenitally narrowed canal is at risk because of both the limited space available for the cord and a greater propensity to age-related spondylotic change.

Acquired cervical central canal stenosis encompasses age-related spondylotic change (most common), ossification of the posterior longitudinal ligament (OPLL), and OLF. Disk degradation results in a loss of disk space height, excess loading of the uncovertebral joints with osteophyte formation, excess facet loading causing hypertrophy, and central buckling of the ligamentum flavum. These processes circumferentially narrow the canal and directly compress the cord, exiting nerves, and the anterior spinal artery. The most common levels of compromise were C3-4 (27%), C4-5 (37%), and C-56 (29%) in a surgical series.[205] This series included patients with spondylosis only and those with OPLL. It is also known that the cross-sectional area of the cervical canal diminishes in both extension and flexion, with greater effects during extension.[44,45] Ventral compression of the cord compromises flow through the arterioles arising from the anterior spinal artery in the ventral sulcus of the cervical cord; dorsal compression reduces perfusion to the central gray matter. Oligodendrocytes are extremely sensitive to ischemic injury; resultant apoptotic cell death may cause the demyelination characteristically observed in CSM.[201] Animal evidence further supports the role of an inflammatory cascade in apoptotic cell death.[206]

IMAGING

Historically, radiographic assessment of cervical anatomic stenosis relied on the anterior-posterior dimension of the central canal as measured from the posterior vertebral body to the spinolaminar line. The normal sagittal diameter from C3 through C7 is considered to be 17 to 18 mm; Edwards and LaRocca noted that a cervical canal with a sagittal diameter of less than 13 mm was at risk for myelopathy; absolute stenosis was defined as being less than 10 mm.[203] The advent of cross-sectional imaging has allowed us to directly measure the diameters and cross-sectional areas of the cervical spinal canal and the cervical cord. MRI has also given us the ability to evaluate physiologic parameters: T2 hyperintensity, T1 hypointensity, gadolinium enhancement, and, with diffusion tensor imaging (DTI), fractional anisotropy (FA), and apparent diffusion coefficient (ADC).

A 2010 study by Naganawa and associates demonstrated good intra- and inter-observer reliability in evaluation of the cross sections of the cervical canal and spinal cord with both CT/myelography and MRI.[207] They noted that dural sac diameter and cross-sectional area measurements were slightly but significantly larger with CT/myelography than fast spin echo T2-weighted MRI; conversely, the diameters and cross-sectional areas of the spinal cord were slightly but significantly larger with MRI. MRI graded the stenosis as slightly, but significantly, more severe than CT/myelography. A 2009 study by Song and associates found no significant difference in inter-observer or intra-observer reliability between CT/myelography and MRI.[208] With its superior spatial resolution, CT/myelography was somewhat better in assessing foraminal stenosis and much better in discriminating bony versus soft tissue lesions. MRI was more reliable in identifying direct nerve root compression (Fig. 15.21).

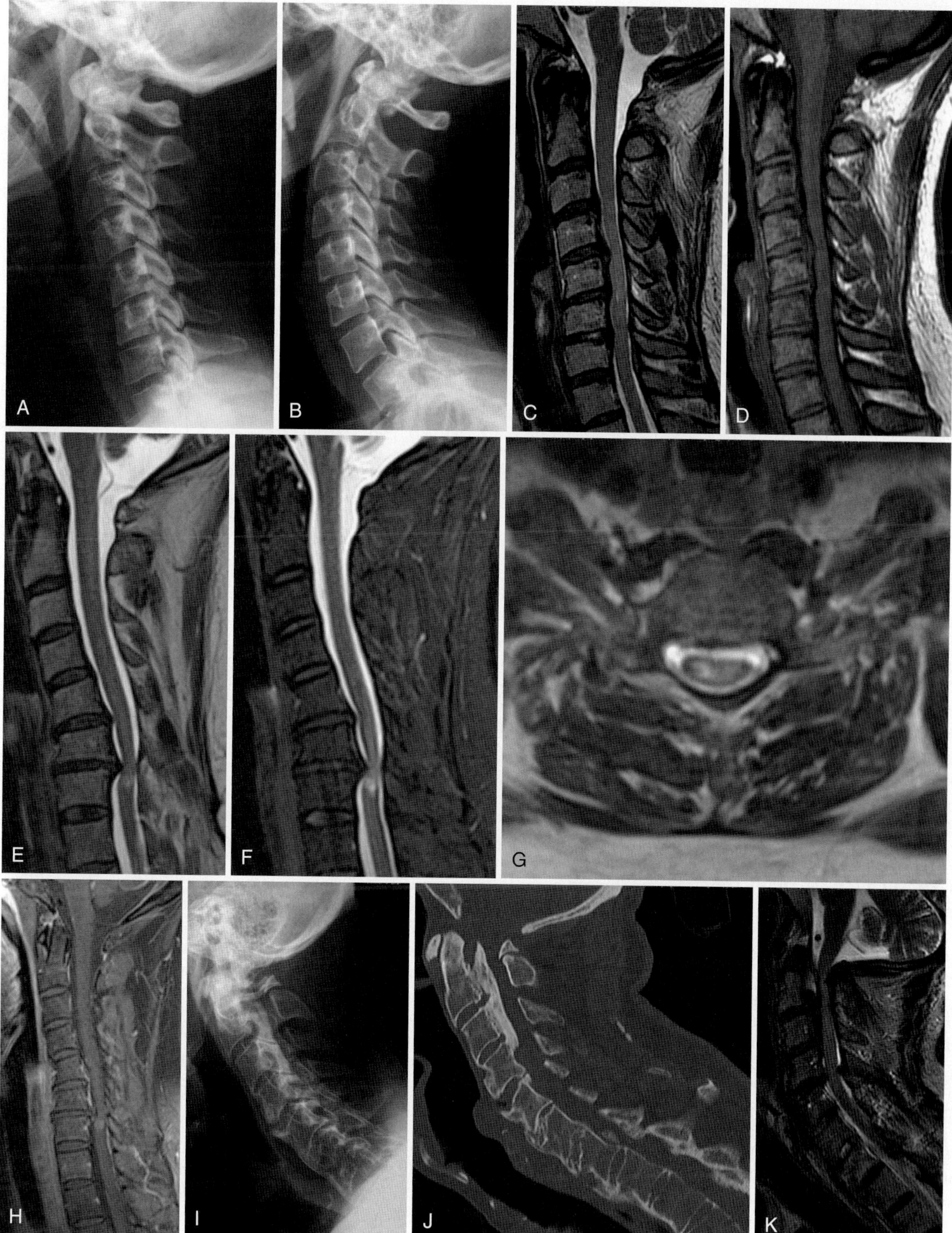

Figure 15.21 Cervical central canal compromise manifest as cervical spondylotic myelography (CSM). A 36-year-old female presents with very subtle bilateral hand incoordination, neck pain, and left arm symptoms. Her lateral radiograph **(A)** shows no lamina posterior to the articular pillar. Compare to a normal lateral radiograph **(B)**. Sagittal T2 **(C)** and T1 **(D)** images show effacement of CSF and cord compression from the C4-C6 interspaces with subtle T2 hyperintensity in the cord at the C5-6 interspace level. Note that no dorsal epidural fat is visible above the C7-T1 level, a typical finding.

A 48-year-old female had intractable upper extremity pain and dysesthesia involving the right lateral forearm. There were also long tract signs. Sagittal T2 **(E)** and T2 with fat saturation **(F)** demonstrate cord deformity at the C6-C7 interspace level, with focal T2 hyperintensity in the right side of the cord, as seen on the axial FSE image **(G)**. Postgadolinium sagittal T1-weighted image with fat saturation **(H)** shows enhancement at the site of T2 hyperintensity, a negative prognostic sign.

A 77-year-old Caucasian male has slowly progressive myelopathy on clinical examination. Lateral radiograph **(I)** demonstrates OPLL in the upper cervical spine; note the coexistent manifestations of DISH. CT sagittal reconstruction **(J)** and sagittal T2 **(K)** images better depict the severe cord deformity at C2.

IMAGING SPECIFICITY

The significant prevalence of asymptomatic cervical central canal stenosis was noted earlier in this chapter. When a population of patients with a clinical diagnosis of CSM is studied, the correlations appear more favorable. The transverse area of the spinal cord as measured by MRI correlates well with the severity of myelopathy and the pathologic changes observed in the cord in CSM.[209] The physiologic parameters of T2 hyperintensity or T1 hypointensity have provided further insight into the evolution of CSM. The several studies addressing these correlates are explored in a review.[210] From these studies we can conclude the following:

1. Intramedullary T2 hyperintensity represents a range of reversible (edema) and irreversible (demyelination, gliosis, cystic necrosis) pathology.
2. Faint and indistinct T2 hyperintensity is more likely to reflect reversible edema.
3. Very intense and well-defined T2 hyperintensity more likely represents fixed gliosis or cystic necrotic change.
4. Intramedullary T1 hypointensity represents irreversible necrosis and myelomalacia.

A 2010 study by Ozawa[211] and a 2011 study by Cho[212] compared CSM patients who exhibited gadolinium enhancement with a nonenhancing control group. The zone of enhancement was always within and smaller than a zone of T2 hyperintensity at the site of maximal compression, with extension caudally. It was typically observed in the posterior or posterolateral cord. There was no correlation of enhancement with preoperative clinical symptoms. Enhancement disappeared in most patients within 1 year of surgical decompression; patients who exhibited preoperative enhancement had a poorer postoperative prognosis than those who did not. Floeth studied 20 CSM patients with FDG-PET in the setting of a single level stenosis at C3/C4 or C4/C5.[213] All the CSM patients showed a significant decrease in 18F-FDG uptake in the lower cord below the stenosis, relative to normal controls. A cohort of these patients also exhibited increased uptake at the level of the stenosis. The patients with increased 18F-FDG uptake at the stenosis had a significantly shorter duration of symptoms, a more precipitous decline in function in the 3 months prior to decompression, and ultimately exhibited significant improvement after decompression. Patients without increased uptake at the stenotic zone did not recover neurologic function after decompression.

Early reports suggest that diffusion tensor imaging may offer greater accuracy in the identification of symptomatic cord compromise than T2 hyperintensity or T1 hypointensity. The measured parameters are fractional anisotropy (FA), mean diffusivity (MD), or apparent diffusion coefficient (ADC). The ADC or MD values reflect overall diffusivity in the tissue irrespective of directional dependence. Anisotropy (directional dependence) of diffusion in white matter tracts results from oriented membrane structure (i.e., axons and myelin). Diminished FA values may reflect loss of directionally oriented membrane structures, increased extracellular edema, or both. Several studies[210] suggest diminished FA is more sensitive in the detection of early cord injury than intramedullary T2 hyperintensity and is better correlated with symptoms. This may assist in the selection of patients for surgical decompression, although additional work remains to be done.

Box 15.7 Cervical Spondylotic Myelopathy: Prognostic Factors for Surgical Decompression

1. Intramedullary T2 hyperintensity diminishes prognosis relative to normal signal.
   a. Intense, focal T2 hyperintensity is a more negative prognostic sign than ill-defined hyperintensity.
   b. Multilevel T2 hyperintensity is a more negative prognostic sign than single level change.
   c. Resolution of T2 hyperintensity postoperatively improves prognosis.
   d. Expansion of T2 hyperintensity postoperatively diminishes prognosis.
2. Intramedullary T1 hypointensity greatly diminishes prognosis.
   a. Evolution of T1 hypointensity postoperatively diminishes prognosis.
3. Intramedullary gadolinium enhancement greatly diminishes prognosis.
4. Increased metabolic activity at the site of compression on 18F-FDG PET improves prognosis over no increased activity.
5. Postoperative residual compression and failure of re-expansion of the cord cross section are negative prognostic signs.

From Maus TP. Imaging of spinal stenosis: neurogenic intermittent claudication and cervical spondylotic myelopathy. *Radiol Clin North Am.* 2012;50:651-679.

IMAGING CORRELATES WITH DECOMPRESSION PROGNOSIS

The ultimate goal of imaging must be to improve the clinical outcomes of patients. In the CSM population, this currently implies the timely and appropriate selection of patients for therapeutic interventions, primarily surgical decompression. There is a large body of literature[210] that has examined the role of imaging in predicting clinical response to surgical decompression; imaging parameters under consideration include the cross-sectional area of the cord, intramedullary T2 hyperintensity, including its degree of intensity and multifocality, intramedullary T1 hypointensity, change or stability of intramedullary signal after decompression, recovery of cord cross-sectional area after decompression, and intramedullary gadolinium enhancement. These are summarized in Box 15.7. Utilization of these findings should assist in the selection and counseling of CSM patients regarding surgical decompression.

OSSIFICATION OF THE POSTERIOR LONGITUDINAL LIGAMENT (OPLL)

Ossification of the posterior longitudinal ligament (OPLL) is a multifactorial disease, whose genetic basis is a defect in the nucleotide pyrophosphatase (NPPS) gene.[201] The prevalence is 1.9 to 4.3% of the Japanese population and approximately 3% of the populations of Korea and Taiwan. It is implicated in up to 25% of North American and Japanese cases of CSM. It has a significant association (up to 50%) with DISH, and some consider it a subtype of DISH. Like age-related causes of structural central canal narrowing, it is often asymptomatic. The ossification is most common in the cervical region, where it causes static narrowing of the canal; repeated impact of the ventral cord on the bony mass contributes to myelopathic injury. Patients may present in their 40s and 50s with pain, chronic myelopathy, or acute neurologic injury after modest trauma. The natural history of the ossification is progression. Close clinical follow-up is warranted.

The ligamentous ossification may be identified on radiographs, CT, and MRI. On lateral radiographs, reduction of the sagittal canal diameter available for the cord by > 60% correlates strongly with myelopathy.[213] The ossification is located from C2-4 in 70% of cases, T1-4 in 15%, and L1-3 in 15%.[214] On CT, the ossification may be classified as segmental (posterior to individual vertebrae, 39%), continuous (bridging across vertebra, 27%), mixed type (29%), and other (ossification posterior to disks, variable sagittal extension, 5%).[215] In addition to documenting the degree of central canal compromise, the CT characteristics of OPLL can suggest dural penetration. CSF leaks are a significant risk in anterior decompression surgery, particularly when the dura is ossified or inseparable from the bony ligamentous mass. On MRI, mature ligamentous ossification is of diminished signal intensity on all sequences; early OPLL may have inhomogeneous signal and exhibit slight enhancement.[215] When mature, there is no enhancement, allowing differentiation from epidural fibrosis. The secondary signal alterations in the cord were described earlier in the chapter.

SYSTEMIC DISEASE CAUSAL OF SPINE/LIMB PAIN

In the context of the very low prevalence of systemic disease as causal of spine or limb pain, this chapter has focused on the mechanical and inflammatory processes involving the articulations of the spine that most commonly provoke axial or radicular pain syndromes and syndromes of neurologic dysfunction. It must be remembered, however, that detection of undiagnosed systemic disease—including stress fractures, infection, spondyloarthropathy, neoplasm, and dural fistula—is the primary role of spine imaging.

STRESS FRACTURES

Stress fractures encompass fatigue fractures, in which normal osseous architecture is subjected to sustained supraphysiologic loads, and insufficiency fractures, in which deficient osseous structure fails under normal load conditions. Insufficiency (osteoporotic) fractures are the most common manifestation of systemic disease to present as back pain. In 2005, an estimated 2 million osteoporotic fractures occurred in the United States in patients > 50 years of age; 27% were vertebral body fractures.[216] This is an underestimate of prevalence, as many vertebral fractures remain asymptomatic. Each vertebral wedge configuration fracture accentuates load on the anterior aspect or adjacent vertebra and increases the annual risk of additional fractures fivefold.[217]

Imaging of vertebral compression fractures begins with weight-bearing radiographs, which provide a low-cost means of assessing change over time with serial images but are relatively insensitive in fracture detection. Radiographic findings include a wedge deformity, most commonly of the superior end plate, which may be accompanied by increased density in the involved end plate in the acute or subacute phase. Chronic deformities often demonstrate remodeled osteophytes. MRI or bone scan are much more sensitive in fracture detection and can better assess acuity. The presence and extent of a marrow edema pattern (T1 hypointense, T2 hyperintense, most conspicuous on STIR or fat-saturated images) can provide an estimate of acuity. The signal abnormality in the marrow tends to be bandlike, paralleling the involved end plate; it may be traversed by a low signal line, adding further confidence to the diagnosis of fracture.

A primary role of imaging in this setting is the characterization of a vertebral fracture as benign or malignant. Malignant lesions are much more likely to exhibit diminished T1 signal throughout the vertebral body. Extension of diminished T1 signal to the vertebral pedicles or posterior elements is relatively specific for malignancy. Paravertebral or epidural mass associated with a fracture is more common in malignant lesions. Posterior bowing of the vertebral body strongly suggests malignancy. Gadolinium enhancement to a level greater than that noted in normal marrow suggests a malignant lesion. Associated disk rupture and retropulsion of a bony fragment without bowing of the posterior margin of the vertebral body suggest a benign lesion. Discrete linear zones of T2 hyperintensity similar to CSF adjacent to the fractured end plate (the fluid sign) are visible in 40% of osteoporotic compression fractures and are a finding of high specificity for a benign fracture.[218] Advanced MRI techniques, such as diffusion sequences or chemical shift imaging, may play a problem-solving role.[219]

In the non-MRI compatible patient, CT can aid in characterization of fractures but is less sensitive to marrow abnormality than MRI. Trabecular preservation within the vertebral body outside the fracture zone suggests a benign process. The ability of CT to display cortical or trabecular destruction or an adjacent soft tissue mass can aid in the diagnosis of a malignant lesion. The fluid sign noted earlier is occasionally visible as a vacuum cleft containing gas under the fractured end plate, marking a benign osteoporotic compression. Bone scans are highly sensitive in fracture detection, but they are of poor specificity in characterization.

Pelvic insufficiency fractures are increasingly recognized as a cause of axial and somatic referred pain experienced in the low back, pelvis, groin, and proximal lower extremities. Postmenopausal osteoporosis is the dominant risk factor, along with pelvic radiation, corticosteroid use, rheumatoid arthritis, and osteomalacia. The role of osteoporosis is emphasized by the marked female predominance of these lesions, with a reported female-to-male ratio of 9:1.[220] Patients are typically in their sixth decade or older. There is often significant morbidity associated with insufficiency fractures. Taillandier and colleagues[220] noted that 50% of their patients did not recover their former level of independence, and in 25% the insufficiency fracture precipitated institutionalization in their elderly study population. Sacral insufficiency fractures are the most common expression of this condition; pubic ramus fractures, parasymphyseal fractures, and para-acetabular fractures have also been described.

Sacral insufficiency fractures were first described by Lourie in 1982.[221] Plain radiographs of the pelvis are relatively insensitive. The most common radiographic finding is a vertical sclerotic band in the sacral ala paralleling the SI joint, representing trabecular compression and callous formation.

Less commonly one may see cortical disruption at the superior or inferior margins of the sacrum or directly visualize a fracture line. These are difficult findings to appreciate in the setting of osteoporotic bone and overlying bowel gas. In Grangier's[222] series, only 25% of patients had typical plain film findings. CT is more sensitive in detecting cortical disruption and the sclerotic margins of the fracture. Axial CT demonstrates the vertical component of the fracture. There is often a horizontal fracture line extending through the sacral body; this may be missed on axial images and will be better identified on coronal CT images. A vacuum phenomenon may also be observed within the fracture.

Technetium bone scan also represents a sensitive means of insufficiency fracture detection. The classic finding is the so-called Honda sign. Increased metabolic activity in bilateral vertical sacral ala fracture lines are bridged by a horizontal line representing a fracture through the sacral body, resulting in a representation of the letter *H*. In Fujii's[223] series, 63% of patients with sacral insufficiency fractures exhibited this sign in toto, with 35% showing a variant thereof such as two vertical lines without a crossbar or a single vertical and horizontal line. In this series, the Honda sign taken with its variants had a 96% sensitivity and 92% positive predictive value for sacral insufficiency fracture.

MRI is more sensitive than CT in the early detection of insufficiency fractures; it will reveal marrow edema (low T1, high T2 signal with gadolinium enhancement) in a pattern typical of insufficiency fracture (Honda sign) before sclerosis or a fracture line can be visualized with CT.[219] Imaging in the coronal plane is preferred; fat-saturated or STIR sequences are mandatory. In Grangier's series, marrow edema was observed in all cases as early as 18 days after symptom onset.[222] Over time, the fracture line will become visible within the zone of marrow edema as a line of diminished signal. Fluid (very high, homogeneous T2 signal) may be detected within insufficiency fractures. The confidence in the diagnosis of sacral insufficiency fracture will be increased by the presence of similar bone lesions in the pubic rami, immediately about the pubic symphysis, and in the para-acetabular region, also typical sites of insufficiency fracture.

SPONDYLOLYSIS

Spondylolysis, or isthmic spondylolisthesis, describes a defect in the pars interarticularis, which may be unilateral or bilateral. It is considered a fatigue fracture occurring within a vulnerable pars; the vulnerability may be related to the distribution of ossification centers within the posterior neural arch, not a deficit in bone quality. Spondylolysis has a familial predisposition. There is a 2-4:1 male-to-female predominance. The incidence of spondylolysis has been estimated at 7% in the U.S. population.[224] Spondylolysis is frequently asymptomatic, but it is a particular clinical issue in adolescent athletes. A retrospective study of lumbar radiographs in more than 4000 athletes demonstrated a 13.9% rate of spondylolysis with concomitant spondylolisthesis in 47%.[224] Spondylolysis occurs most commonly at the L5 level (67%), followed by the L4 level (15% to 20%), and L3 (1% to 2%). It is unusual in the cervical region, where it most often occurs at the C6 level. Spondylolysis is extremely rare in the infant population but appears to develop in childhood or adolescence, with no significant change in its incidence beyond age 20.

Although considered a fatigue fracture, it is unusual in that there is seldom an effective healing response, and the bony defect is persistent. The pars defect is frequently a synovial-lined pseudoarthrosis. Shipley demonstrated that injection of the facet immediately superior to a pars defect showed communication with the pars defect cavity in 30 of 32 facets, with communication to the next most inferior facet in 20 of 32 facets.[225] The presence of synovial fluid in the defect likely contributes to its diminished capacity to heal.

Radiographic findings of spondylolysis are often evident on lateral plain films where a radiolucent band can be directly visualized across the pars interarticularis, with or without a sclerotic margin; there is no role for oblique radiographs. Spondylolisthesis refers to the anterior translation of the vertebral body bearing the spondylolytic defects in relation to the vertebral body below (Fig. 15.22). The degree of spondylolisthesis is graded from I to V based on the percentage of anterior translation relative to the anterior-posterior dimension of the vertebrae: grade I, 0% to 25%; grade II, 26% to 50%; grade III, 51% to 75%; grade IV, 76% to 100%; and grade V, > 100% (spondyloptosis).[219] Most cases of spondylolisthesis are of grade I. A trapezoidal appearance of L5 with a dome-shaped superior end plate of S1 can be observed in chronic spondylolysis with spondylolisthesis.

Computed tomography allows direct visualization of the pars defect interposed between the adjacent facet joints on axial images. Sagittal reconstructions make the defect more obvious. Care must be taken to distinguish between a true pars defect and severe facet arthrosis. CT will also help distinguish between a stress response (sclerosis, hypertrophy) in the contralateral pedicle or pars in a unilateral spondylolysis, and an osteoid osteoma. CT allows characterization of the process as a stress response (sclerosis), an incomplete fracture, or a completed fracture. Fujii and colleagues categorized these types as early, progressive, and terminal.[226] The early stage consists of a narrow fissure with sharp margins; the progressive stage consists of a narrow fissure with less well-defined, rounder margins; and the terminal stage consists of a wide defect with rounded, sclerotic margins. Early stage lesions healed with conservative care, including bracing, more frequently than progressive lesions; no terminal stage lesions healed (see Fig. 15.22).[226]

The defect in the pars interarticularis can be directly visualized on sagittal MRI images. Several ancillary signs have been described on MRI including (1) an increase in the sagittal diameter of the central canal at the level of the pars defect, (2) reactive marrow changes (hypointense T1, hyperintense T2) within the adjacent pedicle, and (3) wedging of the posterior aspect of the associated vertebral body, usually L5.[227] Reactive marrow changes in a vertebral pedicle are not specific for the presence of spondylolysis and may be observed in the presence of adjacent facet arthrosis or synovitis. Hollenberg and colleagues developed an MRI

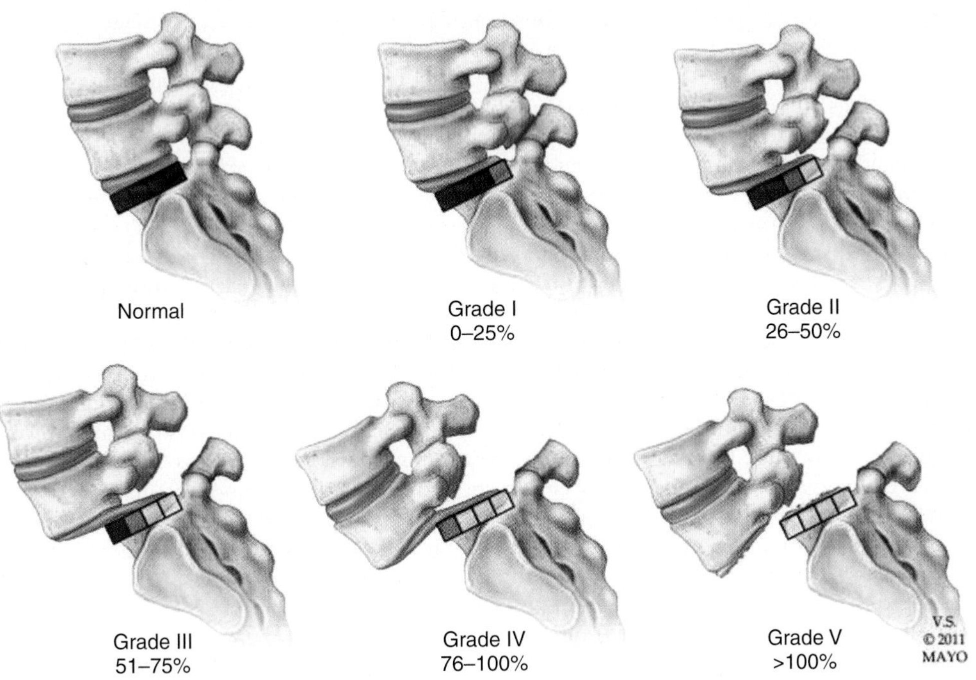

Figure 15.22 Spondylolisthesis, modified Meyerding classification. Modified Meyerding classification of spondylolisthesis: grade I, 0% to 25%; grade II, 26% to 50%; grade III, 51% to 75%; grade IV, 76% to 100%; grade V, greater than 100% (spondyloptosis [falling off]). (From Murthy NS. Imaging of stress fractures of the spine. *Radiol Clin North Am.* 2012;50:799-821.)

Table 15.8 MRI Classification of Spondylolysis

Grade	Description	MRI Features
0	Normal	Normal bone marrow signal No cortical disruption
1	Stress reaction	Bone marrow edema No cortical disruption
2	Incomplete fracture	Bone marrow edema Incomplete fracture through the pars interarticularis
3	Acute complete	Bone marrow edema Complete fracture through the pars interarticularis
4	Chronic complete	No bone marrow edema Complete fracture through the pars interarticularis

From Murthy NS. Imaging of stress fractures of the spine. *Radiol Clin North Am.* 2012;50:799-821, Table 1.

classification of spondylolysis (Table 15.8).[228] A subsequent study comparing CT staging and MRI findings noted that CT-defined early stage lesions all exhibited T2 hyperintensity in the ipsilateral pedicle; terminal stage lesions never exhibited T2 hyperintensity in the pedicle.[228] Nearly 80% of lesions with T2 hyperintensity in the pedicle healed with conservative care.[229]

Spondylolysis has also been assessed with SPECT/CT, although at the cost of radiation dose to a typically young population. Gregory and colleagues assessed the diagnostic value of combining SPECT with CT in the evaluation of spondylolysis.[230] They described four categories of patients: group A: (+) SPECT and (+) CT findings for spondylolysis; group B: (+) SPECT and (−) CT findings for spondylolysis +/− sclerosis of the pars; group C: (−) SPECT and (+) CT findings for spondylolysis; and group D: (−) SPECT and (−) CT findings for spondylolysis. Group A and B patients were felt to have a healing potential with early fatigue fractures or stress responses; group C patients had terminal lesions without healing potential, and group D patients had other pain generators, often the disk.[230] Although adult spondylolysis is often asymptomatic, there is a tendency to develop significant disk failure at the level of the pars defect, which may result in late progression of the degree of vertebral displacement and neural element compromise resulting from foraminal stenosis, which is well demonstrated on sagittal MRI. Spondylolysis patients may then experience axial pain caused by the inflammatory change about the pars defect, diskogenic pain from the failed disk, and radicular pain from secondary foraminal compromise.

Characterization of pars defects sufficient for therapeutic planning requires assessment of both morphologic and physiologic parameters. A stress response in the pars, or an incomplete fracture, may respond to conservative therapy with healing; completed chronic fractures seldom heal and are often asymptomatic. Persistent symptoms in the face of a chronic completed fracture may reflect secondary phenomena of diskogenic pain or radicular pain from foraminal stenosis. The combined morphologic and physiologic characterization can be performed with SPECT/CT or MRI. The interested reader is referred to a far more complete review by Murthy.[219]

SPINE INFECTION

Extradural spinal infections are primarily the result of arterial seeding. In children, the disk and end plate have a rich blood supply; infection occurs initially in the disk itself. In the adult, the disk is avascular; an infection develops in the anterior subchondral vertebral body with secondary spread to the disk, adjacent vertebrae, and subligamentous (deep to the anterior longitudinal ligament) space. Most disk space infections involve two adjacent lumbar vertebrae. Spread from contiguous infection or direct inoculation of the disk (surgery, injections, diskography) is much less common.

Pyogenic disk space infection involves men much more commonly than women (2-3:1) in the fifth to seventh decades of life.[231] Infection is usually unimicrobial, *Staphylococcus aureus* is the most common pathogen, and urinary tract infections are the most common source of seeding.[232] Clinical symptoms may precede radiographic findings by 1 to 8 weeks. Clinical signs of elevated sedimentation rate, white cell count, and C-reactive protein are usually present. Plain films reveal early rarefaction of anterior subchondral bone, followed by a loss of disk space height (at 1 to 3 weeks) with subsequent destructive changes in the vertebral end plates. Late changes include variable amounts of sclerosis, kyphotic deformity from vertebral collapse, and ankylosis. CT in pyogenic diskitis shows early hypodensity in the disk, moth-eaten destruction of the vertebral end plates, inflammatory changes in paravertebral soft tissues, and epidural mass. Scattered gas formation may be observed as well. Extensive gas formation in the central portion of the disk is typical of noninfectious disk degeneration; the disappearance of such a vacuum disk sign may herald infection.

MRI is the preferred imaging modality for the evaluation of diskitis, with a greater than 90% sensitivity and specificity in disease detection.[231,232] It also provides critical anatomic information. Early marrow changes are elevated T2 signal (best observed with fat saturation or STIR), diminished T1 signal, and gadolinium enhancement (Fig. 15.23). There is loss of the crisp dark cortical line of the vertebral end plate. Within the disk, the intranuclear cleft is lost and foci of elevated T2 signal and gadolinium enhancement develop. The paravertebral and epidural soft tissues show diffuse enhancement (phlegmon) or frank abscess formation with zones of hypo-enhancement and increased T2 signal where liquid purulent material is present. The imaging differential diagnosis consists of a Modic type I degenerative change, atypical cartilaginous (Schmorl's) nodes, adjacent metastatic lesions, osteomalacia secondary to osteodystrophy, and pseudoarthroses in patients with ankylosing spondylitis or a Charcot spine. Discrimination from a Modic type I end plate change can be particularly vexing; differential points are presented in Table 15.9. In challenging cases, image-guided biopsy and culture are appropriate.

MRI abnormalities lag behind the clinical syndrome. Imaging may be minimally abnormal early in the disease process and remain quite dramatic even after a gratifying clinical response to antibiotics. In following the short-term efficacy of antibiotic therapy, erythrocyte sedimentation rate (ESR), C-reactive protein (CRP), and white cell count will be more useful than repeated imaging. Follow-up imaging should be reserved for patients in whom there is a clinical concern for continued infection with central canal compromise. Persistently elevated or increasing ESR or CRP at week 4 of antibiotic therapy predicts treatment failure.[233]

Nuclear medicine scans using gallium-67 citrate and technitium-99m diphosphonate are complementary in the evaluation for suspected spondylodiscitis. A series by Hadjipavlou and colleagues demonstrated 100% sensitivity, specificity, and accuracy for the combination of gallium and technetium scans when compared with surgical biopsy results.[234] Gallium may be useful in following resolution of the infection. All nuclear medicine techniques lack anatomic information; they are unable to define the extent of epidural or paraspinal disease or central canal compromise.

Pyogenic epidural abscesses may arise from the contiguous spread of adjacent spondylodiscitis or facet joint infection, but they are most commonly primary, because of the hematogenous dissemination or direct inoculation of the epidural space. *S. aureus* is the most common pathogen; immune compromise, especially diabetes, is common.[231] Emergent MRI is the imaging modality of choice. This will demonstrate a T1 hypointense, T2 hyperintense epidural process with peripheral or heterogenous enhancement, depending on the physical state of abscess versus phlegmon. The midline ventral epidural septum may be violated; most neoplasms respect this structure. Compression of the dural sac is common; severe compromise with neurologic deficit precipitates emergent decompression. Imaging resolution of an epidural abscess more closely parallels the clinical state than in spondylodiscitis.

Pyogenic facet joint infection is uncommon; it is usually the result of hematogenous dissemination, although direct inoculation caused by invasive procedures is reported. Clinical presentation may resemble spondylodiscitis, although most commonly with lateralizing symptoms; the lumbar spine segment is most frequently affected. Bilateral involvement may occur via the space of Okada.[130] CT will demonstrate an erosive process centered on the joint with inflammatory change in adjacent multifidus muscle. MRI will demonstrate marrow edema in the articular processes, a joint effusion, and edematous changes in the multifidus; enhancement in the joint with peripheral enhancement about an adjacent paraspinal or epidural abscess or uniform heterogeneous enhancement within a phlegmon may be noted.

Tuberculosis (TB) remains the most common cause of spinal infection worldwide, and it is of increasing incidence in industrialized societies. Clinical symptoms are usually insidious. Whereas 90% to 100% of patients will have back pain, only 50% will have constitutional symptoms or fever. Tuberculous spondylitis (Pott's disease) arises from hematogenous (arterial) spread of tuberculous bacilli, usually from a pulmonary source. This initially lodges in the anterior subchondral bone. There is early anterior subligamentous extension and then spread to adjacent vertebrae, often multiple, as well as spread across the disk. Neurologic deficit occurs in a moderate number of patients due to epidural extension. Posterior elements tend to be spared. Extensive anterior column destruction with gibbus deformity is characteristic.

Tuberculous spondylitis with diskitis shows disk space narrowing, vertebral osteolysis with collapse, and gibbus deformity on plain films. The thoracolumbar junction is most frequently affected, with less frequent involvement as one ascends the thoracic or descends the lumbar spine.[231] Plain films may not be abnormal until 2 to 5 months after the onset of infection. Paraspinal soft tissue masses caused by subligamentous spread, particularly with calcification, are characteristic. CT will demonstrate the osteolytic changes of spinal tuberculosis earlier than plain films will. It more readily demonstrates epidural involvement, particularly when

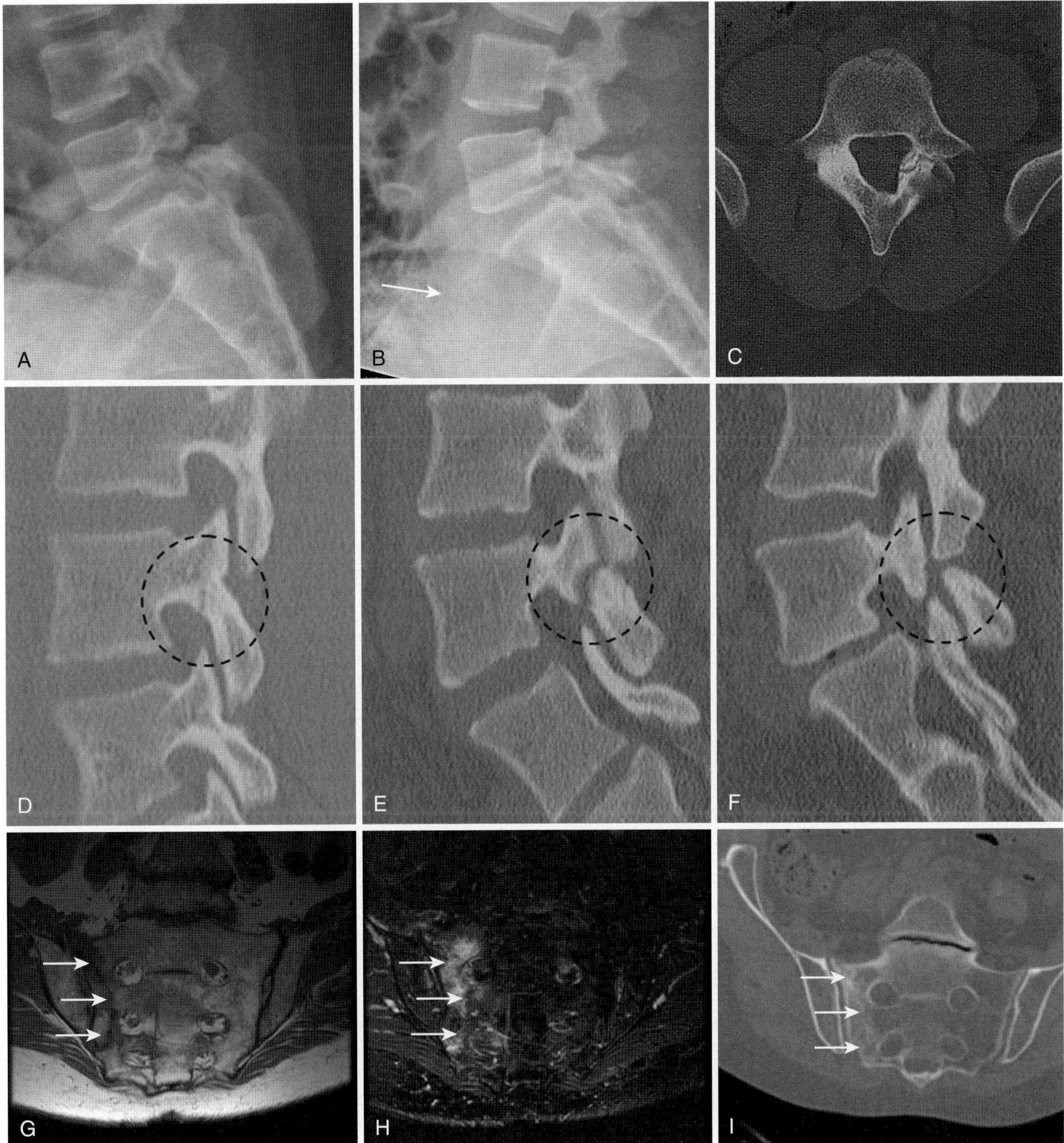

Figure 15.23 Stress fractures. Spondylolysis at L5 is visible on flexion **(A)** and extension **(B)** radiographs. Although there is no translation of L5 on S1, the degree of rotation (12 degrees) qualifies this as unstable. In unilateral spondylolysis, the contralateral pars often shows hypertrophy and sclerosis **(C)**. CT can be used to stage pars fractures as early stage **(D)** with a narrow, sharply marginated fissure; progressive stage **(E)** with a narrow fissure having slightly rounded margins; and terminal stage **(F)** with a wide fissure with rounded margins and sclerosis. Typical sacral stress fracture *(arrows)* demonstrates a low signal fracture line on a coronal T1 image **(G)**, a linear zone of T2 hyperintensity on a STIR image **(H),** whereas CT demonstrates a linear zone of sclerosis **(I)**. The integrity of the neural foramina is better defined on CT. (From Murthy NS. Imaging of stress fractures of the spine. *Radiol Clin North Am.* 2012;50:799-821.)

calcification or bone fragments are visible in the epidural space. Paraspinal involvement is also well demonstrated.

MRI is the primary imaging procedure for the detection of spinal TB. Early changes of tuberculous spondylitis with diskitis are very similar to pyogenic disk space infection, with marrow and disk inflammatory changes consisting of elevated T2 signal, diminished T1 signal, and enhancement. Extensive subligamentous spread of disease suggests TB. Paraspinal abscesses, granulomas, and epidural involvement are common. Epidural involvement may be observed in 60% to 80% of cases.[231]

Table 15.9 Differentiating Spondylodiscitis from Modic Type I End Plate Changes

	Favoring Spondylodiscitis	Favoring Modic Type I End Plate Changes	Pitfall/Comments
Disk Space Signal	T2 hyperintensity	T2 hypointensity or lack of T2 hyperintensity	Severely degenerated disks rarely can be T2 hyperintense (even fluid signal)
Disk Space Enhancement	Present	Absent	Rarely absent in infection; rarely present in Modic I
Disk Space Vacuum Sign	Absent, or only scattered	Often present; large amount of confluent gas on radiographs virtually exclude infection	Gas may be present early in infection, in rare gas-forming bacterial infection, or in rare fistulas with the gastrointestinal tract
Vertebral Body End Plates	End plate destruction	Lack of end plate destruction	Modic I can have end plate irregularity; *CT is very useful here*
Paraspinal, Epidural Spaces	Inflammation or abscess	Absent	Peripherally enhancing disk herniation can be confused for abscess
Location	Anteriorly eccentric	Laterally eccentric: at point of biomechanical stress (e.g., inner aspect of curve)	Both spondylodiscitis and Modic I are often along entire end plate
Fever, Elevated Inflammatory Markers	Present	Absent	Fever is only variably present in spondylodiscitis; inflammatory markers are nonspecific
Short-Term Follow-up	Progression	Stability	If *remote* comparison images are available, even Modic I can show significant progression

From Diehn FE. Imaging of spine infection. *Radiol Clin North Am. 2012*;50:777-798.

A second pattern of tuberculous infection is spondylitis without diskitis (see Fig. 15.23).[235] This describes lytic lesions in the central portions of the vertebral bodies, often multiple, without disk involvement. This pattern of involvement was present in approximately 50% of patients in one large series.[234] Imaging findings consist of discrete, destructive vertebral body lesions. Plain films show well-defined lytic lesions, often multifocal, and with more frequent posterior element and cervical involvement than is observed in tuberculous diskitis. Lytic lesions may exhibit marginal sclerosis on CT, indicating a more indolent lesion than a typical metastatic deposit. These lesions typically enhance peripherally on MRI, often with a cystic central cavity. There may be cortical destruction with an adjacent paravertebral abscess. Because of the greater frequency of multiple lesions, this entity must be distinguished from metastasis, myeloma, or lymphoma.

MRI has significantly advanced the diagnosis of spinal infection, allowing this to be suggested as a likely diagnosis before destructive changes have evolved. The MRI findings remain unspecific, however, and accurate diagnosis and therapy require tissue sampling for histology and culture. Image-guided percutaneous aspiration/biopsy with large caliber bone cutting needles can provide minimally invasive tissue sampling.

INFLAMMATORY SPONDYLOARTHROPATHY

Noninfectious inflammatory disease of the spine includes rheumatoid arthritis (RA) and the seronegative spondyloarthropathies (SpA), of which ankylosing spondylitis is the prototype. These diverse entities have spine involvement in common and may present with axial spine pain.

Rheumatoid arthritis is most common in the cervical spine, sometimes referred to as the fifth limb in RA patients. Symptoms and signs of cervical spine involvement are present in 60% to 80% of RA patients.[236] The most frequent site of involvement is the atlantoaxial articulation. Inflammatory pannus may be seen on MRI as a low T1, high T2 signal-enhancing mass posterior to the dens. This may cause compression of the cervicomedullary junction. The inflammatory change may destroy the transverse and alar ligaments, resulting in atlantoaxial instability in 20% to 25% of RA patients. A distance of greater than 4 mm between the posterior arch of C1 and the cortical surface of the dens on radiographs is abnormal and is most evident in flexion views. The destruction of supporting structures at the craniocervical junction may also result in cranial settling, a vertical migration of the dens into the foramen magnum, with possible compression of the C1 and C2 cranial nerves, the medulla, and vertebral arteries.

The cervical spine below the C1-2 articulations demonstrates erosive arthritis in the uncovertebral and facet joints in RA patients. The inflammatory change can be demonstrated on MRI as increased T2 signal on STIR sequences and gadolinium enhancement on fat-saturated T1 sequences. This results in multilevel instability, with anterior subluxation of successive vertebral bodies in flexion, the so-called step ladder cervical spine, noted in up to 30% of RA patients.[236] Disk space narrowing and end plate sclerosis are common, but this may be a secondary phenomenon to the posterior element instability.

Involvement of the thoracic and lumbar spine in RA is uncommon. Synovitis and erosive change may be present in the facet and costovertebral joints but is inconstant and not well demonstrated. Discovertebral changes may be present,

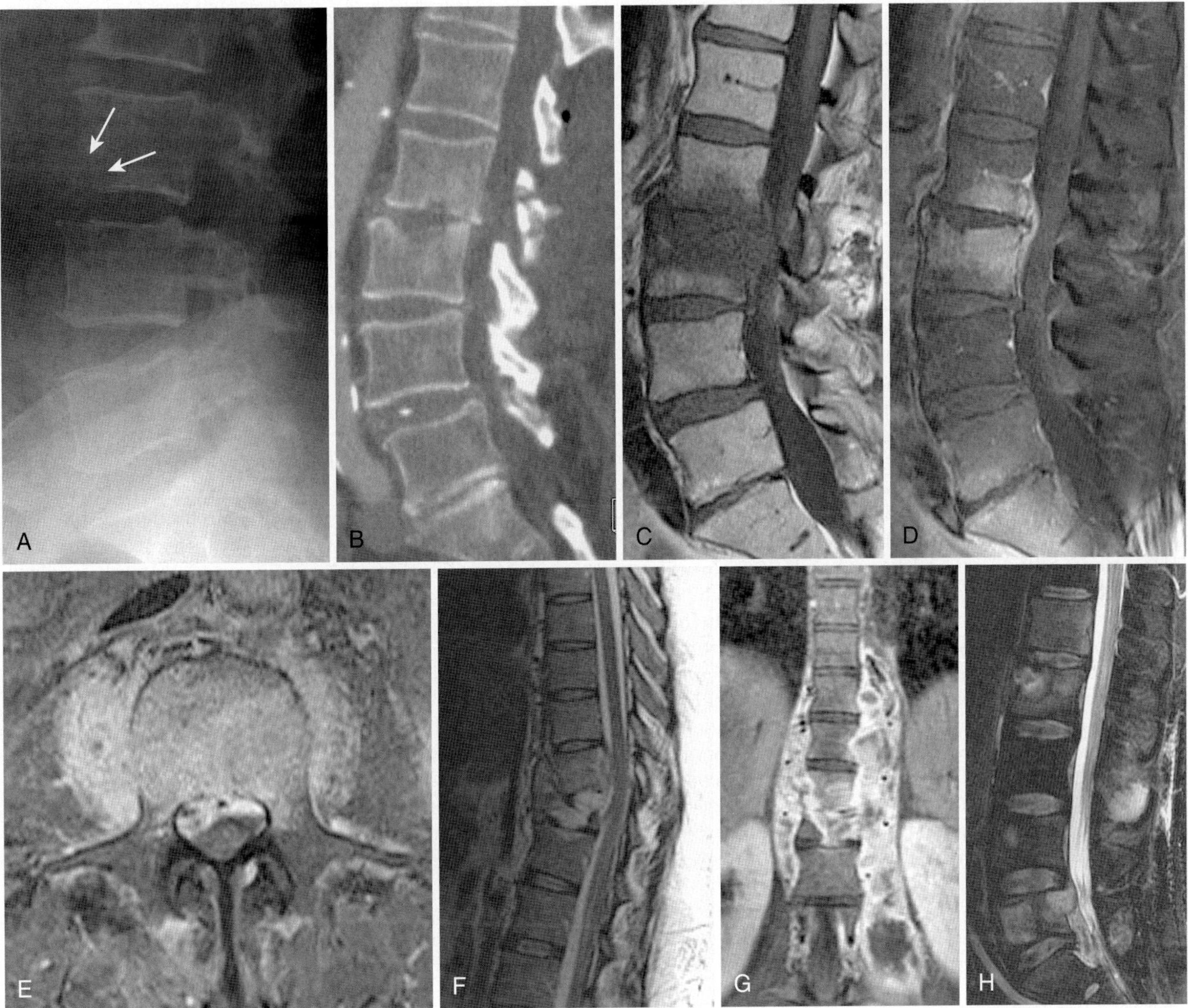

Figure 15.24 Spondylodiscitis. A lateral radiograph **(A)** demonstrates early pyogenic spondylodiscitis manifest as subtle destruction of the anterior inferior aspect of the L3 vertebrae. In another patient, a sagittal CT reconstruction **(B)**, sagittal T1-unenhanced **(C)** and enhanced **(D)** and axial T1-enhanced MRI images **(E)** of a patient with L2-3 pyogenic diskitis. Note loss of disk space height, end plate destruction, low T1 signal and extensive vertebral, epidural, and paraspinal enhancement.

Sagittal T2-weighted MRI **(F)** of a back pain patient without myelopathy demonstrates vertebral destruction with kyphotic deformity; this is tuberculous spondylodiscitis. Coronal T1-enhanced MRI **(G)** in the same patient demonstrates the extensive paraspinal disease typical of Pott's disease. A sagittal T2-weighted MRI **(H)** in another patient with tuberculous spondylodiscitis; note the multiple vertebral lesions with sparing of the disks. This can be confused with metastatic disease. Tissue sampling is essential. (From Maus T. Imaging the back pain patient. *Phys Med Rehabil Clin N Am.* 2010;21:725-766.)

but it is again unclear if these are primary inflammatory lesions or a response to facet instability. The sacroiliac joints may show inflammatory change, but with much less frequency and severity than in ankylosing spondylitis patients.

The seronegative spondyloarthropathies are a group of rheumatoid factor negative inflammatory disease processes affecting the spine and sacroiliac joints, with a unique predilection for entheses. Historically these have included ankylosing spondylitis, psoriatic arthritis, reactive arthritis (formerly known as Reiter's syndrome), and the arthritis associated with inflammatory bowel disease. The categorization of these diseases has evolved, most recently in 2009 with the designation of axial spondylarthritis for the spectrum of disease with axial, as opposed to peripheral, dominance.[237] Axial spondylarthritis requires active sacroiliitis on MRI plus one or more features of spondylarthritis, or human leukocyte antigen B27 (HLA-B27) positivity with two or more features of spondylarthritis. This discussion only encompasses the axial imaging features of the classically defined processes (Fig. 15.24).

MRI is the necessary imaging modality for the assessment of disease activity in the SI joints and spine articulations. MRI or CT can demonstrate the aftermath of disease: joint space narrowing, subchondral erosions, reactive sclerosis, or periarticular fat deposition (a Modic II analog); only MRI can assess active inflammation with T2 hyperintensity (STIR or fat-saturated images) and gadolinium enhancement on fat-saturated T1 images.

Ankylosing spondylitis (AS) is the prototypical seronegative spondyloarthropathy; active disease in the SI joints by MRI criteria is integral to its diagnosis. AS has a prevalence of up to 0.1% in the general population; a very high percentage will be HLA B27 positive. Males dominate by 4:1. The disease involves synovial and cartilaginous joints and entheses (ligament and tendon insertions on bone) with a strong predilection for the axial skeleton. The most common presentation is low back pain with inflammatory features (Calin criteria, 4 out of 5 of insidious onset, age < 40, 3 months persistence, morning stiffness, and pain improved by exercise). Radiating pain mimicking sciatica may be observed in up to 50% of patients.

Imaging findings in AS include sacroiliitis, ultimately bilaterally symmetric and multiple manifestations of spondylitis (see Fig. 15.24). Sacroiliitis is the uniform initial imaging finding. Early plain film findings of sacroiliitis are blurring of the subchondral cortex by small erosions, predominantly on the iliac side of the joint. As the erosions coalesce, the joint space appears widened and ill defined; sclerotic reaction develops in the trabecular bone about both sides of the joint. Over time the joint undergoes ankylosis via direct bony bridging; the joint space is no longer visible and the sclerosis resolves.[238] MRI can detect inflammation in the SI joint in symptomatic patients with normal plain films. Inflammation can be reliably identified with low interobserver variability as high T2 signal on STIR sequences or gadolinium enhancement on fat-saturated T1 images.[239] In patients with recent onset axial low back pain with inflammatory clinical characteristics, SI joint inflammation may be detected by MRI in one third of patients and structural changes in one sixth of patients.[239] Inflammation is initially observed in the iliac side of the joint at its caudal and dorsal aspects, and in the adjacent dorsal entheses.

Spine findings in AS are present in 50% of patients and include osteitis, syndesmophyte formation, discovertebral lesions, and inflammation leading to ankylosis of facet and costovertebral joints.[238] Osteitis is observed at the anterior margins of the discovertebral junction, termed the *Romanus lesion*. On plain films, sclerosis at these sites leads to increased density of the anterior corners of the vertebra, termed the *shiny corners sign*.[238] Remodeling of the anterior margin of the vertebral body as a result of osteitis straightens the normally concave anterior vertebral margin, referred to as "squaring" of the vertebra. These findings are most evident in the lumbar region. MRI is more sensitive to the early detection of osteitis, recognized as diminished T1 and increased T2 signal and enhancement at the anterior vertebral corners.[238] Osteitis at the margins of the discovertebral junctions leads to reactive bone formation in the outer annulus fibrosis, which ultimately bridges the margins of adjacent vertebrae. These vertically oriented bony struts are syndesmophytes. They are distinguished from osteophytes by their vertical orientation and gracile nature; osteophytes are oriented in the horizontal plane and are bulkier. Syndesmophytes are most common at the anterior and lateral aspects of the vertebral body; when long standing, the ossification may involve the anterior longitudinal ligament.

Erosions at the discovertebral junction are termed *Andersson lesions*; this inflammatory destruction of the vertebral end plate with intravertebral disk displacement can progress to pseudarthrosis. End plate destruction is visible on plain films; MRI demonstrates structural and inflammatory change. The inflammatory change will undergo evolution reminiscent of the progression from Modic type 1 to Modic type 2. Over time there is sclerosis and transdiscal ossification leading to ankylosis. The facet and costovertebral joints show similar findings, with initial periarticular erosions followed by sclerosis and ankylosis. Enthesitis of the posterior interspinous and supraspinous ligament attachments ultimately leads to ossification of these structures, visible as a vertical midline bony band on frontal radiographs, the so-called dagger sign. The inflammatory spinal lesions are most common in the midthoracic spine (T7-T8) and in the midlumbar region (L2-3).

AS may also produce changes at the atlanto-axial articulation. Synovitis may result in erosive changes in the dens, although the extent of inflammatory change seldom reaches that noted in RA. Atlanto-axial subluxation may be present. The extensive ankylosis observed in patients with longstanding AS leads to flattening of the lumbar lordosis and exaggeration of the thoracic kyphosis. The rigidity places these patients at risk for catastrophic fracture-dislocations with modest trauma, most commonly with a hyperextension mechanism. The cervical spine is most frequently involved; neurologic deficits are common. Plain film evaluation is difficult because of the osteopenia typical of these patients; the three-column nature of these fractures is best appreciated with CT or MRI. The threshold for use of advanced imaging in the AS patient with trauma should be low. Three-column fractures that do not cause acute neurologic injury or go undetected may be a cause of chronic focal pain as a pseudarthrosis. MRI will show a linear zone of inflammatory change, often through a disk space with extension through the posterior elements. The cortical disruption may be best appreciated on CT. Finally, some AS patients will have findings of dural ectasia (see Fig. 15.24). The thecal sac will be abnormally capacious with diverticular-like outpouchings; there is associated bony erosion in the posterior elements, medial margins of the pedicles, and the posterior vertebral body. These patients may present with a cauda equina syndrome, perhaps related to arachnoiditis.

Psoriatic arthritis (PA) is far less common than AS; it affects 7% of patients with cutaneous psoriasis.[238] Approximately 10% to 25% of patients with moderate to severe skin disease will have abnormal SI joint radiographs. Spondylitis is present in a roughly similar proportion but may or may not coexist with sacroiliitis. Males and females are equally affected.[238] The sacroiliitis is usually bilateral but asymmetric, with a lesser tendency to progress to bony ankylosis. Erosions and foci of reactive sclerosis tend to be larger and more discrete than in AS. The spondylitis in psoriatic arthritis is characterized by asymmetric, coarse paravertebral ossification more resembling osteophytes than syndesmophytes. Vertebral squaring and shiny corners are absent. Facet involvement is infrequent.

Reactive spondylarthritis describes an inflammatory arthropathy, preferentially affecting the heel and large peripheral joints.[238] Sacroiliitis is very common, affecting up to 45% of patients. It is more commonly unilateral or asymmetric than in AS; ankylosis is rare. Spine involvement may be identical to that of PA but more common; the lumbar spine is involved in 30% of RS patients.[238] In the setting of a triggering infection (often chlamydia) and the triad of urethritis, uveitis, and arthritis, the term *Reiter's syndrome* may be applied.

Enteropathic arthritis may also be observed in association with ulcerative colitis or Crohn's disease. The initial presentation of back pain may precede symptoms of gastrointestinal disease. The spondylitis and sacroiliitis noted in association with these conditions are indistinguishable from classic ankylosing spondylitis. Sacroiliitis is usually bilaterally symmetric progressing to ankylosis; spondylitic findings of vertebral squaring, discovertebral lesions, syndesmophytes, and involvement of the facet joints are typical.

SPINE NEOPLASM

Spinal neoplasms are classified by the anatomic compartment from which they arise: extradural, intradural-extramedullary, or intramedullary. Extradural neoplasms arise from the vertebral bodies, within the paravertebral soft tissues, or within the epidural space. These include metastatic lesions, hematologic malignancies, and primary osseous or cartilaginous tumors. Intradural-extramedullary lesions arise within the dural tube but are extrinsic to the spinal cord itself. Lesions in this category include meningiomas, Schwannomas, neurofibromas, and leptomeningeal metastatic disease. Intramedullary lesions are those that arise primarily from the spinal cord or filum terminale. Astrocytomas, ependymomas, and hemangioblastomas make up the majority of these lesions.

Extradural neoplasms are common. MRI provides the best combination of lesion detection, morphologic characterization, and assessment of neural compromise. Nuclear medicine techniques such as technetium bone scan and PET scanning provide high sensitivity to lesion detection and excellent body wide assessment of tumor burden (Fig. 15.25). Nuclear medicine studies will not provide anatomic information regarding compression of neural elements. CT is less sensitive than MRI in lesion detection; plain films are far less sensitive.

Extradural neoplasms may narrow the subarachnoid space (cerebrospinal fluid) as they extrinsically intrude into the spinal canal. They exhibit diminished T1 signal, elevated T2 signal, and gadolinium enhancement on MRI. The unenhanced T1 image is the mainstay of lesion detection; normal adult marrow should be brighter than the intervertebral disks. Fat-saturated T2-weighted images and STIR images provide high sensitivity to lesion detection. Fat-saturated postgadolinium images will also display extradural neoplasm with high sensitivity. On axial images, compression of the thecal sac or exiting nerve roots can be directly displayed. CT and plain films play a role in characterizing primary bone and cartilaginous tumors including malignant lesions such as osteosarcoma, chondrosarcoma, chordoma, and the benign tumors, including hemangioma, osteoid osteoma, giant cell tumor, and aneurysmal bone cyst.

Metastases are the most common extradural spine tumor, and the spinal column is the most common site of osseous metastases. An overwhelming majority of spine metastases are due to prostate, lung, and breast cancer. The thoracic spine is most commonly involved (70%), followed by the lumbar and cervical segments. Involvement of the vertebral body is most common (85%), with less frequent spread to the paravertebral tissues or epidural space. The disks, dura, and the anterior longitudinal ligament are resistant to invasion by metastatic tumor; the posterior longitudinal ligament is more readily involved, as it is penetrated by numerous venous channels. Vertebral body metastases may be blastic (bone forming), lytic (destructive), or mixed. Blastic lesions are observed as ill-defined areas of increased density on plain films or CT; on MRI, blastic lesions will have low T1 and T2 signal with enhancement. Common primary tumors are prostate, carcinoid, or bladder cancer. Lytic metastases show destruction on plain films and CT, and low T1 and variable T2 signal with enhancement on MRI. Lytic metastases are most commonly produced by breast, lung, renal, and thyroid neoplasms. Mixed lytic and blastic lesions are visible in lung, breast, cervical, and ovarian primaries.

Hemangiomas are the most common spine tumor, present in up to 10% to 12% of adults. They are frequently multiple. Typical hemangiomas are benign and of no clinical significance; they are identified by their fatty content on MRI (high T1 and T2 signal) and a corduroy appearance on plain films or CT. This is due to sparse, thickened trabeculae surrounded by fat; on axial images this results in a polka dot appearance.

Osteoid osteomas occur in patients under the age of 30, and they typically present with pain, often nocturnal. Aspirin or nonsteroidal anti-inflammatory drugs (NSAIDs) can usually relieve pain. The lesion consists of a small nidus, less than 1.5 cm in diameter, surrounded by a larger zone of sclerotic reaction or soft tissue inflammation, visible on plain films or CT. The nidus is intensely enhancing on CT, MRI, or bone scan. Ten percent of osteoid osteomas occur in the spine, almost exclusively in the posterior neural arch. The lumbar spine is involved in 59% of spinal osteoid osteomas, the cervical region in 27%, and the thoracic spine in 12%. Lesions larger than 1.5 cm are considered osteoblastomas.

Myeloma is the most common malignant primary tumor of bone; it presents with bone pain in 75% of patients. It is often widespread at presentation. Its imaging appearance can range from discrete destructive lesions to diffuse loss of bone density indistinguishable from osteoporosis on plain films. CT is better able to resolve the discrete destructive lesions in trabecular or cortical bone. The MRI appearance is variable, with diminished T1 marrow signal and gadolinium enhancement in a multifocal or diffuse pattern. Compression fractures are common and they may be indistinguishable from benign osteoporotic fractures. Single focal lesions (plasmacytomas) are expansile and lytic on imaging.

Leukemia may present with spine pain in the setting of diffuse marrow involvement and associated compression fractures. The most common imaging finding is that of diffuse marrow replacement, with osteopenia on plain films and CT, and generalized loss of the normal T1 marrow signal. Normal marrow should always be brighter than disk signal on T1 images. Focal extra-osseous soft tissue masses of leukemic tissue may be present and are termed *chloromas.*

Lymphoma is the great mimic. It can present in the spine as vertebral lesions indistinguishable from metastases, as an epidural soft tissue mass without bone involvement, as a diffuse leptomeningeal process, and as a primary intramedullary lesion.

Intradural-extramedullary neoplasms are situated within the dural sac, widening the subarachnoid space as they displace the cord or cauda equina. Meningiomas typically exhibit a broad base against the dural surface and enhance uniformly. Schwannomas and neurofibromas are indistinguishable on imaging. They may enhance uniformly

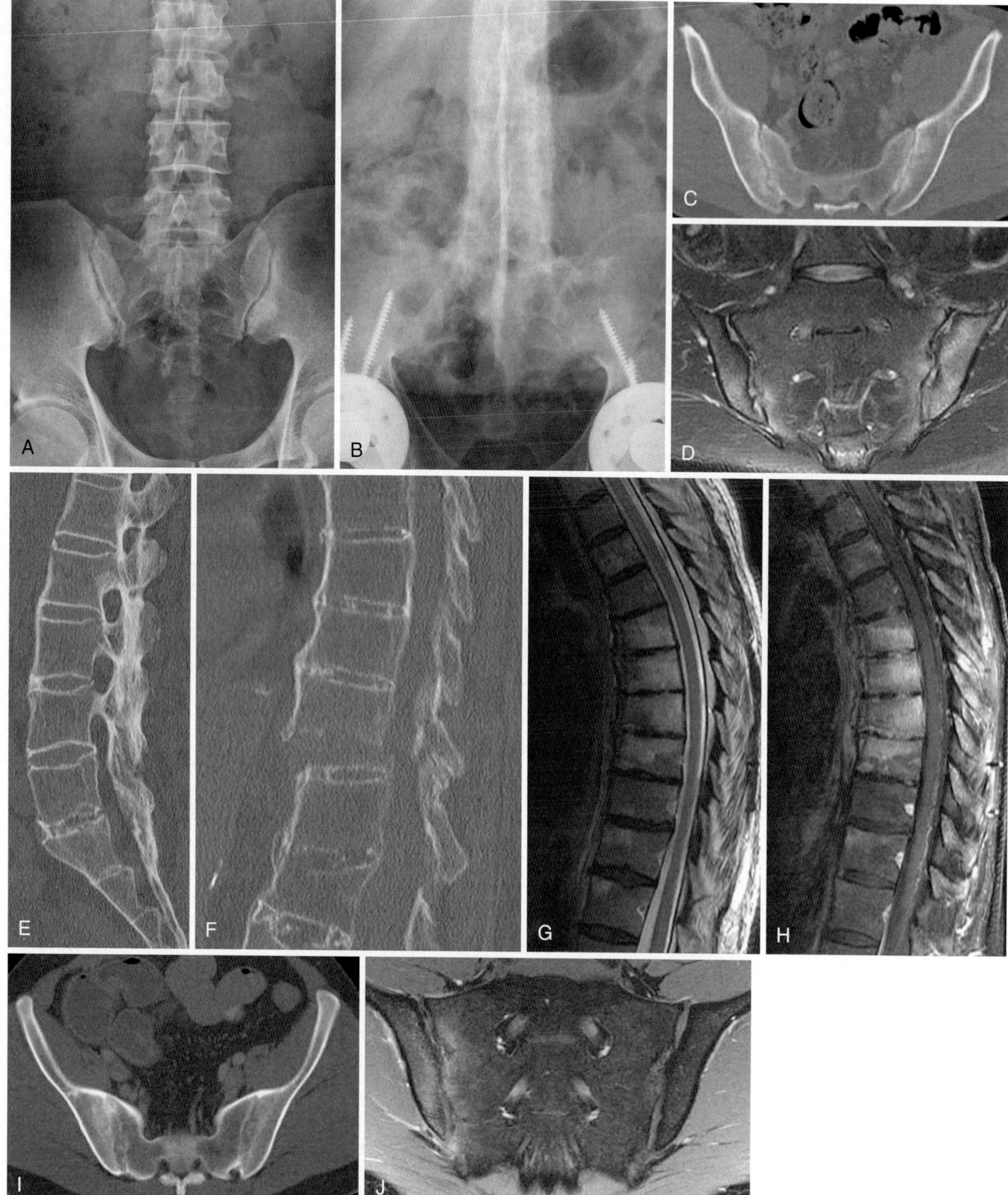

Figure 15.25 Spondyloarthropathy. Changes of sacroiliitis are detectable on radiographs **(A)** as irregularity, erosions, and sclerosis, dominant on the iliac side of the joint. In the end stage of ankylosing spondylitis (AS), the sacroiliac joints are fused and the sclerosis resolves **(B)**; this radiograph also depicts the dagger sign, as the fused spinous processes make a continuous sclerotic structure in the midline. CT **(C)** is more sensitive in the detection of erosions and early sclerotic reaction in AS; this structural change may simply reflect prior disease. Only MRI can detect disease activity **(D)** as demonstrated by the T2 hyperintensity in and about both SI joints in this AS patient. The gracile vertical syndesmophytes bridging lumbar vertebrae and the fused posterior elements are well seen on CT **(E)**; the spine in AS is rendered vulnerable to three-column unstable fractures with modest trauma **(F)**. These situations deserve CT imaging. The spondyloarthropathy of inflammatory bowel disease may present as back pain (T2 sagittal **[G]** and enhanced T1 fat-saturated sagittal **[H]**) with evidence of multifocal inflammatory spondyloarthropathy. The differential diagnosis here is multilevel spondylodiscitis, especially Pott's disease (tuberculosis). Changes of sacroiliitis in inflammatory bowel disease **(I)** may be indistinguishable from AS. Asymmetric sacroiliitis (T1-enhanced, fat-saturated coronal MRI **[J]**) is typical of reactive spondylarthritis (formerly Reiter's syndrome).

or show central zones of cystic degeneration. The classic "dumb-bell" neurofibroma may issue through and widen a neural foramen. They may also occur entirely within the dural sac or in a paravertebral location. Leptomeningeal metastatic disease is most typically seen as enhancement on the surface of the cord or within the roots of the cauda equina. In some cases more discrete small masses may be observed within the cauda equina. CSF cytology remains more sensitive than MRI in the detection of leptomeningeal metastatic disease.

Intramedullary neoplasms are rare entities, but they may present with pain or dysfunction that can mimic degenerative disease. Ependymomas arise from the ependymal cells lining the central canal of the cord. Ependymomas are the most common intramedullary tumor in adults; they are most frequently located in the conus medullaris and filum terminale (myxopapillary ependymoma). Because of their slow growth, they may cause bony erosion and scalloped enlargement of the central canal. MRI demonstrates an enlarged cord or filum terminale with an elevated T2 signal and heterogenous enhancement. Small cysts or hemorrhage are frequent. Astrocytomas are typically low-grade neoplasms, more commonly noted in young patients and in the cervical region. They typically extend over multiple vertebral segments within the cord with poorly defined margins. The cord is enlarged with heterogenous enhancement. The entire cross section of the cord is typically involved. Considerable edema within the white matter of the cord extends cephalad and caudal to the enhancing neoplasm itself. Peritumoral cysts may be present. Hemangioblastomas are rare lesions that typically occur in the cervical and thoracic spine. An intensely enhancing vascular nodule adjacent to the pial surface, often associated with an intramedullary cyst, is typical. About one third of patients with hemangioblastomas will have Von Hippel Lindau syndrome.

SPINAL DURAL ARTERIOVENOUS FISTULA (AVF)

Spinal dural AVFs are the most common form of vascular malformation involving the spine. This lesion merits description in that it may present with pain and progressive neurologic deficit, mimicking neurogenic intermittent claudication; it frequently remains undiagnosed for prolonged periods. In Atkinson's series, the mean delay from symptom onset to diagnosis was 23 months.[240] Patients are frequently subjected to misdirected interventions, including decompressive surgery. When diagnosed, it is treatable with arrest of the progressive neurologic deficit.

Spinal dural AVFs are an acquired lesion, with a fistulous communication within the dura of a root sleeve and intrathecal venous drainage to the venous plexus surrounding the cord. This results in venous hypertension within the cord and ultimately cord dysfunction. The fistula is most commonly in the low thoracic or lumbar spine. It is a lesion of elderly males. Gilbertson's series[241] had a mean age of 62, with a range from 37 to 81; Atkinson's series[240] reported a 4:1 male predominance. Pain was a reported symptom in 53% of patients; many of these patients described a burning, dysesthetic pain in the lower extremities; 15% had low back pain when erect, which worsened with use of the lower extremities. This is typically accompanied by a slowly progressive or stepwise worsening myelopathy, manifest as lower extremity fatigue and weakness. Atkinson's series[240] reported that 69% of patients had upper and lower motor neuron signs; 30% had only lower motor neuron signs.

Imaging findings of dural AVFs have been well described.[242] On CT myelography, abnormally prominent tortuous vessels are present in 100% of cases; this may give the cauda equina a beaded appearance. On MRI, there will be T2 hyperintensity in the cord in nearly 100% of cases (Fig. 15.26). This typically extends over multiple vertebral segments and may be accompanied by cord enlargement in 45% of cases. There may be patchy cord enhancement; these findings may raise a concern for tumor. A differentiating finding is the presence of prominent flow voids or intravascular enhancement caused by the dilated veins, particularly on the dorsal surface of the cord. The T2 hyperintensity in the cord usually involves the low thoracic cord and conus; this does not predict the site of the fistula. Magnetic resonance angiography (MRA) is useful in predicting the site of the fistula (Fig. 15.27)[242] and reducing the scope of spinal angiography, which provides the definite diagnosis. The fistula then may be disconnected surgically or by an endovascular approach.

The goal of diagnosis and therapy is primarily to arrest the progression of the neurologic deficit and possibly improve the current disability. After successful occlusion of the fistula, either surgically or by endovascular embolic techniques, gait improvement was noted in 67% to 80% of patients.[242] Bowel/bladder dysfunction or pain is relieved in only a minority of patients. Worsening of motor symptoms should prompt an imaging investigation for recanalization of the fistula.[242] After successful fistula occlusion, cord enlargement, enhancement, and T2 hyperintensity and the prominent veins about the conus will slowly resolve; T2 hyperintensity and enhancement may persist for up to a year.

CONCLUSION

As a synopsis of the imaging assessment of the patient with spine or limb pain, this chapter has ranged widely over large swaths of pathology and imaging technology. There are enduring themes. The primary role of imaging is to detect systemic disease causal of the patient's pain or neurologic dysfunction; such disease is uncommon. Imaging is currently overutilized to the detriment of patients and society. It has no value in the initial presentation of the patient in the absence of red flag features suggesting systemic disease. The decision to begin imaging should be a reasoned one, considering benefits of improved outcomes versus real risks and harms. The ACR and the ACP have promulgated evidence-based guidelines for imaging use; they should be respected. When imaging occurs, it must be done with a full appreciation of its inherent specificity and sensitivity faults. There is a high prevalence of asymptomatic, age-related change evident on all types of spine imaging; loss of T2 signal in the disk nucleus, anterior and lateral vertebral osteophytes, disk protrusions, and facet and sacroiliac joint arthrosis do not correlate with pain. Imaging performed without axial load and physiologic posture may be insensitive to dynamic lesions.

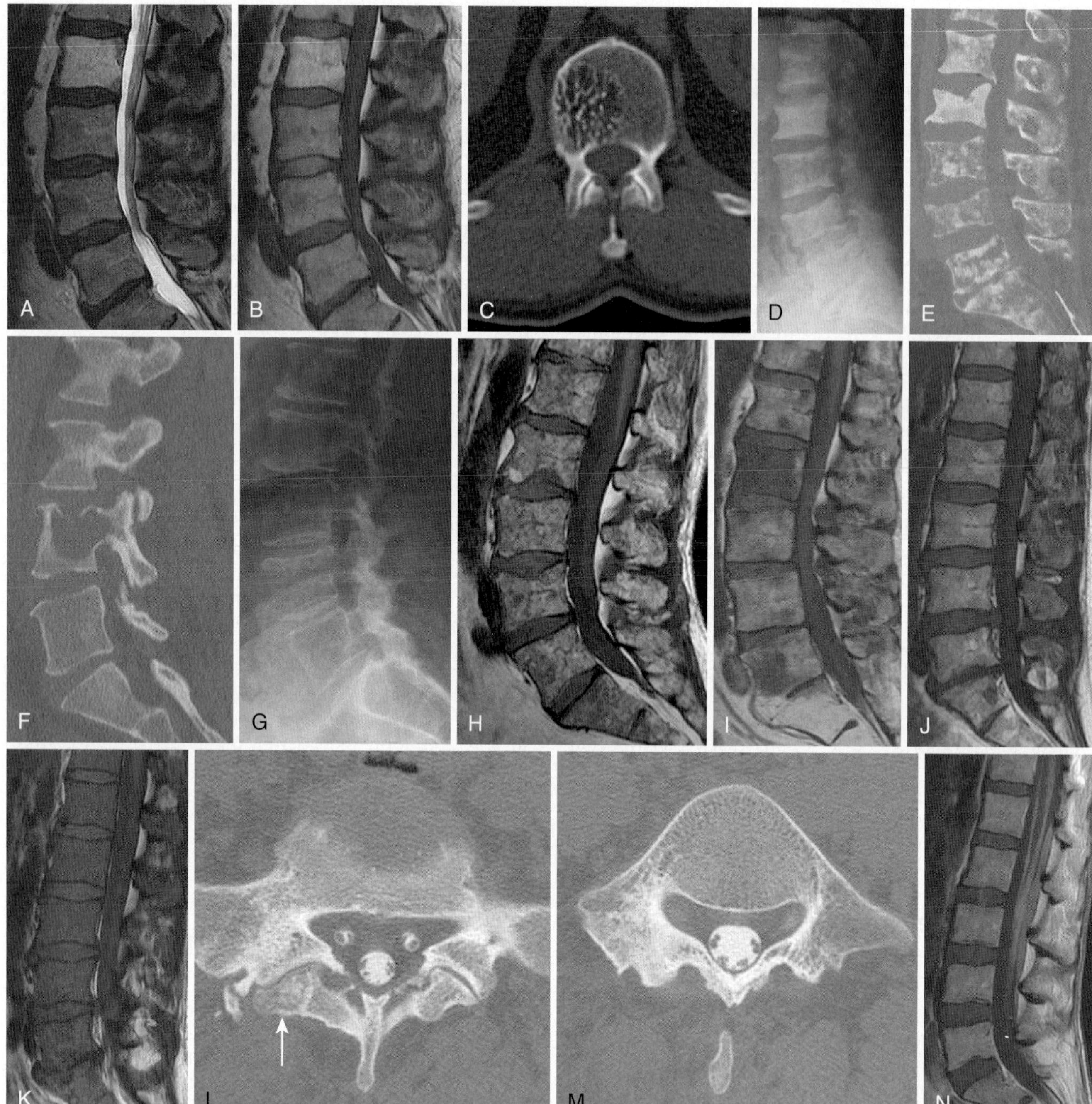

Figure 15.26 Spine neoplasm. Sagittal T2 **(A)** and T1 **(B)** images show a lesion in the L2 vertebral body characterized by increased signal intensity on both sequences, typical of hemangioma, the most common benign spinal extradural neoplasm. A CT image in another patient **(C)** demonstrates the classic CT features of hemangioma: thickened trabeculae surrounding increased marrow fat, resulting in a polka dot appearance. Blastic metastases **(D)** have increased bone density; CT is more sensitive than radiographs **(E)**, particularly in the detection of lytic metastases **(F)**. Myeloma can be challenging to detect on radiographs, mimicking osteoporosis **(G)**; MRI in the same patient **(H)** identifies the myriad of tiny destructive lesions. The MRI T1 sagittal sequence **(I)** typically reveals metastatic disease as focal hypointense lesions, as in this patient with prostate cancer, as the bright signal of normal marrow fat is replaced. When marrow replacement is diffuse, this can be difficult to detect. Normal marrow should always be brighter than adjacent disks. Note that normal marrow in **(J)** is completely replaced 2 years later by leukemia **(K)** when this patient presented with back pain. Osteoid osteoma is a posterior element benign neoplasm causal of pain, often nocturnal and relieved by salicylates. It is visible as a small nidus (*arrow* in **[L]**) with surrounding sclerotic reaction **(M)**. Leptomeningeal metastases or lymphoma may be imaged as diffuse enhancing tissue coating the cord and cauda equina **(N)**.

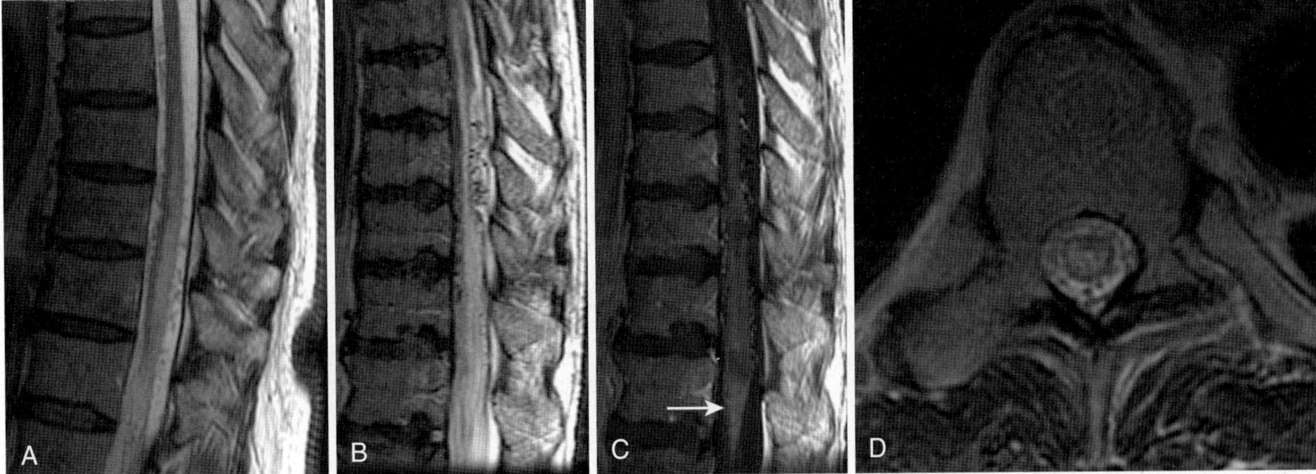

Figure 15.27 Dural arteriovenous fistulae. T2 sagittal MRI images in two patients, **(A)** and **(B)**, both demonstrate enlargement of the conus with multisegmental T2 hyperintensity. Postgadolinium T1 sagittal MRI (**[C]**, same patient as **[B]**) shows intravascular enhancement in the enlarged perimedullary veins and patchy parenchymal enhancement in the conus *(arrow)*. Axial T2 image through the lower thoracic cord **(D)** demonstrates increased T2 signal throughout the substance of the cord, with a dark border of diminished T2 signal at the periphery of the cord. (From Morris JM. Imaging of dural arteriovenous fistula. *Radiol Clin North Am.* 2012;50:823-839.)

Structural alterations detected by imaging are of less significance than physiologic parameters of edema, hyperemia, disruption of blood-nerve barrier, or accelerated metabolism noted with T2 hyperintensity (STIR or fat-saturated images), gadolinium enhancement, or nuclear medicine techniques. Always treat the patient, not the images.

KEY POINTS

- The primary role of imaging is to identify systemic disease; no imaging is indicated in the acute presentation of back or limb pain without "red flag" features.
- All spine imaging has a significant specificity fault: a high prevalence of asymptomatic age-related findings, including disk "degeneration" and facet arthrosis.
- Spine imaging performed without physiologic positioning and axial load may be insensitive to dynamic lesions.
- Imaging correlates poorly with clinical presentation and course.
- Meticulous enumeration of spine segmentation from the skull base caudally is necessary to avoid wrong segment procedures.
- Magnetic resonance imaging (MRI) findings can reasonably predict positive lumbar diskography; the high intensity zone and significant expression of Modic end plate change have high specificity but low sensitivity.
- Imaging cannot identify cervical diskogenic pain.
- Findings of structural arthrosis of the facet or sacroiliac joints (osteophytes, joint space narrowing, sclerosis) have no relationship to pain; physiologic findings (positive bone scan, MRI T2 hyperintensity) may predict pain but have not been tested against an appropriate reference standard.

KEY POINTS—cont'd

- Radicular pain requires both neural compression and an inflammatory response; standard imaging detects only the neural compression.
- There is no relationship among the size, type, or change in disk herniations over time and patient outcomes.
- The imaging natural history of disk herniation is resolution.
- Neurogenic intermittent claudication requires compression at multiple segmental levels or in multiple compartments (central, lateral recess, foraminal) for clinical expression.
- MRI signal changes in the cervical cord can provide prognostic guidance for decompression in the cervical spondylotic myelopathy patient.

SELECTED READINGS

Amrami KA. Imaging of the seronegative spondylarthropathies. *Radiol Clin North Am.* 2012;50:841-854.

Baptiste DC, Fehlings MG. Pathophysiology of cervical myelography. *Spine J.* 2006;6(suppl 6):190S-197S.

Bogduk N, ed. *Practice Guidelines for Spinal Diagnostic Procedures.* San Francisco: International Spine Intervention Society; 2004.

Bogduk N. *Clinical and Radiologic Anatomy of the Lumbar Spine.* 5th ed. Churchill Livingstone Elsevier; San Francisco, USA, 2012.

Carrino JA, Campbell PD Jr, Lin DC, et al. Effect of spinal segment variants on numbering vertebral levels at lumbar MR imaging. *Radiology.* 2011;259:196-202.

Chou R, Fu R, Carrino JA, et al. Imaging strategies for low-back pain: systematic review and meta-analysis. *Lancet.* 2009;373:463-472.

Chou R, Loeser J, Owens D, et al. Interventional therapies, surgery, and interdisciplinary rehabilitation for low back pain: evidence based clinical practice guidelines from the American Pain Society. *Spine.* 2009;34:1066-1077.

Chou R, Qaseem A, Owens DK, et al. Diagnostic imaging for low back pain: advice for high-value health care from the American College of Physicians. *Ann Intern Med.* 2011;154:181-189.

Chou R, Deyo RA, Jarvik JG. Appropriate use of lumbar imaging for evaluation of low back pain. *Radiol Clin North Am.* 2012;50:569-585.

Diehn FE. Imaging of spine infection. *Radiol Clin North Am.* 2012;50:777-798.

Fardon DF, Milette PC. Combined Task Forces of the North American Spine Society, American Society of Spine Radiology, and American Society of Neuroradiology. Nomenclature and classification of lumbar disk pathology: recommendations of the combined task forces of the North American Spine Society, American Society of Spine Radiology, and American Society of Neuroradiology. *Spine.* 2001;26:E93-E113.

Jarvik JG, Deyo R. Diagnostic evaluation of low back pain with emphasis on imaging. *Ann Intern Med.* 2002;137:586-597.

Maus TP. Imaging of spinal stenosis: neurogenic intermittent claudication and cervical spondylotic myelopathy. *Radiol Clin North Am.* 2012;50:651-679.

Maus TP, Aprill CN. Lumbar discogenic pain, provocation diskography, and imaging correlates. *Radiol Clin North Am.* 2012;50:681-704.

Maus TP, Martin DP. Imaging for discogenic pain. In: Kapural L, Kim P, Deer T, eds. *Diagnosis, Management and Treatment of Discogenic Pain.* Philadelphia: Elsevier/Saunders; 2012: 38.

Morris JM. Imaging of dural arteriovenous fistula. *Radiol Clin North Am.* 2012;50:823-839.

Mulleman D, Mammou S, Griffoul I, et al. Pathophysiology of disk-related sciatica, I: evidence supporting a chemical component. *Joint Bone Spine.* 2006;73:151-158.

Mulleman D, Mammou S, Griffoul I, et al. Pathophysiology of disk-related low back pain and sciatica, II: evidence supporting treatment with TNF-alpha antagonists. *Joint Bone Spine.* 2006;73:270-277.

Murthy NS. Imaging of stress fractures of the spine. *Radiol Clin North Am.* 2012;50:799-821.

North American Spine Society. *Evidence-Based Clinical Guidelines for Multidisciplinary Spine Care, Diagnosis and Treatment of Degenerative Lumbar Spinal Stenosis.* Burr Ridge, Ill: North American Spine Society; 2011.

The references for this chapter can be found at www.expertconsult.com.

16

Psychological and Behavioral Assessment

Elizabeth Seng | Robert D. Kerns | Alicia Heapy

Chronic pain presents two broad challenges to proper assessment: the inherently subjective nature of pain complaints and the wide-ranging influence of chronic pain on patients' functioning. These challenges necessitate a systematic approach that involves standardized assessment of multiple domains of functioning through the use of several assessment techniques, including questionnaires, behavioral observation, psychophysiologic measurement, diary data, and reports of significant others. This chapter begins with a brief discussion of the clinical goals of psychological and behavioral assessment of patients with persistent pain, provides a rationale and context for the use of psychological assessment in the practice of pain management, articulates recommendations for the core domains of assessment, and provides an overview of the psychological assessment process. The remainder of the chapter provides specific information about some of the most commonly used psychological and behavioral assessment strategies for general use across chronic pain conditions. Disease-specific measures may also be of interest to clinicians but are not specifically covered in this chapter. Examples include the Oswestry Disability Questionnaire[1] (lower back pain), Western Ontario and McMaster Universities Osteoarthritis Index[2] (osteoarthritis), and the Neuropathic Pain Scale (neuropathic pain).[3]

CLINICAL OBJECTIVES

Psychological and behavioral assessment of pain serves several clinical goals. First, data gathered in the assessment process provide important information about a patient's pain experiences, pain treatment history, current and past emotional and physical functioning, and beliefs about pain. Thorough assessment of the multidimensional nature of a patient's pain experiences not only informs clinicians' treatment planning by identifying problems and intervention targets but also reinforces the multidimensional nature of pain to the patient, which may enhance engagement in future treatment modalities. Second, assessment allows the clinician to identify a patient's strengths and weaknesses and the factors that contribute to the development and maintenance of problems in physical, social, and emotional functioning. This information can direct selection of the treatment modality most likely to correspond to the patient's strengths and the intervention targets most related to the patient's specific functional deficits. Third, assessment allows the clinician to identify comorbid psychiatric or behavioral conditions that may interfere with pain coping and overall adjustment. Fourth, assessment can determine whether the patient is psychologically appropriate and likely to benefit from surgical or invasive procedure if medically indicated. Finally, thorough assessment of a patient's pain complaint and functioning at baseline provides an important benchmark against which the efficacy of future treatments can be measured. Assessment should not stop after the initial visit but should be ongoing throughout the treatment process. This allows identification of new problems, quantifies progress across domains, and facilitates refinement or revision of treatment if necessary. Post-treatment assessment is imperative to evaluate the overall success of the treatment, as well as the differential success of the treatment across various domains of function such as pain intensity and social, emotional, and physical functioning.

USE OF PSYCHOLOGICAL AND BEHAVIORAL ASSESSMENT IN THE PRACTICE OF PAIN MANAGEMENT

Multidimensional psychological and behavioral assessment of a patient with pain can assist a multidisciplinary pain team or treating clinician in several ways. Multidimensional assessment serves as a foundation for planning treatment and subsequent evaluation of treatment outcomes. Psychological and behavioral assessment may also reveal the need for adjunctive psychological treatment of preexisting or emerging psychosocial difficulties that may interfere with medical treatment of the patient's painful condition. Psychological assessment can provide information about the patient's motivation and readiness to engage in treatment, as well as treatment preferences. Finally, psychological assessment can provide data about a patient's suitability for surgical or other invasive procedures under consideration.

When making a request for a psychological and behavioral assessment it is necessary to explicitly state the reasons for the request or pose a question to be answered about the patient or the patient's treatment. It is helpful for the psychologist or behavioral specialist to understand the specific question that the clinician or team is trying to answer about a patient to perform a thorough evaluation and provide meaningful feedback. Although any psychological or behavioral assessment should be multidimensional and include all relevant domains of function, the specific measures used and the areas of most intense focus differ depending on the consultation question.

OVERVIEW OF THE PSYCHOLOGICAL AND BEHAVIORAL ASSESSMENT PROCESS

Ideally, psychological and behavioral assessment of a patient with chronic pain should follow an approach in which hypotheses are generated and tested. The assessment should begin broadly; as problems are identified, the clinician can hypothesize contributing and maintaining mechanisms. The assessment process will be increasingly focused and behaviorally oriented as the hypothesized mechanisms are investigated. Generally, the assessment process begins with a standardized interview that assesses the pain complaint, as well as the patient's physical, emotional, social, and occupational functioning. This allows assessment of the patient's past and present level of functioning and the temporal association of any changes in functioning to the pain complaint. In addition to the information gained in the interview, questionnaires, diaries, behavioral observations, reports by significant others, and medical record information may be used as adjunctive sources of information. Use of multiple adjunctive measures helps avoid the biases or error associated with reliance on a single assessment strategy. Hypotheses about the factors that initiated and maintain problems in adjustment and functioning are generated and refined throughout the assessment process. Ultimately, the validity of hypotheses is tested by examining the patient's response to treatment.

For example, anxiety and fear of pain have been shown to contribute to unfavorable outcomes in persons with chronic pain complaints.[4] Significant functional disability can be associated with fear of pain and further injury, such as behavioral avoidance, muscle deconditioning as a result of reduced activity, muscle hyperreactivity in response to stress, negative and distorted cognitions about the adverse effects of activity, and psychological distress secondary to restricted access to pleasant and rewarding activities. Thus, when an initial interview provides evidence of a significant decline in physical functioning and the presence of anxiety, the process just described becomes a reasonable hypothesis and avenue for more targeted assessment through the use of specific questionnaires, diaries, or reports by significant others. Ultimately, the assessment process should result in a model that describes the patient's specific pain experience; explicate how that patient's beliefs, experiences, strengths, and weaknesses have resulted in the current level of functioning across domains; and provide an individualized treatment plan that uses these hypotheses to target specific factors for intervention.

DOMAINS OF FUNCTIONING

The multidimensional nature of chronic pain necessitates a broad assessment of multiple domains of functioning to provide a valid snapshot of the patient's unique pain experience and meaningfully guide intervention strategies. A useful guide for the assessment process is the Initiative on Methods, Measurement, and Pain Assessment in Clinical Trials (IMMPACT) group consensus statement regarding the core outcome domains that should be assessed, as well as recommended instruments for measuring these domains, when evaluating the efficacy of a pain treatment.[5-7]

These recommendations, though originally generated to aid researchers in increasing comparability across randomized controlled studies of pain treatments, can be useful to the clinician in guiding assessment. The IMMPACT group, which consists of recognized experts drawn from academia, government agencies, and the pharmaceutical industry, recommends assessing the following chronic pain domains: pain, physical functioning, emotional functioning, patient ratings of improvement and satisfaction with treatment, treatment-related symptoms and adverse events, and patient disposition. Additionally, through literature review and expert consensus the group has provided recommendations regarding specific assessment instruments within each domain that are applicable across a diverse range of pain complaints. Most recently, this same group has provided recommendations for the future development of patient-oriented outcome measures that may provide more sensitive and efficient assessment of the key outcome domains relevant to a comprehensive assessment of patients with pain. To date, however, there are no prospective data to support the routine application of such measures in clinical care settings.

OVERVIEW OF ASSESSMENT STRATEGIES

Multiple assessment strategies such as interviews, standardized questionnaires, diaries, behavioral observation, psychophysiologic evaluation, and assessment of family members and significant others are commonly used to investigate and quantify the pain experience and concomitant physical and emotional functioning. The use of multiple, standardized assessment measures is encouraged to obtain comprehensive, valid, and reliable information.

A well-conducted *clinical interview* can be a rich source of information on a patient's pain and pain treatment history, as well as the resulting physical, emotional, behavioral, and cognitive responses.[8,9] The interview also provides an opportunity for clinicians to interact with the patient, establish rapport, and develop an impression of the patient's receptivity to rehabilitation and treatment efforts. Interviews may be standardized or unstandardized. Even when conducting an unstandardized interview it is useful to systematically investigate a prespecified set of domains (Box 16.1 is an example of an interview structure used in the author's [RK] comprehensive pain management clinic).

Questionnaires and *inventories* provide opportunities for focused assessment of specific domains of functioning and quantifying patient responses. Because published questionnaires have typically met standards for reliability and validity, greater confidence can be placed in the information provided by these measures. Questionnaires typically permit quantification of important dimensions of the experience of pain and allow evaluation of within-person change over time. Concurrent administration of measures of multiple domains of functioning can assist in the identification of a patient's relative strengths and weaknesses across these domains, such as identification of patients who report low levels of disability and distress despite an apparently severe level of pain intensity. Questionnaires with normative data offer the added benefit of providing a comparison point for evaluating the status of the respondent relative to others with

Box 16.1 CPMC Clinical Interview Template for Assessment of Pain

Demographics

Age, marital status, race, etc.

Referral Source

Referring MD and service, reason for referral

Behavioral Observations

Noteworthy pain behavior indicative of psychiatric disturbance; otherwise, state "unremarkable"

Pain Complaints and Treatment History

Please ask the patient the location of the pain sites, and then copy and paste questions 1 through 7 for each pain site. If the patient describes a pain site as running through the leg, knee, and foot, check all sites below but evaluate as one pain site. Thus, for a patient who identifies 3 pain sites: lower back region, right hip and leg, and hands, record 3 pain sites here and then complete questions 1 to 7 three times, each time identifying a different pain location "lower back," "hip and leg," and "hand." Qualify when necessary (e.g., left leg only; write this in).

1. LOCATION OF PAIN
   [] Head/face, [] neck, [] shoulder, [] arm, [] hands
   [] Stomach/abdomen, [] upper back, [] lower back, [] hip, [] leg
   [] Knee, [] foot, [] anal, [] genital
   [] Whole body, [] other sites (specify)
2. INTENSITY OF PAIN
   Patients rate their average level of pain over the past week as follows:
   0-----1-----2-----3-----4-----5-----6-----7-----8-----9-----10
   No Pain Worst Possible Pain
   Worst pain gets: Best pain gets: Average pain rating:
3. QUALITY OF PAIN (Do not prompt; use the patient's own words when possible.)
   [] Dull, [] stabbing, [] hot-burning, [] shooting, [] aching
   [] Piercing, [] tingling, [] numb, [] squeezing, [] throbbing
   [] Pulling, [] sharp, [] cramping, [] gnawing, [] heavy
   [] Tender, [] radiating, [] deep
   [] Other (specify)
4. ONSET/DURATION
   Approximate time the pain started:
5. VARIATIONS/PATTERNS/RHYTHMS
   The pain is [] constant, [] intermittent, [] episodic/recurring, [] other (specify)
6. WHAT RELIEVES THE PAIN?
   [] Sitting, [] lying down, [] standing, [] heat, [] cold, [] rest
   [] Distraction, [] exercises, [] movement
   [] Other (specify)
7. WHAT CAUSES OR INCREASES THE PAIN?
   [] Sitting, [] lying down, [] standing, [] heat, [] cold, [] rest, [] exercises
   [] Movement
   [] Other (specify)
8. EFFECTS OF PAIN
   Other associated symptoms: [] nausea, [] vomiting, [] dyspnea
   [] Confusion, [] weakness, [] numbness
   [] Other (specify)
   The pain affect the patient's
   [] Sleep, [] movement, [] energy
   [] Lifestyle, [] personal relationships, [] work, [] emotions
   [] Concentration, [] appetite, [] motivation, [] ADLs, [] IADLs
   [] Other (specify)
9. PATIENT'S PAIN GOAL (Check any appropriate boxes, if appropriate, and add brief descriptors of the patient's goals regarding reduced level of pain intensity and goals related to function, ADLs, quality of life, etc.)
   [] Sleep comfortably, [] comfort at rest, [] comfort with movement
   [] Stay alert, [] perform activity (specify)
   [] Other (specify)
   Acceptable level of pain (0 to 10 scale):
10. PAIN MEDICATIONS (During the interview, determine the current use, dosage, and general effectiveness of *pain medications* to determine the patient's perception of effectiveness.)
11. NONPHARMACOLOGIC METHODS OF PAIN RELIEF AND EFFECTIVENESS (For each method that the patient has used, note which pain sites are involved, past or present use, and effectiveness [yes/no].)
    [] Physical therapy
    [] Surgical interventions
    [] Psychotherapy
    [] Relaxation
    [] Biofeedback
    [] Manual treatments
    [] TENS
    [] Heat application
    [] Cold application
    [] Occupational therapy
    [] Distraction
    [] Exercises, [] stretching
    [] Other (specify)

Relevant Medical History

Significant recent medical history

Psychosocial History and Present Status

Significant mental health and substance abuse history
Current employment status, current living arrangements

ADLs, activities of daily living; CPMC, Chronic Pain Management Clinic; IADLs, instrumental activities of daily living; TENS, transcutaneous electrical nerve stimulation.

similar painful conditions or within similar demographic groups (i.e., age, race/ethnicity, gender). Ultimately, they may provide a more efficient and cost-effective option to more intensive and time-consuming interviews. Following this brief overview of psychological and behavioral assessment strategies, a number of questionnaires and inventories that are frequently used for the assessment of patients with pain in the clinical setting are reviewed.

Diaries offer two advantages over other assessment methods. They allow recording of prospective, day-to-day, or even more frequent information about pain, sleep, and physical and emotional function, thereby eliminating the distortion associated with memory and retrospective recall.[10] Additionally, diaries allow recording of the temporal association between pain and other factors. For example, many sleep diaries collect information about pain intensity scores before sleep, as well as sleep quality and duration.[11] This allows investigation of the relationship between pain and functioning as opposed to examining either factor in isolation. The composition of diaries can vary from those designed to assess a single domain, such as pain intensity, to those that are much more comprehensive and multidimensional. The use of innovative technologies such mobile telephone applications, web-based diaries, and interactive voice response systems is increasingly being promoted as a more efficient strategy for collection of prospective information.[12]

Although pain is a private, subjective experience, it is possible to observe signs that a patient is experiencing pain by direct *behavioral observation*. Patients can communicate that they are experiencing pain and the intensity of their pain through facial expressions, crying, moaning, limping, guarding, and rubbing affected areas. Behavioral observation of patients with chronic pain can provide valuable adjunctive information beyond that gathered with a self-report format and is crucial to the evaluation of those with cognitive or physical limitations that interfere with verbal communication. Behavioral observation methods have been developed for the assessment of patients with a range of painful medical conditions, including cancer pain,[13] rheumatoid arthritis,[14] osteoarthritis,[15] and low back pain.[16] Prkachin and colleagues[17] reported on a method for assessment of pain behavior in the context of clinical evaluation of patients with low back pain. These methods have also been developed and used in studies of pain-relevant communication in partner dyads.[18] To obtain reliable and valid behavioral observation data it is necessary to have a systematic plan for behavioral observation, coding, and interpretation of the data; accordingly, use of these methods requires considerable technological sophistication and expense.[19] The use of behavioral observation methods is commonly limited to the clinical research setting because of the time-intensive and costly nature of these methods.

Reports of families and significant others in the assessment of pain have been strongly encouraged in contemporary models of pain, particularly Fordyce's operant conditioning model[20] and Turk's cognitive-behavioral model,[21] which have specifically encouraged this focus given the hypothesized roles of social contingencies in the perpetuation, if not etiology, of persistent pain and disability and awareness of the frequent negative impact of persistent pain on significant others. In particular, the role of solicitousness in the development and maintenance of pain-related disability has been a topic of a great deal of research. Operant principles specify that when spouses provide solicitous responses to pain behavior, the pain behavior is more likely to occur in the future, even in the absence of continued nociception. Positive or solicitous responses from spouses and family members, contingent on pain behavior, may serve to reinforce the maladaptive behavior and encourage the development and maintenance of pain and pain-related disability. Examples of solicitous behavior examined in the literature include expressions of sympathy or concern for the spouse, physical assistance or performance of a task, and encouraging rest and discouraging activity. A 2006 review summarized the evidence for relationships between marital functioning and chronic pain.[22] In general, spouse solicitousness is significantly related to greater pain intensity, greater frequency of pain behavior, higher levels of disability,[22-24] and increased help-seeking behavior.[23,24] Distracting responses from significant others, meaning responses that are intended to cue engagement in other behavior in an effort to distract from pain, have been found to be positively related to poor outcomes despite the probable intent of these responses to encourage adaptive coping with pain.[22] In addition to global measures of family and marital relationships, numerous questionnaires and inventories,[25-27] diaries,[28] and behavioral observation methods[18] have been developed specifically for the assessment of pain-relevant communication and the impact of pain on family members and significant others.

Psychophysical measures are used primarily to demonstrate the influence of psychological factors on the initiation and maintenance of pain symptoms.[29] For clinicians, psychophysical measures provide evidence that psychological factors are influencing biologic reactions in an individual patient and provide information on the utility of certain types of interventions (e.g., biofeedback). For the patient, evidence that psychological factors are influencing physical responses related to pain can provide direct feedback regarding the successful use of behavioral strategies to manage a pain disorder and increase confidence to engage in these behavioral strategies.[30]

The most common clinical use of psychophysical measures in the treatment of pain occurs primarily during biofeedback treatments. Biofeedback treatments use psychophysical measures to train patients in voluntary modifications of bodily reactions through provision of feedback of physiologic processes.[29] Surface electromyographic (EMG) recordings are the most widely used psychophysical measure in biofeedback for pain disorders because muscle tension is implicated in the majority of musculoskeletal pain disorders. EMG readings typically target specific muscle groups associated with the patient's pain disorder (e.g., trapezius muscle for patients with upper back pain and the erector spinae muscle for patients with lower back pain). Additionally, blood flow is linked to several chronically painful conditions, including migraine headaches and Raynaud's disease. For these conditions, measures of blood flow and peripheral skin temperature (a proxy for peripheral circulation) can be used in biofeedback treatments. Other types of biofeedback include heart rate variability and skin conductance, but more research is required to determine the relationship of these measures to chronic pain disorders and their utility in biofeedback treatment of chronic pain.

SPECIFIC PSYCHOLOGICAL AND BEHAVIORAL ASSESSMENT STRATEGIES

Standardized assessment instruments, often in the form of questionnaires or inventories, are used frequently in the assessment of patients with pain (Table 16.1).[31-54] Questionnaires allow a focused examination of a specific domain such as pain intensity, physical and emotional functioning, or coping beliefs and provide quantitative data that can be used to understand the patient's functioning relative to the general population or other patients experiencing pain.

PAIN INTENSITY

A primary objective in assessing patients experiencing pain is to determine their level of pain intensity. Change in pain

Table 16.1 Overview of Assessment Measures

Measure	Domain	Measure Details	Advantage/Disadvantages
Numerical rating scale (NRS)[31*]	Pain intensity	Single item, written or oral	Demonstrated validity, easy to administer, high completion rate; use of a single item hinders reliability
Verbal rating scale (VRS)[31]		Collection of pain descriptors	Demonstrated validity, easy to administer, high completion rate; may be difficult for persons with poor command of English
Visual analog scale (VAS)[31]		10-cm line with descriptive end points	Demonstrated validity, easy to administer; more likely to be incomplete than the NRS or VRS, and use of a single item hinders reliability
McGill Pain Questionnaire (MPQ)[32*]	Pain quality	Collection of pain descriptors; also assesses location of pain and exacerbating and ameliorating factors	Demonstrated validity; not consistently associated with pain intensity but more consistently associated with psychological distress
Minnesota Multiphasic Personality Inventory, recently revised version (MMPI-2-RF)[33]	Personality	567 true-false items	Most widely used personality measure, uses normative data in scoring; high response burden, difficult to score, requires training to interpret, more information needed regarding validity for chronic pain
Millon Behavioral Health Inventory (MBHI)[34]		150 true-false items	Developed specifically for use in persons with medical conditions, demonstrated validity and reliability; high response burden, scoring time-consuming, not predictive of outcomes in treatment studies of persons with chronic pain
West Haven–Yale Multidimensional Pain Inventory (WHYMPI)[35*] (interference subscale)	Psychosocial impact	52 items, assesses multiple domains	Demonstrated validity and reliability, useful for a variety of pain complaints, widely used; relatively high response burden, scoring time-consuming
Patient-Reported Outcomes Measurement Information System (PROMIS)[36,37] (pain-interference and pain-behaviors item banks)		Item banks (interference = 41 items; behaviors = 39 items)	Standardized bank of items developed by the NIH, demonstrated reliability and initial validity, available in short forms; more information regarding validity needed
Sickness Impact Profile (SIP)[38]		136 items and 24-item brief version for persons with chronic back pain	Demonstrated validity and reliability, responsive to change; full version has high response burden
Pain Disability Index (PDI)[39]	Physical/social role function	49 items, assesses perceived disability in 7 areas	Demonstrated validity and reliability, can identify specific areas of perceived disability; relatively high response burden, scoring time-consuming
Brief Pain Inventory (BPI)[40*]		32-items, short form has 15 items, ultra-brief version (PEG) has 3 items	Widely used, demonstrated validity and reliability, easy to administer, brief versions appropriate for multiple clinical settings; further validity information for PEG warranted
Beck Depression Inventory (BDI)[41*]	Emotional function	21 items, measures depression	Demonstrated reliability and reliability, sensitive to change; somatic items may be associated with pain rather than mood, possible bias in certain populations
Center for Epidemiologic Studies Depression Scale (CES-D)[42]		20 items, measures depression	Demonstrated reliability and validity in a wide variety of ethnic populations, non-English version available; lacks sensitivity and specificity without psychiatric interview
Geriatric Depression Scale (GDS)[43]		30 yes-no questions, measures depression in older adults	Demonstrated reliability and validity, good sensitivity and specificity; has not yet been widely used in chronic pain samples
Pain Anxiety Symptoms Scale (PASS)[44]		53 items, assesses pain-related fear	Demonstrated validity; poor prediction of pain-related disability, relatively high response burden
State-Trait Anxiety Inventory (STAI)[45]		Two 20-item measures of state and trait anxiety	Acceptable psychometric properties, widely used, sensitive to change

Continued on following page

Table 16.1 Overview of Assessment Measures (Continued)

Measure	Domain	Measure Details	Advantage/Disadvantages
Profile of Mood States (POMS)[46]		65-item measure of several dimensions of emotional functioning	Strong psychometric properties, sensitive to change, captures negative and positive dimensions of emotional functioning; high response burden
Symptom Checklist—90 Revised (SCL-90R)[47]		90-item measure of numerous areas of psychological functioning	Demonstrated reliability and validity; normed on psychiatric patients and may not be valid for use in persons with chronic pain, high response burden
Medical Outcomes Study Short Form Health Survey (SF-36)[48]		36-item measure of perceived physical and emotional health	Psychometrically sound, widely used; has not yet been widely used in chronic pain samples
Survey of Pain Attitudes (SOPA)[49]	Pain beliefs and coping	57-item measure of pain-related beliefs; brief forms also available	Psychometrically sound, scores correlated with treatment outcomes and physical and emotional functioning
Pain Stages of Change Questionnaire (PSOCQ)[50]		30-item measure of readiness to change	Demonstrated reliability and validity, predicts completion of treatment, changes in PSOCQ predict changes in "readiness"; may not be predictive of treatment outcomes
Chronic Pain Coping Inventory (CPCI)[51]		64-item measure of use of pain-coping strategies	Psychometrically sound, patient coping strategies found to be associated with outcomes; high response burden
Pain Catastrophizing Scale (PCS)[52]		13-item measure of pain-related catastrophic thoughts	Psychometrically sound, associated with treatment outcomes; further evaluation in clinical samples warranted
Chronic Pain Acceptance Questionnaire (CPAQ)[53]		20-item measure of pain acceptance; 8-item brief form also available	Demonstrated reliability and cross-sectional validity; associated with treatment outcomes, measure is specific to a single type of pain treatment, and further information regarding predictive validity is warranted
Patient Outcome Questionnaire (POQ)[54]	Quality of care	12-item measure of perceived quality of pain treatment	Commissioned by the American Pain Society, demonstrated reliability and internal validity; additional validity studies are needed

*Measure was selected by the Initiative on Methods, Measurement, and Pain Assessment in Clinical Trials (IMMPACT) panel as the preferred measure within a domain.
NIH, National Institutes of Health.

intensity from baseline to after treatment is often the primary outcome measure used in evaluating the efficacy of a given pain treatment. The following measures attempt to quantify the private experience of perceived pain. The *numerical rating scale* (NRS), the *verbal rating scale* (VRS), and the *visual analog scale* (VAS) are the most frequently used measures of pain intensity.[31]

The NRS is a single-item rating scale of pain intensity that can be administered in an oral or written format. Patients are asked to specify their pain on a scale from 0 to 10, with 0 representing "no pain" and 10 representing "the worst pain imaginable" or extreme pain. Although a 0 to 10 scale is most commonly used, ranges of 0 to 20 or 0 to 100 are also used. Farrar and colleagues[55] suggested that a 2-point decrease in the 0 to 10 NRS may be indicative of a clinically important change in pain intensity. Advantages of the NRS include ease of administration and scoring and high rates of completion by respondents.[31,56]

The VRS contains a list of pain descriptors that typically range in intensity from "no pain" to "severe pain." Patients select the descriptor that best characterizes their level of pain from a list that ranges from 4 to 15 descriptors. The descriptors are then assigned a number value based on the intensity level (i.e., no pain = 0, mild = 1, moderate = 2, and severe = 3).[31] Like the NRS, the VRS has demonstrated validity through significant correlations with other measures of pain intensity.[31,56] Although the VRS is an attractive option because it is easy to administer, patients with limited vocabulary or command of English may have difficulty discriminating among the descriptor words, and the selection of descriptors may not adequately describe a respondent's pain, especially when a four-descriptor format is used.[31]

The VAS uses a 10-cm-long line with end points denoting the absence of pain (e.g., "no pain") at one end and extreme pain at the other. Respondents place a mark on the line at the point that best characterizes their pain intensity relative to the end points. Calculation of a pain intensity score is based on the distance from the "no pain" end point to the respondent's mark.

A review by Jensen and Karoly found that all the aforementioned measures demonstrated validity through significant correlations with other pain intensity measures and have comparable responsiveness to changes in pain in the context of pain treatment.[31] Evidence suggests that respondents may prefer VRS and NRS instruments over the VAS and that VAS instruments are more likely than NRS measures to result in missing or incomplete data, possibly because of cognitive or motor disabilities.[31,55] For these reasons, the consensus statement of the IMMPACT committee's review of core measures for chronic pain clinical trials recommends using an 11-point NRS scale to assess pain intensity and the VRS as an adjunct.[5] Although these recommendations were developed for use by clinical researchers, the importance of consistent use of valid, reliable, and understandable measures in clinical practice should not be ignored, and the guidelines provide valuable information for all users of these measures.

The *McGill Pain Questionnaire* (MPQ)[32] is a more lengthy measure designed to assess the quality and affective component of the pain experience, not simply pain intensity. Respondents choose pain descriptors from a list of 78 potential descriptors that fall into 20 pain categories. These descriptors assess four pain domains: sensory, affective, evaluative, and miscellaneous. Within each category the individual descriptors reflect varying degrees of intensity and are assigned corresponding numerical values that reflect this difference. Respondents also highlight the location of their pain on a figure drawing and provide information about the factors that alleviate and aggravate their pain intensity. The MPQ generates three scores: (1) the Pain Rating Index, which is the sum of all words chosen in the available categories (the sum of the value of each subclass can also be obtained); (2) the number of words chosen, a score that reflects the number of words chosen from each of the four categories; and (3) the present pain intensity, a rating of current pain on a scale from 0 (no pain) to 5 (excruciating).[19] The MPQ has been widely used in a variety of pain-focused research and has been translated into several languages, although not all new versions of the scale have been subjected to adequate clinimetric or psychometric testing.[57] A 15-item short-version of the MPQ (SF-MPQ) is also available.[58]

Strengths of the MPQ include demonstrated validity of its subscales through their association with perceived quality of life, ability to discriminate among pain conditions, pain medication use, and sensitivity to the effects of pain treatment.[19] The MPQ scale scores have not shown a consistent association with pain intensity ratings, and a review concluded that the MPQ scales may not measure the same construct as other pain intensity measures do and may be less sensitive than "pure" measures of pain intensity such as the NRS and VRS.[55] The SF-MPQ demonstrated high correlation with the Pain Rating Index of the MPQ and was sensitive to changes produced by pain medications in patients with pain.[59] The IMMPACT committee recommended use of the SF-MPQ as a measure of pain quality and the affective component of pain because these aspects of the pain experience may respond differently to treatment than pain intensity does.[5]

PERSONALITY

The *Minnesota Multiphasic Personality Inventory* (MMPI)[33] is by far the most commonly used objective measure of personality, and it is similarly the most commonly used measure for the evaluation of psychological functioning of patients with pain. A recently revised version, known as the MMPI-2-RF, consists of 338 true-false items that are used to derive scores on: 3 higher-order scales; 9 restructured clinical scales; 8 validity scales; 14 somatic/cognitive and internalizing scales; 11 externalizing, interpersonal, and interest scales; and 5 personality psychopathology scales.[33] The most recent version of the MMPI has several advantages over previous versions: it is based on more modern views of psychopathology, it has fewer items and therefore lower patient burden, and its normative sample is more representative of the U.S. population. Additionally, the restructured clinical scales have reduced intercorrelations with respect to the original scales and have demonstrated validity in predicting pathology with more accuracy while using fewer items than the original scales. However, the MMPI-2-RF has not been examined in patients with chronic pain.

Significant concerns have been raised about the appropriateness of the previous versions of the MMPI (MMPI or MMPI-2) for use in the assessment of patients with chronic pain.[60] Differences observed on the clinical scales between pain and nonpain samples have been demonstrated to more likely reflect disease status than psychological functioning.[61] An extensive research effort has focused on the identification of reliable subgroups of patients with chronic pain based on their MMPI profiles. The sum of this literature suggests that even though reliable subgroups can be identified despite evidence that the subgroups differ in terms of behavioral correlates of the experience of pain, it has yet to be demonstrated in a compelling fashion that the MMPI has value in characterizing patterns of coping with chronic pain over and above data derived from pain-specific measures.[62,63] No information is available to indicate whether these issues have been alleviated (or exacerbated) by the significant revisions of the MMPI-2-RF. Results in patients with chronic pain should be interpreted with caution until further studies are able to validate the MMPI-2-RF in chronic pain populations.

The *Millon Behavioral Health Inventory* (MBHI)[34] was developed to assess the psychological functioning of patients with medical conditions. This 150-item measure contains eight scales designed to assess the respondent's interaction style (e.g., cooperation), six scales that assess the respondent's response to illness (e.g., pain treatment responsivity), and six scales that assess the presence of psychosocial stressors (e.g., social alienation). Questions are posed in a true/false format. A respondent's answers are scored by comparison with the base rate in the normative sample, which consisted of patients with a variety of medical illnesses.

The MBHI has been demonstrated to have substantial reliability and validity indices. It may have advantages relative to the MMPI-2-RF for use in the assessment of patients with pain conditions as a function of its relative brevity and the fact that it was developed and normed on medical as opposed to psychiatric populations. However, to date, studies have failed to demonstrate the predictive validity of the scale in studies of psychological interventions,[64] surgical interventions,[65] or multidisciplinary treatment[66] of patients with chronic pain.

ASSESSMENT OF PSYCHOSOCIAL IMPACT

The *West Haven–Yale Multidimensional Pain Inventory* (WHYMPI)[35] is designed to measure the psychosocial and behavioral aspects of chronic pain and is useful across a variety of pain complaints. It is a 52-item multidimensional self-report instrument that uses 7-point Likert scales. The instrument consists of three sections. Section one includes six scales measuring pain-related interference across several domains, including work and leisure activities, as well as interpersonal relationships, perceived support from spouse or significant other, pain severity and suffering, perceived life control, and negative mood. Section two assesses patient perception of significant others' responses to overt expressions of pain by classifying responses as solicitous, distracting, or negative. Section three measures the frequency with which the patient engages in four clusters of everyday activities, including household chores, social activities, outdoor work, and activities away from home. The WHYMPI takes approximately 10 to 15 minutes to complete and is written at a fifth-grade reading level. Test-retest reliability over 2 weeks ranges from 0.62 to 0.91, and internal reliability coefficients range from 0.70 to 0.90.[35] Several investigative teams have generally replicated the factor structure and psychometric properties of the WHYMPI.[67] Turk and colleagues proposed an empirically derived taxonomy of the WHYMPI that includes three reliable profiles of patients with persistent pain labeled as dysfunctional, interpersonally distressed, and adaptive copers,[68] and these investigators and several other groups have replicated these findings in numerous samples of patients with various pain conditions.[69] The measure has been used in many empirical studies, including clinical trials of psychological and pharmacologic interventions, studies of the psychosocial impact of pain, and studies examining the role of psychosocial factors as contributors to the development and maintenance of persistent pain. The IMMPACT group recommended use of the interference scale of the WHYMPI as an outcome measure in pain clinical trials.[5] The second section of the measures that focus on responses of significant others has been particularly valuable in evaluating the role of such responses as predictors of the severity of pain and pain-related disability and distress.[70]

Three additions to the original version of the scale have enhanced its overall reliability, validity, and clinical utility. Rudy[71] added two items to the life control and interference scales, Okifuji and colleagues[72] proposed alternative instructions for the significant other response section to reduce missing observations, and Bruehl and colleagues[73] developed a scale to detect random responding and malingering. A significant other version of the measure has also been published.[25]

The National Institutes of Health *Patient-Reported Outcomes Measurement Information System* (PROMIS) is a standardized item bank developed by a cooperative group for the purpose of developing psychometrically sound standardized measures to assess patient-reported outcomes. These measures provide information on the domains of physical, mental, and social health across a variety of medical illnesses. Measures for pain currently available in the PROMIS assessment center (www.assessmentcenter.net) include "pain-interference" and "pain-behaviors." The pain-interference item bank includes 41 items, with 4 short forms consisting of 4 to 8 items.[36] The pain-behaviors item bank includes 39 items with a single short form consisting of 7 items.[37] Both measures have demonstrated reliability and validity in psychometric evaluation, were related to other measures of pain-related outcomes, and discriminated among groups of patients with different self-reported health, number of chronic conditions, and number of disabling conditions. Further studies have demonstrated that pain-related measures are higher and global scores of quality of life are lower in clinical pain samples than in samples from the general population.[74] The PROMIS pain-interference and pain-behaviors scales have recently been developed and therefore have only a small body of evidence regarding reliability and validity. Available studies suggest that these scales provide comprehensive, sophisticated, and psychometrically sound measures for pain-related patient-reported outcomes.

The *Sickness Impact Profile* (SIP)[38] measures the degree of disability across 12 domains of functioning. One hundred thirty-six items are used to derive measures of sleep and rest, eating, work, home management, recreation and pastimes, ambulation, mobility, body care and movement, social interaction, alertness behavior, emotional behavior, and communication. These domain scores are combined to produce physical, psychosocial, and total disability scores. The SIP can be self-administered or administered by an interviewer in about 20 to 30 minutes.

An extensive period of development and testing and reports on these efforts support the reliability and validity of the measure. The SIP has been found to be responsive to change during treatment of chronic pain.[75] A brief version consisting of 24 items, called the Roland-Morris Disability Questionnaire, has been developed specifically for use in patients with chronic low back pain.[76,77] This measure has also been shown to have strong evidence of reliability, validity, and responsiveness to change as a function of psychological interventions and is recommended by the IMMPACT group[5] as the preferred measure of physical functioning for evaluating persons with back pain.

PHYSICAL AND SOCIAL ROLE FUNCTIONING

Assessment of physical functioning has been recommended as a core outcome domain in pain clinical trials,[6] and others have suggested that it should perhaps be considered the primary outcome in such trials.[78] Measurement of physical and social role functioning represents a challenge to the field given the broad range of levels of functioning, for example, the range of activities of daily living to the broader domain of health-related quality of life. A variety of strategies have been developed to assess these varying dimensions, and selection of the appropriate measure in the research or clinical setting should take into account the specific population being assessed (e.g., unexplained chronic low back pain, frail elderly) and the purpose of the assessment (e.g., responsivity to change during treatment, comparison to population norms). Three of the most commonly used measures of this domain for the assessment of patients with painful medical conditions are briefly reviewed.

The *Pain Disability Index* (PDI)[39] is a brief measure of pain-related interference in role functioning. The PDI includes seven items assessing perceived disability in each of seven areas of functioning: family/home responsibilities, recreation, social activity, occupation, sexual behavior, self-care, and life support activity. Each item is rated on a 10-point Likert scale (0 = no disability to 10 = worst disability).

The PDI has demonstrated internal consistency values of 0.85 to 0.86 and excellent test-retest reliability.[79] Validity has been demonstrated through its association with the Oswestry Disability Questionnaire (focused specifically on chronic lower back pain),[80] physical functioning tests,[81] and measures of pain intensity.[80]

The *Brief Pain Inventory* (BPI)[40] was originally developed to measure pain intensity and interference in patients with cancer pain, but it has been widely used to assess non–cancer-related pain. A short-form of the BPI containing 15 items is also available. The short form of the BPI has been found to have high internal consistency scores ranging from 0.82 to 0.95 for the severity and interference scales in a sample of patients with arthritis and lower back pain.[82] Demonstration of its reliability and validity and its availability in multiple languages have contributed to it being recommended by the IMMPACT group for use as a measure of physical functioning in pain clinical trials.[5] The PEG is an ultra-brief version of the BPI that consists of three items: (P) pain intensity, (E) enjoyment of life, and (G) general activity. Development studies demonstrated reliability and validity of the PEG comparable to that of the longer BPI.[83]

EMOTIONAL FUNCTIONING

Assessment of the emotional functioning of patients experiencing chronic pain should be conducted in the context of any pain-relevant intervention. The high prevalence of emotional distress in patients with chronic pain conditions, the negative effects of emotional distress on pain and pain-related disability, the inflated health care cost associated with emotional distress in patients with chronic pain, and the influence of emotional distress on participation in pain treatment provide the rationale for this recommendation.[5] The following brief review considers just a few of the many standardized measures of depressive symptom severity, anxiety, and anger, the three most commonly cited and studied emotional concomitants of the experience of persistent pain.

The *Beck Depression Inventory* (BDI)[41] was developed to measure the behavioral manifestations of depression in adolescents and adults and to standardize the assessment of depressive symptom severity for monitoring change over time. In its original form, the BDI consisted of 21 groups of four to five statements describing symptoms in each cluster from low to high. Respondents were instructed to endorse the single item in each group that best describes how they were feeling "right now." The original version was designed to be used in an interview format, but subsequent versions have more commonly been used in a self-report, questionnaire format. In 1978 the full scale was revised to eliminate redundancy among some of the items, and the time frame for assessment was altered to "during the last week, including today." Only four possible responses for each symptom cluster are now included, so scores on the measure range from 0 to 63. In 1996 the BDI-II was published and included revisions of some items and the time frame for assessment to be consistent with the *Diagnostic and Statistical Manual of Mental Disorders,* fourth edition (DSM-IV). Although the BDI-II has advantages in terms of the content of the items and consistency with current diagnostic nomenclature, concerns have been raised about its sensitivity to change during brief periods of time.[84] The 21-item version of the BDI takes about 5 to 10 minutes to complete.

The reliability and several dimensions of validity of the measure have been extensively reported. In a review of 25 years of research with the BDI, Beck and colleagues reported on 25 studies that assessed the internal consistency of the measure.[85] Across psychiatric, healthy, and medically ill samples, indices of internal consistency (alphas) ranged from 0.73 to 0.95. Stability estimates (i.e., test-retest correlations) have consistently been high as well, typically varying in the 0.80 to 0.90 range, depending on the assessment interval and sample. Estimates of validity for psychiatric patients have been assessed by examining the correlation between BDI scores and clinical ratings of depression (e.g., by using the Hamilton Rating Scale for Depression), with validity averaging about 0.72. For nonpsychiatric patients, the average estimate of validity is 0.60. In a review of eight studies of sensitivity to change, Moran and Lambert[86] found that the BDI was sensitive to change as a function of psychotherapy and pharmacotherapy outcome studies. Some evidence suggests a reporting bias for certain populations, including women, adolescents, and elderly persons, although the robustness of these observations is not clear.

The BDI has been used extensively in studies designed to evaluate the efficacy of pharmacologic and nonpharmacologic treatments of chronic pain,[87-91] and there is ample evidence of its sensitivity to change. The results of most studies provide compelling support for use of the BDI in assessing improvements in depressive symptom severity as a function of pain treatment, and it has been recommended as one of the core outcome measures for assessment in pain clinical trials.[5]

The *Center for Epidemiologic Studies Depression Scale* (CES-D)[42] was developed to screen for the presence of depressive illness and to measure levels of symptoms of depression in community samples. The scale's 20 items were selected from existing scales (e.g., BDI, MMPI depression scale, Zung Self-Rating Depression Scale) to represent the major components of depression on the basis of clinical and empirical studies. Respondents are asked to rate the frequency of a given symptom on a 0 (rarely or none of the time) to 3 (most or all of the time) scale with reference to the past week. Four items are worded in the positive direction to partially control for response bias. The CES-D takes about 5 minutes to complete.

Indices of internal consistency (Cronbach's alpha) have been reported to be 0.85 in community samples and 0.90 in psychiatric samples. Split-half reliabilities are also high and range from 0.77 to 0.92. Test-retest correlations over a 6- to 8-week period range from 0.51 to 0.67.[42] Roberts[92] reported that studies of African American and Mexican American respondents revealed similar reliability estimates. The reliability and validity of the measure have also been examined in numerous ethnic populations, and it has been translated into several languages.[42] Overall, high levels of internal consistency have been reported across numerous samples from the general population and patient samples, irrespective of age, gender, race, and geographic location. In a sample of chronic pain patients, the level of internal consistency was found to be 0.90.[93] Indices of criterion-related validity have generally been reported to be moderate to high. For example, correlations between the CES-D and the depression scale of the Symptom Checklist—90 Revised in samples of psychiatric patients have been reported to range from 0.73 to 0.90. Correlations with the Hamilton Rating Scale for Depression in similar samples have ranged from 0.49 to 0.85. Studies of elderly samples have revealed somewhat lower validity estimates.

Investigators have challenged the diagnostic sensitivity of the CES-D.[94,95] Investigators in the pain field have called for modifications of the measure in terms of item content[96] or scale cutoffs for the diagnosis of depression.[95,96] Ultimately, it is fair to say that the measure lacks the sensitivity and specificity for supporting its use in clinical diagnosis without the concurrent use of a psychiatric interview. The CES-D has increasingly been used for the assessment of outcome following pain interventions, and in numerous cases the measure has been demonstrated to be sensitive to change.[97,98]

The *Geriatric Depression Scale* (GDS)[43] was specifically developed to assess depressive symptom severity in older patients and was encouraged by observations that all the other self-report measures of the construct were developed and validated in medically healthy younger adults. These measures suffer from the criticism that they include numerous somatic symptoms that are common in nondepressed elderly patients and that their format for responding may be difficult for some older patients.

The GDS consists of 30 "yes" versus "no" questions; 10 are negatively keyed and 20 are positively keyed. Questions are ordered, with more "acceptable" items presented first. A 15-item short form is also available.[99]

In the original publication, indices of internal consistency (0.94) and split-half reliability (0.94) were extremely high.[43] The GDS demonstrated high correlation with other measures of depression and was successful in discriminating mildly from severely depressed groups in this same study and depressed older patients with arthritis from nondepressed patients with arthritis. Brink and colleagues[100] reported a high degree of sensitivity and specificity in discriminating depressed from nondepressed patients in a separate sample.

This measure seems to have substantial advantages for the assessment of depressive symptom severity in elderly patients. However, additional research in chronic pain samples will be necessary before its use in pain treatment outcome research can be supported.

The *Pain Anxiety Symptoms Scale* (PASS)[44] was designed to assess the cognitive, physiologic, and behavioral domains of pain-related fear. It includes 53 items distributed across four subscales measuring fear of pain, cognitive anxiety, somatic anxiety, and escape and avoidance. Respondents use 0 (never) to 6 (always) scales to endorse the frequency of each of the symptoms. The PASS has been demonstrated to have adequate internal consistency,[44] with indices of internal consistency ranging from 0.81 to 0.89 for each of the four scales and 0.94 for the total scale. Good predictive validity[101] and acceptable criterion validity[102] have also been demonstrated. The PASS has been criticized for its poor prediction of disability relative to other pain-related fear measures,[102] and its factor structure has also been challenged.[103]

The *Spielberger State-Trait Anxiety Inventory* (STAI)[45] was designed to identify and quantify both situational anxiety (state) and dispositional anxiety (trait). The STAI consists of two 20-item self-report inventories of each of these constructs. Respondents rate the degree of agreement to brief statements (e.g., "I feel calm") on 4-point scales ranging from "not at all" to "very much so" in terms of both their present state (state version) and their frequency over time (trait version). There is high concordance between pain and anxiety as measured by the STAI,[104] and it has been widely used in the pain literature. It has acceptable psychometric properties[45,102] and is sensitive to change in anxiety as a function of pain treatment.[105]

The *Profile of Mood States* (POMS)[46] is a self-report measure composed of a list of 65 mood-related adjectives that requires respondents to report the degree to which each feeling or mood state has applied to them over the past week via a 0 (not at all) to 4 (extremely) Likert scale. The scale assesses six dimensions of mood: tension-anxiety, depression-dejection, anger-hostility, fatigue-inertia, vigor-activity, and confusion-bewilderment. The POMS requires only 3 to 5 minutes to administer. It has been recommended for use in pain clinical trials[5] because of its capacity for briefly assessing the multiple dimensions of emotional functioning of patients with pain; its strong psychometric properties, including evidence of its responsiveness to change, especially in analgesic medication trials; and its availability in multiple languages.

Indices of internal consistency (alphas) for the six mood scales ranged from 0.84 for confusion-bewilderment to 0.95 for depression-dejection. Stability estimates (test-retest reliability correlations) ranged from 0.65 for vigor-activity to 0.74 for depression-dejection. Regarding validity, correlations between scales of the POMS and analogous scales from the MMPI-2 were largely in the expected direction and significant, with coefficients ranging from −0.58 to 0.69. The POMS has been used extensively in the pain treatment literature and has been shown to be sensitive to change as a function of pain treatment.[106]

Advantages of the POMS include its ease of administration, its brevity, its development on nonpsychiatric populations, and its design to capture both the negative and positive dimensions of emotional functioning. In particular, since the POMS has scales for three of the most important dimensions of emotional distress in patients with pain (anxiety, depression, and anger), the scale has an explicit advantage over any alternative scale. Within each of these three negative emotions, some items also have an intuitive appeal for capturing the construct in patients with chronic pain. For example, the tension-anxiety scale incorporates items that reflect both somatic and cognitive distress. The depression-dejection scale includes mood descriptors other than sadness that have been observed to be present in a large proportion of patients with chronic pain who meet the criteria for current major depressive disorder but who otherwise deny feelings of depression. Inclusion of an anger-hostility scale is particularly novel and potentially an advantage of the POMS relative to any other comparable instrument. The vigor-activity scale represents a relatively unique opportunity to assess improvements in this key dimension of emotional functioning rather than relying on a reduction in negative mood and symptoms of emotional distress. The fatigue-inertia scale provides an opportunity to measure this common concomitant of the experience of chronic pain, especially when assessing pain treatment in patients with clinical pain conditions in which fatigue is particularly prevalent (e.g., pain in multiple sclerosis). The opportunity to discriminate the effects of a pain intervention on fatigue and anergia, on the one hand, and other symptoms of emotional distress on the other may have particular utility in certain cases. Finally, given concerns about the effects of certain pain medications on cognitive functioning, the bewilderment-confusion scale may also have some benefit.

The *Symptom Checklist—90 Revised* (SCL-90R)[47] requires respondents to rate the extent to which they have been bothered by each of 90 physical or mental health symptoms in the past week. Responses are used to derive nine standardized indices of psychological disturbance labeled somatization, obsessive-compulsive, interpersonal sensitivity, depression, anxiety, hostility, phobic anxiety, paranoid ideation, and psychoticism. A global severity index may also be derived. The reliability and validity of the SCL-90R for the evaluation of psychiatric patients have been extensively reported in a manual for the instrument[47] and elsewhere.[107]

Numerous researchers have criticized the appropriateness of this measure for use in the assessment of patients with chronic pain. For example, Shutty and colleagues[108] were able to identify only five rather than nine reliable factors from the SCL-90R in a sample of chronic pain patients. These investigators also challenged the validity of evaluating patients with chronic pain by using norms developed from samples of psychiatric patients.[109] On the other hand, Jamison and colleagues[110] identified three reliable subgroups of patients with chronic pain by using the SCL-90R. These investigators demonstrated that patients with elevations in the subscales of the measure, relative to those who have a profile consistent with normative data, reported significantly higher levels of disability, sleep disturbance, and emotional distress. Several other investigators have largely replicated these findings. Unfortunately, no data have been published in support of the ability of these subgroups or the individual scales to predict response to pain treatment. Finally, the sensitivity of the SCL-90R to change as a function of treatment has not been adequately demonstrated.

The *Medical Outcomes Study Short-Form Health Survey* (SF-36)[48] was developed as a general measure of perceived health status and is typically self-administered. The measure contains 36 items that are combined to form eight scales: physical functioning, physical role functioning, bodily pain, general health, vitality, social functioning, emotional role functioning, and mental health. Respondents use "yes-no" or 5- or 6-point scales to endorse the presence or degree of specific symptoms, problems, and concerns. Scores on the scales range from 0 to 100, with higher scores indicating better health status and functioning. The measure takes about 10 to 15 minutes to complete. The SF-36 has been extensively validated with large samples from the general population and across several demographic subgroups, including samples of healthy persons older than 65.[111]

Estimates of internal consistency (alphas) for most samples range from 0.62 to 0.94 for the subscales, with most estimates ranging over 0.80. Test-retest coefficients ranged from 0.43 to 0.81 for a 6-month period and from 0.60 to 0.81 for a 2-week period.[106] The SF-36 has been shown to correlate reasonably well with other criterion measures, measures of ability to work, utilization of health care resources, and other clinically meaningful criteria such as "burden of care."[111-114] Factor analysis studies have supported the presence of two distinct factors labeled physical health and mental health functioning, which account for 82% of the measure's variance.[114-116]

In one multisite trial of cognitive-behavioral therapy, exercise, and their combination in patients with Gulf War illness that included chronic, diffuse musculoskeletal pain as a primary feature, each of these treatments was found to be associated with improvements in the mental health–functioning component score.[117] On a more negative note, Rogers and colleagues reported that the SF-36 lacked reliability in the assessment of outcomes following multidisciplinary pain treatment, and they questioned aspects of the measure's validity in discriminating dimensions of functional limitations.[118] Similar concerns about the sensitivity of the SF-36 to change have also been raised.[119] Continued examination of the sensitivity of the SF-36 mental health–functioning component to change as a function of pain interventions is indicated.

PAIN BELIEFS AND COPING

The *Survey of Pain Attitudes* (SOPA)[49] was developed to measure beliefs about chronic pain and included five domains: perceived ability to control pain (control), perceived level of pain-related disability (disability), belief in medical cures for pain (medical cures), belief that others should be solicitous toward them when they are in pain (solicitude), and the importance of medication as a treatment of pain (medication). The measure was later expanded to include two new dimensions: belief in the influence of emotions on pain (emotions) and belief that pain indicates underlying physical damage that necessitates limitation of physical activity (harm).[120,121] The final version of the SOPA has 57 items and uses a 0 (this is very untrue for me) to 4 (this is very true for me) response scale. The SOPA is grounded in cognitive-behavioral theory, which specifies that patients' beliefs about their pain influence important pain-related outcomes, including emotional and physical functioning. A 30-item brief form of the SOPA (the SOPA-B)[122] and a 35-item short version (SOPA-R)[123] are also available.

Internal consistency alphas for the 57-item SOPA scales are good and range from 0.71 (control) to 0.81 (disability), and test-retest stability ranged from 0.63 to 0.68.[121] The shorter version of the SOPA, the SOPA-B, has demonstrated a seven-factor structure consistent with the original measure, adequate internal consistency (ranging from 0.56 [medication] to 0.83 [solicitude]), and strong correlations with the corresponding SOPA scales (0.79 to 0.97).[122] The original factor structure of the SOPA-R has largely been confirmed by other investigators, and the measure has demonstrated good internal consistency (0.65 to 0.84) with the exception of the medication scale (0.49).[124]

The main strength of the various versions of the SOPA is their correlation with clinical treatment outcomes. The disability scale of the SOPA (higher scores indicate higher beliefs that one is disabled) has demonstrated significant correlations with physical and emotional functioning.[121,125,126] The harm scale showed a significant association with reported physical disability, and the medication scale was associated with treatment utilization.[121]

The most frequently used measure of the construct of "pain readiness to change" is the *Pain Stages of Change Questionnaire* (PSOCQ).[50] The PSOCQ measures beliefs about the degree of a patient's personal responsibility for pain control and interest in making behavioral changes to cope with pain. The PSOCQ is a 30-item self-report measure composed of four distinct scales. The precontemplation scale measures the degree to which a patient endorses little personal responsibility for pain control and no interest in making behavioral changes. Contemplation represents an increasing recognition of personal responsibility for pain control and interest in behavioral changes that support pain management. The action scale measures the extent to which patients believe that they are actively learning pain management skills. The maintenance scale quantifies patients' degree of commitment to using self-management strategies in their daily life and a high degree of personal responsibility for pain management.

A review of the empirical literature documents the reliability and criterion and concurrent validity of the measure.[127] Internal consistencies of the four scales range from 0.77 to 0.86, and stability indices range from 0.74 to 0.88. The utility of the PSOCQ, however, hinges on its ability to predict important treatment process variables. Thus far, research has been encouraging. For example, the PSOCQ subscales (i.e., precontemplation, contemplation, action, and maintenance) predict completion of self-management treatment programs[128] and improvements in pain coping during treatment.[129] Furthermore, changes in the PSOCQ during treatment consistent with increased readiness to change, or "forward stage movement," are associated with improvements in pain and physical and emotional functioning.[128-131] The readiness-to-change model, however, has not been without critics. For example, Strong and colleagues[132] challenged the external validity of the PSOCQ and demonstrated that a measure of self-efficacy had greater predictive validity than the PSOCQ.

The *Chronic Pain Coping Inventory* (CPCI)[51] is a 64-item questionnaire designed to assess a patient's use of pain-coping strategies. The questions contained in the scale fall into three broad categories and include eight subscales: wellness-focused or positive coping strategies (exercise, relaxation, task persistence, coping self-statements), illness-focused or negative coping strategies (guarding, asking for assistance, resting) and neutral coping strategies (seeking social support). Respondents report the number of days in the last week that they used each strategy.

In the initial validation, the CPCI subscales demonstrated good internal consistency (0.74 to 0.91) and test-retest reliability (0.65 to 0.90).[51] Spouse report of patient disability and coping skills use was strongly associated with CPCI scales.[51] Other studies have largely confirmed the initially specified eight-subscale factor structure.[133,134]

Studies have found various associations between the CPCI subscales and patient adjustment and outcomes, but overall, illness-focused coping strategies were found to be significantly associated with poorer patient adjustment and outcomes, and wellness-focused strategies were significantly associated with better patient adjustment and outcomes.[133,134] An exception is relaxation, with some studies showing a counterintuitive association between relaxation and higher affective distress and lower pain control[133,135] and another showing no associations between relaxation and any patient adjustment or outcome variable examined.[134] Importantly, even after controlling for pain severity and demographic factors, the CPCI subscales were significant predictors of patient-reported physical functioning, mood, disability, and activity level.[134] A 6-month longitudinal study of patients with low back pain following a work accident demonstrated that higher guarding scores were predictive of prolonged leave from work.[135]

The *Pain Catastrophizing Scale* (PCS)[52] is a 13-item instrument designed to measure the extent to which patients engage in catastrophic thinking regarding their pain. Catastrophic thinking is characterized by thoughts that the pain is horrible and unbearable and that the worst possible outcome of the patient's pain will be manifested. Patients record the frequency with which they experience thoughts and feelings described by items on a 5-point Likert-type scale ranging from 0 (not at all) to 4 (all the time).

Initial scale development used an undergraduate sample[52]; however, the PCS has demonstrated reliability and validity in both nonclinical and clinical samples. Factor analyses tend to identify three subscales: magnification, rumination, and helplessness.[52,136-138] These factors have demonstrated gender invariance[137]; however, evidence from a single study suggests that particularly for African Americans, two subscales of rumination and magnification/helplessness might be more appropriate.[139] Internal consistency coefficients range from 0.60 to 0.91 for subscales and from 0.87 to 0.95 for the full scale.[52,136-138] The PCS has demonstrated validity through its association with catastrophic thought patterns identified through clinical interview,[52] pain severity,[136,138,139] pain interference,[136] pain-related disability,[139] and mood and anxiety symptoms.[136] Furthermore, the PCS has demonstrated discriminant validity from affect[136] and psychological disturbance.[136]

The PCS has demonstrated responsiveness to cognitive, behavioral, and physical activity pain treatments and is considered an important mechanism of changes in these treatments.[140-144] The PCS has also been translated into several languages.[145-149]

The *Chronic Pain Acceptance Questionnaire* (CPAQ)[53] is a 20-item scale designed to measure chronic pain acceptance, or the extent to which a patient accepts the inevitability of chronic pain and engages in activities despite experiencing pain. The recent interest in acceptance and commitment therapy as an effective psychological intervention for chronic pain has precipitated widespread use of the CPAQ.[150] Patients respond to statements of acceptance-related pain beliefs by using a 7-item Likert scale ranging from 1 (never true) to 6 (always true).

The CPAQ has two subscales: engagement in activities and willingness to experience pain.[53] Additional factor analyses have confirmed these two subscales with the scale as published[151] or with minor revision.[152] Internal consistency coefficients of the total scale range from 0.72 to 0.91.[52,151,153] Regarding validity, the CPAQ has been associated with lower pain severity and pain-related disability, less health care and medication use, lower self-reported depressive symptoms, less pain-related anxiety and pain catastrophizing, higher self-efficacy, and lower dysfunctional pain coping and social support interaction styles.[153] The CPAQ has also demonstrated responsiveness to acceptance-based and cognitive-behavioral pain treatment,[151,154] as well as to a yoga-based pain treatment.[155]

The CPAQ is available in an adolescent version[156] and in multiple languages.[157,158] An eight-item version of the CPAQ has demonstrated reasonable reliability (internal consistency coefficients of 0.77 to 0.89) and validity, as evidenced by relationships with pain severity and interference, pain treatment seeking, and depressive and anxious symptoms.[152]

QUALITY OF CARE

The quality of pain care offered to patients can differ substantially by institution, clinician, and individual patient experience. High-quality pain care is thought to improve outcomes of pain treatment through a high-quality patient-provider relationship and faithful administration of validated treatments.[159] Any effort to improve the quality of pain care across a system must first begin with measurement. For this reason, the American Pain Society produced its first *Patient Outcome Questionnaire* (POQ)[54] to assess multiple domains of the quality of patient care. The most recent version of the POQ[160] is a 12-item scale that assesses pain severity; the impact of pain on affect, sleep, and activity; side effects; satisfaction with information provided about pain treatment; shared decision making; and use of nonpharmacologic strategies. Patients circle or check the statement that best applies to their pain management care (e.g., "Were you allowed to participate in decisions about your pain treatment as much as you wanted to?" with responses ranging from 0 [not at all] to 10 [very much so]). In the initial development study, inpatients who had been in the hospital for less than 72 hours were administered the POQ orally to evaluate the first 24 hours of their hospital stay.[160] Overall internal consistency was 0.86. Factor analysis identified five subscales that corresponded with the domains described above, with alphas of 0.63 to 0.83. As with previous versions of the POQ,[54] higher pain severity was associated with higher interference in activities, adverse effects from pain treatments, and affective distress, as well as with lower satisfaction with pain care, thereby providing preliminary evidence for validity.[160] Although initial analyses looked promising, criterion validity analyses were restricted to intercorrelations among POQ subscales. Thus, further evaluation of the validity of the POQ is warranted.

CONCLUSION

This chapter provides an overview of the role of psychological and behavioral assessment in the context of the provision of comprehensive and integrative care to patients with painful medical conditions. Discussion of more general principles that can be used to guide decisions regarding psychological assessment of pain in the clinical setting was followed by a more detailed consideration of some of the most commonly used standardized psychological assessment strategies. This review is designed to serve as a general guide to clinicians who are compelled by the value of more thorough consideration of psychosocial factors in the assessment of patients with pain that may be used to guide and evaluate pain care. Having acknowledged the potential value of such an approach, several relevant issues that may serve as cautionary notes and targets for future research and clinical investigation may be highlighted.

Of particular note are the overall limitations of this field with regard to consideration of the influence of cultural, racial, ethnic, and other aspects of diverse society on the reliability and validity of existing psychological and behavioral assessment methods. Few standardized measures have been evaluated for their use in specific populations. Given a growing awareness and empirical evidence of reliable differences in the experience of pain in patients of different racial/ethnic backgrounds, gender, and age, among other relevant variables,[161] caution is encouraged when using most of the reviewed assessment strategies, and specific consideration of culturally specific norms for the measures is important.

Already emphasized throughout this chapter is the fact that several measures that are frequently used in this field were not originally developed for use in patients with painful conditions, and as a result, the validity of these methods is still subject to concern. The continued development and evaluation of psychological and assessment methods designed specifically for patients with painful conditions and further evaluation of the psychometric properties of these measures are clearly indicated. With increasing appreciation of differences in the experience of pain and its impact on patients with different conditions, specific examination of the psychometric properties in patients with similar disorders is encouraged. Consistent with this observation, the IMMPACT group, for example, though providing recommendations for the use of specific measures to assess the effects of pain treatment, has encouraged the selection of measures that were developed and normed for a specific population (e.g., osteoarthritis patients) when such instruments are available.

Another area for continued work is the importance of developing patient-oriented outcome measures. One example is work that helped identify the types of pain-coping strategies that are commonly used by older patients living in the community.[162] Using a more qualitative approach, these investigators have collected information that may be useful in developing an age-appropriate quantitative measure of pain coping that may be more valid than existing coping measures for this population. Several other investigator groups are currently working on the development and validation of more comprehensive measures for assessing patient-oriented outcomes, and the future availability of these methods promises to provide alternatives to existing methods that may have increased sensitivity to important and meaningful changes in pain and its impact, at least from a patient's perspectives.

One particularly challenging area of ongoing research is the development of reliable and valid strategies for the assessment of pain in patients who are significantly cognitively impaired or otherwise unable to communicate. In the absence of existing reliable methods, clinical scholars have encouraged the use of an array of methods, including reliance on systematic observation and reports from significant others. With a growing population of older patients with significant dementia and younger patients with significant brain injuries, efforts designed to develop reliable and valid strategies for pain assessment in patients with cognitive impairment will continue to be a high priority for clinical investigation.

Clinicians must consider pragmatic issues related to the use of existing methods and measures for the psychological and behavioral assessment of patients with pain in the clinical setting. Response burden is an important factor to consider when selecting measures for use in the clinical setting. Clinicians are encouraged to consider specific objectives of the assessment and the importance of reaching a balance between the desire for more thorough assessment and patient burden. Clinicians should also consider measurement precision, brevity, and cost of the assessment process in making decisions about the use of psychological assessment strategies. As already emphasized, the clinical interview and examination remain the core method for clinical assessment and should not be displaced by the use of questionnaires, diaries, and other methods. Finally, managed care reimbursement methodologies are, of course, critical to consider in most clinical settings.

In closing, the potential value of incorporating assessment methods that permit a more comprehensive evaluation of the psychological and behavioral aspects of the experience of pain has been emphasized. As in most similar contexts, the "devil is in the details," and clinicians and investigators alike are encouraged to consider a range of important issues when designing an assessment approach consistent with their goals and objectives.

KEY POINTS

- Chronic pain is challenging to assess because pain complaints are inherently subjective and pain has a wide-ranging influence on patient functioning.
- Psychological and behavioral assessment of pain serves several clinical goals: (1) providing information about a patient's pain experiences, treatment history, current and past emotional and physical functioning, and beliefs about pain; (2) identifying the patient's strengths and weaknesses; (3) identifying factors that contribute to the development and maintenance of problems in physical, social, and emotional functioning; (4) identifying comorbid psychiatric or behavioral conditions that may interfere with pain treatment; (5) determining whether the patient is psychologically appropriate and likely to benefit from surgery or invasive procedure; and (6) providing a benchmark of the patient's pain and functioning against which the efficacy of treatments can be measured.
- Because of the wide range of clinical goals for psychological and behavioral assessment of pain, when making a request for psychological and behavioral assessment it is necessary to explicitly state the reasons for the request or pose a question to be answered about the patient or the patient's treatment.
- A useful guide for assessment of the multidimensional nature of pain is the Initiative on Methods, Measurement, and Pain Assessment in Clinical Trials (IMMPACT) group consensus statement on the core outcome domains that should be assessed when evaluating the efficacy of a pain treatment and recommended instruments for measuring these domains. The group has encouraged the selection of measures that were developed and normed for a specific population (e.g., low back pain patients) when such instruments are available.

KEY POINTS—cont'd

- The consistency, validity, and reliability of the numerous measurement tools have been noted in the following domains: pain intensity, personality, psychosocial impact, physical and social role functioning, emotional functioning, pain beliefs and coping, and quality of care (see Table 16.1). Several of these tools were not originally developed for use in patients with painful conditions, and their validity has not been tested in specific pain populations.
- Areas for continued research include developing patient-oriented outcome measures, evaluating standard measures in specific populations, and evaluating measures across diverse cultural populations, particularly those with limited communication capability.

SUGGESTED READINGS

American Pain Society Committee on Quality Assurance Standards. American Pain Society quality assurance standards for the relief of acute pain and cancer pain. In: Bond MR, Charlton JE, Woolf CJ, eds. *Proceedings of the VIth World Congress on Pain.* Seattle: IASP Press; 1991.

Beck AT, Ward CH, Mendelsohn M, et al. An inventory for measuring depression. *Arch Gen Psychiatry.* 1961;4:561-571.

Cleeland CS, Ryan KM. Pain assessment: global use of the Brief Pain Inventory. *Ann Acad Med.* 1994;23:129-138.

Dworkin RH, Turk DC, Farrar JT, et al. Core outcome measures for chronic pain clinical trials: IMMPACT recommendations. *Pain.* 2005;113:9-19.

Farrar JT, Portenoy RK, Berlin JA, et al. Defining the clinically important difference in pain outcome measures. *Pain.* 2000;88:287-294.

Jensen MP, Karoly P, Huger R. The development and preliminary validation of an instrument to assess patients' attitudes toward pain. *J Psychosom Res.* 1987;31:393-400.

Jensen MP, Turner JA, Romano JM, et al. Comparative reliability and validity of chronic pain intensity measures. *Pain.* 1999;83:157-162.

Kerns RD, Turk DC, Rudy TE. The West Haven–Yale Multidimensional Pain Inventory (WHYMPI). *Pain.* 1985;23:345-356.

Pollard CA. Preliminary validity study of the Pain Disability Index. *Percept Mot Skills.* 1984;59:974.

Revicki DA, Chen WH, Harnam N, et al. Development and psychometric analysis of the PROMIS pain behavior item bank. *Pain.* 2009;146:158-169.

Spielberger CD, Gorsuch RL, Lushene R. *Manual for the State-Trait Anxiety Inventory.* Palo Alto, Calif: Consulting Psychologists Press; 1970.

Sullivan MJL, Bishop SC, Pivik J. The Pain Catastrophizing Scale: development and validation. *Psychol Assess.* 1995;7:524-532.

Tellegen A, Ben-Porath YS. *MMPI-2-RF (Minnesota Multiphasic Personality Inventory-2 Restructured Form): Technical Manual.* Minneapolis: University of Minnesota Press; 2008.

Turk DC, Dworkin RH, Allen RR, et al. Core outcome domains for chronic pain clinical trials: IMMPACT recommendations. *Pain.* 2003;106:337-345.

Ware JE, Sherbourne CD. The MOS 36-item Short-Form Health Survey (SF-36), I: conceptual framework and item selection. *Med Care.* 1992;30:473-483.

The references for this chapter can be found at www.expertconsult.com.

17 Disability Assessment

Robert D. Rondinelli | Mohammed Ranavaya

INTRODUCTION

Physicians dealing with the evaluation and treatment of patients with chronic painful and disabling conditions can expect to be called on from time to time to formally assess the disability of their patients. Recent estimates indicate that more than 40 to 50 million persons are currently living with potentially disabling conditions,[1] and these numbers are likely to increase in the next few decades with our aging generation of baby boomers. Continued advancements in medical and surgical technologies enable increased survival after catastrophic injuries and illnesses and may help mitigate the disabling consequences of the same, as well as allow an increased prevalence of disability within our society. As the face of our disabled population changes, treating physicians can adapt their practice to better address the needs of patients associated with these changes by gaining greater familiarity with and understanding of the concepts and terminology of disablement and the practices of impairment rating and disability evaluation.

This chapter is intended to provide pain specialists with a practical vocabulary of the terminology and definitions unique to the emerging field of disability medicine, to provide a brief historical and conceptual overview of models of disablement and U.S. disability systems, to familiarize pain specialists with the processes and tools available for impairment rating and disability determination, and to examine the medical-legal pitfalls and ramifications of these clinical activities.

WORKING TERMINOLOGY AND DEFINITIONS

The following terms and definitions are frequently applied to the evaluation and reporting of disablement:

Aggravation: A circumstance or event that permanently worsens a preexisting or underlying and susceptible condition[2]

Exacerbation: A circumstance or event that temporarily worsens a preexisting or underlying and susceptible condition[2]

Apportionment: A determination of the percentage of impairment directly attributable to preexisting or resulting conditions and directly contributing to the total impairment rating derived[2]

Causality: An association between a given cause (an event capable of producing an effect) and effect (a condition that can result from a specific cause) within a reasonable degree of medical probability. Causality requires determining that

- An event took place.
- The claimant experiencing the event has the condition (i.e., pathology, impairment).
- The event could cause the condition (biologic plausibility, etc.).
- Within medical probability the event did cause the condition.[3]

Impairment: A significant deviation, loss, or loss of use of any body structure or function in an individual with a health condition, disorder, or disease[2]

Maximum medical improvement (MMI): The point at which a condition (impairment) has stabilized and is unlikely to change (improve or worsen) substantially in the next year with or without treatment.[2] MMI is thought to occur when the following criteria have been satisfied:

- A sufficient healing period has transpired (usually based on an analysis that includes consideration of the natural course of disease for the specific pathology, which in some cases may be days, months, or rarely even years.
- The medical condition (impairment) has fully resolved or has reached a static and stable status (plateau), after which no further reasonable progress occurs or is expected to occur in the next 12 months toward resolution of the pathology.

MMI does not preclude any deterioration of a condition that is expected to occur with the passage of time (i.e., beyond 12 months), nor does it preclude allowances for ongoing follow-up or maintenance medical care should such care be indicated based on current evidence-based practice generally accepted by the scientific community.[4]

MODELS AND CLASSIFICATION OF DISABLEMENT

MODELS OF DISABILITY

The "medical model" of disability was the paradigm for understanding disablement throughout much of the 19th and 20th centuries, during which causation of disability was directly viewed in terms of the underlying pathology (impairment) arising through illness or disease. Management of disability was closely linked to diagnosis and treatment of the underlying pathology, long considered the purview of the physician examiner, who then became empowered to rate, as well as to diagnose and treat, the disabling condition (impairment).[5,6] Anatomic and physiologic objectivity is the conceptual lynchpin of the medical model of disability. This model worked well for conditions in which the diagnosis was unambiguous and the pathology was well understood and in which treatment strategies and end points were often well established and also clearly understood.[7,8] Today, the medical model still serves as the basis for Social Security disability determinations (see later).

The "social model" of disability grew out of the disability advocacy movement of the 1970s and 1980s and was founded on the notion that society imposes disability on individuals with impairments by failing to address their special needs in terms of priority awareness, environmental access, and infrastructural accommodation for major life activities. The resulting disability was viewed in terms of restrictions imposed on the impaired individual ranging from individual and institutional prejudicial thinking and discrimination, architectural and other physical barriers to access and transportation, educational segregation, and lack of accommodation in the workplace.[6] An understanding of the social model has helped foster strategies to better neutralize social barriers to individuals with impairments, thereby enabling them and minimizing their disability.

The "biopsychosocial model" of disability[9] is now widely accepted as the preferred conceptual model of disablement. It simultaneously recognizes the contributions of medical, social, personal, and psychological determinants of disability. The *biologic* component refers to the physical and mental aspects of an individual's health condition, the *psychological* component recognizes personal and psychological factors that are affecting that individual's functioning, and the *social* component recognizes contextual and environmental factors that may also have an impact on functioning in each particular case.[7,10]

CLASSIFICATIONS OF DISABLEMENT

The most commonly used, contemporary, internationally accepted definitions, terminology, and classification of disablement have been created by the World Health Organization, the origins of which can be traced to the work of Bertillon's *Classification of Causes of Death* (1893), which later was expanded into the *International Statistical Classification of Diseases, Injuries and Causes of Death* (*ICD*).[11] In 1948 the World Health Organization took over this effort, which ultimately led to creation of the *International Classification of Impairments, Disabilities and Handicaps* (*ICIDH*) in 1980.[12] This system applied a model of disablement with four ordinal domains linked in a linear relationship as follows (Fig. 17.1):

Pathology—"a disease or trauma acting at a tissue anatomical or physiological level to potentially alter the structure and/or function of an organ."

Impairment—"any loss or abnormality of psychological, physiological or anatomical structure or function and resulting from a pathology." Impairment occurs at an organ system level.

Disability—"any restriction or lack (resulting from impairment) of ability to perform an activity in the manner or within the range considered normal for a human being." Disability is commonly conceptualized in terms of limitations in activities within one's personal sphere, including mobility (transfers and ambulation) and self-care (activities of daily living [ADLs]).

Handicap—"a disadvantage for an individual that limits or prevents fulfillment of a role that is normal (depending on age, sex, social and cultural factors) for that individual."[12]

There were several shortcomings of the ICIDH system. It was rooted in the medical model of disease, whose limitations are described above. The linearity of the system implies a unidirectional and causal relationship among its elements, which may not always be the case. It inadequately accounted for various modifiers (e.g., personal, environmental) that could influence the magnitude of disability[13]; for example, other work showed that environmental factors play a key role in determining outcomes of disability, which could be studied independently.[14] Subsequent work by the Institute of Medicine (IOM)[15] and the National Center for Medical Rehabilitation Research (NCMRR)[16] expanded on the view that the resulting disability was the product of the individual with an impairment interacting with the environment in each specific case. Additional attention was given to the role of personal modifiers (e.g., lifestyle choices, belief systems, entitlement, and coping abilities) affecting the outcomes of disability for individual cases.[17]

The *International Classification of Functioning, Disabilities and Health: ICF*[18] is depicted in Figure 17.2.

The ICF has replaced the ICIDH and portrays an interactive (as opposed to linear) association between an individual with a health condition, the functional consequences of the impairment, and contextual factors of a personal and environmental nature. The ICF classification system embraces the biopsychosocial model of disease described earlier by taking into account environmental and personal modifiers of functional outcomes in any given case.

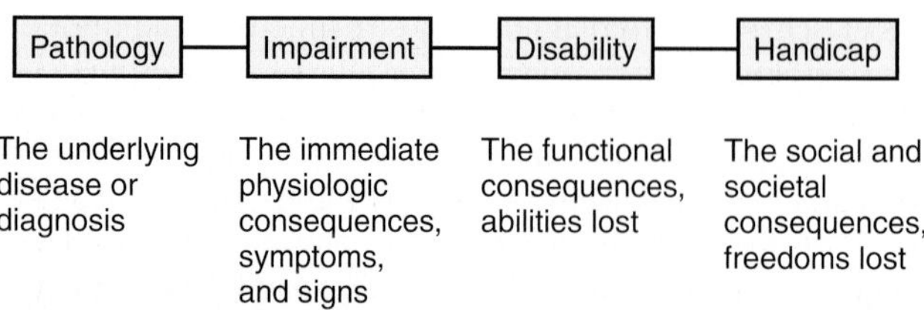

Figure 17.1 World Health Organization's international classification of illness. (Reproduced with permission from World Health Organization. *International Classification of Impairments, Disabilities and Handicaps: A Manual of Classification Relating to the Consequences of Disease*. Geneva: World Health Organization; 1980.)

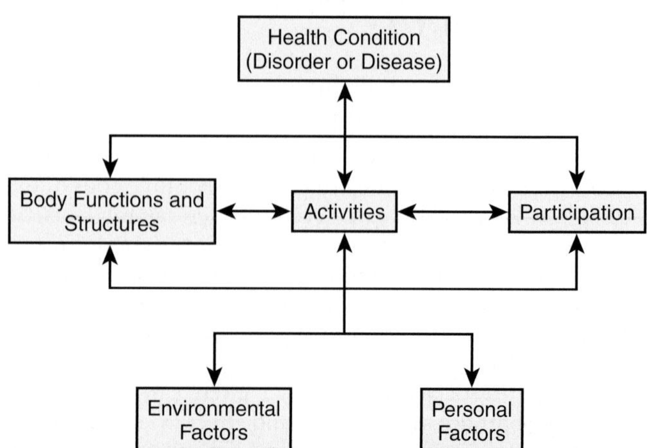

Figure 17.2 Components and interactions of the World Health Organization's international classification of functioning. (Reproduced with permission from World Health Organization. *International Classification of Functioning, Disabilities and Health: ICF*. Geneva: World Health Organization; 2001.)

The components of disablement according to the ICF classification system include the following:

Body functions and body structures: physiologic functions and body parts, respectively
Activity: execution of a task or action by an individual (typically within that person's personal sphere)
Participation: involvement in a life situation (typically within a social sphere)
Impairments: problems in body function or structure such as a significant deviation or loss
Activity limitations: difficulties that an individual may have in executing activities
Participation restrictions: problems that an individual may experience in involvement in life situations

Within this conceptual framework the disabling consequences of impairment may be amplified or mitigated by factors unique to the individual with a health condition, by interaction with the environment, and by personal choice. To illustrate the importance of environmental factors, consider Vignette 1:

Vignette 1

A farmer in rural Iowa suffers a unilateral medium-length transradial amputation of the forearm in a combine accident. He would probably have immediate access to level 1 trauma services on an emergency basis and receive timely and appropriate surgical and medical care to repair and heal the residual limb. He would benefit from rehabilitation and most likely from fitting with a body-powered upper limb prosthesis with an appropriate industrial-grade terminal hook device. With proper training and motivation, he could recapture the majority of his "baseline" functional activities—independent ADLs, household activity, community activity, and work (with some limitations).[19] If need be, he might also be fitted with a myoelectric or cosmetic hand, or both, thereby maximizing his full functional potential. Alternatively, a similar clinical scenario in a "third world" country could have a significantly less favorable functional outcome. Consider a transradial amputation in a local Haitian resident following the devastating earthquake in 2009, where the availability of timely medical and surgical care was compromised by local destruction of the existing medical infrastructure and access to rehabilitative care and adaptive technology was scarce or nonexistent. In such a scenario the less fortunate individual might be left with one functioning upper limb and be destined to manage ADLs with one-handed techniques indefinitely.

To illustrate the importance of personal choice, consider Vignette 2:

Vignette 2

A long-term smoker with advanced chronic obstructive disease has measurable pulmonary impairment as noted by a significant reduction in forced expiratory volume in 1 second (FEV_1) on pulmonary function testing. The probability of the symptoms worsening and a further decline in FEV_1 over time is directly linked to the amount and duration of continued smoking, and consequently, the impairment can be substantially mitigated or worsened simply by making a personal choice to adopt or reject permanent smoking cessation.

Despite its superiority as a classification system, shortcomings of the ICF can be noted. The distinctions between activities and participations are often blurred, and inadequate attention has thus far been given to measures of quality of life (QOL) (e.g., life satisfaction, burden of care) in the model itself.[8]

MEASURING DISABILITY FOR COMPENSATION PURPOSES

Social justice requires that individual group members contribute productively to the common good of the whole. Provisions must be made, however, to exempt this requirement and to support members who are incapable of such productivity by virtue of age, illness, or disability. A related expectation is that individuals who incur loss or disablement as a result of illness or injury are thereby entitled to some compensation for their loss.

Within our social system there exist a number of different disability systems (see later) designed to compensate individuals for such loss. They share a common conceptual and operational platform in which the initial estimate of physical or psychological loss (or both) can be translated into an estimate of functional and economic loss expressed in monetary terms.

By convention, the severity of physical and psychological loss is operationally defined and measured in terms of a *medical impairment rating* at an organ system level that is typically expressed as a percentage of regional loss of the affected body part or parts and that can be further extrapolated to the body as a whole. The severity of functional and hence economic loss associated with this impairment percentage is further estimated in terms of a *disability rating* expressed as a percentage of the economic worth of the "whole person." The disability rating is operationally derived from the impairment percentage and is at once intended to reflect direct economic losses, noneconomic losses, and negative impact on QOL in terms of a monetary sum. The whole person value and the magnitude of awards vary according to the disability system in question, and disability payments may be awarded as a lump sum or on an annuity basis.

The IOM[20] recently developed a generalized model to demonstrate the essential features common to all disability systems. Individuals seeking compensation and meeting the criteria for entitlement must demonstrate losses according to five domains of interest (see Fig. 17.3).

The first of these, *medical impairment*, traditionally carries the most weight for several reasons. It is largely anatomically and physiologically based and hence can readily be measured in objective terms. Objectivity enables codification of the disability and fosters standardization, reliability, and reproducibility of measurement according to some uniform scale. Impairment can be measured and expressed in terms of anatomic or functional losses.

The second domain of interest, *functional limitations*, can be expressed and measured in terms of basic ADLs or instrumental (advanced) activities of daily living (IADLs), or both. ADLs include such basic activities of self-care as feeding, toileting, grooming, bathing, hygiene, and dressing—activities that generally occupy our personal sphere. IADLs require greater cognitive and physical capacity and include

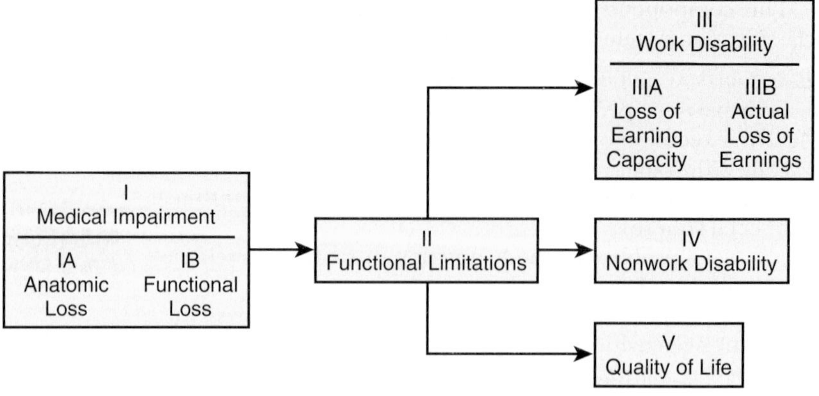

Figure 17.3 Disabling consequences of an injury or disease. (Reproduced with permission from McGeary M, Ford M, McCutchen SR, et al, eds. *IOM Committee on Medical Evaluation of Veterans for Disability Compensation. A 21st Century System for Evaluating Veterans for Disability Benefits. The Rating Schedule.* Washington, DC: National Academies Press; 2007:117.)

such activities as meal preparation, driving, and managing finances, medications, and one's daily routine.

The third domain, *work disability*, can be understood in terms of loss of earning capacity (an actuarial determination of negative impact on employability and earnings brought about by work restrictions because of the impairment and other considerations such as age, baseline employment and earnings history, availability of accommodation and alternative job opportunities, and other local factors). It can also be understood in terms of actual loss of earnings directly attributable to the impairment.

A fourth domain, *nonwork disability*, includes losses in terms of inability to visit friends and relatives and to engage in communal activities, hobbies, or other recreational pursuits because of barriers to access or performance attributable to the impairment.

A fifth domain, *quality of life*, includes losses attributable to diminished life satisfaction and self-esteem and increased burden of care in terms of treatment compliance and caregiver support.

The metrics whereby each of these constructs is defined and measured vary and remain incompletely understood. This is partly due to the persisting confusion in terminology, definitions, and criteria for impairment and disability across the various systems and the continuing emphasis on objective, medically determined impairment as the prime determinant of disablement.[8]

Unfortunately, there is also lack of agreement on the metrics whereby the impairment ratings themselves are determined between and even within the various disability systems of interest. For example, U.S. workers' compensation (WC) jurisdictions show considerable variability in terms of their acceptance or rejection of standard and uniform impairment rating guides, and those that mandate or recommend use of the same vary in the choice of reference; even in the case of the American Medical Association *Guides to the Evaluation of Permanent Impairment* (AMA Guides), the actual edition chosen for reference varies from state to state.[21] The same is true for international use of the AMA Guides, where in many countries (e.g., Australia, the Netherlands, South Africa), the various editions are used for individuals in motor vehicle accidents and with other personal injury claims to determine the severity of injury (a threshold) before access to benefits for general damage (nonpecuniary, noneconomic losses) is granted.[22]

The importance of the impairment rating to cash awards also varies within and between the various disability systems, as a closer examination of the U.S. WC system illustrates. Operationally, the WC system awards cash benefits according to three basic approaches: the first of these, the *impairment approach*, awards benefits in direct relation to the percentage-of-impairment rating; the second, the *loss of earning capacity approach*, requires that the injured worker have an impairment rating but then bases the actual amount of cash benefits on the estimate of associated loss of earning capacity; the third approach, the *actual wage loss approach*, requires the worker to have both an impairment and loss of earning capacity and then bases the amount of cash benefits on demonstration of the actual loss of workers' earnings.[23,24]

The mechanism by which WC cash benefits are awarded is further complicated by distinguishing between various types of injuries as scheduled versus unscheduled. *Scheduled* injuries are those typically affecting the upper or lower extremities and listed as percentage of the extremity; *unscheduled* injuries affect the spine, nervous system, or other organ systems and are awarded as percentage of the "whole person."[24]

Although the impairment rating is the common factor in determination of disability for cash benefits, it is not the sole factor. In practice, however, many jurisdictions implement procedural shortcuts whereby the impairment rating percentage becomes a direct surrogate for the disability rating according to a predetermined formula that multiplies the impairment percentage times a number of weeks' wages (up to a cap) times a percentage (generally ⅔ to ¾) of the average weekly wage (up to a cap) to determine a lump sum payout. The adequacy of applying the impairment rating as an operational surrogate measure of disability continues to be a subject of debate.[20]

Implications for pain sufferers can be noted as follows: the metrics for the medical impairment rating clearly favor and emphasize objective over subjective criteria. Accordingly, painful entities such as headache, fibromyalgia, and low back pain often occur in the absence of objective verifiable pathology or may occur in a setting in which objective clinical findings are most consistent with normal anatomic variation and the aging process and may be of little or no clinical significance to the individual's actual complaints. Impairment ratings in such cases are ineffective, at best, since minimal or no rating percentage is currently allowed for any apparent (and often profound) negative impact that these conditions may be having on ADLs. The disablement and ensuing loss in such cases potentially become more evident if viewed in terms of QOL. Well-respected psychometric instruments are now available to measure QOL; notable examples include the Quality of Well Being (QWB) scale, the WHOQOL-100, and the Quality of Life Index (QLI).[25] Unfortunately, such metrics are not familiar tools to the typical rating physician and are not routinely taken into account by the rating systems per se; consequently, losses in terms of QOL remain largely unaccounted for by the rating practice summarized above.[8]

U.S. DISABILITY SYSTEMS COMPARED (TABLE 17.1)

WORKERS' COMPENSATION

WC law is determined by jurisdictional statutes, which vary from state to state and may differ in terms of the definition of an employee-employer relationship and the exemptions that may apply. WC is a *no-fault* system whereby the injured employee forgoes the right to sue the employer for damages in most cases in exchange for coverage when eligibility requirements are met. A causality determination must be made that the injury or illness *arose out of and in the course of employment* and occurred while the employee was at work and actively participating in work activity (job-related social and recreational activities generally do not qualify). Coverage is established in accordance with jurisdictional statutes, and to qualify for wage loss benefits, the injured employee's condition must persist beyond a statutory waiting period that typically extends from 0 to 7 days; the injury or illness must also be reported to the employer within 30 days of onset and a claim filed within 1 year for disability and 2 years for death.[26,27]

WC benefits include survivor benefits (in the case of death), medical and rehabilitation expenses, and wage loss benefits (typically ⅔ the weekly wages up to a cap). An employee risks forfeiture of benefits if the claim is due to intoxication or substance abuse at the time of injury, for refusal to comply with safety rules and equipment, for incarceration, or for refusal to return to work after being medically cleared to do so.[27]

Disability under WC can be determined to be temporary or permanent, partial or total. Many states have enacted a *second injury fund* whereby employment of individuals with preexisting work-related disabilities is encouraged. Such funds can reduce employer risk (hence cost to ensure) for excessive compensation and medical expenses in such cases.[27]

Physician rating schedules vary among WC jurisdictions, the majority of which require or recommend a version of the AMA Guides.[8,21]

SOCIAL SECURITY

The Social Security Administration (SSA) is the largest U.S. disability system, with an estimated ⅓ to ½ of all persons qualified as disabled being assisted. Coverage is typically extended to persons whose medical disablement renders them unable to "engage in any substantial activity by reason of any medically determinable physical or mental impairment that can be expected to result in death or that has lasted or can be expected to last for a continuous period of not less than 12 months."[27,28]

The SSA offers two separate disability programs: the first, Social Security Disability Insurance (SSDI), extends coverage to disabled workers who have worked in a qualified job for 5 of the 10 preceding years and who are younger than 65 years. SSDI is funded through the Federal Insurance Contribution Act (FICA) payroll tax, with deductions covering Old Age and Social Disability Insurance (OASDI). Benefits are afforded to those considered totally incapacitated and their surviving spouses and children and are provided in the form of a monthly stipend.[27]

The second program, Supplemental Security Income (SSI), provides income for medically indigent persons who suffer from blindness, disability, or old age (>65 years of age). Eligibility is determined according to a means test and also extends to disabled children who demonstrate an inability to function independently and in an age-appropriate fashion. SSI operates as a federal-state partnership that is funded through general revenue (federal and state income tax) and does not require a work history to be eligible.[27,28]

A separate physician rating scale is provided by the SSA.[29]

DEPARTMENT OF VETERANS AFFAIRS

The Veterans Benefits Administration (VBA) within the Department of Veterans Affairs oversees the Compensation and Pensioning (C&P) Service, and all veterans who have received an honorable or general discharge from active military service are eligible for benefits. Entitlement may be *service connected* for injuries or disease incurred or aggravated during the time of active duty or *non–service connected* for conditions determined to be unrelated to active duty. Entitlement is determined by the C&P Service's Adjudication Division.

Disability compensation for eligible veterans is paid out in monthly pensions not subject to state or federal income tax, is adjusted by Congress to reflect changes in cost of living, and varies according to the number of dependents. In the event of death, monthly benefits are payable to the surviving spouse or children. Additional benefits include hospitalization and medical care, orthotic and prosthetic devices, durable medical equipment, and adaptive modifications to home and vehicle.[30]

The *Veterans Administration Schedule for Rating Disabilities* (VASRD)[31] is the required physician rating schedule within the VBA.

FEDERAL EMPLOYEES COMPENSATION ACT

The Federal Employees Compensation Act (FECA) is the federal workers' compensation program, a *no-fault* system in which a federal employee cannot sue the federal government or recover damages under any other statute governing work-related injuries. It is adjudicated by the Office of Workers' Compensation (OWCP) of the U.S. Department of Labor (USDOL) and provides coverage to more than 3 million civilian employees of the U.S. Government, U.S. Postal Service, and Peace Corps. It also covers nonfederal employees such as state and local law enforcement personnel and employees of the Civil Air Patrol. It provides benefits, including ⅔ to ¾ wage loss compensation as a monthly stipend, as well as uncapped medical benefits.[27]

Table 17.1 Graphic Comparison of Major U.S. Disability Systems

	Eligible Individuals	Adjudicating Body	Rating Schedule	Employability Status	Benefits	Maximum Monthly Benefit
Workers' compensation	Nonfederal workers injured out of and in the course of employment	Individual state, jurisdictional statutes	AMA Guides in many states; special schedules in Fla, Minn, Calif Utah has its own supplemental rating guide	Unable to work in one's own occupation or in modified duty if available	Survivor benefits, medical and rehabilitation expenses, wage loss benefits. Tort immunity for the employer	Determined by statute
Social Security	Workers <65 yr or survivors who are or have contributed to the SS Trust Fund (SSDI); needy disabled children, aged, disabled and blind adults (SSI)	Social Security Administration	*Disability Evaluation Under Social Security* (listing of impairments)	Unable to engage in substantial gainful employment that pays $500/mo for >12 mo	Monthly stipend	
Disability insurance	Those covered by a group or individual long-term disability plan after a period of short-term disability defined by the policy	Long-term disability carrier	None	Inability to engage in own occupation up to 2 yrs or in any occupation thereafter, depending on the individual plan	Wage compensation	Generally 60-70% of employment income
Federal Employees' Compensation Act (FECA)	Federal employees, including U.S. Postal Service workers	Office of Workers' Compensation Programs (OWCP) in the U.S. Department of Labor (USDOL)	AMA Guides, 6th ed	Loss of earnings (no schedule loss) because of disability resulting from personal injury sustained while in the performance of duty	66.6-75% of wages, reasonable medical care. Lump sums not available	75% of wages if the worker is married or has dependents
Longshore and Harbor Workers' Compensation Program	Maritime employees such as seamen, longshoremen, harbor workers, ship workers (not seamen)	Office of Workers' Compensation Programs in the U.S. Department of Labor	AMA Guides, 6th ed	Wage loss and schedule loss benefits for injuries arising out of and in the course of employment	Full medical care, death benefits, lump sum awards, 66.6% of weekly wages	200% of the current national average weekly wage
Railroad Workers' and Seamen	Railroad workers and seamen	Railroad Retirement Board	None	Sickness and unemployment benefits from the Railroad Retirement Board	Railroad workers and seamen must pursue action for damages under the Federal Employers' Liability Act	
Black Lung Benefits Program	Coal miners	Office of Workers' Compensation Programs in the U.S. Department of Labor	CXR, PFTs, ABGs, and physical examination	Total disability because of pneumoconiosis		
Veterans Disability Programs	Honorable or general discharge from the armed forces or a survivor of a veteran	Adjudication Division of the Compensation and Pension Service of the Veterans Benefits Administration	*VA Schedule for Rating Disabilities* (VASRD)	Wage loss and schedule loss for the average person unable to follow a substantially gainful occupation	Disability pension, death benefits, hospitalization, medical care, orthotics, prosthetics, durable medical goods, adaptive modifications	$1989 as of 1999

ABG, arterial blood gas anlaysis; CXR, chest x-ray; PFT, pulmonary function test.
Reproduced with modifications from Katz RT, Rondinelli RD. Major U.S. disability and compensation systems graphically compared. *Phys Med Rehabil Clin N Am*. 2001;12:500.

The physician reference guide for FECA is the sixth edition of the AMA Guides.

VARIOUS OTHER DISABILITY PROGRAMS

The *Longshore and Harbor Workers Compensation Act* (LHWCA) covers shoreside maritime employees for occupational disabilities arising during longshore work, ship building, and other shoreside maritime activity. It is a *no-fault* federally administered system under the USDOL. Benefits include full medical care, wage loss compensation of up to ⅔ the weekly wages, death benefits, and lump sum awards. The physician reference guide for the LHWCA is the sixth edition of the AMA Guides.

The *Federal Black Lung Program* provides coverage of coal miners engaged in surface or underground activity for total disability secondary to pneumoconiosis (black lung) arising from employment in and around coal mines. It is administered through the USDOL. The diagnosis of pneumoconiosis must be made with special chest radiographs according to the International Labor Organization (ILO) classification system. Chest radiographs require official interpretation by B-readers, who are physician specialists certified by the National Institute of Occupational Health and Safety according to the ILO system. Claimants must demonstrate total disability from pulmonary causes as documented by pulmonary function test results according to the USDOL.[27]

The *Federal Employers Liability Act* (FELA) provides disability benefits for railroad workers under a potentially adversarial system whereby the claimant must prove negligence on the part of the railroad; it has disadvantages similar to those existing under tort law before no-fault systems. Claimants may recover economic damages, as well as receive compensation for "pain and suffering." Additional benefits may include retirement, sickness, and disability annuity payments.[27]

The *Jones Act* (*Merchant Marine Act*) covers sailors for permanent injury suffered while in service of a ship in navigable waters. The system is potentially adversarial in that the claimant must file suit against the ship's owner; since seamen are regarded as wards of the state, they enjoy liberal treatment by the court system in general and most claims are likely to be settled out of court.[27]

Private disability systems offer long-term disability insurance that is generally available through the workplace. Specific contractual language governs the criteria for eligibility, entitlement, and benefits. The injured party must complete a 90-day waiting period, after which the long-term disability policy takes effect. Such policies may be group policies (more affordable), with coverage of individuals who cannot perform their usual and customary job during a finite period (typically 2 years). Subsequently, disability benefits may continue only if the individual can be determined to be unable to perform *any occupation* according to the definitions and provisions of the policy. Individual policies, though requiring higher premiums, may provide coverage to individuals who cannot continue to perform their own occupation for a more extended period. Private disability generally pays up to 65% of the individual's wages (to a cap) and may have a built-in cost-of-living allowance to adjust for inflation.[27]

AMERICAN MEDICAL ASSOCIATION GUIDES

The process whereby disability determinations are made requires that an initial impairment rating be determined according to standard and specific medical criteria. Since the physician is empowered and charged to render such ratings, the AMA has produced a rating manual to assist physicians in this regard. The AMA Guides is a standardized, objective reference for this purpose that was originally published in 1971 as a compilation of a series of impairment rating articles for different organ systems that were published in the *Journal of the American Medical Association* from 1958 to 1970. It has periodically been updated and revised to the most current of the AMA Guides published in 2008.

The AMA Guides is recognized nationally and globally as the preferred reference for medical impairment ratings. Various editions are required or recommended by statute in the majority of U.S. WC jurisdictions. The sixth edition of the AMA Guides has recently been adopted by 15 of these jurisdictions and is the reference mandated by the USDOL for the various disability systems outlined earlier; it has also been adopted and used internationally in WC and personal injury claims, including 9 of 10 Canadian provinces and all 3 Canadian territories, the Netherlands, Australia, New Zealand, Hong Kong, and Korea.

The sixth edition of the AMA Guides builds on the precedent of the fifth edition of the AMA Guides[32] in placing increasing emphasis on a diagnosis-based approach, with particular emphasis on musculoskeletal impairment ratings of the spine and extremities. Diagnosis-Based Impairment (DBI) grids are provided for each anatomic region (cervical spine, thoracic spine, lumbar spine, and pelvis for the spine; digits and hand, wrist, elbow, and shoulder for the upper extremity; and foot and ankle, knee, and hip for the lower extremity). Each grid has five potential impairment classes (class 0 to 4), consistent with the ICF classification system, and each covers a broad and precise array of diagnoses ranging from soft tissue conditions (nonspecific, chronic, or recurrent), to muscle-tendon and motion segment injuries (sprains, strains, tendinopathy), to ligament, bone, and joint injuries (fractures, dislocations, arthrodesis, etc.). Impairment rating is a two-step process whereby initial assignment to an impairment class requires the rating examiner to identify the most appropriate diagnosis, and each DBI class has an available range of impairment values with an initial "default" midrange value. The rating is then adjusted within range as a second step by using three separate criteria (functional history, examination findings, and clinical test results) to validate the diagnosis and severity of the condition and by using a simple triangulation method to enable a final numerical adjustment upward for less favorable outcomes or downward for more optimal outcomes according to the specific result in each case.[2]

MEDICOLEGAL CONSTRUCTS AND CONSTRAINTS

A pain practitioner in general has unique legal liabilities that include administrative, civil, and criminal liability exposure at both the state and federal level, discussion of which is beyond the scope of this chapter. Alternatively, a brief overview of the interaction between impairment and the disability assessor and the law is indicated. A pain practitioner participating in such evaluation is encouraged to become familiar with the emerging field of disability medicine, which is described as a subspecialty of clinical medical practice that encompasses the identification, prediction, prevention, assessment, evaluation, and management of impairment and disability in both human individuals and populations.[33]

THE INDEPENDENT MEDICAL EXAMINATION

An independent medical examination (IME) is (usually) a one-time evaluation performed by a physician examiner who is not treating the patient or claimant to answer specific questions posed by the referring party, including determination of MMI, impairment rating, and return-to-work restrictions, if applicable.[2]

IMEs are examinations performed by a physician who is not involved in the person's care for the purpose of clarifying medical and job issues. IMEs are performed to provide information to case management and for evidence in hearings and other legal proceedings. IMEs are a component of most WC statutes, although the specifics vary by state and country. They are performed at several stages during the cycle of injury or illness, treatment, rehabilitation, and return to work. The key issues associated with an IME differ from clinical consultations in role and focus. In the WC arena, IMEs may be performed any time there is a dispute, concern, or question regarding the medical treatment or condition of the injured worker. These issues include such topics as the following:

1. Diagnosis, proximate causation, and work-relatedness of an illness or injury
2. Current and proposed medical treatment or diagnostic efforts
3. Appropriate work and general activity level during treatment
4. Stability of the medical condition and status regarding MMI
5. Identification of other nonmedical factors that can have a significant impact on the outcome of the medical condition or treatment
6. Impairment rating and related disability issues under certain circumstances
7. Ability to return to work (fitness for duty) and reasonable accommodation

IMEs can help untangle the complex relationship between pathology (a medical condition or diagnosis), impairment (an anatomic or functional abnormality or loss), limitations in activity (a reduction in ADLs that can be assessed by functional metrics), and restrictions in participation (a reduction in ability to perform socially defined activities or roles).

The opinions set forth in the IME report are expected to be expressed in terms of medical probability versus medical possibility in all cases where the following definitions apply:

Medical possibility: Something could occur as a result of a particular cause (probability of 50% or less).[34]

Medical probability: Something is more likely to occur than not (probability exceeding 50%.[34])

PHYSICIAN TESTIMONY AND LIABILITIES

The IME is a form of expert witness testimony that embraces the important task of assessing claimants' health in accordance with their legal rights, entitlement, and potential for monetary gain. The independent medical examiner, acting as an agent for the consulting party rather than as a patient advocate, also bears the risk of becoming a target for allegations of wrongdoing leveled by a disgruntled claimant.

From a legal perspective, an independent medical examiner or a disability evaluator is essentially an expert witness. Accordingly and until recently, the expert had enjoyed essentially the same type of immunity as any other witness in the judicial process. This immunity from civil liability ran quite deep and included protection from claims of defamation and negligence. The witness immunity can be traced back to 16th-century English common law.[35] The idea behind witness immunity was to ensure that the witness would speak freely when giving testimony.[36] Subsequently, the American courts considered the issue of witness immunity to be so important that it was maintained even when there might be negligence.[37] Traditionally, the argument for such immunity has been that expert witnesses are an important part of the legal system and that in the interest of justice, expert witnesses need to be protected from liability. Several state courts have affirmed the concept of witness immunity for reasons of public policy because without immunity, there would be loss of objectivity and the fear of infinite vexation would have a chilling effect on the witness and a reluctance to testify.[38]

The U.S. Supreme Court in the 1980s confirmed the importance of witness immunity in two cases. In *Briscoe v LaHue*[39] the court noted that a witness who knows that he might be forced to defend a subsequent lawsuit and perhaps pay damages might be inclined to shade his testimony in favor of the potential plaintiff and to magnify uncertainties and thus deprive the finder of the fact (judge or jury) of candid, objective, and undistorted evidence.

In *Mitchell v Forsyth*[40] the U.S. Supreme Court reasoned that witness immunity is important because the judicial process is an arena of open conflict and in virtually every case there is, if not always a winner, at least one loser. The court noted that it is inevitable that many of those who lose will pin the blame on witnesses and would bring suit against them in an effort to relitigate the underlying conflict.

The continuous theme that ran through these cases emphasized that the object of immunity is not to protect those whose conduct is open to criticism but to protect those who would be subject to unjustified and vexatious claims by disgruntled litigants. However, a recent development in the law of liability of expert witnesses in the past 2 decades has caused many cracks in the expert witness armor.

The legal liabilities of an independent medical examiner as an expert witness are mainly grounded in legal theories (referred to in legal parlance as causes of action) of tort law and to some extent in contract law by which the injured party as a plaintiff may bring a lawsuit against a health care provider (Box 17.1). It should be noted that a liability claim against a practitioner can be and is usually brought simultaneously under several legal theories. The plaintiff's hope is to win under any or all of these claims and receive a monetary award from the defendant practitioner.

Box 17.1 Legal Theories of Causes of Action against Independent Medical Examiner Doctors and Expert Witnesses

A. Intentional torts
   1. Assault
   2. Battery
   3. Intentional infliction of emotional distress
   4. False imprisonment
   5. Defamation
   6. Invasion of privacy
   7. Fraud and misrepresentation
   8. Conspiracy
   9. Bad faith
   10. Deceptive trade practices
B. Unintentional torts
   1. Ordinary negligence
   2. Professional malpractice
   3. Failure to warn
   4. Wrongful death
   5. Loss of chance of recovery or survival
   6. Vicarious liability for the acts of others
   7. Negligent referral
   8. Failure to diagnose
   9. Failure to inform
C. Actions under the law of contract
   1. Breach of contract
   2. Breach of warranty
   3. Abandonment
D. Miscellaneous causes of action
   1. Deceptive trade practices
   2. Violation of a statute or regulation

The underlying principle of common law (both law of tort and contracts) is to provide a venue for a person who has suffered damage as a result of an action or inaction by others to seek redress for his or her grievance in the courtroom. Tort law has been described as a great equalizer because it gives the individual an ability to bring a potentially mightier wrongdoer (referred to in legal parlance as a *tortfeasor*) before the bar on a more equal footing for the wrongs that may have been done to the person and secure compensation for the loss. Obviously, the law cannot make tortfeasors undo the injury or harm but makes them pay monetary compensation for both intentional wrongs (e.g., defamation, assault and battery) and unintentional wrongs (e.g., negligence). The law of tort not only shifts the burden of the cost of the injury or damages to the responsible party but also serves to prevent similar harm to other members of society through enforced accountability. The idea is to make the offensive and undesirable behavior costly to the tortfeasor and in principle serves to deter others from engaging in behavior such as the defendant's in the future.[41]

Traditionally, health care providers' liability to their patients arises out of medical malpractice claims. The term *malpractice* refers to any professional misconduct that encompasses an unreasonable lack of skill or unfaithfulness in carrying out professional or fiduciary duties.[42] The law of torts under the theory of negligence is the most common basis for a medical malpractice action against a health care provider. However, under this action the plaintiff must prove that the practitioner had a duty to the patient and breached that duty as a result of which (causation) harm or damage occurred.

Up until recently, medical malpractice actions against IME doctors and expert witnesses failed because of lack of a doctor-patient relationship with the examinee or plaintiff.[43] The continuous theme that ran through the cases across various jurisdictions in the United States was that as long as the IME doctor neither offered nor intended to treat the individual examinee, there was a lack of a doctor-patient relationship that prevented sustaining the medical malpractice cause of action.[44,45] Many potential cases were either not filed because of a prevailing notion among the legal community based on the previous case law or, when filed, were dismissed on pretrial motions from the defendants.[46-48] This has, however, changed significantly in the past 2 decades, with increasing case law from various jurisdictions holding independent medical examiners and expert witnesses accountable for the alleged harm suffered by the plaintiff/examinee. This was initially done under the cause of action of simple negligence and outside the law of torts for medical malpractice.[49]

More recently, at least two state Supreme Courts have allowed civil action against IME doctors to proceed under the traditional medical malpractice theory. Legal commentators have observed that this increasing erosion of immunity from civil action for the independent medical examiner as an expert witness is due to proliferation and growth of the litigation/expert witness industry, as well as to courts' perception of lack of protection of the injured party from unscrupulous witnesses and inadequacy of the traditional safeguards against expert witness malfeasance from potential prosecution for perjury and inadequate cross-examination.

The beginning of this trend of judicial hostility toward expert witness immunity can be traced back to the mid-1990s, when state courts in the United States started holding independent medical examiners and expert witnesses without any doctor-patient relationship accountable to their examinee in ordinary negligence. This trend began in Colorado with the *Greenberg v Perkins*[49] case. Several other jurisdictions have since followed suit. The Virginia Supreme Court in *Harris v Kreutzer*[50] held as a matter of first impression (making a new precedent) that a doctor could be sued for malpractice for negligent performance of mental and physical examination of a party during an IME.

Similarly, the Court of Appeals in Arizona in the *Stanley v McCarver*[51] case found that a formal doctor-patient relationship is not the only source of a doctor's duty toward a patient and that the doctor owed a duty of care to the patient despite the absence of a formal doctor-patient relationship. The Arizona Supreme Court took it a notch further in *Ritchie v Krasner*[52] and allowed medical malpractice to go forward despite no doctor-patient relationship by essentially stating that the court can envision no public benefit in not holding a doctor accountable to a duty to conform to the legal standard of reasonable care.

As can be seen from the above, under the case law of various jurisdictions in the United States, the immunity of expert witnesses (as well as IME doctors), traditionally enjoyed until recently against a variety of legal causes of action, is now rapidly eroding. The news from the other side of the Atlantic is even worse. In a recent decision by the U.K. Supreme Court in the *Devaney S. Jones v Karney* case,[53] expert witnesses were practically stripped of all the immunities that are available to fact witnesses in general. After a lengthy discussion the majority of the *Jones* court concluded that they see no public policy reason to justify immunity for expert witnesses. Even though this recent decision in the United Kingdom has no authority in U.S. jurisprudence, it is nonetheless regarded by some as a persuasive argument.

In summary, pain practitioners should be aware of not only the legal liabilities in the overall practice of their subspecialty but also the additional liabilities entailed with exposure to IMEs and expert witness work. It should be emphasized that even though the recent case law in some jurisdictions has significantly removed the traditional immunity of providers with no doctor-patient relationship with their examinees from medical malpractice claims, in American jurisprudence there still remains a great need for expert medical witness service. Practitioners attracted to disability assessment and inclined to serve as independent medical examiners are encouraged to attend several of the high-quality training programs offered in the United States to independent medical examiners and expert witnesses with the goal of empowering them with the knowledge, skills, and abilities necessary to practice as an independent medical examiner or expert witness in the field of disability medicine.

IMPLICATIONS FOR DISABILITY ASSESSMENT OF INDIVIDUALS WITH CHRONIC PAIN

An important point of this chapter can best be made by drawing into focus the distinction between impairment ratings and disability ratings as they pertain to the issue of pain. As noted above, the construct of impairment is conceptually and operationally grounded in the medical model of disease discussed earlier; impairment is codified and systematically defined according to a predetermined set of objective and measurable criteria for each organ system. Conditions that affect one or more organ systems and manifest themselves in terms of objective, measurable organ system pathology are infinitely ratable according to these organ systems. The painful experience that often accompanies specific pathology can and should be accounted for in some systematic manner and included in such ratings. However, pain can occur in the absence of observed pathology specific to the organ system, and chronic painful conditions transcend the organ system boundaries of the individual and can perhaps best be described and understood in terms of the biopsychosocial model described above.[54]

Global pain or other chronic painful conditions not attributable to any specific organ system pathology according to the impairment rating method alluded to earlier can perhaps be more adequately accounted for by adopting and applying QOL measures. Such metrics have the necessary empirical foundation from which to develop standards for losses in terms of nonvocational function, life satisfaction, and the burden of care and medical compliance needed to maintain optimal function in the presence of chronic pain and other disabling conditions.[25] Such metrics, when applied properly, can and should enable modification of any disability payment as a percent add-on or stand-alone cash award according to the specifications of each disability system. Perhaps the disabling consequences of chronic painful conditions can be more favorably captured in overall disability determinations at the point of final integration of the impairment rating, functional outcomes, and other relevant disability criteria as evidenced through such QOL assessments.[8] Such a shift in emphasis must recognize that a valid disability assessment of pain may require a skill set and applied metrics beyond those typically embodied by the physician disability examiner. Until this ideal can be more closely achieved, the role of pain as a contributor to disability can most properly be accounted for in two separate ways: pain directly affecting impairment can be viewed in terms of the functional outcomes accompanying a specific impairment, as the following Vignette 3 suggests.

Vignette 3

Consider the example of a transradial amputee cited earlier in terms of possible functional results. In a "standard" case with expected medical, surgical, and rehabilitative outcomes and availability of resources, the affected individual should achieve acceptable wound healing and uncomplicated scarification; proximal range of motion should be within functional limits; and fitting of a body-powered prosthesis should be uncomplicated and enable the performance of ADLs bimanually at or near the "baseline" level of ability. A "better than expected" outcome could occur if the amputation was undertaken to correct a preexisting malfunction or painful condition and results in an uncomplicated healing scenario with a better than baseline functional outcome. A less than expected outcome could also occur in the presence of complicated wound healing, painful scarification, or a neuroma making fitting of a prosthetic difficult or ineffective or in the presence of permanent loss of proximal range of motion because of pain, nerve injury, or contracture.

It is now possible, by using the DBI approach outlined earlier for impairment rating as put forward in the sixth edition of the AMA Guides, to modify the "expected" impairment rating upward by means of a functionally based "grade modifier" sensitive to pain and other limiters of function in order to award individuals with additional impairment for pain-associated loss of function.

Alternatively, in cases in which a specific diagnosis is lacking and pain appears to be the primary problem, the sixth edition of the AMA Guides currently offers a "stand-alone" assessment of pain that awards up to 3% loss to the whole person when pain is not effectively rated elsewhere.

Clearly, additional work is needed to perfect our current disability infrastructure and further enhance the relevance, validity, and reliability of medical impairment ratings and to provide alternative metrics to expand and modify disability determinations to properly account for functional losses as a result of chronic pain.

RESOURCES AVAILABLE TO THE PHYSICIAN DISABILITY EXAMINER

A number of educational venues and reference resources are available to enable interested physicians to gain the additional knowledge, expertise, and credentials needed to perform impairment ratings, disability evaluations, and IMEs competently and authoritatively. Such resources include courses,[55,56] certification examinations,[55,56] and several reference texts.[2,57,58]

KEY POINTS

- Maximum medical improvement (MMI) represents a treatment end point (for purposes of case closure) at which a given ratable condition (impairment) has stabilized (is unlikely to change substantially in the next year with or without treatment) and no further improvement in function can be expected.
- The "biopsychosocial model" of disability is currently accepted as the preferred conceptual model of disablement because it simultaneously recognizes three components of disability: the *biologic* component (the physical and mental aspects of an individual's health condition), the *psychological* component (personal and psychological factors that are having an impact on the individual's functioning), and the *social* component (contextual and environmental factors that may also have an impact on functioning) in each particular case.
- The International Classification of Functioning, Disabilities and Health (ICF) of the World Health Organization is the currently accepted classification system of disablement for purposes of health policy and legislation. It has replaced earlier systems to provide more interactive (as opposed to linear) representation between individuals with a health condition, the functional consequences of their impairment, and contextual factors of a personal and environmental nature potentially affecting their disablement. The ICF classification system embraces the "biopsychosocial model" of disease by taking into account environmental and personal modifiers of functional outcomes in a given case.
- Within our society a number of different disability systems exist to compensate individuals for losses. They share a common conceptual and operational platform in which the initial estimate of physical or psychological loss (or both) can be translated into an estimate of functional and economic loss and expressed in monetary terms.
- By convention, the severity of physical and psychological loss is defined and measured in terms of a *medical impairment rating*, which represents a percentage of regional loss of the affected body part or parts and can be extrapolated to the body as a whole. The expected degree of functional and economic loss of the affected individual can be further operationally derived from the impairment percentage as a *disability rating*—a percentage of the economic worth of the "whole person" awarded in terms of a monetary sum that differs for each particular disability system.

KEY POINTS—cont'd

- The metrics for medical impairment rating clearly favor and emphasize objective over subjective criteria. Accordingly, painful entities such as headache, fibromyalgia, and low back pain often occur in the absence of objective verifiable pathology or may occur in a setting in which objective clinical findings are most consistent with a normal anatomic variation and the aging process and have little or no bearing on the individual's actual complaints. Impairment ratings in such cases are ineffective, at best, since minimal or no rating percentage is currently allowed for any apparent (and often profound) negative impact that these conditions may be having on activities of daily living. The disablement and ensuing losses in such cases potentially become more evident if viewed in terms of burden of care and quality of life. Although metrics currently exist to measure losses of the individual in these areas, unfortunately they are not familiar tools to the typical rating physician and are not routinely taken into account by the rating systems per se; consequently, losses and disablement caused primarily by pain remain largely unaccounted for by the rating practice summarized in this chapter.
- A number of U.S. disability systems exist to provide economic and other benefits to claimants experiencing losses because of aging, infirmity, illness, or injury. Chief among these are the Social Security Administration (SSA), federal and state workers' compensation systems, the Veterans Benefits Administration (VBA), personal injury claims, and others. Physicians working within the jurisdictional boundaries of any of these systems must be familiar with the definitions, eligibility requirements, and rating criteria of each particular system and follow the system-specific procedures and rules prescribed in each particular case.
- The American Medical Association *Guides to the Evaluation of Permanent Impairment* (AMA Guides) is a standardized, objective reference for this purpose that was originally published in 1971 and periodically updated and revised to the most current sixth edition published in 2008.
- The AMA Guides is recognized nationally and globally as the preferred reference for medical impairment ratings. Various editions are required or recommended by statute in the majority of U.S. workers' compensation jurisdictions, although it is not directly used in disability determinations by the SSA or in compensation and pensioning by the VBA at present time.
- The *independent medical examination* (IME) is an evaluation performed by a physician examiner who is not treating the patient or claimant in order to answer specific questions posed by the referring party, including determination of MMI, impairment rating, and return-to-work restrictions, if applicable. IMEs may be performed any time there is a dispute, concern, or question regarding the medical treatment or condition

KEY POINTS—cont'd

of the injured worker. These issues include topics such as the following:

1. Diagnosis, proximate causation, and work-relatedness of an illness or injury
2. Current and proposed medical treatment or diagnostic efforts
3. Appropriate work and general activity level during treatment
4. Stability of the medical condition and status regarding MMI
5. Identification of other nonmedical factors that can have a significant impact
6. Impairment rating and related disability issues
7. Ability to return to work (fitness for duty) and need for reasonable accommodation

- Pain practitioners should be aware of not only the legal liabilities in the overall practice of their subspecialty but also the additional liabilities entailed with exposure to IMEs and expert witness work. Practitioners attracted to disability assessment and inclined to serve as independent medical examiners are encouraged to attend several of the high-quality training programs readily available with the goal to empower themselves with the knowledge, skills, and abilities needed to practice as an independent medical examiner or expert witness in the field of disability medicine.
- Additional work is needed to perfect our current disability infrastructure in order to further enhance the relevance, validity, and reliability of medical impairment ratings and provide alternative metrics to expand and modify disability determinations to properly account for functional losses as a result of chronic pain.

SUGGESTED READINGS

American Medical Association. *Guides to the Evaluation of Permanent Impairment.* 6th ed. Chicago: American Medical Association; 2008.

Burton JF Jr. Workers' compensation cash benefits. Part one. The building blocks. *Workers' Compensation Policy Rev.* 2008;8:15-28.

Burton Jr JF. Workers' compensation cash benefits. Part two. Cash benefit systems and criteria for evaluation. *Workers' Compensation Policy Rev.* 2008;8:13-31.

Iezzoni LI, Freedman VA. Turning the disability tide: the importance of definitions. *JAMA.* 2008;299:332-334.

Katz RT, Rondinelli RD. Major U.S. disability and compensation systems graphically compared. *Phys Med Rehabil Clin N Am.* 2001;12:499-505.

Ranavaya ML, Brigham C. International use of the *AMA Guides to the Evaluation of Permanent Impairment.* AMA Guides Newsletter, May/June 2011.

Rondinelli RD. Changes for the new *AMA Guides to Impairment Ratings,* 6th ed. Implications and applications for physician disability evaluations. *PMR.* 2009;1:643-656.

Rondinelli RD, Katz RT, eds. *Impairment Rating and Disability Evaluation.* Philadelphia: Saunders; 2000.

Turk DC, Monarch ES. Biopsychosocial perspective on chronic pain. In: Turk DC, Gatchel RJ, eds. *Psychological Approaches to Pain Management: A Practitioner's Handbook.* 2nd ed. New York: Guilford Press; 2002:3-29.

Wadell G, Burton AK, Aylward M. A biopsychosocial model of sickness and disability. *AMA Guides Newsletter.* May-June 2008:1-20.

WHO. *International Classification of Functioning, Disabilities and Health: ICF.* Geneva: World Health Organization; 2001.

The references for this chapter can be found at www.expertconsult.com.

PART 4

CLINICAL CONDITIONS

CHRISTOPHER L. WU | CHARLES E. ARGOFF, EDITORS

PART OUTLINE

18

Postoperative Pain and Other Acute Pain Syndromes

Marie N. Hanna | Jean-Pierre P. Ouanes | Vicente Garcia Tomas

INTRODUCTION

Untreated postoperative pain can result in unwanted psychological and physiologic effects that may increase morbidity and mortality, compromise quality of recovery, and increase the incidence of chronic pain.[1-4] Although management of postoperative pain has improved tremendously in the last few decades, pain in surgical patients is still undermanaged. In 2000, the Joint Commission on Accreditation of Healthcare Organizations (JCAHO) officially recognized patients' rights in pain management and implemented standards for assessment, monitoring, and treatment of pain.[5] In 2004, the American Society of Anesthesiologists established the Pain Task Force and published clinical practice guidelines to promote standardization of procedures and the use of multimodal analgesia.[6] In 2010, the Department of Health and Human Services and the Institute of Medicine agreed to promote the recognition of pain as a significant public health problem and to encourage pain research, pain care, and pain education in the United States. Pain management is becoming an important ethical responsibility of the medical profession and a focus of the health care system, thus encouraging many institutions to support the proper practice of pain control for surgical patients. Opioids remain the primary analgesic agent for treating moderate and severe pain after surgery; however, in many cases opioid-related side effects may compromise a patient's quality of recovery.

PREVENTIVE ANALGESIA

Preventive analgesia is a method of preventing or attenuating the central sensitization that results from a painful insult and the inflammatory reaction that develops after the insult.[7] Previously, the term "preemptive analgesia" described mainly the timing of pain intervention (i.e., before vs. after the insult). Its use was controversial, and proving its clinical relevance in clinical trials was difficult.[7-9] Recent clinical trials have shown that the effectiveness and duration of pain treatment interventions are clinically relevant in blocking or attenuating the noxious stimuli and decreasing central sensitization to pain.[10] For preventive analgesia to effectively prevent central sensitization and reduce postoperative and chronic pain,[2,11] intensive multimodal analgesic interventions should be used during the perioperative period. Maximum benefit occurs when pain interventions are extended into the postoperative phase.[12] The focus of this chapter is on available pain treatment intervention techniques and drugs for multimodal analgesia in the setting of surgery and trauma.

MULTIMODAL ANALGESIA

Multimodal analgesia involves the administration of two or more analgesic agents by one or more routes that exert their effects via different analgesic mechanisms and ideally act synergistically at different sites in the nervous system, thereby providing superior analgesia with fewer side effects. The concept of a multimodal strategy, including regional analgesia, was introduced more than a decade ago to allow early ambulation, promote better rehabilitation, accelerate recovery, and reduce the length of hospital stay. In the ambulatory surgery setting, evidence has shown great promise for the use of local anesthetics, acetaminophen, and nonsteroidal anti-inflammatory drugs (NSAIDs), among other treatment options, with opioids being reserved as a rescue drug only.[13] Some recent publications have found that NSAIDs and selective cyclooxygenase-2 (COX-2) inhibitors consistently reduce postoperative opioid requirements. Furthermore, the combination of several nonopioid analgesics with opioids delivered by patient-controlled analgesia (PCA) offers advantages over opioids alone.[14,15] Multimodal pain control strategies for certain procedures could become an integral part of clinical pathways to provide effective postoperative analgesia and rehabilitation.[16,17]

PAIN MANAGEMENT OPTIONS

Pain management is an art; a clinician must balance the risks and benefits of each modality to customize treatment based on a patient's specific needs. Many institutions have recognized that suboptimal treatment of acute postoperative pain occurs frequently and have begun to support the development of postoperative pain services, many of which are led by anesthesiologists who have clinical experience in regional anesthesia and knowledge of drug pharmacology to provide surgical patients with an optimal pain treatment plan that minimizes side effects. Even though pain treatment modalities may decrease morbidity, more common outcomes generally include improvement in the quality of recovery and quality of life. Patient satisfaction can be used as an indicator of an effective treatment response to these programs. Options available for the management of postoperative pain include, but are not limited to, various combinations of

Table 18.1 Systemic Opioid and Nonopioid Analgesic Options

Agent	Delivery	Analgesic Ceiling	Side Effects	Comments
Opioids	PO, IV PCA, IM, SQ, NA, PNB, TD (including TD PCA)	No	Induced hyperalgesia, nausea, vomiting, sedation, respiratory depression, pruritus, constipation, urinary retention	Side effects limit full their analgesic potential
Tramadol	PO, IV	Yes (comparable to ibuprofen, 400 mg)	Dizziness, drowsiness, sweating, nausea, vomiting, dry mouth, headache	Also inhibits serotonin reuptake Caution/contraindication in patients taking MAOIs, with seizure history, or with increased ICP Appears to lack side effects of respiratory depression, major organ toxicity, constipation, and dependence
Acetaminophen	PO, IV	Yes	Hepatotoxicity	Coadministration with opioids appears to provide opioid-sparing analgesia but may not reduce opioid-related side effects
NSAIDs	PO, IV, IM	Yes	Renal, GI, platelet inhibition, inhibition of bone healing, inhibition of osteogenesis, cardiovascular	Coadministration with opioids appears to provide opioid-sparing analgesia but may not reduce opioid-related side effects
COX-2 inhibitors	PO	Yes	Renal, cardiovascular, inhibition of bone healing, inhibition of osteogenesis	Coadministration with opioids appears to provide opioid-sparing analgesia but may not reduce opioid-related side effects
Ketamine (low dose)	IV	Yes	No cognitive impairments or psychotomimetic effects seen with dosing of 0.25 mg/kg	May attenuate both postoperative pain and chronic pain; may attenuate opioid-induced hyperalgesia
Gabapentin and pregabalin	PO	Unknown	Dizziness, somnolence, ataxia, memory impairment, weight gain, edema, altered vision	May be useful for acute analgesia and chronic antihyperalgesia, pending further study

COX, cyclooxygenase; ICP, intracranial pressure; IM, intramuscular; IV, intravenous; MAOI, monoamine oxidase inhibitor; NA, neuraxial; NSAID, nonsteroidal anti-inflammatory drug; PCA, patient-controlled analgesia; PNB, peripheral nerve block; PO, per oral; SQ, subcutaneous; TD, transdermal.

systemic and neuraxial opioids, nonopioid analgesics, and regional analgesia (neuraxial and perineural).

SYSTEMIC ANALGESICS

OPIOIDS

Opium and its derivatives are the most commonly used medications for the treatment of acute and chronic pain (Table 18.1). Opioids exert their analgesic effect through μ-opioid receptors. These receptors are located mainly in the central nervous system (CNS), although some are also present in the peripheral nervous system.[18] The therapeutic benefits (and side effects) of morphine, the prototypical opioid analgesic agent, are mediated predominantly through activation of μ-opioid receptors and less likely through the δ- and κ-receptor subtypes.[19] Although opioids do not exhibit an analgesic ceiling effect, the analgesic efficacy of opioids can be limited by the development of adverse effects such as nausea, vomiting, pruritus, ileus, and respiratory depression.

One of the many advantages of opioid analgesics for the treatment of acute postoperative pain is that it can be administered via a number of routes (e.g., subcutaneous, oral, intravenous [IV], intramuscular [IM], intranasal, transmucosal, and neuraxial). This feature enhances the versatility of opioids as a therapeutic agent. For the treatment of moderate to severe postoperative pain, opioids are typically administered parenterally (IV, IM), although there may be wide individual variability in the relationship between opioid dose, serum concentration, and analgesic response in the treatment of postoperative pain.[20] IV administration of opioids is desirable for treating acute postoperative pain because of the rapid and reliable onset of analgesia. Oral administration of opioids is the most common form used for the treatment of mild to moderate postoperative pain or when inpatients have successfully initiated oral intake.

Opioid receptor physiology is complex and regulated by multiple mechanisms that may play a role in the development of opioid receptor tolerance and desensitization. Tolerance and desensitization may contribute not only to a short-term decrease in analgesic efficacy but also to long-term changes in receptor sensitivity.[19,21,22] Desensitization may lead to increased analgesic requirements for a similar pain response.

IV PCA is considered the "gold standard" by which systemic opioids are delivered postoperatively. Unlike traditional "as needed" (PRN) analgesic regimens, IV PCA allows the clinician to compensate for several factors, including the wide interpatient and intrapatient variability in analgesic needs, variability in serum drug levels, and administrative

Table 18.2 Intravenous Patient-Controlled Analgesia Regimens in Adults

Drug Concentration	Bolus Size (Adult)*	Bolus Size (Pediatric)*	Lockout Interval (min)	Continuous Infusion (Opioid Tolerant)†	Continuous Infusion (Pediatric)
Agonist					
Morphine (1 mg/mL)	0.5-2.5 mg	0.01-0.03 mg/kg (max, 0.15 mg/kg/hr)	5-10	0.5-2.5 mg/hr	0.01-0.03 mg/kg/hr
Fentanyl (0.01 mg/mL)	10-20 µg	0.5-1 µg/kg (max, 4 µg/kg/hr)	4-10	20-100 µg/hr	0.5-1 µg/kg/hr
Hydromorphone (0.2 mg/mL)	0.05-0.25 mg	3-5 µg/kg (max, 20 µg/kg/hr)	5-10	0.05-0.25 mg/hr	3-5 µg/kg/hr
Methadone (1 mg/mL)	0.5-2.5 mg		8-20	0.5-2.5 mg/hr	
Meperidine (10 mg/mL)	5-25 mg		5-10		
Alfentanil (0.1 mg/mL)	0.1-0.2 mg		5-10	0.1-0.2 mg/hr	
Sufentanil (2 mcg/mL)	2-5 µg		4-10	2-5 µg/hr	
Agonist-Antagonist					
Nalbuphine (1 mg/mL)	1-5 mg		5-15		
Buprenorphine (0.03 mg/mL)	0.03-0.1 mg		8-20		
Pentazocine (10 mg/mL)	5-30 mg		5-15		

*Bolus doses for adults or children should be titrated and based on clinical evaluation of the patient.
†Continuous infusion is not recommended for opioid-naïve adult patients.

delays, which might result in inadequate postoperative analgesia. The IV PCA device per se has a safety mechanism integrated into its design, although when the negative feedback loop is violated, excessive sedation or respiratory depression may occur.[23,24] Most of the problems related to the use of IV PCA are caused by user or operator error and are not attributable to the device itself.[23]

Variables that can be programmed into an IV PCA device include the demand or bolus dose, lockout interval, and background infusion. Optimal settings for IV PCA administration of opioids for the management of postoperative pain are not known; however, there are general principles that may promote effective postoperative analgesia. The setting for the demand or bolus dose should be sufficient to provide analgesia after multiple self-administered doses; it should not be an excessive dose that may result in adverse effects such as respiratory depression.[25] For opioid-naïve patients, a commonly used demand dose for morphine is 0.5 to 2.5 mg, for fentanyl it is 10 to 20 µg,[23,25] and for hydromorphone it is 0.05 to 0.25 mg (Table 18.2). Commonly used lockout intervals range from 5 to 10 minutes, and varying the interval within this range appears to have no effect on analgesia or side effects.[23,26] The final variable is the continuous or background infusion. Although use of a background infusion was initially thought to provide improved analgesia, especially during sleep, routine use of continuous or background infusions in IV PCA in adult opioid-naïve patients is not recommended because it increases the incidence of adverse effects such as respiratory depression.[23,27] Use of a background infusion in opioid-naïve patients, even if limited to nighttime, does not improve analgesia or sleep patterns.[27-29] However, a background infusion for opioid-tolerant or pediatric patients may be appropriate.

When compared with traditional PRN analgesic regimens, use of IV PCA may be associated with improved patient outcomes, including superior postoperative analgesia, improved patient satisfaction,[30] and possibly decreased risk for pulmonary complications.[30,31] At least two meta-analyses have been conducted to compare IV PCA with PRN administration of opioids. Both meta-analyses demonstrated that the analgesia provided by IV PCA is superior to that achieved with PRN administration. An early meta-analysis of 15 randomized trials in which PRN IM dosing was compared with IV PCA failed to demonstrate a reduction in opioid consumption.[30,31] IV PCA had no obvious economic benefit, although it may be associated with fewer pulmonary complications.[30] In addition, patients tended to prefer IV PCA,[30,31] which may result in greater patient satisfaction.[30-33] Although IV PCA provides no apparent decrease in cost or length of hospital stay, it does reduce demand on the nursing staff, who are required for delivery of IV or IM PRN analgesics. This reduced administration by the nursing staff may indeed have a cost benefit.[34] The incidence of opioid-related side effects, including respiratory depression (0.5%), from IV PCA does not appear to differ significantly from that of other administration routes (e.g., IV, IM, or subcutaneous).[23,30,33,35] Many factors could contribute to the occurrence of respiratory depression with IV PCA, including the use of a background infusion, concomitant use of a sedative or hypnotic agent, advanced age, and the presence of pulmonary disease or sleep apnea.[23,33]

Transdermal delivery of fentanyl, a continuous passive dose, is not indicated for the treatment of acute pain but could be an option for the treatment of chronic cancer pain; it could also be an alternative to oral opioids when patients cannot tolerate oral intake for an extended time. A recent technological development has added the process of iontophoresis to substantially increase dermal penetration capacity and thereby allow in essence a "PCA fentanyl patch."[36] Clinical studies have shown iontophoretic patient-controlled transdermal fentanyl to be superior to placebo and comparable to IV PCA with morphine for the treatment of acute postoperative pain.[37-39]

Table 18.3 Guidelines for Equianalgesic Dosing of Opioid Agonists*

Drug	Parenteral IV/IM (mg)	Oral Dose (mg)
Morphine	10	30
Hydromorphone	1.5-2	6.5-7.5
Fentanyl	0.1	—
Oxymorphone	1-1.1	7-10†
Levorphanol	2-2.3	4
Meperidine	75-100	300-400
Methadone	10	10-20
Codeine	130	200
Oxycodone	—	20-30
Propoxyphene		130-200

*Dosages and range of dosages are approximate and used as an estimate of the calculated dose.
†Immediate- and extended-release forms of oxymorphone are approved by the Food and Drug Administration.
IM, intramuscular; IV, intravenous.

Morphine, in either extended-release or immediate-release form, is still the gold standard for oral opioids. Oxycodone is commonly used alone or in combination with an adjuvant such as acetaminophen. One should be cautious of exceeding the total recommended daily dose of acetaminophen because of hepatic toxicity. Transmucosal fentanyl could be used when acute intense pain is anticipated. With opioid conversion, especially in opioid-tolerant patients, the dose should be decreased by 33% because of incomplete cross-tolerance between drugs.[40]

Tramadol is a centrally acting, synthetic analgesic agent that is structurally related to codeine and morphine. The use of tramadol for postoperative analgesia may confer several advantages over traditional opioids, including the relative lack of respiratory depression, major organ toxicity, constipation, and dependence.[41,42] Common side effects of tramadol include dizziness, drowsiness, sweating, nausea, vomiting, dry mouth, and headache.[42,43]

Conversion from one opioid or one route of administration to another should de done with caution to avoid underdosing or overdosing. A conversion table (Table 18.3) may facilitate equianalgesic conversion; however, it provides only an estimate to assist in initiating the opioid dose.

NONOPIOID ANALGESICS

NONSTEROIDAL ANTI-INFLAMMATORY AGENTS AND ACETAMINOPHEN

NSAIDs and acetaminophen are a diverse group of analgesic compounds that exhibit different pharmacokinetic properties and produce analgesia presumably by inhibiting COX enzymes and the subsequent synthesis of prostaglandins, which are important mediators of peripheral and CNS hyperalgesia.[44] COX has at least two isoforms with different functions. The COX-1 isozyme is constitutively present and mediates platelet aggregation, hemostasis, and gastric mucosal protection. The COX-2 enzyme is upregulated during inflammation and may play a role in nociception. Recently, it has been recognized that the COX-2 enzyme may play an important role in cardioprotection via prostacyclin (PGI_2).[45]

Nonopioid analgesics are used as part of a multimodal analgesic regimen mainly to decrease systemic opioid consumption and improve postoperative pain.[46,47] IV acetaminophen, which has been available in Europe for more than 20 years, was recently approved by the Food and Drug Administration (FDA) in the United States and is quickly gaining popularity for the treatment of acute postoperative pain. The mechanism of pain relief with acetaminophen is still not clear. Acetaminophen rapidly crosses the blood-brain barrier[48,49] and inhibits central prostaglandins via the COX pathways.[50-52] It also triggers the activation of cannabinoid receptors[53,54] and inhibits nitric oxide pathways.[55,56] Acetaminophen has weak peripheral anti-inflammatory activity, limited gastrointestinal effects, and little impact on platelet function.[57] When compared with oral acetaminophen, IV acetaminophen provides faster onset of pain relief, reduces the duration of meaningful pain, and decreases the time to maximal pain relief.[49,58-60] Sinatra and colleagues[61] demonstrated a 33% reduction in morphine consumption over a 24-hour period when IV acetaminophen was delivered at 1 g every 6 hours after orthopedic surgery. Acetaminophen has also been shown to reduce the doses of narcotics required after tonsillectomy and endoscopic sinus surgery.[62]

Acetaminophen is available in rectal, oral, and IV formulations. The peak acetaminophen plasma concentration occurs 3 to 4 hours after a rectal dose, 45 to 60 minutes after an oral dose, and 15 minutes after IV infusion.[60,63,64] The rectal form has been associated with lower and more unpredictable bioavailability, thus making it less favored for acute postoperative pain.[65,66] The dosage for oral and IV acetaminophen in adults is 1 g every 4 to 6 hours, not to exceed 4 g/day. The dose interval should be at least 6 hours in patients with renal insufficiency.[58] Acetaminophen has a known potential for hepatotoxicity with excessive doses, but the risk is extremely low with therapeutic doses.[63] It is considered safe, with an adverse event profile similar to that of placebo.[67-69] Acetaminophen has only limited potential for drug interactions that is independent of the route of administration.[70]

In a qualitative systematic review of analgesic efficacy in relieving acute postoperative pain that assessed reductions in pain intensity scores and opioid consumption,[71] the combination of acetaminophen and NSAIDs was more effective than acetaminophen alone in 85% of relevant studies and more effective than NSAIDs alone in 64% of relevant studies. Several meta-analyses suggest that the use of NSAIDs, COX-2 inhibitors, or acetaminophen in combination with IV PCA does result in an opioid-sparing effect. However, the use of acetaminophen and COX-2 inhibitors does not appear to decrease the relative risk for opioid-related side effects (e.g., postoperative nausea and vomiting [PONV], sedation, pruritus, urinary retention) or adverse events (respiratory depression), whereas the use of nonspecific NSAIDs appears to decrease the relative risk only for some opioid-related side effects (e.g., PONV, sedation).[15,72-75] In terms of pain control, the addition of NSAIDs (multiple dose or infusion only) and COX-2 inhibitors, but not acetaminophen or single-dose NSAIDs, produces significantly lower pain scores postoperatively.[15,72-75]

Although NSAIDs are an integral part of postoperative pain management, their use is limited by several adverse effects (e.g., gastrointestinal bleeding, impaired renal function, inhibition of platelet aggregation, and inhibition of bone healing and osteogenesis). These adverse effects occur because of the general inhibition of COX and prostaglandin formation. The inhibition of platelet function and decreased perioperative hemostasis result from NSAID inhibition of COX-1, which is responsible for the synthesis of thromboxane A_2, a mediator of platelet aggregation and vasoconstriction,[76,77] although the available evidence on the effect of NSAIDs on perioperative bleeding is equivocal.[77,78] High-risk surgical patients (e.g., those with hypovolemia, abnormal renal function, or abnormal serum electrolytes) may be at risk for NSAID-induced renal dysfunction. Prostaglandins dilate the renal vascular beds, and NSAIDs may inhibit these beneficial diuretic and natriuretic renal effects,[79] but euvolemic patients with normal renal function are unlikely to be affected.[80] Although it is not clear whether NSAIDs may also have an adverse effect on bone healing,[81] they may be associated with a higher incidence of gastrointestinal bleeding[78] as a result of NSAID-induced inhibition of cytoprotective gastric mucosal prostaglandins (produced by COX-1 activity).[76]

Traditional NSAIDs block both COX-1 and COX-2 enzymes. The development of selective COX-2 inhibitors was based on the premise that selective inhibition of COX-2 would provide analgesia without the side effects associated with COX-1 inhibition. Although selective COX-2 inhibitors are associated with a lower incidence of gastrointestinal complications[82] and exhibit minimal platelet inhibition even when administered in supratherapeutic doses,[83] recent data indicate that COX-2 inhibitors may be associated with a higher incidence of cardiovascular events such as myocardial infarction.[84] Because COX-2 inhibitors inhibit PGI_2, these agents may actually promote coronary thrombosis via the unopposed action of thromboxane A_2.[45] A meta-analysis of rofecoxib trials indicated that administration of rofecoxib is associated with a 2.3-fold greater risk for cardiovascular events.[84] Unlike rofecoxib, celecoxib was not removed from the market, although some data suggest that celecoxib is also associated with a higher incidence of cardiovascular events.[85-87]

KETAMINE

Ketamine is an *N*-methyl-D-aspartate (NMDA) receptor antagonist and has generally been used as an intraoperative anesthetic agent. Because of its NMDA antagonistic properties, which may attenuate central sensitization (chronic postsurgical pain) and opioid tolerance, ketamine has been re-examined for its potential use in postoperative analgesia.[88] The perioperative administration of low-dose ketamine may be integrated into a multimodal analgesic regimen or used as an adjunct to opioids and local anesthetics to enhance postoperative analgesia and potentially reduce opioid-related side effects.[88-91] In one study of patients undergoing total knee replacement surgery under general anesthesia, ketamine or placebo was given during surgery (0.2 mg/kg followed by 2 μg/kg/min) and through the second postoperative day (10 μg/kg/min). Pain scores were lower at rest and with movement in the ketamine group than in the placebo group at all times. Time to achieve 90 degrees of flexion was shorter in the ketamine group, and the incidence of PONV was lower.[92] A systematic review revealed that perioperative administration of ketamine (vs. control) resulted in lower pain scores and significantly decreased morphine consumption over a 24-hour period, with no difference in morphine-related adverse effects between the groups.[93] However, use of ketamine as an adjunct to IV PCA may not improve postoperative analgesia.[94] Low-dose ketamine infusions do not appear to cause hallucinations or cognitive impairment, and in patients undergoing general anesthesia, the incidence of hallucinations appears to be low and may be independent of benzodiazepine premedication.[93,95,96] Reports of epidural and intrathecal ketamine have been published,[97,98] but neuraxial use of ketamine is discouraged until further safety and neurotoxicity data are available. Although intraoperative IV administration of subanesthetic ketamine in conjunction with general anesthesia may attenuate acute postoperative pain and potentially chronic postsurgical pain, the role of low-dose ketamine in postoperative analgesia remains unclear.[93,99] In addition, it is unclear at this time whether perioperative use of ketamine will result in better long-term recovery or improved functional outcome. Furthermore, evidence is insufficient to show a clear benefit of *S*(+)-ketamine over racemic ketamine.[99]

GABAPENTIN AND PREGABALIN

Gabapentin and pregabalin are analogous in molecular structure to γ-aminobutyric acid. Their use in acute pain models has provided promising preliminary evidence for potential routine use.[100] Their role in preempting chronic hyperalgesia is uncertain.[101] Five studies have shown benefit in acute pain management when an oral dose of 1200 mg gabapentin was administered preoperatively.[102-106] One of these studies also incorporated a limited postoperative dosing course (for 10 days after breast surgery) and reported lower opioid requirements and pain scores with movement.[103] After abdominal hysterectomy, use of gabapentin (400 mg four times a day for 1 day preoperatively and 5 days postoperatively) led to lower pain scores 1 month after surgery, but not in the immediate postoperative period.[107] Somnolence from single-dose gabapentin pretreatment was described only when epidural analgesia was coadministered,[105] thus leading to the possibility that the interaction between gabapentin and local anesthetics may augment the sedative effects.

Based on currently available data, randomized controlled trials, and meta-analyses, there is no clear evidence that the perioperative use of pregabalin reduces postoperative pain scores. The use of pregabalin has a great opioid-sparing effect in the first 24 hours and significantly reduces opioid-related side effects (vomiting).[108] Side effects of pregabalin are sedation, dizziness, and visual disturbance.

In summary,

- Opium and its derivatives are the most commonly used medications for the treatment of acute and chronic pain.
- IV PCA is considered the gold standard by which systemic opioids are delivered postoperatively.
- Transdermal delivery of fentanyl is not indicated for the treatment of acute pain unless the patient cannot tolerate oral intake for an extended time.

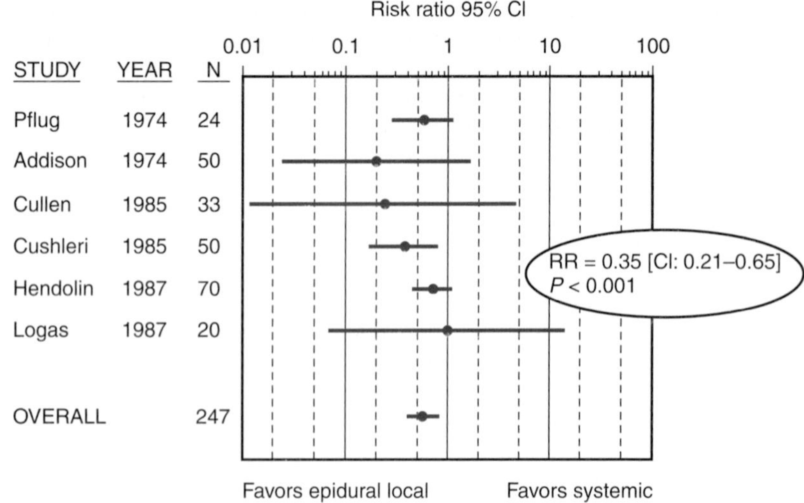

Figure 18.1 Epidural local analgesia versus systemic opioids: pulmonary complications. CI, confidence interval; RR, relative risk. (Redrawn from Ballantyne JC, Carr DB, deFerranti S, et al. The comparative effects of postoperative analgesic therapies on pulmonary outcome: cumulative meta-analyses of randomized, controlled trials. *Anesth Analg*. 1998;86:598-612.)

- Conversion from one opioid or one route of administration to another should be done with caution to avoid underdosing or overdosing.
- The use of NSAIDs, COX-2 inhibitors, or acetaminophen in combination with opioids does result in an opioid-sparing effect.
- The perioperative administration of low-dose ketamine may be integrated into a multimodal analgesic regimen to enhance postoperative analgesia.
- Use of gabapentin and pregabalin for the management of acute pain has shown promising preliminary results.

NEURAXIAL AND PERIPHERAL ANALGESIA

Perioperative neuraxial or peripheral techniques in general provide better analgesia than do systemic opioids. Continuous administration techniques have the advantage of decreasing adverse perioperative pathophysiology and improving patient outcomes, including major morbidity.[109,110]

CONTINUOUS EPIDURAL ANALGESIA

Continuous epidural analgesia may provide a longer duration of analgesia than an individual injection and analgesia superior to that with systemic opioids.[111] Postoperative use of continuous epidural analgesia may be associated with improved patient morbidity by decreasing pulmonary[112-115] (Fig. 18.1), cardiovascular,[112,114-116] and gastrointestinal[117,118] (Fig. 18.2) complications in high-risk patients and after high-risk procedures. However, many factors can affect the overall outcomes of continuous epidural analgesia. Among them are the congruency of epidural catheter location and the surgical incision, the type of analgesic regimen, and whether the epidural is used as part of a multimodal approach.[119,120] Local anesthetics used alone or in combination with opioids will offer better physiologic benefit to the patient than opioid use alone. However, premature discontinuation of epidural analgesia may negate its physiologic benefit. When compared with systemic administration of opioids, local anesthetic–based epidural regimens provide superior analgesia and may decrease opioid-related side effects; epidural infusion of opioids alone may be used to avoid hypotension when sympathetic blockade is a concern.

Postoperative epidural analgesia may be delivered as a fixed continuous infusion or as patient-controlled epidural analgesia (PCEA). Based on the principles of PCA, PCEA allows individualization of postoperative analgesic requirements, reduces drug use, improves patient satisfaction, and provides superior analgesia.[121,122]

The choice of drug for epidural analgesia is usually a local anesthetic with a long duration of action. It should exhibit preferential clinical sensory blockade and cause only minimal impairment of motor function.[123] Another option is a lipophilic opioid (e.g., fentanyl or sufentanil), which allows relatively rapid titration of analgesia, although hydrophilic opioids (e.g., morphine and hydromorphone) may also be used for postoperative analgesia.[124]

Even though clonidine and epinephrine are potentially useful adjuvants, neither is widely used clinically. Clonidine may enhance postoperative analgesia by activating the descending noradrenergic pathway; however, its clinical usefulness is typically limited by the presence of hypotension, bradycardia, and sedation.[125,126] Epinephrine has been shown to improve epidural analgesia and increase sensory block in the postoperative setting.[127]

NEURAXIAL OPIOIDS

Classification of opioids is based on their lipophilic property. Hydrophilic opioids (e.g., morphine and hydromorphone) tend to remain within cerebrospinal fluid (CSF) after neuraxial administration and usually produce a delayed but longer duration of analgesia. They also tend to cause a higher incidence of side effects because of CSF spread, unlike lipophilic opioids (e.g., fentanyl and sufentanil), which tend to provide a faster onset but shorter duration of analgesia as a result of rapid clearance from CSF. Hydrophilic opioids provide analgesia primarily via a spinal mechanism, whereas lipophilic opioids provide analgesia via either a spinal or systemic mechanism.[128,129] Single-shot neuraxial administration of a lipophilic opioid may be appropriate for short-duration analgesia,[130] but single-shot neuraxial administration of a hydrophilic opioid will be appropriate for longer-duration analgesia. The latter may

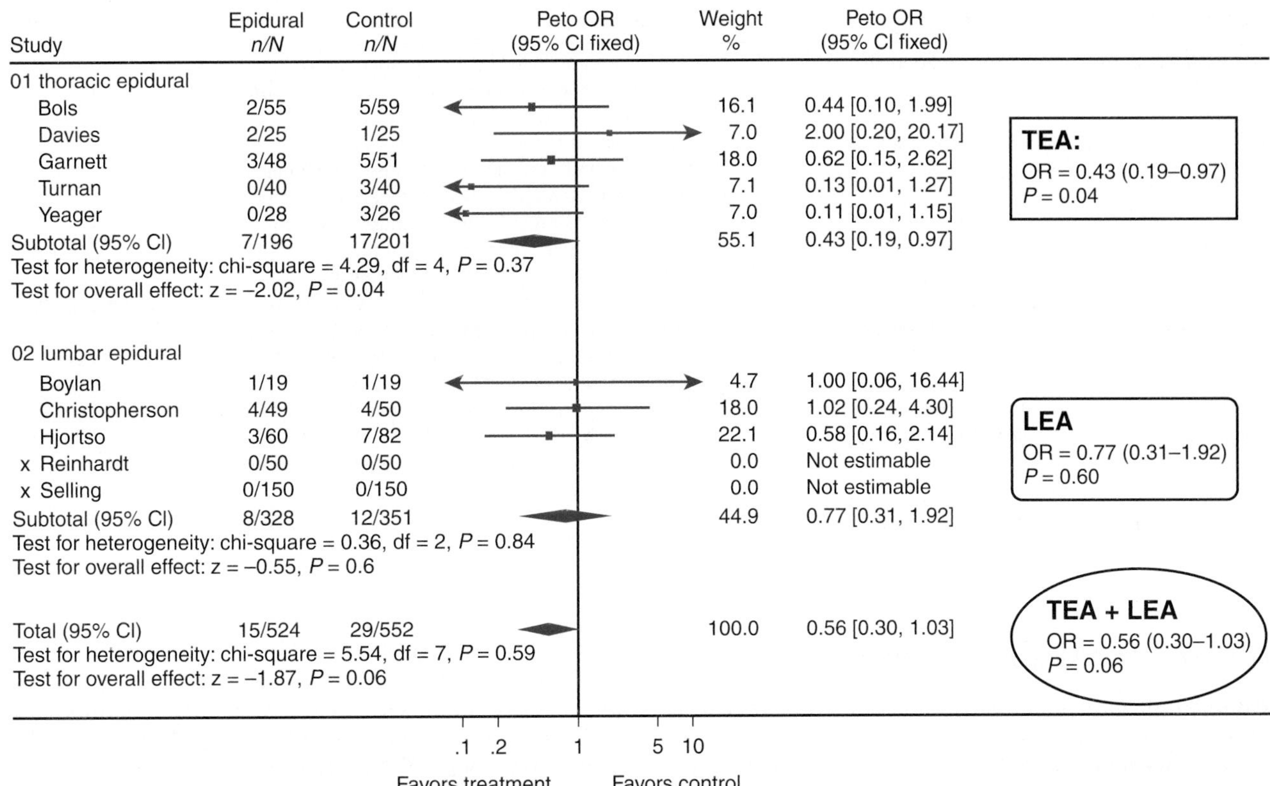

Figure 18.2 Epidural local analgesia versus opioids in patients with myocardial infarction. LEA, lumbar epidural analgesia; OR, odds ratio; TEA, thoracic epidural analgesia. (Redawn from Beattie WS, Badner NH, Choi P. Epidural analgesia reduces postoperative myocardial infarction: a meta-analysis. *Anesth Analg*. 2001;93:853-858.)

provide effective postoperative analgesia in an appropriately monitored setting (Table 18.4).[131] It is essential that the dose of neuraxial opioid be reduced with use in older patients.[132]

Although some studies indicate that the incidence of pulmonary and cardiovascular comorbidity may be lower with neuraxial morphine than with systemic opioids,[133-136] the overall benefit is observed only when compared with intermittent IV doses and not when compared with IV infusion of opioids.[124,137,138] Neuraxial opioids are associated with side effects that could affect patients' quality of recovery. Side effects include nausea and vomiting in more than 50% of patients[139,140] and pruritus in up to 60%,[31] as opposed to 15% to 18% for PCEA with local anesthetic or systemic opioids.[141,142] Other adverse effects include urinary retention in up to 80% of patients and respiratory depression in 0.2% to 1.9%.[140] These side effects are not limited to any specific opioid, and it is not clear whether their incidence is dose dependent. Both early and late respiratory depression can occur with neuraxial opioids. Most reported respiratory depression occurs with morphine because of its hydrophilic nature and cephalic CSF spread.[143] PCEA with combined local anesthetic and neuraxial opioids results in a low incidence of respiratory depression that varies from 0.07% to 0.4%,[144-146] thus making PCEA relatively safe to use in an unmonitored hospital setting.

EXTENDED-RELEASE EPIDURAL MORPHINE

Extended-release epidural morphine (EREM) incorporates new technology in which microscopic particles consisting of numerous morphine-containing vesicles are each separated from adjacent chambers by naturally occurring lipid membranes. EREM provides a longer duration of postoperative analgesia than does traditionally available formulations but without the need for indwelling epidural catheters.[147] Preliminary randomized controlled trials have indicated that EREM provides significant postoperative analgesia for up to 48 hours after hip and abdominal surgery.[41,42] This modality appears to have a dose-dependent relationship for decreased oxygen saturation, with 20- and 25-mg doses being associated with higher rates of desaturation.[41] Clinicians should not freeze, aggressively agitate, or shake the EREM vials. In addition, one should not administer any other agents in the epidural space around the time of EREM administration because an increased peak serum concentration of morphine may result. Side effects of EREM are mainly pruritus and respiratory depression, which requires treatment with opioid antagonists in 12.5% of patients.[147-149]

Neuraxial analgesic agents, given as a single shot or as a continuous epidural infusion, provide effective postoperative analgesia (see Table 18.5). The choice of a particular technique should be made on an individual basis. The risks and benefits of a particular technique should be weighed for each specific patient.

Table 18.4 Neuraxial Analgesic Options and Considerations

Technique	Examples	Considerations and Comments
Neuraxial, lipophilic opioid	Fentanyl, sufentanil	Limited rostral spread after intrathecal injection Respiratory depression unlikely but pruritus possible Safely combined with local anesthetics
Neuraxial, hydrophilic opioid	Morphine, hydromorphone	Rostral spread after neuraxial injection Neuraxial and/or systemic analgesic mechanism Postoperative respiratory monitoring recommended Respiratory depression and pruritus common Limited analgesic mechanism (24 hr) Safely combined with local anesthetics
Continuous epidural analgesia	Combinations of low-concentration local anesthetics and opioids	Fixed-rate infusion, patient-controlled boluses, or combinations of both More efficacious analgesia than IV PCA Follow ASRA guidelines for anticoagulation when used during perioperative anticoagulation
Extended-release epidural opioid	Extended-release epidural morphine	Pruritus and respiratory depression requiring treatment with opioid antagonists Should not administer any other agents in the epidural space

ASRA, American Society of Regional Anesthesia; IV PCA, intravenous patient-controlled analgesia.

PERIPHERAL OR PERINEURAL ANALGESIA

The number of ambulatory procedures performed in North America has increased significantly, and the cost-saving benefit of minimizing patients' hospital stays has gained importance. With the goals of same-day discharge, reduction in hospital length of stay, and improvement in postsurgical outcomes, many anesthesiologists routinely use multimodal analgesia with peripheral techniques. A variety of peripheral regional techniques can be used to enhance postoperative pain control while reducing side effects. Among these techniques are local anesthetic wound infiltration[150,151]; brachial, lumbar, and sacral plexus blocks; and nonepidural truncal blocks (paravertebral, transabdominal, and rectus sheath blocks). Peripheral analgesic techniques are important for facilitating cost savings in ambulatory surgery centers, especially when phase 1 recovery bypass is achieved[152,153] and unplanned admissions are reduced.[152,154] Peripheral regional analgesia delivered as a single injection or as a continuous infusion through a perineural catheter (PNC) provides analgesia superior to that with systemic opioids or epidural analgesia and is associated with minimal side effects,[110,154-158] better rehabilitation,[159,160] and shorter hospital stay.[161] Use of a PNC in the lower extremity provides analgesia equal to that of an epidural with minimal side effects (hypotension, urinary retention, and inability to ambulate).[162] Regardless of location, the analgesia provided through a PNC is superior to that of single-shot blocks, epidural analgesia, intra-articular analgesia, and IV PCA.[162-164]

The number of complex orthopedic procedures such as joint replacement has increased tremendously in the last 2 decades and is expected to continue to increase as the population advances in age.[165] Joint replacement, which is well known to improve a patient's quality of life, typically causes severe pain in the immediate postoperative period and thus interferes with physical rehabilitation. Multimodal analgesia and the use of a PNC as the main techniques for control of pain have been shown to provide better analgesia, earlier passive joint movement,[166] and earlier discharge home with adequate joint movement.[166,167] A large series of hospital patients and outpatients treated with a PNC reported minimal clinician interventions and clinical adverse effects[168,169] during treatment. With adequate instructions and phone access to health care providers, patients were able to manage their pain at home[168,170,171] and remove the PNC without need for a hospital visit. More studies are needed before home use of a PNC becomes a widely applicable standard of care.

Techniques for peripheral single-injection or PNC analgesia vary among practitioners and include a paresthesia technique, peripheral nerve stimulation, and ultrasound-guided regional anesthesia (UGRA). Although evidence regarding the safety of UGRA is currently limited in comparison to what is known about nerve stimulation,[172] it is becoming the technique of choice for most single-injection and continuous-infusion techniques.

Studies have shown that when compared with nerve stimulation, use of UGRA for upper or lower extremity blocks and placement of catheters offers a faster onset of sensory blockade and a greater block success rate. UGRA has also been shown to achieve faster block performance, require fewer needle passes, and induce less block-related discomfort, thus making this technique better received by patients.[173-176]

Local anesthetics are the main analgesics used for peripheral blocks and in continuous-infusion catheters. Drugs with an intermediate duration of action, such as lidocaine and mepivacaine,[177,178] are commonly used for blocks, whereas long-acting drugs such as ropivacaine, bupivacaine, and levobupivacaine are used mainly for continuous infusion.[179] Some data suggest that bupivacaine and levobupivacaine are more potent than ropivacaine[180,181]; therefore, the ropivacaine concentration is often increased to compensate. However, ropivacaine, bupivacaine, and levobupivacaine have provided similar analgesic profiles in human trials.[180,182,183]

Several medications are infrequently added to the local anesthetic to improve perineural analgesia. Although there are reports of opioids being added,[184-186] insufficient evidence is available to draw any conclusion regarding the efficacy of this practice.[187,188] Clonidine has been reported to prolong the duration of perineural analgesia,[159,184,185,189] but randomized controlled studies have failed to demonstrate any clinical benefit.[190-192] Epinephrine is commonly used in blocks to detect inadvertent intravascular injection, but it is rarely used in a continuous infusion because it causes prolonged vasoconstriction.[193-196] Other adjuvants have been reported, but none are currently approved for perineural use in humans because of systemic side effects.[197,198]

In summary,

- Continuous neuraxial techniques provide superior analgesia and better patient outcomes, including those related to major morbidity.
- Many factors affect the overall outcomes of continuous epidural analgesia, including the congruency of epidural catheter location and placement of the surgical incision and the type of analgesic regimen.
- Neuraxial opioids provide postoperative pain control when administered alone or in combination with local anesthetics.
- Peripheral or perineural regional techniques provide pain control superior to that with systemic opioids or epidural analgesia and are associated with minimal side effects.
- Perineural continuous analgesia is beneficial in complex orthopedic procedures and is used as part of multimodal analgesia in the perioperative setting.

BRACHIAL PLEXUS BLOCKS

Nerve conduction in the brachial plexus (Fig. 18.3) can be blocked at many levels to provide anesthesia and postoperative analgesia during and after surgical procedures on the upper extremity (Table 18.5). Use of UGRA may increase the overall success rate when compared with nerve stimulation or other methods.[199] UGRA techniques for the brachial plexus may allow patients to receive the best anesthetic and analgesic effect with less local anesthetic volume and minimal side effects. An analysis of neurologic complications in 1000 UGRA procedures for elective orthopedic surgery showed that the rate of postoperative neurologic symptoms was very similar to that previously reported for traditional techniques.[200] The incidence of nerve injury from a peripheral nerve block (PNB) has been estimated to be 0.4 per 1000 PNBs based on large prospective audits.[201] Use of PNCs or perineural continuous infusion of local anesthetic is being advocated when prolonged analgesia of the arm is needed. PNCs could be used in the hospital setting or in an ambulatory setting as a home PNC. Insertion of a PNC may be facilitated by using paresthesia, nerve stimulation, or ultrasound guidance.[202]

Interscalene Block

The gold standard technique for shoulder and upper arm procedures is the interscalene block (ISB). The interscalene groove is commonly approached through an anterolateral technique. A posterior approach to the brachial plexus remains underused despite its effectiveness in securing a continuous interscalene block (CISB) catheter.[203,204] The interscalene approach typically provides a complete block for the superior and middle trunk, but the inferior trunk is often blocked incompletely, thus making this approach unsuitable for forearm and hand procedures. For elbow procedures, the ISB is frequently supplemented by other nerve blocks such as the intercostobrachial, medial cutaneous and medial antebrachial cutaneous, and ulnar.

A single-injection ISB provides analgesia superior to that of systemic opioids. A reduction in verbal pain scale scores of greater than 50%[205-207] and a reduction in total opioid requirement[205-208] have been reported. CISB for shoulder surgery provides better analgesia than placebo or systemic opioids do and is associated with less opioid consumption and fewer opioid-related side effects.[184,209-213] CISB with perineural infusion of local anesthetic has been shown to benefit patient rehabilitation[214] and can be continued at home with a portable infusion pump.[215] In a randomized controlled study, Ilfeld and colleagues[166] showed that ambulatory CISB with perineural infusion of 0.2% ropivacaine decreased the time until readiness for discharge after total shoulder arthroplasty by allowing good shoulder range of motion and providing adequate pain control without parenteral opioids. When compared with ISB for moderate to severe outpatient shoulder procedures, 2-day CISB provided better pain control, reduced opioid requirements, improved sleep quality, and increased patient satisfaction.[216] In the last decade, the UGRA technique for ISB has become more popular than the nerve stimulator technique. It provides a better block profile, has a faster onset and longer duration, requires fewer needles, and is associated with better patient satisfaction. Moreover, it has not sacrificed patient safety or increased the incidence of neurologic complications.[217-219]

Concomitant phrenic nerve block occurs after brachial plexus block at the interscalene level, especially at the C6 level, because of its close proximity (2 to 4 mm) to the plexus.[220] Blocking the brachial plexus at this level should be considered with great caution if a patient has respiratory insufficiency or chronic obstructive pulmonary disease. Some investigators have shown no difference in hemidiaphragmatic paresis after a reduction in local anesthetic volume of up to 10 mL at the ISB when ultrasound was used.[221] Others are trying to identify the minimum effective local anesthetic volume necessary to provide postoperative analgesia with minimal side effects.[219,222] Although the local anesthetic volume needed for ultrasound-guided ISB may be reduced, the optimal volume for analgesia still remains to be determined. For shoulder procedures, the addition of tramadol or dexamethasone as an adjuvant to local anesthetic prolongs the duration of analgesia.[223,224]

Recently, different ultrasound approaches have been tried in an attempt to block the brachial plexus at the interscalene groove. No difference in block onset time or block quality was observed when intraplexus injection of local anesthetics or periplexus blocks were used.[225] A low approach to the brachial plexus resulted in more distal spread of sensory and motor coverage than when the traditional approach was used.[226]

Supraclavicular Block

The supraclavicular block is considered the spinal of the arm. This block is associated with the greatest blockade of the brachial plexus at the trunk and division level where all the trunks are compact and can be achieved with a single injection of local anesthetic. At lower volumes of

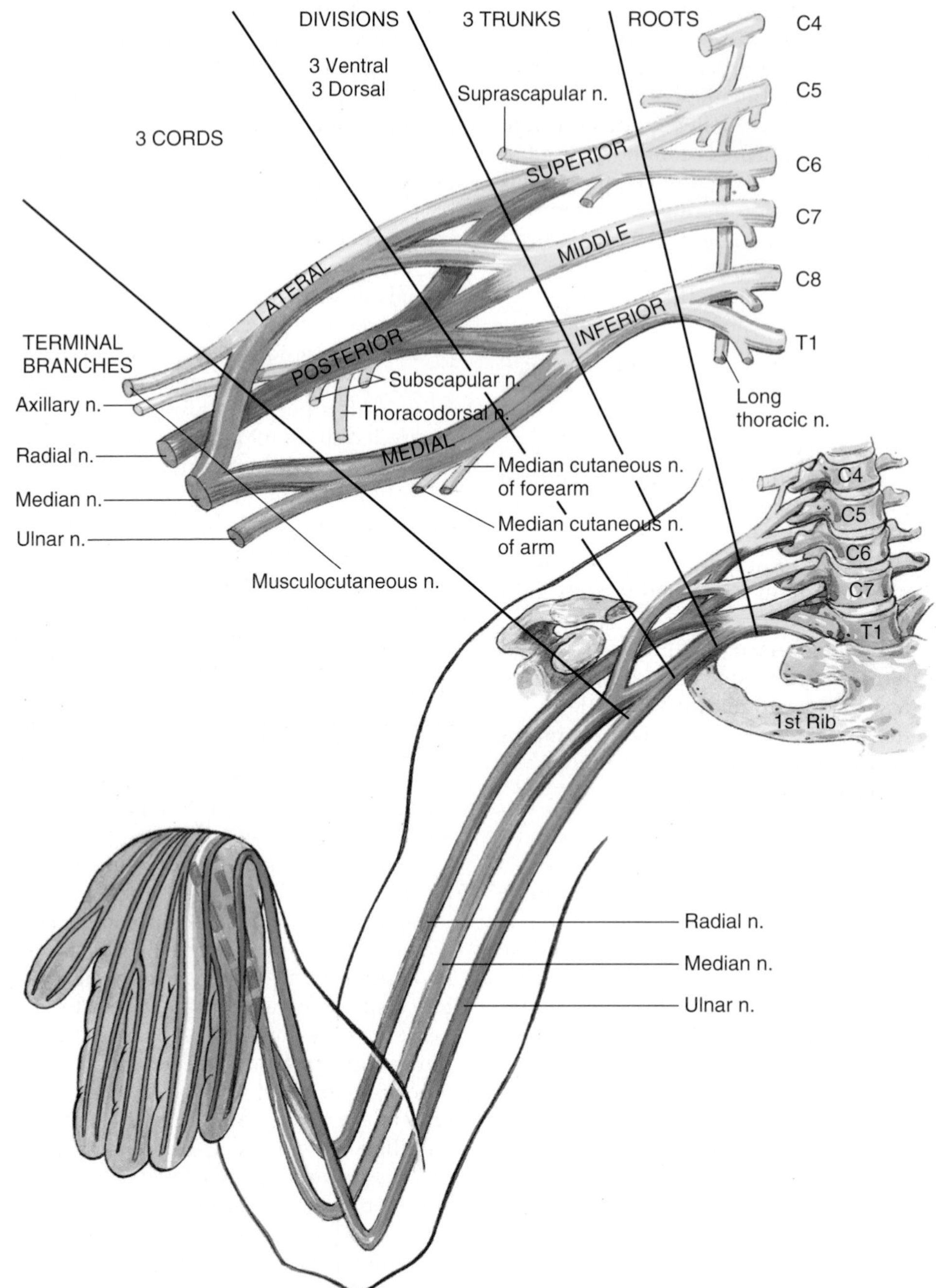

Figure 18.3 Brachial plexus anatomy. (From Brown D. *Atlas of Regional Anesthesia*. Philadelphia: Saunders; 2010.)

local anesthestic, the supraclavicular block misses the dorsal scapular nerve, which arises from the root of C5, and also misses the superficial cervical plexus. Unless the local anesthesic tracks proximally toward the interscalene region, this block may be inadequate for shoulder surgery, but it provides adequate block for upper arm surgery. As with the ISB, supplemental blocks are required for elbow procedures (i.e., intercostobrachial). Of all the brachial plexus blocks, the supraclavicular block has the highest risk for pneumothorax, especially when done with the traditional "plumb bob" technique. Some recent studies have shown that the calculated volume of local anesthetic required for an ultrasound-guided supraclavicular block does not seem to differ from the conventionally recommended volume required for supraclavicular blocks performed with non–ultrasound-based nerve localization techniques.[227] The minimum effective volume of 1.5% lidocaine with 5 µg/mL epinephrine was 32 mL.[228] Multiple studies have confirmed that when UGRA is used, a single injection offers the same clinical profile and analgesic benefit as two injections.[229,230]

Infraclavicular Block

Like the supraclavicular block, the infraclavicular block also approaches the brachial plexus where it is compact

Table 18.5 Upper Extremity Block Considerations

Technique	Agents	Indication	Considerations and Comments
A: Interscalene single injection B: Interscalene continuous infusion	All upper extremity blocks except Bier blocks are amenable to most LAs. Choice of agent based on duration of anesthesia and postoperative analgesia	A: Procedures on the shoulder and proximal aspect of the upper part of the arm and clavicle B: Procedures on the shoulder and proximal aspect of the upper part of the arm requiring prolonged analgesia	Blocks the brachial plexus at the root/trunk level NS- or US-guided techniques Cervical paravertebral approach, lateral approach Inferior trunk is commonly missed (ulnar nerve sparing) Ipsilateral phrenic nerve block expected 100% of the time Intraplexus and periplexus injections have similar clinical profile
A: Supraclavicular single injection B: Supraclavicular continuous infusion	A: Choice of agent based on goal duration of anesthesia and analgesia B: Ropivacaine 0.2% or bupivacaine 0.125% ± opioid	Procedures on the upper extremity (shoulder to hand, depending on volume of the LA)	Blocks the brachial plexus at the trunk/division level NS- or US-guided techniques Described as "the spinal of the arm" Pneumothorax risk higher with the NS technique Superficial cervical plexus and posterior scapular nerve are commonly missed Single injection has similar clinical profile as multiple injections
A: Infraclavicular single injection B: Continuous infusion		Procedures on the midhumerus and below	Blocks the brachial plexus at the division level NS- or US-guided techniques More reliable blockade of the musculocutaneous and axillary nerves than the axillary block Single injection posterior to the axillary artery has similar clinical profile as multiple injections The most stable catheter is in the brachial plexus
A: Axillary single injection B: Continuous infusion		Procedures on the elbow and distal to it	Blocks the brachial plexus at the level of terminal branches NS- or US-guided techniques Targeting individual branches has a clinical profile superior to that of a single injection The musculocutaneous nerve is commonly missed with a single injection
IV regional (Bier)	Lidocaine (0.5%)	Procedures on the forearm and distal to it	Used only for intraoperative surgical pain Need to supplement for postoperative analgesia Risk for LA toxicity if early discontinuation of the tourniquet

IV, intravenous; LA, local anesthetic; NS, nerve stimulator; US, ultrasound.

(Fig. 18.4), at the level of the cords. This block can be used for procedures involving the elbow, forearm, and hand. It is especially useful in patients unable to abduct their shoulder to allow access to the axilla. A single injection or a continuous-infusion catheter placed with this technique provides effective analgesia.[231-234] This approach also results in the most secure catheter insertion site of all brachial plexus blocks. This block has two main approaches—the traditional perivascular infraclavicular approach and the coracoid approach.[235] They provide similar results, but the coracoid approach is associated with less risk for pneumothorax. For outpatient wrist and hand surgery, Hadzic and colleagues[234] compared the use of a chloroprocaine infraclavicular nerve block with general anesthesia induced with volatile agents. They found that general anesthesia with volatile agents led to increased postanesthesia care unit admissions (vs. phase 1 recovery bypass), higher reports of postoperative pain, longer time to ambulation, and longer time to same-day discharge. Chelly and coworkers[231] stated that PNB catheters are probably indicated for implantation procedures after trauma, as well as for open reduction and internal fixation of the hand or digits, although a prospective randomized trial to definitively verify this intuitive concept may be difficult to conduct. Ilfeld and colleagues[233] showed that use of a continuous infraclavicular brachial plexus catheter resulted in less postoperative dynamic pain and opioid consumption and fewer sleep disturbances than did placebo catheter infusion. The surgical procedures performed included open reduction and internal fixation (elbow, radius, or ulna), bony and capsular wrist procedures (carpectomy, capsulodesis, fusion, or shrinkage), metacarpal arthroplasty, suspensionplasty, and ulnar nerve transposition.

An infraclavicular brachial plexus block for regional anesthesia of the lower part of the arm has efficacy comparable to that of other brachial plexus blocks. This block has a lower likelihood of tourniquet pain during surgery and provides more reliable blockade of the musculocutaneous and axillary nerves than does a single-injection axillary block.[236] Many investigators have confirmed that when using UGRA for an infraclavicular block, a single injection

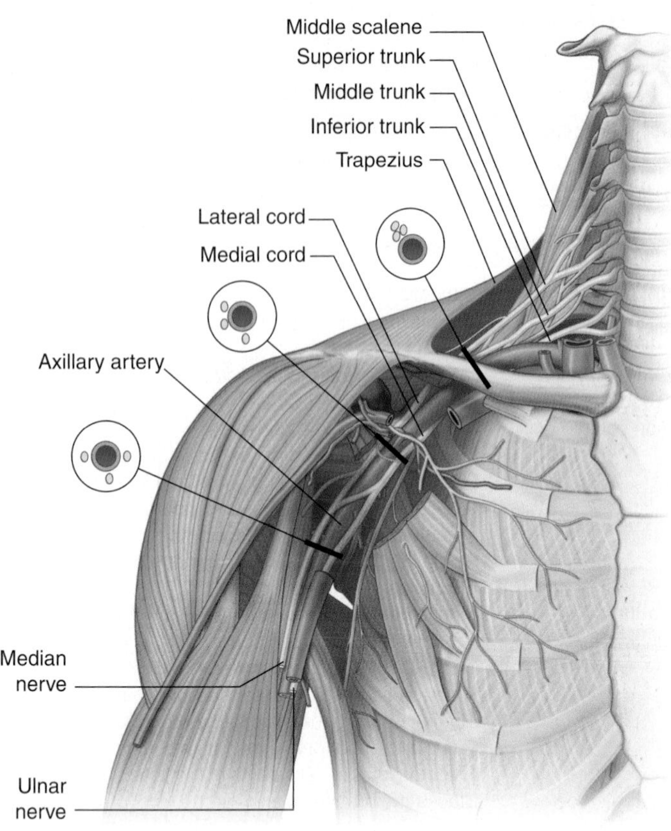

Figure 18.4 Infraclavicular anatomy. (From Wells M. *Local and Regional Anaesthesia in the Emergency Department Made Easy*. Philadelphia: Churchill Livingstone; 2010.)

of local anesthetic posterior to the axillary artery is as effective as multiple injections.[237-239] A randomized comparison of infraclavicular and supraclavicular PNCs for postoperative analgesia showed that local anesthetic infusion via an infraclavicular PNC provides analgesia superior to that via a supraclavicular PNC.[240]

Axillary Block

This block produces the most effective block for all surgical procedures on and distal to the elbow, but it requires supplementation for the tourniquet (intercostobrachial, medial brachial cutaneous, and medial antebrachial cutaneous) if it is to be used as a surgical block. Axillary blocks have been shown to reduce postoperative pain scores by more than 50%, decrease the total in-hospital opioid requirement, and lengthen the time until the first analgesic dose.[241,242] The axillary sheath at this level is often discontinuous, and the block should target the individual terminal branches. A nerve stimulator can be used to identify all the individual components and to obtain a consistently effective block.[243-245] A small study demonstrated that each terminal branch can be targeted under ultrasound guidance with as little as 1 mL of 2% lidocaine with 1:200,000 epinephrine per nerve to provide a fast onset and surgical anesthesia.[246] The traditional transarterial and single-injection techniques can often miss the musculocutaneous nerve (C5-6); therefore, that nerve should be specifically sought and blocked. It can be visualized in the corocobrachialas muscle and traced proximally to the axillary artery under ultrasound guidance.

Intravenous (Bier) Block

The mechanism of IV regional anesthesia (IV RA) is generally accepted to involve diffusion from veins to small nerves and nerve endings after exsanguination. IV regional blocks for the upper extremity, which use a proximal arm tourniquet or double tourniquet, have been well described. IV regional blocks for the lower extremity have been reviewed as well.[247] Traditional IV regional techniques that use a single- or double-tourniquet technique for the lower extremity may carry a high failure rate,[248] in which case supplementation by the surgeon or conversion to general anesthesia is required. Of potential interest, however, is an intercuff technique for IV RA that has been developed for use in knee surgery in an effort to produce better localization and reduce overall dosing requirements.[249,250]

Opioids (other than meperidine, 30 mg or more) are generally considered not to be beneficial when given via the IV regional technique[251]; systemic side effects of meperidine are manifested at the 30-mg threshold. Tramadol, 100 mg, administered as IV RA with lidocaine is associated with a self-limited rash below the tourniquet and does not necessarily confer an analgesic benefit.[252] In addition, tramadol has not been shown to improve block or postoperative analgesic quality when coadministered with ropivacaine.[253]

Less controversial additives to IV RA appear to have the potential to provide intraoperative tourniquet tolerance, postoperative analgesia, or both. Ketorolac can achieve both end points when the tourniquet is applied to both the upper and lower parts of the arm. Its use for this purpose is generally accepted, with no basis at this time for exceeding a 20-mg dose in adults.[251] Clonidine at a dose of 1 μg/kg is accepted to improve tourniquet tolerance and reduce postoperative analgesic requirements with minimal side effects. Dexmedetomidine (0.5 mg/kg) has also shown benefit.[254] Ketamine at a dose of 100 μg/kg has also been shown to improve tourniquet tolerance and reduce postoperative analgesic requirements

Table 18.6 Lower Extremity Block Considerations

Technique	Agents	Indication	Considerations and Comments
A: Lumbar plexus block B: Continuous infusion	All lower extremity blocks except Bier blocks are amenable to most LAs. Choice of agent based on duration of anesthesia and postoperative analgesia	A: Procedures on the hip, thigh, and knee. B: Procedures on the hip, thigh, femur, and knee requiring prolonged analgesia	Reliable way to block the femoral, lateral femoral cutaneous, and obturator nerves with a single injection NS- or US-guided techniques Ensure a quadriceps twitch without a foot twitch and without an obturator (hip adduction) twitch to reduce the chance of unwanted epidural spread Cause weakness of the psoas muscle (hip flexion) and hip adduction The fascia iliaca is the anterior approach for LPB
A: Femoral block B: Continuous infusion	A: Choice of agent based on goal duration of anesthesia and analgesia B: Ropivacaine 0.2% or bupivacaine 0.125% ± opioid	A: Procedures on the anterior aspect of the thigh, femur, and knee B: Procedures on the anterior aspect of the thigh, femur, and knee requiring prolonged analgesia	Simple and easy to perform Commonly combined with sciatic single-injection or catheter techniques NS- or US-guided techniques Preserves hip adduction and psoas-mediated hip flexion
Saphenous nerve		Procedures on the knee and medial aspect of the ankle Saphenous (midthigh) used with knee procedures	Sensory continuation of the femoral nerve Supplies the medial aspect of the leg, ankle, and foot US-guided techniques or subcutaneous infiltration
Obturator nerve		Infrequently used in knee arthroplasty Bilateral obturator is used for urologic procedures	Gives motor branches to the adductors of the thigh, sensory branches to medial part of the thigh, and less than 5% to the knee joint
A: Proximal sciatic approaches B: Continuous infusion		A: Procedures on the hip, posterior aspect of the thigh, and posterior aspect of the knee B: Procedures on the hip, posterior aspect of the thigh, and posterior aspect of the knee requiring prolonged analgesia	Approaches include parasacral, gluteal (e.g., Labat), subgluteal, lateral, and anterior NS- or US-guided techniques Parasacral and gluteal approaches used for hip procedures Subgluteal used for knee procedures Cause hamstring weakness
A: Distal sciatic approaches B: Continuous infusion		A: Procedures below the knee and ankle B: Procedures below the knee and ankle requiring prolonged analgesia	NS- or US-guided techniques Common peroneal and tibial blocked at the bifurcation Avoid hamstring weakness

LA, local anesthetic; LPB, lumbar plexus block; NS, nerve stimulator; US, ultrasound.

in a manner that appears to be more potent than 1 μg/kg clonidine.[255] When compared with plain lidocaine, dexamethasone (8 mg) was recently shown to reduce postoperative analgesic requirements during the first 24 hours after surgery.[256] Given the multiple mechanisms that contribute to postoperative pain, the logical future study would involve a step-function assessment of serial additives and combinations of ketorolac, clonidine or dexmedetomidine, ketamine, and dexamethasone. The coadministered local anesthetic (0.5% lidocaine or 0.1% to 0.2% ropivacaine) is unlikely to influence results with respect to duration of postoperative analgesia beyond the recovery room period.[257]

Complications with IV RA are very uncommon. Seizures have been reported after deflation of the tourniquet with a tourniquet time as long as 60 minutes and with lidocaine at its lowest effective dose (1.5 mg/kg). Several cases of compartment syndrome have also been reported.[258]

In summary,

- Interscalene analgesia is the gold standard technique for shoulder and upper arm procedures. Phrenic nerve paresis is a common side effect.
- Supraclavicular analgesia is considered the spinal of the brachial plexus. It provides an adequate block for upper arm surgery; supplemental blocks are required for elbow procedures. It is associated with a risk for pneumothorax.
- Infraclavicular analgesia can be used for procedures involving the elbow, forearm, or hand. It provides the most secure catheter insertion site.
- Axillary analgesia produces the most effective block for all surgical procedures on the elbow, forearm, and hand. Supplemental blocks are required, especially musculocutaneous.
- IV (Bier) regional analgesia is well described in the upper extremity but used less frequently in the lower extremity.

LOWER EXTREMITY BLOCKS

For patients undergoing surgical procedures on the lower extremity, nerve conduction in the lumbar and sacral plexuses can be blocked at many levels for anesthesia and postoperative analgesia (Table 18.6). The nerve supply to the lower extremity is derived from two nerve plexuses arising from the ventral rami of the spinal nerve roots of the lower

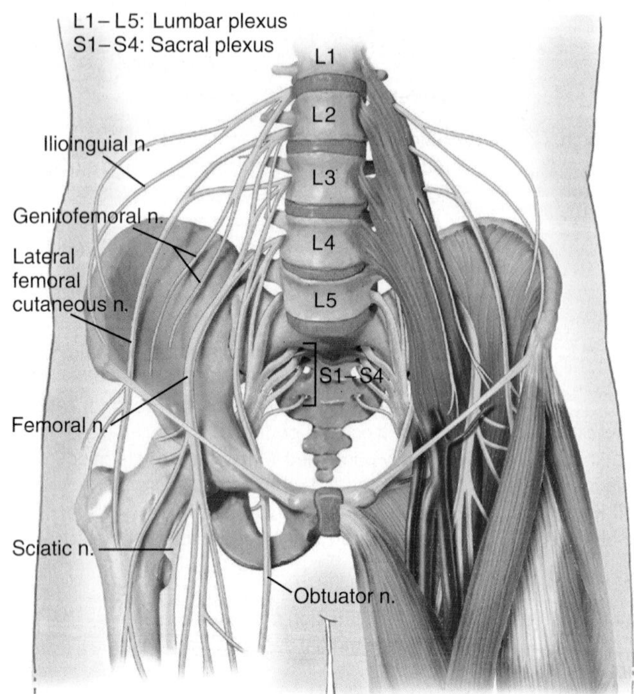

Figure 18.5 Lower extremity anatomy. (Courtesy of Mayo Foundation.)

spinal cord (Fig. 18.5)—the lumbar plexus (L1-4) and the sacral plexus (L4-5, S1-3). The lumbar plexus gives rise to the femoral nerve (L2-4), the obturator nerve (L2-4), the lateral femoral cutaneous nerve (L2-3), and three other branches that supply the inguinal and genital areas (iliohypogastric, ilioinguinal, and genitofemoral nerves). The sacral plexus gives rise to the sciatic nerve (L4-5, S1-3) and provides branches that supply the musculature around the hip and pelvis.

Lumbar Plexus Block

Because the main nerves supplying the hip joint are the femoral and obturator nerves, this block (either single shot or continuous infusion) provides adequate postoperative analgesia for procedures involving the hip joint, including total joint replacement and repair of hip fractures. In a randomized clinical trial of patients undergoing hip hemiarthroplasty under general anesthesia, Turker and colleagues[259] compared the use of continuous infusion from a lumbar plexus catheter with the use of an epidural catheter. They found that patients who received a lumbar plexus catheter had less motor block, ambulated sooner, and experienced significantly fewer overall complications. More than a decade ago investigators reported that for patients undergoing total hip arthroplasty, those who received lumbar plexus single-injection blocks had less pain and less blood loss during and after surgery than did those who did not receive the block.[260] Others reported that in elderly patients with hip fractures, those who received lumbar plexus and parasacral blocks (vs. general anesthesia) exhibited significantly less hypotension during surgery, had fewer intensive care unit admissions (0/30 vs. 11/30), and had a shorter length of hospital stay (7 vs. 14 days).[261]

A lumbar plexus block also provides excellent postoperative analgesia for most invasive knee procedures such as anterior cruciate ligament (ACL) reconstruction, multiligament reconstruction, or total knee arthroplasty (TKA).[262] Matheny and colleagues[263] found that the opioid requirement after arthroscopic ACL reconstruction was 89% lower in the group that received a continuous lumbar plexus block than in those who had IV PCA. However, a femoral nerve block in the groin is much simpler and easier to perform than a lumbar plexus block and provides equally efficacious analgesia for invasive knee procedures[264] in which obturator nerve coverage is not relevant. In a randomized triple-masked trial, Ilfeld and colleagues[167] compared the use of an overnight lumbar plexus catheter with use of the catheter for four nights in patients who had undergone hip arthroplasty. They found that use of the catheter for four nights decreased the time that patients needed to reach discharge criteria by 38% but did not significantly increase ambulation distance.

Femoral Nerve Block

Like the lumbar plexus block, a femoral nerve block provides excellent postoperative analgesia for invasive procedures around the knee (excluding the posterior aspect of the knee). Unlike the lumbar plexus block, a femoral nerve block preserves hip adduction and psoas-mediated hip flexion. A femoral block must often be supplemented with a single-shot or continuous sciatic nerve block for procedures such as TKA[265] or ACL reconstruction with a hamstring autograft.[154] Many randomized controlled studies that have compared UGRA, peripheral nerve stimulation, and loss-of-resistance techniques for the femoral nerve suggest that the ultrasound technique could offer faster onset of sensory loss and longer analgesia with less local anesthetic volume.[266-268]

In the late 1990s, two studies from Europe examined rehabilitation outcomes after total knee replacement when a continuous femoral block (CFB) was used. When compared with IV PCA, CFB led not only to better pain relief but also to significantly better knee flexion, faster achievement of ambulation goals, and overall faster convalescence.[159,160] Patients who received CFB infusions experienced fewer side effects than did epidural patients in both studies, and patients in the CFB groups were discharged home from inpatient rehabilitation units 20% sooner than were patients in the IV PCA groups.[159,160]

In the United States, a similar anesthetic treatment method was applied to patients undergoing total knee replacement.[269] All patients underwent general anesthesia and were randomized to receive IV PCA, epidural infusion, or single-injection femoral-sciatic blocks followed by a continuous femoral infusion. Continuous femoral infusion patients (vs. IV PCA patients) had a 72% reduction in postoperative bleeding ($P = 0.05$), achieved better performance on continuous passive motion, had a 90% decrease in serious complications (including less blood loss), ambulated sooner (2.5 vs. 3.5 days), and had a 20% decrease in the length of hospitalization (4 vs. 5.5 days).[269] In 2010, a meta-analysis of 23 randomized controlled trials showed that a femoral nerve single block or continuous infusion provides better analgesic outcomes after TKA than does IV PCA.[270] A continuous femoral nerve block after TKA was associated with lower opioid consumption and better functional recovery at 6 weeks than periarticular infiltration was.[271]

A continuous femoral nerve block is an acceptable analgesic alternative to a continuous posterior lumbar plexus block for hip arthroplasty when a stimulating PNC is used. However, patients who receive continuous femoral catheters might experience more motor block, thus making ambulation suboptimal.[272]

Fascia Iliaca Block

The fascia iliaca compartment block was mainly described for the pediatric population in 1989[273] and was widely reported to provide good analgesia for hip and knee procedures in adolescents and adults.[274] In 2008, Dolan and colleagues[275] compared the use of UGRA for this block with the traditional fascial loss of resistant (LOR) technique for postoperative analgesia in hip and knee arthroplasty. They found that when compared with the LOR technique, use of UGRA significantly increased the block success rate, especially at the medial aspect of the thigh (95% versus 60%), and increased the percentage of patients in whom the femoral, obturator, and lateral cutaneous nerves were all completely blocked (82% vs. 47%).

Sciatic Nerve Block

Proximal sciatic nerve blocks are most often used as an adjunct to femoral or lumbar plexus blocks for painful procedures around the hip or knee, as discussed earlier,[154] but they can also provide excellent analgesia for all major foot and ankle procedures (especially when a thigh tourniquet is planned).

In patients undergoing TKA, continuous sciatic nerve blocks provide greater analgesia, decrease morphine request, and improve early rehabilitation when compared with the use of single-injection sciatic nerve block or lumbar plexus blocks.[276] Studies that have examined subgluteal continuous sciatic nerve blockade for orthopedic ankle and foot surgery have reported significant reductions in visual analog pain scores.[277,278] Similarly, continuous sciatic nerve blockade has shown significant analgesic benefit in patients undergoing below-knee amputation.[279] Use of a proximal sciatic nerve block for distal foot and ankle procedures is often limited by concerns of hamstring muscle weakness.[280]

Studies that have compared UGRA of the sciatic nerve with peripheral nerve stimulation techniques[281,282] have shown that UGRA has a higher sensory block success rate and requires less local anesthetic and less time to perform. Insufficient data are available to compare the block failure rate and the actual duration of sensory blockade between the two techniques.[174]

Popliteal Fossa Sciatic Nerve Block

The nerve can be blocked from the posterior or lateral approach, although the lateral approach may be superior when there are concerns regarding patient positioning.[283-285] A popliteal fossa block provides effective postoperative analgesia for all foot and ankle procedures (assuming that the saphenous nerve is concomitantly blocked). It also preserves hamstring function, thus facilitating ambulation.[280]

Effectiveness of the popliteal sciatic block for outpatient foot and ankle procedures was demonstrated by McLeod and colleagues.[285] They compared the lateral popliteal fossa block with an ankle block[286] and with subcutaneous infiltration of local anesthetics.[284] The popliteal fossa block provided longer postoperative analgesia.[287] When the UGRA technique is used, blocking the tibial and common peroneal nerves in the popliteal fossa separately at the bifurcation provides a faster onset than does a prebifurcation sciatic block.[288]

Continuous popliteal sciatic nerve catheters were first introduced by Singelyn and colleagues, who described a challenging Seldinger (catheter-over-guidewire) technique for catheter placement and achieved a 92% success rate.[289] Since then, authors have repeatedly found that continuous-infusion nerve blocks lead to excellent analgesic outcomes when compared with single-injection blocks or placebo catheters.[290-292] Ultrasound guidance may reduce the time required for placement of popliteal-sciatic PNCs and result in fewer placement failures than when stimulating catheters are used, but analgesia may be mildly better with successfully placed stimulating catheters.[175] Patient satisfaction with block placement was also higher with ultrasound guidance than with the nerve stimulation technique.[176] Adding continuous femoral catheter infusion of ropivacaine to continuous popliteal catheter infusion improved postoperative analgesia during movement after major ankle surgery. This effect was still present 6 months after surgery.[293]

In summary,

- The nerve supply to the lower extremity comes from the lumbar plexus and the sacral plexus.
- Lumbar plexus analgesia provides excellent postoperative analgesia for most invasive hip and knee procedures. It is considered a high-risk block.
- Femoral nerve analgesia provides excellent postoperative analgesia for invasive knee procedures; it is relatively noninvasive and safe.
- A fascia iliaca block is performed via an anterior approach to the lumbar plexus.
- The sciatic nerve can be blocked at various sites along its course (parasacral, subgluteal, and popliteal) to provide analgesia below the knee joint.

TRUNCAL BLOCKS

Paravertebral, Interpleural, and Intercostal

Among truncal blocks (interpleural/intrapleural, paravertebral/extrapleural, and intercostal analgesia), the most effective technique appears to be the paravertebral block.[294] A paravertebral block provides analgesia presumably via direct somatic nerve, sympathetic nerve, or epidural blockade.[294] A paravertebral block can be administered as a single injection or continuous infusion through a catheter. The analgesia provided by paravertebral catheters is superior to that with placebo and may be equal to that of thoracic epidural analgesia.[295] A systematic review of six trials (152 subjects received extrapleural/paravertebral analgesia; 149 received epidural analgesia) indicated that extrapleural/paravertebral catheters provide analgesia that is equivalent to that of thoracic epidural analgesia at 8 to 12 hours postoperatively.

Evidence for the analgesic efficacy of interpleural analgesia is not as compelling as that for paravertebral catheters. When compared with epidural or paravertebral analgesia, interpleural analgesia provides inferior pain control. Moreover, it does not preserve lung function after thoracotomy or reduce the incidence of postoperative pulmonary complications.[296] A systematic review of eight trials (141 subjects received interpleural analgesia; 134 received saline placebo) indicated that interpleural catheters do not provide analgesia that is significantly superior even to placebo.

Intercostal blocks may be another option for postoperative analgesia for thoracic pain. These blocks may be administered by the surgeon at the end of the open thoracic procedure, but they provide only short-term postoperative analgesia that is limited to the duration of action of the local anesthetic injected. Intercostal blocks may be repeated postoperatively, but at the risk of increasing the incidence of pneumothorax (1.4% per nerve blocked with an overall incidence of 8.7% per patient).[297] Intercostal blocks have not been shown to reduce the incidence of pulmonary complications postoperatively when compared with systemic opioids.[297]

Transversus Abdominis Plane Block

Our current understanding of the transversus abdominis plane (TAP) block and its role in postsurgical pain control is limited by the small number of randomized controlled trials. Improved analgesia was noted in patients undergoing laparotomy for colorectal surgery, laparoscopic cholecystectomy, and open and laparoscopic appendectomy.[298-302] Analgesic outcomes were better when 15 mL or more of local anesthetic was used per side versus smaller volumes.[298,301,303-305] Blocks can be achieved by using anatomic landmarks or by ultrasound-guided techniques. Preincisional timing for injection has yet to be tested in randomized trials.[298,299,302,303,306-309] Reported complications include intraperitoneal injection or hemorrhage, transient femoral nerve palsy, and local anesthetic toxicity.[310-312]

In summary,

- A paravertebral (extrapleural) block may be beneficial for thoracic, breast, and upper abdominal surgery and for the treatment of rib fracture pain.
- When compared with epidural or paravertebral analgesia, interpleural analgesia provides inferior pain control and does not preserve lung function after thoracotomy.
- A TAP block has been shown to reduce pain and analgesic requirements after abdominal surgery.
- Our current understanding of the TAP block and its role in postsurgical pain control is still limited.

CONTINUOUS WOUND INFUSION OF LOCAL ANESTHETICS

The mechanisms of action of local anesthetic wound infusions include blockade of nociceptive transmission from the wound surface, inhibition of the local inflammatory response to surgical injury,[313,314] and spinal cord suppression from systemic absorption of local anesthetics.[315] Recently, special wound infusion catheters have become available that can be placed intraoperatively into the wound under direct supervision of the surgeon to infuse local anesthetics, and use of such a technique is an acceptable option as part of multimodal postoperative analgesia.[316,317]

A systematic review of randomized trials that examined the use of continuous wound catheters in multiple surgical procedures consistently demonstrated analgesic efficacy in terms of reduced pain scores and opioid use for all surgical subgroups examined.[150] A total of 39 randomized controlled trials (1761 patients) were included in the final analysis. Overall, when compared with placebo, local anesthetic infusions resulted in a significant decrease of approximately 33% in pain scores of patients both at rest and with activity. Subgroup analysis confirmed the decreased pain scores in patients undergoing all types of surgical procedures except for abdominal surgery. When compared with subjects given placebo, those who were randomized to receive subcutaneous infusions of local anesthetics demonstrated reduced need for opioid rescue and decreased daily opioid consumption, which may have contributed to a reduction in the incidence of nausea in the continuous wound catheter group (21% vs. 39%, odds ratio = 0.42, 95% confidence interval = 0.27 to 0.67). When compared with epidural morphine, continuous wound infusion with ropivacaine for 48 hours after cesarean delivery was associated with better analgesia, lower incidence of side effects, and shorter hospital stay.[318] PCEA with opioids and local anesthetics was superior to patient-controlled local anesthetic wound infusion for laparotomy. The incidence of side effects was similar in both groups.[319]

INTRA-ARTICULAR ANALGESIA

Intra-articular analgesics have been used for more than 2 decades. Despite the many studies published on intra-articular analgesia, the effect of single-agent intra-articular injections on postoperative pain management remains unclear. Combination therapies have been shown to produce maximum benefit with fewer side effects.[320,321]

Intra-articular Morphine

In the intra-articular region, morphine may act on peripheral receptors[322] and through systemic absorption.[323] Morphine, the most commonly used opioid,[324-326] is used intra-articularly at doses of 1 to 5 mg.[323,327] Reductions in pain intensity occur mainly during the first 6 hours after surgery.[322] The results from a meta-analysis indicated that intra-articular morphine provides a definite but mild analgesic effect.[323] This effect is dose dependent, and the possibility of systemic absorption cannot be excluded. Some investigators have reported that postoperative intra-articular morphine is effective only in patients with moderate or severe pain,[327,328] but others support the idea that inflammation is a prerequisite for the peripheral analgesic effectiveness of opioids.[329]

Local anesthetics are considered effective short-term postoperative analgesics, whereas opioids produce more sustained intra-articular analgesia. A study by Marchal and colleagues[329] revealed that patients who had undergone "low inflammatory surgery" received greater short-term (4 to 8 hours) benefit from intra-articular bupivacaine, whereas those who had undergone "high inflammatory surgery" received greater long-term (24 hours) benefit from intra-articular morphine (5 mg).[329]

Intra-articular meperidine is favored by some practitioners because of its *dual opioid and local anesthetic effect.* In the literature, the dose of intra-articular meperidine varies from 50 to 200 mg.[330] Doses greater than 100 mg (which produce a higher circulating concentration of normeperidine) are associated with a higher incidence of side effects (nausea, vomiting, and somnolence).

Intra-articular NSAIDs

Both ketorolac and tenoxicam have shown efficacy when delivered via the intra-articular route. Two studies have demonstrated improved analgesia and ambulation in patients when ketorolac was combined with either morphine[331] or bupivacaine.[332] It was shown that the addition of ketorolac to continuous intra-articular infusion of ropivacaine and morphine led to lower pain scores and less analgesic consumed after ACL reconstruction than when ketolorac was omitted.[333] Tenoxicam, 20 mg, has been used successfully both as a sole intra-articular analgesic and as an adjunct in combination therapy.[334,335]

Intra-articular Neostigmine and Clonidine

Intra-articular administration of neostigmine (0.5 mg) was shown by Yang and coworkers[336] to provide more pain relief than morphine (2 mg) in patients undergoing knee arthroscopy. Intra-articular neostigmine (0.5 mg) has not been reported to increase PONV.[337] Neostigmine (0.5 mg) and clonidine (1 μg/kg) as sole analgesics have been demonstrated to be superior to tenoxicam (20 mg), and all three individual agents were superior to either morphine (2 mg) or bupivacaine (100 mg) given alone.[338] Clonidine (1 μg/kg) coadministered with bupivacaine provided greater analgesic benefit than did either agent used alone. The combination of clonidine (150 μg) and neostigmine (0.5 mg) was no more effective than either agent given alone, but all intra-articular treatment groups had lower pain scores than did the intra-articular placebo group.[339] Clonidine (150 μg) was found to be equivalent to morphine (2 mg) and superior to placebo, but the combination of clonidine and morphine provided no additional benefit.[340] The analgesic benefits of intra-articular clonidine have been shown to be unrelated to vascular uptake.[341]

Evidence suggests that regional anesthesia might be superior to intra-articular injection of local anesthetics. In a prospective randomized blinded study, Singelyn and colleagues[342] compared the analgesic effects of brachial plexus block, suprascapular nerve block, intra-articular injection of local anesthetics, and a control group for arthroscopic acromioplasty. Patients were observed for 24 hours. No significant difference was observed between the group that received intra-articular local anesthetic injection and the control group. Pain scores were lower in the groups that received suprascapular nerve block and brachial plexus block, but pain relief was better in the latter group. Patient satisfaction scores were higher and opioid use lower in the group that received the brachial plexus block.

In another study it was shown that for ACL repair, epidural or continuous femoral nerve block provided adequate pain relief but that intra-articular infusion of ropivacaine was insufficient to provide pain control.[343] Another prospective randomized controlled study showed that adding an interscalene brachial plexus block to intra-articular and subacromial injection of local anesthetics improved analgesia.[344]

In summary,

- Combination drug therapies for intra-articular analgesia have been shown to produce maximum benefit with fewer side effects.
- Intra-articular morphine provides benefit mainly for highly inflammatory joint surgery.
- Intra-articular meperidine could be favored because of its dual local anesthetic effect.
- Both ketorolac and tenoxicam have shown efficacy when delivered via the intra-articular route.
- Continuous perineural analgesia provides better analgesia than does intraarticular injection of local anesthetics, but it requires strong technical skills.

ACUTE PAIN MANAGEMENT IN SPECIAL POPULATIONS

OPIOID-TOLERANT PATIENTS

Acute pain management is sometimes extremely challenging in opioid-tolerant patients. Tolerant patients could be those who use opioids legitimately for the treatment of chronic pain, those who obtain and use opioid medications illicitly, and those who abuse heroin. An opioid-tolerant patient will be encountered in the acute pain setting after routine operative care or trauma. Drug use among trauma victims is high. Studies have shown that as many as 50% of all trauma victims test positive for drugs other than alcohol.[345,346] Data also suggest that patients with substance use disorders are more likely to have chronic pain conditions, thus further complicating acute pain management.[347,348] Concerns that health care providers might contribute to a patient's opioid addiction and tolerance often lead to the undertreatment of acute pain. However, data suggest that the risk for iatrogenic addiction from the use of opioids for pain management is minimal.[349,350] Regardless of why a patient is opioid tolerant, it is important from both a patients' rights perspective and an ethical perspective to treat pain adequately in the acute phase. Undertreated pain can lead to drug-seeking behavior known as *pseudoaddiction*.[351]

A comprehensive analgesic plan should start in the preoperative period and preferably be discussed with the patient and surgical and nursing teams. The pain treatment regimen should be continued until the morning of surgery. Then multimodal analgesia, including regional analgesia, should be considered.[352] Tolerant patients will sometimes require higher doses of long-acting opioids to achieve adequate analgesia. Patients who abuse opiates typically deny the magnitude of their opioid use and usually report high pain scores.[353] Therefore, it is advisable to base the treatment plan on a functional, objective pain scale that includes ambulation and maintenance of effective deep breathing. It is generally recommended that if a patient was using a long-acting opioid such as methadone or transdermal fentanyl before the trauma or surgery, it be continued after the event or be resumed as soon as possible. In patients who are unable to take oral medications, parenteral dosing with a transdermal patch, scheduled nurse-administered IV or IM injections, or baseline continuous IV infusion is preferred. When converting from oral to parenteral administration, the dose is usually decreased because parenteral administration bypasses gastrointestinal absorption variables and first-pass hepatic effects.[354,355] Caution is needed when using continuous high-dose opioid therapy that causes excessive CNS and respiratory depression. Frequent assessment of the patient is recommended, especially during the early phase of therapy before a stable dose has been reached.

Multimodal analgesia can be used to decrease the total amount of opioid medication that is administered. The use of nonopioid analgesics, including acetaminophen and NSAIDs, can help to decrease the pain from inflammation and reduce the subsequent use of opioids. Ketorolac is particularly useful because it has been shown to decrease morphine use and morphine-related side effects.[356] Use of ketorolac must be weighed against an increased risk for bleeding and potential impairment of bone fracture

acupuncture may also benefit patients with ileus by stimulating the release of endogenous opioids.[394-396] Additionally, the use of cognitive-behavioral approaches may improve patients' coping strategies and thus further reduce the need for opioid medications.[397]

In summary,

- Global aging will increase the annual number of surgical procedures performed in the elderly.
- The available data on pain management in the elderly are limited.
- The use of multimodal analgesia, including regional analgesia, may minimize sedation and cognitive dysfunction.
- Future research should focus on the impact of using continuous regional analgesia (neuraxial and perineural) on quality of recovery after surgery and trauma in the elderly.
- Pain management in the elderly should be taught to all health care providers who interact with these patients.

OBESITY AND OBSTRUCTIVE SLEEP APNEA

In the United States, 20% to 25% of the population are either obese or morbidly obese. Obesity is defined as a body mass index (BMI) greater than 30 kg/m^2 and morbid obesity as a BMI greater than 35 kg/m^2. Obstructive sleep apnea (OSA) is defined as more than five episodes of apnea (cessation of airflow for 10 seconds or longer) per hour. Up to 90% of patients with OSA are obese, and a large percentage of obese patients have OSA.[398] The frequent association between the two conditions makes postoperative care of patients with OSA challenging.[399] When considering pain management options for such patients, one should avoid using sedating medications, and systemic opioids should not be used as a first choice.

Regional analgesic techniques consisting of local anesthetics may be preferable to any opioid use.[400] The literature contains no reports of whether low doses of circulating local anesthetics (delivered via incisional, perineural, or neuraxial techniques) inhibit respiratory drive in these patients. However, IV lidocaine has been shown to depress the ventilatory response to hypoxia in healthy subjects.[401]

The American Society of Anesthesiologists Task Force on Perioperative Management of Patients with Obstructive Sleep Apnea published an article in *Anesthesiology* in 2006 recommending that NSAIDs and multimodal analgesia be the first choice for patients with OSA.[402] Furthermore, they recommended that regional techniques with local anesthetics be considered rather than systemic opioids. If parenteral narcotics are chosen, the patient should be monitored for respiratory depression.[402]

The task force also recommended that opioids be excluded from epidural infusions and that basal infusion of opioids be avoided. Nonopioid analgesics such as tramadol should be considered rather than opioids. The use of NSAIDs and acetaminophen should be optimized with a scheduled dose. Patients with OSA may require careful monitoring and vigilance, especially during the first 24 hours after surgery.

PNBs may be critical components in providing postoperative pain relief to patients who are overweight. This concept was reviewed by Nielsen and colleagues,[403] who prospectively collected observational data on almost 7000 patients receiving 9000 nerve blocks. Their findings indicated that block failure was 1.62 times more likely in obese than in nonobese patients (P = 0.04) and that the unadjusted rate of acute complications was higher in obese patients (P = 0.001). However, when compared with patients with a normal BMI, postoperative pain at rest, unanticipated hospital admissions, and overall satisfaction were similar in overweight and obese patients.[403] Therefore, nerve blocks in overweight and obese patients will probably be more technically complicated and have a higher risk for failure, but PNBs (in the hands of experienced practitioners) are the logical first choice of analgesic technique, pending further study.

In summary,

- The frequent association between obesity and OSA in certain patients makes their postoperative pain management very challenging.
- Encourage the use of multimodal pain regimens, including regional analgesic techniques consisting of local anesthetics.
- Discourage the use of sedating medications and long-acting systemic opioids.

TRAUMA AND CRITICALLY ILL PATIENTS

Extensive tissue injury from trauma causes an immediate, potent, and magnified inflammatory response. Activation of nociceptors not only transmits afferent messages to the dorsal horn of the spinal cord but also initiates the process of neurogenic inflammation. Neurogenic inflammation causes release of neurotransmitters, notably substance P and calcitonin gene–related peptide, which leads to severe vasodilation, as well as plasma leakage of proteins and fluid from postcapillary venules.[404] The magnified inflammatory process frequently results in major morbidity and mortality in trauma patients. Hemorrhagic trauma could lead to generalized ischemia, and reperfusion can contribute to multiple-organ dysfunction, acute lung injury, and acute brain injury.[405,406] Numerous reports point to the inadequacy of pain management in trauma patients, particularly during the evaluation and resuscitation phases of care (Table 18.8).[407-412]

Undertreatment of acute pain in trauma patients may have many causes, including lack of proper pain assessment, especially if the patient cannot report the pain; late or improper administration of analgesics; concerns about hemodynamics; fear that analgesia may interfere with the accurate diagnosis of injuries; the misconception that sleep automatically indicates the absence of pain; unfounded concerns that opioid use in the management of acute pain leads to addiction; and beliefs that trauma patients do not remember painful events.[409,413,414]

Evidence indicates that untreated pain in trauma and critically ill patients has a negative impact on the physiologic stress response to injury and can contribute to the incidence of complications such as pulmonary dysfunction, thromboembolic phenomena, myocardial infarction, decreased immune function, and immobility.[415-417] Furthermore, evidence suggests that acute pain may lead to secondary hyperalgesia, allodynia, and chronic pain by inducing changes in the way that pain signals are transmitted and processed within the CNS.[418-420] Finally, there are reports of depression and post-traumatic stress disorder (PTSD) resulting directly from uncontrolled pain.[421,422] Treating pain properly and early in patients with trauma and critical illness will suppress

Table 18.8 Pain Management Options in Patients after Acute Trauma

Patient Characteristic	Therapy	Considerations and Comments
Primary survey complete, patient hemodynamically stable	Short-acting IV opioid (fentanyl)	Goals of improving patient cooperation and detection of unrecognized injuries Risk for decreased sympathetic tone, with possible vasodilation and hemodynamic decompensation
Patient conscious, hemodynamically unstable	Ketamine, tramadol	Risks with ketamine: dysphoria, agitation, airway secretions Risks with tramadol: sedation, especially if coadministered with other CNS depressants. Not recommended in head trauma patients
Head trauma, need for neurologic assessment	Ultrashort-acting opioids (remifentanil)	Allows rapid neurologic evaluation Effective only as an infusion
Pain related to specific interventions (IV access, DPL, fracture manipulation)	Short-acting and ultrashort-acting opioids, ketamine, dexmedetomidine, nitrous oxide	Opioids are generally more readily available Dexmedetomidine may cause vasodilation and hypotension with the initial bolus Nitrous oxide is contraindicated if the patient potentially has pneumothorax or bowel obstruction
Concern for respiratory depression	Ketamine, dexmedetomidine	Both maintain respiratory drive; ketamine may be a better choice if the patient is hypovolemic or hemodynamically unstable Ketamine's dissociative effects may be dose limiting
Pain likely to exceed 2 days' duration	Perineural catheterization	May need to be accompanied by an intracompartmental pressure monitor (i.e., evaluate for the development of compartment syndrome) Possible risk for infection if the sterile field is disrupted or systemic sepsis ensues Requires certain technical skills
Desire for amnesia related to painful procedures	Midazolam, scopolamine	If analgesic intervention is not possible because of hemodynamic decompensation, induction of amnesia is still commonly indicated

CNS, central nervous system; DPL, diagnostic peritoneal lavage; IV, intravenous.

the production of inflammatory mediators, decrease the catabolic response of pain, improve the lymphocytic immune system, and decrease the incidence of PTSD.[423-427]

EVALUATION OF ANALGESIC NEEDS IN TRAUMA PATIENTS

The prehospital and emergency department evaluation and resuscitation phase of trauma care is a period of severe physiologic stress for the victim. The primary therapeutic goals during this time are to maintain a patent airway, ensure adequate oxygenation and ventilation, support the circulation, and assess global neurologic function.[428,429] Assessment and management of life-threatening injuries take priority above all else, but treatment of pain is not necessarily contraindicated.

Once the patient has been determined to have a stable or hyperdynamic circulation, careful use of short-acting IV opioids such as fentanyl is indicated. Often a patient will become more cooperative once adequate analgesia is achieved, which facilitates further evaluation and detection of previously unrecognized injuries. Such cooperation is particularly important during the evaluation of cervical spine injuries, wherein distracting injuries can contribute to late or missed diagnoses.[430,431] In rare cases, the stress response to pain and associated elevations in catecholamine levels may contribute to the patient's hemodynamic stability, and alleviation of pain may result in hemodynamic decompensation. In such cases, even though analgesic administration may be the proximal cause of the decompensation, the actual cause is generally related to blood loss and hypovolemia, which is responsive to rapid but careful fluid resuscitation.

In a study evaluating the use of fentanyl during air medical transport for trauma, only 4 (2.2%) of 177 patients exhibited reductions in systolic blood pressure to below 90 mm Hg after fentanyl administration, with the lowest in this study being 81 mm Hg. In all cases, systolic blood pressure returned to 90 mm Hg or higher within 3 to 10 minutes.[432] This finding indicates that fentanyl is a safe and effective analgesic in the prehospital setting and that analgesia should not be withheld because of concerns regarding hemodynamic instability in patients who are otherwise stable.

In patients who are conscious but hemodynamically unstable, ketamine or tramadol have been shown to be useful alternatives.[433,434] Nitrous oxide may be available in some clinical settings for the management of pain related to specific procedures, such as establishment of IV access, diagnostic peritoneal lavage, or manipulation of extremity fractures. Nitrous oxide should not be used in patients with pneumothorax.[435,436] If respiratory depression is of concern, dexmedetomidine, a centrally acting α_2-adrenergic agonist that lacks respiratory effects, has been shown to provide effective analgesia and sedation; it produces minimal hemodynamic change when given as an infusion without an initial bolus.[437] If the ability to rapidly evaluate a patient's neurologic status is of primary concern, one can consider an infusion of remifentanil, an ultrashort-acting opioid.[438] Finally, in patients for whom none of these options is available because of hemodynamic instability, drug allergy, or institutional drug availability, an adjuvant agent such as scopolamine or midazolam may be used alone to prevent further compromise of hemodynamic stability. These agents may promote amnesia and minimize the psychological impact associated with uncontrolled pain (see Table 18.8).[439]

During the initial hospitalization time, additional invasive and noninvasive diagnostic studies are performed to identify and further characterize the patient's injuries. Operative management of second-priority injuries such as eye and facial trauma, musculoskeletal and spine injuries, and vascular or visceral trauma may be undertaken at this time.[428,429] Titration of short-acting opioids is recommended.

Although systemic opioids will probably continue to be the primary pain therapy for trauma and critically ill patients, a multimodal approach that includes regional analgesia should also be considered. Intermediate-acting agents such as morphine and hydromorphone are useful for achieving a stable level of analgesia for background pain. IV PCA is a very useful mode of delivery and could be converted to an oral preparation after the patient begins to tolerate oral intake of food. A plan must also be in place to provide additional analgesia for times when a patient may need to undergo procedures or dressing changes that trigger intense exacerbation of pain. In special cases, other adjuncts such as propofol, along with fentanyl, ketamine, or midazolam, may be used to provide adequate analgesia and sedation. Sometimes general anesthesia may be needed.[440]

Spinal or epidural analgesia can be very useful for treating postoperative pain in trauma patients and after procedures such as laparotomy, thoracotomy, or reduction of lower extremity fractures.[441] Continuous epidural analgesia was found to be superior to IV PCA after intra-abdominal surgery.[442] The potential hemodynamic impact of the sympathetic blockade associated with these techniques must be carefully considered. IV crystalloid administration during placement of a spinal anesthetic has been shown to decrease hemodynamic changes.[443]

Depending on the mechanism of injury, one should confirm definitive spine clearance before proceeding with a neuraxial technique. Another consideration, depending on the nature and extent of the patient's injuries, is that patient positioning may factor into the feasibility of these techniques. Finally, one should be alert for the presence of coagulopathy in patients with polytrauma, which would be a contraindication to neuraxial techniques.

Selected peripheral regional analgesic techniques may be useful for the management of pain related to specific sites of injury. For example, paravertebral blocks may be indicated for pain related to rib fractures.[444] Isolated PNBs may also be useful in the management of extremity injuries. These may include femoral and sciatic nerve blocks for knee injuries, popliteal sciatic nerve and saphenous nerve blocks for lower leg injuries, and brachial plexus blocks for upper extremity injuries.[445-448] The use of continuous-infusion PNCs should be considered in patients with more extensive trauma for which the duration of severe pain is expected to be longer than 1 to 2 days.

Peripheral regional techniques not only improve pain and patient satisfaction and decrease side effects related to systemic opioids but also facilitate participation in physical therapy and examination of painful injured extremities.[448,449] The ongoing benefit of perineural and neuraxial catheters must be weighed against the small but real potential for infection if catheters are left in place for long periods.[450]

ANALGESIA FOR TRAUMA IN ALCOHOL-INTOXICATED PATIENTS

Alcohol consumption has a strong association with trauma,[451,452] both accident related and violence related. According to the Insurance Institute for Highway Safety, alcohol is a contributing factor in 50% of all trauma deaths. Patients who are not accustomed to regularly using alcohol are subject to higher risk for an injury immediately after alcohol consumption than are patients who drink more heavily.[453] Furthermore, alcohol abuse is associated with an increased risk for readmission for new trauma.[454]

During the acute phase of injury, administration of sedative or opioid medications places an intoxicated patient at risk for increased CNS and respiratory depression because of the additive effects with alcohol. However, once the acute effects of alcohol intoxication have worn off, a chronic alcoholic patient will demonstrate tolerance to sedative medications, as well as cross-tolerance to opioids. As a result, much higher doses of opioids may be necessary to achieve adequate analgesia. This situation may be particularly problematic if the patient's alcohol abuse history is undocumented and normally adequate doses of opioids are proving to be ineffective. In patients with alcoholic cirrhosis and advanced liver disease, altered metabolism and excretion of drugs will change the dosing of hepatically metabolized medications, including opioid analgesics. In patients with end-stage liver disease, coagulopathy may contraindicate the use of neuraxial and some PNB techniques for pain control. Patients with a history of chronic alcohol abuse also have a twofold increased risk for complications, particularly pneumonia, infection, prolonged hospitalization, and respiratory failure.[455] Pain control in patients with abdominal and thoracic trauma becomes particularly important to promote deep breathing and appropriate pulmonary toilet. Given the increased risk for pneumonia and the known respiratory depressant effects of opioids, one may consider neuraxial or regional techniques in alcoholic patients who undergo exploratory laparotomy or thoracotomy, as long as coagulopathy has been ruled out. Paravertebral nerve blocks can also be considered for the same reasons in chronic alcoholic patients with rib fractures.

ANALGESIA IN PATIENTS WITH HEAD TRAUMA

Acute pain management of head trauma patients presents several unique considerations. First, it is difficult to assess the level of pain in patients with altered mental status. Another concern is that the sedating effects of opioids could interfere with adequate neurologic assessment. As a result, trauma patients with head injuries are less likely to receive opioids than are patients with comparable injuries who have not sustained head trauma.[414] Whether the pain results directly from the head trauma or, more likely, is a result of other injuries, it is important to tailor the analgesic regimen to facilitate ongoing neurologic assessment. To minimize the sedating effects of opioids, analgesic treatments should include the use of nonsedating analgesic agents and opioid-reducing strategies whenever possible. IV acetaminophen (recently approved by the FDA in the United States) is a good choice for mild to moderate pain. NSAIDs such as ibuprofen and ketorolac are best avoided in any patient at risk for intracranial bleeding because of the platelet-inhibiting effects of this drug class. For moderate

Table 18.9 Analgesic Modalities in Patients with Blunt Chest Trauma

Therapy	Pros	Cons	Comments
Opioids	Effective Simple administration Readily available	CNS/respiratory depression, impaired cough reflex, risk for hypoxia and hypoventilation	Patients with multiple rib fractures may have opioid-induced sedation before analgesic efficacy is achieved NSAIDs may improve analgesia and decrease opioid requirement
Continuous epidural analgesia	Better analgesia than IV PCA Improved respiratory function	Hypotension, nausea, pruritus, constipation Technical difficulties (placement, maintenance) Caution with anticoagulation	Advise against simultaneous opioid dosing via epidural and IV PCA in patients with trauma
Paravertebral nerve blocks	Improved respiratory function More hemodynamic stability and better spirometry than with thoracic epidural Ability to use a percutaneous catheter for continuous analgesia	Technical difficulties (placement, maintenance) Caution with anticoagulation Risk for pneumothorax	Excellent alternative to thoracic epidural, especially with unilateral chest trauma
Intercostal nerve blocks	Analgesia comparable to epidural Improved respiratory function	Risk for pneumothorax Multiple blocks often required Risk for local anesthetic toxicity because of large volumes used and increased systemic uptake Limited duration may require repeated injections for single-shot techniques High rate of misplaced catheters because of technical difficulties	Patients may not tolerate palpation of fractured ribs and multiple injections if multiple ribs are fractured
Interpleural catheter analgesia	May be useful when other techniques are contraindicated	Requires the supine position for adequate spread, which has a negative impact on respiratory mechanics Risk for pneumothorax	Conflicting evidence regarding efficacy

CNS, central nervous system; IV, intravenous; NSAIDs, nonsteroidal anti-inflammatory drugs; PCA, patient-controlled analgesia.

to severe pain, shorter-acting opioids such as fentanyl or remifentanil (as an infusion) can be used for the management of background and breakthrough pain in the acute period. IV PCA is a good choice in sufficiently alert patients. A continuous background infusion can be added via IV PCA to provide baseline analgesic requirements. Morphine and hydromorphone have longer half-lives than fentanyl does and can be used in many cases, but the sedating effects may persist longer than the analgesic effects and thus possibly impede neurologic evaluation. In the critical care setting, continuous brief infusions of fentanyl, alfentanil, sufentanil, or ultrashort-acting remifentanil can be used.[456] As a result of their shorter half-lives, these infusions can be temporarily stopped to enable rapid neurologic assessment. Because both morphine and fentanyl have prolonged context-sensitive half-lives with extended infusions, recovery is prolonged after their termination.[457] Longer-acting or sustained-release preparations should be started only after intracranial injury has been definitively excluded or the patient's neurologic status has stabilized.

Paravertebral blocks or catheters may be a better alternative to epidural analgesia in this setting because of the small but real risk of dural puncture associated with an epidural. Dural puncture could result in expansion of an intracranial hematoma or uncal herniation. Continuous nerve block techniques should be considered for the management of coexisting extremity injuries to further reduce opioid requirements.

ANALGESIA IN PATIENTS WITH BLUNT THORACIC TRAUMA

Injuries typically categorized under this heading (Table 18.9) include rib fractures, flail chest, pulmonary and cardiac contusions, disruption of thoracic vessels, hemothorax, pneumothorax, and soft tissue trauma. Motor vehicle accidents and falls account for most of these injuries.[458] Thoracic injuries contribute significantly to trauma-induced morbidity and mortality and lead to 25% of trauma-related deaths.[459] Rib fractures are the most common injury and are seen in 10% of all trauma patients.[460] Thoracic injuries can impair respiratory function directly through physiologic and mechanical changes, such as those seen with pneumothorax, flail chest, and pulmonary contusions. Thoracic injuries can also have indirect effects via increased pain with respiration, commonly seen with multiple rib fractures. These factors lead to splinting during respiration, which increases atelectasis, decreases functional residual capacity, impairs coughing ability, and predisposes patients to pneumonia. Furthermore, these effects can lead to changes in pulmonary ventilation-perfusion matching ($\dot{V}/\dot{Q}$ mismatch) and result in hypoxia.

Because of these latter pain-related sources of morbidity, adequate pain control is of obvious importance, particularly in patients who are breathing spontaneously.

Multiple options exist for the management of pain in patients with blunt thoracic trauma. Traditionally, systemic opioids administered via IV PCA have been the primary means of controlling pain in these patients. The primary disadvantage is that opioids cause CNS and respiratory depression and impair the cough reflex. These factors lead to hypoxemia and further impairment in ventilation.

Continuous epidural infusion (CEI) of a local anesthetic combined with a low-dose opioid has been shown to confer better pain relief than IV PCA and result in increased tidal volume and inspiratory force.[461,462] CEI can be combined with a patient-administered bolus via PCEA to give patients a similar degree of control over their pain management as seen with IV PCA. Hypotension is the most common side effect noted with epidural infusions and is related to local anesthetic–mediated effects on the sympathetic nervous system. Good analgesic results have also been reported with continuous epidural opioid infusions.[463] As with IV opioids, epidural opioids often produce nausea, pruritus, and constipation. In some cases, excessive sedation and respiratory depression occur. If these side effects are seen with epidural infusions of local anesthetic and opioid in combination, one can opt for an epidural infusion of a local anesthetic only. Opioid IV PCA can be added for more precise control of the opioid dose.

Paravertebral blocks provide an alternative to epidural analgesia in patients with unilateral thoracic trauma, which occurs commonly in side-impact motor vehicle accidents and in falls. With paravertebral blocks, local anesthetic injected into the paravertebral space produces an ipsilateral block at multiple dermatomes. For continuous provision of analgesia, a catheter can also be inserted percutaneously or by the surgeon under direct vision during thoracotomy.[464] Paravertebral analgesia has been shown to provide effective pain relief in patients with multiple rib fractures and to improve respiratory parameters and oxygenation.[444] Paravertebral techniques are considered easier to perform than epidural techniques.[294] Catheters could be an option.

Paravertebral blocks have a low incidence of complications, including failure, inadvertent vascular puncture, hypotension, hematoma, epidural or intrathecal spread, pleural puncture, and pneumothorax.[465] Paravertebral blocks are an excellent choice in patients who already have chest tubes inserted on the side of the planned block. Because the sympatholytic effects of paravertebral blocks are typically unilateral, patients who receive these blocks experience hypotension much less frequently than those who receive continuous epidural analgesia, provided that the patient is adequately fluid-resuscitated.[444,466]

Intercostal nerve blocks are another effective option for the management of pain associated with chest trauma and rib fractures. These blocks have been shown to improve oxygenation and respiratory mechanics and offer pain relief that is comparable to that of epidural analgesia.[467,468] The technique is limited by the relatively large doses of local anesthetic required; the relatively high intravascular uptake from the intercostal space increases the risk for local anesthetic toxicity. The most common complication associated with this technique is pneumothorax (occurring at an incidence of 1.4% per individual nerve block and in 5.6% of patients with multiple blocks for multiple rib fractures).[297] Because the duration of analgesia is only 6 to 12 hours, multiple daily injections are often necessary. Even though percutaneously placed intercostal nerve block catheters can deliver effective continuous analgesia, the technical difficulty associated with their placement results in a high rate of misplaced catheters.[469]

Local anesthetics can be delivered via a catheter into the interpleural space; the local anesthetics then diffuse through the parietal pleura to block the intercostal nerves. Interpleural blocks may or may not be as effective as epidural blocks in patients who have rib fractures[470,471] or have undergone thoracotomy.[472,473] Because insertion may be technically difficult, catheters may be misplaced into either the pleura or the chest wall. Pneumothorax is the most common complication of interpleural catheters. Despite these limitations, this technique may be useful for patients in whom other techniques are contraindicated.

In summary,

- The extensive tissue injury in trauma and critically ill patients causes a potent and magnified inflammatory response.
- Untreated pain in trauma and critically ill patients can lead to increased morbidity and mortality.
- The choice of analgesic drug in trauma patients depends on the patient's hemodynamic status and the need to assess CNS function.
- Ketamine, tramadol, and nitrous oxide have been shown to be useful alternatives in patients who are conscious but hemodynamically unstable.
- Selected peripheral regional analgesic techniques may be useful for the management of pain related to specific sites of injury.
- Peripheral regional analgesic techniques can play an important role in analgesia for trauma patients because they can substantially reduce the use of opioids.
- Both perineural and neuraxial continuous techniques are beneficial in blunt chest trauma.

ANALGESIA IN PATIENTS WITH BURN INJURY

Burn injuries cause severe pain that is associated with the injury itself and with the multiple interventions that follow. Thus, patients have background pain that is exacerbated during wound care, dressing changes, and débridement. The level of pain can be difficult to predict. Full-thickness burns involve the destruction of nerve fibers and consequently do not result in pain. Patients with extensive full-thickness burns will experience pain only from tissues at the margins of the burned areas. Patients with partial-thickness burns will have damaged but functioning nerve fibers that are exposed at the surface of the skin. These nerve fibers can transmit severe pain, particularly in response to surface contact. Furthermore, activation of nociceptive and inflammatory mediators can alter the response to additional stimulation and result in hyperalgesia and temporal summation.[474] Pain can persist well beyond the healing period and cause impaired function and psychological problems. Therefore, it is imperative to manage burn pain aggressively.

Table 18.10 Analgesic Modalities in Burn Patients

Therapy	Pros	Cons	Comments
Opioids	Effective for background pain Short-acting opioids (fentanyl, remifentanil) effective for dressing changes	Tolerance develops	Once an adequate baseline established, can be converted to continuous IV infusion or long-acting oral therapy Transdermal absorption is variable because of alterations in tissue perfusion
NSAIDs	Useful adjunct to opioid therapy	Risk for peptic ulcers in predisposed patients	Ibuprofen may improve tissue perfusion and decrease the hypermetabolic response
Ketamine	Provides analgesia while maintaining hemodynamic and respiratory function Multiple routes of administration available May suppress secondary hyperalgesia	Dissociative effects may be unpleasant Agitation	Suitable for repetitive administration (e.g., dressing changes) Dissociative effects attenuated by midazolam, propofol
Clonidine	No respiratory depression	Possible hypotension, sedation	Synergistic effects with opioids
Local anesthetics	Significant opioid-sparing effect when given by the IV route Decreases inflammation at burn sites No respiratory depression	Variable systemic absorption when applied topically Potential for cardiac and CNS toxicity	
Regional analgesia	Useful for management of pain at graft donor sites Effective analgesia Opioid-sparing effects	Risks associated with techniques	Regional analgesic techniques are often not practical in burn patients because the skin overlying the site of the block must be intact and the burn must be contained in the neural distribution of the block

CNS, central nervous system; IV, intravenous; NSAIDs, nonsteroidal anti-inflammatory drugs.

OPIOIDS IN PATIENTS WITH BURN INJURY

Opioids continue to be the primary therapy for the management of background and procedural pain (Table 18.10). Despite the enhanced potency of opioids after acute burn injury,[475] opioid requirements can be quite high. Burns cause substantial changes in metabolism and protein binding, but the pharmacokinetics of IV opioids remains unaltered. Therapy is initiated with small IV boluses, which are titrated to effect. To this end, IV PCA has been shown to be safe and effective.[476] Absorption of IM and transdermal opioids is variable because of decreased tissue perfusion and uptake, which makes these routes unsuitable in this patient population. However, gastrointestinal absorption and emptying appear to be unchanged.[477] Once an adequate baseline opioid requirement is established for the management of background pain, opioids can be given via continuous IV infusion or by equianalgesic enteral formulations of long-acting or sustained-release opioids.

Dressing changes and wound débridement cause brief but intense periods of pain. During such episodes, opioids are the principal therapy, with preference given to fentanyl or short-acting opioids such as alfentanil and remifentanil. These opioids can be administered by a clinical provider or via IV PCA. Opioids whose effects last longer than the duration of the procedure can produce excessive sedation and respiratory depression once the intervention is completed.

NONOPIOID ANALGESICS IN PATIENTS WITH BURN INJURY

NSAIDs can be useful as adjuncts to opioids by decreasing inflammation and opioid requirements. Ibuprofen may improve tissue perfusion after burn injury[478] and may decrease the hypermetabolic response.[479] However, one should be wary of NSAIDs' gastrointestinal side effects, including gastric ulcers, particularly in a patient population already predisposed to stress gastritis. In addition, NSAIDs have been implicated as a contributing cause in renal impairment after burn injury.[480] Acetaminophen may be a better alternative for mild pain in burn patients with normal hepatic function.

Local anesthetics have been used in a variety of ways for burn patients. Topical application has been shown to be effective for the treatment of postburn pain[481] and pruritus.[482] However, local anesthetics pose an increased risk for rapid systemic uptake and toxicity when applied to non-intact skin and can potentially cause seizures[483] or dysrhythmias. Lidocaine, when given by IV infusion, has significant opioid-reducing effects[484] and acts to decrease inflammation at the burn site.[485] Local anesthetics, administered either topically or by local infiltration, have also been used successfully to decrease the pain associated with skin grafting.[486,487]

Ketamine, a dissociative anesthetic, has the advantage of providing analgesia while maintaining stable hemodynamic function and causing minimal respiratory depression. Studies also suggest that ketamine may suppress burn-induced secondary hyperalgesia.[488] Ketamine can be administered via IV or IM injection, as well as by the oral, rectal, or nasal route. The primary clinical use of ketamine has been to provide sedation and analgesia during wound dressing changes and débridement, particularly in children. Ketamine infusion has also been used successfully for long-term sedation and analgesia in a burn patient, with remarkable opioid-sparing effects.[489] Its dissociative effects can be unpleasant for patients, however, and can lead to emergence delirium.

Delirium may be attenuated by preemptive or rescue doses of midazolam or propofol.[490-492]

Clonidine, an α_2-adrenoreceptor agonist, exerts sedative and analgesic effects through its action on the CNS. Clonidine exhibits synergistic effects with opioids and has been used as an adjunct in the management of postoperative pain.[493] Several case studies have reported its successful use in burn patients.[494,495] Clonidine does not cause respiratory depression, and its opioid-sparing effect can be used to decrease opioid-related side effects. One should avoid using clonidine in hemodynamically unstable or hypovolemic patients because of the risk for hypotension.

PERIPHERAL REGIONAL ANALGESIC TECHNIQUES IN PATIENTS WITH BURN INJURY

Patients with burn injuries are generally poor candidates for regional analgesic techniques. In most cases the duration of pain after burn injury is far longer than it is practical to maintain an indwelling PNC. Also, the skin overlying the proposed peripheral block site must be intact to reduce the risk for infection in patients already at high risk for infection and sepsis. In addition, many burns are not limited to the distribution of one or two peripheral nerves that are easily blocked. Hence, the usefulness of these techniques is limited to cases of mild isolated extremity burns. However, nerve blocks have been used successfully in the management of pain at graft donor sites.[496]

PSYCHOLOGICAL SUPPORT AFTER BURN INJURY

Burn trauma can be devastating to a patient both physically and psychologically. Patients can become depressed or have high levels of fear and anxiety, particularly if the degree of injury or disability is severe or if hospitalization is lengthy. The anxiety often revolves around the repeated painful wound treatments that patients must undergo. Evidence has shown a relationship between patients' levels of depression and anxiety and their reported levels of pain.[497] In a study by Van Loey and associates,[498] PTSD developed in as many as 25% of patients after burn injury. Predictors included anxiety, female gender, and severity of injury.

Effective anxiolysis with benzodiazepines such as midazolam, diazepam, and lorazepam has been shown to reduce pain in patients with burn injuries.[499,500] Low doses of antidepressants, including selective serotonin reuptake inhibitors and tricyclic antidepressants, have also been shown to potentiate the analgesic effects of opioids.[501,502] Other therapeutic interventions, including hypnosis, acupuncture, auricular electrical stimulation, massage therapy, biofeedback, mental imagery, and relaxation training, have been used to reduce pain scores in burn patients with mixed results.[413,503,504]

In summary,

- Pain after burn injury can persist well beyond the healing period and result in impaired function and psychological problems.
- IV opioids are still the primary therapy for the management of acute pain and procedural pain in burn injury.
- Absorption of IM and transdermal opioids is variable because of decreased tissue perfusion and uptake.
- Short-acting opioids such as alfentanil and remifentanil are essential for wound débridement.
- Ketamine has the advantage of providing analgesia while maintaining stable hemodynamic function with minimal respiratory depression.
- Regional anesthetic techniques are of limited use in patients with extensive burns but could be used in cases of mild isolated extremity burns.

SUMMARY OF THE CHAPTER

- Adequate postoperative pain control continues to be a public health problem.
- Multimodal analgesia is becoming the standard practice in acute pain management.
- Systemic opioids are still the traditional foundation for the treatment of acute pain in many practices.
- Nonopioid analgesics play a primary role in pain management and result in an opioid-sparing effect.
- Neuraxial and perineural analgesic techniques have established an important role in acute pain management; however, their use is limited by variability in the skills and experience of practitioners.
- Analgesic needs warrant special consideration in patients who have suffered trauma or burn injury and for patients who are elderly, obese, or opioid tolerant.
- Pain management is becoming an important ethical responsibility of the medical profession and the focus of the health care system.

ACKNOWLEDGMENT

Portions of this chapter were transcribed or modified from the chapter "Postoperative Pain and Other Acute Pain Syndromes" authored by Dr. Brian A. Williams and colleagues in *Raj's Practical Management of Pain* (fourth edition).

SUGGESTED READINGS

Abdallah FW, Chan VW, Brull R. Transversus abdominis plane block: a systematic review. *Reg Anesth Pain Med.* 2012;37:193-209.

Buvanendran A, Kroin JS. Multimodal analgesia for controlling acute postoperative pain. *Curr Opin Anaesthesiol.* 2009;22:588-593.

Duggan E, El Beheiry H, Perlas A, et al. Minimum effective volume of local anesthetic for ultrasound-guided supraclavicular brachial plexus block. *Reg Anesth Pain Med.* 2009;34:215-218.

Elia N, Lysakowski C, Tramer MR. Does multimodal analgesia with acetaminophen, nonsteroidal antiinflammatory drugs, or selective cyclooxygenase-2 inhibitors and patient-controlled analgesia morphine offer advantages over morphine alone? Meta-analyses of randomized trials. *Anesthesiology.* 2005;103:1296-1304.

Fredrickson MJ, Kilfoyle DH. Neurological complication analysis of 1000 ultrasound guided peripheral nerve blocks for elective orthopaedic surgery: a prospective study. *Anaesthesia.* 2009;64:836-844.

Gross JB, Bachenberg KL, Benumof JL, et al. Practice guidelines for the perioperative management of patients with obstructive sleep apnea: a report by the American Society of Anesthesiologists Task Force on Perioperative Management of Patients with Obstructive Sleep Apnea. *Anesthesiology.* 2006;104:1081-1093.

Ilfeld BM. Continuous peripheral nerve blocks in the hospital and at home. *Anesthesiol Clin.* 2011;29:193-211.

Joshi GP, Bonnet F, Shah R, et al. A systematic review of randomized trials evaluating regional techniques for postthoracotomy analgesia. *Anesth Analg.* 2008;107:1026-1040.

Loftus RW, Yeager MP, Clark JA, et al. Intraoperative ketamine reduces perioperative opiate consumption in opiate-dependent patients with chronic back pain undergoing back surgery. *Anesthesiology.* 2010;113:639-646.

McGhee LL, Maani CV, Garza TH, et al. The correlation between ketamine and posttraumatic stress disorder in burned service members. *J Trauma.* 2008;64:S195-S198.

Neal JM, Brull R, Chan VW, et al. The ASRA evidence-based medicine assessment of ultrasound-guided regional anesthesia and pain medicine: executive summary. *Reg Anesth Pain Med.* 2010;35:S1-S9.

Ong CK, Seymour RA, Lirk P, et al. Combining paracetamol (acetaminophen) with nonsteroidal antiinflammatory drugs: a qualitative systematic review of analgesic efficacy for acute postoperative pain. *Anesth Analg.* 2010;110:1170-1179.

Practice guidelines for acute pain management in the perioperative setting: an updated report by the American Society of Anesthesiologists Task Force on Acute Pain Management. *Anesthesiology.* 2004;100:1573-1581.

Richman JM, Liu SS, Courpas G, et al. Does continuous peripheral nerve block provide superior pain control to opioids? A meta-analysis. *Anesth Analg.* 2006;102:248-257.

Salinas FV. Ultrasound and review of evidence for lower extremity peripheral nerve blocks. *Reg Anesth Pain Med.* 2010;35:S16-S25.

Wu CL, Fleisher LA. Outcomes research in regional anesthesia and analgesia. *Anesth Analg.* 2000;91:1232-1242.

The references for this chapter can be found at www.expertconsult.com.

19

Prediction and Prevention of Persistent Post-Surgical Pain

Frederick M. Perkins | Julie S. Franklin

Chronic pain as an outcome of surgery is an area of investigation that has received increased attention over the last 15 years.[1-5] Twenty years ago there were a few identified postsurgical pain syndromes, such as post-mastectomy pain syndrome and post-thoracotomy pain syndrome. The problem of persistent postsurgical pain (PPSP) as a more generalized phenomenon has received attention more recently. Cross-sectional quality-of-life surveys[6] reveal that 40% of the population who underwent surgery in the last 3 years reported persistent pain at the surgical site. The risk for PPSP is now commonly discussed with patients before surgery. In addition to the ethical obligation to discuss this risk prospectively, there may be ways to minimize the risk for certain subpopulations of patients. In this chapter we address the extent of the problem of chronic pain following surgery in general and then, by using four specific surgeries as examples, attempt to better understand the effect of patient factors, surgical factors, and analgesic interventions on the risk for PPSP. Among the questions that we will address are the following:

- Can patients at increased risk for the development of PPSP pain be identified prospectively?
- Are there interventions that can be initiated in the preoperative, intraoperative, or immediate postoperative period to minimize the risk for chronic pain?
- What is the relative importance of patient factors, surgical factors, and analgesic factors in the development of chronic pain following surgery?

To discuss these questions in an effective manner, it is necessary to agree on the definitions of the terms used in the discussion. Table 19.1 is a list of definitions of important terms used in this chapter.

Pain is a common phenomenon after surgery. Some degree of postsurgical pain is expected after most surgical procedures. However, the extent of acute postoperative pain is highly variable among individuals undergoing similar surgery.[7] As a generalization, more extensive surgical procedures are associated with greater acute pain. In many studies the extent of acute postoperative pain has been a predictor of PPSP.[2] Consequently, a number of studies have been conducted to address questions that may relate to both acute postoperative pain and PPSP. Does the use of minimally invasive approaches have advantages beyond the acute postoperative period? Does our ability to alter the acute pain experience influence the probability of PPSP? If acute postoperative pain control alters PPSP, how does that happen? What patient factors are predictive of PPSP? We will explore these questions by using the examples of breast surgery, hip surgery, inguinal hernia repair, and thoracotomy.

In a recent review, Katz and colleagues[8] emphasized that the timing of the preemptive intervention needs to correlate with the period of intense nociceptive stimulation and not just be a single intervention of short duration. They suggested that the term "preventive analgesia" would be more useful, and we agree, although it has been pointed out that evidence to support the concept of preventive analgesia is weak.[9] The concept of preemptive analgesia originated with a paper by Clifford Woolf in 1983.[10] The findings of this study, when combined with what is known as wind-up,[11] or increasing pain intensity when a given painful stimulus is delivered repeatedly above a critical frequency, gave rise to the hope that interventions that decrease nociceptive input or block central sensitization would have lasting analgesic benefit. How pain progresses from acute nociceptive pain, to subacute pain, to chronic pain has been reviewed by Devor and Seltzer,[12] who incorporated animal model data and human data. Briefly, persistent acute nociceptive stimulation elicits both pain and activation of sensitization in the spinal cord. In the subacute pain period there is probably some nociceptive stimulation that can maintain the sensitization and pain. In some models and some individuals there does not appear to be any resolution of this sensitization. It is not clear whether some nociceptive input is needed to maintain the sensitization or whether changes in the spinal cord following nerve injury are sufficient to maintain sensitization and thus pain.[13]

FACTORS INFLUENCING THE DEVELOPMENT OF PERSISTENT POSTSURGICAL PAIN

Numerous factors related to the surgery appear to be of importance. First among these is the surgical procedure. Previous reviews have documented that the prevalence of chronic pain varies with the type of surgery, with some surgical procedures such as lower extremity amputation and posterolateral thoracotomy having a high prevalence of chronic pain (greater than 50%). Table 19.2 summarizes the prevalence of chronic pain following many common surgical procedures.[2,14-26] As shown in this table, chronic pain is infrequent following some surgical procedures, such as cataract extraction, but prevalent following other surgical procedures, such as thoracotomy. Additionally, the prevalence of pain may decrease following certain surgeries (hip arthroplasty, lumbar laminectomy for a herniated disk) but increase following other surgeries (thoracotomy, breast surgery). This does not mean that PPSP cannot result from a surgery such as hip arthroplasty, but rather that the majority of patients experience a reduction in pain following the procedure, and a smaller number may have increased pain.

Table 19.1 Definitions

Term	Definition
Central sensitization	Persistent postinjury changes in the central nervous system that result in pain hypersensitivity
Chronic pain	Pain that lasts for more than 3 mo.
Pain	An unpleasant sensory and emotional experience associated with actual or potential tissue damage or described in terms of such damage
Peripheral sensitization	A lowering of the threshold for a stimulus to be felt as painful
Preemptive analgesia	An intervention that is initiated before a nociceptive stimulus. The intervention needs to significantly decrease or eliminate the usual immediate effect of the nociceptive stimulus (e.g., pain, central sensitization)
Preventive analgesia	An intervention that is initiated before a nociceptive stimulus (e.g., surgical incision), and then intervention is continued until the major nociceptive stimulus has abated

Within a given type of operation, a number of surgical approaches may be possible. For thoracotomy, an anterior approach appears to be associated with less acute and chronic pain than the classic posterolateral approach. Additionally, there may be less acute and chronic pain with visually aided thoracoscopic surgery than with the same operation performed as an open procedure.[27] Likewise, laparoscopic inguinal hernia repair is associated with less acute pain and less chronic pain than open inguinal hernia repair is.[28-30] Thus there are data to support the hypothesis that minimally invasive surgical procedures are associated with less chronic pain than the same operations performed as open procedures.

Another factor may be what has been referred to as "volume-dependent outcome." Database studies[31,32] demonstrate that for a number of major high-risk surgeries, outcome is worse when the procedure is performed in a low-volume institution and that a large part of the risk can be attributed to low-volume surgeons. We previously noted that in the case of hernia repair, the lowest prevalence of chronic pain is reported by high-volume hernia centers.[2] The incidence of complications, including chronic pain, following laparoscopic hernia repair has been noted to be greater early in the experience of surgeons.[33,34] This may be analogous to the observation that hernia surgery performed by trainees has a higher incidence of recurrence and chronic pain than the same surgery performed by experienced surgeons.[35]

Adjuvant treatments associated with a number of surgical procedures for cancer may also play a role in the development of PPSP. In particular, radiation therapy for women undergoing breast and axillary surgery is associated with an increased probability of chronic pain.[36] Whether adjuvant

Table 19.2 Prevalence of Chronic Pain and Preprocedure Pain

Surgical Procedure	Prevalence of Chronic Pain	Prevalence of Preoperative Pain
Amputation, lower extremity[2]	Phantom pain, 70% Stump pain, 62%	Very common, chronic, continuous ischemic pain
Arthroplasty, hip[14]	27%	Common, chronic, incident arthritic pain
Arthroplasty, knee[14]	44%	Common, chronic, incident arthritic pain
Cataract with lens implant[15]	<1%	Infrequent
Cesarean section[16]	6%	Common, intermittent, acute labor pain
Cholecystectomy[17]	23%	Common, variable, from acute cholecystitis to chronic vague abdominal pain
Colectomy[18]	28%	Uncommon
Dental, root canal[19]	12%	Common, usually with breakage or infection
Hernia repair, inguinal[20]	12%	Common, incident pain with peritoneal stretch
Lumbar spine surgery for herniated disk[21]	44%	Very common, primary reason for surgery
Mammoplasty, augmentation[22]	20%	Infrequent
Mastectomy plus axillary dissection[2]	30% 50%	Infrequent
Prostatectomy, radical[23]	32%	Infrequent
Sternotomy		
CABG[24]	30%	Common, intermittent, exertional angina
Valve[25]	32%	Infrequent
Thoracotomy[2]		
Posterolateral	50%	Infrequent
VATS	31%	
Vasectomy[26]	20%	Rare

CABG, coronary artery bypass grafting; VATS, video-assisted thoracic surgery.

therapies in the perioperative period affect the risk for chronic postsurgical pain after other cancer surgeries has not yet been determined.

It should be understood that patients vary in their sensitivity to pain and in other factors that may predict the evolution of acute pain to chronic pain. This has been an area of research for many years, with Lasagna and Beecher[7] finding that one third of patients following surgery did not experience significant pain relief with commonly used dosages of morphine. Likewise, in subsequent studies, Lasagna and associates continued to find significant patient variability in response to both surgery and opioids[37] and that patients' reports of pain sensitivity predicted neither the extent of pain nor the response to opioids. A number of more recent studies have investigated the genetic basis of pain variability (see Young and colleagues for a review[38]).

There are also psychological factors, other than pain sensitivity, that appear to predispose certain individuals to experiencing pain. Psychological vulnerability has been found to be a predictor of long-term pain and symptoms following cholecystectomy.[39] Gatchel and coworkers[40] noted a set of psychosocial risk factors for acute back pain to evolve into chronic back pain. It appears that the strongest predictors involve deficits in coping ability, neuroticism, and somatization, although depression and anxiety add a component.[41] Catastrophizing may also be a predictor of PPSP.

The intensity of pain in the postoperative period has been a reproducible predictor of chronic pain following a number of surgeries, including lower extremity amputation, thoracotomy, mastectomy, cholecystectomy, and inguinal hernia surgery.[2] Usually, pain intensity is measured directly with some instrument, but analgesic consumption is also frequently measured as a surrogate algometer. When looking at studies of interventions aimed at decreasing the intensity of acute pain and reducing the prevalence or intensity of chronic pain, there are a number of factors that we believe should be considered.

- What intervention or interventions were implemented?
- When were they initiated relative to the initial nociceptive stimulus?
- How long were the interventions continued?
- Were the interventions effective in decreasing acute pain or acute opioid consumption?
- Were the doses of medication used in a clinically reasonable range?
- Was there a systematic evaluation of pain and symptoms both acutely and chronically?
- What chronic pain was assessed?
- Were the randomization and blinding adequate to eliminate investigator bias?

We will be reviewing studies for some selected surgical procedures in the following sections and will try to identify how some of these factors may have influenced the observed outcome. In particular, specific drugs such as gabapentin or pregabalin[42] have been advocated to decrease the prevalence of PPSP, but the results have been highly variable.

BREAST SURGERY

The majority of studies of chronic pain following breast surgery involve women with cancer. There are also some reports of reasonable quality following augmentation mammoplasty or reduction mammoplasty. Studies of both cancer surgery and augmentation mammoplasty document a significant prevalence of chronic pain following breast surgery (see Table 19.2). Women undergoing cancer surgery also have problems with persistent arm pain following axillary dissection. Radiation therapy and chemotherapy following breast surgery will further increase the prevalence of persistent pain.[2] Careful handling of the intercostal brachial nerves in the axilla appears to decrease the risk for persistent pain.[43] A number of studies now demonstrate that axillary sentinel node biopsy is associated with less persistent pain than primary axillary dissection is. Table 19.3 presents the risk (odds ratio) for persistent pain when sentinel node biopsy is compared with axillary dissection.[43-54] In women with negative pathology on a sentinel node biopsy, arm pain and other arm symptoms are significantly less likely to develop. In women who underwent secondary axillary node dissection, chronic pain was as likely or more likely to develop than in those who underwent primary axillary node dissection.[55]

Breast-conserving surgery has been associated with a higher prevalence of chronic pain than simple mastectomy,[2] but only in studies where persistent pain was assessed as a tertiary, not a primary or secondary, outcome, and this association has not been found consistently. There are no randomized studies on this issue.

Paravertebral block has been advocated as an analgesic technique for breast surgery and the immediate postoperative

Table 19.3 Interventions in Breast Surgery and Risk (Odd Ratio) for Persistent Pain

Experimental Group	Control Group	Odds Ratio	95% Confidence Interval	Study Type	N	Follow-up (mo)	Reference
Sentinel node biopsy	Axillary dissection	0.42	0.34-0.51	RCT	2573	12-24	Veronesi,[44] Purushotham,[45] Fleissig,[46] Del Bianco,[47] Lucci,[48] Fougo[49]
Paravertebral block	General anesthesia	0.10	0.04-0.27	RCT	118	3-6	Kairaluoma,[43] Iohom,[50] Ibarra[51]
Gabapentin	Control	0.52	0.28-0.94	RCT	191	3-6	Fassoulaki,[52] Fassoulaki,[53] Amr[54]

RCT, randomized controlled trial.

period.[56] In 2006 two randomized controlled studies looked at the influence of perioperative paravertebral blockade on persistent pain following breast surgery. Both found a significantly lower prevalence of chronic pain in women who had the block. One[43] was a follow-up study of 60 women who had participated in an acute perioperative pain study.[57] In this study, the prevalence of pain at both 6 and 12 months was significantly lower in the women who had received a block (17% vs. 40% at 6 months and 7% vs. 33% at 12 months). The second study[50] was smaller (29 subjects) and involved placement of a paravertebral catheter preoperatively in patients in the treatment arm. A dose of 10 mL of 0.25% bupivacaine was administered before surgery and every 12 hours for 48 hours. A telephone follow-up inquired about pain 3 months following surgery ("Do you have chronic pain as a result of your breast surgery?"). The paravertebral block group had a significantly lower prevalence of pain at 3 months (0% vs. 80%). There has now been a third study published[51] supporting the use of paravertebral block to decrease the prevalence of PPSP at 4 to 5 months. If the data from these three studies are combined, the calculated odds ratio of preventing PPSP with a paravertebral block is highly significant (see Table 19.3).

A number of randomized controlled studies have investigated perioperative interventions to decrease the prevalence of persistent pain after breast surgery. Romundstad and associates[22] compared a single dose of methylprednisolone (125 mg) with a single dose of parecoxib (40 mg) and placebo in women undergoing augmentation mammoplasty. At 12 months the prevalence of pain at rest in the three groups was 16%, 7%, and 16%, respectively. Evoked pain was found in 16%, 14%, and 29%, respectively. The calculated odds ratio and 95% confidence intervals were 0.49 (0.30 to 0.74) for methylprednisolone versus placebo and 0.40 (0.25 to 0.64) for parecoxib. Fassoulaki and colleagues published two randomized controlled studies of perioperative gabapentin.[52,53] In the first,[52] women received gabapentin, 400 mg three times a day starting the evening before surgery, or mexiletine, 200 mg three times per day, or placebo three times per day. There were no significant differences in pain prevalence or intensity or in analgesic requirement at 3 months, although the character of the pain in the control group tended to be burning rather than throbbing, aching, or stabbing. In the second study,[53] women undergoing breast cancer surgery received a combination of gabapentin, 400 mg four times a day for 10 days starting the evening before surgery, plus EMLA cream (20 g) for 3 days starting the day of surgery, plus intraoperative irrigation of the brachial plexus with 10 mL of 0.75% ropivacaine. The control group underwent placebo administration in each of the interventions. This study found a significantly decreased prevalence of pain at both the 3- and 6-month follow-up in the intervention group (30% vs. 57% at 6 months). The calculated odds ratio for pain at 6 months was 0.32 (0.18 to 0.62). Amr and Yousef[54] randomized patients scheduled for mastectomy plus axillary dissection to receive gabapentin, 300 mg/day, or venlafaxine, 37.5 mg/day, or control (all for 10 days starting the day before surgery). At 6 months' follow-up, pain scores with movement were lower in the venlafaxine group than in the gabapentin or control groups. It is not clear, however, whether gabapentin can reliably alter long-term pain following breast surgery. If the three gabapentin studies are combined (see Table 19.3), there appears to be a benefit, but the dose and duration required to achieve maximal benefit need further investigation, and follow-up at 12 months and longer is needed.

Clearly, there is a need for follow-up studies to confirm these findings on perioperative interventions aimed at reducing persistent pain after breast surgery, but early results suggest utility for these interventions.

INGUINAL HERNIA REPAIR

A number of excellent reviews on post-herniorrhaphy pain have been published.[20,58] The PROSPECT group[59] has recommended that spinal anesthesia not be used routinely because of acute postoperative complications, but to date, no differences in persistent pain have been found between different anesthetic techniques or different postoperative analgesic methods.[60] However, a number of studies have evaluated the effect of different surgical techniques and found differences. These studies include comparison of open hernia repair with mesh and laparoscopic repair with mesh, identification and sectioning of major nerves versus preservation of these nerves, the use of lightweight mesh versus regular mesh, and comparison of open mesh repairs with open nonmesh repairs. Table 19.4 is a summary of the effects of different surgical interventions on the probability of persistent pain.[61-65] These data are presented as odds ratios and 95% confidence intervals. A recent systematic review comparing open hernia repair with laparoscopic

Table 19.4 Interventions in Inguinal Hernia Repair and Risk (Odd Ratio) for Persistent Pain

Experimental Group	Control Group	Odds Ratio	95% Confidence Interval	Study Type	*N*	Follow-up (mo)	Reference
Laparoscopic (primary)	Open	0.66	0.51-0.87	Meta	7161	12-36	O'Reilly[61]
Laparoscopic (recurrent)	Open	0.91	0.14-5.88	Meta	322	6-60	Karthikesalingam[62]
Lightweight mesh	Standard mesh	0.61	0.50-0.74	Meta	2069	6-60	Sajid[63]
Shouldice	Open (other)	0.70	0.40-1.22	Meta	1968	12-60	Amato[64]
Shouldice	Mesh	0.87	0.55-1.39	Meta	1371	3-72	Amato[64]
Nerve sectioning	Nerve identification	0.80	0.60-1.07	Meta	851	6	Wijsmuller[65]

Meta, meta-analysis.

repair[61] found a lower risk for PPSP with a laparoscopic approach for primary, unilateral hernia repair. Repair of recurrent hernias appears to be different, with no benefit found when comparing laparoscopic and open hernia repair.[62] A Cochrane Database review[64] did not find a difference in the prevalence of chronic pain when comparing a Shouldice repair with an open mesh repair or when comparing a Shouldice repair with an open nonmesh repair. A systematic review of nerve preservation versus sectioning found three randomized controlled trials and four cohort trials.[65] Intentional sectioning of the ilioinguinal and iliohypogastric nerves did not alter the probability of persistent pain following hernia repair at 6 months (21% prevalence of pain for nerve sectioning and 23% prevalence for nerve preservation). Lightweight mesh appears to be associated with a lower prevalence of chronic pain than heavyweight mesh does.[63] Use of tissue adhesives rather than sutures to secure the mesh in open hernia repairs is associated with fewer moderate to severe complications at 6 to 12 months.[66] In another study comparing a cyanoacrylate as an adhesive for the mesh with sutures, pain prevalence at 13 months was zero in the adhesive group and 18% in the suture group.[67]

Few analgesic interventions have been reported to be of benefit regarding PPSP. A consensus statement was issued regarding prevention and management of PPSP,[68] but neither anesthetic nor postoperative management was addressed. One study of a single dose of gabapentin given 1 hour before surgery reported lower mean pain intensity at 1, 3, and 6 months' follow-up.[69]

There are some data on which patients are at increased risk for the development of PPSP following hernia repair. Aasvang and colleagues[70] performed detailed somatosensory examinations on patients scheduled for elective, unilateral hernia repair both before and 6 months following surgery. The studies were performed at two hernia centers; one center performed only open mesh repairs, whereas the other center used a laparoscopic transabdominal preperitoneal (TAP) approach and used fibrin glue rather than tacks. They found a significant interaction between pain sensitivity and nerve damage, and nerve damage was strongly associated with the open repair. Patients with a high pain threshold were unlikely to have pain at 6 months regardless of the surgical approach, whereas patients with a low pain threshold who also had documented nerve damage were at high risk of having pain at 6 months. Bittner and coworkers[71] noted that patients undergoing a TAP hernia repair were more likely to report pain at 6 months if they reported pain before the procedure. Together, these studies raise the possibility that patients with increased pain sensitivity or those who already have pain are at higher risk for PPSP.

Surgical treatment of chronic pain following hernia repair has been reviewed recently.[72] Neurectomy of the ilioinguinal, iliohypogastric, genitofemoral, or lateral femoral cutaneous nerve was described in 14 papers, with most reporting good outcomes. However, the reviewers questioned the quality of these studies in terms of methodology, preoperative and intraoperative diagnostic criteria, and follow-up. They also found insufficient data on the effect of removal of mesh or staples to make a recommendation on this. Medical management of persistent post-herniorrhaphy pain is limited to a few case reports.

HIP REPLACEMENT

Total hip arthroplasty (THA) is the most successful treatment of arthritis-induced pain in the hip, but unfortunately, the success rate of treating pain is not 100%, and some patients have worse pain following THA.[14] There are a wealth of data regarding outcomes following THA, including pain, quality of life, and patient satisfaction. Reports include numerous national registries, as well as prospective randomized studies, that looked at various interventions and surgical approaches. A report from the Swedish Hip Arthroplasty Register (nearly 35,000 procedures) documented that mean pain scores on a visual analog scale (VAS) decreased from 62 out of 100 preoperatively to 14 out of 100 at 12-month follow-up and that 88.6% of the patients reported that they were satisfied with the procedure.[73] Predictors of a worse outcome included a preoperative report of pain in multiple joints, older age, and male gender. One finding that has become obvious recently is that the presence of pain at other sites is a major predictor of persistent pain following THA. Wylde and colleagues[14] found an increasingly large odds ratio for persistent pain with an increasing number of other reported pain problems. This was echoed by Liu and associates[74] and supported by data from the Swedish registry.[73] Additionally, mental health has an effect, with depression being associated with a higher probability of persistent pain[14] or worse score on the mental health component of the 36-item Short Form Health Survey (SF-36).[75]

Depression has been associated with worse outcomes and is a predictor of PPSP. Data from the Swedish registry document less of an improvement in mobility and more pain in individuals who had greater anxiety or depression before surgery.[76] Wylde and associates found a statistically significant association between depression and PPSP.[14]

There have been a number of attempts to incorporate minimally invasive surgery into THA. A systematic review[77] found that minimally invasive surgery resulted in less acute postoperative pain and more rapid discharge, but there was no decrease in the prevalence of PPSP.

Since more severe acute pain has been associated with PPSP,[2] there is hope that improved acute pain control will decrease PPSP. Use of local anesthetics has been tried by a number of investigators, but with equivocal benefit. Aguirre and colleagues[78] used continuous wound infusion of ropivacaine for 48 hours and found no difference in rest pain at 3 months, but subjects in the ropivacaine group reported less discomfort to touch and pressure in the area of the wound. One small study compared a single iliofascial injection of L-bupivacaine, clonidine, and epinephrine with a single epidural injection of L-bupivacaine with sufentanil. A statistically significant difference in pain prevalence was observed at 3 months, but no difference at 1, 6, or 12 months.[79] There are no reports of continuous epidural infusions, femoral nerve blocks or infusions, or sciatic blocks decreasing long-term pain following THA.

A single study demonstrated improved pain at 6 months in patients who received a ketamine infusion intraoperatively and then for 24 hours.[80] They noted a morphine-sparing effect in the acute postoperative period and facilitation of rehabilitation for the first month. At 6 months, 8% of the ketamine subjects and 21% of the control group had pain at rest. Acute pain control was not different. Whether the improved outcome at 6 months can be directly attributed to the ketamine infusion or attributed to the improved participation in rehabilitation will need to be determined. One study of incorporating gabapentin (600 mg before surgery and 600 mg after surgery) into a multimodal analgesic regimen showed no benefit on acute or chronic pain.[81]

THORACOTOMY

The prevalence of pain before thoracotomy is generally low (12%), but persistent pain following thoracotomy is a significant problem, with estimates of pain prevalence at 1 year of 50%.[2] The presence of existing pain is thought to be a risk factor for PPSP.[82] A recent review of the subject[83] identified more areas needing answers than having clearly resolved issues.

The use of thoracic epidural analgesia has been advocated,[84] but recent studies have found that a paravertebral block works just as well for acute pain control and has fewer side effects.[85,86] Whether paravertebral blocks are of benefit for long-term pain has not been addressed. Thoracic epidural analgesia may be of benefit. Obata and associates[87] and Senturk and colleagues[88] both found a lower prevalence of PPSP 6 months following thoracotomy in patients who received a continuous infusion of epidural local anesthetic starting before skin incision and continuing throughout the surgery and postoperatively than in patients in whom the infusion was started postoperatively. All the patients in these two studies underwent posterolateral thoracotomy. In contrast, Ochroch and coworkers[82] did not find a significant benefit, but only a minority of their patients (32%) underwent posterolateral thoracotomy. The studies also differed in that Ochroch's group was looking at mean differences in VAS-measured pain, whereas Obata's and Senturk's groups looked at pain prevalence. There were also differences in the amount of local anesthetic in the epidural infusions, with Ochroch's subjects receiving the least local anesthetic.

How the intercostal nerves are handled can make a difference. In a prospective randomized study of 120 patients undergoing posterolateral thoracotomy, pericostal (control group) sutures were compared with intracostal sutures and an intercostal muscle flap.[89] By 6 months postoperatively there were no differences in pain and analgesic use between the groups, but at 3 months the intercostal muscle flap group was using fewer analgesics, and at the 4-week follow-up the intercostal muscle flap group had less pain and was using fewer analgesics.

A single study of low-dose (600 mg) gabapentin preoperatively found no benefit on either acute pain or pain at 3 months.[90] A study in which a low dose of ketamine was added to an epidural infusion also lacked benefit.[91] High-dose remifentanil is associated with increased allodynia and increased pain for up to 6 months.[92]

SUMMARY AND CONCLUSIONS

Based on the data presented in this chapter, we come to a number of conclusions. First, chronic pain following surgery is far from rare. Second, the surgical technique can make a significant difference in the prevalence of PPSP in hernia and breast surgery. Third, the addition of gabapentin appears to be of benefit in the perioperative period for breast surgery, but an optimal dose or duration is not known. Fourth, local anesthetics may be useful in epidural infusions for thoracic surgery or paravertebral blocks for breast surgery, but dosing has not been established. Fifth, individual patient factors are important. Such factors include pain sensitivity (as measured by thermal pain sensitivity), personality factors such as neuroticism and somatization, and the presence of depression or anxiety (or both). The extent to which any of the interventions alter spinal cord sensitization is not clear.

KEY POINTS

- Chronic pain following surgery is not rare and should be discussed as a risk before surgery.
- Minimally invasive surgery performed by experienced surgeons appears to decrease the risk for chronic pain. This is best documented for laparoscopic hernia repair and for sentinel node biopsy.
- For breast surgery, a paravertebral block has been shown to decrease the prevalence of chronic pain.
- For patients undergoing posterolateral thoracotomy, intraoperative plus postoperative epidural analgesia with local anesthetics decreases the prevalence of chronic pain.
- Adjuvant analgesics have not been adequately studied, but gabapentin, ketamine, and venlafaxine have been associated with a lower prevalence of chronic pain.
- Patients vary in their sensitivity to pain and probably in psychological factors that will alter the individual's risk for the development of chronic pain.

SUGGESTED READINGS

Aasvang EK, Gmaehle E, Hansen JB, et al. Predictive risk factors for persistent postherniotomy pain. *Anesthesiology*. 2010;112:957-969.

Aasvang E, Kehlet H. Chronic postoperative pain: the case of inguinal herniorrhaphy. *Br J Anaesth.* 2005;95:69-76.

Johansen A, Romundstad L, Nielsen CS, et al. Persistent postsurgical pain in a general population: prevalence and predictors in the Tromsö study. *Pain.* 2012;153:1390-1396.

Joshi GP, Bonnet F, Shah R, et al. A systematic review of randomized trials evaluating regional techniques for postthoracotomy analgesia. *Anesth Analg.* 2008;107:1026-1040.

Kehlet H, Jensen TS, Woolf CJ. Persistent postsurgical pain: risk factors and prevention. *Lancet.* 2006;367:1618-1625.

Macrae WA, Davies HTO. Chronic postsurgical pain. In: Crombie IK, Croft PR, Linton SJ, et al, eds. *Epidemiology of Pain.* Seattle: IASP Press; 1999:125-142.

Perkins FM, Kehlet H. Chronic pain as an outcome of surgery. *Anesthesiology.* 2000;93:1123-1233.

Poleschuck EL, Dworkin RH. Risk factors for chronic pain in patients with acute pain and their implications for prevention. In: Dworkin RH, Breitbart WS, eds. *Psychosocial Aspects of Pain: A Handbook for Health Care Providers.* Seattle: IASP Press; 2004:589-606.

Wildgaard K, Kehlet H. Chronic post-thoracotomy pain—what is new in pathogenic mechanisms and strategies for prevention? *Tech Reg Anesth Pain Manage.* 2012;15:83-89.

Woolf CJ. Evidence for a central component of postinjury pain hypersensitivity. *Nature.* 1983;308:386-388.

Wylde V, Hewlett S, Learmonth ID, et al. Persistent pain after joint replacement: prevalence, sensory qualities, and postoperative determinants. *Pain.* 2011;152:566-572.

The references for this chapter can be found at www.expertconsult.com.

20 Pediatric Acute Pain Management

Ravi Shah | Amod Sawardekar | Santhanam Suresh

Recognition and treatment of acute pain in children have vastly improved the care of pediatric patients.[1,2] Data emphasizing the efficacy of adequate pain control and decreases in adverse neurohormonal changes have led to better treatment of infants and children.[3-5] Recent advances in pharmacologic therapy and regional anesthetic techniques have helped expand the scope of pediatric acute pain management.[6] In addition, the establishment of pediatric acute pain services has played an important role in ensuring timely and consistent care of children.[7-12]

DEVELOPMENTAL NEUROBIOLOGY OF PAIN

The study of pain in neonates has been a major focus in the field of neuroscience. Nociceptive pathways are well developed even at birth. A study of brain perfusion in response to pain has demonstrated significant changes in perfusion with noxious stimuli versus non-noxious stimuli.[13] Newborn rats appear to have significant proliferation of A and C fibers at the site exposed to pain; a pattern of hyperalgesia appears to develop in these animals.[14] Human neonates exposed to repeated heel sticks may have cutaneous hyperalgesia, which can be reversed with topical local analgesia.[15] Studies in the area of pain in infants and children continue to be published, thus signifying interest in both pediatric pain management and its neurobiology.[16,17]

ASSESSMENT OF PEDIATRIC ACUTE PAIN

Essential to acute pain management in children is assessment of pain.[18] Unlike adults, pediatric patients may be too young, developmentally immature, or unwilling to provide adequate interpretation of their pain.[19] Measures of acute pain in such patients often rely on observer reports, whereas assessment in older children involves self-report measures[20] (see Table 20.1).[17,21-35] Observational pain assessment tools use information about pain-related behavior, such as body movements, facial expression, and vocalizations; physiologic changes such as heart rate and oxygen saturation; and the child's behavioral state. These measures have been designed to assess procedural pain (e.g., Premature Infant Pain Profile [PIPP],[17] Neonatal Facial Coding System [NFCS][21,22]) or postoperative pain (e.g., Children's Hospital of Eastern Ontario Pain Scale [CHEOPS],[36] Toddler-Preschooler Postoperative Pain Scale [TPPPS][28]). The FLACC scale (faces, legs, activity, cry, consolability)[37] is another pain assessment tool that can be used for all ages, including mentally challenged children (see Table 20.2). These scales have been shown to have construct validity and internal and inter-rater reliability despite intrinsic limits in their specificity for pain, such as physiologic parameters, which can vary because of other conditions not associated with pain.[23-27,29-35]

Developmentally appropriate children 5 years and older can typically provide self-reports on one of several validated visual analog (e.g., coloured analogue scale [CAS][31,38]) or faces scales (e.g., Faces Pain Scale—Revised [FPS-R],[24,39,40] Oucher[26]) (Fig. 20.1). McGrath and Hillier[41] developed a separate Facial Affective Scale (FAS) designed to measure pain affect, as distinct from pain intensity. Interestingly, the faces scales anchored with a smiling face produce higher pain ratings than do those anchored with a neutral face.[42] The well-described discordance between an observer's ratings of a child's pain and the child's self-report[43-46] allows the clinician to consider the child's self-report as the "gold standard" whenever it can reliably be obtained.[47]

The majority of pediatric pain assessment measures that have been developed focus on acute, procedure-related pain.[48,49] Alterations in the behavioral and sensory aspects of pain that can habituate when pain becomes chronic may not be captured by these measurement scales.[43] However, a systematic evaluation of chronic pain in children is beyond the scope of this chapter (see Chapter 33).

NONMEDICAL MANAGEMENT OF PEDIATRIC ACUTE PAIN

Management of pain through nonmedical techniques (e.g., environmental and behavioral strategies) has proved effective in modulating pain, both independently and in conjunction with pharmacologic interventions in children.[50-53,54] Cognitive-behavioral therapy (e.g., relaxation, problem solving, cognitive coping skills) and distraction techniques such as deep breathing, cartoon videos, party blowers, and hypnosis have strong empirical support for their efficacy in easing procedure-related pain in children.[55-59] Distraction methods are hypothesized to work by engaging children and redirecting their attention away from the pain, thereby reducing perceived pain intensity and inhibiting the neural activity that underlies pain perception.[60-66] Complementary and alternative medicine techniques such as acupuncture have also been described as potential treatments of acute pain in children.[67,68]

Table 20.1 Clinical Measurements of Pediatric Acute Pain

Age Group	Measure	Type of Measurement	Type of Pain
Neonates and infants	Premature Infant Pain Profile (PIPP) (preterm and full-term neonates)[17]	Behavioral, physiologic; gestational age	Procedural
	Neonatal Facial Coding System (NFCS) (preterm and full-term neonates, infants ≤18 mo)[21,22]		
	COMFORT scale (0-3 yr)[23]	Behavioral, physiologic	Procedural, postoperative
Toddlers and preschoolers	Faces scales[24,25]	Self-report	Procedural, postoperative
	Oucher (≥3 yr)[26]	Self-report	Procedural
	Poker chip tool (4-8 yr)[27]	Self-report	Procedural
	Toddler-Preschooler Postoperative Pain Scale (TPPPS) (1-5 yr)[28]	Behavioral	Postoperative
	Children's Hospital of Eastern Ontario Pain Scale (CHEOPS) (1-7 yr)[29]	Behavioral	Postoperative
	Children's and Infants' Postoperative Pain Scale (CHIPPS) (0-4 yr)[30]	Behavioral, physiologic, alertness, calmness	Postoperative
School-age children and adolescents	Colored analog scale (CAS) (≥5 yr)[31]	Self-report	Procedural, recurrent, chronic
	Visual analog scale (VAS) (≥5 yr)[31,32]	Self-report	Procedural, recurrent, chronic
	Faces Pain Scale	Self-report	Procedural, recurrent, chronic
Non-communicating children, children with cognitive impairment	Non-communicating Children's Pain Checklist—Postoperative Version (NCCPC-PV), Non-Communicating Children's Pain Checklist—R (NCCPC-R)[33,34]	Behavioral	Procedural, postoperative injury, pain related to chronic medical condition
	VAS[35]	Self-report	Procedural

Table 20.2 FLACC Behavioral Pain Scale

Categories	Scoring 0	Scoring 1	Scoring 2
Face	No particular expression or smile	Occasional grimace or frown, withdrawn, disinterested	Frequent to constant frown, clenched jaw, quivering chin
Legs	Normal position or relaxed	Uneasy, restless, tense	Kicking or legs drawn up
Activity	Lying quietly, normal position, moves easily	Squirming, shifting back and forth, tense	Arched, rigid, or jerking
Cry	No cry (awake or asleep)	Moans or whimpers, occasional complaint	Crying steadily, screams or sobs, frequent complaints
Consolability	Content, relaxed	Reassured by occasional touching, hugging, being talked to; distractible	Difficult to console or comfort

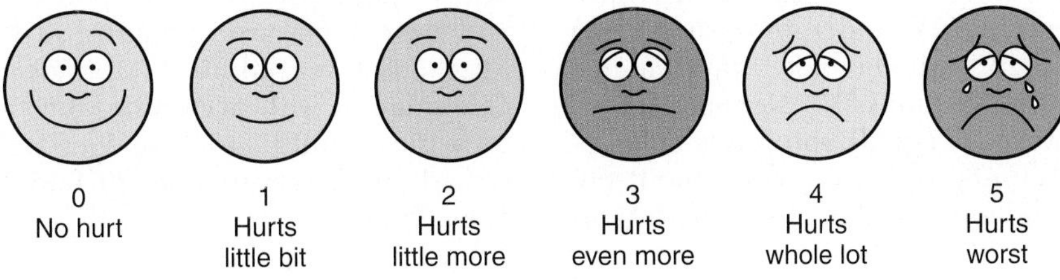

Figure 20.1 Faces Pain Scale.

PAIN TREATMENT MODALITIES

Acute pain in infants and children can be treated with various analgesics.[69] The use of multimodal analgesia is beneficial for the management of pediatric pain.[70] A pain treatment plan is best developed before the patient's surgery, and an important goal is to provide a consistent approach to treating pain with minimal adverse effects.[12,71-74]

MILD ANALGESICS

SUCROSE

Administration of glucose and sucrose orally can provide mild analgesia since opioid peptides in the ventral striatum and cingulate gyrus may play a role in regulating positive responses to energy-rich food sources.[75,76] A Cochran database review suggested that sucrose may be effective in reducing procedural pain in neonates.[77] Doses in the range

Table 20.3 Nonopioid Analgesic Dosing

Medication	Dose (mg/kg)	Dosing Interval (hr)	Maximum Daily Dose (mg/kg)	Maximum Daily Dose (mg)
Acetaminophen (oral)	10-15	4	75	4000
Acetaminophen (IV)	15	6	75	4000
Acetaminophen (rectal)	30-40 as loading dose, 15-20 thereafter	6	75	4000
Ibuprofen	10	6	40	2400
Ketorolac (IV)	0.5	6	2	120

of 0.01 to 0.1 g can be used to reduce procedural pain in infants younger than 6 months.[78]

ACETAMINOPHEN

Acetaminophen is commonly used in children to reduce or eliminate pain. It can be administered via the oral, rectal, and intravenous routes. The rectal and intravenous routes are preferable during the perioperative period. Rectal suppositories require higher dosing and may have variable absorption but can be an effective analgesic for postoperative pain in children. Specifically, an initial rectal dose of 30-40 mg/kg is recommended, followed by subsequent doses of 15-20 mg/kg at 4- to 6-hour intervals. This produces therapeutic plasma levels that may be adequate for managing pain.[79,80] Intravenous acetaminophen has recently been made available in the United States; it has more predictable bioavailability and achieves maximum concentration more rapidly than rectal dosing does.[81]

Dosing in premature and term neonates can be affected by renal and hepatic immaturity. Hepatotoxicity is a potential risk with acetaminophen use and is dose dependent. Though a rare complication, the incidence of hepatic toxicity with higher doses of acetaminophen should be presented cautiously to parents so that injudicious use of the medication is avoided.[82]

NONSTEROIDAL ANTI-INFLAMMATORY DRUGS

Nonsteroidal anti-inflammatory drugs (NSAIDs) are commonly used in children in the perioperative and postoperative periods and can be administered via the oral, intravenous, or intramuscular routes. NSAIDs have been used effectively in children undergoing surgery to reduce postoperative pain and decrease requirements for supplemental pain medications.[83-85] Neonatal clearance of NSAIDs improves with age. Ibuprofen is metabolized by the 2C9 and 2C8 subgroups of cytochrome P-450 (CYP).[86] Ketorolac is commonly used in children and can be administered via the intravenous or intramuscular routes. The clinical significance of the effects of NSAIDs on bleeding remains controversial, which has led to its avoidance by some for procedures such as tonsillectomy. Known side effects, including bleeding, renal toxicity, and gastritis, are more likely to occur with prolonged administration and in the presence of coexisting disease. Despite conflicting views about the use of intravenous ketorolac following orthopedic surgery in animal experiments, a short duration of therapy does not seem to affect bone healing.[87] NSAIDs are excellent adjuvants to opioids for pain relief. In certain surgeries that could lead to postoperative bleeding, it may be wise to avoid using ketorolac[88] (see Table 20.3). A randomized controlled trial of acetaminophen, ibuprofen, and codeine for relief of acute pain in children with musculoskeletal trauma demonstrated that ibuprofen provided the best analgesia among the three study medications.[89]

TRAMADOL

Tramadol is increasingly being used for the control of pain in children.[90,91] The absence of respiratory depression, along with a decrease in postoperative nausea and vomiting, makes it an attractive alternative to conventional opioids.[92] It is metabolized to *O*-desmethyltramadol by CYP2D6.[93] The recommended dose of tramadol is 1 mg/kg orally every 6 hours. Children with significant obstructive sleep apnea may particularly benefit from the use of tramadol as an alternative to intravenous opioids with respect to respiratory compromise.[94]

OPIOID ANALGESICS

Opioids can be used effectively in infants and children, particularly in the postoperative setting and for managing chronic painful conditions, including sickle cell disease, cystic fibrosis,[95] and painful cancer states. Dosing may be achieved via the oral, parenteral, intranasal,[96,97] and epidural routes. Opioids have lower clearance in neonates and infants but reach normal mature values in the first 6 months of life.[98] Opioid-induced respiratory depression may be more pronounced in neonates and infants, whose respiratory reflex responses to airway obstruction and hypoxemia are immature at birth but mature during the first year of life.[99] Opioids are commonly used in combination with acetaminophen or NSAIDs (or both) to achieve multimodal analgesia. Commonly used oral opioids are listed in Table 20.4 and parenteral opioids in Table 20.5.

Intravenous opioids are chosen when patients are unable to take oral medications or require markedly increased pain control. Adverse effects of opioids, including respiratory depression, nausea and vomiting, pruritus, and itching, can be managed effectively, thereby resulting in a favorable postoperative outcome (Table 20.6).[100]

PATIENT-CONTROLLED ANALGESIA

Patient-controlled analgesia (PCA) can be used to provide analgesia to children and adolescents in a controlled autonomous fashion. Several controlled trials support the safety and efficacy of PCA in children older than 6 years.[101] In the

Table 20.4 Oral Opioid Analgesic Dosing Guidelines

Medication	Potency Relative to Morphine	Typical Starting Dose (mg/kg)	Typical Dose (mg if >60 kg)	Dosing Interval (hr)
Morphine	1	0.3	15-20	3-4
Codeine	0.1	0.5-1	30-60	4-6
Hydrocodone	1-1.5	0.1-0.2	5-10	4-6
Oxycodone	1-1.5	0.1-0.2	5-10	4-6
Hydromorphone	5-7	0.04-0.08	2-4	3-4
Methadone	1	0.1-0.2	10	6-12

Table 20.5 Parenteral Opioid Dosing Guidelines

Medication	Loading Dose	Demand Dose	Lockout Time (min)	Continuous Infusion
Morphine	0.05-0.20 (mg/kg)	0.01-0.02 (mg/kg)	5-15	0.01-0.02 (mg/kg)
Fentanyl	0.5-2.0 (μg/kg)	0.2-0.4 (μg/kg)	5-15	0.2-0.4 (μg/kg)
Hydromorphone	1-4 (μg/kg)	2-3 (μg/kg)	5-15	2-3 (μg/kg)

Table 20.6 Management of Opioid-related Side Effects

Adverse Effect	Initial Management	Secondary Management
Pruritus	Benadryl, hydroxyzine	IV low-dose naloxone
Nausea, vomiting	Phenergan	Ondansetron, IV naloxone
Urinary retention	Decrease opioid dose	Urinary catheterization
Respiratory depression	Decrease opioid dose	IV naloxone

IV, intravenous.

pediatric realm, PCA use is commonly extended to include the educated provider of the child, most often the patient's nurse or parent. The use of nurse-controlled or parent-controlled analgesia[102] has been controversial because of safety issues. However, cautious use of PCA, whether it is nurse or parent controlled, can provide excellent pain relief in the postoperative period, even in developmentally delayed children or infants. Morphine, fentanyl, and hydromorphone are commonly used opioids for PCA. A basal infusion may be added to PCA settings to increase analgesia in patients undergoing major surgery. Children likely to experience significant postoperative pain may require additional continuous infusions of adjuvant medications for further pain control. Appendix A is a sample order set for managing PCA in children undergoing spinal fusion, for which we administer continuous epidural analgesia in addition to PCA.

REGIONAL ANESTHESIA

Enthusiasm for the use of regional anesthesia to manage acute pain in children has been increasing. Despite some controversy regarding the performance of regional anesthesia in children under general anesthesia, there is consensus among pediatric anesthesiologists about the importance and use of safely providing a regional anesthetic technique under general anesthesia.[103]

CAUDAL ANALGESIA

One of the most commonly used pediatric regional anesthetic techniques for postoperative analgesia is a caudal block, which is used in children undergoing surgery from the lumbosacral to midthoracic dermatome levels with anticipated moderate postoperative pain. Its popularity originates in part from the readily palpable landmarks and relative ease of placement in infants and children versus adults. A needle with a blunt stylet is passed through the sacrococcygeal ligament into the caudal space. A distinct "pop" is usually felt when the caudal space is entered. Nerve stimulation[104] and ultrasonography[105] have also been described as tools to assist in caudal placement. Local anesthetics include bupivacaine (0.125% to 0.25%) and ropivacaine (0.1% to 0.375%) with 1:200,000 epinephrine at a dose of 1 mL/kg (maximum dosage, 30 mL).

SPINAL ANESTHESIA

Spinal anesthetic techniques have been used, especially in former preterm infants who are undergoing hernia repair as a method to avoid apnea and bradycardia.[106] The procedure can be performed in an awake infant, thereby avoiding exposure to general anesthesia. This technique, though effective, has limitations because of the lack of adequate training to perform this block on a routine basis.[107]

CONTINUOUS NEURAXIAL CATHETERS

Continuous epidural analgesia is a commonly used technique in infants and children.[108] Epidural catheters may be placed in the thoracic, lumbar, or caudal regions. It is also possible to insert a caudal catheter and thread it cephalad to the desired dermatomal level. Bupivacaine and ropivacaine are frequently used local anesthetic solutions. Common additives to these solutions include opioids and α_2-agonists, including fentanyl, morphine, hydromorphone, and clonidine. It is

Table 20.7 Pediatric Epidural Dosing Guidelines

Medication	Initial Bolus	Infusion Solution	Infusion Limits
Bupivacaine	≤2.5-3 mg/kg	0.0625-0.1%	≤0.4-0.5 mg/kg/hr
Ropivacaine	≤2.5-3 mg/kg	0.1-0.2%	≤0.4-0.5 mg/kg/hr
Fentanyl	1-2 μg/kg	2-5 μg/mL	0.5-2 μg/kg/hr
Morphine	10-30 μg/kg	5-10 μg/mL	1-5 μg/kg/hr
Hydromorphone	2-6 μg/kg	2-5 μg/mL	1-2.5 μg/kg/hr
Clonidine	1-2 μg/kg	0.5-1 μg/mL	0.5-1 μg/kg/hr

imperative that standardized dosing parameters for a single injection, as well as for continuous infusion, be used in neonates, infants, and children to avoid local anesthetic–related systemic toxicity.[109] Suggested pediatric dosing regimens are listed in Table 20.7. Patient-controlled epidural analgesia can be used successfully with continuous infusions of local anesthetic and patient-determined boluses, which are delivered to augment analgesia.[110]

PERIPHERAL NERVE BLOCKADE

Peripheral and truncal nerve blocks have played an increasing role in pediatric postoperative pain management.[111,112] In addition, these techniques have been described as an effective means of achieving analgesia in the setting of pediatric trauma.[113] These techniques are typically performed under general anesthesia and increasingly with the use of ultrasound guidance. Head and neck, transversus abdominis plane (TAP), rectus sheath, ilioinguinal/iliohypogastric, and upper and lower extremity blocks are performed frequently to provide analgesia in suitable candidates (Box 20.1).[114-125] Common dosing guidelines for these blocks have been included as a reference point for practitioners (Table 20.8). Multicenter databases such as the Pediatric Regional Anesthesia Network have been created to accumulate valuable information about the frequency of use and complication rates with both neuraxial and peripheral blocks in the pediatric population.[126]

CONTINUOUS PERIPHERAL NERVE BLOCKADE

Continuous peripheral nerve blocks (CPNBs) with ultrasonographic guidance are now more widely used in pediatrics as a way to provide pain relief for an extended duration.[127] CPNBs can not only control pain but may also enable physical therapy in children with chronic regional pain syndromes.[128] They can be placed in various locations to ensure analgesia in site-specific areas.

Brachial plexus catheters are useful for surgical procedures on the elbow, forearm, and hand. Perineural catheter placement in the axillary region can provide pain control, but concerns over catheter sterility and migration exist.[129] Catheters placed in the supraclavicular location are effective and may reduce these concerns.

The TAP block provides somatic analgesia to the anterolateral abdominal wall. Three muscle layers lie lateral to the rectus abdominis: the external oblique, internal oblique, and transversus abdominis. The thoracolumbar nerve roots

Box 20.1 Commonly Performed Peripheral Nerve Blocks in Children

Head and Neck

Supraorbital and supratrochlear[114]
Occipital[115]
Infraorbital[116]
Superficial cervical plexus[117]
Auriculotemporal[118]

Upper Extremity

Brachial plexus[119]
- Interscalene
- Supraclavicular
- Infraclavicular
- Axillary

Elbow
- Median
- Radial
- Ulnar

Wrist
- Median
- Radial
- Ulnar

Lower Extremity

Lumbar plexus
Femoral nerve[120]
Lateral femoral cutaneous[121]
Saphenous
Sciatic nerve[122]
- Infragluteal
- Popliteal fossa

Trunk and Thorax

Intercostal
Ilioinguinal, iliohypogastric[123]
Rectus sheath block[124]
Penile[125]
Transversus abdominis plane block

Table 20.8 Suggested Dosing Guidelines for Local Anesthetics for Peripheral Nerve Blocks

Technique	Dose (mL/kg)	Maximum Volume (mL)
Head and neck blocks	0.1 mL/kg	5 mL
Axillary block	0.2-0.3 mL/kg	15 mL
Infraclavicular block	0.2-0.3 mL/kg	15 mL
Intercostal block	0.05-0.1 mL/kg	5 mL
Rectus sheath block	0.2 mL/kg	10 mL
Ilioinguinal block	0.2-0.3 mL/kg	15 mL
Femoral nerve block	0.2-0.4 mL/kg	15 mL
Sciatic nerve block	0.3-0.5 mL/kg	20 mL
Popliteal fossa block	0.3-0.4 mL/kg	15 mL
Lumbar plexus block	0.3-0.5 mL/kg	20 mL
Penile block	0.1 mL/kg	10 mL
Digital nerve block	0.05-0.1 mL/kg	2-3 mL
Transversus abdominis plane block	0.2 mL/kg/side	15mL/side

(T8-L1) course between the internal oblique and transversus abdominis muscle (TAP plane). A single-injection TAP block with the assistance of ultrasonography can provide relief of pain following abdominal incisions. Placement of a catheter into the TAP plane provides continuous analgesia and decreases supplemental postoperative systemic opioid requirements.[130] The use of continuous TAP catheters in pediatric patients is an alternative to conventional neuraxial catheters.[131] TAP catheters can also provide analgesia in patients with severe spinal deformities that preclude neuraxial anesthesia.[132]

CPNBs are useful in providing lower extremity analgesia for an extended period. Femoral catheters have been used safely and effectively in the pediatric population.[133] Continuous femoral nerve blocks are commonly used to treat pain from surgery on the distal end of the femur and anterior aspect of the knee and have also been used in the treatment of complex regional pain syndrome and cancer-related pain. The proximity of the femoral nerve to major vessels (the femoral vein and artery) makes vessel puncture and hematoma formation potential complications. Risks associated with indwelling catheter placement include infection, nerve damage, and falls as a result of block-induced quadriceps motor weakness.

Continuous sciatic nerve blockade can be used successfully to provide analgesia to the lower extremity in infants and children. It has been shown to have fewer adverse effects than epidural anesthesia in children undergoing major foot and ankle surgery.[134] The sciatic nerve is formed by the L4 to S3 nerve roots and provides innervation to the posterior aspect of the thigh and the distal end of the leg (beyond the knee) with the exception of the calf. The sciatic nerve exits the pelvis through the greater sciatic foramen and then courses deep to the gluteus maximus muscle and distally to the posterior popliteal fossa. There it bifurcates to form the tibial and common peroneal nerves. Sciatic nerve catheters can be placed at the subgluteal or popliteal fossa in children (Fig. 20.2).

Continuous peripheral nerve blocks are evolving as a novel extended analgesic modality in children. The use of ultrasonography can facilitate and confirm placement of the catheter, which may reduce pain and diminish or eliminate the need for opioid medications and their undesirable side effects.

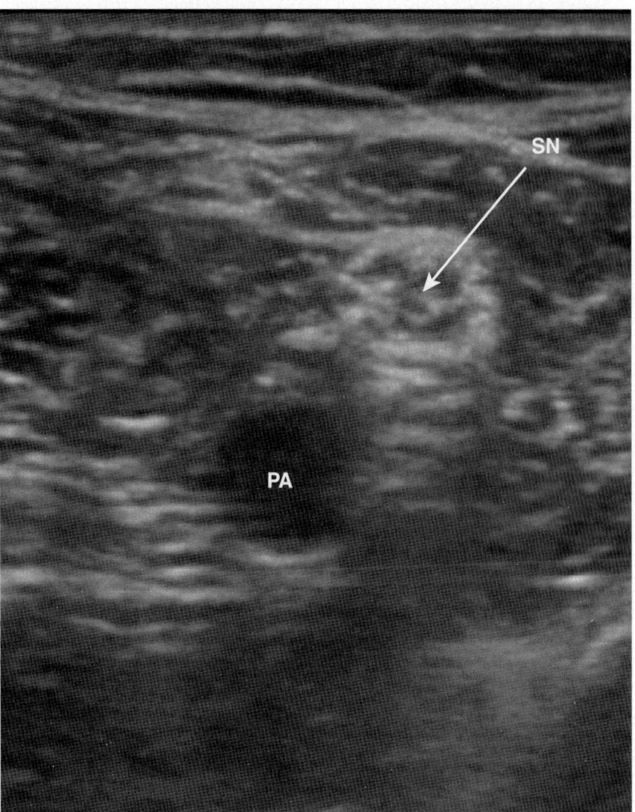

Figure 20.2 Sonographic anatomy of the sciatic nerve at the popliteal fossa *(arrow)*. PA, popliteal artery; SN, sciatic nerve.

CONCLUSION

Acute pain management in children has made significant strides. The addition of medications with better safety profiles and the emerging role of regional anesthesia have clearly improved the care of neonates, infants, and children.[135] Pediatric patients have unique needs, and it is critical that we continue to advance this field through ongoing research and innovation.

KEY POINTS

- Various measures of pain intensity are available for the pediatric population, and selection of the correct scale must be based on the patient's age, development delay, and willingness to provide feedback.
- Nonopioid analgesics, in the forms of acetaminophen and nonsteroidal anti-inflammatory drugs, can provide relief of mild to moderate pain and are administered via the oral, intravenous, intramuscular, and rectal routes.
- Patient-controlled opioid analgesics can be used effectively to control pain and improve patient satisfaction.
- Neuraxial anesthesia can provide reliable effective pain relief after general anesthesia is induced in infants and young children.
- Continuous peripheral nerve blockade provides site-specific analgesia and is being used more commonly in pediatrics.

SUGGESTED READINGS

Anand KJ. Neonatal stress responses to anesthesia and surgery. *Clin Perinatol.* 1990;17:207-214.

Anand KJ, Aranda JV, Berde CB, et al. Summary proceedings from the Neonatal Pain-Control Group. *Pediatrics.* 2006;117:S9-S22.

Birmingham PK, Tobin MJ, Fisher DM, et al. Initial and subsequent dosing of rectal acetaminophen in children: a 24-hour pharmacokinetic study of new dose recommendations. *Anesthesiology.* 2001;87:244-252.

Birmingham PK, Wheeler M, Suresh S, et al. Patient-controlled epidural analgesia in children: can they do it? *Anesth Analg.* 2003;96:686-691.

Butler LD, Symons BK, Henderson SL, et al. Hypnosis reduces distress and duration of an invasive medical procedure for children. *Pediatrics.* 2005;115:77-85.

Chay PC, Duffy BJ, Walker JS. Pharmacokinetic-pharmacodynamic relationships of morphine in neonates. *Clin Pharmacol Ther.* 1992;51:334-342.

Chidambaran V, Sadhasivam S. Pediatric acute and surgical pain management: recent advances and future perspectives. *Int Anesthesiol Clin.* 2012;50:66-82.

Clark E, Plint AC, Correll R, et al. A randomized controlled trial of acetaminophen, ibuprofen, and codeine for acute pain relief in children with musculoskeletal trauma. *Pediatrics.* 2007;119:460-467.

Hicks CL, von Baeyer CL, Spafford PA, et al. The Faces Pain Scale—Revised: toward a common metric in pediatric pain measurement. *Pain.* 2001;93:173-183.

Iyer SB, Schubert CJ, Schoettker PJ, et al. Use of quality-improvement methods to improve timeliness of analgesic delivery. *Pediatrics.* 2011;127:e219-e225.

Krane EJ, Dalens BJ, Murat I, et al. The safety of epidurals placed during general anesthesia. *Reg Anesth Pain Med.* 1998;23:433-438.

Nowicki PD, Vanderhave KL, Gibbons K, et al. Perioperative pain control in pediatric patients undergoing orthopaedic surgery. *J Am Acad Orthop Surg.* 2012;20:755-765.

Polaner DM, Taenzer AH, Walker BJ, et al. Pediatric Regional Anesthesia Network (PRAN): a multi-institutional study of the use and incidence of complications of pediatric regional anesthesia. *Anesth Analg.* 2012;115:1353-1364.

Suresh S, Birmingham PK, Kozlowski RJ. Pediatric pain management. *Anesthesiol Clin.* 2012;30:101-117.

Tsui B, Suresh S. Ultrasound imaging for regional anesthesia in infants, children, and adolescents: a review of current literature and its application to neuraxial blocks. *Anesthesiology.* 2010;112:719-728.

The references for this chapter can be found at www.expertconsult.com.

Appendix A

Sample Patient-Controlled Analgesia Order Set

ANESTHESIA - EPIDURAL [240]

Routine Orders

Routine

	Order	Details
☑	VITAL SIGNS	Routine, PER PROTOCOL, Starting today, Vital Signs per PROTOCOL including Pain Relief and Sedation.
☑	PULSE OX CONTINUOUS IP-NURSING	Routine, CONTINUOUS (BILL EVERY 24 HOURS), Starting today
☑	CARDIAC/RESPIRATORY MONITORING IP UNITS	Routine, CONTINUOUS (BILL EVERY 24 HOURS), Starting today, Consider HR/RR low alarm guidelines as follows: (<2yrs: 100/24; 2-5yrs: 80/20; 6-12 yrs: 70/16; >12yrs 60/12)
☑	NOTIFY PAIN MANAGEMENT TEAM - STAT (#97009)	STAT, AS NEEDED, Starting today, *NOTIFY STAT (Pager #97009) if respiratory rate < 12, SpO2 <92%, patient is cyanotic and/or the patient is unarousable. STOP PCA or PCEA and apply supplemental O2 by mask.
☑	NOTIFY PAIN MANAGEMENT TEAM - APN (#75157) or Anesthesia Resident (#97009)	Routine, AS NEEDED, Starting today, For inadequate analgesia, side effect management, other questions, and to evaluate PCA discontinuation.
☑	NURSING COMMUNICATION - No Additional Sedatives	NO ADDITIONAL SEDATIVES/OPIOIDS TO BE GIVEN DURING EPIDURAL INFUSION UNLESS DISCUSSED WITH ANESTHESIA/PAIN MANAGEMENT TEAM (Pager #75157 APN or pager #97009 Resident).
☑	REFER TO MAR OR KARDEX FOR PCA/EPIDURAL SETTINGS	Routine, ONCE, Starting For 1 Occurrences

Routine PCEA

	Order	Details
☑	NOTIFY PAIN MANAGEMENT TEAM-STAT (#97009)	STAT, AS NEEDED, Starting today, STOP PCEA INFUSION and page Anesthesia if: Systolic Blood Pressure < 60 mmHg in a patient < 1 year old, Systolic Blood Pressure < 70 mmHg in a patient > 1 year old, If the patient or nurse notes increased leg weakness or numbness or signs of local anesthetic toxicity such as ringing in ears, metallic taste in mouth, lip numbness, or slurred speech.
☑	NOTIFY MD/PROVIDER	Routine, AS NEEDED, Starting today, *NOTIFY Primary/Surgical Service if no urine output after 8 hours to evaluate patient for urinary retention. *NOTIFY Pain ManagementTeam (APN or Resident) and Primary/Surgical Service if pressure sores or blisters noted.

Nursing Orders

NURSING - ANESTHESIA - EPIDURAL

	Order	Details
☑	ASSESS PIV	Routine, PER ROUTINE, Starting today, Maintain access during infusion.
☑	INFORMATION SHEETS	*PCA Information Sheets to be given to patient/parents. *Epidural Information Sheets to be given to patient/parents.
☑	NURSING COMMUNICATION - Instructions for Activity	If patient is allowed to ambulate per the service/surgeon's orders, may ambulate ONLY with assistance.
☑	ASSESS	Routine, EVERY SHIFT, Starting today, Assess SKIN in dependent areas for pressure sores and/or blisters.
☑	DRESSING CHECKS - Epidural Catheter	Routine, EVERY SHIFT, Starting today, Assess epidural catheter dressing for signs of infection, soiling, or catheter displacement (fluid leaking into dressing) every shift. If any of these occur, stop infusion and notify Anesthesia Resident (#97009) and Pain Team APN (#75157).

Epidural Only

Epidural (Single Response)

	Order	Details
○	fentanyl-bupivacaine epidural	Epidural, CONTINUOUS
○	cloNIDine-bupivacaine epidural	Epidural, CONTINUOUS

Concurrent Epidural + PCA

Consider using both epidural infusion + PCA continuous and demand for spinal fusion. For pectus repair, consider using both continuous epidural infusion and demand-only PCA. Consider avoiding fentanyl in epidural when also ordering IV PCA.

Epidural (Single Response)

	Order	Details
○	bupivacaine epidural	Epidural, CONTINUOUS
○	cloNIDine-bupivacaine epidural	Epidural, CONTINUOUS

PCA (Single Response)

	Order	Details
○	HYDROmorphone pca 50 mcg/mL (patient < 10 kg)	Intravenous, PCA
○	HYDROmorphone pca 100 mcg/mL (patient >10 kg)	Intravenous, PCA

Medications

Pruritus (Single Response)

Dose range 0.1-0.5 mg/kg/dose, maximum 25 mg/dose.

	Order	Details
○	diphenhydrAMINE (BENADRYL) injection	0.3 mg/kg/dose, Intravenous, EVERY 6 HOURS PRN, Itching, PCA pruritus

Muscle Spasm/ Anxiety (Single Response)

Dose range 0.02-0.04 mg/kg/dose, maximum 5 mg/dose.

	Order	Details
○	diazepam (VALIUM) injection	0.03 mg/kg/dose, Intravenous, EVERY 6 HOURS PRN, Muscle Spasm, Anxiety

Nausea/Vomiting (Single Response)

Dose = 0.1 mg/kg. Maximum 4 mg/dose.

	Order	Details
○	ondansetron (ZOFRAN) injection	0.1 mg/kg/dose, Intravenous, EVERY 6 HOURS PRN, Nausea, Vomiting

Pain (Single Response)

Consider using with spinal fusion, pectus repair, and other painful procedures. Consider dose of 50-100 mg BID.

	Order	Details
○	pregabalin (LYRICA) capsule	Oral, TWICE DAILY, For 6 Doses, For 6 Doses

21 Low Back Pain

Khalid Malik | Honorio T. Benzon

Low back pain (LBP) is the most common cause of pain and disability in modern society, and costs related to disorders that cause LBP amount to billions of dollars each year.[1] Pathologic conditions responsible for LBP are protean, and their precise diagnosis remains elusive. Pain can originate not only from the various components of the spinal column, such as the intervertebral disks (IVDs), vertebral bodies, facet joints, spinal nerve roots (NRs), and surrounding muscles and ligaments, but also from adjacent structures such as abdominal and pelvic viscera. The list of conditions that can produce LBP is exhaustive and includes causes as diverse as degenerative conditions, spinal metastasis, vertebral body fractures, abdominal aortic aneurysm, and chronic pancreatitis. Furthermore, the various disorders causing LBP are often present concomitantly, and their symptoms and signs are frequently analogous. The problem is further confounded by the fact that the tests currently used for diagnosis of these disorders are nonspecific and may show abnormalities in asymptomatic individuals. It is therefore crucial that a thorough clinical evaluation be accompanied by appropriate diagnostic testing to elucidate the cause of the LBP. In this chapter we will discuss the causes of chronic LBP that are pertinent to the practice of pain medicine. The clinical conditions discussed here include lumbar radicular syndrome (LRS), herniated lumbar disk (HD), lumbar spinal stenosis (LSS), internal disk disruption (IDD), and lumbar facet syndrome (LFS). Other significant causes of chronic LBP such as myofascial pain syndrome, spondylosis, spondylolisthesis, spinal instability, and sacroiliac joint dysfunction are discussed elsewhere in this book. Notable but less common causes of LBP such as spinal fractures, malignancies, osteomyelitis, and inflammatory and metabolic conditions such as ankylosing spondylitis and Paget's disease are usually excluded before a patient is evaluated by a pain medicine physician and are beyond the scope of this chapter.

LUMBAR RADICULAR SYNDROME

DEFINITION AND TERMINOLOGY

Pain, paresthesias, and numbness in a typical dermatomal distribution, with or without the accompanying signs of weakness, diminished reflexes, and a positive straight-leg raise (SLR) test, are typically due to pathology or dysfunction of the sensory spinal nerve roots (SSNRs) or dorsal root ganglia (DRGs).[2] Although radicular signs and symptoms are often present in conjunction with axial LBP, LRS is distinctive in its etiology and treatment. The term *lumbar radiculopathy* is frequently used to describe this clinical entity; however, it inappropriately implies the obligatory occurrence of objective signs of NR damage—loss of sensation, muscle weakness, and diminished reflexes.[2] *Lumbar radiculitis* is another term commonly used, although it incorrectly proposes that an inflammatory process is primarily responsible for the radicular signs and symptoms. Another term used, *lumbar radicular pain*, mistakenly assumes pain as being the predominant symptom. Hence, the descriptive term *lumbar radicular syndrome* may be the most accurate in that it correctly suggests a constellation of clinical signs and symptoms of variable etiology secondary to pathology or dysfunction of the SSNRs or DRGs. Although the term *sciatica* is often used synonymously for LRS, this term is more suited to describe pain in the distribution of the sciatic nerve.[3]

PREVALENCE

Epidemiologic studies of low back and lower extremity pain are often inexact in that the conditions producing these symptoms are frequently nonhomogeneous and poorly defined. Although the prevalence and lifetime incidence of LBP are reported variably, its overall occurrence ranges from 13.8%[4] to 31%,[5] and the related health care costs amount to billions of dollars each year.[6] The incidence of radicular symptoms in patients with LBP has been reported to range from 12%[3] to 40%.[4]

ETIOLOGY AND DIFFERENTIAL DIAGNOSIS

Pathologic involvement of SSNRs and DRGs generates ectopic impulses at these locations that are perceived as pain, numbness, and tingling in areas innervated by the affected axons (i.e., a dermatomal distribution) (Fig. 21.1).[2] Pathologic processes that can affect SSNRs and DRGs are diverse, with lesions of the IVDs and degenerative spinal disorders being most prevalent. Neoplastic, infectious, traumatic, metabolic, and vascular lesions involving SSNRs, DRGs, the spine itself, and lumbosacral plexuses can also produce radicular signs and symptoms.[7] Pathologic lesions and entrapment neuropathies involving the sciatic nerve (e.g., piriformis muscle and ischial tunnel syndromes) can generate pain and paresthesias in its distribution and often affect multiple dermatomes.[7] Pain originating in the IVDs and in the sacroiliac and facet joints and pain of myofascial origin can also be referred to the lower extremities. This somatic referred pain is due to interneuronal convergence within the spinal cord. It is nondermatomal, has a deep aching quality, rarely radiates below the knees, and lacks the objective signs of NR involvement.[2] In this chapter we review the two most common causes of radicular pain in the lower extremities, HDs and LSS.

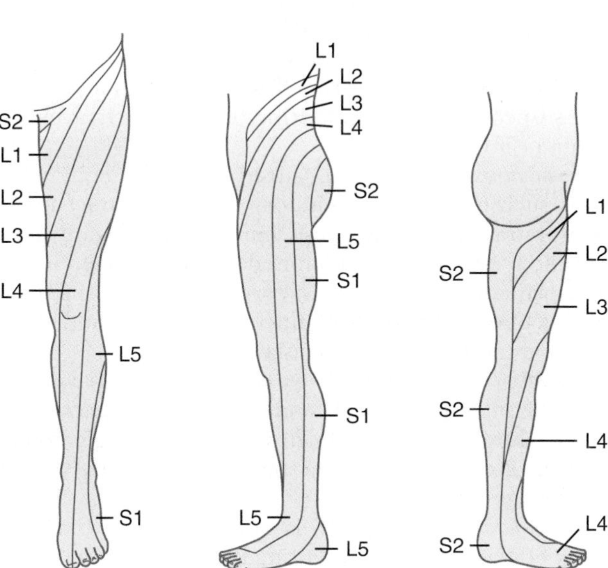

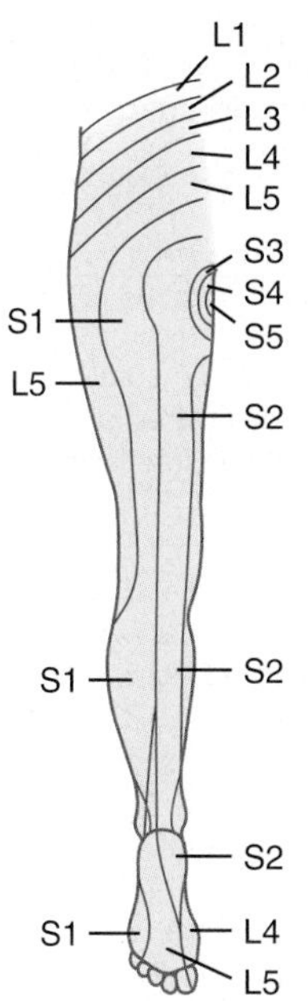

Figure 21.1 Lower extremity dermatomes.

CLINICAL FEATURES

Although pain is the predominant symptom, other symptoms of radicular involvement include paresthesias, numbness, and weakness in the territory of the involved NR. Radicular pain typically travels along a narrow band and has a sharp, shooting, and lancinating quality.[8] Objective signs of gait disturbances, loss of sensation, reduced muscle strength, and diminished reflexes involve the appropriate dermatome. HDs and the degenerative conditions commonly involve the lower lumbar NRs, whereas other, often more sinister causes of LRS involve higher NRs with greater frequency.[9] The following are characteristic features of various lumbar and sacral NR involvement:

- S1: Pain, paresthesia, and numbness of the posterior part of the thigh, calf, and plantar surface of the foot; there may be associated difficulty in toe walking, weakness of plantar flexion, and loss of the plantar reflex.
- L5: Similar symptoms involving the buttock, anterolateral aspect of the leg, dorsal surface of the foot, and great toe, with possible difficulty heel walking (steppage gait) and weakness of ankle and toe extension.
- L4: Radicular symptoms involving the anterior part of the thigh, knee, and upper to medial portion of the leg with weakness of knee extension and a diminished patellar tendon reflex.
- L3 and L2 NRs: Tend to produce symptoms and sensory alterations involving the groin and inner thigh areas.
- Lower sacral NRs: Involvement produces decreased sensation in the buttock and perineal areas (i.e., saddle anesthesia) and autonomic dysfunction, as indicated by bowel and bladder dysfunction, typically urinary retention and constipation followed by incontinence, and sexual dysfunction manifested as loss of erection in men and vaginal anesthesia in women.[10,11]

CLINICAL TESTS OF NERVE ROOT IRRITATION

Several tests can be used to confirm the presence of NR irritation (Box 21.1). Passive SLR with ankle dorsiflexion of the extended lower extremity causes traction on the lower lumbar NRs by pulling them caudally between 1.4 and 4 mm.[12] The radicular nature of the pain is suggested by worsening pain in the radicular distribution caused by such a maneuver. A positive SLR or Lasègue test is therefore suggestive of radicular pathology of the lower lumbar NRs (L4, L5, and S1). Radicular pain in the affected leg when the contralateral asymptomatic leg is similarly raised constitutes a positive crossed straight-leg raise (X-SLR) test. Although a positive SLR test is highly sensitive, X-SLR is more specific for lumbar NR irritation.[13] An increase in back pain during an SLR is typically attributed to lumbar spinal movement and indicates the mechanical nature of the LBP.[14] One exception noted is that centrally, HDs can generate LBP with an SLR because of strain on the anterior theca.[15] The tripod test is a maneuver to confirm a positive SLR test when the patient is sitting—extending the knee and dorsiflexion of the foot with the patient seated. The femoral stretch test places the L2 and L3 NRs under tension and indicates irritation of these NRs; this is tested by bending the knee and extending the hip with the patient in the prone position.

Box 21.1 Tests to Confirm the Presence of Nerve Root Irritation

Straight-leg raise
Straight-leg raise and ankle dorsiflexion of the extended lower extremity
Crossed straight-leg raise
Tripod test
Femoral stretch test

"RED FLAGS" IN THE MEDICAL HISTORY OF A PATIENT WITH LOW BACK AND RADICULAR PAIN

As previously stressed, the list of conditions causing LBP, with or without radicular symptoms, is intimidating. Fortunately, in the vast majority of patients the pain is due to

Table 21.1 "Red Flags" in the Clinical History of Patients with Low Back and Radicular Pain

Red Flag	Implications
Red Flags in the History	
Age younger than 20 yr	Congenital and developmental disorders, spondylolisthesis
Age older than 50 yr	Malignancy, pathologic fractures, infections, AAA
Short-term symptoms of <3 mo	More serious etiology
Trauma	Fractures
Fever, chills, malaise, night sweats, weight loss	Malignancy, osteomyelitis, abscess, fracture
History of cancer, HIV, chronic steroid use, IV drug abuse, immunosuppression	Malignancy, osteomyelitis, abscess, fracture
Unrelenting pain	Malignancy, osteomyelitis, abscess, fracture
Incontinence, saddle anesthesia, bilateral neurologic symptoms	Cauda equina compression
Red Flags in the Physical Examination	
Fever	Malignancy, osteomyelitis, abscess
Motor weakness, diminished reflexes, saddle anesthesia, weak anal sphincter	Cauda equina compression
Spinous process tenderness	Fracture

AAA, abdominal aortic aneurysm; HIV, human immunodeficiency virus; IV, intravenous.

benign, self-limited musculoskeletal conditions, such as muscular sprain or ligamentous strain, and the symptoms typically resolve in 4 to 6 weeks.[16] Indiscriminate diagnostic workup in these patients can be expensive and may produce findings that are unrelated and could be misleading. Hence, the Agency for Health Care Policy and Research (AHCPR) developed guidelines to help identify signs and symptoms—red flags—that indicate the presence of conditions that pose significant threat to life or neurologic function and would require further diagnostic testing (Table 21.1).[16] These conditions include malignancies, infections, fractures, and cauda equina syndrome (CES). The following is the list of "red flags" proposed in the AHCPR Publication 95-0643, published in 1994.[16]

- *Age younger than 20 or older than 50 years*: Patients younger than 20 years have a higher incidence of congenital and developmental anomalies, and those older than 50 years are prone to neoplasms, pathologic fractures, serious infections, and life-threatening extraspinal processes as a cause of their low back and radicular symptoms.[7]
- *Duration of symptoms*: The AHCPR guidelines consider symptoms of less than 3 months' duration as acute and subacute LBP. Chronic pain, or pain greater than 3 months' duration, indicates symptoms of a less serious etiology.
- *History of trauma*: A history of trauma in older patients and those with serious medical conditions may result in bony injury and require further workup.
- *Constitutional symptoms*: A history of fever, chills, malaise, night sweats, and unexplained weight loss should make one suspect a serious underlying disorder such as malignancy or infection.
- *Systemic illness*: A history of cancer, recent bacterial infections such as serious respiratory or urinary tract infections, intravenous drug abuse, immunosuppression (e.g., infection with human immunodeficiency virus), organ transplantation, and chronic corticosteroid use increase the likelihood of pathologic fractures, epidural and vertebral body abscesses, and metastasis.
- *Unrelenting pain*: Pain of benign etiology is typically relieved with rest and in supine position, especially at night. Unrelenting pain from serious pathologic conditions is often worse at night and is unresponsive to rest and analgesics.
- *Cauda equina syndrome*: CES is caused by acute compression of the spinal NRs comprising the cauda equina in the lumbosacral spine. In approximately 10% of patients with symptoms similar to CES, however, the cause is spinal cord compression at higher levels—the thoracic and even the cervical spinal cord.[17] Although CES is rare, with a prevalence of approximately 4 in 10,000 patients with LBP,[18] it is a neurosurgical emergency that requires emergency spinal decompressive surgery.[18] Massive midline disk herniation[10,11] or smaller disk herniation in a previous stenotic spine[19] is the most frequent cause of CES. Rare causes of CES include spinal metastases, hematoma, epidural abscess, traumatic compression, acute transverse myelitis, and abdominal aortic dissection. Almost 70% of patients with CES relate a history of chronic LBP, whereas the rest of the patients have CES as their primary compliant.[19] These patients are typically seen within 24 hours of the onset of their symptoms (Box 21.2), usually with bilateral radicular pain, although pain in one leg is often worse than pain in the other, and less frequently with back pain. The pain is often accompanied by weakness in both feet, gait disturbances secondary to pain and weakness, and abdominal discomfort as a result of urinary retention, which may be followed by overflow urinary incontinence. Objective signs include motor and sensory deficits, diminished reflexes, and a positive SLR test, often in both lower extremities. Of particular importance is diminished sensation in the buttocks and perineum (saddle anesthesia), diminished sphincter tone, and evidence of urinary bladder retention. Imaging of the entire spine, with magnetic resonance imaging (MRI) being the "gold standard," is indicated because of the possibility of spinal cord compression at higher levels.[17] Once the diagnosis is made, treatment involves high-dose intravenous steroids and urgent decompressive surgery to reduce permanent neurologic disability.[19]

DIAGNOSTIC STUDIES

Because of the favorable natural history and often spontaneous resolution of symptoms, in the absence of red flags, diagnostic studies are not typically recommended for low back and radicular pain of less than 4 to 6 weeks' duration.[16,20] In addition, the common presence of abnormal diagnostic findings in asymptomatic individuals[21-23] makes

Box 21.2 Clinical Signs and Symptoms of Cauda Equina Syndrome

Features in the Clinical History

Radicular pain in both lower extremities; pain in one leg may be greater
Isolated low back pain is rare
Complaint of weakness in one or both legs and feet
Gait disturbances because of pain and weakness
Abdominal discomfort as a result of urinary retention

Features in the Clinical Examination

Motor and sensory deficits in the lower extremities
Diminished lower extremity reflexes
Positive straight-leg raise and crossed straight-leg raise tests
Saddle anesthesia
Diminished sphincter tone
Evidence of urinary bladder retention

interpretation of the test results challenging. Diagnostic tests should be used to corroborate the clinical findings and to determine the site of surgical or minimally invasive spinal interventions. Ordering tests selectively and correlating their results with the clinical findings should prevent inappropriate diagnoses and poor outcomes.[16]

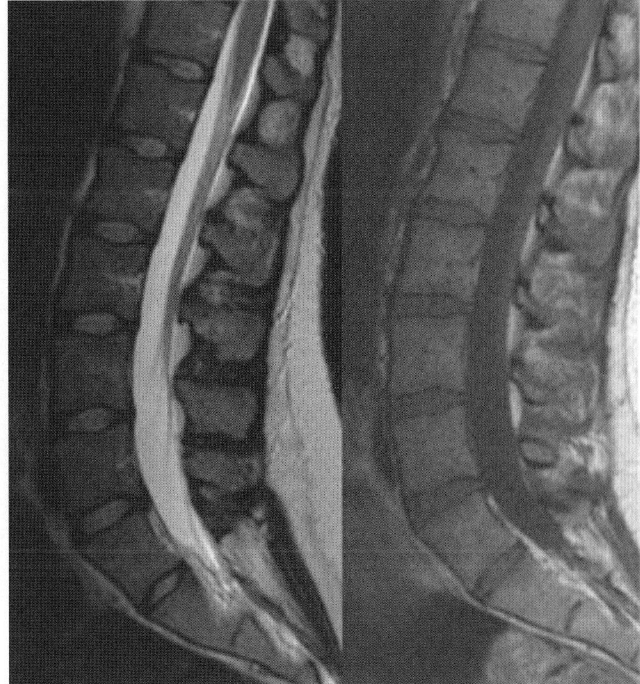

Figure 21.2 Normal T2- and T1-weighted midline sagittal magnetic resonance images of the lumbar spine.

IMAGING STUDIES

- *Magnetic resonance imaging*: MRI is considered the gold standard in determining the etiology of low back and radicular pain (Figs. 21.2 and 21.3). It offers the best resolution of the spinal canal, spinal cord, neural foramina, NRs, and disk spaces and allows evaluation of the entire spine. In patients with a history of previous spine surgery, contrast-enhanced MRI is recommended to differentiate between scar tissue and recurrent disk herniation. Limitations of MRI include a lengthy examination time, claustrophobia, and its effects on metallic objects. It is contraindicated in patients with pacemakers, mechanical heart valves, aneurysm clips, and intraocular foreign bodies.
- *Computed tomography (CT)*: CT scanning is superior to MRI in evaluating bony details of the spine, particularly the facet joints and lateral recesses. When combined with myelography (CT-myelography), the results are comparable to those of MRI in diagnosing spinal canal lesions. It can therefore be used as a substitute when MRI is contraindicated.[24] CT without myelography cannot distinguish between HDs and other intradural lesions such as tumors, and its routine use is therefore discouraged.[24]
- *Plain radiography*: The anteroposterior, lateral, and oblique spinal plain x-ray views are the simplest and most readily available tests that reveal bony abnormalities; however, only diminutive spinal soft tissue details are envisioned (Fig. 21.4). Among the skeletal abnormalities, spinal fractures and deformities are easily appreciated; however, lumbar lordosis, transitional vertebrae, disk space narrowing, and spondylolisthesis are common in asymptomatic individuals,[23] and routine spine roentgenograms are therefore not recommended.[25] Flexion and extension films are used to reveal segmental instability as a source of pain, but there is little correlation between abnormal motion and pathologic instability.[26]

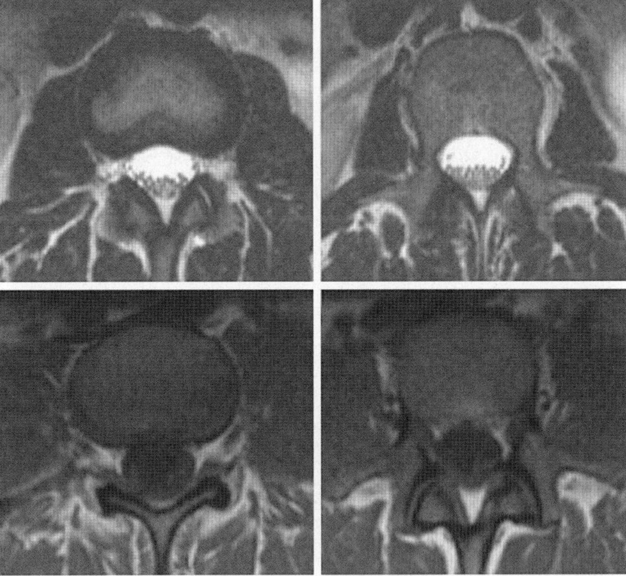

Figure 21.3 Normal T2- and T1-weighted axial transdiscal and interdiscal magnetic resonance images of the lumbar spine.

- *Myelography*: Myelography without CT is useful in detecting lesions in the spinal canal when other studies yield conflicting information, are not available, or are contraindicated.

ELECTRODIAGNOSTIC STUDIES

Electrodiagnostic studies, including electromyography (EMG), nerve conduction velocity (NCV), and somatosensory evoked potentials (SSEPs), are useful in establishing the radicular nature of symptoms when the clinical features of LRS are inconclusive and indistinguishable from the

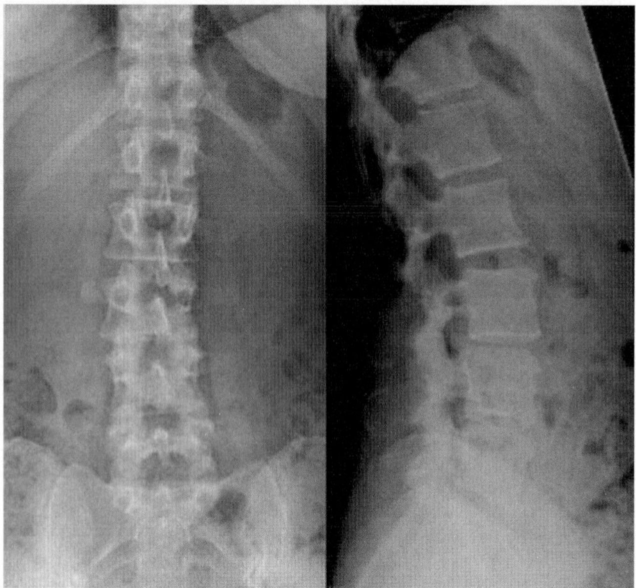

Figure 21.4 Normal anteroposterior and lateral plain x-ray images of the lumbar spine.

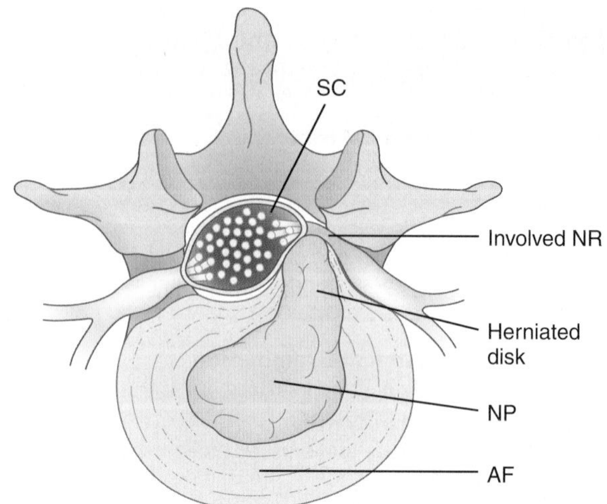

Figure 21.5 Schematic depiction of disk herniation. AF, annulus fibrosus; NP, nucleus pulposus; NR, nerve root; SC, spinal cord.

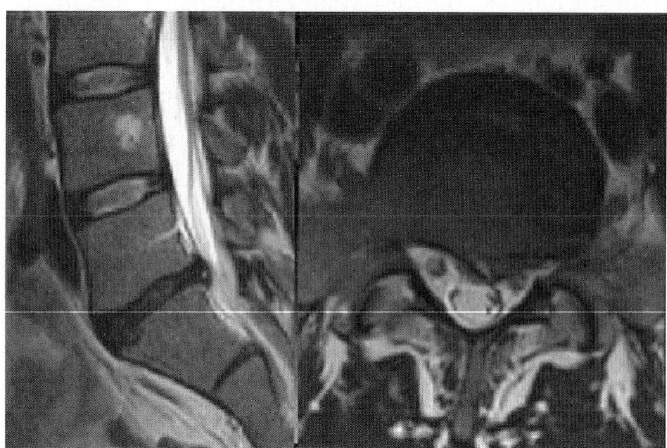

Figure 21.6 T2-weighted sagittal and axial magnetic resonance images of disk protrusion.

symptoms of peripheral neuropathy. In contrast to the imaging studies, combined EMG and NCV results have high diagnostic specificity[27]; however, they give no information on the etiology of LRS and correlate poorly with the anatomic level of the radicular lesions. Routine use of EMG/NCV is therefore not recommended.[20] Use of SSEPs is typically limited to identifying intraoperative nerve injury because the test cannot pinpoint the exact location of nerve dysfunction.

OTHER DIAGNOSTIC TESTS

Various other diagnostic and laboratory tests, such as bone scan, complete blood count, urinalysis, erythrocyte sedimentation rate, C-reactive protein, rheumatoid factor, antinuclear antibodies, and HLA-B27 antigen, are useful when spinal tumors, infections, and rheumatologic disorders are suspected.

HERNIATED LUMBAR DISK

HISTORY AND EPIDEMIOLOGY

Although radicular symptoms have been known since ancient times, they were first attributed to "posterior displacement of the disc" by Goldthwaite in 1911.[28] The incidence of symptomatic HD is estimated to be 1% to 2% in the general population,[4] for which approximately 200,000 lumbar diskectomies are performed each year.[29]

TERMINOLOGY

Disk herniation may be defined as displacement of disk material beyond the confines of the IVD space (Fig. 21.5).[30] Even though the nucleus pulposus (NP) is the predominant component of the herniated material, other disk constituents (e.g., cartilage, bone, and annular tissue) frequently constitute the herniated elements.[31] Although various terms such as *herniated nucleus pulposus*, *ruptured disk*, and *prolapsed disk* have been used to describe this entity, the term *herniated disk* seems to be most appropriate because it conveys the image of displacement of any disk component regardless of the cause.[30] HD is variably classified, typically according to the morphology of the herniated material.[30] A *protruded disk* is present if the neck of the herniated material (i.e., the distance between the edges of the base) is wider than the widest disk diameter in any given plane (Fig. 21.6). *Disk extrusion* is the opposite of disk protrusion; the neck is narrower than the widest disk diameter in any given plane (Fig. 21.7). *Disk sequestration* is a type of disk extrusion wherein no continuity exists between the herniated material and the parent disk. HD is also sometimes classified according to the integrity of the overlying annulus fibrosus (AF). In contrast to *noncontained* herniation, the term *contained* herniation is used when the displaced disk portion is covered by an intact annulus. However, with currently available diagnostic modalities such as CT, MRI, and diskography, the details of the integrity of the annulus are often not identified, and these distinctions are therefore arbitrary. The terms *disk desiccation*, *disk fibrosis*, *disk narrowing*, *disk bulging*, *disk fissuring*, and *disk sclerosis* are often used; these terms, however, suggest degenerative disk processes and do not reflect disk herniation.[30]

PATHOPHYSIOLOGY

Since Mixter and Barr first reported alleviation of lumbar radicular pain after removal of the HD material in 1934,[32] HD is thought to be the most common cause of radicular pain. Although MRI findings of degenerated, bulging, and protruded disks are common, disk extrusion is uncommon in asymptomatic individuals.[21,22] Mechanical compression of the spinal NR by the herniated disk material (see Fig. 21.5) has commonly been acknowledged as the primary factor inducing radicular symptoms. Data from animal studies indicate that compression of the NR impairs its nutrition and can lead to NR ischemia and injury.[33,34] Deformation of the NR by HD fragments is also seen on diagnostic imaging in patients with radicular symptoms. There is, however, no direct evidence of increased mechanical pressure created by the HD. Moreover, clinical studies have demonstrated that only NRs that are exposed to HD material for a prolonged period produce pain on mechanical deformation and that similar NR deformation, not exposed to HD material, produces no pain.[8,35] These observations suggest that mechanisms other than mechanical pressure may be at work in the causation of radicular pain. The presence of inflammatory mediators in the HD material, retrieved from patients at diskectomy, has been demonstrated.[36,37] Additionally, in animal models, application of NP to the NR, and not epidural fat, produced the physiologic and anatomic evidence of radiculopathy.[38] Furthermore, the presence of clinical and electromyographic evidence of radiculopathy has been demonstrated in patients with normal findings on spinal imaging.[39] These observations suggest that factors other than mechanical compression and inflammatory mediators and inflammation may play a major role.

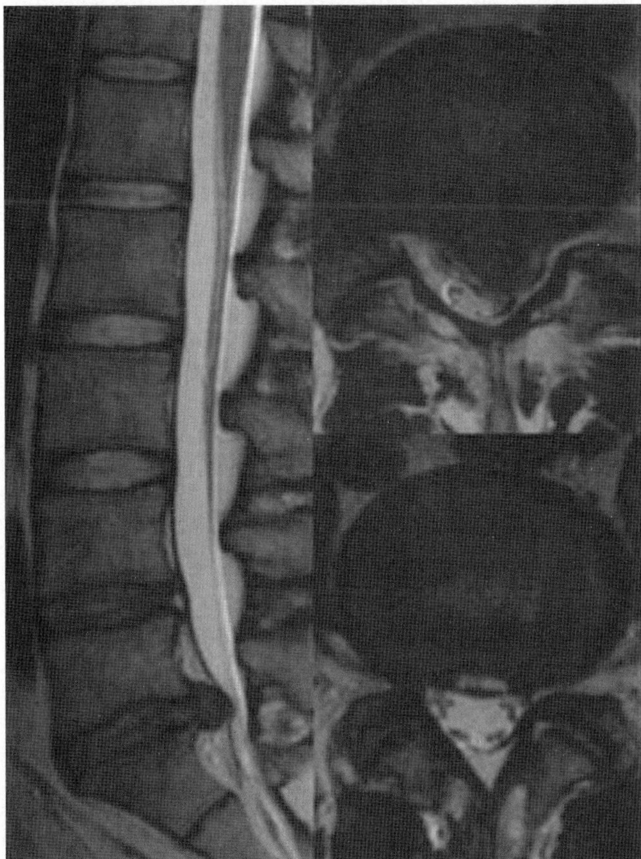

Figure 21.7 T2-weighted sagittal magnetic resonance images of a 31-year-old man with severe axial and lower extremity pain showing two distinct disk pathologies. At the L5-S1 level there is left-sided disk extrusion, and the L4-5 disk shows desiccation and a high-intensity zone; the remaining disks appear normal.

NATURAL HISTORY

The natural history of HD is favorable in that the majority of patients (60%) experience significant resolution of their symptoms within the first few months of their onset. In a smaller percentage of patients (20% to 30%), however, the symptoms fail to improve over time.[40] Clinical improvement is usually accompanied by resolution of the HD on spinal imaging.[41] Large extruded disks have a higher tendency to decrease in size than do smaller disk protrusions and disk bulges.[42] Spontaneous regression is thought to be caused by the phagocytic process, predominated by macrophages, which is most prominent in the outermost layers of the HD material.[43]

CLINICAL CORRELATIONS

Most lumbar disk herniations occur at the lower lumbar levels, with an L4/5 HD being the most common (59%), followed by L5/S1 (30%) and L3/4 (9%) disk hernaition.[19] Herniation at these levels produces the typical radicular signs and symptoms in the affected dermatomes described earlier. Central HDs may, however, produce primarily LBP, which is exacerbated by SLR.[15]

NONOPERATIVE TREATMENT OF HERNIATED DISKS

Because of the favorable natural history of LRS caused by HDs, in the absence of progressive neurologic deficit and red flags in the clinical history, expectant and symptomatic treatment is recommended.[16,20] A wide array of nonoperative treatments are available, and each has claimed success.

- *Medications*: Although opioids, muscle relaxants, and neuroleptics are routinely used for the symptomatic treatment of HDs, there are scant data in the literature to support their use. Nonsteroidal anti-inflammatory drugs (NSAIDs) have been shown to have some efficacy in the management of acute radicular symptoms.[44] Systemic corticosteroids are prescribed, both orally and parenterally, for the treatment of acute disk herniation; however, evidence to support this practice is also lacking.[45,46]
- *Bed rest*: Strict bed rest used to be the hallmark of treatment of acute HDs. However, because of the potentially harmful effects of prolonged bed rest,[47] continuation of activities within the limits permitted by the pain has been reported to result in more rapid recovery and is currently being recommended.[48]
- *Bracing*: Bracing is another method of immobilizing a painful spine, but there is limited evidence in support of the use of lumbar braces versus no treatment.[49]

- *Traction*: Once a mainstay of treatment, traction in either a continuous or intermittent form remains an unproven treatment of HD.[50] Vertebral axial decompression is a newer modality based on traction principles; it also remains untested in the treatment of HD.
- *Acupuncture*: There are a few observational studies that claim acupuncture to be effective in the treatment of chronic LBP; however, its support in the literature for the treatment of acute LBP is lacking.[51]
- *Physical therapy*: Physical therapy techniques for acute low back and radicular pain include active and passive exercises. Although active exercises are claimed to be more effective,[52] the overall role of physical therapy in the treatment of acute HD remains questionable.[53]
- *Psychological treatments*: Behavioral therapy, biofeedback, and other psychological treatments have been shown to have some efficacy in patients with chronic LBP; however, their role in the treatment of HD remains unknown.[54]
- *Miscellaneous treatments*: Chiropractic manipulations, massage therapy, magnets, transcutaneous electrical nerve stimulation, and ultrasound application are often used in the treatment of low back and radicular pain, but their use remains unproven.

INTRASPINAL INJECTIONS

Epidural steroid injections (ESIs) have been used to treat HDs for more than 50 years. Traditionally, a posterior interlaminar (IL-ESI) approach is used. The injectate reaches the site of the HD anteriorly by flowing around the thecal sac. Fluoroscopically guided transforaminal injections (TF-ESIs) have the theoretical advantage of delivering the injectate directly into the anterior epidural space. Fluoroscopic guidance significantly improves the precision with which the injectate is deposited in the epidural space.[55] The literature is replete with case series and uncontrolled studies, both in support of and against the efficacy of ESI. A review of the literature on randomized controlled trials (RCTs) of IL-ESI for sciatica showed four such trials; ESIs were found to be more beneficial than control treatments, especially in the short term.[56] Although no long-term RCTs exist for TF-ESI, it was found to have results superior to those of IL-ESI in one study.[57] ESIs are discussed in detail elsewhere in this book.

PREDICTORS OF OUTCOME WITH NONINVASIVE TREATMENT

There are several predictors of a favorable outcome of conservative treatment (Box 21.3), including a negative X-SLR test, absence of leg pain with spine extension, absence of stenosis on spine imaging, favorable response to ESIs, return of any neurologic deficits within 12 weeks, a motivated physically fit patient with more than 12 years of education, no workers' compensation claims, and a normal psychological profile.[53]

PERCUTANEOUS DISK DECOMPRESSION

Percutaneous disk decompression (PDD) was developed following the success of intradiscal injection of chymopapain for radicular pain from an HD. The positive results of intradiscal chymopapain injections suggested that dissolution of nonherniated intranuclear discal contents may resolve HD symptoms without directly targeting the HD material (Fig. 21.8). Although the HD material causing radicular irritation is directly removed in addition to the nonherniated NP during surgical diskectomy, removal of the nonherniated nuclear tissue during PDD is postulated to reduce intradiscal pressure, which allows inward collapse of the herniated fragment. This has been suggested to be true especially in the presence of an intact AF—a presumed contained disk herniation—with the HD fragment acknowledged as

Box 21.3 Predictors of Favorable Outcomes of Conservative Noninvasive Treatment of Herniated Disks

Negative crossed straight-leg raise test
Absence of leg pain on extension of the spine
Return of neurologic function within 12 weeks of onset
Absence of stenosis on spine imaging
Favorable response to epidural steroid injections
Patient with 12 years of education
Motivated and physically fit patient
Normal psychological profile
Absence of workers' compensation claim

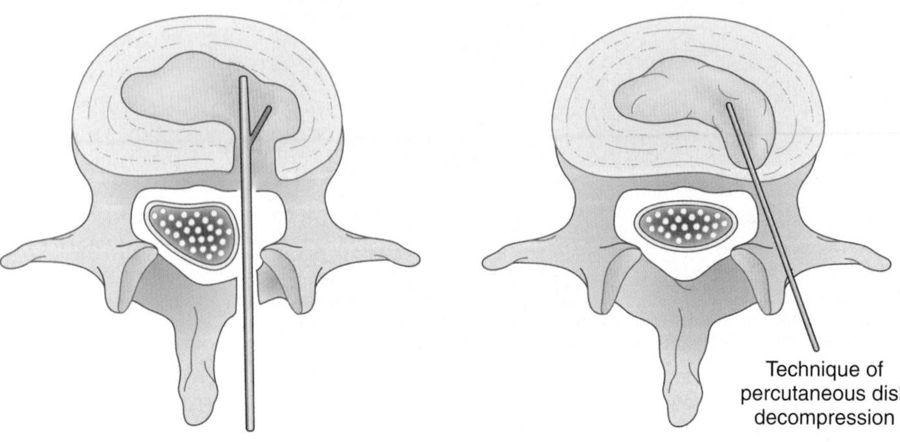

Figure 21.8 Schematic depiction of surgical diskectomy and percutaneous disk decompression.

typically being smaller than 4 mm.[58] Chymopapain injections are now rarely performed in the United States because of complications associated with unintentional injection into the subarachnoid space and the rare occurrence of severe allergic reactions. Based on the principles of joint endoscopy, PDD was initially performed with large-bore endoscopes (7 mm or greater in internal diameter) to remove the intradiscal material. These early endoscopes were cumbersome to operate, with the added risk of trauma to the disk annulus, and were quickly abandoned. The technique of automated percutaneous lumbar diskectomy (APLD) was then introduced, wherein a smaller introducer cannula (2.5 mm) was used and the nuclear material was removed with a suction and cutting technique. Later, a variety of lasers were used to vaporize the nuclear material; these laser disk decompression devices used cannulas smaller than 3 mm in internal diameter and often included a fiberoptic channel for observation. The technique of disk nucleoplasty used a 1.5-mm (17-gauge) introducer needle and bipolar radiofrequency (RF) energy to create small channels in the disk to remove the nuclear material. Proponents of this technique claimed that the procedure provided localized disk ablation with minimal damage to the surrounding tissue. A percutaneous diskectomy technique with the proprietary name of DeKompressor uses 1.5- and 1.0-mm (19-gauge) outer cannulas and a probe that rotates to remove the disk material. A modified intradiscal electrothermal therapy (IDET) catheter (Acutherm) is also available and aims to induce localized thermal lesioning and shrinkage at the base of the HD material.

Despite its use spanning several decades, there is little evidence in the literature to support the use of various PDD techniques. In one study, MRI of patients before and after APLD showed no measurable difference in the size of HDs at 6 weeks.[59] Although animal[60] and cadaver studies[61] have shown a reduction in disk pressure after PDD, there is no evidence of either high intradiscal pressure in patients with HDs or its reduction after disk decompression procedures. The amount of nuclear material removed is also variable in the various PDD techniques, with a range of 4 to 5 g for APLD to 1 g for nucleoplasty and the DeKompressor device; it varies greatly for various laser decompression devices and is unknown for the Acutherm device. No studies have correlated either disk pressure or eventual outcomes with the amount of nuclear material removed, and the optimum amount of disk material that should be removed is unknown. Removing large amounts of disk material has been correlated with disk collapse and accelerated disk degeneration.[62] It is therefore prudent to remove the least amount of disk material possible to achieve the most beneficial results. Removing nuclear contents from within the disk protrusion itself via a more lateral percutaneous approach has also been recommended.[58] Use of smaller-gauge introducer cannulas would limit the annular damage and therefore should be preferred. Diskography followed by a post-diskography CT scan has been used to assess the size and location of the HD and the integrity of the disk annulus; its use before PDD has been linked to improved clinical results.[63] Two randomized trials of APLD showed success rates of 29%[64] and 33%.[65] There are no randomized trials supporting the use of laser disk decompression, nucleoplasty, DeKompressor, and Acutherm, and their use is based mostly on anecdotal reports.

OPERATIVE TREATMENT OF HERNIATED DISKS

Detailed discussion of the various surgical procedures performed for HDs is beyond the scope of this chapter. Classic diskectomy, popularized since the first report on HDs by Mixter and Barr,[32] is the most popular procedure performed for HDs. The essentials of this technique include laminectomy and release of the ligamentum flavum to access the epidural space and remove the HD fragment and annulotomy to remove the nonherniated disk material (see Fig. 21.8). Several variations of this technique exist and differ in the extent to which laminectomy, ligamentum flavum release, and annulotomy are performed during the procedure. The more recent microdiskectomy procedure is less invasive and aims to minimize surgical trauma in order to limit the potential for NR injury and epidural scarring. Although surgery is commonly performed for HDs,[29] there is little high-quality evidence in its support. A prospective, randomized trial comparing surgical with nonsurgical treatment of HDs demonstrated that during the first year, the surgically treated patients had significantly better results (92%) than did the nonsurgically treated patients (61%).[66] However, the results of the surgery deteriorated over time and the difference between the groups became statistically insignificant at 4 years and insignificant at 10 years. This study was criticized for lack of careful randomization, lack of blinding, large number of crossovers to the surgically treated group, insensitive outcome measures, and small sample size.[67] There is one other frequently cited study of operative treatment of HDs, and although this was a major prospective study, it was nonrandomized and observational.[68] The results of this study were similar to those of the previous quoted study at 1 and 5 years; at 10 years, the results of surgical treatment were slightly better (56% vs. 40%, $P = 0.006$), but the incidence of work and disability status remained the same.[68] A more recently published study showed the efficacy of both surgical and nonoperative treatment of lumbar disk herniation. The Spine Patient Outcomes Research Trial (SPORT)[69] showed between-group differences in improvements to be consistently in favor of surgery for all the observation periods, but these differences were small and not statistically significant for their primary outcomes. Patients in both groups were satisfied with their care, with the main benefit of surgery appearing to be more rapid resolution of the disabling pain.

It appeared that the decision to undergo surgery depended on how urgently a patient wished to achieve pain relief in the next 2 to 4 months.[70] The need for surgery in patients with CES appears to be absolute,[19] and it is generally agreed that surgical treatment is necessary in patients with progressive motor deficits. However, other indications for surgery are relative and include intractable pain and poor response to conservative therapy.[71] The lack of consensus and the variability with which these indications are adhered to are supported by a nearly 20-fold difference in surgery rates in otherwise demographically similar populations within the United States.[72] The results of microdiskectomy have been reported to be superior to those of traditional diskectomy.[73] Although patients with sciatica of more than 12 months' duration have been shown to have less favorable results after surgery,[74] the full effects of a potential delay in operative treatment while nonsurgical treatment is attempted remain unknown.

LUMBAR SPINAL STENOSIS

TERMINOLOGY AND ETIOLOGY

Though recognized for some time, modern descriptions of the clinical syndrome and pathologic lesions of LSS first appeared in 1954.[74] LSS is defined as a clinical syndrome consisting of neurogenic claudication or radicular pain secondary to narrowing of the spinal or NR canal and compression of its neural elements.[75] Traditionally classified (Table 21.2) into congenital and acquired types, it is the degenerative variety of the acquired type that is most prevalent. Developmental LSS is either idiopathic in nature or due to rare developmental bone dysplasias such as achondroplasia. Aside from the degenerative type, less common causes of acquired spinal stenosis include metabolic disorders such as Paget's disease, trauma, surgery, spinal tumors, and spinal deformity. Anatomically, LSS can be classified as central spinal canal stenosis, or central stenosis, and as lateral recess and neural foraminal stenosis, or lateral stenosis.[75]

Table 21.2 Classification of Lumbar Spinal Stenosis

Etiologic Classification	
Congenital	Idiopathic Achondroplastic
Acquired	Degenerative Iatrogenic—postsurgical Metabolic—Paget's disease Post-traumatic Deformity—spondylolisthesis
Combined	Congenital with secondary degenerative changes
Anatomic Classification	
Central stenosis	Central spinal canal stenosis
Lateral stenosis	Lateral recess stenosis Neural foraminal stenosis

PATHOPHYSIOLOGY

Acquired degenerative LSS is characteristically the result of disk degeneration and its sequelae. Loss of disk height, disk bulging, facet joint hypertrophy, thickening and redundancy of the ligamentum flavum, and local osteophyte formation are the typical lesions seen in LSS.[76] The degenerative changes causing LSS are most common at the disk level, and one or several vertebral motion segments may be involved (Fig. 21.9). Central stenosis can cause compression of the NRs of the cauda equina, whereas lateral stenosis typically causes compression of the exiting spinal NRs. The L5 NR is most commonly involved (75%), followed by the L4 (15%), L3 (5.3%), and L2 (4%) NRs.[77] The capacity of the lumbar spinal canal is significantly larger during flexion than during extension, and the symptoms of LSS are therefore characteristically worse during lumbar extension.[78] The spinal degenerative changes analogous to LSS are prevalent in older adults[79] and have been shown to frequently be present in asymptomatic individuals.[20,21] Direct compression or ischemia of the neural structures is thought to be primarily responsible for the clinical manifestations of LSS.[80] In contrast to HD, however, the role played by inflammatory changes in the causation of symptoms from LSS is less clear. Degenerative changes that result in spinal stenosis can also give rise to spinal instability (degenerative spondylolisthesis) and spinal deformities (degenerative scoliosis), which can contribute further to spinal narrowing.

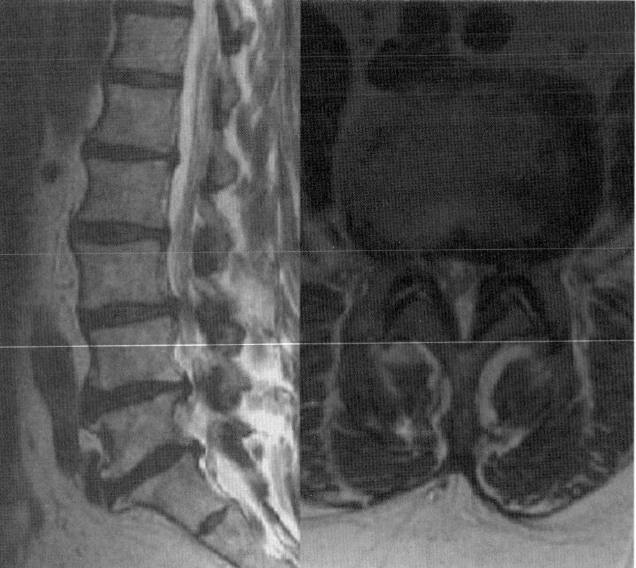

Figure 21.9 T2-weighted sagittal and axial magnetic resonance images of multilevel lumbar spinal stenosis.

CLINICAL CONSIDERATIONS

- *Neurogenic claudication*: The typical manifestations of neurogenic claudication include pain radiating to both lower extremities—posterolateral aspect of the thighs and legs—that is worse with walking and lumbar extension and is relieved by sitting down. The pain is often associated with numbness and heaviness or weakness of the lower extremities. It is essential that these symptoms be distinguished from claudication of vascular origin. The latter possibility must be entertained in the presence of any sign of vascular insufficiency.[81] In contrast to vascular claudication, the pain of neurogenic claudication continues to be present with standing and is eased by walking in a flexed position, such as pushing a walker or a shopping cart.[82]
- *Radicular pain*: Unilateral radicular symptoms unrelated to any activity are a sign of NR involvement; they usually reflect lateral stenosis and can be present with or without symptoms of neurogenic claudication.[83]
- *Axial pain*: Axial pain is more reflective of disk, facet joint, or sacroiliac joint pathology and may indicate spinal instability; it is unlikely to be an exclusive symptom of LSS.[84]
- *Clinical signs*: Patients with LSS tend to walk with a stooped forward gait and often maintain this position while standing—stooped posture—with loss of lumbar lordosis and decreased range of lumbar extension. Because of the slow and chronic nature of progression of the disease, the SLR test is infrequently positive and the sensorimotor deficits are less pronounced. In a study of patients with LSS, a sensorimotor deficit in the lower extremity was seen in 30% of patients (most commonly in the L5 NR distribution), a decreased or absent plantar reflex was present in 43%, and a diminished patellar reflex was noted in 18% of the patients; the SLR test was positive in only 10% to 23%.[85]

DIAGNOSIS

MRI is the most common imaging modality used to detect the pathologic lesions of LSS. It provides the best visualization of the IVDs, ligamentum flavum, central canal, and neural foramina.[86] CT provides better details of the bony abnormalities, especially facet pathology, and superior visualization of the lateral recesses. Lumbar CT-myelography is the imaging technique of choice when MRI is contraindicated or is not available. The value of EMG/NCV and plain radiologic films in detecting LSS is similar to their application for other types of LRS and was discussed earlier. Because of the frequent presence of radiologic abnormalities in asymptomatic individuals with LSS[21,22] and their common occurrence in older adults,[79] it is crucial to correlate the radiologic abnormalities with the clinical findings to make this diagnosis.

NATURAL HISTORY AND TREATMENT OPTIONS

Though at first thought to be unrelentingly progressive,[87] the natural history of LSS is interspersed by intermittent flare-ups and is relatively unchanged over time.[88,89] Because of its seemingly progressive nature and poor prognosis, LSS was treated by early surgical intervention in the past.[87] However, nonsurgical treatments have been shown to be effective and can prevent progression of the patient's symptoms.[89,90] Surgical treatment of LSS typically provides superior control of the symptoms initially,[91] but the benefits seem to decline over time.[92] The prevalence of this condition in older adults and the frequent presence of other comorbid conditions often make these patients unsuitable for invasive treatments. Delaying surgery for a trial of nonsurgical treatment, even with severe stenosis, has been shown to have minimal detrimental effect on the final surgical outcome.[93] In conclusion, in the absence of progressive neurologic deficits or CES (rare in spinal stenosis), surgical treatment is prudent in patients who have failed an appropriate trial of nonoperative treatment.

NONOPERATIVE TREATMENT OF LUMBAR SPINAL STENOSIS

Nonoperative treatments are particularly useful for the acute flare-ups of LSS and include medications, modification of activity, bracing, physical therapy, and ESI.

- *Medications*: Acetaminophen and NSAIDs are often helpful in providing symptomatic relief during acute flare-ups. However, because this condition is chronic, the use of opioid pain medications should be limited to acute exacerbations.[94] Calcitonin has been found to be beneficial in spinal stenosis and is particularly effective for LSS resulting from Paget's disease.[95]
- *Modification of activity*: Avoidance of aggravating activity and relative rest are suggested during acute flare-ups. Nevertheless, because of the potential for deconditioning, strict bed rest is no longer advocated for the treatment of LSS.[94]
- *Bracing*: Rigid lumbar braces extend the spine and may worsen the symptoms of LSS. Lumbar binders are expected to reduce loads across the lumbar spine and may provide symptomatic relief. Nonetheless, to avoid muscle deconditioning and back stiffness, any such braces should be worn for short periods only.
- *Physical therapy*: Flexion-based exercises (e.g., stationary bicycle and inclined treadmill) increase the cross-sectional area of the spinal canal and may improve microcirculation of the neural elements. Such exercises may therefore allow patients to tolerate the exercise programs better and may promote weight loss and cardiovascular fitness.[96] Aquatic therapy is also useful because it stretches the hip flexors and hamstrings and strengthens the core abdominal and trunk muscles.
- *Epidural steroid injection*: IL-ESIs have been shown to be effective, especially in the short term, and may provide symptomatic control of acute exacerbations of neurogenic claudication.[97] Fluoroscopically guided TF-ESIs appear to be better suited for radicular symptoms secondary to LSS and have been shown to have both short- and long-term efficacy.[98,99]

OPERATIVE TREATMENT

Wide laminectomy, performed at the stenotic levels, is the standard procedure for surgical decompression of LSS.[100] It involves broad removal of the spinal laminae and ligamentum flavum extending laterally from pedicle to pedicle. Extensive removal of the posterior spinal elements can result in spinal instability, which can be avoided by preservation of the pars interarticularis and lateral half of the facet joints. Extensive decompressive surgery, as is typically indicated for complex stenosis and degenerative spondylolisthesis, may result in significant spinal instability. The post-decompressive instability may be avoided by spinal fusion, performed with or without instrumentation.[100] Lately, surgical techniques involving minimal decompression, such as laminotomy, fenestration, and laminoplasty, are increasingly being used to preserve spinal stability and avoid post-decompressive fusion. However, these minimally decompressive techniques are accompanied by higher rates of restenosis.

INTERNAL DISK DISRUPTION

Although the role of a herniated IVD as a cause of pain is well established, pain originating from the disk itself is poorly understood and has remained controversial.[101] The various terms used for pain of discal origin have included *discogenic pain, internal disk disruption*, and *painful degenerative disk disease* (DDD). Changes within the disk that are linked to pain may well be a variant of age-related and nonpainful degenerative disk changes. It is therefore vital to understand basic disk anatomy and physiology and normal age-related degenerative disk changes before pathologic changes within the disk that are attributed as being painful are examined.

BASIC INTERVERTEBRAL DISK ANATOMY AND PHYSIOLOGY

The IVD is grossly compartmentalized into the inner NP and the outer rim of the AF (Fig. 21.10). This distinction is most obvious at the lumbar levels and decreases with advancing age. Both the NP and AF are sparsely populated by very distinct cell types that maintain normal disk function and integrity. The NP is inhabited by chondrocyte-like cells that are found in clusters, whereas the AF is populated by fibrocyte-like cells.[102] The composition of the expansively present intercellular matrix is also very different for the NP and AF; the matrix in the NP is jelly-like and has a high concentration of water and proteoglycans, whereas the matrix in the AF is firmer and has a high collagen content. The collagen fibers in the AF are arranged as interlacing lamellae that are firmly attached to the adjacent vertebral bodies.[102] A healthy IVD is able to sustain a substantial amount of physical strain.[103] These compressive forces are borne directly by the NP and are equally distributed to the AF as tensile force.[104] The incompressibility exhibited by a normal NP is largely due to its high water content, maintained in turn by the hydrostatic pressure generated by its high proteoglycan content.[102] A delicate balance exists between the anabolic activities of the NP cells and the catabolic activities of the matrix proteolytic enzymes—matrix metalloproteinases (MMPs)—involved in maintaining the normal NP proteoglycan content.[105] A normal IVD is scantly innervated and is the largest avascular structure in the body. The IVD is innervated by mechanoreceptors, which, like its vascularity, are limited exclusively to the outer third of the AF. A normal NP is completely lacking in innervation and blood supply.[102,106] The outer third of the AF is innervated by plexuses along the anterior and posterior longitudinal ligaments (see Fig. 21.10). The posterior plexus receives its input from the sinuvertebral nerve and gray rami communicans; the latter also contributes mainly to the anterior plexus. The sinuvertebral nerve receives its contributions from the ventral rami and gray rami communicans.[107] A normal disk therefore has rich autonomic connections, which may explain the diffuse and nonspecific nature of pain originating from the disk. The metabolic requirements of the cells in the NP and inner AF are met almost entirely by diffusion to and from capillary plexuses in the adjacent vertebral bodies across the cartilaginous end plate and the outer AF.[108] This arrangement is at best tenuous, and cells in the NP function in a precarious anaerobic environment.[109] Because the IVD also lacks scavenger cells, degradative products of disk macromolecules accumulate over time, which can alter the normal cell and matrix interactions.[110] The state of hydration and thus the compressibility of the NP can therefore be altered by a host of factors that can influence the metabolic activities within the NP and AF.

PATHOPHYSIOLOGY OF DEGENERATIVE DISK DISEASE

Degenerative changes within the disk are commonly seen in asymptomatic individuals, especially with advancing age; however, extensive and often isolated degenerative disk changes are also seen in younger patients with considerable LBP (see Fig. 21.7).[111] Degenerative disk changes may therefore be painless and represent the physiologic consequence of aging, or they could be painful and may be pathologic in nature.[112] A host of factors have been shown to predispose to early and progressive disk degeneration, including genetic predisposition, diminished blood supply from causes such as smoking and vascular insufficiency, increased mechanical stress from repeated heavy lifting, contact sports, obesity, and traumatic injury to the cartilaginous end plate.[113-117] These risk factors may promote degenerative changes within the NP by a host of factors such as dysfunction and decline in viable NP cells,[118] enhanced MMP activity,[119] and increased NP cytokine and proinflammatory mediator content.[120] A reduction in NP proteoglycan content may be followed by diminished NP water and hydrostatic pressure. These changes would make the NP more compressible and expose the AF to direct axial compression.[104] Along with the axial stress, the AF may undergo concomitant degenerative changes with loss of annular collagen. These alterations in the AF would eventually lead to stress failure of the collagen fibers and the development of AF fissures that spread outward toward the periphery.[121] These NP and AF structural changes affect the biomechanical properties of the entire disk and cause it to shrink and become less plastic.[122] Changes in disk dynamics also increase stress on structures adjacent to the disk and may lead to sclerosis, hypertrophic new bone formation, and arthritic changes in the adjacent joints. The various spinal and paraspinal changes have been described as Modic changes in the adjacent vertebral bodies,[123] accelerated degeneration of adjacent disks, hypertrophy and arthritis of the facet joints, sacroiliac joint dysfunction, and paraspinal myofascial syndrome.[124] In addition, stenotic changes within the spinal canal and intervertebral foramina may follow and can cause NR and spinal cord compressive symptoms.[125] Nonetheless, the presence of spinal degenerative changes correlates poorly with the pain experienced by patients.[126]

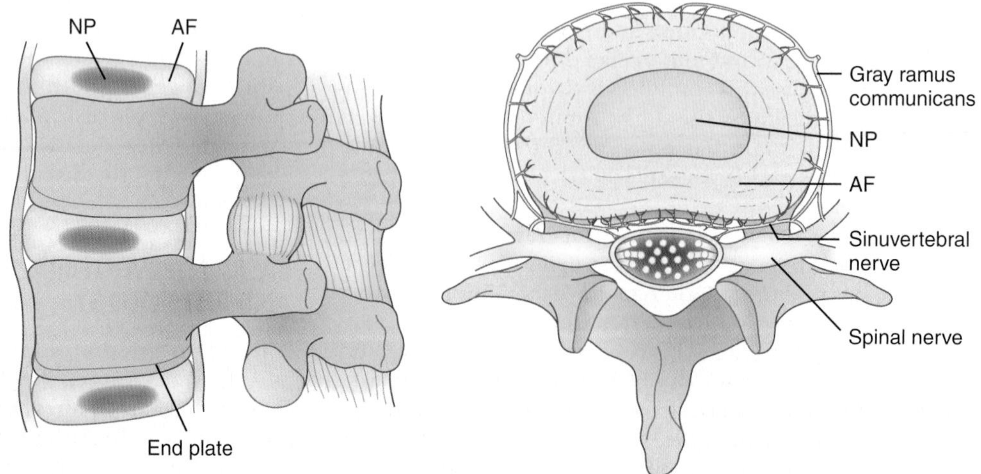

Figure 21.10 Schematic representation of normal intervertebral disk components and innervation. AF, annulus fibrosus; NP, nucleus pulposus.

PATHOLOGY OF INTERNAL DISK DISRUPTION AND DISCOGENIC PAIN

A positive painful response on provocative diskography is subjective in nature, is confounded by a host of psychosocial and somatization influences, and has been a subject of controversy for some time.[127] Yet the pain of positive diskography has been linked to a host of disk lesions and is considered indicative of IDD.[128-135] It is uncertain whether IDD is a distinct disease entity or represents painful, early-onset, and progressive DDD. It is likely that the factors that predispose to early and progressive DDD are also central to the pathologic changes of IDD. Disks from patients with concordant pain on diskography have been shown to contain vascularized granulation tissue zones or fissures that extend from the NP to the outer AF (Fig. 21.11).[133-135] These granulation tissue zones have been correlated with the annular fissures seen on post-diskography CT scans[133] and the high-intensity zones seen on MRI.[134] As mentioned previously, innervation and vascularity in a normal disk are limited to the outer third of the AF.[102,106,107] However, in addition to their highly vascular nature, two types of nerve fibers are found along these AF fissures[133]: nerve fibers that accompany the neovascularization are possibly vasoregulatory, and free nerve endings that are high in substance P and penetrate deep into the inner AF and NP and are most likely nociceptors.[129,130] These zones of granulation tissue also show an abundant mononuclear cell infiltrate and exhibit strong expression of nerve growth factors, which may contribute to nerve ingrowth and accelerate degeneration of the disk.[132,135] These disks also produce a significant amount of proinflammatory mediators,[131] which can sensitize the neonociceptors and thus maintain a state of hyperalgesia within the affected disk. These hyperalgesic disks can cause chronic pain that is worse with mechanical stress (axial loading) and produce a painful response with minimal stimulation on diskography (i.e., a chemically sensitized disk).[136] The presence of annular fissures, nociceptive innervation of the inner AF and NP, and inflammatory mediators and cells, along with the abundance of sympathetic connections at the spinal cord level, provide a substrate for the origin of discogenic pain.

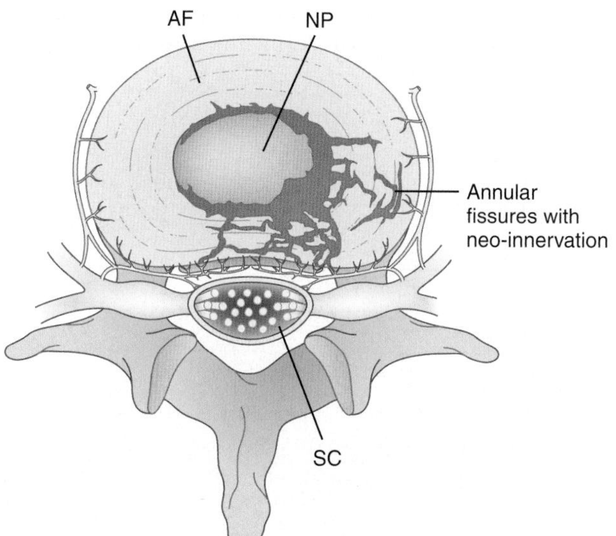

Figure 21.11 Schematic depiction of lesions of internal disk disruption. AF, annulus fibrosus; NP, nucleus pulposus; SC, spinal cord.

HISTORICAL BACKGROUND

The concept of the IVD as a source of pain is relatively old and was espoused as early as 1947.[137] The term *internal disk disruption*, however, was not used until 1986[138] and was based on the observation that disks that produce pain on diskography—initially used exclusively to demonstrate an HD—often appear morphologically intact on plain x-ray imaging. The diagnosis of IDD was initially based almost entirely on a subjective pain response generated during provocative diskography. The validity of a positive provoked pain response on diskography, however, was seriously challenged in a study published by Holt in 1968 that showed a false-positive rate of 37%.[139] Although the methodology of Holt's study was later seriously criticized[140] and a study by Walsh and associates showed a false-positive rate of 0%,[141] Carragee and colleagues[127] have continued to criticize the diagnostic significance of a positive pain response on diskography. More stringent criteria for positive diskograms were later adopted to reduce the false-positive rates; such criteria included a concordant pain response, the presence of at least one disk level with no pain on disk provocation ("control disk"), and evidence of disk disruption on post-diskography CT (i.e., one or more tears extending to the outer annulus).[142] Pressure diskography using manometry during disk provocation was also introduced to identify disks that are painful with minimal stimulation. This technique has been suggested to improve the specificity of diskography.[143] However, no test is available to date that can objectively detect the aforementioned pathologic lesions of IDD.

CLINICAL FINDINGS

Pain originating from the disk can be acute or chronic, either from an acute tear of the disk or from the chronic lesions characteristic of IDD. A study performed by Schwarzer and colleagues[144] showed that in a group of patients with axial chronic LBP, the incidence of IDD was as high as 40% when all the criteria of discogenic pain suggested by the International Spine Intervention Society[142] were fulfilled. These authors also claimed that the study population represented the general public and therefore advocated that the incidence of IDD was significantly higher in patients with chronic axial LBP. In another study by Hyodo and associates,[145] 73% of the patients with severe acute LBP obtained greater than 70% pain relief after the intradiscal injection of local anesthetic. This study also proposed that the incidence of discogenic pain was equally high in patients with severe acute LBP. In both studies the incidence of discogenic pain was highest in patients who were younger than 40 years and when the pain was located primarily in the low back and buttock region. It has also been proposed that pain of discogenic origin is precipitated by a torsion injury in the low back region and exacerbated by axial loading, such as occurs with prolonged sitting and standing. Moreover, the pain is often referred to the lower extremities in a nondermatomal distribution.[146]

DIAGNOSIS

Spinal imaging frequently shows degenerative disk changes in asymptomatic individuals[111,126] and is therefore of limited value in the diagnosis of IDD. IDD is frequently referred to as "black disk disease,"[147] which is due to the loss of signal intensity on T2-weighted MRI and signifies desiccation of the NP (see Fig. 21.7). However, it is a change representative of early DDD and may not be painful. A high-intensity zone on MRI of the posterior disk annulus (Fig. 21.7) has been shown to indicate the presence of a tear in the posterior disk annulus and has been correlated closely with the pain of diskography and pathologic IDD lesions.[134] Several authors have attempted to correlate the results of diskography with the radiologic features of DDD, and concordance has ranged from 55%[148] to almost 100%.[149] A concordant pain response to disk provocation, in the presence of a nonpainful or nonconcordant pain response at another disk level and coupled with morphologic abnormalities seen on the post-diskography CT scan (i.e., tears extending to the outer third of the AF), currently remains the only means of diagnosing IDD.

TREATMENT

Treatment of IDD and painful DDD is mainly palliative in nature, similar to that described for HD and LSS. Among the many minimally invasive treatment options available, several disk-heating modalities have been introduced. Among these, IDET has attained significant attention. IDET involves thermal lesioning of the posterior disk annulus by a percutaneously placed heating coil.[150] This technique was founded on shrinkage of collagen by the application of heat to the joint capsule and ligaments during arthroscopy.[151] The mechanism of proposed IDET effect is contraction of the annular collagen and coagulation of the neonociceptive fibers. The true nature of IDET and its reported benefits, however, is unknown.[152] Outcome studies of IDET are also mixed, with efficacy reported as ranging from minimal benefit[153] to highly successful.[150] Complete removal of the painful disk and arthrodesis of the adjacent vertebral bodies—spinal fusion—should theoretically relieve the pain of discogenic origin. However, the results of spinal fusion for discogenic pain are mixed, and serious doubts have been raised about its efficacy.[154] Spinal fusion has also been linked to loss of spinal mobility and accelerated adjacent spinal level disk degeneration. Artificial disk replacement surgery, or disk arthroplasty, was introduced to obviate some of the problems associated with spinal fusion surgery. The initial outcome studies of disk arthroplasty showed that the results were no better than those of spinal fusion surgery, and several unanswered questions remain regarding device longevity, complication rates, and long-term effects.[155] Currently available treatments of discogenic pain are therefore mainly symptomatic, with questionable efficacy and several possible associated complications. These treatments are also generally unable to restore or prevent further deterioration of disk architecture and function.

FUTURE DIRECTIONS

The future for the diagnosis and treatment of pain of discogenic origin is uncertain. Although understanding of the pathologic processes responsible for discogenic pain has improved, accurate knowledge of the differences between a painful and a painless degenerated disk remains indefinite, and early and objective diagnosis of IDD remains elusive. Biologic treatments such as gene therapy,[156] tissue engineering, and stem cell transplantation,[157] though currently being investigated, are experimental, with diminutive clinical application. To be successful, early application of treatment modalities that can retard further disk degeneration and therefore development of the related spinal syndromes is needed.

LUMBAR FACET SYNDROME

ANATOMY

The lumbar facet joints (LFJs), or lumbar zygapophyseal joints, are synovial joints with an articular surface, synovial membrane, fibroadipose meniscoid, and fibrous capsule.[158] These paired joints are located dorsally at the junction of the lamina, pedicle, and base of the transverse process. Each joint is composed of two—superior and inferior—articular processes stemming from the corresponding vertebrae. The orientation of facet joints is distinct at the lumbar, thoracic, and cervical levels. The medial branch (MB) of the posterior primary ramus courses over the base of the superior articular process (SAP) at its junction with the transverse process to innervate the facet joint at the same vertebral level and the vertebral level below. Each facet joint therefore receives innervation from the MB at the same vertebral level and from the vertebral level above (Fig. 21.12). The course of the MB is relatively fixed as it originates from the dorsal ramus, proximally at the base of the SAP, and as it passes under the mamillo-accessory ligament, at the caudal edge of the SAP.[159] The L5 dorsal ramus passes over the sacral ala at the base of the sacral SAP.[159] The fibrous capsule and the synovium of the facet joints are richly innervated by nociceptive fibers.[160]

HISTORICAL BACKGROUND

Goldthwait first proposed LFJs as a potential source of pain in the early 1900s,[28] and the term *facet syndrome* was introduced by Ghormley as early as 1933.[161] Several investigators

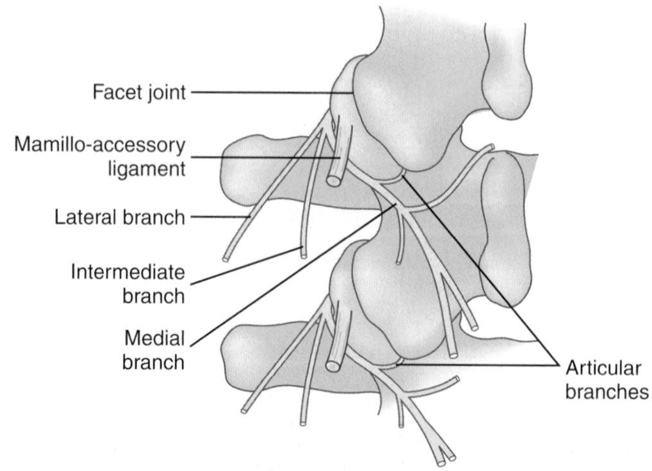

Figure 21.12 Schematic representation of facet joint innervation.

Box 21.4 Pathologic Lesions That Can Cause Lumbar Facet Syndrome

Systemic inflammatory arthritides
- Rheumatoid arthritis
- Ankylosing spondylitis

Degenerative arthritic changes
Villonodular synovitis
Synovial cysts
Infections
Microtrauma
- Microfractures
- Capsular and cartilaginous tears

Meniscoid and synovial entrapment
Joint subluxation

have since reproduced pain in the low back and proximal leg region by injecting hypertonic saline (a physiologic irritant) into the facet joints.[162-164] Relief of pain in patients with chronic LBP by intra-articular injections of local anesthetic and steroids was first reported by Mooney and Robertson in 1976.[163]

PATHOPHYSIOLOGY

The exact cause of pain originating from LFJs is often undetermined. Pathologic lesions such as systemic inflammatory arthritides (e.g., rheumatoid arthritis and ankylosing spondylitis), synovitis, synovial cysts, and infections (Box 21.4) are rare known causes of pain originating from LFJs.[165] Microtrauma, including microfractures and capsular and cartilaginous tears, have been observed on postmortem studies but are undetected by routine imaging studies.[166] The role of these injuries in causing chronic LBP, however, remains unknown. Meniscoid and synovial entrapment and joint subluxation have also been proposed as potential causes of pain.[167] Degenerative arthritic changes are often accepted as a frequent source of LFS, but these changes are observed in symptomatic and asymptomatic individuals with equal frequency, and their correlation with diagnostic facet joint injections is poor.[168] Degenerative changes in the facet joints frequently accompany degenerative changes in the disks and neural canals, and their contribution to patients' overall pain is often undetermined.

DIAGNOSIS

The typical features of LFS include unilateral or bilateral LBP, which is frequently referred to the groin, hip, or thighs but infrequently radiates below the knee joints (Box 21.5).[169] The pain is often exacerbated by arching or twisting movements and with prolonged standing or sitting and is reportedly relieved by forward flexion, rest, and walking. Painful limitation of low back extension, lack of neurologic findings, a negative SLR test, and localized tenderness over the facet joints have all been described as typical findings on physical examination. Other investigators, however, report lack of consistent clinical findings in patients who respond positively to diagnostic facet joint injections.[170] Although correlation between arthritic findings on imaging studies and pain relief from diagnostic injections has been suggested,[171]

Box 21.5 Clinical Features of Lumbar Facet Syndrome

Low back pain
Pain referred to the groin, hip, and posterior aspect of the thigh but rarely below the knees
Pain exacerbated by twisting and extension of the low back region but relieved by forward flexion
Pain with prolonged sitting or standing and relieved by rest and walking
Localized tenderness over the facet joints
Lack of neurologic signs
Normal straight-leg raise test

no imaging findings or radionuclide scans reliably predict facet joints as a source of pain.[172] Though controversial, the analgesic response to targeted, low-volume, intra-articular local anesthetic injections or MB blocks (MBBs) currently remains the only accepted standard for diagnosing pain originating from the LFJs.[169,170,173]

DIAGNOSTIC INJECTIONS FOR LUMBAR FACET SYNDROME

The suspected painful joints typically injected are either the joints found most tender on physical examination or, in the absence of any localizing signs, the lowermost LFJs—L5/S1 and L4/5—because these joints are deemed most commonly affected.[170] Fluoroscopic guidance with use of a coaxial needle insertion technique is considered essential for intra-articular needle placement. The injectate volume is generally kept lower than 2 mL. Larger injectate volumes can cause capsular injury, and leakage of contrast material into the neural foramina and epidural space may result in loss of diagnostic specificity. Before injection of a local anesthetic, a small volume of contrast medium (0.2 to 0.3 mL) may be injected to adequately delineate the joint space and to localize the correct intra-articular needle tip position. MBBs are performed by injecting a small volume (<1 mL) of local anesthetic at the junction of the transverse process and the SAP—the "eye of the Scottie dog" (Fig. 21.13)—and have been shown to have equal diagnostic sensitivity.[170] Injection of a small volume of contrast medium is often done before injection of local anesthetic for an MBB to confirm correct needle placement and to rule out intravascular needle tip location. MBBs are especially useful if joint entry cannot be obtained, as is often the case with severely degenerated joints and in patients after spinal surgery. MBBs are also the preferred diagnostic injections before RF MB rhizotomy because they allow direct testing of the nerves targeted for subsequent neurotomy. Avoidance or use of only short-acting systemic analgesics and resumption of routine activities after the diagnostic injection facilitate evaluation of the pain response from the procedure. The use of local anesthetics of different duration on two separate occasions—double comparative blocks—with the patient reporting pain relief that corresponds to the duration of the local anesthetic used, is considered to be a more specific diagnostic test. The prevalence of LFS in patients with chronic LBP as determined by a single set of diagnostic injections has been reported to vary from 7.7% to as high as 75%.[173] Prevalence rates of

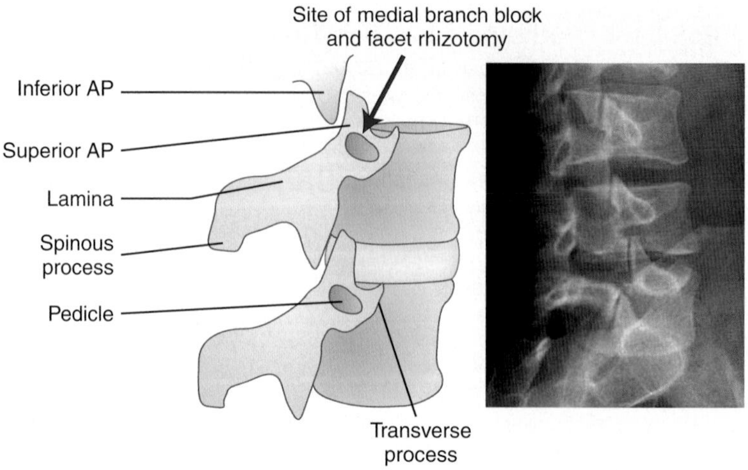

Figure 21.13 Oblique view of the lumbar spine. The schematic representation of the outline of a "Scottie dog" can be appreciated. The parts of the dog include the transverse process (the nose), pedicle (the eye), pars interarticularis (the neck), superior articular process (AP) (the ear), inferior AP (the front leg), lamina (the body), and spinous process (the leg).

15% to 40% are reported when more stringent double comparative blocks are used.[173] In addition to the wide variation in prevalence, a placebo response rate of almost 40% is reported when single diagnostic blocks are used.[174] Double comparative blocks are therefore highly recommended for appropriate diagnosis of LFS and to avoid the unacceptably high false-positive response rate obtained with single blocks.

THERAPEUTIC LUMBAR FACET JOINT INJECTIONS

Therapeutic lumbar facet joint injection (LFJI) of steroids and local anesthetics is a commonly performed pain management procedure. Based on the practice of intra-articular injection of steroids into painful knees and shoulders, intra-articular lumbar facet steroid injections were first performed by Mooney and Robertson in 1976.[163] However, no scientific studies have documented capsular inflammation in LFS, and the use of steroids, along with the typical dosages used—20 to 30 mg of methylprednisolone per joint—is entirely empirical. Confirmation of LFS by using diagnostic blocks before therapeutic LFJI is rarely practiced.[175] Observational studies report long-term (greater than 6 months) success rates of therapeutic LFJI to be in the range of 18% to 63%.[173] Long-term pain relief, however, is also reported after intra-articular facet injections of local anesthetics and saline.[176] The few prospective controlled trials conducted on this topic have been seriously criticized[173] and have failed to show the efficacy of therapeutic LFJI.[173,176]

FACET DENERVATION

Facet denervation, also referred to as facet rhizotomy, neurotomy, or ablation, is accomplished by lesioning of the MB at the same vertebral level and one vertebral level above (see Fig. 21.12). Although chemical neurolysis and cryoablation have been used, thermal RF ablation is the most frequently used technique for facet rhizotomy. Because the distal circumferential radius of the RF lesion generated is shorter than the more proximal circumferential radius, an RF lesion is performed by placing the electrode along the path of the nerve, parallel to the base of the SAP.[177] Optimal electrode position is confirmed radiologically and by sensory and motor testing before creation of the lesion. The size of RF electrodes used has varied from 22 to 18 gauge, with temperatures ranging between 80° C and 90° C, and the duration of RF lesioning has varied between 60 and 90 seconds. Larger probe size and longer duration of lesion creation tend to produce larger lesions with a greater likelihood of thermally injuring the target nerve. Routine use of 18-gauge electrodes with a 1-cm exposed tip and a lesioning duration of 120 seconds at 80° C has been recommended by some authors.[178] Apart from the several observational studies reporting the efficacy of RF ablation for LFS, three RCTs of its efficacy are available. Two of these trials demonstrated improvement in chronic LBP following the procedure, whereas the third showed no such benefit.[178]

SUMMARY

- Syndromes causing low back and radicular pain include herniated disk, spinal stenosis, internal disk disruption, facet syndrome, sacroiliac joint dysfunction, and myofascial pain syndrome.
- "Red flags" in the medical history of a patient with low back pain may indicate serious pathology and include age younger than 20 or older than 50 years, history of trauma, constitutional symptoms, and systemic illness.
- Most patients with a herniated disk experience significant resolution of their symptoms.
- Nonoperative treatment, including epidural steroid injections, should be tried initially in patients with a herniated disk. Although the initial results from surgery are promising, the long-term results appear to be similar to those of nonoperative treatment.
- Transforaminal epidural steroid injections (TF-ESIs) are associated with central nervous system injuries, including paraplegia. Digital subtraction angiography and nonparticulate steroids should be used for cervical TF-ESIs. For lumbar approaches, either a nonparticulate steroid or a steroid with smaller particles should preferably be used.
- Neurogenic claudication, the hallmark of spinal stenosis, should be distinguished from vascular claudication. Conservative management should be used since the benefits from surgical treatment appear to decrease with time.
- The presence of a high-intensity zone indicates an annular tear. The role of diskography is controversial, and the indication for intradiscal electrothermal therapy is limited.

- Facet denervation after diagnostic medial branch blocks may be an effective treatment of facet syndrome.
- The complexity of low back pain could also be attributed to the frequent presence of psychosocial issues in these patients and the lack of adequate diagnostic tests and effective treatments.
- A thorough clinical evaluation with recognition of the specific signs and symptoms of the different low back pain syndromes, their correlation with findings from available diagnostic tests, and the application of proven therapeutic interventions could provide relief for patients with low back pain and help reduce costs.

SUGGESTED READINGS

Arnoldi CC, Brodsky AE, Crock HV. Lumbar spinal stenosis and nerve root entrapment syndromes: definitions and classification. *Clin Orthop Relat Res.* 1976;115:4-5.

Atlas SJ, Keller RB, Wu YA, et al. Long-term outcomes of surgical and nonsurgical management of sciatica secondary to a lumbar disk herniation: 10 year results from the Maine lumbar spine study. *Spine.* 2005;30:927-935.

Bigos S, Bowyer O, Braen G, et al. Acute low back problems in adults. Clinical Practice Guideline. Number 14. AHCPR Publication No. 95-0643 December 1994.

Buckwalter JA. Aging and degeneration of the human intervertebral disc. *Spine.* 1995;20:1307-1314.

Crock HV. Internal disk disruption: a challenge to disk prolapse fifty years on. *Spine.* 1986;11:650-653.

Fardon DF, Milette PC. Nomenclature and classification of lumbar disk pathology. *Spine.* 2001;26:E93-E113.

Frymoyer J. Back pain and sciatica. *N Engl J Med.* 1988;318:291-300.

Jensen MC, Brant-Zawadzki MN, Obuchowski N, et al. Magnetic resonance imaging of the lumbar spine in people without back pain. *N Engl J Med.* 1994;331:69-73.

Mixter WJ, Barr JS. Rupture of the intervertebral disk with involvement of the spinal canal. *N Engl J Med.* 1934;211:210.

O'Connell JER. Sciatica and the mechanism of the production of clinical syndrome in protrusions of the lumbar intervertebral discs. *Br J Surg.* 1943;30:315-317.

Peng B, Hao J, Hou S, et al. Possible pathogenesis of painful intervertebral disk degeneration. *Spine.* 2006;31:560-566.

Renfrew DL, Moore TE, Kathol ME, et al. Correct placement of epidural steroid injections: fluoroscopic guidance and contrast administration. *AJNR Am J Neuroradiol.* 1991;12:1003-1007.

Saal JA. Natural history and nonoperative treatment of lumbar disk herniation. *Spine.* 1996;21(24S):2S-9S.

Weber H. Lumbar disk herniation: a controlled, prospective study with ten years of observation. *Spine.* 1983;8:131-140.

Weinstein JN, Tosteson TD, Lurie JD, et al. Surgical versus nonoperative treatment for lumbar disk herniation. *JAMA.* 2006;296:2441-2450.

The references for this chapter can be found at www.expertconsult.com.

22 Neurosurgical Approaches to Pain Management

Ahmed M. Raslan | Kim J. Burchiel

Neurosurgeons have a long history of surgically treating pain, particularly cancer pain. The notion that sectioning pain pathways could achieve pain control was first introduced by Spiller and Martin in 1912.[1] This was followed by the development of a whole array of surgical procedures aimed at interrupting ascending pain signals throughout different parts of the central nervous system.

Two approaches are used when targeting the brain or spinal cord to treat pain. The first, a nondestructive approach, uses either electrical stimulation of brain targets, which is thought to modulate the process of pain perception, or pharmacologic agents, which are introduced into the ventricular or intrathecal spaces to target pain-modulating receptors. Targets for electrical stimulation include the peripheral nerves, spinal cord, thalamic nuclei, periventricular gray (PVG) matter, periaqueductal gray (PAG) matter, and motor cortex. Currently, the pharmacologic agent of choice for intrathecal or intracerebroventricular (ICV) injection is morphine or other opiates. In general, nondestructive procedures are used for non–malignant-type pain; however, intrathecal opioids are also used for the treatment of cancer pain.

The second, a destructive approach, is used with the goal of interrupting signals that lead to perception of pain at various levels. Neuroablation can be performed on cellular complexes, such as nuclei or gyri, or on tracts with the aim of either disrupting the ascending sensory signals or destroying the limbic pathways involved in the emotional processes associated with pain. Neurosurgical procedures for pain can be performed at the level of the nerve, spinal cord, brainstem, or cerebrum and are considered ablative or neuromodulatory. Spinal cord neuromodulatory procedures fall into two subcategories: electrical and pharmacologic. These procedures are performed by anesthesiologists and neurosurgeons and are discussed elsewhere in this textbook.

We present three broad categories of neurosurgical procedures for pain: (1) cerebral neuroablation (e.g., dorsomedial thalamotomy and the caudalis dorsal root entry zone [DREZ] procedure), (2) spinal neuroablation (e.g., cordotomy, extralemniscal myelotomy, and trigeminal tractotomy), and (3) cerebral neuromodulation (electric: motor cortex stimulation [MCS] and deep brain stimulation [DBS]; and pharmacologic: ICV opioids).

CEREBRAL NEUROABLATION

Historically, many procedures fall into this category, including mesencephalotomy, pontine tractotomy, and hypophysectomy. We focus on procedures that we believe are more than what could be considered of purely historical significance.

MEDIAL THALAMOTOMY

Stereotactic thalamic neuroablative surgery for pain is relatively safe with respect to deep brainstem structures, and because of the wide involvement of many thalamic nuclei in pain processing, it has been considered a part of the pain surgery armamentarium.[2] The first structure targeted for neuroablation was the ventral caudal (Vc) nucleus, as defined by Hassler[3]; however, it was soon recognized that neuroablation of the Vc nucleus was associated with significant deafferentation pain phenomena. The work of Mark and colleagues led to the belief that targeting the medial thalamic nuclei was more effective in managing pain.[4] Nuclear targets for neuroablative medial thalamotomy are (1) the centralis lateralis, (2) centrum medianum, and (3) parafascicularis. Several pain syndromes, including cancer pain, central and peripheral deafferentation pain, spinal cord injury, malignancy, arthritis, and the neurogenic pains associated with Parkinson's disease,[5] have been successfully treated by medial thalamotomy. Frank and coauthors reported the overall success rate of medial thalamotomy to be 52%,[6] with cancer pain being the main condition treated. Jeanmonod and coworkers[7] and Young and colleagues[8] used radiofrequency and Gamma Knife treatment, respectively, and reported a 60% success rate in achieving pain control. The ideal target lying between the three main medial thalamic nuclei (listed above) has yet to be determined, although the centrum medianum nucleus is the most frequently targeted. DBS of the medial nuclei does not usually produce a conscious sensory response, and lesioning does not induce sensory loss. The published literature on medial thalamotomy is inconsistent regarding the target, guidance technique, patient population, and lesioning method used. Therefore, the actual success rate of medial thalamotomy is difficult to assess. However, in general, the procedure is considered to be effective in treating nociceptive pain, with recent data pointing to some success in relieving neuropathic pain.

STEREOTACTIC CINGULOTOMY

Cingulotomy refers to stereotactic lesioning of the anterior cingulate gyrus. Le Beau performed the first open cingulectomy to treat intractable pain in 1954.[9] It is believed that cingulotomy causes relief by altering a patient's emotional reaction to painful stimuli through interruption of the

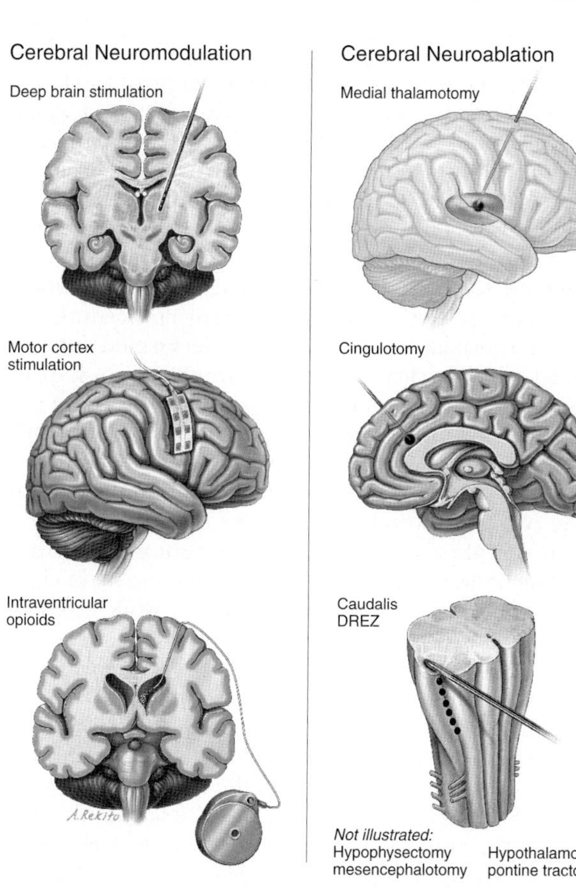

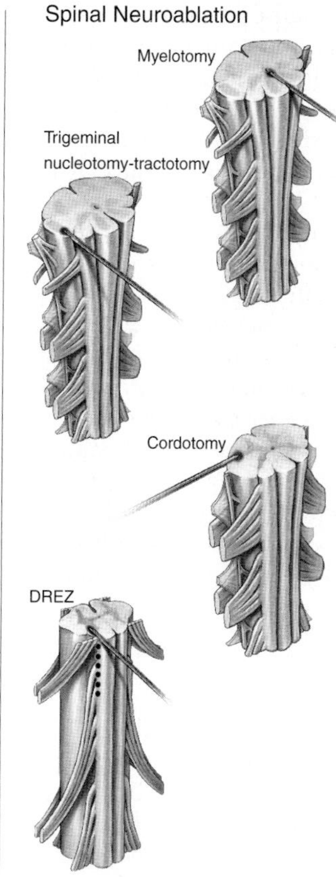

Figure 22.1 Diagrammatic representation of cerebral neuromodulation and neuroablation procedures and spinal neuroablation procedures. DREZ, dorsal root entry zone. (Adapted with permission from © Springer-Verlag 2007, Raslan AM, McCartney S, Burchiel KJ. Management of chronic severe pain: cerebral neuromodulatory and neuroablative approaches. *Acta Neurochir Suppl.* 2007;97:17-26; and Raslan AM, McCartney S, Burchiel KJ. Management of chronic severe pain: spinal neuromodulatory and neuroablative approaches. *Acta Neurochir Suppl.* 2007;97:33-41. With kind permission from Springer Science and Business Media.)

Papez circuit[10] and increasing tolerance to the subjective and emotional feelings of pain.[11,12] Cingulotomy is performed with standard stereotactic protocols, usually under general anesthesia. Bilateral lesions are made in the anterior aspect of the cingulate gyrus, and success of the procedure is directly related to the extent of ablation of the cingulum (Fig. 22.1).[1] A suitable stereotactic cingulotomy candidate is a terminally ill patient with widespread metastatic disease that has extended to the musculoskeletal system, where intrathecal or intraventricular administration of opiates is difficult. Emotional factors associated with pain would favor selection of a stereotactic cingulotomy procedure. Of note, stereotactic cingulotomy has been used to treat nonmalignant pain with a success rate of approximately 25%.[13] Stereotactic cingulotomy involves the ablation of sufficient anterior cingulate gyrus volume, which is usually achieved by producing at least two lesions with a wide–surface area, noninsulated tip electrode. The procedure is generally safe with few and minor side effects. Pillay and Hassenbusch reported on a series of 12 patients in which 7 had satisfactory pain relief.[14] Cingulotomy is rarely used today, mainly because of its narrow indication, advances in the medical management of terminal cancer patients, and the widespread use of neuroaugmentive procedures.

CAUDALIS DORSAL ROOT ENTRY ZONE (BRAINSTEM LEVEL)

Following the introduction of stereotaxis in the 1960s, the use of open ablative brain and brainstem surgery was almost abandoned. Siqueira first reported performance of the caudalis DREZ procedure in two patients.[15] Gorecki, Nashold, and colleagues at Duke University[16,17] later adopted the technique and expanded its indications. In the caudalis DREZ procedure, the caudal portion of the spinal trigeminal nucleus, along with the overlying trigeminal tract, is destroyed. Similar to spinal DREZ surgery, the objective is to destroy the cells of second-order neurons thought to be hyperactive in trigeminal deafferentation pain, thereby achieving pain relief (see Fig. 22.1). The main indications for the caudalis DREZ procedure are ophthalmic postherpetic neuralgia and trigeminal anesthesia dolorosa. In cases of neuropathic facial pain in which all other medical and surgical modalities are ineffective, the caudalis DREZ procedure may represent a last resort. The procedure is rarely performed, and potential risks include ipsilateral limb ataxia and weakness.

SPINAL NEUROABLATION

The first report of surgical disruption of spinal pain pathways was presented by Spiller and Martin in 1912.[1] They sectioned the anterolateral quadrant of the spinal cord with the intention of interrupting transmission of pain signals via the spinothalamic tract (anterolateral system) and relieving pain on the contralateral side of the body, caudal to the lesion.[1]

Several decades ago, open surgical sectioning of the spinothalamic tract (anterolateral cordotomy) to control pain was a common procedure in many neurosurgical centers. The procedure was used mainly to treat somatic nociceptive pain, usually from cancer. However, factors such as the debilitated state of cancer patients resulting in poor tolerance of open spinal cord surgery, together with high complication rates, meant that the procedure was not an ideal solution to the problem of cancer pain.

Currently, spinal cord targets for destructive procedures to treat pain include (1) the *spinothalamic tract* (anterolateral column), where destruction can alleviate somatic nociceptive pain below the level of the neck (e.g., anterolateral cordotomy); (2) *trigeminal spinal nucleus*, which is disrupted to treat trigeminal neuropathic pain (e.g., trigeminal tractotomy-nucleotomy ["caudalis DREZ"]); (3) *midline ascending polysynaptic visceral pain pathway*, which is used to treat visceral pain, particularly pelvic pain (i.e., midline myelotomy); and (4) the DREZ, primarily to treat deafferentation pain in the upper extremity (i.e., DREZ procedure) (see Fig. 22.1). The role of each of these procedures in contemporary surgical pain management will be reviewed.

ANTEROLATERAL CORDOTOMY

Anterolateral cordotomy refers to lesioning, sectioning, or other disruption of the lateral spinothalamic tract (LST), which is located in the anterolateral quadrant of the spinal cord. The procedure was historically performed in the upper thoracic spine via an open posterior approach and, less commonly, high in the cervical spine.[18] The spinal cord anterolateral ascending pain transmission system carries information about pain and temperature from one side of the body. The tract is formed by the central processes of nociceptive neurons in the dorsal horn that cross the spinal cord in the anterior commissure, ascend in the anterolateral column to the brainstem, and relay in the thalamus. Lesions of the anterolateral tract produce a contralateral deficit in pain and temperature sensation two to five segments below the level of the cordotomy. Fibers in the LST have a somatotopic arrangement, with the sacral segments arranged posterolaterally and the cervical segments anteromedially.[19] The corticospinal (pyramidal) tract lies posterior to the LST with white matter in between. The ventral spinocerebellar tract overlies the LST, and a lesion that damages the spinocerebellar tract may cause ipsilateral ataxia of the arm. Autonomic pathways for vasomotor and genitourinary control and reticulospinal fibers that subserve ipsilateral automatic respiration are also part of the anterolateral quadrant of the spinal cord. A patient with hemibody somatic cancer pain localized caudal to the cervical and upper thoracic area represents the best candidate for a cordotomy procedure.[20]

From the beginning of the 20th century until the late 1960s to early 1970s, cordotomy was an open procedure undertaken at the mid to high thoracic levels since these sites largely avoided the complications of upper limb ataxia and sleep apnea.[21] Introduction of the minimally invasive percutaneous approach for cordotomy by Mullan, Rosomoff, and their colleagues mitigated some of the neurologic risks and made it possible for the procedure to be performed on patients in poor general health.[22,23] In the mid-1980s and early 1990s, advances in opioid pharmacology, as well as the introduction of reversible and testable neuroaugmentive techniques, reduced the perceived need for spinal destructive procedures for pain control and led to a major reduction in the number of cordotomies performed by neurosurgeons worldwide. However, these neuroaugmentive procedures were expensive, particularly given the short life expectancy of many of the candidates, and were not uniformly effective.

Kanpolat and coworkers first introduced the concept of computed tomography (CT)-guided cordotomy, which allowed a safer, selective, and more effective procedure.[24-26] In 1995, Fenstermaker and associates[27] performed anterior CT-guided lower cervical cordotomy through the disk space to avoid sleep apnea (a modification of Gildenberg and colleagues' anterior low cervical percutaneous cordotomy).[28] CT-guided cordotomy is typically performed as a percutaneous procedure via a lateral approach to the spinal cord at the level of C2. However, the anterior cervical transdiscal approach can also be used, and in a recent clinical study this approach was used to control cancer pain in six of eight patients with pulmonary-pleural malignancy while avoiding sleep apnea.[29]

Today, the CT-guided cordotomy procedure involves lumbar puncture and injection of a water-soluble dye into the patient's intrathecal space. After 30 minutes, a cervical CT scan is performed. This and subsequent scans are used to direct the cordotomy electrode into the anterolateral quadrant of the ipsilateral spinal cord. The electrode is insulated throughout the entire shaft except the tip (2 mm in length and 0.3 to 0.4 mm in diameter). After measurement of the skin-dura distance and local anesthesia of the lateral cervical region, an electrode is introduced from the lateral side of the neck opposite the C2 foramen into the anterolateral quadrant of the spinal cord. To ensure complete entry into the spinothalamic tract (while avoiding the corticospinal tract), electrophysiologic testing is essential. Radiofrequency lesions are performed until adequate hypoesthesia is achieved in the contralateral hemibody or at least in the region of pain. CT-guided cordotomy has a higher success rate than do more traditional approaches, as well as fewer complications. Control of cancer pain is reportedly achieved in more than 95% of cases. Procedural complications may include weakness, hypotension, dysesthesia, mirror-image pain, ataxia, incontinence, and sleep apnea. However, contemporary CT-guided cordotomy complications tend to be both minor and transient.[30]

A recent evidence-based review concluded that the case for cordotomy is somewhat unique among all cancer pain procedures in that it has the most supportive evidence.[31] In that review the GRADE system of recommendation was used, and a recommendation for cordotomy was given. The GRADE system produces recommendations that are independent of the level of evidence.[32]

TRIGEMINAL TRACTOTOMY-NUCLEOTOMY (SPINAL LEVEL)

Sensory information from the 5th, 7th, 9th, and 10th cranial nerves is carried by the trigeminal tract and branches into the trigeminal tract spinal nucleus and extended caudally into the spinal cord to C2.[33] The trigeminal tract is considered a target for surgically treating facial pain,[34] and the history of procedures directed to this target is similar to cordotomy in that initial open procedures evolved toward less invasive stereotactic operations. Crue and colleagues and Hitchcock developed a stereotactic technique to lesion the trigeminal tract and nucleus via radiofrequency that was named trigeminal nucleotomy.[35,36] As with CT-guided cordotomy, CT is used when performing the trigeminal tractotomy-nucleotomy (TR-NC) procedure today. Indications include anesthesia dolorosa, post-herpetic neuralgia, neuropathic facial pain, facial cancer pain, and either glossopharyngeal or geniculate neuralgia.[26,37] The procedure can be considered, in some ways, a mini–caudalis DREZ procedure. The nucleus caudalis DREZ operation involves the same concept as the TR-NC procedure but includes destruction of the substantia gelatinosa (Rexed laminae II and III) of the nucleus caudalis. Pain relief from TR-NC is reported to be complete or satisfactory in 80% of cases. Complications include ataxia from injury to the spinocerebellar tract (usually temporary) and contralateral hypoalgesia if the spinothalamic tract is included in the lesion.[26,36-38]

EXTRALEMNISCAL MYELOTOMY

The extralemniscal myelotomy (ELM) procedure was first described by Hitchcock, who initially aimed to destroy the decussating fibers of the spinothalamic tract in the anterior commissure of the spinal cord to control pain in the neck and both arms.[39] ELM was achieved by creating a lesion in the central medullary region at the cervicomedullary junction. Unexpectedly, it was noted that the ELM procedure also seemed to control pain caudal to the level of the lesion. Schvarcz added the term "extralemniscal" to "myelotomy" because of the contention that the lesion incorporated an ascending polysynaptic nociceptive pathway.[40] Subsequently, the presence of such a tract has been confirmed anatomically. Several authors have now presented reports of midline "punctuate" ELM via open procedures to interrupt this pathway at various spinal cord levels. The polysynaptic ascending pathway is thought to carry visceral nociceptive information and lies deep to the midline dorsal column.[41-43] The concept of CT guidance, previously applied to cordotomy and TR-NC procedures, has also been applied to ELM by Kanpolat and colleagues, thus developing the image-guided ELM procedure used today.[37]

ELM is currently conceived as a pain control procedure for pain of visceral origin, including patients with pelvic malignancy, or for cancer pain in the lower part of the trunk and lower extremities with a predominant visceral pain component. The procedure appears to be safe; however, pain relief results are not as good as those achieved with cordotomy and TR-NC procedures.[18]

DORSAL ROOT ENTRY ZONE LESIONS

With introduction of the gate control theory in the 1960s, attention was drawn to the spinal dorsal horn as the initial physiologic substrate for pain modulation.[44] The dorsal horn and DREZ were then reconsidered as targets for both neuromodulation (spinal cord stimulation) and neuroablation. In 1972, Sindou[45] first attempted cervical DREZ destruction for neuropathic deafferentation pain in the upper extremity secondary to brachial plexus avulsion. Nashold and associates soon followed and introduced the use of radiofrequency lesions to perform DREZ disruption.[46] Laser and ultrasound have also been used to damage the DREZ.[47,48] When large-fiber afferents (touch, position sense) in peripheral nerves or dorsal roots are altered, there is a reduction in the inhibitory control of the dorsal horn.[49] This situation is presumed to result in excessive firing of the dorsal horn neurons, which is thought to be the cause of deafferentation pain and hence able to be controlled by DREZ lesioning.[50] The technical details of the procedure and its variants are beyond the scope of this chapter, but DREZ lesioning is performed as an open surgical procedure under general anesthesia and oftentimes accompanied by intraoperative neurophysiologic monitoring. Surgical candidates are patients with brachial plexus avulsion, Pancoast's tumor with brachial plexus invasion combined with a good general condition and reasonable life expectancy, pain caused by spinal cord or cauda equina lesions, and pain accompanying spasticity after plexus or cord injury.[45] A general prerequisite for the DREZ procedure is a lack of functional use of the limb where the DREZ procedure is performed since complete sensory denervation of the limb will render it functionless even if there is residual motor power. When patients are carefully selected and the lesions accurately performed, the success rate can be as high as 90% (with follow-up success rates reported for up to 4 years). Complications and side effects include cerebrospinal fluid (CSF) fistula, meningitis, ataxia, increased neurologic deficits, and dysesthesias.[51]

CEREBRAL NEUROMODULATION

ELECTRICAL NEUROMODULATION

DEEP BRAIN STIMULATION

Pool first observed and reported on the analgesic effects of septal stimulation in the frontal and lateral forniceal columns while performing psychosurgery in the 1950s.[52] Heath and Mickle and Pool and colleagues subsequently reported the pain-relieving effect of septal and near-septal stimulation in nonpsychiatric patients.[53,54] Mazars and coauthors and Reynolds first reported pain relief from thalamic stimulation in 1960.[55,56]

Neurostimulation of the brain to relieve pain was thus introduced decades before what has become the main contemporary indication for DBS—treatment of movement disorders.[57] However, these early reports only set the stage for the eventual applications of DBS for pain relief. In the mid-1960s, Melzack and Wall's gate theory[44] provided the logical rationale for DBS of the sensory thalamus to control pain. Shortly afterward, Reynolds reported on the analgesic effect of focal brain stimulation in rats (stimulation-produced analgesia).[56] In the early 1970s, Hosobuchi and associates[58,59] and Richardson and Akil[60,61] were the first to report on stimulation of the human thalamus and PVG and PAG matter for pain control. Even though stimulation of the thalamic sensory nuclei produced paresthesias in painful areas, consistent pain relief was not achieved. Similar results were produced by stimulation of the internal capsule.[62,63] Stimulation of the PVG and PAG typically did not produce paresthesias but did induce a sense of "warmth." Higher-intensity PVG/PAG stimulation produced unpleasant and sometimes overwhelming sensations such as impending doom or terror. The centromedian-parafascicular complex was also targeted by Andy[64] as a stimulation site to treat pain, and this stimulation likewise did not produce paresthesias.

Despite reports describing the use of DBS to treat chronic pain in the 1970s and early 1980s, data to support the technique never reached contemporary evidentiary standards. The use of DBS for pain control has failed to gain much acceptance in the neurosurgical community, and the use of DBS electrodes as pain control implants has never achieved U.S. Federal Drug Administration (FDA) approval. The lack of data to support the procedure is due, in part, to the small number of patients treated, inconsistent target localization, heterogeneity of the pain diagnoses treated, and failure to mount a prospective randomized trial that was sufficiently powered to answer the question of efficacy. The mechanism of pain relief by DBS is poorly understood but appears to be dependent on the site. The thalamus and PVG/PAG were the most commonly[65] targeted sites for DBS implants for pain. Hosobuchi and colleagues[58] suggested that the pain-relieving effect of PVG and PAG stimulation might involve endogenous opioid receptors based on their studies in which it was found that the pain-relieving effect of DBS could be reversed by naloxone. Evidence to support this mechanism of action of PAG/PVG DBS is inconsistent. Some investigators supported the concept whereas others disagreed. Currently, it is postulated that the pain-relieving effect of PAG/PVG DBS is due to activation of multiple supraspinal descending pain modulatory systems, both opioid and nonopioid.[66] Pain relief resulting from stimulation of the ventral posterolateral (VPL) nucleus and ventral posteromedial (VPM) nucleus (Vc nucleus in the European Hassler terminology), the major sensory nuclei of the thalamus, is poorly understood. Inhibition of spinothalamic tract neurons[67] and activation of dopaminergic mechanisms have both been proposed.[68] The most accepted hypothesis is that thalamic stimulation activates the nucleus raphe magnus of the rostroventral medulla, which results in activation of a suprasegmental descending endogenous pain inhibition system.[66]

Meticulous patient selection, with classification of the pain (i.e., nociceptive or neuropathic) combined with informed DBS target selection, should help improve the outcome of DBS for pain. Clinical case series (class III evidence) observations suggest that PVG/PAG stimulation seems to be more effective in treating somatic nociceptive pain. This is consistent with the proposed opioid-mediated effect of PAG/PVG stimulation.[69] It has also been suggested that VPL and VPM (Vc) stimulation is more effective in treating neuropathic pain, a gate theory–based concept.[69] In the absence of controlled trials to prove efficacy, any definitive conclusions regarding the ideal target for any particular pain syndrome remains elusive. Furthermore, many patients have mixed neuropathic/nociceptive pain, which suggests that the DBS target to control pain should be individualized according to the patient. Some authors have even suggested placing two electrodes simultaneously in the sensory thalamic nucleus (Vc) and in the PVG.[70] For some pain syndromes (e.g., thalamic infarction–induced pain), target selection is simpler given that thalamic stimulation is not possible.[70] Chronic *neuropathic* pain conditions treated by DBS have included anesthesia dolorosa, post-stroke pain, thalamic pain, brachial plexus avulsion, post-herpetic neuralgia, post-cordotomy dysesthesia, spinal cord injuries, and peripheral neuropathy pain. *Nociceptive* pain conditions treated by but not limited to DBS have included failed back surgery syndrome, osteoarthritis, and cancer pain.[71]

DBS for chronic pain is similar to DBS for other indications (movement disorders) in that surgeons have a number of targets that are applicable to the general problem (see Fig. 22.1). DBS target locations are often *indirectly* derived from the Schaltenbrand and Bailey atlas or measured *directly* from the patient's CT or magnetic resonance imaging scans. The location of these targets can be confirmed intraoperatively by macrostimulation, microelectrode mapping, or intraoperative imaging. To best judge the benefits of stimulation and help fine-tune stimulation parameters following final electrode implantation, a trial period of approximately 1 week is often a prerequisite. Complications of DBS for pain relief are similar to those for movement disorders. Typically, they are related to either (1) brain injury from bleeding or inadvertent trauma as a result of electrode insertion, (2) infection, (3) hardware failure, and (4) transient site-specific side effects related to overstimulation or unintentional stimulation of neighboring areas. The later might produce diplopia, seizures, nausea, paresthesias, or headaches.

Overall, DBS surgery is a safe procedure with a relatively low chance of complications or unintended neurologic sequelae. However, data to support its efficacy are sparse. Currently, DBS for pain control is an extraordinary treatment that may be applicable to only a few chronic pain conditions. DBS implantable hardware is not approved by the FDA for pain control procedures, and many insurance carriers will not authorize implantation. Given the tremendous interest in and application of DBS for movement disorders, whether DBS for pain will be substantially resurrected at some point remains to be seen.

MOTOR CORTEX STIMULATION

In 1954, Penfield and Jasper observed that stimulation of the precentral (motor) gyrus elicited sensory responses when the corresponding portion of the adjacent postcentral gyrus had previously been resected.[72] They treated burning pain on one side of the body by postcentral gyrectomy, and when the pain recurred, they performed precentral gyrectomy, which then controlled the pain. Independently, in 1955 White and Sweet attempted surgical resection of the postcentral gyrus for relief of central pain and reported 13% pain relief.[73] It was not until 1971, after publication of the gate theory in 1965, that Lende and coworkers re-explored the motor cortex as a potential site for pain control. In an attempt to treat central neuropathic facial pain[74] they performed two cases of precentral and postcentral gyrectomy of the facial cortex. These reports formed the basis for establishing a linkage between the precentral and postcentral areas and pain control surgery.

By the 1980s, the cumulative failure of other procedures, both modulatory and destructive, to fundamentally alter neuropathic pain made it clear that the development of an innovative methodology to surgically treat pain was critically needed. Exploration of the motor area as a target site was well under way. Hardy and associates stimulated the rat medial prefrontal cortex with a resultant significant elevation in nociceptive response latency.[75,76] Hosobushi implanted electrodes in subcortical somatosensory areas for control of dysesthetic pain, and from this study it was concluded that somatosensory stimulation could be effective in the treatment of leg pain.[77] In 1991, Tsubokawa and coworkers first introduced epidural stimulation of the motor cortex as an option to treat central deafferentation pain. His group had tried postcentral gyrus (sensory) stimulation and found that it was either ineffective or exacerbated the pain. They demonstrated that epidural MCS inhibited abnormal thalamic neuronal burst activity and increased regional blood flow to the cortex and thalamus.[78] Primarily, Tsubokawa and colleagues used MCS for central deafferentation pain syndromes such as post-stroke pain.[78,79] The mechanism of action of MCS is still poorly understood; however, the work of Garcia-Larrea, Peyron, and coworkers[80-82] has shed some light on its mechanism of action. Positron emission tomography and electrophysiologic studies have demonstrated that MCS increases blood flow to the ipsilateral thalamus, cingulate gyrus, orbitofrontal cortex, insula, and the brainstem, with some correlation between increased thalamic and brainstem blood flow and efficacy of pain relief. The increased blood flow to the ipsilateral sensory thalamus was greater than that to the motor (ventrolateral) thalamus. It did not appear that an intact somatosensory system was absolutely necessary for the clinical benefits to be realized, an important discovery allowing the use of this technology for stroke and other deafferentation states.[80-82] As with many forms of chronic stimulation, habituation seems to occur, which is more likely with the use of high-frequency stimulation. The patient selection process for MCS is of paramount importance (as it is for all pain-relieving surgeries), and in this case, the debate continues. Neuropathic pain is more responsive than nociceptive pain to this form of therapy. Attempting to predict the best candidates for MCS can be challenging, and Yamamoto and colleagues introduced a pharmacologic classification of post-stroke patients based on their pain relief response to escalating doses of both intravenous thiamylal and morphine. They concluded that patients with a good response to thiamylal or ketamine and a poor response to morphine were the best candidates for MCS.[83] Several neurogenic pain syndromes have been treated by MCS, including thalamic pain, bulbar post-stroke pain (which typically occurs with "Wallenberg's syndrome"), facial neuropathic and deafferentation pain, and phantom and brachial plexus avulsion pain.[84,85] Treatment of central post-stroke pain following thalamic infarction or thalamic or putaminal bleeding by MCS was reported by Tsubokawa and colleagues to achieve good to excellent pain control in 65% of cases (follow up >12 months), with no seizures observed.[78,79] Katayama and associates extended the indications to include bulbar pain secondary to "Wallenberg's syndrome" and reported on four patients initially treated by VPL thalamic stimulation that resulted in increased pain. Three other patients were later treated by MCS, with greater than a 60% reduction in pain in two patients and greater than 40% in one patient.[86] Treatment of neuropathic facial pain appears to be one of the most promising indications for MCS, which may be related to the breadth of facial representation over the motor cortex. Several reports include neuropathic facial pain treatment by MCS. Raslan, Ebel, Herregodts, Meyerson, Nguyen, Rainov, and their colleagues all treated trigeminal neuropathic pain with MCS and reported pain relief in approximately 60% of patients for periods of up to 12 months.[85,87-92] Peripheral deafferentation pain, as well as brachial plexus avulsion pain, has also been treated by MCS, with variable results. Movement disorders are an active area of ongoing MCS research.[84] MCS has been shown to produce improvement in the symptoms of thalamic hand syndrome, action tremors, intention myoclonus, and Parkinson's disease.

MCS involves the implantation of epidural electrodes over the motor cortex (see Fig. 22.1), which can be localized by either (1) radiologic landmarks of the central sulcus, (2) intraoperative somatosensory evoked potentials with observation of "phase reversal" over the central sulcus, (3) intraoperative stimulation of the cortex with concurrent electromyographic monitoring of the relevant muscle groups contralaterally, and more recently, (4) use of neuronavigation systems to localize either the central sulcus or the precentral gyrus. Some authors even recommend the use of functional magnetic resonance imaging for targeting, especially with infarctions involving the motor cortex.[93] A trial period of MCS is usually required followed by implantation of a permanent system if the trial produces adequate relief. Complications of MCS include intraoperative seizures, stimulator pocket infection, epidural bleeding, subdural effusion, and "tolerance" to stimulation with diminished analgesia over time.

CEREBRAL NEUROMODULATION: PHARMACOLOGIC

INTRAVENTRICULAR OPIOIDS

Studies showing the direct analgesic effects of opioids applied in the ventricular region and around the medulla of the central nervous system[94,95] led to the work of Leavens and coworkers in 1982,[96] in which human ICV use of morphine was first reported. The profound analgesic response to intrathecal morphine coupled with its widespread clinical use for lower body pain suggested the need for more rostral injection sites to control pain involving the head, neck, and upper extremity regions. Even though cervical intrathecal opioid injection sometimes resulted in respiratory depression, it was possible to deliver a small amount of ICV morphine without respiratory dysfunction or dysautonomia. Opioid receptors are abundant around the wall of the third ventricle and aqueduct, as well as in the PVG and PAG. In Leavens and colleagues' 1982 report, 1 mg of morphine was used to treat patients with intractable cancer pain and resulted in profound analgesia and no respiratory depression or neurologic changes.[96] In a report on 82 patients, Lazorthes and associates recommended nine specific guidelines for the ICV use of morphine: (1) chronic pain secondary to inoperable malignant tumors in patients with terminal cancer; (2) pain not relieved by medical treatment and, in particular, the development of serious side effects from using oral or systemic morphine; (3) intractable bilateral, midline, or diffuse pain not appropriate for percutaneous or open surgical interruption of nociceptive pathways; (4) chronic pain of somatic nociceptive origin (neurogenic pain was a contraindication); (5) upper body pain secondary to cervicothoracic cancer; (6) chronic pain of the lower half of the body (subdiaphragmatic) only after failure of or contraindication to conventional intrathecal spinal opioid administration; (7) absence of general risks for complications, such as coagulation disturbances, cutaneous infection, and septicemia; (8) informed consent from the patient and family; and (9) the presence of a favorable domestic environment (e.g., physician, nurse, or family) for ambulatory surveillance and chronic ICV morphine treatment. The authors recommended that when the topography of the pain involved a transitional area (e.g., lower thoracic, diaphragmatic, or upper abdominal region), ICV morphine could be indicated if the patient failed a more standard intrathecal morphine trial.[97]

Surgically, the technique for implanting a chronic ICV morphine infusion system involves placement of a catheter into the lateral ventricle near the foramen of Monro to deliver drug near target receptors in the periaqueductal parenchyma of the midbrain (see Fig. 22.1). The analgesic latency of ICV morphine administration is between 15 and 30 minutes, and the effect lasts for a mean of 28 hours. Excellent or good pain relief rates range from greater than 50% to 97%, and side effects include somnolence, nausea, confusion, and respiratory depression, which are usually transient. Finally, Lazorthes and coauthors reported tolerance in 3 of 82 patients.[97]

The increased effectiveness of oral opioids has diminished the necessity for ICV morphine administration. However, the technique remains relatively simple and effective and is a viable option for patients with intractable pain of malignant etiology, following oral opioid failure, and when pain is diffuse or cephalic in topography.[98]

SUMMARY

Neurosurgical procedures to treat intractable pain have gone through an evolutionary process, dictated in part by technological advances, scientific discovery, and changes in the survival rates of chronic pain patients, especially those with cancer pain. Irreversible ablative procedures are used much less frequently today, yet on occasion they remain the procedures of choice. Depending on the physiologic substrate and pain topography, multiple brain and spinal cord regions can be targeted to treat chronic pain. Today, neuromodulation by either electrical stimulation or pharmacologic manipulation is generally the preferred approach to treat chronic pain.

KEY POINTS

- Neurosurgical treatments of intractable pain are usually reserved as last options for the treatment of intractable pain.
- These interventions can be either ablative or neuromodulatory, which in turn could be divided into pharmacologic and electrical.
- Neurosurgical procedures can be done at either a spinal or cerebral level. Spinal spinothalamic ablation (cordotomy) is the most studied and performed neurosurgical ablative procedure, and it is very effective in treating unilateral somatic cancer pain.
- Opioid use has limited the indications for ablative procedures, but there are still defined but limited indications for spinal ablative procedures that are confined to cancer-related pain.
- Spinal neuromodulation (i.e., spinal cord stimulation and intrathecal opioid devices) are used widely for chronic spinal pain.
- Cerebral ablation of pain pathways or centers is rarely done at present. However, cerebral neuromodulation procedures such as deep brain stimulation and motor cortex stimulation have limited indications and utility that are usually related to central pain and neuropathic pain.

ACKNOWLEDGMENT

The authors thank Shirley McCartney, Ph.D., for editorial assistance.

SUGGESTED READINGS

Hosobuchi Y. Combined electrical stimulation of the periaqueductal gray matter and sensory thalamus. *Appl Neurophysiol.* 1983;46:112-115.

Kanpolat Y. Percutaneous cordotomy, tractotomy, and midline myelotomy: minimally invasive stereotactic pain procedures. In: Fisher W, Burchiel K, eds. *Seminars in Neurosurgery: Pain Management for the Neurosurgeon.* Vol. 2/3. New York: Thieme Medical; 2005:203-219.

Lazorthes YR, Sallerin BA, Verdie JC. Intracerebroventricular administration of morphine for control of irreducible cancer pain. *Neurosurgery.* 1995;37:422-428.

Raslan AM, Cetas JS, McCartney S, et al. Destructive procedures for control of cancer pain: the case for cordotomy. *J Neurosurg.* 2011;114:155-170.

Tsubokawa T, Katayama Y, Yamamoto T, et al. Chronic motor cortex stimulation for the treatment of central pain. *Acta Neurochir Suppl.* 1991;52:137-139.

The references for this chapter can be found at www.expertconsult.com.

23 Cancer Pain

Vandana Sharma | Oscar de Leon-Casasola

BACKGROUND

Cancer pain is a result of cancer growth in human tissues or the pain produced by any of the therapies implemented to treat it. Ideal management starts with a thorough assessment via the history and physical examination, as well as the judicious use of diagnostic testing in an attempt to define the pathophysiologic components involved in the expression of pain to implement optimal analgesic therapy. Adequate pain control can be achieved in the great majority of patients with the implementation of aggressive pharmacologic treatment consisting of the use of opioids and adjuvants.[1,2] With the implementation of these strategies, 90% to 95% of patients may achieve adequate pain control.[3] Consequently, 5% to 10% of patients will need some form of invasive therapy. Thus, when following specific guidelines, the great majority of patients with cancer-related pain may expect adequate pain control in the 21st century. Control of pain and related symptoms is a cornerstone of cancer treatment in that it promotes an enhanced quality of life, improved functioning, better compliance, and a means for patients to focus on matters that give meaning to life.[4] In addition to their salutary effects on quality of life, mounting evidence suggests that good pain control influences survival.[5,6]

EPIDEMIOLOGY

Approximately 6.35 million new cases of cancer are diagnosed annually worldwide, half of which originate in developing nations[7] and 1.04 million occur in the United States alone.[8] Mortality is high; one in five deaths in the United States is a result of cancer, which means about 1400 cancer-related deaths per day.[9,10] The morbidity is equally concerning inasmuch as up to 50% of patients undergoing treatment of cancer and up to 90% of patients with advanced cancer have pain.[11] Most (65%) cancer pain is due to involvement of organic structures by tumor, notably bone, neural tissue, viscera, and others. Up to 25% of cancer pain is due to therapy, including chemotherapy, radiotherapy, and surgery, and the rest of "cancer pain" is accounted for by common chronic pain syndromes, including back pain and headaches, which might have been exacerbated by the ongoing growth or treatment of cancer.[12] As new therapeutic regimens are introduced for the treatment of cancer, it is expected that cancer patients will be living longer and potentially experiencing pain as a result of cancer disease itself or therapies implemented for its control for longer periods.

Anorexia, fatigue, and pain are the most common symptom associated with cancer.[13,14] Significant pain is present in up to 25% of patients undergoing active treatment and in up to 90% of patients with advanced cancer.[11,15-19] According to several studies, including a survey of oncologists in the Eastern Cooperative Oncology Group (ECOG) and a survey of 1103 consecutive admissions to a U.S tertiary care cancer hospital, 73% of patients in active treatment admitted to having pain, with 38% reporting severe pain.[20] Despite the availability of simple, cost-effective treatments,[21] inadequately controlled pain remains a significant problem. This is important because of the negative influence of pain on patients' performance status.

Performance status, as measured by the ECOG and Karnofsky scales (Table 23.1), is a global rating of patients' overall functional status. When performance status is low, as is often the case when pain is severe, patients may find it difficult to tolerate the chemotherapy recommended; indeed, they may not be considered candidates for chemotherapy. Further benefits of good pain management often include improvement in nutrition, rest, and mood, all of which contribute to quality of life and have the potential to influence the outcome of antineoplastic therapy.

ASSESSMENT OF PAIN INTENSITY

Questionnaires have been used to aid in standardizing patients' assessment. Ideally, this assessment is completed by patients before their evaluation. The Wisconsin Brief Pain Inventory (BPI)[22] and the Memorial Pain Assessment Card[23] are becoming increasingly well accepted. The characteristics of the different assessment tools are noted in the following outline:

1. *Wisconsin BPI*:
   a. It is a fifteen-minute questionnaire that can be self-administered.
   b. It includes several questions about the characteristics of the pain, including its origin and the effects of previous treatments.
   c. It incorporates two valuable features of the McGill Pain Questionnaire, a graphic representation of the location of the pain and groups of qualitative descriptors. Severity of pain is assessed by a series of visual analog scale (VAS) scores that quantify pain at its best, worst, and on average. The perceived level of interference with normal function is quantified with a VAS also.
   d. Preliminary evidence suggests that the BPI is cross-culturally applicable and is useful, particularly when patients are not fit to complete a more thorough or comprehensive questionnaire.

Table 23.1 Methods of Assessing Performance Status

	ECOG Scale*		Karnofsky Scale†
0	Fully active, able to carry out all predisease performance without restriction	100	Normal; no complaints, no evidence of disease
1	Restricted in physically strenuous activity but ambulatory and able to carry out light or sedentary work (e.g., light housework, office work)	90	Able to carry out normal activity; minor signs or symptoms of disease
2	Ambulatory and capable of all self-care but unable to work; up and about more then 50% of waking hours	80	Normal activity with effort; some signs or symptoms of disease
3	Capable of only limited self-care, confined to bed or chair more than 50% of waking hours	70	Cares for self; unable to carry out normal activity or to do active work
4	Completely disabled, cannot carry on any self-care. Totally confined to bed or chair	60	Requires occasional assistance but is able to care for most needs
5	Dead	50	Requires considerable assistance and frequent medical care
		40	Disabled, requires special care and assistance
		30	Severely disabled, hospitalization indicated; death not imminent
		20	Very sick, hospitalization necessary; active supportive treatment necessary
		10	Moribund; fatal processes; progressing rapidly
		0	Dead

*Oken MM, Creech RH, Tormey DC, et al, Toxicity and response criteria of the Eastern Cooperative Oncology Group. *Am J Clin Oncol.* 1982;5:649-655.

†Schag CC, Heinrich RL, Ganz PA. Karnofsky performance status revisited: reliability, validity, and guidelines. *J Clin Oncol.* 1984;2:187-193.

2. *Memorial Pain Assessment Card:*
   a. It is a simple, efficient, and valid instrument that provides rapid clinical evaluation of the major aspects of pain experienced by cancer patients.[23]
   b. It is easy to understand and use and can be completed by experienced patients in 20 seconds.
   c. It consists of a two-sided, 8.5- × 11-inch card that is folded so that four separate measures are created.
   d. It features scales intended for measurement of pain intensity, pain relief, and mood and a set of descriptive adjectives.
3. *Edmonton staging system:*
   a. It is performed by health care providers.
   b. It was developed to predict the likelihood of achieving effective relief of pain in cancer patients.[24,25]
   c. The system's originators provided validation that treatment outcome can be accurately predicted according to five clinical features (neuropathic pain, movement-related pain, recent history of tolerance to opioids, psychological distress, and a history of alcoholism or drug abuse).
   d. Staging requires only 5 to 10 minutes and no special skills are needed to complete it.
   e. Its value lies in prospective identification of potentially problematic patients, thereby further legitimizing clinical research on control of symptoms by introducing better standardization and improving our ability to critically assess the results of various therapeutic interventions in large population of patients.
4. *Pediatric cancer pain assessment:* This includes Beyer's The Oucher, Eland's color scale–body outline, Hester's poker chip tool, McGrath's faces scale, and others.[26-29]
5. *Numerical rating scale (NRS) or VAS:*
   a. Pain is often assessed on an 11-point NRS from 0 (no pain) to 10 (worst pain imaginable).
   b. The VAS is a 10-cm line without markings from no pain to worst pain; patients mark their pain score and a measurement in centimeters defines their level of pain.

Evaluation of pain should be integrated with a detailed oncologic, medical, and psychosocial assessment. The initial evaluation should include an evaluation of the patient's feelings and attitudes about the pain and disease, family concerns, and the patient's premorbid psychological history. A comprehensive but objective approach to assessment instills confidence in patients and family that will be valuable throughout treatment. A comprehensive evaluation of patients with cancer pain includes the following:

- The *reason for the visit* is determined to ensure appropriate triage (e.g., patients with severe pain because of bowel obstruction may need to be sent to the emergency center for urgent treatment).
- An *oncologic history* is obtained to gain knowledge of the context of the pain problem and includes diagnosis and stage of the disease; a history of therapies implemented, including a list of the chemotherapeutic agents used, types of surgery, site of radiotherapy, and outcome (including side effects); and the patient's understanding of the disease process and prognosis.
- The *pain history* should include any premorbid chronic pain and, for each new pain site, its onset and evolution, site and radiation areas, pattern (constant, intermittent, or unpredictable), intensity (best, worst, average, current)

on VAS scales, quality, exacerbating and relieving factors, interference of the pain with usual activities, neurologic and motor abnormalities (including bowel and bladder continence), vasomotor changes, and current and past analgesics (use, efficacy, side effects). Previous analgesic use, efficacy, and side effects should be cataloged. Prior treatments of pain should be noted (radiotherapy, nerve blocks, physiotherapy, etc.).

- The *medical record and radiologic studies* should be reviewed. Many of the treatments of cancer may cause pain themselves (chemotherapy- and radiotherapy-induced neuropathy or postoperative pain syndromes such as post-thoracotomy and post-mastectomy pain syndrome), and many specific cancers may cause well-established pain patterns as a result of known probable sites of metastasis, including (1) metastasis of breast cancer to long bones, the spine, chest wall, brachial plexus, and spinal cord; (2) metastasis of colon cancer to the pelvis, hips, lumbar plexus, sacral plexus, and spinal cord; and (3) metastasis of prostate cancer to long bones, the pelvis, hips, lung, and spinal cord.
- The *psychosocial history* should include marital and residential status, employment history and status, educational background, functional status, activities of daily living, recreational activities, support systems, health and capabilities of the spouse or significant other, and past history of (or current) drug or alcohol abuse.
- The *medical history* (independent of the oncologic history) should include coexisting systemic disease, exercise intolerance, allergies to medications, medications in use, previous illness and surgery, and a thorough review of systems, including the following:
  - General (anorexia, weight loss, cachexia, fatigue, weakness, insomnia)
  - Neurologic (sedation, confusion, hallucination, headache, motor weakness, altered sensation, incontinence)
  - Respiratory (dyspnea, cough, pneumonia)
  - Gastrointestinal (dysphagia, nausea, vomiting, dehydration, constipation, diarrhea)
  - Psychological (irritability, anxiety, depression, dementia)
  - Genitourinary (urgency, hesitancy, hematuria)
- The *physical examination* must be thorough, although at times it is appropriate to perform a focused examination of particular problems. In patients with spinal pain and known or suspected metastatic disease, a complete neurologic examination is mandatory.
- A *care team meeting* should be arranged if applicable.
- The need for *further studies* should be determined.
- Formulate a *clinical impression* (*diagnosis*). Multiple diagnoses usually apply, and it is optimal to use the most specific known diagnosis, such as somatic pain from a vertebral metastasis, severe pain in a patient with metastatic non–small cell carcinoma of the lung, and neuropathic pain from a paravertebral mass invading the nerve root as it exits the vertebral foramen. Nausea and vomiting with severe weight loss and fatigue, as well as constipation, should be identified.
- *Formulate recommendations* (*plan*) *and alternatives* for each problem. For instance, with respect to the examples just presented in formulating a clinical impression, one could perform magnetic resonance imaging (MRI) of the spine, add a controlled-release opioid administered daily and transmucosal fentanyl citrate for breakthrough pain, implement therapy with a combination of a tricyclic antidepressant and an anticonvulsant with instructions on titration, prescribe an antiemetic before meals and as needed for nausea, prescribe a bowel stimulant and bulk-forming compound twice daily for constipation, and evaluate in 2 weeks to determine the need for a short course of steroid therapy.
- *Call an oncologist or the primary care provider*, or both, if applicable. Have a discussion with the referring physician, primary care provider, and/or oncologist to establish short- and long-term plans.
- Conduct an *exit interview*.
  - Explain the probable cause of the symptoms in terms that the patient can understand.
  - Discuss the prognosis for relief of symptoms, management options, and specific recommendations. In addition to writing prescriptions, oral and written instructions must be provided. Educational material regarding medications, pain management strategies, or procedures should also be provided. Potential side effects and their management should be discussed.
  - Arrange for follow-up with clinic contact information.
  - Dictate a summary of the evaluation to the referring and consulting physicians.

CLASSIFICATION OF CANCER PAIN

TIME RELATED

ACUTE PAIN

Acute pain is frequently associated with sympathetic hyperactivity and heightened distress.[30] It is often temporally associated with the onset or recrudescence of primary or metastatic disease, and its presence should motivate the clinician to aggressively seek its cause and adjust the pharmacologic therapeutic scheme.

SUBACUTE PAIN

Some patients experience subacute pain for 4 to 6 weeks after a major surgical procedure. This type of pain is largely undertreated and deserves special attention because it may affect the patient's ability to perform activities of daily living after discharge from the hospital.

CHRONIC PAIN

Treatment of pain of a chronic nature mandates a combination of palliation, adjustment, and acceptance. With time, biologic and behavioral adjustment to the symptoms occurs, and hopefully the associated symptoms will be blunted. Chronic pain with superimposed episodes of acute pain (breakthrough pain) is probably the most common pattern observed in patients with ongoing cancer pain.

INTENSITY

Consistent use of measurements of pain intensity aids in monitoring a patient's progress and may serve as a basis for interpatient comparisons. High pain scores may alert the clinician to the need for more aggressive treatment or hospitalization (or both) for rapid control of symptoms via intravenous patient-controlled analgesia (IV PCA) or for antineuropathic medications with a rapid titration protocol.

PATHOPHYSIOLOGY

A mechanistic approach is useful when formulating the initial treatment plan, as suggested in the example above.

Somatic pain is described as a constant, well-localized pain often characterized as aching, throbbing, sharp, or gnawing. It tends to be responsive to opioids and nonsteroidal anti-inflammatory drugs (NSAIDs—cyclooxygenase-2 inhibitors) and amenable to relief by interruption of proximal pathways via neural blockade when indicated.

Visceral pain originates from injury to organs. This pain is transmitted by fibers that travel along the sympathetic nervous system.[31] Visceral pain is characteristically vague in distribution and quality and is often described as a deep, dull, aching, dragging, squeezing, or pressure-like sensation. When acute, it may be paroxysmal and colicky and can be associated with nausea, vomiting, diaphoresis, and alterations in blood pressure and heart rate. Mechanisms of visceral pain include abnormal distention or contraction of smooth muscle walls (hollow viscera), rapid capsular stretch (solid viscera), ischemia of visceral muscle, serosal or mucosal irritation by algesic substances and other chemical stimuli, distention and traction or torsion on mesenteric attachments and the vasculature, and necrosis.[32] The viscera, however, are insensitive to simple manipulation, cutting, and burning.[31] Visceral involvement often produces referred pain[33,34] (e.g., shoulder pain of hepatic origin).

Neuropathic pain is defined as pain caused by injury or irritation to some element or elements of the nervous system. Examples of neuropathic pain syndromes include tumor growth around nerve structures; postsurgical pain syndromes such as post-thoracotomy, post-mastectomy, post–radical neck dissection, and post-hepatectomy pain; or pain induced by chemotherapeutic agents affecting peripheral nerve structures. Chemotherapeutic agents associated with this problem include vinca alkaloids (vincristine, vinblastine), cisplatin, paclitaxel (Taxol), docetaxel (Taxotere), vinorelbine (Navelbine), and bortezomib (Velcade). Neuropathic pain is often resistant to standard analgesic therapies and frequently requires an approach using combinations of opioids, tricyclic antidepressants, anticonvulsants, oral or topical local anesthetics, corticosteroids, *N*-methyl-D-aspartate (NMDA) blockers, and others.

TEMPORAL ASPECTS OF PAIN

CONSTANT PAIN

Such pain is most amenable to drug therapy administered around the clock, contingent on time rather than symptoms. It is best managed by long-acting analgesics or, in selected cases, infusion of analgesics.

BREAKTHROUGH PAIN AND INCIDENT PAIN

Breakthrough pain that is related to a specific activity, such as eating, defecation, socializing, or walking, is referred to as incident pain. Incident pain is best managed by supplementing the preventive around-the-clock regimen with analgesics that have a rapid onset of action and a short duration. Once a pattern of incident pain is established, escape or rescue doses of analgesics can be administered in anticipation of the pain-provoking activity. Breakthrough pain that occurs consistently before the next scheduled dose of around-the-clock opioids is called end-of-dose failure (plasma concentrations fall below minimum effective analgesic concentrations) and is ideally managed by reducing the intervals between doses. In contrast, increasing the doses of long-acting opioids under these circumstances may increase the incidence of side effects. Under a strict definition, breakthrough pain is pain that may occur at any time during the day; it increases to a high intensity very rapidly and has duration of 30 to 45 minutes. Consequently, it is important to recognize the differences among these three types of breakthrough pain to implement adequate therapy.

INTERMITTENT PAIN

This type of pain is very unpredictable and can best be managed by the administration of potent analgesics with a rapid onset and short duration as needed.

SPECIFIC CANCER PAIN SYNDROMES

METASTASES

Bone tumor infiltration or bone metastasis is cited as the most common cause of cancer pain[35] and is most often seen with stage IV carcinoma of the prostate, breast, thyroid, lung, or kidney.[35,36] The pain is usually constant, dull, achy or deep, and often intense with movement or weight bearing. Approximately 25% of patients with bone metastases experience pain. Pressure and chemical irritation of nerve endings in the periosteum may cause pain.[37,38] It is noteworthy that greater than 50% decalcification must occur before osseous lesions are visible on plain radiographs.[39] Thus, a bone scan (isotope scanning, scintigraphy) is preferred for detecting most bone metastases.[35] Nonetheless, with primary bone tumors, thyroid cancer, and multiple myeloma, plain films are considered to be more sensitive.[40] Neoplastic changes must be differentiated from changes related to infection, trauma, or degeneration because treatment differs, even in patients with cancer.

Prostaglandin E_2 (PGE_2) and other cytokines are elaborated by osseous metastases. These cytokines are thought to contribute to pain by sensitization of peripheral nociceptors. NSAIDs and steroids are postulated to reduce pain from bony metastases by inhibition of the cyclooxygenase pathway of arachidonic acid breakdown, thus decreasing the formation of PGE_2. As deposits enlarge, stretching of the periosteum, pathologic fractures, and perineural invasion contribute to the pain, and requirements for analgesics increase. Palliative radiation therapy is used successfully to relieve pain emanating from bony metastases. However, pain relief may not be seen in 100% of cases. Thus, other forms of therapy may need to be implemented.

Vertebral body metastases are associated with carcinoma of the lung, breast, and prostate. Localized paraspinal, radicular, or referred pain within the dermatomal distribution of the affected nerve structure is usually the first sign of metastasis to the spine. It is often manifested as severe local, dull, steady, aching pain and is frequently exacerbated by movement and weight bearing. On physical evaluation, local midline tenderness may be present, as well as corresponding neurologic changes associated with either nerve compression or epidural–spinal cord compression. Invasion of the second cervical vertebra may result in pain referred to the occiput, and C7-T1 invasion may produce interscapular pain.[41]

BASE OF SKULL METASTASIS

Metastasis to the base of the skull is usually accompanied by headache and a spectrum of neurologic findings, especially when the cranial nerves are involved. Symptomatic metastasis to the skull is usually, but not always, a late finding.[42] Plain radiography, scintigraphy, and computed tomography (CT) are helpful for the diagnosis of bony disease, whereas MRI and lumbar puncture are useful in evaluating soft tissues and detecting leptomeningeal disease, respectively.[43]

Musculoskeletal pain in the form of myofascial pain is frequently seen in cancer patients.[44] Patients with bone metastases and those with post–radical neck dissection syndrome are frequently affected by this condition. Stress, anxiety, muscle overuse to compensate for the lack of bone support, or the absence of other muscles resected during cancer surgery may play an important role in the development of this condition. Thus, treatment should be multidisciplinary and include pharmacologic therapy, trigger point injections, and physical rehabilitation with the use of orthotic devices as needed.

LEPTOMENINGEAL METASTASIS, MENINGEAL CARCINOMATOSIS

These conditions are frequently seen with primary malignancies of the breast and lung and with lymphoma and leukemia; it is secondary to diffuse infiltration of the meninges. About 40% of patients have headache or back pain, presumably caused by traction on the pain-sensitive meninges or traction on cranial or spinal nerves or secondary to raised intracranial pressure.[45,46] Headache is the most common initial complaint; it is characteristically unrelenting and may be associated with nausea, vomiting, nuchal rigidity, and changes in mental status.[46] Neurologic abnormalities may include seizures, cranial nerve deficits, papilledema, hemiparesis, ataxia, and cauda equina syndrome. The diagnosis may be suggested by the T2 phase of MRI, and it is usually confirmed via lumbar puncture and cerebrospinal fluid (CSF) analysis, which typically shows elevated protein and decreased glucose, as well as malignant cells.[47] The natural history of patients with leptomeningeal metastasis is a gradual decline and death over a period of 4 to 6 weeks, although survival is often extended to 6 months or more when radiation therapy or intrathecal chemotherapy (or both) is instituted.[48] Steroids may be useful in the management of headache,[43] as well as the neuropathic pain associated with spinal cord and nerve involvement.

SPINAL CORD COMPRESSION AND PLEXOPATHIES

Spinal cord compression is usually heralded by pain in the presence of neurologic changes. An urgent radiologic workup is mandatory in patients with neurologic deficits, particularly motor weakness, bandlike encircling pain, or incontinence. Prompt treatment in the form of radiotherapy or spinal stabilization and high-dose IV steroids may limit the neurologic morbidity.[49]

Plexopathies are the result of tumor growth around nerve plexuses in the upper or lower extremity. Cervical plexopathy is most commonly due to local invasion by head and neck cancer. Symptoms include aching preauricular, postauricular, or neck pain. Brachial plexopathy is most commonly caused by upper lobe lung cancer (Pancoast syndrome or superior sulcus syndrome), breast cancer, or lymphoma. Pain is an early symptom that usually precedes the neurologic findings by up to 9 months.[50,51] The lower cord of the plexus (C8-T1) is affected most frequently, and pain is usually diffuse and aching and radiates down the arm, often to the elbow and medial (ulnar) aspect of the hand.[52,53] When the upper part of the trunk is involved (C5-6), pain is generally found in the shoulder girdle and upper portion of the arm and radiates to the thumb and index finger. Horner's syndrome, dysesthesias, progressive atrophy, and neurologic impairment (weakness and numbness) may occur. Brachial plexus invasion may be associated with contiguous spread to the epidural space.[49,54-56] Lumbosacral plexopathy may be due to local soft tissue invasion or compression from tumors of the rectum, cervix, or breast, sarcoma, and lymphoma; pain is usually the initial symptom in 70% of such patients.[57] The pain is usually described as aching or pressure-like and only rarely is dysesthetic.[57] Depending on the level involved, pain is referred to the low back region, abdomen, buttock, or lower extremity.[57,58] This medical problem must be differentiated from spinal cord invasion or cauda equina syndrome, for which urgent diagnosis and treatment are mandatory. Clinical experience shows that brachial plexopathies respond better to medical therapy with opioids, tricyclic antidepressants, and anticonvulsants, whereas lumbosacral plexopathies may require early intervention with intrathecal opioid, bupivacaine, and clonidine therapy.

PAIN ASSOCIATED WITH CANCER TREATMENT

Oral mucositis typically occurs within 1 to 2 weeks of the initiation of chemotherapy. This condition is most common with the use of methotrexate, doxorubicin, daunorubicin, bleomycin, etoposide, 5-fluorouracil, and dactinomycin.[59] Mucositis is often most severe when chemotherapy is combined with radiation treatments involving the head and neck region. Treatment may require hospitalization for IV PCA opioid therapy. Ambulatory care may necessitate transdermal opioids, local anesthetics, or doxepin swishes.

Painful polyneuropathy occurs most commonly with vincristine (motor and sensory involvement), vinblastine, paclitaxel, docetaxel, a platinum derivative (predominantly sensory involvement), vinorelbine, and bortezomib.[60] Symptoms commonly include burning dysesthetic pain in the hands and feet. The majority of these patients will respond to medical therapy with opioids, tricyclic antidepressants, and anticonvulsants. However, the small number of patients who do not achieve adequate pain control with this strategy will usually show a significant response to the use of spinal cord stimulation.

Postsurgical chronic pain syndromes are most common after mastectomy, thoracotomy, radical neck dissection, nephrectomy, and amputation.[61] The clinical characteristics generally include aching, shooting, or tingling pain in the distribution of peripheral nerves (e.g., intercostobrachial, intercostals, cervical plexus), with or without skin hypersensitivity. One study suggested that the incidence of post-mastectomy pain was higher after conservative surgery than after modified radical mastectomy (33% vs. 17%).[62] In this same study, 25% of patients experienced postoperative phantom breast pain. The exact incidence of postsurgical pain syndromes is unclear but appears to be in the 25% to 50% range by some estimates.[61] Medical therapy with opioids, tricyclic antidepressants, and anticonvulsants is successful in the great majority of patients. Those who fail pharmacologic therapy will benefit from intrathecal therapy (post-thoracotomy, post-mastectomy syndromes), spinal cord stimulation (post-thoracotomy, post-mastectomy syndromes), or even peripheral subcutaneous nerve stimulation (post–radical neck dissection, post-thoracotomy syndromes).

Headache is present in 60% of patients with a primary or metastatic brain tumor, half of whom classify it as their primary complaint.[63] It is typically steady, deep, dull, and aching with moderate intensity and is rarely rhythmic or throbbing. It is usually intermittent and may be worse in the morning and with coughing or straining. Symptoms often improve with radiation therapy, NSAIDs, or corticosteroids.[64-66]

Cervicofacial pain syndromes are most common in patients with head and neck cancer. The head and neck are richly innervated by contributions from cranial nerves V, VII, IX, and X and the upper cervical nerves, so the pain varies in character. When cranial nerves are involved, the symptoms represent those of trigeminal, glossopharyngeal, or intermittent neuralgia, with sudden, severe lancinating pain radiating to the face, throat, or ear, respectively. The pain may be accompanied by dysesthesias, trigger points, and impaired swallowing, breathing, and phonation. Pharmacologic therapy with opioids, tricyclic antidepressants, and anticonvulsants is useful in the great majority of these patients. In those whom pharmacologic therapy fails, radiofrequency lesioning of the sphenopalatine or gasserian ganglion may be useful.

Radiation therapy may be associated with both acute and chronic pain syndromes. Acutely, mucositis and cutaneous burns may be seen. Chronically, postradiation syndromes include osteoradionecrosis, myelopathy, plexopathy, soft tissue fibrosis, and the emergence of new secondary neurogenic tumors.

TREATMENT

The goal of treatment of cancer pain is to relieve the pain by modifying its source, interrupting its transmission, or modulating its influence at brain or spinal cord sites. This can be achieved with single therapy or combinations of the following available modalities:

A. Antineoplastic treatment
B. Pharmacologic management
   1. NSAIDs
   2. Opioids
   3. Adjuvant analgesics
      a. Antidepressants
      b. Anticonvulsants
      c. Oral local anesthetics
      d. Corticosteroids
      e. NMDA antagonists
      f. α_2-adrenergic antagonists
      g. Topical analgesics
   4. Interventional pain management
      a. Continuous parenteral infusion of opioids
      b. Neuraxial analgesia—epidural or intrathecal infusions
      c. Vertebroplasty or kyphoplasty
      d. Nerve blocks: local anesthetic nerve blocks and neurolytic nerve blocks
      e. Spinal cord stimulation, peripheral nerve stimulation, or peripheral subcutaneous nerve stimulation
   5. Behavioral pain management
   6. Other interventions such as aromatherapy, relaxation, and herbal medications
   7. Home-based and hospice care

ANTINEOPLASTIC TREATMENT

The most effective form of treatment of any cancer-related pain is treatment of the cancer itself, which in the majority of cases will reduce or eliminate the pain. Once diagnosed, the pathologic process responsible for pain can often be altered by surgical resection, external beam radiation therapy (targeted fractioned or single-dose therapy, hemibody or total-body irradiation),[67,68] radionuclide (e.g., strontium 89, samarium) chemotherapy,[69] hormonal treatment,[70] and even whole-body or limb hyperthermia.[71] The majority of patients require some form of primary analgesic therapy even when pursuing antitumor therapy.

PHARMACOLOGIC MANAGEMENT

Control of pain involves three basic principles: modifying the source of the pain, altering the central perception of pain, and blocking transmission of the pain to the central nervous system. In addition, any new pain in a patient with cancer is assumed to be progression or recurrence of disease until proved otherwise.

Oral analgesics are the mainstay of therapy for patients with cancer pain. An estimated 70% to 95% of patients can be rendered relatively free of pain when straightforward guideline-based principles are applied in a thorough, careful manner.[1,2,72]

The World Health Organization has developed a three-step ladder approach to the management of cancer pain that relies exclusively on the administration of oral agents and is usually effective.[18,72,73] However, this approach lacks the mechanistic approach that may be more effective in decreasing the side effects of drugs that may not necessarily be effective against some types of pain, such as anticonvulsants as first-line agents for neuropathic pain syndromes. When more conservative therapies produce inadequate results, escalating doses or alternative therapies should be sought. The role of more invasive forms of analgesia, ranging from parenteral analgesics to neural blockade or neuromodulation, should be considered judiciously.

Before initiation of therapy, assessment of problems and setting realistic goals that are acceptable to the patient should be established along with a treatment plan and contingencies.

The noninvasive route should be maintained as long as possible for reasons that include simplicity, maintenance of independence and mobility, convenience, and cost. Treatment should be directed toward relief of pain and suffering, which includes consideration of all aspects of function (e.g., disturbances in sleep, appetite, mood, activity, posture, and sexuality), and attention should be paid not only to the physical but also to the emotional, psychological, and spiritual aspects of suffering.

For a specific description of the different agents that may be used for pharmacologic noninvasive therapy, please refer to Chapters 36 to 42.

INTERVENTIONAL PAIN MANAGEMENT

When a comprehensive trial of pharmacologic therapy fails to provide adequate analgesia or leads to unacceptable side effects, consideration should be given to alternative treatments.

CONTINUOUS SUBCUTANEOUS INFUSION OF OPIOIDS

This modality was frequently used in the past and proved to be effective.[74,75] However, the advent of IV PCA therapy and long-term IV lines such as peripherally inserted indwelling central catheter (PIC) lines have made it somehow obsolete in this population of patients.

INTRAVENOUS INFUSION OF OPIOIDS WITH PATIENT-CONTROLLED ANALGESIA DEVICES

The most frequent indication for this form of therapy is severe pain and the need to rapidly titrate opioids in the hospital setting to achieve adequate pain control. Moreover, in the ambulatory setting, this modality is indicated for patients in whom the oral route is not available because of gastrointestinal obstruction, malabsorption, uncontrolled nausea and vomiting, or dysphagia or when the requirement for opioids is large because of tolerance. Some modifications in the implementation of this therapy have been used once the patient is no longer able to control the device. Thus, nurse- or family-controlled analgesia is an acceptable alternative in these circumstances. Consequently, patients will need to be treated in a controlled environment such as hospice or at home with the help and monitoring of family members. In such circumstances visiting nursing services will be required.

INTRASPINAL ANALGESIA

Neuraxial analgesia is achieved by the epidural or intrathecal administration of an opioid alone (very rarely) or in combination with other agents such as bupivacaine, clonidine, or ziconotide. With the use of neuraxial analgesia, pain relief is obtained in a highly selective fashion without motor, sensory, and sympathetic effects, thus making these modalities highly adaptable to the home care environment.[76-79] At its inception, the principle of neuraxial opioid therapy was that introducing minute quantities of opioids in close proximity to their receptors (substantia gelatinosa of the spinal cord) achieves high local concentrations.[80,81] Thus, neuraxial analgesia was potentially superior to that achieved when opioids were administered by other routes, and since the total amount of drug administered is reduced, side effects were minimized. Currently, the biggest advantage is the ability to use multiple agents to target neuropathic, somatic, and visceral components.

In general, patients with a survival expectancy of longer than 3 months will be candidates for intrathecal therapy with a permanent intraspinal catheter and an implanted subcutaneous pump. Conversely, patients with a survival expectancy of less than 3 months will require epidural therapy with an implanted system (the Du Pen epidural catheter or the Sims epidural Port-a-Cath) connected to an external pump with PCA capabilities. Either way, patients will need a trial with an epidural catheter placed at the site where nociception is being processed in the spinal cord. At Roswell Park Cancer Institute, we conduct this trial on an outpatient basis, and if successful, we proceed to implant the permanent device. For this purpose, we suggest the following protocol:

Epidural Trial

- Catheter position: dermatomal specific under fluoroscopic guidance
    1. Opioids:
        - Morphine: 0.1 (60 mg) to 0.2 (120 mg) mg/mL
        - Hydromorphone: 0.03 (20 mg) to 0.12 (80 mg) mg/mL
    2. Bupivacaine: 1 to 2 mg/mL
    3. Clonidine: 3 to 5 μg/mL
    4. Total volume: 600 mL
- Determining epidural opioid doses:
    1. If the patient is receiving more than 300 μg/hr of fentanyl, 1200 mg/day of morphine sulfate (MS), 600 mg/day of oxycodone, or 160 mg/day of methadone:
        - Hydromorphone: 0.12 mg/mL
    2. If the patient is receiving between 100 and 300 μg/hr of fentanyl or equivalent dose:
        - Hydromorphone: 0.06 mg/mL
    3. If the patient is receiving less than 100 μg/hr of fentanyl or equivalent dose:
        - Hydromorphone: 0.03 mg/mL
- Basal infusion: 2 mL/hr
- No bolus during the first 72 hours, then 2 mL every 10 minutes
- The goal is to determine patient requirements
- Trial for 7 days as an outpatient

If the patient had a successful trial, defined as a reduction in pain of greater than 80%, we proceed to implant an intrathecal system if indicated by the survival expectancy. We suggest the following protocol to achieve a success rate higher than 80%:

- Conditions for success:
    1. Place the tip of the intrathecal catheter in the dermatome corresponding to the area of nociception
    2. For severe somatic pain, combinations of local anesthetics and an opioid will be needed
    3. For neuropathic pain:
       Place the tip of the catheter below L3-4: initial therapy with an opioid and clonidine
       Place the tip of the catheter above L1-2: initial therapy with an opioid and bupivacaine

The doses and drugs that we use in our practice are as follows[82]:

Drug	Range of Doses
Morphine	1.0-20 mg/day
Hydromorphone	0.5-25 mg/day
Sufentanil	10-100 µg/day
Bupivacaine	6-20 mg/day
Clonidine	250-2000 µg/day

Thus, compounding by a trained pharmacist will be needed. The goal is to concentrate these drugs to twice the daily dose so that the pumps may be programmed to deliver 0.5 mL/hr. In this way, patients will need pump refills monthly, and it will not be a burden on their quality of life by having to come frequently to the pain specialist's office. The steps that we use to implement the therapy are as follows:

- Step 1:
  1. Opioid plus bupivacaine:
     - MS, 3 to 25 mg/day, or hydromorphone, 0.5 to 15 mg/day (25 mg of MS per day = 4 mg of hydromorphone per day)
     - Bupivacaine: 6 to 20 mg/day
  2. Opioid plus clonidine:
     - Clonidine: 250 to 2000 µg/day
- Step 2: Opioid plus bupivacaine plus clonidine
- Step 3: At this point, ziconotide
- If the patient's insurance does not pay for hydromorphone, bupivacaine, or clonidine, the use of morphine plus ziconotide may be an alternative. However, limitations include the following:
  1. Trials are unpredictable because ziconotide may not be administered in the epidural space. Consequently, the patient will need to undergo a trial once the implanted system is in place
  2. Patients may not allow you to carry out a titration protocol over a 4- to 6-week period:
     - The starting dose is 2.4 µg/day with weekly increases of no more than 2.4 µg/day
     - Therapeutic effects are not usually seen until a dose of 10 µg/day is reached
- Other issues to consider when initiating ziconotide include the following:
  3. Rinse the pump with 2 mL of the 25-µg/mL solution three times
  4. Start low and go slow:
     - Slower titration is tolerated better
     - Initiate therapy at a dose of 2.4 µg/day (0.1 µg/hr) and titrate to patient response
     - Titration increments should not be more than 2.4 µg/day and ideally should be implemented every week
     - Maximum recommended dose: 19.2 µg/day (0.8 µg/hr)

If triple therapy with an opioid, bupivacaine, and clonidine at optimal doses is not working, troubleshooting the system is a must. In doing so, consider the following:

- Pump: The computer program analysis for volume and the volume present within the pump need to be within 10% of each other; otherwise, pump or system failure (e.g., obstruction) should be suspected.
- Catheter: A myelogram will be needed to determine whether obstruction is present and the position of the tip of the catheter. When performing a myelogram through the diagnostic port of the pump, remember that this port accommodates only a 25-gauge Huber needle. Moreover, consider the following:
  1. The dead space of the catheter when injecting contrast medium
  2. The need for a bolus dose after the study is completed

In a recently published multicenter prospective randomized clinical trial by Staats and coauthors in which intrathecal therapy was compared with continued medical management, a slight trend toward better analgesia was noted in the intrathecal group (not statistically significant), but an improved side effect profile and increased survival were seen in the intrathecal group.[83] There is also a report from the MD Anderson group in abstract form in which significant improvement in pain scores (NRS score of 7.6 to 4.8) and oral intake (morphine equivalent drug dose [MEDD] of 300 vs. 80) was documented following intrathecal opioid pump implantation.[84]

The cost of implementing intrathecal therapy is initially high because of equipment acquisition cost. In contrast, the cost of implementing long-term epidural therapy is low. Two studies evaluated the cost of implementing therapy with these two modalities. These analyses show a "break-even" point at approximately 3 months.[85,86] Thus, epidural therapy becomes very expensive after 3 months, which is one of the reasons to limit its use in patients with survival expectations of less than 3 months.

A consensus panel published current practice data on intrathecal medication management. A survey of 413 physicians managing 13,342 patients showed a variety of medications being used in the intrathecal pump, including morphine (48%); morphine and bupivacaine (12%); hydromorphone (8%); morphine and clonidine (8%); hydromorphone and clonidine (8%); morphine, clonidine, and bupivacaine (5%); morphine and baclofen (3%); and others (<3%). Other drugs mentioned included fentanyl, sufentanil, ziconotide, meperidine, methadone, ropivacaine, tetracaine, ketamine, midazolam, neostigmine, droperidol, and naloxone.[87]

NERVE BLOCKS

LOCAL ANESTHETIC NERVE BLOCKS

Local anesthetic injections can be implemented for diagnostic or therapeutic purposes, or for both.[88-97]

Diagnostic blocks help characterize the underlying mechanism of pain (nociceptive, neuropathic, sympathetically mediated) and discern the anatomic pathways involved in pain transmission. Their main indication is as a preliminary intervention conducted before a therapeutic nerve block or other definitive therapy. This helps the clinician determine the potential for subsequent neurolysis if indicated. Although the results often have good predictive value, they are not entirely reliable.

Therapeutic injections of local anesthetics, with or without a corticosteroid, into trigger points may provide lasting relief of myofascial pain.[92]

Epidural steroid–local anesthetic injections are unlikely to provide long-lasting relief for neuropathic pain of neoplastic origin. However, they will produce significant analgesia in patients who may not tolerate rapid titration of antineuropathic medications.

Local anesthetic injections administered into sympathetic ganglia may contribute to lasting pain relief in patients with complex regional pain syndrome (CRPS) type 2, a condition frequently seen in cancer patients.[93-95] This syndrome may arise as a result of tumor invading into nervous system structures (e.g., brachial or lumbosacral plexopathy), postsurgical pain syndromes, or chemotherapy-induced peripheral neuropathy. Local anesthetic blockade of the stellate ganglion or lumbar sympathetic chain has been used with some success to temporarily relieve pain in these patients.

NEUROLYTIC BLOCKS

Neurolytic blocks have played an important role in the management of intractable cancer pain. This modality should be offered when pain persists despite the implementation of aggressive comprehensive medical management or when drug therapy produces unwanted and uncontrollable side effects. Patient selection is essential, and some of the important variables to consider include (1) the severity of the pain, (2) pain that is expected to persist despite chemotherapy or radiotherapy, (3) pain that cannot be modified by less invasive or risky means, (4) a clinical picture that the pain is somatic or visceral in origin, and (5) a short life expectancy.

Alcohol and phenol are the two agents commonly used to produce chemical neurolysis. Ethyl alcohol is a pungent, colorless solution that readily can be injected through small-bore needles and is hypobaric with respect to CSF. For peripheral and subarachnoid blocks, alcohol is generally used undiluted (referred to as 100% alcohol, dehydrated alcohol, or absolute alcohol), whereas a 50% solution is used for celiac plexus blocks. The alcohol should not be exposed to ambient room temperature for a long period because absorbed moisture dilutes it. Alcohol injection is typically followed by intense burning pain and occasionally erythema along the targeted nerve distribution.

Phenol is fairly unstable at room temperature. Its shelf half-life is about 1 year when refrigerated and kept away from light. Phenol can be used in 3% to 15% concentrations and with saline, water, and glycerol or radiologic contrast agents. It is relatively insoluble in water, and as a result, concentrations in excess of 6.7% will result in a suspension at room temperature without adding glycerin to increase its solubility in water. Phenol with glycerin is hyperbaric in CSF but is so dense that even when warmed, it is difficult to inject through needles smaller than 20 gauge. Phenol has a biphasic action: its initial local anesthetic action produces subjective warmth and numbness, which usually gives way to chronic denervation over a day's time. The hypoalgesia after phenol is not as dense as after alcohol, and the quality and extent of analgesia may fade slightly within the first 24 hours of administration, particularly when used for epidural neurolysis.

The use of subarachnoid (intrathecal) injections of alcohol or phenol for the management of intractable cancer pain has significantly decreased in the United States since polypharmacy intrathecal analgesia was implemented. Because alcohol and phenol destroy nervous tissue indiscriminately, careful attention to selection of the injection site, volume and concentration of injectate, and selection and positioning of the patient are essential to avoid neurologic complications,[98,99] a risk that is responsible for the decrease in its use. Most authorities agree that neither alcohol nor phenol offers a clear advantage except to the extent that variations in baric properties may facilitate positioning of the patient.[100,101] With the exception of perineal pain treatment, alcohol is usually preferred for intrathecal neurolysis since most patients are unable to lie on their painful side, as required for intrathecal phenol neurolysis. In an analysis of 13 published series documenting treatment with intrathecal rhizolysis in more than 2500 patients, Swerdlow reported that 58% of the patients obtained "good" relief, "fair" relief was observed in an additional 21%, and in 20% of patients "little or no relief" was noted.[100] The average duration of relief is estimated to be 3 to 6 months, with a wide range of distribution. Reports of analgesia persisting 1 to 2 years are fairly common.[102] In representative series using alcohol ($n = 252$) and phenol ($n = 151$), a total of 407 and 313 blocks were performed, respectively.[103,104] In these two series, neither motor weakness nor fecal incontinence occurred, and of eight patients with transient urinary dysfunction, incontinence persisted in just one.

Subarachnoid neurolysis can be performed at any level up to the midcervical region, above which the risk for spread of drug to the medullary centers and the potential for cardiorespiratory collapse increase.[105] A hyperbaric phenol saddle block is relatively simple to perform and is particularly suitable for many patients with a colostomy and urinary diversion.

Until recently, epidural neurolysis was performed infrequently. The results were inferior to those obtained with subarachnoid blockade, presumably because the dura acts as a barrier to diffusion, thereby resulting in limited contact between the drug and targeted nerves.[102,106]

PERIPHERAL AND CRANIAL NERVE BLOCKS

Peripheral nerve blockade has a limited role in the management of cancer pain.[97] Blockade of the ganglion of Gasser, within the foramen ovale at the base of skull or its branches, may be beneficial for facial pain.[107] However, the indications in patients with tumor-related pain are truly minimal because a neuropathic pain component is usually present. Thus, the risk for deafferentation pain is significantly increased with chemical neurolysis. Again, the use of intraspinal therapy by means of an implanted cervical epidural catheter or intraventricular opioid therapy has become a better option for these patients.[108,109]

VERTEBROPLASTY

Many cancer patients with metastatic vertebral compression fractures (VCFs) or osteoporotic VCFs have movement-related back pain. Percutaneous vertebroplasty (PV) is a minimally invasive procedure that involves injection of bone cement (usually polymethylmethacrylate [PMMA]) into the fractured vertebral body to alleviate the pain and hopefully enhance structural stability. This procedure is performed by placing needles under biplanar fluoroscopic guidance via a unipedicular or bipedicular approach. PMMA mixed with sterile barium is injected in a careful, controlled manner to avoid unintended spread of cement into the spinal canal or into veins within the affected vertebra. Injection is stopped as soon as cement starts approaching the posterior third of the vertebral body. Four studies evaluated the efficacy of PV in patients with vertebral fractures. Two of them found no differences between the treatment and placebo groups.[110,111] The third study reported better pain relief on the first postoperative day, but no difference from placebo thereafter,[112] and the fourth study reported significant pain control at 1 week and 1 month, but *not* at 3, 6, and 12 months.[113] It therefore appears that PV is a questionable alternative for patients with vertebral fractures.

SPINAL CORD STIMULATION

This technique has been used successfully for refractory neuropathic chronic pain states in patients with chronic nononcologic pain. There is a lack of studies evaluating its use for cancer pain states. However, at Roswell Park Cancer Institute we have used it successfully in patients with CRPS type 2, such as those with postsurgical pain syndromes, chemotherapy-induced peripheral neuropathy, and postradiation nerve injury. Patient selection is very important in the cancer population because MRI at this point is contraindicated after this device is placed and medical oncologists rely on this study to monitor the progress of disease in these patients.

NEUROSURGICAL PALLIATIVE TECHNIQUES

Neurosurgical palliative techniques have fallen into less favor as more medications and reversible, titratable, lower-risk techniques have largely replaced these procedures. Pituitary ablation entails destruction of the gland by injecting a small quantity of alcohol through a needle positioned transnasally under light general anesthesia. This technique is effective in relieving pain originating from disseminated bony metastases, particularly those secondary to hormone-dependent tumors (breast and prostate). Commissural myelotomy has been reported to be efficacious in relieving cancer pain refractory to more conservative therapy.[114] Percutaneous cordotomy produces a thermal lesion within the substance of the spinal cord and reliably relieves unilateral truncal and lower limb pain.[115,116] As with pituitary ablation, a high degree of skill and expertise is necessary, but the pain relief is often profound and the rigors of a major neurosurgical procedure are avoided.

BEHAVIORAL INTERVENTIONS

Several behavioral pain management techniques have been used in patients with cancer, including hypnosis, relaxation, biofeedback, sensory alteration, guided imagery, and cognitive strategies.[117] Relaxation and imagery training significantly reduce VAS scores in patients in whom mucositis develops after bone marrow transplantation.[118] This training is probably most effective for patients who have no significant psychological or psychiatric problems[117] and for insightful psychology-minded patients.

HOME-BASED AND HOSPICE CARE

For years, hospice has been regarded as a place where people go to die, but in its purest form, it is a philosophy of care that is "a blend of clinical pharmacology and applied compassionate psychologic care."[119-121] In the United States, hospice care has been developed primarily as a home-based service, with a minority of institutions offering short inpatient stays to stabilize refractory symptoms and provide respite for overwhelmed families.

The principles of home-based pain management are in most respects similar to those that apply to ambulatory and inpatient pain management. Differences generally relate to the recognition that further curative therapy is futile rather than that care is being provided at home. No compromise in quality of care based on where it is delivered is justified.

Hospice care is comfort oriented and focuses specifically on alleviating symptoms rather than necessarily treating their underlying cause. Factors that influence the selection of home treatment are advanced incurable disease, realization and acceptance of the appropriateness of palliative care (care directed at preserving comfort and quality of life rather than curing the tumor and extending life), and a desire to die in familiar surroundings. Many difficulties associated with providing intensive palliative care at home can be reconciled by education and orientation of the family, and such care can be performed in coordination with health care institutions, home care nursing, and laboratory and pharmacy services.

SUMMARY

Acute and chronic pain is highly prevalent in cancer patients. Inadequate assessment and treatment of pain and other distressing symptoms may interfere with antitumor therapy and markedly detract from quality of life. Even though a strong focus on control of pain is important independent of disease stage, it is a special priority in patients with advanced disease who are no longer candidates for potentially curative therapy.

Though rarely eliminated, pain can be controlled in the vast majority of patients with the implementation of an aggressive comprehensive medical management strategy. In the small but significant proportion of patients whose pain is not readily controlled with noninvasive analgesics, a variety of alternative invasive and noninvasive measures, when selected carefully, are also associated with a high degree of success. To this end, it is very reassuring to conclude that at this point we have the appropriate tools to adequately treat cancer-related pain in close to 100% of patients.

KEY POINTS

- Uncontrolled acute or chronic pain still affects 40% to 45% of patients afflicted with cancer. Despite the availability of a multitude of simple cost-effective pain treatments, inadequately controlled pain remains a significant problem in cancer patients.
- Cancer-related pain is mostly due to invasion of organic structures by the tumor (directly or by metastasis), is related to cancer treatment (surgery, chemotherapy, radiation therapy), or in a small minority, is due to chronic pain syndromes.
- Various standardized questionnaires can be used in pain clinics to assess pain intensity. Furthermore, a comprehensive patient assessment can be done by performing a thorough history and complete physical examination, along with subsequent analysis of diagnostic studies, which will lead to an appropriate diagnosis in virtually all patients.

KEY POINTS—cont'd

- Cancer pain can be classified on the basis of various pain parameters, such as time, intensity, pathophysiology of the pain, and temporal aspect of the pain or by the evolution of various cancer pain syndromes.
- Cancer pain can be adequately controlled in the majority of patients (≈95%) with aggressive pharmacologic treatment, with only a minority requiring invasive therapy. Treatment of cancer pain should be directed toward relief of pain and suffering and improvement in function and the psychological aspects of cancer diagnosis and pain.
- Oral and transdermal opioid analgesics are the mainstay of therapy for pain in cancer patients. Other adjuvant analgesics can be added to oral opioids for adequate control of pain if neuropathic pain is present. When oral pharmacotherapy fails, alternative modalities can be considered, including subcutaneous opioid infusion, intravenous patient-controlled analgesia with opioids, neuraxial opioids, and invasive procedures such as intrathecal pump implantation, peripheral nerve radiofrequency lesions, and neurolytic procedures.
- Patients with a survival expectancy of longer than 3 months are generally considered candidates for intrathecal therapy with a permanent intraspinal catheter and an implanted subcutaneous pump. Patients with a survival expectancy of less than 3 months will require epidural therapy with an implanted system. Before either neuraxial procedure, an epidural catheter trial is conducted to assess the need for implantation of the permanent device.
- Behavioral therapy has an important role in the treatment of pain. In patients with advanced or incurable disease, palliative therapy for control of pain and preservation of quality of life with home-based and hospice care can be undertaken.
- Overall, with judicious use of the various modalities available, including noninvasive oral and intravenous pharmacologic therapy combined with invasive therapy when needed, control of cancer pain is possible in the vast majority of patients.

SUGGESTED READINGS

Bedder MD, Burchiel KJ, Larson A. Cost analysis of two implantable narcotic delivery systems. *J Pain Symptom Manage.* 1991;6:368.

Buchbinder R, Osborne RH, Ebeling PR, et al. A randomized trial of vertebroplasty for painful osteoporotic vertebral fractures. *N Engl J Med.* 2009;361:557-568.

Cervero F. Visceral pain. In: Dubner R, Gebhart GF, Bond MR, eds. *Proceedings of the VI World Congress on Pain.* Amsterdam: Elsevier; 1988:216.

Ferrell BR, Wisdon C, Wenzl C. Quality of life as an outcome variable in management of cancer pain. *Cancer.* 1989;63:2321.

Kallmes DF, Comstock BA, Heagerthy PJ, et al. A randomized trial of vertebroplasty for osteoporotic spinal fractures. *N Engl J Med.* 2009;361:569-579.

Klazen CAH, Lohle PNM, de Vries J, et al. Vertebroplasty versus conservative treatment in acute osteoporotic vertebral compression fractures (Vertos II): an open-label randomized trial. *Lancet.* 2010;376:1085-1092.

Perkins FM, Kehlet H. Chronic pain syndromes after surgery: a review of predictive factors. *Anesthesiology.* 2000;93:1123-1133.

Portenoy RK. Cancer pain: epidemiology and syndromes. *Cancer.* 1989;63:2307.

Ropusing R, Hansen KL, Andersen MO, et al. Twelve-month follow-up in forty-nine patients with acute-semiacute osteoporotic vertebral fractures treated conservatively or with percutaneous vertebroplasty. *Spine.* 2010;35:478-482.

Staats P, Smith TJ, Deer T, et al. Randomized comparison of intrathecal drug delivery system (IDDS) + comprehensive medical management (CMM) vs. CMM alone for unrelieved cancer pain. *J Clin Oncol.* 2002;20:4040-4049.

24 Neuropathic Pain Syndromes

Robert W. Hurley | Omar H. Henriquez | Christopher L. Wu

INTRODUCTION

Neuropathic pain comprises a wide range of heterogeneous conditions. Various types of neuropathic pain may have distinct pathophysiologic causes and different clinical signs and symptoms. Despite the diversity of conditions classified as "neuropathic pain," many potentially share common underlying mechanisms of nociception, including neuronal hyperexcitability, but others may not. This may in part explain why certain analgesic agents are relatively effective for a wide range of neuropathic pain states but why notable exceptions exist that appear to be resistant to conventional "neuropathic" pain therapy. A group has been assembled to address the inconclusive research on "neuropathic" pain and to operationalize and specify definitions and criteria for conditions that are to be referred to as neuropathic pain (Box 24.1).[1] This work should lead to a more reductionist approach to the study of neuropathic pain and to effective therapies for specific disease processes.

In this chapter we focus on some of the more common states of "neuropathic" pain as defined by the sensitive but nonspecific definition of the International Association for the Study of Pain (IASP). These conditions include complex regional pain syndrome (CRPS), post-herpetic neuralgia (PHN), painful diabetic peripheral neuropathy (DPN), and human immunodeficiency virus (HIV) painful sensory neuropathy.

COMPLEX REGIONAL PAIN SYNDROME

The term *complex regional pain syndrome,* which denotes both types 1 and 2, originated from a history of different names appointed by individuals who made particular observations.

Box 24.1 Updated Definition of Neuropathic Pain

IASP Definition: 1994[2]

"pain initiated or caused by a primary lesion or dysfunction in the nervous system"

Revised Research and Clinical Definition: 2007[1]

"pain arising as a direct consequence of a lesion or disease affecting the somatosensory system"

IASP, International Association for the Study of Pain.

In 1864 Silas Weir Mitchell made an important observation of Civil War soldiers when he noticed that they suffered from burning pain and muscle atrophy at the sites of their injuries. He called this "causalgia," which is derived from the Greek words *kausis* (burning) and *algos* (pain). In 1900 at a lecture in Germany, Paul Sudeck stated that this syndrome could not only extend from the initial insult but also had an inflammatory component. The name Sudeck's dystrophy was applied in his honor. Half a century passed before the discovery that invasive procedures that block the sympathetic nervous system provide further relief of pain symptoms. Because of the success of these methods, Evans renamed the syndrome "reflex sympathetic dystrophy." Over the years cases arose in which patients lacked a trophic component, sympathetic involvement was absent, or there was no evidence of reflex involvement. These exceptions led to a meeting in 1993 by the IASP at which the term "*complex regional pain syndrome*" was formulated and subsequently published the following year.[2] The most commonly used clinical diagnostic criteria for CRPS types 1 and 2 are low in specificity but high in sensitivity, which has led to overdiagnosis of the pain syndrome.[3] This in turn has made it difficult to obtain accurate epidemiologic data for CRPS or to perform rigorous studies of the pathologic state. In 2007, research criteria (also known as the Budapest criteria) were published that included objective signs of pathology characteristic of patients with CRPS[4] (Box 24.2). These criteria had good specificity and sensitivity. Although they were initially intended for research use, many physicians prefer them to the less stringent original criteria.

PATHOPHYSIOLOGY

There are two types of CRPS, known as type 1 and type 2 (Box 24.3). They differ in that type 2 has evident nerve injury whereas type 1 assumes an injury to the nerve or nerves. A consistent finding in both types of CRPS is the discrepancy between the severity of the symptoms and the severity of the inciting injury. In addition, symptoms have the propensity to spread in the affected limb in a pattern not restricted to the specific nerve's area of innervation. CRPS is characterized by intense burning pain with resultant hyperalgesia or allodynia. It may be associated with local edema and autonomic involvement, such as changes in skin color and sweating and increased or decreased skin temperature in the affected area. There may also be trophic changes in the skin, hair, and nails in the affected site (see Box 24.3). Although many questions concerning the pathophysiology

Box 24.2 Difference between the IASP Criteria and the Budapest Criteria for the Diagnosis of CRPS

IASP Criteria for the Diagnosis of CRPS*

1. Presence of an initiating noxious event or reason for immobilization
2. Disproportional pain, allodynia, or hyperalgesia from a known inciting event
2. Sign or symptom of any evidence showing edema, skin changes, blood flow, or abnormal sudomotor activity in the region of the pain
4. No other condition that would otherwise explain the degree of pain or dysfunction

Budapest Criteria for Diagnosis of CRPS*

1. Presence of continued disproportional pain from the known inciting event
2. Must report at least one symptom in three of the following four categories:
   - Sensory: hyperesthesia, allodynia
   - Vasomotor: temperature asymmetry, changes in skin color
   - Sudomotor/edema: edema, changes in sweating, sweating asymmetry
   - Motor/trophic: decreased range of motion, motor dysfunction (tremor, weakness, dystonia), trophic changes (hair, nail, skin)
3. Must report at least one sign in two or more of the following categories at the time of evaluation:
   - Sensory: hyperalgesia to pinprick, allodynia to touch or joint movement
   - Vasomotor: temperature asymmetry, color asymmetry
   - Sudomotor/edema: edema, asymmetrical sweating, sweating changes
   - Motor/trophic: decreased range of motion, motor dysfunction, trophic changes
4. No other condition that would otherwise explain the degree of pain or dysfunction

*If seen without any major nerve damage, the diagnosis is CRPS type 1; if seen with evidence of nerve damage, the diagnosis is CRPS type 2.
CRPS, complex regional pain syndrome; IASP, International Association for the Study of Pain

Box 24.3 Difference between CRPS Type 1 and Type 2

CRPS Type 1 (Reflex Sympathetic Dystrophy)*

1. The presence of an initiating noxious event or a cause of immobilization
2. Continuing pain, allodynia, or hyperalgesia with which the pain is disproportionate to any inciting event
3. Evidence at some time of edema, changes in skin blood flow, or abnormal sudomotor activity in the region of the pain
4. This diagnosis is excluded by conditions that would otherwise account for the degree of pain and dysfunction

CRPS Type 2 (Causalgia)†

1. The presence of continuing pain, allodynia, or hyperalgesia after a nerve injury, not necessarily limited to the distribution of the injured nerve
2. Evidence at some time of edema, changes in skin blood flow, or abnormal sudomotor activity in the region of the pain
3. This diagnosis is excluded by the existence of conditions that would otherwise account for the degree of pain and dysfunction

*Criteria 2 to 4 must be satisfied.
†All three criteria must be satisfied.
CRPS, complex regional pain syndrome.

of this syndrome are still unanswered, three main principles remain at the core of CRPS: abnormalities in both somatosensory and sensory pathways as well as sympathetic nervous system involvement.

SOMATOSENSORY ABNORMALITIES

Inciting injury to either the upper or lower extremity is an important trigger of CRPS. Studies have shown that changes in cutaneous innervation of the injured extremities take place even when no nerve injury is found. In one recent study, skin biopsy samples were obtained from the affected limbs of patients with CRPS type 1. A lower density of C and A fibers was found in the affected limbs than in the unaffected limbs, which led to sensory deficits in the affected limbs.[5] Brain plasticity is another important factor found to be associated with somatosensory abnormalities. Data suggest that patients with CRPS have decreased activity in the somatosensory cortex of the affected side.[6] These patients also tend to have tactile mislocation because of somatotopic reorganization, which was found to be directly correlated with hyperalgesia.[7] Changes occurring within the primary somatosensory (SI) cortex are dependent on pain and have been shown to be reversible after recovery from the pain.[8]

SENSORY PATHWAYS (CENTRAL NERVOUS SYSTEM SENSITIZATION, PERIPHERAL SENSITIZATION, INFLAMMATION)

Central sensitization occurs when pain perception increases because of constant firing of painful stimuli to the central nervous system. Neuropeptides such as substance P and bradykinin are released in response to nociceptive stimuli and activate *N*-methyl-D-aspartate (NMDA) receptors, which together lead to hyperalgesia and allodynia.[9] Peripheral sensitization is the counterpart of central sensitization. When a nerve injury occurs, multiple proinflammatory factors such as glial cell activation, substance P, bradykinin, tumor necrosis factor-α, interleukin-1β, prostaglandin E_2, and nerve growth factor are activated, which results in increased nociceptive sensitivity and a decreased threshold for firing of nociceptive stimuli.[10] Together, central and peripheral sensitization results in the allodynia and hyperesthesia seen in patients with CRPS. There are other important factors in the inflammatory pathway, such as the role of nuclear factor NFκB upstream in the proinflammatory pathway observed in animal studies.[11]

ALTERED SYMPATHETIC NERVOUS SYSTEM FUNCTION

Involvement of the sympathetic nervous system is thought to be responsible for the limbs in patients with CRPS becoming cool, blue, and painful secondary to vasoconstriction as a result of excessive outflow from the sympathetic nervous system. In an animal study, rats with chronic postischemic pain that had norepinephrine injected into their hind paws experienced increased nociceptive firing, thus supporting the notion that pain can be sympathetically maintained.[12] However, this provides little evidence in support of sympathetic maintenance of CRPS pain. Coupling of sympathetic neurons may occur not only to nociceptive afferents but also to non-nociceptive mechanosensitive or cold-sensitive neurons. Sympathetic afferent coupling, considered the cause of sympathetically maintained pain, occurs in cutaneous and deep somatic tissues, but during the acute event of CRPS, the deep somatic tissues are of greater importance.[13] Although coupling occurs in some patients with CRPS, a subset of patients with clinically identical CRPS have sympathetically independent pain. These patients exhibit little to no response to sympathetic blockade either pharmacologically with phentolamine or via interventional blockade of the sympathetic ganglia.

EPIDEMIOLOGY

Multiple studies of CRPS type 1 have shown that the male-to-female ratio ranges between 1:2 and 1:4, thus suggesting that females are at higher risk for development of the syndrome.[14,15] However, the male-to-female ratio for most other pain syndromes is similar. A retrospective, cross-sectional analysis study showed that the male-to-female ratio was 1:4 and that the most common initiating events were bone fractures, sprains, and trauma.[15] Outcomes of the disease tended to be worse in patients with upper extremity injuries than in those with lower extremity injuries, injuries other than fractures, and "cold" (commonly chronic) CRPS rather than "warm" (acute) CRPS.[11] Other risk factors that contribute to the development of CRPS are age, workplace, and type of injury. The average age of patients ranges between 16 and 79 (median range, 41.6), with a higher incidence in the older population. Patients with motor nerve damage were found to be at higher risk for CRPS than those with sensory nerve damage. Fracture has been reported to be the most common initiating injury.[16] The incidence of job-related injuries leading to CRPS was as high as 76%,[17] which may indicate a psychosocial or secondary gain component in reporting of this pain. Studies report that CRPS develops in patients with a family history of CRPS at a higher incidence and younger age, thus suggesting that CRPS may have a genetic component.[18] Another study showed that siblings of patients in whom CRPS developed before 50 years of age had a threefold increased risk for development of the syndrome.[19] Psychological factors such as depression, personality disorders, and anxiety have no correlation with CRPS patients, which suggests that there is no specific type of CRPS personality.[20]

CLINICAL FEATURES

The pain must be greater in proportion to the inciting event. There must be at least one symptom in three of the following four categories: sensory (hyperesthesia/allodynia), vasomotor (changes in temperature or sweating in the affected limb in comparison to the normal limb), sudomotor/edema, and motor/trophic (demonstration of weakness, decreased range of motion, or trophic changes in hair, nails, or skin). At least one sign must be present at the time of evaluation in two or more of the following four categories: sensory, vasomotor, sudomotor/edema, and motor/trophic. There must be no other diagnosis that better explains the patient's signs and symptoms.[21] This is different from the criteria proposed in 1993 by the IASP (see Box 24.3). A recent study in which the validity of CRPS was evaluated by comparing the Budapest criteria in patients with CRPS and in those with neuropathy showed that the IASP criteria had a sensitivity of 1.0 and a specificity of 0.4 and the Budapest criteria had a clinical sensitivity of 0.99 and a specificity of 0.68.[22] The newly revised criteria are also divided into clinical and research. The research criteria contain more inclusions, which allows a specificity of 0.96.[23]

The current IASP taxonomy also divides CRPS into CRPS 1 (formerly known as reflex sympathetic dystrophy) and CRPS 2 (formerly known as causalgia).[24] The distinction between CRPS 1 and 2 is the presence of a definable nerve lesion in patients with CRPS 2.[25] The signs and symptoms for both conditions are clinically indistinguishable and include sensory changes (allodynia, hyperalgesia, and hypoalgesia), edema, temperature abnormalities, and changes in sweating (see Box 24.3). Pain is the principal feature in both CRPS 1 and CRPS 2. In patients with CRPS the associated clinical signs are typically out of proportion to the inciting injury. Patients describe a burning, deep-seated ache that may be shooting in nature along with associated allodynia or hyperalgesia.[26] Pain occurs in 81.1% of patients meeting the CRPS criteria.[3] Patients also frequently complain of sensory abnormalities such as hyperesthesia in response to the typical mechanical stimuli encountered in day-to-day activities (such as dressing) involving the affected limb.

In CRPS 2 (i.e., CRPS with associated major nerve injury), patients often report hyperesthesia around the injured nerve in addition to electric shock–like sensations, shooting pain, and allodynia. Symptoms indicative of vasomotor autonomic abnormalities (including color changes) occurred in 86.9% of patients; temperature instability occurred in 78.7%. Sudomotor symptoms of hyperhidrosis and hypohidrosis were reported in 52.9%. Trophic changes in skin, nail, or hair pattern were reported in 24.4%, 21.1%, and 18%, respectively. Edema was reported in 79.7%, with decreased range of motion in 80.3% and motor weakness in 74.6%.[3]

DIAGNOSIS

There is currently no "gold standard" test for the diagnosis of CRPS. A very thorough history and physical examination are essential for evaluation and diagnosis. Patients with this condition will have the signs and symptoms mentioned previously. Physical examination must be performed to establish the sensory, motor, trophic, sudomotor/edema, and autonomic changes. Sensory changes such as allodynia may be evaluated by light touch and the application of warm/cold temperature to the affected area. Autonomic dysfunction may be confirmed by the presence of asymmetry in temperature and color. Trophic changes may be manifested as changes in skin, nails, and hair in the affected limb. Motor activity may be evaluated by examining motor strength and range of motion. Sudomotor/edema changes may be assessed by dragging a smooth object over the affected and unaffected limb, with the wetter limb allowing a smoother drag than the drier limb.[25] Common diagnostic tools used for diagnosis of CRPS include quantitative sensory testing, tests of autonomic function, and imaging for trophic changes.

QUANTITATIVE SENSORY TESTING

Such testing includes the use of standardized psychophysical tests of the sensory and motor systems, thermal sensation, thermal pain, and vibratory thresholds to assess the function of large-fiber, myelinated small-fiber, and unmyelinated small-fiber afferents. Patients with CRPS may have impaired paradoxical heat sensations, mechanical detection thresholds, mechanical pain thresholds to pinprick stimuli and blunt pressure, allodynia, and pain summation with the use of continuous pinprick stimuli.[27] There is currently no definitive diagnostic sensory pattern in patients with CRPS, but this test can aid in distinguishing other neuropathies from CRPS.

TESTS OF AUTONOMIC FUNCTION

Thermoregulation and sudomotor regulation are the main systems tested in patients with CRPS for disorders in autonomic function. Thermoregulation is tested by using the thermoregulatory sweat test (TST) and infrared thermography or thermometry. The TST assesses calorimetric precipitation from a specific region of the body by adding a solution that changes color when enough heat is generated to produce sweat.[28] Infrared thermography is direct visualization of the change in temperature of the affected site, and in infrared thermometry, a device is used to measure temperature through detection of infrared energy. Changes in temperature in patients with CRPS versus those with other types of pain had a sensitivity of 76% and a specificity of 94%.[29] Sudomotor regulation is tested by using the quantitative sudomotor axon reflex test (QSART), which measures sweat output from various regions of the skin.[28]

TROPHIC CHANGES

Three-phase bone scintigraphy (TPBS) is a very valuable test for detection of CRPS. Although joint and bone alterations are not part of the IASP inclusion criteria, they are very important in the outcome of the syndrome.[13] TPBS detects alterations in periarticular bone metabolism, particularly increased bone metabolism, by detecting increase uptake of a periarticular tracer, which occurs predominantly within the first year. TPBS is low in sensitivity but high in specificity.[30] Magnetic resonance imaging of the affected limb has also been used for detection of CRPS but has high sensitivity (97%) and low specificity (17%).[31]

TREATMENT

Management of CRPS has been complicated by scant knowledge of the etiology of the disease, which has resulted in few targeted therapies. Most of the medications initiated as first-line therapy have been investigated for other non-CRPS neuropathic pain conditions and then applied to the treatment of CRPS, with mixed success. The historical approach to therapy for CRPS still remains a multimodal, multidisciplinary methodology. The predominant therapeutic modalities for the care of CRPS patients include physical therapy, pharmacologic agents, and interventional procedures.

PHYSICAL AND OCCUPATIONAL THERAPY

Physical and occupational therapy for restoration of function and improvement of limbs affected by CRPS has been studied widely. Physical exercises such as isometric strengthening, active range of motion, myofascial release, and stress loading are all tools that aid in restoring functional capacity of the affected limb.[32] Other methods of therapy are currently under study. In a large controlled study in which tactile acuity and pain on application of a tactile stimulus were measured in patients with CRPS and mirror images were used to show the reflection of the unaffected limb during the stimulus, a decreased two-point discrimination threshold and decreased pain acuity were observed.[33] This suggests that therapies that improve functional restoration of the affected limb may improve the outcome of CRPS.

PHARMACOLOGIC THERAPY

Membrane Stabilizers

Medications such as gabapentin and pregabalin have been shown to be effective in relieving neuropathic pain.[34,35] CRPS is considered neuropathic pain and gabapentin is presumed to be effective in treating it, yet there are very limited studies showing its specific efficacy for CRPS. In a randomized double-blind, placebo-controlled crossover study in which patients were treated for two 3-week periods with 2 weeks in between, gabapentin had minimal effect on pain but it significantly reduced patients' sensory deficits.[36] Although there is no clear evidence of efficacy for gabapentin, these neuroleptic medications are the first-line therapy for neuropathic pain and are thus considered first-line therapy for CRPS.

Corticosteroids

A large part of the pathophysiology in CRPS is the acute inflammatory process that occurs after an inciting event (see "Pathophysiology"). Because of this inflammatory course, corticosteroids have been used for treatment. In a recent randomized controlled trial comparing prednisolone with piroxicam, patients were given either medication for 1 month, and their shoulder-hand syndrome scores (measuring pain, distal edema, passive humeral abduction, and external rotation) were determined. In the prednisolone group, 83.3% showed improvement, and in the piroxicam group, only 16.7% improved. The shoulder-hand syndrome score in the steroid group was significantly lower than that in the piroxicam group.[37]

Antidepressants

These drugs have not been studied for use specifically with CRPS, but they have been widely studied for the control of neuropathic pain, and because CRPS is considered neuropathic pain, they are used in pain management.

Antidepressants such as tricyclic antidepressants (TCAs) and selective serotonin-norepinephrine reuptake inhibitors (SSNRIs) have been used to control neuropathic pain effectively. In a recent Cochrane review, TCAs were found to be effective in treating neuropathy, with a number needed to treat (NNT) of 3.6 and a relative risk (RR) of 2.1. Venlafaxine, an SSNRI, was also found to be effective, with an NNT of 3.1 and RR of 2.2.[38] Further studies to investigate the drugs' ability to specifically target CRPS are warranted. A recent study showed that the combination of gabapentin and nortriptyline was a more effective therapy than either medication alone for neuropathic pain (including CRPS).[39]

Opioids

Studies on the effects of opioids directly on CRPS are lacking, although some have shown opioids to improve neuropathic pain when used in high doses.[40] However, a double-blind, placebo-controlled trial studying the efficacy of sustained-release morphine in CRPS patients for a total treatment of 8 days showed that it was ineffective in decreasing pain, but the study had many limitations.[41] Substantial challenges to using opioid therapy for nonmalignant pain include nausea, constipation, cognitive impairment, tolerance, and hyperalgesia,[42] and therefore it should be used only until other therapies can be initiated. Studies of these medications in the CRPS population are lacking, and more are needed to demonstrate the efficacy of opioids.

Ketamine

Ketamine is an NMDA receptor antagonist. The NMDA receptor is a major part of the central sensitization that occurs in patients with CRPS (see "Pathophysiology"). Ketamine can be administered topically, orally, intranasally, or parentally in subanesthetic (analgesic) doses or in high doses to produce ketamine coma. A double-blind, randomized, placebo-controlled, parallel-group trial studying the effects of subanesthetic intravenous dosing of ketamine for 4 days in CRPS patients showed decreased levels of pain, but the pain progressively increased from the 1st week after infusion to the 12th week. In patients undergoing ketamine infusion, minor and rare side effects such as nausea, vomiting, and psychomimetic effects developed.[43] In another nonrandomized open-label trial in which chronic CRPS patients refractory to standard therapies were treated with anesthetic doses of ketamine for 5 days, the pain improved significantly for 6 months, but 79.3% relapsed back to baseline after the 6-month period.[44] The topical form of ketamine has also been shown to decrease allodynia and hyperalgesia in response to pinprick stimuli,[45] but this has not been well validated.

Bisphosphonates

Bone resorption at the site of inflammation in the affected limb contributes to the pain in CRPS. The use of bisphosphonates to decrease osteoclast overactivity has shown promise in its pain-reducing effects. In an 8-week randomized, double-blind, placebo-controlled study, alendronate was used in patients with post-traumatic CRPS type 1. This drug improved spontaneous pain, tolerance to pressure, and extremity range of motion.[46] However, other trials have shown no reduction in CRPS-related pain.

INTERVENTIONAL TREATMENT

Sympathetic Nerve Block

The most common sympathetic nerve blocks are the stellate ganglion and lumbar sympathetic blocks for treatment of CRPS of the upper and lower extremities, respectively. Multiple modalities have been studied for their ability to disrupt the sympathetic pathway through these nerve plexuses, including local anesthetics, chemical neurolysis, and radiofrequency ablation. In a study in which both stellate ganglion and lumbar sympathetic blocks were performed with local anesthetic and normal saline on each subject, it was observed that the decreased pain that each experienced was almost identical, but the duration of decreased pain was longer when patients received the local anesthetic block.[47] In a small randomized study in which radiofrequency neurolysis was compared with chemical neurolysis, the pain decreased from baseline, but no significant difference was seen between the two methods.[48] Although sympathetic blocks provide a significant reduction in pain by blocking the sympathetic pathway of the pathophysiologic stages in CRPS, their greatest limitation is that they provide only short-term relief in the vast majority of treated patients. This means that patients must continue to frequently undergo sympathetic blocks, which most often places them on maintenance therapy. This form of therapy should be performed to provide enough pain relief so that patients are able to perform physical therapy exercises for functional restoration and multidisciplinary therapy, but not as a sole therapeutic modality.

Spinal Cord Stimulation

A spinal cord stimulator is a generator containing leads that are placed in the dorsal aspect of the spinal cord within the level that innervates the area causing pain. Most patients have been managed with standard medical therapy and some treated surgically before undergoing spinal cord stimulation (SCS). In a randomized trial, patients with CRPS were separated into two groups: SCS with physical therapy and physical therapy only.[49] This study showed that SCS provided significant improvement in pain for the first 2 years.[50] Unfortunately, there was no amelioration in quality of life or functionality in the group undergoing SCS with physical therapy, although this study was seriously flawed because of excessive patient dropout.[51] SCS has been used widely for the control of intractable pain, but further research is needed to verify its impact on CRPS.

Intrathecal Treatments

Baclofen and ziconotide administered intrathecally have been examined for the treatment of CRPS. Baclofen is a γ-aminobutyric acid receptor agonist. It is currently used as a muscle relaxant and has been indicated for muscle spasticity and dystonia. A single-blind, placebo run-in, dose escalation study of CRPS patients with dystonia showed that intrathecal baclofen was very effective in decreasing dystonia and pain, as well as in improving quality of life, as indicated in a 12-month follow-up.[52] Ziconotide is a very potent drug made from the toxin of sea snail venom and works by blocking chemicals that transmit pain signals. Intrathecal administration of this drug has great potential in reducing edema, trophic changes, and pain in these patients.[53] However, it is associated with a nearly 100% side effect profile.

POST-HERPETIC NEURALGIA

PHN is neuropathic pain that arises from herpes zoster (HZ—shingles) in a dermatome distribution. This form of pain is very debilitating and leads to poor quality of life and poor functional status at home and in society. Control of pain is difficult, with multiple interventions being required. There are multiple risk factors for the development of HZ and subsequent PHN. It is essential to understand the risk factors, pathophysiology, and diagnostic approach to PHN to delve into the various pharmacologic and interventional treatments available.

EPIDEMIOLOGY AND RISK FACTORS

Varicella is a viral infection that may lead to varicella zoster (chicken pox) on first exposure and subsequently remains in a latent phase for the majority of lifetimes. HZ develops secondary to reactivation of varicella virus from its latent state. Varicella virus is kept in a latent state by the body's cell-mediated immunity. When there is a decrease in cell-mediated immunity, the risk for reactivation and subsequent HZ increases. Cell-mediated immunity may decrease with age, HIV infection, cancer, and immunosuppressive therapy as used for transplant patients.[54] The incidence of HZ in the United States is approximately 500,000 cases per year, or approximately 2 cases per 1000 persons. The lifetime risk for the development of HZ is 10% to 20%, but this number increases with age. Patients older than 75 years have an incidence of 10 cases per 1000 persons per year.[55] In patients older than 85 years, 50% would have had at least one episode of HZ.[56]

PHN pain that persists after the acute phase of the disease is seen in approximately 10% to 20% of patients infected with HZ. The incidence of PHN developing from HZ also increases with age. Patients older than 70 years with HZ have a 50% risk for the development of PHN, whereas it rarely develops in patients younger than 40 years.[57] There are many risk factors for the development of PHN, and among them are increased age, greater severity of the rash during the acute phase, female gender, and greater acute pain severity.[58] In an epidemiologic study of patients with PHN in the Ferrara University Dermatology Unit, Italy, from the years 2000 to 2008, males had an earlier age at onset than females did, and 72% of the patients were older than 45 years. The sites most commonly observed to have been affected were ophthalmic in 32%, thoracic in 16.5%, and facial in 16%.[59] The correlation of PHN developing after the first episode of HZ was reviewed in a prospective study in which patients were monitored for 12 months. It was concluded that 3 months after appearance of the HZ rash, the risk for development of PHN was 1.8%. In patients older than 60 years, the risk for development of PHN and the severity of the pain were higher.[60]

In recent years, administration of varicella vaccine has become very popular. However, some data suggest that these vaccines may lead to an increase in the incidence of HZ secondary to a reduced opportunity for subclinical boosting, which results in an extreme reduction in the incidence of varicella from the immunizations.[61] In contrast, administration of zoster vaccine has been proven to decrease the incidence of HZ and PHN. In a randomized, double-blind, placebo-controlled trial of the zoster vaccine, the incidence of PHN decreased by 66.5% ($P < 0.001$) and the incidence of HZ decreased by 51.3% ($P < 0.001$).[62] The zoster vaccine has shown great promise in preventing HZ and PHN in patients older than 60 years.

PATHOPHYSIOLOGY

Varicella zoster is the primary infection that leads to chicken pox. After the primary infection, the virus remains dormant within one of the sensory nerve ganglia, the most common of which are the trigeminal and thoracic ganglia; these are also the sites where most of the cutaneous dermatomes are involved. The cell-mediated immune system keeps the virus dormant in the latent phase. Progression from the latent phase to reactivation of the virus leads to the development of HZ and subsequently PHN in some patients.[63] During the reactivation phase of varicella-zoster virus (VZV), destruction of neurons and satellite cells occurs because this is the site of replication for the virus.[64] VZV traveling along the affected sensory nerves leads to evasion of the host immune system and spreads from cell to cell until its characteristic unilateral dermatome rash is produced. Spread of the virus and its destruction of neurons occurs before development of the rash.[65] Studies in postmortem patients have led to the conclusion that reactivation and replication of VZV result in inflammatory changes within the sensory neurons that it disturbs, which causes pain. This mechanism may help explain the findings of loss of cells, myelin, and axons, fibrosis of the affected ganglion, and atrophy of the dorsal horn in postmortem patients.[66]

The previously mentioned mechanism contributes to the two primary pathophysiologic mechanisms of PHN pain: sensitization (hyperexcitability) and deafferentation.[67] These mechanisms describe not only peripheral nerve pain but also central nerve pain. Following nerve injury, nociceptive receptors in the peripheral and central nervous systems become sensitized, which means that the threshold for firing of action potentials after a certain stimulus is lowered. This causes the nerve to become hyperexcitable and leads to allodynia without sensory loss.[67] Deafferentation pain arises from the neuronal destruction and loss of afferent neurons that occur after the virus reactivates and subsequently produces the inflammatory response within the affected nerve. The loss of afferent neurons leads to spontaneous activity centrally, which results in pain in areas where there is sensory loss. Neural sprouting is initiated in an attempt to reconnect the former C-fiber receptors, a process that leads to hyperalgesia with allodynia.[67] The sympathetic nervous system is also thought to play a role in PHN by stimulating a vasoconstrictive response during the inflammatory process that results in decreased intraneural blood flow, hypoxia, and endoneural edema.[68]

DIAGNOSIS

Post-herpetic neuropathy is principally a clinical diagnosis. The typical clinical scenario involves a patient complaining of persistent pain that is within a certain dermatome and affects the region that the dermatome innervates in a unilateral fashion.[69] The acute phase of HZ is characterized as a maculopapular vesicular rash that crusts over after 1 to 2 weeks and results in a burning sensation, hyperesthesia, itching, and severe pain. Prodromal symptoms that may occur 1 to 5 days before the rash include headache, fever, malaise, abnormal skin sensation, and photophobia.

PHN may occur 2 weeks after the presence of HZ and is the chronic form of the disease. This is a very debilitating pain that consists of burning, dysesthesia, pruritus, and allodynia or paresthesia of the affected dermatomal region. The pain usually decreases or resolves within 6 months after exposure, but in some cases it may last years.[70]

TREATMENT

Therapy for HZ can be separated into the acute phase (shingles) and the chronic phase (PHN). In the acute phase of the disease process, the first-line medications that have proved to significantly decrease the length of disease are antiviral medications such as acyclovir, famciclovir, and valacyclovir. Three randomized controlled trials that measured the efficacy of these agents when initiated within the first 72 hours of disease onset concluded that they were all effective in increasing the rate of healing and decreasing pain.[71-73] Another study showed that valacyclovir resulted in faster complete resolution than acyclovir did (44 vs. 51 days, respectively).[74] In addition, a study comparing famciclovir with valacyclovir showed no statistically significant difference.[71] When deciding which agent to use, it is important to consider the amount of administration and cost (Table 24.1). Unfortunately, data on the administration of antiviral medications for prevention of PHN are inconsistent. Other medications that may be used to control the pain of acute HZ are acetaminophen, nonsteroidal anti-inflammatory agents, tramadol, and opioids.[54] Studies and randomized trials comparing opioids, TCAs, and membrane stabilizers for treatment of the acute pain from HZ are lacking, but they are still recommended as adjunctive therapy for refractory severe pain.[54] The addition of corticosteroids with antiviral medications has proved effective in relieving the intensity of the pain of shingles, but not the duration of the disease process.[75] Furthermore, corticosteroid administration did not aid in preventing the development of PHN, as shown in a recent Cochrane review study.[76] Interventional therapy for the treatment of acute HZ has proved effective in relieving the pain but not in preventing the development of PHN. A randomized trial in which patients older than 50 years with HZ were given standard therapy versus standard therapy and one epidural injection of methylprednisolone, 80 mg, with bupivacaine, 10 mg, showed that after 1 month, patients in the epidural injection group experienced a significant reduction in pain.[77]

ANALGESIC THERAPY

PHN is a neuropathic pain historically refractory to many forms of therapy. PHN therapies have been separated into analgesic medications (e.g., topical, membrane stabilizers, opioids), interventional procedures (such as sympathetic blocks, intrathecal injections, or surgical interventions), and preventive therapy with the zoster vaccine. Nontraditional PHN therapies such as cognitive and physical therapy have also proved beneficial. As with most other chronic pain disorders, a multimodal therapeutic plan leads to an optimal chance of success.

Medications such as gabapentin, pregabalin, tramadol, and topical lidocaine are considered first-line treatments because they have been shown to be most well tolerated by the (commonly elderly) patient population. Other medications shown to help in patients with PHN are TCAs and SSNRIs, opioids, and topical capsaicin cream (Table 24.2).

Table 24.1 Antiviral Medications for Acute Herpes Zoster

Medications	Recommended Dosages	Side Effects	Prices
Acyclovir	800 mg 5 times a day for 7-10 days	Nausea, vomiting, diarrhea, constipation, decreased appetite, headache, joint pain	$90.98 for 90 tablets
Valacyclovir	1000 mg 3 times a day for 7 days	Nausea, vomiting, diarrhea, constipation, abdominal pain and cramping, headache, tremors	$203.98 for 30 tablets
Famciclovir	500 mg 3 times a day for 7 days	Headache, nausea, vomiting, fatigue, pruritus	$351 for 30 tablets

Table 24.2 Efficacy and Side Effects of Analgesic Medications for Post-herpetic Neuropathy

Medications	Number Needed to Treat (NNT)	Side Effects
Anticonvulsants		
Gabapentin	4.3	Diarrhea, dizziness, drowsiness, dry mouth, tiredness, somnolence
Pregabalin	4.9	Blurred vision, changes in sexual function, constipation, dizziness, drowsiness, dry mouth
Topical		
Lidocaine	2	Mild skin irritation
Capsaicin	3.6	Major skin irritation and burning
Tricyclic antidepressants	2.64	Dizziness, drowsiness, dry mouth, headache, impotence, nausea, nightmares, pupil dilation, sensitivity to sunlight, sweating, tiredness
Opioids		
Tramadol	4.76	Constipation, dependence, dizziness, drowsiness, increased sweating, loss of appetite, nausea
Oxycodone	2.64	
Morphine	2.64	

The therapeutic modality chosen is patient specific and depends on a thorough history and physical examination.

Topical Medication

A 5% lidocaine patch and 4% to 10% lidocaine cream are widely used topical forms. A randomized, two-treatment period, vehicle-controlled, crossover study showed that a lidocaine patch is effective in controlling PHN pain from allodynia. At the end of the study, 78.1% of subjects enjoyed the lidocaine patch treatment phase and only 9% liked the placebo patch treatment phase.[78,79] The lidocaine patch is also very safe because of minimal systemic absorption. It is also used safely with other medications based on studies showing no significant drug-drug interaction. The most common side effect reported has been mild skin irritation.[80]

Topical capsaicin in cream or high-concentration patch form has shown promise in treating PHN pain. The first application of the cream leads to exacerbation of the burning sensation, but with time, application leads to desensitization of the nerve root endings and decreases the hyperalgesia. In a 4-week, double-blind study, patients were randomized to receive a high-concentration topical capsaicin patch or placebo. The study showed that the high-strength capsaicin patch relieved pain in 64% of patients at the 6-week mark as compared with 25% taking placebo.[81]

Anticonvulsants

Gabapentin has been used widely as a first-line therapeutic agent for PHN. A quantitative systematic review of randomized controlled trials indicated that the pooled NNT for gabapentin was approximately 4.4.[82] Another study, a randomized, double-blind, parallel-group trial of 9 weeks' duration, showed that gabapentin was just as effective as nortriptyline but was tolerated better. The pain score after 9 weeks of gabapentin treatment declined by 43% and sleeping improved by 52%.[83] The dosage may be titrated up to effect to 1800 mg/day to a maximum of 3600 mg/day.[84] Pregabalin has an identical site of action as gabapentin and is as efficacious in the treatment of PHN. It has the drawback of being on patent (and therefore more expensive) but can be better tolerated by patients because of its greater bioavailability, which results in twice-a-day dosing in comparison to the three-times-daily dosing required for gabapentin.[85]

Antidepressants

TCA medications have been the first-line therapy for neuropathic pain. In a recent randomized, double-blind, parallel-group trial of 9 weeks' duration, patients with PHN who received nortriptyline had a 47.6% reduction in pain with sleeping scores improved from baseline.[83] A quantitative systematic review of analgesic therapy for PHN noted a significant analgesic benefit with TCAs for the treatment of PHN pain, with the pooled data showing an NNT of 2.6 (95% confidence interval = 2.1 to 3.5).[82] The efficacy of amitriptyline in providing relief of pain in patients with PHN was studied by comparing nortriptyline with amitriptyline. The results showed that both these drugs provided adequate pain relief in 67% of patients. Although they are both equally effective, patients tolerated nortriptyline better because of its fewer side effects.[86]

Venlafaxine is another antidepressant medication with good potential. It is classified as an SSNRI and provides relief of neuropathic pain by increasing the amount of serotonin and norepinephrine and inhibiting their reuptake. This drug has been shown to have fewer side effects than TCAs.[87] Venlafaxine has yielded improvements in neuropathic pain such that 56% of patients had greater than a 50% reduction in pain in comparison to a placebo group (34%; $P < 0.01$) in a double-blind, randomized, placebo-controlled trial.[88] Venlafaxine must be used in doses exceeding a total daily dose of 200 mg/day to inhibit norepinephrine reuptake; doses below this level will only inhibit serotonin reuptake and have no analgesic benefit.

Opioid Medications

Although opioids are considered effective in overall pain management, their efficacy in controlling neuropathic pain is still controversial. In a double-blind, crossover, 4-week study of sustained-release oxycodone, 20 to 60 mg, for moderate to severe pain in patients with PHN, the response rate for pain relief was 58% versus 18% for placebo.[89] Another study reported that the administration of 10 mg oxycodone to a patient already taking pregabalin did not enhance the pain relief obtained,[89] thus demonstrating that oxycodone at low doses is not as effective as administration at higher doses. Morphine was also found to be beneficial in managing the pain of PHN. It was shown that a combination of morphine and gabapentin improved neuropathic pain in patients with PHN more than did either one of them alone.[90] These data suggest that opioids at high doses are of therapeutic value in relieving pain in patients with PHN.

Tramadol

Tramadol is a weak μ-receptor agonist medication with properties that increase release of serotonin and inhibition of norepinephrine reuptake. This medication has been effective in treating neuropathic pain with an NNT of 4.8.[91] In a multicenter, randomized, double-blind, parallel-group study involving 127 outpatients treated with tramadol or placebo for 6 weeks, the tramadol group showed significantly reduced pain in compared to the placebo group. Quality of life in the tramadol group was also improved.[91]

Combination Therapy

Many studies have combined medications to achieve the greatest efficacy with the least dosage and increased tolerability of the medications. In a double-blind, double-dummy, crossover trial in which patients with neuropathic pain took gabapentin or nortriptyline as monotherapy or combination therapy, combination therapy was shown to be better than monotherapy, although each medication was effective in relieving neuropathic pain.[39] The combination of gabapentin and morphine has also been widely researched. Gabapentin in combination with morphine was more effective than either medication alone.[90]

INTERVENTIONAL THERAPY

Interventional therapy for the pain of PHN includes nerve blocks, intrathecal injections, and SCS. Interventional therapies are not considered to be a first-line choice, but they should be considered in a multimodal management approach for the treatment of PHN.

Sympathetic Nerve Blocks

The role of sympathetic nerve blocks is to provide relief of pain during the development of HZ, provide relief of PHN pain, and prevent the development of PHN from HZ. Unfortunately, most of the data attempting to prove the efficacy of sympathetic nerve blocks in these three main roles come from retrospective studies and are consequently limited. Thus, the use of sympathetic nerve blocks remains controversial. In a small, randomized study based on retrospective data in which bupivacaine was compared with saline solution, there was evidence of reduced duration of acute HZ pain in patients with sympathetic nerve blocks.[68] Another retrospective study concluded that sympathetic nerve blocks provided temporary short-term pain relief in 41% to 50% patients with PHN.[92]

Neuraxial Blocks

Epidural injections, paravertebral injections, and intrathecal steroid injections have all been used for temporary relief of pain from PHN, with successful short-term results. Epidural steroid injections have been proved to effectively reduce pain in the acute phase of PHN, but most research has focused on its effects in preventing progression of HZ to PHN. In a study performed in Italy, 600 patients older than 55 years with HZ were administered bupivacaine and methylprednisolone through an epidural catheter versus intravenous administration of prednisolone and acyclovir until they were pain free. After 1 year, the incidence of PHN was 22% in patients receiving intravenous prednisolone and acyclovir as opposed to 1.6% in those receiving bupivacaine and methylprednisolone through an epidural catheter.[93] The efficacy of paravertebral blocks in preventing PHN was assessed in a single-center randomized study of patients with HZ given either the standard therapy of oral antivirals and pain medications or a series of four paravertebral injections with bupivacaine and methylprednisolone in addition to standard therapy. The study concluded that after 12 months, the incidence of PHN with standard therapy alone was 16% as compared with 2% in the paravertebral block group. Although it seems that paravertebral blocks are effective in preventing PHN, larger multicenter trials are still required.[94] Another promising procedure for the relief of PHN pain is intrathecal methylprednisolone. A study in which 279 patients with intractable PHN pain for more than 1 year were given either intrathecal methylprednisolone with lidocaine, lidocaine alone, or no therapy concluded that the group receiving methylprednisolone with lidocaine experienced a significant reduction in pain in comparison to the groups receiving lidocaine alone or no therapy.[95] Unfortunately, these data have never been replicated and clinical experience has not corresponded to the positive results that the authors obtained. Although this method of management of intractable PHN may have been effective in this single study, its association with adhesive arachnoiditis has and should limit its application.

Spinal Cord Stimulation

A study followed 28 patients refractory to conservative therapies after placement of a spinal cord stimulator. Twenty-three of the 28 patients had significant improvement in pain, and many stopped using their adjuvant oral medications. The pain relief was long lasting.[96] Further trials, including cost-effectiveness data, are needed to determine the role of SCS in the treatment of PHN pain.

DIABETIC NEUROPATHY

EPIDEMIOLOGY AND RISK FACTORS

The definition of diabetic neuropathy as proposed by the San Antonio Consensus Statement is "demonstrable disorder, either clinically evident or subclinical in the setting of diabetes without other causes of peripheral neuropathy."[97] The diabetic neuropathies are collectively considered a diverse, complex disease that affects many components of the nervous system and exhibits varied clinical manifestations. They can be classified into two main categories: generalized neuropathies versus focal or multifocal neuropathies. Generalized neuropathies include acute sensory neuropathy, chronic sensorimotor distal polyneuropathy (DPN), and autonomic neuropathy. Focal and multifocal neuropathies include cranial, truncal, focal limb, and proximal motor neuropathy (amyotrophy), as well as chronic inflammatory demyelinating polyneuropathy.[98]

The prevalence and incidence of DPN have been very difficult to verify given the inconsistencies in clinical diagnostic criteria, variability in patient populations, and wide range of physiologic techniques. The World Health Organization estimated that 150 million people had diabetes in the year 2000, and this number was expected to increase to 366 million by the year 2030.[99] It has been estimated that approximately 56% of patients with DPN will complain of pain that affects their quality of life.[100] In earlier studies, the prevalence of lower limb pain ranged from 6% to 27%, and DPN affected men and women equally.[101] A study conducted in the United Kingdom involved 356 diabetic patients, most of whom had type 2 diabetes, and included a structured questionnaire with physical examination. Chronic sensorineural diabetic peripheral neuropathy (CSDPN) was diagnosed in almost half the patients, but only a third of them complained of pain that had been present for at least 1 year. The prevalence rate for DPN in this study was 16% as opposed to 5% for chronic neuropathic pain in a similar population without diabetes. It is also important to note that in this study 12.5% of patients with DPN did not report symptoms to their physicians and the 39% who reported pain did not obtain treatment of their pain, which suggests that DPN is undertreated.[102] A cross-sectional descriptive study reported the prevalence of DPN in patients with diabetes mellitus type 2 to be 26%. The prevalence of diabetic patients suffering from CSDPN was found to be 44%.[103] A multicenter study recently conducted in Belgium included 1111 diabetic patients, types 1 and 2, and estimated the prevalence of CSDPN and DPN.[104] The study was performed with the NeuroPEN device, which tests for pain and monofilament perception, and based on studies is able to identify CSDPN with confidence.[105] The duration of diabetes in this population was greater in patients with type 1 than in those with type 2, 16 versus 11 years, respectively. The study concluded that the prevalence of CSDPN was 43% and was higher with type 2 (51%) than with type 1 (26%) diabetes. The prevalence of lower limb neuropathic pain was 14%, again higher with type 2 (18%) than with type 1 (6%).[104] According to these and other studies, the prevalence of DPN may be estimated to be 15% to 20% in type 2 diabetics and approximately 5% in type 1 diabetics with an incidence rate of 2% per year.[106]

Risk factors for DPN have been widely studied in an effort to prevent its development. The most commonly reported risk factors are age and duration of diabetes.[107] Other risk factors associated with DPN are arterial hypertension[101] and impaired glucose tolerance (IGT).[108] In a study examining patients with neuropathy of unknown origin, 36% of patients had IGT, 77% of whom had painful neuropathy.[109] Other risk factors shown to have a relationship with the presence of DPN are obesity with low high-density lipoprotein cholesterol and high plasma triglyceride levels.[104] Genetic factors are also considered risk factors based on a study by Galer and colleagues[100]; 56% of patients with DPN also had first- or second-degree relatives suffering from DPN.

PATHOPHYSIOLOGY

Diabetic neuropathy is theorized to occur by three mechanisms: the polyol pathway, microvascular damage, and glycosylation end-product theories. These three models most likely act simultaneously, but there may also be some overlap between them.[110] Neurotrophic factors and neuronal membrane ion channel dysfunction may likewise play a role in DPN.

The polyol pathway theory proposes that increased blood glucose leads to elevated glucose concentrations within nerve endings. Through a series of reactions, the glucose is converted into sorbitol via the polyol pathway involving aldose reductase and elevation of the fructose level. The high sorbitol and fructose levels subsequently lead to a decrease in sodium-potassium adenosine triphosphatase (Na^+,K^+-ATPase) activity. Activation of the aldose reductase–depleting cofactor NADPH (reduced nicotinamide adenine dinucleotide phosphate) leads to decreased nitric oxide and glutathione, which inhibits the buffer against oxidative injury and vasodilation and results in chronic ischemia.[110] In the microvascular damage theory, thickening of the capillary basement membrane along with endothelial cell hyperplasia leads to neuronal ischemia and infarction.[110] The glycosylation end-product theory proposes that interference in axonal transport results in decreased nerve conduction velocity because of chronic hyperglycemia, which results in deposition of advanced glycosylation end products around peripheral nerves. These end products may also produce NADPH (which activates NADPH oxidase) and thereby contribute to the formation of hydrogen peroxide and increased oxidative stress. Nerve growth factors are important in the repair of nerve structure and function after an injury. Low levels of these neurotrophic factors correlate with diabetic neuropathy in animal models. Other factors associated with diabetic neuropathy are abnormal calcium channel activity contributing to cellular injury and death and sodium channel dysfunction playing a role in the genesis of painful neuropathy.[111]

CLINICAL FEATURES

Acute sensorimotor neuropathy often occurs in association with periods of poor metabolic control such as uncontrolled glycemic levels or the development of ketoacidosis. This form of neuropathy is very rare.[98] The most common form of peripheral neuropathy is CSDPN, as seen in more than 80% of patients with DPN. Patients with CSDPN typically complain of distal, symmetrical burning pain that usually involves the feet initially and gradually moves upward in a symmetrical fashion. This is due to damage to longer nerves, a phenomena known as length-dependent diabetic polyneuropathy.[112]

DPN causes neuropathic pain as a result of the involvement of small nerve fibers,[113] and diagnosis is achieved through a diligent history and physical examination. One study showed that clinical neurologic examination, including questionnaires, was 23% sensitive and 93% specific in diagnosing DPN.[114] Another recent study concluded that development of the DN4 questionnaire has improved diagnostic performance, with a sensitivity of 83% and specificity of 90% in patients with a neuropathic pain score greater than 4 out of 10.[115] The initial symptoms in up to 50% of patients with DPN are highly nociceptive and include burning pain, electric or stabbing sensations, paresthesias, hyperesthesias, and deep aching pain, which are typically worse at night. Upper extremity involvement is rare.[96] Physical examination of the lower limbs typically shows sensory loss of vibration, pressure, pain, and temperature perception and absent ankle reflexes. Loss of touch and pin sensation typically occurs before loss of proprioception and vibration and is caused by the involvement of large-diameter fibers.[112] This is evaluated with 10-gauge monofilament and tuning fork tests.[105] Gait ataxia may occur with severe neuropathy. In addition, signs of peripheral autonomic dysfunction can be observed, including a warm or cold foot, distended dorsal foot veins, dry skin, and calluses under pressure-bearing areas.[98] It is important to note that the diagnosis of DPN is a diagnosis of exclusion and that multiple pathologies may mimic this form of neuropathy. The differential diagnosis should include peripheral vascular disease, restless legs syndrome, Morton's neuroma, vitamin B_{12} deficiency, hypothyroidism, and uremia.[98,112]

Autonomic neuropathy is a common pathology that may occur in patients with chronic diabetes types 1 and 2. This form of neuropathy may be present at any stage of the disease, but it most often affects patients who have had the disease for more than 20 years.[116] The parasympathetic, sympathetic, and enteric nerves are affected, and myelinated and unmyelinated nerves are affected and damaged. The condition is considered to be irreversible, but cardiac sympathetic dysinnervation has been shown to revert with tight glucose control.[117] It affects multiple organ systems, including the cardiovascular, genitourinary, sudomotor, gastrointestinal, and endocrine systems. Some clinical manifestations include resting tachycardia, orthostatic hypotension, distal anhidrosis, bladder dysfunction, erectile dysfunction and female sexual dysfunction, severe constipation, diarrhea, and dysmotility syndrome.[118] In addition, because of the loss of sympathetic tone, vasodilation occurs and leads to pooling of blood in the lower extremities. This has been proposed to cause osteopenia and is related to the development of Charcot's neuroarthropathy.[119]

Multifocal neuropathies comprise a wide spectrum of neuropathies, including diabetic amyotrophy, truncal neuropathies, cranial neuropathies, and mononeuropathies. Diabetic amyotrophy most often occurs in type 2 diabetics and is characterized by subacute pain and asymmetrical weakness and atrophy of the proximal lower limb muscles. There may also be involvement of the upper limb muscles and distal end of the lower extremity, but this is rare.[120] Mononeuropathies most commonly involve the ulnar, median, and common peroneal nerves secondary to nerve ischemia because these nerves are more susceptible to injury from compression. Cranial nerve involvement may be present but is extremely rare.[120]

TREATMENT OPTIONS

Treatment of DPN has been widely studied and includes the use of TCAs and SSNRIs, anticonvulsants, opioids, and other modalities. Treatment options can be viewed as approaches either to prevent the development of DPN or to alleviate its symptoms. As is true for all chronic pain syndromes, a multimodal approach is the most effective therapy for DPN, with the primary aim often focusing on protecting the lower limbs from damage caused by sensory loss or on relieving pain to enhance the quality of life and functionality of each patient.

GLYCEMIC CONTROL

Hyperglycemia and insulin deficiency are associated with the pathogenesis of DPN. It appears that glycemic control is one of the most effective treatments to slow progression of the disease and delay its onset.[1] In a study conducted by the Diabetes Control and Complications Trial Research Group, a total of 1441 patients with insulin-dependent diabetes mellitus (726 of whom had no retinopathy and 715 had mild retinopathy) were monitored for 6.5 years after random assignment to intensive external insulin pump therapy or three or more daily insulin injections. The study concluded that in the group without retinopathy, intensive therapy reduced the risk for development of DPN by 76% in comparison to conventional therapy. In the retinopathy group, intensive therapy decreased progression by 54%. The study also showed that progression of microalbuminuria in both groups was reduced by 39%, albuminuria by 54%, and clinical neuropathy by 60% with intensive insulin therapy.[121] Thus, tight glycemic control contributes to a delayed onset and slowed progression of DPN.

ANTICONVULSANTS

Gabapentin has been used as first-line therapy for neuropathic pain and has been shown to provide mild relief of pain in patients with DPN. In a randomized, double-blind, placebo-controlled, 8-week trial comparing gabapentin and placebo, it was concluded that daily pain in the gabapentin-treated patients decreased from 6.4 to 3.9 versus a decrease in the placebo group from 6.5 to 5.1. Patients in the gabapentin treatment group also had improved sleep.[122] Another trial comparing the efficacy of gabapentin for DPN used three different forms of recording pain, including the visual analog scale (VAS), present pain intensity (PPI), and McGill Pain Questionnaire (MPQ) completed before and after therapy. Only the MPQ showed statistical improvement in pain with gabapentin treatment versus placebo.[123] Gabapentin has an NNT of 3 for overall neuropathic pain. Use of gabapentin for DPN had no effect on quality of life, but it did yield improvements in sleep and mental health.[123] A systematic review of the literature on the treatment of DPN from 1960 to 2008 recommended that pregabalin be used if medically appropriate before gabapentin. Gabapentin and valproic acid should be considered as alternative therapies for DPN.[124] A randomized controlled trial comparing pregabalin with placebo in patients with DPN for 1 to 5 years showed that 46% of the patients taking a dosage of 300 mg/day, 48% taking 600 mg/day, and 18% taking placebo had greater than a 50% reduction in pain.[125] In a 12-week randomized, double-blind, multicenter, placebo-controlled trial using a fixed dose of 100 mg/day for 1 week and 600 mg/day for 11 weeks in one group and flexible doses of 150, 300, 450, and 600 mg/day in the other group concluded that both treatments were superior in reducing neuropathic pain in comparison to the group receiving placebo.[126] The NNT is 4 for a 50% reduction in pain at a dosage of 600 mg/day. Thus, pregabalin has been shown to be effective in providing relief of neuropathic pain in patients with DPN.

ANTIDEPRESSANTS

Multiple antidepressant medications, including TCAs and SSNRIs, have been used for general neuropathic pain with positive results. In one study in which nortriptyline and fluphenazine were given in combination and compared with placebo, the group receiving combination therapy had 63% more patients with greater than a 50% reduction in VAS scores for pain.[127] The NNT for TCAs in patients with DPN was 1.3, as recorded by five randomized trials that established its effectiveness in treating neuropathic pain in those with DPN.[38] In addition, combination therapy with gabapentin has increased the effectiveness of treating PHN and DPN pain.[39] In a multicenter, double-blind, randomized, placebo-controlled study in which patients were treated with venlafaxine, those patients taking low dose venlafaxine (75mg) had 32% reduction from their baseline VAS scores after 6 weeks, and those taking high dose venlafaxine (150-225mg) had 50% reduction after 6 weeks with an NNT of 4.5.[88] Duloxetine is another SSNRI that has shown promise in relieving neuropathic pain from DPN. Multiple studies have demonstrated duloxetine to be more effective than placebo.[128,129] In a randomized, double-blind, crossover clinical trial comparing duloxetine with amitriptyline after a 6-week treatment concluded that both were effective in treating DPN. The duloxetine group had a 59% reduction in VAS scores with good pain relief, a 21% reduction with moderate pain relief, and a 9% reduction with mild pain relief. Duloxetine was also better tolerated than amitriptyline.[130]

OPIOIDS AND TRAMADOL

Many studies have shown that opioid medications decrease pain in patients with DPN. The fear of dependency on and addiction to these drugs warrants close observation; opioid medication should be administered only if the patient's condition is unresponsive to nonopioid therapy (Fig. 24.1). Of these agents, tramadol, morphine sulfate, and oxycodone consistently decrease pain from DPN. An open, randomized comparative study of gabapentin versus tramadol and acetaminophen showed that the combination of tramadol and acetaminophen was just as effective in relieving DPN pain as gabapentin.[34] In a randomized, double-blind, placebo-controlled crossover study using tramadol, the group receiving tramadol experienced relief from polyneuropathy symptoms such as pain, allodynia, and paresthesia (NNT of 4.3).[131]

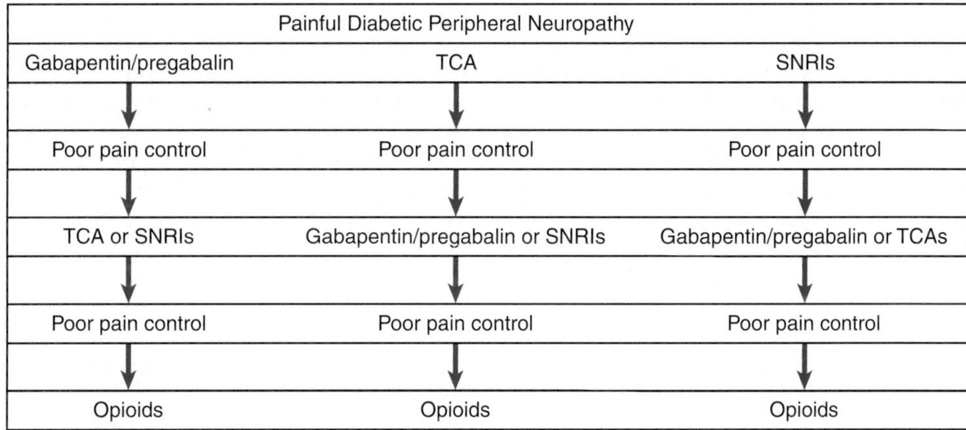

Figure 24.1 Treatment algorithm for painful diabetic peripheral neuropathy. TCA, tricyclic antidepressant; SNRI, serotonin-norepinephrine reuptake inhibitor.

Oxycodone has also been shown to be effective in treating neuropathic pain in patients with DPN. In a multicenter, randomized, double-blind, placebo-controlled study comparing controlled-release oxycodone with placebo, it was concluded that pain scores in the groups receiving oxycodone and placebo were 4.1 and 5.3, respectively.[132] This suggests that oxycodone is mildly effective in relieving neuropathic pain in patients with DPN. Another study that added oxycodone to the regimen of diabetic patients already taking gabapentin for neuropathic pain concluded that use of the combination of these drugs relieved pain more than when gabapentin was used alone.[133] There are limited data on the use of morphine monotherapy in diabetic patients with neuropathy. A crossover study investigating morphine and gabapentin used as either monotherapy or combination therapy showed that the addition of morphine to gabapentin was more effective with lower doses of each medication.[90]

NMDA RECEPTOR ANTAGONISTS

The NMDA receptor plays an important role in processing nociceptive and chronic pain. Thus, antagonizing its actions may reduce neuropathic pain. One of the most common NMDA receptor antagonists is dextromethorphan. This drug has been examined in past studies, and it was shown to be efficacious in providing relief of pain in diabetic patients suffering from neuropathy. One study demonstrated that the pain in DPN patients had been reduced by 33% and that 68% of patients receiving dextromethorphan had more than moderate pain relief.[134] A study comparing dextromethorphan with placebo showed a 27% reduction in neuropathic pain in diabetic patients, with higher efficacy achieved with increased doses.[135] Also, it is worthwhile to note that both these studies showed efficacy of dextromethorphan for DPN but not for PHN.

OTHER INTERVENTIONS

Topical anesthetics have been deemed safe to use because of their lack of drug interactions, decreased side effects, and lack of titration required. Capsaicin cream (0.075%) has been shown to decrease neuropathic pain with an NNT of 6.6.[136] In addition, 5% lidocaine–medicated plaster has been demonstrated to be as effective as capsaicin, amitriptyline, gabapentin, and pregabalin, as shown in a systemic review study comparing the efficacy of each of these drugs in patients with DPN.[137] Because oxidative stress may play an important role in the pathogenic mechanisms of diabetic neuropathy, the use of antioxidants such as α-lipoic acid may have some beneficial effect in the treatment of diabetic neuropathy. A meta-analysis showed that treatment with α-lipoic acid, 600 mg intravenously for a 3-week course, provided effective relief of neuropathic pain and improved neuropathic deficits.[138] A more current study reported significant improvement in neuropathic pain with a 600-mg daily intravenous dose for 5 weeks (NTT of 2.7).[139] Other treatment forms have been suggested for DPN based on its pathophysiology, such as glycation inhibitors, aldose reductase inhibitors, and growth factors, but further research in these areas is necessary.[140]

HIV-RELATED PAIN SYNDROMES

EPIDEMIOLOGY

It is estimated that more than 65 million people worldwide are infected with HIV.[141] With the development and widespread use of highly active antiretroviral therapy (HAART) and the resultant decrease in opportunistic infections of the central nervous system, polyneuropathy has become the most prevalent neurologic complication associated with HIV infection.[142] This disease affects the patient's immune and nervous systems. As the patient progresses through different stages of the disease, a variety of neurologic complications arise that are directly or indirectly related to HIV infection.[143] Although symptomatic neuropathy occurs in 10% to 35% of individuals seropositive for HIV, pathologic abnormalities exist in almost all those with end-stage acquired immunodeficiency syndrome (AIDS).[142] A systematic review in which multiple studies were compiled in the hope of determining the incidence and prevalence of neuropathy in HIV-infected patients found a high level of variation across all the studies. The prevalence of neuropathy ranged from 1.2% to 69.4%. The rate of development of neuropathy per 100 person-years in HIV patients ranged from 0.7 to 39.7, with a greater risk for neuropathy in older patients and those with more advanced disease.[144]

Multiple neurologic deficits occur with HIV infection, but the two most common forms of HIV-related sensory neuropathy (HIV-SN) are distal sensory polyneuropathy (DSP) and antiretroviral toxic neuropathy (ATN). DSP is due to the viral infection itself, whereas ATN is due to medical treatment of the viral disease. The more common of the two disorders is DSP. The most common risk factors for the development of HIV-SN before the introduction of HAART were older age and advanced disease states (such as high plasma viral load and low $CD4^+$ cell count).[145] After initiation of HAART, risk factors for the development of neuropathy became more ambiguous and included older age, $CD4^+$ count lower than 50 cells/mm, nutritional deficit, use of dideoxynucleoside reverse transcriptase inhibitors, and exposure to protease and alcohol.[146]

CLINICAL FEATURES

Although these HIV-SN disorders may represent two distinct entities,[147] the clinical syndrome and pathophysiologic manifestation of the two disorders are almost indistinguishable. The time course of the illness and, in the case of ATN, the temporal relationship to commencement of antiretroviral therapy represent the primary differentiating characteristic. The onset of DSP can occur in either the subacute or chronic phase or following the development of an AIDS-defining illness. The clinical manifestations of ATN can appear within the first week to 6 months after the initiation of antiretroviral therapy and may subside after its cessation.

The clinical features of HIV-SN are dominated by painful dysesthesia, allodynia, and hyperalgesia. Its onset is often gradual, and it most commonly begins with bilateral lower extremity involvement. The neuropathy progresses in a length-dependent fashion with a worsening gradient of disease from distal structures to those more proximal. The dysesthesia commonly involves the soles of the feet first and progresses proximally; when the symptoms encompass the dermatomes of the knee, the patient will frequently report finger involvement. The first symptoms noted are often numbness or burning sensations following a diurnal cycle, with the pain being worse at night. Shortly thereafter, patients will report allodynia (a stimulus previously not found to be noxious is perceived as painful) and hyperalgesia (a lower pain threshold) of the involved structures. As a result, wearing shoes and walking become painful and the patient's gait becomes antalgic. There is minimal subjective or objective motor involvement, and pain is typically limited to the intrinsic muscles of the foot. In addition to the sensory findings, physical examination reveals a diminution or loss of ankle reflexes.

DIAGNOSTIC STUDIES

There is currently no gold standard for the diagnosis of DSP. In addition, the optimal combination of diagnostic studies has yet to be defined. The disease process remains primarily a clinical diagnosis.[148] The neuropathy may be secondary to many other physiologic processes for which blood work must be obtained for exclusion, such as vitamin B_{12} deficiency, diabetes mellitus, hypothyroidism, IGT, and syphilis.[148] In a nonrandomized, cross-sectional study, HIV patients with axonal peripheral neuropathy who were taking neurotoxic nucleoside analogues had their acetylcarnitine serum levels measured. Patients suffering from neuropathy while taking nucleoside analogue medications had a deficiency in acetylcarnitine and were nutritionally deficient.[149] Although the level of acetylcarnitine may be used for the diagnosis of ATN, more studies are necessary. Nerve conduction studies are not necessary for the diagnosis of DSP and will show an axonal, length-dependent, sensory polyneuropathy. Needle electromyograms are of no great benefit because the findings are usually normal, but they may show chronic denervation and reinnervation.[150] Punch skin biopsy specimens from the distal end of the calf and proximal part of the thigh may be used to detect small-fiber neuropathy by measuring intraepidermal nerve fiber density.[147] The lower the intraepidermal density, the greater the likelihood of DSP symptoms developing and the greater the neuropathic pain level. Epidermal nerve fiber density may be used as a quantitative marker in clinical trials of neurodegenerative agents and also to predict the likelihood of symptoms developing in an asymptomatic patient.[151] Dorsal root ganglion (DRG) neuronal loss has been reported, although the reduction is more modest than distal axon loss.[152]

PATHOPHYSIOLOGY

DSP and ATN are clinically similar but have a distinct pathophysiology. The exact mechanism of the disease process is not fully understood, but it is hypothesized that there are multiple mechanisms at work that eventually cause axonal injury. The peripheral and central nerve toxicity related to HIV infection may be due to cytokine-mediated effects because HIV does not infect axons or Schwann cells. The gp120 protein is an HIV-associated protein thought to play a key role in pathogenesis by way of ligation of chemokine receptors located on glial cells and neurons.[153] It may also play a role on chemokine receptors related to Schwann cell–to-neuron interaction.[154] Damage to axons occurs secondary to the inflammatory reaction in the nerve and surrounding tissues, which eventually leads to the characteristic pain seen in DSP. This hypothesis has been supported by animal studies in which gp120 was found to produce pain in rats when administered epineurally into the sciatic nerve[155] and intradermally into the paw.[156] The indirect causes of DSP pain are thought to be mediated by inflammatory injury. They can be divided into peripheral and central mechanisms. The peripheral hypothesis proposes that the pain results from the spontaneous activity of uninjured pain-transmitting or C fibers after injury to adjacent fibers. Inflammatory mediators released by macrophages may further sensitize these fibers. The central hypothesis involves an alteration in ion channels in the DRG combined with changes in the spinal cord dorsal horn that result in "central sensitization."[157]

ATN primarily occurs as a result of the use of nucleoside reverse transcriptase inhibitors and typically ensues within a year of beginning treatment or in patients with preexisting peripheral neuropathy.[158] The mechanism for ATN is currently unknown, but mitochondrial dysfunction as a result of abnormal mitochondria in Schwann cells and axons has been shown to play a role. Data have also shown that the depletion of mitochondrial DNA seen in AIDS patients treated with NRTIs leads to increased levels of serum lactate and increased cell death.[159] In recent years, some of the protease inhibitor medications, more specifically, indinavir, ritonavir, and saquinavir, have led to an increased risk for mitochondrial toxicity that is partly due to their enhanced ability to penetrate within the neural compartments.[160]

TREATMENT

No medication is currently approved by the Food and Drug Administration for the treatment of HIV-SN. Most of the therapeutic modalities available have been tested and approved for other neuropathic pain (PHN and DPN). The therapeutic approach for HIV-SN first involves removing or reducing the dosage of the antiretroviral medication whenever possible. Also, the patient's metabolic and nutritional status must be optimized to exclude alternative explanations for the neurologic symptoms (see "Diagnostic Studies") before initiating any other forms of therapy. Many different medications have been studied for the treatment of this form of neuropathic pain without any great success. Intranasal peptide T did not show any effectiveness in a randomized double-blind multicenter study in which patients with HIV-SN received either placebo or 6 mg/day of peptide T.[161] One medication that has been proved to be effective in relieving pain is recombinant human nerve growth factor, but it does not provide any evidence of neuroregeneration.[162] Acetyl-L-carnitine (ALCAR) increases neurotrophic support of sensory neurons, as demonstrated in a double-blind, parallel-group, placebo-controlled, multicenter study. The groups were divided into those receiving placebo and those receiving ALCAR intramuscularly for 14 days followed by ALCAR orally for 42 days. The group receiving ALCAR had significant improvement in pain.[163] Erythropoietin, a hematopoietic growth factor, was shown to prevent axonal degeneration in cells that had been exposed to HIV gp120 protein, but further studies are needed.[164] Amitriptyline and mexiletine have proved effective in relieving neuropathic pain in patients with DPN and PHN. Unfortunately, they did not prove to be more beneficial for HIV-SN than placebo in a randomized, double-blind study.[165] Other medications such as duloxetine and venlafaxine, both SSNRIs, have been approved for the treatment of DPN, but further research is required to demonstrate their efficacy in relieving pain in patients with HIV-SN. Gabapentin has been shown to be effective in treating all types of neuropathy, including HIV-SN pain. In a placebo-controlled trial in which patients were treated with gabapentin (1200 to 3600 mg/day) or placebo for 4 weeks and then an open trial for 2 weeks, the group receiving gabapentin experienced improvement in pain by 44% and improvement in sleep by 49% when compared with the placebo group, with the most statistically significant side effect being somnolence.[166] Pregabalin is also very effective in relieving neuropathic pain. A recent randomized, double-blind, placebo-controlled, 14-week parallel-group trial testing the efficacy of pregabalin showed that there was no benefit in taking pregabalin over placebo.[167] Lamotrigine, 300 mg/day, was found to significantly reduce pain in patients with DSP and ATN in a randomized controlled trial.[168] Topical medication has also been studied for HIV-SN, including 5% lidocaine and high-dose capsaicin cream. In a randomized controlled trial, 5% lidocaine cream was shown to be ineffective in treating HIV-SN pain.[169] A double-blind, multicenter, randomized trial using high-dose capsaicin cream demonstrated pain relief in patients with HIV-SN.[170]

SUMMARY

Despite the diversity of conditions and pathophysiology characterized by neuropathic pain, many of the underlying treatment options are comparable but not identical. Traditional systemic analgesic agents, such as antidepressants, anticonvulsants, local anesthetics, and opioids, are typically the mainstay of treatment of neuropathic pain, although the efficacy of individual classes of agents varies with the specific type of neuropathic pain. Few high-quality trials are available as interventional options for the treatment of neuropathic pain. Clinicians should be aware of the paucity and support the use of traditional interventional options in some cases.

KEY POINTS

- The most commonly used clinical diagnostic criteria for complex regional pain syndrome (CRPS) types 1 and 2 have low specificity but high sensitivity, which has led to overdiagnosis of this pain syndrome.[3]
- In 2007, research criteria (also known as the Budapest criteria) were published that included objective signs of pathology characteristic of patients with CRPS[4] (see Box 24.2).
- Psychological factors such as depression, personality disorders, and anxiety have no correlation with CRPS patients, which suggests that there is no specific type of CRPS personality.[20]
- A double-blind, randomized, placebo-controlled, parallel-group trial studying the effects of subanesthetic intravenous dosing for 4 days in patients with CRPS showed decreased levels of pain but a progressive increase in pain from the 1st week after infusion to the 12th week. Minor and rare side effects such as nausea, vomiting, and psychomimetic effects developed in patients treated with ketamine infusion.[43]
- In a randomized trial patients with CRPS were separated into two groups: spinal cord stimulation (SCS) with physical therapy and physical therapy only.[49] This study showed that SCS provided significant improvement in pain for the first 2 years.[50]
- The acute phase of herpes zoster is characterized by a maculopapular vesicular rash that crusts over after 1 to 2 weeks and leads to a burning sensation, hyperesthesia, itching, and severe pain. Prodromal symptoms that may occur 1 to 5 days before the rash include headache, fever, malaise, abnormal skin sensation, and photophobia. Post-herpetic neuralgia may occur 2 weeks after the presence of herpes zoster and is the chronic form of the disease.
- Medications such as gabapentin, pregabalin, tramadol, and topical lidocaine are considered first-line treatments because they have been shown to be most well tolerated by the (commonly elderly) patient population.

KEY POINTS—cont'd

Other medications shown to help in relieving the pain associated with post-herpetic neuralgia are tricyclic and serotonin-norepinephrine reuptake inhibitor antidepressants, opioids, and topical capsaicin cream (see Table 24.2).

- The initial symptoms in up to 50% of patients with painful diabetic peripheral neuropathy are highly nociceptive and include burning pain, electric or stabbing sensations, paresthesias, hyperesthesias, and deep aching pain, which are typically worse at night. Upper extremity involvement is rare.[96]
- The rate of development of neuropathy per 100 person-years in patients infected with human immunodeficiency virus (HIV) ranged from 0.7 to 39.7, with a greater risk for neuropathy in older patients and those with more advanced disease.[144]
- Lamotrigine, gabapentin, and topical capsaicin are effective in the treatment of HIV-associated neuropathic pain, but amitriptyline, topical lidocaine, and pregabalin are ineffective.

SUGGESTED READINGS

Backonja M, Beydoun A, Edwards KR, et al. Gabapentin for the symptomatic treatment of painful neuropathy in patients with diabetes mellitus: a randomized controlled trial. *JAMA.* 1998;280:1831-1836.

Boureau F, Legallicier P, Kabir-Ahmadi M. Tramadol in post-herpetic neuralgia: a randomized, double-blind, placebo-controlled trial. *Pain.* 2003;104:323-331.

Bruehl S. An update on the pathophysiology of complex regional pain syndrome. *Anesthesiology.* 2010;113:713-725.

Dworkin RH, Johnson RW, Breuer J, et al. Recommendations for the management of herpes zoster. *Clin Infect Dis.* 2007;44(suppl 1):S1-S26.

Gilron I, Bailey JM, Tu D, et al. Morphine, gabapentin, or their combination for neuropathic pain. *N Engl J Med.* 2005;352:1324-1334.

Gilron I, Bailey JM, Tu D, et al. Nortriptyline and gabapentin, alone and in combination for neuropathic pain: a double-blind, randomised controlled crossover trial. *Lancet.* 2009;374:1252-1261.

Harden RN, Bruehl S, Perez RS, et al. Validation of proposed diagnostic criteria (the "Budapest Criteria") for complex regional pain syndrome. *Pain.* 2010;150:268-274.

Kemler MA, Barendse GA, van Kleef M, et al. Spinal cord stimulation in patients with chronic reflex sympathetic dystrophy. *N Engl J Med.* 2000;343:618-624.

Kieburtz K, Simpson D, Yiannoutsos C, et al. A randomized trial of amitriptyline and mexiletine for painful neuropathy in HIV infection. AIDS Clinical Trial Group 242 Protocol Team. *Neurology.* 1998;51:1682-1688.

Moseley GL, Wiech K. The effect of tactile discrimination training is enhanced when patients watch the reflected image of their unaffected limb during training. *Pain.* 2009;144:314-319.

Oxman MN, Levin MJ, Johnson GR, et al. A vaccine to prevent herpes zoster and postherpetic neuralgia in older adults. *N Engl J Med.* 2005;352:2271-2284.

Rowbotham MC, Goli V, Kunz NR, et al. Venlafaxine extended release in the treatment of painful diabetic neuropathy: a double-blind, placebo-controlled study. *Pain.* 2004;110:697-706.

Simpson DM, McArthur JC, Olney R, et al. Lamotrigine for HIV-associated painful sensory neuropathies: a placebo-controlled trial. *Neurology.* 2003;60:1508-1514.

Treede RD, Jensen TS, Campbell JN, et al. Neuropathic pain: redefinition and a grading system for clinical and research purposes. *Neurology.* 2008;70:1630-1635.

Tyring S, Barbarash RA, Nahlik JE, et al. Famciclovir for the treatment of acute herpes zoster: effects on acute disease and postherpetic neuralgia. A randomized, double-blind, placebo-controlled trial. Collaborative Famciclovir Herpes Zoster Study Group. *Ann Intern Med.* 1995;123:89-96.

van Rijn MA, Munts AG, Marinus J, et al. Intrathecal baclofen for dystonia of complex regional pain syndrome. *Pain.* 2009;143:41-47.

The references for this chapters can be found at www.expertconsult.com

25 Pain in Selected Neurologic Disorders

Randall P. Brewer | Melanie B. Smith

Chronic pain is an accompaniment of many neurologic disorders. Although chronic pain may be the defining feature in certain neurologic disorders, neurologists and primary care practitioners often focus mainly on treatments aimed at addressing the primary neurologic condition (disease-based treatments). Thus, it is important for pain specialists to acquire a pathophysiologic understanding of the specifics of the pain that accompanies these conditions and embark on treatment strategies to complement disease-based treatments and improve the quality of life of affected individuals. Common neuropathic pain disorders are given specific attention in the chapter on neuropathic pain syndromes (see Chapter 24, which includes discussions on complex regional pain syndrome, post-herpetic neuralgia, and diabetic peripheral neuropathy). Another neuropathic pain syndrome, phantom pain, is specifically addressed in Chapter 26. The neuroanatomic basis and pathophysiology underlying the pain associated with these disorders have been detailed in Chapters 8 through 10.

The pain symptoms accompanying neurologic disorders are remarkably similar despite the varied causes of neurologic conditions. The details of advanced therapeutic strategies are covered in the chapters describing classes of pharmacologic and interventional management techniques. The discussion here focuses on the prevalence, symptoms, and characteristics of a selection of neurologic disorders characterized by or having symptomatic pain as a dominant feature during the course of the illness. Although it is not possible to include every disorder in which pain is a feature, this chapter includes those that pain specialists are likely to encounter at some frequency during the course of their practice in the management of chronic pain. Because of the success that leaders in the field of pain medicine have achieved in the recognition of pain, information on the pain associated with each disorder discussed in this chapter may be worthy of a more detailed dissertation (see the reference list for detailed reviews of each disorder in the literature, when available).

The pain associated with neurologic disorders may be broadly characterized as occurring in two basic forms: (1) neuropathic pain resulting from a pathologic entity or lesions in the central or peripheral nervous system and (2) pain occurring as a secondary feature of the neurologic disorder as a result of nervous system dysfunction. The former category is widely accepted as neuropathic pain, as defined by the International Association for the Study of Pain in 1994.[1] Lesions associated with the development of chronic neuropathic pain typically involve damage or dysfunction along the small-fiber peripheral nervous system, spinothalamic pathways within the spinal cord, medial lemniscus and trigeminal pathways in the brainstem, and thalamocortical pathways to the parietal cerebral cortex of the brain. Thus, the location of the neuropathic pain in a given disorder typically follows the neuroanatomic substrate as defined by the location of the lesion or lesions causing the condition. The pain complaints are characterized by numerous pain descriptors, such as burning, shooting, stabbing, aching, and shocklike, along with accompanying sensory phenomena such as numbness and tingling. The pain accompanying these disorders is often a combination of constant and intermittent pain experiences. Additionally, the pain typically has components of stimulus-dependent and stimulus-independent pain. As defined in Chapter 24, stimulus-dependent phenomena include allodynia, hyperalgesia, and hyperpathia. Attention to the dominant pain description, type, and nature of the evoked (stimulus-dependent) pain subtypes allows the clinician to adjust treatment strategies accordingly.

Secondary pain syndromes that arise from nervous system dysfunction may include components of neuropathic or nociceptive pain. Examples of secondary pain syndromes include myofascial pain secondary to spasticity, muscle cramps, and regional myofascial dysfunction. Musculoskeletal pain may stem from bone and joint disorders precipitated or aggravated by paralysis, falls, generalized immobility, and spasticity. Immobility predisposes to decubitus ulcers, disordered intestinal motility, osteoporosis (vertebral compression fractures), and focal peripheral nerve entrapment. During the clinical evaluation of a neurologic patient with chronic pain, it is important to distinguish pain that is a direct result of the neurologic disorder from pain that may be secondary to the accompanying disability or primary disease process. Prevention and treatment of secondary sources of pain require constant diligence and periodic reassessment by the treating pain specialist. Table 25.1 summarizes the types of pain syndromes common in patients with neurologic disorders.

PERIPHERAL NERVOUS SYSTEM DISORDERS

The peripheral nervous system is composed of motor and sensory axons of the anterior horn cells (motor fibers) and dorsal root ganglia (sensory fibers), peripheral autonomic ganglia and their axons, and peripheral ganglia of the gastrointestinal tract. Pain is frequently a dominant symptom in the course of development of peripheral nervous system disorders, especially those that affect the "small fibers" of

Table 25.1 Pain Syndromes in Neurologic Disorders

Primary Disorder	Pain Location	Pain Descriptors	Examples of Secondary Pain Types
Peripheral neuropathy	Stocking-glove distribution	Burning, tingling, stabbing, dysesthesias	Ischemia (diabetes, vasculitis), musculoskeletal, visceral (autonomic neuropathy)
Spinal cord disorders	Radicular, transitional zone pain, deafferentation pain	Constant burning, tingling, aching, evoked shooting pain	Decubitus ulcers, musculoskeletal (spine, osteoporosis), spasticity related, visceral (dysautonomia), secondary neuropathic
Brain and brainstem lesions	Contralateral extremities, ipsilateral face (brainstem)	Aching, burning, dysesthesias, sharp	Musculoskeletal (frozen shoulder), decubitus ulcers, spasticity-related secondary neuropathic
Basal ganglia disorders	Trunk, extremities	Aching, squeezing, gnawing	Musculoskeletal, secondary neuropathic

Table 25.2 Painful Peripheral Neuropathies

Classification by Cause	Examples
Metabolic disorders	Diabetes mellitus, vitamin deficiency (thiamine, vitamin B_{12}), uremia
Toxins	Ethanol, heavy metals (arsenic, lead), industrial solvents
Drug induced	Chemotherapy, isoniazid, antiretroviral therapy
Trauma	Complex regional pain syndrome type 2, neuromas, postamputation pain, peripheral nerve trauma
Entrapment	Peroneal, ulnar, median (carpal tunnel syndrome), posterior tibial (tarsal tunnel syndrome)
Autoimmune	Connective tissue disorders, vasculitis, paraneoplastic disorders, Guillain-Barré syndrome, chronic inflammatory demyelinating polyneuropathy
Infectious	Lyme disease, spirochetal infection, herpes zoster, cytomegalovirus infection
Hereditary	Familial amyloid polyneuropathy, Fabry's disease

the sensory peripheral nervous system. These fiber types (Aδ and C) are characterized by slower axonal conduction and conveyance of the sensory modalities of nociception, warmth, and cold. Injuries to spinal nerve roots, dorsal root ganglia, and peripheral nerves are characterized by sensory and motor dysfunction according to the site or sites of pathologic involvement. The symptoms of peripheral nervous system disorders are thus characterized by neuropathic pain described as numbness, tingling, and shooting or stabbing pain. Of the most common peripheral nervous system disorders, pain from peripheral neuropathies is frequently encountered in the clinical practice of pain medicine. The most common peripheral neuropathy, diabetic peripheral neuropathy, is delineated in Chapter 24. Table 25.2 includes a general classification of painful neuropathies; a few specific examples are discussed in the following sections.

AUTOIMMUNE PERIPHERAL NERVOUS SYSTEM DISORDERS

Autoimmune peripheral nervous system disorders include the neuropathies caused by connective tissue diseases, systemic vasculitis, and autoimmune disorders of peripheral myelin. Neuropathic pain may precede the diagnosis of systemic or focal vasculitis or occur during the course of established disease. When neuropathy precedes the diagnosis of vasculitis, the absence of more severe systemic symptoms may delay the diagnosis.[2] Inflammation leading to ischemia of focal peripheral nerves may result in the clinical syndrome of mononeuropathy multiplex. This syndrome is characterized by pain, numbness, and weakness in the distribution of multiple peripheral nerves. The peripheral nerves most commonly affected include the ulnar, median, and peroneal nerves. Dysfunction in the territories of these nerves will typically occur at sites of peripheral nerve entrapment and at sites distal from locations usually associated with peripheral entrapment. Distal symmetrical polyneuropathy (DSP) may also occur in the setting of vasculitis and connective tissue disease. DSP is characterized by numbness, tingling, and pain in a characteristic symmetrical stocking-glove distribution. Symptoms typically begin in the feet and consist of burning, aching, and dysesthesias. Not uncommonly, asymmetry of progression of DSP leads to a consideration of autoimmune vasculitis and may assist in the clinical diagnosis.

Acute inflammatory demyelinating polyneuropathy, known as Guillain-Barré syndrome, occurs at an annual incidence of approximately 1.11 per 100,000 person-years, with a 20% increase every decade after the first decade of life.[3] Paresthesias or dysesthesias typically precede the development of weakness, which proceeds in an ascending pattern. Contemporary treatment strategies have limited the disability associated with the disorder, but a small proportion of patients may have resulting disability and chronic pain. During the acute phase of the illness, pain is often a prominent symptom. A review of pain in patients with Guillain-Barré syndrome has highlighted the importance of recognizing the primary components of pain and secondary pain syndromes.[4] Deep aching, throbbing pain in the low back region associated with radiation into the lower extremities is typically the most excruciating and disabling pain during the acute episode. A positive straight-leg raise test may accompany the acute pain. Accompanying the low back and radicular pain, myofascial pain may coincide with the development of muscle spasm, cramping, and muscular tenderness. Stabbing, shocklike, or electric pain may be present in the extremities and face. Ectopic impulses caused by acute nerve root inflammation may be the pathologic mechanism associated with the acute neuropathic pain component in Guillain-Barré syndrome. Chronic neuropathic pain may actually persist beyond treatment of and recovery from the paralytic disorder in a small proportion of patients.[4] The autonomic nervous system dysfunction present in Guillain-Barré syndrome may lead to the development of headaches, cardiovascular instability, and visceral pain secondary to ileus and urinary retention.

Treatment of primary neuropathic pain in Guillain-Barré syndrome includes the use of antineuropathic agents in addition to immune-based therapy for the primary disease. Antineuropathic agents commonly used include tricyclic antidepressants, anticonvulsants, and opioids (oral and parenteral, when necessary). In severe cases, epidurally administered local anesthetics or opioids may be of benefit in the acute stage. Treatments beneficial for secondary pain syndromes include muscle relaxants (e.g., baclofen, tizanidine) for acute myofascial pain and supportive measures for the acute dysautonomia (e.g., intravenous fluid administration, stool softeners, urinary drainage).

HUMAN IMMUNODEFICIENCY VIRUS–RELATED NEUROPATHIES

Nervous system complications of human immunodeficiency virus (HIV) type 1 infection have been reviewed by Price.[5] Peripheral neuropathic pain is recognized as a common accompaniment of HIV infection. Neuropathic pain may complicate any stage of the infection and result in disordered sleep and ambulation, disability, and psychosocial distress. It is estimated that 35% of patients infected with HIV experience symptomatic DSP whereas as many as 67% of patients infected with HIV may experience asymptomatic DSP when evaluated neurologically.[6] The peripheral neuropathic pain syndromes characteristic of HIV infection are summarized in Table 25.3.

During the acute course of seroconversion, acute inflammatory demyelinating polyneuropathy may develop and cause numbness, weakness, and peripheral neuropathic pain. The disorder may be the initial manifestation of HIV seroconversion. Its course may be similar to that of Guillain-Barré syndrome, though with a higher incidence of more severe weakness, atrophy, and profound sensory loss. Treatment of moderate to severe cases uses the standard strategies for the treatment of Guillain-Barré syndrome (e.g., immunotherapy, antineuropathic agents, epidural infusions). The acute polyneuropathy associated with seroconversion typically resolves with mild, if any, residual sequelae of neuropathic pain. The chronic form of the disorder, chronic

Table 25.3 Peripheral Nervous System Pain in Human Immunodeficiency Virus Infection

Stage of Disease	Pain Syndrome
Early	Acute inflammatory demyelinating polyneuropathy
Intermediate	Antiretroviral neurotoxicity Chronic inflammatory demyelinating polyneuropathy Autoimmune vasculitic mononeuropathy multiplex HIV-induced sensory axonal polyneuropathy
Late	Antiretroviral neurotoxicity HIV-induced sensory axonal polyneuropathy Cytomegalovirus polyradiculopathy Cytomegalovirus mononeuropathy multiplex Neurosyphilis

inflammatory polyneuropathy, appears in the intermediate to late stages of the disease. It is manifested as neuropathic pain associated with more severe sensory loss, weakness, and gait disturbance.

With the advent of successful antiretroviral therapy, long-term survival rates for those with HIV infection have increased, and as a result, there has been an associated increase in the incidence of chronic neuropathic pain attributable to the treated disease, as well as the treatments. In addition to the neuropathies associated with primary HIV infection, antiretroviral agents may be neurotoxic. In particular, the dideoxynucleoside family of nucleoside analogue reverse transcriptase inhibitors has been shown to have specific peripheral neurotoxic effects.[7] Antiretroviral-induced neuropathies are manifested by distal dysesthesias, burning, tingling, and shooting pains. This antiretroviral-induced polyneuropathy can be distinguished from HIV polyneuropathy in that it occurs more abruptly with more rapid progression and is often more painful. Antiretroviral polyneuropathy occurs in 26% to 66% of patients, but the symptoms often improve with drug cessation or reduction.[6] Allodynia may be experienced during ambulation and can be debilitating. Difficulty with sleep is a common accompaniment secondary to allodynia and spontaneous dysesthesias.

A distal symmetrical HIV-induced sensory axonal polyneuropathy may occur in the intermediate or late stages of infection. The polyneuropathy is manifested as burning pain, numbness, and evoked dysesthesias beginning in the lower extremities, with variable progression to upper extremity involvement. Similar to the antiretroviral neuropathies, allodynia may impair sleep and ambulation. Another intermediate-stage phenomenon, vasculitic mononeuropathy multiplex, may coexist with other peripheral nervous system symptoms of HIV infection. Symptoms of vasculitic neuropathy are similar to those that characterize the connective tissue disorders. Pain, numbness, dysesthesias, and motor symptoms are multifocal and asymmetrical. They often persist despite treatment of the primary disease.

During the course of the illness, especially if untreated or refractory to treatment, opportunistic infections may contribute to the neurologic symptoms. Cytomegalovirus infection may give rise to progressive polyradiculopathy or mononeuropathy multiplex, or both. The polyradiculopathy is characterized by the development of pelvic and lower extremity radicular pain and urinary retention and may progress to cauda equina syndrome. Rapid progression with ascending paralysis, central nervous system involvement, and death occurs in untreated cases.[8] Reactivation of other latent nervous system infections such as neurosyphilis, herpes simplex virus, and toxoplasmosis has been well characterized in advanced HIV and may lead to neuropathic peripheral or central pain syndromes.

Treatment of HIV-related peripheral neuropathy and neuropathic pain follows the usual course of management of neuropathic pain syndromes in general. However, in contrast to other neuropathic syndromes, such as postherpetic neuralgia and diabetic peripheral neuropathy, the neuropathic pain associated with HIV and HIV-related neuropathies has proved difficult to treat. In particular, the antiepileptic drug lamotrigine has been shown to be of benefit in refractory cases.[9]

IDIOPATHIC SENSORY POLYNEUROPATHY

A significant number of patients will exhibit symptoms of peripheral neuropathic pain in a characteristic stocking-glove distribution without a definable causative agent. The disorder is estimated to occur in approximately 25% of those 65 years and older and in as many as 50% of those 85 and older. In many cases the disorder is characterized by loss of peripheral pain and temperature sensation. However, in a significant proportion of cases, complaints of burning, tingling, and symptoms of restless legs syndrome may predominate. This syndrome may be associated with difficulty ambulating, falls, and a reduction in quality of life.[10] It is hypothesized that age-related changes in the peripheral nervous system may contribute to the development of age-related idiopathic sensory neuropathy. As is true for other sensory neuropathies, the symptoms are typically worse at night. This may lead to disrupted sleep and failed attempts at restoring sleep with therapy aimed toward minimizing insomnia. In most cases, physical examination reveals evidence of loss of pain and temperature sensation distally in the lower extremities. In more severe cases there may be loss of large-fiber sensation, with deficits in vibration and joint position sense. It is imperative to exclude vitamin deficiencies, insulin resistance, and incipient diabetes mellitus in the evaluation of these patients. Therapy is aimed toward achieving restorative sleep and minimizing awakenings secondary to pain. An antineuropathic agent, such as a tricyclic antidepressant or anticonvulsant given at bedtime, represents common first-line therapy. An open-label study using topical 5% lidocaine has demonstrated improvement in symptoms over baseline without significant adverse effects.[11]

SUBACUTE SENSORY NEURONOPATHY

Sensory neuronopathy is a rare disorder characterized as an autoimmune response to antigens found on cells in the dorsal root ganglia. The disorder may also result from the effects of drugs or neurotoxins (cisplatin or pyridoxine). It is characterized by ataxia and sensory loss, frequently with painful dysesthesias beginning in the lower extremities and rarely in the upper extremities, trunk, or facial region. This disorder is slowly progressive and may not improve following immunotherapy aimed at removal of paraneoplastic or autoimmune antibodies. Sensory neuronopathy has most commonly been associated with small cell cancer of the lung, Sjögren's syndrome, and the presence of anti-Hu antibodies. In addition to immunotherapy aimed at treatment of the primary disorder or tumor resection (if relevant), the goal of symptomatic therapy is reduction of the neuropathic pain components and prevention of a secondary pain syndrome through limb protection and ambulatory assistive devices. When the disorder is associated with toxin or drug exposure, treatment is typically limited to supportive measures and treatment of any neuropathic pain components.[12]

TABES DORSALIS

Perhaps once the most commonly encountered chronic neuropathic pain condition, neurosyphilitic involvement of the dorsal root entry zone represents a classic neurologic pain disorder. The disorder is characterized by "lightning pain" involving the lower extremities. Similar pain may occur in the trunk, thorax, and abdomen. Tabetic pain may occur for brief periods (seconds or minutes) or last for several days. Occasionally, visceral involvement predominates, known as "visceral crises." These crises are characterized by attacks of epigastric or pelvic pain accompanied by nausea and vomiting. Physical examination is remarkable for loss of sensory modalities distally in the lower extremities. There may also be significant ataxia, hypotonia, and dysautonomia. The neuropathologic hallmark of tabes dorsalis is inflammatory infiltrates along the dorsal roots with degeneration of the posterior columns. Therapy involves standard antibiotic therapy to eradicate the *Treponema pallidum* organism. Antineuropathic agents such as anticonvulsants and tricyclic antidepressants are used for symptomatic therapy. Argyll Robertson pupils (miotic pupils that are unresponsive to light but react with accommodation) are usually present. Though characteristic of the disorder, the classic finding of Charcot's joints is the result of deep anesthesia caused by the disorder. Even though it is an important secondary complication of the neurologic syndrome, once the disorder has reached the stage of profound joint hypoalgesia, the protective mechanism of pain (and therefore the need for aggressive therapy) has been severely attenuated.

PAIN ASSOCIATED WITH SPINAL CORD DISORDERS

Disorders of the spinal cord are commonly associated with pain. The causes and locations of the spinal cord disorders typically determine the need for surgical or medical management of the primary condition. Pain may be a prominent element in the manifestation of certain spinal cord disorders (e.g., acute spinal cord injury) or occur as a late effect of the disease or therapy (e.g., radiation treatment, tumor resection). The characteristics of the pain experience, variable findings, and secondary pain generators are common to all disorders of the spinal cord. In an effort to highlight the aspects of the pain associated with disorders of the spinal

Table 25.4 Pain in Spinal Cord Disorders

Type of Pain	Syndrome
Neuropathic	Transitional ("end zone") pain Deafferentation pain Radicular pain Cauda equina Syringomyelia (may include facial pain) Peripheral entrapment (ulnar, peroneal, median)
Nociceptive	Traumatic spinal instability Spondylotic arthropathy (facet syndrome) Osteoporosis (compression fractures), aseptic necrosis Musculoskeletal overuse (rotator cuff syndrome, joint pain), pressure sores, decubitus ulcers
Visceral	Autonomic dysreflexia, bladder atony, intestinal inertia

cord, a few selected examples are discussed in the following sections. Table 25.4 summarizes the pain syndromes associated with spinal cord disorders.

SPINAL CORD INJURY

The incidence of traumatic spinal cord injury is difficult to establish since rates of 236 to 1009 per million new cases each year have been reported. Cripps and colleagues[13] estimated the incidence of traumatic spinal cord injury in North America to be 39 new cases per million inhabitants per year and 15 new cases per million inhabitants per year in Western Europe. Longitudinal studies of patients with spinal cord injury have noted that 23% of persons with spinal cord injury report pain at 6 weeks; the proportion of patients with pain increases to 41% the year following the injury.[14] After the acute injury, pain is commonly located at the site of spinal trauma. During the weeks to months in recovery, several patterns of pain may emerge. The pattern of pain is somewhat dependent on the extent of spinal cord injury, as well as details regarding any concomitant nerve root injuries that may have occurred as a result of the initial injury. Typically, patients with partial spinal cord lesions associated with moderate or mild neurologic deficits may have severe, debilitating neuropathic pain as a major sequela. Plexus and nerve root avulsions associated with the initial injury often give rise to a distinct focus of neuropathic pain, which must be independently assessed and treated.

The most dominant pain type following spinal cord injury is central neuropathic pain. The neuropathic pain emanates from the area of injury and extends variably into areas of sensory loss. The pain may be more intense from the transition of complete sensory loss to normal sensation. This is known as "end-zone pain" or "transitional pain" and may be associated with severe allodynia, hyperalgesia, and spontaneous attacks of intense lancinating pain. Commonly, the pain follows a single root distribution or multiple root distributions. In the areas with sensory loss, there may be deafferentation pain characterized by constant burning and aching. With lesions above the midthoracic level, the presence of pain caused by spasticity in the upper or lower extremities may predominate. Intense muscular spasms, jerks, and hypertonicity will commonly be associated with neuropathic pain complaints. The patient may have numerous regions of ongoing musculoskeletal pain, either resulting from the initial traumatic episode or aggravated by chronic disability.

The pain associated with spinal cord injury impairs quality of life in these individuals. It is significantly associated with disordered sleep, exercise, work, and activities of daily living. It may impair the patient's ability to engage in social, recreational, and self-care activities. Treatment of pain following spinal cord injury tends to be directed toward the type of pain experience and tolerability of the agent relative to the patient's medical history. Antineuropathic drugs such as gabapentin and other antiepileptics, tricyclic antidepressants, and topical local anesthetics may be of assistance in amelioration of the symptoms of neuropathic pain. Pain related to spasticity and myofascial pain are usually treated with oral muscle relaxants such as baclofen. In patients intolerant of or resistant to oral baclofen, intrathecal baclofen has proved efficacious in the control of chronic lower extremity spasticity. A retrospective study found the addition of intrathecal morphine to baclofen to have variable results in pain relief.[15] Musculoskeletal pain associated with the initial trauma or with emerging disorders may respond to local anesthetic or corticosteroid injections, nonsteroidal anti-inflammatory drugs, and opioids.

SYRINGOMYELIA

Syringomyelia involves cavitation in the central canal of the spinal cord. It may have a post-traumatic (especially following hematomyelia), congenital (associated with Arnold-Chiari malformation), or postinfectious (associated with arachnoiditis) cause or may be associated with intramedullary spinal cord tumors. Post-traumatic syringomyelia involves the presence of new neurologic deficits above a previous level of paraplegia or quadriplegia. Increased levels of sensory loss, spasticity, and progressive atrophy may accompany increasing levels of neuropathic pain. Dissociated sensory loss describes the loss of pain and temperature sensation resulting from involvement of the crossing of spinothalamic second-order neurons, with sparing of dorsal column function. Worsening spasticity is attributable to increasing involvement of the descending corticospinal tracts. Atrophy and fasciculations indicate involvement of the anterior horn cell columns by the syrinx.

The pain associated with syringomyelia is generally neuropathic in nature. Patients with a cervical syrinx will have pain and numbness along multiple cervical root distributions (arm pain and dysesthesia) and often describe burning that may be associated with significant allodynia and hyperalgesia. Pain and temperature sensory loss may be associated with unrecognized trauma. Extension of the syrinx into the upper cervical region may be associated with ipsilateral facial pain caused by involvement of the descending trigeminal tract and nucleus. Thoracic syringomyelia will be manifested as neuropathic pain in a trunk or abdominal distribution, dissociated distal sensory loss, spasticity, and urinary retention. Lower thoracic syringomyelia will exhibit symptoms of dysfunction of the conus medullaris, with prominent sacral neuropathic pain and urinary retention.

Treatment of syringomyelia may involve neurosurgical drainage of the syrinx or surgical resection of a spinal cord tumor (when present), or both. Syrinx drainage is primarily performed to limit neurologic progression; however, alleviation of central pain following drainage of the syrinx is not uncommon.[15] Medical treatment of the central neuropathic pain associated with syringomyelia is often associated with only partial efficacy and a high frequency of treatment refractoriness. Treatment modalities include anticonvulsants, antidepressants, local anesthetics, spinal cord stimulation, and intrathecal drug administration.[16]

MULTIPLE SCLEROSIS

Multiple sclerosis is a relapsing, remitting, and chronic progressive disorder involving central nervous system demyelinization. The disease is characterized by acute exacerbations of neurologic deficits. These exacerbations are associated with acute inflammation of central myelin. Areas of prominent involvement include the optic nerves, periventricular white matter, brainstem, and spinal cord. Estimates have suggested that more than 50% of patients who have the chronic form of multiple sclerosis also experience chronic pain.[17] Because of the chronic nature of the disorder and multiple sites of neurologic involvement, a multidisciplinary approach is recommended for optimizing outcomes.[18] Box 25.1 summarizes the pain conditions associated with multiple sclerosis.

Trigeminal neuralgia has a well-known association with brainstem demyelination in those with multiple sclerosis. Sharp, lancinating facial pain may occur spontaneously or may be evoked by tactile stimulation. An uncommon finding in the idiopathic disorder, trigeminal sensory loss is more common in patients with multiple sclerosis. During acute exacerbations of multiple sclerosis, patients may have significant axial spine pain or radicular pain caused by demyelination along the dorsal root entry zones. Cervical demyelination may be associated with acute neck pain and electric shock–like pain along the axial spine (Lhermitte's phenomenon). Following an acute exacerbation, patients may typically be left with a neurologic deficit that could include spasticity, ataxia, and sensory loss. Following acute transverse myelitis, patients with persistent neurologic deficits often have lingering central neuropathic pain. The pattern of the neuropathic pain is similar to that described for spinal cord injury. Elements of deafferentation pain, end-zone pain, and chronic radicular pain may be present concomitantly or individually in a patient with multiple sclerosis.

The types of secondary pain experienced by patients with multiple sclerosis include chronic myofascial pain related to spasticity and sleep deprivation, chronic headaches, and musculoskeletal pain related to disability. With the increasing burden of disease, it is likely that the intensity, locations, and complexity of the pain in multiple sclerosis progress, along with the neurologic disorder. The pain has a significant impact on psychosocial functioning, daily activities, mood, and sleep.[19,20]

Treatment of chronic pain in multiple sclerosis involves alleviation of the primary neuropathic pain with a contemporary pharmacologic regimen and referral for specific immunotherapy during periods of acute exacerbation. Concomitant myofascial pain may be treated effectively with oral muscle relaxants such as baclofen and tizanidine. The use of intrathecal baclofen for chronic lower extremity spasticity is recognized as an effective therapy in patients with an incomplete response to oral therapy. When intrathecal baclofen and morphine are combined, the pain and spasticity in multiple sclerosis can be effectively treated long-term.[21] In ambulatory patients, a regular exercise regimen may be of benefit in alleviating diffuse myofascial pain symptoms. Concomitant sleep disorders and depression should be addressed and treated by nonpharmacologic means (e.g., sleep hygiene measures, cognitive-behavioral therapy if required) and pharmacologic modalities when appropriate.

Box 25.1 Pain Conditions Associated with Multiple Sclerosis

Neuropathic Pain

Acute transverse myelitis
Acute radicular pain
Chronic myelopathy (deafferentation pain, transitional pain, radicular pain)
Focal peripheral neuropathies (secondary to disability)

Myofascial Pain

Spasticity secondary to myelopathy
Regional myofascial pain (overuse syndromes, posture and gait disorders)
Diffuse myofascial pain (chronic fatigue, sleep deprivation)

Musculoskeletal Pain

Overuse syndromes (wheelchair-bound patients)
Accelerated osteoporosis because of immobility

Headaches

PAIN IN NEUROMUSCULAR DISORDERS

Neuromuscular disorders describe a heterogeneous group of neurologic conditions associated with diseases of the peripheral motor nerves, neuromuscular junction, muscles (muscular dystrophies, myopathies), and anterior horn cells. In a large series of patients with postpolio syndrome, a large proportion of patients (80%) reported muscular and joint pain.[22] The common feature in these conditions is the notable loss of muscle power and tone and the presence of muscular atrophy. Syndromes with slow progression over time are characterized by disorders of ambulation, which may lead to chronic disability and incapacitation. With progression of the disease, there may be concomitant musculoskeletal pain associated with the loss of neuromuscular support of the axial spine and pelvic and shoulder girdles. As is common in other chronic pain syndromes, the pain may be associated with significant psychosocial distress and with mood and sleep disorders. In patients with neuromuscular disorders, muscle and joint pain predominates. Patients with mixed peripheral nervous system disorders may also have a component of neuropathic pain. In addition, neuropathic pain may be incited by peripheral nerve entrapment, which may be considered to be a secondary pain disorder caused by chronic disability and loss of muscular protection over sites of neural compression.

BRAIN CENTRAL PAIN SYNDROMES

In addition to lesions of the spinal cord, lesions of the brain or brainstem may lead to neuropathic central pain. Tumors, vascular malformations, inflammatory diseases (postinfectious encephalomyelitis, meningitis abscess), intracerebral hemorrhage, and stroke may be associated with the development of chronic pain, which therefore depends chiefly on the site of the lesion in the central nervous system, not on the size of the lesion or the specific pathology. The neuroanatomic substrate for brain central neuropathic pain involves a lesion along the somatosensory pathways in the brainstem trigeminothalamic pathways, medial lemniscus, thalamus, thalamocortical projections, and somatosensory cerebral cortex. The classic and most characteristic central neuropathic pain condition is central post-stroke pain.

Central post-stroke pain is estimated to occur in approximately 10% of individuals after the first year following a stroke. Post-stroke pain was characterized by Dejerine and Roussy (in 1906) following lesions of the somatosensory thalamus.[23] Post-stroke pain typically coexists with a concomitant contralateral sensory deficit. The pain may emerge weeks or even months following the initial vascular event. The pain may be described as diffuse burning or aching, interspersed with episodes of spontaneous lancinating or sharp pain. Remarkably, there may be a very mild motor deficit in comparison to the significant pain and hemihypoesthesia. Patients with brainstem infarctions, particularly lateral medullary infarcts (Wallenberg's syndrome), may also be affected with central neuropathic pain. Ipsilateral neuropathic facial pain may coexist with contralateral sensory deficits and central neuropathic pain.[24]

Recognition of central neuropathic pain following a lesion of the central nervous system is important to minimize the disability and disruption in quality of life that may accompany a chronic, yet static neurologic disorder. Attention to secondary pain disorders such as a frozen shoulder following stroke, decubitus ulcers, and muscular spasticity is important in assessment of the pain. Pharmacologic management of central post-stroke pain often provides incomplete or partial results. Antidepressants may be indicated for treatment of the neuropathic pain in addition to a concomitant mood disorder. Antiepileptics and tricyclic antidepressants may be of benefit for the relief of lancinating sharp pain and constant burning pain. Centrally acting muscle relaxants such as baclofen or tizanidine are important adjuvant therapies when a concomitant pain syndrome is produced by muscular spasticity. The pharmacologic management of central post-stroke pain has recently been reviewed.[25]

PAIN IN MOVEMENT DISORDERS

Movement disorders are characterized as slowly progressive disorders of the motor system that have the primary component of dysfunction in the execution of normal motor function—hence the term *movement disorders.* Clinical symptoms of movement disorders involve abnormalities in gait, coordination, fine motor control, and muscular tone. Movement disorders may be the result of dysfunction in numerous deep brain regions known as the basal ganglia. These regions include the globus pallidus, putamen, caudate nucleus, substantia nigra, subthalamic nucleus, and motor nuclei of the thalamus. Certain movement disorders are characterized by dysfunction secondary to neuronal loss in specific brain regions, such as the loss of dopamine-producing cells in the substantia nigra in patients with idiopathic Parkinson's disease. Loss of important components of motor system control in the movement disorders may lead to secondary dysfunction in other deep brain nuclei because of the loss of specific inhibitory or facilitatory neural input. Causes of movement disorders include genetic syndromes, toxin- and drug-induced disorders, post-traumatic states, and post-stroke syndromes. However, the cause of most movement disorders remains elusive, but improved understanding of acquired genetic factors coupled with environmental influences has enhanced our understanding of the pathogenesis of many of the movement disorders.

PARKINSON'S DISEASE

First described by James Parkinson in 1817, Parkinson's disease is a slowly progressive movement disorder characterized by resting tremor, rigidity, and bradykinesia. The incidence of idiopathic Parkinson's disease ranges from 5 to 20 per 100,000 persons per year. It typically occurs in older individuals with a variable pattern of progression. It may progress over a decade and result in rigid immobility or assume a more indolent course of slow progressive loss of motor control over several decades. The symptoms of Parkinson's disease have been ameliorated by the advent of dopaminergic agents, which significantly improve the symptoms of bradykinesia and rigidity.

With progression of the disease, patients typically have significant motor fluctuations with "on" periods of relative ease of movement interspersed with "off" periods of rigidity, bradykinesia, and tremor. It is during the off periods when many patients with Parkinson's disease experience pain. The pain may be described as muscular tightness and cramping. Accompanying pain symptoms may also take the form of restless legs syndrome and peripheral dysesthesias. It is estimated that pain occurs in more than 50% of patients with Parkinson's disease.[26] Treatment of the underlying pain involves obtaining a careful history of the motor fluctuations and accompanying sensory phenomena. The motor symptoms are best treated with dopaminergic agents, whereas the sensory manifestations may require treatment with antineuropathic agents such as anticonvulsants or tricyclic antidepressants.[27] Secondary pain complaints may be proactively managed by symptomatic treatment of arthralgias, management of concomitant osteoarthritis, and prevention of falls.

DYSTONIA

Dystonia describes a heterogeneous group of movement disorders characterized by disordered control of muscle groups. It is typically related to the simultaneous contraction of agonist and antagonist muscle groups. Dystonias are classified according to the extent of neuromuscular involvement—focal, segmental, multifocal, or generalized. Causes of dystonia include several hereditary syndromes and postinfectious, post-traumatic (usually following peripheral nerve trauma), and idiopathic forms. Clinical examples of syndromes of dystonia include those characterized by abnormal posturing of the trunk (torsion dystonia) or head and neck (cervical dystonia). Pain is a prominent feature of the dystonias and occurs as a result of sustained muscle contraction (intracellular acidosis). In most cases, treatment of dystonia includes dopaminergic agents, anticholinergic agents, muscle relaxants (e.g., baclofen), and benzodiazepines. In focal dystonias, especially idiopathic cervical dystonia, the use of locally injected botulinum toxin has resulted in significant symptomatic benefit and is the first-line therapy.[28]

KEY POINTS

- The primary goal of the pain evaluation in neurologic patients is discernment of the type of the most disabling pain.
- Pain is classified as nociceptive, neuropathic, or visceral. Nociceptive pain includes myofascial pain and musculoskeletal pain. Treatment options are determined principally by the predominant type of pain.
- Central or peripheral nervous system disorders may cause chronic pain.
- Pain is probably the principal and most disabling feature in idiopathic small-fiber peripheral neuropathies.
- Residual pain in patients with spinal cord injury is neuropathic, with a combination of central and peripheral neuropathic pain features.

KEY POINTS—cont'd

- Other causes of pain with spinal cord injury, such as joint pain, myofascial pain, and visceral pain, are very common because of comorbid conditions.
- Neuromuscular disorders are uncommonly accompanied by neuropathic pain; nociceptive pain and myofascial pain are more common.
- Brainstem lesions are a very disabling source of neuropathic pain in patients with small lesions.
- Spasticity is a major source of myofascial pain in central disorders and is treated primarily with muscle relaxants.
- Many movement disorders are associated with mixed pain types: myofascial pain, spasticity, musculoskeletal pain, and neuropathic pain.

SUGGESTED READINGS

Frese A, Husstedt IW, Rangelstein EB, et al. Pharmacologic treatment of central post-stroke pain. *Clin J Pain.* 2006;22:252-260.

Goetz CG, Tanner CM, Levy M, et al. Pain in idiopathic Parkinson's disease. *Mov Disord.* 1986;1:45-50.

Petland B, Donald SM. Pain in the Guillain-Barré syndrome: a clinical review. *Pain.* 1994;59:159-164.

Price RW. Neurologic complications of HIV infections. *Lancet.* 1996;348:445-452.

Simpson DM, McArthur JC, Olney R, et al. Lamotrigine for HIV-associated painful sensory neuropathies, a placebo-controlled trial. *Neurology.* 2003;60:1508-1514.

Todor DR, Mu HT, Milhorat TH. Pain and syringomyelia: a review. *Neurosurg Focus.* 2000;8:E11.

Yuki N, Hartung H. Guillain-Barré syndrome. *N Engl J Med.* 2012; 366:2294-2304.

Zoons E, Dijkgraaf MGW, Dijk JM, et al. Botulinum toxin as treatment for focal dystonia: a systematic review of the pharmaco-therapeutic and pharmaco-economic value. *J Neurol.* 2012;259:2510-2526.

The references for this chapter can be found at www.expertconsult.com

Phantom Limb Pain

26

Lone Nikolajsen | Jeanette S. Springer | Simon Haroutiunian

INTRODUCTION

The phenomenon of phantom limbs has probably been known since antiquity, but the first medical descriptions were not published until the 16th century. Historically, Silas Weir Mitchell (1829-1914) is credited with coining the term *phantom limb*, and more than anyone else, Mitchell brought phantom limbs to the attention of the medical community (for a historical review, see Finger and Hustwit[1]). Tragically, over the past several decades, wars and land mine explosions in many parts of the world have been responsible for numerous cases of traumatic amputation. In Western countries, the main reasons for amputation are diabetes and peripheral vascular disease in elderly people. The mechanisms underlying pain in amputees are still not fully understood, and although a large number of treatments have been suggested, the results of treatment are often poor. Phantom phenomena may also occur following the amputation of other body parts, such as the breast and rectum, but the present chapter focuses on the clinical characteristics, mechanisms, possible preventive measures, and treatment of phantom pain after limb amputation.

It is useful to distinguish between several elements of the phantom complex:

- Phantom pain: painful sensations referred to the missing limb
- Phantom sensation: any sensation in the missing limb except pain
- Stump pain: pain referred to the amputation stump

There is an overlap between these elements, and in the same individual, phantom pain, phantom sensations, and stump pain often coexist.

CLINICAL CHARACTERISTICS OF PHANTOM LIMB PAIN

PREVALENCE

The prevalence of phantom pain shows great variability in the literature. Early studies reported figures in the range of 2% to 4%, but most recent studies agree that 60% to 80% of patients experience phantom pain following amputation (see Table 26.1 for details). The prevalence is probably not influenced by age in adults, gender, side, or level and cause (civilian versus traumatic) of the amputation.[2-5] However, a recent prospective study of 85 amputees showed that female gender and upper limb amputation were associated with a higher risk for phantom pain.[6] Phantom pain is less frequent in very young children and congenital amputees.[7-9]

TIME COURSE

Prospective studies in patients undergoing amputation, mainly because of peripheral vascular disease, have shown that the onset of phantom pain is usually within the first week after amputation.[3,10-12] The appearance of phantom pain may, however, be delayed for months or even years.[13] The prevalence of phantom pain often remains the same over the years, but the severity and intensity of phantom pain attacks generally decrease with time.

INTENSITY AND FREQUENCY

Although phantom pain is present in 60% to 80% of amputees, the number of patients with severe pain is substantially smaller and in the range of 5% to 15%. In a prospective study of lower limb amputees, the mean intensity of pain 6 months after amputation was 22 (range, 3 to 82) on a visual analog scale (VAS, 0 to 100).[11] Similar results were found in another prospective study.[10] The pain is usually intermittent and only a few patients are in constant pain. Episodes of pain attacks are most often reported to occur daily or at daily or weekly intervals.[7,12-15]

LOCALIZATION AND CHARACTER

Phantom pain is primarily localized to the distal parts of the missing limb. In upper limb amputees, pain is normally felt in the fingers and palm of the hand, and in lower limb amputees, it is generally experienced in the toes, foot, or ankle.[5,11,16,17] Phantom pain is often described as shooting, pricking, and burning. Other terms used are stabbing, pricking, pins and needles, tingling, throbbing, cramping, and crushing. Some patients have vivid descriptions, such as "a hammer is slammed at my calf" and "ants are crawling around inside my foot."[11]

FACTORS AFFECTING PHANTOM LIMB PAIN

PREAMPUTATION PAIN

Some retrospective studies have pointed to preamputation pain as a risk factor for phantom pain.[2,18,19] Houghton and colleagues found a significant relationship between preamputation pain and phantom pain in the first 2 years after amputation in vascular amputees, but in traumatic amputees, only phantom pain immediately after the amputation was related to preamputation pain.[2] The relationship between preamputation pain and phantom pain

Table 26.1 Selected Studies on the Prevalence of Phantom Pain, Phantom Sensations, and Stump Pain

Author	Year	No. of Amputees	Amputees with Phantom Pain (%)	Amputees with Phantom Sensations (%)	Amputees with Stump Pain (%)
Ewalt et al.	1947	2284	2	95	—
Henderson and Smyth	1948	300	4	—	—
Parkes	1973	46	61	—	13
Jensen et al.	1983	58	72	84	57
Sherman and Sherman	1984	2694	78	—	—
Sherman and Sherman	1985	764	85	—	58
Houghton et al.	1994	176	78	82	—
Wartan et al.	1997	526	55	66	56
Nikolajsen et al.	1997	56	75	—	—
Smith et al.	1999	92	63	80	76
Ehde et al.	2000	255	72	79	74
Kooijman et al.	2000	72	51	76	49
Lacoux et al.	2002	40	33	93	100
Ephraim et al.	2005	914	80	—	68
Hanley et al.	2006	57	62	—	57
Richardson et al.	2006	52	79	100	52
Schley et al.	2008	96	45	54	62
Bosmans and Geertzen	2010	85	32	—	—
Desmond and MacLachlan	2010	141	43	—	43
Byrne	2011	60	58	78	53

Modified from Nikolajsen L. Phantom limb. In: Koltzenburg M, McMahon S, Tracey I, et al, eds. *Wall & Melzack's Textbook of Pain*. 6th ed. Philadelphia: Elsevier; 2013.

has also been confirmed by prospective studies.[10,11,16] In a prospective study by Nikolajsen and associates, a relationship between preamputation pain and phantom pain was found 1 week and 3 months after the amputation. However, phantom pain never developed in some patients with severe preamputation pain, whereas severe phantom pain developed in others with only modest preoperative pain.[11]

Another question is to what extent the pain experienced before amputation may "survive" as phantom pain. In a retrospective study by Katz and Melzack, 68 amputees were questioned about preamputation pain and phantom pain from 20 days to 46 years after amputation.[17] Fifty-seven percent of those who had experienced preamputation pain claimed that their phantom pain was a replicate of the pain that they had before the amputation. The number of patients with similar descriptions of preamputation pain and phantom pain was, however, much lower in two prospective studies.[11,16] In the study by Nikolajsen and associates, the character and localization of pain were recorded before and at specific time intervals after the amputation. Although 42% of patients claimed that their phantom pain was a replicate of the pain that they experienced before the amputation, the degree of similarity between preamputation and postamputation descriptions of pain was not higher in patients who claimed similarity than in those who claimed no similarity between phantom pain and preamputation pain.[11] Thus, retrospective memories about pain should be judged carefully. It is likely that the pain experienced preoperatively may resemble the phantom pain in some patients, but this is not the case in the vast majority of patients.

PSYCHOLOGICAL FACTORS

Amputation of a limb is a traumatic experience, and many amputees exhibit a range of psychological symptoms such as depression, anxiety, grief, and self-pity. In a survey of 914 amputees, depressive symptoms were shown to be a significant predictor of the intensity of phantom pain.[20] As in other chronic pain conditions, coping strategies influence the experience of pain.[21,22] Passive coping strategies, especially catastrophizing, are associated with phantom limb pain.[23,24] Other psychosocial factors, such as social support, also play an important role in the adjustment to phantom pain.[22,25]

OTHER FACTORS

Phantom pain may be modulated by several other internal and external factors such as attention, distress, coughing, urination, and manipulation of the stump. It is unclear whether the use of a functionally active prosthesis, as opposed to a cosmetic prosthesis, reduces phantom pain.[7,26-28]

Both experimental and clinical studies have shown that there is a significant genetic contribution to the development of chronic pain, including neuropathic pain after nerve injury.[29-31]

It has been claimed that phantom pain may be provoked by spinal anesthesia in lower limb amputees.[32] However, Tessler and Kleiman prospectively investigated 23 spinal anesthetics in 17 patients with previous lower limb amputations and found that phantom pain developed in only 1 patient but resolved in 10 minutes.[33]

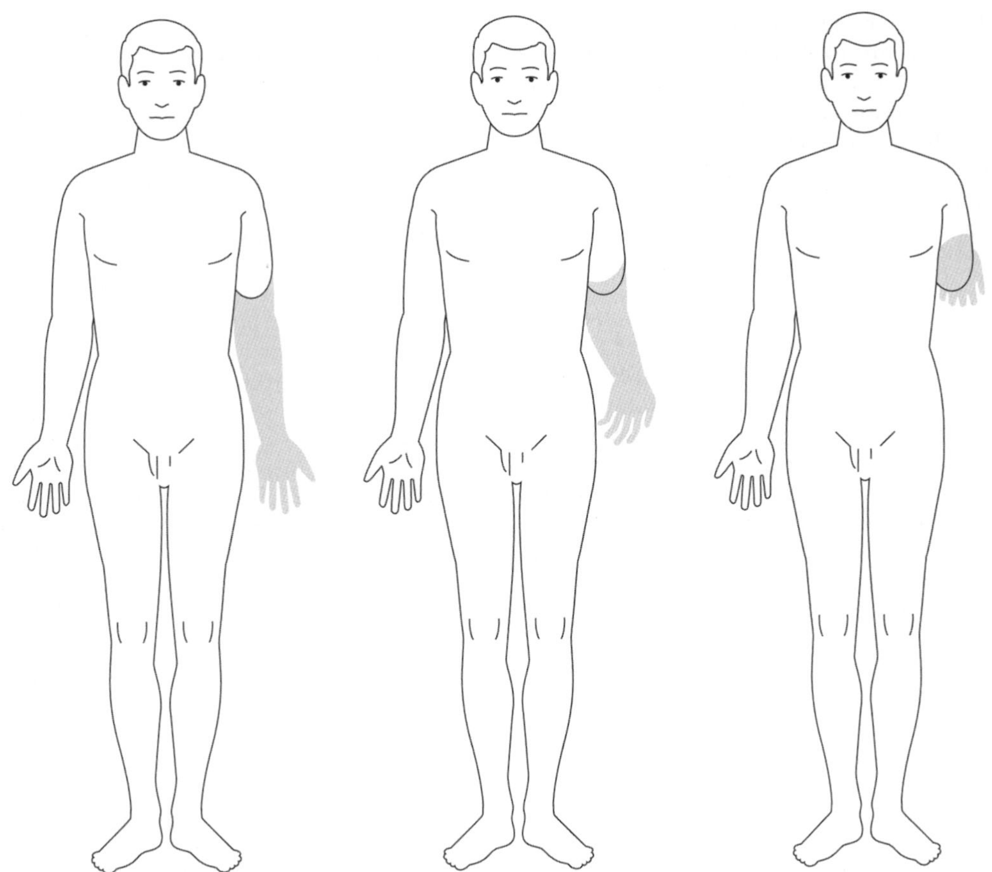

Figure 26.1 This figure illustrates telescoping, a phenomenon in which the phantom hand or phantom foot gradually approaches the amputation stump.

PHANTOM SENSATIONS

Phantom sensations are more frequent than phantom pain and are experienced by nearly all amputees (see Table 26.1 for details). Phantom sensations do not usually pose a major clinical problem; however, more than 30% of amputees may find these sensations moderately to severely bothersome.[34] The two phenomena are strongly correlated. In a study by Kooijman and associates, phantom pain was present in 36 of 37 upper limb amputees with phantom sensations but in only 1 of 17 without phantom sensations.[7] Similar to phantom pain, nonpainful sensations usually appear within the first days after amputation.[13] Immediately after amputation, the phantom limb often resembles the preamputation limb in shape, length, and volume. Over time, however, the phantom fades, with sensation of the distal parts of the limb disappearing. For example, upper limb amputees may feel their hand and fingers, and lower limb amputees may feel their foot and toes. Telescoping (shrinkage of the phantom) is reported to occur in about a third of patients. The phantom gradually approaches the amputation stump and eventually becomes attached to it (Fig. 26.1).

STUMP PAIN

Stump pain is common in the early postamputation period.[3,35] In a prospective study that included 54 lower limb amputees, all patients experienced some stump pain in the first week after amputation, with a median intensity of 15.5 (range, 0 to 61) on a 0 to 100 VAS.[11] Stump pain can, however, persist beyond the stage of postsurgical healing. The prevalence of chronic stump pain varies in the literature, but severe pain is probably seen in only 5% to 10% of cases (see Table 26.1 for details).

Stump pain may be described as pressing, throbbing, burning, squeezing, or stabbing.[16] Some patients have spontaneous movements of the stump ranging from slight, hardly visible jerks to severe contractions. Careful sensory examination of the amputation stump may reveal areas with sensory abnormalities such as hypoesthesia, hyperalgesia, or allodynia.[36]

Stump pain and phantom limb pain are strongly correlated. In a survey of 648 amputees, Sherman and Sherman found that stump pain was present in 61% of amputees with phantom pain but in only 39% of those without phantom pain.[37] Similar results have also been found in more recent studies.[12-14]

MECHANISMS OF PHANTOM PAIN

The mechanisms underlying phantom limb pain are not completely understood. However, it is now clear that nerve injury is followed by a number of morphologic, physiologic, and chemical changes in both the peripheral and central nervous system and that all these changes are likely to play a role in the induction and maintenance of phantom limb pain.[38] The first events are likely to occur in the periphery, which subsequently generates a cascade of events that sweep more centrally until cortical brain structures are finally recruited. The involvement of cortical structures may be responsible for the complex and vivid characteristics of certain phantom phenomena.[39] The following three sections present a brief overview of peripheral, spinal, and supraspinal mechanisms.

PERIPHERAL MECHANISMS

Both experimental and clinical studies confirm that mechanisms in the periphery (i.e., in the stump or in dorsal root ganglion [DRG] cells) play a role in the phantom limb concept. Following a nerve cut, the formation of neuromas is seen universally. Such neuromas show abnormal spontaneous and evoked activity after mechanical or chemical stimulation. The ectopic and increased spontaneous and evoked activity from the periphery is assumed to be the result of an increased and also de novo expression of sodium channels.[40,41]

Percussion of the stump or of the identified stump neuromas induces stump and phantom pain. In a classic microneurographic study of two amputees, Nyström and Hagbarth showed that tapping of neuromas was associated with increased activity in afferent C fibers and increased phantom pain sensation.[42] Consistent with these findings, a more recent study showed that there is an inverse correlation between phantom pain intensity and pressure pain threshold of the stump early after amputation.[43] Injection of local anesthetic into the stump may reduce or abolish the phantom pain and tap-evoked pain temporarily.[44]

It has been claimed that surgical removal of a neuroma abolishes phantom pain. For example, Sehirlioglu and colleagues retrospectively studied 75 lower limb amputees who underwent neuroma removal and reported that all patients were free of any pain symptoms after a mean follow-up period of 2.8 years.[45] However, in a prospective study of six patients, pain was relieved in only two following surgical neuroma removal.[46]

Several studies have indicated the important role of DRG neurons in the mechanism of phantom pain. DRG cells exhibit dramatic changes in the expression of different sodium channels following axonal transection.[47] Cell bodies in the DRG show abnormal spontaneous activity and increased sensitivity to mechanical and neurochemical stimulation.[48] In the study by Nyström and Hagbarth,[42] local anesthesia of neuromas abolished tap-induced afferent discharges and tap-induced accentuation of phantom pain, but spontaneous pain and recorded spontaneous activity were unchanged; these findings are consistent with the generation of activity in DRG cells.

The sympathetic nervous system may also play an important role in generating and particularly in maintaining phantom pain. Sympatholytic blocks can abolish or reduce phantom pain,[49] and in patients with pain relieved after sympatholytic blockade, the pain can be rekindled by injection of noradrenaline into the skin.[50] Long after limb amputation, injection of epinephrine around a stump neuroma is reported to be intensely painful.[51] Lin and associates showed in 20 patients that perineuronal administration of norepinephrine results in a dose-dependent increase in pain, which was partially reversed by pretreatment with phentolamine.[52] Catecholamine sensitivity may also be manifested in the skin, with a cooler extremity on the amputated side, and it has been suggested that the intensity of phantom pain is inversely related to the skin temperature of the stump.[53]

SPINAL MECHANISMS

Clinical observations indicate that spinal factors are involved in the generation of phantom limb pain. For example, phantom limb pain may appear or disappear following spinal cord neoplasia. Aydin and colleagues described a woman who suffered from phantom limb pain following lower limb amputation at the age of 5 years. At the age of 65 years, the pain gradually disappeared, parallel to the evolution of cauda equina compression because of an intraspinal tumor. The phantom limb pain gradually reappeared after surgical removal of the tumor.[54]

A very large number of experimental studies support the importance of spinal factors. After nerve injury there is an increase in the general excitability of spinal cord neurons, where C fibers and Aδ afferents gain access to secondary pain-signaling neurons. Sensitization of dorsal horn neurons is mediated by release of glutamate and neurokinins. This sensitization may manifest itself in several ways, including reduced flexion reflex thresholds in response to noxious mechanical and thermal stimulation in the limb contralateral as well as ipsilateral to the injury, increased persistent neuronal discharges with prolonged pain after stimulation (wind-up phenomena), and expansion of peripheral receptive fields.[55]

Some amputees show abnormal sensitivity to pressure and to repetitive stimulation of the stump with a von Frey filament. The pharmacology of spinal sensitization involves increased activity in *N*-methyl-D-aspartate (NMDA) receptor–operated systems, and many aspects of the central sensitization can be reduced by NMDA receptor antagonists.[56] In human amputees, stump or phantom pain evoked by repetitive stimulation of the stump can be reduced by the NMDA antagonist ketamine.[57]

SUPRASPINAL MECHANISMS

Amputation produces a cascade of events in the periphery and in the spinal cord. It is reasonable to assume that these changes will eventually sweep more centrally and alter neuronal activity in cortical and subcortical structures. Also, the phantom limb concept with its complex perceptual qualities and its modification by various internal stimuli (e.g., attention, distraction, or stress) shows the phantom image to be a product of the brain.

Animal studies have demonstrated functional plasticity of the primary somatosensory cortex after amputation. After dorsal rhizotomy, a lowered threshold to evoked activity in the thalamus and cortex can be demonstrated, and adult monkeys display cortical reorganization in which the mouth and chin invade cortices corresponding to the representation of the arm and digits that have lost their normal afferent input.[58,59]

Studies in humans using different cerebral imaging techniques have also documented cortical reorganization after amputation.[60] In a series of studies, Flor's group has shown a correlation between phantom pain and the amount of reorganization in the somatosensory cortex.[61,62] Birbaumer and associates studied the effect of regional anesthesia on cortical reorganization in upper limb amputees and found that brachial plexus blockade abolished pain and reorganization in three of six amputees.[63] Huse and coworkers showed in a small group of amputees that cortical reorganization and pain were reduced during treatment with morphine.[64] In contrast to cases of traumatic amputation, in a group of four patients with congenital absence of a limb without a phantom, Reilly and Sirigu demonstrated that the motor cortex does not contain a representation of the missing limb in this patient group.[65]

Changes have also been observed at subcortical levels. Using neuronal recording and stimulation techniques, it was shown that thalamic neurons, which do not normally respond to stimulation, begin to respond and show enlarged somatotopic maps in amputees.[66] In addition to functional plasticity, structural alterations also follow amputation. Draganski and colleagues demonstrated a decrease in the gray matter of the thalamus in 28 amputees. The decrease was correlated with the time span after the amputation and explained as a structural correlate of the loss of afferent input.[67,68]

PREVENTION

The idea of using perioperative analgesic interventions to prevent the development of phantom limb pain was prompted by the observations that (1) phantom pain is in some cases a replicate of the pain experienced before the amputation and (2) pain before the amputation increases the risk for postamputation phantom pain. These observations led to the theory that preamputation pain creates an imprint in memorizing structures of the central nervous system and that such an imprint could be responsible for persistent pain after amputation.[69]

EPIDURAL INTERVENTIONS

Bach and associates carried out the first study on prevention of phantom pain: 25 patients were randomized to receive either epidural bupivacaine and morphine for pain relief for 72 hours before the amputation (11 patients) or conventional analgesics (14 patients). All patients underwent spinal or epidural analgesia for the amputation, and both groups received conventional analgesics to treat postoperative pain. Blinding was not described. After 6 months the incidence of phantom pain was lower in patients who had received the preoperative epidural blockade.[70]

Jahangiri and coworkers examined the effect of perioperative epidural infusion of diamorphine, bupivacaine, and clonidine on postamputation stump and phantom pain. Thirteen patients received the epidural treatment 5 to 48 hours preoperatively and for at least 3 days postoperatively. A control group of 11 patients received opioid analgesia on demand. All patients underwent general anesthesia for the amputation. The incidence of severe phantom pain was lower in the epidural group 7 days, 6 months, and 1 year after amputation. The study was not randomized or blinded.[71]

Nikolajsen's group carried out a randomized, double-blind, placebo-controlled study in which 60 patients scheduled for lower limb amputation were randomly assigned to one of two groups: a blockade group that received epidural bupivacaine and morphine before and during the operation (29 patients) and a control group that received epidural saline by the same regimen and oral or intramuscular morphine preoperatively (31 patients). Both groups underwent general anesthesia for the amputation, and all patients received epidural analgesics for postoperative pain management. Patients were interviewed about preamputation pain on the day before the amputation and about stump and phantom pain after 1 week and 3, 6, and 12 months. The median duration of the preoperative epidural blockade (blockade group) was 18 hours. After 1 week, 51.9% in the blockade group and 55.6% in the control group reported phantom pain. Subsequently, the figures (blockade/control) were 82.4%/50% at 3 months, 81.3%/55% at 6 months, and 75%/68.8% at 12 months (difference not significant). The intensity of stump and phantom pain and consumption of opioids were also similar in the two groups at all four postoperative interviews.[72]

In a retrospective review of 150 amputees, no difference was found in the incidence of phantom pain 24 months after the amputation in those who had received epidural, spinal, or general anesthesia for the amputation.[73]

In a recent study, Karanikolas and colleagues described 65 patients undergoing lower limb amputation who were assigned to five treatment groups in a prospective randomized trial: (1) preoperative and postoperative epidural analgesia and epidural anesthesia for surgery; (2) preoperative intravenous patient-controlled analgesia (PCA), postoperative epidural analgesia, and epidural anesthesia for surgery; (3) preoperative and postoperative intravenous PCA and epidural anesthesia for surgery; (4) preoperative and postoperative intravenous PCA and general anesthesia for surgery, and (5) controls—conventional analgesia and general anesthesia. Epidural analgesia or intravenous PCA was initiated 48 hours preoperatively and continued for 48 hours postoperatively. At the 6-month follow-up, the prevalence of phantom limb pain was significantly lower in groups 1 (7.7%), 3 (30.7%), and 4 (23%) than in group 5 (75%), thus showing that perioperative management may affect the phantom pain outcome.[74]

PERIPHERAL REGIONAL ANESTHESIA

The effect of perineural or intraneural blockade on phantom pain was examined in a few studies. Fisher and Meller introduced a catheter into the transected nerve sheath at the time of amputation and infused bupivacaine for 72 hours in 11 patients. Phantom pain did not develop in any patients during a 12-month follow-up.[75] Two retrospective studies have found negative and positive effects, respectively, of a similar treatment.[76,77] Pinzur and associates prospectively randomized 21 patients to receive a continuous postoperative infusion of either bupivacaine or saline at the transected end of the sciatic or posterior tibial nerve but failed to find any difference between the two groups with regard to the incidence of phantom pain after 3 and 6 months.[78]

Lambert and associates compared two techniques of regional analgesia: 30 patients were randomized to treatment via an intraoperatively placed perineural catheter for intraoperative and postoperative administration of bupivacaine or epidural bupivacaine and diamorphine started 24 hours before the amputation and continued for 3 days postoperatively. All patients underwent general anesthesia for the amputation. The preoperative, perioperative, and postoperative epidural pain treatment was not superior to the intraoperative and postoperative perineural pain treatment in preventing phantom pain since the incidence of phantom pain was similar in the two groups after 3 days and 6 and 12 months.[79]

In a recent study, interesting results have been reported following a prolonged infusion of local anesthetics via a perineural catheter. Seventy-one patients received a perineural infusion of 0.5% ropivacaine for a median period of 30 days (range, 4 to 83 days) after the amputation. The infusion of ropivacaine was discontinued at regular intervals but restarted if the intensity of phantom pain exceeded 1 on a 5-point verbal scale. The incidence of severe to intolerable phantom pain was only 3% after 12 months.[80]

SYSTEMIC INTERVENTIONS

A few studies have examined the effect of medical interventions in the perioperative and postoperative period. In an observational open study with historical controls, Dertwinkel and colleagues suggested that intravenous ketamine infused intraoperatively and for 72 hours after amputation could reduce phantom pain.[81] A randomized, double-blind trial including 45 patients found no effect of a similar treatment.[82]

In another double-blind study, 19 patients with acute traumatic amputation of the upper extremity were randomized to either oral memantine, 20 to 30 mg daily, or placebo for 4 weeks after amputation. All patients received continuous postoperative brachial plexus analgesia. Memantine treatment reduced phantom pain after 4 weeks and 6 months, but not after 12 months.[83]

Nikolajsen and associates randomized 46 lower limb amputees to either oral gabapentin or placebo for the first 30 days after amputation. The first dose of 300 mg gabapentin or placebo was given on the first postoperative day, and the dosage was gradually increased until a maximum of 2400 mg/day was reached. The intensity, frequency, and duration of phantom pain attacks were recorded daily in the first 30 days and after 3 and 6 months. The intensity of stump pain was also recorded and sensory testing of the stump was performed. The two treatment groups were similar in almost all outcome parameters. Thus, early and prolonged treatment with gabapentin did not seem to reduce the incidence of phantom pain.[84]

In conclusion, perioperative interventions, such as epidurals, other nerve blocks, and systemic treatments, are effective in the treatment of immediate postoperative stump pain. However, it is evident that more well-designed controlled trials are necessary to further evaluate the potential for different perioperative treatment regimens to reduce chronic phantom pain (for a review of studies on the prevention of phantom pain see Ypsilantis and Tang[85]).

TREATMENT

Treatment of chronic pain after amputation, in particular, treatment of phantom pain, represents a major challenge to the clinician. There is not much evidence from randomized trials to guide clinicians in treatment, and most studies dealing with phantom pain suffer from major methodologic limitations: samples are small, randomization and blinding are either absent or inappropriate, controls are often lacking, and follow-up periods are short. Halbert and colleagues performed a systematic literature search (Medline 1966 to 1999) to determine the optimal management of phantom pain. The authors identified 186 articles, but after exclusion of letters, reviews, descriptive trials without intervention, case reports, and trials with major methodologic errors, only 12 articles were left for review.[86] The most recent Cochrane systematic review on pharmacologic management of phantom limb pain[87] resulted in just 13 eligible studies with a total of 255 amputees. The authors' conclusion was that data from the studies included were not sufficient to support any particular medication for established phantom limb pain. Table 26.2 shows selected studies on the treatment of phantom pain.

MEDICAL TREATMENT

TRICYCLIC ANTIDEPRESSANTS

At least two studies have examined the effect of tricyclic antidepressants on phantom pain. In one study, 39 patients were randomized to receive either amitriptyline or active placebo during a 6-week trial period. The dosage of amitriptyline was increased until the patient reached the maximum tolerated dose of 125 mg/day. However, the study showed no effect of amitriptyline on pain intensity or secondary outcome measures such as satisfaction with life.[88] In the other study, 49 traumatic amputees were randomized to receive amitriptyline (mean dose of 55 mg/day), tramadol (mean dose of 448 mg/day), or placebo for 1 month. The administration of tramadol and placebo was blinded; amitriptyline was given nonblinded as an open comparison. Nonresponders (less than 10-mm pain relief on a VAS from baseline to day 3) were switched to the alternative active treatment, that is, tramadol to amitriptyline treatment and vice versa. Placebo nonresponders were switched to tramadol or amitriptyline. Both tramadol and amitriptyline had almost abolished stump and phantom pain at the end of the treatment period.[89]

GABAPENTIN AND PREGABALIN

The effect of gabapentin on established phantom limb pain has been examined in two studies. Bone's group examined the effect of gabapentin in a double-blind crossover study that included 19 patients with phantom pain. The dose of gabapentin was titrated in increments of 300 mg to the maximum dosage of 2400 mg/day. After 6 weeks of treatment, gabapentin was better than placebo in reducing phantom pain.[90] Smith and associates administered gabapentin or placebo for 6 weeks to 24 amputees in a double-blind, crossover fashion with a maximum dose of 3600 mg/day. Gabapentin did not decrease the intensity of pain significantly, but the participants rated the decrease in pain as more meaningful during the treatment period with gabapentin.[91] Thus far, the effect of pregabalin on phantom pain has not been examined in controlled trials.

Table 26.2 Selected Studies on Medical Treatment of Phantom Pain

Reference	Randomization	Blinding	No. of Patients	Intervention	Effect on Phantom Pain
Tricyclic antidepressants					
Robinson et al., 2004	+	+	39	A (n = 20): amitriptyline up to 125 mg/day for 6 wk B (n = 19): active placebo	–
Wilder-Smith et al., 2005	+	+ (–)	94	A (n = 30): amitriptyline (mean, 55 mg/day) for 1 mo B (n = 33): tramadol (mean, 448 mg/day) C (n = 31): placebo	+
Gabapentin					
Bone et al., 2002*	+	+	19	Gabapentin/placebo for 6 wk, 1-wk washout period; maximum dose of gabapentin, 2400 mg/day	+
Smith et al., 2005*	+	+	24	Gabapentin/placebo for 6 wk, 5-wk washout period; maximum dose of gabapentin, 3600 mg/day	+/-
Opioids					
Huse et al., 2001*	+	+	12	Oral morphine/placebo for 4 wk, 1–2-wk washout period; maximum dose of morphine, 300 mg/day	+
Wu et al., 2002*	+	+	32	Infusion of morphine/lidocaine/diphenhydramine over 40 min on 3 consecutive days	+ (morphine)
Wu et al., 2008*	+	+	60	Oral morphine/mexiletine/placebo for 8 wk, washout period of 1 wk; mean dose of morphine, 112 mg/day; mean dose of mexiletine, 933 mg/day	+ (morphine)
NMDA receptor antagonists					
Nikolajsen et al., 1996*	+	+	11	Infusion of ketamine/placebo over 45 min, washout period of 3 days	+
Eichenberger et al., 2008*	+	+	20	Infusion of ketamine/ketamine and calcitonin/calcitonin/placebo over 1 hr, washout period of 2 days	+ (ketamine)
Nikolajsen et al., 2000*	+	+	19	Oral memantine/placebo for 5 wk, washout period of 4 wk; dose of memantine, 20 mg/day	–
Maier et al., 2003	+	+	36	A (n = 18): memantine (30 mg/day) for 4 wk B (n = 18): placebo	–
Wiech et al., 2004*	+	+	8	Oral memantine/placebo for 4 wk, washout period of 14 days; dose of memantine, 30 mg/day	–
Local/regional injections					
Casale et al., 2009*	+ (?)	+	8	Injection of bupivacaine/saline into contralateral painful muscle areas	+
Cohen et al., 2011	–	– (+)	17	Sympathetic blocks with bupivacaine	+
Wu et al., 2011*	+	(+)	14	Injection of botulinum toxin type A/ lidocaine + methylprednisolone into the stump	–

A, B, and C refer to the different arms in studies with a parallel design.
*Crossover design.
NMDA, *N*-methyl-D-aspartate.
Modified from Nikolajsen L. Phantom limb. In: Koltzenburg M, McMahon S, Tracey I, et al, eds. *Wall & Melzack's Textbook of Pain*. 6th ed. Philadelphia: Elsevier; 2013.

OPIOIDS

Failure to provide efficient pain relief should not be accepted until opioids have been tried. In a placebo-controlled, crossover study that included 12 patients, a significant reduction in phantom pain was found during a 4-week treatment phase with oral morphine.[64] In another randomized, double-blind, active placebo-controlled, crossover study, 31 amputees received a 40-minute infusion of lidocaine, morphine, or diphenhydramine. When compared with placebo, morphine reduced both stump and phantom pain, whereas lidocaine reduced only stump pain.[92] The same group examined the effect of oral treatment with morphine, mexiletine, or placebo in 60 amputees during an 8-week treatment period. Postamputation pain was significantly reduced during treatment only with morphine.[93]

NMDA RECEPTOR ANTAGONISTS

The effect of NMDA receptor antagonists has been examined in different studies. In a double-blind, placebo-controlled, crossover trial, intravenous ketamine reduced pain, hyperalgesia, and wind-up–like pain in 11 amputees with stump and phantom pain.[57] Eichenberger and colleagues studied the effect of a 1-hour infusion of ketamine alone, a combination of ketamine and calcitonin, calcitonin alone, and placebo in 20 amputees with phantom pain. Ketamine alone significantly reduced phantom pain. Its combination with calcitonin provided no additional effect, and calcitonin alone had no effect on pain.[94] Four other trials have examined the effect of memantine, an NMDA receptor antagonist available for oral use. In all studies, memantine was administered in a blinded, placebo-controlled, crossover fashion to patients with established stump and phantom pain. Memantine at doses of 20 or 30 mg/day failed to have any effect on spontaneous pain, allodynia, and hyperalgesia.[95-98]

OTHER DRUGS

Calcitonin significantly reduced phantom pain when used intravenously in the early postoperative phase in one study.[99] However, a more recent study found no effect of such a treatment.[94] A large number of other treatments, such as dextromethorphan, topical application of capsaicin, intrathecal opioids, various anesthetic blocks, injections of botulinum toxin, and topiramate, have been claimed to be effective in relieving phantom pain, but none of them have proved to be effective in well-controlled trials with a sufficient number of patients. In a recent controlled trial of botulinum toxin versus lidocaine/methylprednisolone injections, neither of the treatments reduced the intensity of phantom limb pain at up to 6 months' follow-up.[100] In another recent study with a crossover design, phantom pain was attenuated by injection of bupivacaine into the contralateral painful muscle areas under study.[101] Sympathetic blocks may also reduce phantom pain, but only for a limited time after the injection.[49]

NONMEDICAL TREATMENT

A recent survey of treatments used for phantom pain revealed that after pharmacologic treatment, physical therapy was the treatment modality most often used.[102] Physical therapy involving massage, manipulation, and passive movements may prevent trophic changes and vascular congestion in the stump. Other treatments, such as transcutaneous electrical nerve stimulation (TENS), acupuncture, biofeedback, and hypnosis, may in some cases have a beneficial effect on stump and phantom pain. A recent Cochrane systematic review[103] failed to find any controlled study on the effectiveness of TENS for the treatment of phantom pain and stump pain. It has been suggested that mirror therapy can reduce phantom pain.[104,105] In a larger clinical trial of 80 amputees, however, Brodie and associates failed to find any significant effect of mirror treatment.[106] Flor's group demonstrated that sensory-discriminative training involving the application of stimuli to the stump reduced pain in five upper limb amputees.[107] The advantage of most of the aforementioned methods is the absence of side effects and complications and the fact that the treatment can easily be repeated. However, most studies are mainly observational.

SURGICAL AND OTHER INVASIVE TREATMENTS

Surgery on amputation neuromas and more extensive amputations previously played important roles in the treatment of stump and phantom pain. Today, stump revision is performed only in cases of obvious stump pathology; in properly healed stumps there is almost never any indication for proximal extension of the amputation because of pain. In a recent prospective study of patients with neuropathic pain, including phantom pain, pain was relieved in only two of six patients following surgical neuroma removal.[46] The results of other invasive techniques such as dorsal root entry zone lesions, sympathectomy, and cordotomy have generally been unfavorable, and most of them have been abandoned. Surgery may produce short-term pain relief, but the pain often reappears. Spinal cord stimulation and deep brain stimulation may be used for the treatment of phantom limb pain.[108,109] Because the methods are invasive and associated with considerable cost, they should be used only for carefully selected patients. Until more clinical data become available, guidelines in analogy with the pharmacologic regimens used for other neuropathic pain conditions are probably the best approximation, especially for the treatment of stump pain.[110] A combination of medical and nonmedical treatment may be advantageous, and in general, treatment should be noninvasive. Surgery on the peripheral or central nervous system is always associated with further deafferentation and therefore an increased risk for persistent pain.

SUGGESTED READINGS

Alviar MJ, Hale T, Dungca M. Pharmacologic interventions for treating phantom limb pain. *Cochrane Database Syst Rev.* 2011;12:CD006380.

Birbaumer N, Lutzenberger W, Montoya P, et al. Effects of regional anesthesia on phantom limb pain are mirrored in changes in cortical reorganization. *J Neurosci.* 1997;17:5503-5508.

Borghi B, D'Addabbo M, White PF, et al. The use of prolonged peripheral neural blockade after lower extremity amputation: the effect on symptoms associated with phantom limb syndrome. *Anesth Analg.* 2010;111:1308-1315.

Brodie EE, Whyte A, Niven CA. Analgesia through the looking-glass? A randomized controlled trial investigating the effect of viewing a "virtual" limb upon phantom limb pain, sensation and movement. *Eur J Pain.* 2007;11:428-436.

Eichenberger U, Neff F, Sveticic G, et al. Chronic phantom limb pain: the effects of calcitonin, ketamine, and their combination on pain and sensory thresholds. *Anesth Analg.* 2008;106:1265-1273.

Flor H, Elbert T, Knecht S, et al. Phantom-limb pain as a perceptual correlate of cortical reorganization following arm amputation. *Nature.* 1995;375:482-484.

Flor H, Nikolajsen L, Jensen TS. Phantom limb pain: a case of maladaptive CNS plasticity? *Nat Rev Neurosci.* 2006;7:873-881.

Maier C, Dertwinkel R, Mansourian N, et al. Efficacy of the NMDA-receptor antagonist memantine in patients with chronic phantom limb pain—results of a randomized double-blinded, placebo-controlled trial. *Pain.* 2003;103:277-283.

Nikolajsen L, Hansen CL, Nielsen J, et al. The effect of ketamine on phantom pain: a central neuropathic disorder maintained by peripheral input. *Pain.* 1996;67:69-77.

Nikolajsen L, Ilkjaer S, Christensen JH, et al. Randomised trial of epidural bupivacaine and morphine in prevention of stump and phantom pain in lower-limb amputation. *Lancet.* 1997;350:1353-1357.

Nikolajsen L, Ilkjaer S, Kroner K, et al. The influence of preamputation pain on postamputation stump and phantom pain. *Pain*. 1997;72:393-405.

Nikolajsen L, Finnerup NB, Kramp S, et al. A randomized study of the effects of gabapentin on postamputation pain. *Anesthesiology*. 2006;105:1008-1015.

Sherman RA, Sherman CJ. A comparison of phantom sensations among amputees whose amputations were of civilian and military origins. *Pain*. 1985;21:91-97.

Wilder-Smith CH, Hill LT, Laurent S. Postamputation pain and sensory changes in treatment-naive patients: characteristics and responses to treatment with tramadol, amitriptyline, and placebo. *Anesthesiology*. 2005;103:619-628.

Ypsilantis E, Tang TY. Pre-emptive analgesia for chronic limb pain after amputation for peripheral vascular disease: a systematic review. *Ann Vasc Surg*. 2010;24:1139-1146.

The references for this chapter can be found at www.expertconsult.com.

27 Central Post-stroke Pain Syndrome

Richard L. Harvey

INTRODUCTION AND HISTORICAL CONTEXT

Central post-stroke pain (CPSP) syndrome is uncommon after stroke and occurs in only about 8% of patients. However, because of the common occurrence of stroke, CPSP is a major central neuropathic pain. The pain originates from the stroke lesion itself, which induces neuroplastic changes that result in disordered central nervous system (CNS) processing within the distributed sensory network. The first note of CPSP is attributed to Adolf Wallenberg in 1895 when he described a case of lateral medullary stroke, or *Wallenberg's syndrome.*[1] His case involved a 38-year-old man who suffered "vertigo without loss of consciousness." Wallenberg reported that the man "developed pain and hyperesthesia of the left side of his face and body, hypoesthesiae of the right half of the face, and loss of pain and temperature sensitivity in the right extremities and right half of the torso."[1,2] In 1906, Dejerine and Roussy described a case of intractable pain following a thalamic stroke, which was then named the *thalamic syndrome.*[3] Symptoms included persistent hemianesthesia, mild hemiataxia, severe persistent often intolerable pain unresponsive to treatment, and choreoathetoid movements,[4] all found on the hemiplegic side of the body. In 1911, Head and Holmes,[5] by using controlled stimuli in patients with spontaneous pain following stroke, determined that cortical lesions could not cause such pain without involvement of the thalamus.

Davison and Schick[6] published 11 clinical-pathologic cases of spontaneous pain in 1935 that were associated with lesions in the thalamus, spinal cord, peripheral nerves, and cerebral cortex. It became clear from this review and other case studies that spontaneous pain may follow various lesions in the CNS. Riddoch[7] wrote a summary of these findings and defined central pain as being spontaneous and associated with an over-reaction to stimulation as a result of lesions within the CNS. In 1969, Cassinari and Pagni determined that CPSP can result from a lesion anywhere along the spinothalamic and thalamocortical pathways[8] and that involvement of these pathways is necessary for the development of CPSP. However, it must be recognized that pain does not always result from these lesions. Currently, it is recognized that cortical, subcortical, thalamic, and lateral brainstem strokes can all cause CPSP, in addition to sensory changes and impaired motor control and weakness, but pain is not always a necessary outcome.

CLINICAL DIAGNOSIS

Pain from any cause is common after stroke and occurs at an incidence of 14% to 43% in the acute and subacute stages of recovery.[9,10] Among the many causes of post-stroke pain, CPSP is a less common etiology. More frequently, pain after stroke is a result of musculoskeletal processes, including hemiplegic shoulder pain, arthritis, myofascial disorders, and tendonitis. For this reason, the diagnosis of CPSP cannot be made without eliminating other possible causes of localized pain. In addition to the musculoskeletal causes, others include gout, deep vein thrombosis, complex regional pain syndrome, and painful spasms. Painful diabetic neuropathy is another form of neuropathic pain that can be seen in patients with stroke because of the close association between diabetes and cerebrovascular disease, but this pain is peripheral rather than central. Pain occurs in diabetic neuropathy with damage to Aδ and C fibers.[11] Diabetic neuropathy is often accompanied by bilateral pain, whereas CPSP is almost always unilateral, and both conditions may occur simultaneously in patients with stroke. Although these two forms of neuropathic pain may respond to similar treatment, because of subtle differences in response to therapy, a careful diagnosis is critical.

In clinical practice, therefore, CPSP is a diagnosis of exclusion. The incidence of CPSP in patients with stroke is 8% in general and 9% after thalamic hemorrhage,[12] but there is only a 5% incidence of moderate to severe pain. Onset of CPSP in the first days following the stroke is rare, but 63% of patients will have pain within the first month after stroke onset[13] and nearly all the rest within a year.[14]

Typically, a patient with CPSP will complain of severe pain on the side of the body contralateral to the lesioned hemisphere associated with sensory changes in the painful region. In the case of a lateral medullary stroke, the pain can be located in areas of sensory loss, which include the ipsilateral face and contralateral body. The pain associated with CPSP can be spontaneous or evoked. Spontaneous pain in some cases is episodic, whereas in others it may be continuous.[15] Spontaneous pain is most commonly described as burning (47% to 59%) or aching (30% to 41%), often deep within the painful body area. Less commonly, a patient may complain of lacerating pain (7% to 26%) or pricking pain (6% to 30%).[13,14] When pain is evoked, it can be caused by a nociceptive source that induces pain out of proportion to the stimulus (hyperpathia). Bovie and colleagues found that 59% of patients with CPSP had hyperalgesia in the painful region on pinprick testing, 37% had hypoalgesia, and only

4% had a normal pinprick sensation.[16] Patients with stroke lesions in the thalamus are more likely to report that pinprick sensation is hyperalgesic.

Pain can also be evoked by non-nociceptive sources (allodynia), but the actual clinical response to different nonpainful stimuli can vary. Most patients will have some allodynia on examination, but as many as a third will have none. Of those with allodynia, the majority will experience pain with limb movement (70%), although some find that movement relieves the pain (19%). Thermal and tactile stimulation can evoke pain or reduce it as well. Nearly half of patients will have pain with cold stimuli (48%), but a few find that cold reduces their discomfort (7%). A warm stimulus was found to increase pain in 22% and reduce it in another 30%. Frequently, patients will find that emotions increase pain (19%), and 37% achieve relief of pain with rest.[13]

Just over half (52%) of patients with CPSP have no hemiplegia, and only 37% have moderate hemiplegia. Severe hemiplegia is less commonly associated (11%). On the other hand, ataxia is present in 62%, but choreoathetosis is found in only about 4%.[14]

Establishing a definitive diagnosis of CPSP is difficult and requires a thorough clinical assessment, elimination of other causes of the pain, and cranial imaging to confirm the presence of an appropriate brain lesion. Klit and associates[17] recommended that definitive criteria for CPSP require that the patient have a history of stroke with an associated lesion on imaging and that the pain have a plausible anatomic distribution both by history and physical examination. Before confirming the diagnosis of CPSP, other possible causes of the pain must be excluded (Box 27.1).

Box 27.1 Diagnostic Criteria for Central Post-stroke Pain Syndrome

Exclusion of other probable causes of the pain
Pain with a distinct neuroanatomically plausible distribution
A history suggestive of stroke
Indication of a distinct neuroanatomic distribution by clinical examination
Indication of a relevant vascular lesion by imaging

From Klit H, Finnerup NB, Jensen TS. Central post-stroke pain: clinical characteristics, pathophysiology, and management. *Lancet Neurol.* 2009;8:857-868.

PATHOPHYSIOLOGY

In lecture II of a series of lectures published in 1906 under the title "The Integrative Action of the Nervous System," C.S. Sherrington introduced the division of sensory systems into an *exteroceptive pathway* and an *interoceptive pathway*.[18,19] The exteroceptive pathway begins with receptors in the skin and muscle that transmit stimuli external to the body. This pathway can transmit both nociceptive and non-nociceptive stimuli, with the nociceptive stimuli traveling along the spinothalamocortical tracts. Fibers in this conventional pathway ascend along the lateral spinothalmic tract through brainstem and terminate in the ventrolateral (VL) thalamus. Fibers from the VL thalamus terminate in both the primary (SI) and secondary (SII) somatosensory cortices in the anterior parietal region. Additional fibers ascend from the VL thalamus to the motor cortex (M1) in the precentral gyrus.

The interoceptive pathway, in contrast, responds to signals originating within the body, such as the viscera, and travels along a distinct pathway called the lamina I spinothalmocortical tract (Fig. 27.1). This pathway manages afferent signals that transmit information about the physiologic condition of the entire body and thereby modulates homeostasis, visceral pain, and thermoregulatory activity.[20] Fibers along this tract ascend to the ventromedial thalamus, which then provides a rich supply of afferent input to the insular cortex. The lamina I system also has input to the periaqueductal gray and parabrachial nucleus, which send signals to the anterior cingulate cortex via the medial thalamus. This input influences the emotional state of the individual. The insular cortex modulates this by providing inhibitory feedback to the periaqueductal gray and parabrachial nucleus (see Fig. 27.1). Lesions along either the exteroceptive or interoceptive pathway can result in reduced or altered sensation.

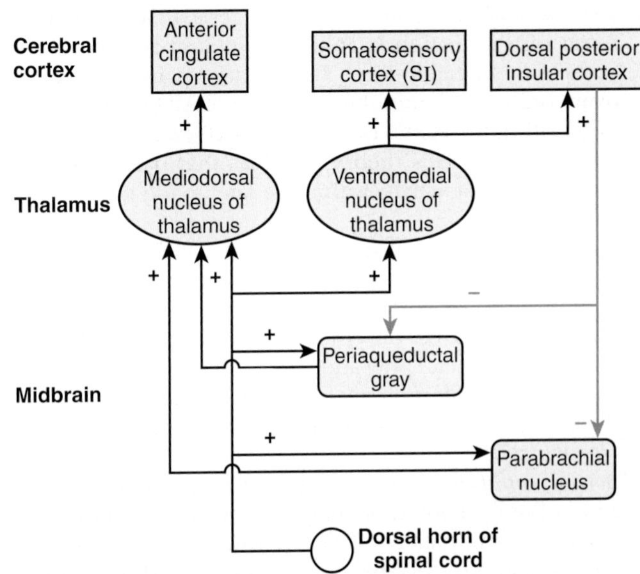

Figure 27.1 The lamina I spinothalamocortical sensory (interoceptive) pathway, which has a role in modulating thermoregulatory activity, homeostasis, and visceral pain. Afferent signals reach the anterior cingulate gyrus via brainstem nuclei (periaqueductal gray and parabrachial nucleus) and the medial dorsal thalamus. The anterior cingulate gyrus along with the rest of the limbic system regulates the emotional state of the individual. Afferent information also reaches the insular cortex through the ventromedial thalamus, which in part functions as a negative feedback to the brainstem nuclei. Disruption of these connections plays an important role in central pain. (From Harvey RL. Central poststroke pain syndrome. *Top Stroke Rehabil.* 2010;17:163-172.)

The pathophysiology of CPSP has not been clarified but probably results from maladaptive neuroplastic changes within the CNS that result in aberrant sensory perception. CPSP can be considered a kind of "deafferentation phenomenon" because lesions are located within the spinothalamocortical pathway and probably resulting in maladaptive alterations in synaptic facilitation and inhibition. Less likely would be a type of "release phenomenon" in which lesions of the lemniscal pathway carrying nonpainful sensation leave the pain pathways and unbalanced pain signals are transmitted to the cortical centers.[21] Because lemniscal injury is neither critical nor necessary for the development of CPSP, this later theory lacks much scientific support.[15,16] Theories on the cause of CPSP are dependent on several concepts: first is that injury to the spinothalamocortical tracts is necessary; second, that the pain is a result of late neuroplastic changes within CNS; and third, that pain perception is linked closely to the emotional state of the individual and the behavioral drive that signals a homeostatic imbalance.[20] For example, disruption of the negative feedback loop to the midbrain homeostatic structures (see Fig. 27.1) might lead to unopposed afferent input to the anterior cingulate gyrus. Activity in the cingulate gyrus is associated with emotional distress. The current theories for CPSP follow.

Central disinhibition: This theory suggests that CPSP is a result of a reduction in inhibitory neural activity at the cortical or thalamic level. In addition, pain may derive from reduced γ-aminobutyric acid (GABA) concentrations within the spinal cord or cerebral levels.

Central excitation: This theory proposes that pain is due to abnormal burst activity within the lateral and medial thalamic nuclei.

Thermosensory inhibition: In this theory, CPSP is proposed to be due to loss of descending inhibitory control from the interoceptive cortical structures, including the dorsal posterior insula on brainstem homeostatic sites such as the periaqueductal gray and parabrachial nucleus, which in turn will result in unabated thermoregulatory drive to the medial thalamus and the anterior cingulate cortex (see Fig. 27.1).

Abnormal central modulation: This theory suggests that there is a loss of central non-noxious temperature fibers along the lamina I spinothalamocortical pathway above the motor decussation. Loss of fibers in this tract would disrupt the capability of the CNS to modulate temperature perception, which could cause symptoms of allodynia.

Loss of aminergic modulation: If there is a general reduction in adrenergic and serotonergic modulation within the CNS, the function of the afferent pathways may be altered and result in greater perception of pain.

Alteration of the N*-methyl-d-aspartate (NMDA)-glutamate system*: Thalamocortical excitability might be enhanced by increased glutaminergic NMDA stimulation and result in changes consistent with long-term potentiation that enhance the perception of pain.

These different proposed mechanisms may all be involved in the development of CPSP, or different mechanisms may be involved. For example, some of the theories listed were formulated by considering the pharmacology of medications that have shown efficacy in treating CPSP, including their inhibitory, excitatory, or modulating effects on CNS activity. It is important to note that because there are a number of medications with different pharmacologic mechanisms and no single medication is completely effective, it is likely that CPSP has multiple physiologic causes associated with neuropharmacologic changes at multiple locations. In any one patient, multiple pain-inducing mechanisms may also be at play. This not only complicates our understanding of the etiology of CPSP but also complicates management as well.

Box 27.2 Pharmacologic Management of Central Post-stroke Pain Syndrome

Membrane stabilizers: carbamazepine, intravenous lidocaine
Aminergic agents: amitriptyline, fluvoxamine, duloxetine (a study showed a trend toward improved pain scores[21])
Antiglutaminergic agents: ketamine, lamotrigine (a study showed a reduction in pain scores but no clear effect on evoked pain[22])
γ-Aminobutyric acid agonists: oral baclofen may be efficacious
N-type calcium channel blockers: pregabalin, possibly gabapentin

PHARMACOLOGIC MANAGEMENT

Use of medication for the treatment of CPSP is part of the overall comprehensive approach to pain management, which also includes physical conditioning, modification of functional task performance, supportive counseling, and behavior modification. Thus, pharmacology is not used in isolation, especially since the clinical response to treatment with medications is literally "fifty-fifty." That is, at best only about half the patients will derive any benefit from the medications prescribed, and those who do will have only about 50% relief of their symptoms. Medications useful in managing CPSP fall into five categories: membrane stabilizers, aminergic agents, glutamate antagonists, GABA agonists, and N-type calcium channel blockers (Box 27.2).[23] When medications are used, it is recommended that one class be tried at a time and if one class fails, a medication from a different class be used for the next trial.

MEMBRANE-STABILIZING AGENTS

Anticonvulsants and antiarrhythmic agents provide a neural membrane-stabilizing effect that may have a tempering effect on CPSP. Carbamazepine was tested by Leijon and Bovie (along with amitriptyline and placebo) in a double-blind, three-phase, placebo-controlled crossover trial. Each of the three drugs was administered in a randomized manner over a period of 4 weeks separated by a 1-week washout in patients with CPSP.[24] Carbamazepine had a modest, but not statistically significant, effect in reducing pain scores in 36% of patients with CPSP versus a 7% reduction during the placebo phase. Side effects of carbamazepine included vertigo, tiredness, and gait disturbance. Phenytoin has not been well studied for CPSP, but in a small study in which eight subjects had central pain associated with thalamic injury, three had improved pain scores and three others had worse pain. Intravenous lidocaine has the capacity to reduce pain associated with stroke, as demonstrated in a randomized, double-blind, crossover trial of lidocaine, 5 mg/kg administered over a 30-minute period; 62.5% of patients with central pain from spinal cord injury or stroke experienced a reduction in spontaneous pain and brush-induced or mechanical allodynia for 45 minutes following drug infusion.[25] When placebo was given, only 37.5% of subjects had any reduction in spontaneous pain, and evoked pain was not affected. In another small case series, Edmonson and colleagues used intravenous boluses of lidocaine, 50 to 100 mg given over a 2-minute period. The four patients with CPSP reported reduced pain within 12 hours of drug administration.[26] Lightheadedness is common during and after lidocaine infusion. Mexiletine is an oral antiarrhythmic similar to lidocaine but was not well tolerated in a clinical trial. Oral doses of mexiletine of between 400 and 800 mg daily improved pain in 30% to 88% of patients, but many stopped taking the medication because of side effects, including nausea, dyspepsia, chest pain, and tiredness.[25-27] Thus, antiarrhythmic agents may have some efficacy in relieving CPSP, but the currently available drugs are impractical for clinical use. Presently, of the membrane-stabilizing agents, carbamazepine has the best, albeit limited efficacy.

AMINERGIC AGENTS

The aminergic agents include antidepressant medications that modify norepinephrine and serotonin centrally. Leigon and Bovie studied amitriptyline, a tricyclic antidepressant, in the placebo-controlled crossover trial mentioned in the last section.[24] Given at a maximum dose of 75 mg daily, amitriptyline resulted in a reduction in pain scores in 67% of patients versus 7% during the placebo phase ($P < 0.05$) and outperformed carbamazepine in comparison. Patients experienced only mild side effects, including tiredness and dry mouth. An open-label trial of the serotonin-specific reuptake inhibitor fluvoxamine (25 to 125 mg) given over a period of 2 to 4 weeks resulted in 31 subjects experiencing a mean pain reduction of 22% on a visual analog scale ($P < 0.01$).[28] Chronic stroke patients did not fare as well as those who were within 1 year of stroke onset. Duloxetine, a mixed serotonin and norepinephrine reuptake inhibitor, has also been studied in a randomized placebo-controlled trial lasting 8 weeks.[21] At doses of 60 to 120 mg daily in patients with either stroke- or spinal cord–related pain, there was a trend toward improved pain scores on a visual analog scale, but a significant reduction in brush ($P = 0.035$) and cold ($P < 0.001$) allodynia. The pain disability index was not different between groups, but patients taking duloxetine had significant improvement in the bodily pain domain of the 36-item Short-Form Health Survey (SF-36). Duloxetine was associated with more somnolence. In all these studies on aminergic agents, the reduction in pain was independent of any effects on depression. Presently, amitriptyline is recommended as the drug of first choice from the adrenergic class for treatment of CPSP.

ANTIGLUTAMINERGIC AGENTS

Glutamine is a potent stimulator of NMDA receptors and calcium channels. Ketamine is an NMDA receptor antagonist that by blocking the action of glutamine postsynaptically has the effect of possibly inducing long-term depression in cortical and subcortical regions. After receiving intravenous ketamine, 48% of subjects with CPSP experienced an average 40% reduction in pain, with the effect lasting less than an hour after the infusion ended.[29] Oral and transdermal administration of ketamine has not been studied. Dextromethorphan, also an NMDA receptor antagonist, failed to show any efficacy in CPSP after administration of a standard oral dose.[30] Higher dosing schedules have not been studied. Lamotrigine reduces release of glutamine presynaptically by acting as a voltage-dependent sodium channel blocker. In a double-blind, placebo-controlled, crossover trial, 30 subjects with CPSP were given 200 mg of lamotrigine or placebo in 8-week treatment phases separated by a 2-week washout. The results showed a reduction in visual analog pain scores by a mean value of 2 points, but no clear effect on evoked pain.[22] The side effects of lamotrigine were minor and included rash and worse pain. Lamotrigine is therefore a reasonable choice from the glutaminergic class for the treatment of CPSP.

GABA AGONISTS

Thiopental is a potent $GABA_A$ agonist in the barbiturate class. Yamamoto and colleagues showed a statistically significant reduction in pain in 56% of patients with CPSP.[29] In another trial of intravenous propofol (a $GABA_A$ agonist), pain was reduced in more than 70% of subjects with CPSP and in patients with other forms of central pain, although it was ineffective for peripheral neuropathic pain.[31] Baclofen is a $GABA_B$ agonist and was studied for treatment of CPSP in a case series by Tiara and others.[32] A bolus of intrathecal baclofen was given to five subjects, and some pain reduction was achieved in four of them. Another trial of oral baclofen given to patients who responded to an intrathecal infusion was not effective. Long-term use of intrathecal baclofen via an implanted pump has not been studied. Intrathecal midazolam has been shown to cause a transient reduction in central pain in one patient with spinal cord injury, but it has not been similarly tested in subjects with CPSP.[33] The GABA agonists have limited use for CPSP, but oral baclofen may be efficacious in some cases.

N-TYPE CALCIUM CHANNEL BLOCKERS

Gabapentin and pregabalin, drugs that are structural analogs of GABA, are commonly used to treat central pain. They have a unique mechanism of action, however, most likely associated with impairment of transmembrane trafficking of voltage gated N-type calcium channels by binding to the $\alpha_2\delta$ subunit of the channel protein.[34] Vranken and colleagues studied 40 subjects with central pain, 12 of whom had strokes. Subjects were randomized to either pregabalin, 150 to 600 mg daily, or placebo. Those receiving pregabalin had a mean reduction in visual analog score by 2.5 points with no corresponding reduction after placebo.[35] Pregabalin was also associated with improved SF-36 pain scores, but there was no reduction in pain-related disability. Gabapentin has yet to be studied for CPSP, but one study did demonstrate a significant reduction in brush allodynia and pinprick hyperalgesia, but no change in spontaneous pain, after experimental intradermal injection of the irritant capsaicin.[36] Pregabalin and gabapentin are agents worthy of trial from this class, but they are clinically often limited by side effects in patients with post-stroke pain.

NONPHARMACOLOGIC APPROACHES

TRANSCUTANEOUS ELECTRICAL NERVE STIMULATION

In a single small study assessing the efficacy of transcutaneous electrical nerve stimulation (TENS) for CPSP, 15 subjects with CPSP underwent TENS treatment consisting of high- and low-frequency stimulation applied to either the side of body, ipsilateral or contralateral to the pain.[37] The results of this study were mixed in that four subjects (27%) experienced clinically important pain relief by an average of 42%, five experienced a transient increase in pain, and the remaining six had no change in their pain characteristics.

DEEP BRAIN STIMULATION

Several clinical trials and case studies have described the use of deep brain stimulation (DBS) for CPSP; however, these reports present conflicting information on efficacy. Owen and others implanted deep electrodes in 15 patients into both the ventroposterolateral (VPL) thalamus and the periventricular gray (PVG) regions with an externalized stimulator.[38] Following trial stimulation, a fully implanted system was placed if the subject responded to the use of one or both electrodes. Seventy percent of the patients with either cortical or subcortical stroke responded positively to DBS with a reduction in visual analog score by 42% to 54%. In contrast, Rasche and colleagues studied the use of DBS in patients with various causes of central pain, including some with CPSP. These patients also received implants in both the VPL thalamus and PVG region. Among the 11 stroke survivors implanted, only 2 (18%) had any relief, and many of the nonresponders had an increase in pain.[39] Current evidence suggests that placement of the electrode in the PVG region might be preferred because stimulation in this area has been shown to reduce low-frequency field potentials in the thalamus in association with pain relief.[40] A recent case study reported a patient with a right temporoparietal lesion who had significant pain relief after DBS of the PVG region. This patient's pain relief was also associated with normalization of sensory testing, including resolution of allodynia and improved sensory discrimination.[41] Although PVG implantation seems to show better efficacy than VPL implantation in the CPSP literature, implantation within the centromedian thalamic nuclei, also involved in the motivational-affective components of pain, may be another option worth exploring further in clinical trials.[42]

MOTOR CORTEX STIMULATION

Motor cortex stimulation (MCS) involves the surgical implantation of a surface electrode usually over the dura covering the precentral gyrus, contralateral to the area of pain. The electrode is connected to a pacemaker-like pulse generator implanted subcutaneously over the chest wall.[43] Direct implantation of the electrode in the subdural space over the M1 cortex or within the central sulcus has been tried as well.[44] Selection of the precentral gyrus rather than the postcentral gyrus was determined by the early work of Tsubokawa and others, who found better pain relief with MCS than with stimulation of the primary sensory cortex.[45] Using the epidural approach, they achieved a 67% to 73% response rate to MCS, defined as at least a 50% reduction in visual analog scale score.[45,46] Acceptable pain relief lasted beyond a year in many patients following implantation, although some experienced recurrence of pain after a few months. In another study, MCS achieved a mean 83% reduction in visual analog score in the 32 subjects who reported reduced pain, 11 of whom had pain following stroke.[47] Katayama and associates achieved greater than a 60% reduction in pain for at least 2 years in nearly half of patients with CPSP in whom an MCS device had been implanted.[48] In a recent review of the efficacy of MCS for chronic pain, Fontaine and associates noted that among all causes, 54% of patients will have a good response to MCS, with the best responders being those with CPSP and trigeminal neuralgia.[49] MCS implantation is not without complications, including infection (5.7%), hardware failure (5.1%), and postoperative seizures (12%), but there have not been any cases of chronic epilepsy.[49]

Canvero and Bonicalzi described several clinical factors that predict success with MCS after implantation of the device.[50] Patients with CPSP have the best outcomes with MCS if they have intact or nearly intact motor function.[48] A normal thermal sensory threshold in the painful body region is also a predictor of clinically relevant pain relief.[51] Pain relief following presurgical intravenous infusion of ketamine or barbiturate predicts a better response to MCS than if pain relief is achieved with an intravenous infusion of morphine.[29] A positive response to intravenous infusion of propofol can also be used to identify candidates for MCS.[43,50,52] Pain relief following repetitive transcranial magnetic stimulation (rTMS) can have predictive value for success with MCS.[50,53-55] Given the invasive nature of epidural cortical stimulators, it has been recommended that these clinical variables be used for patient selection before electrode implantation.

An alternative to epidural implantation might be noninvasive cortical stimulation. rTMS uses a magnetic coil to provide electromagnetic pulses over the cranial surface that induce local currents in the underlying cortex and, as noted, can predict outcomes with MCS. When used as a treatment modality for central pain, both low- and high-frequency rTMS has shown some efficacy in reducing pain, at least transiently.[52-54,56,57] Providing several sessions of rTMS can result in longer-lasting pain relief. As with MCS, rTMS is targeted to the motor cortex contralateral to the pain, which provides better pain reduction than does stimulation of the SI cortex, supplementary motor area, or premotor area.[50] Individuals with lesions in the thalamic region show a better response to rTMS than do subjects with brainstem strokes.[58] A critical limitation of rTMS is that the pain relief is at best transient and lasts just a few hours. Additional clinical trials using various rTMS stimulation parameters and TMS combined with pharmacology may reveal methods to achieve potent and prolonged pain relief in patients with CPSP.[59]

Transcranial direct current stimulation (tDCS) uses a low-voltage (1 mA) direct current between two electrodes, one over the motor cortex and the other over the contralateral orbit. No clinical trials using tDCS have been published for the treatment of CPSP, but this modality has shown efficacy in patients with fibromyalgia and central pain after spinal cord injury.[60,61] Future studies using tDCS with anodal stimulation over the motor cortex, contralateral to the side of pain, may demonstrate utility, and it could prove to be more clinically practical than rTMS because tDCS could potentially be used at home with proper patient education.

It is presently unclear how stimulation of the motor cortex reduces pain in patients with CPSP. Tsubokawa and colleagues suggested that central pain is a result of aberrant plastic changes in the inhibitory receptive fields of the sensory cortex such that non-noxious input can stimulate nociceptive neurons centrally. Thus they have proposed that MCS blocks these aberrant connections either through orthodromic stimulation via motor neuron pathways to the SI cortex or through antidromic stimulation of sensory fibers that project from the SI cortex.[46] Garcia-Larrea and others were not able to support this concept with positron emission tomography (PET). In their study, regional blood flow during MCS was increased primarily in the VL thalamus, a thalamic region described earlier that has rich connections with the M1 cortex and postcentral regions.[62] The PET findings demonstrated no increased regional blood flow in M1 or SI during stimulation of the motor cortex. Similarly, Goto and colleagues used diffusion tensor imaging to evaluate white matter fiber tract integrity in patients with CPSP[63] and found that patients with intact thalamocortical tracts had a better response with rTMS targeted to the motor cortex than did subjects lacking integrity of these fibers. PET scanning also demonstrates increases in regional blood flow within other structures in association with MCS, including structures such as the medial thalamus, anterior cingulate gyrus, upper brainstem, and contralateral insular cortex. These structures make up portions of the lamina I spinothalamocortical (interoceptive) pathway, which has a significant role in pain processing as discussed previously (see Fig. 27.1). It seems plausible, then, that MCS might reduce CPSP via orthodromic and antidromic stimulation of the thalamus via the thalamocortical pathways, which may have a neuromodulating effect on pain-processing structures, including the anterior cingulate, brainstem structures, and insular cortex.[44,63] Some have proposed that MCS works via GABA mediation because patients who respond to an intravenous propofol infusion ($GABA_A$ agonist) also respond well to MCS. It is also possible that MCS modulates pain through descending cortical spinal pathways that connect to dorsal horn structures.[63]

MCS is currently available only for off-label use in the United States for the treatment of central pain, but growing evidence of potential long-term efficacy that is superior to pharmacologic management might bring it to the forefront of clinical practice, at least as one option among many of the current choices available.

KEY POINTS

- Central post-stroke pain (CPSP) is an uncommon, but significant, complication of stroke and is one of the most frequent causes of central pain syndrome. Although several options for clinical management are available, they may not result in optimal clinical outcomes.
- A well-coordinated pain management program using interdisciplinary techniques is the preferred setting for treating CPSP.
- Current recommendations for the first line of pharmacologic treatment of CPSP include amitriptyline, lamotrigine, and pregabalin or gabapentin. Baclofen and the selective serotonin reuptake inhibitors may also have a potential secondary role in treatment.
- Motor cortex stimulation applied noninvasively or with epidural implantation of a stimulating electrode may have a role when patients are carefully selected through well-studied presurgical and surgical protocols.

SUGGESTED READINGS

Boivie J, Leijon G, Johansson I. Central post-stroke pain: a study of the mechanisms through analysis of the sensory abnormalities. *Pain.* 1989;37:173-185.

Bowsher D. Central pain: clinical and physiological characteristics. *Neurol Neurosurg Psychiatry.* 1996;61:62-69.

Craig AD. How do you feel? Interoception: the sense of the physiological condition of the body. *Nat Rev Neurosci.* 2002;3:655-666.

Fregni F, Freedman S, Pascual-Leone A. Recent advances in the treatment of chronic pain with non-invasive brain stimulation techniques. *Lancet Neurol.* 2007;6:188-191.

Jonsson AC, Lindgren I, Hallstrom B, et al. Prevalence and intensity of pain after stroke: a population based study focusing on patients' perspectives. *J Neurol Neurosurg Psychiatry.* 2006;77:590-595.

Katayama Y, Fukaya C, Yamamoto T. Poststroke pain control by chronic motor cortex stimulation: neurological characteristics predicting a favorable response. *J Neurosurg.* 1998;89:585-591.

Kumar G, Soni CR. Central post-stroke pain: current evidence. *J Neurol Sci.* 2009;284:10-17.

Leijon G, Boivie J. Central post-stroke pain: a controlled trial of amitriptyline and carbamazepine. *Pain.* 1989;36:27-36.

Leijon G, Boivie J, Johansson I. Central post-stroke pain—neurological symptoms and pain characteristics. *Pain.* 1989;36:13-25.

Tsubokawa T, Katayama Y, Yamamoto T, et al. Chronic motor stimulation for the treatment of central pain. *Acta Neurochir Suppl.* 1991;52:137-139.

Tsubokawa T, Katayama Y, Yamomoto T, et al. Chronic motor cortex stimulation in patients with thalamic pain. *J Neurosurg.* 1993;78:393-401.

Vestergaard K, Andersen G, Gottrup H, et al. Lamotrigine for central post-stroke pain: a randomized controlled trial. *Neurology.* 2001;56:184-190.

Vranken JH, Dijkgraaf MGW, Kruis MR, et al. Pregabalin in patients with central neuropathic pain: a randomized, double-blind, placebo-controlled trial of a flexible-dose regimen. *Pain.* 2008;136:150-157.

Vranken JH, Hollmann MW, van der Vegt MH, et al. Duloxetine in patients with central neuropathic pain caused by spinal cord injury or stroke: a randomized double-blind, placebo-controlled trial. *Pain.* 2011;152:267-273.

Yamamoto T, Katayama Y, Hirayama T, et al. Pharmacological classification of central post-stroke pain: comparison with the results of chronic motor cortex stimulation therapy. *Pain.* 1997;72:5-12.

The references for this chapter can be found at www.expertconsult.com.

28 Spinal Cord Injury Pain

R. Norman Harden | Amy J. Kirsling | Katrina M. Thomas | Robert P. Yezierski

The chronic pain associated with injury or disease of the central nervous system (CNS) represents a long-standing puzzle, presents a significant challenge to scientific and health care communities, and is consequently a significant barrier to optimal rehabilitation and quality of life in these patients. The mystery of how a lesion in systems that mediate pain perception can actually produce pain continues to baffle those searching for an underlying mechanism. The evidence that we have clearly points to a complicated and heterogeneous pathophysiology and, as in all chronic disease, involvement of psychosocial components. Because therapy for pain from spinal cord injury (SCI) is challenging, it is clear that a more comprehensive understanding of the mechanisms of disease (treatment targets) is crucial. This chapter focuses on clinical identification of the mechanisms and subsets of this condition, its pathobiology, and the current (rather weak) evidence base for treatments.[1,2]

PREVALENCE AND INCIDENCE

Pain is a frequent consequence of paraplegia and tetraplegia following both complete and incomplete spinal cord lesions.[1] The development of pain after SCI was first described over 100 years ago, and currently more than 600,000 individuals in the United States live with SCI, with approximately 11,000 new such injuries occurring per year.[1,3,4] Historically, the loss of sensory, motor, bowel, bladder, and sexual function was viewed as the most significant consequences of SCI. However, the onset and presence of pain directly relate to the ability of patients to regain optimal levels of function and quality of life, and unmanaged pain may be a principal cause of the failure of optimal rehabilitation.[4,5] An early study reported that 37% of SCI patients with cervical or high thoracic lesions would trade relief of pain for any chance at regaining motor function.[6] In one survey, 11% of respondents reported that pain rather than loss of motor function prevented them from working.[1,7] In another study, 37% of patients experiencing SCI pain rated the pain as "very difficult to deal with" (rating it from 7 to 10 on a scale from 0 to 10).[5] These and many other studies lend support to the pervasive and negative impact of pain on function and quality of life following SCI.[1]

Historical prevalence analyses of any type of pain after SCI have found it to range from 34% to 96% (approximate mean of 67%) in studies published between 1947 and 1991. More recent studies using more comprehensive pain assessment strategies indicate that the overall prevalence of all types of SCI pain ranges from 70% to 80%.[5,8,9]

CLASSIFICATION/TAXONOMY

Clinical observations suggest that the variety of pain syndromes associated with SCI together with the lack of a unified taxonomy has been the principal impediment to not only accurate epidemiologic studies but also effective clinical research.[4,10-12] The International Spinal Cord Injury Pain classification was proposed after review by major SCI and pain organizations and validation using vignettes. In this system, the type of SCI pain is classified as nociceptive (visceral, musculoskeletal, or other) or neuropathic (resulting from a disease or lesion of the somatosensory nervous system). Neuropathic pain following SCI is further classified as neuropathic pain directly related to the SCI (at-level or below-level pain, where level refers to the neurologic level of injury) or other neuropathic pain (indirectly related or unrelated to the SCI).[1,13,14] The SCI Pain Task Force of the International Association for the Study of Pain has proposed a similar taxonomy, which represents a further step toward a mechanism-based classification. This taxonomy is divided into three tiers. In the first tier, pain is divided into nociceptive pain (i.e., pain attributable to non-neurogenic tissue damage) and neuropathic pain (i.e., pain attributable to damage to peripheral or central nervous tissue, or both).[15,16]

The most straightforward and logical classification scheme for clinical assessment simply categorizes pain below the lesion (true "central pain" phenomena), pain at the level of the lesion (most like radiculopathic/neuropathic), and pain above the lesion (often called "musculoskeletal" in the literature). Another important source or cause of pain in clinical diagnosis is pain evoked in a viscus ("visceral pain"). In one study of the incidence and prevalence of different types of pain in a cohort of 100 patients, musculoskeletal pain (above the lesion, 59%) was the most common type, followed by at-level (41%) and below-level (34%) neuropathic pain. Visceral pain (5%) was the least common.[4,17] The mean time until onset of any type of SCI pain was 1.6 years. The shortest onset times were recorded for at-level pain (1.2 years) and pain above the level of injury ("musculoskeletal," 1.3 years). Below-level neuropathic pain (1.8 years) and visceral pain (4.2 years) developed later.[17] The delayed onset of pain can potentially cause some confusion for patients who believe that the onset of sensations corresponds to neurologic recovery and thus may present a minor clinical difficulty for physicians who are aware of the reality that these sensations may represent the development of a pathologic condition that complicates the day-to-day management of patients.[4]

Among all types of SCI pain, below-level pain (central pain) is the most common (23% to 52%) and could be the most difficult to treat.[6,11,17-25] Below-level pain is described as the "most severe or excruciating" of all SCI pain reported.[17,18]

Often accompanying below-level pain is autonomic dysreflexia, which is a potentially life-threatening condition triggered by sensory input below the lesion (spasticity, sympathetic nervous system afferent input). Symptoms associated with autonomic dysreflexia include increased or decreased blood pressure and pulse, headache, and a risk for cerebral hemorrhage, cardiovascular collapse, and seizures.

At-level pain is also common (12% to 42%) and "severe" and can likewise be quite difficult to treat.[17,26] Pain at the level of the lesion may result not only from damage to peripheral nerves near the site of entry into the cord but also from damage to central neural elements and tracts; thus, the pain mechanisms associated with this type of pain are probably various and complicated.[17,26]

Above-level pain generators are common (60%) and heterogeneous, such as those of "ergonomic" pathology secondary to overuse of the shoulders and arms causing myofascial pain in the shoulder joints from wheelchair use, or "crutch palsy" as a result of mechanical compression of nerves from orthotics. Above-level pain may also be due to mechanics such as secondary changes following fractures and fixation. Above-level pain is important to identify because it is often the easiest to treat effectively.[17,26]

Visceral pain is usually manifested as dull or cramping abdominal sensations that may be associated with nausea and autonomic reactions. The pain may be related to bowel, bladder, or kidney dysfunction or distention but may also represent a neuropathic type of pain. It is not known whether there is a central component responsible for visceral pain, but damage to central afferent terminals is known to have peripheral consequences. Because SCI patients may not have the typical signs of abdominal illness, a high index of clinical suspicion should be maintained, which requires careful examination whenever any new pain or changes in existing pain occur. Increases in spasticity, pain at any location, or an autonomic reaction may be the only indication of abdominal organ dysfunction. Autonomic dysfunction may complicate the management of SCI patients with a lesion above the splanchnic outflow (sixth thoracic level).[15] At-level and below-level allodynia, hyperalgesia (evoked pain), and spontaneous pain historically represent the primary targets of both basic and clinical research.[1,10,11]

PATHOLOGY AND MECHANISMS

SCI pain is related to the nature of the lesion, damage to neurologic structures, secondary pathophysiologic changes in surviving tissue (neural and non-neural tissue), and associated psychosocial syndromes.[1] Because pain is a significant consequence of SCI, it is crucial to understand the mechanisms involved to target therapy more efficiently. Experimental models reveal crucial insights related to the potential mechanisms responsible for pain following SCI.[1,27,28] These models and methods try to explain a complicated series of anatomic and functional changes seen in spinal and supraspinal locations. There are many similarities between the cellular and chemical events that occur after SCI and those that follow peripheral nerve injury. Furthermore, neuropathic lesions are easier to study (both with animal models and clinically), and there is considerably more evidence in the treatment of neuropathies.[29,30] Thus, because of the absence of much useful evidence on the treatment of SCI pain, we must often extrapolate mechanisms and therapy from the more extensive peripheral neuropathy literature.[4,31,32]

Traumatic or ischemic damage to the spinal cord triggers a dynamic cascade of molecular, biochemical, anatomic ("plasticity"), and cellular responses. These events in turn produce physiologic changes at both the spinal and supraspinal level that contribute to the onset of dysesthetic sensations, prominently pain.[27,29,33] With evolution of the concept of the "central injury cascade" and its role in initiation and maintenance of SCI pain, there has been good progress in determining certain characteristics of each step involved. Injury to the spinal cord ultimately results in abnormal sensory processing in most cases. Contributing to this are changes in the level of neuronal excitability (the "irritable focus"), denervation supersensitivity (and loss of diffuse noxious inhibitory controls), inactivation or activation of cellular signaling pathways, and glial-neuronal interactions.[27,33] Cord injuries obviously cause structural damage but can also lead to reorganization of the spinal and supraspinal circuits that integrate process and transmit sensory information. There are also changes in the supralesional centers and their chemical mediators that maintain the balance between inhibition and excitation.[1,24,34] Primary and secondary events also ultimately result in afferent dysesthesias and efferent modulation, which result in pathologic changes in the initiation, perception, and maintenance of injury-induced pain.[1,8,33] There is an expectation that the completeness (as in surviving tracts) or level of injury should correlate with the onset and type of pain. However, despite a hypothetical correlation between incomplete as well as thoracolumbar lesions and a higher incidence of pain, studies have not identified any other consistent predictors.[20,35,36] One very significant problem in understanding and studying pain in SCI is the vagaries of the clinical designations of "completeness." The American Spinal Injury Association (ASIA) system, though superficially useful in physiatric practice, is not helpful in determining the actual physiologic status of cord structures.[37] Thus, clinically "complete" lesions by ASIA criteria are rarely physiologically or anatomically complete in the sense that there are often surviving tracts (afferent and efferent) and frequently intact and disinhibited sympathetic chains. Reliance on the ASIA system for research categorization is a dead end. Research cannot progress, particularly treatment research, without a surviving tract and functional status subset analysis by formal psychophysical and biometric measurements.[33]

Central pain can be characterized as spontaneous or evoked, persistent or intermittent, and localized or diffuse. A significant number of patients report pain sensations such as "burning," "shooting," "radiating," "ice-like," "squeezing," and "stabbing." There may be allodynia, hyperalgesia, paresthesias, and various dysesthesias, sometimes evoked in "numb" areas. The pain can summate with repeated stimuli (wind-up) and linger with prolonged aftersensations.[1,38] Pain may be evoked or worsen with many peripheral sensory stimuli such as touch, vibration, and cold. It may arise from visceral or somatic structures or be evoked by infections, sudden noises, jarring movements, and distention of visceral structures, as well as by various affective conditions.[11,27] Evoked pain can be dramatic and typically persists long after the stimulation ceases (aftersensation). All these features are consistent with so-called central sensitization/augmentation of cerebral sensory processing.[39] Spontaneous pain varies greatly in character and is aggravated by stress and emotion, especially anxiety. It can be provoked or exacerbated by auditory, visual, olfactory, and visceral stimuli. Thus, when evaluating pain, it is critical to assess intensity, sensory signs and symptoms, physical and emotional triggers, mood, sociologic situations, and the quality of life of patients.[27]

Multiple hypotheses have been advanced to explain central pain, including the loss of spinal inhibitory mechanisms, the presence of pattern generators (irritable focus) within the injured cord, sensitization of supraspinal relay nuclei, synaptic plasticity (rewiring), activation of spinal and supraspinal microglia and astrocytes, changes in cellular signaling pathways at spinal and supraspinal sites, involvement of irritative or excitatory generators of the spinothalamic and lemniscal pathways, and loss of thermosensory inhibitory control over pain pathways (one type of diffuse noxious inhibitory control). There is also a possible contribution from altered gene expression.[1,33,40-51]

Another challenge in researching abnormal sensations following SCI is the development of experimental models of injury that are consistent with the pathologic pain characteristics seen in humans.[52] A number of models have been developed, including mechanical trauma, isolated lesions, complete transection, chemical lesions, and ischemic injury.[40,53-57] The events that follow SCI are dynamic, progress rostrally and caudally from the core of the lesion, and affect spinal, subcortical, and cortical structures.[27] Since there is a broad spectrum of pathophysiologic changes initiated by SCI, it is a challenge to identify which events have a causal relationship with the onset of pain and which are merely secondary consequences of the injury process in the evolution of pain. In human SCI, a variety of critical methods are available for studying and quantifying psychophysical function. Examples of these methods include thermal quantitative sensory testing (QST; small fibers, lateral spinothalamic tracts), vibration QST (large fibers, dorsal columns), and sympathetic skin response.[33]

Evidence of dysesthesia or pain responses at the level of spinal lesions has been provided by animal models of excitotoxicity, ischemia, and contusion injury.[40,43,57-62] The excitotoxic model simulates the elevation in excitatory amino acids that occurs after injury.[1,63,64] The most common experimental model is the weight drop or contusion model, and it is believed to be the most clinically relevant but is difficult to use in studies of sensory function because of hind limb paresis or paralysis interfering with behavioral responses. Although the contusion model has many characteristics in common with the human injury, it has been challenged as an inappropriate model for study of the altered sensation following injury. An alternative approach involves selected spinal lesions (such as cord hemisection) alone or combined with other interventions.[1,55,65-68] These various experimental models produce distinct pathologic or behavioral changes (or both) that appear to be relevant to human SCI, create opportunities to study mechanisms, and may prove useful in drug screening.[1,69,70]

Critical events in the aftermath of experimental SCI include a transient elevation in excitatory amino acids and the production of a variety of potentially toxic mediators such as endogenous opioids (dynorphin), prostaglandins, cytokines, nitric oxide, and reactive oxygen compounds.[33] Other consequences of SCI include upregulation of mRNA for tumor necrosis factor-α and dynorphin and activation of transcription and nuclear factors.[71-74] Activation of the NF-κB family of transcription factors is significant since it has a role in inducing more than 150 genes involved in inflammatory, proliferative, membrane excitatory, and cell death responses.[75]

Within the first 15 minutes after SCI, cell membranes start to break down and the phospholipase, arachidonic acid, and eicosanoid cascades are activated.[76] Reactive oxygen species are destructive by-products of these injury cascades.[77-79] There are significant increases in intracellular calcium.[80,81] Calcium is directly involved in multiple intracellular signaling pathways (including pain sensitization).[1,82] One hour after SCI, DNA microarray analysis has identified changes in the mRNA levels of 165 genes involved in regulating transcription factors, inflammatory processes, cell survival, and membrane excitability.[4,83] Within hours of injury, ion shifts result in cellular swelling and local edema, expansion of the extracellular space, loss of integrity of the blood–spinal cord barrier, and sustained depolarization in damaged cells. This collection of cellular and molecular events can have a profound impact on the functional state of spinal neurons and ultimately promote the onset of chronic pain. Since there are many possible contributing factors and processes, it is not likely that events occur in a uniform, orderly, or sequential manner.[27]

Descending influences may be involved in the at-level pain phenomena, such as pathways emanating from the rostral ventromedial (RVM) medulla.[84-86] The abnormal firing of sensory neurons reaches RVM neurons and completes a spinobulbospinal feedback loop that increases the hyperexcitability of neurons in the spinal cord.[1] Central sensitization and synaptic plasticity in the CNS are thought to contribute to acute and potentially persistent pain, although most research in this regard has been done on peripheral neuropathic pain.[1,33,87-89] Central sensitization is thought to involve changes in the excitability of spinal neurons and eventually in the development of spinal and potentially supraspinal pain generators and amplifiers.[33,90]

Despite evidence supporting the hypothesis that cellular or axonal damage predisposes an individual to both at-level and below-level pain, it may be clinically important to distinguish between these regionally distinct categories of pain. It is interesting to point out that SCI pain may be reported in a progressive sequence from at-level to below-level pain, thus implying that the two clinical entities interact. This suggests the possibility that the abnormal neural activity (spinal or supraspinal) associated with at-level pain predisposes an individual to the development of below-level pain (SCI-type central pain). Importantly, the hypothetical influence of abnormal activity in gray matter nuclei may also influence the development of below-level pain after specific white matter damage.[1]

Following complete spinal transection, pain is reported below the injury with common descriptions such as "uncomfortable sensations," "tightness," or "burning." Severe pain may also follow hemisection.[1] One of the most illustrative conditions that give rise to central pain is syringomyelia.[91] More than half of patients with delayed-onset central pain after a spinal injury have syringomyelia, and it appears that the pathophysiologic changes in spinal tissue surrounding the syrinx itself are responsible for the pain.[92] Damage to Lissauer's tract by root avulsion can also cause very intense and difficult-to-treat pain syndromes.[1,93]

Pathologic damage to the central cord is particularly prominent following vertebral dislocation, an injury that compresses the spinal cord and destroys gray matter, typically with variable white matter involvement. In contrast, surgical interruption or compression of long spinal pathways usually involves only portions of the gray matter either directly or by disruption of the blood supply to injured segments.[94] The gray matter damage resulting from these types of lesions more often results in pain. However, when central damage to the cord is minimized by making superficial lesions in one anterolateral column, prolonged contralateral hypoalgesia is produced without chronic pain, allodynia, or hyperalgesia.[4,65,95]

One of the challenges in studying below-level pain is finding a behavioral measure that effectively engages the neuronal substrates thought to be involved in producing this type of pain. It is generally agreed that below-level pain has spinal as well as supraspinal (including thalamic and cortical) components. Therefore, to effectively evaluate below-level pain, it is necessary to use a behavioral measure that engages both these components. At present, behavioral measures that use operant tasks as the basis for behavioral responses are the only outcome measures that meet these criteria. For this reason, to effectively study below-level pain one must use an operant behavioral task. Unlike reflex responses, these tasks require cortical processing, an important component required for below-level pain. One difficulty in studying pain conditions in SCI is selection of suitable behavioral measures. For example, if the assumption is that to experience below-level pain the cortex must be engaged, the behavioral measures selected to be used in evaluating this type of pain must produce cortical activation. An example paradigm to test this would be through operant testing that requires cortical processing of afferent input, decision making based on environmental cues, and adapting behavior in response to nociceptive stimuli.[96] An example of an error in this regard would be to consider segmental reflex responses below the lesion as relevant in evaluating below-level pain.[33]

Gray matter damage appears to be an important factor in the development of below-level pain. A recent clinical study in patients with and without below-level pain showed that a common pathologic feature in patients with below-level pain was the involvement of lesions that included a central core of spinal gray matter.[1,97] Although reduced temperature and pain sensations have been used to support the involvement of damaged spinothalamic connections in the development of central pain, recent evidence has shown that neuronal hyperexcitability is also important in the development of below-level pain. Furthermore, loss of spinothalamic function did not appear to predict this type of pain.[98] This work complements previous magnetic resonance imaging findings showing that patients with below-level pain have larger gray matter lesions than do patients without pain.[97] Additional evidence supporting this conclusion comes from studies showing that anterolateral cord lesions result in evoked pain caudal to the spinal injury only when gray matter is involved and the fact that spontaneous pain behavior can be elicited with spinal lesions restricted to the gray matter.[57,99] Below-level pain may therefore be expressed when portions of supraspinal sensory processing targets are deprived of input from the classic pain pathways and then indirectly activated by other sources of alternative input from a dysfunctional neuronal core (i.e., pain-generating mechanism) rostral to the site of injury.[27,33]

Although the condition of pain after SCI is believed to originate from abnormal activity in the spinal cord, there is also support for the involvement of supraspinal structures, such as the diencephalon, that receive abnormal input from the injured cord. The contribution of this input, together with the effects of deafferentation (secondary to the death of spinal projection neurons), sprouting of undamaged fibers, and functional unmasking of nonfunctional local circuits, could contribute to the development of focal generators or amplifiers of abnormal discharges at supraspinal sites.[100,101] Two reports describing elevated blood flow in thalamic nuclei (possibly reflecting changes in metabolic demand and the functional state of thalamic neurons) lend support to thalamic involvement in supraspinal responses to SCI.[102,103] Complementing these observations are descriptions of changes in the concentration of metabolites (determined with in vivo magnetic resonance spectroscopy) in the ventral posterolateral nucleus of patients with and without SCI pain and reports of dysrhythmic thalamic activity in hyperreflexic rats following SCI. [29,104] Changes in the excitability of thalamic neurons represent a potential source of abnormal activity, as well as a site for amplification of incoming information from the spinal cord. Thus, below-level neuropathic pain may be expressed when portions of supraspinal targets are deprived of input from the spinothalamic and other spinal pathways and are activated by abnormal (spontaneous or evoked) activity from levels of the spinal cord above the level of injury.[4]

One factor that remains unclear in the mechanism of below-level pain is the precise role of spinal influences (i.e., abnormal activity near the site of the lesion—the penumbral region) in the maintenance of this type of pain. The transient relief of below-level pain in humans following the application of local anesthetic to the proximal stump of a spinal lesion or removal of segments of cord (cordectomy) rostral to the site of injury suggests that the presence of a spinal generator plays a significant role in maintaining chronic below-level pain. Thus, the supraspinal changes secondary to deafferentation and the emergence of a spinal generator of abnormal activity are two significant events that potentially contribute to the development and maintenance of below-level pain.[4,42]

Although the majority of SCI pain research has focused on spinal mechanisms of enhanced sensitivity, the potential role of descending (supraspinal) modulation (both facilitatory and inhibitory) should not be ignored. Given that neurokinin-1 receptor (NK1R)-expressing lamina I neurons represents the spinal effector of a bulbospinal projection system involving μ receptor–expressing neurons in the RVM medulla, one can speculate that this feedback system contributes to the condition of SCI pain, similar to the mechanism proposed following peripheral nerve and tissue damage.[32,84,105-108] The fact that RVM neurons undergo significant functional changes following spinal injury suggests that this region contributes to a central pain–generating mechanism following spinal injury.[109] Accordingly, experiments targeting lamina I NK1R-expressing neurons with the neurotoxin saporin conjugated to substance P showed that elimination of these neurons significantly reduced the onset and severity of injury-induced at-level spontaneous pain behavior.[4,110]

A critical factor in the initial onset of at-level behavioral changes in response to mechanical and thermal stimuli is believed to be loss of inhibitory tone within the injured cord.[40,111,112] Loss of spinal inhibition enhances the recruitment of surrounding neurons and spread of abnormal at-level sensations, including pain. The second condition involves emergence of a "pattern-generating mechanism" (spinal and supraspinal). This hypothesis led to the conclusion that not all postinjury pain is due to noxious input; some may be due to changes in the firing patterns, including burst activity and long afterdischarges, of neuronal pools adjacent to a site of injury.[41] Results consistent with a "pattern-generating" mechanism include (1) the existence of focal regions of hyperactivity in the spinal cord region surrounding the site of injury (penumbral region) and thalamus of spine-injured patients, (2) the effectiveness of cordectomy and local anesthetics in alleviating pain when delivered to the injured cord, and (3) sensitization and prolonged afterdischarges of spinal sensory neurons following SCI injury.[42,52,111,113-121]

Patients with central pain can be studied with neurometabolic techniques such as single-photon emission computed tomography (SPECT), positron emission tomography (PET), functional magnetic resonance imaging (fMRI), and magnetic resonance spectroscopy (MRS), which together with pharmacologic dissection can be helpful in classifying patients according to the pathophysiologic mechanism or mechanisms responsible for producing the central pain. In PET studies patients with chronic pain show a decrease in thalamic activity.[122] These findings may be compatible with the decrease in thalamic neuronal activity between bursts observed in patients with central pain secondary to spinal injury. Cesaro and colleagues, in a SPECT study using an amphetamine tracer, found hyperactivity in the thalamus contralateral to the pain.[123] In another SPECT study, Canavero and associates observed hypoactivity in the parietal cortex of a patient with central pain, thus suggesting that under normal conditions the cortex exerts an inhibitory control over thalamic structures.[124] Consistent with this, four patients with central post-stroke pain (two with hyperpathia) exhibited hyperactivity in the thalamus contralateral to the hyperpathic side. Pattany and colleagues used proton magnetic spectroscopy to study alterations in metabolites resulting from injury-induced functional changes in thalamic nuclei following SCI.[29] In patients with pain the concentrations of *N*-acetylinositol and myoinositol were different from those without pain, thus suggesting anatomic and functional changes in the region of the thalamus. Recently, there has been a focus on cortical and biochemical changes associated with pain following SCI. Using spectroscopy measurements from the brain and processing involving wavelet-based feature extraction, it was possible to identify biochemical changes that distinguish control subjects from subjects with SCI, as well as to subdivide the SCI group into those with and without chronic pain. Thalamic changes appeared to be linked more strongly to SCI, whereas changes in the anterior cingulate cortex and prefrontal cortex appeared to be specifically linked to the presence of pain.[125] Cortical reorganization related to central pain following SCI was observed with fMRI, consistent with the changes in regional brain anatomy and connectivity observed with diffusion tensor imaging.[126,127]

Studies have also demonstrated increased frontal blood flow, cortical expression of cholecystokinin (CCK) and opioid peptides, functional changes in thalamic neurons, and cortical neuronal death following SCI, all of which could contribute to the central mechanism responsible for the onset of pain.[52,104,128-135] Throughout the midbrain there are changes in the expression of CCK (an endogenous opioid antagonist) and several isoforms of protein kinase C (an enzyme that phosphorylates opioid receptors and makes them unavailable for binding).[136,137] These studies demonstrate that following SCI, multiple chemical and anatomic changes (plasticity) take place in the endogenous pain control system. These changes affect cortical structures involved in pain processing and affective motivational/reward areas and begin to provide an explanation for the effects on opioid ligands, receptors, and second messengers. Initiation of the process of synaptic plasticity probably involves glial elements, especially activation of microglia.[138] Microglia may be a target for preventing and treating SCI pain.[139]

The role of the sympathetic nervous system in causing or maintaining SCI pain is very poorly understood, but the fact that many types of SCI injury may spare and perhaps disinhibit the paravertebral sympathetic chain, as well as the awareness of sympathetic dysregulation with cervical and high thoracic injuries ("autonomic dysreflexia"), suggests that this is an area that should be studied.[140]

The pervasive psychosocial factors associated with SCI pain are not well studied. In a study of 42 patients with SCI pain, anger, "negative cognitions," and less acceptance of the condition were found to be related to greater pain severity, as in most chronic pain conditions.[141] The level of the lesion, completeness of the injury, surgical fusion or instrumentation, and (in this study) veteran status were not associated with pain severity. The authors concluded that "overall, psychosocial factors, not physiological factors, were most closely associated with the experience of pain" and that treatment should be directed at the emotional and cognitive sequelae of chronic SCI pain.[140-142]

TREATMENT

At present, because a proven long-term effective treatment of central pain is not available, the strategy for treatment is to consider multiple treatment modalities by extrapolating from similar diseases, especially neuropathy, to systematically determine the best approach for an individual patient.[143] There are varieties of treatment modalities.[30] The realistic goal of treatment of SCI pain is to reduce the intensity of the pain to a tolerable level with interventions that have acceptable risk and cost. In brief, tricyclic antidepressants, gabapentin, and pregabalin are considered first-line drugs (see Table 28.1). Mixed serotonin-noradrenaline (and dopamine) reuptake inhibitors may be considered when tricyclic antidepressants are not tolerated. Opioids, including tramadol, are considered second-line treatments. In refractory cases, implantation treatment of central pain may be considered, but the risk and cost of these unproven

Table 28.1 Therapeutic Considerations

Mild to moderate pain	Simple analgesics (e.g., NSAIDs or "Weak Opioids")
Excruciating, intractable pain	Opioids and adjunctive medications, psychotherapy and rehabilitation techniques; later, more experimental interventions
Regional inflammation or swelling and edema	Steroids, systemic or targeted (acutely), or NSAIDs (chronically); later, immunomodulators
Depression, anxiety, insomnia	Sedatives, analgesic antidepressants/anxiolytics with analgesic properties (e.g., TCAs), and psychotherapy. Consider SNDRIs
Significant allodynia or hyperalgesia	Anticonvulsants (e.g., gabapentinoids, Na^+ channel blockers), TCAs; consider NMDA receptor antagonists. Baclofen?
Significant osteopenia and regional trophic changes	Calcitonin or bisphosphonates
Profound vasomotor disturbance associated with pain in the region affected	Calcium channel blockers, sympatholytics, and/or blocks

These very general and hypothetical pharmacotherapy guidelines are not supported by evidence (because there are no randomized controlled trials of note or drugs approved by the Food and Drug Administration for pain from spinal cord injury); rather, they are often extrapolated from related diseases for which the evidence base is somewhat better, such as neuropathy (e.g., see Harden[30]). These general guidelines do not supplant the education and experience of a skilled physician after careful analysis of the individual case.

NMDA, *N*-methyl-D-aspartate; NSAID, nonsteroidal anti-inflammatory drug; SNDRI, serotonin-noradrenalin-dopamine reuptake inhibitor; TCA, tricyclic antidepressant.

(Modified with permission from Harden R. Neuropathic pain. In: von Roenn JH, Paice JA, Preodor ME, eds. *Current Diagnosis & Treatment of Pain*. Chicago: McGraw-Hill; 2006:122-135.

approaches are of concern. Alternative strategies that may complement existing treatments include comprehensive educational, cognitive, and behavioral approaches, as well as the full array of pain rehabilitation techniques.[1,144-146]

Repeated doses of the antiepileptic agent gabapentin alleviated chronic hypersensitivity in spinally injured rats.[1,67] Gabapentin and pregabalin had strong evidence of effectiveness in treating SCI pain (five good randomized controlled trials), and these drugs should be considered in most clinical scenarios.[142] The anticonvulsants lamotrigine and pregabalin have been found to improve spontaneous and evoked pain.[147,148] Other antiepileptics have not been studied properly but may be considered in selected cases if the risk-benefit ratio is appropriate.

Opioids are very frequently used empirically, and there is some evidence of short-term benefit.[142] However, the chronic nature of SCI pain makes the use of long-term, high-dose opioid therapy questionable. The specter of opioid-induced allodynia and hyperalgesia (unproven, especially in SCI pain) and other concerns suggest that patients being considered for opioid therapy should be selected carefully and monitored closely.

After SCI, functional and anatomic changes occur in the serotonergic (5-hydroxytryptamine [5-HT]) pathways.[149-151] At-level pain is facilitated by the 5-HT_3 receptor, and additional studies have shown reduced pain behavior and excitability of dorsal horn neurons after spinal transplantation of 5-HT precursor cells.[152-154] The use of antidepressants, especially the tricyclic and heterocyclic compounds (which have the added advantage of blocking Na^+ channels), has some support in the literature, particularly in patients with concomitant depression and empirical use over the years. Any type of Na^+ channel blocker may prove useful in some clinical scenarios.[2,22] If a patient has pain, depression, anxiety, or insomnia (or any combination), it is very logical to use these agents as first-line drug therapy.[33]

In animal models, spontaneous pain represented by excessive grooming behavior and the spatial threshold hypothesis were investigated by using three drugs that target different aspects of secondary injury: agmatine (*N*-methyl-D-aspartate [NMDA] receptor antagonist, nitric oxide synthase inhibitor), interleukin-10 (IL-10, anti-inflammatory), and cyclosporine (immunosuppressant).[155] Despite their different mechanisms of action, in excitotoxic, ischemic, or traumatic models of CNS injury, each drug has demonstrated neuroprotective effects by suppressing abnormal neuronal activity and reducing the spread of injury-induced tissue damage.[156] When compared with saline, agmatine, IL-10, and cyclosporine delayed the onset of excessive grooming, reduced grooming severity and the grooming area, and decreased the area of neuronal loss in the spinal cord. Treating the excessive grooming behavior after onset with the same drugs still reduced the grooming area, grooming severity, and neuronal loss in the spinal cord when compared with saline treatment. There is evidence that these medications attenuate ischemic damage, prevent the development of segmental hypersensitivity, and reduce chronic pain from SCI in humans.[1,157,158] Basic science suggests that NMDA receptors and other excitatory amino acid receptors contribute to allodynia and hyperalgesia, thereby implying that drugs that manipulate these conditions may have clinical value.[15,159-161] There is currently no NMDA receptor antagonist that is logistically pragmatic for human use. It is reasonable to consider memantine, dextromethorphan, or a trial of low-dose ketamine, but these agents should be considered "experimental" and presented to the patient as such until there is evidence.[1]

Sex, strain, and gonadal hormones also exert significant influences on the onset and progression of spontaneous pain behavior following SCI.[162] Severe pain behavior develops in animals treated with estradiol, whereas those treated with progesterone have a delayed onset and attenuated severity and progression of such behavior.[162] The fact that sex, strain, and hormonal effects influence the temporal profile of pain behavior and, more importantly, the longitudinal spread of neuronal damage following injury suggests an additional level of complexity of the endogenous neuroprotective and neurodegenerative mechanisms in the CNS. Consistent with these observations are other reports in which age, sex, and strain factors were found to contribute to differences in the prevalence and severity of pain following SCI.[20,163,164] Unraveling the key components of the complex variables associated with SCI may help researchers identify critical therapeutic targets and develop novel strategies for controlling spinal injury and its clinical consequences.[33]

As the results of the aforementioned studies suggest, there is a critical distance of neuronal loss along the longitudinal axis of the cord that when exceeded, leads to the expression of pain-related behavior.[155,162] Neuroprotective interventions that limit the spread of neuronal loss result in the prevention or delayed onset of this behavior. These studies thus support a neuroprotective hypothesis of SCI pain and point to the possibility that neuroprotective strategies targeting selected components of the spinal injury cascade may be useful in the prevention or treatment of pain conditions associated with SCI.[1] Until evidence is available, practical approaches in the clinic may be simple nutraceutical interventions such as vitamin C and bioflavonoids, which certainly meet the risk-benefit analysis.

The concept of a pain-generating mechanism after SCI is bolstered by the existence of hyperactivity, sensitization, and prolonged afterdischarges in spinal sensory neurons following SCI,[43,111,117,130,165] which has led to empirical pharmacologic approaches to the treatment of this condition. For example, lidocaine and ketamine, which reduce the transmission of cell membrane excitability and glutamate activation, have been shown to be effective in reducing SCI pain. Subarachnoid lidocaine, a potent nonselective sodium channel blocker, relieved SCI pain.[15,22,116] In a double-blind crossover trial, the effect of intravenous lidocaine on different components of neuropathic pain was studied in 16 patients with post-stroke pain ($n = 6$) or SCI pain ($n = 10$). The results showed a short-term benefit in spontaneous pain and in mechanical allodynia and hyperalgesia, but not in thermal allodynia or hyperalgesia.[22,131]

Baclofen and propofol are effective in increasing pain modulation or inhibition.[33,158,166-168] Intrathecal baclofen has been shown to reduce the musculoskeletal pain associated with spasticity, but its impact on neuropathic or central pain per se is questionable.[142] Propofol, a γ-aminobutyric acid (GABA) A receptor agonist, has shown some benefit in preliminary studies.[15,166] Cannabinoids also showed conflicting evidence in improving spasticity-related pain.[142]

Anecdotal interventional treatment strategies for different types of SCI pain include surgery, intrathecal pharmacology, and axial and deep brain stimulation; however, there is no definitive evidence at this time, and none of these strategies can currently survive a risk-benefit or cost-benefit analysis. There is very little literature that addresses non–drug-related therapies for SCI pain, but there is an abundance of evidence for general rehabilitation of victims of SCI.[4] A study of transcranial electrostimulation treatment demonstrated that pain decreased in the treatment group by 51% in comparison to sham-treated subjects. Interestingly, an elevation in salivary cortisol levels in this trial was associated with pain relief in the stimulation phase.[140,169,170]

A characteristic of SCI pain that has been consistently documented is its detrimental impact across multiple quality-of-life domains, including life satisfaction, mood, social reintegration, and physical health. Despite the multiple non–drug-related treatment strategies used to manage different aspects of the biopsychosocial disease that is SCI, there are currently no proven treatments.[22,23,171] In the absence of evidence, the risk-benefit analysis suggests that rehabilitation-based interdisciplinary treatments should always be included in the empirical management of SCI pain.

CONCLUSION

The pain associated with spinal injury does not have a simple or single mechanism. It is more probable that in any given case several components of the central injury cascade contribute to the development and maintenance of different pain states or phenotypes.[27] Continued research directed toward understanding specific components of the spinal injury cascade, as well as the neuroplastic changes initiated in the brain and spinal cord, may provide a better understanding of the spinal and supraspinal mechanism or mechanisms responsible for this condition and soon lead to the development of more effective therapeutic approaches. Currently, an approach that includes the best available data for drug therapy, complemented by humanitarian empirical trials informed by evidence from related diseases and, most importantly, a thoughtful interdisciplinary approach to non–drug-associated therapy, is the most likely to lead to effective pain management and optimal functional rehabilitation.[4,22,142]

KEY POINTS

- Pain above the level of the lesion is often mechanical or musculoskeletal and postural. Mechanisms include myofascial pain (e.g., overuse of the shoulder with a wheelchair), nerve compression (e.g., "crutch palsy"), and seating and position problems.
- Pain at the level of the lesion is usually some mixture of proximal peripheral nerve injury (neuropathic, radiculopathic) and central pain (such as damage to the nerve entry zone, Rexed laminae I and II), as well as damage to long tracts causing ectopic generators to arise in the afferent pain pathways and dysfunction of descending inhibitory pathways.
- Pain below the level of the lesion is "true central pain" and is also probably due to ectopic generators, loss of inhibition, demodulation, and central sensitization.
- It is critical to determine as much as possible about the mechanism and location of the pain generators (history, physical examination, psychophysical testing, and imaging) because these are the therapeutic targets.
- All chronic pain is biopsychosocial, and it is critical to embrace the psychosocial dysfunction in SCI pain since these features are often easier to treat effectively than the biomedical targets.

KEY POINTS—cont'd

- Because there is very little evidence to guide the treatment of SCI pain, it is critical to understand its mechanisms since this leads logically to treatment decisions that are often based on data extrapolated from related conditions (e.g., if the putative mechanisms are predominately consistent with neuropathic pain, selection from the pallet of proven antineuropathic medications is logical as early empirical choices).
- Non-drug-related therapies from rehabilitation medicine, which meet the test of risk versus benefit, should be considered.

SUGGESTED READINGS

Finnerup NB, Gyldensted C, Fuglsang-Fredericksen A, et al. Sensory perception in complete spinal cord injury. *Acta Neurol Scand.* 2004;109:194-199.

Finnerup NB, Baastrup C. Spinal cord injury pain: mechanisms and management. *Curr Pain Headache Rep.* 2012;16:207-216.

Hains BC, Waxman SG. Activated microglia contribute to the maintenance of chronic pain after spinal cord injury. *J Neurosci.* 2006;26:4308-4317.

Melzack R, Loeser JD. Phantom body pain in paraplegics: evidence for a central "pattern generating mechanism" for pain. *Pain.* 1978;4:195-210.

Nepomuceuno C, Fine PR, Richards JS, et al. Pain in patients with spinal cord injury. *Arch Phys Med Rehabil.* 1979;60:4.

Norrbrink Budh C, Kowalski J, Lundeberg T. A comprehensive pain management programme comprising educational, cognitive and behavioural interventions for neuropathic pain following spinal cord injury. *J Rehabil Med.* 2006;38:172-180.

Rintala DH, Loubser PG, Castro J, et al. Chronic pain in a community-based sample of men with spinal cord injury: prevalence, severity, and relationship with impairment, disability, handicap, and subjective well-being. *Arch Phys Med Rehabil.* 1998;79:604-614.

Siddall PJ, Yezierski RP, Loeser J. Taxonomy and epidemiology of spinal cord injury. In: Yezierski RP, Burchiel K, eds. *Spinal Cord Injury Pain: Assessment, Mechanisms, Management.* Vol. 23. Seattle: IASP Press; 2002:15.

Siddall PJ, McClelland JM, Rutkowski SB, et al. A longitudinal study of the prevalence and characteristics of pain in the first 5 years following spinal cord injury. *Pain.* 2003;103:249-257.

Teasell RW, Mehta S, Aubut JA, et al. A systematic review of pharmacologic treatments of pain after spinal cord injury. *Arch Phys Med Rehabil.* 2010;91:816-831.

Werhagen L, Hultling C, Molander C. The prevalence of neuropathic pain after non-traumatic spinal cord lesion. *Spinal Cord.* 2007;45:609-615.

Widerstrom-Noga EG, Turk DC. Types and effectiveness of treatments used by people with chronic pain associated with spinal cord injuries: influence of pain and psychosocial characteristics. *Spinal Cord.* 2003;41:600-609.

Woolf CJ. Central sensitization: implications for the diagnosis and treatment of pain. *Pain.* 2011;152(3 suppl):S2-S15.

Wrigley PJ, Press SR, Gustin SM, et al. Neuropathic pain and primary somatosensory cortex reorganization following spinal cord injury. *Pain.* 2009;141:52-59.

Yezierski RP. Spinal cord injury: a model of central neuropathic pain. *Neurosignals.* 2005;14:182-193.

Yezierski RP, Burchiel K, eds. *Spinal Cord Injury Pain: Assessment, Mechanisms, Management.* Vol. 23. Seattle: IASP Press; 2002.

The references for this chapter can be found at www.expertconsult.com.

29 Chronic Widespread Pain

Meredith C.B. Adams | Daniel Clauw

Chronic widespread pain presents challenges to patients, clinicians, and researchers in both diagnosing and treating its complex manifestations. As with many pain disorders, clinicians identified a grouping of symptoms, and the scientific community has attempted to develop sensitive and specific diagnostic criteria. This process has evolved recently to reflect an improved understanding of the disease process and the challenge of accurately diagnosing fibromyalgia (FM) in the clinical setting. Moreover, the complex pathophysiology obscures both the etiology and treatment options for this centrally mediated disease. Myofascial pain syndrome (MPS) is frequently found under the same umbrella as FM. They have separately struggled for recognition in the medical arena despite being fairly common in every contemporary society and exacting a moderately severe toll on the patients who suffer from them.

Explanations for this situation are varied but may relate to obscure belief systems on the part of physicians regarding the nature of the conditions themselves. Similarly, FM and MPS are painful and impair the ability of the affected person to function normally. Both are assessed subjectively, with some semi-objective clinical signs. Both can be associated with patient behavior that makes clinicians worry that something is being missed. Neither has a specific laboratory test that unequivocally defines the condition, like many of the disease states along the spectrum of central sensitization. Both seek simple instruments that are robust to change, with clinical improvement. Until relatively recently, neither had medications approved by the U.S. Food and Drug Administration (FDA) specifically indicated for treatment of its symptoms. Both FM and MPS cause mild to moderate dysfunction in the majority of patients, but with new understanding of the pathophysiology and improved diagnostic criteria, there have been changes in the field in the last several years.

Nevertheless, these conditions are easily distinguished from each other on the basis of medical history, physical examination, and even some laboratory findings. Therefore, it is even possible to identify patients who have both conditions at the same time. This chapter attempts to summarize the current status of these disorders with respect to their clinical features, epidemiology, pathogenesis, and management.

MYOFASCIAL PAIN SYNDROME

DIAGNOSTIC CRITERIA

The combined work of Kellgren, Travell, and Simons has influenced the development of proposed criteria for the diagnosis of MPS[1-4] (Box 29.1). It is described as a painful regional syndrome characterized by the presence of an active trigger point (TrP) in a skeletal muscle. The implications of an active TrP are that the examiner should expect to find spot tenderness with deep palpation over the TrP. Stimulation of these TrPs should result in concordant pain. Moreover, there should be concomitant referral of pain to a zone of reference within the affected muscle. A latent TrP has been defined as one for which there is no passive experience of spontaneous pain but pain is still inducible by manipulating the TrP. Manipulation of the TrP is generally achieved by digital pressure, a flick across the muscle, or penetration by a needle. This stimulation typically induces a "twitch" response, which can be felt as a palpable taut band that restricts normal excursion of the affected muscle.

The problem for investigators trying to validate diagnostic criteria for MPS has been that experienced clinicians have not been able to demonstrate a high level of agreement when applying the Simons and Travell criteria to serially blinded patients versus disease controls or healthy controls.[5-8] Moreover, even experienced clinicians need to standardize their examination techniques and approach for proper interpretation of the findings. When this was done immediately before performing blinded examinations, the results were much more reproducible.[5] The most reproducible clinical features from among the Simons and Travell[3] criteria were finding a tender spot (the TrP) in the proximal or distal third of an affected skeletal muscle, referral of pain to a zone of reference, and reproduction of the patient's usual pain. Much poorer reliability was associated with eliciting local tenderness, palpating a taut band, and documenting the local twitch response.

A telling series of two tables has been provided by Simons and colleagues.[1] The first table summarizes the inter-rater reliability (κ values) from four clinical studies for various critical examination procedures used in diagnosing MPS. The second compares the relative difficulty of performing or interpreting these test procedures versus the relative importance of these tests in diagnosing MPS confidently. The tests considered more important in making the diagnosis are also the ones most difficult to perform or interpret.

Part of the problem may have been that there are so many muscles in the body that have the potential to be affected by MPS; examination techniques need to be adapted for each muscle. Clinicians who are skilled in diagnosing MPS must have an adequate knowledge of neuromuscular anatomy and function, plus a high level of manual dexterity and trained sensory discrimination in their hands. In addition, these skills must account for the common distortions in ideal anatomy by patients' neglect of their physical conditioning and the development of overlying layers of adipose tissue. If every MPS patient had the "ideal body" with well-defined

Box 29.1 Validity of Findings on Physical Examination for Documenting Myofascial Pain Syndrome*

The strongest examination findings are
- A tender spot (trigger point) in an affected muscle
- Referral of pain to a zone of reference
- Reproducibility of the patient's usual pain

Poorer reliability was associated with
- Eliciting local tenderness
- Palpating a taut band
- Documenting the local twitch response

*When experienced clinicians standardized their examination techniques and their approach to interpretation of the findings before participating in a blinded examination.

Adapted from Gerwin RD, Shannon S, Hong CZ, et al. Interrater reliability in myofascial trigger point examination. *Pain*. 1997;69:65-73.

musculature, the anatomic challenge might be less onerous. Some muscles are particularly difficult to evaluate because they are under other muscles (e.g., piriformis deep to the gluteal muscles of the buttocks). The muscles in the lower extremities seem to be more problematic in this regard than those in the trunk and upper extremities.

A study design patterned after that used to develop the 1990 American College of Rheumatology (ACR) research classification criteria for FM[9] has been proposed to validate diagnostic criteria for MPS involving muscles of the upper part of the torso.[10] Application of this protocol by teams of experts (a Delphi and a blinded examiner) at two centers in different countries confirmed the historically observed outcome that there was poor agreement ($\kappa = 0.21$ to 0.35) on the diagnosis between pairs of examiners based on the standard examination approaches.[11] Primarily, this discrepancy resulted from examination of the healthy controls by the blinded examiner when a very high proportion exhibited a taut band, an area of tenderness, a local twitch response, a jump sign, and even referral of pain. Moreover, the most specific discriminators of patients with MPS from healthy controls were painfully restricted range of motion, muscle strength limited by pain, the skin rolling test, and the pressure pain threshold according to algometry. A second component of the study involved the use of validated questionnaire instruments that examined subjective pain, dysfunctional sleep, physical function, anxiety, and depression. Significantly, the questionnaire instruments were more consistently effective in distinguishing individuals with MPS from healthy controls than were the examination measures. Of particular interest were the findings of sleep dysfunction, anxiety, and depression in MPS patients, all of which challenge the long-standing notion that myofascial pain is primarily a "peripheral" pain disorder. Further analysis of these data will probably result in recommendation of a combined diagnostic profile for MPS that involves elements from the medical history, validated questionnaire instruments, and musculoskeletal examination.

Although there are certainly critics of the Simons and Travell clinical criteria for the diagnosis of MPS, it is generally agreed by physicians treating patients with musculoskeletal pain that such a condition does exist. A national survey of 1663 American Pain Society members[12] resulted in 403 completed surveys being returned. The participants responded to questions about the legitimacy of MPS as a unique condition, whether they considered it to be distinct from FM, and which signs or symptoms were important for its diagnosis. Of the respondents, 88% indicated that MPS is a legitimate diagnosis and 81% believed that it is distinct from FM. When examined by specialty, the perception of legitimacy ranged from 50% to 100%, with osteopaths and orthopedic surgeons (poorly sampled at only 0.5% and 1.2% of the respondents, respectively) reporting the lowest legitimacy (50% to 60%) and anesthesiologists and physiatrists, who accounted for 67% of the respondents, indicating higher than 90% legitimacy for MPS. The latter groups were generally (83%) convinced that MPS is distinct from FM. When asked about which findings were essential in making the diagnosis of MPS, the respondents showed strong support for regional pain, the presence of TrPs, normal findings on neurologic examination, and pain that decreases with local injection. The respondents considered irrelevant or placed much less importance on finding palpable nodules, a local twitch response, and decreased range of muscle motion.

As advocates of the MPS construct strive for uniformity in their approach to diagnosis, there is also value in striving for uniform and logical terminology. If the essence of the condition is conceptualized, it is the TrP. Many authors have referred to this construct as a "myofascial TrP," as though there were some other type of TrP. It has been suggested that the term used be simply "TrP" because the term "myofascial" adds nothing of significance. This has already become the editorial policy of the *Journal of Musculoskeletal Pain*.

PREVALENCE ESTIMATES

The prevalence of MPS in the general population is uncertain. This information is difficult to obtain because there are as yet no validated diagnostic criteria for the condition. Thus, it has not been possible to confidently seek out the disorder on a large scale with screening survey instruments.

In a study designed to document the prevalence of MPS in a general internal medicine practice, Skootsky and coworkers[13] screened 201 patients and more thoroughly evaluated 172 who visited an academic health care center for various reasons; 54 patients whose symptoms included musculoskeletal pain were retained for additional testing. Patients with pain conditions clearly unrelated to MPS were eliminated. The remaining patients underwent a detailed TrP examination guided by body pain diagrams that had been completed by the patients. When a muscle was found to contain a TrP, it was digitally compressed for 5 to 20 seconds to see whether that maneuver would intensify the pain. The diagnosis of MPS was made when the patient exhibited regional pain intensified by digital pressure and the referral pattern corresponded with established referral maps. Sixteen patients (30% of 54, 8% of 201) in this academic general internal medicine practice satisfied criteria for the diagnosis of MPS. As shown in Figure 29.1*B*, this would be slightly higher than the reported prevalence of FM (about 6%) in an academic internal medicine practice.[14]

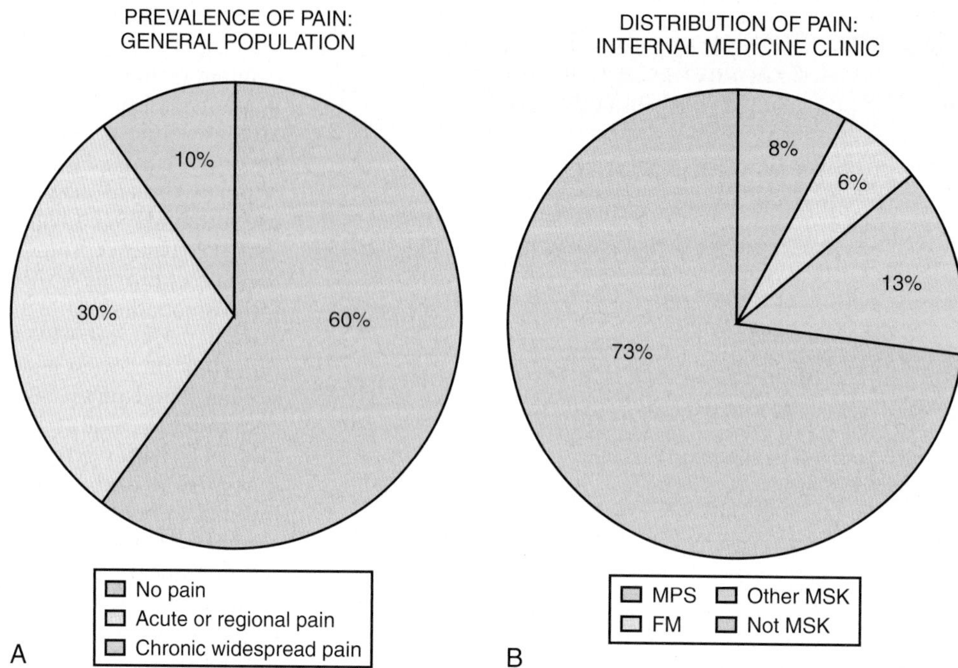

Figure 29.1 Prevalence of pain in the general population (**A**) and in an academic internal medicine clinic (**B**). FM, fibromyalgia; MPS, myopathic pain syndrome; MSK, musculoskeletal.

RELATED SYNDROMES

MPS taxonomy encompasses target areas of dysfunction as well. Specifically, two areas of the body that deserve special attention are the muscles of mastication[15] and the muscles of the pelvis.[16-18]

Dentists typically diagnose and manage temporomandibular joint disorder, now considered part of the spectrum of temporomandibular disorders; it is also referred to by some as myofascial pain dysfunction (MPD) syndrome. Fricton's classic study[15] of MPD identified 164 patients with this condition from among 296 with pain in the head and neck. In the patients with MPD, there was tenderness in at least one muscle of mastication, referral of the pain to an expected zone of reference, and frequent comorbid conditions such as postural or emotive factors. In most cases (66%) the symptoms emerged gradually, but in others there was a history of antecedent dental work or a motor vehicle accident.

The muscles of the pelvis can contribute to pain that can be confused with low back pain or with female organ pathology that can be manifested as urethral pain, vulvodynia, or dyspareunia.[16-19] Pelvic area muscles with MPS (e.g., piriformis, iliopsoas, obturator internus) can refer pain to pelvic structures and cause dysfunction, or they can compress nerves (sciatic nerve, pudendal nerve), which then results in the symptoms.

PROPOSED PATHOGENESIS

Even though many theories on the etiology of MPSs have been proposed, researchers have not yet developed a definitive pathway. Briefly, it has been suggested that predisposing factors, such as body asymmetry and poor posture, can conspire with mechanical stressors, radiculopathy,[20,21] nutritional inadequacies, endocrine dysfunction, or anger or other psychological factors to initiate the symptoms of MPS.

Exploration of the TrP via needle electromyography in a rabbit model of MPS[7] and in symptomatic humans[22] has led to the finding of spontaneous electrical activity (SEA).[23] In a controlled research study, an electromyographer found this SEA phenomenon significantly more often when probing with an electromyographic needle in the location of a human TrP site than in the location of a control site.[24] When researchers demonstrated that local infusion of phentolamine eliminated this SEA phenomenon and the pain, it was speculated that the TrP had the characteristic adrenergic dependency of the muscle spindle.[22,23,25] Others have argued that the TrP is anatomically located at a neuromuscular junction.[24-26] Thus, the evidence seems to support a spinal reflex that could involve the spindle and neuromuscular junction within the muscle, the spinal cord, and the radicular nerves that connect the muscle to the cord.

The most dramatic demonstration of objective abnormalities in MPS has come from microanalysis of interstitial fluid samples obtained from human skeletal muscle TrPs.[27,28] The concentrations of proteins, bradykinin, calcitonin gene–related peptide, substance P (SP), tumor necrosis factor-α, interleukin-1β (IL-1β), serotonin, and norepinephrine were found to be significantly higher in this fluid. Local ischemia is suggested by a lower than normal pH in the region of the TrP ($P < 0.01$).

MANAGEMENT APPROACHES

The trend of therapeutic recommendations for MPSs favors the use of a systematic, comprehensive, multidisciplinary approach to treatment.[1,3,29,30] It has been emphasized that important components of such a program should include the services of an experienced provider who has made an accurate diagnosis, has identified predisposing and perpetuating factors, and makes strategic use of both physical modalities and medications of proven efficacy. These recommendations appear to be surprisingly confident interventions for a condition whose very diagnosis is plagued by uncertainty.

A simple physical intervention that is often at least temporarily effective involves repeatedly applying a cold spray over the TrP in line with the involved muscle fibers, followed by gentle massage of the TrP and stretching of the affected muscle.[1,3] Observing dramatic therapeutic success with this procedure had the effect of generating belief in the MPS concept on a broader scale. It is also potentially educational for patients as a technique to abort progression of future attacks at an early stage by applying their own local stretch and massage. On the other hand, it is acknowledged that this approach is more readily applied to a superficial muscle, such as the trapezius fibers around the neck, than to a more deeply positioned muscle, such as the piriformis or iliopsoas muscles of the pelvis.

The skills of an experienced physical therapist can be used to teach better posture, body mechanics, and relaxation techniques and to provide TrP massage, postisometric relaxation, reciprocal inhibition, and other manual modalities.[1,3]

A more invasive approach to therapy is local injection or dry needling of the TrP.[1,3,29] Even though the pain of MPS in a given muscle can be eliminated by local anesthesia of the relevant sensory and motor nerves, this approach provides only temporary relief. The more lasting approach is referred to as TrP injection. After the symptomatic (active) TrP has been identified, small amounts of local anesthetic can be injected into the muscle via short jabs of the needle into the location of the TrP.

It is believed that local anesthetic offers no long-term benefit but does make the procedure less uncomfortable. Many practitioners argue in favor of dry needling because the overall results are similar and the patient is not placed at risk of being sensitized to an adverse reaction from the anesthetic.[31] The effectiveness of the needling procedure is explained by local structural damage to the TrP as a result of repeated passes of the needle. It is less clear whether scar tissue formation in the area represents an impediment to recurrence or a nidus favoring it. Typically, several local needling applications over a period of weeks or months are needed to achieve a cure. The required course is recognized to be substantially longer when MPS is complicated by the comorbidity of FM.[6] Some have found additional usefulness in the injection of botulinum toxin,[32] but others have failed to demonstrate a significant effect in controlled clinical trials.[33]

Therefore, it seems likely that MPS is a legitimate clinical construct that has not been fully elucidated, partly because MPS is challenging to diagnose but more importantly because diagnostic criteria have not yet been validated. This is not likely to change until experts in the field feel the need for validated criteria and put their collective efforts to the task so that the results will be more universally accepted. Until this is accomplished, MPS will remain in a form of clinical and scientific limbo. Once validated diagnostic criteria are developed, the next steps would be possible—to conduct epidemiologic, pathologic, and therapeutic studies. The outcomes of such studies would substantially advance the field, both scientifically and in the arena of public opinion.

FIBROMYALGIA

DIAGNOSTIC CRITERIA

The ACR developed research criteria for the classification of FM syndrome based on the results of a multicenter research study in 1990 (Table 29.1). The scientific community quickly accepted these criteria with a broad application for epidemiologic, biologic, and therapeutic studies. The ACR research classification required only two components for diagnosis: a history of widespread pain (i.e., located in all four quadrants of the body and axial) for at least 3 months and allodynia in response to digital pressure (defined as pain with 4 kg of pressure) at 11 or more of the 18 anatomically defined tender points (Table 29.2). The research diagnostic criteria demonstrated moderate sensitivity (88.4%) and specificity (81.1%) for FM against control patients. The study design included pain-free individuals and patients with other painful conditions as the control groups.

Table 29.1 American College of Rheumatology Criteria for Research Classification of Fibromyalgia

Criterion	Description
1. History	Chronic, widespread (four quadrants) soft tissue pain for 3 mo
2. Examination	Pain (1+ or greater in severity) induced by 4 kg of digital palpation pressure at 11 of 18 anatomically defined tender points (see Table 29.2)
3. 1 and 2 are true	When 1 and 2 are true, sensitivity and specificity for FMS >80%

FMS, fibromyalgia syndrome.

Adapted from Wolfe F, Smythe HA, Yunus MB, et al. The American College of Rheumatology 1990 criteria for the classification of fibromyalgia. Report of the Multicenter Criteria Committee. *Arthritis Rheum*. 1990;33:160-172.

Table 29.2 Eighteen Anatomically Defined Tender Points in Fibromyalgia Syndrome

Number	Official American College of Rheumatology Bilateral Tender Point Sites
1, 2	Occiput—suboccipital muscle insertions
3, 4	Low cervical—anterior aspects of the C5-7 intertransverse spaces
5, 6	Trapezius—midpoint of the upper border
7, 8	Supraspinatus—origins above the scapular spine, near the medial border
9, 10	Second rib—upper lateral surface of the second costochondral joint
11, 12	Lateral epicondyle—2 cm distal to the epicondyles
13, 14	Gluteal—upper outer aspect of the buttock, anterior fold of the muscle
15, 16	Greater trochanter—posterior to the trochanteric prominence
17, 18	Knees—medial fat pad, just proximal to the medial condyle

Adapted from Wolfe F, Smythe HA, Yunus MB, et al. The American College of Rheumatology 1990 criteria for the classification of fibromyalgia. Report of the Multicenter Criteria Committee. *Arthritis Rheum*. 1990;33:160-172.

The tender points in FM are conceptually and anatomically different from the TrPs that define MPS. FM tender points are symmetrically distributed throughout the body, whereas TrPs have a more random distribution. In contrast to MPS, these tender points are not limited to muscular locations but also include other soft tissue structures and do not refer or radiate pain to other locations. The ACR's research criteria unknowingly created several problems. Researchers developed these criteria to standardize research identification of FM. The research classification identified 18 anatomically defined tender points (see Table 29.2) where patients with FM have allodynia in response to digital pressure. Unfortunately, clinicians appropriated these criteria for clinical diagnosis. Many providers did not follow the intent or structure of the criteria, which made the diagnosis of FM even more complicated.

Primary care physicians diagnose the majority of cases of FM rather than subspecialists. Consequently, many physicians either rigidly (and inappropriately) applied the research criteria or simply rejected their face validity. Accordingly, few providers consistently identified and applied 4 kg of pressure to all 18 designated areas. They used symptom-based diagnostic criteria that focused on fatigue, cognitive impairment, and somatic symptoms, which were excluded in the original research criteria. Moreover, an additional problem with the criteria is that patients with improved symptoms and examination findings no longer met the classification.

Twenty years after the initial research classification was developed, the FM research community recognized the growing need for clinical diagnostic criteria that reflect the spectrum of FM and practical components of clinical diagnosis. The objective was to develop a screening tool with wide applicability that could be used to diagnose and assess the severity of the FM symptoms. Researchers evaluated patients in whom FM was previously diagnosed by using the widespread pain index (WPI) and categorical scales. The new criteria used these categorical scales to assess patients' cognitive symptoms, unrefreshing sleep, fatigue, and other somatic symptoms. The ACR used these categorical scales to develop a severity scale. Finally, they combined the severity scale with the WPI to stratify disease severity in patients with FM (Box 29.2).

PREVALENCE ESTIMATES

FM has been found in all ethnic groups studied to date; it is not limited to affluent or industrialized nations. With prevalence estimates ranging from 2% to almost 12% in the general population, it must be viewed as a common medical condition.[34] Its prevalence increases with age, most dramatically in women, with a peak in the fifth to seventh decade (7.4% to 10%). Middle-aged women are four to seven times more likely to be affected than men of similar age. This was another unintended consequence of the 1990 ACR criteria—by using the same tenderness threshold in men and women even though we now understand that women are substantially more tender than men, these criteria overestimate the prevalence of FM in men. By contrast, the sex distribution of childhood FM is almost equal (probably

Box 29.2 American College of Rheumatology Preliminary Diagnostic Criteria for Fibromyalgia and Measurement of Symptom Severity

Criteria

A patient satisfies the diagnostic criteria for fibromyalgia if the following three conditions are met:

1. Widespread pain index (WPI) score >7 and symptom severity (SS) scale score >5 or WPI score of 3 to 6 and SS scale score >9
2. Symptoms present at a similar level for at least 3 months
3. No disorder present that would otherwise explain the pain

Ascertainment

1. WPI: note the number of areas in which the patient has had pain over the last week. In how many areas has the patient had pain? The score will be between 0 and 19:
   Shoulder girdle, left hip (buttock, trochanter), left jaw, left upper part of back
   Shoulder girdle, right hip (buttock, trochanter), right jaw, right lower part of back
   Upper part of arm, left upper part of leg, left side of chest or neck
   Upper part of arm, right upper part of leg, right side of abdomen
   Left lower part of arm, left lower part of leg
   Right lower part of arm, right lower part of leg
2. SS scale score:
   Fatigue
   Waking unrefreshed
   Cognitive symptoms

For the each of the three symptoms above, indicate the level of severity over the past week according to the following scale:
   0= No problem
   1= Slight or mild problems, generally mild or intermittent
   2= Moderate: considerable problems, often present and/or at a moderate level
   3= Severe: pervasive, continuous, life-disturbing problems

Considering somatic symptoms in general, indicate whether the patient has the following*:
   0= No symptoms
   1= Few symptoms
   2= Moderate number of symptoms
   3= Great deal of symptoms

The SS scale score is the sum of the severity of the symptoms (fatigue, waking unrefreshed, cognitive symptoms) plus the extent (severity) of somatic symptoms in general. The final score is between 0 and 12.

*Somatic symptoms that might be considered are muscle pain, irritable bowel syndrome, fatigue or tiredness, difficulty thinking or remembering, muscle weakness, headache, pain or cramps in the abdomen, numbness or tingling, dizziness, insomnia, depression, constipation, pain in the upper part of the abdomen, nausea, nervousness, chest pain, blurred vision, fever, diarrhea, dry mouth, itching, wheezing, Raynaud's phenomenon, hives or welts, ringing in the ears, vomiting, heartburn, oral ulcers, loss of or change in taste, seizures, dry eyes, shortness of breath, loss of appetite, rash, sun sensitivity, hearing difficulty, easy bruising, hair loss, frequent urination, painful urination, and bladder spasms.

because girls do not appear to be more tender than boys until after puberty), and many children outgrow their symptoms.[35] About 15% of patients seen in rheumatology clinics are classified as having FM, whereas the prevalence of FM is about 6% in other practice settings. In 1997, the annual direct cost of care for the average FM patient in the United States was estimated to be more than $2000.[36] Multiplied by the 6 million U.S. patients with FM, this figure predicts an annual direct cost of more than $12 billion.

In a study designed to examine the prevalence of FM in a midwestern community,[34] Wolfe and associates found that about 60% of the general population in their study did not currently have pain. About 30% of the general population had acute or regional pain (the latter would include MPS), and about 10% had chronic widespread pain (the category for FM). Follow-up examination revealed that about 2% of the general population (all within the 10% in the chronic widespread pain subgroup) met criteria for the classification of FM, but the patients who reported having regional pain were not examined to confirm the presence of MPS (Fig. 29.1*A*). In 2008, the National Arthritis Data Workgroup used these data with the population census data to extrapolate an estimated 5 million Americans with FM. The ability to accurately generalize the estimated 2% prevalence of FM in Wichita, Kansas, to the broader U.S. and international populations is uncertain.[37] FM poses a diagnostic challenge, as well as a management flow quandary, for many providers. The proposed clinical flow would stratify these patients for improved management (Box 29.3).

Little is known about the incidence of FM, but risk factors for its development may include physical trauma, a febrile illness, or a family history of FM; these factors may not be mutually exclusive. A narrowed cervical canal may be an important risk factor for the development of chronic pain following a whiplash injury.[38]

CLINICAL FEATURES

The clinical manifestations of FM are usually more complex than body pain alone. Associated symptoms (comorbidities) often require further investigation and specific management. For example, patients describe disordered sleep, fatigue, cognitive dysfunction, dizziness, headaches, psychological distress, depression, anxiety, chest pains, dysesthesia in the hands, cold intolerance, restless legs, and irritable bowel or irritable bladder syndrome. These comorbid symptoms clearly contribute to the suffering experienced by patients with FM. As a result, dysfunctional behavioral patterns and disability develop in affected individuals.

COGNITIVE DYSFUNCTION

People with FM frequently complain of diminished cognitive function. This ranges from difficulty concentrating when reading a book to short-term memory deficits. Research has suggested that FM patients perform poorly on a range of cognitive tasks[39] and exhibit premature cognitive aging, with the main evidence of abnormality being derived from distraction or multitasking experiments.

AFFECTIVE DISTRESS

Before FM was better understood as a condition of central sensitization, patients with this condition were often suspected of having a psychiatric disorder. Indeed, the frequencies of depression and anxiety in patients with FM were each found to be about 40% at the time of diagnosis of FM,[40] but that left 60% who were not actively depressed or anxious. Depression also occurs with rheumatoid arthritis (20% to 30%), cancer, and other chronic conditions (14% to 33%). In these settings the psychological comorbidities are believed to result from the pain and physical limitations imposed by the disease. The same could be true for FM.

Box 29.3 Proposed Plan for Screening and Comprehensive Care of Patients with Fibromyalgia

Phase 1: Pain Screening and Primary Care

Phase 1 involves a simple screening questionnaire that the receptionist for a primary care health professional (primary care physician [PCP], chiropractor, nurse practitioner, physician assistant, general practitioner, general internist) would give to every patient entering the waiting room until all the primary care professional's regular patients had been assessed (see Fig. 29.2). Thereafter, it may be given only to new patients. When the PCP reviews the form of a patient with pain (question 1 answered "yes"), a decision about the symptom's distribution would be made (localized pain, regional pain, widespread pain). A second decision would be whether to initiate care for the patient's symptoms or refer the patient for further care of this problem.

Phase 2: Comorbidity Screening and Secondary Care

Based on findings on the screening material, a patient identified as having widespread pain would be examined by the PCP or referral physician to make the diagnosis (fibromyalgia [FM] if it applies). The next stage would be screening for comorbid conditions by a well-informed and willing PCP or consultant (rheumatologist, neurologist, pain specialist, internist, physiatrist). The patient would begin an exercise program and counseling with a professional specifically trained to provide advanced care for FM. Problems found in counseling (e.g., marital, financial, psychiatric) would spin off to an experienced specialist (e.g., counselor, psychologist, psychiatrist, disability advisor, financial counselor).

Phase 3: Comorbidity Screening and Tertiary Care

Based on second-line screening for comorbid conditions, care would begin for the additional diagnoses. This phase may invoke referral to tertiary subspecialty care (e.g., cardiologist, gastroenterologist, neurologist, neurosurgeon, physical therapist, psychiatrist, physiatrist, obstetrician-gynecologist, urologist). This care would be integrated with follow-up by the primary care resource.

Phase 4: Long-Term Primary Care and Follow-up Assessment

The primary or secondary health care professional would continue to monitor the patient over time and assess the status of care for pain and comorbid conditions. There would be monitoring for side effects to medications and for new problems intruding on the continuity of the FM that might or might not be related to it. In this phase it is important to not assume that every new symptom in a patient with FM is a component of the FM. Health care providers will need to know what is and is not expected with FM.

Phase 1: Screening Questionnaire

Instructions: Answer Yes or No to each of the following questions. If you answer No to question 1, you are done. You do not need to read any of the other questions. When you are done, please return the completed questionnaire to the office clerk.

Yes No

☐ ☐ 1. Have you had body pain for at least three months?

☐ ☐ 2. Was your body pain one of your reasons for coming to the doctor today?

Instructions: If you answered Yes to question 1, mark a slanted line across the line below to indicate how severe your pain has been over the past two weeks.

No pain ——————————————— Severe pain

Instructions: If you answered Yes to question 1, use a pencil or pen to mark darkly on the body diagrams the locations of your pain during the last week.

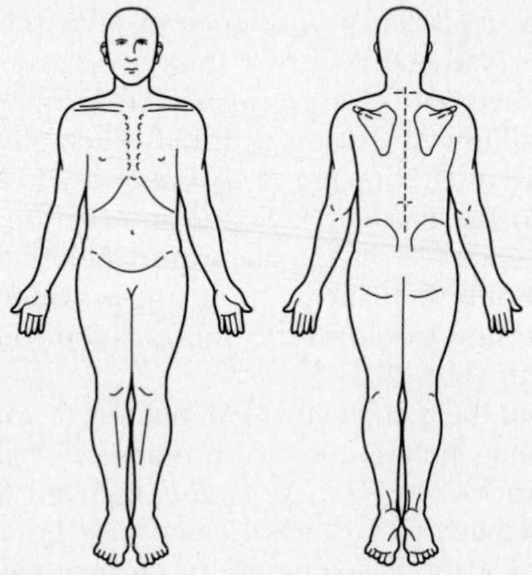

Below this line is for office use only. Please do not mark below this line.

• Physician interpretation [check one]:

__ Localized __ Regional __ Widespread Soft Tissue Pain

• Optional examination findings [indicate values]:

Total Tender Point Count ____ TPI ____ APT ____

• Referral: ___ Yes ___ No To __________

Figure 29.2 Screening questionnaire for chronic widespread pain as seen in fibromyalgia syndrome (FM). The findings supportive of FM would be chronic pain from question 1, the relative severity of the pain from question 3, and widespread pain from question 4. Each question could also be applied to other categories of soft tissue pain, and patients with localized or regional musculoskeletal pain, if present, would be identified by the body pain diagram. APT, average pain threshold; TPI, tender point index.

Sexual abuse in childhood is no longer a viable hypothesis for the primary cause of FM.[41]

INSOMNIA

Most FM patients experience chronic insomnia. Some have difficulty falling asleep (initial insomnia), but most awaken feeling distressingly alert after only a few hours of sleep (midinsomnia) and are then unable to sleep soundly again until it is almost morning (terminal insomnia). People with FM typically awaken in the morning feeling painfully stiff, cognitively sluggish, and unrefreshed by their sleep. It is surprising that these chronically sleep-deprived individuals have difficulty napping during the day.

STIFFNESS

The morning stiffness experienced by most FM patients is remarkable because it lasts so long and is so severe. The typical stiffness of osteoarthritis usually lasts 5 to 15 minutes, whereas that of patients with inflammatory rheumatoid arthritis is 30 minutes to 2 hours. By comparison, the stiffness of FM patients typically lasts 45 minutes to 4 hours. The best clinical correlate with morning stiffness in FM is pain, so patients may not be clearly distinguishing these seemingly different symptoms.

FATIGUE

Approximately 80% of patients with FM complain of fatigue. Consequently, a large proportion of individuals who meet the criteria for FM also meet the criteria for chronic fatigue syndrome. The differential diagnosis of fatigue is difficult because it must include various sleep disorders, chronic infections, autoimmune disorders, psychiatric comorbidities, and neoplasia. Fatigue may also result from residual levels of sedating medication, such as tricyclic antidepressant drugs or other sedatives often used to treat the insomnia associated with FM.

IRRITABLE BOWEL SYNDROME AND DYSPEPSIA

Irritable bowel syndrome (IBS) and benign dyspepsia are common gastrointestinal conditions that occur in 30% to 50% of patients with FM. A feature common in both FM and IBS may be central sensitization. These conditions may be synergistic with respect to patients' perception of their illness and have a modulating effect on the clinical outcome. A common differential diagnosis is lactose intolerance, which can cause intermittent cramping, diarrhea, and flatulence. A simple litmus test of feces will often show acidic pH when lactose intolerance is the cause of the diarrhea.

INTERSTITIAL CYSTITIS, PAINFUL BLADDER SYNDROME, AND FEMALE URETHRAL SYNDROME

Roughly 60% of FM patients experience urinary urgency and nocturia on a regular basis, and there is a high rate of bidirectional comorbidity between interstitial cystitis/painful bladder syndrome and FM. Up to 12% of FM patients also fulfill the diagnostic criteria for female urethral syndrome,[42] which is defined as the presence of urinary frequency, dysuria, suprapubic discomfort, and urethral pain despite sterile urine. Many patients report having been treated with antibiotics frequently for culture-negative urinary tract infections. Intensive investigations often fail to disclose a specific cause. Eliminating certain dietary substances such as caffeine or alcohol from the patient's diet can sometimes be helpful. Self-report questionnaire instruments have been developed to facilitate screening for this condition in FM patients (see Fig. 29-1).[43]

RELATED SYNDROMES

Conversely, FM can develop in patients with other chronic diseases during the course of their symptoms. For want of better terminology, in the setting of another painful condition or inflammatory disorder, the FM condition has been referred to as secondary FM. This terminology is not intended to imply that the FM is caused by the other condition, but the terminology is entrenched and serves a purpose. Secondary FM may not be clinically distinguishable from primary FM,[9] but increasingly, there are laboratory findings that can be used to distinguish these FM subgroups.[44]

As examples of secondary FM, almost 30% of patients with rheumatoid arthritis, 40% of patients with systemic lupus erythematosus, and 50% of those with Sjögren's syndrome have concomitant FM. Patients with a rheumatic disease and FM seem to experience articular pain disproportionate to their synovitis. This must be considered when treating the rheumatic condition because increasing the dosage of antirheumatic medications in the absence of active inflammation may have little effect on the pain amplified by FM. The best results are obtained by treating each condition separately.

Patients with a rheumatic disease and concomitant FM should be warned that a transient increase in FM symptoms may occur with each decrease in glucocorticoid dosage (steroid withdrawal FM), so the usual FM therapy may need to be increased transiently. This is a surprising phenomenon because glucocorticoid is not helpful in treating primary FM. To avoid interference with a steroid taper by emergent FM, it is best to decrease the dosage of the glucocorticoid used to treat the rheumatic disease in graduated steps at about 2-week intervals. The rate of the taper depends on the current dosage.

Infectious and inflammatory conditions that seem to be associated with FM include hepatitis C, tuberculosis, syphilis, and Lyme disease. The prevalence of overlap may depend on the prevalence of the infectious disease in the community. An academic practice in a Lyme-endemic area evaluated 788 patients with apparent infection for a mean of 2.5 years.[45] Of those with Lyme disease, 20% met the criteria for FM. The symptoms of FM developed 1 to 4 months after infection, often in association with Lyme arthritis. The signs of Lyme disease generally resolved with antibiotic therapy, but the FM symptoms often persisted. The largest subgroup of the 788 patients did not have Lyme disease, but they did meet the criteria for FM or chronic fatigue syndrome.

PATHOGENESIS

Patients with FM have a constellation of symptoms, but the most common is pain. Before the advent of research techniques such as quantitative sensory testing and functional neuroimaging, many believed that FM and chronic widespread pain had primarily a psychosocial origin with little "organic" basis. However, patients with FM demonstrate reliably augmented sensory processing that was initially thought to be confined to the sensation of pain (i.e., hyperalgesia or allodynia) but is now known to include hypersensitivity to other sensory stimuli such as auditory stimulation.[46,47] Functional magnetic resonance imaging (MRI) studies have corroborated this finding of hyperalgesia or allodynia in that multiple studies have now shown that FM patients display increased neuronal activation in comparison to controls when the same low-intensity stimulus is applied to both groups.[48] These imaging studies also provide a theoretical basis for globally augmented sensory processing in FM since the area of the brain that most consistently exhibits increased activity in FM and most other chronic pain states is the insula, a region involved in polysensory integration. Even though multiple mechanisms to assess alterations in pain perception are used, the pressure pain threshold (rather than heat or electrical stimuli) response has the closest relationship with the clinical features of FM and other chronic pain states.

Patients with FM have also been found to have altered levels of biomarkers associated with pain, specifically glutamate and SP.[49] Harris and colleagues' recent work using proton spectroscopy to evaluate insular glutamate elevations in patients with FM demonstrated higher mean levels than in controls.[50,51] Although such techniques do not allow simple patient testing, the findings support the distinct biologic identity of FM. Endogenous opioid levels are elevated relative to controls, thereby providing a potential mechanism for the lack of responsiveness to opioid therapy in patients with FM. Objectively, this has been demonstrated through positron emission tomography (PET)-derived μ-receptor occupancy.[52,53]

Abnormalities in neurochemical mediators of central nervous system (CNS) nociceptive function are clearly present in ways consistent with the patterns of symptoms. The role of neurochemicals as neurotransmitters and modulators of the nociceptive process has been studied extensively in animals.[54] It is believed that these agents participate in descending inhibition of nociception. This line of reasoning has led to the measurement of neurotransmitter levels in biologic fluids obtained from FM patients. Several major classes of biochemical participants in the nociceptive process are the biogenic amines (e.g., serotonin, norepinephrine, dopamine), excitatory amino acids (e.g., glutamic acid, glutamine, aspartic acid, asparagine, glycine, arginine), neurokinins (e.g., SP, calcitonin gene–related protein, arginine vasopressin, neuropeptide Y), nerve growth factor (NGF), and probably nitric oxide. The biogenic amines are generally considered to be antinociceptive, whereas the excitatory amino acids, SP, NGF, and perhaps even nitric oxide would more likely be pronociceptive.

Moldofsky and Walsh[55] were the first to suggest that serotonin (5-hydroxytryptamine [5-HT]) might be involved in the pathogenesis of FM, both in failing to attenuate persistent pain and in failing to correct the chronic deficiency in slow-wave sleep. They found a clinical correlate between FM pain and the plasma concentration of tryptophan.

Moreover, the serum and cerebrospinal fluid (CSF) of FM patients were found to exhibit low concentrations of tryptophan.[56,57] Early findings of a low serum concentration of 5-HT[58] have been supported by other investigators.[59] Levels of 5-HT have not yet been reported in the CSF of FM patients, but levels of its immediate precursor, 5-hydroxytryptophan (5-HTP), and its metabolic product, 5-hydroxyindole acetic acid (5-HIAA), have been studied. In FM, both were found to have lower than normal CSF concentrations relative to the CSF of healthy normal controls.[57] In addition, 5-HIAA was measured in 24-hour urine samples of patients with FM and compared with the results from healthy normal controls.[57] Even the numbers of active FM tender points correlated with the concentration of 5-HT in FM sera.[60]

The role of α-adrenergic agonists such as norepinephrine in the antinociception system of FM patients may be similar to that of 5-HT, but a number of unique features of this biogenic amine have attracted attention.[61] The concentration of 3-methoxy-4-hydroxyphenyl-glycol (MHPG), the inactive metabolite of norepinephrine, is significantly lower than normal in FM CSF.[57] The concentration of homovanillic acid, the inactive metabolite of dopamine, was found to be significantly lower than normal in FM CSF.[57] This finding, which would imply low CNS levels of dopamine in FM, was complemented by a study of the role of dopamine receptors in the function of the hypothalamus and pituitary in FM.[62]

The neuropeptide SP is an 11–amino acid peptide that has several important roles in the process of nociception. Activated, small, thinly myelinated Aδ- and C-fiber afferent neurons respond to noxious peripheral stimuli by releasing SP into laminae I and V (Aδ) and lamina II (C fiber) of the spinal cord dorsal horn. With random interstitial diffusion, SP or its C-terminal peptide fragment makes contact with its neurokinin-1 (NK1) effector receptor. The mechanism of action of SP in the dorsal horn of the spinal cord is not entirely clear, but it appears to not be a signal transporter, as is glutamic acid. Rather, SP apparently facilitates nociception by arming or alerting spinal cord neurons to incoming nociceptive signals from the periphery.

Vaeroy and associates,[63] working in Norway, were the first to recognize that the concentration of SP was elevated (average threefold increase) in the CSF of FM patients in comparison to healthy controls. Their findings have now been reproduced in three other clinical studies.[64,65] The biologic relevance of SP in CSF to the pain of primary FM is still uncertain. An important question is whether an elevated CSF SP level is unique to FM. An earlier report[66] indicated that CSF SP concentrations are lower than normal in various chronic painful conditions. For example, CSF SP levels were found to be lower than normal in patients with diabetic neuropathy[67] and chronic low back pain.[66]

The elevated CSF SP level in FM has prompted much speculation about the cause. NGF was known to stimulate the production of SP in small, afferent, unmyelinated neurons. It was therefore an exciting development to have found elevated levels of NGF in the CSF of primary FM patients, but not in those with FM and an associated painful inflammatory condition (secondary FM).[44] This suggests that there may be different mechanisms for the elevated SP level in primary FM and in FM associated with inflammatory diseases.[9] In primary FM, the elevated CSF SP level seems to be induced by NGF, whereas in secondary FM the cause may be inflammation in the periphery.

Another approach to understanding the cause of FM has been through genetic studies. About a third of FM patients have reported that another family member, usually a female, has a similar, chronic pain condition or has already been given the diagnosis of FM. Published studies have documented familial patterns. Some have predicted an autosomal dominant mode of inheritance for FM,[68,69] and evidence for this has increased. In a study by Yunus and coworkers,[70] a linkage of FM with the histocompatibility locus was examined by the sibship method. A complete genome scan of families with two or more FM-affected members has been undertaken[71] by using samples of DNA from a large number of multicase FM families for comparison of clinical and laboratory genotypic features. Meanwhile, several candidate genes have been proposed to directly explain the specific metabolic abnormalities that have been consistently observed in FM. A study of 80 multicase FM families has already examined markers spanning the genomic regions for the following: the serotonin transporter (HTTLPR, three regional markers) on chromosome 17, the serotonin receptor 2A (HTR2A, three regional markers) on chromosome 13, and the histocompatibility locus antigen (HLA, two regional markers) region on chromosome 6.[72] No evidence for linkage was found in the HTTLPR region. Families with an older age of onset were linked to the HLA region (logarithm of the odds [LOD] = 3.02, P = 0.00057), thus suggesting an immune-mediated pathogenesis. In the HTR2A region, the results indicated a moderately strong linkage to families with a younger age of onset, less severe pain, lower levels of depression, and absence of IBS (LOD = 5.56, P = 0.000057). The HTR2A genome is polymorphically imprinted, so the issue of parent of origin will need to be considered in future studies. Bioinformatics mining and further sequencing of genes in the HTR2A region will help identify specific polymorphisms for further clinical association testing.

Another appealing gene candidate as a causative factor in FM would be the enzyme catechol-*O*-methyltransferase (COMT), which physiologically inactivates catecholamines such as dopamine, norepinephrine, and endorphins, as well as catecholamine-containing drugs. Polymorphism (actually dimorphism) in the gene encodes for variations in COMT enzyme activity. The COMT gene exists in two forms, L and H, which make copies differing by a single amino acid (either methionine or valine) at the variable site. This small variation has a large effect on the activity of COMT. Subjects with the LL phenotype, who have two copies of the methionine version, make threefold to fourfold less COMT than do those with the HH variant, which contains valine at the variable site. The significance of COMT polymorphism (LL, LH, or HH) in FM was assessed by Gursoy and colleagues.[73] Sixty-one patients with FM and 61 demographically matched healthy controls were included in the study. Although no significant difference was found between LL and LH separately, the LL and LH genotypes together were more highly represented in FM syndrome than in the healthy normal control groups ($P = 0.024$). In addition, the prevalence of HH genotypes in FM was significantly lower than that in the control groups ($P = 0.04$).

The much higher prevalence of FM in women has led to speculation regarding gender-specific causes. For example, in an epidemiologic study of a midwestern community,[34] the curves representing pain thresholds (sensitivity to a pressure stimulus) in men and women consistently showed lower values for women. Because the examination component of the ACR criteria for FM involves the response to a fixed pressure stimulus of 4 kg, it is not surprising that these criteria have identified more women than men with multiple sclerosis. Understanding of the mechanisms responsible for this gender-related difference in pain thresholds is incomplete. Measurements of female hormones have not been very fruitful. One possible explanation is that men normally synthesize substantially more 5-HT in their brains than women do.[74]

Many symptoms of FM resemble those observed in patients with hormone deficiencies. This observation has led to the study of neuroendocrine function in FM.[75] Subsets of patients with FM exhibit functional abnormalities in the hypothalamic-pituitary-adrenal (HPA) axis, sympathoadrenal (autonomic nervous) system, hypothalamic-pituitary-thyroid axis, hypothalamic-pituitary-gonadal axis, or hypothalamic–pituitary–growth hormone axis.[76] In FM patients, the HPA axis exhibits an exaggerated adrenocorticotropic hormone (ACTH) response to insulin-induced hypoglycemia or stressful exercise. Despite this dramatic rise in serum ACTH level in FM, the level of cortisol did not rise commensurately. Mediators that regulate the HPA axis include corticotropin-releasing factor, serotonin, norepinephrine, SP, and IL-6.[77,78]

Growth hormone was identified as a target because of its production during delta-wave sleep (stages 3 and 4, non–random eye movement sleep), which many FM patients fail to achieve normally. An alternative means of monitoring growth hormone production has been to measure the plasma levels of insulin-like growth factor type I (IGF-I, previously known as somatomedin C), which has a long half-life. An age-adjusted deficiency of IGF-I has been documented in FM.[79] In addition, administration of human growth hormone to FM patients was effective in reducing the severity of FM symptoms.[80]

The reasons why these endocrinopathies would be associated with a chronic pain syndrome are not entirely clear. It may be that CNS abnormalities in the availability of biogenic amines such as serotonin, norepinephrine, and/or dopamine are responsible for the abnormal regulation of the neuroendocrine system.[57] These systems interact and are interdependent, so in susceptible individuals a partial failure of one system may lead to subtle malfunctions in others.

Moreover, immune function abnormalities have been identified as early as the 1980s.[81] This foundation has been expanded to additional markers. An early epidemiologic search for serum antinuclear antibodies disclosed that almost a third of FM patients exhibit low titers of these autoantibodies,[82] but more recent reports have reduced this figure to 14%[83] or to as low as 8.8% in FM versus 8.9% in patients with osteoarthritis.[84] There have been intermittent reports of lymphocyte immune abnormalities in people with FM, but the outcomes of these studies were variable and hard to interpret in light of the clinical picture.[81] More recently, two studies have critically evaluated the possible role of cytokines in patients with FM.[85,86] Serum IL-8 and IL-6 levels from in vitro–stimulated peripheral blood mononuclear cell cultures were significantly higher in the FM sample. The serum IL-8 level was most dramatically elevated in FM patients who were also depressed, but it also correlated with pain intensity and the duration of FM symptoms. Its production in vitro is stimulated by SP, which may help explain the elevated levels of both these cytokines, even in different fluid compartments, in FM patients. It is therefore of interest that IL-6 has been successfully administered to people with FM and found to substantially modulate the severity of FM-related symptoms.[77]

In summary, the pathogenesis of FM was shaped by the recognition of allodynia as a manifestation of abnormal central nociceptive processing. This has redirected the collective view of FM. This revised perspective pointed research on this condition in a new direction, specifically toward the study of central sensitization. Some abnormalities found in FM, namely, the low 5-HT and elevated SP levels, are logically consistent with a pain amplification syndrome. The extent to which these mechanisms are unique to FM will be critical in determining the direction of future research.

MANAGEMENT APPROACHES

The objectives of FM treatment are to reduce pain, improve sleep, restore physical function, maintain social interaction, and re-establish emotional balance. A reasonable community objective might be to reduce the need for expensive health care resources. To achieve these goals, patients will need a combination of social support, education, physical modalities, and medication.

ADEPT

It is reasonable to view treatment approaches in categories, and sometimes an acronym can help the physician remember them. For that purpose, a six-step outline of therapy has been developed; *ADEPT living* stands for attitude, diagnosis, education, physical modalities, treatment with medication, and living.

ATTITUDE

Attitude refers to the preparation, or frame of mind, that each participant brings to the therapeutic interaction. Clinicians must be prepared to accept FM as a real condition that exerts a tremendous impact on the patient's life. From the patient's perspective, it will be important to realize that FM is just one of hundreds of conditions of concern to the health care provider. Additionally, the initial symptoms for different medical conditions can be very similar, therapy for FM is still experimental, and the physician's time with each patient is necessarily limited. The attitudes of family members, employers, policy makers, and politicians all have an important impact on the patient's condition.

DIAGNOSIS

The correct diagnosis should be made not only to identify FM but also to disclose any comorbid medical conditions. If the patient has concomitant hypothyroidism, diabetes mellitus, or renal insufficiency, the approach to management will also need to accommodate these other conditions. For example, when rheumatoid arthritis and FM are evident in the same patient, treatment is more successful when both conditions are treated as though the other were not present.

EDUCATION

Education is crucial to the management of FM. Understanding is power when it comes to maintaining a proper attitude, adapting to limitations, and taking an active role in the therapeutic program. Several studies have examined the effects of cognitive-behavioral therapy (CBT) on outcome in FM and demonstrated positive effects on pain scores, pain coping, pain behavior, depression, and physical functioning.[87] Such gains are often maintained for several months after completion of the therapy, and periodic booster sessions may prolong the benefits. Some clinicians, regarded as providing an environment for learning discontent, have viewed support groups negatively. On the other hand, joining a resource-oriented support group can help FM patients come to terms with a complicated illness.

PHYSICAL MODALITIES

A variety of physical modalities have been proposed as interventions for FM and can logically be segregated into two categories—those that patients can accomplish for themselves and those that require active participation by a trained therapist. At home, patients can pace their usual activities by setting a clock to time the necessary work activity and then balance the work time with an equal period of rest. Progressive exercise, heat applied as a shower or bath, and Jacobson relaxation techniques can all be used as self-directed therapies with minimal cost.[87]

Aerobic exercise was among the first nonpharmacologic strategies advocated for FM patients, with convincing evidence of benefit.[87] Its goals are to maintain function for everyday activities and to prolong life through cardiovascular fitness. Low-impact exercise, with an intensity sufficient to challenge aerobic capacity, can also reduce pain, improve sleep, balance mood, improve stamina, instill new perspectives, restore cognition, and facilitate a sense of well-being.[88] Patients who can exercise sustain a less negative impact of FM in their lives. Other recent studies have shown benefit in quality of life and pain in patients involved in exercise programs alone.[89] However, one should be aware that high levels of exertion can temporarily worsen the pain and result in fear of movement (kinesophobia), especially in this patient population. When the diagnosis of FM is first made, the patient is usually deconditioned and has already learned to fear the pain induced by exercise. When prescribing exercise for FM patients, the clinician should begin with low-intensity exercise, such as walking in place in a swimming pool, and minimize eccentric muscle contractions.[90] Continuation of the exercise program will be facilitated by a gradual reduction in pain. Other physical therapies, including yoga,[91] Pilates,[92] and tai chi,[93] have been found to be effective in reducing the pain associated with FM. However, other alternative and complementary methods, including Reiki, provided no benefit.[94]

Most patients report benefit from heat in the form of dry or moist heat. Many find that a hot bath or shower can be more effective than analgesic medication for headache, body pain, and stiffness. The application of heat can relax muscles, facilitate exercise, and improve the sense of well-being. Cold application is preferred by some. Light massage that gradually progresses to deep sedative palpation of large body surfaces can reduce muscle tension, but its influence on body pain usually lasts only 1 or 2 days.

TREATMENTS

Cognitive-Behavioral Therapies

Numerous psychological therapies have been found to be beneficial for relief of pain in those suffering from chronic widespread pain, including FM. In a recent randomized controlled trial (RCT)[95] it was found that telephone-based CBT was beneficial in health care–related quality outcomes. In this study 442 patients with chronic widespread pain were randomized to receive 6 months of telephone CBT, graded exercise, combined intervention, or treatment as usual. Patients receiving CBT with or without exercise did better than those undergoing standard medical treatment. Those who combined CBT with exercise improved to the greatest degree. These improvements in quality of life were long lasting and the interventions were cost-effective by using telephone instead of face-to-face CBT. Attention modification has also been very successful in altering the perception of pain in patients with chronic widespread pain. Attention bias refers to the phenomenon whereby patients identify with information that reinforces their focus on their painful condition. The goal of attention modification is to interrupt this negative and self-reinforcing cognitive cycle. In a recent RCT, the Attentional Modification Paradigm (AMP), in which patients completed two 15-minute AMP sessions per week for 4 weeks, was used to facilitate such changes in attentional pain biases.[96] Those in the AMP program reported statistically significant and substantial reductions in several individual difference variables relative to those in the control condition, and a greater proportion experienced clinically significant reductions in pain.

Pharmacotherapies

Recent developments regarding FM therapy relate to new medications being developed and tested specifically for this condition. Three medications are currently approved by the FDA for the treatment of pain related to FM—the amine reuptake inhibitors duloxetine and milnacipran and the membrane stabilizer pregabalin—although many medications are used with varying success in off-label fashion. The theoretical background relating these agents to FM has been based on various biochemical or physiologic abnormalities found in FM[33,97,98] and known to be important contributors to the pathogenesis of pain. One approach to the therapeutic goals of pharmaceutical therapy would be to say that FM has three main domains (or symptoms) that represent targets for therapeutic intervention, such as pain, insomnia, and depression, but others could be substituted as well.

Nonsteroidal Anti-Inflammatory Drugs

It seems logical that analgesics such as nonsteroidal anti-inflammatory drugs (NSAIDs) should be an important component of a multimodal treatment program for a painful condition such as FM, but NSAIDs have not been shown to be effective as monotherapy for this condition. Perhaps the more important role of such agents is to contribute synergy with other medications because it is very likely that some of the central sensitization seen in conditions such as FM is probably being driven by peripheral nociceptive input. For example, there is evidence that acetaminophen slightly enhances the benefit achieved from tramadol therapy[99]—hence the development of tramadol-acetaminophen tablets.

Local Anesthetics

Lidocaine infusions have not generally been found to provide supplemental benefit in addition to oral amitriptyline intake on pain outcomes.[100] However, a recent study of 68 FM patients with MPS and 56 FM patients with regional joint pain showed that peripheral TrP injections and hydroelectrophoresis ameliorated FM pain and increased pain thresholds at sites distant from the therapeutic interventions, thus providing further evidence that painful peripheral stimuli contribute to the perpetuation of central augmentation.[101]

Opioids

Although opioids are prescribed for the treatment of FM, clinical experience and empirical evidence indicate that they are not effective in ameliorating this condition.[102] Thus, the risk for tolerance, opioid-induced hyperalgesia, addiction, and prescription drug diversion is not justified by the insignificant therapeutic benefit. When patients are taking an opioid, it is recommended that proactive treatment be undertaken to manage the anticipated side effects, such as constipation and pruritus. The aim of opioids in severe cases and those refractory to all conservative medical and psychological therapies should not be merely pain relief but rather clear improvement in physical function. If improvement in function is not achieved, these agents must be discontinued and not restarted. A therapeutic trial with a defined end point and defined target dose must be discussed with the patient in advance of starting opioid-based therapy. If the physician and patient engage in opioid therapy, a clear behavioral contract needs to be signed by both parties.

Serotonin

In vivo synthesis of 5-HT can be augmented by the administration of 5-HTP, which benefits from one-way kinetics in conversion to 5-HT. It is effective in the treatment of FM at a dosage of 100 mg three times daily[103] and is available over the counter in the United States. Tropisetron is a 5-HT_3 antagonist that has been subjected to controlled study in Europe for the treatment of FM.[104] A responder group that exhibits a rapid and steady decrease in pain intensity has been distinguished from a nonresponder group that showed almost no response. There seems to be a bell-shaped dose-response curve; the best effects are seen in patients receiving 5 mg tropisetron (39% responder rate), but that effect is lost at higher dosages. Treatment with tropisetron is well tolerated, limited mainly by gastrointestinal side effects. A randomized, double-blind, placebo-controlled trial of dolasetron, an intravenously administered 5-HT_3 receptor antagonist, found that patients with FM experience significant pain relief at 3 months of therapy, but this benefit was not long lasting.[105] Recent work has suggested that the drug cyclobenzaprine, which was shown to be effective for FM several decades ago, might work in part by blocking 5-HT_{2a} receptors.

Amine Reuptake Inhibitors

Tricyclic antidepressant drugs are effective at a low dose (10 to 150 mg) and improve sleep and enhance the effects of analgesics. The largest experience is available for amitriptyline in very low doses (10 to 25 mg) given at night to improve sleep. A combination of fluoxetine and amitriptyline was found to be more effective than either agent alone.[106] However, in another study neither amitriptyline nor nortriptyline had any greater benefit than placebo did.[107] Selective serotonin reuptake inhibitor (SSRI) drugs were developed for the treatment of depression; however, in the usual antidepressant dosages these agents are effective as monotherapy for depression, and in very high dosages (fluoxetine, 80 mg/day), for relief of FM pain.[108] This analgesic effect may be non–serotonin selective at these high doses. The analgesic effects of the tricyclic drugs, not apparent with normal dosages of SSRIs, have suggested that the small contribution from inhibition of the norepinephrine transporter might be critical to their pain-relieving effect. In the tricyclic class there is a large—up to 900-fold—difference between norepinephrine reuptake inhibition activity and that of serotonin.

Another class of amine reuptake inhibitors includes the selective serotonin-norepinephrine reuptake inhibitors (SSNRI), which have been developed to achieve better balance between inhibition of the reuptake of serotonin and norepinephrine. One class (exemplified by duloxetine) exhibits almost equivalent activity serotonin-norepinephrine reuptake inhibitor [SNRI] whereas the other class (norepinephrine selective reuptake inhibitor [NSRI] exemplified by milnacipran) exhibits potent inhibition of norepinephrine reuptake. Duloxetine has antidepressant activity, which may be an important reason for choosing it to treat FM patients who are depressed (about 40% of FM patients are depressed). In dosages of 60 to 120 mg once daily in the morning, duloxetine can be effective in controlling FM body pain, regardless of whether the patient is depressed.[109-111] It is well tolerated by most FM patients. Nausea, dry mouth, constipation, diarrhea, and anorexia are reported more frequently with active drug than with placebo. The adverse effects can be lessened by starting the drug at a low dosage (30 mg in the morning) and gradually increasing it as tolerated, such as increasing the morning dosage by 30 mg every week. The most common target dose is 60 mg in the evening; however some have noted efficacy at higher doses.

Tramadol is a medication with mixed action. It inhibits reuptake of serotonin and norepinephrine in combination with weak μ-opioid agonism. It reduces the impact of pain on FM patients.[112] As monotherapy, it significantly reduces the severity of the pain experienced but is not helpful for insomnia or depression. In combination with acetaminophen, substantial synergy has been noted.[99] Nausea and dizziness can be limiting at first in about 20% of patients, but initiating therapy with just one tablet at bedtime for 1 to 2 weeks can reduce the frequency of this adverse effect and allow a progressive increase in dosage by about one tablet every 4 days to full therapeutic levels. A typical maintenance dosage for FM is 300 to 400 mg/day in three to four divided doses, concomitant with acetaminophen at 2 to 3 g/day in divided doses. Milnacipran, an SSNRI with threefold greater selectivity of norepinephrine over serotonin, has been shown to be effective and durable in reducing the pain of FM in two RCTs and the pooled analysis of these studies.[114] Benefit has been shown for a 1-year period with few adverse events; the most common have been nausea, headache, and constipation.[113,114]

Substance P

Because the SP level is markedly elevated in the spinal fluid of FM patients, it has been thought to be involved in the pathogenesis of FM. Discovery and characterization of the SP receptor (NK1 receptor) gave rise to the development of NK1 receptor blockade drugs to provide new treatment options. Unfortunately, the potent NK1 antagonists that were developed failed to exhibit much analgesic efficacy in FM or other chronic pain conditions.[115]

N-Methyl-D-Aspartate Agonists

The pain amplification of central sensitization can be inhibited or attenuated by *N*-methyl-D-aspartate (NMDA) receptor antagonists. Two NMDA receptor antagonists, ketamine and dextromethorphan, have been studied in patients with FM and were both found to exhibit beneficial effects on spontaneous pain and allodynia.[116] In the case of ketamine, about 50% of FM patients benefited in an open trial. The concept of FM subgroups was advanced by these findings because ketamine clearly identified responsive and unresponsive subjects from among otherwise comparable FM patients. The usefulness of ketamine as a therapeutic agent for FM has been limited by the fear of adverse effects, such as psychological disturbances (e.g., feelings of unreality, altered body image perception, modulation of hearing and vision), dizziness, anxiety, aggression, and nausea. Furthermore, a more recent trial that examined the long-term analgesic benefit of intravenous ketamine infusions found no benefit on discontinuation of ketamine or 8 weeks following the discontinuation,[117] and therefore the benefit of intravenous ketamine infusion may be restricted to its predictive value for dextromethorphan or oral ketamine therapy.

$\alpha_2\delta$ Ligands

Some drugs initially developed as anticonvulsants have the potential to raise the threshold for pain fiber depolarization, as they do for central neurons to reduce seizure activity. Pregabalin and gabapentin are ligands for the $\alpha_2\delta$ subunit of voltage-gated calcium channels.[118,119] These compounds have been shown to have anti-hyperalgesic/anti-allodynic, anxiolytic, and anticonvulsant activity in animal models. They reduce the release of several neurochemicals, including glutamate, norepinephrine, and SP. Pregabalin was found to be effective in reducing the severity of body pain, improving quality of sleep, and reducing fatigue in FM patients.[120] Pregabalin is available in the United States but is scheduled as a controlled substance because of its mild anti-anxiolytic activity. In therapeutic dosages (300 to 600 mg/day in two or three divided doses), it is well tolerated. Adverse effects can include dose-related dizziness and somnolence, which resolve despite continuous therapy with the drug. This observation suggests that it is helpful to start at a low dosage and increase it gradually (perhaps weekly) to help the patient adapt. One approach is to start with 100 to 150 mg at bedtime and increase the nighttime dosage weekly to 300 to 450 mg before adding a smaller morning dosage to achieve 450 to 600 mg/day. Weight gain (5 to 10 lb) and peripheral edema occur in 6% to 12% of patients, without any evidence of an effect on the heart or kidneys. Gabapentin has similarly been shown to be effective in FM patients.[121]

Sodium oxybate, a metabolite of γ-aminobutyric acid (GABA), exhibits sedative-hypnotic activity. It influences both presynaptic and postsynaptic $GABA_B$ receptors. This scheduled drug is already approved by the FDA for the treatment of narcolepsy with cataplexy and excessive daytime sleepiness. It is beneficial in managing the insomnia of FM,[122] but it is also effective in reducing the pain of FM.[123] In a small, randomized, placebo-controlled clinical trial of FM patients,[124] oxybate was shown to significantly increase total sleep time, enhance slow-wave sleep, reduce alpha intrusion into slow-wave sleep, decrease nighttime awakenings, reduce daytime fatigue, and increase the production of growth hormone. It was also observed to decrease the severity of the perceived pain significantly and reduce the tender point index. A more recent study has supported these findings.[125] In therapeutic dosages (3 to 6 g/day in two divided doses at night), oxybate was well tolerated, as illustrated by the high rate of study completion. Nausea (15%) and dizziness (7%) were the most common oxybate dose-related adverse events but generally resolved with continued therapy. In a more recent RCT, it was found to reduced pain, fatigue, and sleep disturbance and improve functionality in patients with FM.[126] The strong efficacy of this compound in FM, coupled with recent work showing that GABA levels are low in the insula of individuals with FM,[127] has rekindled interest in the use of GABA agonists for FM and other chronic pain states, although safety issues will probably preclude γ-hydroxybutyrate from being the compound that is used with any frequency.

Strategic Polypharmacy and Newer Therapeutic Agents

The use of specific combinations of the newer therapeutic agents, or strategic polypharmacy, has been proposed for the management of FM.[128] It should be pointed out, however, that there are no published data on the consequences of combining drugs that are effective as monotherapy. The critical principles of this concept for FM are that complementary medications should be from different drug classes, have different mechanisms of action, and not be synergistic for any serious adverse effect. For an FM patient whose two most prominent symptoms are pain and depression, the use of duloxetine would be appropriate, and it might be chosen as first-line monotherapy. Duloxetine or milnacipran can be used to treat pain in an FM patient even if depression is not present because these drugs and other classes of antidepressants subsequently shown to have analgesic properties (e.g., tricyclics) have generally been found to be equally effective for pain regardless of whether depression is present.[109] In an FM patient with pain and insomnia, the use of pregabalin or a tricyclic would be logical. Obviously, either of these drugs could be used to treat the pain even if insomnia were not present. In an FM patient with three prominent symptoms (e.g., pain, insomnia, depression), the use of either pregabalin or a low-dose tricyclic in combination with duloxetine would be appropriate and safe. Because there is little published research experience with such a regimen, it must be considered clinically experimental, tailored to the individual patient, and carefully monitored for safety. Despite the lack of good data to support this, most clinicians and researchers experienced in the treatment of FM believe that it is important to use combinations of drug and nondrug therapies to achieve the best overall improvements.

PROCEDURAL INTERVENTIONS

Surgical interventions for FM pain are not indicated or recommended, and the search for a surgical panacea has resulted in unnecessary or potentially harmful surgical care of patients with chronic widespread pain, including FM. Other noninvasive procedures have been examined for efficacy in the population with chronic widespread pain. Transcranial magnetic stimulation (TMS) of the prefrontal cortex can cause changes in acute pain perception and alleviation of depression.[129,130] In a recent RCT, the authors recruited 20 patients with FM and randomized them to receive 4000 pulses at 10-Hz TMS (n = 10) or sham TMS (n = 10) treatment for 10 sessions over a 2-week period along with their standard medications, which were fixed and stable for at least 4 weeks before starting the sessions. Patients who received active TMS had a mean 29% (statistically significant) reduction in pain symptoms in comparison to their baseline pain. Sham TMS participants had a 4% change in daily pain from their baseline pain. At 2 weeks after treatment, there was significant improvement in depression symptoms in the active group in comparison to baseline.[131] TMS was well tolerated, with few side effects; however, this treatment is rarely covered by insurance and can therefore place a substantial financial burden on the patient.

OTHER COMORBID CONDITIONS

Management of other specific symptomatic domains in FM deserves separate attention.

DYSFUNCTIONAL SLEEP

Since the original description of dysfunctional sleep in people with FM, it has been clear that this symptom should be a focus of therapy. Nonetheless, management of insomnia in patients with FM remains nonspecific and empirical. The sedating tricyclic biogenic amine reuptake drugs, such as amitriptyline and cyclobenzaprine, have been the most commonly prescribed medications for FM insomnia. They are not ideal for this role because they cause a number of adverse effects and are subject to tachyphylaxis, but a 1-month holiday from all biogenic amine reuptake inhibitors can restore effectiveness.[132] Because SSRIs, SNRIs, and NSRIs are sometimes so stimulatory that they can interfere with sleep, they should be taken in the morning. Even though the use of benzodiazepines is not generally recommended for FM since these drugs impair slow-wave sleep, newer hypnotic drugs, such as zopiclone and zolpidem, improve sleep in FM—albeit without correcting the disturbed sleep pattern seen on the electroencephalogram and without any measurable influence on FM pain.[133] Rebound (withdrawal insomnia) with zolpidem is problematic but can be avoided if patients use the drug no more than three times weekly (alternate days). Two medications used more recently in the FM setting—pregabalin and oxybate—will probably meet the needs for this indication because they are effective for both pain and sleep disturbances.[124,134,135] In addition, both actually correct the non–rapid eye movement sleep pattern abnormalities seen with FM.

FATIGUE AND DAYTIME TIREDNESS

Fatigue in FM is probably the direct result of chronic insomnia. In addition, a small subpopulation of FM patients are sufficiently depressed to make the usual activities of daily life seem overwhelming. Overlap of FM with medical conditions such as sleep apnea, hypothyroidism, diabetes, chronic infection, or anemia can also drain energy, so they should be included in the differential diagnosis. Mild exercise can reduce fatigue in patients with FM. Pharmacologic therapy for fatigue in FM will increasingly rely on the improved rest that can be achieved with medication therapy. It seems unwise to treat the daytime fatigue of FM with stimulants such as caffeine or ephedrine derivatives because the exhausted brain will eventually require restorative rest.

DYSAUTONOMIA

Orthostatic hypotension may respond to liberal intake of water, increased dietary salt, the use of compressive stockings, or a combination of these measures, but occasionally, the addition of a mineralocorticoid will be required.[136] Patients may benefit from avoiding the effects of caffeine and nicotine. Mild cardiac rhythm dysautonomia may be viewed more as a marker of FM than as a comorbid condition requiring intervention.

IRRITABLE BOWEL SYNDROME

Treatment of IBS in FM patients relies on general measures that include dietary adaptations such as avoiding caffeine, alcohol, fat, or specific foods that can be identified as worsening the symptoms. Depending on the predominant form of IBS (constipation predominant, diarrhea predominant, or a combination of constipation and diarrhea) experienced by the patient, somewhat selective symptomatic medications can be used. Pain can be treated with antispasmodic agents and tricyclics. For the diarrhea-predominant form, classic antidiarrheal agents such as loperamide and diphenoxylate can be used. In refractory cases, cholestyramine or antibiotics can be considered. Alosetron (Lotronex) is indicated for severe cases of diarrhea-predominant IBS, but there is a black box warning regarding the use of this potent 5-HT_3 receptor antagonist. It can cause ischemic colitis and serious complications of constipation, such as hospitalization, blood transfusion, surgery, and death. Distribution of this drug is restricted to prescription by physicians who have been specifically trained in its use. For the constipation-predominant form of IBS, a diet high in fiber and osmotic laxatives such as lactulose, psyllium (Metamucil), and sorbitol or magnesium preparations can be helpful. Sometimes four prunes per day will facilitate a more normal stool consistency. Tegaserod maleate (Zelnorm) had been used for this purpose for some time, but it has been withdrawn from the market because of liver toxicity.

INTERSTITIAL CYSTITIS, PAINFUL BLADDER, AND FEMALE URETHRAL SYNDROME

Treatment of irritable bladder or urethral syndrome in patients with FM includes general measures and medication. It is important to maintain high fluid intake, avoid foods that irritate the bladder (fruits, fruit juices, coffee), and perform pelvic floor exercises regularly. Medications that can be helpful include antispasmodics, muscle relaxants, urinary anesthetics, and tricyclic agents. Interstitial cystitis may or may not be related to the FM.

ACKNOWLEDGMENT

Portions of this chapter were transcribed or modified from the chapter "Myofascial Pain Syndrome and Fibromyalgia Syndrome" by I. Jon Russell in the fourth edition of *Raj's Practical Management of Pain.*

SUMMARY

Despite our evolving understanding of the disease process and increased therapeutic options, patients with chronic widespread pain continue to present a diagnostic and management challenge. The disparate range of symptoms found in patients with chronic widespread pain and the multitude of associated comorbid conditions in the patient population contribute to the diagnostic difficulties in an increasingly overburdened health care system. Moreover, the most successful treatment modalities require significant personal changes in behavior and lifestyle by patients, which creates a substantial barrier to implementation. Even FM's diagnostic criteria are controversial, with researchers and clinicians working to develop a working definition to help identify these patients. The most recent collaboration resulted in the development of preliminary diagnostic criteria that address symptom severity (see Box 29.2).

The clinical manifestations of FM include cognitive dysfunction, affective distress, insomnia, stiffness, musculoskeletal pain, and fatigue. These nonspecific symptoms have contributed to both the diagnostic and therapeutic challenge of managing FM. Associated comorbid conditions include chronic fatigue syndrome, IBS, interstitial cystitis, rheumatoid arthritis, systemic lupus erythematosus, and Sjögren's syndrome. This diverse clinical picture complicates both the diagnostic specification and the burden of individual patient suffering.

The evolution of the pathogenesis of FM is being clarified through molecular studies, sensory testing, and other testing modalities, including functional MRI and PET. Abnormalities in neurochemical biomarkers are being recognized as being associated with FM. Immunologic changes are also being identified through work with interleukins and cytokines. Genetic markers (COMT gene) and gender may also play a role in the development of these chronic widespread pain syndromes. The composite result of these novel investigative approaches is an emerging spectrum of identifiable biochemical and functional changes that contribute to chronic widespread pain.

Treatment modalities are aligning into a multidisciplinary paradigm that includes multiple recent drug developments, cognitive-behavioral modalities, physical therapy, and exercise programs. Recent changes in FDA-approved pharmacotherapies include the use of pregabalin, as well as the amine reuptake inhibitors duloxetine and milnacipran. Implementation of therapeutic agents is frequently tailored to the patient's individual symptoms and comorbid conditions (e.g., osteoarthritis vs. insomnia). Ultimately, the most successful treatment outcomes result from multimodal therapy that relies heavily on patient involvement and investment (physical therapy, exercise regimens, CBT).

KEY POINTS

- The objectives of treatment of fibromyalgia (FM) are to reduce pain, improve sleep, restore physical function, maintain social interaction, and reestablish emotional balance. To achieve these goals, patients will need a combination of social support, education, physical modalities, and medication.
- Patients with FM demonstrate reliably augmented sensory processing, which was initially thought to be confined to the sensation of pain (i.e., hyperalgesia, allodynia) but is now known to include hypersensitivity to other sensory stimuli.
- Patients with FM have also been found to have altered levels of biomarkers associated with pain, specifically, glutamate and substance P.
- Three medications are currently approved by the Food and Drug Administration for the treatment of pain related to FM: the amine reuptake inhibitors duloxetine and milnacipran and the membrane stabilizer pregabalin.
- Myofascial pain syndrome is defined as a painful regional syndrome characterized by the presence of an active trigger point in a skeletal muscle.

SUGGESTED READINGS

Branco JC, Cherin P, Montagne A, et al. Longterm therapeutic response to milnacipran treatment for fibromyalgia: a European 1-year extension study following a 3-month study. *J Rheumatol.* 2011;38:1403-1412.

Crofford LJ, Rowbotham MC, Mease PJ, et al. Pregabalin for the treatment of fibromyalgia syndrome: results of a randomized, double-blind, placebo-controlled trial. *Arthritis Rheum.* 2005;52:1264-1273.

Dadabhoy D, Crofford LJ, Spaeth M, et al. Biology and therapy of fibromyalgia: evidence-based biomarkers for fibromyalgia syndrome. *Arthritis Res Ther.* 2008;10:211.

Geisser ME, Strader DC, Petzke F, et al. Comorbid somatic symptoms and functional status in patients with fibromyalgia and chronic fatigue syndrome: sensory amplification as a common mechanism. *Psychosomatics.* 2008;49:235-242.

Geisser ME, Palmer RH, Gendreau RM, et al. A pooled analysis of two randomized, double-blind, placebo-controlled trials of milnacipran monotherapy in the treatment of fibromyalgia. *Pain Pract.* 2011;11:120-131.

Jones KD, Clark SR. Individualizing the exercise prescription for persons with fibromyalgia. *Rheum Dis Clin North Am.* 2002;28:419-436, x-xi.

Jones KD, Clark SR, Bennett RM. Prescribing exercise for people with fibromyalgia. *AACN Clin Issues.* 2002;13:277-293.

Short EB, Borckardt JJ, Anderson BS, et al. Ten sessions of adjunctive left prefrontal rTMS significantly reduces fibromyalgia pain: a randomized, controlled pilot study. *Pain.* 2011;152:2477-2484.

Simons LS. *Myofascial Pain and Dysfunction: The Trigger Point Manual. Vol. 1. Upper Half of Body.* Baltimore: Williams & Wilkins; 1999.

Travell JG, Simons DG. *Myofascial Pain and Dysfunction: The Trigger Point Manual.* Philadelphia: Lippincott Williams & Wilkins; 1992.

Wolfe F, Smythe HA, Yunus MB, et al. The American College of Rheumatology 1990 criteria for the classification of fibromyalgia. Report of the Multicenter Criteria Committee. *Arthritis Rheum.* 1990;33:160-172.

The references for this chapter can be found at www.expertconsult.com.

30 Headache Management

Stephen D. Silberstein

INTRODUCTION

Headache is a problem that has plagued humans since the beginning of recorded time. It is one of the most common medical complaints and accounts for more than 18 million outpatient visits per year in the United States. More than 1% of physician's office visits and emergency department visits are primarily for headache.[1,2] In 1988, the International Headache Society (IHS) published a formal classification system for the diagnosis of headache disorders,[3] which has since been updated and improved (International Classification of Headache Disorders, second edition [ICHD-2]).[4] The IHS classification system (Box 30.1) continues to divide headache into primary and secondary disorders. In a primary headache disorder, headache itself is the illness and no other etiology is diagnosed. In a secondary headache disorder, headache is attributed to an identifiable structural or metabolic abnormality.

INSTRUMENTS AND SCALES IN HEADACHE

Headaches can severely interfere with daily functioning and productivity.[5,6] Research has demonstrated that improvement in symptoms and quality of life (QOL) are not perfectly correlated: symptoms may improve, but function may not.[7] Consequently, it is important to embrace instruments that measure QOL. Instruments that assess migraine disability can improve headache care by facilitating physician-patient communication and guiding treatment decisions. Various headache scales are in use. The scales can be divided into two main groups: scales that measure the impact of a single migraine attack (with or without therapy) over a 24-hour period and scales that measure the impact of migraine over a span of weeks or months. The first group of scales has been used in randomized, placebo-controlled trials; they are highly sensitive to acute treatment effects.[8] The second group of scales has been chosen to compare results in randomized trials.[9]

Scales that measure the impact of an acute attack include (1) QOL (Migraine-Specific Quality-of-Life Questionnaire [MQoLQ] and Quality of Life Questionnaire [MSQ Version 2.1]) and (2) headache impact and disability (Headache Needs Assessment [HANA] Survey). Scales that measure long-term impact are (1) QOL (Migraine-Specific Quality-of-Life [MSQOL] Scale), (2) headache impact (Headache Impact Test [HIT], Headache Impact Questionnaire [HimQ], and Henry Ford Hospital Disability Inventory [HDI]), and (3) migraine disability (Migraine Disability Assessment [MIDAS]).

SCALES THAT ASSESS QUALITY OF LIFE

QOL is influenced by environmental, economic, social health–related, spiritual, and political factors. The fundamental domains of instruments that measure QOL include physical, psychological, and social areas. Both generic and disease-specific measures have been used to measure QOL. The most commonly used generic scales are the Medical Outcomes Study (MOS) instrument, which includes the 20-Item Short-Form Health Survey (SF-20),[10] the SF-36, and the SF-12.[11] Other generic QOL scales used in headache studies include the Sickness Impact Profile,[12] the Nottingham Health Profile,[13] and the Psychological General Well Being Index.[14] The specific QOL scales for migraine fall into two broadly defined categories: those that measure QOL in a single migraine attack (MQoLQ and MSQ Version 2.1) and those that measure the QOL over a period of weeks or months (MSQOL).

MIGRAINE-SPECIFIC QUALITY-OF-LIFE QUESTIONNAIRE

The MQoLQ is a questionnaire that assesses the short-term decrements in QOL associated with acute migraine headache attacks.[15] This questionnaire evaluates QOL impairment in the 24-hour period following the onset of a migraine headache. The questionnaire is self-administered and is completed quickly and easily. The MQoLQ consists of 15 items with five domains: (1) work functioning, (2) social functioning, (3) energy/vitality, (4) migraine headache symptoms, and (5) feelings and concerns. There are three items within each domain. The response option for each of the items is on a 7-point scale, with 1 indicating maximum impairment of QOL and 7 indicating no impairment. Each domain has a maximum score of 21 and a minimum score of 3. The scores were compared between migraine-free and migraine periods. The construct validity of the questionnaire was established by showing that there are significant relationships between subjects' 24-hour MQoLQ scores and other indices of clinical migraine headache such as headache severity, limitation of activity, number of associated migraine symptoms, global change in migraine symptoms, and migraine duration.[15] The ability of the MQoLQ to capture within-subject change in QOL was evaluated by comparing QOL scores during a "migraine-free" period with MQoLQ scores 24 hours after migraine onset.[8] The MQoLQ should be applicable to all adults suffering from episodic migraine headache. It was designed primarily for use in clinical trials to assess migraine management and to be responsive to subject changes in QOL in the 24 hours following the onset of a migraine headache. The MQoLQ

Box 30.1 International Headache Society Criteria (ICHD-2)

Migraine

Migraine without aura
Migraine with aura
Childhood periodic syndromes that are commonly precursors of migraine
Retinal migraine
Complications of migraine
- Chronic migraine
- Status migrainosus

Tension-Type Headache

Infrequent episodic tension-type headache
Frequent episodic tension-type headache
Chronic tension-type headache

Cluster Headache and Other Trigeminal Autonomic Cephalalgias

Cluster headache
Paroxysmal hemicrania
Short-lasting unilateral neuralgiform headache attacks with conjunctival injection and tearing

Other Primary Headaches

Primary stabbing headache
Primary cough headache
Primary exertional headache
Primary headache associated with sexual activity
Hypnic headache
Primary thunderclap headache
Hemicrania continua
New daily persistent headache
Headache attributed to head and/or neck trauma
Headache attributed to cranial or cervical vascular disorders
Headache attributed to nonvascular intracranial disorders
Headache attributed to a substance or its withdrawal
Headache attributed to infection
Headache attributed to a disorder of homeostasis
Headache or facial pain attributed to a disorder of the cranium, neck, eyes, ears, nose, sinuses, teeth, mouth, or other facial or cranial structure
Headache attributed to a psychiatric disorder
Cranial neuralgias and central causes of facial pain

ICHD-2, International Classification of Headache Disorders, second edition.

assesses subjective well-being and daily ability to function, in addition to measuring the typical associated symptoms of migraine, such as nausea, photophobia/phonophobia, and head pain. The 24-hour MQoLQ should not be used to measure global QOL between headache episodes.

QUALITY-OF-LIFE QUESTIONNAIRE (MSQ VERSION 2.1)

The MSQ is a disease-specific QOL instrument with three hypothesized scales; it has been developed, tested, and revised.[16] The MSQ (version 2.1) was structured similar to older versions of the MSQ (versions 1.0 and 2.0). The revised 14-item MSQ (version 2.1) consists of 7 items in the role-restrictive dimension that measure the degree to which performance of normal activities is limited by migraines, 4 items in the role-preventive dimension that measure the degree to which performance of normal activities is interrupted by migraines, and 3 items in the emotional function dimension that measure the emotional effects of migraine.[16] The MSQ dimensions had low to modest correlations with the two component scores of the SF-36 and were modestly to moderately correlated with migraine symptoms. The validation was structured in three separate analyses applied to 267 subjects.[17] The MSQ provides clinicians, researchers, and those who fund health care a measurement tool to assess health-related QOL. The questionnaire was designed to be completed quickly and easily in a self-administered form. This study suggested that the mean MSQ (version 2.1) scores 6 to 12 points higher (indicating better QOL).

MIGRAINE-SPECIFIC QUALITY-OF-LIFE SCALE

The MSQOL is used to assess a migraine patient's QOL over a long period (average of 3 weeks). It is a valid and reliable self-administered measure and a useful tool in clinical migraine research.[18] The information that MSQOL provides can add important information about migraine's impact on QOL and the potential benefits of therapeutic interventions. This questionnaire has 25 items, with each question having four answers. The general format and scoring are 1, very much; 2, quite a lot; 3, a little; and 4, not at all. The total score is then transferred to a scale of 0 to 100, with a higher number representing a better QOL. For the MSQOL, Cronbach's alpha was 0.92, thus suggesting that the items are tapping into a single concept. The MSQOL has the potential to provide valuable information on a migraineur's QOL and be a useful adjuvant measure when assessing long-term treatment outcomes.

SCALES THAT ASSESS HEADACHE IMPACT AND DISABILITY

Headache impairs physical, social, and emotional functioning, but a diagnosis cannot always be made despite the availability of helpful tools. One reason for this is poor patient-physician communication. If the impact that headaches are having on a person's life can be communicated adequately to the physician, the likelihood of appropriate management will increase.[19] Impact and disability instruments are scored differently and have different interpretations. Generally, the impact is scaled in a positive direction, with higher scores reflecting better QOL (i.e., lower impact). For disability measures, higher scores reflect greater limitation of activity (i.e., higher impact). Measurement of headache-related disability, together with assessments of pain intensity, headache frequency, tiredness, alterations in mood, and cognition, can be used to assess the impact of migraine on sufferers' lives and on society.[20] The tools currently used for assessing headache impact are the HIT and HIT-6, HimQ, HANA Survey, and HDI or Henry Ford Hospital Questionnaire. These scales, when used properly, can improve communication between patients and physicians, assess migraine severity, and act as outcome measures to monitor treatment efficacy. Impact tools are also used, along with other clinical assessments, to produce an individualized treatment plan.[20] Disability measures assess impairment in role functioning (i.e., reduced ability to function in defined roles, such as paid work).[6] The disability instruments used are the HDI and the MIDAS.

HEADACHE IMPACT TEST

The HIT is a tool that measures headache's impact on a person's ability to function on the job, at home, and in social situations. The HIT was developed by the psychometricians who developed the SF-36 health assessment. HIT was designed for greater accessibility (on the Internet at www.headachetest.com and www.amlhealthy.com and as a paper-based form known as HIT-6). HIT-6 is a practical test that consists of six questions. A patient can complete the test in less than 2 minutes. HIT-6 assesses disability over a 4-week period. The range of scores is 36 to 78. Higher scores signify greater impact of disability. A score of 60 or higher indicates a severe impact (the headache stops family, work, school, or social activities), a score between 56 and 59 indicates a substantial impact, a score between 50 and 55 signifies some impact, and a score below 49 denotes no impact.[21] The availability of this test on the Internet, with feedback provided, makes it a useful tool to help headache sufferers understand the burden of their migraines and seek appropriate management.

HEADACHE IMPACT QUESTIONNAIRE

The HimQ measures pain and limitations in activity over a 3-month period. This instrument was the precursor to the MIDAS instrument (see disability scales). The HimQ score is derived from four frequency-based questions (i.e., number of headaches, missed days of work, missed days of chores, or missed days of non–work-related activity) and four summary measures of the average experience across headaches (i.e., average pain intensity and average reduced effectiveness when having a headache at work, during household chores, and in non–work-related activity).[22,23] This scale was validated after assessing the pain and limitations in activity in a population-based sample of 132 migraine headache sufferers enrolled in a 90-day daily-diary study who completed the HimQ at the end of the study. Previous studies of the validity of retrospective pain and disability reporting were mixed.[22,24-31] Study participants completed the HimQ in person and then completed daily diaries for 90 days. The HimQ was developed to identify headache sufferers who have the greatest need for medical care. Self-administered questionnaires can adequately capture information to rate pain severity.

HEADACHE NEEDS ASSESSMENT SURVEY

The HANA questionnaire was designed to assess two dimensions (frequency and bothersomeness) of migraine's impact.[32] Seven issues related to living with migraine were used as ratings of frequency and bothersomeness. Validation studies were performed in a Web-based survey, a clinical trial responsiveness population, and a retest reliability population. Headache characteristics (e.g., frequency, severity, and treatment), demographic information, and the HDI were used for external validation. The HANA can be used in medical practice groups (e.g., headache centers, managed care groups) as a screening tool to detect potential problems. Scores from the scale are compared before and after treatment to determine the headache's impact. Primary care physicians could use the HANA to screen patients with migraine for further evaluation. Once identified, those with severe migraine may be candidates for further evaluation and immediate treatment. The HANA has several advantages in that it can (1) select who should be treated, (2) increase productivity by adequately treating headaches, and (3) identify the need for aggressive treatment without the usual slow advancement through stepped-care algorithms. This brief, self-applied questionnaire may be a useful screening tool to evaluate migraine's impact. The two-dimensional approach to patient-reported QOL allows individuals to weight the impact of both frequency and bothersomeness of chronic migraine (CM) on multiple aspects of daily life.

HENRY FORD HOSPITAL DISABILITY INVENTORY

The HDI is useful in assessing the impact of headache and its treatment on daily living.[33-36] It is a paper-and-pencil instrument that probes the functional and emotional effects of headache on everyday life. The HDI is a 25-item headache disability inventory, with each item requiring a "yes" (4 points), "sometimes" (2 points), or "no" (0 points) response. Thus, a maximum score of 100 points reflects severe self-perceived headache disability. The scale is easy to complete and simple to score and interpret. The HDI has high internal consistency, reliability, and good content validity; the long-term (2 month) test-retest stability of the HDI was robust.[33,34] The test-retest reliability for the beta-HDI was acceptable for the total score and functional and emotional subscale scores.[33] Scales of this nature help investigators understand headache's impact on everyday life. Thus, the HDI can be used to (1) assess the impact of headache on the patient's daily living, (2) monitor the effect of therapeutic intervention, and (3) plan for a global approach to coping with headache with the patient's involvement.

MIGRAINE DISABILITY ASSESSMENT QUESTIONNAIRE

The MIDAS questionnaire (Fig. 30.1) was developed to measure headache-related disability and improve doctor-patient communication about the functional consequences of migraine. The questionnaire was based on five disability questions that focus on lost time in three domains: schoolwork or work for pay; household work or chores; and family, social, and leisure activities.[37] This scale can be used by physicians, nurses, pharmacists, and alternative practitioners. It is easy to complete and takes only a few minutes. The MIDAS questionnaire has demonstrated reliability,[38] as reported in two separate population-based studies, one in the United States and one in the United Kingdom, and validity by using a 3-month daily-diary study as the "gold standard."[39] Scores on the MIDAS are highly correlated with physician judgments about the severity of illness and need for treatment.[40] This instrument is scored as follows: 5 to 10 indicates little or no disability, 10 to 20 indicates moderate disability, and higher than 20 denotes severe disability. The MIDAS questionnaire is an important part of a package of educational, investigative, and therapeutic measures and could play a major role in improving the care of patients with migraine and other types of headache.[20,41-48] A randomized, placebo-controlled trial showed that the MIDAS grade provides a basis for selecting initial treatment in stratified care.[49]

MIGRAINE

Migraine is a chronic neurologic disease characterized by episodic attacks of headache and associated symptoms. "Migraine" is derived from the Greek word "hemicrania" (Galen ≈200 A.D).[50] The diagnosis is based on retrospective reporting of headache characteristics and associated symptoms.[51] The revised IHS diagnostic criteria for headache disorders[3] (ICHD-2) provide the criteria for a total of seven subtypes of migraine.[4]

Instructions: Please answer the following questions about ALL your headaches you have had over the last 3 months. Write your answer in the box next to each question. Write zero if you did not do the activity in the last 3 months.

1 On how many days in the last 3 months did you miss work or school because of your headache? [ ]
2 How many days in the last 3 months was your productivity at work or school reduced by half or more because of your headaches? (Do not include days you counted in question 1 where you missed work or school.) [ ]
3 On how many days in the last 3 months did you not do household work or go to school because of your headache? [ ]
4 How many days in the last 3 months was your productivity in household work reduced by half or more because of your headache? (Do not include days you counted in question 3 where you did not do household work.) [ ]
5 On how many days in the last 3 months did you have a headache? (If a headache lasted more than 1 day, count each day.) [ ]

Total days [ ]

A On how many days in the last 3 months did you have a headache? (If a headache lasted more than 1 day, count each day.) [ ]
B On a scale of 0-10, on average how painful were these headaches (where 0 = no pain at all and 10 = pain as bad as it can be). Once you have filled in the questionnaire, add up the total number of days from questions 1-5 (ignore A and B). [ ]

Grading system for the MIDAS questionnaire:

Grade	Definition	Score
I	Little or no disability	0-5
II	Mild disability	6-10
III	Moderate disability	11-20
IV	Severe disability	21+

Figure 30.1 MIDAS questionnaire. (From Stewart WF, Lipton RB, Dowson AJ, et al. Development and testing of the Migraine Disability Assessment (MIDAS) Questionnaire to assess headache-related disability. *Neurology*. 2001;56:S20-S28.)

EPIDEMIOLOGY

The prevalence of migraine is similar and stable in Western countries and the United States.[52] Three large-scale population-based studies have been conducted in the United States, one in 1989,[53,54] one in 1999,[55,56] and one in 2004.[57,58] The first American Migraine Study[53] found that the prevalence of migraine was 17.6% in women and 6% in men. Two follow-up studies, the American Migraine Study II and the American Migraine Prevalence and Prevention Study (AMPPS), provided results identical to the first, thus indicating that the prevalence of migraine has been stable in the United States, at least over the last 15 years.[58]

Before puberty, the prevalence of migraine is approximately 4%[58]; after puberty, it increases more rapidly in girls than in boys. It increases until approximately 40 years of age and then declines. Prevalence is lowest in Asian Americans, intermediate in African Americans, and highest in Caucasians.[6] In the United States, the prevalence of migraine decreases as household income increases.[6,53,56]

Migraine decreases sufferers' QOL. The World Health Organization (WHO) ranks migraine among the world's most disabling medical illnesses.[59] Approximately 28 million Americans have severe, disabling migraine headaches.[55] Migraine's cost to employers is approximately $13 billion per year, and annual medical costs exceed $1 billion.[6] Instruments to quantify migraine disability include the MIDAS[39] and the HIT.[21]

DESCRIPTION OF THE MIGRAINE ATTACK

The migraine attack can consist of premonitory, aura, headache, and resolution phases. Premonitory symptoms occur in 20% to 60% of migraineurs, hours to days before onset of the headache. They may include psychological, neurologic, constitutional, or autonomic features, such as depression, cognitive dysfunction, and bouts of food craving.[60]

AURA

The migraine aura consists of focal neurologic symptoms that precede, accompany, or (rarely) follow an attack. Aura usually develops over a period of 5 to 20 minutes; lasts less than 60 minutes; can be visual, sensory, or motor; and may involve language or brainstem disturbances.[3] Headache usually follows within 60 minutes of the end of the aura. Patients can have multiple aura types: most patients with a sensory aura also have a visual aura.[61] Simple auras include scotomata (loss of vision), simple flashes (phosphenes), specks, geometric forms, and shimmering in the visual field. More complicated visual auras include teichopsia or fortification spectra (the characteristic aura of migraine), metamorphopsia, micropsia, macropsia, zoom vision, and mosaic vision. Paresthesias are often cheiro-aural: numbness starts in the hand, migrates up the arm, and jumps to involve the face, lips, and tongue.[51,62] Weakness is rare, occurs in association with sensory symptoms, and is unilateral.[63] Apraxia, aphasia, agnosia, states of altered consciousness associated with déjà vu or jamais vu, and elaborate dreamy, nightmarish, trance-like, or delirious states can occur.[60]

HEADACHE PHASE

The median migraine attack frequency is 1.5 per month.[53] The typical headache is unilateral, of gradual onset, throbbing (85%),[64] moderate to marked in severity, and aggravated by movement.[3] Pain may be bilateral (40%) or start on one side and become generalized. It lasts 4 to 72 hours in adults and 2 to 48 hours in children.[3]

Anorexia is common. Nausea occurs in almost 90% of patients, whereas vomiting occurs in about a third.[65] Sensory hypersensitivity results in patients seeking a dark, quiet room.[51,65] Blurry vision, nasal stuffiness, anorexia, hunger, tenesmus, diarrhea, abdominal cramps, polyuria, facial pallor, sensations of heat or cold, and sweating may occur. Depression, fatigue, anxiety, nervousness, irritability, and impairment of concentration are common. Symptom complexes may be generated by linked neuronal modules.[66]

FORMAL DIAGNOSTIC CRITERIA

The IHS subdivides migraine into migraine with aura (Box 30.2) and migraine without aura (Box 30.3).[4] To diagnose migraine without aura, five attacks are needed. No single feature is mandatory, but recurrent episodic attacks must be documented.[3] Migraine persisting for more than 3 days defines "status migrainosus."[3,4] Migraine occurring 15 or more days per month is called CM by the ICHD-2 (Box 30.4).[67]

Migraine with aura is subdivided into typical aura, prolonged aura, hemiplegic migraine, basilar-type migraine, and migraine with acute-onset aura. The IHS classification now allows the association of aura with other headache types. Prolonged aura lasts from 1 hour to 1 week, and persistent aura lasts for more than 1 week (but resolves); if neuroimaging demonstrates a stroke, a migrainous infarction has occurred.

Box 30.2 Diagnostic Criteria for Migraine with Aura

A. At least 2 attacks fulfilling criteria B to E
B. Fully reversible visual and/or sensory and/or speech symptoms but no motor weakness
C. Homonymous or bilateral visual symptoms, including positive features (i.e., flickering lights, spots, lines) or negative features (i.e., loss of vision), and/or unilateral sensory symptoms, including positive features (i.e., visual loss, pins and needles) and/or negative features (i.e., numbness)
D. At least one of the following:
   1. At least one symptom developing gradually over a period of 5 or more minutes and/or different symptoms occurring in succession
   2. Each symptom lasting between 5 and 60 minutes
E. Headache that meets criteria B to D for migraine without aura begins during the aura or follows the aura within 60 minutes
F. Not attributed to another disorder

MIGRAINE VARIANTS

Basilar-type migraine aura is characterized by brainstem symptoms: ataxia, vertigo, tinnitus, diplopia, nausea and vomiting, nystagmus, dysarthria, bilateral paresthesia, or a change in level of consciousness and cognition.[3] It should be considered when patients have paroxysmal brainstem disturbances. Some have suggested that hemiplegic migraine should be diagnosed if weakness is present.[63]

Ophthalmoplegic migraine is due to an idiopathic inflammatory neuritis.[68] There is enhancement of the cisternal segment of the oculomotor nerve, followed by resolution over a period of several weeks as the symptoms resolve.

Hemiplegic migraine can be sporadic or familial.[51] Attacks are frequently precipitated by minor head injury.[63] Familial hemiplegic migraine (FHM) is an autosomal dominant, genetically heterogenous disorder with variable

Box 30.3 Diagnostic Criteria for Headache without Aura

A. At least 5 attacks fulfilling criteria B to D
B. Headache attacks lasting 4 to 72 hours and occurring less than 15 days/mo (untreated or unsuccessfully treated)
C. Headache with at least 2 of the following characteristics:
   1. Unilateral location
   2. Pulsating quality
   3. Moderate or severe intensity
   4. Aggravated by or causing avoidance of routine physical activity (i.e., walking or climbing stairs)
D. During headache at least one of the following:
   1. Nausea and/or vomiting
   2. Photophobia and/or phonophobia
E. Not attributed to another disorder

Box 30.4 Revised International Headache Society Criteria for Chronic Migraine

A. Headache on 15 or more days per month for at least 3 months
B. Patient has had at least 5 attacks fulfilling criteria B to D for *migraine without aura* (see Box 30.3)
C. On 8 or more days per month for at least 3 months headache has fulfilled C1 and/or C2 below, that is, has fulfilled the criteria for pain and associated symptoms of migraine without aura
   1. Has at least 2 of the characteristics in a to d:
      a. Unilateral location
      b. Pulsating quality
      c. Moderate or severe pain intensity
      d. Aggravated by or causing avoidance of routine physical activity (e.g., walking or climbing stairs)
   And at least 1 of characteristics a or b:
      a. Nausea and/or vomiting
      b. Photophobia and/or phonophobia
   2. Treated and relieved by triptans or ergot before the expected development of C1 above
D. No medication overuse and not attributed to another disorder

penetration. FHM includes attacks of migraine without aura, migraine with typical aura, and episodes of prolonged aura, fever, meningismus, and impaired consciousness.[69] Headache may precede the hemiparesis or be absent. The onset of hemiparesis may be abrupt and simulate a stroke. In 20% of unselected FHM families, patients have cerebellar symptoms and signs (nystagmus, progressive ataxia). All have mutations in *CACNA1A*.[70]

TREATMENT

Migraine varies widely in its frequency, severity, and impact on patients' QOL. A treatment plan should consider not only the patient's diagnosis, symptoms, and any coexistent or comorbid conditions but also the patient's expectations, needs, and goals.[71] Migraine treatment begins with making a diagnosis,[51] explaining it to the patient, and developing a treatment plan that takes into account any coincidental or comorbid conditions.[72] Comorbidity indicates an association between two disorders that is more than coincidental.

Conditions that occur in migraineurs with a higher prevalence than would be expected include stroke, myocardial infarction, angina, patent foramen ovale (aura), epilepsy, Raynaud's syndrome, and affective disorders (depression, mania, anxiety, and panic disorder). Possible associations include essential tremor, mitral valve prolapse, and irritable bowel syndrome.

Pharmacologic treatment of migraine may be acute (abortive) or preventive (prophylactic), and patients with frequent, severe headaches often require both approaches. Acute treatment attempts to relieve or stop the progression of an attack or the pain and impairment once an attack has begun. It is appropriate for most attacks and should be used a maximum of 2 to 3 days per week. Preventive therapy is given, even in the absence of a headache, in an attempt to reduce the frequency, duration, or severity of attacks. Additional benefits include improving responsiveness to acute attack treatment, improving function, and reducing disability.

PHARMACOTHERAPY FOR ACUTE MIGRAINE HEADACHE

Acute treatment can be specific (ergots and triptans) or nonspecific (analgesics and opioids). Nonspecific medications control the pain of migraine and other pain disorders, whereas specific medications are effective for migraine (and certain other) headache attacks but are not useful for non–headache-related pain disorders. Triptans are effective for mild, moderate, and severe migraine attacks.[73]

The choice of treatment depends on attack severity and frequency, associated symptoms, coexistent disorders, previous treatment response, and the medication's efficacy and potential for overuse and adverse events (AEs). A nonoral route of administration and an antiemetic should be considered when severe nausea or vomiting is present.[74] Injections provide rapid relief. Headaches can be stratified by severity and disability (using the MIDAS or the HIT). Analgesics are used for mild to moderate headaches.[74] Triptans and dihydroergotamine (DHE) are first-line drugs for severe attacks and for less severe attacks that do not adequately respond to analgesics.[74] Patients with moderate or severe headaches and moderate or severe disability (based on the MIDAS) who were stratified to treatment with a triptan did better than patients given aspirin and metoclopramide.[75]

Early intervention prevents escalation and may increase efficacy.[76] Triptans can prevent the development of cutaneous allodynia, and cutaneous allodynia predicts triptans' effectiveness.[77] Before deciding that a drug is ineffective, at least two attacks should be treated. It may be necessary to add an adjuvant or change the dose, formulation, or route of administration. If the response is inadequate, the headache recurs, or AEs are bothersome, a change in medication may be needed. Limiting acute treatment to 2 to 3 days a week can prevent medication overuse headache (MOH). When headaches are very frequent, early intervention may not be appropriate.

All treatments occasionally fail; therefore, rescue medications (opioids, neuroleptics, and corticosteroids) are needed. They provide relief but often limit function because of sedation or other AEs.

PREVENTIVE TREATMENT

Preventive therapy is given in an attempt to reduce the frequency, duration, or severity of attacks. Additional benefits include improving responsiveness to acute attack treatment, improving function, and reducing disability. Preventive treatment may avert episodic migraine's progression to CM and result in reductions in health care cost. Silberstein and colleagues retrospectively analyzed resource utilization information in a large claims database. The addition of migraine preventive drug therapy to therapy that consisted of only an acute medication was effective in reducing resource consumption. When the 6 months after the initial preventive medication was compared with the 6 months preceding preventive therapy, office and other outpatient visits with a migraine diagnosis decreased 51.1%, emergency department visits with a migraine diagnosis decreased 81.8%, computed tomography (CT) scans with a migraine diagnosis decreased 75.0%, magnetic resonance imaging (MRI) with a migraine diagnosis decreased 88.2%, and other migraine medication dispensing decreased 14.1%.[78]

Preventive medications reduce attack frequency, duration, or severity.[51,79] According to the U.S. Headache Consortium Guidelines,[80] as recently revised,[81] indications for preventive treatment include the following:

- Recurring migraine that significantly interferes with the patient's QOL and daily routine despite acute treatment
- Failure of, contraindication to, or troublesome AEs from acute medications
- Acute medication overuse
- Very frequent headaches (>1/wk) (risk for CM or medication overuse)
- Patient preference
- Special circumstances such as hemiplegic migraine; frequent, very long, or uncomfortable auras; or attacks with a risk for permanent neurologic injury

Prevention is not being used to the extent that it should be. Results from the American Migraine Study I and II and the Philadelphia Phone Survey 2 demonstrated that migraine preventive therapy is underused: only 13% of all migraineurs currently use preventive therapy to control their attacks.[58] In the American Migraine Study II, 25% of all people with migraine, or more than 7 million people, experienced more than three attacks per month, and 53% of those surveyed reported either having severe impairment because of their attacks or needing bed rest.[56] According to the AMPPS, 38.8% of patients with migraine should be considered for (13.1%) or offered (25.7%) migraine preventive therapy.[82]

Preventive medication groups include β-adrenergic blockers, antidepressants, calcium channel antagonists, serotonin antagonists, anticonvulsants, and nonsteroidal anti-inflammatory drugs (NSAIDs). The choice is based on efficacy, AEs, and coexistent and comorbid conditions. The drug chosen is started at a low dose and increased slowly until therapeutic effects develop or the ceiling dose is reached. A full therapeutic trial may take 2 to 6 months. Acute headache medications should not be overused. Women of childbearing potential should be on adequate contraception.

Preventive treatment is often recommended for only 6 to 9 months, but until now no randomized, placebo-controlled trials have been performed to investigate migraine frequency after preventive treatment has been discontinued. Diener and associates[83] assessed 818 migraine patients who were treated with topiramate for 6 months to see the effects of discontinuation of topiramate. Patients received topiramate in a 26-week open-label phase. They were then randomly assigned to continue this dose or switch to placebo for a 26-week, double-blind phase. The mean increase in number of migraine days was greater in the placebo group (1.19 days in 4 weeks, 95% confidence interval [CI] = 0.71 to 1.66, $P < 0.0001$) than in the topiramate group (0.10, −0.36 to 0.56, $P = 0.57$). Patients in the placebo group had a greater number of days on acute medication than did those in the topiramate group (mean difference between groups of −0.95, −1.49 to −0.41, $P = 0.0007$). Sustained benefit was reported after topiramate was discontinued, although the number of migraine days did increase. These findings suggest that patients should be treated for 6 months with the option to continue to 12 months. If headaches are well controlled, medication can be tapered and discontinued. Dose reduction may provide a better risk-to-benefit ratio.

Behavioral and psychological interventions used for prevention include relaxation training, thermal biofeedback combined with relaxation training, electromyography biofeedback, and cognitive-behavioral therapy.[84]

Coexistent diseases have important implications for treatment. In some instances, two or more conditions may be treated with a single drug. If individuals have more than one disease, certain categories of treatment may be relatively contraindicated.

The preventive medications with the best documented efficacy are divalproex, topiramate, and the β-blockers. The choice is based on a drug's proven efficacy, the physician's informed belief about medications not yet evaluated in controlled trials, the drug's AEs, the patient's preferences and headache profile, and the presence or absence of coexisting disorders.[51] The drug chosen should have the best risk-to-benefit ratio for the individual patient and take advantage of the drug's side effect profile.[85,86] An underweight patient would be a candidate for one of the medications that commonly produce weight gain, such as a tricyclic antidepressant (TCA); in contrast, one would try to avoid these drugs and consider topiramate when the patient is overweight. Tertiary TCAs that have a sedating effect would be useful at bedtime for patients with insomnia. Older patients with cardiac disease or patients with significant hypotension may not be able to use TCAs, calcium channel blockers, or β-blockers but could use divalproex or topiramate. Athletic patients should use β-blockers with caution. Medications that can impair cognitive functioning should be avoided when patients are dependent on their faculties.[85,86]

Comorbid and coexistent diseases have important implications for treatment. The presence of a second illness provides therapeutic opportunities but also imposes certain therapeutic limitations. In some instances, two or more conditions may be treated with a single drug. However, there are limitations to using a single medication to treat two illnesses. Giving a single medication may not treat two different conditions optimally: although one of the two conditions may be treated adequately, the second illness may require a higher or lower dose, and therefore the patient is at risk for the second illness not being treated adequately. Therapeutic independence may be needed should monotherapy fail. Avoiding drug interactions or increased AEs is a primary concern when using polypharmacy. For some patients, a single medication may adequately manage any comorbid conditions. However, this is likely to be the exception rather than the rule. Polytherapy may enable therapeutic adjustments based on the status of each illness. TCAs are often recommended for patients with migraine and depression.[87] However, appropriate management of depression often requires higher doses of TCAs, which may be associated with more AEs. A better approach might be to treat the depression with a selective serotonin reuptake inhibitor or selective serotonin-norepinephrine reuptake inhibitor and treat the migraine with an anticonvulsant. Migraine and epilepsy[88] may both be controlled with an antiepileptic drug, such as topiramate or divalproex sodium. Divalproex and topiramate are the drugs of choice for a patient with migraine and bipolar illness.[89,90] When individuals have more than one disease, certain categories of treatment may be relatively contraindicated. For example, β-blockers should be used with caution in a depressed migraineur, whereas TCAs or neuroleptics may lower the seizure threshold and should be used with caution in an epileptic migraineur.

Although monotherapy is preferred, it is sometimes necessary to combine preventive medications. Antidepressants are often used with β-blockers or calcium channel blockers, and topiramate or divalproex sodium may be used in combination with any of these medications. Pascual and colleagues[91] found that combining a β-blocker and sodium valproate could lead to increased benefit in patients with migraine previously resistant to either drug alone. Fifty-two patients (43 women) with a history of episodic migraine with or without aura and previously unresponsive to β-blockers or sodium valproate monotherapy were treated with a combination of propranolol (or nadolol) and sodium valproate in an open-label fashion. Fifty-six percent had greater than a 50% reduction in migraine days. This open trial supports the practice of combination therapy. Controlled trials are needed to determine the true advantage of this combination treatment in patients with episodic migraine and CM.

SUMMARY

Migraine is an extremely common neurobiologic headache disorder that is due to increased central nervous system excitability. It ranks among the world's most disabling medical illnesses. Diagnosis is based on the headache's characteristics and associated symptoms. The economic and societal impact of migraine is substantial. It affects sufferers' QOL and impairs work, social activities, and family life. There are many acute and preventive migraine treatments on the market. Acute treatment is either specific (triptans and ergots) or nonspecific (analgesics). Disabling migraine should be treated with triptans. Increased headache frequency is an indication for preventive treatment. Preventive treatment decreases migraine frequency and improves QOL. More treatments are being developed, which provides hope to the many sufferers whose migraines are still uncontrolled.

CHRONIC DAILY HEADACHE

Chronic daily headache (CDH) refers to headache disorders experienced very frequently (15 or more days per month), including those associated with medication overuse (MOH). CDH can be divided into primary and secondary varieties.[92] Primary CDH is not related to a structural or systemic illness. Population-based studies in the United States, Europe, and Asia suggest that 4% to 5% of the general population have primary CDH[93-95] and that 0.5% have severe headaches on a daily basis.[96,97] In population samples, chronic tension-type headache (CTTH) is the leading cause of primary CDH.[98] CDH patients account for the greatest number of consultations in headache subspecialty practices.[99] They often overuse medication, which may play a role in initiating or sustaining the pattern of pain. Anxiety, depression, and other psychological disturbances may accompany the headaches.[99]

Once secondary headache (including MOH) has been excluded, frequent headache sufferers are subdivided into two groups based on headache duration. When headache duration is less than 4 hours, the differential diagnosis includes cluster headache, paroxysmal hemicrania, idiopathic stabbing headache, hypnic headache, and short-lasting unilateral neuralgiform headache with conjunctival injection and tearing (SUNCT syndrome). When headache duration is longer than 4 hours, the major primary disorders to consider are CM (see Box 30.4), hemicrania continua (HC), CTTH (Box 30.5), and new daily persistent headache (NDPH).[99] CM, NDPH, and HC are primary CDH disorders that are now included in the second IHS classification.[4] Transformed migraine (TM) is similar but not identical to CM.[4]

CM (see Box 30.4) has been called TM.[100] Most patients with this disorder are women, 90% of whom have a history of migraine without aura. Patients often report a process of transformation characterized by headaches that become more frequent over a period of months to years, with the associated symptoms of photophobia, phonophobia, and nausea becoming less severe and less frequent. A pattern of daily or nearly daily headaches often develops that phenomenologically resembles a mixture of tension-type headache (TTH) and migraine. That is, the pain is often mild

Box 30.5 Diagnostic Criteria for Tension-Type Headache

Infrequent Episodic Tension-Type Headache (IHS Diagnostic Criteria)

A. At least 10 previous headache episodes fulfilling criteria B to E listed below. Number of days with such headache less than 1 day/mo (<12 days/yr)
B. Headache lasting from 30 minutes to 7 days
C. At least 2 of the following pain characteristics:
   1. Pressing or tightening (nonpulsating) quality
   2. Mild or moderate intensity (may inhibit but does not prohibit activities)
   3. Bilateral location
   4. No aggravation by walking stairs or similar routine physical activity
D. Both of the following:
   1. No nausea or vomiting (anorexia may occur)
   2. Photophobia and phonophobia are absent or one but not the other is present
E. Not attributed to another disorder

Frequent Episodic Tension-Type Headache

A. At least 10 episodes fulfilling criteria B to E. Number of days with such headache is 1 day/mo and less than 15 days/mo for at least 3 months (≥12 days and <180 days/yr)
B. Headache lasting from 30 minutes to 7 days
C. At least 2 of the following pain characteristics:
   1. Pressing or tightening (nonpulsating) quality
   2. Mild or moderate intensity (may inhibit but does not prohibit activities)
   3. Bilateral location
   4. Not aggravated by walking stairs or similar routine physical activity
D. Both of the following:
   1. No nausea or vomiting (anorexia may occur)
   2. Photophobia and phonophobia are absent or one but not the other may be present
E. Not attributed to another disorder

Chronic Tension-Type Headache (IHS Diagnostic Criteria)

A. At least 10 episodes fulfilling criteria B to F. Fifteen or more days/mo with such headache for at least a 3-month period (≥180 days/yr)
B. Headache lasting hours or may be continuous
C. At least 2 of the following pain characteristics:
   1. Pressing or tightening quality
   2. Mild or moderate severity (may inhibit but does not prohibit activities)
   3. Bilateral location
   4. Not aggravated by walking stairs or similar routine physical activity
D. Both of the following:
   1. No more than one of the following: photophobia, phonophobia, or mild nausea
   2. No moderate or severe nausea and no vomiting
E. No medication overuse
F. Not attributed to another disorder

IHS, International Headache Society.

to moderate and is not always associated with photophobia, phonophobia, or gastrointestinal features. Other characteristics of migraine, including aggravation by menstruation and other trigger factors, as well as unilaterality and gastrointestinal symptoms, may persist. Attacks of full-blown migraine superimposed on a background of less severe headaches occur in many patients. The term TM has been used to refer to this process. The term CM is now being used by the IHS, in part because a history of transformation is often missing.

DRUG OVERUSE AND MEDICATION OVERUSE (REBOUND) HEADACHE (BOX 30.6)

MOH was previously called rebound headache, drug-induced headache, and medication misuse headache. Patients with frequent headaches often overuse analgesics, opioids, ergotamine, and triptans. Although stopping the acute medication may result in the development of withdrawal symptoms and a period of increased headache, subsequent improvement in headache usually occurs.[101-105] Many primary CDH patients who were withdrawn from ergotamine and analgesics and given no further therapy no longer had daily headaches, although about 40% still had episodic migraine attacks.[95,106]

DEFINITION AND CLASSIFICATION OF MEDICATION OVERUSE HEADACHE

In 1988 the IHS used the term "drug-induced headache" for MOH.[3] Overuse is now defined in terms of treatment days per month (see Box 30.6).

The epidemiology of MOH is uncertain. In European headache centers, 5% to 10% of patients have drug-induced headache. One series of 3000 consecutive headache patients reported that 4.3% had drug-induced headaches.[107] Experience in the United Kingdom (P. Goadsby, personal communication) suggests that drug-associated headache is more common than the literature suggests. In American specialty headache clinics, as many as 80% of patients with primary CDH were reported to use analgesics on a daily or nearly daily basis.[95] Other headache clinics have reported a smaller percentage but a majority nonetheless.[108] In India, in contrast, medication overuse is less common.[109]

Box 30.6 Headache Attributed to Medication Overuse

A. Headache present on more than 15 days/mo
B. Regular overuse for more than 3 months of one or more acute or symptomatic treatment drugs as defined under subforms of 8.2.
   1. Ergotamine, triptans, opioids, *or* combination analgesic medications on 10 or more days/mo on a regular basis for more than 3 months
   2. Simple analgesics *or* any combination of ergotamine, triptans, analgesics, and opioids on 15 days/mo or more on a regular basis for more than 3 months without overuse of any single class alone
C. Headache has developed or markedly worsened during medication overuse

Diener and colleagues[110,111] summarized 29 studies that included 2612 patients with chronic MOH. Migraine was the primary headache in 65% of patients, TTH in 27%, and mixed or other headaches (i.e., cluster headache) in 8%. Women had more drug-induced headache than men did (3.5:1; 1533 women, 442 men). This ratio is slightly higher than one would expect because of the usual gender differences in migraine frequency. The mean duration of primary headache was 20.4 years. The mean admitted time of frequent drug intake was 10.3 years in one study, and the mean duration of daily headache was 5.9 years. Results from headache diaries show that the number of tablets or suppositories taken daily averaged 4.9 (range, 0.25 to 25). Patients averaged 2.5 to 5.8 different pharmacologic components simultaneously (range, 1 to 14).[111]

A prospective study of 98 patients investigated the pharmacologic features, such as the mean critical duration until onset of MOH, mean critical monthly intake frequency, and mean critical monthly dosages, as well as the specific clinical features of MOH, after the overuse of different acute headache drugs.[111] In this study, triptan overuse far outnumbered ergot overuse. This reflects the fact that despite high cost, triptans have become widely used (and overused) and suggests that they are about to become the most important group causing MOH. Unlike patients who suffer from MOH following ergot or analgesic overuse, migraine patients (but not TTH patients) with triptan-induced headache did not describe the typical tension-type daily headache but rather a migraine-like daily headache (a unilateral, pulsating headache with autonomic disturbances) or a significant (and pure) increase in migraine attack frequency. Furthermore, the delay between frequent medication intake and the development of daily headache was shortest with triptans (1.7 years), longer with ergots (2.7 years), and longest with analgesics (4.8 years). Intake frequency (single dosages per month) was lowest for triptans (18 single dosages per month), higher for ergots (37 single dosages per month), and highest for analgesics (114 single dosages per month). Hence, triptans not only cause a different spectrum of clinical features but can also result in MOH faster and with lower dosages than needed with other substance groups.[112]

In addition to exacerbating the headache disorder, drug overuse has other serious effects. Overuse of acute drugs may interfere with the effectiveness of preventive headache medications. Prolonged use of large amounts of medication may cause renal or hepatic toxicity in addition to tolerance, habituation, or dependence. (Tolerance refers to decreased effectiveness of the same dose of an analgesic, which often leads to the use of higher doses to achieve the same degree of effectiveness. Habituation and dependence are, respectively, the psychological and physical need to repeatedly use drugs.)

EPIDEMIOLOGY

In population-based surveys using the Silberstein-Lipton criteria, primary CDH was found to occur in 4.1% of Americans, 4.4% of Greeks, 3.9% of elderly Chinese, and 4.7% of Spaniards. Population-based estimates for the 1-year prevalence of CTTH are 1.7% in Ethiopia,[113] 3% in Denmark,[114] 2.2% in Spain,[115] 2.7% in China,[97] and 2.2% in the United States.[96]

Scher and coworkers,[96] using a validated computer-assisted telephone interview, ascertained the prevalence of CDH in 13,343 individuals aged 18 to 65 years in Baltimore County, Maryland. Those reporting 180 or more headaches per year were classified as having frequent headache. Three mutually exclusive subtypes of frequent headache were identified: TM, CTTH, and unclassified frequent headache. The overall prevalence of CDH was 4.1% (5.0% in women, 2.8% in men; 1.8:1 female-to-male ratio). Prevalence was highest in the lowest educational category for both men and women. More than half (52% of women, 56% of men) met the criteria for CTTH (2.2%), almost a third (33% of women, 25% of men) met the criteria for TM (1.3%), and the remainder (15% of women, 19% of men) were unclassified (0.6%). Overall, 30% of women and 25% of men who were frequent headache sufferers met the IHS criteria for migraine (with or without aura). On the basis of chance, migraine and CTTH would co-occur in 0.22% of the population; the fact that TM occurred in 1.3% of this population would suggest that their co-occurrence is more than random.

Castillo and associates[115] sampled 2252 subjects older than 14 years in Cantalucia, Spain. Overall, 4.7% had CDH. According to the criteria of Silberstein and colleagues,[99] none had HC, 0.1% had NDPH, 2.2% had CTTH, and 2.4% had TM. Nineteen percent of CTTH patients and 31.1% of TM patients had a history of acute medication overuse. Eight patients had a previous history of migraine without aura and now had primary CDH with the characteristics of TTH only. These headaches met the criteria for CM but could have been migraine and coincidental CTTH.

Wang and associates[97] looked at the characteristics of primary CDH in a population of elderly Chinese (older than 65 years) in two townships on Kinmen Island. Seventy-seven percent of the eligible population (1533 of 2003) participated. Sixty patients (3.9%) had CDH. Significantly more women than men had primary CDH (5.6% and 1.8%, $P <$ 0.001). Of the patients with primary CDH, 42 (70%) had CTTH (2.7%), 15 (25%) had CM (1%), and 3 (5%) had other CDH. Only 23% of patients had consulted a physician for headache in the previous year.

Lu and colleagues[116] conducted a two-stage population-based headache survey of subjects 15 years or older in Taipei, Taiwan. Subjects who had experienced CDH in the past year were identified, interviewed, and followed up. CDH was defined as a headache frequency of greater than 15 days a month with a duration of more than 4 hours per day. Of the 3377 participants, 108 (3.2%) fulfilled the criteria for CDH, with a higher prevalence in women (4.3%) than in men (1.9%). TM was the most common subtype (55%), followed by CTTH (44%). Thirty-four percent of the CDH subjects overused analgesics.

The gradual evolution of the definition of CM has resulted in varying conclusions drawn from prevalence studies. Two reviews that defined chronic headache as being present on 15 or more days per month estimated its global prevalence to be 3% to 4%.[117,118] A systematic review from 2010 focused on 12 worldwide, population-based incidence and prevalence studies that determined rates of CM with either the Silberstein-Lipton criteria for TM[100,119,120] or the current ICHD-2R criteria for CM.[121] The prevalence of CM in these studies ranged from 0.0% to 5.1% (initial estimates of these rates were typically in the range of 1.4% to 2.2%) and varied by WHO-defined geographic regions, as well as by gender.[121] These estimates are imperfect because of the heterogeneity of definitions applied across studies and the lack of data from certain regions. Nevertheless, the target population is equally well defined by both the Silberstein-Lipton TM criteria and the ICHD-2R term CM, so the data presented are likely to give a reasonably accurate global perspective. The prevalence of CM in this systematic review also suggests that this condition represents approximately half of all cases of chronic primary headache. In further population-based studies—HUNT 2 and HUNT 3, published in 2011—the age-adjusted prevalence of CM was consistently 0.5% throughout an 11-year follow-up period.[122]

RISK FACTORS (BOX 30.7)

Wang and associates[97] ascertained that significant risk factors for CDH included analgesic overuse (odds ratio [OR] = 79), a history of migraine (OR = 6.6), and a Geriatric Depression Scale–Short Form score of 8 or higher (OR = 2.6). At follow-up, patients with persistent primary CDH had a significantly higher frequency of analgesic overuse (33% vs. 0%, $P = 0.03$) and major depression (38% vs. 0%, $P = 0.04$).

Granella and colleagues[123] found that risk factors associated with the evolution of migraine without aura into TM included head trauma (OR = 3.3), analgesic use with every attack (OR = 2.8), and long duration of oral contraceptive use.

Scher and coworkers[124] described factors that predict CDH onset and remission in an adult population. CDH was more common in women (OR = 1.65 [1.3 to 2.0]), those previously married (OR = 1.5 [1.2 to 1.9]), those with obesity (body mass index >30) (OR = 1.27 [1.0 to 1.7]), and those with less education. Obesity, high baseline headache frequency, high caffeine consumption, habitual daily snoring, and stressful life events were significantly associated with new-onset CDH.[125] Having less than a high school education was associated with a threefold increased risk for CDH (OR = 3.56 [2.3 to 5.6]).

Bigal and colleagues,[126] in a clinic-based study, looked for risk factors associated with CDH and its subtypes. TM without MOH (vs. episodic migraine) was associated with allergies, asthma, hypothyroidism, hypertension, and daily caffeine consumption.

Box 30.7 Risk factors for Chronic Daily Headache

- High headache frequency
- Female gender
- Obesity (body mass index >30)
- Snoring
- Stressful life events
- High caffeine consumption
- Acute medication overuse
- Depression
- Head trauma
- History of migraine
- Less than a high school education

Zwart and associates[127] examined the relationship between analgesic use at baseline and the subsequent risk for chronic pain (≥15 days/mo) and analgesic overuse in a population-based study. In total, 32,067 adults reported the use of analgesics from 1984 to 1986 and at follow-up 11 years later (1995 to 1997). The risk ratios for chronic pain and for analgesic overuse in the different diagnostic groups (i.e., migraine, nonmigrainous headache, and neck pain) were estimated in relation to analgesic consumption at baseline. Individuals who reported using analgesics daily or weekly at baseline had a significantly increased risk of having chronic pain at follow-up. The risk was most evident for CM (relative risk [RR] = 13.3, 95% CI = 9.3 to 19.1), intermediate for chronic nonmigrainous headaches (RR = 6.2, 95% CI = 5.0 to 7.7), and lowest for chronic neck pain (RR = 2.4, 95% CI = 2.0 to 2.8). In subjects with chronic pain associated with analgesic overuse, the RR was 37.6 (95% CI = 21.3 to 66.4) for CM, 14.4 (95% CI = 10.4 to 19.9) for chronic nonmigrainous headaches, and 7.1 for chronic neck pain (95% CI = 5.5 to 9.2). The RR for chronic headache (migraine and nonmigrainous headache combined) associated with analgesic overuse was 19.6 (95% CI = 14.8 to 25.9) versus 3.1 (95% CI = 2.4 to 4.2) for those without overuse. Analgesic overuse strongly predicts chronic pain and chronic pain associated with analgesic overuse 11 years later, especially in those with CM.

Although data on the natural history of patients with CM is not available (because of the 10- to 15-year time scale that would be required for a population-based study of this condition), information from the AMPPS on the clinical evolution of this condition was published in 2011.[128] Longitudinal data over a 3-year period were analyzed to determine rates of CM remission and to assess predictors of remission via logistic regression models. Three hundred eighty-three individuals who had CM in 2005 were identified and evaluated in 2006 and 2007. Among individuals with CM at baseline, 52.7% continued to report this condition for at least 1 year of follow-up. The study also found that 34% had persistent CM (defined as CM across all 3 years), whereas only 26% had remission of CM (defined as fewer than 10 headache days per month).[128] Over a 2-year period the individuals with persistent CM demonstrated increased disability, whereas those with remission showed decreased disability. Predictors of remission included a lower baseline headache frequency (15 to 19 headache days per month vs. 25 to 31 headache days per month; OR = 0.29, 95% CI = 0.11 to 0.75) and the absence of allodynia (OR = 0.45, 95% CI = 0.23 to 0.89).

TREATMENT

OVERVIEW

Patients with CDH can be difficult to treat, especially when the disorder is complicated by medication overuse, comorbid psychiatric disease, low tolerance of frustration, and physical and emotional dependency.[94,129] We recommend the following steps. First, exclude secondary headache disorders; second, diagnose the specific primary headache disorder (CM, CTTH, HC, or NDPH); and third, identify comorbid medical and psychiatric conditions and exacerbating factors, especially medication overuse. Limit acute medications (with the possible exception of long-acting NSAIDs). Patients should start taking preventive medication (to decrease reliance on acute medication), with the explicit understanding that the drugs may not become fully effective until medication overuse has been eliminated.[51] Some patients need to have their headache cycle terminated.[51] Patients need education and continuous support during this process. Outpatient detoxification options, including outpatient infusion in an ambulatory infusion unit, are available. If outpatient treatment proves difficult or is dangerous, hospitalization may be required.[92,130]

Two separate studies in Europe and the United States showed that topiramate at a dose of 100 mg daily was effective as preventive therapy for CM.[131,132] The key difference between the two studies was that patients were allowed to take acute rescue medication as usual in the European trial[131] but not in the U.S. trial.[132] Remarkably, the benefits of topiramate extended to the subgroup of patients who were overusing acute medications, as demonstrated by the significant reductions in mean monthly migraine days in this group versus the placebo group.

The Phase III Research Evaluating Migraine Prophylaxis Therapy (PREEMPT 1 and 2) multicenter randomized clinical trials were conducted to evaluate the efficacy and safety of botulinum toxin type A as prophylactic treatment in adults with CM. A total of 1384 patients with CM were enrolled across trials.[133-135] Patients were stratified into groups according to whether they were overusing acute headache medications at baseline and were randomly assigned in a 1:1 ratio to treatment with either botulinum toxin type A or placebo injections. A total dose of 155 units of botulinum toxin type A was administered to 31 sites in seven head and neck muscles.[133-135] The PREEMPT study results demonstrated significant improvement at the population level in multiple measures of headache symptoms, as well as improvement in patients' functioning, vitality, psychological distress, and overall health-related QOL, in response to treatment with botulinum toxin type A.

Three studies have evaluated the safety and efficacy of occipital nerve stimulation (ONS) for the treatment of CM. They indicated that ONS could potentially be an effective treatment of patients with drug-refractory CM.[136-138]

In some cases, CDH reverts to episodic headache when preventive medication is initiated and acute medications are limited. In other cases, only moderate or no improvement may occur. Zeeberg and coworkers[139] described the treatment outcomes of patients withdrawn from medication overuse. They studied 337 outpatients in whom MOH was diagnosed and who were treated and dismissed from the Danish Headache Centre in 2002 and 2003. A 46% decrease in headache frequency from the first visit to dismissal was noted ($P < 0.0001$). Patients with no improvement 2 months after complete drug withdrawal (n = 88) subsequently responded to pharmacologic or nonpharmacologic prophylaxis (or both) with a 26% decrease in headache frequency as measured from the end of withdrawal to dismissal. At dismissal, 47% of patients were being maintained on prophylaxis. In this population, about half of MOH patients benefited from drug withdrawal alone.[139]

PROGNOSIS

The AMPPS was published in 2011.[128] Among individuals with CM at baseline, 52.7% continued to report this condition for at least 1 year of follow-up. The study also found that 34% had persistent CM (defined as CM across all 3 years), whereas only 26% had remission of CM (defined as fewer than 10 headache days per month).[140] Over 2 years the individuals with persistent CM demonstrated increased disability, whereas those with remission showed decreased disability. Predictors of remission included a lower baseline headache frequency (15 to 19 headache days per month vs. 25 to 31 headache days per month; OR = 0.29, 95% CI = 0.11 to 0.75) and the absence of allodynia (OR = 0.45, 95% CI = 0.23 to 0.89). In addition, retrospective analysis suggests that there may be periods of stable drug consumption and periods of accelerated medication use. Patients treated aggressively generally improve. There are no literature reports of spontaneous improvement of rebound headache, although this may happen. We performed follow-up evaluations on 50 hospitalized primary CDH drug overuse patients who were treated with repetitive intravenous DHE and became headache free.[141] Once detoxified, treated, and discharged, most patients did not resume daily analgesic or ergotamine use. Seventy-two percent continued to show significant improvement at 3 months, and 87% continued to show significant improvement after 2 years. This would suggest at least 70% improvement at 2 years in the initial group (35 of 50) if allowance is made for patients lost to follow-up.

Our 2-year success rate of 87% is consistent with the long-term success rates reported in the literature.[141] In a series of 22 papers published between 1975 and 1999, the success rate of withdrawal therapy (often accompanied by pharmacologic or behavioral intervention, or both) for patients overusing analgesics, ergotamine, or both was between 48% and 91%, with the rate being reported as 77% or higher in 10 papers.[102,103,106,123,142-147]

TENSION-TYPE HEADACHE

Epidemiologic studies of the general population have shown that TTH is the most common type of headache, with a lifetime prevalence of 69% in men and 88% in women.[148] TTHs can begin at any age, but onset during adolescence or young adulthood is most common. The prognosis of patients with frequent episodic TTH (ETTH) and CTTH was favorable in a Danish follow-up to a cross-sectional headache study that included 549 persons. Among 146 subjects with frequent ETTH and 15 with CTTH at baseline, 45% experienced infrequent or no TTH (remission), 39% had frequent ETTH, and 16% experienced CTTH (poor outcome) at follow-up. A poor outcome was associated with baseline CTTH, coexisting migraine, sleeping problems, and single state.[149]

CLINICAL FEATURES AND ASSOCIATED DISORDERS (SEE BOX 30.5)

ETTH is now classified as either infrequent (<1 day/mo or 12 days/yr) or frequent (>1 but <15 days/mo or >12 but <180 days/yr). The IHS criteria for TTH require that patients experience at least 10 previous headaches, each lasting 30 minutes to 7 days (median, 12 hours) and with at least two of the following characteristics: a pressing or tightening (nonpulsating) quality, mild to moderate intensity, bilateral location, and no aggravation with physical activity. In addition, the patient should not have nausea or vomiting or a combination of photophobia and phonophobia. ETTH occurs less than 15 days per month, whereas CTTH occurs 15 or more days per month.[150] The pain is a dull, achy, nonpulsatile feeling of tightness, pressure, or constriction (vise-like or hatband-like), and it is usually mild to moderate, in contrast to the moderate to severe pain of migraine. The intensity increases with headache attack frequency.[151] Most patients have bilateral pain, but the location varies considerably within and between patients and can involve the frontal, temporal, occipital, or parietal regions, alone or in combination, and can change locations during an attack.[152] An occipital location is less common than a frontal or temporal location. Some patients have neck or jaw discomfort or have frank problems with their temporomandibular joint.[153,154]

The onset of TTH is gradual, often occurring after or during stress, and the pain is typically worse late in the day. There is no prodrome. The pain is usually a nagging, tight, or vise-like bilateral pressure that is located in the forehead, the temples, or the back of the head. It may radiate to the neck and shoulders. There are no associated autonomic or gastrointestinal symptoms except for occasional anorexia. The frequency of ETTH ranges from 2 to 12 days per month, with a median of 6 days per month. The headaches may be associated with menstruation.[150,155]

Twenty-five percent of TTH patients also have migraine.[156] What we call ETTH may be two distinct disorders. The first disorder may be mild migraine. The second may be a pure TTH that is not associated with other features of migraine (nausea, photophobia, or sensitivity to movement) or with attacks of severe migraine.[4] The fact that sumatriptan is effective for the TTH that migraineurs experience but not for the TTH that nonmigraineurs experience supports this concept.[157]

Patients with ETTH are no different from controls in terms of stress, depression, anxiety, emotional conflicts, sleeping problems, and fatigue. Patients with CTTH are often depressed.[155]

DIFFERENTIAL DIAGNOSIS

Migraine is the headache disorder most frequently confused with TTH. Both can be bilateral, nonthrobbing, and associated with anorexia. Migraine is more severe, often unilateral, and frequently associated with nausea. Idiopathic intracranial hypertension, brain tumor headache, chronic sphenoid sinusitis, and cervical, ocular, and temporomandibular disorders need to be considered.[150,155]

EVALUATION

Most patients with a long history of unchanged ETTH do not require extensive evaluation if they have normal findings on neurologic examination and are otherwise healthy. Patients with CTTH should be evaluated with CT or MRI, even if the results of general and neurologic examination are normal. A metabolic screen, complete blood count, electrolytes, and kidney and thyroid function studies are also appropriate.[155]

MANAGEMENT

TTH patients usually self-medicate with over-the-counter analgesics (aspirin, acetaminophen, NSAIDs), with or without caffeine. If these medications are not effective, prescription NSAIDs or combination analgesic preparations can be used. Narcotics and combination analgesics that contain sedatives or caffeine should be limited because overuse may cause dependence. Symptomatic medication overuse can cause ETTH to convert to CTTH. Patients with both migraine and TTH benefit from specific migraine medication, such as sumatriptan or DHE (see Boxes 30.5 and 30.6).[150,155]

Preventive therapy should be administered when a patient has frequent headaches that produce disability or may lead to symptomatic medication overuse. Medications used for prevention of TTH include antidepressants, β-blockers, and anticonvulsants. Antidepressants, the medication of first choice, should be started at a low dose and increased slowly every 3 to 7 days. An adequate trial period of at least 1 to 2 months must be allowed. The addition of biofeedback therapy or β-blocking agents may improve its therapeutic benefit.[150,155]

PROGNOSIS AND FUTURE PERSPECTIVES

ETTH is a benign recurrent condition that usually improves with time. Some patients, however, progress to CTTH, especially when analgesic overuse is present. The prognosis of patients with CTTH is controversial because many studies include patients with more severe headaches and coexisting conditions, such as migraine and psychiatric disorders.

CLUSTER HEADACHE AND OTHER TRIGEMINAL AUTONOMIC CEPHALGIAS (BOX 30.8)

The short-lasting primary headache syndromes may be conveniently divided into those that exhibit marked autonomic activation and those without autonomic activation. This group includes cluster headache (episodic or chronic), paroxysmal hemicrania (episodic or chronic), and SUNCT syndrome.

PATHOGENESIS AND PATHOPHYSIOLOGY

The pathogenesis of cluster headache involves the trigeminovascular system, as demonstrated by a marked increase in the level of calcitonin gene–related peptide in the cranial venous circulation during attacks.[158] Activation of the parasympathetic system has been corroborated by the finding of dramatically elevated levels of vasoactive intestinal polypeptide during attacks[158] with robust ipsilateral autonomic features. Cluster events are probably related to alterations in the circadian pacemaker, which may be due to hypothalamic dysfunction. Attacks increase following the beginning and end of daylight saving time, and there is loss of the circadian rhythm for blood pressure, temperature, and hormones, including prolactin, melatonin, cortisol, and β-endorphins. Evidence for the role of the hypothalamus in the pathogenesis of cluster headache has come from functional and morphometric neuroimaging. Using positron emission tomography, May and colleagues demonstrated marked activation in the ipsilateral ventral hypothalamic gray matter during nitroglycerin-induced acute cluster

Box 30.8 Cluster Headache

A. At least 5 attacks fulfilling criteria B to E
B. Severe or very severe unilateral orbital, supraorbital, and/or temporal pain lasting 15 to 180 minutes if untreated
C. Headache accompanied by at least 1 of the following:
   1. Ipsilateral conjunctival injection and/or lacrimation
   2. Ipsilateral nasal congestion and/or rhinorrhea
   3. Ipsilateral eyelid edema
   4. Ipsilateral forehead and facial sweating
   5. Ipsilateral miosis and/or ptosis
   6. Sense of restlessness or agitation
D. Attacks having a frequency from 1 every other day to 8 per day
E. Not attributed to another disorder

Episodic Cluster Headache

A. Attacks fulfilling the above criteria A to E for *Cluster Headache*
B. At least two cluster periods lasting 7 to 365 days and separated by pain-free remission periods of 1 month or longer

Chronic Cluster Headache

A. Attacks fulfilling criteria A to E for *Cluster Headache*
B. Attacks recurring longer than 1 year without remission periods or with remission periods lasting less than1 month

Paroxysmal Hemicrania

A. At least 20 attacks fulfilling criteria B to F
B. Attacks of severe unilateral orbital, supraorbital, or temporal pain lasting 2 to 30 minutes
C. Headache accompanied by at least 1 of the following:
   1. Ipsilateral conjunctival injection and/or lacrimation
   2. Ipsilateral nasal congestion and/or rhinorrhea
   3. Ipsilateral eyelid edema
   4. Ipsilateral forehead and facial sweating
   5. Ipsilateral miosis and/or ptosis
D. Attacks having a frequency higher than 5 per day for more than half of the time, although periods with lower frequency may occur
E. Attacks prevented completely by therapeutic doses of indomethacin
F. Not attributed to another disorder

Episodic Paroxysmal Hemicrania

A. Attacks fulfilling criteria A to F for *Paroxysmal Hemicrania*
B. At least two attack periods lasting 7 to 365 days and separated by pain-free remission periods of 1 month or longer

Chronic Paroxysmal Hemicrania

A. Attacks fulfilling criteria A to F for *Paroxysmal Hemicrania*
B. Attacks recurring more than 1 year without remission periods or with remission periods lasting less than 1 month

headache attacks.[159] Neurogenic inflammation, dysfunction of the carotid body chemoreceptor, an imbalance in central parasympathetic and sympathetic tone, and increased responsiveness to histamine have been proposed as the cause of cluster headache.[160]

EPIDEMIOLOGY AND RISK FACTORS

With an incidence of 0.01% to 1.5% in various populations, the prevalence of cluster headache is lower than that of migraine or TTH. Men have a higher prevalence than women do, and African American patients have a higher prevalence than Caucasian patients do. Recent evidence suggests a progressively decreasing male preponderance: the male-to-female ratio based on the year of onset in Manzoni's study[161] decreased from 6.2:1 in the 1960s to 2.1:1 in the 1990s.[162] A family history of cluster headache is rare. The most common form of cluster headache is episodic cluster. The rarest form is chronic cluster headache without remissions, with only about 1% of patients suffering from this variety of cluster. Cluster headache can begin at any age but generally commences in the late twenties. Cluster headache rarely begins in childhood, and it develops in only about 10% of patients when they are in their sixties.[160,163]

CLINICAL FEATURES AND ASSOCIATED DISORDERS

Patients with cluster headache have multiple episodes of short-lived but severe, unilateral, orbital, supraorbital, or temporal pain. At least one of the following associated symptoms must occur: conjunctival injection, lacrimation, nasal congestion, rhinorrhea, facial sweating, miosis, ptosis, and eyelid edema. Episodic cluster consists of headache periods of 1 week to 1 year, with remission periods lasting at least 14 days, whereas chronic cluster headache has either no remission periods or remissions that last less than 14 days.[160,163]

The pain of a cluster attack increases to excruciating levels rapidly (within 15 minutes). The attacks often occur at the same time each day and frequently awaken patients from sleep. If the condition is left untreated, the attacks usually last from 30 to 90 minutes, but they may last as long as 180 minutes. The pain is deep, constant, boring, piercing, or burning in nature and located in, behind, or around the eye. It may radiate to the forehead, temples, jaws, nostrils, ears, neck, or shoulders. During an attack, patients often feel agitated or restless and feel a need to isolate themselves and move around. Gastrointestinal symptoms are uncommon. A small subset of patients experience a typical migraine aura before a cluster headache attack.[164] Attack frequency varies from one every other day to eight per day, with cluster periods lasting a week to a year. Remissions between cluster periods generally last from 6 months to 2 years. Most patients have one or two cluster periods per year that last 2 to 3 months, with one to two attacks per day.[160]

Peptic ulcer disease is the only known associated medical disorder. Secondary cluster-like headache may be due to structural lesions near the cavernous sinuses.[160,163]

DIFFERENTIAL DIAGNOSIS

The differential diagnosis of cluster headache includes chronic paroxysmal hemicrania, migraine, trigeminal neuralgia, temporal arteritis, pheochromocytoma, Raeder's paratrigeminal syndrome, Tolosa-Hunt syndrome, sinusitis, and glaucoma.[160] Raeder's syndrome has characteristics similar to cluster headaches. It may be associated with severe pain, unilateral and supraorbital distribution, and an associated partial Horner syndrome. It is distinct from cluster headache in that there are no distinct attacks and the pain is constant.

EVALUATION

No studies have addressed the need for testing in patients with cluster-like headache. In most cases a careful history is all that is needed to make the diagnosis. MRI of the head is justified only for atypical cases or those with abnormal findings on neurologic examination (except when the abnormality is Horner's syndrome).

MANAGEMENT

Patients with cluster headaches should avoid alcohol and nitroglycerin, yet other dietary and drug restrictions have little effect. Pharmacologic treatment of cluster headaches is divided into acute and preventive therapy, and recommendations are based mainly on uncontrolled trials.[160,163] Because oral preparations are absorbed slowly, they are not recommended for acute attacks. Effective acute treatments that provide a rapid onset of action include oxygen, sumatriptan, DHE, and (perhaps) topical local anesthetics. Inhaled oxygen, 7 to 10 L/min for 10 minutes following onset of the headache, is 70% effective and is often the first choice of treatment. Parenteral injections of sumatriptan or DHE provide significant relief in about 80% of patients. An intranasal local anesthetic provides relief for some patients.[160,163]

Most patients with cluster headache require preventive treatment because each attack is too short in duration and too severe in intensity to treat with only acute medication. In addition, ergotamine, DHE, sumatriptan, and oxygen may just postpone rather than abort the attack. Preventive therapy for cluster headache includes ergotamine, calcium channel blockers, lithium, corticosteroids, divalproex, topiramate, melatonin, and capsaicin. Occasionally, indomethacin is effective. If medical therapy fails completely, surgical intervention may be beneficial in psychologically stable patients with strictly unilateral chronic cluster headache. The surgery consists of neuronal ablative procedures directed toward the sensory input of the trigeminal nerve and autonomic pathways and is effective in 75% of patients.[165] Gamma knife radiosurgery was reported to be effective in six medically recalcitrant cluster headache patients, but delayed radiation necrosis can occur.[166] Deep brain (hypothalamic) stimulation has been reported to be effective for intractable chronic cluster headache.[167] Since cluster headache is a chronic headache disorder that may last for the patient's lifetime, the prognosis is guarded. Drug therapy may help convert some patients from chronic to episodic cluster headache.[160]

Deep brain stimulation of the posterior hypothalamus (hDBS) and ONS along the greater occipital nerve have been introduced and evidence is accumulating. Deep brain stimulation was developed on the basis of findings of activation in the posterior part of the lateral portion of the hypothalamus.[168] Both hDBS and ONS have thus far resulted in positive outcomes in patients with drug-resistant chronic cluster headache (about a 50% reduction in attacks), but long-term studies have revealed that a positive outcome, especially with ONS, may take week to months of stimulation to be reached, thus pointing at long-term brain alterations in pain processing as a mechanism.[169-172] With both hDBS and ONS the pain and autonomic symptoms return to baseline levels when the stimulator is turned off.[169-172] So far no predictors of treatment response have been found, and greater occipital nerve block does not predict ONS response.[173]

SPHENOPALATINE GANGLION STIMULATION

In 2010 Ansarinia and coauthors described the acute effect of external electrical stimulation in eight patients with cluster headache, of whom four achieved complete freedom from pain, three achieved a reduction in pain, and one had no change.[174] More sophisticated systems have been developed, and an ongoing European multicenter study is now testing the effect of an electrode implanted directly in the sphenopalatine fossa very close to the sphenopalatine ganglion (SPG). The preliminary results are very promising; there appears to be a significant preventive effect in addition to an acute abortive effect. The side effects have been limited, so the therapy looks promising for severely affected chronic cluster headache patients; however, long-term studies are needed. Furthermore, important insight in the pathophysiology of cluster headache and the mechanisms of SPG stimulation can be achieved.

CHRONIC PAROXYSMAL HEMICRANIA (SEE BOX 30.8)

Chronic paroxysmal hemicrania resembles cluster headache in character but is distinguished by its dramatic responsiveness to indomethacin therapy. The pathophysiology of chronic paroxysmal hemicrania is unknown. The changes in intraocular pressure that occur during attacks suggest autonomic dysfunction, and the periodicity of this disorder suggests a central generator.[175] In contrast to cluster headache, chronic paroxysmal hemicrania is a rare disorder that affects women more than men (ratio of approximately 7:1). Its prevalence is approximately 2% that of cluster headache.[175]

Like patients with cluster headache, those with chronic paroxysmal hemicrania have severe unilateral headaches associated with unilateral nasal stuffiness, lacrimation, conjunctival eye tearing, ptosis, and eyelid edema. Headaches average 13 minutes in duration and occur an average of 11 times per day. Occasionally, patients experience a continuous dull ache between attacks. Ten percent of patients can trigger attacks by flexing, rotating, or pressing the upper portion of the neck.[175] Typically, no remissions occur. Rarely, a patient has episodic paroxysmal hemicrania with remissions that last weeks or months. Patients may evolve from the episodic to the chronic form of the illness. By definition, chronic and episodic hemicrania is responsive to indomethacin. No other medical or psychiatric disorders have been associated with chronic paroxysmal hemicrania.[175]

DIFFERENTIAL DIAGNOSIS

The differential diagnosis of chronic paroxysmal hemicrania is similar to that for cluster headache. In addition, patients with "jabs and jolts syndrome" occasionally resemble those with chronic paroxysmal hemicrania. A rare headache disorder called SUNCT syndrome should be considered, although these headaches are much shorter in duration (15 to 30 seconds) and occur much more frequently (many times per hour) than those of chronic paroxysmal hemicrania.

EVALUATION

When evaluating a patient with chronic paroxysmal hemicrania, a trial of indomethacin is necessary to establish the diagnosis. Brain imaging with MRI or CT should be undertaken to exclude symptomatic causes of apparent chronic paroxysmal hemicrania. The treatment of choice is indomethacin (in a dose of up to 200 mg/day). Aspirin may also be beneficial, but it does not usually afford complete relief. Chronic paroxysmal hemicrania may last indefinitely, but the indomethacin requirement may be reduced over time. Temporary remissions and spontaneous cures have been described. Selective prostaglandin synthesis inhibitors, or indomethacin-like drugs without the gastrointestinal side effects of the current NSAIDs, are in development and may be beneficial.

SUMMARY

Headache is a problem that has plagued humans since the beginning of recorded time. Headaches can severely interfere with daily functioning and productivity. Migraine is a chronic neurologic disease characterized by episodic attacks of headache and associated symptoms. The migraine attack can consist of premonitory, aura, headache, and resolution phases. The IHS subdivides migraine into migraine with aura and migraine without aura. Migraine varies widely in its frequency, severity, and impact on patients' QOL. Pharmacologic treatment of migraine may be acute (abortive) or preventive (prophylactic), and patients with frequent, severe headaches often require both approaches. CDH refers to headache disorders experienced very frequently (15 or more days per month), including headaches associated with medication overuse. The major primary disorders to consider are CM, HC, CTTH, and NDPH. MOH was previously called rebound headache, drug-induced headache, and medication misuse headache. Patients with frequent headaches often overuse analgesics, opioids, ergotamine, and triptans. Patients with CDH can be difficult to treat. First, exclude secondary headache disorders; second, diagnose the specific primary headache disorder; and third, identify comorbid medical and psychiatric conditions. Limit acute medications. Patients should start taking preventive medication, with the explicit understanding that the drugs may not become fully effective until medication overuse has been eliminated. TTH is the most common type of headache, with a lifetime prevalence of 69% in men and 88% in women. ETTH is now classified as either infrequent (<1 day/mo or 12 days/yr) or frequent (>1 but <15 days/mo or >12 but <180 days/yr). Patients with TTH usually self-medicate with over-the-counter analgesics, with or without caffeine. Preventive therapy should be administered when a patient has frequent headaches that produce disability or may lead to symptomatic medication overuse. Cluster headache and other trigeminal cephalgias are short-lasting primary headache syndromes that may be conveniently divided into those that exhibit marked autonomic activation and those without autonomic activation. This group includes cluster headache, paroxysmal hemicrania, and SUNCT syndrome. Patients with cluster headache have multiple episodes of short-lived but severe unilateral, orbital, supraorbital, or temporal pain. Chronic paroxysmal hemicrania resembles cluster headache in character but is distinguished by its dramatic responsiveness to indomethacin therapy.

SUGGESTED READINGS

Dodick DW, Turkel CC, DeGryse RE, et al. OnabotulinumtoxinA for treatment of chronic migraine: pooled results from the double-blind, randomized, placebo-controlled phases of the PREEMPT clinical program. *Headache.* 2010;50:921-936.

Hartmaier SL, Santanello NC, Epstein RS, et al. Development of a brief 24-hour migraine-specific quality of life questionnaire. *Headache.* 1995;35:320-329.

Headache Classification Committee. The International Classification of Headache Disorders. 2nd ed. *Cephalalgia.* 2004;24:1-160.

Lipton RB, Bigal M, Diamond M. Migraine prevalence, disease burden and the need for preventive therapy. *Neurology.* 2007;68:343-349.

Lipton RB, Bigal MD, Hamelsky S, et al. Headache: epidemiology and impact. In: Silberstein SD, Lipton RB, Dodick DW, eds. *Wolff's Headache and Other Head Pain.* 8th ed. New York: Oxford University Press; 2008:45-62.

Lipton RB, Cady RK, O'Quinn S, et al. Sumatriptan treats the full spectrum of headache in individuals with disabling IHS migraine. *Headache.* 1999;40:783-791.

Lipton RB, Scher AI, Silberstein SD, et al. Migraine diagnosis and comorbidity. In: Silberstein SD, Lipton RB, Dodick DW, eds. *Wolff's Headache and Other Head Pain.* 8th ed. New York: Oxford University Press; 2008:153-176.

Magis D, Allena M, Bolla M, et al. Occipital nerve stimulation for drug-resistant chronic cluster headache: a prospective pilot study. *Lancet Neurol.* 2007;6:314-321.

Natoli JL, Manack A, Dean B, et al. Global prevalence of chronic migraine: a systematic review. *Cephalalgia.* 2010;30:599-609.

Schwedt TJ, Dodick DW, Trentman TL, et al. Response to occipital nerve block is not useful in predicting efficacy of occipital nerve stimulation. *Cephalalgia.* 2007;27:271-274.

Silberstein SD. Migraine. *Lancet.* 2004;363:381-391.

Silberstein SD, Holland S, Freitag F, et al. Evidence-based guideline update: pharmacologic treatment for episodic migraine prevention in adults: report of the Quality Standards Subcommittee of the American Academy of Neurology and the American Headache Society. *Neurology.* 2012;78:1337-1345.

Stewart WF, Lipton RB, Dowson AJ, et al. Development and testing of the Migraine Disability Assessment (MIDAS) Questionnaire to assess headache-related disability. *Neurology.* 2001;56:S20-S28.

Ware J Jr, Kosinski M, Keller SD. A 12-Item Short-Form Health Survey: construction of scales and preliminary tests of reliability and validity. *Med Care.* 1996;34:220-233.

Ware JE, Bjorner JB, Kosinski M. Practical implication of item response theory and computerized adaptive testing: a brief summary of ongoing studies of widely used headache impact scales. *Med Care.* 2000;38:73-82.

The references for this chapter can be found at www.expertconsult.com.

31 Dental and Facial Pain

Noshir R. Mehta | Steven J. Scrivani | Egilius L.H. Spierings

Because of the complex anatomy and specialized sensory innervation of the head and neck, craniofacial pain disorders merit special consideration. Many craniofacial syndromes are unique and represent a clinical diagnostic challenge. This chapter presents an introduction to practical issues regarding assessment and treatment of common craniofacial pain disorders in accordance with the diagnostic classification scheme of the International Headache Society (IHS) (Boxes 31.1 to 31.3).[1]

PAIN CAUSED BY PATHOLOGY OF THE HEAD, FACE, AND ORAL CAVITY

The specialized structures of the head and face have a rich sensory innervation supplied by the trigeminal system, lower cranial nerves, and upper cervical roots. Accordingly, pain is one of the most prominent symptoms of disease in this area. In most cases the acute pain symptoms closely correlate with other signs and symptoms of disease. However, correlation between pain and other symptoms may not be evident in a number of more complex, chronic pain problems, particularly those involving the masticatory system.[2]

DENTAL PAIN

Tooth pulp has a specialized and possibly exclusively nociceptive innervation.[2,3] In contrast, periodontal tissues are innervated by a wide variety of sensory afferents. Dentin and pulp are closely related and function as a unit. In other words, all procedures performed on dentin are essentially performed on dentin and pulp, the pulpodentinal complex.[2]

Dental pain is usually well localized, and the quality of the pain can range from a dull ache to severe electric shocks, depending on the specific etiology and extent of disease (Box 31.4). Dental pain is typically provoked by thermal or mechanical stimulation of the damaged tooth. Clinical and radiographic findings of dental decay, tooth fracture, or abscess drainage may confirm the source of dental pain.

DENTIN SENSITIVITY

Exposed dentin (open cavities, exposed cervical dentin) is markedly sensitive to changes in temperature, to touch, and to sweets. When exposed, dentin is stimulated (cold, sweet, touch); a sharp pain of short duration is experienced immediately following stimulation. "Conduction of pain" through dentin has received quite a lot of attention both clinically and in research. Treatment of sensitive dentin has attracted the attention of industry, and quite a few products are commercially available. Through the years, hundreds of methods have been advocated for the treatment of sensitive dentin, thus showing that no method is really effective.

PULP INFLAMMATION AND PAIN

The duration of pain is commonly used as a clinical yardstick for determining whether the symptoms are caused by sensitive dentin or pulp inflammation. If a cold test results in pain that lasts for a few seconds, the cause is considered to be sensitive dentin. Lingering pain is taken as an indication of pulp inflammation. This clinical yardstick is crude and inexact, but no better method exists. So if the pain lasts beyond seconds or lingers when the stimulus is removed, it is considered an indication for endodontic intervention. Pulp inflammation as a result of dental caries (decay) needs to be treated surgically and medically with routine dental restorative or endodontic therapy (or both).

Pulp inflammation, if left untreated, will spread apically and the inflammatory process will extend outside the apical foramen. Therefore, in the late stages of pulp inflammation, there is no border between pulp and periapical inflammation, and symptoms from the two types of processes can be mixed.

PERIAPICAL INFLAMMATION AND PAIN

Bacterial by-products seep out through the apical foramen and create a local response to the canal infection. The periapical inflammation does not cause symptoms during most of its existence. There appears to be a balance between the infection and defense forces. It is important to keep this in mind when examining a patient in pain. A radiolucent area does not equal pain. The patient's history, including findings on clinical examination and radiographs, determines the need for therapy. All the classic symptoms of inflammation are involved in an exacerbated periapical inflammation—pain, swelling, redness, and lack of function. The tooth is tender to percussion and periapical palpation. To make the tooth free of symptoms, the infection has to be removed, which involves cleaning the root canal with antiseptic irrigants. Occasionally, a periapical inflammation flares up before radiographic signs are visible. These teeth are extremely painful and tender to percussion, and neither the patient nor the clinician has any problem localizing such teeth. Usually, treatment of a periapical flare-up does not require the use of antibiotics. Root canal cleaning and, when appropriate, drainage of an abscess through the canal or through an incision take care of the infection. This rids the patient of pain. If the patient has fever and malaise or an abscess develops, the use of antibiotics is necessary.

Acute dental pain typically responds to local treatment (e.g., ice packs and reduced mechanical stimulation) or to systemic nonsteroidal anti-inflammatory drugs (NSAIDs).

Box 31.1 International Headache Society Classification of Headache Disorders II

- 14 Categories
- Primary headaches: 1-4
- Secondary headaches: 5-12
- Cranial neuralgias, central and primary facial pain, and other headache disorders: 13-14

Box 31.2 Headache or Facial Pain Attributed to Disorders of the Cranium, Neck, Eyes, Ears, Nose, Sinuses, Teeth, Mouth, or Other Facial or Cranial Structures (11.1-11.8)

11.2—Neck
 Cervicogenic headache
11.3—Eyes
 Acute glaucoma
 Latent or manifest squint
 Ocular inflammatory disorders
11.5—Sinus disorders ("sinus headache")
11.6—Teeth, jaws, or related structures
11.7—Temporomandibular joint disorders

Opioid analgesics are also occasionally indicated, depending on the extent of objective pathology. Opioids should be used only short-term and in combination with NSAIDs. In many cases, treatment with antibiotic agents is appropriate and palliative until a definitive dental intervention is performed.

DISORDERS OF THE PERIODONTIUM (PERIODONTAL DISEASE)

Chronic periodontal disease is an immune-mediated inflammatory process initiated by pathogenic oral microorganisms[4] that results in either focal or generalized areas of destruction of the tooth-supporting structures and surrounding bone. Chronic periodontitis is not generally a chronically painful disorder. Typically, patients may notice gingival sensitivity and tenderness or gingival enlargement because of inflammation and bleeding with brushing or probing examination. There is loss of gingival attachment around the necks of and soft tissue pocketing around the roots of the tooth with loss of bone support, which may result in tooth sensitivity, tenderness, and mobility. In the presence of an acute infection in the periodontal tissues, tenderness to the touch, erythema, and bleeding may be evident. An acute periodontal abscess may cause swelling and purulence (Table 31.1). When inflammation or infection (i.e., acute pericoronitis) occurs in the soft tissue or bone around an erupting or partially erupted tooth (particularly third molars, otherwise known as "wisdom teeth"), similar signs and symptoms may be seen, with pain being a primary symptom.

Box 31.3 Cranial Neuralgias, Central and Primary Facial Pain, and Other Headaches (13.1-13.19)

13.1—Trigeminal neuralgia
13.2—Glossopharyngeal neuralgia
13.3—Nervus intermedius neuralgia
13.4—Superior laryngeal neuralgia
13.5—Nasociliary neuralgia
13.6—Supraorbital neuralgia
13.7—Other terminal branch neuralgias
13.8—Occipital neuralgia
13.9—Neck-tongue syndrome
13.12—Constant pain caused by compression, irritation, or distortion of cranial nerves or upper cervical roots by structural lesions
13.13—Optic neuritis
13.14—Ocular diabetic neuropathy
13.15—Head or facial pain attributed to herpes zoster postherpetic neuralgia
13.16—Tolosa-Hunt syndrome
13.17—Ophthalmoplegic "migraine"
13.18—Central causes of facial pain
 Anesthesia dolorosa
 Central post-stroke pain
 Facial pain attributed to multiple sclerosis
 Persistent idiopathic facial pain
 Burning mouth syndrome

Box 31.4 Dental and Oral Surgical Conditions

- Dentoalveolar pathology
  - Pulpal
  - Periodontal
- Odontogenic and nonodontogenic pathology
- Trigeminal neuralgia and "equivalents"
- Headache and neck pain
- Temporomandibular disorders
- Oral mucous membrane disease
- Oral manifestations of systemic disease
- Neuropathic pain (persistent idiopathic facial pain)
- Burning mouth/tongue syndrome

The pain of periodontal disorders is also generally responsive to NSAIDs, opioid analgesic agents, or combination analgesic agents. An acute abscess may also have to be locally incised and drained. Areas of generalized periodontitis may be treated by tooth scaling and curettage of the gingival pocket and possibly by local or systemic antibiotic therapy.

ORAL MUCOUS MEMBRANE DISORDERS

Diseases of the oral mucosa are numerous and due to a variety of local and systemic causes. Typically, these diseases are accompanied by pain and oral mucosal lesions, including vesicles, bullae, erosions, erythema, or red and white patches (Box 31.5). Pain may be a symptom of the primary disease process, secondary to an associated process (i.e., infection),

Table 31.1 Odontogenic Pain

Diagnosis	Pulpitis	Periodontal Pain	Cracked Tooth	Dentinal Pain
Diagnostic features	Spontaneous and/or evoked deep/diffuse pain in compromised dental pulp. Pain may be sharp, throbbing, or dull	Localized deep continuous pain in compromised periodontium (e.g., gingiva, periodontal ligament) exacerbated by biting or chewing	Spontaneous or evoked brief sharp pain in a tooth with a history of trauma or restorative work (e.g., crown, root canal)	Brief, sharp pain evoked by different kinds of stimuli to the dentin (e.g., hot or cold drinks)
Diagnostic evaluation	Look for deep caries and recent or extensive dental work. Pain provoked/exacerbated by percussion and thermal or electrical stimulation of the affected tooth. Dental radiographs helpful (periapical)	Tooth percussion over compromised periodontium provokes pain. Look for inflammation or abscess (e.g., periodontitis). Apical dental radiographs helpful (bitewings, periapical)	Presence of a tooth fracture may be detectable on radiographs. Percussion should elicit pain. Dental radiographs are helpful (periapical taken from different angles)	Exposed dentin or cementum because of recession of the periodontium. Possible erosion of dentinal structure. Cold stimulation reproduces the pain
Treatment	Medication: NSAIDs, nonopiate analgesics	Medication: NSAIDs, nonopiate analgesics, antibiotics, mouthwashes	Medication: NSAIDs, nonopiate analgesics	Medication: mouthwash (fluoride), desensitizing toothpaste
	Dentistry: remove carious lesion, tooth restoration, endodontic treatment or tooth extraction	Dentistry: drainage and débridement of the periodontal pocket, scaling and root planing, periodontal surgery, endodontic treatment or tooth extraction	Dentistry: depends on the level of the tooth fracture-restoration; treatment or extraction of the tooth	Dentistry: fluoride or potassium salts, tooth restoration, endodontic treatment
				Patient education on diet, tooth brushing force and frequency, proper toothpaste

NSAIDs, nonsteroidal anti-inflammatory drugs.

Box 31.5 Common Painful Mucosal Conditions

Infections

Herpetic stomatitis
Varicella zoster
Candidiasis
Acute necrotizing gingivostomatitis

Immune/Autoimmune

Allergic reactions (toothpaste, mouthwashes, topical medications)
Erosive lichen planus
Benign mucous membrane pemphigoid
Aphthous stomatitis and aphthous lesions
Erythema multiforme
Graft-versus-host disease

Traumatic and Iatrogenic Injuries

Factitial, accidental (burns: chemical, solar, thermal)
Self-destructive (rituals, obsessive behavior)
Iatrogenic (chemotherapy, radiation)

Neoplasia

Squamous cell carcinoma
Mucoepidermoid carcinoma
Adenocystic carcinoma
Brain tumors

Neurologic

Burning mouth syndrome, glossodynia
Neuralgias
Postviral neuralgias
Post-traumatic neuropathies
Dyskinesias and dystonias

Nutritional and Metabolic

Vitamin deficiencies (B_{12}, folate)
Mineral deficiencies (iron)
Diabetic neuropathy
Malabsorption syndromes

Miscellaneous

Xerostomia secondary to intrinsic or extrinsic conditions
Referred pain from esophageal or oropharyngeal malignancy
Mucositis secondary to esophageal reflux
Angioedema

Table 31.2 Temporomandibular Disorders

Diagnosis	TMJ Articular Disorders	Muscle Disorders	Myofascial Disorders
Diagnostic features	Pain localized in the pre-auricular area during jaw function. Usually presence of a painful click or crepitus during mouth opening. Limited opening (<35 mm), deviated or painful jaw movements	Tenderness of the masticatory muscles. Dull, aching pain exacerbated by jaw function or palpation	Diffuse dull or aching pain affecting multiple groups of muscles of the head and neck region, as well as other parts of the body
Diagnostic evaluation	Internal derangement of the TMJ with abnormal function of the disk-condyle complex and/or degeneration of the joint surface. Palpation is painful. Possible joint swelling in acute phases. MRI, CT, etc., of the joint may rule out tumors and advanced degenerative stages	Tenderness during palpation of the masticatory muscles and tendons. Possible limited range of jaw movement and during passive stretching examination. Can be associated with a parafunctional habit (bruxism—early morning pain)	Presence of trigger or tender points in one or more groups of muscles. Pain can radiate to distant areas with stimulation or not of the trigger points. Rule out the presence of lupus erythematosus
Treatment	Patient education and self-care Medication: NSAIDs, nonopiate analgesics	Patient education and self-care Medication: topical and systemic NSAIDs, nonopiate analgesics, muscle relaxants, antidepressants (usually TCAs), anxiolytics, anticonvulsants, BTX, trigger point injections, vapocoolant spray	Same as for muscle disorders
	Physical therapy: exercise program	Physical therapy: TENS, massage, exercise program	
	Occlusal splints Oral maxillofacial surgery: arthrocentesis, arthroscopic surgery, open surgery	Occlusal splints Cognitive-behavioral: biofeedback, relaxation, coping skills	

BTX, botulinum toxin; CT, computed tomography; MRI, magnetic resonance imaging; NSAIDs, nonsteroidal anti-inflammatory drugs; TCAs, tricyclic antidepressants; TENS, transcutaneous electrical nerve stimulation; TMJ, temporomandibular joint.

or related to damaged oral mucosa (i.e., mouth movements, chewing foods, thermal, chemical). The pain is often treated with both systemic and local analgesic agents.

DISORDERS OF THE MAXILLA AND MANDIBLE

Numerous disorders of the bony substrate of the jaws can be associated with pain. These disorders are generally classified as being of odontogenic or nonodontogenic origin, cystic, cystic- or tumor-like, or benign or malignant (either primary or metastatic disease). There are often additional findings on the history or physical examination that warrant further evaluation (i.e., swelling, mass, discoloration, numbness, weakness, bleeding, drainage, tooth loss or mobility). Pain can be treated symptomatically until a definitive diagnosis is established and definitive therapy is initiated (Table 31.2).

SALIVARY GLAND DISORDERS

Disorders of the three pairs of the major salivary glands (parotid, submandibular, and sublingual) and the many hundreds of minor salivary glands within the oral cavity may also produce pain as a primary or associated complaint. These disorders are often accompanied by other signs and symptoms (including swelling, drainage, cervical adenopathy, or generalized symptoms of systemic infection), depending on the etiology of the disorder. Disorders of the parotid gland can extend locally to produce otologic symptoms or cranial nerve (V, VII, or IX) involvement. Disorders of the submandibular gland may result in symptoms of impaired swallowing or impairment of cranial nerves V, IX, and XII (Box 31.6).

Box 31.6 Salivary Gland Disease

- Inflammatory
- Noninflammatory
- Infectious
- Obstructive
- Immunologic (Sjögren's syndrome)
- Tumors
- Others (red herrings)

BURNING MOUTH/TONGUE DISORDER (ORAL BURNING)

Burning mouth/tongue disorder (BMD) is an idiopathic pain condition of the oral mucous membranes. It can be focal (inside of the lips or tongue) or generalized and is typically described as a constant, bilateral painful burning sensation. BMD generally affects middle-aged or older women and has been attributed to numerous oral disorders (e.g., mucous membrane disease, Sjögren's syndrome/dry mouth, fungal infections) and systemic diseases (e.g., vitamin deficiencies, diabetes mellitus, immune connective tissue disorders, vasculitides). More recent evidence suggests that BMD is more likely a neuropathic pain disorder of either peripheral or central origin. Some recent taste-testing data and functional brain imaging studies seem to support this hypothesis (Table 31.3).[5-10] Current treatments of BMD focus on this hypothesis and the use of both topical (oral mucosa) and systemic

Table 31.3 Trigeminal Neuropathic Pain Disorders

Diagnosis	Trigeminal Neuralgia	Deafferentation Pain	Acute and Post-Herpetic Neuralgia	Burning Mouth Syndrome
Diagnostic features	Brief severe lancinating pain evoked by mechanical stimulation of the trigger zone (pain free between attacks). Generally unilateral, affects the V2/V3 areas (rarely V1). Possible pain remission periods (for months/years)	Spontaneous or evoked pain with a prolonged aftersensation following tactile stimulation. Trigger zone caused by surgery (tooth extraction) or trauma. Positive and negative descriptors (e.g., burning, nagging, boring)	Pain associated with herpetic lesions, usually in the V1 dermatome. Spontaneous pain (burning and tingling), but may be manifested as dull and aching. Occasional lancinating evoked pain	Constant burning pain of the mucous membranes of the tongue, mouth, hard palate, soft palate, or lips. Usually affects women older than 50 years
Diagnostic evaluation	MRI for evidence of tumor or vasocompression of the trigeminal tract or root (cerebropontine angle). Rule out MS, especially in young adults	Etiologic factors such as trauma or surgery in the painful area. Order MRI if the area is intact to rule out peripheral or central lesions	Small cutaneous vesicles (AHN) or scarring (PHN), usually affecting V1. Loss of normal skin color. Corneal ulceration can occur. Sensory changes in affected area (e.g., hyperesthesia, dysesthesia)	Rule out salivary gland dysfunction (xerostomia) or tumor, Sjögren's syndrome, candidiasis, geographic or fissured tongue, and chemical or mechanical irritation. Nutrition and menopause
Treatment	Medication: anticonvulsants (e.g., carbamazepine, gabapentin), antidepressants (e.g., amitriptyline, nortriptyline, desipramine), nonopiate analgesics, BTX. Combination of baclofen and anticonvulsants can produce good results	Medication: anticonvulsants (e.g., carbamazepine, gabapentin), antidepressants, nonopiate analgesics, topical agents (e.g., lidocaine 5% patches)	Medication: acyclovir (acute phase), anticonvulsants, antidepressants, nonopiate analgesics, topical agents (e.g., lidocaine 5% patches)	Medication: anticonvulsants, benzodiazepines, antidepressants, nonopiate analgesics, topical agents (e.g., lidocaine, mouthwashes)
	Surgery: microvascular decompression of the trigeminal root, ablative surgery (e.g., rhizotomy, Gamma Knife)	Surgery: ablative surgery (e.g., rhizotomy, Gamma Knife)	Surgery: ablative surgery (e.g., rhizotomy, Gamma Knife)	Cognitive-behavioral: biofeedback, relaxation, coping skills

AHN, acute herpetic neuralgia; BTX, botulinum toxin; MRI, magnetic resonance imaging; MS, multiple sclerosis; PHN, post-herpetic neuralgia.

antineuropathic pain medications (see Chapters 24 and 38); however, there is little evidence that such treatments are effective for BMD.

SINUS DISORDERS

Patients frequently describe their facial pain problem as a "sinus headache." However, sinus disorders do not cause chronic headaches, and the clinician should look for a more specific cause of the pain symptoms in such cases.[11] Diseases of the nose and paranasal sinuses typically cause acute pain associated with multiple other symptoms that are generally related to the specific nasal or sinus disease (i.e., allergic, inflammatory, infectious) (Table 31.4). Acute dentoalveolar pathology of the maxillary posterior teeth can often be accompanied by signs and symptoms consistent with sinus disease. In addition, acute dentoalveolar inflammation or infection (dental abscess) can cause secondary maxillary sinus inflammation or infection. These disorders are typically acute in nature but can become chronic. This condition is often confused with other facial pain and headache disorders.

DISORDERS OF THE EYE AND EAR

Because numerous disorders can cause pain in and around the eye and ear, patients need to be evaluated for any primary ophthalmologic or otologic disease. Very often pain in and around these structures is also associated with a variety of other craniofacial and headache syndromes (Boxes 31.7 to 31.9).

TUMORS

Numerous intracranial and extracranial tumors can cause oral cavity, oropharyngeal, facial, and head pain as a primary symptom. Cancers of the upper aerodigestive tract, jaws, base of the skull, and neck may all be accompanied by pain along with other associated signs and symptoms. In addition, numerous intracranial tumors and lesions (i.e., vascular malformations) can be manifested as facial pain and headache. These are primarily tumors of the cerebellopontine angle; however, various primary brain neoplasms and metastatic disease have been associated with facial pain and headache. Headache and facial pain of

Table 31.4 Paranasal, Periocular, Periauricular, and Head and Neck Cancer Pain

Diagnosis	Paranasal Sinus Pain	Periocular Pain	Periauricular Pain	Head and Neck Cancer Pain
Diagnostic features	Bilateral or unilateral throbbing, pressure, or pain in the frontal area exacerbated by leaning forward or palpitation over the sinus	Pain or tenderness with or without eye movements, deep orbital pain, referred pain	Diffuse aching or sudden pain with or without an aural discharge (e.g., otitis media)	Variety of symptoms. Pain may be due to tumor, nerve compression, secondary infection, secondary myofascial pain, deafferentation, radiotherapy, chemotherapy
Diagnostic evaluation	History of chronic allergies, frequent URIs, sinusitis, headaches of various types, sinus surgery Refer to ENT for endoscopic and/or CT study (e.g., sinus opacification)	Examine the eyelids, lacrimal function, conjunctiva, sclera. Ophthalmoscopy and ophthalmology referral. Rule out primary headache, temporal arteritis, orbital pseudotumor	The area is innervated by multiple cranial and cervical nerves, so complete functional and structural examination is necessary (e.g., inspect the tympanic membrane, TMJ, and myofascia). CT and MRI invaluable for mastoiditis and cholesteatoma	Complete evaluation by multidisciplinary team, CT, MRI, endoscopy, biopsy, and surveillance. Treatment coordination by oncologist
Treatment	ENT evaluation/treatment	Proper ophthalmologic evaluation and treatment	Proper ENT evaluation and treatment	Oncologist evaluation and treatment
	Medication: sinusitis—topical decongestants, systemic antibiotics Chronic sinus pain—NSAIDs, nonopiate analgesics, topical agents (lidocaine spray), anticonvulsants, antidepressants, BTX	Medication: NSAIDs, nonopiate analgesics. systemic antibiotics, topical corticosteroids, BTX across the forehead and glabellar areas in selected cases	Medication: NSAIDs, nonopiate analgesics, systemic antibiotics, topical corticosteroids, BTX in selected cases	Medication: anticonvulsants, antidepressants, opiate or nonopiate analgesics, topical agents, muscles relaxants
	Surgery	Surgery	Surgery	Surgery: ablative surgery

BTX, botulinum toxin; CT, computed tomography; ENT, ear, nose, and throat; MRI, magnetic resonance imaging; NSAIDs, nonsteroidal anti-inflammatory drugs; TMJ, temporomandibular joint; URI, urinary tract infection.

Box 31.7 Headache and Facial Pain Syndromes with Eye Pain

- Cluster headache and cluster-tic syndrome
- Paroxysmal hemicrania
- SUNCT syndrome
- Trigeminal neuralgia
- Sphenopalatine neuralgia (Sluder's neuralgia)
- Ice pick headache
- Ice cream headache
- Hypnic headache
- Eye pain, headache, and lung cancer
- Nonorganic pain and headache (psychosomatic and psychiatric disorders)

SUNCT, *s*hort-lasting, *u*nilateral, *n*euralgiform headache attacks, *c*onjunctival injection, *t*earing.

Box 31.8 Red Flags for a Patient with Eye Pain

- New visual acuity defect, color vision defect, or visual field loss
- Relative afferent pupillary defect
- Extraocular muscle abnormality, ocular misalignment, or diplopia
- Proptosis
- Lid retraction or ptosis
- Conjunctival chemosis, injection, or redness
- Corneal opacity
- Hyphema or hypopyon
- Iris irregularity
- Nonreactive pupil
- Fundus abnormality
- Recent ocular surgery (<3 months)
- Recent ocular trauma

unknown origin should warrant careful evaluation for an underlying occult tumor (see Boxes 31.7 and 31.8).[12-14]

Patients with facial pain or headache should undergo a comprehensive medical history and careful physical examination with particular attention paid to the cranial neurologic examination. Consideration should be given to obtaining appropriate imaging studies, including computed tomography (CT), magnetic resonance imaging (MRI), and magnetic resonance angiography.

TEMPOROMANDIBULAR DISORDERS

Temporomandibular disorders (TMDs) are defined as a subgroup of craniofacial pain problems that involve the

Box 31.9 Structural Lesions and Facial Pain

- Multiple sclerosis plaques
- Tumors of the cerebellopontine angle
- Schwannomas
- Chiari malformations
- Midbrain lesions
- Pontine hemorrhage
- Vascular malformations
- Skull base tumors
- Small cell carcinomas
- Salivary gland tumors
- Oral cancers
- Carotid/vertebral disease

temporomandibular joint (TMJ), masticatory muscles, and associated head and neck musculoskeletal structures.[15] Patients with TMDs most frequently have pain, limited or asymmetrical mandibular motion, and TMJ sounds.[16,17] The pain or discomfort is often localized to the jaw, TMJ, and muscles of mastication. Common associated symptoms include ear pain and stuffiness, tinnitus, dizziness, neck pain, and headache. In some cases the onset is acute and the symptoms are mild and self-limited. In other patients, a chronic TMD with persistent pain develops in association with physical, behavioral, psychological, and psychosocial symptoms similar to those of patients with chronic pain syndromes in other areas of the body (e.g., arthritis, low back pain, chronic headache, fibromyalgia, chronic regional pain syndrome),[18-20] all requiring a coordinated interdisciplinary diagnostic and treatment approach.

At least three distinct and separate dysfunctions that can create or affect the symptoms described by patients with a TMD are recognized[21]:

1. **Muscle disorders (myofascial pain disorder [MPD]).** MPD is related to muscle dysfunction, which often leads to muscle spasms, pain, and dysfunction. This type of dysfunction can occur in any skeletal muscle. The triggering area lies in the fascial coverings and attachment zones of the muscles, hence the term *myofascial.*
2. **Temporomandibular joint articular disorders (TMJDs).** TMJDs are related to specific problems in the TMJs. These problems may range from joint sounds to locking, pain, and degenerative changes in the joints themselves. Invariably, muscle dysfunction is a secondary effect of true TMJDs.
3. **Cervical spinal dysfunction (CSD).** This syndrome is related to the spinal column, the vertebrae, the ligaments, and muscles related to them. The majority of symptoms not directly related to the jaw muscles are triggered or affected by CSD syndrome.

Common associated signs and symptoms of TMDs that need to be evaluated are headache, facial pain, eye pain, ear symptoms, TMJ symptoms, neck pain, and arm and back symptoms.

HEADACHE

Symptoms of bilateral head and facial pain involve multiple postural muscles or the muscles of mastication. The pain is dull and aching in quality with a chronic or persistent temporal pattern.[22,23] It is typically moderate in intensity, and patients often exhibit daily symptoms that can wax and wane in severity. Exacerbations of pain are often provoked by functional use of the affected muscles. Morning headaches may be related to nocturnal bruxism, sleep disorders, or both.[23,24] Increasing pain during the day may be related to muscle use or maintenance of head posture.[23,24]

FACIAL PAIN

Pain in the sides of the mandible and pain described by the patient as "sinus" pain in the zygomatic or orbital area may also have a musculoskeletal origin.[25] Daytime clenching and acute or chronic stress, combined with a reduction in dental vertical dimension (height) related to loss of posterior teeth, can create muscle trigger points or muscle fatigue. This is particularly noticed by the patient after meals and reported as "a heavy and tired feeling" in the jaw muscles. Facial pain related to sinus and other pathologic conditions is discussed later in the chapter.

EYE PAIN

TMDs frequently include pain symptoms that involve the eye and periorbital region.[26-28] The pain is typically referred from other muscular sites, including the suboccipital region. Orbital pain symptoms are often described as unilateral, constant, and "boring." This is frequently seen in patients with a history of trauma or chronic upper cervical vertebral subluxation or nerve root impingement related to the occiput and atlantoaxial region. In addition, entrapment of the greater occipital nerve at the occiput level can also produce this type of pain, which is often diagnosed as occipital neuralgia. It may frequently be amenable to physical medicine along with changes in head posture and mandibular position.

EAR SYMPTOMS

Pain, stuffiness, and tinnitus may have a musculoskeletal etiology.[29-34] Mandibular posture related to the maxilla affects the masticatory elevator muscles. The medial pterygoids are intimately related in the left-to-right balance of the mandible on tooth closure. The tensor tympani and tensor palati are actually one muscle with a raphe that wraps around the hamular notch of the maxilla. Improper growth of the maxilla during development may affect eustachian tube function and contribute to middle ear infections in children and stuffiness and changes in ear pressure in adults.

Tinnitus and other types of sounds may also have a musculoskeletal etiology. Specifically, cervical factors and mandibular postural factors have been seen in subjects with tinnitus. A combination of physical medicine and dental mouth guard therapy has been effective in some patients with a history of trauma or childhood growth affecting proper expansion of the maxilla. Ear pain that is sharp and jabbing on movement of the mandible is frequently seen in patients with internal derangement of the TMJ. This type of pain is generally unilateral and ipsilateral to the joint in question. Ear pain and symptoms such as stuffiness in the absence of positive otologic findings are among the most common reasons for evaluation of dental- and maxillomandibular-related imbalance. Treatment can often alleviate the symptoms completely or reduce their impact on the patient in conjunction with standard medical intervention.[29-34]

TEMPOROMANDIBULAR JOINT SYMPTOMS

Pain and sounds are very common with TMDs.[35,36] The pain is typically unilateral and may be related to trauma or bruxism in the presence of missing posterior teeth; it can result in injury or anterior disk displacement without reduction and subsequent "locking" of the TMJ. Treatment often includes a combination of dental, medical, physical medicine, and mouth guard therapy plus stress management through biofeedback relaxation.

NECK PAIN

Neck stiffness and pain are commonly part of the umbrella of TMDs.[37-39] Trauma, habitual posturing, and musculoskeletal tension will chronically affect the cervical area and create pain, stiffness, and trigger points in the muscles of the head and neck. It is well documented that the trigeminal and cervical nerve systems are interactive in the maintenance of head, neck, and jaw posture.[39,40] Examination of dental factors in patients with chronic neck pain is important[41,42] because studies examining the relationship between maxillomandibular position and the cervical spine have shown that loss of vertical dimension of the teeth and a deep bite can adversely affect cervical muscle function and lead to chronic stiffness, pain, and a reduction in range of motion.[42]

ARM AND BACK SYMPTOMS

Patients with TMJDs will often also have other musculoskeletal findings, including shoulder pain and pain radiating down the arm that may or may not be accompanied by tingling or numbness. Physical examination may reveal positive signs of thoracic outlet syndrome, costoclavicular syndrome, vertebral subluxation or nerve impingement of the brachial plexus of nerves, and even previously undiagnosed rotator cuff injuries.[41] Treatment requires a thoughtful multimodal approach to the various areas affected.

ETIOLOGY

In 1934, Costen, an otolaryngologist, evaluated 13 patients with pain in or near the ear, tinnitus, dizziness, a sensation of ear fullness, and difficulty swallowing.[43] He observed that these patients had many missing teeth and, as a result, their mandibles exhibited overclosure. The patients seemed to improve when their missing teeth were replaced and the proper vertical dimension of the occlusion was restored. The malocclusion and improper jaw position were perceived to be the cause of both "disturbed function of the temporomandibular joint" and the associated facial pain. Thereafter, the emphasis of treatment was on altering the affected patient's occlusion.

More recently, advances in the understanding of joint biomechanics, neuromuscular physiology, autoimmune and musculoskeletal disorders, and pain mechanisms have resulted in changing concepts of the etiology of TMDs. These disorders are now considered multifactorial in etiology, with biologic, behavioral, environmental, social, emotional, and cognitive factors alone or in combination contributing to development of the signs and symptoms of TMDs.[15,16,44]

Box 31.10 Temporomandibular Joint Articular Disorders

11.1.1—Congenital or developmental
- Aplasia
- Hypoplasia
- Hyperplasia
- Neoplasia

11.7.1.1—Disk derangement disorders
- Disk displacement with reduction
- Disk displacement without reduction

11.7.1.2—Temporomandibular joint dislocation

11.7.1.3—Inflammatory disorders
- Capsulitis, synovitis
- Polyarthritides

11.7.1.4—Noninflammatory disorders
- Primary osteoarthritis
- Secondary osteoarthritis

11.7.1.5—Ankylosis

11.7.1.6—Fracture

Various forms of trauma to the TMJ structures (ligaments, articular cartilage, articular disk, bone) can lead to intra-articular biochemical alterations that have been demonstrated to produce oxidative stress and the generation of free radicals. Subsequent inflammatory changes in synovial fluid with the production of a variety of proinflammatory cytokines can then lead to altered functioning of normal tissues and degenerative disease in the TMJ.[45-49]

Genetic marker studies involving catecholamine metabolism and adrenergic receptors suggest that certain genetic polymorphisms (e.g., in the catechol-*O*-methyl transferase [*COMT*] gene) might be associated with the changes seen in pain responsiveness and pain processing in patients with chronic TMDs.[50-52]

Differences in pain modulation between women and men with TMDs have been reported; women have been observed to demonstrate decreased thresholds to noxious stimuli and more hyperalgesia. In addition, in women with TMDs, some studies suggest that the affective component of pain may be enhanced during the low-estrogen phase of the menstrual cycle.[53-55]

Functional brain-imaging studies demonstrating changes in cortical circuitry support the concept that TMDs are very similar to other chronic pain disorders and may be related to abnormal pain processing in the trigeminal system.[56-58] In particular, muscle pain disorders appear to be associated with little, if any, abnormality of the muscles or peripheral tissues and may represent a central sensitization pain-producing process.

Finally, numerous biobehavioral studies support a connection between chronic TMDs and comorbid psychopathology (anxiety and depression disorders, post-traumatic stress disorder, and childhood physical, sexual, and psychological abuse).[59-65]

TMDs fall into the 11th major category of the IHS classification (see Box 31.2).[1] The American Academy of Orofacial Pain has expanded on this IHS classification and subdivided TMDs into TMJDs and muscle disorders (Boxes 31.10 and 31.11).[15]

Box 31.11 Masticatory Muscle Disorders

11.7.2.1—Local myalgia
11.7.2.2—Myofascial pain
11.7.2.3—Centrally mediated myalgia
11.7.2.4—Myospasm
11.7.2.5—Myositis
11.7.2.6—Myofibrotic contracture
11.7.2.7—Neoplasia

COMMON CLINICAL TEMPOROMANDIBULAR JOINT ARTICULAR DISORDERS

Disk derangement disorders and articular disk displacement are by far the most common TMJDs and are characterized by abnormal position of the articular disk in relation to the head of the condyle or temporal fossa. Disk displacement usually starts with the presence of a "clicking or popping" sound in the TMJ on opening and closing the mouth. Pain is typically an initial symptom as long as full function is present. Disk displacement is usually anterior or anteromedial in nature, although posterior and lateral displacement has been described in the literature. This may be related in part to the thinnest discal attachments being on the lateral pole of the condyle, as well as the medial direction of pull by the lateral pterygoid and inward direction of condylar movement during mouth opening.[66] Disk displacement therefore clinically suggests torn or stretched collateral discal ligaments that bind the disk to the condyle.

In disk displacement with reduction, a clicking sound on mouth opening and closing may be present. The term *reduction* is used to describe the misaligned disk temporarily coming back (or slipping back) to its proper interposition between the condyle and fossa during full opening (Figs. 31.1 and 31.2). On closing the mouth, the disk is again displaced as the teeth come closer together. This repetitive ongoing displacement on opening and closing produces a reciprocal noise (clicks) and is hence termed *reciprocal clicking*. This stage may actually represent a physiologic accommodative stage without any need for therapy other than discussion regarding its anatomic significance. With progression to the next stage, intermittent "locking" takes place as a result of the momentary impedance of the disk to the travel path of the condyle. This occurs as a sequela of a chronic clicking condition in subjects who tend to clench and grind their teeth at night (nocturnal parafunction) and have missing posterior teeth with subsequent overclosure of their bite. The teeth act as the doorstop for the TMJs and support the ultimate position of the TMJ on full closure. Good dental vertical dimension without shift on closure is essential in reducing the risk factors for progression (Fig. 31.3). Bite appliance therapy has been shown to be effective in relieving muscular[67-70] and disk displacement problems.

Disk displacement without reduction is sometimes referred to as a "closed lock." This suggests that the disk has been permanently displaced and the disk's shape has been permanently changed such that it physically prevents the condyle of the mandible from translating to a full open position (Fig. 31.4). Jaw opening is limited to 22 to 25 mm, with pain and deviation of the mandible to the side of the lock. As a result, chewing capability is reduced because of pain, inflammation at the affected joint, and possible changes in the normal occlusion or "bite." MRI of the TMJ is the "gold standard" for assessing soft tissue details of the articular

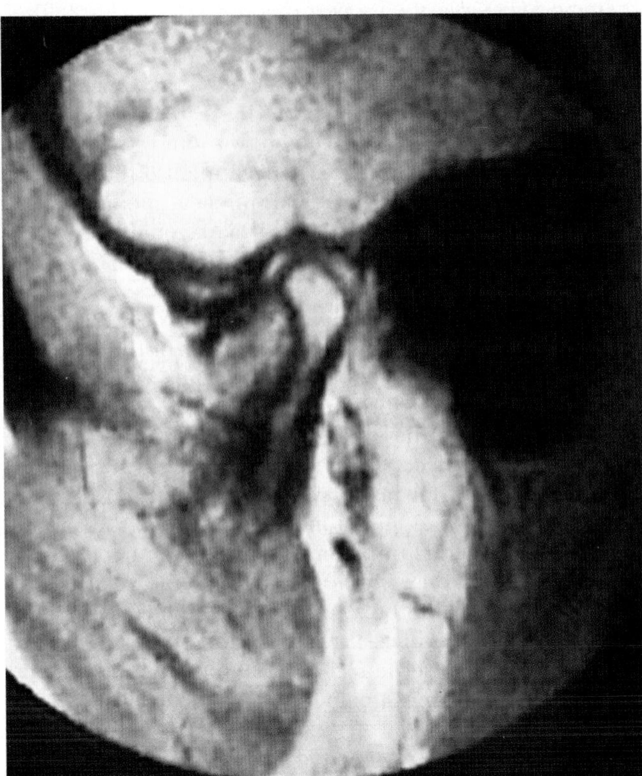

Figure 31.1 Magnetic resonance image of an anteriorly displaced disk that lies at the 10-o'clock position with respect to the head of the condyle with the teeth together.

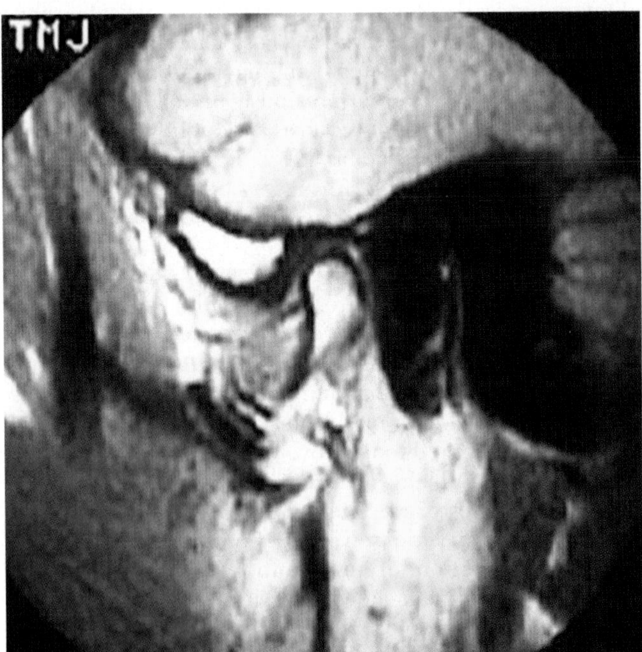

Figure 31.2 Opening movement with a clinical "click" sound allows the disk and condyle from the image in Figure 31.1 to assume a normal open position. TMJ, temporomandibular joint.

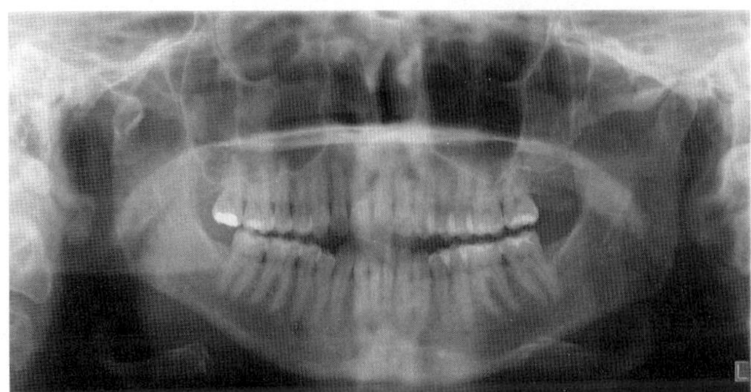

Figure 31.3 Panoramic radiograph showing a displaced right subcondylar fracture with premature tooth contact on the right and an open bite on the left.

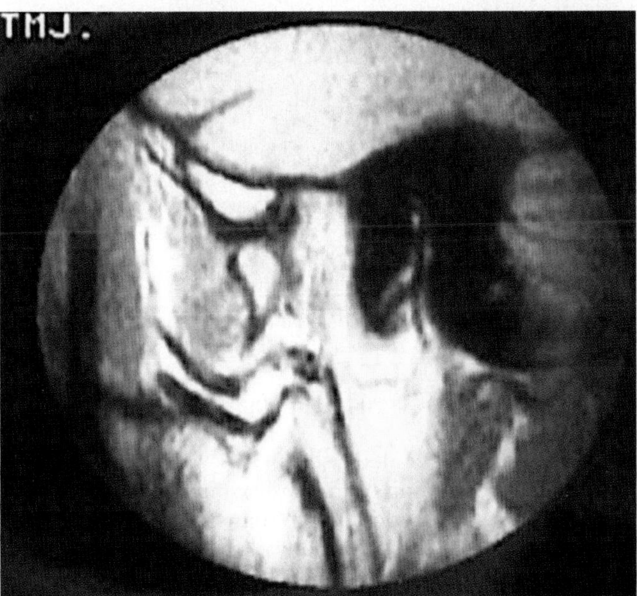

Figure 31.4 Anterior disk displacement without reduction. The disk is folded in front of the head of the condyle, thereby preventing full opening of the mandible.

cartilage and its displacement, whereas hard tissue CT scans are generally done to assess chronic osteoarthritic or bony changes.[71,72]

TMJ dislocation is also known as open lock or condylar subluxation when the condyle translates beyond the anterior eminence of the articular fossa with subsequent trapping in this open-mouth position. Chronic hypertranslation can usually be managed by the subject physically manipulating the jaw. If the condition is chronic, the subject knows to relax the jaw-closing muscles and slip the condyle back into position. The most common subluxation occurs during yawning or opening the mouth widely. If the problem is related to trauma or to sudden acute translation, the subluxation is considered to be an acute dislocation and requires medical intervention in which the muscles are relaxed by anesthetics or analgesics followed by manual manipulation of the joint with a downward and backward motion. Follow-up with anti-inflammatory medication, ice, and rest or a dental appliance may be necessary until the acute stage subsides.[73]

Inflammatory disorders, including capsulitis and synovitis, are relatively common in the TMJ secondary to macrotrauma or microtrauma, irritation, or infection. These disorders may be manifested as pain on function and inflammation with extreme tenderness on palpation of the TMJ. MRI may show effusions on the T2-weighted signal and an inability to completely bring the teeth together accompanied by pain in the ear. Joint inflammation may also be a result of polyarthritis of systemic origin, which is generally secondary to connective tissue diseases.

OSTEOARTHRITIS (NONINFLAMMATORY)

Primary osteoarthritis is a degenerative condition of the joints characterized by hard tissue abrasion and degradation of the articular surface of the condyle related to overload. It is frequently seen in patients with a long history of missing teeth or maloccluded dentures. This process is generally slow, is not associated with symptoms of pain during the early stages, and may remain relatively benign over the life of the individual. Primary osteoarthritis is usually identified by radiographic screening of hard tissue (e.g., dental panoramic image), a tomograph or dental CT scan, or the presence of grating (crepitus) noises in the joint during movement (Figs. 31.5 and 31.6).

Secondary osteoarthritis is usually identified by a history of a single previous event such as trauma or infection or may result from rheumatoid arthritis. An idiopathic degenerative condition primarily affecting adolescent girls is termed condylysis. It involves sudden lysis of the condyle that creates a rapid change in the bite of the individual with a shift of the jaw and resultant open bite that is notable by the subject. The etiology of condylysis is not clear, but it has been known to be associated with rheumatoid arthritis in young girls.[47,48,73]

Ankylosis is usually related to trauma to the joint with subsequent bleeding and restricted mandibular movement; the ankylosis may be fibrous or bony in nature. Fibrous ankylosis generally occurs in the upper joint compartment as a result of adhesions forming after joint bleeding and prolonged immobility. Limited jaw opening (usually one to two fingers placed horizontally between the central incisors) is typically present. Bony ankylosis has no movement associated with it. Both conditions may require surgical release followed by postsurgical mobilization techniques.

FRACTURE

Trauma to any part of the face may result in bony fractures of the condylar neck, condylar head, body of the mandible, and maxilla and temporal fossa and may result in a reduction in opening, pain, and fibrosis of the bony ankylosis if untreated. Uncomplicated (nondisplaced) fractures require no immediate treatment as long as function is not compromised.

COMMON CLINICAL MUSCLE DISORDERS

LOCALIZED MYALGIA

Masticatory muscle injury can occur as a result of acute muscle strain or direct trauma. Soft tissue injury results in bleeding, inflammation, and swelling, which causes myalgia, muscle spasm, muscle splinting, or myositis.[74] Myofascial trigger points may develop in many locations within the

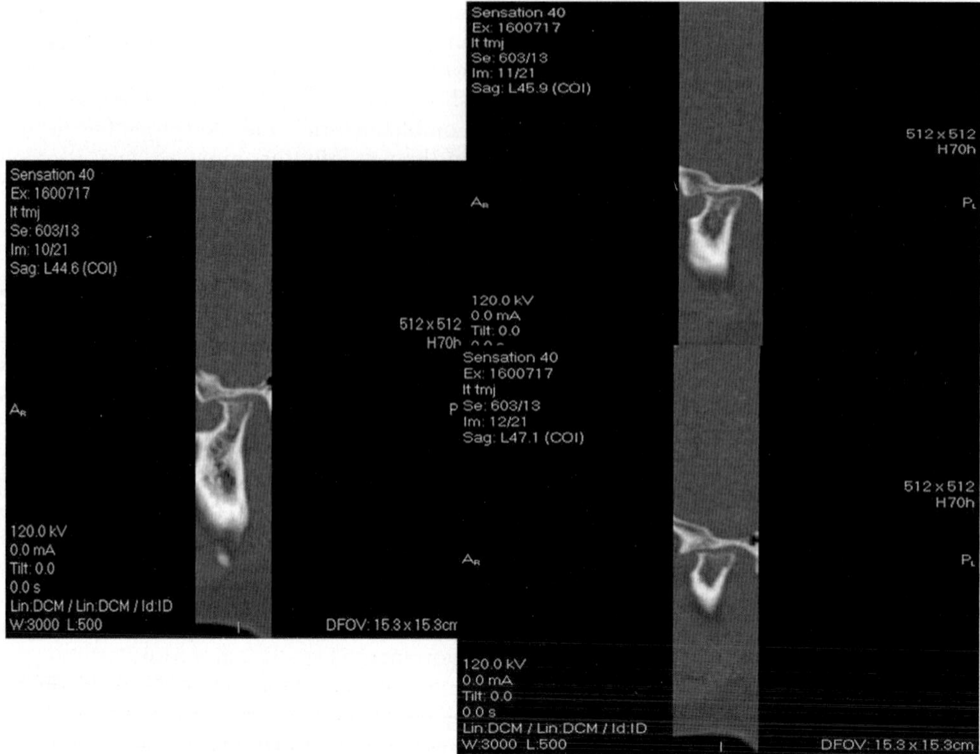

Figure 31.5 Sagittal computed tomography scan showing severe degenerative osteoarthritis.

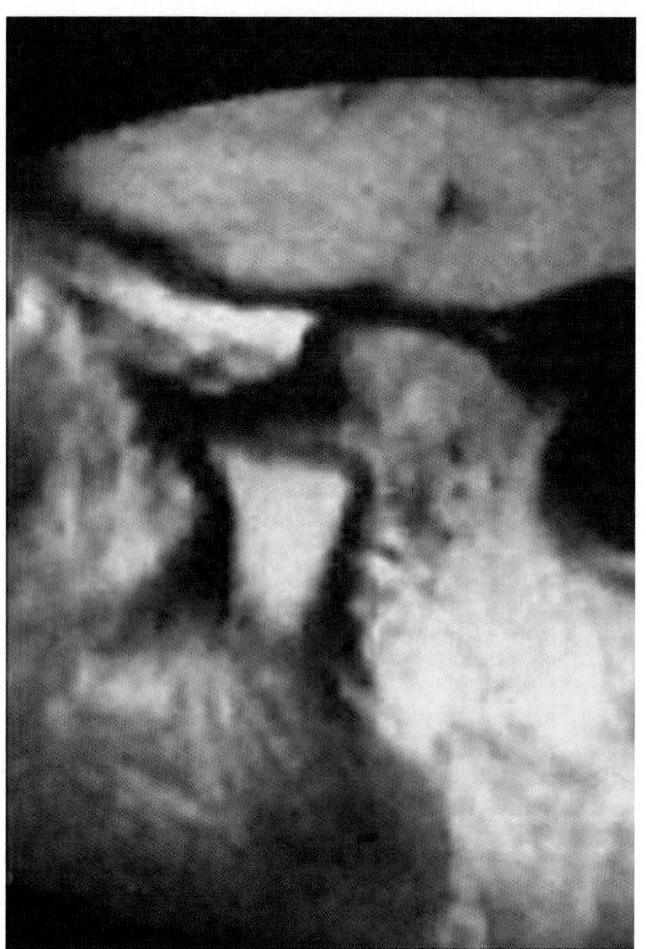

Figure 31.6 Magnetic resonance image of a degenerative joint. The disk is folded in front of the head of the condyle, thereby preventing full opening of the mandible.

muscle and are considered[75,76] to be the primary source of the muscular pain.

Injury results in a deep sharp ache on contraction of the muscle. Depending on the area of injury, the pain may emanate from the tendon attachments (tendonitis), fascial component (myofascitis), or body of the muscle (myospasm and myositis). The temporalis tendon attachment to the coronoid process is the most frequent site of masticatory tendonitis. In the presence of acute or chronic internal derangement of the TMJ complex, the muscles that support and move the joints can be secondarily affected. Protective muscle splinting is used to prevent further injury to the joint. Immobilization of the injured joint is frequently seen with anterior disk displacement without reduction (closed lock). Splinting of the masticatory elevator muscles is maintained until the joint is healed.

Myalgia secondary to injury to the cervical spine can affect the masticatory muscles and result in headaches and facial pain. Once the masticatory muscles are secondarily involved, they affect mandibular position. Mandibular dysfunction results from masticatory muscle involvement and in tightening of the muscles of the cervical spine, thereby perpetuating the cycle. Consequently, a significant proportion of TMD patients also have a history of cervical injury, and treatment of this craniofacial and cervical syndrome requires that both the jaw and neck be treated in a multidisciplinary manner.[77]

Muscle disorders may occur secondary to rotation, fixation, fusion, or injury to or locking of the facets of the cervical, thoracic, lumbar, and sacral vertebrae. The history, physical examination, and radiographic evaluation will elucidate the acuteness and severity of the vertebral problem. Disk herniations can secondarily affect the cervical muscles through protective splinting, which may eventually

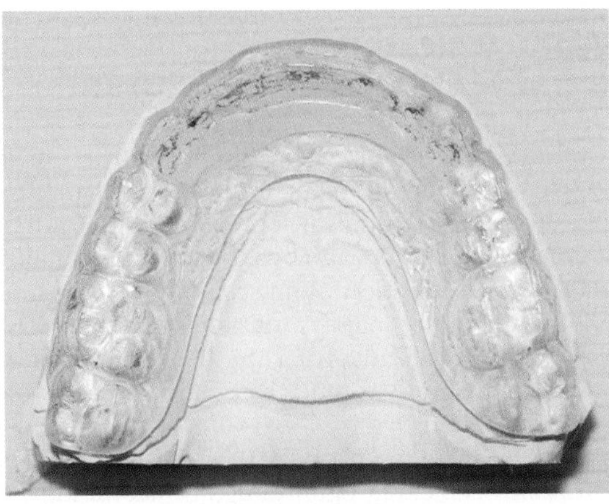

Figure 31.7 A maxillary dental night guard with anterior contact to reduce bruxism forces helps unload teeth and allows muscles and nerves to relax. The guard is usually made of dental acrylic.

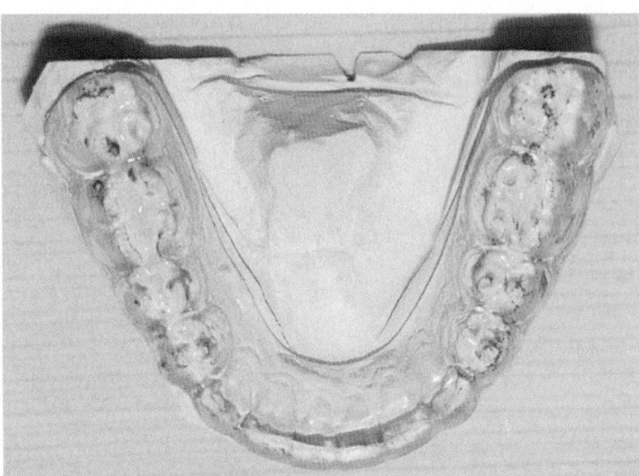

Figure 31.8 Lower hard full-coverage bite plate usually worn during the day by patients with maxillomandibular dysfunction. Contact is generally bilateral and equal.

lead to chronic postural changes. Nerve impingement and nerve root injuries can also affect muscle function. Cervical problems are frequent comorbid conditions seen in TMD patients.[77-79] A reduction in the space between the posterior spine of the atlas and the base of the occiput[79] may cause pain by compression of suboccipital tissues. The pain will be perceived as a headache starting from the back of the head.[77-79]

ORAL PARAFUNCTION

Oral parafunction includes bruxism, clenching, lip biting, thumb sucking, and any other oral habit not associated with mastication, deglutition, and speech. Bruxism and clenching are the most common of the parafunctional activities and have a prevalence of up to 90% in the general population.[80,81] In most patients, parafunction occurs in a milder intermittent form and does not require treatment. Whether moderate or severe, bruxism and clenching can damage oral structures and cause wear of the teeth, breakdown of the periodontium in the presence of inflammation, and internal derangement and muscular dysfunction.[82]

Studies on bruxism and clenching have reported excessive force occurring for extended periods (normal tooth contact during a 24-hour period is about 20 minutes and takes place during chewing and swallowing).[82,83] Parafunctional forces exceed normal masticatory forces, with the resultant force vector being primarily horizontal. Under such conditions, damage is likely to occur to the teeth and periodontium (Figs. 31.7 and 31.8). Ironically, most treatments are designed to protect the occlusion in function rather than in parafunction. The detrimental effects of parafunction will cause breakdown of the weakest structure, which may include the teeth, periodontium, TMJ, or muscles. The patient can therefore have both tooth and joint pathology.[81-83]

Bruxism and clenching have been explained historically by theories of occlusion but to date have yet to be substantiated by research. Nocturnal bruxism is currently classified as a sleep disorder, the duration and intensity of which vary nightly depending on emotional stress and activities of the individual before sleep. Sleep studies have shown that bruxism occurs during body movement and the rapid eye movement stage of sleep and during the transition from a deeper to a lighter stage of sleep.[84]

Numerous studies have been done on the personality characteristics of "bruxers."[84-87] People who clench and grind their teeth have been shown to exhibit higher degrees of anxiety, aggressiveness, and hostility. The conclusions of these and other studies have confirmed an emotional etiology of diurnal (daytime) parafunction,[80-83,84,88] which includes lip biting, nail biting, thumb sucking, clenching, and habitual bruxism. The pathologic effects are the same as those for nocturnal parafunction.

MYOFASCIAL PAIN DISORDER AND MUSCLE TRIGGER POINTS

A myofascial trigger point is defined as a hyperirritable locus within a taut band of skeletal muscle that is located in muscular tissue or in its associated fascia or tendon. The spot is painful on compression and can evoke characteristic referred pain and autonomic phenomena.[74,75] Active trigger points may cause pain spontaneously or during movement. Latent trigger points, which affect nearly half the population by early adulthood,[76] are not usually painful but create weakness and restriction of movement in a muscle. These trigger points can be activated by sudden overloading contraction, viral infection, cold temperature, fatigue, and increased emotional stress. Because of the complex nature of myofascial trigger points and their common presence in patients with acute and chronic muscle dysfunction, an understanding of their clinical features is necessary. According to Travell and Simons,[76] myofascial trigger points have seven clinical features:

- Local tenderness over the trigger point
- Referred pain, tenderness, and autonomic phenomena
- Palpable taut band associated with the trigger points
- A local twitch response of a trigger point that is usually present in a palpable taut band
- Perpetuation of trigger points
- A therapeutic effect when stretching a muscle with trigger points
- Weakness and fatigability of muscles afflicted by trigger points

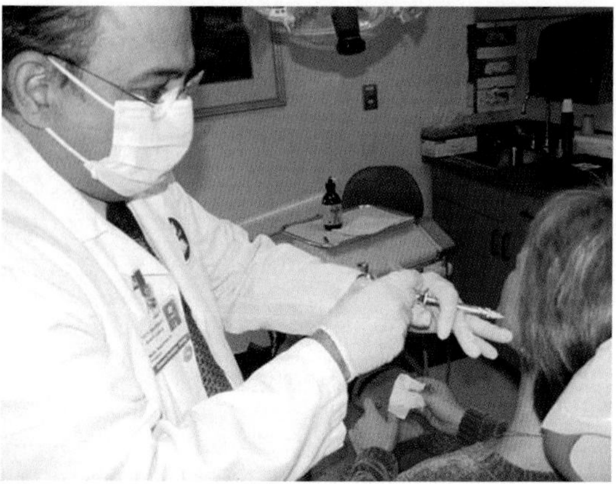

Figure 31.9 Trigger point injection for a trigger point of the masseter.

Myofascial pain often refers pain to the head and neck and is considered by some to constitute tension-type headaches. Myofascial pain and trigger points of the masticatory muscles can send pain to the eyes, ears, TMJ, and teeth, depending on the specific muscles. The pain is usually a dull or intense ache that varies but is strongly related to posture or muscle activity and can generally be localized by the patient on a diagrammatic representation of the body. The muscles of posture and mastication are commonly affected by trigger points. The pain may occur in the same dermatome, myotome, or sclerotome. Satellite trigger points may occur within the pain reference zone. Clinically, there is restricted movement with pain on passive stretching, and strong contraction will dramatically increase the pain. Resistive testing reveals weakness as a result of protective splinting.

Trigger points are palpated by rubbing the fingertip lightly along the long axis of the muscle. If present, a taut band will be located first, and then the more sensitive trigger point. Applying pressure on a trigger point elicits a grimace or an involuntary sound from the patient, a response called the "jump sign." Snapping palpation of the taut band will produce a local twitch response, which confirms the presence of the trigger point. Final confirmation is achieved with reproduction of the patient's pain by digital pressure.[76]

Treatment of myofascial trigger points includes spraying the involved muscle with ethyl chloride or fluoromethane followed by stretching, hot compresses, and range-of-motion exercises. Trigger point injections of procaine (0.5% solution in saline) or lidocaine (2% without epinephrine) have also been used commonly (Fig. 31.9), along with botulinum toxin (Botox) more recently. Other techniques involve ischemic compression for 30 to 60 seconds and acupressure. Pharmacological treatments include analgesics, muscle relaxants, antidepressants, and NSAIDs. Physical therapy modalities such as myofascial release and craniosacral techniques, including postural correction and exercise, have also been effective in the management of myofascial trigger points. Stress, nutritional, and hormonal factors should also be addressed (Fig. 31.10).[86]

In the case of the masticatory muscles, occlusal appliances may be used.[88] Dental guards or appliances have been found to be effective in reducing muscle symptoms and trigger points in mandibular elevators.

GENERAL MANAGEMENT OF TEMPOROMANDIBULAR DISORDERS

The overall management goals mimic those for other orthopedic or rheumatologic disorders. In patients with craniofacial and cervical disorders, reduction of functional maxillomandibular forces and occlusal loading, stabilization of the TMJ, and relaxation of muscles allow easier function of the joint. Since the majority of patients with TMDs have a chronic pain history involving the head and neck, multidisciplinary management tends to be more successful than individual treatments.

Currently, management of TMDs consists of a combination of home self-care, counseling, physiotherapy, pharmacotherapy, jaw appliance therapy, physical medicine, behavioral medicine, and surgery (see Table 31.2). Surgery is performed only to treat structural anatomic pathology that is producing pain and dysfunction. Surgical procedures include arthrocentesis, arthroscopy, open arthrotomy, and combined joint and reconstructive jaw procedures.

NEUROPATHIC PAIN SYNDROMES

Neuropathic pain syndromes result from pathology in the peripheral or central nervous system. These disorders are particularly common in the head and neck, probably because of the dense and specialized sensory innervation of this region. For practical purposes, craniocervical neuropathic pain disorders can be divided into two main groups: (1) trigeminal neuralgia (TN) and (2) a more heterogeneous group of neuralgic disorders termed "painful posttraumatic trigeminal neuropathy" (PTN) (see Box 31.3).

TRIGEMINAL NEURALGIA

TN is a well-recognized disorder characterized by brief paroxysms of severe, unilateral, electric pain in the trigeminal region. TN has an incidence of 4 per 100,000.[89,90] The condition is most common in people older than 50 years, and women are affected only slightly more often than men[90,91]; however, TN has no geographic or ethnic preference. The pain with TN typically consists of "lightning bolts" of momentary pain that radiate within the second or third trigeminal divisions. In individual patients, the attacks are stereotyped in that they typically recur with the same intensity and in the same distribution. Despite the severity of TN pain, however, most patients are symptom free between attacks, and most have normal clinical sensory findings between pain episodes.[91-95] Many TN patients demonstrate a discrete (<10 mm) sensory "trigger zone" in the oral mucosa or perioral skin; light touch or thermal stimulation within the trigger zone evokes a TN pain attack. Although a trigger zone is not a requirement for TN, the presence of a trigger zone is pathognomonic for the diagnosis of TN. White and Sweet[96] emphasized that TN has five major clinical features:

- The pain is paroxysmal.
- The pain is confined to the trigeminal distribution.
- The pain is unilateral.
- The findings on bedside clinical sensory examination are normal.

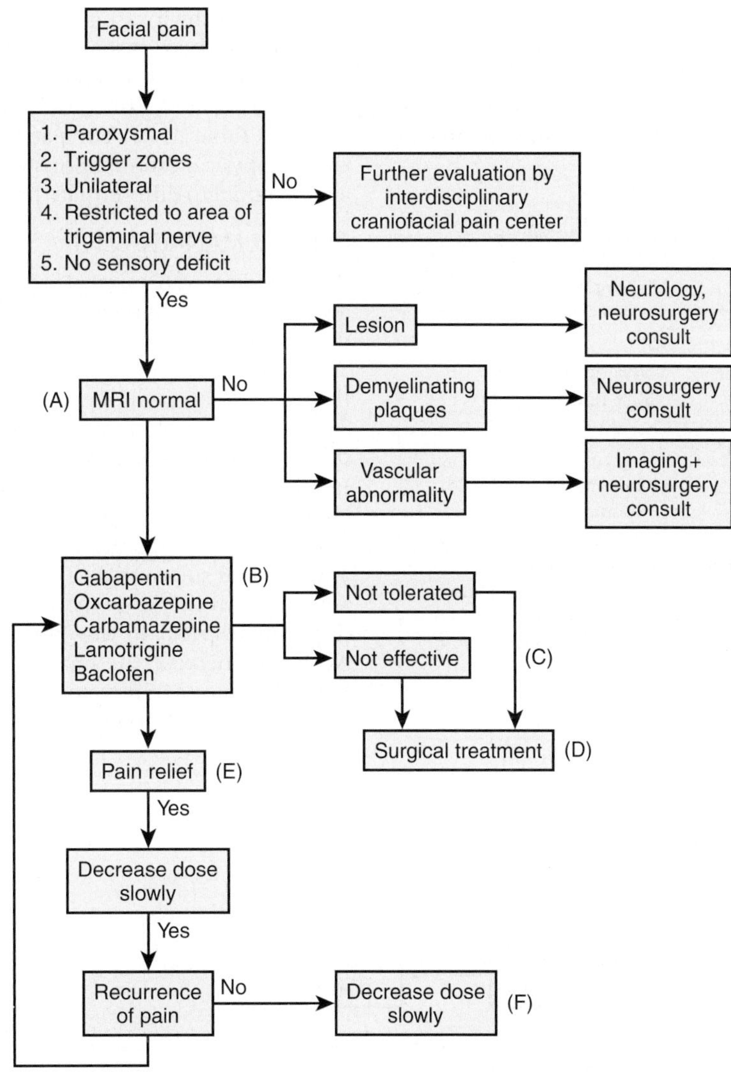

A. MRI of the brain, brainstem, and base of the skull. Further diagnostic studies are performed when physical examination or MRI findings are abnormal.

B. Medication is titrated progressively until pain is relieved or adverse effects occur. Often, a second AED is added early if single therapy is ineffective.

C. Drug allergy, idiosyncratic reaction, laboratory abnormalities, intolerable or dangerous side effects, patient preference.

D. Local anesthetic trigeminal nerve blocks are performed in some patients as part of further diagnostic evaluation prior to surgical therapy.

E. Dosages of medications can be tapered slowly if the patient remains pain free after several weeks to months of pharmacological therapy.

F. Further decrease in dosage of medication is predicated on the patient's pain history. Many patients may need to be maintained on pharmacotherapy for prevention.

Figure 31.10 Facial pain diagnostic and treatment algorithm. AED, antiepileptic drug; MRI, magnetic resonance imaging.

- The pain may be provoked by light touch on the face (trigger zones).

These criteria were incorporated, largely unchanged, into the official research diagnostic criteria published by the International Association for the Study of Pain and the IHS (see Box 31.3).[1] TN appears to result from a chronic partial injury to the trigeminal sensory nerve root as it enters the brainstem.[92-95,98-101] Consistent with this view is the presence of a separate disease process affecting the trigeminal nerve roots in 5% to 10% of patients with TN symptoms. This is generally multiple sclerosis or a benign tumor (schwannoma, meningioma) in the cerebellopontine angle. These cases are usually termed *symptomatic trigeminal neuralgia*. In the remaining majority of TN cases, imaging studies and laboratory tests are negative. These cases are usually termed *idiopathic trigeminal neuralgia*. Despite the idiopathic label, increasing evidence documents that subtle forms of chronic nerve root injury (such as compression by a vascular loop) produce trigeminal root irritation in these cases.

In summary, the diagnosis of TN is based on a clinical history consistent with widely accepted, specific diagnostic criteria (Table 31.5). For patients that meet the criteria, a careful physical examination and cranial imaging studies are also essential to differentiate primary from symptomatic TN.

Table 31.5 Diagnosis of Trigeminal Neuralgia

Diagnosis	History
Spontaneous Onset	
Trigeminal neuralgia type 1	>50% episodic pain
Trigeminal neuralgia type 2	>50% constant pain
Trigeminal Injury	
Trigeminal neuropathic pain	Unintentional, incidental trauma
Trigeminal deafferentation pain	Intentional deafferentation
Symptomatic trigeminal neuralgia	Multiple sclerosis
Post-herpetic neuralgia	Trigeminal herpes zoster outbreak
Atypical facial pain*	Somatoform pain disorder

*Cannot be diagnosed by the history alone.

CLINICAL MANAGEMENT

Both medical and surgical treatments are available to manage the severe pain attacks of TN. The present authors use a diagnostic and management algorithm for TN (Fig. 31.11). The patients should initially undergo a trial of medical therapy with an antiepileptic drug (AED) (Boxes 31.12 and 31.13). A series of clinical trials over the past 50 years have demonstrated that oral AEDs are effective for TN, with gabapentin, baclofen, or carbamazepine being the initial drug of choice. The AED dosage should be increased progressively to therapeutic "anticonvulsant" levels. Single-drug AED therapy provides substantial relief from the recurrent attacks of facial pain in the large majority of TN patients. If a patient does not respond to single-AED therapy, adding a second AED may increase the chance for a therapeutic response. Lack of response of the patient to AEDs warrants a search for other causes of the patient's pain.

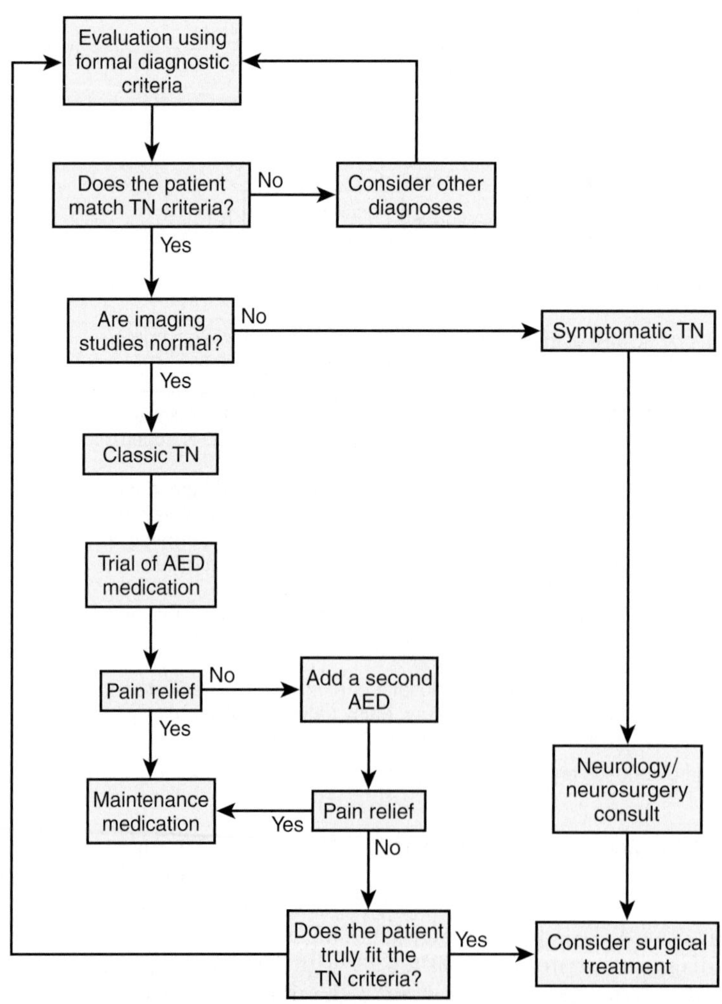

Figure 31.11 Algorithm for the evaluation and management of trigeminal neuralgia (TN). AED, antiepileptic drug.

Box 31.12 Anticonvulsants

- Phenytoin (Dilantin)
- Carbamazepine (Tegretol)
- Baclofen (Lioresal)*
- Clonazepam (Klonopin)
- Gabapentin (Neurontin)
- Lamotrigine (Lamictal)
- Topiramate (Topamax)
- Oxcarbazepine (Trileptal)
- Tiagabine (Gabitril)
- Levetiracetam (Keppra)
- Zonisamide (Zonegran)
- Pregabalin (Lyrica)

Box 31.13 Pharmacological Effect and Mechanism of Pain Relief

- CBZ: Na channel
- OXC
- CLO: GABA
- BAC: $GABA_B$
- GBP: Na, Ca channel
- LTG: Na channel, inhibit GLU
- TOP: Na channel, GABA, AMPA
- TGB: GABA RI
- Suppress spontaneous ectopic neuronal activity
- Reduce neuronal hypersensitivity
- Segmental inhibition of signaling

AMPA, α-amino-3-hydroxy-5-methyl-4-isoxazolepropionate; BAC, baclofen; CBZ, carbamazepine; CLO, clonazepam; GABA, γ-aminobutyric acid; GBP, gabapentin; GLU, glutamate; LTG, lamotrigine; Na, sodium; OXC, oxcarbazepine; TGB, tiagabine; TOP, topiramate.

Surgical options are also available for patients in a variety of clinical situations. Three procedures are commonly recommended:

- Percutaneous retrogasserian radiofrequency lesion[102-104]
- Posterior fossa microvascular decompression[105-107]
- Gamma Knife radiotherapy[108,109]

These procedures substantially reduce or eliminate pain attacks in as many as 90% of patients with TN.

ATYPICAL TRIGEMINAL NEURALGIA

Many authors use the diagnosis "atypical TN"[110,111] to describe cases in which the clinical findings do not fully meet the standard diagnostic criteria for TN. However, there is general agreement that patients with atypical TN are less responsive to AEDs and surgical intervention than are patients with "standard" TN.[112-118] It is reasonable to assume that the TN is probably neither homogeneous nor unique, but the general diagnosis of atypical TN seems misleading since the term does not identify a meaningful subset of TN patients who could be examined more closely. Nonetheless, the clinical problem of atypical TN is a real one because patients with complex facial pain disorders often have a spectrum of symptoms, some of which may be quite similar to the TN criteria.

PAINFUL POST-TRAUMATIC TRIGEMINAL NEUROPATHY

In a significant number of patients, chronic facial pain develops following trauma to sensory nerves in the craniocervical region.[119,120] These cases are distinct from TN and are usually grouped according to the nature and location of the painful nerve damage (neuralgia). We usually classify this group under the heading "painful PTN." Patients with PTN exhibit chronic or recurrent pain in the area of the previous nerve injury, numbness, dysesthesias, and chronic burning sensations. Diagnostic evaluations rule out any other cause of pain. Most craniocervical neuralgias meet these general PTN criteria, although individual clinical features vary depending on the specific syndrome. Common examples of craniocervical neuralgias include post-herpetic neuralgia, inferior alveolar neuralgia following mandibular third molar extraction, and infraorbital neuralgia following maxillary trauma.

Patients with PTN pose a significant clinical challenge since the symptoms of PTN respond poorly, if at all, to the AEDs or surgical therapies commonly used for TN. The general approach to the clinical management of PTN is similar to that for other forms of neuropathic pain and is discussed in Chapter 24.

CONCLUSION

Pain syndromes that involve the face are very common in clinical practice. Many facial pain syndromes are also unique given the complex anatomy and specialized sensory innervation of the head, face, and neck. These syndromes represent a clinical diagnostic challenge and deserve special attention. The common descriptive terms for facial pain complaints are frequently misleading. Clinicians should be comfortable distinguishing painful conditions that arise from structural pathology, headache syndromes, oral and facial structures, TMJDs, MPDs, and primary cranial neuralgias.

KEY POINTS

- Pain syndromes that involve the face, head, and neck are very common in clinical practice. These syndromes are often unique and deserving of special attention.
- The common descriptive terms for cranial pain symptoms are frequently misleading. To avoid confusion, pain clinicians should be familiar with the International Headache Society's diagnostic criteria for head and neck disorders. Clinicians should be comfortable distinguishing painful conditions that arise from structural pathology, headache syndromes, myofascial pain disorders, and primary neuralgias.
- Clinicians should be familiar with the clinically relevant features of craniocervical anatomy and the distinctive neurobiology of pain transmission in this region.
- Chronic/recurrent pain syndromes are extremely common in the head and neck, and myofascial pain

KEY POINTS—cont'd

disorders are among the most common causes of pain and dysfunction in this group. Myofascial syndromes overlap with several common diagnoses, including temporomandibular joint myofascial pain dysfunction syndrome, tension headache, and most cases of occipital neuralgia. Clinicians should be aware of the diagnostic features, potential causes, and exacerbating factors for such disorders. They should also understand how these factors are associated with the various multidisciplinary options currently recommended for treatment.

- Clinicians should be aware of the unique anatomy and physiology of the temporomandibular joint and how jaw position and dental occlusion can contribute to myofascial pain symptoms.
- Bruxism and sleep disorders are common contributors to craniocervical pain that occurs in the morning.
- Bite appliances in conjunction with stress management and physical therapy may be a viable treatment option for patients with craniofacial and myofascial pain.
- Trigeminal neuralgia is a unique neurogenic disorder. Patients who meet the clinical diagnostic criteria for trigeminal neuralgia may benefit substantially from anticonvulsant drugs or surgical therapy. Patients with other forms of neurogenic facial pain have a poorer prognosis.

SUGGESTED READINGS

de Leeuw R. *Orofacial Pain: Guidelines for Assessment, Diagnosis and Management.* 4th ed. Chicago: Quintessence; 2008.

de Leeuw R, Albuquerque RJ, Andersen AH, et al. Influence of estrogen on brain activation during stimulation with painful heat. *J Oral Maxillofac Surg.* 2006;64:158-166.

Dworkin SF, Sherman J, Mancl L, et al. Reliability, validity, and clinical utility of the research diagnostic criteria for Temporomandibular Disorders Axis II Scales: depression, non-specific physical symptoms, and graded chronic pain. *J Orofac Pain.* 2002;16:207-220.

Israel HA, Langevin CJ, Singer MD, et al. The relationship between temporomandibular joint synovitis and adhesions: pathogenic mechanisms and clinical implications for surgical management. *J Oral Maxillofac Surg.* 2006;64:1066-1074.

Laskin DM. Temporomandibular disorders: a term past its time? Guest editorial. *J Am Dent Assoc.* 2008;139:124-128.

Milam SB, Schmitz JP. Molecular biology of temporomandibular joint disorders: proposed mechanisms of disease. *J Oral Maxillofacial Surg.* 1995;53:1448-1454.

Nackley AG, Tan KS, Fecho K, et al. Catechol-*O*-methyltransferase inhibition increases pain sensitivity through activation of both beta2- and beta3-adrenergic receptors. *Pain.* 2007;128:199-208.

Scrivani SJ, Keith DA, Mathews ES, et al. Stereotactic differential radiofrequency thermal rhizotomy for the treatment of trigeminal neuralgia. *J Oral Maxillofac Surg.* 1999;57:104-111.

Ship JA, Grushka M, Lipton JA, et al. Burning mouth syndrome: an update. *J Am Dent Assoc.* 1995;126:842-853.

Solberg WK. Epidemiology, incidence and prevalence of temporomandibular disorders: a review. In: *The President's Conference on the Examination, Diagnosis and Management of Temporomandibular Disorders.* Chicago: American Dental Association; 1983:30-39.

The International Classification of Headache Disorders. 2nd ed. *Cephalalgia.* 2004;24(suppl 1):9-160.

Travell JG, Simons DG. *Myofascial Pain and Dysfunction: The Trigger Point Manual.* Vol. 1. *The Upper Extremities.* Baltimore: Williams & Wilkins; 1983.

Wright EF, Syms III CA, Bifano SL. Tinnitus, dizziness, and nonotologic otalgia improvement through temporomandibular disorder therapy. *Mil Med.* 2000;165:733-736.

Young RF, Vermulen S, Posewitz A. Gamma knife radiosurgery for the treatment of trigeminal neuralgia. *Stereotact Funct Neurosurg.* 1998;70(suppl 1):192-199.

The references for this chapter can be found at www.expertconsult.com.

Visceral Pain

32

Klaus Bielefeldt | G.F. Gebhart

Chronic visceral pain is very common. Abdominal pain is among the main reasons for physician visits, with more than 12 million consultations occurring each year in the United States.[1] Patients with visceral pain present unique challenges because the pain is often poorly localized and is associated with strong autonomic reactions and changes in visceral function. Pain management, in turn, may further alter visceral function, with opioid effects on the gastrointestinal tract providing a good example. These unintended treatment effects on visceral function can exacerbate the pain or lead to additional discomfort, thus showing that rational and effective pain management needs to be based on an understanding of the anatomic and physiologic basis of visceral function *and* pain.

PHYSIOLOGIC BASIS OF VISCERAL SENSATION AND PAIN

ANATOMY AND PHYSIOLOGY OF VISCERAL AFFERENT PATHWAYS

Most viscera arise from midline structures and thus receive bilateral innervation. As a result, visceral stimuli activate both hemispheres of the brain, with a predominance of the left side in most right-handed individuals.[2,3] In addition, organs in the chest cavity and most viscera within the abdomen receive dual afferent innervation, with vagal and spinal nerves conveying sensory input to the central nervous system (Fig. 32.1). Although vagal fibers do not reach the pelvic organs, the distal part of the colon, bladder, prostate, and uterus also have a complex sensory innervation, with afferents projecting through the thoracolumbar (hypogastric) and lumbosacral (pelvic) nerves to the spinal cord.

The vagus nerve is predominantly composed of afferent fibers (≥80%) that project via the nodose and jugular ganglia to the nucleus of the solitary tract in the brainstem. Spinal afferents pass through prevertebral (sympathetic) ganglia to the dorsal root ganglia and send their endings to the dorsal horn and central gray matter of the spinal cord. Information about noxious stimuli is relayed rostrally through the spinothalamic tract. In addition, postsynaptic dorsal horn neurons within the central gray send their central processes through the medial aspect of the dorsal columns, a pathway that has only recently been recognized as being uniquely important in visceral pain.[4]

Most physiologic studies characterizing the properties of visceral sensory pathways rely on responses to defined mechanical stimuli. Vagal afferents form a relatively homogeneous group that is activated by low-intensity mechanical stimuli and encodes stimulus intensity over a wide range. The low threshold of activation is consistent with the presumed role of these sensory pathways in the regulation of physiologic processes. In contrast, two classes of mechanosensitive spinal afferents can be distinguished by their response characteristics: low-threshold fibers are similarly activated by low-intensity stimuli and continue to encode stimulus intensity over a wide range, whereas high-threshold fibers are activated by intense, potentially noxious intensities of mechanical stimuli. Thus, spinal high-threshold fibers resemble specialized nociceptors that have been described and characterized best in the skin, thus suggesting that they play a primary role in visceral nociception.[5,6] However, because mechanosensitive visceral afferents encode stimulus intensity over a wide range and can become sensitized after a visceral insult, it is likely that both low- and high-threshold mechanosensitive afferents can contribute to visceral pain conditions. Finally, most visceral sensory neurons are polymodal, which means that they respond to multiple stimulus modalities, including endogenous and exogenous chemicals contained in luminal contents, temperature (heat or cold), and stretch.

MUCOSAL SIGNALING AND VISCERAL SENSATION

In the airways, gastrointestinal tract, and urinary bladder, nerve fibers are found in close proximity to epithelial cells, which often exhibit specializations consisting of secretory vesicles on the basal surface.[7-9] This structural organization and functional studies suggest that visceral epithelial cells function as an interface between chemical or mechanical stimuli and the nervous system. The best example is serotonin released from enteroendocrine cells in the gastrointestinal tract. The gut is the major source of this signaling molecule and contains 95% of the body's serotonin. Much of this serotonin is stored in specialized enteroendocrine (enterochromaffin) cells and can be released by chemical or mechanical stimuli to activate intrinsic and extrinsic neurons.[7] Within the urinary tract, epithelial cells release adenosine triphosphate, which acts on purinergic receptors (P2X receptors) and is involved in normal micturition, as well as in bladder pain.[10] Finally, bladder epithelial cells also express the capsaicin receptor transient receptor potential vanilloid-1 [TRPV1]), an ion channel that is activated by acid, temperature, endogenous lipid mediators, and the pungent substance (capsaicin) contained in hot peppers. Animals with a targeted deletion of this channel display altered micturition behavior, again pointing to the importance of epithelial cells in visceral sensation.[11]

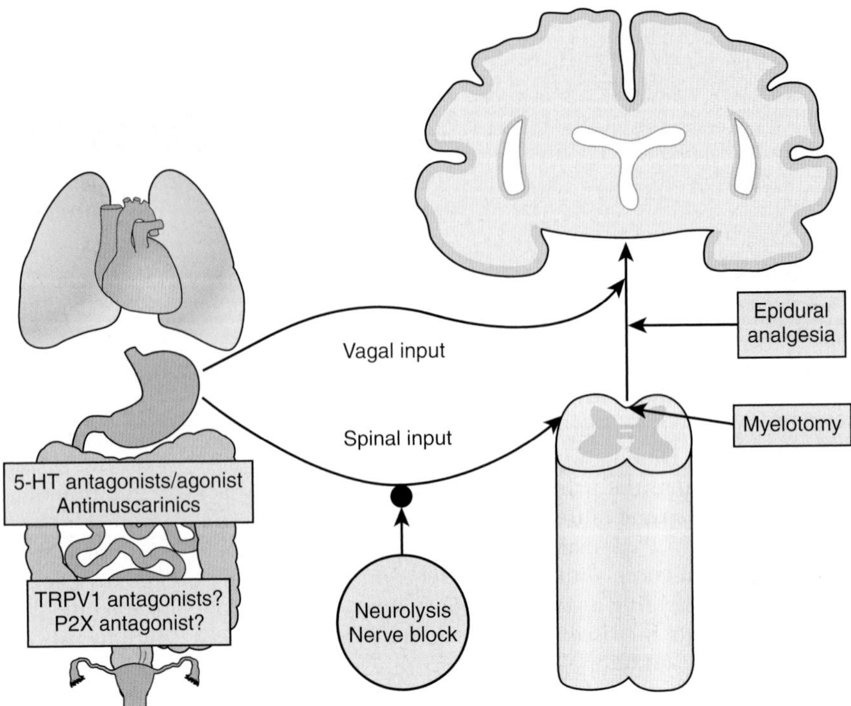

Figure 32.1 Schematic description of visceral innervation and potential targets for analgesic therapy. As indicated by the arrows, most viscera receive dual sensory innervation with vagal and spinal afferents. Current symptomatic treatment of peripheral targets relies largely on agents interfering with intestinal contractility. However, the capsaicin receptor (transient receptor potential vanilloid-1 [TRPV1]) and purinergic P2X receptors constitute promising targets for the treatment of visceral pain. Neurolytic block, myelotomy and epidural analgesia all target spinal afferent pathways involved in relaying visceral pain.

SENSITIZATION OF VISCERAL AFFERENT PATHWAYS

Visceral afferents can become sensitized in response to inflammation or injury. The release of mediators, such as prostaglandins or bradykinin, rapidly alters the properties of ion channels and thereby leads to an increase in neuron excitability. In addition, cytokines and growth factors may trigger transcriptional changes that affect the properties of sensory neurons through changes in gene expression. The increased peripheral input (*peripheral sensitization*) may secondarily alter sensory processing in the central nervous system (*central sensitization*), with both contributing to visceral pain syndromes. One easily recognized consequence of sensitization of visceral afferent pathways is increased tenderness to palpation over a larger area than normal.[12] Both peripheral and central mechanisms contribute to the increased sensitivity and expanded areas of referral, both of which are common in patients with irritable bowel syndrome, dyspepsia, and interstitial cystitis.

CENTRAL PROCESSING OF VISCERAL SENSATION AND PAIN

Vagal afferents project to the nucleus of the solitary tract and from there via the parabrachial nucleus and ventromedial thalamus to the insular cortex.[13] They form many connections with the hypothalamus, supraoptic nucleus, anterior cingulate cortex, and amygdala, which is essential for autonomic and emotional responses to visceral stimulation.[14,15] Spinal afferents also project to the thalamus but are preferentially found in the ventral posterolateral nucleus, which is connected to cortical areas, including the insula. The lateral components primarily serve discriminative functions associated with pain perception (e.g., location and intensity), whereas the medial thalamic nuclei, the main target of vagal input, are more closely linked to the emotional and autonomic responses triggered by pain. Consistent with the bilateral innervation of organs originating from midline structures, most visceral stimuli activate both cerebral hemispheres, albeit with a preferential activation of one—mostly the left—side.[2,16,17] Studies using functional brain imaging have not demonstrated striking differences in the processing of visceral and nonvisceral pain. However, visceral pain preferentially activates the perigenual portion of the anterior cingulate cortex, whereas nonvisceral pain is primarily represented in the midcingulate cortex. The physical proximity or even overlap between processing of visceral pain and emotion in the perigenual portion of the anterior cingulate cortex provides a potential explanation for the stronger emotional response to painful visceral than to nonvisceral stimuli.[18-20]

VISCERAL PAIN STIMULI

Visceral events that can produce conscious sensation or acute pain in humans include traction on the mesentery, distention of hollow organs, strong contractions of muscle layers surrounding such hollow organs, ischemia, and chemical irritants.[12,21] Routine endoscopic interventions have established that cutting or burning—two clearly noxious stimuli when applied to the skin—are not perceived when applied to viscera, thus setting visceral apart from nonvisceral sensation. Because of its sensitizing influences on sensory pathways, visceral inflammation can trigger pain or increase the excitability of visceral afferent pathways (e.g., enhancing low-threshold input into a noxious range), which can become chronic (e.g., chronic pancreatitis). Finally, though not studied in as much detail, malignancies can trigger chronic pain as a result of direct effects of the tumor on afferent nerves (e.g., nerve compression, release of chemicals) or as a result of indirect effects such as distention of a hollow organ.[22]

CLINICAL IMPLICATIONS

Current evidence suggests that spinal afferents primarily serve the discriminatory function of nociception, encoding location and intensity of visceral pain. Thus, treatment strategies, such as regional block or surgical dissection, generally target spinal afferent pathways.

Unilateral nerve blocks are often ineffective, which is partly due to the fact that most viscera receive bilateral innervation and are innervated by two sets of nerves.

Visceral pain is a complex experience associated with strong emotional and autonomic reactions. The emotive component of visceral pain is at least in part due to the central projections of spinal *and* vagal sensory pathways, both of which can activate the perigenual area of the anterior cingulate cortex, an area closely associated with emotional processing. The complex innervation of most viscera by spinal and vagal afferent pathways provides an explanation for the often only partial or temporary effects of regional blocks.

Impaired function of viscera, such as decreased transit of material in the gut, may significantly contribute to pain due to distension or strong contractions of visceral muscles or the composition of luminal contents. Thus, effective pain management needs to combine analgesic therapies with treatment strategies targeting specific visceral function.

REGIONAL BLOCK AND NEURAL ABLATION

Surgical and nonoperative approaches have been developed to perform transient nerve blocks or more permanently destroy the sensory pathways involved in visceral pain. In view of concerns about the irreversible nature of nerve ablation or neurolysis, most studies targeting visceral sensory pathways have involved patients with inoperable cancer and a relatively short life expectancy. Because these patients are typically seen in advanced stages of their disease with poor performance status, surgical denervation plays only a minor role in treatment. Chemical neurolysis, generally performed with high concentrations of ethanol, can achieve comparable results without subjecting patients to the risk associated with an operation. Since the first description by Kappis nearly 100 years ago,[23] several techniques have been developed to optimize the targeted delivery of neurolytic agents or minimize the likelihood of adverse effects, or both. Most of these approaches use imaging methods, such as fluoroscopy, ultrasound, or computed tomography (CT). However, despite this wealth of literature, few systematic studies have addressed the efficacy, outcomes, or adverse effects of these interventions. Problems assessing the effects of visceral pain management with peripheral blocks are further confounded by differences in type, concentration, and amount of the neurolytic agent, primarily ethanol; differences in both definition and measurement end points; and differences in follow-up time. Only five randomized controlled trials comparing ablative therapies with conventional pharmacologic pain management have been published.[24-28] All but one of them showed at least transiently improved pain levels and a concomitant decrease in opioid use. A recently conducted meta-analysis concluded that at least for pancreatic cancer, the pain relief achieved with neurolytic blocks is comparable to that achieved with conventional analgesic therapy but may be associated with fewer side effects.[29]

CELIAC PLEXUS AND SPLANCHNIC NERVE BLOCK

Spinal afferents innervating organs in the upper part of the abdomen traverse the celiac plexus, with two distinct ganglia located caudal to the origin of the celiac artery. The afferents travel centrally behind the crura of the diaphragm in the splanchnic nerves. The traditional dorsal approach uses the 12th rib and spinal process of the first lumbar vertebra as landmarks.[30,31] With the patient in the prone position, a needle is advanced about 7 cm lateral to the midline at a 30- to 45-degree angle and tilted slightly cranially to reach the lateral wall of the body of the first lumbar vertebra. The needle is then moved anteriorly by about 2 cm. If aspiration does not yield return of blood, water-soluble contrast material (3 to 5 mL), often mixed with a local anesthetic, is injected under fluoroscopic control. To better directly target the celiac plexus, the needle can be placed about 2 cm more anterior, which requires piercing the diaphragmatic crura and positions the needle close to the anterolateral aspect of the aorta. Severely ill patients with respiratory compromise and patients with significant ascites or recent abdominal surgery often poorly tolerate being in the prone position for the time required to complete this procedure. Therefore, an anterior approach has been developed in which the needle is advanced from the epigastric area toward the body of the first lumbar vertebra. If the appropriate position is confirmed, the neurolytic agent, generally phenol or ethanol, is administered. Current approaches rely mostly on the tissue destructive properties of ethanol, which is used in concentrations between 50% and 99% and volumes between 20 and 50 mL per injection. Injections are generally performed bilaterally to effectively destroy the afferent pathways. A recent report suggested that radiofrequency ablation may provide an alternative to chemical neurolysis.[32] Although this approach has since been adopted by others, well-designed studies on visceral pain syndromes are still missing.

Various imaging techniques have been used with the intent of improving the efficacy of neurolysis and decreasing the potential for adverse effects. The celiac ganglia are too small to allow direct visualization with CT or transabdominal ultrasound. Using endoscopic ultrasonography, the scanner can be brought into close proximity to the plexus. However, the ganglia do not differ in echogenicity from surrounding structures, thus again not allowing direct imaging of the target structure. Therefore, all these approaches rely on identifying the celiac artery as the main landmark. CT allows guidance of the needle to the target area and three-dimensional reconstruction of the area affected by the neurolytic agent based on the spread of radiopaque contrast material.[33] Although ultrasound allows real-time guidance without exposure to radiation, air in the overlying structures often interferes with sound penetration and imaging, thus limiting its utility in patients undergoing celiac plexus block.[34] Endoscopic ultrasound with an endoscopically advanced needle has been used successfully. Close inspection may identify tumor infiltration as a negative prognostic criterion and hence help in appropriate patient selection.[35] In addition, ethanol injection alters the echogenicity of the affected tissue, thus allowing direct visualization of spread of the neurolytic agent.[36] Only one trial directly compared the endoscopic and conventional transcutaneous approaches for celiac plexus block, and it suggested superiority of the endoscopic approach.[37]

SURGICAL NERVE ABLATION

One randomized controlled trial and several small case series have used surgical approaches to ablate the celiac ganglia or splanchnic nerves. The direct visualization during surgical exploration allows targeted injection of neurolytic agents into the celiac plexus if curative resection cannot be performed.[38] Because of advances in preoperative imaging, fewer patients currently undergo exploratory laparotomy, thus limiting the number of patients in whom an intraoperative celiac plexus block might be performed. With the advent of minimally invasive surgery, thoracoscopic resection of splanchnic nerves has been reported. As is true for the less invasive procedures, approaches have not been standardized, with unilateral and bilateral resection with or without vagotomy being performed to achieve pain control in these patients.[39-41]

EFFICACY OF NEURAL BLOCK AND ABLATION

Differences in patient selection, techniques, and outcome measures complicate comparison of published results. A meta-analysis published in 1995 concluded that nearly 90% of patients with various malignancies experienced good pain relief for about 3 months after the procedure.[31] Even though most case series report similar results, it is important to determine whether ablative therapy actually improves pain control or quality of life (or both) over that of conventional treatment involving the systemic use of analgesic substances. Two small randomized controlled trials demonstrated similar pain control but fewer adverse effects as a result of opioid consumption in patients treated with neurolytic blocks.[24,28] Subsequent studies have pointed to a slight advantage of ablative treatment over pharmacotherapy. Intraoperative celiac plexus block with 50% ethanol led to stable pain levels in patients with inoperable pancreatic cancer, whereas patients receiving saline injection as control experienced a significant increase in pain scores during follow-up. This improvement in pain control was associated with significantly lower use of opioids.[38] In a post hoc analysis, patients with significant pain lived longer than controls did if they underwent celiac plexus block. However, there was no overall survival benefit when the comparison involved use of the original study design as a template for the analysis. Three subsequent trials comparing neurolytic celiac plexus block with analgesic therapy confirmed better pain relief after ablative therapy. In two studies, the improvement was transient, with progressive recurrence of pain after about 1 to 2 months.[25,26] Most patients still required opioids, albeit in lower dosages than needed by controls in the two smaller studies.[25,26] A recent study by Wong and coworkers did not confirm this decrease in opioid consumption.[27] Consistent with the results shown by Kawamata and colleagues, their results also demonstrated that appropriate dosing of opioids achieves good pain control and a comparable quality of life that does not differ between treatment groups.[26] None of these investigations demonstrated a significant effect of neurolytic plexus block on patient survival.

Because cancer progression may affect the efficacy of ablative procedures, one small study randomly enrolled patients to receive early or late neurolytic blocks, with stages being defined by the use of low or high dosages of opioids, respectively.[42] Although both groups reported better pain control than medically treated controls did, there were no significant differences between the groups.

A randomized controlled trial reported better pain control after bilateral splanchnic nerve blockade than after celiac plexus blockade.[43] This assessment was based on a more significant decrease in pain intensity from baseline scores rather than a difference in the primary end point—pain measured by visual analog scale. Thus, confirmatory studies are needed to establish whether splanchnic nerve destruction is indeed superior to neurolysis of the celiac plexus. De Cicco and associates used CT scanning to examine the spread of contrast material injected before the neurolytic agent.[33] In their retrospective study, the pattern was a good predictor of pain control, with optimal results being achieved in patients in whom the contrast agent spread bilaterally above and below the origin of the celiac artery. However, case series using CT guidance do not report better response rates than when the conventional approach is used.[33,34,44] The more recently introduced endoscopic ultrasonography allows visualization of the area of interest during injection of the neurolytic agent. Only one small and underpowered study compared this approach with CT guidance and reported better results with endoscopic ultrasonography.[45] Published case series reveal results that fall within the range achieved with other techniques.[36,46]

Similarly, the results of surgical interventions with neurolytic or neuroablative therapy remain inconclusive. Although the only randomized controlled trial demonstrated good pain relief and a decrease in opioid consumption,[38] a case series evaluating different palliative operations for pancreatic cancer did not confirm the decrease in opioid use after celiac plexus block.[47] Smaller case series report improved pain control in about 60% to 80% of patients after thoracoscopic splanchnicectomy performed unilaterally or bilaterally with or without vagotomy.[39-41,48-52] Poor definition of end points, limited assessment of analgesic effects, lack of appropriate control groups, and the fact that comparable results were obtained with a variety of often quite different approaches clearly demonstrate the need for appropriately designed studies. Splanchnicectomy reduces opioid requirements in comparison to systemic pharmacotherapy, but not in comparison to celiac plexus block.[41,52] Overall, the current data suggest acceptable pain relief with at least a transient decrease in opioid requirements[29] but do not support the superiority of one ablative approach over another. Thus, the choice that patients and physicians face should primarily focus on the available expertise when selecting one technique over another.

NERVE BLOCK OR ABLATIVE THERAPY FOR BENIGN DISORDERS

As described earlier, the pain relief after a neurolytic block is often transient, which decreases the enthusiasm to use such approaches in patients with benign disorders and long life expectancy. Therefore, less information is available about the efficacy of nerve blocks in such patients. Several case series combining about 400 patients with chronic pancreatitis have been published, thus making this the largest patient group with benign diseases. Initial response rates varied between 30% and 90%, with limited follow-up in the majority of cases.[32,37,40,45,51,53-56] Because of concerns about the use of neurolytic agents, the largest series combined bupivacaine with triamcinolone.[54] Although about half the patients reported an initial benefit, sustained responses after 24 weeks were seen in only 10%. Though commonly practiced, a recently completed randomized controlled trial showed no additional benefit of triamcinolone, with response rates of about 15% 1 month after celiac plexus block with bupivacaine.[57] Moore and coauthors reported the results of stellate ganglion and paravertebral blocks with bupivacaine in 59 patients with refractory angina, a thoracic visceral pain, secondary to coronary artery disease.[58] About 60% of the patients experienced pain relief for more than 2 weeks. However, the benefit was transient and most patients required multiple interventions to maintain some benefit. Interestingly, the limited experience with differential neuraxial blocks suggests that primary visceral pain was present only in about a fifth of patients with chronic pancreatitis, with the majority experiencing "central pain," defined as persistent pain despite surgical anesthesia through the epidural administration of lidocaine.[59] Overall, the data highlight the complex etiology of chronic pain syndromes in patients with benign disorders and do not support the routine use of ablative therapies in these patients.

ADVERSE EFFECTS OF NEUROLYTIC BLOCKS

Transient pain is the most common side effect reported when ethanol is used as the neurolytic agent. Although the use of local anesthetic before the ethanol injection decreases the incidence of this adverse effect, at least 10% to 30% of patients experience significant pain within the first hours after the procedure.[34,44,46,60] The destruction of sympathetic efferent pathways causes vasodilation of the splanchnic vessels, which results in hypotension in up to 20% of patients.[25,44,46] Similarly, the unopposed parasympathetic drive can lead to diarrhea, which again is reported by about a fifth of patients.[24,25,46,60] All these problems can generally be managed medically with appropriate premedication, hydration, postprocedural observation, and appropriate symptomatic therapy. More significant adverse effects are rare but have been reported for all the different approaches.

The posterior approach may traverse the kidney, as well as the pleural space, thereby potentially leading to hematuria or pneumothorax.[30,31,60] The anterior approach requires advancing the needle through the liver, stomach, and colon. Although this is largely inconsequential, clinically relevant perforation can occur and may be difficult to diagnose because of the neurolytic block and often concomitantly administered analgesia.[61] Therefore, all patients should be well hydrated, receive an intravenous fluid bolus before performance of the nerve block, and remain under observation for at least 2 to 4 hours after the procedure. Delivery of neurolytic agents in close proximity to major vessels is another potential source of complications. In all cases, aspiration should ensure that the needle is not inside a vessel before the neurolytic agent is injected. However, indirect effects, such as mesenteric venous thrombosis, may occur rarely despite these precautions.[62] Spread of the neurolytic agent within the retroperitoneal space with injury to the lumbar nerves has been reported.[31] Paraparesis is the most feared and mostly irreversible complication that is thought to be caused by injury to the nutrient vessels supplying the spinal cord.[30,31] Even though sufficiently powered studies addressing the likelihood of these adverse effects are not available, current evidence suggests that the incidence does not differ between the different approaches.[36,46,52]

CLINICAL IMPLICATIONS

Neurolytic celiac or splanchnic nerve block is a moderately effective method to decrease pain in patients with intra-abdominal malignancies, and has been best studied in patients with pancreatic cancer. The benefit is often transient, and may decrease the need for opioids, but does not affect life expectancy or quality of life compared to conventional pain management. Adverse effects occur in about 20% of patients, are largely minor and transient and can be managed by appropriate medical therapy. Approaches using different imaging techniques or even direct operative visualization do not seem to affect outcome or the incidence of side effects.

SPINAL TREATMENT TARGETS FOR VISCERAL PAIN

Epidural block or pharmacotherapy and surgical myelotomy can be performed to treat chronic visceral pain syndromes. Two aspects unique to visceral pain syndromes warrant some specific discussion of spinal treatment targets. First, preliminary studies suggest that patients with ischemic heart disease may derive significant benefit from epidural blocks. Second, unlike nonvisceral pain, which is primarily relayed to supraspinal sites via the spinothalamic tract, functional and neuroanatomic studies have convincingly demonstrated that a dorsal column ascending pathway plays an important role in visceral pain.[63,64] Only few studies have systematically evaluated the clinical efficacy of these approaches over long periods, thus limiting the ability to fully assess their therapeutic value at this point.

EPIDURAL ANALGESIA AND VISCERAL PAIN

Spinal drug delivery through epidural catheters allows the administration of opioids and other agents without a significant risk for systemic adverse effects. Acute or chronic epidural drug delivery alleviates visceral pain in patients with malignant disorders and in some patients with benign disorders.[59,65] Interestingly, high thoracic epidural anesthesia significantly improved angina in patients with refractory pain as a result of coronary artery disease and decreased documented episodes of cardiac ischemia as judged by ST-segment depression.[66,67] A recent study provided further insight into the underlying mechanism by demonstrating improved cardiac perfusion during high epidural analgesia, probably as a result of a concomitant block of the sympathetic pathways.[68] Because of limited information about the use of epidural analgesia for visceral pain, safety issues remain largely unaddressed. However, it is likely that the incidence and nature of adverse effects will be similar to the previously reported complication rate with epidural drug delivery, which is addressed in more detail in Chapters 18 and 43.[69-71]

SPINAL CORD STIMULATION AND VISCERAL PAIN

Recently, several case reports described significant improvement in severe visceral pain with spinal cord stimulation. The largest series compiled data from a total of 70 patients with refractory thoracic, abdominal, or pelvic pain syndromes.[72] Less than 10% did not respond to the temporarily implanted electrodes; responders were offered a permanent device, which was surgically implanted and led to maintenance of improvement with lower opioid requirements in the majority of patients. Though promising, no prospectively designed trial has been published, and assessment of long-term results was based on physician rather than patient reporting.

MYELOTOMY AND VISCERAL PAIN

Since its introduction about 20 years ago, midline myelotomy has been used to treat patients with refractory pain from visceral malignancies.[73] The nature of this intervention as a "rescue" treatment in patients who failed other therapies limits the ability to judge its clinical efficacy. No randomized controlled trials have determined its efficacy or adverse effects in comparison to optimized standard treatment. Case series are typically limited to patients with advanced malignancies and have reported improved pain control in about 60% of patients, with symptoms recurring in up to half of the patients.[74-76]

CLINICAL IMPLICATIONS

While systematic studies have not specifically addressed the efficacy of epidural drug delivery in patients with chronic visceral pain syndromes, currently available data support its use in patients with refractory pain due to ischemic heart disease. Initial data on spinal cord stimulation are promising, but require confirmation through well-designed prospective trials. As is true for all ablative therapies, midline myelotomy appears to provide only partial and transient pain relief. In the absence of more conclusive studies, myelotomies should be reserved for patients with intractable pain due to terminal disease.

MECHANISM-ORIENTED PHARMACOTHERAPY FOR VISCERAL PAIN

Visceral pain is often associated with abnormalities in organ function, such as constipation, nausea, cardiac failure, or dysuria. These abnormalities may cause pain or contribute to pain caused by the pain syndrome or its treatment. Thus, evaluation of patients with visceral pain syndromes should always go hand in hand with appropriate functional evaluation of the affected organ system.

SEROTONIN AND GASTROINTESTINAL PAIN MANAGEMENT

As described earlier, the gastrointestinal tract contains 95% of the body's serotonin (5-hydroxytryptamine [5-HT]), where it is involved in many different functions. Different serotonin receptors are found on neurons, smooth muscle, and epithelial cells. The ligand-gated 5-HT_3 receptor has been found on vagal and spinal afferents and is involved in visceral sensation, including the perception of nausea.[77,78] Metabotropic 5-HT receptors exert more complex effects on gut function because they act on multiple targets, including muscle and nerve cells, with limited studies suggesting that 5-HT_4 agonists and 5-HT_1 antagonists may decrease visceral sensation in experimental animals and healthy volunteers.[79-81] Currently, selective 5-HT_3 receptor antagonists and 5-HT_4 receptor agonists are available for clinical use. Although there is some experience with other serotonin receptor blockers, this experience is limited to mostly demonstrating physiologic changes in healthy controls or short-term effects in patients with mild abdominal discomfort. Antidepressants alter serotonin signaling, mainly by inhibiting the reuptake mechanism that terminates the effect of the released serotonin, and are commonly used in patients with various pain syndromes, including those with visceral pain. In view of their significant impact on central processing, it is not possible to clearly attribute effects to the peripheral changes in serotonin signaling.

CLINICAL EFFICACY OF SEROTONIN AGONISTS AND ANTAGONISTS

The 5-HT_3 antagonist alosetron has been used successfully in patients with functional bowel disease characterized by abdominal pain and diarrhea.[82-85] However, the effect is relatively modest, with a recent meta-analysis showing a small odds ratio (1:8) favoring the active agent over placebo, which translates into a number needed to treat of about 7.[86] Other 5-HT_3 receptor antagonists, such as ondansetron, play an important role in the treatment of severe nausea and vomiting but do not affect visceral pain.[77] Tegaserod, a 5-HT_4 agonist, significantly accelerates gastrointestinal transit and alleviates symptoms of constipation, including the associated discomfort and pain.[87,88] Using global improvement scores, currently available data suggest a relatively low odds ratio (2.0) favoring tegaserod over placebo, with a number needed to treat of about 7.[89] Both agents have been removed from the market in the United States because of safety concerns.

Many studies have addressed the impact of antidepressants on visceral pain, with most focusing on gastrointestinal disorders. Even though individual studies have discrepant results, recent meta-analyses suggest improvement in functional gastrointestinal disorders, but not as clearly improvement in pelvic pain.[90,91] One large trial examined the effect of amitriptyline in patients with interstitial cystitis without showing benefit over placebo.[92] At least for selective serotonin reuptake inhibitors, the improvement was primarily due to changes in global assessment scores rather than pain. Considering the potential impact of psychiatric comorbidity as a confounder, one recent study examined the effect of citalopram in nondepressed patients with irritable bowel syndrome and did not demonstrate any benefit.[93] Only one serotonin-norepinephrine reuptake inhibitor, venlafaxine, has been examined for visceral pain and was not found to be superior to placebo.[94]

ADVERSE EFFECTS OF SEROTONIN AGONISTS AND ANTAGONISTS

The most common side effect of alosetron and related agents is constipation, which is reported by 20% to 40% of patients.[89] Alosetron has been linked to ischemic colitis, a potentially fatal disease, which led to its withdrawal from the market.[86] It is currently available only under a restricted access program with stringent monitoring. Tegaserod has been associated with ischemic events and was similarly removed from the market.

SMOOTH MUSCLE RELAXANTS AND VISCERAL PAIN

Stretch and tension are adequate stimuli for visceral sensation and correspond to distention of a hollow viscus or contraction of the tunica muscularis.[21] Visceral muscle is morphologically and functionally distinct from striated muscle, thus potentially allowing the use of pharmacologic interventions that may not significantly affect striated muscle. Several strategies have emerged or are currently under investigation. Most rely on blockade of muscarinic receptors, the main excitatory signaling mechanism between parasympathetic neurons and visceral smooth muscle. Less commonly used strategies use agonists for α-adrenergic receptors or L-type calcium channel blockers to affect the contractility of visceral smooth muscle. The latter two approaches have largely been used in healthy volunteers, showed only limited efficacy in small studies involving patients with different painful disorders, and carry a significant risk for adverse effects, primarily symptomatic hypotension.[95-100] Therefore, the discussion of spasmolytic agents will focus on muscarinic receptor antagonists, with the best evidence emerging from studies performed in patients with functional diseases of the gastrointestinal tract.

CLINICAL EFFICACY OF SMOOTH MUSCLE RELAXANTS

Two recently published meta-analyses concluded that when compared with placebo, patients receiving anticholinergic drugs are twice as likely to report an overall benefit, including pain relief.[101,102] However, many of the patients experienced relatively mild pain at baseline and achieved only moderate pain relief in comparison to placebo.[90]

ADVERSE EFFECTS OF SMOOTH MUSCLE RELAXANTS

About 10% of patients experience largely minor adverse effects, mainly because of effects on the mucous membranes, urinary tract, and eye, such as dry mouth, urinary retention, and accommodation problems. Based on the mechanisms of action, anticholinergic drugs are contraindicated in patients with known glaucoma and should be avoided in patients with micturition problems.

BOTULINUM TOXIN AND VISCERAL PAIN

The clinical use of botulinum toxin has expanded significantly beyond its initial target—spastic motor disorders of skeletal muscles.[103] Around 20 years ago it was shown to affect smooth muscle as well and led to symptomatic improvement in patients with achalasia.[104] Because anecdotal evidence has suggested a decrease in pain independent of its effect on muscle activity, botulinum toxin has increasingly been used to treat various pain syndromes, presumably by directly altering peripheral transmitter release from nociceptive afferent nerve terminals.[105] Essentially, all the studies focusing on patients with visceral pain are case series. Frequently, patients have associated impairment of visceral function, such as dysphagia, gastroparesis, or voiding dysfunction.

CLINICAL EFFICACY OF BOTULINUM TOXIN

Few studies have focused on pain and systematically examined changes in pain intensity after treatment with botulinum toxin. In patients with various esophageal motility disorders characterized by pain, injection of botulinum toxin into the distal end of the esophagus significantly improved pain scores from severe to mild in about two thirds of patients for about 5 months.[106] In a smaller case series of patients suffering from diffuse esophageal spasm with severe chest pain, endoscopically guided injection of botulinum toxin along the tubular esophagus resulted in nearly complete alleviation of pain for 6 months.[107] Limited results on the effects of this neurotoxin on other areas of the gastrointestinal tract suggest potential benefit in disorders associated with pain.[108] In the urinary tract, botulinum toxin has been used successfully to treat voiding disorders. Although a case series suggested some effect in patients with interstitial cystitis, an idiopathic disorder characterized by pelvic pain, urinary urgency, and increased frequency of micturition, a recently completed randomized controlled trial did not confirm its superiority over placebo.[109,110]

ADVERSE EFFECTS OF BOTULINUM TOXIN

The generally low dosages of locally injected botulinum toxin do not cause systemic side effects. Adverse effects are largely limited to transient pain or infectious complications at the injection site. Injection in close proximity to striated muscle, most notably sphincteric muscle of the bladder or rectum, may lead to transient incontinence.

κ-OPIOIDS AND VISCERAL PAIN

Opioids are potent analgesics for nonvisceral as well as visceral pain. However, μ-opioid receptor agonists commonly cause gastrointestinal side effects such as nausea, vomiting, and constipation. Especially in patients with gastrointestinal disorders, these unwanted effects may become dose limiting. In addition, the rise in opioid use for chronic pain has led to increasing concern about the use of these agents for benign disorders. Because peripheral visceral afferents express κ-opioid receptors, κ-agonists were developed to take advantage of their analgesic properties and the lower likelihood of adverse effects.[111] Animal and acute studies in human volunteers demonstrated increased thresholds to painful visceral stimuli, consistent with a potential analgesic effect.[112,113] However, central effects with significant dysphoria limit the use of κ-agonists to peripherally acting agents.

CLINICAL EFFICACY OF κ-OPIOID AGONISTS

A single small study reported κ-agonist–induced pain relief in patients with chronic pancreatitis who were refractory to μ-opioid agonists. However, the patients were studied acutely after only a single administration of the agonist.[114] Several randomized controlled trials examined the effects of fedotozine, a κ-opioid agonist, in patients with chronic abdominal pain secondary to functional disorders over a period of at least 6 weeks. Although an overall benefit was reported, the effect was rather small in comparison to placebo.[115-117] On-demand therapy with asimadoline, a peripherally acting κ-opioid agonist, did not affect pain severity in patients with irritable bowel syndrome.[118]

ADVERSE EFFECTS CAUSED BY κ-OPIOID AGONISTS

Randomized controlled trials did not report a significantly higher incidence of adverse effects after the administration of peripherally acting κ-opioid agonists than after placebo.[89]

AGENTS TARGETING THE $\alpha_2\delta$ CALCIUM CHANNEL SUBUNIT

Voltage-sensitive calcium channels play an important role in neuronal excitability. Gabapentin and pregabalin have been developed as anticonvulsive agents. Because changes in neuronal excitability contribute to peripheral and central sensitization, both agents have been used in patients with chronic visceral pain. In healthy volunteers and patients with irritable bowel syndrome, the agents blunted acute pain triggered by rectal distention.[119,120]

CLINICAL EFFICACY OF AGENTS TARGETING THE $\alpha_2\delta$ SUBUNIT

Despite changes in acute pain sensitivity, pregabalin was not superior to placebo during a 2-week course of treatment in patients with irritable bowel syndrome.[120] In contrast, a recent study showed improved pain control and decrease opioid use in patients with chronic pancreatitis treated with pregabalin.[121]

ADVERSE EFFECTS OF AGENTS TARGETING THE $\alpha_2\delta$ SUBUNIT

Even though gabapentin and pregabalin were well tolerated without serious adverse events, patients reported problems with cognition and balance, often stating that they felt as though they were drunk.

CLINICAL IMPLICATIONS

The improved understanding of normal visceral function and sensation has led to the development of new therapeutic strategies. In the gastrointestinal tract, muscarinic receptor antagonists and serotonin receptor agonists and antagonists alter function and may improve discomfort associated with functional disorders. Antidepressants are commonly used and may lead to some improvement of global symptoms score, likely in part due to their effect on often coexisting psychiatric illnesses. A recent study in patients with chronic pancreatitis suggests some efficacy of pregabalin in visceral pain. Several targeted treatments are currently under development using drugs that interact with purinergic receptors and members of the family transient receptor potential channels (TRPV1 or TRPA1).

SUGGESTED READINGS

Arcidiacono PG, Calori G, Carrara S, et al. Celiac plexus block for pancreatic cancer pain in adults. *Cochrane Database Syst Rev.* 2011;3:CD007519.

Camilleri M. Treating irritable bowel syndrome: overview, perspective and future therapies. *Br J Pharmacol.* 2004;141:1237-1248.

De Schepper HU, Cremonini F, Park M-I, et al. Opioids and the gut: pharmacology and current clinical experience. *Neurogastroenterol Motil.* 2004;16:383-394.

Gottsch H, Miller J, Yang C, et al. A pilot study of botulinum toxin for interstitial cystitis/painful bladder syndrome. *Neurourol Urodyn.* 2011;30:93-96.

Houghton LA, Fell C, Whorwell PJ, et al. Effect of a second-generation $\alpha_2\delta$ ligand (pregabalin) on visceral sensation in hypersensitive patients with irritable bowel syndrome. *Gut.* 2007;56:1218-1225.

Kuiken SD, Tytgat GN, Boeckxstaens GE. Review article: drugs interfering with visceral sensitivity for the treatment of functional gastrointestinal disorders—the clinical evidence. *Aliment Pharmacol Ther.* 2005;21:633-651.

Ladabaum U, Sharabidze A, Levin TR, et al. Citalopram is not effective therapy for non-depressed patients with irritable bowel syndrome. *Clin Gastroenterol Hepatol.* 2010;8:42-48.

Olesen SS, Bouwense SAW, Wilder-Smith OHG, et al. Pregabalin reduces pain in patients with chronic pancreatitis in a randomized, controlled trial. *Gastroenterology.* 2011;141:536-543.

Ruepert L, Quartero AO, de Wit NJ, et al. Bulking agents, antispasmodics and antidepressants for the treatment of irritable bowel syndrome. *Cochrane Database Syst Rev.* 2011;8:CD003460.

Strigo IA, Duncan GH, Boivin M, et al. Differentiation of visceral and cutaneous pain in the human brain. *J Neurophysiol.* 2003;89:3294-3303.

Wong GY, Schroeder DR, Carns PE, et al. Effect of neurolytic celiac plexus block on pain relief, quality of life, and survival in patients with unresectable pancreatic cancer: a randomized controlled trial. *JAMA.* 2004;291:1092-1099.

The references for this chapter can be found at www.expertconsult.com.

Pediatric Chronic Pain Management

33

Santhanam Suresh | Ravi Shah

Chronic pain in children is an undertreated entity that is commonly ignored. Over the last decade, several studies in the literature have addressed pain in children and its measurement and management.[1,2] In this chapter we discuss common chronic pain syndromes in children along with their assessment, diagnosis, and management (Box 33.1). Recurrent or persistent pain is seen in 5% to 10% of children. One study demonstrated that 96% of children aged 9 to 13 years experienced some form of acute pain over the previous month, with 78% experiencing headaches, 57% experiencing recurrent pain, and 6% experiencing chronic persistent pain.[3]

ASSESSMENT OF CHRONIC PAIN IN CHILDREN

Assessment of children with chronic pain starts with a biopsychosocial perspective to take into account the multiple factors that can influence the child's pain experience. Multidimensional models elaborate various biologic, developmental, temperamental, cognitive-behavioral, affective, social, and situational factors that may both shape the child's pain experience and influence the pathways by which they exert their effects.[3-5] Each domain may become a target of assessment and intervention. Several developmentally sensitive validated instruments are now available to measure the varied aspects of children's pain[6] (Table 33.1).

Two standardized interviews for school-age and adolescent children and their parents provide comprehensive yet practical evaluations of the child's chronic pain—the Children's Comprehensive Pain Questionnaire (CCPQ)[7] and the Varni-Thompson Pediatric Pain Questionnaire (VTPPQ).[8] These interviews separately assess both the child's and parents' experience of the pain problems with open-ended questions, checklists, and quantitative pain-rating scales. Some studies suggest potential limitations of these self-report measures because of cultural or cognitive differences among children.[9] Additionally, the Pain Behavior Observation Method is a 10-minute observational pain behavior measure that can be used in children with chronic pain who may have difficulty with self-report measures because of age or cognitive limitations.[10] Studies have supported the use of electronic versus paper pain diaries in children with chronic pain; electronic diary use was shown to be feasible[11] and resulted in greater compliance and accuracy in diary recording than did traditional paper diaries in children with recurrent pain.[12]

The well-documented comorbidity between pediatric chronic pain and psychiatric disorders,[13,14] particularly internalizing disorders such as depression and anxiety,[15-18] obligate the clinician to screen for these disorders. The Children's Depression Inventory (CDI)[19] is a widely used self-report questionnaire for assessing depression in children 7 to 17 years of age. The Beck Depression Inventory-II can be used with adolescents[20] because some items on the CDI may be less age appropriate for older adolescents. It is important to assess for anxiety symptoms because pain-related disability is associated with anxiety sensitivity, a stable predisposition to fear of anxiety-related sensations,[21] and pain-related avoidance behavior in children as well as adults with chronic pain.[22-24] The Children's Anxiety Sensitivity Index (CASI)[25] is the only instrument thus far developed to assess this characteristic in children, and the Pain-Anxiety Symptoms Scale (PASS)[26] was developed for adults to assess fear of pain but has been used in children as young as 8 years.[24] A recent study suggested that the CASI is a better predictor of health-related quality of life than pain intensity in children with chronic pain.[27]

Several well-validated self-report questionnaires assess anxiety in children (see Table 33.1). Two instruments, the Self-Report for Child Anxiety Related Disorders (SCARED)[28] and the Spence Children's Anxiety Scale (SCAS),[29] include subscales that distinguish among specific anxiety disorders listed in the *Diagnostic and Statistical Manual of Mental Disorders*, Fourth Edition (DSM-IV). The Multidimensional Anxiety Scale for Children (MASC)[30] and the Revised Children's Manifest Anxiety Scale (RCMAS)[31] include subscales that focus on other dimensions of anxiety. These subscales include physical symptoms, social and separation anxiety, and harm avoidance (the MASC) and physiologic symptoms, worry and oversensitivity, and concentration factors (the RCMAS); both also include social desirability items to detect inconsistency or randomness in reporting. The SCAS and SCARED provide both child and parent forms of the instrument, which allows examination of the convergence or lack thereof between the child's and parent's assessment of the child's anxiety symptoms. The State-Trait Anxiety Inventory for Children (STAIC)[32] provides a state version, which measures situation-specific anxiety, and a trait form, which assesses anxiety symptoms that are stable across situations.

Factors that are closely linked with a child's ability to function with chronic pain, such as perceived stress[33-35] and coping,[36-38] can assist in planning behavioral interventions. The Pain Coping Questionnaire (PCQ),[39] Pain Response Inventory (PRI),[40] and Pain Catastrophizing Scale for Children (PCS-C)[41] assess pain-specific coping strategies. The Response to Stress Questionnaire (RSQ) has been used to assess coping with abdominal pain but also has other versions that target other stressors, such as social stress.[42]

Box 33.1 Chronic Pain in Children: Common Diagnoses

Neuropathic pain
- Complex regional pain syndrome type 1
- Peripheral nerve injuries
- Postamputation pain
- Deafferentation pain

Headache

Chest pain

Chronic illness
- Sickle cell crisis
- Cystic fibrosis
- Collagen vascular disease (e.g., juvenile rheumatoid arthritis, systemic lupus erythematosus)

Recurrent abdominal pain

Pelvic pain

Back pain

Cancer-related pain

Identification and modification of maladaptive coping responses constitute core elements of cognitive-behavioral approaches for treating pediatric chronic pain. For example, if the child endorses a catastrophizing coping style, which is an established risk factor for poor adaptation to chronic pain,[43-45] this coping style can become a target of treatment.

The ability to function in tasks of daily living is a critically important outcome measure to assess when treating children and adolescents with chronic pain. Frequently, pain cannot be completely relieved and the child must learn to accept, cope, and adapt to the pain to enable participation in normal developmental activities and tasks, such as going to school, participating in extracurricular activities, and developing and sustaining social relationships. Several measures have been developed to assess the child's functional abilities, as well as quality of life. For example, the Pediatric Migraine Disability Scale (PedMIDAS) measures headache-related disability in children with chronic pain.[46] This six-question tool assesses school, recreational, and social areas of participation and disability, domains relevant to all children with chronic pain. The Child Activity Limitations Interview (CALI)[47] assesses the impact of recurrent pain on children's daily activities as a way to identify appropriate targets for treatment. Additionally, the Functional Disability Inventory (FDI),[48-50] developed to assess illness-related disability in children and adolescents, is a useful tool for evaluating the functional status of pediatric patients with chronic pain, a particularly important concern in children with pain disorders associated with psychological factors and pain-associated disability syndrome.[51] Pain-related disability increases with age and as sex differences emerge in adolescence, with more girls than boys reporting pain-related functional disability.[52]

Quality of life can also be assessed in children and adolescents with chronic pain and as an index of treatment progress,[53-55] with one study finding that the quality of life of children with recurrent headaches is similar to that of children with rheumatoid arthritis or cancer.[56] The Quality of Life Pain–Youth (QLP-Y)[57] was developed to address quality-of-life issues particular to chronic pain. The Child Health Questionnaire, both child (CHQ-CF87) and parent reports (CHQ-50),[58] as well as the PedsQL,[59] are measures that may be used to assess general quality of life in children with chronic pain and have the advantage that the scores obtained on these instruments can be compared with standardized samples of scores obtained by children with other medical illnesses.

Other instruments that may further elucidate the psychological factors contributing to a child's behavioral adaptation to chronic pain include the Children's Somatization Inventory (CSI),[60] which measures a child's propensity to somatization, and the Harter Scales of Perceived Competence,[61-63] which assess a child's judgment about his or her capabilities in important domains such as school performance, peer relationships, and athletic abilities. The child's own judgment of his or her competencies in these domains is useful in understanding other factors that may contribute to the child's functioning.[64] For example, children with chronic pain who rate themselves as low on social and academic competency may have multiple reasons to avoid returning to school.

Parental or family issues that could impede or support a child's progress with treatment are also important to assess. The Family Environment Scale (FES)[65] and the Family Adaptation and Cohesion Scales II (FACES II)[66] have been used to assess family characteristics, whereas the Family Crisis-Oriented Personal Evaluation Scale (F-COPES)[67] assesses the family's problem-solving and coping efforts in relation to a challenging situation, such as having an ill child. At times the parents themselves may require psychiatric treatment to assist them in their efforts to help in their child's rehabilitation. The Symptom Checklist 90–Revised (SCL-90-R)[68] is a useful screen for parental psychiatric symptoms, and the Medical Outcomes Short-Form 36-Item Health Survey[69] can be used to assess parental adaptive functioning, as well as disabilities.

Scharff and colleagues[70] attempted to identify specific subgroups of pediatric chronic pain patients. Identifying subgroups of adults with chronic pain has proved useful in identifying patients' coping efforts and determining appropriate psychological interventions. For example, the West Haven–Yale Multidimensional Pain Inventory (WHYMPI)[71] has been used to identify clinical subgroups of adult chronic pain patients—"adaptive copers," who have good coping and supportive relationships; "dysfunctional copers," who have poor coping skills and are highly stressed; and the "interpersonally distressed," who have inadequate social support.[72] These three subgroups have been found in diverse adult populations with chronic pain and are associated with different outcomes in behaviorally based pain treatment programs. Although all three groups were found to benefit from a behavioral intervention, the dysfunctional copers benefited the most, with lower pain scores, decreased impact of the pain on their lives, and decreased depression and negative thoughts.[73] Scharff and colleagues[70] identified similar subgroups in a population of 117 children with various types of chronic pain conditions: a high-functioning group, a disabled and low-functioning group, and a group with family dysfunction. These strongly resemble the subgroups identified by Turk and Rudy[72] in adult chronic pain patients. Although findings from this study were preliminary and need to be interpreted cautiously, such efforts to

Table 33.1 Methods for Assessment of Chronic Pain in Children and Adolescents

Pain Measure	Disability or Quality of Life	Stress and Coping	Anxiety	Depression	Family and Parental Functioning	Other Behavioral Measures
Varni-Thompson Pediatric Pain Questionnaire (PPQ) Ages: 5-18	Functional Disability Inventory (FDI) Ages: 8-17 (plus parent form)	Children's Hassles Scale (CHS) Ages: 8-17	Multidimensional Anxiety Scale for Children (MASC) Ages: 8-19	Children's Depression Inventory (CDI) Ages: 7-17	Family Environment Scale (FES) Ages: Adult	Children's Somatization Inventory (CSI) Ages: 8-18 (plus parent form)
Children's Comprehensive Pain Questionnaire (CCPQ) Ages: 5-19	Child Health Questionnaire (CHQ) Ages: 5+ (plus parent form)	Response to Stress Questionnaire (RSQ) Ages: 11+ (plus parent form)	Self-Report for Childhood Anxiety-Related Disorders (SCARED) Ages: 9-18 (plus parent form)	Beck Depression Inventory-II Ages: 13+	Family Adaptation and Cohesion Scale II (FACES-II) Ages: Adult	Harter Scales of Perceived Competence for Children Ages: 4-12
Pain diary (written, electronic) Ages: 8+	Pediatric Quality of Life Inventory Generic Core Scales (PedsQL 4.0) Ages: 5-18 (plus parent report ages 2-18)	Pain Coping Questionnaire (PCQ) Ages: 8-18	Spence Children's Anxiety Scale (SCAS) Ages: 8-12 (plus parent form)		Family Crisis-Oriented Personal Evaluation Scales (F-COPES) Ages: Adult	
Pain Behavior Observation Method Ages: 6-17	Quality of Life Pain—Youth (QLP-Y) Ages: 12-18	Pain Response Inventory (PRI) Ages: 8-19	Revised Children's Manifest Anxiety Scale (RCMAS) Ages: 6-19		Symptom Checklist-90–Revised (SCL-90-R) Ages: 13+	
Non-Communicating Children's Pain Checklist (NCCPC-R) Ages: 2-adult	Pediatric Migraine Disability Assessment Scale (PedMIDAS) Ages: 6-18	Pain Catastrophizing Scale (PCS) Ages: 8-16	State-Trait Anxiety Scale for Children (STAIC) Ages: 9-12		Medical Outcomes 36-Item Short Form Health Survey (MOS-SF-36) Ages: Adult	
	Children's Activity Limitations Scale (CALI) Ages: 8-16		Childhood Anxiety Sensitivity Index (CASI) Ages: 7-12 Pain-Anxiety Symptoms Scale (PASS) Ages: 8-adult			

Box 33.2 Pediatric Questionnaire Components

1. Developmental level
2. Understanding of pain
3. Pain and medical treatment history
4. Interactions with others in relation to pain
5. Affect and behavior
6. Impact of pain on functional abilities
7. Family environment and stress
8. Coping skills
9. History of psychiatric illness
10. Medical problems

distinguish subgroups of children with chronic pain should serve to provide targeted treatments to improve the care of pediatric patients with chronic pain.

Therefore, thorough baseline and ongoing assessment is essential to guide interventions for chronic pain and evaluate the child's response to treatment. Core elements of assessment include comprehensive evaluation of the child's pain problem and screens for psychiatric comorbidity and functional status (Box 33.2). More intensive screening of the child's perceived stress and competencies and the parents' and family's functioning adds valuable information to treatment planning, especially in a child with long-standing pain problems that have not responded to previous treatment efforts.

PSYCHOLOGICAL PAIN MANAGEMENT METHODS

A rehabilitative approach that emphasizes improving the child's and family's ability to cope with a chronic condition characterizes the course of most chronic pain treatment programs for children. The focus shifts from the narrow goal of pain reduction, which might be used in the treatment of acute pain, and broadens to decrease pain-related emotional and behavioral disability, thereby increasing the child's functional status.[51,74,75] Psychological pain management methods are directed toward increasing the child's and family's understanding of the child's pain and its treatment, including factors that may reduce or exacerbate the child's pain, and enhancing cognitive and behavioral coping skills so that pain-related discomfort and disability are reduced. Research on the use of psychological therapies has focused mostly on clinical trials in children with headache.[76,77] In a meta-analysis conducted to evaluate the efficacy of behavioral interventions for pediatric chronic pain, Eccleston and coworkers[76] concluded that "There is strong evidence that psychological treatment, primarily relaxation and cognitive behavioural therapy, are highly effective in reducing the severity and frequency of chronic pain in children and adolescents." Additionally, findings by Logan and colleagues suggest that interdisciplinary pediatric pain rehabilitation may facilitate increased willingness to self-manage pain, which is associated with improvements in function and psychological well-being.[78]

A few promising psychological treatments have also been used for children with disease-related chronic pain, including sickle cell disease,[79-81] recurrent abdominal pain,[82-85] complex regional pain syndrome (CRPS) type 1,[86] musculoskeletal pain,[87,88] and juvenile primary fibromyalgia syndrome,[89,90] and further support the probable efficacy of cognitive-behavioral approaches to pediatric pain management. Although there is evidence to support the use of single behavioral treatment modalities for the treatment of pediatric chronic pain, such as the use of thermal biofeedback and relaxation for recurrent pediatric headache,[91] most treatment programs include a diverse array of techniques that treat chronic pain by modifying children's cognitive, affective, and sensory experiences of pain, their behavior in response to pain, and environmental and social factors that influence the pain experience. Education about chronic pain and problem solving for improving the child's functional status is central to the child and family assuming an active role in managing chronic pain. Cognitive techniques are targeted at modifying the child's thoughts about the pain, in particular, to increase a sense of predictability and control over the pain, to alter memories about painful experiences,[92] and to reduce negative cognitions about pain, especially "catastrophizing."[93] Decreasing somatic preoccupation, pain-related rumination,[94] and passive coping and learning to accept that the pain may persist[95] are also key interventional goals in the psychological management of pain.[38]

Techniques to alter the sensory aspects of chronic pain include relaxation training, biofeedback, imagery, and hypnosis. Interventions aimed at modifying situational factors that exacerbate chronic pain and disability include contingency or behavioral management methods, modification of activity and rest cycles, and exposure to situations previously avoided because of pain.[74,95] Few component analyses have been conducted to determine which psychological therapies may be most essential in the management of pediatric chronic pain, but it is likely that for most chronic pain conditions, a combination of modalities will provide the best opportunity to effect the desired change. Changes in the emphasis of various behavioral components may present the opportunity to individualize treatment for the specific child by taking into account developmental, psychological, parental, and family factors, which may provide a way to tailor specific treatment to a child.

There is growing acknowledgment of parents' crucial role in successful rehabilitation of children with chronic pain, and thus they are increasingly becoming involved as active partners in their child's treatment.[74,83,96] Parental interactions with their child related to pain and the family characteristics of children with chronic pain that may be associated with the development of maladaptive coping with pain are areas of active research.[97-99] Particular types of parental behaviors have been shown to influence a child's ability to cope with pain. For example, parental attention has been associated with increased symptoms in children with recurrent abdominal pain.[100] Walker and colleagues[100] found that girls with functional abdominal pain are more vulnerable than boys to the symptom-reinforcing effects of parental attention. Interestingly, although the children with pain rated parental distraction as a helpful strategy, their patients rated distraction as having greater potential for a negative impact on their child than attention. Such findings help guide behavioral interventions for children with chronic pain and their families because parents' beliefs in the most effective pain management strategies need to be targeted in any intervention designed to increase the functional abilities of children with chronic pain.

Several methods for the delivery of psychological interventions for recurrent or chronic pain in children have been shown to be effective, including those that involve intensive inpatient[96,101] or outpatient[74,82] treatment; those that are self-administered,[102] school based,[103,104] Internet-based,[105] or CD ROM based[106]; and those that involve minimal clinic contact with home-based practice.[107,108] The variety of methods for delivery of these interventions offers opportunities to reach a broad population of children with chronic pain, thus increasing the potential to reach many more children than can be treated in specialized pediatric pain treatment centers. Optimally, the child's school and other caretakers are included in the treatment team to ensure a consistent and comprehensive approach to the child's pain and disability. For example, if a child's pain management involves strategies to cope with stress and headache at school, the school nurse can prompt the child to use these strategies rather than defaulting to having the parents pick the child up from school to rest at home (see Brown[109] for a review of school issues related to pediatric pain). Complementary therapies such as massage and acupuncture are increasingly available to children seen in chronic pain clinics, but there is limited literature thus far to document the efficacy of these treatments in pediatric patients.[110]

The complex nature of chronic pain in children creates many challenges in regard to its assessment and treatment, but this same complexity can be exploited to provide the most efficacious methods for pain control and functional rehabilitation. Multidimensional assessment provides the foundation for optimal pain management and functional rehabilitation of chronic pain in children. Psychological interventions include a diverse array of techniques that treat chronic pain by modifying children's cognitive, affective, and sensory experiences of pain, their behavior in response to pain, and environmental and interactional factors that influence the pain experience. Without addressing the factors that may contribute to pain and pain-related disability, medical treatment of a child's chronic pain may result in poorer outcomes. Research informed by multidimensional models of pediatric chronic pain can guide investigators in efforts to identify effective pain treatments, as well as the individual children for whom they work best. Finally, the lessons learned about optimal management of pain in children need to be practiced to the fullest extent possible so that the incidence of their suffering and disability may be diminished. For further reviews of psychological interventions for pediatric chronic pain, see McGrath and Holahan,[111] Hillier and McGrath,[112] and Eccleston and coworkers.[76]

CHRONIC PAIN SYNDROMES

We briefly discuss the diagnosis and management of some common chronic pain syndromes diagnosed in pediatric patients referred to chronic pain clinics. The introduction of multidisciplinary pediatric pain clinics has allowed children to be seen in a single office visit by a number of consultants who are able to provide service for the child and develop a comprehensive pain management plan. Our clinic includes an anesthesiologist specialized in pain management, a child psychologist with a special interest in pain, a physical therapist, a complementary medicine practitioner (including message therapy and acupuncture therapy), and a specialist in biofeedback. This comprehensive approach reduces the need for multiple visits and exposes our patients to a multimodal therapeutic approach.[113]

Common pain syndromes in children include CRPS type 1, headache, abdominal pain, chest wall pain, back pain, pelvic pain, and cancer-related pain. We address each of these conditions with a specific emphasis on accepted current therapy.

COMPLEX REGIONAL PAIN SYNDROME TYPE 1

CRPS 1, or reflex sympathetic dystrophy (RSD) as it was originally called, is a complex syndrome consisting of pain, allodynia, hyperalgesia, and possible loss of function. The International Association for the Study of Pain (IASP) has defined CRPS 1 as "A continuous pain in a portion of an extremity after trauma, which may include fracture but does not involve major nerve lesions and is associated with sympathetic hyperactivity."[114] CRPS 1 is a common reason for referral to a pediatric pain clinic. It is seen more commonly in the lower extremity,[115] and most of the children involved are female, many of whom have endured minor trauma before the development of chronic pain.[116,117] Though reported in a 2½-year-old girl,[118] it is generally seen in children older than 9 years and more frequently in girls 11 to 13 years of age.[86,119] Early recognition and management are the major factors in improving outcome and preventing resistant CRPS.[120] Management by an experienced multidisciplinary team is recommended. Because psychosocial factors play an important role, psychological evaluation and cognitive-behavioral treatment should be provided in an expeditious manner.[7]

The mechanisms that generate neuropathic pain (NP) are varied and complex. Injuries to peripheral nerves may involve crush, transection, compression, demyelination, axonal degeneration, inflammation, ischemia, or other processes. The primary loci of increased irritability following peripheral nerve injury may be at several levels in the nervous system, including axonal sprouts or neuroma, the dorsal root ganglia, the dorsal horn of the spinal cord, or sites more rostral in the central nervous system.[121,122] Central neural causes and peripheral small-fiber neuropathy have been implicated in the mechanisms leading to NP. NP rarely keeps the subject from harm because it involves the erroneous generation of impulses.[86]

EVALUATION OF NEUROPATHIC PAIN

History

A detailed history of the nature of the injury, the type and duration of the pain, relieving and aggravating factors, and dependence on medications is mandatory before evaluation.

Physical Evaluation

A thorough and systematic neurologic examination should be performed. Complete evaluation of motor, sensory, cerebellar, cranial nerve, reflex, cognitive, and emotional functioning is important. A concerted effort must be made to rule out a rare but possible malignancy or central degenerative disorder.

Sympathetically mediated pain is often diagnosed by clinical and diagnostic criteria based on responses to sympathetic blocks. However, the diagnosis of sympathetically mediated pain cannot be based on responses to sympathetic blocks alone.

The *strength* of the extremity should be evaluated on several occasions. It is important to compare it with the strength in the contralateral extremity because CRPS 1 can occur in both extremities at the same time.

Allodynia is excruciating pain that can be produced by innocuous stimuli such as stroking (e.g., stroking the skin with a feather). This is very characteristic of NP. Tactile allodynia in the absence of skin problems is a classic diagnostic criterion for NP.

Hyperalgesia is an increased sensitivity to pain. Hyperalgesia to cold is seen more frequently than hyperalgesia to warmth.[123] The distribution is not generally restricted to particular dermatomes, as in an adult, and commonly occurs along a glove-and-stocking distribution.

Nerve conduction studies may provide some insight into the location and type of nerve injury.[124] However, the use of invasive electromyography may not be acceptable to children.

Quantitative sensory testing (QST) with thermal and vibration sensations and thermal pain detection thresholds in the affected limbs can be compared with data from normal healthy children. The patient's rating of pain and quality of pain can be assessed. Mechanical static allodynia and dynamic allodynia can be measured. Quantitative thermal and vibration detection thresholds can be measured. Although this involves cumbersome equipment, bedside QST may have a greater role in the diagnosis of CRPS 1 in children and adolescents.[125]

Bone scans may be helpful in the diagnosis of CRPS 1. Although there are not enough data on their diagnostic accuracy in children, they are nevertheless performed in children and adolescents with CRPS 1. A decrease in isotope uptake is noticed with CRPS 1.[126]

Box 33.3 International Association for the Study of Pain Diagnostic Criteria for Complex Regional Pain Syndrome

1. Presence of an initiating noxious event or cause of immobilization
2. Continuous pain, allodynia, or hyperalgesia in which the pain is disproportionate to any known inciting event
3. Evidence at some time of edema, changes in blood flow, or abnormal sudomotor activity in the region of pain
4. Diagnosis excluded by the existence of other conditions that would otherwise account for the degree of pain and dysfunction

Adapted from Bruehl S, Harden RN, Galer BS, et al. External validation of IASP diagnostic criteria for complex regional pain syndrome and proposed research diagnostic criteria. International Association for the Study of Pain. Pain. *1999;81:147-154.*

Diagnosis

Diagnosis of CRPS 1 in children is usually based on symptoms and signs (Box 33.3). The characteristics of the pain and sensory, motor, and sudomotor changes may vary among patients[86]; also, differences between NP and nociceptive pain can be noted (Table 33.2). A test with phentolamine has been used to confirm the diagnosis and to predict the response to sympathetic blockade.[127] Bone scans may offer some information about CRPS 1. Disturbed vascular scintigraphy with increased pooling in the initial phase and hyperfixation on bone scintigraphy may denote the presence of CRPS 1. The IASP criterion for CRPS 1 is applicable to children and adolescents (see Box 33.3). Classic signs and symptoms of the various stages of CRPS 1 are presented in Table 33.3.[114]

TREATMENT OF NEUROPATHIC PAIN

Management of NP (Box 33.4) can be frustrating for the caregiver, as well as the patient. No single therapy can uniformly provide relief to these patients. Management depends largely on the response to various clinical measures. Titration of medications is limited by the presence of side effects and complications. One of the primary goals is to return the child to a functional state and to school. Definitive resolution of the pain is not always possible. Most management techniques have been extrapolated from work done in adult patients.[128] It is imperative to build trust with the patient and the parents. Family dynamics are important

Table 33.2 Differences Between Neuropathic and Nociceptive Pain

Characteristic	Neuropathic Pain	Nociceptive Pain
Description of pain	Burning, lancinating, pins and needles	Varied
Tactile allodynia	Present	Absent
Duration and intensity of pain	Increases with duration	Decreases
Opioid resistant	Present	Absent
Use of tricyclic antidepressants	Useful	Not useful

Table 33.3 Symptoms and Changes in Stages of Chronic Regional Pain Syndrome Type 1

Characteristic	Acute	Dystrophic	Atrophic
Pain	Hyperpathic, burning	Chronic	
Blood flow	Increased	Decreased	No change
Temperature	Increased	Decreased	No change
Hair and nail growth	Increased	Decreased	Chronic change
Sweating	Decreased	Increased	No change
Edema	None	Brawny edema	Wasted muscles, atrophic skin
Color	Red	Cyanotic	Atrophic

because the added burden of familial disharmony or parental abuse can worsen the symptoms. There seems to be a greater propensity for enmeshment in these families. The algorithm shown in Figure 33.1 is used by our pain clinic.[129]

Psychological and Behavioral Therapy

Behavioral measures are extremely useful in the management of NP. Family therapy often helps family members cope with the situation.[130] We generally advocate consultation with a medical psychologist during the initial visit to the pain clinic. Several techniques, including biofeedback, visual guided imagery, and structured counseling, have been shown to assist in the development of adequate coping skills.[131] Participation in a day program for acute psychological intervention has been valuable for some of our patients, specifically those with significant psychiatric co-illness. See earlier for more detailed explanations of various psychological interventions.

> **Box 33.4 Management of Neuropathic Pain**
>
> **Nonpharmacological Treatment**
>
> Hypnosis, biofeedback, visual guided imagery
> TENS, physical therapy, occupational therapy
> Individual and family therapy (day program if required)
>
> **Pharmacological Therapy**
>
> Acetaminophen, NSAIDs
> Tricyclic antidepressants (e.g., amitriptyline, nortriptyline, doxepin); start at low doses, 0.1 mg/kg, and advance slowly
> Anticonvulsants (gabapentin, pregabalin, carbamazepine, phenytoin, clonazepam), systemic local anesthetics (mexiletine, lidocaine)
> Serotonin and norepinephrine reuptake inhibitors
> Opioids (morphine, methadone given orally, intravenously, or via regional technique [epidural or intrathecal], especially in cancer patients)
>
> **Regional Blockades for Chronic Pain**
>
> Epidural, subarachnoid and sympathetic plexus, peripheral catheter blockade
> Sympathetic blockade for CRPS 1
> Continuous catheter techniques may be used for 5 to 7 days
> Epidural and subarachnoid block for cancer patients: left in place for longer periods by tunneling subcutaneously
> Neurolytic blockade for cancer
>
> CRPS, complex regional pain syndrome; NSAIDs, nonsteroidal anti-inflammatory drugs; TENS, transcutaneous electrical nerve stimulation.

Physical Therapy

Physical therapy is geared toward adequate functional ability of the child. Transcutaneous electrical nerve stimulation (TENS) is widely used, and its efficacy has been studied in adults as well as children; therapeutic benefits with TENS in children with RSD have been reported by Kesler and colleagues.[132] We use TENS extensively in our practice, along with physical therapy, which consists of both active and passive physical modalities. The physical therapy program is geared toward individual patients, and the goal is to allow the child to participate in as many activities as possible. It may be necessary to have input from a pediatric physical therapist or occupational therapist for adequate management. Other commonly used modalities include desensitization, warm and cold baths, massage therapy, and heat therapy. Such modalities, when used in conjunction with active physical modalities, can help ameliorate the pain symptoms.[133]

Medical Therapy

Most of the work in children has been extrapolated from the experience in adults. It is best to start with nonsteroidal anti-inflammatory drugs (NSAIDs) in moderate doses, followed by other medications (see Box 33.4). There are certain differences between adult and pediatric patients:

1. Symptoms of NP may differ in children and adults.
2. The response to medications may be different.
3. There may be unrecognized toxicity to medications.

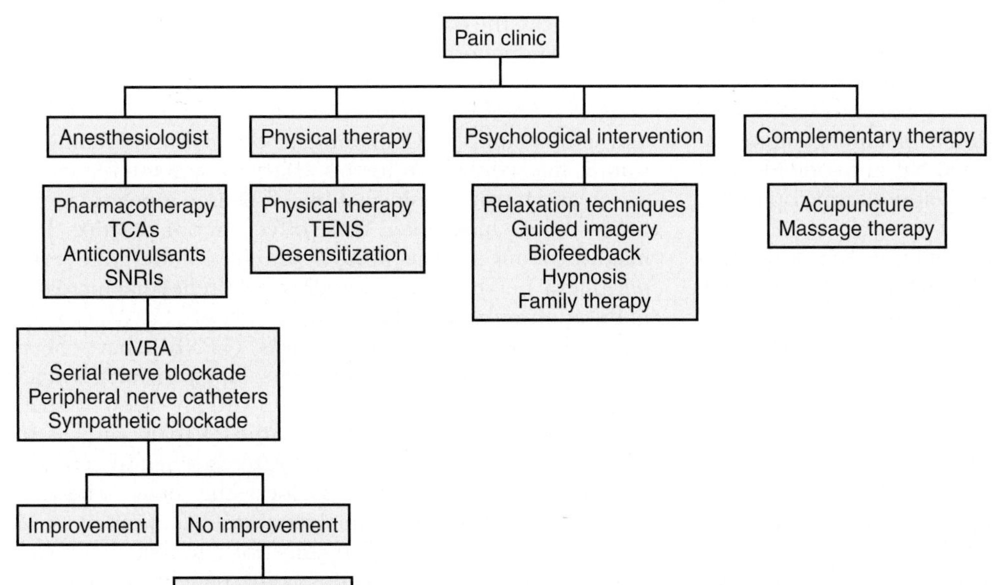

Figure 33.1 Algorithm for the management of chronic regional pain syndrome type 1. IVRA, intravenous regional anesthesia; SNRIs, serotonin norepinephrine reuptake inhibitors; TCAs, tricyclic antidepressants; TENS, transcutaneous electrical nerve stimulation.

Tricyclic Antidepressants. Adults are frequently prescribed tricyclic antidepressants (TCAs) for the management of NP.[134] Despite the lack of adequately controlled studies in pediatric patients, TCAs are widely prescribed for several forms of NP.[135] Because amitriptyline may cause sedation, it is our practice to use nortriptyline, which appears to have less sedative and fewer anticholinergic side effects. Thorough examination of the cardiovascular system is necessary before instituting TCA treatment because of associated tachydysrhythmia and other conduction abnormalities of the heart, particularly prolonged QT syndrome.[136,137]

Anticonvulsants. Anticonvulsant medications have been used for several years to manage NP.[138] Although carbamazepine and oxcarbazepine have been used extensively to treat NP,[139-143] the introduction of gabapentin and pregabalin has revolutionized the world of pain medicine.[140-143] Despite the lack of controlled trials in children to demonstrate the efficacy of either drug, both of these voltage-gated calcium channel blockers have been used in our clinic with promising results.[144] More controlled trials need to be conducted to better determine the dosing and efficacy of this class of drugs in children with CRPS 1. An important side effect that we have noted in our clinic setting is the potential for increased somnolence, as well as the potential for weight gain in children taking pregabalin. This is important to consider, especially when treating adolescent girls, who happen to be the majority of this cohort.

Selective Serotonin Reuptake Inhibitors and Serotonin-Norepinephrine Reuptake Inhibitors. Despite the lack of proven efficacy of the use of selective serotonin reuptake inhibitors in the management of pain in children and adolescents, they are occasionally used to treat psychological comorbidity, including depression associated with pain.[145] More recently, serotonin-norepinephrine reuptake inhibitors have been introduced and used successfully to treat NP, especially in patients with psychological comorbidity.[146]

Opioids. Opioids can be helpful in the management of NP, especially for cancer-related NP (see later). Arner has shown that several types of NP are resistant to the effects of opioids.[127] Opioids should be titrated in a graded fashion to optimize the effect. Sedation is a side effect that may be desirable, especially in cancer-related NP, and in some cases it may need to be antagonized with the addition of amphetamines.[147] For children with non–cancer-related NP, non–opioid-based techniques are generally exhausted before starting opioids.

Systemic Vasodilators. Several patients with RSD have benefited from the use of vasodilators such as prazosin, nifedipine, and phenoxybenzamine. However, overwhelming adverse effects of orthostatic hypotension often offset the efficacy of this therapy.

Regional Anesthesia and Sympathetic Blocks. A common treatment of these syndromes is to interrupt the apparent pathologic reflexes by performing sympathetic blocks (Box 33.5). Regional anesthesia, though used often in adults for the diagnosis and management of CRPS, is generally introduced in children after pharmacological and cognitive-behavioral management has been exhausted.[148] In severe cases, regional anesthesia is used to introduce a physical therapy regimen. In this section we discuss the different regional techniques that are used in children for the management of CRPS.

Box 33.5 Regional Anesthesia for Complex Regional Pain Syndrome Type 1

- Intravenous regional anesthesia—guanethidine, bretylium, lidocaine-ketorolac
- Epidural analgesia (continuous)
- Intrathecal analgesia
- Sympathetic chain blocks
  - Stellate ganglion blocks
  - Lumbar sympathetic blocks
- Brachial plexus catheters
- Sciatic nerve catheters

Central neuraxial blockade is used in children with severe pain to facilitate the introduction of physical therapy. An indwelling epidural catheter is placed in the lumbar or cervical area and infused with a low-concentration local anesthetic solution, which allows better cooperation from the patient and the parents to introduce a physical therapy regimen.[23] In addition, intrathecal analgesia has been reported to be an effective method for treating refractory CRPS 1 in children.[149,150]

Bier block has been used for mild to moderate cases of CRPS 1 as a primary modality for providing analgesia and sympathetic blockade.[127] Although a myriad of substances have been used to provide a Bier block, a local anesthetic in combination with either an α_2-agonist or an NSAID appears to produce better results. In our case series of children who received intravenous regional anesthesia with lidocaine and ketorolac, we demonstrated a marked improvement in symptoms and the ability to perform physical therapy.[129]

Peripheral nerve blocks are used to facilitate physical therapy while providing a sympathectomy and have become more plausible, especially with the use of ultrasound guidance.[148] Serial peripheral nerve blocks may be performed. With serial blocks, the patient's pain relief often outlasts the duration of conduction blockade, which may be due to reduced central sensitization, as well as interruption of the circuit established between the nociceptor, central nervous system, and motor unit.[151] Concomitant corticosteroid administration may contribute to this effect via anti-inflammatory action and by suppressing ectopic discharge in neural membranes.[152] We have noted these effects in our practice. The majority of our patients with NP who have undergone serial peripheral nerve blocks experience pain relief that increases in duration with each block.

Continuous peripheral nerve blocks (CPNBs) have been reported to be effective in both controlling pain and facilitating physical therapy in children with CRPS.[153] Despite such reports, limited data exist regarding the feasibility, safety, and efficacy of CPNBs in children.[154] After perineural catheter placement, a dilute solution of local anesthetic is infused with the view of providing analgesia while allowing physical activity. The catheter is left in place for 4 to 5 days; this can be done on an inpatient basis, or the patient may be sent home with a portable infusion device. We prefer sciatic nerve

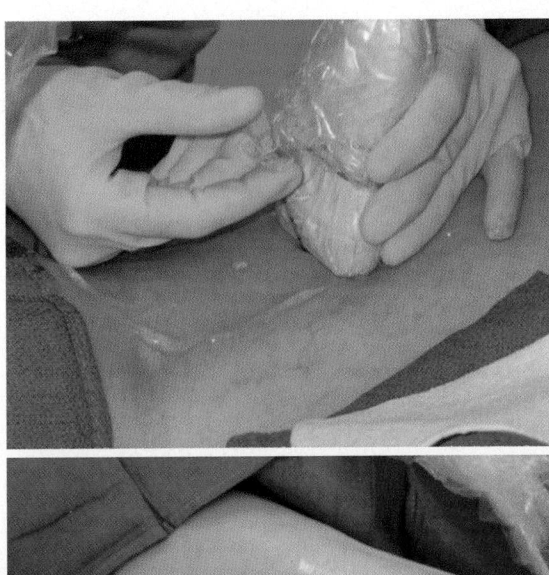

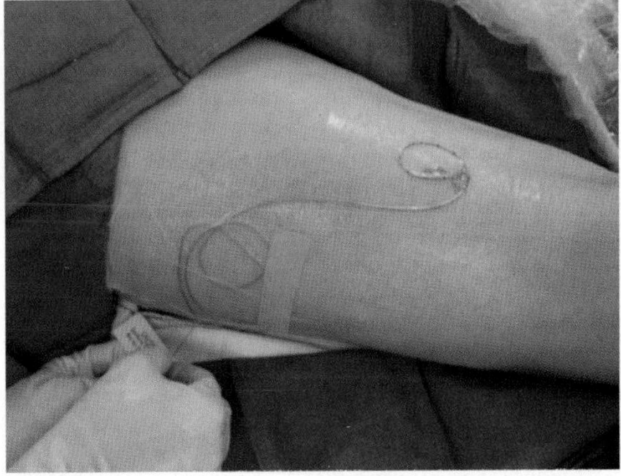

Figure 33.2 Sciatic nerve catheter for the management of complex regional pain syndrome type 1.

catheter placement for the lower extremities (see Fig. 33.2) and interscalene or infraclavicular brachial plexus catheters for the upper extremities. Concurrent physical therapy is indicated to improve range of motion and function. We institute physical therapy at the time of provision of a nerve block to enhance the patient's experience with therapy.

Sympathetic blockade is used in children after exhausting the aforementioned techniques. A stellate ganglion block may be performed under ultrasound guidance for upper extremity CRPS (see Fig. 33.3), and a lumbar sympathetic block is performed under fluoroscopic guidance for lower extremity CRPS.[155] A crossover trial of fluoroscopically guided lumbar sympathetic blocks demonstrated a decrease in allodynia and pain intensity when compared with intravenous injection of lidocaine in adolescents with CRPS.[156]

Neuromodulation via spinal cord stimulation, though commonly performed in adults for refractory cases of CRPS, is very rarely used in the pediatric setting.[157,158] Spinal cord stimulation has been reported to achieve favorable outcomes in adolescents with therapy-resistant CRPS.[159] The use of peripheral nerve stimulators, however, is gaining ground in the pediatric setting and may benefit children with refractory CRPS.

PROGNOSIS OF NEUROPATHIC PAIN

Varni and colleagues[160] reported uniform improvement in their series of patients who endured a prolonged course of physical therapy and inpatient rehabilitation. Ashwal and associates[161] concluded that the prognosis of childhood CRPS

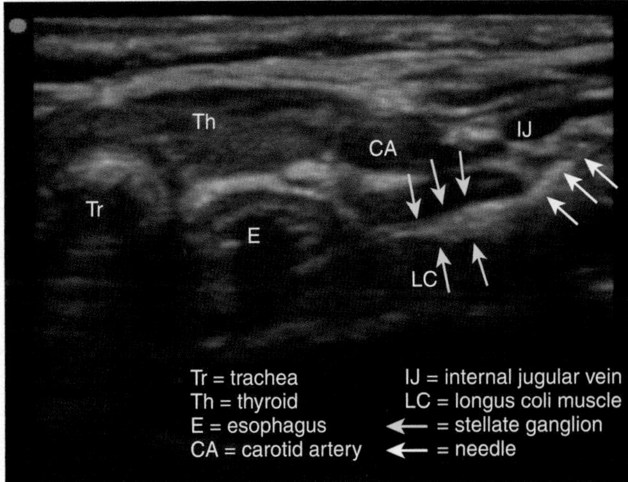

Figure 33.3 Image of ultrasound-guided stellate ganglion blockade.

is more favorable than that of adult CRPS. NP can be puzzling and frustrating and requires a strong alliance with the family and the patient. A multidisciplinary algorithmic management approach involving the use of available techniques can be helpful. The use of physical therapy and psychological management must be stressed while managing these patients.

HEADACHES IN CHILDREN

Headaches are a common finding in children and adolescents. Few physicians discussed headaches in children until 1873, when William Henry Day, a British pediatrician, devoted a chapter to the subject of headaches in his book *Essays on Diseases in Children.*[162] In 1967, Freidman published the data available in *Headaches in Children.*[163] These books provided an impetus to the many subsequent papers dealing with headaches in children. Many child care providers do not believe that children have an appreciable number of headaches. In a study of 9000 children in Sweden, Bille[164] reported migraine headaches in 3.9% of children younger than 12 years and a 6.8% incidence of nonmigrainous headaches daily. This translates to a greater number of school days lost from absenteeism because of the debilitating nature of the headaches. A more recent study by Bille[165] demonstrated that almost 40% of these children with headaches in childhood progress to a headache-free state in adulthood. A 2010 survey of middle schools in the Chicago area demonstrated the presence of headaches in a large percentage of all schoolchildren.[166]

Most headaches in children are linked to either organic or nonorganic causes and may be deemed acute or chronic based on the duration of the headaches. Chronic daily headache is classified as headaches that occur at least 15 times monthly for a period of 3 months and can last for more than 4 hours daily.[167]

EVALUATION OF HEADACHE

A thorough history and physical examination help determine the nature of the headache. Specific questions about neurologic symptoms such as ataxia, lethargy, seizures, or visual impairment should be asked. Other medical conditions such as hypertension, sinusitis, and emotional disturbances must

Box 33.6 Pathophysiology of Headache

Pain-Sensitive Headache

Extracranial
- Skin
- Subcutaneous tissue
- Muscles
- Mucous membranes
- Teeth
- Larger vessels

Intracranial
- Vascular sinuses
- Larger veins
- Dura surrounding the veins
- Dural arteries
- Arteries at the base of the brain

Pain-Insensitive Headache

Brain
Cranium
Most of the dura
Ependyma
Choroid plexus

be evaluated. Physical examination, including a thorough neurologic examination and blood pressure measurement, is mandated for children with headaches. Neuroimaging may be required and a lumbar puncture might be advised in some cases. Benign intracranial hypertension or idiopathic intracranial hypertension is a constellation of symptoms and signs that includes headaches, diplopia, tinnitus, and eye pain. These conditions usually have normal imaging results.[167] Although a diagnostic lumbar puncture may be needed in some settings, patients with chronic daily headaches may be prone to post–lumbar puncture headaches.[167]

PATHOPHYSIOLOGY OF HEADACHE

A headache is modulated by extracranial as well as intracranial structures (Box 33.6).

CLASSIFICATION OF HEADACHE

Classification of headaches is based on the presumed location of the abnormality, its origin, its pathophysiology, or the symptom complex that the patient has (Box 33.7).

EVALUATION OF HEADACHE

Comorbid symptoms are associated with headaches. The most common comorbidity is sleep deprivation. Delayed sleep is a frequent disorder seen in children with headaches. Many also have symptoms of dizziness, which may be associated with postural hypotension and tachycardia (postural orthostatic tachycardia syndrome).[168] Orthostatic hypotension should be treated by increasing fluid intake, and in some cases, a β-blocker may be needed. A history of a new-onset severe headache, pain that awakens a child from sleep, headaches associated with straining, changes in chronic headache patterns, or the presence of a headache accompanied by nausea or vomiting suggests a more pathologic origin of the headache and must be carefully evaluated (Box 33.8).

It is imperative to evaluate any relevant neuroimaging studies before the patient's appointment in the pain clinic.

Box 33.7 Classification of Headaches: Differential Diagnosis

Acute headache
- Systemic illness
- Subarachnoid hemorrhage
- Trauma
- Toxins such as lead or carbon monoxide
- Electrolyte imbalances
- Hypertension

Acute recurrent headache
- Migraine

Chronic progressive headaches
- Organic brain disease
- Ventriculoperitoneal shunt malfunction

Chronic nonprogressive headache
- Functional in quality

Mixed headache

Box 33.8 Evaluation for Headache

General Physical Examination

Blood pressure, postural hypotension
Careful skin examination for café au lait spots, adenoma sebaceum, hypopigmented lesions, petechiae

Neurologic Examination

Cranial circumference measurement
Bruit on auscultation of the cranium
Tenderness in the sinuses or presence of occult trauma indicating a battered child
Funduscopic examination—optic atrophy, papilledema
Cranial nerve examination for the presence of damage
Mental status
Alteration in language skills
Alteration in gait
Cranial nerve examination

Laboratory Tests

Electroencephalography—very nonspecific
Computed tomography scan, especially with contrast enhancement—may be useful in determining vascular abnormalities
Magnetic resonance imaging—best for delineating abnormalities in the sella turcica, posterior fossa, temporal lobes
Lumbar puncture helpful in determining acute infectious causes
Psychological tests to determine whether the headache has a psychological basis
Tilt test—if postural hypotension is present (postural orthostatic tachycardia syndrome)
Angiography (venous or arterial) if intracranial pathology is suspected.

After establishing that the headaches are not secondary to any intracranial pathology, the following information is obtained:

1. Neurologic status, including a complete neurologic examination.
2. Physical status of the patient (i.e., is the patient actively mobile?).

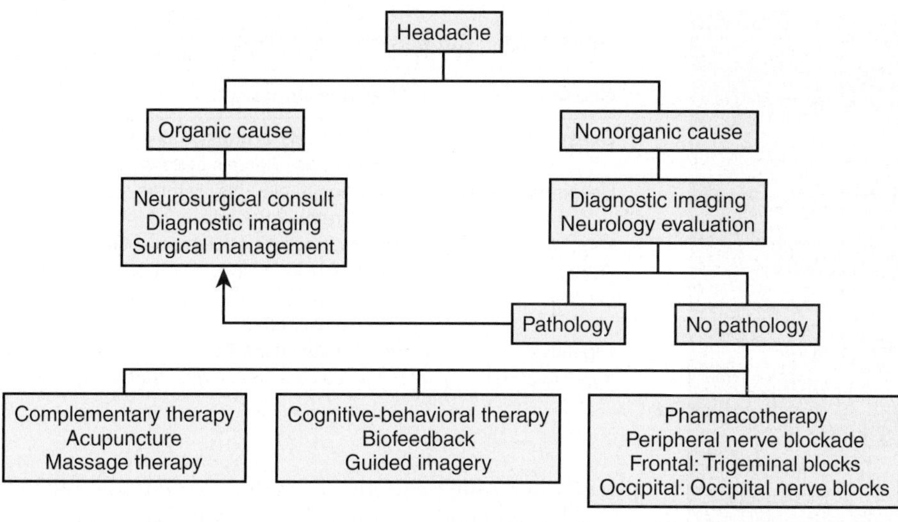

Figure 33.4 Algorithm for the management of headache. If the patient experiences nausea, vomiting, or other signs of increased intracranial pressure, neurosurgical consultation should be obtained.

3. Does the headache prevent the child from performing normal activities (e.g., interacting with others, participating in sports)?
4. Is there a history of school absenteeism?
5. What is the child's interaction with the parents and siblings at home?
6. Are there any factors that relieve the headache?
7. Has the child been taking any medications for pain? Has there been any improvement at all in the clinical characteristics of the pain?
8. Are any postural changes associated with the headaches? Is there diurnal variation in the headaches?
9. The family history is crucial in these children; a family history of migraine is suggestive of childhood migraine.

After careful evaluation and classification of the type of headache, treatment is initiated in stepwise fashion. We use the algorithm shown in Figure 33.4 for the management of headaches.

Patients with migraine headaches are frequently managed by neurologists and are referred to the pain clinic only in refractory cases.[169] We have intervened by providing peripheral nerve blocks for headaches. A trigeminal nerve block for frontal headaches and occipital nerve blocks for persistent occipital pain have been shown to be effective in children.[170]

A tension-type headache is perhaps the most common type of headache that we see in our pain clinic. These patients frequently complain of debilitating frontotemporal or frontoparietal headaches. The headache results from contraction of the temporalis muscle and tension on the scalp muscles.[171] Management of tension-type headaches includes the use of relaxation techniques, as well as biofeedback. These patients frequently benefit from the routine use of nonsteroidal agents.[172] In addition, caffeine has been described as an effective adjuvant to nonsteroidal drugs in treating childhood headaches.[173]

Children occasionally have persistent neuropathic headaches. This commonly occurs in those who have undergone ventriculoperitoneal shunt revision or surgical decompression for a Chiari malformation. After cognitive-behavioral therapy we have attempted to use serial peripheral nerve blocks in these patients. This includes trigeminal nerve blocks for frontal headaches and occipital nerve blocks for occipital headaches. An ultrasound-guided approach to the occipital nerve allows easy access to the C2 nerve root, thereby providing a more robust blockade than can be achieved with a peripheral subcutaneous injection.[174] Local anesthetic is injected with or without a small dose of steroid to provide analgesia.

ABDOMINAL PAIN IN CHILDREN

Abdominal pain is a frequently encountered problem in infants, children, and adolescents. When evaluating abdominal pain, it is imperative that all organic causes be eliminated. Functional abdominal pain (FAP) is defined as pain unrelated to an identifiable organic gastrointestinal disorder.[175] Once a diagnosis of FAP is established, cognitive-behavioral therapy along with family-centered therapy has proved effective.[176] Several authors have described an affective component of FAP.[177] Furthermore, Walker and associates suggested that children with FAP are at increased risk for the development of chronic pain in adulthood.[178] This may be due to mechanisms linked to heightened central sensitization.[179] Amitriptyline has been described as an effective treatment of FAP in children, although a randomized prospective trial demonstrated no significant difference between control and amitriptyline.[180]

We demonstrated the efficacy of serial nerve blocks in children with abdominal pain, particularly those in whom NP develops after abdominal surgery. The use of serially performed ultrasound-guided rectus sheath blocks or transversus abdominis plane blocks has decreased abdominal pain in our cohort.[181] By blocking the thoracolumbar nerve roots, complete analgesia is provided to the anterior abdominal wall (see Fig. 33.5).

Ilioinguinal neuralgia following hernia repair is an underreported cause of abdominal pain in older children and adolescents[182] and is probably secondary to major dissection during surgery. TENS may be helpful and peripheral nerve blocks can be used to manage pain. Serial ultrasound-guided ilioinguinal nerve blocks have been demonstrated to be effective.[183] A perineural catheter may be left in place in severe cases.

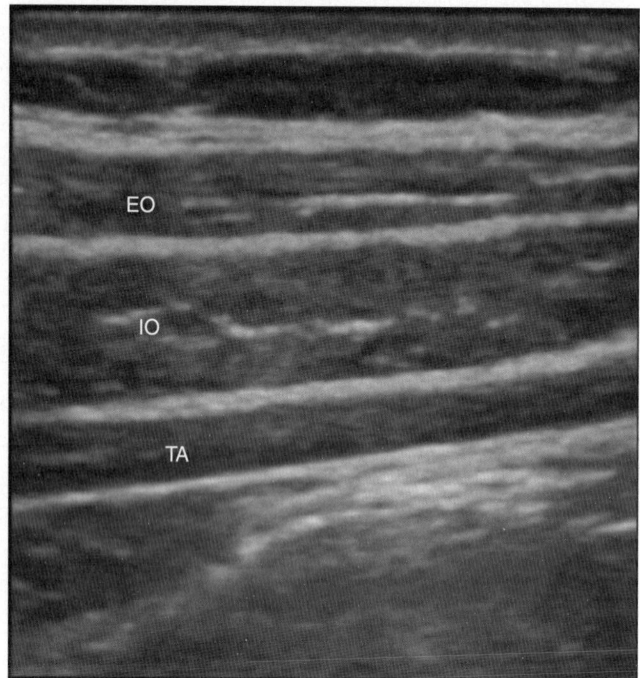

Figure 33.5 Sonographic anatomy of the transversus abdominis (TA) plane. EO, external oblique muscle; IO, internal oblique muscle.

CHEST PAIN IN CHILDREN

Chest pain is a common symptom in older children and adolescents. A study conducted in Belgium reported a greater preponderance in males.[184] Most children encountered in the emergency department complain of chest tightness with pain located lateral to the sternum. In a study of 96 patients with a mean age of 13 years, 37% were noted to have idiopathic chest pain. A major life event, such as a family divorce or death of a relative, was a significant factor predisposing to chest pain in more than 30% of these children.[185]

CAUSES OF CHEST PAIN

The most common causes of chest pain include chest wall pain (64.5%) and cardiac (5%), respiratory (13%), gastrointestinal (3%), psychological (9%), and traumatic causes (5%). After cardiac causes are ruled out with an electrocardiogram and a careful physical examination, other causes of chest pain should be considered.[186] Each has similar initial symptoms, although the diagnostic workup may be different, depending on the physical findings (Table 33.4).

Table 33.4 Causes of Chest Pain

Cause	Manifestations
Chest wall pain	Musculoskeletal chest wall pain, costochondritis, Tietze's syndrome
Respiratory disease	Pneumonia, pleuritis, asthma, upper respiratory infection
Psychogenic	Anxiety, depression, hyperventilation
Traumatic	Soft tissue injury, pneumothorax
Cardiac	Carditis, arrhythmia, mitral valve prolapse, ischemia
Digestive	Esophagitis, gastritis
Miscellaneous	Sickle cell disease, cystic fibrosis related

Chest Wall Pain

This is often seen in teenagers and is manifested as acute pain along the costal margin. The most common chest wall pain is secondary to costochondritis.[186] The diagnosis is made by eliciting pain along the costochondral margin with deep pressure. Other chest wall pain syndromes include Tietze's syndrome[187] and slipping rib cage syndrome.[187] Management usually consists of the use of NSAIDs. We have seen several patients with slipping rib cage syndrome who have not had relief despite surgical resection of the slipping rib. We use cognitive-behavioral therapy, as well as alternative therapies, including acupuncture and massage therapy, for these children. In addition, we have successfully placed intercostal nerve blocks under ultrasound guidance and achieved good relief in children with severe, recurring chest wall pain. Serial blocks are performed with adequate resources available for biofeedback and massage therapy to allay any pain-associated anxiety.

Pulmonary Causes

The most common respiratory emergencies manifested as acute chest wall pain occur in children with acute asthma attacks, who may have primarily chest pain without actual respiratory embarrassment. Other common causes include bronchial pneumonia and respiratory illnesses, including severe lower respiratory tract illnesses. Management includes treating the respiratory illness with antibiotics or anticholinergics and inhaled bronchodilators.

Cardiac Causes

Cardiac causes of chest pain are probably the most compelling reasons for a good diagnostic workup. The most common cardiac causes of chest pain include mitral valve prolapse and the presence of dysrhythmias. Workup may include echocardiography, electrocardiography, and in some cases, Holter monitoring for diagnosis. It is important to address the pain in an expeditious manner.

Abdominal Causes

Gastroesophageal reflux is the most common abdominal cause of continued chest pain in children. In addition, the presence of eosinophilic esophagitis should be ruled out by upper endoscopy because it can usually be treated.

Psychogenic Causes

Usually, there is a family history of intercurrent cardiac illness, including a recent myocardial infarction in an older family member or possibly the death of a family member from cardiac causes that can lead to chest wall pain. In most cases, adequate family therapy should be offered.[188] With the increasing diagnostic methodologies available, the diagnosis is far more accurate in these children than several decades ago.

BACK PAIN

Back pain is a common problem in adults and is now becoming a significant health issue in children.[189-192] With high-impact sports that involve a greater degree of stress on the back muscles, such as gymnastics, children seem to have a higher degree of injuries to their back.[193] Common back problems include spondylolysis,[194] spondylolisthesis, disk degeneration, disk herniation,[195,196] tumors of the spinal cord, and other diseases, including sickle cell disease. Classic symptoms of herniation may be seen, including radicular symptoms. Management in children is usually conservative with an emphasis on exercise for the back. We have found that a small segment of these children may require a lumbar epidural steroid injection. Alternative medicine, including massage therapy and acupuncture, is used extensively for the management of children and adolescents with back pain. These therapies are especially effective when the pain has a myofascial component.

PELVIC PAIN

Pelvic pain is often reported in female adolescents.[197] A thorough history has to be obtained, including a history of sexual activity. Children with a history of sexual abuse have a greater preponderance of chronic pelvic pain.[198] Though not common, a subpopulation of these adolescent girls have a history of endometriosis. This could lead to severe pelvic pain and may need to be treated more aggressively than the occasional pelvic pain. Alteration of the ovulatory cycles with birth control pills, as well as the use of strong NSAIDs, should be implemented in these patients. We have had success with the use of active massage therapy and physical therapy as adjuncts for the management of these patients.

CANCER-RELATED PAIN

Cancer remains the second leading cause of death in children. Cancer is diagnosed in more than 12,000 children annually, and 2200 children die each year of this disease.[199] Pain is a common symptom during different phases of cancer treatment. The incidence of cancer-related pain in children at the time of diagnosis is estimated to be 75%, with ongoing pain affecting 50%.[200,201] However, the incidence of pain at the terminal phase of disease is likely to be higher than 89%.[202] Cancer pain in children is due to several reasons: (1) cancer-related pain (e.g., solid tumor or bony metastatic tumors), (2) pain caused by treatment (e.g., mucositis or surgical pain), and (3) NP secondary to tumor invasion or surgery. Pain caused by treatment and procedural pain are cited as the most frequent types of pain experienced by children with cancer.[203]

Management of pediatric cancer-related pain must be individualized, and caregivers must be empathetic to family needs and concerns. Although more than most pain complaints can be managed by implementation of the World Health Organization (WHO) cancer pain ladder paradigm, a significant number of children may require additional therapies or techniques for pain management because of escalating or intractable pain. Only allopathic techniques are discussed in this section. The pediatric doses for most medications are off-label recommendations; dosing is based on the current pediatric clinical literature.

ORAL MEDICATIONS

Most pain management is achieved with oral maintenance dosing. Around-the-clock scheduling is supplemented with as-needed analgesic doses for breakthrough pain. Oral techniques include sublingual and transmucosal applications for breakthrough and procedural pain.

Sublingual application of morphine is as effective as intravenous morphine for pediatric postoperative pain.[204] Because sublingual administration avoids hepatic first-pass dosing, it is comparable to intravenous administration. Sublingual morphine may be a suitable alternative to intravenous morphine for pain control in children with cancer-related pain if enteral tolerance or intravenous access is limited. Sublingual buprenorphine, 5 to 7 μg/kg per dose, has demonstrated similar analgesic efficacy as intravenous morphine, 150 μg/kg.[205] Oxycodone concentrate prepared as 20 mg/mL is appropriate for sublingual application, but small changes in volume can mean large changes in dose. When using this concentrated formulation, an increment of 0.1 mL (from 0.2 to 0.3 mL) constitutes a 50% increase in dose; an additional 0.1-mL increase (from 0.2 to 0.4 mL) represents a 100% increase or doubling of the dose administered. Thus, prescribing dosing increments that are less than 5 mg may result in variation in the actual amount of oxycodone concentrate delivered. Oxycodone concentrate is not recommended for use in small children.

Intravenous preparations administered by the transmucosal route have been tried with some success. Oral administration of the intravenous formulation of fentanyl can achieve a pharmacokinetic distribution similar to that of oral transmucosal fentanyl citrate (OTFC) lozenges, but there is much interpatient variability. OTFC lozenges have been used for breakthrough pain and procedural pain in children. Oral mucositis pain treated with 200-μg OTFC lozenges is tolerated but ineffective in adult cancer patients.[206] The effective oral dosage range for postoperative pain management is 10 to 15 μg/kg for buccal application.[207] Schechter and colleagues[208] found 15 to 20 μg/kg of OTFC to be effective for pediatric procedural pain, but a third of the children experienced vomiting. Transmucosal oxycodone, 200 μg/kg, provides relief similar to 10 μg/kg of OTFC for procedure-related pain.[209]

Tablets designed for buccal delivery aim to enhance bioavailability and drug uptake and speed the onset of pain relief. Hepatic first-pass effects are avoided.[210] Studies on fentanyl effervescent buccal tablets have revealed pain relief onset times of 10 to 15 minutes. The efficacy of the system is dependent on pH because higher plasma levels are achieved at a lower pH. Another benefit of the technique is its discrete nature since the tablets are held between the cheek and gum without telltale evidence of drug intake. The buccal tablet is designed for faster onset than with oral or transmucosal delivery, so it is particularly useful in the management of breakthrough pain and may be helpful in cases of anticipated incident pain or potentially noxious activity. This formulation may be an alternative route of administration for those with an inability to swallow medications because of dysphagia or a history of pill aversion.

INTEGUMENTARY APPLICATIONS

Transdermal Delivery Systems

Transdermal delivery systems of analgesics and adjuvants can be effective for chronic pain. The ideal characteristics of a transdermal delivery system include low molecular weight, lipophilicity, high potency, and reliable patch adhesion.[211] The drug's solubility in the adhesive, its diffusion coefficient, and its permeability coefficient also play major roles in the time to steady-state release into the skin.[212] Release rates of the agent are dependent on the drug concentration and type of matrix used. A steady-state skin flux is required to yield consistent rates of drug release at zero-order kinetics. Several transdermal systems are available for opioids, α_2-agonists, and anesthetics.[213]

Fentanyl. Transdermal fentanyl was approved for use in children in 2002.[213,214] A prospective study has cited improvement in pain and quality of life in children 2 to 16 years of age who had established opioid requirements for cancer and chronic noncancer pain.[214] In pediatric oncology studies, 75% to 90% have reported that transdermal fentanyl therapy is "good" or "very good" for the relief of cancer-related pain. These findings suggest that transdermal fentanyl is effective and acceptable to children and their families.[214,215]

Buprenorphine. Transdermal buprenorphine has been used for the treatment of nociceptive pain and NP. Buprenorphine is a long-acting partial μ-opioid agonist with antagonist action at κ-opioid and δ-opioid receptors. Reversal of respiratory depression and sedation from this mixed agonist-antagonist is difficult to achieve with naloxone.[216,217] Patients with previous opioid use have experienced up to a 30% dose reduction in analgesic requirements. Pediatric tolerance is associated with marked ventilatory reduction with buprenorphine in comparison to morphine and would warrant close observation for the initial 24 hours of use.[218]

Clonidine. Transdermal application of clonidine has been the most studied mode of delivery of α_2-agonists. Transdermal clonidine is well studied in adults, but it is a difficult-to-use modality for the management of acute or chronic pain. Although neuraxial clonidine has a place in cancer and chronic pain management, transdermal clonidine has limited evidence of analgesic efficacy or opioid sparing.[219] However, transdermal application does appear to increase the release of enkephalin-like substances and may therefore be an agent enhancer in balanced analgesia techniques.[220]

Lidoderm Patch

The 5% lidocaine patch is a topical peripheral analgesic that has been approved by the U.S. Food and Drug Administration (FDA) for the treatment of post-herpetic neuralgia.[221] It has been used for nociceptive pain and NP in noncancer patients. This technique may be of use for malignancy-induced peripheral nerve disease. Unlike other transdermal delivery systems, which work by systemic uptake, the lidocaine contained in the patch penetrates the skin to act locally on damaged or dysfunctional nerves and soft tissue under the skin.[221] Each 10- × 14-cm 5% lidocaine patch contains 700 mg of lidocaine in an aqueous base. It should be applied to intact skin only because of the risk for possible systemic uptake. The patch is applied directly on or beside the area of pain. Patches can be cut before removal of the release liner to fit the targeted area. The recommended use is a 12-hour-on, 12-hour-off dosing schedule. It should be used with caution in patients taking oral local anesthetic antiarrhythmic drugs, such as mexiletine, to prevent additive effects. Patients sensitive to amide local anesthetics, such as bupivacaine or ropivacaine, should not use the lidocaine patch. The 5% lidocaine patch has not been studied in children.

Topical Local Anesthetic

Eutectic Mixture of Local Anesthetics. Four percent tetracaine gel and a eutectic mixture of local anesthetics (EMLA)—lidocaine and prilocaine—as a cream or patch have proved effective in relieving pain in children undergoing cancer-related procedures.[222,223] Studies in children 3 to 21 years of age have shown these commercial preparations to be beneficial in diminishing the pain associated with lumbar puncture, venipuncture, and central port accessing.[224] These preparations should not be used in premature infants because of the risk for local anesthetic toxicity. Plasma concentrations of lidocaine and prilocaine were well below the toxic level for each agent. Moderate plasma lidocaine levels (4.5 to 7.5 μg/mL) may cause restlessness, dizziness, blurred vision, or tremors. At high levels (>7.5 μg/mL), lidocaine can produce generalized tonic-clonic seizures.[225] Buccal application of EMLA has not led to local anesthetic toxicity. A study in 12 subjects showed peak concentrations at 40 minutes for lidocaine and prilocaine; the maximum concentration measured in any subject was 418 ng/mL for lidocaine and 223 ng/mL for prilocaine, each below toxic plasma levels.[226] Methemoglobinemia from prilocaine has been reported with the application of EMLA onto newly regenerated postburn or abraded skin.[227] An occlusive dressing was also used in both cases. Methemoglobin levels below 3% are nontoxic, but skin cyanosis may occur. Levels above 3% can be associated with agitation and levels higher than 50% result in coma, seizures, arrhythmias, and acidosis.[228] Adverse effects of EMLA include transient skin blanching, erythema, urticaria, allergic contact dermatitis, irritant contact dermatitis, hyperpigmentation, and purpura.

Liposome-Encapsulated Lidocaine. Another option for topical pain control before venipuncture is 4% liposomal lidocaine (L-M-X4), an over-the-counter topical local anesthetic that poses no risk for methemoglobinemia because it does not contain prilocaine. Both 4% tetracaine gel and 4% liposomal lidocaine are effective within 30 minutes of application.

Compounding Topicals

Creams and gels applied topically to the skin target the primary site of pain and discomfort. Pluronic lecithin organogel (PLO) is a poloxamer used for topical delivery that has a bioavailability of 10% to 60%.[229] The advantage of using topical medications is that a high concentration of the drug is deposited exactly where it is needed, and purportedly little drug is taken up systemically. This would reduce or eliminate the usual side effects of these medications when taken orally. With a prescription, compounding pharmacies can locally prepare selected agents into topical preparations not currently available on the open market. However, variation in concentration and sterility and lack of FDA regulatory control require that caution be used with these agents. Death has resulted from the use of PLO preparations.[229] Commonly compounded agents for topical application include NSAIDs (e.g., aspirin, ketoprofen), membrane stabilizers (e.g., amitriptyline, clonidine, gabapentin, lidocaine), muscle relaxants (e.g., cyclobenzaprine [Flexeril], baclofen), and antibiotics (e.g., amoxicillin, clavulanate). Topical application of clonidine has been shown to be beneficial in children with cancer. Successful use of topical clonidine ointment in a child with herpetic neuralgia after bone marrow transplantation relieved the associated pain, pruritus, and insomnia.[230]

PARENTERAL MEDICATIONS

Subcutaneous Infusions

Subcutaneous infusions are considered equivalent to intravenous infusions once a plasma steady state is achieved. Up to 5 mL/hr can be absorbed by subcutaneous infusion, thus making this route of delivery feasible for pediatric cancer pain management.[231] This technique should be considered when oral management is not practical but long-term opioid requirements have been substantiated. Success of this technique is dependent on patient selection, ongoing home health care support, and choice of analgesic drug. Highly concentrated solutions are well tolerated and allow lower infusion rates. Opioid concentrations of up to 30 mg/mL have been used in adults and tolerated for up to 7 days, with rotation of the site of delivery every 72 hours.[232] Patient-controlled analgesia (PCA) can be delivered by subcutaneous infusion if intravenous access is not possible. Access via small-caliber needles, such as a 27-gauge butterfly needle, or access with as large as a 22-gauge tunneled intravenous catheter can be maintained in situ for the infusion. Combined techniques of subcutaneous and intravenous infusion may be indicated when venous access is limited but titration of individual agents is needed.

Intravenous Infusions

Outpatient use of intravenous opioids and adjuvants is indicated for gastroenteric intolerance, escalating pain inadequately controlled with adjusted oral medications, or intolerable side effects from oral agents. Intravenous access via peripheral catheters or central ports and catheters is often used in situ for chemotherapy or nutrition. Because of limited access, coadministration of analgesics with parenteral nutrition should be considered to limit interruption of access and control the risk for infection. Trissel and coworkers[233] studied the compatibility of parenteral nutrition solutions with selected drugs during simulated Y-site administration. They reported that parenteral nutrition solutions are compatible with many agents, including opioids, for 4 hours at 23° C. Morphine, fentanyl, hydromorphone, and oxymorphone are compatible via a filter with total parenteral nutrition. Despite visual compatibility testing, admixtures of analgesics into nutritive solutions are not advised. Delivery of the analgesic drug at a Y site in the central catheter system is best.

Neuraxial Delivery System

The WHO has advocated a three-step ladder approach designed to provide adequate analgesia for most adults with cancer-related pain; however, only 60% of adults achieve satisfactory pain control. Children with solid tumor disease compounded by extension of the neoplasm to peripheral nerves or nerve roots at the neuraxis are more likely to require massive opioid doses than are children with nonsolid tumors (e.g., leukemia).[234] It has been proposed that hyperalgesia and NP are associated with reduced opioid antinociception and contribute to the massive dose requirements. Systemic morphine doses as high as 518 mg/kg/hr have been cited in the pediatric literature.[235] The use of neuraxial (epidural and intrathecal) analgesia is indicated for the management of cancer pain when other routes are impractical or yield intolerable side effects. Retrospective reviews of adult and pediatric populations suggest that neuraxial (epidural or intrathecal) infection is a rare occurrence. A review by Strafford and colleagues[236] revealed no serious complications in 1620 general pediatric subjects who underwent short-term epidural catheterization. Bacterial colonization of caudal and lumbar epidural catheters in children has been studied prospectively. Kost-Byerly and associates[237] found a 35% colonization rate of epidural catheters and an 11% occurrence of local inflammatory changes when catheters remained in situ for up to 5 days (mean duration, 3 days). No clinical evidence of epidural abscess was found, but no reports in the literature have identified the risk factors for epidural infection.[65,238] Fine and coworkers[239] noted that epidural infection is rare in adult immunocompromised cancer patients.

Long-standing epidural analgesia is effective and safe for the spectrum of cancer-related pain, as well as for terminally ill patients, but proper management of infection risk and strict catheter care are imperative. Tunneling of epidural catheters is done to decrease the likelihood of infection, improve catheter stability, and aid patient mobility during prolonged administration of neuraxial analgesia. One case report noted a 15-year-old child who received 5 months of effective analgesia until his disease-related demise.[240] A percutaneously inserted tunneled catheter connected to an externalized pump is a feasible technique for prolonged care (Figs. 33.6 to 33.9). Use of a 0.2-μm filter, regular changing of the pump tubing, and weekly or biweekly dressing site

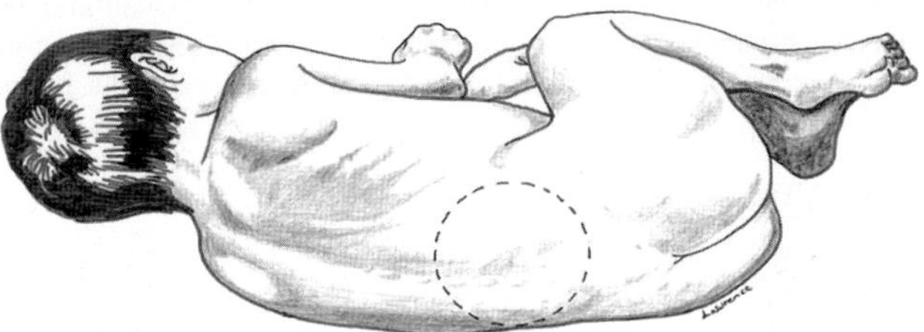

Figure 33.6 Positioning for epidural placement in a child.

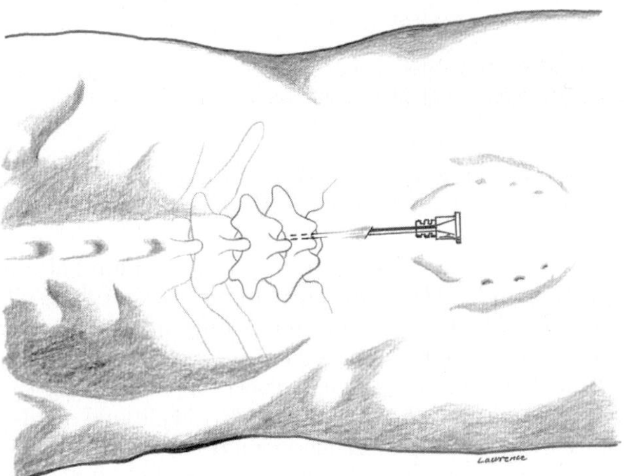

Figure 33.7 Percutaneous placement of an epidural.

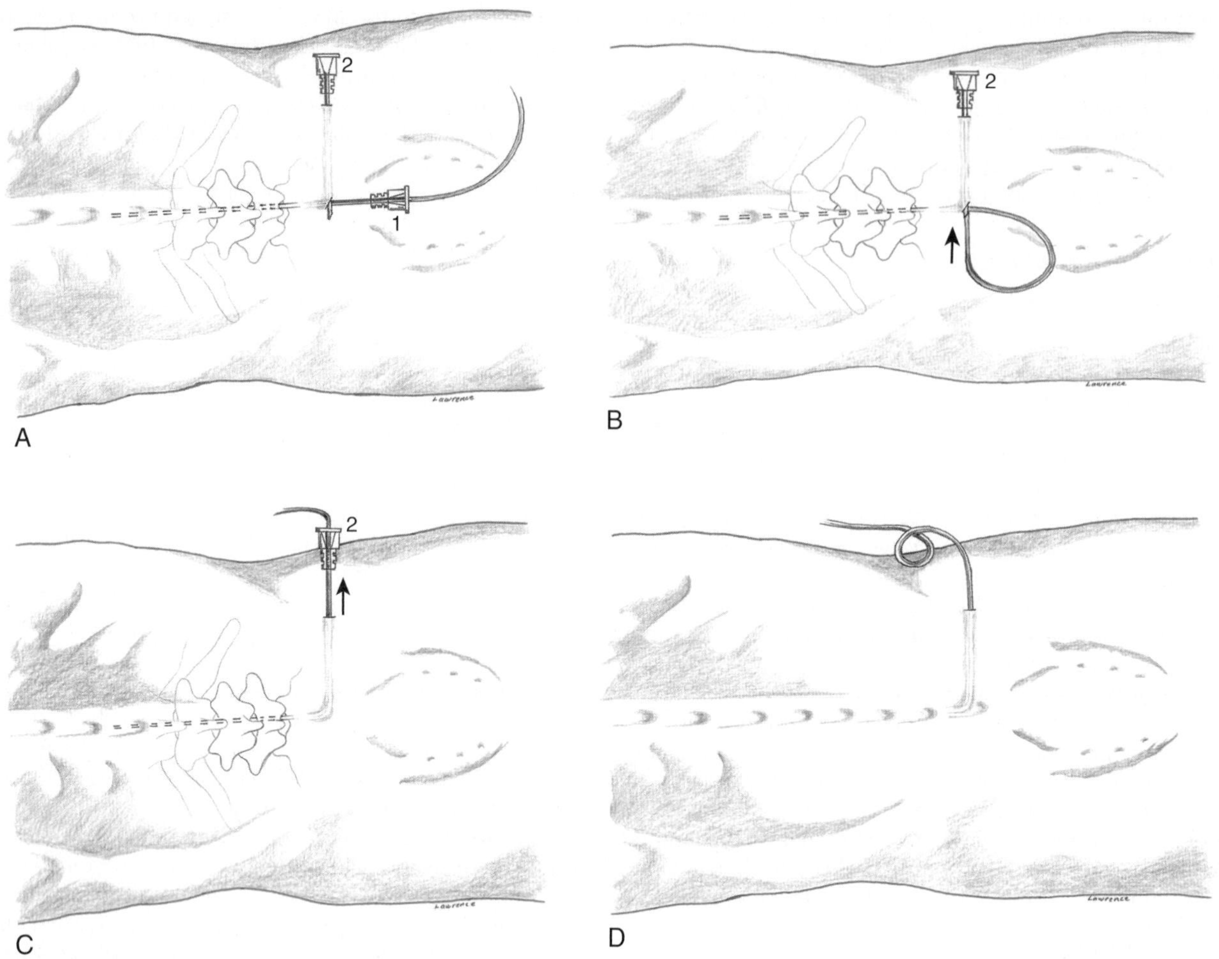

Figure 33.8 **A,** The epidural catheter is threaded and the second needle is tunneled to exit the initial (first needle) entry site. This is performed before removal of the first needle to avoid shearing of the catheter. **B,** The second needle acts as a trocar. This step can be repeated for a longer tunneled section that can be brought to the anterior. **C,** The first needle is removed and the catheter is threaded in retrograde fashion into the tip of the second needle and exits the hub. **D,** The second needle is then withdrawn.

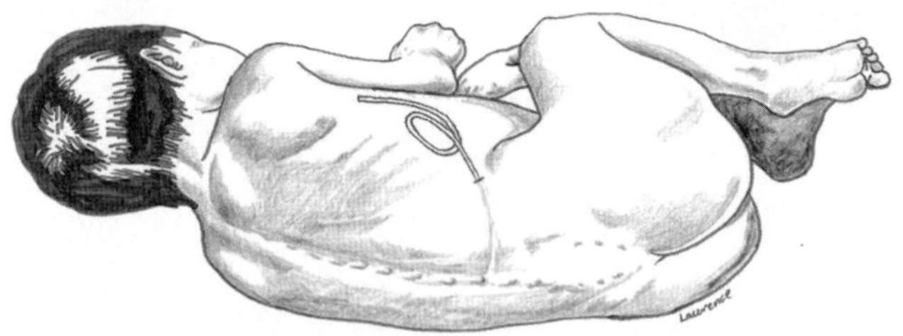

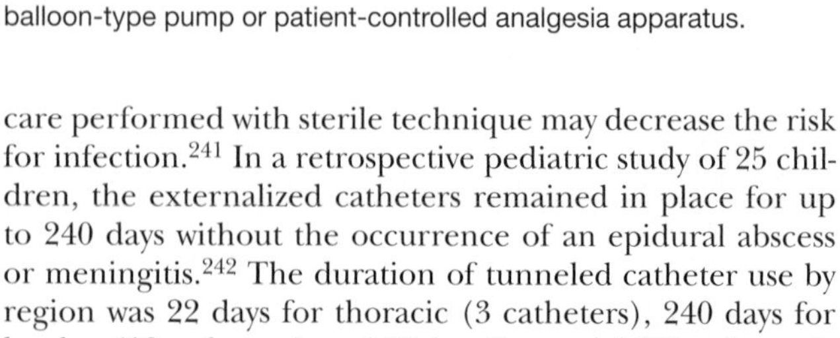

Figure 33.9 The externalized catheter can be connected to a balloon-type pump or patient-controlled analgesia apparatus.

care performed with sterile technique may decrease the risk for infection.[241] In a retrospective pediatric study of 25 children, the externalized catheters remained in place for up to 240 days without the occurrence of an epidural abscess or meningitis.[242] The duration of tunneled catheter use by region was 22 days for thoracic (3 catheters), 240 days for lumbar (12 catheters), and 42 days for caudal (10 catheters).

Tunneled epidural catheters placed in patients with cancer and coexisting NP may have a higher likelihood of infection. Patients with non–cancer-related NP appear to have a higher rate of neuraxial infection than do patients with chronic noncancer pain. Hayek and colleagues[243] reviewed 260 accounts of tunneled epidural use in 218 adult patients with NP or nociceptive pain. Because of superficial infection or suspected infection, 34 catheters were removed; 33 of those removed were in the NP group. In addition, 24 patients had infections in the epidural space confirmed by positive catheter tip cultures or epidural fluid lavage; 23 of these patients were in the NP group.[243] The duration of catheter use was not ruled out as a contributing factor because those with NP had their catheters indwelling for a significantly longer time (28 days) than did those in the somatic pain group (16.5 days).

The risks and benefits of tunneled epidural analgesia in patients with cancer and coexisting NP should be weighed closely. It is recommended that totally implanted systems be considered for patients with NP.[243] The signs and symptoms of epidural infection include fever, escalating back pain, back or neck ache, magnetic resonance imaging evidence of inflammation, and an elevated sedimentation rate, C-reactive protein level, and white blood cell count.[243] Superficial infection may include local tenderness, erythema, subcutaneous phlegmon, and exudates at the exit site. The presence of an epidural abscess is confirmed by aspiration of exudates, an epidurogram with dye loculation at the catheter tip or retrograde flow, positive culture of the catheter tip, or positive culture of epidural lavage material.[243] Removal of the epidural catheter is indicated in those with temperatures of 39° C or higher and if any of the aforementioned signs and symptoms are present.[237] Superficial infections are treated with a 7- to 14-day course of antibiotics. Epidural abscess management includes 6 weeks or more of intravenous antibiotics with or without neurosurgical drainage of the epidural abscess.[237,243]

Analgesia via the neuraxial route is associated with less sedation and fewer adverse effects because significantly smaller doses of opioids are used. Spinal opioids provide selective pain blockade without sympathetic nervous system blockade.[244] The more hydrophilic or hydrophobic opioids have limited uptake in epidural fat and its vasculature and yield greater rostral spread in cerebrospinal fluid (CSF) than do hydrophobic lipophilic opioids such as fentanyl. Intrathecal opioids bypass the bloodstream and have direct CSF spread. The onset of action of intrathecal morphine is 15 to 45 minutes.[244] Delayed respiratory depression is a concern with spinal opioids. Gregory and coworkers[245] noted that peak morphine levels in the medulla coincided with peak ventilatory depression 6 hours after lumbar intrathecal injection. Nichols and colleagues[246] injected 0.020 mg/kg of morphine into the intrathecal space at the L4-5 interspace; this showed the greatest depressed ventilatory response to carbon dioxide at 6 hours that persisted for up to 18 hours, and infants 4 to 12 months of age responded in similar fashion to children 2 to 15 years old. Other side effects do not appear to be dose dependent and include nausea, vomiting, pruritus, and urinary retention. However, side effects are worse with intrathecal than with epidural opioids.[247] The incidence of nausea and vomiting in cancer patients is lower when repeated epidural dosing is used.[247]

The more commonly used adjuvants to improve pain and decrease opioid requirements include local anesthetics and α_2-agonists. The literature has consistently documented appreciable pain control when clonidine is administered by the intravenous and neuraxial routes as an adjuvant to opioid or local anesthetics.[248] The benefits of clonidine as an adjuvant include the following: (1) reduction in the amount of opioid required for analgesia and thus a probable decrease in side effects because of opioids; (2) titrated sedation and anxiolysis without additive respiratory depression when given in combination with opioids; and (3) vasodilation and improved circulation of the cerebral, coronary, and visceral vascular beds.[248]

Continuous intravenous infusion of clonidine has been cited as a safe adjuvant for control of pain in adult and pediatric populations, but the question of long-term impact on neurobehavioral function has been raised. The amount of opioid required by patients experiencing procedural pain was found to be reduced by 30%. Hemodynamic stability was maintained within normal limits because patients experienced less than a 10% change in mean blood pressure. Clonidine has the further advantage of producing sedation associated with only small reductions in minute ventilation and has no effect on hypercapnic or hypoxic respiratory drive.[249,250]

PAIN IN TERMINAL ILLNESS

There has recently been a surge in treatment modalities for pain, and treatment of children is now part of a cure-oriented and technology-based health care system. Recently, with the involvement of facilities such as hospices, the care of terminally ill children has been based on the same philosophy as that for adults.[251,252] Pain can be a significant problem in children who require terminal care. When some children with a life-threatening illness have a significant setback, there may be no firm criteria to stop treatment and direct palliative care.

Alternative novel methods for providing analgesia have been used by our pain service for children who do not have intravenous access. Nebulized opioids[253] or transdermal delivery systems have been used to offset pain in children with intractable pain. Adverse effects associated with the long-term use of opioids include tolerance and withdrawal. Careful rotation of opioids, along with the judicious use of other adjuvants such as *N*-methyl-D-aspartate (NMDA) receptor antagonists, should be considered in the care of children and adolescents.

Several approaches to pain management can be taken depending on the state of the patient, involvement of the disease process, and general state of the caregivers. PCA has been widely used in our institution for homebound patients with terminal cancer. Smaller, more user-friendly pumps have been devised for easy programming and less frequent changing. In patients who do not have venous access, we recommend the use of subcutaneous PCA. Other drugs are useful for terminally ill children. NSAIDs and steroids are particularly helpful in the management of bone pain from metastasis. Carbamazepine, gabapentin, pregabalin, and TCAs are useful for the management of NP. Hypnosis, biofeedback, and distraction techniques can be used effectively in children who are not heavily sedated.

A child's view of death is very different from that of an adult. There is a consistent progression of the conceptual aspects of death as children grow older. A school-age child finally understands the permanence of death. Home care may be useful for the family to cope with the grief and sorrow. It also allows other siblings to spend some time with the loved one. A home care coordinator should be available for the management of any adverse conditions. Knowing the family helps the coordinator understand the goals of the family. One basic tenet of hospice care is to enable the patient to lead a full life, of the best quality, for whatever time is remaining. Cooperation between the family and caregiver should allow the child to die with as much dignity as possible. It is the responsibility of the home coordinator to provide the caregivers with enough information about the management of pain.

Targeted and titrated delivery of antinociception is becoming a reality as more receptor-specific agents are devised. More pediatric studies are needed to substantiate the use of the agents and techniques discussed for the management of cancer-related pain in children and adolescents. Regardless of how creative advancements in pain management may become, patient safety must be first. Novel applications of older agents have broadened the armamentarium of pediatric anesthesiologists and pain management specialists.

CONCLUSION

Chronic pain in children is an under-recognized entity. Early diagnosis and intervention are helpful in ensuring adequate recovery. A dedicated cognitive-behavioral therapy program is a helpful adjunct to medical management and physical therapy. Complementary therapy, including massage, acupuncture, and biofeedback, can be used to reduce pain and decrease the need for additional pain medication. Interventional techniques, including serial nerve blocks, can be helpful in refractory cases. A dedicated pain treatment center facilitates adequate and early management of pain in children to ensure rapid recovery to normal function. Future research in the paradigms for managing chronic pain in children needs to be conducted to shape treatment strategies and develop novel approaches to caring for this challenging group of patients.

KEY POINTS

- Assessment of pain in children involves a multidisciplinary approach specifically tailored to the biomedical, psychological, and social elements of each patient and family.
- Psychological interventions can treat pain effectively by modifying the child's cognitive, affective, and sensory experiences of pain; behavior in response to pain; and environmental and interactional factors that influence the pain experience.
- Management of pediatric complex regional pain syndrome includes physical therapy, pharmacological therapy, regional and sympathetic blockade, neuromodulation, and psychological interventions.
- Headaches in children should be evaluated carefully to determine their cause before initiating treatment.
- Management of headache includes pharmacological therapy, cognitive-behavioral therapy, peripheral nerve blocks, and complementary therapy.
- Functional abdominal pain is best treated with cognitive-behavioral therapy, antidepressants, and serial rectus sheath or transversus abdominis plane blocks.
- Noncardiac chest wall pain may be treated with nonsteroidal anti-inflammatory drugs, cognitive-behavioral therapy, and complementary techniques, including acupuncture and message therapy. Nerve blocks may be used in refractory cases.
- Common causes of pediatric back pain include spondylolysis, spondylolisthesis, disk degeneration, disk herniation, tumors of the spinal cord, and other diseases, including sickle cell disease.
- Management of pediatric cancer-related pain is individualized and based on family needs and concerns.
- Pain can pose a significant problem in children who require terminal care. Approaches to pain management are based on the state of the patient, involvement of the disease process, and general state of the caregivers.

SUGGESTED READINGS

Aram L, Krane EJ, Kozloski LJ, et al. Tunneled epidural catheters for prolonged analgesia in pediatric patients. *Anesth Analg.* 2001;92:1432-1438.

Claar RL, Walker LS. Functional assessment of pediatric pain patients: psychometric properties of the Functional Disability Inventory. *Pain.* 2006;121:77-84.

Dadure C, Motais F, Ricard C, et al. Continuous peripheral nerve blocks at home for treatment of recurrent complex regional pain syndrome I in children. *Anesthesiology.* 2005;102:387-391.

Eccleston C, Jordan AL, Crombez G. The impact of chronic pain on adolescents: a review of previously used measures. *J Pediatr Psychol.* 2006;31:684-697.

Hunfeld JA, Perquin CW, Duivenvoorden HJ, et al. Chronic pain and its impact on quality of life in adolescents and their families. *J Pediatr Psychol.* 2001;26:145-153.

Konijnenberg AY, de-Graeff-Meeder ER, van der Hoeven J, et al. Psychiatric morbidity in children with medically unexplained chronic pain: diagnosis from the pediatrician's perspective. *Pediatrics.* 2006;117:889-897.

Lee BH, Scharff L, Sethna N, et al. Physical therapy and cognitive-behavioral treatment for complex regional pain syndromes. *J Pediatr.* 2002;141:135-140.

Logan DE, Carpino EA, Chiang G, et al. A day-hospital approach to treatment of pediatric complex regional pain syndrome: initial functional outcomes. *Clin J Pain.* 2012;28:766-774.

McGrath PA. Pain in the pediatric patient: practical aspects of assessment. *Pediatr Ann.* 1995;24:26-128.

Nyame YA, Ambrosy AP, Saps M, et al. Recurrent headaches in children. An epidemiological survey of two middle schools in inner city Chicago. *Pain Pract.* 2010;10:214-221.

Olsson GL, Meyerson BA, Linderoth B. Spinal cord stimulation in adolescents with complex regional pain syndrome type I (CRPS-I). *Eur J Pain.* 2008;12:53-59.

Saps M, Hudgens S, Mody R, et al. Seasonal patterns of abdominal pain consultations among adults and children. *J Pediatr Gastroenterol Nutr.* 2013;56:290-296.

Varni JW, Rapoff MA, Waldron SA, et al. Chronic pain and emotional distress in children and adolescents. *Dev Behav Pediatr.* 1996;17:154-161.

Walker LS, Dengler-Crish CM, Rippel S, et al. Functional abdominal pain in childhood and adolescence increases risk for chronic pain in adulthood. *Pain.* 2010;150:568-572.

Wolfe J, Grier HE, Klar N, et al. Symptoms and suffering at the end of life in children with cancer. *N Engl J Med.* 2000;342:326-333.

Zernikow B, Dobe M, Hirschfeld G, et al. Please don't hurt me!: a plea against invasive procedures in children and adolescents with complex regional pain syndrome (CRPS). *Schmerz.* 2012;26:389-395.

The references for this chapter can be found at www.expertconsult.com.

34 Management of Pain in Older Adults

Carrie Stewart | Pat Schofield | Rachael Gooberman-Hill | Sonal Mehta | M. Cary Reid

INTRODUCTION

The population is aging, with demographic shifts resulting in a significant increase in the proportion of adults 65 years and older.[1] The rising prevalence of many long-term conditions, of which pain is a frequent symptom, is strongly associated with advancing age.[1] Persistent pain, which exists beyond the expected healing time, often has no identifiable physical cause[2] and is reported by around 50% of community-dwelling older adults and up to 80% of nursing home residents.[3] In addition to increasing age,[4] factors associated with the development of persistent pain include sex, with women being more likely than men to report persistent pain[5,6]; low income[7]; and mental health conditions such as depression and anxiety.[8] Obesity is a leading risk factor for development of the painful condition osteoarthritis,[9] which affects as many as half of all older adults.[10,11] Cancer-related pain is also prevalent in older adults, with cancer being the second leading cause of death in this population.[12] Research indicates that advancing age is a strong risk factor for undertreatment of cancer-related pain.[13] In contrast, acute pain, a sign of injury or disease, is often treatable or even curable.

Unrelieved persistent pain in later life has many debilitating consequences, including psychological distress, social isolation, impaired sleep quality, physical disability, and increased risk for falls, as well as loss of independence.[3,14,15] Optimizing pain management is important, but in older adults this process can be complex. Consideration of an older patient's functional capacity is essential when formulating a management plan. Cognitive deficits are common in later life and must be considered, especially in relation to the patient's ability to reliably report pain.[14] The presence of obstacles to the identification, assessment, and management of pain in older adults[16] underscores the importance of paying extra attention when providing pain care to older patients. This chapter provides the reader with an overview of current thinking regarding the assessment and management of persistent pain in older adults and describes challenges that health care providers may encounter when delivering pain care to older patients.

PHYSIOLOGIC FUNCTION AND AGING

Anatomic and physiologic changes are considered a normal part of the aging process. Such changes are progressive, but concomitant injury or disease can rapidly worsen the health status of older individuals. Age-related changes in both pharmacokinetics (alteration of absorption, distribution, metabolism, and excretion of drugs) and pharmacodynamics (drug-related adverse side effects) necessitate a modified approach to pain management in older patients.[17] Renal impairment is quite common and leads to increased half-lives of medications that are excreted by the kidneys.[18] In addition, hepatic function can decline and thereby reduce arterial hepatic blood flow and increase the elimination time for hepatically metabolized drugs.[18] Reductions in dose strength and the frequency of analgesic dosing are necessary to decrease the risk for toxicity. Older age is also associated with a change in the volume of distribution. Total body fat increases and total body water decreases, which translates into higher peak plasma concentrations for water-soluble drugs and prolonged half-lives for lipid-soluble drugs.[18]

Both the peripheral and central nervous systems are affected by aging. There is a reduction in β-endorphin content and γ-aminobutyric acid (GABA) synthesis in the lateral thalamus and a reduced concentration of GABA and serotonin receptors. Speed of processing nociceptive stimuli and both C- and Aδ-fiber function also decrease with age,[19] which can lead to corresponding reductions in older adults' ability to sense and respond to "first or initial pain." As a result, older adults may have greater susceptibility to burns and other injuries such as lacerations because they are not as likely to sense the initial pain and do not respond (e.g., removing the hand) as quickly as younger adults.

ASSESSING PAIN IN OLDER ADULTS

Although accurate assessment of pain is the critical first step in the pain management process, this step can challenge even seasoned clinicians. The presence of sensory and cognitive deficits, older patients' beliefs that pain is a natural part of the aging process, patient (or caregiver) misconceptions about the meaning of pain, and language and cultural issues can all operate as barriers to effective assessment. Barriers to assessment also occur at the provider level. For example, the belief that pain is an expected part of the aging process can lead to underassessment of pain. Inadequate provider training is likewise a commonly endorsed barrier to effective pain assessment.[20] Furthermore, older adults typically have multiple symptoms and medical conditions, which leave health care providers little time to address pain in the context of a busy office visit. The implications of these barriers are described in subsequent sections of this chapter. Recognizing these challenges and addressing them are important first steps in the assessment and management of pain in older adults.

Older patients should be asked routinely about pain at each visit, but because many older adults will not admit to experiencing "pain," they should also be queried about the presence of ache, discomfort, or burning sensations. The following section outlines age-appropriate assessment tools for use with both cognitively intact and cognitively impaired older adults.

ASSESSMENT TOOLS

A wide range of assessment tools are available for use in older adults, many of which have been well validated (Box 34.1). Unidimensional pain scales (e.g., those that assess pain intensity only) are feasible for use in the context of a busy clinical encounter. Examples include the verbal pain descriptor (none, mild, moderate, or severe) and numerical rating scales (0 to 5 or 0 to 10), the Pain Thermometer, and the Faces Pain Scale, all of which have been validated for use in older populations, including individuals with mild to moderate cognitive impairment.[18] However, it is important to remember Melzack's famous quote: "To describe pain solely in terms of intensity is like specifying the visual world only in terms of light flux, without regard to pattern, color, texture and the many other dimensions of the visual experience."[21] Using instruments that capture the multidimensional experience of pain, including its impact on function, is therefore strongly encouraged. In terms of multidimensional measures, the Brief Pain Inventory[22] and Geriatric Pain Measure[23] are both appropriate for use in geriatric pain populations. The McGill Pain Questionnaire (MPQ) is another useful measure of pain quality that provides a list of 78 descriptors of pain from which the user can pick words that can later be summed to yield a sensory, effective, and evaluative overall pain score.[21] This well-validated measure has been translated into many languages, thus making it particularly appropriate for cross-cultural use. A short-form of the MPQ is also available. The Short-Form MPQ (SF-MPQ) correlates well with the original MPQ and is more practical for use in the clinical setting.[24]

Box 34.1 Pain Assessment Tools for Older Persons

Unidimensional Pain Scales

Verbal pain descriptor (none, mild, moderate, severe)
Numerical rating scale (0 to 5 or 0 to 10)
Pain Thermometer
Faces Pain Scale

Multidimensional Scales

Brief Pain Inventory
Geriatric Pain Measure
McGill Pain Questionnaire (MPQ); Short-Form MPQ (SF-MPQ)

Measurement Tools in Older Patients with Cognitive Impairment

Doloplus, Doloplus-2
Pain Assessment Checklist for Seniors with Limited Ability to Communicate (PACSLAC)

ASSESSING PAIN IN OLDER PATIENTS WITH COGNITIVE IMPAIRMENT

Assessment of pain in older patients with cognitive impairment requires the use of a triangulated approach that includes self-report, caregiver report, and direct observation. Patient self-report can include responses to questions such as "How much pain do you have now" and the use of reliable self-assessment tools such as the visual analog scale or Faces Pain Scale.[25] The same scale should be used to reassess the pain to determine the effects of treatment over time.

Types of behavior that suggest underlying pain include facial expressions (grimacing, frowning), vocalizations (noisy breathing), changes in activity patterns (eating, sleeping), changes in mental status (confusion, irritability), body movements (guarding, bracing), and interpersonal interactions (aggressive, disruptive, social withdrawal).[26] Numerous observational tools are available and can help providers assess pain in older patients who are unable to communicate verbally. Recent systematic reviews[27-29] have identified at least 10 behavioral assessment tools for measuring pain in older adults with cognitive impairment. Most of the scales, with the exception of the Doloplus, have been used only in small studies, and there is limited evidence of the instruments' validity and reliability.[29] The most promising scales for both practice and research appear to be the Pain Assessment Checklist for Seniors with Limited Ability to Communicate (PACSLAC), Abbey, and Doloplus-2.[29]

PHARMACOLOGIC MANAGEMENT OF PERSISTENT PAIN IN OLDER PATIENTS

Analgesic medications constitute the primary treatment used by physicians when managing older adults with persistent pain,[30] and it is the most commonly reported method used by older persons with a persistent pain condition.[31] For example, in one study of older black and non-Hispanic white adults with osteoarthritis, more than 80% of both groups reported regular use of prescription and over-the-counter (OTC) pain medications.[31]

Barriers to effective pharmacologic management of pain in older adults are diverse and include age-related physiologic changes (described earlier), which often dictates altering the dose and frequency of analgesic administration. Most older adults with a persistent pain disorder have multiple chronic conditions such as diabetes, hypertension, and osteoporosis, and they must be taken into account when formulating a treatment plan. Many older adults experience polypharmacy (defined as the use of multiple medications, with five or more being a typical threshold criterion), which frequently complicates the pharmacologic management of pain.[32] Various patient sociodemographic factors can also operate as barriers. Although adequate social support enhances adherence to medication,[33] many older adults live alone with limited social support. In addition, many older adults cannot afford the high cost of certain pain medications. Furthermore, substantial numbers of older adults lack the necessary skills to read and process basic health

Box 34.2 Pharmacologic Management of Pain in Older Adults

Nonopioids
- Acetaminophen
- Nonsteroidal anti-inflammatory drugs (use in selected cases and with caution)

Opioids

Adjuvants
- Antidepressants (nortriptyline, desipramine)
- Selective norepinephrine reuptake inhibitors (duloxetine, venlafaxine)

care information, including understanding instructions on pill bottles, information present on patient handouts, and clinicians' instructions about the side effects of medications.[34] Low health literacy can lead to problems with medication adherence, such as taking too much or too little pain medication.

In older adults with persistent pain, commonly prescribed analgesic agents include nonopioids, opioids, and adjuvant therapies (Box 34.2). Issues related to the safety and efficacy of these three analgesic classes are summarized briefly in the following sections.

NONOPIOIDS

Acetaminophen is the most commonly prescribed analgesic for the treatment of mild to moderate persistent pain in older adults because of its low cost and overall safety profile.[18] One meta-analysis found that up to 4 g of acetaminophen daily was modestly effective in reducing pain in comparison to placebo, with a standardized mean difference of −0.13 (95% confidence interval [CI] = −0.22 to −0.04).[35] With respect to safety, acetaminophen toxicity is the leading cause of acute liver failure in the United States.[36] Unintentional overdose remains the major cause of acetaminophen-induced hepatotoxicity, and the vast majority of affected individuals report having taken acetaminophen to treat pain.[36] Nonsteroidal anti-inflammatory drugs (NSAIDs) continue to be one of the most commonly prescribed and consumed analgesic agents, particularly as OTC products. One meta-analysis examining the efficacy of oral NSAIDs reported an effect size of 0.29 (95% CI = 0.22 to 0.35) for pain reduction.[37] Although oral NSAIDs are widely considered to be more effective pain relievers than acetaminophen, NSAID use has significant limitations in the form of renal, gastrointestinal (GI), and cardiovascular toxicity, particularly in older patients. When compared with younger patients, older patients are at increased risk of experiencing GI complications in the form of peptic ulcer disease and GI bleeding.[18] Use of either cyclooxygenase-2 (COX-2)-selective inhibitor NSAIDs (e.g., celecoxib) or nonselective NSAIDs is associated with increased risk for myocardial infarction, stroke, and mortality.[38] These safety concerns led the American Geriatrics Society to generate an updated pain management guideline that recommends the use of nonselective or selective NSAIDs in highly selected cases only and with "extreme caution."[18] Given the risks associated with oral NSAID use, increasing attention has focused on the development and testing of topical NSAIDs. Two topical NSAIDs have been approved for use by the U.S. Food and Drug Administration (both are diclofenac preparations), and a number of trials testing other topical NSAID formulations are currently under way.[39] Although no long-term studies have been published, preliminary evidence suggests that topical NSAIDs produce fewer side effects and are better tolerated than oral NSAIDs.[40] The COX-2 inhibitors do not appear to be more efficacious than nonselective NSAIDs, and there are no data that they are better tolerated. The promise of reducing GI toxicity is also still questionable.

OPIOIDS

The short-term efficacy of opioids has been established in older adults for conditions such as osteoarthritis and painful neuropathies.[41] In one meta-analysis,[41] positive effect sizes were demonstrated for reductions in pain (effect size = −0.56, $P < 0.001$) and physical disability (effect size = −0.43, $P < 0.001$). However, the studies included in the meta-analysis were short-term (most lasted 8 weeks or less), and most excluded older adults with comorbidity, thus raising questions about the long-term efficacy and safety of opioids in typical older patients (i.e., those with multiple chronic conditions and taking multiple prescription medications). Though well accepted as a means of treating both acute and cancer pain, opioid analgesics remain controversial in the treatment of persistent non–cancer-related pain.[42] Solomon and colleagues used Medicare claims data to examine the safety of selective and nonselective NSAIDs versus opioids for nonmalignant pain.[43] Patients receiving selective NSAIDs or opioids experienced more adverse cardiovascular outcomes than did nonselective NSAID users. Although both nonselective and selective NSAID users had similar risk for fractures, opioid users were found to have a significantly increased risk for fractures, adverse events requiring hospitalization, and all-cause mortality.[43] Study limitations included concerns about an inability to control for certain confounders (e.g., OTC analgesic use, functional status, cognitive deficits) and an inability to quantify the risk associated with distinct patterns of analgesic use. Despite these limitations, the findings provide strong support for additional studies to quantify both the risks and the benefits of opioid use (vs. other types of analgesics) when treating persistent pain disorders in older adults.

ADJUVANT AGENTS

Commonly administered adjuvants include both antidepressants and anticonvulsants, and they are typically prescribed to treat neuropathic pain. Tricyclic antidepressants such as nortriptyline and desipramine are effective for the treatment of diabetic neuropathy and post-herpetic neuralgia.[44] Although the use of low doses can mitigate the occurrence of side effects, many older adults experience treatment-limiting anticholinergic side effects in the form of dry mouth, urinary retention, and constipation, as well as increased risk for falls. Duloxetine, a selective serotonin-norepinephrine reuptake inhibitor (SSNRI), has also been shown to be effective in the treatment of diabetic neuropathy[45] and to have a superior safety profile relative to the tricyclic antidepressants.[46] Venlafaxine, also an SSNRI, has been shown to be effective in lowering pain levels in patients with painful diabetic neuropathy.[47] Nausea is a commonly reported side effect with both SSNRI agents. Anticonvulsants (pregabalin and gabapentin) may be useful in treating neuropathic pain disorders in older adults.[48] However, side effects in the form of sedation, confusion, and peripheral edema can limit the use of these medications in older patients.

PRACTICE RECOMMENDATIONS

For many classes of pain-relieving medications, older patients have been shown to have increased analgesic sensitivity.[18,32] However, it is important to remember that older adults constitute a highly heterogeneous group, so dosing guidelines need to be based on careful consideration of a patient's pain, its impact on functional status, and the patient's comorbid conditions and other factors (e.g., polypharmacy and sociodemographic and health literacy issues). There are currently no geriatric-specific dosing guidelines. Since advancing age is associated with a greater incidence of treatment side effects,[18] the adage "start low and go slow" is a reasonable rule of thumb when initiating a trial of an analgesic in older patients. This does not mean that one should "start low and stay low," which can contribute to undertreatment.[49] Sustained-release analgesic preparations are recommended for continuous pain, along with the use of short-acting agents to treat pain flares and breakthrough pain. Although long-acting agents are more convenient (and probably associated with greater adherence), there is no evidence that they provide better pain relief.

If treatment goals are not being met and the patient is tolerating the therapy, advancing the dose is reasonable before prescribing another therapy.

NONPHARMACOLOGIC AND SELF-MANAGEMENT APPROACHES TO MANAGING PERSISTENT PAIN

A range of nonpharmacologic pain management (NPM) modalities are available and should be considered when managing pain in older patients.[14] Strategies popular among older adults include exercise, the application of heat or cold, and nutritional supplements.[14,50,51] The American Geriatrics Society guideline recommends NPM as an adjunctive treatment to pharmacologic management.[5] The guideline specifically advises practitioners to consider recommending exercise, cognitive-behavioral therapy (CBT), and patient education for long-term pain management.[5] Complementary and alternative approaches such as massage, transcutaneous electrical nerve stimulation, or acupuncture may be initiated on a trial basis to find strategies that offer short-term relief in the event of pain flare-ups.[5] Fear of pain can result in avoidance of movement and consequentially reduced physical function, which exacerbates the pain experience.[52] With regular moderate exercise, older adults can increase physical function, slow physical deterioration, and improve joint range of motion.[53] Prescribed exercise should be individualized, be supervised for those with either severe pain or significant physical disability, and include flexibility, strength, and endurance exercises.[5] Poor coping skills and negative beliefs about pain and its management make managing persistent pain difficult regardless of patient age.[54] CBT is a psychological therapy that aims to promote and reinforce self-management and positive health behavior and pain beliefs.[53] CBT is recommended for older adults with persistent pain disorders and can be provided as a structured, professionally led program that can be delivered on an individual or group basis, face to face or online.[5] However, the limited number of providers skilled in delivering CBT may restrict the availability of this particular therapy.[55]

Most older adults express a willingness to try new strategies and voice preference for self-delivered strategies that promote independence and control.[56] An increasing number of papers on the management of persistent pain in older adults have been published, and there is increasing awareness that self-management of persistent pain is a viable strategy for older populations.[57] The American Geriatrics Society guideline[5] recommends encouraging older patients to locate information about self-help strategies and participate in pain education to increase awareness of pain treatments and skills important in pain management, such as goal setting.[5] Pain self-management is a patient-centered process that involves the acquisition, practice, and execution of skills needed to respond to and control pain and its associated symptoms. Successful and optimized pain management requires that older patients be confident and able to manage the everyday symptoms and consequences of pain.[58-60] To achieve this, older patients must adopt responsibility for managing their pain, along with support from others.[61] Identifying older patients who are already effective self-managers and those who would benefit from additional support remains a difficult area, however. Self-efficacy, or confidence in one's ability to self-manage pain, is an important psychological predictor of an individual's capability for effective self-management[58] and can be assessed in the clinical setting.[62] Other factors, such as pain beliefs, attitudes, and motivation, also influence participation in self-management.[63] For older patients who require additional support, a variety of materials and interventions are available, including professional or lay-led group courses (delivered in person or online), educational resources (i.e., workbooks, leaflets, and CDs), and self-help groups. The efficacy of self-management programs for older adults that specifically focus on generalized management of persistent pain remains controversial,[64] with some reviews suggesting little patient benefit.[65] Conversely, disease-specific programs, such as those developed for arthritis, have demonstrated more consistent benefit, including moderate reductions in pain and enhanced psychological well-being.[66,67] Decisions on how best to support older patients' self-management will largely be determined by what is available and accessible to the patient locally, but to the extent possible, older patients should be encouraged to choose between available formats and select individual strategies that best meet their needs.

Older patients' use of NPM and self-management strategies varies extensively, and barriers include a lack of advice and support from their primary care providers, affordability of and access to certain strategies, and the pain management attitudes of professionals, older patients, and their caregivers.[56,68,69] It is important that clinicians discuss NPM and self-help strategies with older patients. These strategies can improve quality of life and reduce pain and the associated impact of pain on daily life through the adoption of positive pain behavior and coping responses.[59,60] Although many strategies may appear harmless, unknown risks may exist. For example, some dietary supplements or herbal remedies may pose a risk to older patients when taken with particular pharmacologic agents.[18] It is therefore imperative that clinicians ascertain the full extent of their older patients' pain and pain management experiences and consider cultural, lifestyle, and socioeconomic factors that may influence these experiences. This must be done in a manner that identifies the use of risky NPM strategies that have the potential to cause harm but still encourages patients to play an active role in the management of their pain.

OTHER IMPORTANT BARRIERS TO SUCCESSFUL PAIN MANAGEMENT IN OLDER PATIENTS

PATIENT AND PROVIDER BELIEFS AND ATTITUDES ABOUT AGING AND PAIN

Certain beliefs that older patients and providers have about pain and pain treatments may negatively influence their expectations, behavior, and decisions regarding treatment recommendations (at the provider level) and engagement or adherence (at the patient level). As noted, many older individuals believe that pain is a natural part of getting older.[70] Previous studies have also demonstrated that some older adults believe that pain only gets worse over time,[71] whereas others believe that treatment of pain is not likely to provide any meaningful benefit.[72] Beliefs such as these can lead to stoicism or acceptance of the status quo. Although relatively little research has examined whether these beliefs are associated with specific health behaviors, it is likely that such beliefs can negatively affect an older patient's willingness to seek treatment or adhere to a recommended treatment plan. Indeed, one study found that participants who endorsed the belief that nothing can be done for one's arthritis were significantly less likely to have a regular physician.[73] This finding suggests that beliefs about persistent pain can negatively affect an older patient's treatment-seeking behavior. Previous research has also shown that some older adults endorse beliefs about pain medications that may decrease their willingness to engage in or adhere to pharmacologic interventions.[42] For example, some older adults use pain medications sparingly because of a fear of addiction or dependence.[74] Older patients' caregivers, often a spouse or an adult child, can also voice fears about the possibility of addiction in older patients.[42] Finally, some older adults believe that the use of pain medication invariably results in harmful side effects.[42] Older adults with pain who endorse this belief report minimizing medication use except when the pain is "very bad."[75]

From the perspective of health care providers, practitioners may also approach pain as though it were an inevitable symptom associated with the aging process and give older patients advice such as "what do you expect, you're just getting older."[76] Other research has documented that health care providers are often reluctant to prescribe opioid medications for older patients with non–cancer-related pain because of fear of causing patient harm.[42] Other provider barriers include the absence of objective methods of determining whether a patient is experiencing pain[42] and fear of contributing to addiction or dependence.[77] Although clinicians should remain vigilant about the possibility of misuse or abuse of opioid agents in all patients irrespective of age, it is important to note that advancing age is associated with a significantly decreased risk for opioid misuse or abuse.[78] Indeed, some authors suggest that underuse of opioids in older populations constitutes a bigger problem.[79]

SENSORY IMPAIRMENT

Sensory impairment is common in older adults and can have a negative impact on the management of pain. As many as 30% of older adults experience visual impairments in the form of cataracts, macular degeneration, and diabetic retinopathy, which can make reading prescription labels or participating in recommended exercise programs difficult.[80] Use of good lighting in patient examination rooms, asking older patients to wear eyeglasses to appointments, and providing reading material in large font can help mitigate the negative impact of poor vision on pain care. Hearing impairments are also common.[81] As many as 40% of adults 75 years and older experience hearing problems as a result of conductive or sensorineural hearing loss (or both).[82] Hearing problems can make it hard to communicate a treatment plan during a clinical encounter (e.g., discussing the risks and benefits of a given analgesic). Use of handheld amplifiers, speaking slowly while facing older patients directly to allow lip reading, and providing written instructions can help decrease the negative impact of hearing loss when managing pain in older adults with hearing deficits.

COGNITIVE IMPAIRMENT

Pain in older patients with cognitive impairment is common, under-recognized, and undertreated.[83,84] Cognitively impaired older patients have been shown to receive significantly less opioid and nonopioid analgesia than cognitively intact older adults.[84-86] Numerous barriers exist to providing appropriate analgesia to this group, both at the patient level and at the provider level. Cognitively impaired older patients have been shown to under-report pain.[87] Communication is a major challenge to both assessing and managing pain in this patient population. Short-term memory impairment can alter the interpretation of pain and the response to treatment modalities and thereby potentially lead to increased doses of analgesics and associated side effects.[88] Manifestation of pain in cognitively impaired older patients can also vary, from behavioral disturbances such as lethargy and physical aggression to more expected reactions such as groaning and grimacing.[89,90]

For health care providers, a diagnosis of cognitive impairment creates additional challenges to assessing pain in older adults. Studies have documented a failure to assess for pain[84,91] and provider lack of trust in actual reports of pain by this vulnerable population.[87] Provider fear of precipitating medication-induced adverse effects and exacerbating underlying clinical conditions also leads to undertreatment.

General principles for pharmacologic management of pain in cognitively impaired older patients include a collaborative assessment of pain; administration of around-the-clock analgesics; frequent reassessment of the verbal, behavioral, and functional responses to treatment; and timely titration of analgesics.[92,93] Reviewing side effect profiles of the pharmacologic agents, starting with low doses, and initiating a prophylactic bowel regimen with opioid use are equally important strategies.

In addition to pharmacologic management, nonpharmacologic therapies should be instituted concurrently, including physical techniques, such as repositioning, use of heat and cold, massage, transcutaneous electrical stimulation, and therapeutic touch, as well as behavioral modifications such as distraction, relaxation, and guided imagery. Research evaluating their use in the cognitively impaired population is limited; however, based on their efficacy in cognitively intact older adults, their general use can be inferred in this population. Choosing the appropriate complementary therapy should be individualized inasmuch as the level of cognitive impairment may limit the use of certain interventions, particularly behavioral modifications. Sensory techniques such as music and art therapy represent emerging approaches in NPM that are being piloted in older adults with cognitive impairment.[94]

PROVIDING PAIN CARE TO OLDER PATIENTS WHO BELONG TO AN ETHNIC MINORITY GROUP

Pain assessment and management take place in increasingly multiethnic settings. Pain specialists may find themselves providing pain care to recent immigrants or long-standing minority groups or may work in societies that are not their "own." Appreciating cultural diversity in older patients' pain beliefs and behavior can help in providing appropriate and acceptable pain care.

Older adults who are members of ethnic minorities face particular barriers to adequate pain management. Older members of some ethnic minority groups have a higher prevalence of certain forms of persistent pain, may be less inclined to seek help for their pain, and are less likely to receive adequate intervention.[95,96] Reasons for the established disparities in pain management are complex but include socioeconomic disadvantage, discriminatory health care systems, and pain beliefs and behavior. Beliefs and behavior are further affected by factors such as acculturation, time since migration and sex. Socioeconomic disadvantage and broader discriminatory systems are not easily addressed by providers. However, in their clinical practice, providers are well positioned to improve pain assessment and management for members of ethnic minority groups.

Cultural variation in how patients understand and communicate their pain has been well documented. A classic study by Zborowski suggested that members of American ethnic groups (i.e., Italian, Jewish, Irish, and "Old American") exhibit different emotional responses to pain and have varying attitudes to pain medication.[97] More recent research continues to draw similar conclusions about diverse ethnic groups.[98] Although such work highlights differences, it is important not to use reports of diversity as a basis for stereotyping members of different ethnic groups in practice. Stereotyping has the potential to obscure individual variation and to foster discriminatory practices.

As a framework to help providers conceptualize older patients' culturally informed views about illness and pain, several models are useful, including the "health belief model" and the "explanatory model" (EM). The health belief model focuses on individual patients' views about their health, as well as barriers to and facilitators of illness behavior.[99] The EM hails from medical anthropology.[100,101] The EM approach highlights the different views of health and illness held by older patients and providers because all individuals possess their own EM, which includes a person's views about health and behavior. An approach using an EM places more emphasis on cultural and social factors than the health belief model does. Treatment is more likely to be appropriate when a patient's EM accords with that of the provider, but providers can take steps to understand the content of a patient's EM. Since EMs are socially and culturally grounded, a person's EM can change over time for a number of reasons, including migration or other experiences through the course of life. Within a pain management context, finding out about a patient's EM would mean asking open questions about the patient's views on the origins and cause of the pain, the meaning and impact of the pain, and the patient's views about appropriate treatment and treatment goals. Attempts to systematize the elicitation of patients' EMs have not provided a single "recipe" of questions because appropriate questions will depend on the context and goals of the health care encounter. However, when assessing and managing pain, it is important to understand that highlighting these general areas by an EM approach may be critical in achieving shared decisions and acceptable pain care.

Although language and ethnicity are not synonymous, some older members of ethnic minorities may need additional help in communicating or the services of interpreters ("translators") within health care. Recent and older immigrants may find health care challenging if they do not achieve competence in the dominant language and may rely on family or friends as means of accessing health care.[102] The presence of an interpreter may influence a consultation, not only because of the accuracy of language translation but also because of social roles in the health care interaction, which may be influenced by age, sex, and position in a social hierarchy. Interpreters are invaluable in assisting health care providers to work with patients to facilitate effective, acceptable care. Building good relationships with interpreters may help health care providers in this context.

KEY POINTS

- A wide range of validated tools are available to assess pain in older adults, including those with cognitive impairment.
- A multidimensional approach to pain management is imperative, just as in younger patients.
- Providers need to be aware of and work to address barriers that often occur in assessing and managing pain in this age group, such as physical and cognitive impairment and social and cultural issues.
- The full range of available pharmacologic and nonpharmacologic pain management approaches should be considered.

KEY POINTS—cont'd

- Although increased analgesic sensitivity occurs with advancing age, older adults constitute a highly heterogeneous group, so dosing guidelines need to be based on a careful consideration of an older patient's pain, its impact on functional status, and the patient's comorbid conditions and other factors (e.g., polypharmacy).
- Providers are strongly encouraged to support older patients' efforts to become active participants in their own care.

SUGGESTED READINGS

Altman RD, Hochberg MC, Moskowitz RW, et al. Recommendations for the medical management of osteoarthritis of the hip and knee 2000 update: American College of Rheumatology Subcommittee on Osteoarthritis Guidelines. *Arthritis Rheum.* 2000;43:1905-1915.

American Geriatric Society. Pharmacological management of persistent pain in older persons. *J Am Geriatr Soc.* 2009;57:1331-1346.

Anderson KO, Green CR, Payne R. Racial and ethnic disparities in pain: causes and consequences of unequal care. *J Pain.* 2009;10:1187-1204.

Bruckenthal P, Reid MC, Reisner L. Special issues in the management of chronic pain in older adults. *Pain Med.* 2009;10:S67-S78.

Buffum MD, Hutt E, Chang VT, et al. Cognitive impairment and pain management: review of issues and challenges. *J Rehabil Res Dev.* 2007;44:315-330.

Chodosh J, Morton SC, Mojica W, et al. Meta-analysis: chronic disease self-management programs for older adults. *Ann Intern Med.* 2005;143:427-438.

Christo PJ, Li S, Gibson SJ, et al. Effective treatments for pain in the older patient. *Curr Pain Headache Rep.* 2011;15:22-34.

Eccleston C. Role of psychology in pain management. *Br J Anaesth.* 2001;87:144-152.

Edwards CL, Fillingim RB, Keefe F. Race, ethnicity and pain. *Pain.* 2001;94:133-137. Available at http://www.ncbi.nlm.nih.gov/pubmed/11690726.

Ersek M, Turner JA, Cain KC, et al. Results of a randomized controlled trial to examine the efficacy of a chronic pain self-management group for older adults. *Pain.* 2008;138:29-40.

Ferrell BA, Fine PG, Herr KA. Strategies for success: pharmacologic management of pain in the older adult. *Monthly Prescribing Reference Supplement.* October 2010:1-14.

Ferrell BA, Stein WM, Beck JC. The Geriatric Pain Measure: validity, reliability and factor analysis. *J Am Geriatr Soc.* 2000;48:1669-1673.

Fine PG. Treatment guidelines for the pharmacological management of pain in older persons. *Pain Med.* 2012;13:S57-S66.

Haas M, Groupp E, Muench J, et al. Chronic disease self-management program for low back pain in the elderly. *J Manipulative Physiol Ther.* 2005;28:228-237.

Helme RD, Gibson SJ. The epidemiology of pain in elderly people. *Clin Geriatr Med.* 2001;17:417-431.

Lansbury G. Chronic pain management: a qualitative study of elderly people's preferred coping strategies and barriers to management. *Disabil Rehabil.* 2000;22:2-14.

Melzack R. The McGill Pain Questionnaire: major properties and scoring methods. *Pain.* 1975;1:277-299.

Papaleontiou M, Olkhovskaya Y, Moore AA, et al. Outcomes associated with opioid use in the treatment of chronic non-malignant pain among older persons. *J Am Geriatr Soc.* 2010;58:1353-1369.

Schofield P. Assessment and management of pain in older adults with dementia: a review of current practice and future directions. *Curr Opin Support Palliat Care.* 2008;2:128-132.

Schofield P, Clarke C, Jones D, et al. Chronic pain in later life: a review of current issues and challenges. *Ageing Health.* 2011;7:551-556.

Solomon DH, Rassen JA, Glynn RJ, et al. The comparative safety of analgesics in older adults with arthritis. *Arch Intern Med.* 2010;170:1968-1978.

Tan G, Jensen MP, Thornby JI, et al. Validation of the Brief Pain Inventory for chronic nonmalignant pain. *J Pain.* 2004;5:133-137.

Warsi A, Lavalley MP, Wang PS, et al. Arthritis self-management education programs: a meta-analysis of the effect on pain and disability. *Arthritis Rheum.* 2003;48:2207-2213.

Zwakhalen SMG, Hamers JPH, Abu-Saad HH, et al. Pain in elderly people with severe dementia: a systematic review of behavioral pain assessment tools. *BMC Geriatr.* 2006;6:3-18.

The references for this chapter can be found at www.expertconsult.com.

35 Managing Pain during Pregnancy and Lactation

Geeta Nagpal | James P. Rathmell

Almost all women will experience pain during pregnancy. Common musculoskeletal conditions can cause severe pain in an otherwise uncomplicated pregnancy. Some women will enter pregnancy with preexisting painful disorders, and management of the ongoing pain and painful exacerbations can be challenging. This chapter reviews the common painful musculoskeletal conditions of pregnancy and an approach to the management of chronic pain during pregnancy and in breastfeeding mothers.

USE OF MEDICATIONS DURING PREGNANCY

Medical management of pregnant patients should begin with attempts to minimize the use of all medications and use nonpharmacologic therapies whenever possible. When opting for drug therapy, the clinician must consider any potential for harm to the mother, the fetus, and the course of the pregnancy. The degree of protein binding and lipid solubility of the medication, the speed of maternal metabolism, and molecular weight all affect placental transfer of medications from mother to fetus. With the exception of large polar molecules (such as heparin and insulin), as well as ionized molecules (glycopyrrolate), almost all medications will reach the fetus to some degree.

Approximately 3% of newborns will have a significant congenital malformation.[1] Only 25% of fetal malformations have a known genetic cause, and just 2% to 3% have a clear environmental link, such as maternal medication exposure during organogenesis.[2] One of the major limitations in evaluating any medication's potential for causing harm to a developing human fetus is the degree of species specificity for congenital defects. A classic example of such specificity is the drug thalidomide; nonprimate studies revealed no teratogenic effects, but severe limb deformities occurred in human offspring when thalidomide was prescribed during pregnancy.[3]

The most critical period for minimizing maternal drug exposure is during early development, from conception through the 10th menstrual week of pregnancy (the 10th week following the start of the last menstrual cycle). Drug exposure before organogenesis (prior to the fourth menstrual week) usually causes an all-or-none effect—the embryo either does not survive or develops without abnormalities.[4] Drug effects later in pregnancy typically lead to single- or multiple-organ involvement, developmental syndromes, or intrauterine growth retardation.[2] Certain medications may not influence fetal organ development directly but have the potential to influence the physiology of pregnancy adversely. For example, nonsteroidal anti-inflammatory drugs (NSAIDs) may delay the onset of labor, decrease amniotic fluid volume, or place a newborn at risk for pulmonary hypertension or renal injury.

The U.S. Food and Drug Administration (FDA) has developed a five-category labeling system for all approved drugs in the United States (Table 35.1). This labeling system rates the potential risk for teratogenic or embryotoxic effects based on available scientific and clinical evidence. It is important to note that the FDA classification system has been revised to address neonatal influences other than teratogenicity. For example, ibuprofen is associated with decreased amniotic fluid and constriction of the ductus arteriosus. In fact, many NSAIDs used to be class B before 30 weeks and class D after 30 weeks. More recently, this has changed to class C before 30 weeks and class D thereafter. Because few medications have undergone large-scale testing during human pregnancy, most are category C, which indicates incomplete knowledge of the potential for benefit and harm with drug therapy. More specifically, our present knowledge about the adverse effects of uncontrolled pain, as well as the risks associated with administering medications during pregnancy, remains incomplete, and the physician is left to weigh the risks against the benefits of instituting pharmacologic therapy for each individual.

USE OF MEDICATIONS IN BREAST-FEEDING MOTHERS

The same physicochemical properties that facilitate transplacental drug transfer affect drug accumulation in breast milk. High lipid solubility, low molecular weight, minimal protein binding, and the un-ionized state all facilitate excretion of medications into breast milk. The neonatal dose of most medications obtained through breastfeeding is 1% to 2% of the maternal dose.[5] Even with minimal exposure via breast milk, neonatal drug allergy and slower infant drug metabolism must be considered.[6] Only small amounts of colostrum are excreted during the first few postpartum days; thus, early breastfeeding poses little risk to an infant whose mother received medications during delivery.[7]

Most breast milk is synthesized and excreted during and immediately following breastfeeding. Taking medications after breastfeeding or when the infant has the longest interval between feedings and avoidance of long-acting medications will minimize drug transfer via breast milk.[8] However, effective treatment of chronic pain often necessitates the

Table 35.1 FDA Pregnancy Risk Classification for Pain Management Medications

FDA Classification	Definition	Examples
Category A	Controlled human studies have indicated no apparent risk to the fetus. The possibility of harm to the fetus seems remote.	Multivitamins
Category B	Animal studies have not indicated fetal risk or animal studies have indicated teratogenic risk, but well-controlled human studies have failed to demonstrate a risk.	Acetaminophen Caffeine Metoprolol Prednisolone, prednisone
Category C	Studies have indicated teratogenic or embryocidal risk in animals, but no controlled studies have been conducted in women; there have been no controlled studies in animals or humans.	Aspirin, ketorolac Butorphanol, nalbuphine* Codeine, fentanyl, hydrocodone, methadone, meperidine, morphine, oxycodone, oxymorphone* Ibuprofen, naproxen, indomethacin† Fluoxetine, duloxetine Gabapentin, pregabalin Lidocaine, mexiletine Nifedipine Propranolol Sumatriptan
Category D	There has been positive evidence of human fetal risk, but in certain cases the benefits of the drug may outweigh the risks involved.	Amitriptyline, imipramine Diazepam Paroxetine Phenobarbital Phenytoin Valproic acid
Category X	There has been positive evidence of significant fetal risk, and the risk clearly outweighs any possible benefit.	Ergotamine

*All opioid analgesics are FDA risk category D if used for prolonged periods or in large doses near term.
†All nonsteroidal anti-inflammatory drugs are FDA risk category D after 30 weeks' gestation.
FDA, U.S. Food and Drug Administration.
Adapted from the Food and Drug Administration website. Available at www.fda.gov/Drugs/DrugSafety. Last accessed August 12, 2012.

use of long-acting medications, particularly long-acting opioids. To aid physicians in drug selection and to provide advice to lactating mothers, the American Academy of Pediatrics has categorized medications in relation to the safety of ingestion by breastfeeding mothers[9] (Table 35.2). Although many common pain medications are listed as category 3 (compatible with breastfeeding), psychotropic medications, which are used frequently for the treatment of chronic pain, are category 2, for which the effects are unknown and caution is urged.

MEDICATIONS COMMONLY USED FOR PAIN MANAGEMENT

NONSTEROIDAL ANTI-INFLAMMATORY DRUGS

NSAIDs have both analgesic and anti-inflammatory properties and are commonly used for musculoskeletal pain.[10] Although the exact mechanism of action is uncertain, NSAIDs decrease pain by acting as nonselective inhibitors of cyclooxygenase and thereby inhibiting prostaglandin synthesis.[10] During pregnancy, prostaglandins modulate many key processes, including stimulating uterine activity, maintaining patency of the fetal ductus arteriosus (essential for adequate in utero blood flow), and promoting fetal urine production (which contributes to the level of amniotic fluid in the second and third trimesters). As expected, alteration of prostaglandin metabolism then has varied effects on the pregnancy, depending on the timing and duration of use. For example, short-term use of indomethacin in the second trimester is effective for the treatment of pain caused by degenerating fibroids; use for long periods (more than 48 hours) in the third trimester has been associated with narrowing of the ductus arteriosus[11,12] and oligohydramnios.[13] To complicate this picture further, aspirin, the prototypical NSAID, is used in a therapeutic manner in low doses (80 to 160 mg/day) to decrease the incidence of pregnancy complications in certain high-risk groups but is associated with premature narrowing of the ductus arteriosus at higher doses.[14] Therefore, NSAID use in pregnancy must be carefully planned to achieve the proposed benefit and avoid fetal risk. In general, if NSAID use is indicated, the duration should be short (less than 48 hours) in the absence of monitoring of fetal ductus flow and amniotic fluid volume. All NSAID use for pain should be discontinued by 34 weeks' gestation to prevent pulmonary hypertension in the newborn.[15]

NSAIDs are among the most frequently used drugs during the first trimester of pregnancy.[16,17] Over-the-counter use of these medications is very common in this population. With their use so common, many women may not realize that there is a potential for deleterious effects on them or their developing fetuses. Furthermore, as the age of first-time

Table 35.2 Classification of Maternal Medication Use during Pregnancy

Classification	Definition	Examples
Category 1	These medications should not be consumed during lactation. Strong evidence exists that serious adverse effects on the infant are likely with maternal ingestion of these medications during lactation.	Ergotamine
Category 2	Effects on human infants are unknown, but caution is urged.	Amitriptyline, desipramine, doxepin, fluoxetine, imipramine, trazodone Diazepam, lorazepam, midazolam
Category 3	These medications are compatible with breastfeeding.	Carbamazepine, phenytoin, valproate Atenolol, propranolol, diltiazem Codeine, fentanyl, methadone, morphine, propoxyphene Butorphanol Lidocaine, mexiletine Acetaminophen Ibuprofen, indomethacin, ketorolac, naproxen Caffeine

Adapted from American Academy of Pediatrics Committee on Drugs. Transfer of drugs and other chemicals into human milk. *Pediatrics*. 2001;108:776-789.

mothers increases, more women are likely to take NSAIDs for conditions such as joint and musculoskeletal pain. The effects of fetal exposure to NSAIDs in the third trimester are well documented, and they are associated with premature narrowing of the ductus arteriosus, which can lead to pulmonary hypertension in the newborn. However, there is controversy regarding the risk associated with maternal exposure and other congenital anomalies.[18]

There is no role for the routine use of NSAIDs for pain other than that related to rheumatologic disease or uterine fibroids. In the largest published series of NSAID use during pregnancy to date, Ostensen and Ostensen[19] detailed a series of 88 women with rheumatic disease and compared the outcomes of 45 who received NSAID therapy during pregnancy with the outcomes of 43 who were not treated during pregnancy. The most common agents used were naproxen (23/45) and ibuprofen (8/45). NSAIDs were most frequently used during the first and second trimesters because many patients stopped therapy once pregnancy was recognized; many of the rheumatic conditions remitted later in pregnancy. They found no significant differences in pregnancy outcome (duration of pregnancy and labor, vaginal delivery rate, maternal bleeding requiring transfusion, or incidence of congenital anomalies) or the health status of offspring at long-term follow-up (ranging from 6 months to 14 years). The authors concluded that NSAID therapy limited to periods of active rheumatic disease until weeks 34 to 36 did not adversely affect the neonate.[19] It is of note, however, that women with rheumatic disease have poor pregnancy outcomes in general, so these outcome data should not be applied to the general obstetric population.

More recently, Ofori and colleagues[18] published a case-control study of the risk for congenital anomalies in pregnant users of NSAIDs. Using a population-based pregnancy registry from 1997 to 2003 in Quebec, they identified 93 births with congenital anomalies in 1056 women (8.8%) who filled prescriptions for NSAIDs in the first trimester of pregnancy versus 2478 in 35,331 (7%) women who did not. They concluded that there may be a greater risk of NSAID users having children with congenital anomalies, particularly those related to cardiac septal closure.

Despite the physiologic effects of NSAIDs, the results of the Collaborative Perinatal Project suggested that first-trimester exposure to aspirin does not pose appreciable teratogenic risk,[20] nor does ibuprofen or naproxen, the most commonly used NSAIDs. Patients who conceive while taking NSAIDs can be reassured that this will not impair the outcome of the pregnancy. However, NSAIDs can interfere with implantation and placental circulation. In a population-based cohort study, the risk for miscarriage was 1.8 (95% confidence interval [CI] = 1.0 to 3.2) with any NSAID use and increased to 8.1 (95% CI = 2.8 to 23.4) if used for more than 1 week around the time of conception.[21]

Aspirin has well-known platelet-inhibiting properties and, theoretically, may increase the risk for peripartum hemorrhage. Neonatal platelet function is inhibited for up to 5 days after delivery in aspirin-treated mothers.[22] Although low-dose aspirin therapy (60 to 80 mg/day) has not been associated with maternal or neonatal complications, higher doses appear to increase the risk for intracranial hemorrhage in neonates born before 35 weeks' gestation.[13] Low-dose aspirin has been used to improve pregnancy outcomes in women with both preeclampsia and antiphospholipid antibodies.[23] However, as with other NSAIDs, aspirin crosses the placenta. Even though it has not been implicated in causing congenital abnormalities, it has been associated with an increased risk for vascular disruptions, particularly gastroschisis.[23,24] Data from two retrospective meta-analyses suggest that there may be a twofold to threefold increased risk for gastroschisis with aspirin exposure.[24,25] However, reassuring data from more than 30,000 women enrolled in randomized, controlled trials of low-dose aspirin versus placebo have not shown any significant risk for intraventricular hemorrhage, other neonatal bleeding, or poor pregnancy outcomes.[23]

Box 35.1 Guidelines for Use of NSAIDs during Pregnancy

- Consider nonpharmacologic management or acetaminophen use first.
- Consider use of a mild opioid or opioid-acetaminophen combination analgesic.
- Continue aspirin or other NSAID if the symptoms cannot be controlled nonpharmacologically or with acetaminophen alone.
- Institute close fetal monitoring during the second trimester. If high doses of NSAIDs are required, periodic fetal ultrasound, including fetal echocardiography, should be used to monitor amniotic fluid volume and patency of the ductus arteriosus.
- Discontinue NSAID use after weeks 34 to 36 to reduce the risk for peripartum bleeding, neonatal hemorrhage, and persistent fetal circulation.

NSAID, nonsteroidal anti-inflammatory drug.

Ketorolac is an NSAID available for oral and parenteral administration. According to the manufacturer's prescribing information,[26] ketorolac did not cause birth defects in the offspring of pregnant rabbits. However, ketorolac administration during labor did lead to dystocia in rodents. Ketorolac shares the platelet-inhibiting properties of other NSAIDs.[27] Although ketorolac has not undergone evaluation for its effects on the fetal ductus arteriosus or renal vasculature, it is likely to have effects similar to those of other NSAIDs. Until more information is available, it may be prudent to choose the more extensively studied NSAIDs for use during pregnancy.

Based on our clinical experience and a review of the available literature, we have formulated guidelines for the use of NSAIDs during pregnancy (Box 35.1). NSAID use in pregnancy must be planned carefully to achieve benefit and avoid fetal risk. In general, if NSAID use is indicated, the duration should be short (48 hours) in the absence of monitoring of fetal ductus flow and amniotic fluid volume. Chronic use of NSAIDs should be avoided in pregnancy, especially in the third trimester. Before the 24th week of pregnancy, NSAIDs should be used with caution. It is preferable to use both low-dose and short–half-life NSAIDs.

Because of the antiplatelet properties of NSAIDs, many anesthesiologists are concerned about the risk for epidural hematoma formation as a result of epidural catheter placement. To date, there are no outcome studies on which to base recommendations. There is no evidence that low-dose aspirin therapy or the use of other NSAIDs increases the risk for epidural hematoma formation following spinal or epidural placement.[28] As part of our routine history and physical examination of parturients, we screen for any evidence of bleeding diathesis or easy bruising and, in their absence, proceed with epidural placement without further laboratory testing. This practice is consistent with the guidelines published by the American Society of Regional Anesthesia.[29]

In breastfeeding women, salicylate transport into breast milk is limited by its highly ionized state and high degree of protein binding. Caution should still be exercised if more than occasional or short-term aspirin use is contemplated during lactation because neonates have very slow elimination of salicylates.[30] High-dose aspirin can lead to rashes, platelet abnormalities, and bleeding in nursing infants. The American Academy of Pediatrics considers diclofenac, flufenamic acid, ibuprofen, indomethacin, naproxen, ketorolac, piroxicam, and tolmetin to be compatible with breastfeeding.[9] Both ibuprofen and naproxen are also minimally transported into breast milk and are considered compatible with breastfeeding[9]; these agents are generally better tolerated than indomethacin.[31] Little information is available on the safety of maternal ketorolac use during lactation. One study found that ketorolac concentrations ranged from 1% to 4% of maternal serum levels in breast milk.[32] Analysis of breast milk in 10 women given ketorolac, 10 mg orally every 6 hours for 4 days, resulted in clinically insignificant levels that the nursing infant would be exposed to.[32] Taking into account the bioavailability of ketorolac after oral administration, this would probably result in neonatal blood levels between 0.16% and 0.40% of the maternal dose. The American Academy of Pediatrics considers ketorolac to be compatible with breastfeeding.

Acetaminophen is a analgesic and antipyretic drug used frequently by pregnant women. It provides similar analgesia without the anti-inflammatory effects seen with NSAIDs. Acetaminophen has no known teratogenic properties, does not inhibit prostaglandin synthesis or platelet function, and is hepatotoxic only in extreme overdosage.[13,33] As with most drugs, there are no controlled studies in pregnant women in the first trimester. In animal studies, acetaminophen has not demonstrated fetal risk. Data obtained from 88,142 patients in the Danish National Birth Cohort (1996 to 2003) who had information on acetaminophen use during the first trimester of pregnancy indicated that ingestion of acetaminophen during pregnancy is not related to an overall increased prevalence of congenital abnormalities or to an increased prevalence of the most frequent abnormalities.[34] If persistent pain demands use of a mild analgesic during pregnancy, acetaminophen appears to be a safe and effective first-choice agent. Acetaminophen does enter breast milk, although maximal neonatal ingestion would be less than 2% of a maternal dose.[35] Acetaminophen is considered compatible with breastfeeding.[9]

OPIOID ANALGESICS

Many women of childbearing age are prescribed opioids for the management of intermittent or continual pain. In the United States, more than half of pregnancies are unplanned, which can lead to fetal medication exposure before a woman knows that she is pregnant. Much of our present knowledge about the effects of chronic opioid exposure during pregnancy is derived from the study of opioid-abusing patients.[36-38] Chronic opioid use in pregnancy is associated with low birth weight and decreased head circumference, although the contribution of comorbid conditions, including polysubstance abuse and smoking, is not clear. Enrollment and compliance with methadone therapy for opioid dependence improve birth weight and prolong gestation, thus supporting the role of therapy during gestation.

Until recently there was no evidence to suggest a relationship between exposure to any of the opioid agonists or agonist-antagonists during pregnancy and large categories of major or minor malformations. The Collaborative Perinatal Project monitored 50,282 mother-child pairs and studied exposure to codeine, propoxyphene, hydrocodone, meperidine, methadone, morphine, and oxycodone.[20] Only codeine was found to have an association with malformation (respiratory), but this has not been confirmed by other studies. No evidence was found for either agent to suggest a relationship to large categories of major or minor malformations. In spring 2011, a study by Broussard and colleagues used data gathered from the National Birth Defects Prevention Study (1997 to 2005), which consisted of an ongoing multisite, population-based, case-control study of more than 30 types of major structural birth defects.[39] They reported that opioid treatment from 1 month before pregnancy through the first trimester was associated with a greater risk for conoventricular septal defects, atrioventricular septal defects, hypoplastic left heart syndrome, spina bifida, and gastroschisis. Codeine and hydrocodone represented 69% of all reported exposures. However, these results should be interpreted with caution because some sample sizes were borderline and further investigation is necessary. It is important to understand that the increased relative risk for a rare birth defect with exposure to medications usually translates into only a modest absolute increase in risk above baseline. All opioid analgesics are now teratogenic risk category C *when used for a short time.* It is critical that health care providers weigh the risks and benefits when prescribing opioids to pregnant women or to those of childbearing age.

It is important to note that all opioid medications are risk category D *when used for long periods* during pregnancy. This increased risk warning is due to the potential for neonatal opioid dependence when mothers are treated with opioid medications for prolonged periods during pregnancy. Abrupt cessation of opioids by an opioid-dependent patient late in pregnancy can precipitate fetal withdrawal in utero, which is characterized by fetal tachycardia and fetal death.[40] Therefore, pregnant women who are opioid dependent, regardless of whether use is prescription or illicit, should not undergo acute withdrawal late in pregnancy without careful fetal monitoring. The general recommendation is to offer continuation of narcotic medication (for prescription use) or opioid substitution therapy such as methadone or buprenorphine plus entry into treatment programs for women using illicit drugs.[41-43] Additional benefits of treatment programs include improved prenatal care, higher birth weight, and reduction of infectious risk to the neonate.

Neonates exposed to opioid medications in utero can develop dependence and manifest withdrawal symptoms in the first few days of life, known as neonatal abstinence syndrome (NAS). Although NAS is characterized by irritability and increased tone in mild cases, severe neonatal withdrawal is associated with poor feeding and seizures.[44] NAS occurs in 30% to 90% of infants exposed to heroin, methadone, or buprenorphine in utero[37,38,42,45] when mothers are treated for illicit opioid use. Patients requiring methadone for the treatment of chronic pain tend to require lower doses of methadone, and their infants have a lower incidence of NAS, approximately 11%.[46] Most infants who undergo narcotic withdrawal are symptomatic by 48 hours postpartum, but there are reports of withdrawal symptoms beginning 7 to 14 days postpartum.[37] Neonates with prenatal exposure to opiates for long periods may require very slow weaning (as slow as a 10% reduction every third day) to prevent withdrawal symptoms.[47] The American Academy of Pediatrics considers methadone to be compatible with breastfeeding.[9]

Recognition of infants at risk for NAS and institution of appropriate supportive and medical therapy typically result in little short-term consequence to the infant.[48,49] The long-term effects of in utero opioid exposure are unknown. Chasnoff considered the environmental and socioeconomic factors that influence child development and concluded that no definite data demonstrate long-term developmental sequelae from in utero opioid exposure.[50]

Buprenorphine, a partial μ-opioid agonist and κ-opioid antagonist, is currently used for office-based treatment of opioid dependence but is increasing in use for the treatment of chronic pain.[51,52] Obstetricians and anesthesiologists will therefore encounter patients treated with buprenorphine with increasing frequency. This drug's low intrinsic receptor efficacy results in a ceiling effect and diminished risk for overdose when compared with methadone.[43] Although methadone has been used for more than 40 years for the treatment of opioid dependence, buprenorphine has recently been advocated as first-line therapy.[42] The literature reporting use of buprenorphine in pregnancy remains limited, but buprenorphine has been found to be superior to methadone in reducing signs of withdrawal in newborns, thus requiring less medication and hospitalization time for the babies. In a randomized, double-blind trial comparing 175 women and infants treated with methadone versus buprenorphine, infants who had prenatal exposure to buprenorphine required significantly less morphine for the treatment of NAS, a significantly shorter period of NAS treatment, and significantly shorter hospitalization than did those with prenatal exposure to methadone. However, there was no difference in the number of neonates requiring NAS treatment, in peak NAS scores, in head circumference, or in any other neonatal or maternal outcome.[43,53] In buprenorphine-maintained patients, though, acute pain can be difficult to treat because of the partial antagonist activity at the μ receptor. Whereas treatment of opioid dependence requires only once-daily dosing, opioid-dependent patients with mild pain who are receiving buprenorphine may attain analgesia simply by splitting the same daily dose into intervals of every 6 hours.[54]

According to the drug manufacturer's insert, buprenorphine is not recommended during breastfeeding; however, it appears to be safe.[42] Because of low levels in breast milk, as well as poor oral bioavailability in infants, an infant is exposed to about 1% to 1.4% of the maternal weight-adjusted dose. Breast milk–induced addiction appears to be unlikely, and there is no reason to time breastfeeding to avoid peak levels of buprenorphine. The amount of buprenorphine in milk may not be sufficient to prevent neonatal withdrawal, and treatment of the infant may be required.[55]

Fentanyl is one of the most common parenteral opioid analgesics administered during the perioperative period. As with all opioid analgesics, administration of fentanyl to the mother immediately before delivery may lead to respiratory depression in the newborn.[56] Maternal administration of fentanyl or other opioids may also cause loss of the normal variability in fetal heart rate. Loss of fetal heart rate variability can signal fetal hypoxemia, so administration of opioids during labor may deprive obstetric caregivers of a useful tool for assessing fetal well-being.[57]

Table 35.3 Oral Analgesics for Treating Pain during Pregnancy*

Drug	How Supplied	Equianalgesic Oral Dose (mg)	FDA Risk Category
Acetaminophen	—	325-, 500-mg tablets; 500 mg/15 mL elixir	B
Codeine	60	15-, 30-, 60-mg tablets; 15 mg/5 mL elixir	C†
Acetaminophen with codeine	—	300 · 15-, 300 · 30-, 300 · 60-mg tablets; 120·12/5 mL elixir	C†
Hydrocodone	60	—‡	C†
Acetaminophen with hydrocodone	—	500 · 2.5-, 500 · 5-, 500 · 7.5-, 660·10-mg tablets; 500·7.5/15 mL elixir	C†
Oxycodone	10	5-mg tablets; 5 mg/5 mL elixir	C†
Acetaminophen with oxycodone	—	325 · 5-, 500 · 5-mg tablets; 325 · 5/5 mL elixir	C†
Morphine	20	15-, 30-mg tablets; 10, 20 mg/5 mL elixir	C†
Hydromorphone	2	2-, 4-, 8-mg tablets; 5 mg/5 mL elixir	C†

*There is wide variability in the duration of analgesic action from patient to patient. All the oral agents listed are generally started with dosing every 4 to 6 hours. The dosing interval can then be adjusted as needed to maintain adequate analgesia.
†All opioid analgesics are FDA risk category D if used for prolonged periods or in large doses near term.
‡No oral formulation of hydrocodone alone is available in the United States.
FDA, U.S. Food and Drug Administration.

Meperidine undergoes extensive hepatic metabolism to normeperidine, which has a long elimination half-life (18 hours). Repeated dosing can lead to accumulation, especially in patients with renal insufficiency.[58] Normeperidine causes excitation of the central nervous system manifested as tremors, myoclonus, and generalized seizures.[59] Significant accumulation of normeperidine is unlikely in a parturient who receives single or infrequent doses; however, meperidine offers no advantages over other parenteral opioids.

Although mixed agonist-antagonist opioid analgesic agents are widely used to provide analgesia during labor, they do not appear to offer any advantage over pure opioid agonists. In a blinded randomized comparison of meperidine and nalbuphine during labor, the two agents appeared to provide comparable analgesic effects, as well as similar neonatal Apgar and neurobehavioral scores.[60] Use of nalbuphine[61] or pentazocine[62] during pregnancy can lead to NAS. Nalbuphine may also cause a sinusoidal fetal heart rate pattern after maternal administration, thereby complicating fetal assessment.[63]

Low-affinity opioid agonists, such as tramadol (Ultram), are being used with increasing frequency, in part because of a perceived lessening of the abuse and addiction potential. There is no evidence that acute use of tramadol for labor analgesia has any advantages over more traditional opioids. According to the manufacturer's prescribing information, no drug-related teratogenic effects were observed in the progeny of rats treated orally with combination tramadol and acetaminophen at 1.6 times the maximum human daily dose. However, at this dose embryo and fetal toxicity consisted of decreased fetal weight and increased supernumerary ribs.[64] Tramadol administered intramuscularly to mothers in labor reaches the neonate almost freely, thus confirming a high degree of placental permeability. The neonate already possesses the complete hepatic capacity for metabolism of tramadol into its active metabolite,[65] but renal elimination of the active tramadol metabolite M1 is delayed, in line with the slow maturation process of renal function in neonates. Neonates born to women who are chronically taking tramadol during pregnancy carry a risk for withdrawal. No studies have compared the relative rate of NAS with tramadol versus other opioid analgesics. Breastfeeding is of unknown risk when the mother is taking tramadol.

Table 35.4 Analgesics for Moderate to Severe Pain during Pregnancy*

Drug	Equianalgesic Parenteral Dose	Equianalgesic Oral Dose
Fentanyl	50 µg	—
Hydromorphone	1 mg	2-4 mg
Morphine	5 mg	30-60 mg
Meperidine	50 mg	150-300 mg

*There is wide variability in the duration of analgesic action from patient to patient. All the parenteral agents listed are generally started with dosing every 3 to 4 hours and the oral agents every 4 to 6 hours. The dosing interval can then be adjusted as needed to maintain adequate analgesia.

Postoperative analgesia for most pregnant women undergoing nonobstetric surgery can be provided readily with narcotic analgesics (Tables 35.3 and 35.4). Fentanyl, morphine, and hydromorphone are all safe and effective alternatives when a potent opioid is needed for parenteral administration. There are a range of safe and effective oral analgesics—for mild pain, acetaminophen alone or in combination with hydrocodone is a good alternative; for moderate pain, oxycodone alone or in combination with acetaminophen is effective; and more severe pain may require morphine or hydromorphone, both of which are available for oral administration.

Narcotic analgesics can also be administered into the intrathecal or epidural compartments to provide postoperative analgesia. Such neuraxial administration of hydrophilic agents (e.g., morphine) greatly reduces the total postoperative opioid requirements while providing excellent analgesia.[66] Spinal or epidural delivery of opioids can be used to minimize maternal plasma concentrations, thereby reducing placental transfer to the fetus or exposure of breastfeeding infants.

Opioids are excreted into breast milk. Pharmacokinetic analysis has demonstrated that breast milk concentrations of codeine and morphine are equal to or somewhat higher than maternal plasma concentrations.[67] Use of meperidine by breastfeeding mothers via patient-controlled analgesia (PCA) has resulted in significantly greater neurobehavioral depression of the breastfeeding newborn than seen with equianalgesic doses of morphine.[68] After absorption from the infant's gastrointestinal tract, opioids contained in ingested breast milk undergo significant first-pass hepatic metabolism. Morphine undergoes glucuronidation to inactive metabolites,[67] whereas meperidine undergoes *N*-demethylation to the active metabolite normeperidine.[69] The half-life of normeperidine is markedly prolonged in newborns,[70] so regular breastfeeding leads to accumulation and the resultant risk for neurobehavioral depression and seizures. The American Academy of Pediatrics considers the use of many opioid analgesics, including codeine, fentanyl, methadone, morphine, and propoxyphene, to be compatible with breastfeeding.[9] There are insufficient data to determine the safety of buprenorphine with breastfeeding; however, excretion of buprenorphine into breast milk is minimal.[71]

LOCAL ANESTHETICS

Few studies have focused on the potential teratogenicity of local anesthetics. Lidocaine and bupivacaine do not appear to pose significant developmental risk to the fetus. In the Collaborative Perinatal Project,[20] only mepivacaine was found to have any suggestion of teratogenicity; however, the number of patient exposures was inadequate to draw conclusions. Animal studies have found that continuous exposure to lidocaine throughout pregnancy does not cause congenital anomalies but may decrease neonatal birth weight.[72] Continuous exposure to local anesthetics is unusual but might be seen with the frequent use of local anesthetic patches or creams, which are used for post-herpetic neuralgia and other neuropathic pain states.

Neither lidocaine nor bupivacaine appears in measurable quantities in breast milk after epidural local anesthetic administration during labor.[7] Intravenous infusion of high doses (2 to 4 mg/min) of lidocaine for suppression of cardiac arrhythmias has led to minimal levels in breast milk.[73] Based on these observations, continuous epidural infusion of dilute local anesthetic solutions for postoperative analgesia should result in only small quantities of drug actually reaching the fetus. The American Academy of Pediatrics considers local anesthetics to be safe for use in nursing mothers.[9]

Mexiletine is an orally active antiarrhythmic agent with structural and pharmacologic properties similar to those of lidocaine. This agent has shown promise in the treatment of neuropathic pain. Mexiletine is lipid soluble and crosses the placenta freely. There are no controlled studies in humans of mexiletine use during pregnancy. However, studies in rats, mice, and rabbits involving doses of up to four times the maximum daily dose in humans have demonstrated an increased risk for fetal resorption but not teratogenicity.[74] Mexiletine appears to be concentrated in breast milk, but based on expected breast milk concentrations and average daily intake of breast milk, the infant would receive only a small fraction of the usual pediatric maintenance dose of mexiletene.[75] Mexiletine is rated risk category C by the FDA, and its use should be undertaken cautiously during pregnancy. The American Academy of Pediatrics considers the use of mexiletine to be compatible with breastfeeding.[9]

STEROIDS

Corticosteroids may be used commonly in pregnant patients with autoimmune disease, as well as in those with premature rupture of membranes. There is variability in placental metabolism and transplacental passage of steroids, depending on the preparation.[10] Most corticosteroids cross the placenta, although prednisone and prednisolone are inactivated by the placenta,[2] whereas dexamethasone and betamethasone do not undergo significant metabolism.[10] Fetal serum concentrations of prednisone are less than 10% of maternal levels. In 145 patients exposed to corticosteroids during their first trimester of pregnancy, no increase in malformations was seen.[20] The use of corticosteroids during a limited trial of epidural steroid therapy in a pregnant patient probably poses minimal fetal risk (see further discussion later in this chapter).

In a mother who is breastfeeding, less than 1% of a maternal prednisone dose appears in the nursing infant over the next 3 days.[76] This amount of steroid exposure is unlikely to affect infants' endogenous cortisol secretion.[76]

BENZODIAZEPINES

Benzodiazepines are among the most frequently prescribed of all drugs and are often used as anxiolytic agents, for the treatment of insomnia, and as skeletal muscle relaxants in patients with chronic pain.[77] First-trimester exposure to benzodiazepines may be associated with an increased risk for congenital malformations. Diazepam may be associated with cleft lip or cleft palate,[78] as well as with congenital inguinal hernia.[79] However, epidemiologic evidence has not confirmed the association of diazepam with cleft abnormalities; the incidence of cleft lip and palate remained stable after the introduction and widespread use of diazepam.[80] Epidemiologic studies have confirmed the association of diazepam use during pregnancy with congenital inguinal hernia.[80] Benzodiazepine use immediately before delivery also increases the risk for fetal hypothermia, hyperbilirubinemia, and respiratory depression.[81]

Two other benzodiazepines have been evaluated for teratogenicity. Chlordiazepoxide has been reported to produce a fourfold increase in congenital anomalies, including spastic diplegia, duodenal atresia, and congenital heart disease.[82,83] However, a study of more than 200,000 Michigan Medicaid recipients did not support these earlier findings.[84] Instead, this study found a high co-prevalence of alcohol and illicit drug use in patients receiving benzodiazepines. Benzodiazepine use alone did not appear to be a risk factor for congenital anomalies. Oxazepam use during pregnancy has also been associated with congenital anomalies, including a syndrome of dysmorphic facial features and central nervous system defects.[85] In addition to the risk for teratogenesis, neonates who are exposed to benzodiazepines in utero may experience withdrawal symptoms immediately after birth.[86]

In a breastfeeding mother, diazepam and its metabolite desmethyldiazepam can be detected in the infant's serum for up to 10 days after a single maternal dose. This is due to the slower metabolism in neonates than in adults.[87] Clinically, infants who are nursing from mothers receiving diazepam may exhibit sedation and poor feeding.[87] It appears most prudent to avoid any use of benzodiazepines during organogenesis, near the time of delivery, and during lactation.

ANTIDEPRESSANTS

Antidepressants are often used for the management of migraine headaches, as well as for analgesic and antidepressant purposes in chronic pain states. Although they are an effective therapy in nonpregnant patients, the most commonly used medications of this class are FDA category C or D. Selective serotonin reuptake inhibitors (SSRIs) have become the mainstay for the treatment of depression and are widely prescribed. As with most medications, increased use has been associated with increased reports of adverse effects in pregnancy and the neonate. Though initially thought to be safe in early pregnancy, unpublished epidemiologic reports from GlaxoSmithKline have raised concern that paroxetine, one of the most widely prescribed antidepressants, may be associated with an increase in malformations, particularly cardiovascular malformations, when used in the first trimester.[88] This recent retrospective epidemiologic study of 3581 pregnant women exposed to paroxetine or other antidepressants during the first trimester suggested that paroxetine has an increased risk for overall major congenital malformations relative to other antidepressants (odds ratio [OR] = 2.20; 95% CI = 1.34 to 3.63). The risk for cardiovascular malformations was also increased with the use of paroxetine versus other antidepressants (OR = 2.08; 95% CI = 1.03 to 4.23); 10 of the 14 infants with cardiovascular malformations had ventricular septal defects. In addition, use late in pregnancy has recently become a concern, with reports of NAS, including jitteriness or seizures[89] and pulmonary hypertension, occurring in the newborn.[90] These data initiated a re-evaluation of the risks and benefits of SSRIs during pregnancy and raised the FDA risk category from B to C. It is important to note that although the relative risk for adverse outcomes has increased, the incidence of malformations (1% to 3%) and pulmonary hypertension (0.5% to 1%) remains low, whereas the presence of severe depression in pregnant women is high (15%). As with all medications, the risk associated with no medication must be carefully weighed against the risk related to treatment; there are many women who will need to keep taking their antidepressant throughout pregnancy, and the low incidence of adverse outcomes remains reassuring.

Although tricyclic antidepressants have had a more limited role in the treatment of depression, they can be of benefit in patients with chronic pain. Amitriptyline, nortriptyline, and imipramine are all rated risk category D by the FDA. Desipramine and all other conventional antidepressant medications are category C.[91] Amitriptyline is teratogenic in hamsters (encephaloceles) and rats (skeletal defects).[13] Imipramine has been associated with several congenital defects in rabbits, but not in rats, mice, or monkeys.[92] Although there have been case reports of human neonatal limb deformities after maternal use of amitriptyline and imipramine, large human population studies have not revealed an association with any congenital malformation, with the possible exception of cardiovascular defects after maternal imipramine use.[13] There have been no reports linking maternal desipramine use with congenital defects. Withdrawal syndromes have been reported in neonates born to mothers taking nortriptyline, imipramine, and desipramine, with symptoms including irritability, colic, tachypnea, and urinary retention.[13]

Amitriptyline, nortriptyline, and desipramine are all excreted into human milk. Pharmacokinetic modeling has suggested that infants are exposed to about 1% of the maternal dose.[93] In a critical review of the literature regarding the use of antidepressants during breastfeeding, Wisner and colleagues concluded that amitriptyline, nortriptyline, desipramine, clomipramine, and sertraline are not found in quantifiable amounts in nurslings and reported no adverse effects; they recommended use of these agents as the antidepressants of choice for breastfeeding women.[93] Fluoxetine is also excreted into human milk and has a milk-to-plasma ratio of about 0.3. No controlled studies are available to guide fluoxetine therapy during lactation[13]; however, colic and high infant serum levels have been reported.[94] Maternal doxepin use has also been associated with elevated plasma levels of the metabolite *N*-desmethyldoxepin and respiratory depression in a nursing infant.[95] The American Academy of Pediatrics considers all antidepressants to have unknown risk during lactation.[9]

Duloxetine, a selective serotonin-norepinephrine reuptake inhibitor (SSNRI), is representative of a new class of drug that combines inhibition of serotonin and norepinephrine reuptake. Duloxetine is efficacious for depression and neuropathic pain and may have particular efficacy for diabetic neuropathy. Duloxetine is FDA pregnancy category C, a class indicating potential risks and benefits. Neonates born to mothers receiving SSRI or SSNRI drugs may have a withdrawal reaction, as discussed earlier. Although the relative risks and benefits of breastfeeding when a woman is receiving duloxetine have not been fully evaluated, the manufacturer advises against its use during breastfeeding.

ANTICONVULSANTS

A number of anticonvulsant medications are used in chronic pain management. However, most data on the risk for major malformation in fetuses of mothers taking anticonvulsants are derived from the treatment of epilepsy. Although epilepsy itself is not associated with an increased risk for congenital malformations, some theoretical risk may exist. Nonetheless, data from anticonvulsant use in epileptic women are used to assess the risk associated with the same medications when used for pain conditions. Recently, the American Academy of Neurology and the American Epilepsy Society subcommittee undertook a systematic review of the evidence for teratogenic potential and perinatal outcomes in pregnant women taking antiepileptic medication.[96,97] The review found that exposure to valproic acid, especially in the first trimester, contributes to neural tube defects, facial clefts, and possibly hypospadias. They also found that neonates of women taking anticonvulsants were also more likely to be small for gestational age and have lower Apgar scores. Treatment with valproic acid is more likely to be associated with a major congenital malformation than is treatment with carbamazepine or lamotrigine. There is a possible dose relationship for the development of congenital malformations when valproic acid is taken during the first trimester. Though not consistent throughout all the studies, a dose of valproic acid greater than 1000 mg daily may be associated with the greatest risk for malformations.

In the same review, carbamazepine was associated with an increased risk for cleft palate, but this was not confirmed by another study focusing specifically on carbamazepine and using the EUROCAT (European Surveillance of Congenital Anomalies) database. Although this study did not find an association between carbamazepine and clefts, it did find an association with spina bifida.

Data suggest that topiramate (Topamax) increases the risk for cleft lip and cleft palate in babies born to women who use the medication during pregnancy.[98] Its use has also been linked to low birth weight.[99] The FDA has recently changed its pregnancy category from C to D.

Gabapentin is a newer anticonvulsant that is being used for the treatment of neuropathic pain syndromes. Little information exists about the safety of gabapentin in pregnant women, and thus far, the Gabapentin Registry Study has not shown an increased risk for adverse maternal and fetal events.[100] In their prescribing information, the manufacturer[101] has reported a series of nine women who received gabapentin during their pregnancies. Four women elected termination of their pregnancy, four had normal outcomes, and one neonate had pyloric stenosis and an inguinal hernia. Insufficient data exist to counsel patients regarding the fetal risk associated with gabapentin use during pregnancy.

A drug similar to gabapentin is pregabalin, which combines anticonvulsant activity and affinity for the γ-aminobutyric acid receptor. The main applications of pregabalin are for the treatment of pain associated with diabetic neuropathy and post-herpetic neuralgia. Pregabalin is listed as FDA pregnancy risk category C, but the risk during breastfeeding is unknown.

Patients contemplating childbearing who are taking anticonvulsants should have their pharmacologic therapy critically evaluated. Those taking anticonvulsants for neuropathic pain should strongly consider discontinuation during pregnancy, particularly during the first trimester. Consultation with a perinatologist is recommended if continued use of anticonvulsants during pregnancy is being contemplated. Frequent monitoring of serum anticonvulsant levels and folate supplementation should be initiated, and maternal α-fetoprotein screening may be considered to detect fetal neural tube defects.

The use of anticonvulsants during lactation does not seem to be harmful to infants. Phenytoin, carbamazepine, and valproic acid appear in small amounts in breast milk, but no adverse effects have been noted.[13] No data exist on the use of gabapentin during lactation.

ERGOT ALKALOIDS

Ergotamine can have significant therapeutic efficacy for the episodic treatment of migraine headaches. However, even low doses of ergotamine are associated with significant teratogenic risk, and higher doses have caused uterine contractions and spontaneous abortion.[91] During lactation, ergot alkaloids are associated with neonatal convulsions and severe gastrointestinal disturbances.[13] Occasionally, methylergonovine is administered systemically to treat uterine atony and maternal hemorrhage immediately after delivery. This brief exposure is not a contraindication to breastfeeding.[102]

CAFFEINE

Caffeine is a methylxanthine often used in combination with analgesics for the management of vascular headaches. It is readily absorbed from the gastrointestinal tract and crosses the placenta such that concentrations in the fetus are similar to maternal plasma levels.[103] Early studies of caffeine ingestion during pregnancy suggested an increased risk for intrauterine growth retardation, fetal demise, and premature labor,[104] but more recent studies do not.[105] Although the data against caffeine use in pregnancy are not strongly compelling, most obstetricians recommend that pregnant women limit caffeine intake to less than 300 mg/day. To date, there is no evidence for birth defects related to caffeine.[106]

Caffeine use is also associated with certain cardiovascular changes. Ingestion of modest doses of caffeine (100 mg/m^2, a dose similar to that found in two cups of brewed coffee) by caffeine-naïve subjects produces modest cardiovascular changes in the mother and fetus, including increased maternal heart rate and mean arterial pressure, increased peak aortic flow velocity, and decreased fetal heart rate.[107] The modest decrease in fetal heart rate and increased frequency of fetal heart rate accelerations may confound the interpretation of fetal heart tracings. Caffeine ingestion is also associated with an increased incidence of tachyarrhythmia in the newborn, including supraventricular tachyarrhythmia, atrial flutter, and premature atrial contractions.[108] Many over-the-counter analgesic formulations contain caffeine (typically in amounts of 30 to 65 mg per dose), and use of these preparations must be considered when determining total caffeine exposure.

Moderate ingestion of caffeine during lactation (up to two cups of coffee per day) does not appear to affect the infant. Breast milk usually contains less than 1% of the maternal dose of caffeine, with peak breast milk caffeine levels appearing 1 hour after maternal ingestion. Excessive caffeine use may cause increased wakefulness and irritability in the infant.[109]

SUMATRIPTAN

Sumatriptan is a selective serotonin agonist that has achieved widespread use because of its efficacy in the treatment of migraine headaches. It has been associated with fetal malformations in rabbits, but not in rats.[110] Limited data in humans have not demonstrated any strong teratogenic effects.[91,111] Sumatriptan is advantageous in the treatment of migraine headaches in pregnancy because it does not share uterine contractile properties with ergotamine and would probably not have abortifacient effects.[112] Beginning in January 1996, Glaxo Wellcome established a registry to prospectively evaluate the risk associated with sumatriptan use during pregnancy.[113] The accumulated evidence from the Sumitriptan Pregnancy Registry and other studies suggests that this drug is a safe therapeutic option for the treatment of migraine attacks in pregnant women. Sumatriptan is labeled risk category C by the FDA.

A minimal amount of sumatriptan is excreted into breast milk, and it is considered safe for breastfeeding. The use of sumatriptan during lactation has not been well studied. One study of a single 6-mg subcutaneous dose of sumatriptan given to lactating women found total breast milk sumatriptan level to be only 0.24% of the maternal dose. Because sumatriptan is poorly absorbed from the infant's gastrointestinal tract, only 14% of the drug ingested by the fetus would be bioavailable. Even this minor exposure could be largely avoided by expressing and discarding all milk for 8 hours after injection.[114]

β-BLOCKERS

Propranolol and other β-blockers are used for chronic prophylaxis against migraine and nonmigraine vascular headaches. Most of the studies on β-blocker use during pregnancy involve women being treated for hypertension, as opposed to migraine prophylaxis, and hypertension itself may increase the risk for small-for-gestational-age fetuses.[115] A 2009 Cochrane review looking at β-blocker use for mild to moderate hypertension during pregnancy found that the effect of β-blockers on perinatal outcome is unclear.[116] There is no evidence that propranolol is teratogenic. Fetal effects noted with maternal consumption of propranolol include decreased weight, potentially because of a modest decrease in maternal cardiac output with consequent diminished placental perfusion.[117] Patients should be aware that fetal toxicity can result in complications, including intrauterine growth retardation, hypoglycemia, bradycardia, and respiratory depression.[117] Longer-acting agents should lead to less fluctuation in both maternal and fetal blood concentrations and perhaps less fluctuation in the drug's effects on fetal heart rate. The FDA rates all β-blockers as class C with the exception of atenolol, which is rated class D.

In a lactating mother, propranolol doses of up to 240 mg/day appear to have minimal neonatal effects. The average neonatal exposure at this maternal dose is less than 1% of the therapeutic dose.[118] Atenolol is concentrated in breast milk but still results in subtherapeutic levels in the infant.[119]

EVALUATION AND TREATMENT OF PAIN DURING PREGNANCY

We have been asked to consult on numerous patients with uncontrolled pain during the course of pregnancy. Frequently, severe pain was arising from an extreme form of one of the more common musculoskeletal pain syndromes of pregnancy. Thus, a working knowledge of the painful musculoskeletal conditions that occur during pregnancy is essential. We also discuss evaluation of back pain and migraine headaches during pregnancy because these are among the most common problems encountered in practice. Although sickle cell pain crisis is less common, it provides a good example of the approach to managing chronic recurrent pain during the course of pregnancy.

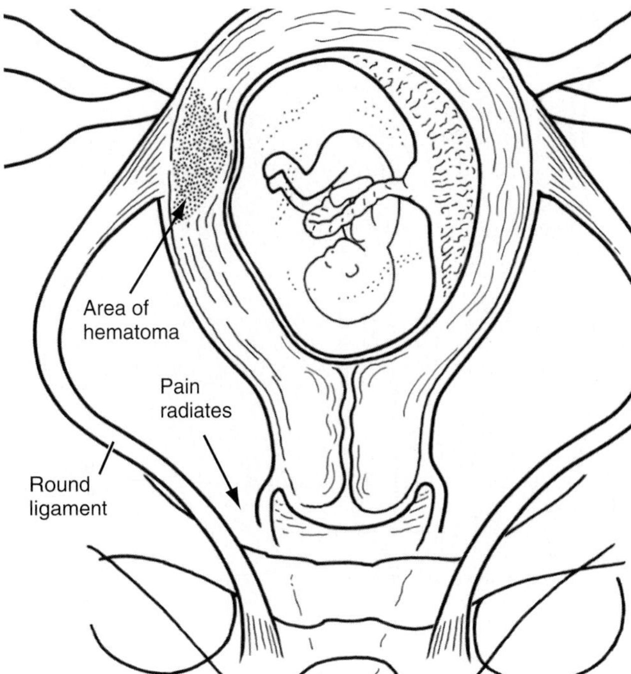

Figure 35.1 Abdominal pain and tenderness arising from stretch and hematoma formation in the round ligament usually develop between 16 and 20 weeks' gestation and radiates to the pubic symphysis. (Adapted with permission from Chamberlain G. ABC of antenatal care. Abdominal pain in pregnancy. *Br Med J.* 1991;302:1390-1394.)

ABDOMINAL WALL AND LIGAMENTOUS PAIN

Abdominal wall pain during pregnancy typically results in prompt evaluation by an obstetrician. One of the most common causes of abdominal pain early in pregnancy is miscarriage, which is manifested as abdominal pain and vaginal bleeding. Unruptured ectopic pregnancy and ovarian torsion may cause vague hypogastric pain and suprapubic tenderness. Once these conditions, which require the immediate attention of an obstetrician, have been ruled out, myofascial causes of abdominal pain should be considered.

The round ligaments stretch as the uterus rises in the abdomen. If the pull is too rapid, small hematomas may develop in the ligaments (Fig. 35.1). This usually begins at 16 to 20 weeks' gestation, with pain and tenderness being localized over the round ligament and radiating to the pubic tubercle.[120] Treatment is bed rest and local warmth, along with oral analgesics in more severe cases.

Less common is abdominal pain arising from hematoma formation within the sheath of the rectus abdominis muscle (Fig. 35.2). As the uterus expands, the muscles of the abdominal wall become greatly overstretched. Rarely, the rectus muscle may dehisce or the inferior epigastric veins may rupture behind the muscle. Severe pain localized to a single segment of the muscle often follows a bout of sneezing. A diagnosis of rectus hematoma is made when the localized pain is exacerbated by tightening the abdominal muscles (raising one's head in the supine position). Ultrasonography can be helpful in confirming the diagnosis. Conservative management consisting of bed rest, local heat, and mild analgesics is often all that is needed.

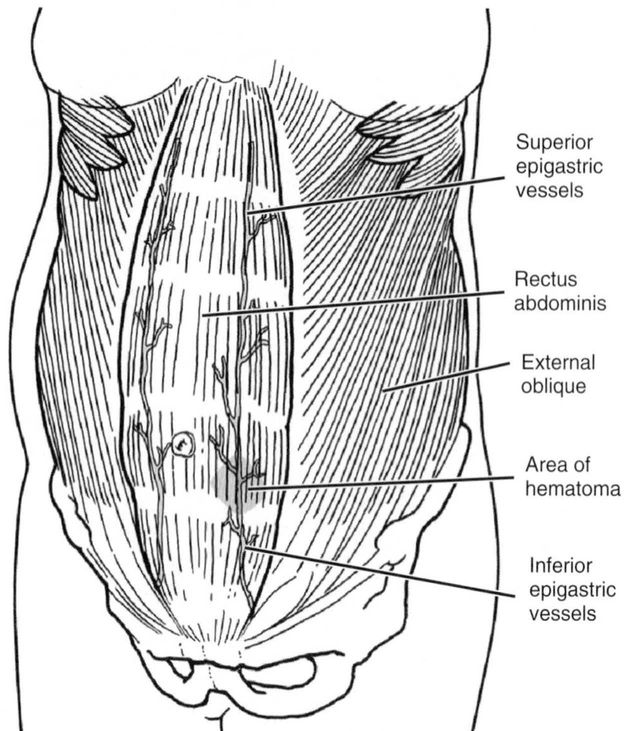

Figure 35.2 Stretch of the abdominal wall in pregnancy can lead to tearing of the rectus abdominis muscle or inferior epigastric veins and formation of a painful hematoma within the rectus sheath. The pain is well localized, can be severe, and often starts after a bout of coughing or sneezing. (Adapted with permission from Chamberlain G. ABC of antenatal care. Abdominal pain in pregnancy. *Br Med J.* 1991;302:1390-1394.)

HIP PAIN

Two relatively rare conditions, osteonecrosis and transient osteoporosis of the hip, both occur with somewhat greater frequency during pregnancy.[121] Although the exact cause is not known, high levels of estrogen and progesterone in the maternal circulation and increased interosseous pressure may contribute to the development of osteonecrosis.[122] Transient osteoporosis of the hip is a rare disorder characterized by pain and limitation of motion of the hip and osteopenia of the femoral head.[123] Both conditions are associated with hip pain during the third trimester, which may be sudden or gradual in onset. Osteoporosis is easily identified, with plain radiography demonstrating osteopenia of the femoral head and preservation of the joint space. Osteonecrosis is best evaluated with magnetic resonance imaging (MRI), which will demonstrate changes before they appear on plain radiographs. Both conditions are managed symptomatically during pregnancy. Limited weight bearing is essential with transient osteoporosis of the hip to avoid fracture of the femoral neck.[123]

PELVIC GIRDLE PAIN

CAUSATIVE FACTORS AND CLINICAL FEATURES

Pelvic girdle pain is a clinical syndrome consisting of pain localized to the posterior iliac crest and gluteal fold over the anterior and posterior elements of the bony pelvis. The syndrome has been called by many other terms, including symphysis pubis dysfunction, pelvic joint insufficiency, pelvic girdle relaxation, and posterior pelvic pain.[124] This pain entity is distinct from pregnancy-related low back pain (Box 35.2). The pain is often described as stabbing, sometimes burning in the region of the sacroiliac joints, and can extend anteriorly to the region of the pubic symphysis. Radiation patterns can include the groin, perineum, and posterior aspect of the thigh in a nondermatomal pattern. The location of pain can change during the course of pregnancy. Onset can take place from the first trimester to 1 month postpartum, although most regard the third trimester to be the peak of symptoms. In most patients the symptoms subside by 6 months after delivery. The incidence is difficult to establish given the various diagnostic criteria used. Some report the incidence to be between 16% and 25%.[125,126]

Box 35.2 Signs and Symptoms of the Syndrome of "Pelvic Girdle Pain"

- A history of time- and weight-bearing–related pain in the posterior of the pelvis, deep to the gluteal area
- A positive "posterior pelvic provocation test" (see Fig. 35.4)
- A pain drawing with well-defined markings of stabbing pain in the buttocks distal and lateral to the L5-S1 area, with or without radiation to the posterior portion of the thigh or knee, but not to the foot (see Fig. 35.5)
- Free movement in the hips and spine and no nerve root symptoms
- Pain when turning in bed

Adapted with permission from Ostgaard HC, Zetherstrom G, Roos-Hanson E, et al. Reduction of back and posterior pelvic pain in pregnancy. *Spine*. 1994;19:894-900.

The etiology of pelvic girdle pain remains unclear but is probably multifactorial with mechanical, hormonal, and genetic influences. Mechanical factors relate to separation of the pubic symphysis during pregnancy. Hormonal changes include elevated levels of progesterone and relaxin. Genetic influence is based on the epidemiologic finding of an increased prevalence in first-degree relatives.

BACK PAIN

CAUSATIVE FACTORS AND CLINICAL FEATURES

Pregnancy-related low back pain is characterized by pain in the lumbar region. Fifty percent of women will experience low back pain during their pregnancy, and it is commonly looked on as a normal part of pregnancy.[127] In a third of pregnant women, back pain is a severe problem that compromises normal everyday activity.[128] The pain resembles the low back pain of the nonpregnant state and is often described as dull and aching in nature. There can be a limitation in range of motion of the lumbar spine, and the pain is exacerbated by both forward flexion and palpation of the erector spinae muscles.[129]

As with pelvic girdle pain, the etiology of pregnancy-related low back pain is probably multifactorial. The lumbar lordosis becomes markedly accentuated during pregnancy to balance the anterior weight of the womb and may represent a mechanical cause of the pain.[130] Endocrine changes

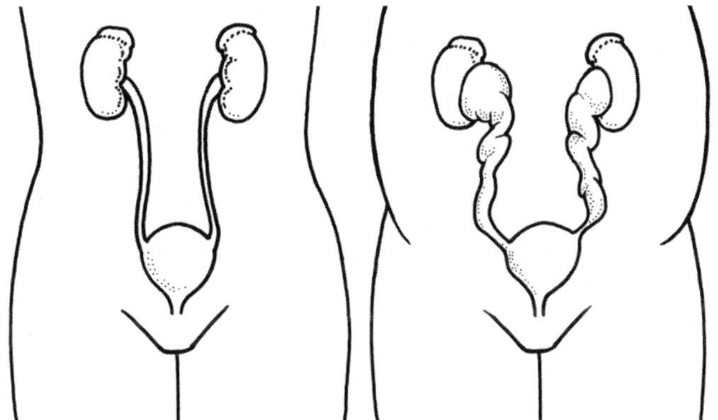

Figure 35.3 Elevated progesterone levels and pressure from the expanding uterus lead to dilation of the ureters in pregnancy. Stasis in the urinary tract can lead to pyelonephritis. (Adapted with permission from Chamberlain G. ABC of antenatal care. Abdominal pain in pregnancy. *Br Med J*. 1991;302:1390-1394.)

during pregnancy may also play a role in the development of back pain. Relaxin, a polypeptide secreted by the corpus luteum, softens the ligaments around the pelvic joints and cervix to allow accommodation of the developing fetus and facilitate vaginal delivery. This laxity may cause pain by allowing an exaggerated range of motion.[131]

The onset of low back pain is usually around the 18th week of pregnancy, with peak intensity occurring between the 24th and 36th weeks.[129] However, the pain can start as early as the first trimester or as late as 3 weeks postpartum. Sixteen percent of women with pregnancy-related back pain report persistent pain 6 years later, thus suggesting that pregnancy is a risk factor for persistent low back pain.[132] Although radicular symptoms often accompany low back pain during pregnancy, herniated nucleus pulposus has an incidence of only 1 in 10,000.[133] Pregnant women do not have an increased prevalence of lumbar disk abnormalities.[134] Direct pressure of the fetus on the lumbosacral nerves or lumbar plexus has been postulated as the cause of radicular symptoms.

EVALUATION OF PATIENTS WITH BACK AND PELVIC GIRDLE PAIN

Evaluation of pregnant patients with low back pain and pelvic girdle pain must begin with a thorough history and physical examintation.[135] The aim is to exclude other causes of pain because obstetric complications (preterm labor, abruption, degeneration of uterine fibroids, round ligament pain, and chorioamnionitis) may also be manifested as low back pain.[136,137] Urologic disorders, including hydronephrosis, pyelonephritis, and renal calculi, may likewise result in low back discomfort.[138] Major morphologic changes occur in the collecting system of pregnant women, including dilation of the calices, renal pelvis, and ureters[139] (Fig. 35.3). The physical examination should include complete back and neurologic evaluations. Particular attention should be directed toward the pelvis and sacroiliac joints during the examination. Posterior pelvic pain (sacroiliac dysfunction) can often be distinguished from other causes of low back pain based on the physical examination (Figs. 35.4 and 35.5 and Table 35.5; also see Box 35.2). A positive straight-leg raise test (typical low back pain with or without radiation to the ipsilateral lower extremity) during physical examination

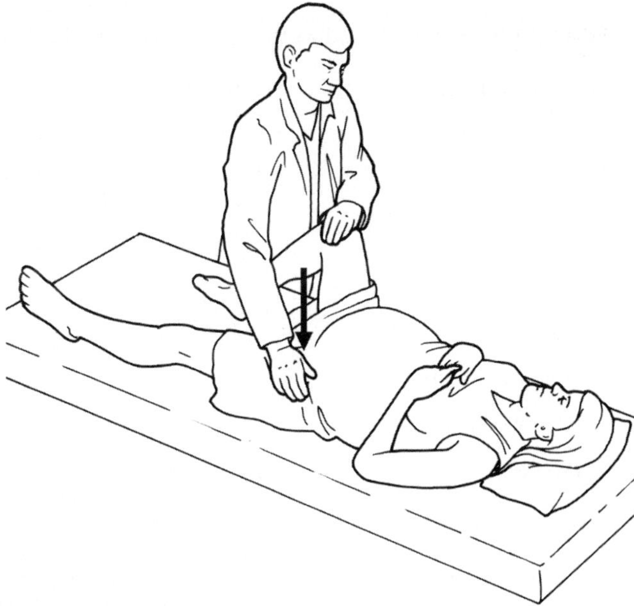

Figure 35.4 The posterior pelvic provocation test. (Adapted with permission from Ostgaard HC, Zetherstrom G, Roos-Hanson E, et al. Reduction of back and posterior pelvic pain in pregnancy. *Spine*. 1994;19:894-900.)

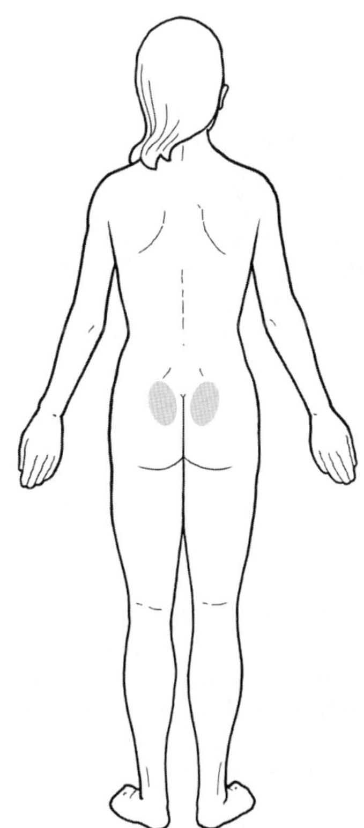

Figure 35.5 Areas where pain is felt when the posterior provocation test is performed in women with posterior pelvic pain. (Adapted with permission from Ostgaard HC, Zetherstrom G, Roos-Hanson E, et al. Reduction of back and posterior pelvic pain in pregnancy. *Spine*. 1994;19:894-900.)

Table 35.5 Sacroiliac Subluxation: Criteria for Diagnosis and Common Confirmatory Signs

Criterion or Sign	Description
Diagnostic Criterion	
Sacral pain	The pain is usually unilateral and, in some cases, radiates to the buttock, lower part of the abdomen, anterior medial aspect of the thigh, groin, or posterior aspect of the thigh.
Positive Piedallu's sign	Forward flexion of the lower part of the back results in asymmetrical movement of the posterior superior iliac spines (PSISs), with one PSIS becoming higher than the other.
Positive pelvic compression	Pain in the sacral area is provoked by direct bilateral downward pressure on the ASISs.
Asymmetry of the anterior superior iliac spine (ASIS)	The ASISs should be examined with the patient in the supine position to eliminate the effect of leg length discrepancy; with sacroiliac subluxation, one ASIS will be higher than the other.
Confirmatory Signs	
Straight-leg raise	Passive raising of the patient's leg with the knee extended and the patient in the supine position causes pain, usually at the end range.
Flexion block	With the patient in the supine position, the knee is flexed to 90 degrees and then passively pressed toward the chest; flexion is blocked to half the expected range on the painful side.
Positive Patrick's test	Placing one heel on the opposite knee in the recumbent position and simultaneously rotating the leg outward provokes pain.
Pain at Baer's point	A point of acute tenderness is found just to the side and below the umbilicus on the painful side, which is about a third of the way between the umbilicus and ASIS.

Adapted with permission from Daly JM, Frame PS, Rapoza PA. Sacroiliac subluxation: a common, treatable cause of low back pain in pregnancy. *Fam Pract Res J*. 1991;11:149-159.

is consistent with sacroiliac subluxation or a herniated nucleus pulposus. Unilateral loss of knee or ankle reflex or the presence of a sensory or motor deficit is suggestive of lumbar nerve root compression.

X-ray imaging techniques such as computed tomography (CT) are not ideal in pregnancy. However, pregnancy is not an absolute contraindication to radiographic evaluation. Radiation exposure during pregnancy leads to concerns about resultant congenital anomalies, mental retardation, and increased risk for subsequent cancers.[140] No detectable growth or mental abnormalities have been associated with fetal exposure to less than 10 rads; the dose received during a typical three-view spinal series typically does not exceed 1.5 rads.[141] Plain radiographs will contribute vital information primarily when fracture, dislocation, and destructive lesions of the bone are suspected.

MRI has revolutionized diagnostic imaging during pregnancy; it has proved to be effective and reliable in the diagnosis of many structural abnormalities.[142] Although MRI appears to be safe during pregnancy, no long-term studies have examined the safety of fetal exposure to intense magnetic fields during gestation.[143] Schwartz[141] presented a thorough and insightful review of neurodiagnostic imaging of pregnant patients. Practical guidelines for the use of radiographic studies in the evaluation of pregnant patients are given in Box 35.3.

Electromyography and nerve conduction studies (collectively referred to as EMG) serve as good screening tests in a patient with a new onset of low back pain accompanied by sensory or motor symptoms. When the clinical findings are confusing, EMG can aid in differentiating peripheral nerve lesions, polyneuropathies, and plexopathies from single radiculopathies. However, false-negative results on EMG are common, especially in the case of a herniated nucleus pulposus causing compression of a single nerve root.[144]

PREVENTION AND TREATMENT

Few of the commonly used strategies to prevent low back pain during pregnancy are universally effective. Patients who were instructed in basic lifting techniques experienced significantly less backache than did a control group who did not receive similar instruction.[145] Aerobic exercise can be prescribed safely throughout pregnancy[145]; however, maintenance of good physical conditioning may not alter the incidence of back pain during pregnancy.[146] Nonetheless, the American College of Obstetricians and Gynecologists recommends specific muscular conditioning exercises to promote good posture and prevent low back pain during pregnancy.[147]

Treatment of pregnancy-related low back and pelvic girdle pain begins with education on the common causes of pain during pregnancy. Back care classes that focus on anatomy, ergonomics, correct posture, and relaxation techniques are available.[148] If the pain remains poorly controlled, referral to a physical therapist for instruction in body mechanics and low back exercises may be beneficial. In a recent Cochrane review of the treatment of low back pain, pregnancy-specific exercise programs, physiotherapy, and acupuncture added to the usual prenatal care appeared to reduce back pain more than just the usual prenatal care. When compared with each other, acupuncture may be more effective than physiotherapy. Participation in water gymnastics programs also reduced the number of back pain–related work absences.[149]

Although the incidence of herniated nucleus pulposus during pregnancy is low, radicular symptoms are common and often accompany sacroiliac subluxation and myofascial pain syndromes. Use of epidural steroids outside pregnancy remains controversial.[150] The strongest evidence for efficacy of epidural steroids appears to be in patients with symptoms attributable to acute disk pathology.[151] Although the risk to the fetus following a single epidural dose of

Box 35.3 Guidelines for Use of Neurodiagnostic Imaging in Pregnant Patients

- Determine the necessity for a radiologic examination and the risks involved.
- If possible, perform the examination only during the first 10 days after menstruation; if the patient is pregnant, delay the examination until the third trimester or preferably postpartum.
- Determine the most efficacious use of radiation for the problem.
- Use magnetic resonance imaging if possible.
- Avoid direct exposure to the abdomen and pelvis.
- Avoid contrast agents.
- Do not avoid radiologic testing purely for the sake of pregnancy. Remember that you are responsible for providing the best possible care for the patient. The risk to the pregnant patient of not having an indicated radiologic examination is also an indirect risk to the fetus.
- If significant exposure is incurred by a pregnant patient, have a radiation biologist (usually stationed in the radiology department) review the radiology examination history carefully so that an accurate dose estimate can be ascertained.
- The decision to terminate pregnancy because of excessive radiation exposure is an extremely complex issue. Because any increased risk for malformations is considered to be negligible unless radiation doses exceed 0.1 to 0.15 Gy (10 to 15 rads), the amount of exposure that an embryo or fetus would probably receive from diagnostic procedures is well below the level at which a therapeutic abortion should be considered.
- Consent forms are neither required nor recommended. The patient should be informed verbally that any radiologic examinations ordered during pregnancy are considered necessary for her medical care. She should also be informed that the risk to the fetus from computed tomography or plain film radiography is very low and that there is no known risk to humans with magnetic resonance imaging. Having the patient sign a consent increases the perceived risk and adds needlessly to her concerns during and after the examination.

Adapted with permission from Schwartz RB. Neurodiagnostic imaging of the pregnant patient. In: Devinsky O, Feldmann E, Mainline B, eds. *Neurologic Complications of Pregnancy*. New York: Raven Press; 1994:243-248.

a corticosteroid appears to be low, it is our opinion that epidural steroids should be reserved for parturients with a new onset of signs (e.g., unilateral loss of deep tendon reflex, sensorimotor change in a dermatomal distribution) and symptoms consistent with lumbar nerve root compression. In such patients, we believe that it is reasonable to proceed with epidural steroid treatment before obtaining imaging studies. Resolution of the radicular symptoms after epidural steroid treatment may well obviate the need for imaging studies.

Guided local anesthetic injection into the sacroiliac joint or pubic symphysis can have diagnostic and therapeutic value. As mentioned previously, most clinicians wish to limit exposure to ionizing radiation during pregnancy. Surface ultrasound can be used to aid entry into the sacroiliac joint. Relief after an intra-articular injection is indicative only of intra-articular pathology. Extra-articular pathologies contributing to pelvic girdle pain such as strain of the superficial long sacroiliac joint ligament are unlikely to improve after an intra-articular injection.

Treatment options during pregnancy are limited by the presence of and potential hazard to the fetus. After delivery, the majority of women do have improvement in their symptoms within a few months. Nonpharmacologic treatment modalities used during pregnancy include physical therapy with pelvic tilt exercises, rotational manipulation of the sacroiliac joint, water gymnastics, transcutaneous electrical nerve stimulation (TENS), and acupuncture.[149] With use of a TENS unit during pregnancy, there is a theoretical concern about inadvertent induction of labor through the use of certain acupuncture points, as well as fetal cardiac conduction disturbances with passage of current through the fetal heart. Limited data suggest that TENS is safe during pregnancy. A recent Cochrane review on the use of TENS for treatment of pain during labor found no deleterious effects on the mother or fetus.[152] Given the theoretical concerns, one recommendation for the use of TENS during pregnancy is to keep the current density low and avoid certain acupuncture points.[153]

MIGRAINE HEADACHE DURING PREGNANCY

CAUSATIVE FACTORS AND CLINICAL FEATURES

The clinician is often confronted with the occurrence of headache during pregnancy because recurring headaches most commonly take place during the childbearing years. Migraine can be a disabling disorder and is more prevalent in women than men, which is thought to be due in part to the influence of female sex hormones.[154] Migraine headaches vary with female reproductive events, including menarche, menstruation, oral contraceptives, pregnancy, and menopause.[155] Eighty percent of female migraineurs report an onset of migraine from the age of 10 to 39 years, thus suggesting that sex hormones do play a significant role in pathogenesis.[156] They typically improve in the first trimester of pregnancy, when there is a sudden and sustained increase in estradiol levels.[157] In fact, 50% to 80% of patients who suffer from migraines experience a significant reduction in frequency or total cessation of migraine attacks during pregnancy. However, women with headaches persisting into the second trimester are less likely to improve thereafter.

Migraine headaches rarely begin during pregnancy, but if they do, they typically occur during the first trimester. Many clinicians believe that headaches initially occurring during pregnancy should generate a thorough search for potentially serious causes.[91,158] One report of nine women with migraine-like headaches during pregnancy found that four were severely thrombocytopenic, two met the criteria for preeclampsia, and one had a threatened abortion.[158] The literature is replete with reports of intracranial pathology that mimicked migraines during pregnancy, including strokes, pseudotumor cerebri, tumors, aneurysms, arteriovenous malformations, and cerebral venous thrombosis.[91] Metabolic causes of headache during pregnancy include illicit drug use (most notably cocaine[159]), antiphospholipid antibody syndrome, and choriocarcinoma.[160]

EVALUATION

Patients with their first severe headache during pregnancy should be evaluated aggressively. Only when secondary causes of headache in pregnancy, including head trauma, cerebral venous thrombosis, preeclampsia, intracranial or subarachnoid hemorrhage, ischemic stroke, vasculitis, and dehydration, have been ruled out should primary headache be diagnosed in pregnant women. The first step is a detailed history and neurologic examination. Focal neurologic abnormalities, papilledema, and seizures in the setting of headache warrant further investigation. Diagnostic suggested tests for new-onset headache during pregnancy include urinalysis, blood chemistries, hematologic studies, liver function tests, and coagulation studies.[156] Brain imaging is also an important component of the workup. MRI without gadolinium enhancement is safe in all trimesters and should be the modality of choice during pregnancy.[156] In a patient with a sudden onset of the "worst headache of my life," subarachnoid hemorrhage should be ruled out.[91] If CT of the brain is negative for hemorrhage, a lumbar puncture should be performed and the spinal fluid evaluated for subarachnoid blood. Progressively worsening headaches in the setting of sudden weight gain should suggest preeclampsia or pseudotumor cerebri. The triad of elevated blood pressure, proteinuria, and peripheral edema points toward preeclampsia; hyperreflexia and elevated serum uric acid are also found in patients with preeclampsia.

TREATMENT AND PREVENTION

In pregnant women with a history of migraines before pregnancy and normal neurologic findings, the therapeutic challenge is to achieve control of the headaches while minimizing risk to the fetus. Nonpharmacologic techniques, including relaxation, biofeedback, and elimination of certain foods, often suffice for treatment. Marcus and colleagues[161] demonstrated a significant reduction in headache that continued throughout pregnancy and at the 1-year follow-up when a combination of relaxation training, thermal biofeedback, and physical therapy exercises was used.

If pharmacologic therapy appears to be warranted, acetaminophen with or without caffeine is safe and effective.[162] A drawback with acetaminophen is the potential for medication overuse and rebound headache, which could lead to the development of chronic daily headaches. Ibuprofen and naproxen are the most commonly used NSAIDs for abortive management of migraines; however, they are risk category C before 30 weeks and risk category D in the third trimester. The short-term use of mild opioid analgesics such as hydrocodone, alone or in combination with acetaminophen, also appears to carry little risk (see Table 35.3). When oral analgesics prove ineffective, hospital admission and administration of parenteral opioids may be required (see Table 35.4).

Until more information is available on the safety of sumatriptan during pregnancy, it should be used only after other strategies have failed. Triptans are the most used abortive agents in nonpregnant patients, but they are rarely used during pregnancy. There are pregnancy registries for both sumatriptan and naratriptan to track pregnancy outcomes after exposure to these medications. At this time there does not seem to be an increased incidence of teratogenicity or adverse pregnancy outcomes with use in the first trimester. Ergot preparations should be avoided during pregnancy and lactation. They are known to cause prolonged and markedly increased uterine tone and impaired placental flow leading to fetal distress or spontaneous abortion.

A history of three to four incapacitating headaches per month warrants consideration of prophylactic therapy.[162] If the frequency of the headache or headaches is less than three to four per month but they are severe and unmanageable with acute therapies, prophylactic therapy should be considered to prevent dehydration of the mother, which could cause fetal distress. Daily oral propranolol or atenolol is a reasonable choice, although patients should understand that their use is associated with small-for-gestational-age infants.[163] Longer-acting agents should lead to less fluctuation in maternal and fetal blood concentrations and perhaps less fluctuation in drug effects on the fetal heart rate. Based on this theoretical advantage, we prefer to use long-acting agents (e.g., atenolol or sustained-release propranolol).

Although antidepressants are effective as prophylactic therapy in nonpregnant patients, the most commonly used medications in this class (imipramine, amitriptyline, and nortriptyline) are all FDA category D. The SSRIs are category B or C and can be used with caution, especially if comorbid depression is present. There are very limited data, which has led most physicians to avoid these medications. Limited anecdotal experience with calcium channel blockers (verapamil, nifedipine, and diltiazem are all FDA class C) or minidose aspirin (80 mg/day) suggests that they may be effective prophylactic agents during pregnancy.[91,162]

MIGRAINE AND LACTATION

Postpartum headaches are common and can occur in 30% to 40% of all women.[155] Most take place in the first week, and about 50% of those who experience relief of their migraine during pregnancy have recurrence a short time after delivery. This phenomenon may be secondary to the rapid ovarian withdrawal of progesterone and estradiol. Lactation can inhibit ovulatory cycles during the puerperium and is characterized by increased levels of prolactin and low levels of estradiol. In mothers of bottle-fed infants, the hormonal cycle is restored rapidly, which may contribute to it being a main risk factor for postnatal recurrence of migraine.[164]

PAIN IN PREGNANT PATIENTS WITH SICKLE CELL DISEASE

CAUSATIVE FACTORS AND CLINICAL FEATURES

Sickle cell disease is an inherited multisystem disorder. The presence of abnormal hemoglobin in red blood cells leads to the cardinal features of the disease, namely, chronic hemolytic anemia and recurrent painful episodes. Vaso-occlusive crisis is the most common maternal complication noted in parturients with sickle cell hemoglobinopathies.[165] The vaso-occlusive crises follow a characteristic pattern of recurrent sudden attacks of pain, usually involving the abdomen, chest, vertebrae, and extremities. One prospective study has demonstrated that the clinical course of women with sickle cell disease is not adversely affected by their pregnancy as measured by the rate of painful episodes over a 100-day period.[166] The rate was constant before, during, and after the first and subsequent pregnancies. Painful episodes occurred at some time during the course of 50% of pregnancies.

Most crises during pregnancy are vaso-occlusive and often precipitated by urinary tract infection, preeclampsia or eclampsia, thrombophlebitis, or pneumonia. Clinically, the individual will describe pain in the bones or joints but may also perceive the soft tissues as being affected. Visceral pain is also common and may be related to events in the liver or spleen. Painful episodes can be variable in severity and duration, with most episodes lasting from 3 to 5 days.[167]

EVALUATION

Because laboratory evaluation is nonspecific, the diagnosis of vaso-occlusive crisis begins with exclusion of other causes of the painful episode, particularly occult infection.[165] Complete assessment and acute management of sickle cell crises in pregnancy have been reviewed by Martin and coworkers.[168]

TREATMENT

Management of vaso-occlusive crisis during pregnancy is primarily supportive and symptomatic. A 2009 Cochrane review of interventions for treating a sickle cell crisis during pregnancy attempted to assess the effectiveness and safety of commonly used treatment regimens, including red cell transfusion, oxygen therapy, intravenous hydration, analgesic drugs, and steroids; there are no randomized clinical trials on this topic, in part because pregnant women tend to be excluded from clinical trials.[169] Most clinicians begin management with aggressive hydration to increase intravascular volume and decrease blood viscosity.[168] Supplemental oxygen is essential in patients with hypoxemia. Partial exchange transfusions to reduce polymerized hemoglobin S remain an integral part of the management of sickle cell disease[170]; prophylactic transfusion may reduce the incidence of severe sickling complications during pregnancy.[171]

Education about how pregnancy interacts with sickle cell disease can help reduce depression or anxiety and often decreases the pain that the patient is experiencing. Biofeedback has been shown to reduce the pain of sickle cell crises and the number of days that analgesics are taken.[172] Physical therapy techniques (e.g., exercise, splinting, local application of heat) can also be helpful.[173] TENS may be helpful when the pain is isolated to a limited region.[174]

The severity of the pain dictates the pharmacologic approach to managing sickle cell pain. Although nonopioid analgesics may suffice, oral or parenteral opioids are often required (see Tables 35.3 and 35.4). Acetaminophen remains the nonopioid analgesic of choice during pregnancy. Although NSAIDs can be useful adjuncts, particularly for controlling bone pain, they should be used cautiously during pregnancy. Oral analgesic combinations containing acetaminophen and hydrocodone or another opioid with weak to moderate potency can be added for more severe pain.

In a hospitalized patient with severe sickle cell pain, potent opioid analgesics administered intravenously may be necessary to control the pain adequately (see Table 35.4). Morphine sulfate is well tolerated and effective for control of severe sickle cell pain[175]; fentanyl and hydromorphone provide reasonable alternatives for patients who cannot tolerate morphine. Administration of morphine via a PCA device allows patients a sense of control over their illness. Weisman and Schechter[176] noted that significantly higher doses of opioids may be necessary for control of the pain of vaso-occlusive crisis than for control of postoperative pain. In our practice we aggressively treat individuals with severe sickle cell pain with potent opioids administered via PCA (most often using morphine). As the pain of vaso-occlusive crisis begins to resolve, patients are transitioned to a long-acting oral opioid (such as sustained-release morphine). This approach allows earlier ambulation and hospital discharge. All opioids are then tapered over the following 7 to 10 days.

The use of regional anesthesia has not been formally studied in sickle cell disease. There are case reports describing epidural analgesia for the treatment of sickle cell crisis during pregnancy in parturients with pain localized to the trunk or lower extremities.[177,178] This technique offers the theoretical advantage of increased microvascular blood flow while providing pain relief without opioids.

ACUTE PAIN IN OPIOID-DEPENDENT PATIENTS

Acute pain in pregnant patients is most often encountered during labor and delivery. Both pain control and withdrawal symptoms are mediated through the μ-opioid receptor. Therefore, narcotic pain medication requires availability of the μ-opioid receptor, which in opioid-dependent patients is also occupied by opioid agonist therapy for dependence. No randomized or controlled studies are available to determine whether anesthetic needs differ in opioid-dependent and control patients. One descriptive study found that 24% of opioid-dependent women had difficulty with labor analgesia and 74% had difficulty with postcesarean analgesia.[179] These statistics may overestimate the difficulty in pain control because it was not clear that treatment of opioid dependence was adequate before the treatment of acute pain. When opioid dependence is untreated and combined with acute pain, opioid needs reflect the combined therapies rather than treatment of pain alone. Although no randomized clinical trials have been performed, we have found that epidural analgesia with a standard dose of local anesthetic and low-dose opioid (e.g., 0.625% bupivacaine with fentanyl, 2 μg/mL) provides adequate intrapartum analgesia.

Intrathecal or epidural analgesia using only opioids may not be effective in reducing the need for systemic narcotics. Sustained administration of μ-opioid agonists by any route can induce both opioid tolerance and abnormal pain that is similar to neuropathic pain.[180] Though previously attributed to pharmacologic tolerance, patients maintained on methadone may experience opioid-induced hyperalgesia, a paradoxical effect mediated in part by the neurotransmitter *N*-methyl-D-aspartate and possibly by the novel neuropeptide dynorphin.[181] Interestingly, dynorphin may be an important mediator of chronic neuropathic pain, a common complaint in opioid-dependent patients.

No trials have investigated opioid use and pain control after vaginal or abdominal delivery in opioid-tolerant patients. Recently published guidelines for the treatment of acute pain in patients maintained on methadone or buprenorphine provide a reasonable approach until more data are available.[54] Patients maintained on methadone for opioid dependence should have their methadone continued at the same dose in addition to standard-dose opiates as needed for acute pain. Use of nonopioid analgesics should be included, but additional opioid medication should not be withheld. This additional short-acting opioid medication can be discontinued gradually as clinically indicated. If patients are unable to tolerate oral medication, methadone can be administered intramuscularly or subcutaneously in two to four divided doses.

Patients maintained on buprenorphine pose a more difficult dilemma in the postoperative period. As a combined opioid agonist-antagonist, continued administration of buprenorphine can block the μ-mediated analgesic effect of additional short-acting opioids.[182] It is of note that although nonpregnant patients receive a combination of buprenorphine and naloxone, monotherapy with buprenorphine is prescribed during pregnancy to avoid naloxone exposure by the neonate.[183] Pain control options, in addition to nonopioid analgesics, include the following[54]: (1) adding short-acting opioids with the realization that larger doses may be needed; (2) dividing the daily dose of buprenorphine into 6-hour intervals, which can take advantage of the short-term analgesic effect of buprenorphine; and (3) discontinuing buprenorphine and initiating methadone at 30 mg/day, with increasing titration in 5- to 10-mg intervals daily to alleviate withdrawal symptoms. In this way, short-acting opioids can be used for pain and methadone can be used to prevent withdrawal, with less direct antagonism at the μ-opioid receptor. This approach is best attempted with the help of an addiction specialist because restarting the buprenorphine after the acute pain has resolved can precipitate withdrawal if not carefully managed. In general, buprenorphine should be restarted only when patients have mild withdrawal symptoms (not before) to prevent antagonistic effects at the μ-opioid receptor.

CONCLUSION

Many physicians find themselves apprehensive about treating pain in pregnant patients. Evaluation and treatment are limited by the relative contraindication of radiography in the workup and the risks associated with pharmacologic therapy during pregnancy. Nonetheless, familiarity with common pain problems, as well as the maternal and fetal risks associated with pain medications, can allow the pain physician help women achieve a more comfortable pregnancy. A single health care provider should be designated to coordinate the specialist evaluations and incorporate their suggestions into a single integrated plan of care.

KEY POINTS

- Medical management of pregnant patients should begin with attempts to minimize the use of all medications and use nonpharmacologic therapies whenever possible.
- The most critical period for minimizing maternal drug exposure is during early development, from conception through the 10th menstrual week of pregnancy
- Most breast milk is synthesized and excreted during and immediately following breastfeeding. Taking medications after breastfeeding or when the infant has the longest interval between feedings and avoidance of long-acting medications will minimize drug transfer via breast milk.
- There is no role for the routine use of nonsteroidal anti-inflammatory drugs (NSAIDs) for pain other than that related to rheumatologic disease or uterine fibroids.
- All NSAIDs used for pain should be discontinued by 34 weeks' gestation to prevent pulmonary hypertension in the newborn.
- All opioid analgesics are teratogenic risk category C *when used for a short time* and risk category D *when used for long periods* during pregnancy.
- For opioid-dependent parturients, buprenorphine has been found to be superior to methadone in reducing signs of withdrawal in newborns, thus requiring less medication and hospitalization time for the babies.
- Benzodiazepines should be avoided during organogenesis, near the time of delivery, and during lactation.
- Fifty percent of women will experience low back pain during their pregnancy, and it is commonly considered a normal part of pregnancy.
- Although the incidence of herniated nucleus pulposus during pregnancy is low, radicular symptoms are common and often accompany sacroiliac subluxation and myofascial pain syndromes.
- Migraine headaches rarely begin during pregnancy, but if they do, they typically occur during the first trimester.
- Patients suffering their first severe headache during pregnancy should be evaluated aggressively, and only when secondary causes of headache in pregnancy have been ruled out should primary headache be diagnosed in pregnant women.
- Postpartum headache is common and can occur in 30% to 40% of all women. Most occur in the first week, and about 50% of those who experience relief of their migraine during pregnancy have recurrence a short time after delivery.
- Vaso-occlusive crisis is the most common maternal complication noted in parturients with sickle cell hemoglobinopathies.
- Evaluation and treatment of parturients with pain are limited by the relative contraindication of radiography in the workup and the risks associated with pharmacologic therapy during pregnancy.

SUGGESTED READINGS

Alto W, O'Connor A. Management of women treated with buprenorphine during pregnancy. *Am J Obstet Gynecol.* 2011;205:302-308.

American Academy of Pediatrics Committee on Drugs. Transfer of drugs and other chemicals into human milk. *Pediatrics.* 1989;84:924-936.

Gutke A, Ostgaard H, Oberg B. Predicting persistent pregnancy related low back pain. *Spine.* 2008;33:386-393.

Jones H, Kaltenbach K, Heil S. Neonatal abstinence syndrome after methadone or buprenorphine exposure. *N Engl J Med.* 2010;363:2320-2330.

Kanakaris NK, Roberts CS, Giannoudis PV. Pregnancy related pelvic girdle pain: an update. *BMC Med.* 2011;9:15.

Martí-Carvajal AJ, Peña-Martí GE, Comunián-Carrasco G, et al. Interventions for treating painful sickle cell crisis during pregnancy. *Cochrane Database Syst Rev.* 2009;1:CD006786.

Mattick RP, Kimber J, Breen C, et al. Buprenorphine maintenance versus placebo or methadone maintenance for opioid dependence. *Cochrane Database Syst Rev.* 2008;2:CD002207.

Menon R, Bushnell C. Headache and pregnancy. *Neurologist.* 2008;14:108-119.

Nappi R, Albani F, Sances G, et al. Headaches during pregnancy. *Curr Pain Headache Rep.* 2011;15:289-294.

Ofori B, Oraichi D, Lais L, et al. Risk of congenital anomalies in pregnant users of non-steroidal anti-inflammatory drugs: a nested case-control study. *Birth Defects Res B Dev Reprod Toxicol.* 2006;77:268-279.

Ostensen M, Ostensen H. Safety of nonsteroidal antiinflammatory drugs in pregnant patients with rheumatic disease. *J Rheumatol.* 1995;23:1045-1049.

Rebordosa C, Kogevinas M, Horváth-Puho E, et al. Acetaminophen use during pregnancy: effects on risk of congenital abnormalities. *Am J Obstet Gynecol.* 2008;198:178:e1-e7.

Safra MJ, Oakley GP Jr. Association between cleft lip with and without cleft palate and prenatal exposure to diazepam. *Lancet.* 1975;2:47-80.

Vermani E, Mittal R, Weeks A. Pelvic girdle pain and low back pain in pregnancy: a review. *Pain Pract.* 2010;10:60-71.

Winder A, Johnson S, Murphey J, et al. Epidural analgesia for treatment of sickle cell crisis during pregnancy. *Obstet Gynecol.* 2011;118:495-497.

The references for this chapter can be found at www.expertconsult.com

PART 5

PHARMACOLOGIC, PSYCHOLOGICAL, AND PHYSICAL MEDICINE TREATMENTS

ROBERT W. HURLEY | DENNIS C. TURK, EDITORS

PART OUTLINE

Major Opioids and Chronic Opioid Therapy

36

Megan H. Cortazzo | David Copenhaver | Scott M. Fishman

Derivatives from the opium plant have been described as analgesics and used for pain control since 3500 BC. It was not until 1806 that a pure opioid substance was isolated. This substance was called "morphine," named after the Greek god Morpheus.[1] Since that time the opium plant has yielded other derivatives, and synthetic analogues of morphine have been produced for medicinal use. The use of opioid medications in the United States has fluctuated because of a variety of factors, including but not limited to production, availability, governmental regulation, and physician and societal attitudes. Over the last 20 years the prescribing pattern of opioids has escalated significantly for a number of reasons. The increased trend in prescription writing has been accompanied by a concordant rise in the incidence of diversion and abuse, as well as an increase in the incidence of complications, including overdose and death. Over the past decade, evidence for a sustained benefit of opioids in alleviating chronic pain has remained weak and inadequate, although evidence of risk associated with use of the drugs has clearly escalated. This change in which evidence of the efficacy of opioids has not changed whereas risk has increased should have a significant impact on treatment decisions based on risk-benefit analysis. The goal of this chapter is to review clinically relevant aspects of selected opioids, including side effects and pharmacology, and review current consensus on rational opioid prescribing.

GENERAL CONSIDERATIONS OF OPIOID ADMINISTRATION

OPIOID RECEPTORS

Multiple systems are involved in the modulation of pain perception, including the endogenous opioid system. The natural endogenous opioids include the endogenous peptides—β-endorphins, enkephalins, and dynorphins. Since the discovery of opioid receptors in the central nervous system (CNS) in 1973, the body of literature describing their function and location has grown immensely.[2,3] Opioid receptors have integral roles in the endogenous antinociceptive system and, accordingly, are located throughout the central and peripheral nervous systems. The best described opioid receptors are labeled mu (μ), kappa (κ), and delta (δ) and are prominently located in the CNS, particularly in the dorsal horn of the spinal cord,[4] as well as on dorsal root ganglia and peripheral nerves.[5,6] The three opioid receptors identified, μ, κ, and δ, belong to a superfamily of guanine (G) protein–coupled receptors located at presynaptic and postsynaptic sites in the CNS and peripheral tissues.[7]

The μ-opioid receptor modulates input from mechanical, chemical, and thermal stimuli at the supraspinal level. The κ receptor is similar to the μ receptor in that it influences thermal nociception but, in addition, it also modulates chemical visceral pain. The δ receptor influences mechanical and inflammatory pain.[8] An opioid agonist such as morphine binds with an opioid receptor to produce analgesia, as well as undesired side effects, such as respiratory depression and constipation, largely via interaction with the μ receptor. In a study using knockout mice that lacked the μ receptor, it was found that they have no response to morphine with respect to analgesia, respiratory depression, constipation, or physical dependence.[9]

DISTRIBUTION, METABOLISM, AND EXCRETION

The amount of opioid required to produce analgesia has significant interindividual variability. Factors responsible for this variability include opioid receptor individuality, as well as variations in opioid absorption and clearance. Such individual variability requires careful titration of an opioid to the desired response. The onset, duration, and intensity of analgesia depend on the delivery of drug to the target and on the length of time that the receptor is occupied. The number of receptors occupied and the length of time that the opioid activates its target receptor depend on the perfusion, plasma concentration, pH, and permeability coefficient of the drug.[10]

The metabolic pathway for each opioid is based on the molecular variables of the specific opioid. Opioids with hydroxyl groups, such as morphine and hydromorphone, undergo hepatic metabolism via uridine diphosphate glucuronosyltransferase (UGT) enzymes. UGT adds a glucuronic acid moiety to form glucuronide metabolites (hydromorphone 3-glucuronide [H3G], morphine 6-glucuronide [M6G], and morphine 3-glucuronide [M3G]). These metabolites are then excreted through the kidneys. Patients with renal impairment are particularly prone to deleterious effects from metabolite accumulation.[11]

The cytochrome P-450 (CYP) system contains two polymorphic isoforms that metabolize certain opioids. The first CYP isoform, responsible for the biotransformation of codeine, oxycodone, and hydrocodone, is 2D6. It is estimated that up to 10% of white individuals lack this enzyme, thus making them "poor metabolizers" of certain opioids and providing another cause for the high interindividual variability seen in patients treated with opioids.[11] The 3A4 isoform of the CYP system is involved in the biotransformation of fentanyl and methadone to their inactive forms.[12] Because some other drugs also interact with 3A4 isoenzymes, the metabolism of methadone and fentanyl can be problematically decelerated or accelerated. For example, macrolide antibiotics inhibit the enzyme, which decreases the clearance of methadone and fentanyl, whereas anticonvulsants such as phenytoin induce the activation of this enzyme system and increase the clearance of methadone and fentanyl.[13,14] Excretion of most opioid metabolites is via the kidneys, but some of the glucuronide conjugates are excreted in bile, and methadone is excreted primarily in feces.[11]

The study of pharmacogenomic polymorphisms is important in understanding the interindividual variability in analgesic effects. Opioid-related therapies have a multiplicity of genetic factors that influence the metabolism and clearance of specified opioids. As we look to the future, the use of regulator-approved pharmacogenomic assays may be advantageous in identifying many of these variant alleles. Understanding pharmacogenomic polymorphisms will most assuredly play a role in the everyday clinical decision making for management of acute and chronic pain. As safety and patient care benefit from detailed knowledge of specified polymorphisms, this science will most likely be incorporated into the standard of care for physicians.[15]

ADMINISTRATION

Multiple routes of administration are one of the many clinically useful characteristics of opioids. Administration can range from intrathecal, intravenous, or oral to rectal, sublingual, buccal, intranasal, or transdermal. Depending on the clinical situation, one route may be more advantageous than another. For example, a patient who requires continuous opioid delivery but is unable to take medications orally may benefit from a transdermal delivery system, such as is currently available in a transdermal patch containing fentanyl. Fentanyl is also available as a rapid-onset transmucosal delivery product. Neuraxial routes of opioid delivery are widely used in perioperative and postoperative care, as well as for terminally ill patients.

The goal of effective opioid therapy for chronic pain is to provide sustained analgesia over regular intervals.[16] This requires consideration of a number of factors, including knowledge of equianalgesic dosages between opioids and the pharmacologic properties and side effects of specific opioid agents. Pain in opioid-tolerant patients is particularly challenging because typical dosages for opioid-naïve patients do not apply and exact opioid requirements may require careful titration.

Whether fixed dosing is better than as-needed (PRN) dosing is controversial, with each method having advantages in particular situations. With fixed dosing there is consistent opioid delivery, which can theoretically reach steady-state levels.[17] Presumably, this avoids the peak-and-trough effect that can be associated with on-demand dosing and may prevent the delays in delivery that can occur with on-demand schedules. One problem for opioid-naïve patients who receive fixed doses of opioids that have longer half-lives is that they may experience excessive side effects or toxicity because of the difficulty in predicting the exact opioid requirement and potential accumulation. For example, morphine may take less than 24 hours to reach steady-state levels, whereas methadone can take up to 1 week. When there is a need to assess a patient's analgesia threshold, PRN dosing of an opioid with a short half-life may be used, or conservative fixed dosing of opioids that have a short half-life, supplemented by PRN "rescue" dosing, may be used.

Analgesic therapy with long-acting opioids (LAOs) offers convenient dose intervals that can attain safe, effective, steady-state levels. Several controlled-release opioids are available, including morphine (MS Contin, Oramorph SR, Kadian), oxycodone (OxyContin), fentanyl (Duragesic patch), and oxymorphone. Methadone can be used as an LAO, but it poses specific issues and concerns for clinicians distinct from those of other opioids (see later discussion). Methadone has a faster onset and longer analgesic effect than many other opioids do and may be ideal in some situations. However, these effects may also limit its use. Methadone is not specifically formulated for sustained release like other LAOs, which essentially release a short-acting opioid (SAO) throughout the drug's passage through the gastrointestinal (GI) tract. Methadone simply has an intrinsically longer plasma half-life than other typical opioids do, such as hydromorphone (Dilaudid) and morphine, and can therefore be advantageous in patients with GI motility issues such as short gut syndrome.

Although sustained- and immediate-release opioid preparations have made the oral route a practical option, some cancer patients are unable to tolerate oral delivery.[18] In such cases, transdermal, buccal, rectal, intravenous, or subcutaneous infusions are often a practical alternative option. With infusion, the first-pass effect is eliminated, thereby potentially offering some advantages. When compared with the oral route, there may be faster onset of analgesia with uncomplicated access. When compared with the intramuscular route, administration is often less painful and may be safer in patients with bleeding disorders or reduced muscle mass.

ADVERSE EFFECTS

The most commonly encountered side effects associated with opioids include constipation, nausea, vomiting, sedation, urinary retention, pruritus, and respiratory depression. Any of these side effects can significantly limit therapy, but tolerance to them usually ensues shortly after initiation of opioids. However, constipation is a major exception because it does not resolve with the prolonged use of opioids. Particular attention should be given to older adults and patients with hepatic or renal insufficiency. Tolerance and physical dependency are also commonly associated with opioid therapy. These are pharmacologic properties related to opioids that are frequently misinterpreted as indicators of addiction. Addiction is also a potential risk associated with opioid use (see later discussion). Physicians should anticipate any or all of these adverse effects, remain vigilant throughout therapy, and monitor patients closely, particularly when initiating therapy and escalating opioid doses.

CONSTIPATION

The most common side effect of opioid administration is constipation, and unfortunately, tolerance to it does not generally develop. Constipation can cause significant discomfort, nausea, and emesis. The underlying mechanism of opioid-induced constipation is thought to be decreased gastric motility related to opioid binding to highly concentrated opioid receptors located in the antrum of the stomach and the proximal part of the small bowel.[19,20] There is limited evidence that certain opioids at equianalgesic doses produce more or less constipation than others. Because the transdermal route bypasses initial exposure to the GI tract, transdermal fentanyl has been postulated to produce less constipation than orally administered opioids.[21-23] However, current data are not convincing, particularly since transdermal opioids are well known to result in significant constipation that requires aggressive laxative therapy, irrespective of whether they produce less constipation than oral agents do.

When initiating any opioid, it is important to prescribe medications to concomitantly maintain regular bowel motility. Treatment of opioid-induced constipation should include an active laxative such as senna, lactulose, or bisacodyl; passive agents such as stool softeners or fiber-based bulking agents may be ineffective because they rely on triggering gastric motility, which in the case of opioids is usually inhibited. Alternatively, use of an adjunctive agent with a side effect profile that includes diarrhea, such as misoprostol, can coexist well with constipating opioids. However, misoprostol should be used with caution in females of childbearing age because it can initiate uterine contractions and miscarriage.[24,25]

Methylnaltrexone, a quaternary derivative of naltrexone, contains a permanently charged tetravalent nitrogen atom and therefore cannot cross the blood-brain barrier.[26,27] Methylnaltrexone is an antagonist at the μ receptor. It blocks the peripheral actions of opioids while sparing their central analgesic effects and reverses the slowing of bowel motility that can often occur with opioid-related therapy. Methylnaltrexone was approved by the U.S. Food and Drug Administration (FDA) in 2008 as an indication for opioid-induced constipation. Alvimopan, which was also approved in 2008 by the FDA, functions as a peripherally acting μ-opioid antagonist with limited ability to cross the blood-brain barrier. Alvimopan can treat constipation without affecting analgesia or precipitating withdrawal. The primary indication for this medication is in patients to avoid postoperative ileus following partial large or small bowel resection with primary anastomosis.[26,27]

NAUSEA AND EMESIS

Nausea and vomiting are frequently seen in patients who take opioids, but it is usually a transient side effect that often only lasts 2 to 3 days. The underlying mechanism of nausea and vomiting appears to be related to several causative factors. One is activation of receptors in the brainstem site that produces afferent input to the medullary chemoreceptor trigger zone, which is responsible for afferent input to the emetic center of the brain. These areas are dense in neurotransmitter receptors that correspond to the antiemetic agents used clinically. A potential cause of nausea is stimulation of receptors in the vestibular apparatus.[28,29] Another underappreciated cause of opioid-related nausea is constipation, which will often respond to treatments that increase motility.

In evaluating a patient who reports nausea and vomiting while taking opioids, one should determine important history-related factors involved in the genesis of nausea, such as the time of the last bowel movement, whether it worsens with movement, or whether there is a temporal relationship between opioid ingestion and the onset of nausea. The choice of antiemetic agent depends on the historical aspects surrounding the reported side effect. Patients who experience nausea when they are more ambulatory may be more likely to have vestibule-related nausea. In such cases, drugs such as meclizine, promethazine, or scopolamine may be useful in relieving this type of induced nausea. Droperidol, prochlorperazine, ondansetron, or hydroxyzine may have greater benefit for nausea that is not associated with movement, a type of nausea thought to be related to chemoreceptor trigger zone–associated activation.[30,31] One should also ensure that reversible metabolic causes, intracranial pathology, or other factors such as medications are not the origin of the nausea or emesis before it is attributed solely to opioids.

Several approaches can be taken when treating opioid-induced nausea and vomiting. An antiemetic may be added, often choosing an agent that offers secondary benefits such as promotility, sedative, antipruritic, anxiolytic, or antipsychotic effects, depending on the needs of the individual patient. Another option to reduce the frequency and severity of side effects is to decrease the opioid dose to the minimum acceptable dose that will still achieve adequate analgesia. Based on the observation that tolerance to opioid-induced nausea accrues rapidly, the dose that had previously been reduced may be titrated upward slowly to increase analgesia without inducing nausea. If the nausea is protracted, one may consider changing to a different opioid. The emetogenic response to opioids is idiosyncratic, and therefore a different opioid may not produce nausea.[32]

PRURITUS

Opioid-induced pruritus occurs more frequently with opioids delivered by the intravenous or neuraxial route than with oral administration. Tolerance to pruritus usually develops fairly quickly, but in rare cases it can be more persistent. The underlying mechanism of pruritus appears to be related to release of histamine, which activates C-fiber itch receptors on C fibers that are distinct from pain-transmitting C fibers. Clinically, pruritus is often limited to the face and perineum but can become generalized and severe. Treatment includes antihistamines, but the therapeutic effect may be related more to sedation than to a direct antihistaminergic effect.[32] In patients receiving intrathecal or intravenous morphine who have significant pruritus that is unresponsive to antihistamines, low dosages of nalbuphine, a μ-receptor antagonist and κ-receptor agonist, may effectively reduce pruritus without reversing the analgesia.[33,34]

SEDATION

Opioid-naïve patients or those chronically taking opioids who are undergoing dose escalation often experience sedation and drowsiness. Sedation is usually temporary as patients accommodate to the new medication or new dose, and it has been demonstrated that patients maintained on a stable dose of opioids for 7 days rarely have psychomotor impairment.[35-37] The importance of this fact cannot be overemphasized because patients are increasingly being prescribed opioids for cancer- and non–cancer-related pain. Patients and others may question whether it is safe to operate a motor vehicle while taking opioids. This is a controversial issue, and strong arguments can be made on both sides. Some physicians may recommend taking no precautions, whereas others may counsel their patients to never drive while taking opioids. Emerging evidence is not completely clear on this issue, but some studies have suggested that patients managed with long-term opioid therapy may be alert enough to drive safely.[38,39] However, it seems prudent to restrict driving, at least for 1 week or longer at the onset or with dose escalation of an opioid regimen.

Sedation that persists despite an adequate adjustment period to the opioid dose can become as problematic as the pain itself. In such cases, lowering the dose of opioid to the minimal acceptable analgesic level, increasing (widening) the dosing interval, or changing to another opioid that may not be as sedating may be considered.[32] It is important to consider additional causes of sedation such as other medications (e.g., benzodiazepines, antiemetics, tricyclics, muscle relaxants), renal or hepatic dysfunction leading to accumulation, or progression of the patient's primary disease state itself. If the sedation is thought to be secondary to accumulating levels of the drug or its metabolites, changing to a different agent that is not as dependent on renal clearance or does not have active metabolites, such as fentanyl, may reduce the sedation. In patients with continued unremitting sedation after limiting CNS depressants, attempting opioid dose reduction, and excluding all other underlying causes, psychostimulants may be useful (e.g., amphetamines, modafinil).

RESPIRATORY DEPRESSION

One of the most serious concerns and feared complications of opioid prescribing is respiratory depression. The underlying mechanism of respiratory depression is μ-receptor–induced depression of brainstem centers that subserve respiratory drive.[40] It has long been recognized that depressed respiratory drive may occur more rapidly in patients who have received combined intrathecal-epidural and oral or intravenous opioids. Although there is minimal evidence to support this claim, recognizing that this is a possible risk often supports an acceptable risk management–oriented approach to opioid administration. In addition, combining opioids with other sedating drugs can hasten respiratory depression. This is particularly important in view of the escalating rates of unintended overdose deaths associated with opioids, many involving multiple drugs that include additional respiratory depressants such as benzodiazepines. Clinically, the patient manifests sedation as the first sign of respiratory depression, which can pose a problem in detection during the evening hours when the patient is sleeping. Because respiratory depression can occur after the administration of epidural and intrathecal opioids and is often delayed and does not appear until approximately 12 hours after injection, the signs of sedation may be lost during sleep. Therefore, it is advisable to use alarmed pulse oximetry in patients in whom clinical suspicion is warranted.[32]

Pain is a powerful physiologic stimulant of respiratory drive and opposes the respiratory depressant effects of opioids. In patients in whom pain relief is anticipated from a nonopioid analgesic treatment (e.g., neurolytic procedure, radiation therapy, adjuvant analgesics, surgery), a reduction in opioid dose may be required.[40]

If a patient cannot be aroused and opioid-induced respiratory depression is suspected, the specific opioid receptor antagonist naloxone should be administered. Care must be taken when giving naloxone to patients who have been taking opioids for longer than 1 week or to older adult patients because severe withdrawal symptoms, seizures, and severe pain can be induced. Administration of naloxone has also led to congestive heart failure in susceptible patients. Naloxone is often packaged in an ampule containing 0.4 mg, which can then be diluted in 10 mL of normal saline and administered as 0.5-mL boluses (0.02 mg/0.5 mL) every 2 minutes.[40]

OPIOIDS AND IMMUNOLOGIC EFFECTS

Opioids have been suggested to play a role in the incidence of infection in heroin addicts and act as a contributing factor in the pathogenesis of human immunodeficiency virus.[27,41,42] Of note, despite the suggestion that exogenous opioids may cause immunosuppression, endogenous opioids such as endorphins promote immunoactivation.[27] Inhibitory effects on antibody and cellular immune responses, natural killer cell activity, cytokine expression, and phagocytic activity have all been implicated with acute and chronic opioid administration.[27,41] Furthermore, it has been noted that peripheral immune cells express opioid receptors and this allows intricate communication between cells and cytokines.[27,41] Opioid-induced alteration of immune function can be categorized into central and peripheral components. It has been postulated that central opioid receptors mediate peripheral immunosuppression via the hypothalamic-pituitary-adrenal axis and autonomic nervous system.[27,41,42] Interestingly, severe chronic pain in and of itself has been suggested to be associated with a reduction in immune function.[27,41,42]

OPIOIDS AND HORMONAL CHANGES

The oral, intravenous, and intrathecal routes of administration of chronic opioid therapy have been well described to alter hormonal effects in both men and women.[27] Mendelson and colleagues found that in illicit drug users, serum hormones that were altered by opioid administration subsequently returned to normal following suspension of the drug.[43] Hormones disrupted by opioids are not relegated to testosterone (both total and free) but also include estrogen (estradiol), luteinizing hormone, gonadotropin-releasing hormone, dehydroepiandrosterone, adrenocorticotropin, corticotropin-releasing hormone, and cortisol.[27,44-48] Opioid-related endocrinology research focuses on androgen hormones because of the well-described symptomatic side effects. Sexual dysfunction (erectile dysfunction, decreased libido), depression, and fatigue are some of the many side effects that men may experience when prescribed chronic opioid therapy.[27,44,45] Many of the aforementioned side effects have been correlated with hypogonadism. Symptoms such as depression and sexual dysfunction are not relegated just to men; women can experience such side effects as well.[27,44,45] Women also experience dysmenorrhea and potentially reduced bone mineral density. Testosterone levels likewise appear to be reduced in women and may have some correlation with body mass index.[27,44-47]

OPIOID-INDUCED SLEEP DISTURBANCES

A considerable amount of study on the effects of chronic opioid therapy on sleep is still needed. Despite the paucity of data, some research suggests that opioids increase the number of shifts in sleep-waking states and reduce total sleep time, sleep efficiency, delta sleep, and rapid eye movement (REM) sleep.[27,49-51] In various studies it is difficult to separate the effect of opioids on sleep from those of comorbid condition (e.g., cancer, addiction or dependence, postoperative pain). Research suggests that γ-aminobutyric acid (GABAergic) signaling via inhibition of acetylcholine release in the medial pontine reticular formation is the primary focus for disruption of sleep by opioids.[27,49-51] Morphine has been demonstrated to reduce REM sleep. The resulting disruption in sleep architecture affects the state of arousal during wakefulness.[27,49-51]

OPIOID TOLERANCE AND PHYSICAL DEPENDENCE

There are substantial differences that distinguish tolerance, dependence, and addiction from each other. Unfortunately, these concepts are frequently misunderstood. In 2001, the American Pain Society, American Academy of Pain Medicine, and American Society of Addiction Medicine approved definitions of addiction, physical dependence, and tolerance in the hope of reducing misguided treatment of patients who require opioids for pain treatment. In a patient who is chronically administered opioids, it should be anticipated that physical dependence and tolerance will develop, but the maladaptive changes in behavior witnessed in patients with addiction (see later discussion) should not necessarily follow.[52]

TOLERANCE

The term *opioid tolerance* is often used to describe the phenomenon that occurs when a fixed dose of an opioid results in decreasing analgesia, thus requiring higher doses of medication to achieve the same or less effect over time.[32] The mechanisms responsible for this phenomenon are not entirely understood, but the *N*-methyl-D-aspartate (NMDA) receptor has been demonstrated to be involved.[53,54] The clinical usefulness of NMDA receptor involvement has yet to be determined fully, but nonhuman studies have continued to promulgate the potential for using NMDA receptor antagonists in conjunction with opioids to attenuate tolerance and physical dependence.[55,56] A subpopulation of dorsal horn neurons expressing NMDA receptors and treated with high-dose morphine have been shown to have enhanced NMDA receptor–mediated activity.[55] Furthermore, μ-receptor antagonist and NMDA receptor antagonist treatment of this subpopulation has attenuated the increased activity.[55] Another study has demonstrated that in "morphine-tolerant" rats treated with an NMDA receptor antagonist, the morphine-induced tolerance reversed.[56] The relevance of these findings at the bedside have, to date, not been clear.

Human studies on the effect of the NMDA receptor on tolerance have been less promising. There has been great hope that NMDA receptor antagonists such as ketamine or dextromethorphan might potentiate the analgesic effect of opioids, but not much convincing evidence has emerged from replicated trials.[57,58] In a double-blind controlled clinical trial comparing morphine and a combination of morphine and dextromethorphan, statistical differences in analgesia or dose were not seen between groups.[59] Nonetheless, basic concepts continue to support the understanding that the NMDA receptor is a key component in the development of opioid-induced tolerance. In particular, ketamine continues to be a drug of major interest because of its potential to improve opioid performance through preventing tolerance and enhancing opioid-induced analgesia.[60-62]

When it is suspected that a patient has become tolerant to one medication, the cause may be opioid tolerance, but it may also relate to increased pain, which requires adjustment in dosing. The need for dose escalation in a patient treated with chronic opioids should always stimulate consideration that the underlying disease may be progressing. When opioid-induced tolerance is present, opioid rotation can be performed. This is based on the clinical observation that patients often have intraindividual analgesic responses to different opioids and that improved analgesia with fewer side effects may occur when a different opioid is used.[63] Although the full mechanism of this phenomenon is not completely understood, it is usually thought to occur because of incomplete tolerance, possibly related to differing μ-opioid and other opioid receptor affinities of one opioid versus another. When opioid rotation is performed in an opioid-tolerant as opposed to an opioid-naïve patient, equal analgesic doses may not be necessary. The patient may respond with analgesia to half the equianalgesic dose, and if not, the dose may be titrated to an adequate analgesic effect that is less than would be expected by calculation of equianalgesic conversion from standard formulas. This is a potentially useful phenomenon whereby the overall opioid requirement of the patient may be reduced, thereby achieving an opioid-sparing effect.

PHYSICAL DEPENDENCE AND WITHDRAWAL

Physical dependence is a physiologic state that occurs when a medication is abruptly stopped and a withdrawal syndrome results. It is *not* synonymous with addiction. This separation of physical dependence and addiction is supported by evidence of two distinct anatomic areas within the CNS that are involved in physical dependence versus addiction. Noradrenergic neurons within the locus coeruleus are implicated in the maintenance of dependence and development of withdrawal, whereas the ventral tegmental dopaminergic area and orbitofrontal glutamatergic projections to the nucleus accumbens are particularly thought to subserve addiction.[60,64] It has been shown that drugs of abuse such as heroin, cocaine, nicotine, alcohol, phencyclidine, and cannabis initiate their habit-forming actions by activating a common reward pathway in the brain.[65] There is also evidence for the involvement of noradrenergic neurons in the development of withdrawal. Not only do norepinephrine levels change in the brain following opioid dependence, but the administration of an α_2-agonist such as clonidine or a β-antagonist such as propranolol also attenuates many of the symptoms of opioid withdrawal but does not reverse addiction.[66]

The clinical manifestations of opioid withdrawal usually begin with irritability, anxiety, insomnia, diaphoresis, yawning, rhinorrhea, and lacrimation. If it progresses without intervention, a flu-like condition develops, with chills, myalgia, fever, abdominal cramping, nausea, diarrhea, tachycardia, and other features of a heightened adrenergic state occurring. Though uncomfortable for patients, it is self-limited and lasts approximately 3 to 7 days. Opioid withdrawal may occur in patients who abruptly discontinue opioids or who have relative discontinuation because of taking SAOs after accommodating to the longer plasma half-life of LAOs.[32]

It is usually possible to taper patients from opioids to prevent withdrawal symptoms. Although faster tapering can be accomplished without the advent of withdrawal symptoms, if time allows, few patients will be symptomatic if the dose is decreased by 10% to 20% every 48 to 72 hours over a prolonged period (usually 2 to 3 weeks, depending on the dose).[67] If, however, symptoms of withdrawal develop during discontinuation or taper, clonidine, 0.2 to 0.4 mg/day, may be used to decrease discomfort.[68] Clonidine is often maintained for 4 days during taper of an SAO and for 14 days during taper of an LAO. Once opioids have been discontinued, clonidine can be tapered over a period of approximately 1 week.[32]

ADDICTION

Opioids are associated with addiction at a rate that is high enough to be a significant concern; however, the exact rate of addiction as a result of therapeutic opioid use is controversial. Opioid addiction is a disorder characterized by opioid use that results in physical, psychological, or social dysfunction (or a combination of these), as well as continued use of the opioid despite the dysfunction. Neurobiologic evidence has suggested that this phenomenon may be subserved by positive reinforcement and sensitization of the dopaminergic system in the brain, which may explain the continued seeking of a substance destructive to the patient's life.[69] Patients who are receiving an inadequate dose of opioid medication may engage in drug-seeking behavior to obtain more pain medication for relief of pain, which can be mistaken for the drug-seeking behavior associated with addiction. Physicians are often challenged to distinguish true addiction from undertreated pain because on the surface, undertreated pain may appear similar to addiction because of features such as drug seeking and self-escalation. However, unlike addiction, with increased doses of opioids, an undertreated patient experiences pain relief and improved function. Whereas undertreated pain should resolve when the patient obtains adequate analgesia, true addictive behavior does not. Addiction exists in direct contradistinction to what is seen in a patient with undertreated pain who goes through dose escalation. With opioid addiction, the aberrant behavior not only continues despite an increase in opioid but is also usually further stimulated and promoted by increased exposure to the addicting drug. It is difficult to make a prospective diagnosis of addiction because there is no single behavior or diagnostic test that can confirm the diagnosis. The Committee on Pain of the American Society of Addiction Medicine has defined addiction in the context of pain treatment with opioids as a persistent pattern of dysfunctional opioid use.[70] Patient behavior may be used cumulatively to support the diagnosis of addiction, but absolute conclusions cannot always be made, particularly without longitudinal information over extended periods. Many types of behavior may indicate the possibility of addiction to some degree (Box 36.1).

Nonadherence to opioid therapy may be related to many possibilities, including adverse effects, forgetfulness, incompatibility with lifestyle, and confusion about the drug regimen. It may rarely be related to aberrant behavior such as diversion or drug abuse, and an astute physician will maintain a position of vigilance without feeling compelled to reach immediate conclusions. If a physician chooses to pursue pain treatment with an abusable drug in a patient at risk for addiction, collaboration with an addiction specialist or addiction psychiatrist is advised to ensure that the necessary resources to support an appropriate risk management program are available. Such resources are usually far greater than those available to the average prescriber, and without the necessary resources to ensure safety, prescribing should not begin. As always, high vigilance and tempered judgment are required.

The prevalence of addiction, abuse, or dependence in patients with chronic pain is not known exactly but is

Box 36.1 Aberrant Behavior Indicative of Addiction

Behavior *Less* Indicative of Addiction

Expresses anxiety or desperation over recurrent symptoms
Hoards medications
Takes someone else's pain medications
Aggressively complains to the physician for more drugs
Requests a specific drug or medication
Uses more opioids than recommended
Drinks more alcohol when in pain
Expresses worry over changing to a new drug, even if it offers potentially fewer side effects
Takes (with permission) someone else's prescription opioids
Raises the dose of opioids on one's own
Expresses concern to the physician or family members that pain might lead to the use of street drugs
Asks for a second opinion about pain medications
Smokes cigarettes to relieve pain
Has used opioids to treat other symptoms

Behavior *More* Indicative of Addiction

Buys pain medications from a street dealer
Steals money to obtain drugs
Tries to get opioids from more than one source
Performs sex for drugs
Sees two physicians at once without them knowing
Performs sex for money to buy drugs
Steals drugs from others
Prostitutes others for money to obtain drugs
Prostitutes others for drugs
Forges prescriptions
Sells prescription drugs

From Passik SD, Kirsh KL, Donaghy KB, et al. Pain and aberrant drug-related behaviors in medically ill patients with and without histories of substance abuse. *Clin J Pain*. 2006;22:173-181.

estimated to range from 3% to 19%.[71] Treating chronic pain in a person with a history of addiction is challenging but is not an absolute contraindication. Nonetheless, responsible prescribers of opioids must ensure that the appropriate resources for safe use are in place before initiating treatment. If appropriate risk management is not available, treatment should not be started. Moreover, treatment should not be started unless it can be terminated when necessary.

Although a low percentage of the population with chronic pain appears to have an addiction problem, the remainder of the population has been shown to receive suboptimal analgesia because of prescribers' fears of patient misuse of the opioid.[72] A growing debate has emerged that focuses on understanding how opioids should be used in the setting of substantial rates of chronic pain while balancing the imperative for vigilant use of opioids with sufficient risk management for acceptable safety.

SELECTED OPIOIDS

Although therapeutic options to provide analgesia continue to emerge, opioids remain the "gold standard" of currently available analgesics. Despite the widespread use of opioids for the treatment of acute and chronic pain, controversy exists over whether opioids should be used for the treatment of chronic nonmalignant pain. There are proponents on each side of the controversy, and part of the fear of prescribing opioids stems from an inaccurate understanding of appropriate outcomes for prescribing opioids and the risk for abuse or side effects. Although opioids can be a useful tool to provide adequate analgesia for patients, fear of the development of addiction, dependence, or untoward side effects often precludes physicians from prescribing opioids.[73] If it is decided to initiate opioid therapy in patients with chronic nonmalignant pain, the decision should be based on a well–thought-out rationale for treatment, with clear end points in mind.

SAOs are generally used for acute pain, whereas LAOs are prescribed for patients with chronic pain syndromes. Because SAOs have relatively brief peak serum blood levels of active analgesic metabolites, using them to treat persistent baseline chronic pain will require frequent dosing. This roller coaster effect is thought to promote nonoptimal pain-related behavior, which is why LAOs have been considered more appropriate in such cases. However, science has not clearly demonstrated such an advantage.

SAOs are often combined with other analgesics such as acetaminophen, nonsteroidal anti-inflammatory drugs (NSAIDs), or aspirin, which may offer drug-sparing effects because less medication may be used. Although combination opioids may help reduce potential opioid-related side effects and toxicity, there is a potential for harm to major organs from the nonopioid components (e.g., acetaminophen, NSAIDs, aspirin). When using combination opioids, physicians must be aware of renal and liver function problems, as well as the potential harm that could occur to the GI system. Patients must be educated about the risks of taking other analgesics such as acetaminophen, NSAIDs, and aspirin in conjunction with the combination opioids. Moreover, physicians must also consider that the compounded nonopioid drug is likely to have a ceiling effect beyond which it is no longer efficacious. Because opioids induce tolerance and have no ceiling effect, the pharmacologically appropriate need for increased opioid may inadvertently push the dose of a combination drug to appropriate levels of the opioid component but to toxic levels of the nonopioid agent. Although reviewing all available opioids is beyond the scope of this chapter, we will review the most commonly used opioids for pain management. Minor opioids such as hydrocodone are discussed in Chapter 37.

CODEINE

Codeine is an alkaloid found in very low concentrations in opium; it is now derived from morphine. Codeine is frequently administered in combination with acetaminophen, butalbital, and caffeine.[68] It has been shown to be an effective analgesic for chronic nonmalignant pain, but with limitations.[74] It is a weak μ-opioid agonist and has a half-life of 2.5 to 3 hours. The major metabolic pathway leads to glucuronidation of codeine to codeine 6-glucuronide, with a minor metabolic pathway catalyzed by the polymorphically expressed enzyme CYP2D6 through *N*-demethylation of codeine to norcodeine and *O*-demethylation of codeine to morphine.[10] Evidence has suggested that the analgesic effects of codeine rely on its conversion to morphine, and patients with genetic variations in the enzymes needed to make this conversion may find codeine to be less effective.[75] The genetic polymorphism of CYP2D6 is responsible for the variable response to the medication. Patients with the genotype CYP2D6 PM (poor metabolizers) do not achieve adequate analgesia with codeine. In addition, certain medications that inhibit CYP2D6, such as quinidine, paroxetine, fluoxetine, and bupropion, can alter the phenotype of normal patients with normal genetics and thus decrease the therapeutic analgesic effect of codeine.[76] Urinary excretory products of codeine include codeine (70%), norcodeine (10%), morphine (10%), normorphine (4%), and hydrocodone (1%).[68] This may be important to remember when interpreting the urine toxicology screens of patients taking codeine.

MORPHINE

Morphine, a hydrophilic phenanthrene derivative, is the prototypical opioid against which all other opioids are compared for equianalgesic potency. Because of its hydrophilic nature, it exhibits delayed transport across the blood-brain barrier, thus delaying its onset of action. Conversely, it has a longer duration of action, 4 to 5 hours, than its plasma half-life of 2 to 3 hours.[25] Metabolism of morphine to its two major metabolites, M6G and M3G, occurs mainly in the liver (see Table 36.1). Although the parent compound produces analgesia and side effects, M6G may also produce some analgesia along with some adverse effects. M6G accounts for 5% to 15% of morphine's metabolites and is a μ- and δ-agonist, which accounts for its analgesic effects. It has been demonstrated that M6G does not exert antinociceptive effects in knockout mice lacking the μ receptor.[77]

M3G, which accounts for 50% of morphine's metabolites, does not appear to possess opioid agonism but may produce effects that oppose morphine's analgesic actions, such as allodynia, hyperalgesia, myoclonus, and seizures.[10] Oral administration of morphine has been shown to result

Table 36.1 Selected Opioids: Oral Bioavailability, Half-Lives, Duration of Action, and Metabolites

Opioid	Availability (%)	Half-Life (hr)	Duration of Action (hr)	Metabolites
Morphine	10-45	2-3	4-5	M6G, M3G
Oxycodone (OxyContin)	60-80	4.5	12	Oxymorphone, noroxycodone
Methadone	60-95	8-80 (average, 27)	6-8	—
Hydromorphone	24	2.3	3-4	H3G
Oxymorphone (Opana ER)	10	9 ± 3	12	O3G, 6-hydroxyoxymorphone

H3G, hydromorphone 3-glucuronide; M3G, morphine 3-glucuronide; M6G, morphine 6-glucuronide; O3G: oxymorphone 3-glucuronide.

in higher levels of M3G and M6G than achieved with the intravenous, intramuscular, or rectal routes, which bypass hepatic metabolism.[78] Chronic administration of morphine ultimately results in higher circulating levels of M3G and M6G metabolites than the parent compound.[79] It has been found that patients receiving chronically high morphine doses metabolize morphine to hydromorphone and test positive for hydromorphone on urine toxicology screens.[80] This is of critical importance in patients using morphine for chronic pain who undergo urine drug screening.

Although extrahepatic metabolism of morphine has been shown to occur in gastric and intestinal epithelia, morphine should be used with caution in patients with decreased hepatic function, such as those with cirrhosis.[10] In addition, glucuronides have been shown to undergo deconjugation back to the parent compound by colonic flora and to be reabsorbed as morphine.[10] Morphine metabolites are excreted by the kidneys, so caution should also be taken when prescribing morphine to patients with renal impairment because accumulation of M6G and M3G can be toxic. Currently available forms of morphine include short- and long-acting preparations. Short-acting agents may be compounded for almost any route of administration, and long-acting preparations generally use specialized sustained-release matrix technology, such as found in MS Contin, Kadian, Oramorph SR, and Avinza.

OXYCODONE

Oxycodone is a semisynthetic opioid that is closely related to morphine. It has been available for analgesia since 1917, when it was introduced into clinical practice in Germany.[81] It is processed from thebaine, an organic compound found in opium. Like morphine, currently available forms of oxycodone include short- and long-acting preparations. Short-acting oxycodone may be used alone (e.g., Roxicodone) or may be compounded with acetaminophen (e.g., Percocet, Roxicet, Endocet) or aspirin (e.g., Percodan). Long-acting oxycodone preparations are designed for oral administration and involve the use of specialized sustained-release technology (e.g., OxyContin and similar generics).

Oxycodone has high bioavailability, 60%, when compared with morphine, which has a bioavailability of 33%, thus making oxycodone almost twice as potent as morphine.[68] Oxycodone is a prodrug that undergoes hepatic metabolism via the CYP2D6 isoenzyme, whereby it is converted into its active metabolite oxymorphone, a μ-opioid agonist, and its inactive metabolite noroxycodone. Oxymorphone is reportedly often undetectable and is 14 times more potent than the parent compound.

Similar to codeine, there is genetic polymorphism in 10% of the population, which accounts for significant variation in the metabolism of oxycodone. This variation explains why some patients require higher than usual doses of oxycodone to achieve analgesia. Another factor to be considered when prescribing oxycodone is whether other potential competitors of the CYP2D6 isoenzyme are being prescribed. Such interacting medications include neuroleptics, tricyclic antidepressants, and selective serotonin reuptake inhibitors (SSRIs). Cases of serotonin syndrome have been described in the literature when SSRIs and oxycodone were used concomitantly.[81,82]

MEPERIDINE

The use of meperidine for analgesia has been declining recently because of its potential for neurotoxicity. It is a weaker μ-opioid agonist than morphine with 10% of its potency, more rapid onset, and a shorter duration of action.[79] The half-life of meperidine is 3 hours, and it is hepatically demethylated to its neurotoxic metabolite normeperidine, which has a half-life of 12 to 16 hours. Normeperidine has been well documented to cause CNS hyperactivity and seizures.[25] Excretion of normeperidine is via the kidneys; therefore, caution should be taken when administering meperidine to patients with renal impairment or those prone to CNS hyperactivity. Initially, the toxic effects may be seen as subtle changes in mood that can progress to naloxone-irreversible tremors, myoclonus, and seizures. Chronic administration of meperidine to patients with normal renal function and administration of meperidine in conjunction with SSRIs, monoamine oxidase inhibitors, tramadol, and methadone can also result in neurotoxic side effects.[79]

HYDROMORPHONE

Hydromorphone has strong affinity for the μ receptor. It is a hydrogenated ketone analogue of morphine and can be formed by *N*-demethylation of hydrocodone.[83] Hydromorphone is similar to morphine in that it is hydrophilic and has a comparable duration of analgesia, but it differs with respect to side effects and potency. Pruritus, sedation, nausea, and vomiting occur less frequently. Furthermore, hydromorphone is five times more potent than morphine

Table 36.2 Equianalgesic Doses of Opioids

Opioid	Oral Equianalgesic Dose (mg)
Buprenorphine	0.3
Oxymorphone	1.5
Butorphanol	2
Hydromorphone	2
Oxycodone	7
Hydrocodone	10
Morphine	10
Methadone	10-20
Tramadol	40
Propoxyphene	43-45
Codeine	80
Meperidine	100

when administered orally (see Table 36.2) and seven times more potent when administered parenterally. Though essentially hydrophilic, it is 10 times more lipophilic than morphine. This lipophilicity may be an advantage when treating patients who are unable to take oral medications and cannot maintain intravenous access, such as is in hospice environments. It can be given subcutaneously at a dose of 10 or 20 mg/mL; this route delivers approximately 80% of the dose absorbed through intravenous delivery.[83] The onset of analgesia occurs in 30 minutes after oral administration and 5 minutes after intravenous administration, with peak analgesic effects occurring within 8 to 20 minutes.[84]

Hydromorphone is metabolized in the liver to H3G and, like its parent compound, is excreted renally. Similar to M3G, H3G lacks analgesic effect but may be an active metabolite that potentiates neurotoxic effects such as allodynia, myoclonus, and seizures.[10] Production of H3G is relatively low, so the risk for neurotoxic side effects is relatively low, except in patients with renal insufficiency, in whom H3G may accumulate.[79]

FENTANYL

Fentanyl is a highly lipophilic agent with high affinity for the μ-opioid receptor. It is 75 to 125 times more potent than morphine and has a faster onset of action.[79] Because of its higher potency, smaller quantities of the medication can be delivered to the patient relative to other opioids. Even though fentanyl is considered to be a short-acting medication, its lipophilic nature allows long-acting transdermal and very rapid-onset transmucosal administration for the treatment of chronic and acute pain, respectively.[79] Although there are other minor pathways, fentanyl undergoes hepatic biotransformation via CYP3A4 *N*-dealkylation to norfentanyl. Its half-life and onset of action vary greatly by route of administration. (Transmucosal fentanyl undergoes first-pass metabolism and has an onset of action within 5 to 10 minutes.)

A transdermal fentanyl patch is used by some patients with chronic pain or with pain related to cancer. Transdermal fentanyl has been used for acute postoperative pain but may be associated with hypoventilation.[85] Transdermal patches are typically placed on a hairless part of the body that is flat and free of any defects that could interfere with adherence of the patch. Patients should be advised to avoid submerging the patch in hot water or placing a heating pad over the area because this influences absorption. Patients report local skin erythema or irritation as the most common side effect.[86]

Transdermal fentanyl is an alternative choice for patients who have significant GI issues, such as persistent emesis, chronic nausea, or "short gut" syndrome, or for those believed to be at risk of diverting oral medications. Use of the patch offers the opportunity to have patients return the old patches for inspection at the time of prescription refill. Theoretically, transdermal delivery may induce less constipation than oral opioids because it avoids direct exposure to the GI tract, but this is questionable in light of the common finding of significant constipation in almost all who use transdermal opioids.

Unlike other LAOs, transdermal fentanyl may be challenging to titrate because of variation in individual patient characteristics, such as skin perspiration, skin temperature, fat stores, and muscle bulk.[10] The rate of achieving therapeutic serum levels can be variable (ranging from 1 to 30 hours with a mean of 13 hours). Because of the wide variation in reaching therapeutic levels, a short-acting oral analgesic or intravenous patient-controlled analgesia may be necessary to address breakthrough pain while the transdermal opioid effect is ramping up or to prevent withdrawal symptoms if rotation from another opioid has occurred. Achieving steady-state levels may require up to 6 days, and the amount of SAO needed after a steady state is attained will help determine whether the dose of fentanyl must be increased.[10] If the patch is removed, however, it may take up to 16 hours for serum fentanyl concentrations to drop by 50%.

Oral transmucosal fentanyl has a more rapid onset of analgesia than do other SAOs and offers some special advantages. Because it is transmucosal, it avoids the GI tract and first-pass hepatic metabolism and has a rapid onset of action, within 10 to 15 minutes. One study compared intravenous morphine with transmucosal fentanyl in an acute postoperative setting and demonstrated similar onset of analgesia.[87] Transmucosal fentanyl can be beneficial for patients with acute breakthrough pain. To date, a major limitation in using this route has been cost.

METHADONE

Methadone may be an attractive choice for analgesia because of several of its unique properties, but it also has many features distinguishing it from other opioids that have raised its potential for adverse outcomes. Recently, methadone has become the most common opioid found to be related to unintended overdose deaths in the United States. Thus, the need for caution with this drug should be self-evident. On the positive side of the methadone risk-benefit profile, its attributes include no known neurotoxic or active metabolites, high absorption and bioavailability, and multiple receptor activities, including μ- and δ-opioid agonism, NMDA antagonism, and serotonin reuptake blockade. Methadone has been shown to have a bioavailability that is approximately threefold that of morphine.[88,89] In patients who require high-dose LAOs, methadone appears to be a theoretical second-line choice despite of the lack of accumulation of neurotoxic metabolites that induce myoclonus, hallucinations, seizures, sedation, and confusion.

Unfortunately, it is methadone's unique pharmacokinetics and pharmacodynamics that render its effects somewhat unpredictable.

Methadone is structurally unrelated to other opioid-derived alkaloids. It is a racemic mixture of two enantiomers, the D isomer (*S*-methadone) and L isomer (*R*-methadone). *R*-Methadone accounts for its opioid receptor affinity and thus its opioid effect. Animal studies have demonstrated that methadone has lower affinity than morphine for the μ receptor.[90] This may explain why methadone may have fewer μ-opioid–related side effects than morphine. Methadone, however, has higher affinity for the δ receptor than morphine does.[91]

Methadone has a slow but variable elimination half-life that averages approximately 27 hours, which may be related to its lipophilicity and extensive tissue distribution.[89] The delayed clearance of methadone is the basis for its use in maintenance therapy. Surprisingly, although methadone may be efficacious for purposes of opioid maintenance therapy since it potentially prevents withdrawal symptoms for 24 hours or longer, its analgesic half-life is shorter than 24 hours, usually found to range from 6 to 8 hours. This discrepancy is related to its biphasic elimination. The alpha elimination phase lasts 8 to 12 hours and correlates with the period of analgesia, which lasts approximately 6 to 8 hours. The beta elimination phase ranges from 30 to 60 hours and is responsible for preventing withdrawal symptoms; this property is exploited in maintenance therapy.[79]

Methadone has multiple drug interactions related to inducers or inhibitors of the CYP system, particularly the 2D6 and 3A4 subtypes.[92] Because these interactions are not commonly seen with other opioids, drug interactions with methadone may not be as readily anticipated or detected. In addition to interacting with drugs, 3A4 is an auto-inducible enzyme, which accounts for the fact that methadone can bring about its own metabolism and increase its clearance with prolonged use.[90]

Other issues affecting methadone absorption and accumulation are gastric and urinary pH. Decreased gastric pH, such as in patients taking proton pump inhibitors, results in increased rates of methadone absorption. Renal failure and hemodialysis do not alter the excretion of methadone; however, as urinary pH increases, methadone clearance in urine decreases. Urine pH higher than 6 can reduce methadone clearance from 30% to almost 0% and thereby result in increased circulating levels.[90] Most methadone is eliminated in feces.[10] Another source of methadone's potential metabolic instability relates to its avid protein binding. Acute changes in protein binding may lead to sudden increases or decreases in circulating methadone levels.[90]

The difference between methadone and other LAOs is that methadone's duration of effect is intrinsically long acting, whereas most other LAOs are sustained-released forms based on compounding technology. It is beneficial in patients with impaired GI absorption. In addition, methadone is available as a powder, which allows it to be formulated for almost any route of administration. Methadone pills can be broken and cut in half, and it is also available as a liquid elixir (1 or 10 mg/mL). This avoids having to crush pills, which offers a potential advantage in patients with gastrostomy tubes. In addition, because methadone elixir has a low-concentration formulation, careful and precise titration of methadone can be performed to achieve adequate analgesia.[90]

One of the most disturbing aspects of methadone use in the United States has been the reported increase in methadone-related deaths.[93,94] Although the mechanism for these deaths is not exactly clear, many appear to be related to overdose and drug interactions. In some cases, overdose may be related to misunderstanding the standard conversion rates for methadone from other opioids. Contrary to conventional wisdom, methadone appears to be more potent (milligram for milligram) in patients whose treatment is being switched to methadone from high doses of other opioids. Although standard conversion tables may suggest that the ratio of conversion from morphine to methadone may be from 1:1 to 1:3, these ratios were taken from studies on acute pain or normal controls. Many of these conversion tables were developed more than 20 years ago, far before recent increases in methadone use as a chronic analgesic. In cases in which much higher pre-switch dosages are converted to methadone, the appropriate morphine-to-methadone ratio may range from 1:5 to 1:20 or higher. Obviously, such a counterintuitive dosing phenomenon leads to the potential for overdose.

Another possible source of methadone-related mortality includes torsades de pointes arrhythmias, which have been reported in some patients.[95] Although a prospective study has demonstrated QT prolongation on electrocardiogram in patients taking methadone, it was also concluded that the magnitude of the increase is less than that with other antiarrhythmic drugs and is not higher than the QT widening caused by other drugs such as tricyclic antidepressants.[96] Use of methadone requires awareness of possible QT prolongation and the possible additive effect that other QT-prolonging agents may have when combined with methadone. Table 36.1 shows the oral bioavailability, half-lives, duration of action, and metabolites of selected opioids. Table 36.2 shows the equianalgesic doses of different opioids.

Methadone must be used with significant knowledge of the special properties that predispose it to substantial risk. Slow dosing titration and careful monitoring are essential to safe use. If this and all other elements of safe prescribing of opioids are not possible, the drug should not be prescribed.

RATIONAL OPIOID PRESCRIBING

Opioids work for some pain but not all. They may be problematic for many and even life-threatening for some, but knowing who is susceptible is not always clear. Treatment of substantial pain may necessitate the use of opioid-related medications. Opioids are not the first choice, nor should they necessarily be the last choice in the pain management armamentarium. A detailed diagnosis with a thorough history and physical examination and an essential focus on risks and benefits will drive the selection of specified analgesic treatments. Nonopioid treatments will often be the initial choice. The decision to use opioid therapy has undergone intense scrutiny as the public health epidemic of prescription drug abuse has been elevated to a national discussion. The importance of risk management with focal attention on the risk-benefit ratio for safe use of opioids underscores the serious potential for opioid abuse and overdose death that has been well documented through approximately 15 years of retrospective data. A history of psychiatric comorbidity and a history of substance abuse are known variables suggestive of increased risk for abuse and unintentional overdose death. A full discussion of the safe use of opioids is beyond the scope of this chapter but can be found in other resources, such as the White House Office of the National Drug Control Policy and the National Institute on Drug Abuse (http://www.medscape.org/viewarticle/770687 and http://www.medscape.org/viewarticle/770440 [as of 10/2012]), Boston University (http://www.opioidprescribing.com [as of 10/2012]), the National Institutes of Health (http://www.opioidrisk.com [as of 10/2012]), and the Federation of State Medical Boards (http://www.fsmb.org/cme/ [as of 10/2012]).

Before the initiation of opioid therapy, a detailed evaluation is necessary. This evaluation must include risk stratification, assessment of functional activity, a thorough review of the patient's medical history with special attention paid to previous experience with opioid analgesics, and a review of other related comorbid factors, including previous substance abuse; mental illness; hepatic, renal, or pulmonary dysfunction; or sleep apnea. Informed consent is a critical element of opioid treatment that requires patient education on the benefits and risks associated with treatment. The expectations and responsibilities on the part of the patient must be clarified early. Monitoring for and management of opioid-induced side effects are imperative. The use of opioid agreements, urine drug screens, and well-defined boundaries of care must be considered in advance of initiating treatment, as well as an exit strategy if treatment fails to be successful for any variety of reasons.

Should the patient be opioid naïve, low-dose SAOs such as propoxyphene, hydrocodone, or oxycodone may be initiated and carefully titrated to establish an opioid requirement. Because of the rapid clearance and brief half-life of SAOs, toxic accumulation of the medications is less likely than with LAOs. The severity and duration of the patient's pain should help guide whether PRN or fixed dosing is required. In patients with acute pain secondary to an injury or surgery for which rapid healing is expected, PRN dosing is reasonable. However, in patients with the expectation of prolonged recovery or with chronic pain and significant baseline or persistent pain, opioids may be administered in fixed-dosing intervals, as well as in PRN intervals for breakthrough pain. Scheduled dosing decreases clock-watching anxiety and reinforcement of pain behavior. If a patient is able to tolerate an SAO and its side effects, consolidation of the daily opioid requirement into an equianalgesic LAO regimen may be an appropriate step.

Although opioids may be excellent analgesics, they are often used as second-line treatment of chronic pain, mainly because chronic pain may respond to nonopioid treatments that might carry fewer risks. When other pharmacologic, rehabilitative, or interventional procedures are not appropriate or are unsuccessful, chronic opioid therapy should be considered. It is not uncommon to combine opioid treatment with other modalities, including psychological treatment and physical rehabilitation. Simultaneously, interventional pain procedures and adjunctive analgesics may be useful as well.

The effectiveness of opioid therapy for certain types of chronic pain, such as neuropathic pain, remains controversial. Because antidepressants and anticonvulsants have been shown to provide less than 50% pain relief on average, opioids have been used for the treatment of chronic neuropathic pain despite their narrow therapeutic window.[97] When treating neuropathic pain, it has been shown that opioid potency may be relatively lower than that for other conditions. The basis of this seems to be secondary to changes that occur in the endogenous opioid system after nerve injury. It appears that endogenous peptide levels and opioid receptor density decrease in nociceptive pathways.[98] It also appears that GABAergic tone decreases after nerve injury and that the inhibitory effect of morphine on dorsal horn neuron projections after nerve injury is reduced in comparison to its effect on noninjured nerves.[99] Despite these findings, there is evidence in the literature that opioids are efficacious for neuropathic pain; a trial demonstrated that combining gabapentin and morphine for the treatment of neuropathic pain was superior to either alone.[100]

In forms of chronic pain unrelated to nerve injury that have not responded well to other treatments, opioid therapy has been shown to be more effective than placebo or antiinflammatory medications alone in reducing pain. However, studies have struggled to show substantial improvement in overall functioning with opioid therapy. In a meta-analysis comparing analgesia and function in subjects taking opioids, NSAIDs, or placebo, there was no statistical difference among the groups with regard to improved function. It should be noted, however, that this study did not use adjunctive medications or physical therapy.[101] This emphasizes the point that although opioids may be effective, if used as the sole agent for changing all the primary and secondary effects of chronic pain, they may not be effective enough. The importance of a multidisciplinary approach to the treatment of chronic pain syndromes cannot be overstated.

The use of opioids requires a comprehensive strategy, including consideration of other potentially effective therapies that have less risk. Rational prescribing also requires consideration of all potential risks associated with the treatment and should include a plan to avoid or deal with these risks.

CONSIDERATIONS FOR OPIOID PRESCRIBERS

In response to a surging public health crisis regarding the misuse of prescription drugs, the Obama Administration in 2011 developed the Prescription Drug Abuse Prevention Plan through the Office of National Drug Control Policy (ONDCP). The ONDCP plan entails specialized efforts with regard to monitoring, proper medication disposal, enforcement, and education.[102] In fact, education of patients, parents, and youth is a key element of focus for the White House–implemented drug abuse prevention plan. Equally important is education of prescribing physicians and providers of care. In 2012 the Federation of State Medical Boards of the United States revised and expanded the book *Responsible Opioid Prescribing: A Clinician's Guide.* The revised guide reviews the new data on opioid risk and toxicity, including high rates of unintended overdose deaths, that were not available when the first edition was written in 2006. It offers clinicians strategies to reduce the risk for addiction, abuse, and diversion of opioids.[103] Moreover, the revised edition includes but is not limited to defined strategies for patient evaluation that includes risk assessment, treatment plans that incorporate functional goals, periodic review and monitoring of patients, documentation, informed consent, and termination strategies for chronic opioid therapy.[103] It also emphasizes the special care that is needed when using methadone and treating children and adolescents, as well as prescriber responsibilities for consumer education on the safe use of opioids. The use of defined risk stratification methods by prescribers of chronic opioid therapy has become paramount. Gourlay and colleagues endorsed taking a universal precautions approach and suggested that addiction can only be elucidated on a behavioral prospective basis.[104]

TREATMENT END POINTS

Because pain is a subjective experience, using "pain relief" as a treatment end point is a subjective and nontestable marker of therapeutic success or failure. One of the most feared consequences of chronic opioid therapy is drug addiction, which as discussed earlier, is compulsive use of an opioid that causes dysfunction and continued use of the opioid despite the dysfunction (i.e., negative impact on or harm to the patient's life). Because effective analgesia should improve function and because of fear of the side effect of addiction, which hinges on dysfunction, a major focus of chronic opioid therapy should be on functional improvement as an objective end point. It is expected that patients who are treated carefully and judiciously with opioids and achieve analgesia should have functional gains. This is in contradistinction to an addict, who becomes impaired by substance abuse as manifested by dysfunction. The challenge for physicians treating chronic pain with opioids is to devise a system of objective markers that distinguish function from dysfunction and that emphasize a wide spectrum of therapeutic goals.

Several markers of functional improvement can be used in patients treated chronically with opioids. Several standardized functional measurements (e.g., the 36-Item Short-Form Health Survey [SF-36], Oswestry Disability Index [ODI]) can be used to subjectively measure the reduction in pain with supportive and objective evidence of improvement in functional status and effect on quality of life. However, psychological and social factors, as well as the status of coexistent disease, may influence the perception of pain, suffering, and entitlement and can alter the overall assessment.[105-109] Unfortunately, not all of these parameters will improve concomitantly or proportionately following the initiation of opioid therapy. If factors related to psychological and physical reconditioning have not been addressed, pain perception and reduction of pain after a trial of an opioid may be less than optimal.

Determining effective treatment end points during an opioid trial may require flexibility in considering the many possible variations in efficacy and functional gain. A central question that may be useful at the beginning of an opioid trial is "What do you need to do with this medicine that you cannot do now?" What follows should be the creation of a list of reasonably attainable functional goals that cover multiple domains of the patient's life. Equally important in documenting this list is the process by which the goals will be attained and how the patient plans to document progress toward each functional goal for the clinician on every subsequent follow-up visit. Each goal is monitored regularly and adjusted on the basis of progress. Expectations may need to be reduced if goals are not being met or may be advanced as the patient improves.

One approach to determining whether a patient is benefiting from opioid therapy is to gather collateral information from others involved in the patient's care and life. Input from physical and occupational therapists, psychologists, family members, and caregivers may prove invaluable. Evidence of improved function may include gains in employment, increased activities of daily living, and socializing with family and friends. On the contrary, if a patient becomes dysfunctional in employment or in social or private life, concerns about possible medication-related deterioration should be raised, including addiction. However, decreased function is not pathognomonic of addiction. It may be related to other factors beyond a patient's control, such as sedation, cognitive impairment, or other external causes. If these or other external problems are not the cause of a patient's deteriorating mental or physical health, it may be helpful to consider seeking additional support in the form of a multidisciplinary program or referral to other specialty providers, such as psychologists, social workers, psychiatrists, or addiction specialists.

It remains controversial whether subjective relief without objective evidence of improved quality of life is sufficient to justify the chronic use of opioids. Pain reduction is a subjective variable. Its use as an assessment tool for therapeutic success represents only a single aspect of adequate chronic opioid therapy. For example, consider a patient with significant disability related to pain that is rated 6 on a pain severity scale of 1 to 10. Although opioid therapy may not be successful in significantly reducing subjective pain scores, this does not signify treatment failure. In fact, despite no reported reduction in pain scores, objective signs of return to work and increased physical activity clearly demonstrate that treatment has improved the patient's quality of life. Conversely, if an opioid trial is characterized by subjective reports of marked pain relief but there are no observable functional gains and possibly even signs of persistent sedation with decreased physical activity, voluntary unemployment, dysfunctional interpersonal relationships, or diminished physical activity, the physician must consider why the patient would regard this as a positive outcome and attempt to resolve any underlying conditions or misunderstandings.

As noted by the Federation of State Medical Boards, a critical aspect of safe opioid management is documentation of a patient's care, including current functional status on initial evaluation and throughout follow-up.[106] Documentation not only requires clarity of events but should also offer transparency about the physician's decision process, particularly in regard to risk-benefit considerations, choices, and plans for risk management. Vigilance for decreased function is important; this may help reveal problems such as addiction, progressive disease, or pain unresponsive to opioids.

Another critical issue to consider before and during the course of treatment is when to discontinue opioid therapy if the treatment is deemed to be ineffective. Many factors must be considered before a treatment is considered to be a failure, including inadequate dosing, inappropriate dosing schedule, improper drug delivery route, opioid-insensitive pain, side effects limiting dose escalation, and social and psychological issues.

The appropriate duration of effective opioid therapy remains controversial. Currently, there are no clear guidelines and consensus on this issue. The efficacy of treatment related to adverse effects and progression of the underlying disease must be considered fully when formulating decisions regarding the length of treatment, and these factors must be reconsidered on a regular basis. Once opioid therapy has been initiated, it may be difficult to know whether pain would be present without opioid therapy unless the opioids are tapered.

KEY POINTS

- Opioid drugs have been used for control of pain for thousands of years.
- Opioids may be reliable and potent analgesics, but they do not work for all pain, for everyone, or for every condition, and they may pose serious risks.
- The evidence for sustained benefits of opioids in relieving chronic pain is weak and inadequate, whereas evidence of risk associated with use of the drugs is significant.
- Modulation of pain perception is controlled by multiple systems, including the endogenous opioid system.
- The most common side effect of opioid administration is constipation, and unfortunately, tolerance to it does not usually develop.
- Opioids are associated with addiction at a rate that is high enough to be a significant concern; however, the exact rate of addiction because of therapeutic opioid use is controversial.
- A growing debate has emerged that focuses on understanding how opioids should be used for chronic pain while balancing the imperative for vigilant use of opioids with sufficient risk management for safety.
- Methadone has many features that distinguish it from other opioids, including heightened risk and significant life-threatening adverse outcomes.
- Methadone has recently been found to be the most common opioid to be related to unintended overdose death in the United States.
- Opioid therapy has undergone intense scrutiny as the public health epidemic of prescription drug abuse has been elevated to a national discussion.
- Focal attention on the risk-benefit ratio for safe use of opioids underscores the serious potential for opioid abuse and overdose death, which has been well documented through approximately 15 years of retrospective data.
- A detailed diagnostic assessment with a thorough history and physical examination, as well as an essential focus on risks and benefits, will drive the selection of specified analgesic treatments.

KEY POINTS—cont'd

- The increased risk for abuse and unintentional overdose death requires increased risk management, including risk assessment, treatment plans that incorporate functional goals, periodic review and monitoring of patients, documentation, informed consent, and termination strategies for chronic opioid therapy.
- A thorough history of psychiatric comorbid conditions and a history of substance abuse are important elements of safe prescribing.
- Once opioid therapy has been initiated, it may be difficult to know whether pain would be present without opioid therapy unless the opioids are tapered.

SUGGESTED READINGS

American Academy of Pain Medicine, American Pain Society, American Society of Addiction Medicine. Definitions related to the use of opioids for the treatment of pain: a consensus document from the American Academy of Pain Medicine, the American Pain Society, and the American Society of Addiction Medicine, 2001. Available at http://www.ampainsoc.org/advocacy/opioids2.htm.

Chou R, Fanciullo GJ, Fine PG, et al. Clinical guidelines for the use of chronic opioid therapy for chronic noncancer pain. *J Pain.* 2009;10:113-130.

Federation of State Medical Boards of the United States. Model policy for the use of controlled substances for the treatment of pain, 2004. Available at www.fsmb.org/pdf/2004_grpol_Controlled_Substances.pdf.

Fishman SM. *Responsible Opioid Prescribing: A Clinicians Guide.* 2nd ed. Washington, DC: Waterford Life Sciences; 2012.

Fishman SM, Wilsey B, Mahajan G, et al. Methadone reincarnated: novel clinical applications with related concerns. *Pain Med.* 2002;3:339-348.

Gourlay DL, Heit HA, Almahrezi A. Universal precautions in pain medicine: a rational approach to the treatment of chronic pain. *Pain Med.* 2005;6:107-112.

Jannetto P, Bratanow N. Pharmacogenomic considerations in the management of pain: review. *Genome Med.* 2010;2:66.

Mahajan G, Fishman SM. Major opioids in pain management. In: Benzon HT, Raja SN, Molloy RE, et al, eds. *Essentials of Pain and Regional Anesthesia.* Philadelphia: Elsevier Churchill Livingstone; 2005:94-105.

Prescription Drug Abuse. The White House. Available at http://www.whitehouse.gov/ondcp/prescription-drug-abuse. Accessed 6/18/2012.

Ramsin B, Trescot A, Datta S, et al. Opioid complications and side effects. *Pain Physician.* 2008;11:S105-S120.

Soin A, Cheng J, Brown L, et al. Functional outcomes in patients with chronic nonmalignant pain on long-term opioid therapy. *Pain Pract.* 2008;8:379-384.

Stoelting RK, Hillier S. Opioid agonists and antagonists. In: Stoelting RK, Hillier SC, eds. *Handbook of Pharmacology and Physiology in Anesthetic Practice.* 2nd ed. Philadelphia: Lippincott, Williams & Wilkins; 2006:78-117.

Trescot A, Helm S, Hansen H, et al. Opioids in the management of chronic non-cancer pain: an update of American Society of the Interventional Pain Physicians' (ASIPP) guidelines. *Pain Physician.* 2008;11:S5-S62.

Wilsey BL, Fishman SM. Minor and short-acting opioids. In: Benzon HT, Raja SN, Molloy RE, eds. *Essentials of Pain and Regional Anesthesia.* Philadelphia: Elsevier Churchill Livingstone; 2005:107-112.

The references for this chapter can be found at www.expertconsult.com.

37 Minor and Short-Acting Analgesics, Including Opioid Combination Products

Steven P. Stanos | Mark D. Tyburski | Sagar S. Parikh

The use of naturally occurring plant material for the relief of pain dates back to early times. Advances in antipyretic and analgesic medications began in the late 1800s with the development of salicylic acid, antipyrine, phenacetin, and acetaminophen (APAP).[1] These basic medications are still used today to various degrees in both over-the-counter (OTC) and prescription preparations—the minor analgesics salicylic acid and APAP are widely marketed and heavily consumed. Minor analgesics for acute and chronic pain include a number of prescription and OTC agents, which may be useful in isolation or as adjuvants in a more comprehensive multimodal pharmacologic approach. Adjuvants refer to agents that enhance the effect of other medications but may not be fully effective when used alone. A population survey has reported that the use of OTC medications, many of which include minor analgesics, account for the most common method of relieving pain (53%). This is closely followed by physical exercise (52%) and prescription medications (35%).[2]

The minor analgesics reviewed in this chapter include oral APAP, opioid combination preparations, tramadol, steroids, and caffeine, as well as topical compounds and delivery systems (Box 37.1). See the chapters in this text that discuss opioids, anticonvulsants, antidepressants, and nonsteroidal anti-inflammatory drugs (NSAIDs) for complete information on these topics (Chapters 36, 38, 39, and 40). Additional combination OTC formulations with minor analgesics include convenience combinations—those that contain aspirin, APAP, or ibuprofen plus other remedies such as nasal decongestants, antihistamines, cough suppressants, or antacids. These medications are useful for treating the sequelae of a primary illness (e.g., cold and flu symptoms, insomnia, cough) and any pain symptoms that may coexist.[3]

Prescribing habits regarding the use of analgesics for the treatment of various musculoskeletal conditions continue to evolve. Caudill-Slosberg and colleagues[4] compared prescribing habits between 1980 and 1981 with those between 1999 and 2000 and demonstrated a significant increase in patients receiving prescriptions for acute and chronic musculoskeletal pain. Increases were seen in the use of NSAIDs and cyclooxygenase-2 (COX-2) agents, as well as more potent opioids, including combination opioid preparations containing APAP and NSAIDs.

Minor analgesics are used widely, with reported prevalence rates of twice-weekly use of approximately 8.7% for prescription drugs and 8.8% for OTC analgesics. Analgesics have been found to be the largest selling group of OTC medications in a number of population studies.[5] Daily use was more common for prescribed analgesics, whereas OTC analgesics were used a few times per week.[6,7] Among prescription and OTC medications, APAP, ibuprofen, and aspirin were the most commonly used (17% to 23% of the population).[8] Use of analgesics, many of which include minor agents, accounts for a significant amount of health care dollars. In a recent population study, analgesic cost ranked second behind diagnostic imaging in expenditures for the treatment of acute low back pain.[7] Chronic use of prescription and OTC analgesics (i.e., aspirin, non–aspirin-containing NSAIDs, and APAP) may continue for longer than 1 year. In the same survey, approximately 2.3 million adults reported using non–aspirin-containing NSAIDs and 2.6 million used APAP on a frequent basis for longer than 5 years.[9] This widespread use occurs despite general knowledge of the increased risk for gastrointestinal (GI), renal, and cardiac toxicity with short-term and chronic use. Unfortunately, the perception remains that as a class of medications, OTC and prescription NSAIDs are relatively safe. This misbelief leads to frequent inappropriate use and the potential for serious adverse events.[10] The increased availability and marketing of OTC agents has probably contributed to patient misuse, with consumers still being unaware of the potential catastrophic risks associated with their use—60% of people cannot identify the active ingredient in their analgesics, and 40% of Americans believe that OTC drugs are too weak to cause significant harm.[11]

The use of OTC and prescription analgesics is not only confined to the outpatient setting. Significant use of these agents in nursing home facilities was reported in a group of Medicare beneficiaries during 2001. Patients averaged 8.8 unique medications per month, including 2.9 OTC medications. Of these subjects, 70% used nonopioid OTC analgesics and 19.0% used nonopioid prescription analgesics.[12]

SPECIFIC DRUGS

MINOR OPIOIDS

In this chapter, minor opioids are defined as analgesic combination products with codeine, hydrocodone, or oxycodone. These products continue to account for a large percentage of prescriptions written for chronic nonmalignant pain. Combination opioid analgesics—compounds containing APAP or anti-inflammatory medications—make up a significant

Box 37.1 Minor Analgesics

Minor opioids and combination products
Acetaminophen
Tramadol
Oral steroids
Caffeine and combination products
Topical medications (analgesics, rubefacients, local anesthetics, cooling agents, heating agents)
Over-the-counter convenience products

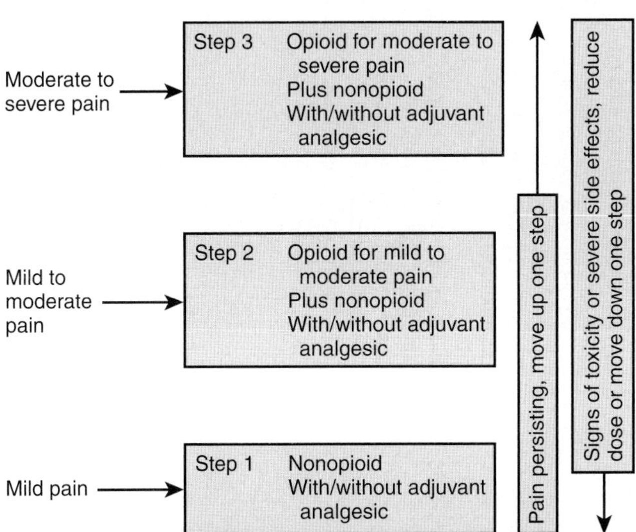

Figure 37.1 World Health Organization analgesic ladder. (Adapted from World Health Organization: *Cancer Pain Relief*. Geneva: World Health Organization; 1990.)

amount of opioids prescribed by primary care physicians[13] and pain specialists. Combination analgesics are advocated in several treatment guidelines, including the three-step analgesic ladder of the World Health Organization (step 2)[14,15] (Fig. 37.1). Since the 1990s, the use of minor analgesic combinations containing oxycodone and hydrocodone has continued to increase, whereas the use of those containing codeine has declined. Clinic type (e.g., primary care, spine center, pain center), geographic, and socioeconomic variables may also affect prescribing practices.[16]

Opioid analgesics as a class can be categorized into three chemical groups: (1) synthetic phenylpiperidines (e.g., meperidine, fentanyl), (2) synthetic pseudopiperidines (e.g., methadone, propoxyphene), and (3) naturally occurring alkaloids derived directly from the poppy seed (e.g., heroin, morphine, codeine) and their semisynthetic derivatives (e.g., hydromorphone, oxycodone, oxymorphone).[17] This chapter reviews codeine, oxycodone, hydrocodone, and tramadol, all natural or synthetic opioids used in isolation or in combination forms for the treatment of mild to moderate pain (Tables 37.1 and 37.2).

PHARMACOKINETICS AND PHARMACODYNAMICS

An understanding of pharmacokinetics and pharmacodynamics is essential for appropriately prescribing minor opioid analgesics, interpreting related toxicology screens, and appreciating the potential mechanisms for adverse side effects. In general, medications are primarily metabolized by the cytochrome P-450 (CYP) and glucuronidation pathways. Opioid analgesics, like any medication, may be metabolized by the CYP drug-metabolizing enzyme system 2D6. Genetic polymorphism of CYP2D6 may lead to variability in enzyme breakdown and clinical effectiveness of the medication. Deficiency of CYP2D6 may be seen in whites (7%) and those of Asian descent (1%).[18] These enzyme systems can be induced (activated) or inhibited by various agents, including drugs, alcohol, and cigarette smoke, as well as by endogenous substances. Inducers are agents that activate the CYP enzyme system and thereby lead to increased metabolism and reduced drug effect. Inhibitors may impair the CYP enzyme system and thus limit metabolism of the drug and increase the effect of the drug. Although pharmacokinetic drug-drug interactions may affect serum levels of a drug, this may be subclinical in most patients, with significant interactions occurring rarely in vivo in only about 10% to 15% of patients.[19] Patients' response to individual opioids may vary markedly. Recent evidence has supported more than one mechanism for μ-opioid analgesic reactions, which may be related to receptor polymorphism.[20]

Morphine, hydromorphone, and oxymorphone are not metabolized by CYP but are metabolized by uridine diphosphate glucuronosyltransferase (UGT) enzymes. Except for morphine and codeine, UGT enzymes metabolize medications primarily to inactive metabolites. Morphine is converted into large quantities of relatively inactive morphine-3-glucuronide (M3G) and smaller quantities of the active metabolite morphine-6-glucuronide (M6G). M6G is 50 times more potent than morphine. M3G may account for central nervous system (CNS) toxicity, including lowering of seizure thresholds.[21] Equianalgesic oral doses of the various minor opioid combination products and morphine are listed in Table 37.3.

CODEINE

Along with morphine and thebaine, codeine (methylmorphine) is a naturally occurring opium alkaloid derivative. A weak analgesic, codeine is similar in structure to morphine but has affinity for the μ-opioid receptor that is 300 times lower. Classically, codeine is thought to be metabolized by *O*-demethylation to its primary active metabolite morphine by the CYP2D6 enzyme.[22] Studies have demonstrated that only a small percentage of the total dose (3%)[23] is converted by CYP2D6 to morphine. Approximately 80% is directly glucuronidated by uridine diphosphate glucuronosyltransferase 2B7 (UGT2B7) enzyme to codeine-6-glucuronide (C6G), an additional active metabolite. The remaining inactive metabolites are primarily norcodeine (2%) and normorphine (2.4%).[24] Nonfunctional CYP2D6 renders codeine ineffective, perhaps because of genetic mutations or deletions[25] or pharmacologic inhibition.[26] Effects of codeine not related to the formation of morphine include cognitive impairment,[27] sedation, dizziness, euphoria and dysphoria, headache, blurred vision,[28] and prolongation of GI transit time.[29] The average half-life of codeine is 2.5 hours.

Efficacy

When used alone, codeine is typically prescribed in doses of 30 to 60 mg every 4 to 6 hours, with onset of analgesia taking place in 30 to 60 minutes and the duration of effect lasting 4 to 6 hours.

Table 37.1 Minor and Short-Acting Opioids

Class	Name	Adult Dose	Half-Life (Onset)	Mechanism of Action	Other
Natural opium alkaloids	Codeine with acetaminophen (APAP) or acetylsalicylic acid (ASA) (Tylenol No. 2, No. 3, No. 4; Empirin No. 3, No. 4; Capital with Codeine; Aceta with Codeine; Fioricet with Codeine; Fiorinal with Codeine)	PO: 15-60 mg q4h (max daily APAP-ASA dose, 4 g)	2.5-3.5 hr (30-60 min)	Opioid agonist activity at multiple receptors—μ (supraspinal analgesia, euphoria), κ (spinal analgesia and sedation), δ (dysphoria, psychotomimetic effects)	Compared with morphine—decreased analgesia, constipation, respiratory distress, sedation, emesis, and physical dependence; increased antitussive effects
Phenanthrene derivatives	Hydrocodone plus ASA or APAP (Lortab, Lortab ASA, Vicodin, Norco, Vicoprofen, ZTuss, P-V-Tussin, Tussafed HC)	PO: 5-10 mg q4-6h (max dose, 4 g)	3.8 hr (10-30 min)	Opioid agonist activity at multiple receptors—μ (supraspinal analgesia, euphoria), κ (spinal analgesia and sedation), δ (dysphoria, psychotomimetic effects)	Compared with morphine-equivalent analgesia—respiratory depression and physical dependency; equivalent antitussive effects
	Oxycodone (with or without APAP or ASA) (OxyIR, Roxicodone) Oxycodone plus ASA (Percodan, Endodan, Roxiprin) Oxycodone plus APAP (Percocet, Endocet, Tylox, Roxicet, Roxilox)	PO: 5-30 mg q4-6h (4-g max dose of ASA/APAP); sustained release: 10/10-160 mg q12h	2-5 hr (10-15 min)	Opioid agonist activity at multiple receptors: μ (supraspinal analgesia, euphoria), κ (spinal analgesia and sedation), δ (dysphoria, psychotomimetic effects)	Compared with morphine— more potent analgesia, constipation, antitussive effects, respiratory depression, sedation, emesis, and physical dependence
Diphenylheptane derivative	Propoxyphene, with or without APAP (Darvon, Darvon-N) Propoxyphene plus APAP (Darvocet A500, Propacet 100)	PO: 65 mg q4h (max, 390 mg/day); napsylate, 100 mg q4h (max, 600 mg/day)	6-12 hr (15-60 min)	Opioid agonist activity at multiple receptors: μ (supraspinal analgesia, euphoria), κ (spinal analgesia and sedation), δ (dysphoria, psychotomimetic effects)	Compared with morphine — less analgesia, sedation, emesis, respiratory depression, and physical dependence

Table 37.2 Opioid Combination Products

Drug Class	Drug Name	Trade Name	Available Dose	Typical Dose	Comments	Half-Life
Para-aminophenol derivatives/natural opium alkaloids	Acetaminophen/ codeine phosphate	Tylenol with Codeine elixir; Tylenol with Codeine No. 2, No. 3, No. 4.	(120/12 mg)/5 mL liquid; 300/15 mg, 300/30 mg, 300/60 mg (tablets)	Elixir—children <3 yr, safe dose not established; 3-6 yr, 5 mL (1 tsp) 3-4 times daily; 7-12 yr, 10 mL 3-4 times daily; adults, 15 mL q4h; tablets and capsules, 15-60 mg codeine q4-6h	Codeine phosphate, max, 360 mg daily; acetaminophen, max, 4000 mg daily	Acetaminophen, 1-4 hr; codeine, 2.5-3 hr
			650/30 mg (tablets)	30-60 mg codeine q4-6h	Codeine phosphate, max, 360 mg daily; acetaminophen, max, 4000 mg daily	Acetaminophen, 1-4 hr; codeine, 2.5-3 hr
Acetylsalicylic acid/ natural opium alkaloids	Aspirin/codeine phosphate	Empirin with Codeine No. 3, No. 4	325/30 mg, 325/60 mg (tablets)	1-2 tablets q4h	Codeine phosphate, max, 360 mg daily	Aspirin, 2.5-3.5 hr; codeine, 2.5-3 hr
Para-aminophenol derivatives/ phenanthrene derivatives	Hydrocodone bitartrate/ acetaminophen	Vicodin, Lorcet-HD, Lortab, Norco, Maxidone, Anexsia	2.5/500 mg, 5/500 mg, 7.5/325 mg, 7.5/500 mg, 7.5/650 mg, 7.5/750 mg, 10/325 mg, 10/500 mg, 10/650 mg, 10/660 mg, 10/750 mg (tablets)	1-2 tablets q4-6h	Dosage typically limited by acetaminophen, max, 4000 mg daily	Hydrocodone, 3.5-4.1 hr
	Oxycodone/ acetaminophen	Percocet, Endocet, Tylox, Roxicet, Roxilox	5/325 mg, 7.5/325 mg, 5/500 mg (Tylox), 7.5/500 mg, 10/325 mg, 10/650 mg (tablets); 5/500 mg (caplets; Roxicet); 5/325 mg/ 5 mL (solution) (Roxicet)	1-2 tablets q4-6h	Acetaminophen, max, 4000 mg daily	Acetaminophen, 1-4 hr; oxycodone, 3.1-3.7 hr
Acetylsalicylic acid/ phenanthrene derivates	Oxycodone/ aspirin	Percodan, Endodan, Roxiprin	4.8/325 mg (tablet)	1 tablet q4-6h	Aspirin, max, 4000 mg daily	Aspirin, 2.5-3.5 hr; oxycodone, 3.1-3.7 hr
Propionic acid/ phenanthrene derivatives	Hydrocodone bitartrate/ ibuprofen	Vicoprofen	7.5/200 mg (tablet)	1 tablet q4-6h	Marketed for short-term management of acute pain; NSAIDs may increase risk for serious cardiovascular thrombotic events, myocardial infarction, stroke	Hydrocodone, 3.5-4.1 hr; ibuprofen, 4-6 hr
	Oxycodone/ ibuprofen	Combunox	5/400 mg (tablet)	1-2 tablets q4-6h	Max dosage of ibuprofen, 2400-3200 mg daily	Oxycodone, 3.1-3.7 hr; ibuprofen, 1.8-2.6 hr
Diphenylheptane derivatives	Propoxyphene HC1/APAP		65/650 mg (tablet)	1 tablet q4-6h	Structurally related to methadone; propoxyphene HC1, max, 390 mg daily	Propoxyphene, 6-12 hr; norpropoxyphene, 30-36 hr; acetaminophen, 1-4 hr
	Propoxyphene HC1/aspirin/ caffeine	Darvon Compound 65	65/389/32.4 mg (tablet)	1-2 tablets q4-6h	Structurally related to methadone; propoxyphene HC1, max, 390 mg daily	Propoxyphene, 6-12 hr; norpropoxyphene, 30-36 hr; aspirin, 2.5-3.5 hr, caffeine, 3-6 hr
	Propoxyphene napsylate/ acetaminophen	Darvocet-N 50, Darvocet-N 100, Darvocet A500, Propacet 100	50/325 mg (N 50), 100/650 mg (N 100), 100/500 mg (A500) (tablets)	1-2 tablets q4-6h	Structurally related to methadone; propoxyphene napsylate, max, 600 mg daily	Propoxyphene, 6-12 hr; norpropoxyphene, 30-36 hr; acetaminophen, 1-4 hr

NSAIDs, nonsteroidal anti-inflammatory drugs.

Table 37.3 Combination Analgesics for Mild to Moderate Pain

Agent	Onset (min)	Duration of Action (hr)	Equianalgesic Oral Dose (mg)*	DEA Schedule
Oxycodone combinations	10-15	4-6	30†	II
Hydrocodone combinations	30-60	4-6	30	III
Codeine combinations	30-60	4-6	130	III
Propoxyphene combinations	15-60	4-6	130	IV
Tramadol combinations	60	6-7	100	Not scheduled

*Doses reflect the opioid component only and are equianalgesic to 30 mg morphine.
†Doses for moderate to severe pain not necessarily equivalent to 30 mg morphine.
DEA, U.S. Drug Enforcement Agency.
From Gutstein HB, Akil H. Opioid analgesics. In: Hardman JG, Limbird LE, Gilman AG, eds. *Goodman and Gilman's The Pharmacological Basis of Therapeutics*. 10th ed. New York: McGraw-Hill; 2001:569-619.)

Codeine has been shown to be an effective cough suppressant (10 to 120 mg/day) and is present in a number of OTC cold and cough convenience preparations.[30] However, codeine's potential opioid analgesic effect has long been questioned. Houde's classic study in the 1960s reported the analgesic effects of codeine (32 mg) to be no more than that of 650 mg of aspirin, although both were more effective than placebo.[31] The number needed to treat (NNT), or the number of patients needed to receive the medication to achieve at least 50% pain relief, with 60 mg codeine has been reported to be 16.7,[32] which has led to its widespread use as a combination analgesic.

Codeine (10 to 60 mg) is more commonly prescribed in combination with APAP (400 to 1000 mg), aspirin, or NSAIDs such as ibuprofen (400 mg). A systematic review of codeine and APAP trials for acute non–cancer-related pain concluded that the benefit over codeine alone is only modest (5%).[33] A systematic review of trials of APAP alone or in combination with codeine noted efficacy in patients prescribed APAP plus 60 mg codeine versus APAP alone. At doses higher than 60 mg, there was diminishing incremental analgesia with increasing dose and a higher incidence of side effects (e.g., constipation, nausea, and sedation).[34] A head-to-head study of codeine (30 mg) plus APAP (300 mg) and hydrocodone (7.5 mg) plus APAP (500 mg) showed significant relief of moderate to severe acute (6 hours) postoperative pain in comparison to placebo, but the analgesia was no greater than that achieved with hydrocodone-APAP.[35]

PROPOXYPHENE (DEXTROPROPOXYPHENE)

Propoxyphene (dextropropoxyphene) is a mild synthetic opioid originally synthesized in the 1950s and primarily marketed in its hydrochloride form as Darvon (65 mg; maximum, 400 mg/day), as propoxyphene napsylate (Darvocet-N 50, Darvocet-N 100), and in Europe, as co-proxamol (32.5 mg dextropropoxyphene plus 325 mg paracetamol). By the late 1960s, propoxyphene was the most widely prescribed analgesic in the United States.[36] Reports of propoxyphene overdoses led to warnings by the U.S. Food and Drug Administration (FDA) in 1978 and a subsequent reduction in use.[37] Use of propoxyphene continued for a number of years, primarily in older adults, because of its perceived safety profile.[38] However, Smith[39] suggested that its analgesic activity is lower than that of aspirin. Propoxyphene's major metabolite norpropoxyphene has fewer CNS effects than propoxyphene does but accumulates in cardiac tissue, thereby leading to a local anesthetic effect and prolongation of action potentials, in some cases fatal torsades de pointes.[40] Because of the increasing number of fatal overdoses of co-proxamol and limited evidence supporting its efficacy versus APAP for acute and chronic pain, the British government announced the gradual withdrawal of co-proxamol from British markets in January 2005.[41] As a result of increasing public outcry from patient advocacy groups and recommendations by an FDA advisory board group, propoxyphene was voluntarily removed from the U.S. market in 2011 (Propoxyphene: withdrawal—risk of cardiac toxicity. Available at www.fda.gov/Safety/MedWatch/SafetyInformation/.../ucm234389.ht. Accessed August 28, 2012). It is interesting to note that at the time of its withdrawal from the market, a survey showed that 68% of pain medicine practitioners saw patients who were prescribed propoxyphene by their primary care physicians.[42]

OXYCODONE

Oxycodone is a semisynthetic opioid analgesic derived from the opium alkaloid thebaine. Human studies have demonstrated it to have analgesic potency 1.5 times that of morphine after oral administration.[43] A number of active metabolites have been proposed to contribute to the clinical pharmacokinetics of oxycodone. One theory supports 3-*O*-demethylation by CYP2D6 to oxymorphone. Oxymorphone is a potent μ-opioid ligand with two to five times higher receptor affinity than morphine has. Though potent, oxymorphone accounts for only 10% of oxycodone metabolites. Oxymorphone has been available for a number of years for parenteral and rectal use and was reformulated and released in an immediate-release (IR) and extended-release (ER) schedule II formulation. In vitro studies have shown that *O*-demethylation of oxycodone accounts for 13% of its oxidative metabolism. Oxidation of oxycodone primarily occurs via *N*-demethylation by CYP3A4/5 to noroxycodone, which is the most abundant circulating metabolite in human studies. Unfortunately, noroxycodone has weak affinity for μ-opioid receptors.[44]

In vivo, oxycodone has potent μ-opioid receptor effects, but data suggest that the intrinsic antinociceptive effects may be additionally mediated by κ-opioid receptors.[45] This has led some to consider oxycodone an ideal medication for opioid rotation in patients not responsive to morphine, a classic μ-opioid receptor agonist.[46,47] Recent studies have proposed non-CYP2D6 metabolites (noroxycodone, noroxymorphone, noroxycodols, oxycodols) as additional substances responsible for its μ-opioid receptor binding and analgesic effects.[48] Animal studies have recently demonstrated conflicting gender-related differences in female versus male rats when examining the antinociceptive effects of oxycodone.[49]

HYDROCODONE

Hydrocodone is similar in structure to codeine but is six to eight times more potent.[50] Hydrocodone is a prodrug and undergoes CYP2D6 metabolism to hydromorphone and CYP3A4 metabolism to noroxycodone. Hydrocodone is less potent than morphine by receptor affinity and demonstrates a relative analgesic potency of 0.59 in comparison to morphine. The discrepancy between hydrocodone's binding affinity and potency versus that of morphine is possibly the result of active hydrocodone metabolites or the intrinsic efficacy of receptor activation, which is more efficient for hydrocodone than for morphine.[51] Hydrocodone is marketed as a combination product with APAP, ibuprofen, and aspirin.

Efficacy

The hydrocodone-ibuprofen combination product was introduced in the United States in 1997 as a fixed dose of hydrocodone (7.5 mg) and ibuprofen (200 mg) and has demonstrated efficacy for acute postoperative pain.[52] Neither hydrocodone (7.5 mg) nor ibuprofen (200 mg) given alone was superior to placebo, thus supporting the concept of analgesic synergy between the two agents. Similar findings were demonstrated in patients with acute low back pain[53] and postoperative obstetric and gynecologic pain.[54] Hydrocodone-APAP (7.5, 200 mg), one and two tablets, was compared with a fixed-dose combination of codeine (30 mg) and APAP (300 mg). The two-tablet dose of combination hydrocodone-APAP was more effective than the one-tablet dose and one or two tablets of the fixed codeine-APAP combination.[55]

In 2010, more than 139 million prescriptions for hydrocodone combination products (APAP, ibuprofen) were dispensed in the United States (Drug Enforcement Administration. Hydrocodone, June 2011. Available at: www.deadiversion.usdoj.gov/drugs_concern/hydrocodone.pdf. Accessed June 11, 2012.). Hydrocodone-APAP combination products are classified as schedule III controlled substances. Pure hydrocodone is schedule II but is not presently commercially available in the United States (Code of Federal Regulations. Title 21: Food and Drugs Part 1308; Schedules of Controlled Substances 1308.13; Schedule III, June 2012.). Because of high rates of misuse and abuse of hydrocodone products, the U.S. House of Representatives is considering legislation that would reclassify all products containing hydrocodone from schedule III to schedule II. As a result of increasing reported toxicity of APAP in combination opioid and OTC products, the U.S. FDA has mandated a reduction in APAP in combination opioid products by 2014. Reformulations of these products will include a maximum of 300 mg of APAP (Abbott Laboratories, 2012). Commonly prescribed hydrocodone-APAP combination products presently include 10, 7.5, and 5 mg hydrocodone and 325, 500, 750 mg APAP, with ranges between 5 and 10 mg hydrocodone and 325 and 750 mg APAP (Hydrocodone Bitartrate/Acetaminophen Tablets, package insert, Mallinckrodt, Inc., St. Louis).

Pipeline hydrocodone formulations in development include an ER hydrocodone product (hydrocodone bitartrate ER capsules [Zohydro], Zogenix, Inc., San Diego. Available at www.zpgenix.com/index/php/products/zx002. Accessed June 11, 2012) and a tamper-resistant (Teva Pharmaceuticals) long-acting formulation. A "tamper-deterrent" pure hydrocodone product with approximately 45 mg hydrocodone is also in development (Teva Pharmaceuticals).

ACETAMINOPHEN

APAP (paracetamol) and APAP combination products (i.e., containing opioids) are commonly prescribed as a minor analgesic for acute and chronic pain (see Table 37.2). The American College of Rheumatology and similar European professional colleges have recommended it as first-line pharmacologic therapy for osteoarthritis (OA).[56,57] Prescription APAP is available as an opioid-containing combination product (e.g., codeine, hydrocodone, oxycodone), whereas OTC preparations may be combined with pseudoephedrine or dextromethorphan as convenience drugs.

MECHANISM OF ACTION AND DESCRIPTION

APAP (paracetamol) is a *p*-aminophenol analgesic that was introduced in the late 1800s in Germany, a product of the rapidly developing chemical industry. Newly synthesized compounds included synthetic antipyretics and analgesics such as acetophenetidin (phenacetin), antipyrine (phenazone), and acetylsalicylic acid (ASA; aspirin).[58] Paracetamol, the active metabolite of phenacetin, was found to demonstrate less intense GI side effects, which led to its use as an analgesic. Paracetamol was formally introduced in the United States in the 1950s, and though found in the 1960s to have hepatotoxic effects with unintentional misuse and overdose, it became one of the most widely used OTC and combination prescription analgesics worldwide.

Although APAP has been in use since the 1890s, its pharmacologic mechanism of action remains unclear. Generally, it has known analgesic and antipyretic activity with no known peripheral anti-inflammatory or platelet effects. Its antipyretic activity may be secondary to blockade of prostaglandin (PG) production and inhibition of PG endoperoxide H_2 synthase and COX centrally. APAP may block COX activity by reducing the active form of COX to an inactive form, but with only limited effects in the GI tract and peripherally at sites of inflammation, thus contributing to a lower GI side effect profile than that of NSAIDs.[59] Also, recent studies have suggested that its central analgesic qualities may be related to decreased activation of a subtype of endogenous opioid peptide, β-endorphin.[60]

APAP is available in oral and rectal formulations and is rapidly absorbed from the GI tract, mainly the small intestine.[61] APAP has a half-life ($t_{1/2}$) of between 1.25 and 3 hours and serum therapeutic levels of 10 to 30 μg/mL. Twenty-five percent of the dose undergoes first-pass metabolism in the liver. Up to 90% of APAP is metabolized in the liver via glucuronidation and sulfate conjugation to nontoxic metabolites. The remaining 10% undergoes oxidative metabolism via the CYP system (CYP2E1 and CYP1A2), which is responsible for formation of the potentially hepatotoxic and nephrotoxic metabolite *N*-acetyl-*p*-benzoquinoneimine (NAPQI; Fig. 37.2). This minor pathway becomes more critical when

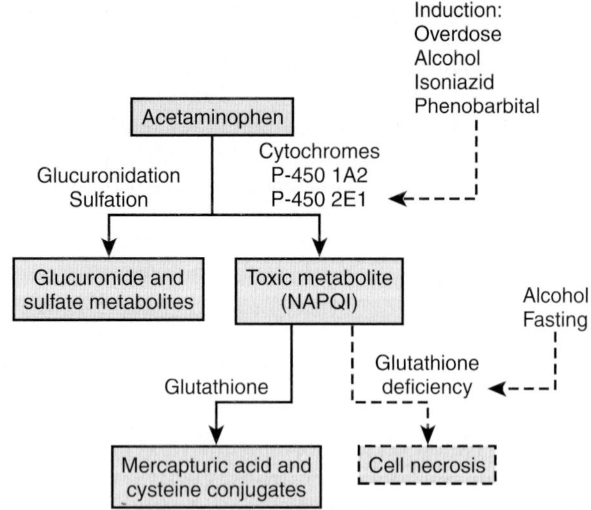

Figure 37.2 Metabolism of acetaminophen. NAPQI, *N*-acetyl-*p*-benzoquinoneimine. (From Barkin RL. Acetaminophen, aspirin, or ibuprofen in combination analgesic products. *Am J Ther*. 2001;8:433-442.)

the enzyme system responsible for sulfonation and glucuronidation becomes saturated with doses higher than 150 mg/kg, thereby increasing the total fraction of NAPQI. Approximately 85% of the dose is excreted in urine within 24 hours of oral dosing. NAPQI is itself detoxified by conjugation with glutathione.[62] Case reports have suggested that clinical situations characterized by low glutathione levels (e.g., chronic hepatitis C, malnourishment, human immunodeficiency virus infection, cirrhosis) may place these patients at greater risk for adverse events from APAP. However, one study found no significant evidence that these populations are at higher risk for APAP toxicity.[63] There are few clinically significant pharmacokinetic interactions with therapeutic doses of APAP. Although case reports have attributed an elevated international normalized ratio (INR) to APAP and oral anticoagulant drug interactions,[64] randomized controlled studies have found no evidence of clinically significant changes in the INR.[65] Even though studies have demonstrated an association, there is no clear evidence of cause and effect.[66]

RISKS AND PRECAUTIONS

APAP-induced toxicity is often associated with liver and renal dysfunction. APAP hypersensitivity reactions are rare, but severe reactions are possible. In general, chronic administration of APAP may cause depletion of glutathione stores and hence lead to greater production of the hepatotoxic and nephrotoxic metabolite NAPQI. Current recommendations for a maximum daily dosage of APAP are approximately 4 g/day in adults and 75 mg/kg/day in infants and children[67] (Box 37.2). Unintentional liver injury, such as hepatic necrosis or acute liver failure from self-medication with OTC and prescription APAP products, can develop with dosages exceeding 4 g/day.

The serum alanine transaminase (ALT) level may be elevated with acute use of recommended doses of APAP. Watkins and Seeff[68] studied healthy adults given 4 g of APAP for 14 days. They found that 31% to 44% of the study subjects, which included patients taking APAP and various

Box 37.2 Acetaminophen Dosing Considerations

Dosing for Mild Pain

- 325-1000 mg PO, per rectum, q4-6h
- Maximum dose: 1 g/dose; 4 g/24 hr
- American Liver Foundation: patients should not exceed 3 g/day for any prolonged period*

Renal Impairment

- Adjust dose frequency
- Creatine clearance (CrCl) = 10-50 mL/min, q6h; CrCl < 10 mL/min, q8h

Hepatic Impairment

- Use with caution
- Consider decreasing the dose, monitor liver function, avoid chronic use

Counseling Patients

Acetaminophen (APAP) in over-the-counter products:

- Regular-strength APAP products commonly contain 325 mg/tablet
- Extra-strength APAP products commonly contain 500 mg/tablet

*Based on a recent study by Watkins and Seeff.[68]

opioid-APAP combination products, demonstrated elevations to three times the upper limit of normal (typically considered clinically significant). Opioids were found to have no additional effect on ALT levels. Elevated liver function is not routinely seen with chronic use and is thought to occur because of cellular adaptation.[68] This APAP tolerance may be characterized by possible downregulation of CYP bioactivation and increases in glutathione production by liver hepatocytes.[69]

The concomitant use of alcohol and APAP resulting in increased risk, lower threshold for hepatic and renal toxicity, or both remains controversial and has been reported primarily in retrospective reviews and case reports.[70] Acute and chronic alcohol use contributes to drug-induced hepatotoxicity via induction of CYP2E1 and NAPQI formation.[71] Enhanced ethanol-related toxicity was demonstrated only in patients at high risk with APAP levels above 300 mg/mL, a level far above the package insert recommendation for no more than three alcoholic beverages daily.[72] When consumed with APAP, ethanol may block the formation of NAPQI.[73] Other inducers of hepatic isoenzymes CYP2E1 and CYP1A2 that are commonly used for pain management include carbamazepine, oxcarbazepine, barbiturates, and phenytoin[74] (Box 37.3). Most importantly, the risk for APAP-induced hepatotoxicity may be increased in patients with alcoholic hepatic disease, viral hepatitis, or alcoholism because of a reduction in glucuronide conjugation and subsequent depletion of glutathione reserves.

Chronic APAP prescribing should be avoided in patients with renal disease, although the exact mechanism of injury is unknown and may be relevant only in patients with preexisting renal compromise or systemic disease.[75] Patients with a history of salicylate hypersensitivity characterized

Box 37.3 Serotonergic Drugs

Serotonin (5-HT) Reuptake Inhibitors

Paroxetine, sertraline, fluoxetine, fluvoxamine, citalopram
Venlafaxine, milnacipran, duloxetine
Clomipramine, imipramine
Tramadol, meperidine, fentanyl, methadone, dextromethorphan, dextropropoxyphene

Serotonin Precursors

5-Hydroxytryptophan, L-tryptophan

5-HT$_{1A}$ Antagonists

LSD, dihydroergotamine, bromocriptine, buspirone

Serotonin Releasers

Amphetamine, MDMA ("ecstasy")

Monoamine Oxidase Inhibitors

Tranylcypromine, phenelzine, nialamide, isoniazid, iproniazid, isocarboxazid
Pargyline, selegiline, procarbazine
Moclobemide

Adapted from Gillman PK. A review of serotonin toxicity data: implications for the mechanisms of antidepressant drug action. *Biol Psychiatry.* 2006;59:1046-1051.

by drug-induced urticaria have demonstrated 11% cross-reactivity to APAP.[76] APAP use has been shown to be associated with hypertension in two large prospective studies in women.[77,78] Similar studies in healthy men failed to show an association with use of APAP and hypertension.[79] Analgesics, in general, may modestly affect blood pressure via a number of mechanisms, primarily through kidney or systemic COX-2 inhibition of PGs, which leads to an imbalance between the vasodilators PGI_2 and PGE_2 and the vasoconstrictors $PGF_{2\alpha}$ and thromboxane A_2. These effects on PG synthesis are greater with NSAIDs than with APAP.[80]

CLINICAL USE

Although a number of guidelines have recommended APAP as a first-line agent, its advantages over NSAIDs in managing OA-related pain remain controversial. A double-blind trial of paracetamol, 4 g/day, for 1 month found it to be as effective as both analgesic and anti-inflammatory doses of ibuprofen in patients with knee OA.[81] More recent studies have demonstrated the efficacy of both a traditional NSAID (diclofenac)[82] and a COX-2 inhibitor (celecoxib)[83] versus APAP in hip and knee OA cohorts. A Cochrane database review of the use of APAP for the chronic pain of OA found the drug to be less effective than NSAIDs in terms of pain reduction scores, although the superiority of NSAIDs over APAP appeared to be more evident in OA patients with more severe pain. Both the NSAID and APAP groups had similar efficacy with regard to functional status.[84] Recent evidence has suggested that APAP may retain anti-inflammatory action comparable to that of NSAIDs in patients with knee OA. Brandt and associates[85] performed a pilot study of 30 subjects in whom OA of the knee was diagnosed and showed that treatment with APAP results in similar significant decreases in mean total knee effusion volume (measured by magnetic resonance imaging) as does treatment with NSAIDs.

Table 37.4 Affinity of Tramadol and Selected Compounds for Opioid Receptors

	K_i Values (mmol/L)		
Drug	**μ Receptor**	**δ Receptor**	**κ Receptor**
Morphine	0.00034	0.092	0.66
Dextropropoxyphene	0.034	0.38	1.22
Codeine	0.2	5.1	6.0
Tramadol	2.1	57.6	42.7
Imipramine	3.7	12.7	1.8

Note: lower K_i = higher binding affinity.
K_i, constant of inhibition.
From Hennies HH, Friderichs E, Schneider J. Receptor binding, analgesic and antitussive potency of tramadol and other selected opioids. *Arzneimittelforschung*. 1988;38:877-880.

TRAMADOL

Tramadol, (±)cis-2-[(dimethylamino)methyl]-1-(3-methoxyphenyl)-cyclohexanol hydrochloride, is a synthetic racemic mixture typically used for its centrally acting analgesic properties. However, clinical and basic science studies have described numerous mechanisms of action at central and peripheral sites. Tramadol is classified as a weak synthetic opioid with mild serotonin and norepinephrine reuptake–inhibiting effects.[86,87]

MECHANISM OF ACTION AND DESCRIPTION

The most well-studied mechanism of action of tramadol is its weak affinity for opioid receptors, the most significant of which involves the μ receptor. However, tramadol-induced analgesia is only partially inhibited by the opiate antagonist naloxone, thus suggesting additional non–opioid-related analgesic mechanisms.[88] Tramadol also displays an inhibitory effect on the central neuronal norepinephrine and serotonin (5-HT) reuptake systems. More recently, noted actions include a local anesthetic effect, anti-inflammatory effects in rat experimental models, and reduction of substance P levels in human synovial fluid.[89,90] Although α_2-agonist activity has also been reported, concentrations in the range of 10 to 100 μmol/L do not bind significantly to α_2-adrenergic receptors.

OPIOID RECEPTORS

Tramadol's affinity for the μ receptor appears to be approximately 10 times weaker than that of codeine, 60 times weaker than that of dextropropoxyphene, and 6000 times weaker than that of morphine[88] (Table 37.4). The active *O*-demethylated metabolite M1 has 300 times higher affinity for the μ receptor than the parent compound does and is up to six times more potent in producing analgesia.[91]

CENTRAL NEURONAL ACTIONS

Multiple actions affecting the descending inhibitory pain pathways have been reported.[92,93] The first system involves neurons originating in the periaqueductal gray matter in the midbrain that synapse at the nucleus raphe magnus, from which fibers then project to the spinal cord. Inhibition of 5-HT reuptake may contribute to inhibition of pain. Another pathway originates at the locus coeruleus in the pons, with fibers projecting to the spinal cord. The norepinephrine released from this pathway inhibits pain responses at the spinal cord via an α-adrenergic mechanism.

Activation of these descending pain inhibition pathways stimulates interneurons that inhibit the transmission of painful stimuli in the dorsal horn by the action of endogenous opioids. Opioid receptor activity has been proposed to be mediated by the dextrorotatory (+) enantiomer as opposed to the levorotatory (−) enantiomer.[94] The (−) enantiomer is approximately 10 times more potent than its (+) counterpart in the inhibition of norepinephrine uptake, and the (+) enantiomer is approximately 4 times more potent than the (−) enantiomer in the inhibition of 5-HT uptake. M1 retains higher affinity for the μ-opioid receptor (300 to 400 times) and possesses greater analgesic activity than the parent compound does. The M1 (+) enantiomer acts at the μ receptor, whereas the M1 (−) enantiomer mainly inhibits reuptake of norepinephrine[92,93] (Table 37.5).

Formulations include IR and sustained-release (SR) oral forms (SR, dosing every 12 hours; ER, dosing every 24 hours); injectable solutions for subcutaneous, intravenous, spinal, or intramuscular administration; and a rectal formulation. SR formulations are available in a number of countries worldwide, but only the ER formulation is currently available in the United States. In addition, an orally disintegrating tablet version of tramadol (Ralivia FlashDose) for the treatment of moderate to moderately severe pain is under development.[95] Tramadol is currently recommended for the treatment of moderate to moderately severe pain in patients unresponsive to previous oral therapies or who have a contraindication to COX-2–selective or COX-2–nonselective NSAIDs.[9]

HISTORY

Tramadol has been available in Germany since 1977, where it remains one of the most widely prescribed analgesics. Before its U.S. release in 1995, clinical[96] and epidemiologic studies[97] suggested that tramadol demonstrates low abuse potential, which led the Drug Abuse Advisory Committee to recommend FDA approval of tramadol as a nonscheduled analgesic.[98] Current studies continue to support the low abuse potential of tramadol. A postmarketing survey has demonstrated limited evidence of tramadol use–related dependence, withdrawal, and abuse.[99] Another study assessing the prevalence of abuse compared tramadol with NSAIDs and hydrocodone-containing analgesics in patients with chronic non–cancer-related pain.[100] This study used an abuse index that identified subjects according to the following behavior: (1) increased doses without physician approval, (2) used for purposes other than intended, (3) demonstrated an inability to stop use, and (4) experienced withdrawal. The percentage of subjects who scored positive (at least one of the four types of behavior) during a 12-month period was 2.5% for NSAIDs, 2.7% for tramadol, and 4.9% for hydrocodone.

FORMULATIONS

Currently available oral formulations of tramadol include 50-mg scored IR tablets, SR tablets and capsules (every-12-hour dosing available worldwide but not in the United States), two ER once-daily tablets (Ultram ER and Ryzolt [Purdue Pharma]), and combination tablets consisting of tramadol, 37.5 mg, plus APAP, 325 mg.[101] The SR preparations are available in strengths of 50, 100, 150, and 200 mg taken on a twice-daily schedule. ER tramadol hydrochloride tablets (Ultram ER) are available in 100-, 200-, and 300-mg strengths taken on a once-daily basis. The bioavailability of Ultram ER, 200 mg, relative to tramadol, 50-mg IR formulation every 6 hours, is approximately 85% to 90%. Steady-state plasma concentrations of tramadol and M1 are achieved within 4 days of once-daily dosing. Important pharmacokinetic parameters of the 200-mg ER formulation include a time of maximum concentration (T_{max}) of 12 and 15 hours for tramadol and the M1 metabolite, respectively, as compared with a T_{max} of 1.5 and 1.9 hours for tramadol and the M1 metabolite, respectively, with the 50-mg IR formulation[101] (Table 37.6).

Once-daily ER Ultram was formulated to counter the need for doses of IR tramadol hydrochloride (Ultram) every 6 hours, improve compliance, and decrease sleep interruptions because of more stable serum concentrations. The bioavailability of ER tramadol is comparable to that of IR tramadol and demonstrates steady-state bioequivalence

Table 37.5 Affinity between Tramadol, Two Enantiomers, and Its Active Metabolite M1, Opioid Receptors, and Inhibition of Serotonin and Norepinephrine Reuptake

	Affinity for Opioid Receptors (K_i, mmol/L)			Reuptake Inhibition	
Product	μ	δ	κ	Norepinephrine	Serotonin
(±) Tramadol	2.1	57.6	42.7	0.78	0.9
(+) Tramadol	1.3	62.4	54.0	2.51	0.53
(−) Tramadol	24.8	213	53.5	0.43	2.35
(+) M1	0.0034				
Morphine	0.00034	0.092	0.57	Inactive	Inactive
Imipramine	3.7	12.7	1.8	0.0066	0.021

K_i, constant of inhibition.
Modified from Grond S, Sablotzki A. Clinical pharmacology of tramadol. *Clin Pharmacokinet*. 2004;43:879-923; and Mattia C, Coluzzi F. Tramadol. Focus on musculoskeletal and neuropathic pain. *Minerva Anestesiol*. 2005;71:565-584.

(area under the plasma drug concentration–vs.-time curve and maximum concentration [C_{max}] values) when compared with IR tramadol administered four times daily.[101] ER tramadol (200 mg) has a longer T_{max} (tramadol, 12 hours; M1 metabolite, 15 hours) than IR tramadol does (tramadol, 1.5 hours; M1 metabolite, 1.9 hours) but reaches steady-state plasma concentrations (tramadol and M1) within 4 days with once-daily dosing.

ER tramadol (100, 200, 300 mg) was found to be superior to placebo in average change from baseline pain from 1 through 12 weeks in a randomized trial of OA of the knee. The average ER tramadol dose was 276 mg/day.[102]

Tramadol hydrochloride ER tablets (Ryzolt, Purdue Pharma L.P., Stamford, Conn, 2009) contain both IR and ER characteristics (100, 200, and 300 mg). Ryzolt is indicated for the management of moderate to moderately severe chronic pain in adults who require around-the-clock treatment of their pain for an extended period. The median time to peak plasma concentrations of tramadol and M1 after multiple doses of 200-mg tablets is about 4 and 5 hours, respectively. Steady state is achieved after 2 days with a relative bioavailability of approximately 95% with 200 mg of Ryzolt versus IR tramadol, 50 mg every 6 hours (Ryzolt Package Insert, Purdue Pharma L.P., 2009).

PHARMACOKINETICS

The maximum serum concentration of oral tramadol is reached in approximately 2 hours.[103] Its mean bioavailability after a single dose is 68%,[104] and this increases to 90% to 100% after multiple doses. Mean bioavailability after intramuscular administration is 100% and after rectal administration is 78%. Tramadol is 20% bound to plasma proteins and crosses the placenta.[105] Metabolism is primarily hepatic via the CYP enzyme system. Tramadol is excreted by the kidneys (90%) and in feces (10%). Biotransformation in the liver creates 23 metabolites; the primary metabolite is *O*-desmethyltramadol (M1).[106] Polymorphism of the CYP2D6 isoenzyme in the liver (present in approximately 7% to 10% of whites) may cause attenuation of analgesia in poor metabolizers. Such patients may require higher loading doses and more rescue analgesia.[107] The elimination $t_{1/2}$ of tramadol is 5 to 6 hours and that of M1 is approximately 8 hours. Adjustments in dosage are required for patients with hepatic and renal failure and for geriatric patients (Table 37.7).[108] Bioequivalence has been demonstrated between IR and SR-ER formulations[91] (see Table 37.6).

Table 37.6 Pharmacokinetic Properties of Immediate- and Extended-Release Tramadol and Its M1 Metabolite

	Tramadol		M1 Metabolite	
Pharmacokinetic Parameter	Ultram ER	Ultram IR	Ultram ER	Ultram IR
C_{max} (μg/L)	335	383	95	104
C_{min} ((μg/L)	187	228	69	82
T_{max} (hr)	12	1.5	15	1.9

MANAGEMENT CONSIDERATIONS

For improved tolerability of tramadol, various titration regimens have been proposed (Table 37.8). An alternative example of a titration schedule for the IR 50-mg tablets in patients with moderate to moderately severe chronic pain is as follows:

1. Start at 25 mg/day and titrate in 25-mg increments as separate doses every 3 days to reach 100 mg/day (25 mg four times daily).
2. Increase the total daily dose by 50 mg as tolerated every 3 days to reach 200 mg/day (50 mg four times daily).
3. After titration, tramadol, 50 to 100 mg, can be administered as needed for pain relief every 4 to 6 hours, not to exceed 400 mg/day.

Patients with moderately severe pain who need more immediate pain control may benefit from a more aggressive dosing schedule. In this case, the increased risk for adverse events associated with higher initial doses must be clearly discussed and acceptable. In this subset of patients, tramadol, 50 to 100 mg, may be administered as needed every 4 to 6 hours, not to exceed 400 mg total per 24-hour period.

The initial recommended dose of tramadol SR formulations is 50 to 100 mg twice daily. Titration to doses of 150 to 200 mg twice daily pending side effect tolerability and

Table 37.7 Primary Kinetic Parameters of Tramadol*

	Young Healthy Volunteers		Older Healthy Volunteers			
Parameter	IV (*n* = 10)	PO (*n* = 10)	PO (*n* = 12; age = 65-75 yr)	PO (*n* = 8; age >75 yr)	Patients With Renal Failure (IV, *n* = 12)	Patients With Hepatic Failure (PO, *n*= 10)
T_{max} (hr)	—	1.9	2.0	2.1	—	1.9
C_{max} (μg/L)	409	290	324	415	894	433
AUC (μ/L × hr)	3709	2488	2508	3854	7832	7848
$t_{1/2}\beta$ (hr)	5.2	5.1	6.1	7.0	10.8	13.3
TC (L/hr)	28.8	42.6	47.6	29.5	16.8	16.3

*Depending on the patient's age and hepatic and renal failure.

AUC, area under the plasma drug concentration-versus-time curve; TC, total clearance; C_{max}, maximum plasma concentration; $t_{1/2}\beta$, elimination half-life; T_{max}, time necessary to reach the maximum plasma concentration.

From Mattia C, Coluzzi F. Tramadol. Focus on musculoskeletal and neuropathic pain. *Minerva Anestesiol*. 2005;71:565-584.

efficacy of pain relief as needed may be carried out. Tramadol ER dosage recommendations include an initial dose of 100 mg daily, with upward titration by 100 mg every 5 days to a maximum daily dosage of 300 mg.

RISKS AND PRECAUTIONS

When compared with traditional opioid analgesics, tramadol retains a more favorable side effect profile and may be associated with a lower risk for addiction with chronic use.[109]

Common Side Effects

The most commonly reported side effects include nausea, vomiting, dizziness, fatigue, sweating, dry mouth, drowsiness, sedation, and orthostatic hypotension. The incidence of side effects has been reported to be as high as 16.8% in patients with chronic pain complaints. Controlled-release formulations may produce a lower incidence of side effects (6.5%).[110]

Despite its improved side effect profile and early consideration as an alternative to pure μ-opioid receptor agonist medications, reports of overdose and fatality have led to a change in the package insert information that includes a contraindication in patients with a past or present history of addiction or dependence on opioids.[97] Other more severe side effects include angioedema,[111] bleeding complications because of the increased effect of oral anticoagulants,[112] and serotonin toxicity.[113-115]

Tramadol and Serotonin Toxicity (Serotonin Syndrome)

Concomitant use of tramadol with other serotonergic medications (e.g., selective serotonin reuptake inhibitors [SSRIs], monoamine oxidase inhibitors [MAOIs], and serotonin-norepinephrine reuptake inhibitors [SNRIs]; Box 37.4) has been associated with case reports of serotonin toxicity.[116,117] Given the fact that a number of medication classes commonly used for management of pain may predispose patients to mild to severe symptoms of serotonin toxicity, a review to gain a more clear understanding of serotonin toxicity and serotonin syndrome is in order.

Definition

Serotonin toxicity is an iatrogenic drug-induced toxidrome, a group of signs and symptoms occurring together with a particular type of chemical poisoning. Life-threatening serotonin toxicity, though rare, is usually precipitated by ingestion of MAOIs and SSRIs and leads, in some cases, to hyperpyrexia and death.[118] The pathophysiology remains unclear but may involve overstimulation of 5-HT_{1A} and 5-HT_2 receptors in the brain. Serotonin toxicity has been described by Gillman and Whyte as a triad involving neuromuscular hyperactivity, autonomic hyperactivity, and altered mental status (Table 37.9).[115]

Sternbach proposed criteria for serotonin syndrome in one of the earlier published comprehensive reviews of serotonin syndrome.[113] In 2000, Radomski and associates[114] published an updated review of the subject with revised diagnostic criteria (Table 37.10).

Mechanisms of Serotonin Toxicity. Serotonin toxicity may be related to the mechanisms and potency of drugs. Tricyclic antidepressants (TCAs) exhibit a 100-fold variability in affinity for the serotonin transporter in humans. Overdose of amitriptyline alone does not precipitate serotonin toxicity.[119] More potent TCAs, such as clomipramine, may actually have more potent serotonergic effects clinically and in overdose. In overdoses of SSRIs or SNRIs such as with venlafaxine alone, 15% of individuals exhibit moderate serotonin toxicity without life-threatening symptoms or pyrexia.[120] Although venlafaxine has less potency than amitriptyline at the receptor level, it precipitates serotonin toxicity more frequently than SSRIs do (30% vs. 15%). This may be related to mechanisms other than inhibition of serotonin reuptake.[121] Trazodone and nefazodone differ from TCAs and SSRIs in that they are primarily 5-HT_{2A} antagonists. Neither exhibit serotonergic side effects, nor do they induce signs of serotonin toxicity in overdose.[118]

A number of other pharmacologic agents, including illicit substances, enhance 5-HT activity and must be considered in

Table 37.8 Sample Tramadol Dosing Schedules

Tramadol Dose (mg)	Day
Chronic Pain	
25 qAM	1
25 bid	2
25 tid	3
25 qid	4
50 qAM, 25 noon, 25 afternoon, 50 qhs	5-7
50 qid	8-10
50-100 qid	11-X
Acute or Subacute Pain	
50 q6h	1-3
100 q6h	4-X

Box 37.4 Agents That Increase Risk for Acetaminophen Hepatotoxicity through Cytochrome P-450 (CYP) Induction

CYP1A2

Barbiturates
Bupropion (possible)
Caffeine
Carbamazepine
Charcoal-broiled food
Cruciferous vegetables
Dihydralazine
Isoniazid
Phenytoin
Primidone
Rifampin
Ritonavir
Sulfinpyrazone

CYP2E1

Ethanol
Isoniazid

Adapted from Barkin RL. Acetaminophen, aspirin, or ibuprofen in combination analgesic products. *Am J Ther*. 2001;8:433-442.

the workup for possible serotonin toxicity (e.g., buspirone, ergot alkaloids, amphetamine, cocaine, TCAs, MAOIs[122]; see Box 37.3).

CLINICAL USE OF TRAMADOL FORMULATIONS

Earlier reports evaluating the effectiveness of tramadol for varied painful conditions yielded conflicting results. In comparative studies of acute pain, oral tramadol was found to have efficacy similar to that of propoxyphene in a postoperative pain study and comparable efficacy as codeine for pain related to dental surgery.[123] However, tramadol hydrochloride, 50 and 100 mg, was found to have efficacy similar to that of placebo for pain after total hip arthroplasty[124] but provided analgesia inferior to that of hydrocodone-APAP in an emergency room acute musculoskeletal pain cohort consisting of fracture, sprain-strain, and contusion.[125]

More recent clinical and evidence-based practice has found tramadol to be useful for a wide range of painful conditions, including OA,[126] postamputation phantom limb and residual limb pain,[127] postoperative pain reduction after arthroscopic knee surgery,[128] and cancer-related pain.[129] Guidelines for the pharmacologic management of OA have recommended tramadol for patients who fail to achieve analgesia with APAP, COX-2 inhibitors, or NSAIDs.[56,130]

Table 37.9 Clinical Triad of Serotonin Toxicity

Parameter	Manifestations
Neuromuscular hyperactivity	Tremor, clonus, myoclonus, hyperreflexia
Autonomic hyperactivity	Diaphoresis, fever, tachycardia, tachypnea, mydriasis
Altered mental status	Agitation, excitement, confusion

A 2004 Cochrane collaboration review of tramadol for neuropathic pain identified a number of eligible trials, including two comparing tramadol with placebo,[131,132] one comparing tramadol with clomipramine,[133] and one comparing tramadol with morphine for cancer pain.[134] Tramadol was found to be effective for the treatment of neuropathic pain based on this limited number of short-term studies (4 to 6 weeks). The NNT for tramadol in relieving neuropathic pain states (3.5) was similar to that for other commonly used medications—2.4 for TCAs, 2.5 for carbamazepine, and 3.7 for gabapentin.

TRAMADOL-ACETAMINOPHEN

A number of different strengths of combination tramadol and APAP compounds are available in the United States and Europe. The combination takes advantage of the potential synergy between the two compounds demonstrated in animal and human models, with an initial onset of analgesia with APAP (20 minutes) followed by tramadol (approximately 50 minutes).[135] A meta-analysis of dental pain has demonstrated that the combination of APAP plus tramadol has a similar rapid onset of efficacy as paracetamol alone, but levels of analgesia are maintained for a longer period than with tramadol alone.[136] Tramadol-APAP combination products contain less tramadol by dose (in the United States, 37.5 vs. 50 mg) and relatively less APAP (325 vs. 500 mg [extra-strength APAP]) and thus may lower the potential incidence of organ toxicity (liver) when taken within the range of recommended doses.[91] Tramadol-APAP combination products have demonstrated efficacy for acute and chronic pain conditions.[137] Combination tramadol, 37.5 mg, plus APAP, 325 mg, may provide analgesia equivalent to that of codeine and APAP in patients with chronic OA, but with greater tolerability.[138] The most common treatment-related adverse events include somnolence, nausea, and constipation with a mean dosage of 4.1 tablets daily.[139] Figure 37.3 illustrates NNT data from

Table 37.10 Spectrum of Serotonin Syndrome

Mild State of Serotonin-Related Symptoms	Serotonin Syndrome (Full-Blown Form)		Toxic States
Single symptom may predominate	At least four major or three major and two minor of the following:		Coma
Most common are	Major	Minor	Generalized tonic-clonic seizures
Tremor	Mental symptoms:	Restlessness	Fever (may exceed 40° C)
Myoclonus	Impaired consciousness	Insomnia	Disseminated intravascular coagulation and renal failure
Diaphoresis and shivering	Elevated mood	Incoordination	
	Neurologic symptoms:	Dilated pupils	
	Myoclonus	Akathisia	
	Tremor	Tachycardia	
	Shivering	Tachypnea, dyspnea	
	Rigidity	Diarrhea	
	Hyperreflexia	Hypertension, hypotension	
	Vegetative symptoms:		
	Fever		
	Sweating		

Coincident with the addition of or an increase in a known serotonergic agent. Clinical features were not an integral part of the underlying psychiatric disorder before commencing the serotonergic agent. Other causes (e.g., infectious, metabolic or endocrine, substance abuse or withdrawal) have been ruled out. A neuroleptic drug has not been started or increased in dosage before onset of the signs and symptoms listed.
From Gnanadesigan N, Espinoza RT, Smith R, et al. Interaction of serotonergic antidepressants and opioid analgesics: is serotonin syndrome going undetected? *J Am Med Dir Assoc*. 2005;6:265-269.

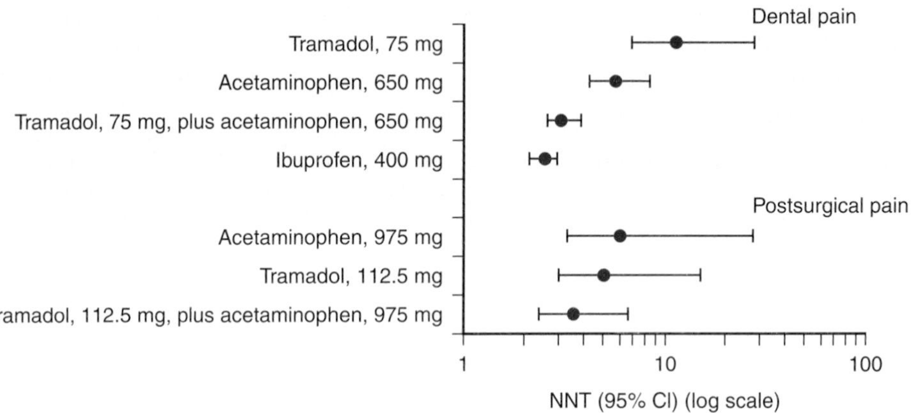

Figure 37.3 Meta-analysis evaluating a tramadol-acetaminophen combination for moderate to severe postoperative pain. CI, confidence interval; NNT, number needed to treat. (From Edwards JE, McQuay HJ, Moore RA. Combination analgesic efficacy: individual patient data meta-analysis of single-dose oral tramadol plus acetaminophen in acute postoperative pain. *J Pain Symptom Manage.* 2002;23:121-130.)

a meta-analysis evaluating the efficacy of a tramadol-APAP combination for moderate to severe postoperative pain.[140]

ORAL STEROIDS

The first glucocorticoid was isolated in 1935. This naturally occurring corticosteroid, cortisone, was later synthesized in the laboratory in 1944. Four years later, Hench and colleagues at the Mayo Clinic were able to obtain a portion of the total 9 g of synthetic cortisone available from Merck for clinical trial use. They injected this "compound E" (cortisone) into patients with rheumatoid arthritis. Accounts describe the treatment of multiple patients with 100-mg injections, with astonishing results—patients experienced dramatic pain reduction and remarkable improvement in their functional mobility. Reports noted that one of their formerly totally bedridden patients was able to get out of bed and tried to dance. However, when the supplies ran out just 1 week later, all the treated patients went into remission.[141] This report led not only to the widespread use of cortisone for the treatment of rheumatologic conditions but also earned Hench a joint award (along with Kendall and Reichstein) of the Nobel Prize in Medicine and Physiology in 1950. As oral steroid preparations evolved, their use increased in addition to injection therapy as a method of producing systemic levels for chronic treatment regimens. Pulsed dosing schedules are now routinely used for disease management and episodic flares of a wide range of conditions, including rheumatic, pulmonary, dermatologic, neurologic, ophthalmologic, hematologic, and endocrine disorders. Exogenous glucocorticoid administration has been shown to have a suppressive effect on the hypothalamic-pituitary-adrenal (HPA) axis. Some believe that this can occur in as few as 5 days when using high supraphysiologic doses, whereas at physiologic doses this may not occur for 3 to 4 weeks. Thus, a tapered dosing schedule is typically recommended when treatment exceeds 2 to 3 weeks.[142] The use of steroids for the treatment of painful conditions is largely based on the premise that there is an inflammatory role in the mediation of pain.[143] Chronic oral steroid therapy is used for the treatment of rheumatologic inflammatory conditions (e.g., rheumatoid arthritis, polymyalgia rheumatica, Crohn's disease), as well as cancer pain. In addition, oral steroids are commonly used in short-term or pulsed dosing schedules for conditions such as complex regional pain syndrome (CRPS), rheumatoid arthritis flares, gouty or OA flares, painful radiculopathy, bursitis, carpal tunnel syndrome, and other acute or chronic musculoskeletal conditions.[144-146]

MECHANISM OF ACTION AND DESCRIPTION

Adrenocortical steroids such as prednisone, methylprednisolone, and dexamethasone act by inhibiting multiple cellular mechanisms, including accumulation of inflammatory cells at sites of inflammation, macrophage phagocytosis, lysosomal enzyme release and synthesis, and release of mediators of inflammation. In regard to their ability to attenuate pain responses, this action is probably related to their strong anti-inflammatory action. Steroids suppress or prevent cell-mediated immune responses and decrease or prevent tissue response to the inflammatory process. The mechanisms for reduction of cancer pain are thought to be secondary to inhibition of PG synthesis and reduction in peritumor and perineural edema by decreasing capillary permeability.[143]

Oral prednisone is readily absorbed in the GI tract. It is highly protein bound (up to 70% to 90%) and is distributed widely in a variety of tissues. The plasma $t_{1/2}$ of prednisone is 3.4 to 4 hours, with a biologic $t_{1/2}$ of 18 to 36 hours. It is metabolized in the liver to its active metabolite prednisolone, which is further metabolized to inactive compounds. The active metabolite and inactive compounds are excreted in urine, and the drug is not removed by hemodialysis.[147] The pharmacodynamics of commonly used glucocorticoids is presented in Table 37.11.

Prednisone tablets are available in multiple dosage forms ranging from 2.5- to 50-mg tablets. Other glucocorticoids commonly prescribed for painful conditions include methylprednisolone (Medrol Dosepak) and dexamethasone (Table 37.12). The Medrol Dosepak consists of 21 4-mg tablets taken in a tapering fashion from 6 tablets on day 1 to 1 tablet on day 6. See Box 37.5 for common glucocorticoid dosing schedules.

RISKS AND PRECAUTIONS

In general, long-term administration at physiologic replacement doses does not lead to adverse effects. Similarly, short-term dosing at supraphysiologic levels typically does not cause adverse effects. Many have recommended a tapering dose schedule to avoid glucocorticoid withdrawal, which can occur in as few as 5 days at high supraphysiologic doses or in 3 to 4 weeks at physiologic doses.[142] Suppression of the HPA

Table 37.11 Pharmacodynamics of Common Glucocorticoids

Agent	Equivalent Glucocorticoid Dose (mg)	Relative Glucocorticoid Activity	Relative Mineralocorticoid Activity*	Relative Half-Life in Plasma (hr)	Biologic Half-Life (hr)
Cortisone	25	0.8	0.8	0.5	8-12
Cortisol	20	1	1	1.5-2	8-12
Methylprednisolone	4	5	0.5	>3.5	18-36
Prednisolone	5	4	0.6	2.1-3.5	18-36
Prednisone	5	4	0.6	3.4-3.8	18-36
Triamcinolone	4	5	0	2->5	18-36
Dexamethasone	0.75	20-30	0	3-4.5	36-54
Betamethasone	0.6	20-30	0	3-5	36-54

*Clinically—sodium and water retention, potassium depletion.

Adapted from Jacobs JWD, Bijlsma JWJ. Glucocorticoid therapy. In: Kelly W, Harris E, Ruddy S, et al, eds. *Kelly's Textbook of Rheumatology.* 7th ed. Philadelphia: Saunders; 2005, Table 57-1.)

Table 37.12 Commonly Prescribed Oral Glucocorticoids

Agent	Trade Name	Available Dose Form
Methylprednisolone	Medrol	2-, 4-, 8-, 16-, 24-, 32-mg tablets
Prednisone	Deltasone, Sterapred	2.5-, 5-, 10-, 20-, 50-mg tablets
	Prednisone Intensol (oral concentrate)	5 mg/mL
Dexamethasone	Decadron	0.25-, 0.5-, 0.75-, 1.5-, 4-, 8-mg tablets
	Decadron elixir (oral concentrate)	0.5 mg/5 mL

Box 37.5 Common Glucocorticoid Dosing Schedules

Prednisone taper—prednisone, 10-mg tablets
- 3 tablets PO bid × 4 days, 2 tablets PO bid × 3 days, 1 tablet PO bid × 3 days

Medrol Dosepak—methylprednisolone, 4-mg tablets
- Day 1: 2 tablets before breakfast, 1 tablet after lunch and dinner, and 2 tablets at bedtime (total = 6 tablets). If given later in the day, may take all 6 tablets at once or in divided doses
- Day 2: 1 tablet before breakfast, 1 tablet after lunch and dinner, and 2 tablets at bedtime
- Day 3: Same as day 2, except 1 tablet at bedtime
- Day 4: 1 tablet before breakfast, after lunch, and at bedtime
- Day 5: 1 tablet after breakfast and at bedtime
- Day 6: 1 tablet after breakfast

Dexamethasone taper—dexamethasone, 8-mg tablets
- Tapering schedule over 7 days: 64, 32, 24, 16, 8, 8, 8 mg

axis can persist for up to 12 months after cessation of prolonged corticosteroid therapy, and supplementation may be required during periods of physiologic stress such as surgery, acute blood loss, or infection. Because of the depression and prevention of cell-mediated immune responses, oral corticosteroids are not well tolerated by patients with immunocompromised states, whether acute or chronic. However, they do play an adjuvant role in the management of cancer pain.[148] In such cases, new pain complaints in cancer patients or palliative care patients must be monitored vigilantly because in the presence of opioid analgesics and corticosteroid therapy, symptoms may be less severe and related to a new diagnosis, such as appendicitis.[149]

A population-based study examining more than 2400 patients maintained on long-term oral glucocorticoid therapy found that side effects are associated with cumulative and average doses in a dose-dependent fashion. The study allowed the use of varied glucocorticoid preparations and converted them into a prednisone-equivalent dose. The most common side effects, with approximate prevalence, included weight gain (70%), skin bruising (53%), sleep disturbance (45%), mood symptoms (42%), cataracts (15%), acne (15%), and fractures (12%). An increasing daily dosage was more significantly associated with fractures and sleep disturbance than was an increased duration of use.[150]

Use of prednisone during pregnancy is schedule D during the first trimester and schedule C in the second and third trimesters (Table 37.13). First-trimester exposure to systemic corticosteroids (category C) has been associated with intrauterine growth retardation and an increased incidence of cleft lip, with or without cleft palate. If necessary, the maternal benefits of short courses of oral corticosteroids may outweigh the fetal risks when given beyond the first trimester.[151]

CLINICAL USE

Oral corticosteroids have a limited role in the treatment of painful conditions. They may be useful in the treatment of acute painful inflammatory conditions, including CRPS, carpal tunnel syndrome, rotator cuff arthropathy–adhesive capsulitis, and painful cervical or lumbar radiculopathy.

Table 37.13 FDA Pregnancy Categories for Drugs

Category	Description
A	No fetal risk in controlled studies
B	No risk to the human fetus despite possible animal risk or no risk in animal studies but human studies lacking
C	Human risk cannot be ruled out. Animal studies may or may not show risk.
D	Evidence of risk to the human fetus

FDA, U.S. Food and Drug Administration.

Steroids have been and continue to be administered by multiple routes for the treatment of CRPS. After early reports of success with systemic steroids,[152] Christensen and coworkers[146] studied 23 patients and reported that 30 mg/day of oral prednisone is significantly better than placebo based on their stated clinical outcome measures. Braus and colleagues[153] studied the effects of methylprednisolone, 32 mg/day for 2 weeks, followed by a taper over 2 weeks, for the treatment of CRPS in post-stroke patients. This randomized study showed a significant clinical improvement in the steroid-treated patients at 4 weeks. A recent investigation of the effects of chronic methylprednisolone treatment on the rat CRPS type 1 model (tibia fracture) has revealed that glucocorticoids reverse hindpaw edema and warmth after fracture, with persistent effects occurring after discontinuation of treatment. However, glucocorticoid treatment has no effect on the allodynia, hindpaw unweighting, or periarticular bone loss observed after tibia fracture.[154]

The use of minor analgesics in the cancer pain population is common. The most commonly used opioid co-analgesics are NSAIDs and APAP, but up to 39% of cancer patients take various types of corticosteroids, with dexamethasone being the most common formulation. These patients have a wide range of conditions, with breast, lung, and colorectal cancer topping the list. This cross-sectional study did not specifically determine whether each adjuvant medication was given specifically for control of pain as opposed to other diseases, but other studies have documented the usefulness of corticosteroids for the rational polypharmacy of cancer pain management.[148,155,156] Efficacy has been demonstrated for neuropathic pain caused by tumor compression (malignant compression of the spinal cord or brachial or lumbosacral plexus), tumor-induced bone pain, and hepatic capsule distention secondary to liver metastases.[143,157] In addition to NSAIDs and disease-modifying antirheumatic drugs, low-dose oral corticosteroids may also be helpful in managing joint symptoms caused by chemotherapy-induced arthropathy.[158]

Despite the lack of many directed controlled clinical trials, corticosteroids are frequently prescribed in an adjunctive role for palliation and control of the side effects of chemotherapy; therefore, these agents may play a dual role in selected patients. Many believe that corticosteroids may help in preventing chemotherapy-induced nausea and emesis and hypersensitivity reactions. In addition, they may also help ameliorate asthenic symptoms and fatigue, as well as stimulate appetite.[145,159]

The use of oral glucocorticoids in the form of methylprednisolone or prednisone burst or taper is common practice in the acute treatment of disk herniation with radicular pain complaints. Despite a significant increase in studies evaluating the efficacy of fluoroscopically guided epidural steroid injections,[160] there is a paucity of reports on the usefulness of oral or systemic corticosteroids in this pain population. In the only prospective, double-blind, randomized controlled trial evaluating the use of oral corticosteroids for the treatment of radicular pain, a tapering dose of dexamethasone over a 7-day period was not superior to placebo for early or long-term relief of lumbosacral radicular pain. Dexamethasone, however, was superior to placebo in reducing stretch-invoked pain during the straight-leg raise test. This study did allow the concurrent use of meperidine, oxycodone, and APAP for analgesia.[161] Systemic dexamethasone taper via the intramuscular route has been studied to a limited degree, with conflicting results.[162,163] The rationale for the use of oral corticosteroids is based on the observance that proinflammatory mediators and neurosensitizing chemicals are released from the damaged intervertebral disk.[164,165] One study suggested that epidurally administered glucocorticoids do not appear to have a negative effect on spontaneous resorption of disk herniations.[166]

With most musculoskeletal injuries there is a close relationship between injury and pain. Therefore, individual treatments in a comprehensive management program may serve dual purposes—reducing inflammation to control local damage and concurrently reducing pain. Although few trials have evaluated the efficacy of oral corticosteroids for musculoskeletal injuries, clinical practice reveals that their use is widespread. A questionnaire-based study involving 99 physicians at a national sports medicine conference found that 59% of the physicians prescribe oral corticosteroids for musculoskeletal injuries, with prednisone being the most commonly used.[167] The study did not differentiate whether the medication was being prescribed specifically for pain or for its anti-inflammatory properties, but prescriptions were written for acute and chronic conditions equally.

Although the mainstays of treatment of carpal tunnel syndrome include neutral wrist splints, ergonomic evaluation and modification of biomechanics, oral NSAIDs, steroid injections, and surgical release of the transverse carpal ligament, there is evidence to suggest that oral corticosteroids may play a role in the short-term management of patients with mild to moderate symptoms and in those not interested in or awaiting surgical release of the transverse carpal ligament. Studies have examined varied dosing and duration-of-treatment regimens with prednisolone (10 days to 3 weeks, doses of up to 25 mg daily); the results suggest that regardless of dosing, the global symptom score is improved in patients treated with oral corticosteroid versus placebo.[144]

Short-term dosing of oral prednisolone at variable doses has been studied for adhesive capsulitis. Binder and associates[168] used 10 mg daily for 4 weeks, followed by 5 mg daily for 2 weeks. Night pain was significantly lower in the treatment group at 8 weeks. However, by 5 months this difference had resolved. Over the total 8-month period, no difference was found in pain at rest or with movement, range of motion, or the cumulative recovery curve between the oral steroid group and the control group, which received no specific therapy. Other studies have evaluated a 3-week

Table 37.14 Components of Caffeine-Containing Over-the-Counter Medications

Name	Caffeine (mg)	Acetaminophen (mg)	NSAID (mg)
Excedrin Tension Headache	65	500	N/A
Excedrin Migraine	65	250	250 ASA
Goody's Extra Strength Headache Powder	32.5	260	520 ASA

ASA, acetylsalicylic acid; N/A, not applicable; NSAID, nonsteroidal anti-inflammatory drug.

course of 30 mg prednisolone daily and reported a significant reduction in pain and disability, improved active range of motion, and better participant-rated improvement at 3 weeks. By 6 weeks, the improvements were still evident, but none of the values were statistically significant; at 12 weeks, the placebo group was favored.[145]

The use of oral corticosteroids for the treatment of rheumatoid arthritis has been studied since 1949, when Hench and coworkers[169] showed efficacy of the treatment in an uncontrolled trial. Although oral corticosteroids may show beneficial effects with respect to radiologic progress of the disease,[170] they are more commonly used during episodes of symptomatic flares to control pain or as bridge therapy with slower-acting agents.[171,172] A meta-analysis evaluating the effectiveness of low-dose prednisolone versus placebo and NSAIDs found that low-dose prednisolone (<15 mg daily) has greater effect than placebo and NSAIDs on joint tenderness and pain.[172]

CAFFEINE

Caffeine is an important adjuvant compound used in combination with OTC and prescription analgesics. Caffeine exhibits antinociceptive effects and analgesic properties when used in combination with opioid analgesics.[173] Caffeine combination products have been studied for a number of pain conditions, including headache,[174] oral surgery,[175] low back pain,[176] and postpartum-related pain.[177] Caffeine (65 to 130 mg) was shown to increase the potency of other analgesics by 40%.[178] OTC headache medications typically include 65 or 32.5 mg caffeine combined with APAP, 250 to 500 mg, and/or ASA, 250 to 520 mg (Table 37.14).

MECHANISM OF ACTION AND DESCRIPTION

Caffeine, a methylxanthine, is a nonselective adenosine receptor antagonist that blocks multiple adenosine receptors (A1, A2A, A2B, and A3) in peripheral tissues and the CNS.[179,180] Centrally, caffeine may increase dopamine and norepinephrine, as well as act as a vasoconstrictor of vessels, thereby contributing to its analgesic effect in certain headache conditions.[181] A recent animal study using a fixed dose of aspirin, APAP (paracetamol), and caffeine demonstrated increased secretion of norepinephrine and a reduction in dopamine in rat striatal tissue.[182]

CLINICAL USE

Studies examining the relationship between dietary caffeine intake and chronic low back pain have yielded conflicting results.[183,184] One review that included more than 10,000 patients in 30 trials found that caffeine is successful as an adjuvant for analgesia. Without the combination of caffeine, 40% higher doses of aspirin, APAP, or salicylamide would have been required to achieve equivalent analgesia. When used for the treatment of nonmigrainous headache, 65 mg of caffeine was found to be as effective as 648 mg of APAP.

TOPICAL MEDICATIONS

Prescription and OTC topical medications for pain, including topical analgesics, counterirritants, heat and cold preparations, and patches, constitute a growing area of development in pain management. In the previous decade alone, topical analgesics accounted for approximately 6% of the growing U.S. analgesic market.[185] In addition, a smaller evolving niche market of compounding pharmacies—those that provide the unique service of customized compounding of various creams and gels for topical use—has broadened the use of topical medications for analgesia. Commonly used medications include ketamine, lidocaine, gabapentin, cyclobenzaprine, and various NSAIDs.[186]

The use of topical analgesics may be a viable option for patients because of safety concerns of NSAIDs in the popular media and scientific literature.[187] The FDA's black box warnings of prescription and OTC NSAIDs, including COX-2 inhibitors,[188] may have led to renewed interest in safer pharmacologic alternatives to oral medications. In general, topical preparations have considerably less potential for systemic adverse effects and organ toxicity. Interestingly, a recent meta-analysis of randomized placebo-controlled trials for OA found topical NSAIDs to be more effective than oral nonselective NSAIDs and COX-2 inhibitors and second to intra-articular steroid injections, as measured by patient-perceived improvement during the first 2 to 3 weeks following treatment.[189] Commonly prescribed topical medications include the following: lidocaine 5% patches, indicated for post-herpetic neuralgia (PHN)[190]; topical TCAs, including doxepin and amitriptyline, for neuropathic pain states[191,192]; topical NSAIDs, including diclofenac; and counterirritants and vanilloid receptor agonists, such as capsaicin, for neuropathic pain.[193] This section reviews various prescription-strength and OTC topical medication classes, including analgesics, anesthetics, counterirritants, and hot or cold products used commonly for the treatment of acute and chronic pain conditions (Table 37.15).

METHODS OF DELIVERY

Topical agents may potentially achieve a similar level of efficacy as oral formulations without the associated systemic side effects. Some evidence has shown that topically delivered agents can accumulate to therapeutic concentrations within

Table 37.15 Topical Medications

Class	Ingredients
Counterirritants (rubefacients)	Capsaicin, 0.025%, 0.075%, 0.1%; camphor; salicylic acid; trolamine salicylate; poison ivy; marsh tea; benzyl nicotinate
Local anesthetics	Benzocaine; lidocaine 5% patch, ointment; EMLA—lidocaine 2.5%/ prilocaine 2.5%
Cooling agents	Menthol, peppermint oil
Heating agents	Iron, charcoal, table salt, water (ThermaCare heat wrap)

Box 37.6 Benefits and Limitations of Analgesia by Cutaneous Delivery

Benefits

First-pass metabolism, other variables associated with the gastrointestinal tract (e.g., pH, gastric emptying time) avoided[195-197]
Reduced side effects, minimization of drug concentration peaks and troughs in blood[197,198]
Ease of dose termination in case of untoward side effects
Delivery can be sustained and controlled over a prolonged period[199,200]
Direct access to the target site[201]
Convenient, painless administration[195,196]
Improved patient acceptance, adherence to therapy[202-204]
Ease of use—may reduce overall health treatment cost[205,206]
Provides a viable solution for treatment when oral dosing not feasible (e.g., in unconscious or nauseated patients)[197]

Limitations

Diffusion across the stratum corneum occurs only with molecules smaller than 500 Da[207]
Topical agents must have both aqueous and lipid solubility[208]
Both intraindividual and interindividual variability in skin permeability, as well as between healthy and diseased skin, causes variable efficacy[209,210]
Skin enzymes can cause metabolism before cutaneous absorption, thereby reducing drug potency[211]
Localized skin irritation (e.g., erythema, edema) can be common
Da, dalton.

From Brown MB, Martin GP, Jones SA, et al. Dermal and transdermal drug delivery systems: current and future prospects. *Drug Deliv.* 2006;13:175-187.

the local tissues to which they have been applied while maintaining low serum levels and subsequently resulting in less organ toxicity. Box 37.6 lists the benefits and limitations of dermal and transdermal delivery systems.[194-215]

Topical agents can be delivered by passive and active methods. Passive methods involve application of drugs to the skin (e.g., ointments, creams, gels, patches) and may include modified systems that enhance the driving force of the agent through the skin. These systems include thermodynamic and permeability enhancers, such as penetration enhancers, prodrugs, and liposomes. Passive methods currently on the market are usually well tolerated but are limited by skin irritation, poor adhesion, and limitation in size because of practical cosmetic issues.[194] Active methods use modalities to facilitate the distribution of medication.

"Topical" versus "Transdermal"

"Topical" and "transdermal" are distinct modes of delivery of medication to the skin. Both delivery methods must traverse the stratum corneum, the major barrier to delivering treatment. Transdermal methods deliver medication through percutaneous absorption, with the goal of achieving similar therapeutic systemic levels as active oral preparations do. Transdermal pharmacotherapies can be administered distal to the site of injury (e.g., SR nicotine and clonidine patches, long-acting fentanyl delivery systems). In contrast, topical agents use cutaneous delivery to target the site of application specifically. The sites of action of topical agents are the soft tissues and peripheral nerves underlying the site of application.[216] Serum levels generally remain relatively low with topical agents, and systemic side effects or drug-drug interactions are consequently more unlikely.[216]

The vehicle in which the active ingredient or ingredients are delivered can affect the skin penetration depth and absorption rate into the epidermis.[216] Primarily, penetration of topical modalities is limited by the relatively dense stratum corneum, a layer of flattened dead cells or keratinocytes covering the live epidermis.[217,218] Once past this relatively impermeable barrier, analgesics may access cutaneous nociceptors, including unmyelinated C fibers of the epidermal layer. Below the epidermis, the dermal layer also contains nociceptive fibers, along with fibroblasts, connective tissue, blood vessels, hair follicles, and glands.[218]

Animal models have suggested that the variability in transcutaneous absorption rates between topical agents is probably derived from their ability to negotiate the superficial layer of skin.[219] Ideally, the most effective topical agent will have a low molecular weight (less than 500 Da)[217] and both hydrophobic features to transverse the stratum corneum and hydrophilic components to penetrate the predominantly aqueous epidermis.[219,220] Occlusive dressings and specialized delivery agents may also help improve penetration.[220] Lecithin organogels are biocompatible jelly-like phases composed primarily of hydrated phospholipids and organic liquid.[221] Poloxamer-lecithin organogel (PLO) is a commonly used vehicle that includes a viscosity-enhancing agent that facilitates oil-in-water preparations and is used by a number of compounding pharmacies.[222] PLO also includes lecithin and propylene glycol, which help disperse the drug more uniformly. Additionally, polyethylene glycol and limonene[223] have been used as topical penetration enhancers to increase the absorption rate of NSAIDs by up to 75-fold.[220]

Modalities

Active delivery of medication may be enhanced by the use of physical modalities, including iontophoresis and phonophoresis.[224] Iontophoresis is the migration of charged particles across biologic membranes under an electric field, usually applied transcutaneously.[225] This method, generally under the direction of a physical therapist or other health care professional, uses low-level current to enhance the permeability of the topically applied agent (e.g., corticosteroid,

Table 37.16 Topical Nonsteroidal Anti-inflammatory Drugs

Formulation	Active Ingredient	Brand	Strength
Ointment	Indomethacin		10%
Solution (lotion)	Diclofenac	Pennsaid	1.5%
Cream	Diclofenac	Voltaren Emulgel	1%
	Ibuprofen	Dolgit (5%)	5%, 10%, 15%
	Benzydamine	Difflam	3%
	Salicylic acid	Fostex	2%
Spray	Indomethacin		1%, 4%
Patch/plaster	Diclofenac/diclofenac epolamine (DHEP)		65- to 180-mg plaster, 1% patch
	Flurbiprofen	TransAct	40-mg patch
Gel	Piroxicam	Feldene	0.5%
	Diclofenac	DDA Emulgel	1%/1.16%
	Felbinac	Traxam	3%
	Eltenac		0.1%, 0.3%, 1%
	Ketoprofen	Powergel, Tiloket gel	15%
	Indomethacin		1%
	Naproxen sodium	Naprosyn gel	10%
	Ibuprofen		1%
	Salicylic acid	Keralyt gel	3%
Drops	Ketorolac	Acular	0.2%
	Flurbiprofen	Ocufen	0.03%
	Suprofen	Profenal	1%
	Diclofenac	Voltaren	0.1%
Foam	Ketoprofen		15%
	Felbinac	Traxam	3%

Adapted from Vaile JH, Davis P. Topical NSAIDs for musculoskeletal conditions. A review of the literature. *Drugs*. 1998;56:783-799.

NSAID). Phonophoresis involves migration of drug through the skin via an ultrasound transducer. Phonophoresis is commonly used in the treatment of musculoskeletal conditions to enhance the delivery of topical NSAIDs to inflamed tissues.[226]

TOPICAL TREATMENT: CLINICAL TRIAL EVIDENCE

Nonsteroidal Anti-inflammatory Drugs

Topical NSAIDs are more widely used and studied in Europe than in the United States. Several proposed peripheral mechanisms of their analgesic activity include inhibition of PGE synthesis, the lipoxygenase pathway, and excitatory amino acids, as well as modulation of G protein–mediated signal transduction.[216] A large variety of topical NSAID formulations are available commercially (Table 37.16).

Pharmacokinetic data suggest that topically applied NSAIDs can result in enhanced local concentrations without significant toxic systemic levels. Heyneman and colleagues[220] reviewed single- and multiple-dose NSAID absorption studies. Collectively, these studies indicated that following topical administration of NSAIDs, peak plasma levels are less than 10% of the concentrations obtained from oral dosing (range, 0.2% to 8.0%), with total systemic absorption from topical application being only 3% to 5% of the oral route. The time to achieve C_{max} following topical application ranged from 2.2 to 23 hours, approximately 10 times longer than the time required for the equivalent oral dose. Topical NSAIDs generally achieve steady-state concentrations within 2 to 5 days of repeated application.[220]

Furthermore, penetration studies have indicated that topically applied NSAIDs reach therapeutic concentrations below the site of application.[220] A two-way crossover design assessed the levels of subcutaneous and muscle absorption of 800 mg of oral ibuprofen versus 16 g of 5% ibuprofen gel applied to the thigh.[227] Microdialysis probes inserted 25 to 30 mm into the muscle found average values of 63.5 ± 90.3 and 213.4 ± 117 ng/hr/mL of ibuprofen for the oral and topical routes, respectively. Ibuprofen concentrations in the dermis were 22.5-fold greater when delivered topically; mean values of ibuprofen in subcutaneous tissue were 731.2 ± 605.0 and 176.6 ± 122.9 ng/hr/mL for the topical and oral routes, respectively.[227] Another study of 100 patients who underwent knee arthroscopy evaluated ketoprofen concentrations in intra-articular tissue following a single application of a 30-mg plaster, multiple applications of plaster over a 5-day period, or a 50-mg oral dose.[228] The median C_{max} levels in the cartilage with topical and oral administration were 568.9 and 85.7 ng/g, respectively (a 6.8-fold difference). In contrast, plasma values were 18.7 ng/mL for topically administered ketoprofen and 2595.3 ng/mL for the oral route. Overall, when administered by a topical route, ketoprofen levels were 30-fold greater in cartilage than in plasma.[228]

Relative to all other topically administered drugs, NSAIDs have accumulated the largest amount of clinical evidence for their use.[216] A meta-analysis by Moore and associates[229] considered 86 randomized controlled trials of NSAIDs for the treatment of pain conditions. This review included a total of 10,160 patients. Following 1 to 2 weeks of topical application, placebo-controlled trials demonstrated the benefit of NSAIDs for the treatment of acute pain conditions, such as soft tissue trauma, sprains, and strains, as well as for chronic pain conditions, such as OA and tendinitis.

Overall, the NNT was 3.9 for acute pain conditions—more specifically, 2.6 for ketoprofen, 3.5 for ibuprofen, and 4.2 for piroxicam. For chronic pain conditions, the NNT was 3.1 (range, 2.7 to 3.8). Side effects encountered for all the pain conditions studied were minimal; topical NSAIDs rarely induced local skin reactions (3.6%) or adverse systemic effects (<0.5%).[229] Similarly, a smaller meta-analysis of 26 double-blind, placebo-controlled trials by Mason and coworkers[230] found that topical NSAID treatment is safe and effective for acute pain after 1 week of application.

Osteoarthritis and Topical Nonsteroidal Anti-inflammatory Drugs

A meta-analysis of randomized controlled trials assessed the efficacy of topical NSAIDs relative to placebo or oral formulations for the treatment of OA.[231] When compared with placebo, a positive treatment effect was observed for topical NSAIDs only during weeks 1 and 2 of treatment, with effect sizes of 0.41 (95% confidence interval [CI], 0.16 to 0.66) and 0.40 (95% CI, 0.15 to 0.65), respectively. In contrast, even during the first week, topical NSAIDs were found to provide analgesia inferior to that of oral versions, and topical agents induced more local side effects. The authors concluded that no trial evidence has supported the benefit of NSAIDs over placebo in treating OA after 2 weeks of application and even suggested that current practice guidelines on OA that advocate the use of topical NSAIDs[56,232,233] be revised.[231] However, two recent randomized, controlled trials of topical diclofenac solution for the treatment of pain secondary to knee OA reported benefit at 4 and 12 weeks of application.[234,235] As measured by Western Ontario and McMaster Universities (WOMAC) OA index scores, relative to baseline the study group had a 42.9% decrease in pain at 4 weeks and a 45.7% decrease after 12 weeks as opposed to 26.9% and 33.3% decreases in pain for the vehicle control groups, respectively. Measurements of physical function, stiffness, and pain on walking indicated similar benefit of topical diclofenac over placebo in both studies. Probably because of the skin penetration enhancer dimethyl sulfoxide (DMSO), 30 of 84 patients in the 4-week study group and 68 of 164 patients in the 12-week study group reported skin irritation (typically dryness), which led to discontinuation by 5 patients in each of the treatment groups.[234,235]

Diclofenac

Various novel NSAID patches and plasters have been developed that confer more constant, continuous delivery of a standardized dose of analgesic, although individual skin variability affects the actual amount absorbed. Galer and colleagues[236] conducted a multicenter, randomized, parallel-design trial to assess the efficacy of a topical diclofenac patch for the treatment of pain from sports-related soft tissue injuries such as sprains, strains, and contusions. A 1.3% diclofenac epolamine or placebo patch was applied twice daily onto 222 patients for 2 weeks. The study group achieved statistically significant differences in pain intensity from placebo on clinic visits at day 3 ($P = 0.036$) and day 14 ($P = 0.044$) following initiation of treatment, but not on day 7. Forty percent of participants given placebo reported adverse events, whereas 34% of the study group patients reported side effects.[236] A similar study comparing a diclofenac patch (140 mg diclofenac sodium) and placebo applied within 3 hours of blunt, soft tissue trauma-type injury found a statistically significant analgesic effect over placebo ($P < 0.0001$) as measured by tenderness produced by pressure and the time required to for the pain to resolve at the site of injury ($P < 0.0001$). Adverse events, most commonly local cutaneous reactions, were experienced at a similar frequency by both groups.[237]

Topical 1.5% diclofenac solution (Pennsaid) is presently approved in Canada and Europe for the treatment of OA. Topical 1.5% diclofenac in a carrier containing DMSO solution applied three times daily demonstrated efficacy when compared with vehicle-controlled solution and placebo in patients with OA of the knee. Adverse effects included skin irritation (36%), most commonly skin dryness, which led to discontinuation in only 6% of cases.[234] A similar study of knee OA found that a 1.5% diclofenac solution (40 drops, four times daily) resulted in improvements in pain, physical function, patient global assessment, stiffness, and pain on walking.[235]

Ketoprofen

Topical ketoprofen has been suggested to demonstrate more favorable physicochemical properties than other available NSAIDs, including greater lipophilicity and more rapid absorption.[238] Some studies have demonstrated plasma ketoprofen levels to correlate with measures of efficacy in a postoperative orthopedic cohort for up to 12 hours of oral dosing. Another study found variability in serum levels of topical ketoprofen (20%) in a PLO-based formulation after a single application, with a low rate and extent of systemic absorption (approximately 0.5%).[239] A placebo-controlled study of patients with pain from an ankle sprain assessed the analgesia achieved over a 2-week period by the application of a 100-mg topical ketoprofen patch.[240] Significantly less spontaneous pain was observed in the study group than in the control group during all visits (days 3 to 4, 7 ± 1 and 14 ± 2). Most notably, there was a 49.9- ± 20.2-mm (−73%) decrease in pain from baseline at day 7 ± 1 for patients given the ketoprofen patch as compared with a 37.6- ± 24.3-mm (−57%) decrease in patients given a placebo patch. The intergroup difference in pain relief was significant ($P = 0.0007$), but the difference in adverse events was not. Thirty-one percent of the study group and 24% of the control group experienced adverse events.[240] A similar study with a topical ketoprofen patch, 100 mg, demonstrated efficacy for symptomatic tendinitis, with a reduction in pain occurring after 1 week in the treatment group (−38.4 ± 25.6 mm) versus placebo (−25.8 ± 24.5 mm).[241]

Ketoprofen, an arylpropionic acid derivative, has been associated with an increasing number of case reports describing contact allergic and photosensitization skin reactions in Europe and Asia.[242,243] The unique photoallergy may be related to the benzophenone structure of ketoprofen.[244] Caution or avoidance of use may be necessary during periods of significant skin exposure to sun.

NEUROPATHIC PAIN AND TOPICAL ANALGESICS

Mechanisms of action for neuropathic pain include spontaneous discharges of peripheral or central neurons, spontaneous ectopic electrical activity mediated by abnormal expression and upregulation of Na^+ channels or peripheral sensitization via Na^+ channel phosphorylation in injured

Table 37.17 Topical Counterirritants and Hot and Cold Preparations

	Ingredients (%)				
Product	Methyl Salicylate	Menthol	Camphor	Capsaicin	Other
Icy Hot Balm	29	7.6			
Ben-Gay Ultra Strength	30	10	4		
Ben-Gay patch		1.4			
Salon Patch				0.025	
Mineral Ice		2			
Capzasin-HP				0.1	
Flexall Ultra Plus	10	16	3.1		
Aspercreme					Trolamine salicylate, 10

peripheral nerves, demyelination, or discharges in cell bodies in the dorsal root ganglion.[245] This all results in longer depolarizations in specific Na^+ channels and increases in the release of neurotransmitters. Sodium channel blockers bind rapidly to open channels and limit their accessibility, thereby ultimately reducing neurotransmitter release.

Commonly used topical agents for neuropathic pain are amitriptyline, ketamine, lidocaine, and capsaicin (described later). As mentioned previously, along with commercially available products are pharmacy-compounded preparations, which unlike the former, lack the support of controlled trials and are potentially variable in preparation without established safety. Compounded preparations include gabapentin, ketamine, nifedipine, and TCAs. Commercially available and studied products include capsaicin cream, 5% lidocaine patch, lidocaine/prilocaine topical cream, and doxepin. In a double-blind, randomized, placebo-controlled 3-week study, topical 2% amitriptyline, topical 1% ketamine, and a combination of the two achieved a reduction in pain scores (in patients with CRPS type 2, painful diabetic neuropathy, or PHN) by 1 to 1.5 units. In addition, blood concentrations revealed no significant systemic absorption.[246]

Lidocaine patches work by binding to and blocking sodium channels, which theoretically reduces the pain signal. In a randomized, double-blind vehicle-controlled, 3-week efficacy study with use of the neuropathic pain scale, 5% lidocaine patch was found to effectively treat all neuropathic pain qualities.[247] It was also found to significantly improve pain levels and quality of life in patients with diabetic neuropathy.[248]

TOPICAL COUNTERIRRITANTS AND HOT OR COLD PREPARATIONS

An increased understanding of nociceptor physiology, including a greater understanding of thermosensation, has been spurred by the identification of proteins called vanilloid receptors, detectors of noxious heat, and the subsequent identification of a new family of thermosensation receptors, the transient receptor protein (TRP) channel family.[249] The vanilloid receptor (TRPV1) is a nonselective cation receptor activated by capsaicin, the pungent agent found in chili peppers. TRPV1 is also activated by heat (>43° C) and decreased pH and enhanced by bradykinin and nerve growth factor.[250] The TRPV2 receptor, which is 50% identical to TRPV1, may mediate high-threshold noxious heat (>52° C). TRPV3 is activated by increased temperature (>31° C) and is expressed

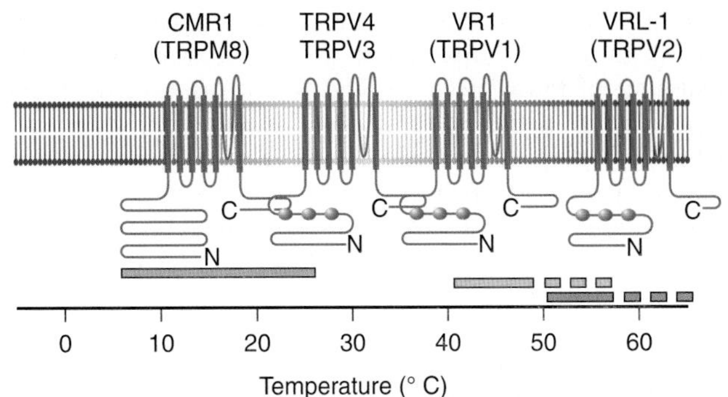

Figure 37.4 Transient receptor protein (TRP) family receptors and their thermosensitivity. (From Tominaga M, Caterina MJ. Thermosensation and pain. *J Neurobiol.* 2004;61:3-12. With permission.)

in the skin, tongue, and nervous system, where it may act as a "warm sensitive neuron."[250] Another TRPV receptor, the cold- and menthol-sensitive receptor (CMRI), has been identified and may help us better understand cold thermosensation and the development of targeted cold-producing analgesics. Pharmacologic studies of menthol have suggested possible κ-opioid receptor effects, thereby contributing additional analgesic properties to the substance.[251]

Review and Physiology

Counterirritants such as capsaicin, camphor, menthol, and garlic represent a category of analgesics that excite and subsequently desensitize nociceptive sensory neurons (Table 37.17).[252] Although many of the group's members have had a long history of common medical use, it was not until recently that their molecular mechanisms of action were elucidated. All these pungent plant derivatives act on the TRP superfamily, a group of structurally similar, thermosensitive ion channels. As noted earlier, members include TRPV1 (also called vanilloid receptor subtype 1 [VR1]), TRPV3, TRPM8, and TRPA1,[253] which are activated by capsaicin, camphor, menthol, and garlic, respectively (Fig. 37.4).[252] These thermosensitive receptors detect a wide range of temperatures, from noxious heat to extreme cold, as well as other stimuli, including heat, protons, lipids, changes in extracellular osmolarity or pressure (or both), and depletion of intracellular Ca^{2+} stores.[254] These proteins are expressed in primary sensory neurons, as well as in other tissues. On activation of TRP receptors, release of calcitonin gene–related peptide, substance P, and other inflammatory neurotransmitters is induced, and local irritation and inflammation ensue.[255] This can lead to two types of desensitization: acute or "pharmacologic" desensitization, characterized by a diminished response during constant agonist application, and a longer period of tachyphylaxis, or "functional" desensitization, characterized by desensitization to other stimuli such as chemicals, pressure, or temperature.[252]

Capsaicin

As early as the 19th century the selective effects of capsaicin on sensory nerve fibers were recognized.[218] The spicy ingredient in chili peppers has been used to relieve neuropathic pain, uremic pruritus, and bladder overactivity, as well as to provide analgesia.[256] Capsaicin has been recommended in a number of treatment guidelines for the treatment of OA.[233] Currently, nonprescription creams, lotions, and patches containing 0.025% to 0.075% capsaicin by weight are available for the treatment of musculoskeletal and neuropathic pain.[257] The mechanism of action of capsaicin is characterized by a paradoxical biphasic pharmacologic action on sensory neurons. An initial excitatory phase (pain and inflammation), mediated by activation of the TRPV1 receptor, is followed by a secondary analgesic phase that has been attributed to long-term desensitization of nociceptors and depletion of substance P.[258] A systematic review of topical capsaicin for the relief of musculoskeletal pain pooled the results of three double-blind, placebo-controlled trials with a total of 368 patients.[259] After 4 weeks of treatment with 0.025% capsaicin or plaster, the mean response rate (percentage of patients with at least 50% pain relief) was 38% (range, 34% to 42%), and the placebo response rate was 25% (range, 17% to 37%). The NNT was 8.1, and approximately a third of patients experienced local, treatment-related adverse events.[259] An older meta-analysis reported that capsaicin cream provides better pain relief of OA pain than placebo does (odds ratio, 4.36; 95% CI, 2.77 to 6.88).[260] However, products with low concentrations of capsaicin require multiple applications to provoke desensitization of nerves,[256] which may be problematic for daily use because of potential adverse application effects such as burning or irritation of the eyes or other mucous membranes if not adequately removed from the hands after application.[218] Additionally, burning and pain on application reduce patient adherence and may adversely limit efficacy.[218,256] The combination of topical capsaicin (0.025%) with 3.3% doxepin provided more rapid analgesia than did treatment with either of these two agents independently.[261] For neuropathic pain, topical capsaicin was compared with oral amitriptyline and found to be similar in analgesia and improvements in daily activities, with lower side effects noted in the capsaicin group.[262] Most recently, Qutenza, a high-concentration capsaicin (8%) patch, has been approved for use in patients with PHN. Its mechanism of action is thought to be due to a reduction in TRPV1 expression and a decrease in the density of epidermal nerve fibers in the application area.[263] When compared with a control 0.04% capsaicin patch, Qutenza was shown to achieve higher reductions in pain levels for 12 weeks (32% vs. 24% reduction).

Camphor

Camphor is derived from the wood of the camphor laurel tree (*Cinnamomum camphora*). Historically, the sweet-smelling compound has had many medicinal applications, including use as a decongestant, cough suppressant, and antipruritic agent.[252] OTC camphor-containing balms have also been used to provide analgesia. Recent studies have implicated three receptors in camphor's mechanism of action: TRPV3, the capsaicin receptor TRPV1, and the garlic receptor TRPA1.[252]

Menthol

In contrast, menthol—the component that confers the mint smell and flavor to the *Mentha* species—is often included in eutectic formulations of local anesthetic agents.[251] Anecdotally, menthol induces tingling and cooling sensations when applied topically. Menthol confers analgesia through its Ca^{2+} channel–blocking actions. In addition to binding TRPM8,[253,257] menthol binds κ-opioid receptors and thus may confer an additional opioid analgesic effect.[251] Furthermore, similar to other terpenes, menthol is an effective topical permeation enhancer for water-soluble drugs, such as the TCA imipramine.[264]

Salicylates

Topical rubefacients containing salicylates, another type of counterirritant, have an unidentified mechanism of action.[262] It is thought that analgesia is conferred by a mode different from that of NSAIDs, yet salicylates are often found in many topical preparations. Further randomized, clinical trial evidence for salicylates has been systematically reviewed by Mason and coworkers.[265] Three double-blind, placebo-controlled trials examined topical salicylates for the treatment of acute musculoskeletal pain. The study groups exhibited significantly better reductions in pain than did the placebo group (relative benefit, 3.6; 95% CI, 2.4 to 5.6; NNT, 2.1; range, 1.7 to 2.8). The long-term efficacy data and adverse events reported were poor for chronic musculoskeletal pain, but information from six double-blind, placebo-controlled trials indicated a relative benefit versus control of 1.5 (range, 1.3 to 1.9; NNT, 5.3; range, 3.6 to 10.2).

CONCLUSION

Analgesics play an important role in the treatment of many acute and chronic pain conditions. They represent the first line of agents in the World Health Organization's analgesic ladder and range from OTC convenience medications to adjuvants for the treatment of musculoskeletal, arthritis, spine-related, and cancer pain conditions. Though considered relatively safe in comparison to many other prescription-strength medications, minor analgesics must be used with caution. Side effects and adverse events related to common use and misuse of these medications include liver toxicity (APAP); GI, renal, and cardiac toxicity (NSAIDs and COX-2 inhibitors); and physiologic dependence, tolerance, and addiction (combination opioid analgesics and tramadol products).

Topical analgesics (e.g., patches, creams, solutions) represent a growing area of development in pain management because of their relative ease of application, potential for reduced systemic side effects, and lowered risk for end-organ damage. Advancements in pharmaceutical delivery systems may also aid in the development and more widespread use of various OTC and prescription-strength topical compounds. The pain clinician should be cognizant of the vast array of ingredients found in various OTC topical analgesics and counterirritants, including capsaicin, menthol, camphor, and methylsalicylates.

KEY POINTS

- Regular use of over-the-counter analgesic medications is a common method used by patients to relieve various pain-related conditions.
- Minor opioid analgesics include propoxyphene, hydrocodone, oxycodone, and tramadol, individually and in combination products.
- Patients' responses to individual opioids and opioid combination products may vary significantly. This is probably explained by opioid receptor polymorphisms, differences in pharmacokinetics, and genetic variation related to enzymatic breakdown by hepatic metabolic systems.
- True serotonin toxicity and serotonin syndrome are rare, but potentially deadly conditions seen in the field of pain management. They are characterized clinically by changes in mental status and autonomic and neuromuscular hyperactivity.
- The use of over-the-counter and prescription-strength topical preparations represents a growing area of development in pain medicine, with significantly less potential for systemic adverse effects and organ toxicity than noted with oral formulations.
- When compared with other topically administered medications, topical nonsteroidal anti-inflammatory drugs have accumulated the largest amount of clinical evidence for their use in relieving acute versus chronic musculoskeletal conditions.

SUGGESTED READINGS

Attal N, Bouhassira D. Mechanisms of pain in peripheral neuropathy. *Acta Neurol Scand Suppl.* 1999;173:12-24.

Cicero TJ, Inciardi JA, Adams EH, et al. Rates of abuse of tramadol remain unchanged with the introduction of new branded and generic products: results of an abuse-monitoring system, 1994-2004. *Pharmacoepidemiol Drug Saf.* 2005;14:851-859.

Gillman PK. A review of serotonin toxicity data: implications for the mechanisms of antidepressant drug action. *Biol Psychiatry.* 2006;59:1046-1051.

Grond S, Sablotzki A. Clinical pharmacology of tramadol. *Clin Pharmacokinet.* 2004;43:879-923.

Julius D. The molecular biology of thermosensation. In: Dostrovsky JO, Carr DB, Koltzenburg M, eds. *Proceedings of the Tenth World Congress on Pain. Progress in Pain Research and Management.* Vol 24. Seattle: IASP Press; 2003:63-70.

Mason L, Moore RA, Edwards JE, et al. Topical NSAIDs for acute pain: a meta-analysis. *BMC Musculoskelet Disord.* 2004;5:10.

McCleane G. Topical application of doxepin hydrochloride, capsaicin and a combination of both produces analgesia in chronic human neuropathic pain: a randomized, double-blind, placebo-controlled study. *Br J Clin Pharmacol.* 2000;49:574-579.

Pasternak GW. Molecular biology of opioid analgesia. *J Pain Symptom Manage.* 2005;29(suppl 5):S2-S9.

Pendleton A, Arden N, Dougados M, et al. EULAR recommendations for the management of knee osteoarthritis: report of a task force of the Standing Committee for International Clinical Studies Including Therapeutic Trials (ESCISIT). *Ann Rheum Dis.* 2000;59:936-944.

Wilcox CM, Cryer B, Triadafilopoulos G. Patterns of use and public perception of over-the-counter pain relievers: focus on nonsteroidal anti-inflammatory drugs. *J Rheumatol.* 2005;32:2218-2224.

The references for this chapter can be found at www.expertconsult.com.

38 Antidepressants as Analgesics

Howard S. Smith | Charles E. Argoff | Gary McCleane

The second half of the 20th century saw the introduction of a range of therapeutic agents that were shown to have an antidepressant effect. Among these agents were those with a tricyclic chemical structure, which led to their classification as tricyclic antidepressants (TCAs). Even before their introduction into clinical practice, the concept of a link between depression and pain was obvious, and the possibility that this link was causal encouraged the use of antidepressants for patients who exhibited features of both pain and depression.

In 1962, Kuipers reported a case series in which the TCA imipramine was used in patients with "nonarticular rheumatism" and in whom 60% to 70% experienced pain relief.[1] Similarly, Scott reported a double-blind trial in patients with rheumatoid arthritis, osteoarthritis, and ankylosing spondylitis in whom imipramine provided significantly more pain relief than placebo did.[2] In both these reports it was postulated that the pain relief produced is secondary to mood elevation rather than an intrinsic analgesic effect of the antidepressant. It is now recognized that the pain relief apparent with the use of antidepressants can be independent of any alteration in mood caused by the drug,[3] although it has been noted with, for example, doxepin treatment that a reduction in pain is intimately associated with a reduction in depression.[4]

Therefore, the focus of this chapter is on the potential pain-reducing capability of drugs otherwise associated with the treatment of depression. However, pain rarely exists in isolation, and any muscle relaxation, mood enhancement, or improvement in the quality and duration of sleep, all of which are potential effects of antidepressant use, is often a welcome accompaniment of any pain relief that is produced.

Dharmshaktu and coworkers[5] reviewed the efficacy of antidepressants as analgesics, and Häuser and colleagues[6] performed a systematic review and meta-analysis of the role of antidepressants in the management of fibromyalgia (FM).

CLASSIFICATION OF ANTIDEPRESSANTS

Antidepressants are currently classified partly on the basis of their chemical structure and partly according to their primary in vivo effects (Box 38.1).

TRICYCLIC ANTIDEPRESSANTS

The structures of some TCAs are shown in Figure 38.1.

ANALGESIC MECHANISM OF ACTION

In 1987, Max and colleagues demonstrated that TCAs possess analgesic effects independent of their effects on moods.[3] Later, it was found that the analgesic effects of TCAs tend to occur more rapidly (a week or less after initiating TCA therapy), at lower serum blood levels, and at lower doses than those used for antidepressive effects. It is now clear that the TCAs have a number of diverse effects that contribute to their analgesic effect (Table 38.1). The extent to which each individual TCA exerts these effects differs, which may account for differences in the effectiveness and propensity to cause side effects when members of this class of drugs are used. As noted later in this chapter, not all the proposed modes of action of TCAs are the result of central effects, with a number of possible peripheral actions now becoming apparent.

Serotonergic Effect

The presence of a descending bulbospinal inhibitory influence on spinal neural activity has been well defined in animal models of antinociception. When 5-hydroxytryptamine (5-HT) antagonists are administered, the antinociceptive effect of TCAs is inhibited.[7] Similarly, when central 5-HT systems are depleted with the use of *p*-chlorophenylalanine, the antinociceptive effects of TCAs are again reduced.[8-11] Some tricyclics interfere with serotonin reuptake into nerve terminals.[12-14] In addition, some TCAs alter binding of serotonin to receptors on neural tissue.[15,16] Although this evidence exists in the animal literature, the contribution of 5-HT to the antinociceptive effects of TCAs and its role in the anti-hyperalgesic or anti-allodynic properties of TCAs in humans have not been established.

Noradrenergic Effect

In a similar fashion to the serotonergic effect of TCAs, the descending bulbospinal noradrenergic inhibitory influence is thought to be important in their analgesic effect. Depletion of central norepinephrine systems with α-methyl *p*-tyrosine inhibits the antinociceptive actions of TCAs,[8-11] and α-adrenoreceptor antagonists also have the same effect.[17-19] Specifically, when phentolamine, a nonspecific α_1- and α_2-adrenoreceptor antagonist, is administered with a TCA, antinociception is inhibited.[20] However, when the α_1-adrenoreceptor antagonist prazosin is coadministered with the TCA amitriptyline in mice, antinociception is observed. Conversely, when amitriptyline is coadministered with the α_2-adrenoreceptor antagonist RX821002, antinociception is observed,[18] thus suggesting that TCAs derive at least part of their antinociceptive effect by interacting with α_2 adrenoreceptors rather than α_1 receptors.

Opioidergic Effect

The noradrenergic effects of TCAs are thought to be the primary mechanism of action of this drug class, but other indirect actions may also be important. When clomipramine

Box 38.1 Classification of Antidepressants

Monoamine Oxidase Inhibitors

- Harmaline
- Iproclozide
- Iproniazid
- Isocarboxazid
- Moclobemide
- Nialamide
- Selegiline
- Toloxatone
- Tranylcypromine

Dopamine Reuptake Inhibitors

- Amineptine
- Bupropion

Serotonin-Norepinephrine Reuptake Inhibitors

- Duloxetine
- Milnacipran
- Nefazodone
- Venlafaxine

Selective Serotonin Reuptake Inhibitors

- Alaproclate
- Citalopram
- Escitalopram
- Etoperidone
- Fluoxetine
- Fluvoxamine
- Paroxetine
- Sertraline
- Zimeldine

Selective Serotonin Reuptake Enhancer

- Tianeptine

Tricyclic Antidepressants

- Amitriptyline
- Clomipramine
- Desipramine
- Dothiepin
- Doxepin
- Imipramine
- Iprindole
- Lofepramine
- Nortriptyline
- Opipramol
- Protriptyline
- Trimipramine

Tetracyclic Antidepressants

- Amoxapine
- Maprotiline
- Mianserin
- Mirtazapine

is administered to rats in the formalin test, the opioid antagonist naloxone can completely antagonize the antinociceptive effect of that TCA.[20] Similarly, administration of the delta (δ)-opioid antagonist naltrindole with antidepressants shifts the antinociceptive dose-response curves to the right, thus suggesting inhibition of the antinociceptive effects of TCAs, whereas administration of the enkephalin catabolism inhibitor acetorphan with the antidepressants dothiepin, amitriptyline, or sibutramine enhances their antinociceptive effects.[21] Chronic antidepressant administration can modify opioid receptor densities[22] and increase opioid levels in certain brain regions.[23,24] The alterations seen with opioid receptor antagonists may represent a direct action of TCAs on opioid receptors; however, this is unlikely given the lack of TCA affinity in opioid receptor binding assays.

N-Methyl-D-Aspartate Receptor Effect

Reynolds and Miller observed that desmethylimipramine and imipramine both prevent the Ca^{2+} influx into cultured cortical neurons of the rat produced by *N*-methyl-D-aspartate (NMDA). They also noted that other TCAs had a similar but less intense effect.[25] Others have observed that antidepressants bind to the NMDA receptor complex[25,26] and that chronic administration of antidepressants alters NMDA binding characteristics.[27] There is considerable debate on the importance of an NMDA effect in regard to the analgesic effect of antidepressants.[28]

Adenosine Receptor Effect

Adenosine is known to produce analgesia,[29] and antidepressants inhibit the uptake of adenosine in neuronal preparations.[30] The antinociceptive effect of antidepressants is inhibited by adenosine receptor antagonists.[31-33] Adenosine receptors have both peripheral and central representation (see later discussion).

Sodium Channel Effect

Sodium channel blockade may contribute to the analgesic efficacy of antidepressants.[34] Amitriptyline appears to be the most potent TCA in its ability to block sodium channels, with doxepin and imipramine following (all were superior to bupivacaine) and then desipramine (less effective than bupivacaine), and nortriptyline was one of the least effective TCAs in blocking sodium channels.[35] Sudoh and associates concluded that *N*-methyl doxepin is a potent Na^+ channel blocker and a long-acting local anesthetic for rat sciatic nerve blockade.[36]

Although amitriptyline is more potent than bupivacaine in a subcutaneous infiltration model[37] and in an intrathecal administration model in rats and sheep,[38] when amitriptyline was evaluated for ulnar nerve blockade in healthy human volunteers, it was found to be less effective than bupivacaine, contrary to the results of a large number of animal studies.[39] This may be due to the thicker nerve sheaths present in humans than in rats, which presents more of a barrier for amitriptyline to penetrate into the nerve.[39,40] Local anesthetics and TCAs both bind more tightly to the inactivated state of the sodium channel.[41] Thus, neural blockade with amitriptyline (like local anesthetics) is use dependent.[42]

Potency is extremely difficult to assess because of differences in agents, different routes of administration, different

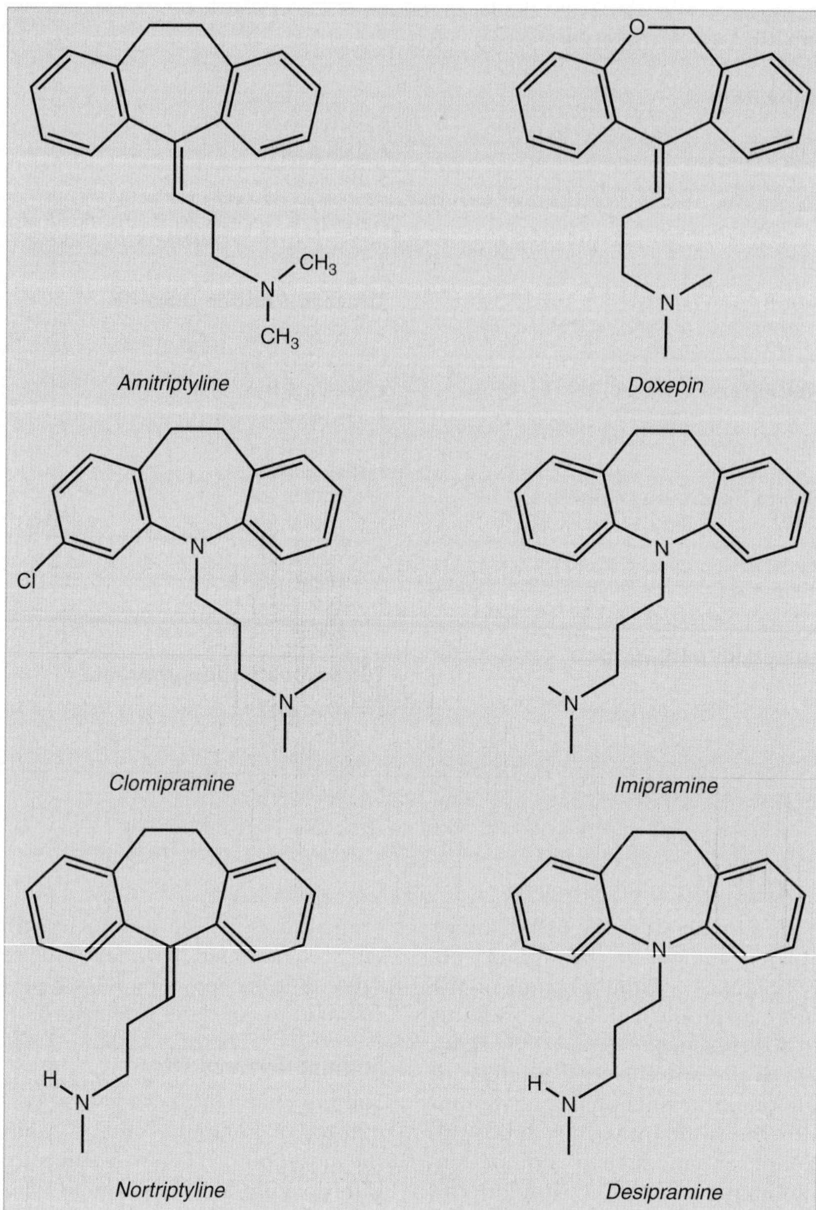

Figure 38.1 Tricyclic antidepressants.

environments, different species, different sodium channels, and different measurements.

Rats differ from sheep and humans, topical administration differs from intrathecal and perineural application, and motor function differs from proprioception and nociception. However, in an effort to present a very rough idea of local anesthetic potency, *N*-phenylethyl amitriptyline is about 50 times as potent as lidocaine, amitriptyline is about 8 times as potent as lidocaine, and bupivacaine is about 4 times as potent as lidocaine. However, *N*-phenylethyl amitriptyline appears to have a narrow therapeutic index.[43] *N*-Methyl amitriptyline is similar to amitriptyline but has a much longer duration of action.[38] Furthermore, *N*-methyl amitriptyline appears to exhibit significant differential blockade (i.e., selective block of a specific [pain-transmitting] nerve fiber group), greater than that achieved with amitriptyline, bupivacaine, and lidocaine in sheep.[38]

Table 38.1 Mode of Action of Tricyclic Antidepressants

Effect	Mode of Action
Serotonergic	Interferes with serotonin reuptake Alters serotonin binding to receptors
Noradrenergic	Interacts with α_2 adrenoreceptors
Opioidergic	Modifies opioid receptor densities Increases opioid levels in some brain areas
N-Methyl-D-aspartate (NMDA) receptor	Binds to the NMDA receptor complex Alters NMDA binding characteristics
Adenosine receptor	Inhibits adenosine uptake
Sodium channel	Blocks sodium channels
Calcium channel	Increases densities of L-type calcium channels
Other receptors	Inhibits histaminic, cholinergic, muscarinic, and nicotinic receptors

Since amitriptyline blocks persistently open sodium channels at low plasma concentrations, because of its significantly longer half-life, it may have utility in the perioperative period. Lidocaine has been demonstrated to be effective for chronic neuropathic pain states[44] and has also been shown to diminish acute postoperative pain, as well as facilitate return of normal bowel function[45]; preclinical evidence also seems to support this notion. Amitriptyline demonstrates antinociceptive effects in experimental mouse models of pain states.[46] Additionally, amitriptyline in combination with morphine had better analgesic effects than did morphine alone.[46]

Calcium Channel Effect

Although acute treatment with an antidepressant has no observable effect on calcium channels, chronic treatment with citalopram and chlorprothixene (but not imipramine) increases the density of L-type calcium channels. It also has an antinociceptive effect, with this effect being nullified by administration of nifedipine.[47]

Other Effects

Antidepressants also interact with histaminergic, cholinergic muscarinic, and cholinergic nicotinic receptors in an inhibitory manner.[28] However, individual antidepressant agents may differ markedly in their potency at different receptors. These interactions may contribute to the side effects of the antidepressants (e.g., dry mouth, sedation, urinary retention). These important side effects are discussed in the following sections.

ANIMAL STUDIES OF ANTINOCICEPTIVE EFFECTS

Because of the many proposed pharmacologic effects of TCAs, one would expect them to have an antinociceptive effect. A number of studies have confirmed that this class of antidepressants does have this property. For example, Abdel-Salam and colleagues[48] have shown that antidepressants, including those in the TCA class, display antinociceptive properties in a rat tail electrical stimulation assay, and others have shown that chronic administration decreases self-mutilation in the rat autotomy test,[49,50] produces an antinociceptive effect in the formalin test,[51,52] and has similar action in a hot plate test.[53]

Ardid and Guilbaud[54] confirmed that both acute and chronic administration of TCAs (e.g., clomipramine, amitriptyline, desipramine) has an antinociceptive effect in a rat mononeuropathy model. This effect on neuropathic pain has been substantiated in other studies.[55,56]

Some of the TCAs also seem to possess anti-inflammatory effects. For example, when imipramine is administered on a chronic basis to rats that are then exposed to carrageenan, which induces intense inflammation, the local inflammatory response normally observed is significantly reduced.[57] Similarly, clomipramine reduces carrageenan-induced skin inflammation in a dose-dependent fashion, as well as decreases the prostaglandin E_2–like biologic and immunologic activity and substance P concentration in the inflammatory exudate.[58] When both amitriptyline and imipramine are administered on a chronic basis to rats with adjuvant-induced arthritis, behavioral tests suggest that they both induce antinociception.[59]

HUMAN EXPERIMENTAL PAIN

Even with a single 100-mg dose of imipramine, verbal pain ratings and the amplitude of somatosensory evoked cerebral potentials in response to suprathreshold intradermal electrical stimuli are reduced significantly, more than in subjects taking placebo.[60] Similarly, a single oral dose of desipramine has been shown to increase subjective pain thresholds and the nociceptive withdrawal reflex threshold in response to percutaneous electrical stimulation of the sural nerve.[61] Poulsen and associates[62] examined the effect of a single oral dose of 100 mg of imipramine on pain detection and tolerance thresholds to heat and pressure, thresholds of the quadriceps femoris muscle withdrawal reflex to single and repeated electrical stimulation of the sural nerve, and continuous pain ratings during the cold pressor test in 12 healthy volunteers. They found that imipramine significantly increases pain thresholds to heat and pressure, as well as the pain tolerance threshold and reflex threshold to single electrical stimulation. Pain ratings during the cold pressor test and pain detection thresholds in response to heat and pressure were unaltered.[62] These studies have suggested that TCAs can have a differential hypoanalgesic effect in different human experimental pain tests.

TRICYCLIC ANTIDEPRESSANTS IN CLINICAL PAIN MANAGEMENT

Historically, TCAs were used for human pain management before their modes of action as analgesics were elucidated. The fact that they can reduce pain and independently elevate mood, as well as normalize sleep patterns and cause muscle relaxation, is an additional potential benefit of their use. In no human field of use is the evidence for an analgesic effect of TCAs greater than in neuropathic pain conditions. A significant body of evidence underpins the use of TCAs for a number of specific neuropathic pain conditions, and because the features of neuropathic pain are not dependent on the causal disease or neural irritation, it is widely accepted that the evidence for analgesia in specific conditions is strong enough to allow uniform use for any condition manifesting the symptoms of neuropathic pain.

Post-herpetic Neuralgia

A prototypical neuropathic pain condition involving neural irritation and destruction makes post-herpetic neuralgia (PHN) a particularly difficult condition to treat. With established PHN, palliation rather than cure is the only prospect. Perhaps in no other condition have TCAs made such an impact. Evidence has suggested that amitriptyline,[63-66] nortriptyline,[67] and desipramine[68] are among the TCAs that can usefully alleviate the suffering associated with PHN. As an example of potential efficacy, Watson and coworkers reported "good to excellent" pain relief in 16 of 24 patients studied,[63] and Max and coauthors[66] reported that 47% of 58 patients studied in their randomized controlled trial obtained "moderate or greater" pain relief with amitriptyline. Interestingly, in a study comparing amitriptyline with the tetracyclic antidepressant maprotiline (which has a predominantly noradrenergic effect), Watson and associates[64] noted that "amitriptyline relieves some patients with postherpetic neuralgia. Many patients suffer side effects and better therapies are necessary." Incidentally, the pain relief produced by amitriptyline was greater than that apparent after maprotiline.

Watson and coworkers[67] compared the effect of nortriptyline and amitriptyline and found both to have an analgesic effect but that nortriptyline was associated with fewer side effects. Kishore-Kumar and colleagues[68] examined the effect of desipramine on PHN and confirmed an analgesic effect. They stated that "other antidepressants—notably amitriptyline—are known to ameliorate postherpetic neuralgia, but those agents are often toxic." Almost 2 decades after this study, amitriptyline is still considered a frontline agent and arguably the preferential first therapeutic agent for the treatment of PHN.

Painful Diabetic Neuropathy

Again, strong evidence exists for pain relief with TCAs in patients with painful diabetic neuropathy (PDN). Amitriptyline,[3,69] desipramine,[69-71] clomipramine,[71] imipramine,[72-74] and nortriptyline[75] have all been shown to have an analgesic effect in patients with PDN.

In terms of comparative efficacy, Max and associates[69] found that desipramine and amitriptyline are equally efficacious, whereas Sindrup and coworkers[71] found that clomipramine tends to produce better pain relief than desipramine does. When the dose-response relationship is considered, Sindrup and colleagues[74] found that imipramine is associated with such a relationship. Although a dose-response relationship is also noted when clomipramine is used, this does not seem to be the case with desipramine.[71]

Painful Mononeuropathy and Polyneuropathy

Some evidence exists for an analgesic effect of clomipramine in the treatment of painful mononeuropathy and polyneuropathy pain. Langohr and associates[76] compared treatment with clomipramine and acetylsalicylic acid in a blinded crossover study and were able to show a greater analgesic effect during the clomipramine treatment phase.

Pain Associated with Spinal Cord Injury

Not all studies examining the effect of TCAs on neuropathic pain have produced a positive result. Cardenas and coworkers[77] studied 84 patients with pain from a spinal cord injury (SCI) who were randomized to receive amitriptyline or an active placebo, benztropine mesylate. No significant differences in measured pain parameters were found between the treatment groups or when comparing pretreatment and treatment periods. This evidence is in contrast to that presented by others who have suggested a beneficial effect of TCAs on SCI pain, although their evidence is based on case reports rather than blinded, placebo-controlled trials.[78,79] In contrast to the negative response in studies of SCI pain, Leijon and Boivie[80] reported a useful analgesic effect when amitriptyline is used in patients with central post-stroke pain.

Fibromyalgia

Although the use of TCAs in patients with FM is widespread, consideration of the evidence supporting their use is difficult, largely because FM is a complex disorder with a spectrum of symptoms and signs. From a broad perspective, there can be little doubt that antidepressants do improve the symptoms of FM in some patients.[81] O'Malley and colleagues[82] undertook a meta-analysis of studies that examined the effect of antidepressants in patients with FM. They calculated that the odds ratio for improvement with antidepressant therapy was 4.2 (95% confidence interval, 2.6 to 6.8). They concluded that antidepressant therapy has a positive effect on sleep, fatigue, pain, and well-being, but not on trigger points. They also found that in only one of the five studies that measured depression scores was there a correlation between improvement in symptoms and depression scores.[81] When TCAs are specifically considered, Arnold and associates[83] concluded from their meta-analysis that TCAs produce the largest improvement in sleep quality, with modest improvement found in measures of stiffness and tenderness.

In terms of the number of patients who can improve with antidepressant treatment, Carette and coworkers[84] found that after 1 month of treatment of FM, 21% were improved (as opposed to 0% with placebo) and that after 6 months of treatment, the proportion had increased to 36% and 19%, respectively.

Osteoarthritis

Historically, an analgesic effect of TCAs was first noted in patients with joint pain.[1] Limited evidence has suggested that TCAs can reduce joint pain caused by osteoarthritis.[59]

Low Back Pain

Although a diagnosis of low back pain is extremely wide and nonspecific and encompasses a wide range of different problems, it does represent a significant clinical problem for many practitioners. A single report of a randomized, controlled trial involving the use of doxepin in patients with low back pain suggested that it can reduce pain and decrease indices of depression.[85]

Cancer-Related Neuropathic Pain

TCAs seem to exert an analgesic effect on a range of painful conditions, but Mercadante and colleagues[86] reported that amitriptyline failed to produce any pain relief in 16 patients with advanced cancer who had features of neuropathic pain. However, their study numbers were small, the neuropathic pain may not have been present in isolation given the diagnosis of cancer, and any neuropathic pain arising in association with cancer could have been emanating from a diverse number of neural structures irritated by tumor deposits.

Human Immunodeficiency Virus–Related Sensory Neuropathy

TCAs do not seem to be effective in relieving this condition.[87]

COMPARATIVE STUDIES

Morello and associates[88] studied 28 patients with PDN in a crossover study comparing the effect of amitriptyline and gabapentin. They found that the pain relief produced by the TCA is of similar magnitude and quality to that obtained with gabapentin.

OVERALL EFFECTIVENESS

One way of displaying the potential efficacy of any agent is to consider the number needed to treat (NNT; Table 38.2). In terms of analgesic medication, this represents the number of patients who need to take the treatment to obtain a 50% or greater reduction in their pain.

Table 38.2 Number Needed to Treat When Using Tricyclic Antidepressants for Pain

Condition	NNT
Painful diabetic neuropathy	3.0
	3.4
	1.3
Post-herpetic neuralgia	2.3
	2.1
	2.2
Atypical facial pain	2.8
Central pain	1.7

Data from McQuay HJ, Tramer M, Nye BA, et al. A systematic review of antidepressants in neuropathic pain. *Pain*. 1996;68:217-227; Collins SL, Moore R, McQuay HJ, et al. Antidepressants and anticonvulsants for diabetic neuropathy and postherpetic neuralgia: a quantitative systematic review. *J Pain Symptom Manage*. 2000;20:449-458; and McQuay HJ, Moore RA. Antidepressants and chronic pain. *BMJ*. 1997;314:763-764.

SELECTIVE SEROTONIN REUPTAKE INHIBITORS

TCAs have analgesic potential for various pain conditions and a diverse range of pharmacologic actions, but these actions can also increase their propensity to cause side effects. It was hoped that with the advent of antidepressants with more specific modes of action, analgesia would still be associated with their use and the potential to produce side effects would be reduced.

When the antinociceptive effect of selective serotonin reuptake inhibitors (SSRIs; Fig. 38.2) were examined in a mouse hot plate pain test, fluvoxamine induced a dose-dependent antinociceptive effect, whereas fluoxetine and citalopram induced only a weak antinociceptive effect.[89] Escitalopram failed to elicit any antinociceptive effect. The antinociceptive effect of these three SSRIs was not blocked by the opioid antagonist naloxone. In contrast, again using a mouse hot plate test, paroxetine produced an antinociceptive effect that was inhibited by naloxone, thus suggesting that this SSRI may act not only via its serotonergic effect but also via an interaction with the opioidergic system.[90] In the same study, paroxetine-induced antinociception was inhibited by the 5-HT_3 antagonist ondansetron, but not by the 5-HT_2 receptor antagonist ketanserin.

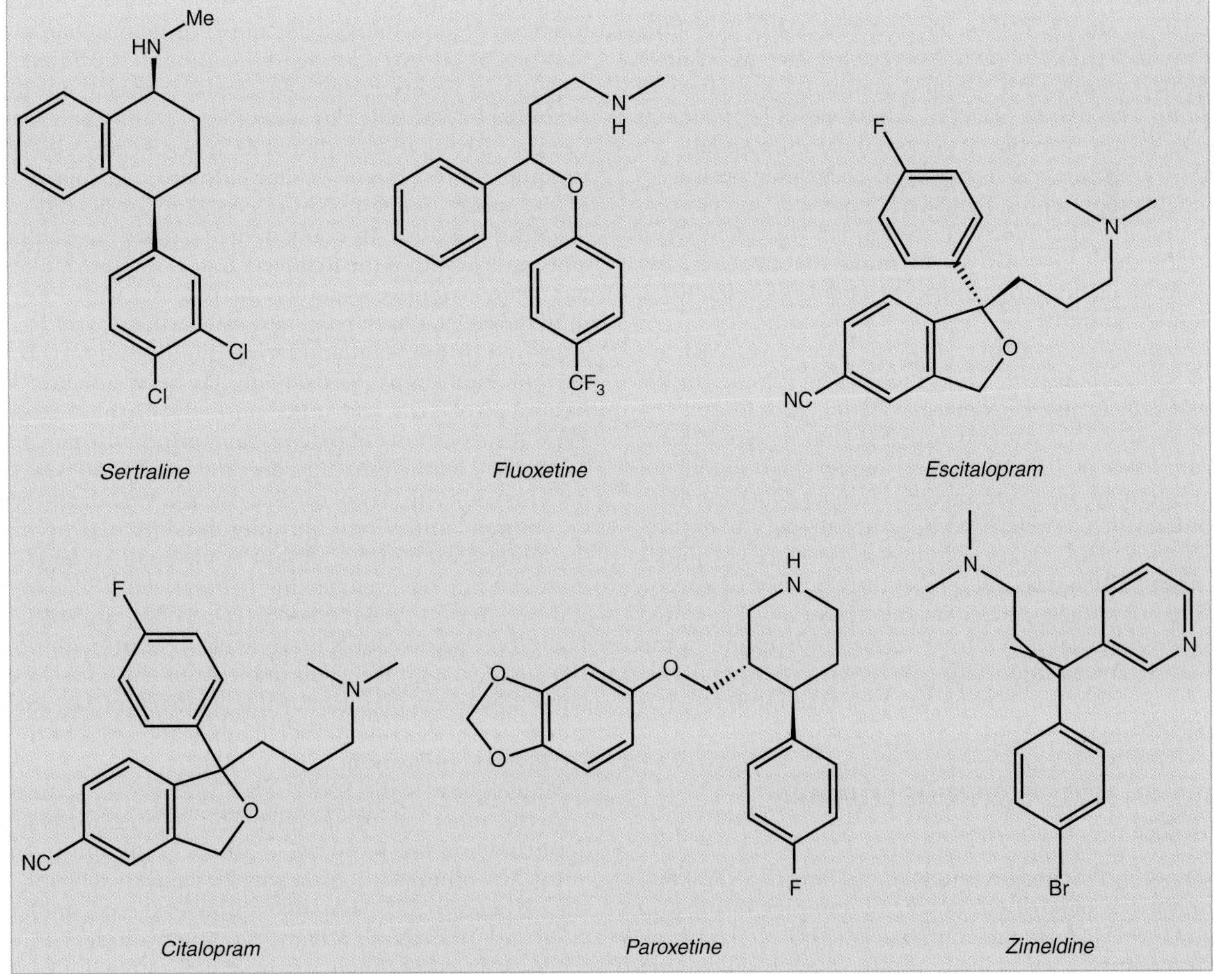

Figure 38.2 Selective serotonin reuptake inhibitors.

When considering the overall results from studies, it has been calculated that the NNT for one patient to obtain a 50% reduction in pain is 5 for paroxetine and 15.3 for fluoxetine.[91] This leads to the conclusion that evidence for the effectiveness of SSRIs in pain management is limited, at best.[92,93]

SELECTIVE SEROTONIN REUPTAKE INHIBITORS AND HUMAN PAIN

Painful Diabetic Neuropathy

A number of studies have examined the effect of SSRIs on PDN. Sindrup and colleagues[94] compared the effects of paroxetine and imipramine. Paroxetine did produce pain relief, but less than that obtained with imipramine. On the other hand, use of paroxetine was associated with fewer side effects than occur with imipramine.[94] Max and associates[69] compared the effect of amitriptyline, desipramine, fluoxetine, and placebo in patients with PDN. When subjects were considered in terms of the percentage of those who derived moderate or greater pain relief, the results were 74% in those receiving amitriptyline and 61%, 48%, and 41%, respectively, in those receiving desipramine, fluoxetine, and placebo. Citalopram has also been studied and found to be relatively effective with few side effects.[95]

Fibromyalgia

A number of studies have suggested that SSRIs have little effect on FM pain. In one, Norregaard and associates[96] studied 22 patients with FM and compared the effect of citalopram with that of placebo. After 8 weeks of treatment (4 weeks taking placebo, 4 weeks taking citalopram), no changes were observed in any pain parameter measured, nor in depression scores. Similarly, Anderberg and coworkers[97] found no difference with citalopram treatment when the results were analyzed on an intent-to-treat basis, but there were reductions in pain and well-being scores in those completing the study.

Although in general the analgesic effects of SSRI are limited and inconsistent, when higher doses are used, the analgesic effects may be somewhat better. Arnold and colleagues showed that patients with FM who received fluoxetine at doses of 45 mg/day or higher had significant improvement in the Fibromyalgia Impact Questionnaire (FIQ) total score, as well as in FIQ pain, fatigue, and depression scores.[98] This makes intuitive sense since at higher doses most SSRI agents will inhibit the reuptake of norepinephrine somewhat. Nakajima and coworkers presented data suggesting that an increase in norepinephrine in the spinal cord plays an important role in the anti-hyperalgesic effects of not only norepinephrine reuptake inhibitors but also SSRIs.[99]

SEROTONIN-NOREPINEPHRINE REUPTAKE INHIBITORS

Serotonin-norepinephrine reuptake inhibitors (SNRIs; Fig. 38.3) selectively block the reuptake of norepinephrine and serotonin (5-HT). Milnacipran blocks 5-HT and norepinephrine reuptake with equal affinity, whereas duloxetine has a 10-fold selectivity for 5-HT and venlafaxine a 30-fold selectivity for 5-HT.[100]

ANIMAL PAIN STUDIES

The probable effects of drugs in humans can often be predicted by testing them on specific animal pain models. However, there may be species differences in response; in human clinical practice, mixed pain states are common, whereas animal models are based on specific pain types.

When formalin is applied to animal paws, a two-stage response is observed that can be measured electrophysiologically or by behavioral observation. Both duloxetine (an SNRI) and citalopram (an SSRI) attenuate the second phase of the formalin response.[101] When compared with venlafaxine and milnacipran, duloxetine attenuates the second phase of this test more significantly.[102]

In the tail flick test (a test of acute nociception), duloxetine has minimal effect,[101-103] whereas in the hot plate test, some antinociceptive response with duloxetine is observed.[101,103] In the chronic nerve constriction injury model of neuropathic pain, venlafaxine[104] and duloxetine[101] both have a significant antinociceptive effect.

CLINICAL PAIN MANAGEMENT

Duloxetine is the first antidepressant to have a specific pain indication in the United States—treatment of PDN.[105] SNRIs may also be useful for other conditions.

Duloxetine and venlafaxine are antidepressants with both serotonergic and noradrenergic reuptake–inhibiting properties (SNRIs). In the treatment of PDN, duloxetine has been demonstrated to be more efficacious than placebo at doses of 60 and 120 mg/day, although the higher dose appears to be associated with similar efficacy but greater side effects. The side effect profile of duloxetine seems to be more favorable than that of TCAs, especially with respect to anticholinergic and cardiac side effects. Nausea is one of the more common side effects but can be reduced by lowering the dose. In many patients, nausea is self-limited and resolves within the first several weeks of use. Duloxetine has been extensively studied in patients with PDN, FM, musculoskeletal back pain, and osteoarthritis and has been approved by the Food and Drug Administration (FDA) for all four indications. Venlafaxine has been effective in the treatment of PDN and other polyneuropathies except for PHN. A small subset of patients demonstrated abnormalities in cardiac conduction; thus, precautions should be taken in patients with a history of cardiac disease. Venlafaxine should be tapered rather than abruptly discontinued because of the potential for a withdrawal syndrome. At doses lower than 150 mg/day, venlafaxine behaves more like an SSRI; at doses above 150 mg, it behaves more like an SNRI agent. Therefore, pain relief is more likely to occur with doses of 150 mg/day or greater. This point should be taken into consideration when prescribing this medication for analgesic purposes. Venlafaxine is not currently approved by the FDA for any pain indication.

Milnacipran is the SNRI (also referred to as an NSRI) with the most balanced activity on inhibition of norepinephrine and 5-HT reuptake. Milnacipran and its metabolites are eliminated primarily by renal excretion, with approximately 55% of milnacipran excreted unchanged in urine, 19% as a carbamoyl-*O*-glucuronide conjugate, 8% as *N*-desethyl milnacipran, and the remainder of the administered dose as other minor metabolites, all of which are inactive.[106]

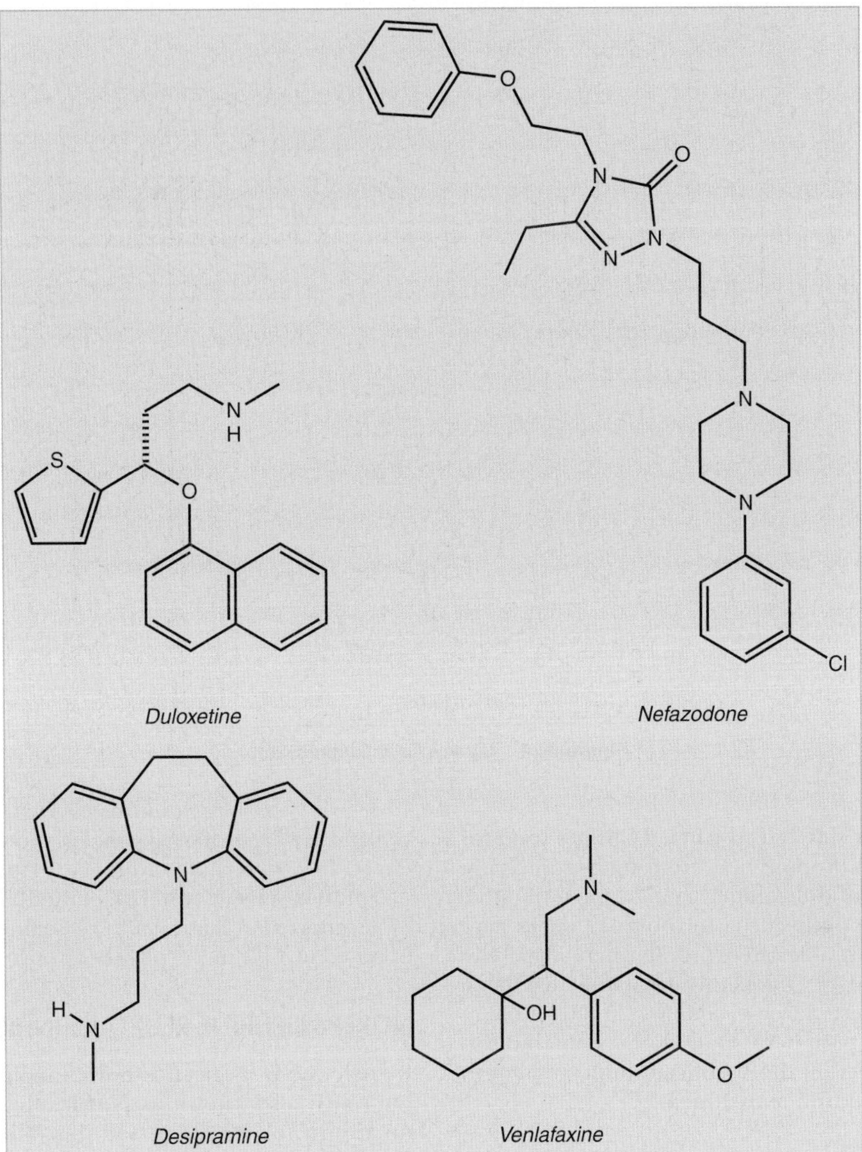

Figure 38.3 Serotonin-norepinephrine reuptake inhibitors.

Desvenlafaxine, or *O*-desmethylvenlafaxine, is the major active metabolite of the SNRI venlafaxine.[107,108] Like venlafaxine, desvenlafaxine selectively inhibits neuronal uptake of serotonin and norepinephrine and has little affinity for muscarinic, cholinergic, histaminergic H_1, and α_1-adrenergic receptors.[109] Desvenlafaxine has been shown to be active in preclinical in vitro and in vivo models used to predict antidepressant efficacy[110]; however, there are no robust trials of desvenlafaxine for pain relief. Desvenlafaxine succinate is well absorbed following oral administration, with a mean terminal-phase elimination half-life of approximately 9 to 11 hours.[111]

Few published data are available regarding milnacipran, which has been approved by the FDA in the United States only for FM. In a small randomized study, patients treated with milnacipran were shown to have a greater reduction in pain than were placebo-treated patients with FM.[112,113] In a published case report, milnacipran was reported to successfully manage trigeminal neuralgia in a 64-year-old patient.[114] The SNRIs have differing activity in both the serotonergic and noradrenergic systems.[115,116] Table 38.3 compares effects on the serotonergic system relative to the noradrenergic system for multiple SNRIs.

Table 38.3 Serotonin-Norepinephrine Reuptake Inhibitors

Agent	Selectivity Potency Ratio (5-HT/NE)
Venlafaxine (Effexor)	30:1
Desvenlafaxine (Pristiq)	14:1
Duloxetine (Cymbalta)	5-10:1
Milnacipran (Savella)	1:1.6-3

5-HT, serotonin; NE, norepinephrine.

Painful Diabetic Neuropathy

It is well established that duloxetine reduces the pain associated with diabetic neuropathy.[117-119] Bearing in mind the

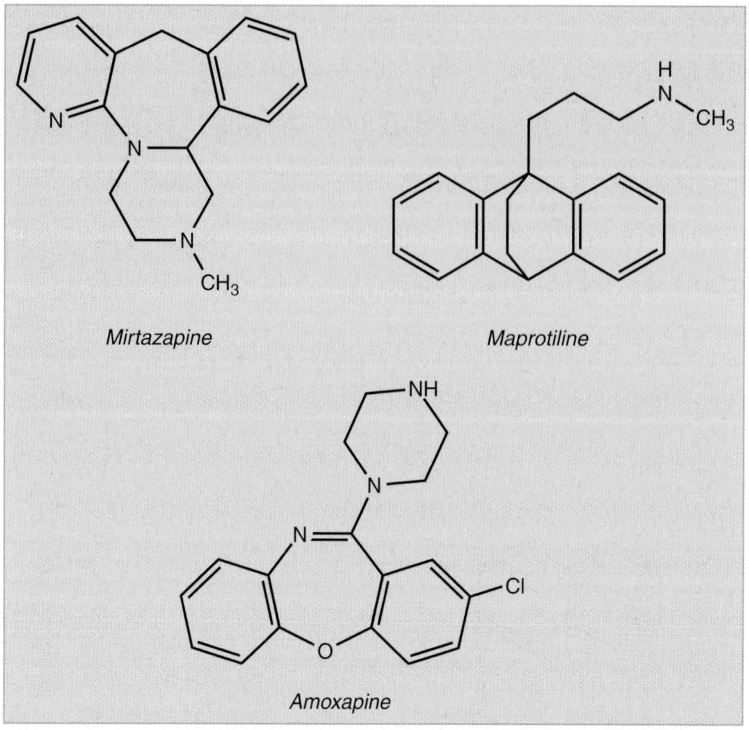

Mirtazapine

Maprotiline

Amoxapine

Figure 38.4 Tetracyclic antidepressants.

relatively high risk for side effects when TCAs are used for the treatment of PDN, dropout rates from studies are as low as 12% with the use of duloxetine,[117] and long-term studies examining the use of this drug for up to 52 weeks have shown that it has a favorable safety profile when taken over this prolonged period.[118] Duloxetine treatment has been associated with modest adverse changes in glycemia in patients with diabetic peripheral neuropathic pain, but this does not have an effect on the significant improvement in pain observed with duloxetine treatment.[120]

Fibromyalgia

Traditionally, TCAs have been used for the treatment of FM. However, their side effect profiles often reduce compliance. Conversely, the SSRIs have a more acceptable side effect profile but are relatively ineffective. The SNRIs, however, combine a relatively low risk for side effects with a relatively high chance of alleviating symptoms.

In a number of large studies, duloxetine has been found to be efficacious, not only in terms of pain reduction but also for many of the other problematic complaints associated with this condition.[119,121] For example, in a study of 207 subjects, Arnold and colleagues[121] found that duloxetine significantly reduces pain, number of tender points, and stiffness scores while significantly increasing the tender point pain threshold when compared with placebo. Furthermore, measures of quality of life were improved by active treatment. In an even larger study of 354 patients with FM, Arnold and associates[122] confirmed their previous findings and also showed that the beneficial effects of duloxetine therapy are independent of its effect on mood.

These positive effects with duloxetine therapy seem to be reproduced by other SNRIs, with milnacipran[112,123] and venlafaxine[124] also having been shown to have a positive effect. In Vitton and coworkers'[123] study of the use of milnacipran in subjects with FM, of the 125 enrolled in the study, 37% reported at least a 50% reduction in pain intensity (as opposed to 14% in the placebo group).

NOREPINEPHRINE REUPTAKE INHIBITORS

Reboxetine is a selective norepinephrine reuptake inhibitor (NRI; also known as NARI). Reboxetine has little or no affinity for serotonin and dopamine uptake sites or for muscarinic and histaminergic receptors and is no less effective for depression than the TCAs and SSRIs.[125,126] Limited clinical data point to reboxetine being a poorly effective stand-alone analgesic.[127,128]

TETRACYCLIC ANTIDEPRESSANTS

Limited evidence for an analgesic effect of tetracyclic antidepressants (Fig. 38.4) exists. When amitriptyline is compared with the tetracyclic antidepressant maprotiline in patients with PHN, even though maprotiline displays analgesic properties, those of amitriptyline are more pronounced.[74] In animal nociceptive models, mirtazapine exhibits antinociceptive properties with evidence of an antinociceptive effect in the hot plate chronic nerve constriction model of neuropathic pain and in the second phase of the formalin response.[101]

MONOAMINE OXIDASE INHIBITORS

Renowned for their multiple side effects, drug interactions, and necessity for a tyramine-free diet when used, monoamine oxidase inhibitors (Fig. 38.5) have no place in pain management. Little evidence exists for any analgesic effect.[129]

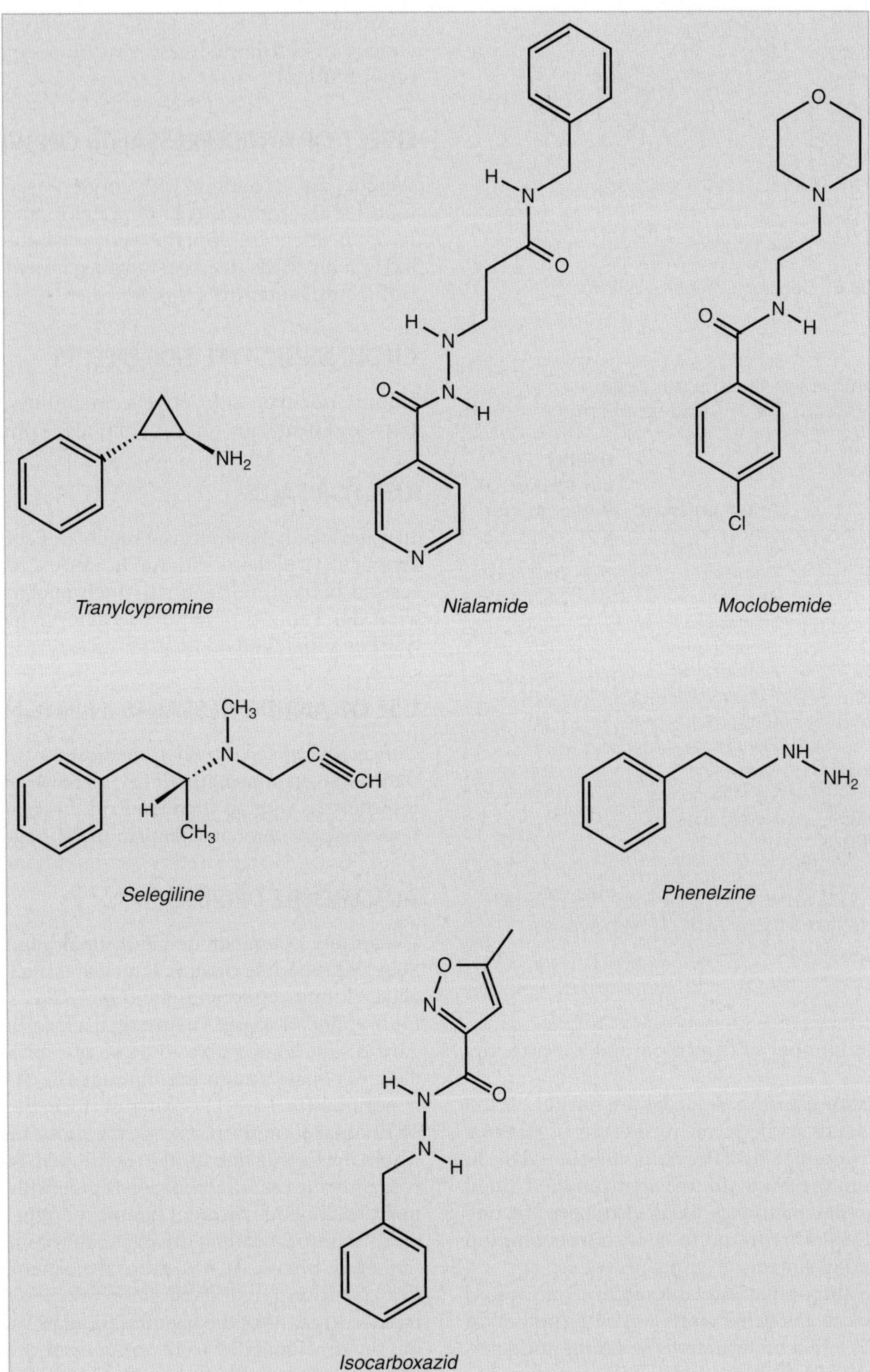

Figure 38.5 Monoamine oxidase inhibitors.

DOPAMINE REUPTAKE INHIBITORS

Though classified as a dopamine reuptake inhibitor (Fig. 38.6), bupropion also has noradrenergic activity. Evidence of an analgesic effect is limited, although Semenchuk and colleagues[130] found that 73% of subjects with neuropathic pain studied in their placebo-controlled trial obtained pain relief with bupropion treatment.

ANTIDEPRESSANTS: SAFETY AND SIDE EFFECTS

The safety of antidepressants can be considered both from the perspective of normal use and in overdose. Buckley and McManus[131] provided an interesting insight into the potential dangers of antidepressants when taken in overdose.

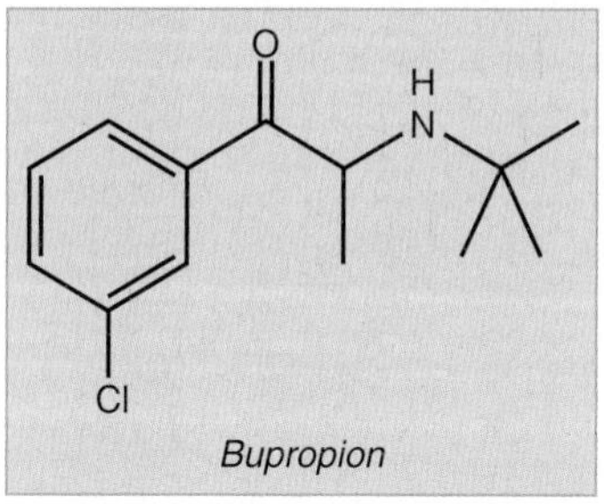

Bupropion

Figure 38.6 Dopamine reuptake inhibitor.

Table 38.4 Numbers of Deaths per Million Prescriptions of Antidepressants

Class of Antidepressant	Antidepressant	Deaths per Million Prescriptions
Tricyclic antidepressants (TCAs)	Desipramine	200.9
	Dothiepin	53.3
	Amitriptyline	38.0
	Imipramine	2.8
	Clomipramine	12.5
	Nortriptyline	5.5
Selective serotonin reuptake inhibitors (SSRIs)	Fluvoxamine	3.0
	Citalopram	1.9
	Fluoxetine	0.9
	Paroxetine	0.7
Serotonin-norepinephrine reuptake inhibitors (SNRIs)	Venlafaxine	13.2
	Nefazodone	0

Data from Buckley NA, McManus PR. Fatal toxicity of serotonergic and other antidepressant drugs: analysis of United Kingdom mortality data. *BMJ*. 2002;325:1332-1333.

They calculated the number of deaths per million prescriptions (Table 38.4).

The implications for use of these drugs are obvious. Careful consideration needs to be given to the use of desipramine if there is any danger that the drug may be taken in overdose. The data in the study cited[131] are from the United Kingdom, but a similar picture is likely elsewhere. In one study in Virginia, TCAs were found to be the most common antidepressants used in suicide attempts.[132]

In terms of overall comparative tolerability, one would expect that the newer antidepressants would be tolerated better than the TCAs. In a meta-analysis reviewing the tolerability of TCAs and SSRIs (when used for the treatment of depression), Arroll and coworkers[133] found that the number needed to harm—in this case the number of subjects receiving the treatment—for one subject to need to drop out because of side effects was calculated to be 5 to 11 for TCAs and 21 to 94 for SSRIs. In sharp contrast, Wilson and Mottram[134] studied the use of antidepressants in older depressed patients and concluded that "…TCA-related drugs are comparable to SSRIs in terms of tolerability," but they did note that the use of TCAs is associated with an increased risk for dry mouth, drowsiness, dizziness, and lethargy when compared with SSRIs.

Among the SSRIs, it seems that fluoxetine has a greater chance of causing adverse gastrointestinal effects than do other SSRIs.[135]

EFFECT OF ANTIDEPRESSANTS ON WEIGHT

Weight gain is common with antidepressants. When they are used for the treatment of depression, mood alteration may have an effect on appetite and well-being. TCAs are more likely than SSRIs to cause weight gain (which may interfere with compliance).[136]

CHOLINERGIC-TYPE SIDE EFFECTS

Cholinergic-type side effects, including dry mouth, sedation, and urinary retention, may also complicate TCA use.

RISK FOR FALLS

In a study of U.S. veterans, French and colleagues[137] showed that of 2212 patients with hip fractures, 70% had taken medication before the fracture, which may have contributed to their fall. Patients were twice as likely to have taken a TCA or SSRI as a matched control.

USE OF ANTIDEPRESSANTS IN PREGNANCY

Concern always exists when medication is taken during pregnancy. It seems that neither TCA nor SSRI use during pregnancy is associated with an increased risk for major fetal malformation, but poor neonatal adaptation has been reported.[138]

AUTOMOBILE DRIVING

Use of any potentially sedative medication leads to concern about its use while driving. Ramaekers[139] concluded that after acute dosing of sedating antidepressants (e.g., amitriptyline, imipramine, doxepin, mianserin), a measure of driving ability gave results comparable to those of individuals whose blood alcohol concentration was 0.8 mg/mL. When treatment was continued for 1 week, driving performance returned to that of the placebo group, except for those taking mianserin, in whom the driving impairment continued. It was also noted that concomitant use of a benzodiazepine with an antidepressant makes driving impairment significant. When SSRIs are considered, no impairment in driving ability has been noted.[140] Consequently, when a TCA is given, the patient should be warned to avoid driving until stabilization with a fixed dose of the TCA has occurred. Also, the patient should be warned of the potential for driving ability to be influenced over the longer term when the TCA is taken with other sedative medication.

SELECTIVE SEROTONIN REUPTAKE INHIBITORS AND NONSTEROIDAL ANTI-INFLAMMATORY DRUGS

De Jong and colleagues[141] studied 15,445 new users of antidepressants with or without use of nonsteroidal anti-inflammatory drugs (NSAIDs). They counted the number of first prescriptions of peptic ulcer drugs, with or without an NSAID, from day 2 after starting until 10 days after commencement of an antidepressant. In the 691 individuals given TCAs who were not taking NSAIDs, the incidence of peptic ulcer drug request was 0.051. In the SSRI-only group (1181 subjects), the incidence was 1.2. When an SSRI was taken with an NSAID (86 subjects), the incidence of peptic ulcer drug request was 12.4% as opposed to 2.5% in the TCA-NSAID cohort. This would suggest that some caution needs to be taken when SSRIs are given to patients taking NSAIDs.

PARADOXICAL PAIN

We have seen that strong evidence exists for a useful analgesic effect of TCAs . However, two studies have provided interesting and thought-provoking insight into the possibility that perhaps TCAs can produce pain symptoms as well as relieve them. In the first study, Esser and Sawynok[55] studied rats with a chronic constriction injury involving the lumbar nerve roots that produced features of neuropathic pain. When amitriptyline was administered systemically, thermal hyperalgesia was completely reversed in the injured paw. It also produced an anti-hyperalgesic effect on that side but had no effect on mechanical allodynia. However and of more importance, systemic administration of amitriptyline produced hyperesthesia on the contralateral (uninjured) side. In the second study, Esser and coworkers[56] again looked at a rat neuropathic pain model and found that amitriptyline reduced thermal hyperalgesia on the injured side but had no effect on allodynia. They again noted contralateral hyperesthesia with the use of amitriptyline. The significance of these results for human use of TCAs is not known but warrants investigation.

POSSIBLE ANALGESIC EFFECT WHEN APPLIED TOPICALLY

PERIPHERAL MODE OF ACTION

Thus far discussion has revolved around the use of antidepressants by the oral route of administration. Unfortunately, such systemic use also produces systemic side effects, which particularly with the TCAs, may reduce patient compliance.

Earlier we reviewed the potential modes of action of TCAs when given as oral analgesics, including effects on the serotonergic and noradrenergic pathways, on sodium and potassium channels, and on adenosine, NMDA, and opioid receptors. Not all these potential pharmacologic targets, however, have exclusively central representation.

ADENOSINE RECEPTORS

At peripheral nerve terminals in rodents, adenosine α_1-receptor activation produces antinociception by decreasing cyclic adenosine monophosphate (cAMP) levels, whereas adenosine α_2-receptor activation produces pronociception by increasing cAMP levels in the sensory nerve terminals. Adenosine α_3-receptor activation produces pain behavior as a result of the release of histamine and 5-HT from mast cells and subsequent actions on the sensory nerve terminal.[142] Caffeine acts as a nonspecific adenosine receptor antagonist. When caffeine and amitriptyline are administered systemically, the normal effect on thermal hyperalgesia is blocked. When amitriptyline is administered into a neuropathic pain site, an anti-hyperalgesic effect is recorded, but not when it is administered into the contralateral paw. This anti-hyperalgesic effect is blocked by caffeine,[143] thus suggesting that at least part of the effect of peripherally applied amitriptyline is mediated through peripheral adenosine receptors.

SODIUM CHANNELS

Sudoh and colleagues[144] administered various TCAs by a single injection into rat sciatic notches. They measured the duration of complete sciatic nerve blockade and compared it with the duration provided by bupivacaine. They found that amitriptyline, doxepin, and imipramine produce a longer complete sciatic nerve block than bupivacaine does whereas trimipramine and desipramine produce a shorter block. Nortriptyline and maprotiline failed to produce any block. When the effect of topical application of amitriptyline was compared with that of lidocaine, amitriptyline was found to produce longer cutaneous analgesia than lidocaine did.[144] These studies therefore suggest that from a mode-of-action perspective, TCAs could well have an analgesic effect when applied peripherally.

ANIMAL EVIDENCE OF ANTINOCICEPTIVE EFFECTS

Neuropathic Pain

When amitriptyline is applied to rodent paws made neuropathic by a chronic nerve constriction injury, an antinociceptive effect is observed. When amitriptyline is applied to the contralateral paw, no antinociceptive effect is observed in the paw on the injured side.[55,56,143] When desipramine and the SSRI fluoxetine are considered, desipramine has a similar antinociceptive effect when applied topically, whereas fluoxetine does not.[145]

Formalin Test

It seems that when amitriptyline[146,147] and desipramine[145] are coadministered peripherally with formalin, both the first- and second-phase responses are reduced. When amitriptyline is administered peripherally along with formalin, Fos immunoreactivity in the dorsal region of the spinal cord is significantly lower than in animals in which formalin is administered alone.[148]

Visceral Pain

Using a noxious colorectal distention model in the rat, Su and Gebhart[149] have shown that the antidepressants imipramine, desipramine, and clomipramine reduce the response to noxious colorectal distention by 20%, 22%, and 46%, respectively, when compared with control-treated animals.

Thermal Injury

Thermal hyperalgesia is produced by exposing a rodent hindpaw to 52° C for 45 seconds. Locally applied amitriptyline at the time of thermal injury produces anti-hyperalgesic and analgesic effects, depending on the concentration used. When amitriptyline is applied after the injury, the analgesic but not the anti-hyperalgesic effect is retained.[150]

HUMAN PAIN

Human evidence of an analgesic effect with the topical application of TCAs is limited. A small randomized, placebo-controlled trial (RCT) of 40 subjects with neuropathic pain of mixed cause showed a reduction of 1.18 on a 0 to 10 linear visual analog scale (LVAS) score relative to placebo use with the application of 5% doxepin cream. Minor side effects were seen in only three subjects.[151] A larger RCT involving 200 subjects, again with neuropathic pain of mixed cause, suggested that 5% doxepin cream reduces LVAS scores by approximately one relative to placebo and that time until effect is about

2 weeks. Again, side effects were minor and infrequent.[152] A pilot study examining the effect of topical amitriptyline application failed to produce any pain relief, but the maximum duration of therapy was 7 days,[153] and therefore the study may have been terminated before the time to maximal effect had been reached. Case studies of a useful reduction in pain when 5% doxepin cream is applied topically in subjects with complex regional pain syndrome type 1[154] and when doxepin is used as an oral rinse in patients with oral pain as a result of cancer or cancer therapy[155] have been reported.

Although the results of studies in humans of an analgesic effect with topical doxepin are interesting, more research is needed to verify this and other effects of TCAs when administered by this method. The evidence would suggest that topically applied doxepin has a local effect and that the consequences of systemic administration and systemic side effects can be substantially reduced.

CONCLUSION

There is compelling evidence of an antinociceptive effect when TCAs are used in animal pain models. This is substantiated by the recognition that TCAs have a number of effects that could account for their antinociceptive properties, including serotonergic and noradrenergic effects; actions on opioid, NMDA, and adenosine receptors; and actions on sodium and potassium channels. The results of animal studies, a large number of human clinical studies, and extensive and long-term use of TCAs in clinical practice suggest that these agents have a pain-reducing potential for various pain conditions, including neuropathic pain and pain associated with FM.

The analgesic effect seen when TCAs are used is present only to a slight degree with SSRIs, although their side effect potential is substantially less. The more recently introduced SNRIs appear to have a more favorable side effect profile than the TCAs do, along with many of their analgesic effects. It could be argued, therefore, that SNRIs should be the first choice when an antidepressant is chosen to treat pain and that TCAs should be reserved for use when there is therapeutic failure with an SNRI.

The potential for a peripheral mode of action of TCAs may allow them to be used as topical analgesics, with the reassurance that at least some of their effects are local. Thus, it is possible that systemic side effects can be avoided.

KEY POINTS

- Tricyclic antidepressants (TCAs) possess analgesic effects independent of their effects on moods. The analgesic effects tend to occur more rapidly, at lower serum blood levels, and at lower doses than those used for antidepressive effects.
- The mechanisms of analgesia of TCAs include serotonergic (interferes with reuptake of serotonin), noradrenergic (interaction with α receptors), opioidergic, and adenosine receptor (inhibits reuptake of adenosine) effects. They also block the sodium channel and have anti-inflammatory properties.

KEY POINTS—cont'd

- Antidepressants interact with histaminergic, cholinergic muscarinic, and cholinergic nicotinic receptors in an inhibitory manner. These interactions contribute to the side effects of the antidepressants.
- TCAs are effective in patients with post-herpetic neuralgia and painful diabetic neuropathy; nortriptyline and amitriptyline are equally effective, with nortriptyline having fewer side effects.
- Evidence supporting the use of TCAs for fibromyalgia is difficult because the disease is a complex disorder with a spectrum of symptoms and signs. However, antidepressants seem to improve the symptoms of fibromyalgia in some patients.
- The side effect profiles of TCAs often reduce compliance, whereas the selective serotonin reuptake inhibitors (SSRIs) have a more acceptable side effect profile but are relatively ineffective. The serotonin-norepinephrine reuptake inhibitors (SNRIs) combine a relatively low risk for side effects with a relatively high chance of alleviating symptoms.
- At doses of less than 150 mg/day, venlafaxine behaves more like an SSRI; at doses above 150 mg, it behaves more like an SNRI. It should gradually be discontinued because of the potential for a withdrawal syndrome.
- Neither TCA nor SSRI use during pregnancy is associated with an increased risk for major fetal malformation, but poor neonatal adaptation has been reported.
- No impairment in driving ability has been noted with SSRIs. For TCAs, the patient should be warned to avoid driving until stabilization with a fixed dose of the TCA has occurred. They should also be warned when the TCA is taken with other sedative medications.

SUGGESTED READINGS

Butterworth JF, Strichartz GR. Molecular mechanisms of local anesthesia: a review. *Anesthesiology.* 1990;72:711-734.

Derry S, Gill F, Phillips T, et al. Milnacipran for neuropathic pain and fibromyalgia in adults. *Cochrane Database Syst Rev.* 2012;3:CD008244.

Dick IE, Brochu RM, Purohit Y, et al. Sodium channel blockade may contribute to the analgesic efficacy of antidepressants. *J Pain.* 2007;8:315-324.

Fillion G, Fillion MP. Modulation of affinity of post-synaptic receptors by antidepressant drugs. *Nature.* 1981;292:349-351.

Häuser W, Wolfe F, Tölle T, et al. The role of antidepressants in the management of fibromyalgia syndrome: a systematic review and meta-analysis. *CNS Drugs.* 2012;26:297-307.

Max MB, Culnane M, Schafer SC, et al. Amitriptyline relieves diabetic neuropathy pain in patients with normal or depressed mood. *Neurology.* 1987;37:589-596.

Max MB, Schafer SC, Culnane M, et al. Amitriptyline, but not lorazepam, relieves postherpetic neuralgia. *Neurology.* 1988;38:1427-1432.

Saarto T, Wiffen PJ. Antidepressants for neuropathic pain. *Cochrane Database Syst Rev.* 2005;3:CD005454.

Scott WA. The relief of pain with an antidepressant in arthritis. *Practitioner.* 1969;202:802-807.

The references for this chapter can be found at www.expertconsult.com.

39

Membrane Stabilizers for the Treatment of Pain

Robert W. Hurley | Brian E. McGeeney | Charles E. Argoff

Multimodal medical management of cancer- and non–cancer-related pain can involve the use of nonopioid medications, as well as opioid medications. Nonopioid medications, often referred to as adjuvant medications, can take the form of amine reuptake inhibitors, such as the tricyclic antidepressants (TCAs); neuronal membrane stabilizers, such as the sodium and calcium channel–blocking anticonvulsants; nonsteroidal anti-inflammatory drugs (NSAIDs); topical analgesics; and muscle relaxants. The neuronal membrane stabilizers and data associated with their use for primarily neuropathic pain (NP) are discussed in this chapter.

Based on extensive studies, NP appears to result from a cascade of multiple mechanisms following tissue injury.[1] In broad terms, neural plasticity following nerve injury may result in peripheral nerve fibers communicating abnormal input to the central nervous system (CNS), which in turn may remodel CNS signaling. NP has a heterogeneous origin and may involve both the central and peripheral neural pathways following injury. Although neuroplasticity may help facilitate recovery, unfortunately, this is not always the case, and in fact, the downstream impact of the neuromodulatory changes associated with neuroplasticity, including abnormal stimulation or decreased inhibitory activity, may result in enhanced pain processing. Chronic pain develops when this neural stimulation continues beyond the range of expected healing and the triggering stimulus is no longer present. Moreover, ion channel functioning is affected as well by changes in signaling. Sodium and calcium channels play a fundamental role in the propagation of hyperexcitability in central and peripheral neurons.[2] Accumulation of excessive or misplaced ion channels can lead to ectopic, spontaneous firing of sensory nerves and dorsal root ganglion cell bodies and result in hyperexcitability of the primary afferents and pain.

Research into the physiologic source and pharmacologic management of NP led to a focus on sodium and calcium channel blockade.[3,4] Clinically available agents that act on these ion channels include the membrane-stabilizing agents typically used for the treatment of epilepsy. Many of these agents have been tried with varying success in patients with pain. Multiple classes of medications that fall under the membrane stabilizer classification are beneficial in the treatment of pain (Table 39.1). These agents include the antiepileptic/anticonvulsants, local anesthetics, TCAs, and antiarrhythmic medications. As a group, they inhibit the development and propagation of ectopic discharges. The primary agents used for NP include antiepileptic/anticonvulsants, local anesthetics, and the TCAs, which are discussed in a separate chapter. Gabapentin and pregabalin, also anticonvulsants, are discussed separately under calcium channel modulators because their mechanism of action differs from that of the other agents typically used for epilepsy.

The effectiveness of medications for pain relief is often determined by using one of several standard outcome measures, each of which assesses the change in average daily pain intensity score on a 10-cm (100-mm) visual analog scale (VAS) or a 11-point Likert (0, no pain; 10, worst possible pain) numeric rating scale (NRS). Patients who report pain relief of 30% or greater (moderate benefit) are considered to have experienced a clinically meaningful result; patients who report pain relief of 50% or greater are considered to have experienced substantial benefit. An often-used tool to allow comparison between different drugs and diseases and more precisely judge the efficacy of an agent is the number needed to treat (NNT).[5,6] The NNT is the number of patients needed to be treated with a particular drug to obtain one patient with a defined degree of relief. Usually, the parameter "NNT for greater than 50% pain relief" is used because it is easily understood and seems to be related to relevant clinical effect.[5] The number needed to harm (NNH) is the number needed to treat with a certain drug before a patient experiences a significant side effect. The NNH of several drugs used for pain management is not yet known. Drugs with a low NNT/NNH ratio are superior to the drugs with a high NNT/NNH ratio.

CALCIUM CHANNEL MODULATORS

The first-line treatment agents recommended for NP include the calcium channel modulators.[7] The intracellular free calcium ion concentration is only 1 in 10,000 that of the extracellular environment, and influx of calcium through calcium channels has important depolarizing effects on neurons. Voltage-gated calcium channels can be divided into high-voltage–activated (HVA) and low-voltage–activated (LVA) channels. Electrophysiologic characteristics allow division into HVA and LVA channels, depending on the threshold of activation. The HVA group is further divided into types L, P/Q, N, and R.[8] These groups require large membrane depolarization and are mainly responsible for entry of calcium and release of neurotransmitter from presynaptic nerve terminals. Low-voltage channels, such as the T type, regulate firing by participating in bursting and intrinsic oscillations. The spike and wave discharges from the thalamus with absence seizures are dependent on T-type calcium channels; these discharges are inhibited by valproic acid or ethosuximide. The N-type HVA calcium channels are thought to be largely responsible for release of neurotransmitter at

Table 39.1 Membrane Stabilizers for Pain

Membrane Stabilizer	Mechanism	Side Effects
Carbamazepine	Na channel blockade	Sedation, dizziness, gait abnormalities, hematologic changes
Oxcarbazepine	Na channel blockade	Hyponatremia, somnolence, dizziness
Lamotrigine	Stabilizes slow Na channel; suppress release of glutamate from presynaptic neurons	Rash, dizziness, somnolence
Gabapentin/pregabalin	Binds to $\alpha_2\delta$ subunit of voltage-gated Ca channel	Dizziness, sedation
Valproic acid	Na channel blockade; increases GABA	Somnolence, dizziness, gastrointestinal upset
Topiramate	Na channel blockade; potentiates GABA inhibition	Sedation, kidney stones, glaucoma
Mexiletine	Na channel blockade	Nausea, blurred vision
Lacosamide	Na channel blockade	Dizziness, nausea, double vision, headache

GABA, γ-aminobutyric acid.

Table 39.2 Dosing Recommendations for Neuropathic Pain

Membrane Stabilizer	Initial Dosage	Titration	Max Therapeutic Dosage
Carbamazepine	100-200 mg BID	Increase by 200-mg increments gradually	1200 mg QD
Oxcarbazepine	600 mg daily BID	Increase by 300 mg	1200-1800 mg TID
Lamotrigine	25-50 mg QHS	Increase by 50 mg every 1-2 wk	300-500 mg QD
Gabapentin*	100-300 mg QHS	Increase by 100-300 mg or 100-300 mg TID every 1-7 days as tolerated	3600 mg (1200 TID)
Gabapentin GR	300 mg QHS	Day 1, 300 mg; day 2, 600; days 3-6, 900; days 7-10, 1200; days 11-14, 1500, then 1800	1800 mg QHS
Pregabalin*	50 mg TID or 75 mg BID	Increase to 300 mg daily after 3-7 days, then by 150 mg/day every 3-7 days as tolerated	600 mg QD (200 mg TID or 300 mg BID)
Valproic acid	250 mg BID	Increase by 250 mg weekly	500 mg BID
Topiramate	50 mg QHS	Start at 50 mg BID after 1 wk, then increase 100 mg BID after 7 days	100 mg BID
Mexiletine	150 mg QD	Increase to 300 mg in 3 days and then 600 mg	Maximum: 10 mg/kg daily

*Reduce if impaired renal function.
BID, twice daily; QHS, at bedtime; QD, daily; TID, three times daily.

synaptic junctions and become inactivated rather quickly. The P/Q-type calcium channel is so named because it was first described in the Purkinje cells of the cerebellum. The T-type channel, named after the transient currents elicited, starts to open with weak depolarization, near resting potential. L-type channels are found in high concentration in skeletal muscle and in many other tissues, such as neuronal and smooth muscle, where it has been most studied. The voltage-gated calcium channel is composed of five polypeptide subunits and is the target of many drugs. Calcium channels consist of an α protein, along with several auxiliary subunits; the α protein forms the channel pore.

GABAPENTIN (NEURONTIN, GRALISE, HORIZANT)

The calcium channel modulators that are used for the treatment of NP, such as gabapentin and pregabalin, bind to the $\alpha_2\delta$ subunit of L-type voltage-gated calcium channels, and such binding results in decreased release of glutamate, norepinephrine, and substance P.[9,10] Though structurally derived from the inhibitory neurotransmitter γ-aminobutyric acid (GABA), neither gabapentin nor pregabalin bind to or have activity at the GABA receptor. They also have no effect on the uptake or metabolism of GABA.

The standard initial dose of gabapentin is dependent on the particular gabapentin formulation used. For the first available preparation of gabapentin (Neurontin), it is 100 to 300 mg daily. Although the U.S. Food and Drug Administration (FDA)-approved dose of this preparation for the treatment of post-herpetic neuralgia (PHN) (the only painful condition for which this preparation is indicated) is 1800 mg, many clinicians will proceed with a gradual increase to a maximum of 3600 mg/day administered in three divided doses (Table 39.2). To minimize the consequence of certain adverse effects such as sedation and dizziness, the initial dose is often given at bedtime. After 2 to 5 days, the dose is increased to 300 mg twice daily and, after another 2 to 5 days, to 300 mg three times daily thereafter. Subsequently, the dose can be increased by 300 to 600 mg every other week as tolerated until an effective dosage is obtained or the maximum daily dose is reached. The main dose-limiting side effects are fatigue, somnolence, and dizziness, which are often attenuated by gradual dose titration. Although gabapentin has few drug interactions, a reduced dosage is necessary in patients with renal insufficiency. However, starting dosages of gabapentin often do not provide immediate pain relief, and the slow titration requirements may result in adequate pain relief taking up to 2 months to achieve when given as immediate-release gabapentin, although when given as the extended-release formulation, therapeutic doses can be reached in approximately 2 weeks.

Gabapentin has many uses in patients with multiple pain conditions. Studies have been performed on patients being treated for PHN, complex regional pain syndrome (CRPS), painful diabetic neuropathy (PDN), and other forms of NP, as well as for pain of controversial etiology, including opioid-induced hyperalgesia.[11-13] In one study, patients with PHN being treated with opioids, TCAs, or both were identified and divided into two groups: 113 receiving gabapentin and 116 receiving placebo, in addition to their current baseline pain treatment regimen. For a period of 8 weeks patients were maintained on their respective therapies, with a 4-week titration of gabapentin to a maximum dose of 3600 mg/day. The results indicated that the patients who received gabapentin had a decrease of nearly 2 points in their VAS score for pain, as opposed to a decrease of just 0.5 in the placebo-treated patients ($P < 0.001$). Along with a decrease in pain, patients also reported improvement in their 36-Item Short-Form Health Survey (SF-36) quality-of-life scores and noted improved functionality and feeling better with more restful sleep at night.

The analgesic effect of gabapentin in patients with PDN has also been evaluated.[11] A randomized, double-blind, placebo-controlled (RCT) multicenter trial demonstrated a decrease of 2.5 in the VAS score in patients receiving gabapentin, up to 3600 mg/day, versus a decrease of 1.4 in patients in the control group ($P < 0.001$).[11] As with the PHN study, patients also had a favorable change in their SF-36 scores, with more restful sleep at night and overall improvement in functioning.

Gabapentin has also been studied in patients with lumbar spinal stenosis. In a pilot study, both patient groups received "standard care," including physical therapy, lumbosacral bracing, and NSAIDs.[14] The treatment group also received gabapentin, 900 to 2400 mg, administered in three divided doses. After 4 months, patients who received gabapentin reported improvement in pain scores, increased walking distance, and decreased sensory and motor deficits. These results suggest that in the appropriate setting, gabapentin may provide symptomatic benefit for certain patients with lumbar spinal stenosis. In a double-blind, randomized, placebo-controlled 8-week trial, patients enrolled included those with CRPS, PHN, radiculopathy, post-laminectomy syndrome, post-stroke syndrome, phantom limb pain, and other NP syndromes. Gabapentin was initially started at 900 mg/day for 3 days and then increased to a maximum of 2400 mg/day at the end of week 5. The conclusion of the study showed that gabapentin reduced pain and improved certain quality-of-life measures in these patients.[15] Gabapentin has also been found to be effective in reducing the pain associated with multiple sclerosis, specifically, the paroxysmal pain with a throbbing, pricking, and cramping quality rather than the dull, aching pain experienced by patients with multiple sclerosis.[16] Of interest is that gabapentin appears to improve the analgesic efficacy of opioids in patients with NP.[17]

In studies of gabapentin for postamputation pain and phantom limb pain, it was found to be less effective than for other NP states. Nikolajsen and colleagues[18] administered gabapentin to patients following limb amputation and found no effect on postamputation or phantom limb pain. In a small cohort-control study, gabapentin was found to be effective for the treatment of chemotherapy-induced, painful peripheral neuropathy.[19] However, an earlier, larger RCT found no benefit with gabapentin therapy for the same condition.[20]

Combination therapies for NP have also proved successful. In a crossover RCT, patients received daily active placebo, sustained-release morphine, gabapentin, or a combination of gabapentin and morphine for 5 weeks. Fifty-seven patients underwent randomization (35 with PDN and 22 with PHN) and 41 completed the trial. Mean daily pain at the maximally tolerated dose of the study drug was reduced from 5.72 at baseline to 4.49 with placebo, 4.15 with gabapentin, 3.70 with morphine, and 3.06 with the gabapentin-morphine combination ($P < 0.05$ for the combination vs. placebo, gabapentin, and morphine).[17] In an extremely important and well-performed trial, combination therapy with gabapentin and the TCA nortriptyline was found to be highly effective in the treatment of NP resulting from diabetes and varicella zoster.[21] Although this study was not designed to examine the manner of interaction (e.g., drug-drug synergism vs. simple additivity), the results are highly suggestive of a synergistic analgesic effect. Patients achieved greater pain relief with a combination of low dosages of gabapentin (600 mg orally three times daily) and nortriptyline (50 mg orally at bedtime) than with either medication given alone at high doses. Importantly, patients receiving combination therapy had good analgesia without the significant side effects experienced by those treated with monotherapy. This trial, supported by the Canadian Institutes of Health, is a rare study in that the investigators had no influence from pharmaceutical companies and two inexpensive generic medications were studied.

A new gastric-retentive formulation of gabapentin (Gralise) has recently been approved by the FDA for PHN. It is intended to provide a simpler dosing paradigm than needed with the traditional generic gabapentin through the use of a polymer-based technology that allows gastric retention of the pill for extended delivery of the active medication. In a blinded RCT examining the analgesic benefit of single-day versus twice-a-day dosing in patients with PHN, the gastric-retentive formulation, when given twice per day, was more effective than placebo with an NNT of 5.9.[22] The single-day dosing was not significantly different from placebo and had an NNT of 7.3,[23] although a more recent multicountry RCT showed a significant improvement in pain after a single dose of 1800 mg given in the evening.[24] Another formulation of gabapentin, gabapentin enacarbil (Horizant), has been developed and was initially approved for the treatment of restless legs syndrome. It is an actively transported prodrug form of gabapentin that allows twice-a-day dosing because of increased stability in bioavailability in comparison to the standard formulation of gabapentin. In a recent RCT, this prodrug formulation was found to be effective in the treatment of PHN when given twice per day.[25] This drug is now approved by the FDA for the treatment of PHN as well as restless leg syndrome.

PREGABALIN (LYRICA)

Pregabalin, like gabapentin, is used for the treatment of NP and acts by binding to the $\alpha_2\delta$ subunit of L-type voltage-gated calcium channels, which results in decreased neuronal excitation. With respect to NP, pregabalin is approved by the FDA for the treatment of PHN, PDN, and spinal cord injury–associated pain. Initial pregabalin dosing is 150 mg/day given in two or three divided doses or 25-50 mg given at bedtime in elderly patients. Upward dose titration can be completed after 3 to 7 days to 300 mg/day and subsequently increased to a maximum dose of 600 mg/day within 2 weeks of initiation. Similar to gabapentin, dosing of pregabalin must be decreased in patients with reduced kidney function. Advantages of pregabalin over gabapentin include a more rapid onset of pain relief; linear pharmacokinetics with low intersubject variability[26]; fewer dose-related side effects, thereby allowing faster upward dosage titrations; and twice-daily versus three times a day dosing. Additionally, maximum benefit often occurs after 2 weeks of treatment at target doses of 300 to 600 mg/day versus up to 2 months in gabapentin-treated patients.

In patients with PHN, a trial that included 370 patients was conducted to evaluate doses of 150, 300, or 600 mg/day versus placebo.[27] The RCT demonstrated reduced mean pain scores and improvement in sleep interference. Patients responded at all dosages, with the greatest response noted with 600 mg/day. Patients responded as early as the first week, and beneficial effects were sustained throughout the 13-week study duration. Adverse effects were generally mild to moderate, and 13% of patients withdrew from the study, most commonly because of dizziness or somnolence.

In a randomized, double-blind study, the effects of pregabalin on PDN were evaluated.[28] A total of 395 patients were randomized to receive 150, 300, or 600 mg/day. In patients who received 600 mg/day, 46% reported greater than 50% improvement in pain scores from baseline, and the NNT to achieve this response was 6.3. Pregabalin also improved pain-related sleep interference and was well tolerated overall, with an NNH of 10.3 in patients treated with 600 mg/day.

Pregabalin was evaluated in a 12-week multicenter study in patients with central NP secondary to spinal cord injury.[29] A total of 137 patients were randomized either to a flexible-dose regimen of 150 to 600 mg/day or to placebo and were allowed to continue an existing stable pain regimen. Pregabalin was found to be significantly more effective in relieving central NP than placebo was.

Pregabalin has also been studied for use in patients with "refractory" NP of various origins.[30] A 15-month open-label study was conducted in 81 patients with PHN and PDN refractory to treatment, including gabapentin, a TCA, and a third medication (e.g., other anticonvulsant, opioid, specific serotonin reuptake inhibitor, tramadol). Patients took 150 to 600 mg/day for 3-month intervals and then had a 3- to 28-day "drug holiday." As evaluated by VAS scores, patients had a clinically meaningful and sustained reduction in pain intensity during the treatment cycle, with return of pain during "drug holidays." In patients with an unsatisfactory response to other medications, pregabalin may be considered as an adjunctive therapy.

The advantage of pregabalin is its early response and favorable side effect profile.[31] The most common adverse effects include somnolence and dizziness, and they occur more frequently with higher doses. When discontinuing pregabalin, it should be tapered down gradually over at least a 1-week period to minimize symptoms, including insomnia, nausea, headache, and diarrhea.

ZONISAMIDE (ZONEGRAN)

Zonisamide is indicated as adjunctive therapy for partial seizures in adults and became available in the United States in 2000. It acts by blocking T-type calcium channels and sodium channels; its action also increases release of GABA. The initial dose is 100 mg/day for 2 weeks with increases of 200 mg/wk to a target of 600 mg/day. There have been case reports on its usefulness for post-stroke pain and headache. A randomized, double-blind, placebo-controlled pilot study of the efficacy of zonisamide for the treatment of PDN revealed that pain scores on the VAS and Likert (psychometric response) scales decreased more in the zonisamide group than in the placebo group, but these differences did not reach statistical significance.[32] Side effects included ataxia, decreased appetite, rash, and renal calculi (as a result of the carbonic anhydrase inhibitor effect). Zonisamide is contraindicated in those with sulfonamide allergy because it is a sulfonamide derivative, and the drug is approximately 40% bound to plasma proteins. Children have an increased risk for oligohidrosis and susceptibility to hyperthermia. The exact role of zonisamide in the management of patients with NP is yet to be elucidated, and further research is needed.

ZICONOTIDE (PRIALT)

Ziconotide is a ω-conopeptide (previously known as SNX-111) that is administered intrathecally because of its peptidic structure. It is derived from the venom of a marine snail (genus *Conus*). Ziconotide blocks calcium influx into N-type calcium channels in the dorsal horn laminae of the spinal cord, thus preventing afferent conduction of nerve signals.[33] Administration is via an intrathecal infusion pump, and dosing should be started low, at a recommended dose of 2.4 μg/day (0.1 μg/hr). Because of a lag time, it should be titrated up slowly at intervals of no more than two to three times per week to a recommended maximum of 19.2 μg/day.[33] Ziconotide does not cause tolerance, dependence, or respiratory depression, and adverse effects primarily involve the CNS and include dizziness, ataxia, confusion, and headache.

Ziconotide has been evaluated in randomized, double-blind, placebo-controlled trials for severe, chronic, treatment-refractory pain in patients with or without cancer.[34] Patients experienced a significant improvement in mean pain scores and global pain relief. The response rate was higher in patients receiving a maximum of 21.8 μg/day; however, pain relief was accompanied by a high incidence of adverse effects that resulted in frequent interruptions of the trial. A slow titration schedule with a lower maximum infusion rate was associated with significantly lower dropout rates but also resulted in a more modest treatment effect. At the conclusion of one trial, nearly 90% of patients elected to continue receiving ziconotide. Rare, but serious adverse effects include hallucinations; thus, ziconotide is not recommended for use in patients with a history of psychosis. Elevations in creatine kinase (CK) were noted in some studies to be related to ziconotide. The etiology remains unclear, and CK levels should be monitored periodically.

The role of ziconotide in the management of chronic pain has yet to be fully elucidated. Currently, ziconotide is approved for the management of severe chronic pain in patients in whom intrathecal therapy is warranted and who are intolerant of or refractory to other treatments, including intrathecal opiates; however, this medication should be used cautiously because of its poor side effect profile.

NIMODIPINE (NIMOTOP)

Nimodipine has been shown to decrease the dose of morphine needed for relief of cancer pain in 9 of 14 patients.[35] In a colorectal surgery population, concomitant calcium channel blocker therapy did not decrease opioid requirements.[36] Nimodipine taken concurrently with antiretroviral medications demonstrated a trend toward improvement or stabilization of human immunodeficiency virus (HIV)-associated neuropathy when compared with placebo.[37]

SODIUM CHANNEL BLOCKERS

Sodium channel blockers are used as primary therapy or adjunctive treatment of processes such as trigeminal neuralgia (TN), CRPS, PDN, radicular extremity pain, chemotherapy-induced peripheral neuropathy, and PHN. When using these agents, as with all membrane stabilizers, it is crucial to be knowledgeable of the proper dosages, toxicities, and their effects when coadministered with other drugs. As a general rule, the dose should be titrated to patient comfort within safety standards.

When neurons are depolarized and approaching an action potential, the voltage-gated sodium channels quickly change conformation in response and permit the flow of sodium ions. Activation of sodium channels (and other voltage-gated ion channels) derives from the outward movement of charged residues because of an altered electrical field across the membrane. Sodium channels play an essential role in the action potentials of neurons and other electrically excitable cells. The flow of sodium ions is terminated by inactivation of the channel in a few milliseconds (fast inactivation). Sodium channels can cycle open and close rapidly, which may result in seizures, NP, or paresthesias. The structure of the channel is essentially a rectangular tube, with its four walls formed from four subunits, the four domains of a single polypeptide. A region near the N-terminus protrudes into the cytosol and forms an inactivating particle. It has been demonstrated that a short loop of amino acid residues, acting as a flap or hinge, blocks the inner mouth of the sodium channel and results in fast inactivation.[38] The highly conserved intracellular loop is the inactivating gate that binds to the intracellular pore and inactivates it within milliseconds. Site-directed antibody studies against this intracellular loop have prevented this fast inactivation.

The voltage-gated sodium channel can be divided into an α subunit and one or more auxiliary β subunits. At least nine α subunits have been functionally characterized—$Na_v1.1$ through $Na_v1.9$.[39] The sodium channels 1.2, 1.8, and 1.9 are preferentially expressed on peripheral sensory neurons, where they are important in nociception and may be a future target for channel-specific analgesics.[40] Seven of the nine sodium channel subtypes have been identified in sensory ganglia, such as the dorsal root ganglia and trigeminal ganglia. $Na_v1.7$ is also present in large amounts in the peripheral nervous system. $Na_v1.2$ is expressed in unmyelinated neurons and $Na_v1.4$ and $Na_v1.5$ are muscle sodium channels. Sodium channel mutations that cause well-recognized syndromes have been described. A mutation in $Na_v1.4$ is responsible for hyperkalemic periodic paralysis, and an inherited long QT syndrome can be caused by a mutation in $Na_v1.5$.

Increased expression of sodium channels has been demonstrated in peripheral and central sensory neurons in patients with NP; it is one mechanism for the observed hyperexcitability of pain pathways.[41] Anticonvulsants that modulate the gating of sodium channels are phenytoin, lamotrigine, carbamazepine, oxcarbazepine, and zonisamide, with some evidence for topiramate and valproic acid. It is important to note that at clinical concentrations, the sodium channel is only weakly blocked when hyperpolarized. When the neuronal membrane is depolarized, there is a much greater inhibition of the channel. Binding of the channel by anticonvulsants is slow in comparison to local anesthetics. The slow binding of anticonvulsants ensures that the kinetic properties of normal action potentials are not altered. Generally, anticonvulsants have no role in the treatment of acute pain, although they have demonstrated efficacy in chronic pain conditions. Interestingly, local application of phenytoin and carbamazepine has an antinociceptive effect that is more potent than that of lidocaine.[42] It has been demonstrated that phenytoin, carbamazepine, and lamotrigine bind to a common recognition site on sodium channels, and it is probably the result of their two phenol groups, which act as binding elements.[43] At normal resting potentials, these medications have little effect on action potentials. In addition to the fast current of the open channel, there is also a persistent sodium current. This current, carried by persistent openings, is a small fraction of the fast current but may have an important role in regulating excitability. There is evidence that a number of anticonvulsants, such as phenytoin, valproate, and topiramate, also act by blocking the persistent sodium current, which is separate from the fast sodium current.

SODIUM CHANNEL–MODULATING ANTICONVULSANTS

PHENYTOIN (DILANTIN)

In addition to the widespread use of phenytoin for seizures, it was the first anticonvulsant to be used for NP, with a 1940s report on its use for TN. Phenytoin is known for its nonlinear metabolism, which is manifested as marked increases in plasma level with small increases in dose after saturation of metabolism. Around 95% of a phenytoin dose is excreted as metabolites from the cytochrome P-450 system. The initial dosage of phenytoin is 100 mg two to three times daily. It has primarily been used for the treatment of diabetic neuropathy; however, because of the mixed results of its efficacy and high side effect and medication interaction profile, it has fallen into disuse. Phenytoin provides pain relief by blocking sodium channels, thereby preventing the release of excitatory glutamate and inhibiting ectopic discharges.

Trials have been performed to investigate the efficacy of phenytoin for diabetic neuropathy, with conflicting results.[44] Intravenous phenytoin has been studied in the pain management setting. Doses of 15 mg/kg have provided relief of acute pain when administered over a 2-hour period. Side effects of phenytoin include slowing of mentation and somnolence, with nystagmus and ataxia occurring in some patients. Among the epileptic drugs, phenytoin is unique in the development of facial alterations, including gum hyperplasia and coarsening of facial features. Fosphenytoin, an intravenously administered prodrug that converts to phenytoin, is used by some to avoid long dosing intervals or initial burning at the injection site.

Phenytoin activates the cytochrome P-450 enzyme system in the liver, and hence careful assessment of co-therapy is warranted. For example, phenytoin decreases the efficacy of methadone, fentanyl, tramadol, mexiletine, lamotrigine, and carbamazepine. As a result, dosages of these medications should be adjusted accordingly. Coadministration with antidepressants and valproic acid could lead to an increased blood concentration of phenytoin, thereby lowering the subsequent doses required for effect in patients. Currently, most would not use phenytoin for the treatment of NP except perhaps in refractory situations.

CARBAMAZEPINE (TEGRETOL)

Carbamazepine has been used in the United States since the 1980s to treat partial and generalized tonic-clonic seizures. Carbamazepine was first approved by the FDA for the treatment of TN, not for epilepsy. In addition to its anticonvulsant and TN indications, it is used frequently for bipolar disorder. It was one of the first anticonvulsants studied for the relief of NP. The analgesic properties of carbamazepine were first reported in 1962.[45] It is chemically related to the TCAs; reports have included studies of its use for PHN, PDN, post-stroke pain, and pain in Guillain-Barré syndrome. The initial dosage of carbamazepine is 100 to 200 mg twice daily, titrated to effect, with typical dose ranges of 300 to 1200 mg/day administered in two divided doses. Common maintenance doses are 600 to 800 mg.

Common side effects include drowsiness, dizziness, and nausea and vomiting, which can often be limited by slow titration. Carbamazepine is associated with very deleterious side effects, including pancytopenia (necessitating a complete blood count and monitoring while being treated with this therapy), Stevens-Johnson syndrome, and toxic epidermal necrolysis.

Carbamazepine is considered to be the pharmacologic treatment of choice for TN, a sharp severe facial pain in one or more of the distributions supplied by the trigeminal nerve.[46] Although the pathology of this process has not been fully determined, the majority of cases are thought to be caused by compression of the trigeminal nerve at the pontine origin of the nerve by an aberrant loop of an artery or vein.

With an NNT of lower than 2, carbamazepine is the most studied treatment of TN, and many studies have highlighted its usefulness.[46] One study noted the effect of carbamazepine in 70 patients with TN and reported a 68% decrease in pain episodes and a 58% decrease in the severity of pain. Research from other studies has noted a verbal response of "excellent" or "good" by patients on initiation of therapy for 2 weeks.[47] Additionally, the positive effect of carbamazepine on TN has been tested by crossover, placebo, and controlled double-blinded studies[48]; yet even with these positive results, TN is a disease process that in many patients is difficult to treat completely, with multiple agents often being required.

Carbamazepine has also been investigated for use in pain states caused by diabetes mellitus. Its application in animals resulted in a decrease in hyperalgesia in response to various stimuli. This agent has been shown to be more beneficial than placebo in the human diabetic patient population.[44] Carbamazepine therapy, when compared with a combination of nortriptyline and fluphenazine in patients with PDN, was found to be equally effective with fewer side effects.

Patients maintained on carbamazepine therapy should have blood tests done every 2 to 4 months because of increased risk for the development of agranulocytosis and aplastic anemia with this agent. Studies have noted that the NNH for severe adverse effects was 24 and for minor adverse effects, such as sedation, was 3.[46]

OXCARBAZEPINE (TRILEPTAL)

Oxcarbazepine, the keto-analogue of carbamazepine, was developed to preserve the membrane-stabilizing effects of carbamazepine while minimizing minor adverse effects such as sedation and serious, life-threatening reactions. A major advantage of oxcarbazepine is that monitoring of plasma drug levels and hematologic profiles is not generally necessary. Similar to carbamazepine, oxcarbazepine blocks sodium channels; it does not affect GABA receptors.

Significant hyponatremia (sodium <125 mmol/L) may develop during treatment with oxcarbazepine. This typically occurs during the first 3 months, with sodium levels normalizing within a few days of discontinuing the drug. Monitoring of sodium levels should be performed when instituting oxcarbazepine therapy. Frequently reported adverse effects of oxcarbazepine include dizziness, somnolence, and nausea and vomiting, which are generally well tolerated.

In a randomized, placebo-controlled trial lasting 16 weeks, oxcarbazepine was evaluated in patients with PDN.[49] Patients were treated with 300 mg and titrated to a maximum dose of 1800 mg/day. Oxcarbazepine-treated patients reported less pain on the VAS, global improvement, and less sleep disturbances because of pain.

The superior side effect profile of oxcarbazepine over carbamazepine has led to its increased use. In several countries, oxcarbazepine is now the drug of choice for TN. Oxcarbazepine was also found to be effective in treating TN in patients who had no positive response to carbamazepine.[50]

LAMOTRIGINE (LAMICTAL)

Lamotrigine received FDA approval in 1994; it is used as an adjunctive agent for partial seizures and as monotherapy for partial and generalized seizures. Like other agents discussed in this section, lamotrigine is an agent that blocks sodium channels in actively firing nerves. It has no effect on sensation in the native, normally functioning nervous system.

Unique to lamotrigine is the fact that in addition to acting as a sodium channel blocker, the drug prevents release of glutamate, an excitatory transmitter involved in pain propagation. Adverse events such as dizziness, somnolence, and cognitive impairment occur with lamotrigine.[51] There is little dose-dependent toxicity, so monitoring of laboratory values is not necessary. The most concerning side effect is rash, which is known to occur more often with rapid titration; it can be manifested as Stevens-Johnson syndrome.[52] The risk for rash is similar to that with phenytoin or carbamazepine, 5% to 10%. Enzyme-inducing drugs reduce the serum level of lamotrigine. Lamotrigine has no effect on liver enzymes, is metabolized via glucuronidation, and is 55% protein bound with a half-life of 30 hours. It needs slow titration, at least 4 to 6 weeks.

A major use for lamotrigine is in patients with TN. Although carbamazepine has been advocated as the first-line therapy for TN, it is not always effective in these patients. Lamotrigine has been investigated in this patient model for use as a coadministered drug and as a substitute for carbamazepine.[53] Twenty-one patients with TN who received no benefit from carbamazepine therapy were treated with lamotrigine. In a population of 7 men and 14 women, 14 of the patients noted significant to complete relief of their symptoms after the institution of lamotrigine therapy, and the remaining 7 patients had no benefit.[44] Recently, lamotrigine was compared directly with carbamazepine for the treatment of TN and found to be effective in fewer patients than carbamazepine was (70% vs. 90%); however, those who did have benefit with lamotrigine received greater pain relief and suffered fewer adverse effects (especially hematologic, renal, and liver) than those who had benefit in relieving pain with carbamazepine.[54] The use of lamotrigine may therefore be indicated for carbamazepine-resistant TN, or it could be trial-tested before carbamazepine. Lamotrigine may also play a role in the prevention of TN symptoms. This positive result has been seen in follow-up in a group of 15 patients with TN being treated with lamotrigine. In this review,[55] 73% of patients were free of their painful symptoms at the conclusion of the study. Subsequent interval follow-up revealed a continued positive result, with no change in pain scores reported by patients. As a result of these studies, lamotrigine may have a role in the prevention of TN in susceptible patients.

Lamotrigine has also been evaluated for lumbar radicular pain resulting from intervertebral disk herniation. In a 4-week open-label trial it was found to provide pain relief and increased range of motion, but only at high doses (400 mg/day).[56] It has also been evaluated in the PDN population. Lamotrigine for diabetic neuropathy was investigated in two randomized, double-blind, placebo-controlled trials with a total of 360 patients. In patients receiving 400 mg, a reduction in pain intensity score versus placebo was observed in one of the two studies. Doses of 200 and 300 mg did not demonstrate any benefit.[57] A group of 15 patients with diabetes (types 1 and 2 combined in the study)-induced peripheral neuropathy were treated in an open study. They were tested with brush and cold stimuli for allodynia and pinprick for hyperalgesia. On completion of the study, patients were tested and reported improvement of pain in all settings, and their relief persisted as noted during the subsequent 6-month interval follow-up.

In one RCT, lamotrigine (300 mg/day) was found to significantly reduce pain in patients with distal sensory polyneuropathy (DSP) but not in those with antiretroviral toxic neuropathy (ATN) associated with HIV disease.[58] HIV-associated neuropathy is believed to be on the rise, concomitant with the increase in the number of patients in whom the virus is being diagnosed. Patients with distal sensory peripheral neuropathy associated with HIV infection were subjected to a placebo-controlled, randomized, double-blind study to identify the benefit of lamotrigine therapy. Although both placebo- and lamotrigine-treated patients had a decrease in pain, the rate of decrease was more rapid in the lamotrigine group. Patients administered antiretrovirals and lamotrigine, however, were noted to have slower pain relief than those treated with lamotrigine without the antiretroviral agents. In a subsequent larger trial, it was found to be effective for both DSP- and HIV ATN-related pain.[59] The effect of lamotrigine as adjunctive therapy was also studied in 220 patients with a variety of NP conditions uncontrolled by monotherapy.[60] This randomized, double-blind, placebo-controlled study evaluated the efficacy and tolerability of lamotrigine in addition to gabapentin, a TCA, and a nonopioid analgesic. The study included patients with PDN, PHN, traumatic or surgical nerve injury, incomplete spinal cord injury, TN, multiple sclerosis, and HIV-associated peripheral neuropathy. Lamotrigine was generally well tolerated but did not demonstrate effective pain relief as evaluated by pain score or the use of rescue medication.

Lamotrigine has not been found to be effective in the treatment of chemotherapy-induced peripheral neuropathy,[61] nor has it been found to be beneficial in treating the central pain related to multiple sclerosis.[62]

TOPIRAMATE (TOPAMAX)

Topiramate has multiple mechanisms of action and broad use for seizure disorders. Topiramate blocks voltage-sensitive sodium channels, limits sustained repetitive firing, and binds to $GABA_A$ receptors to enhance GABA activity through non–benzodiazepine– and non–barbiturate–related mechanisms. It increases the opening frequency of chloride ion channels in $GABA_A$ receptors and can block α-amino-3-hydroxy-5-methyl-4-isoxazolepropionate (AMPA)-kainate glutamate receptors by acting as a negative modulator of glutamate at this receptor. Topiramate reduces the activity of L-type calcium channels and is a carbonic anhydrase inhibitor. Topiramate exhibits linear pharmacokinetics over its dose range and has a half-life of 19 to 25 hours. Its oral bioavailability is about 85% and it is not affected by food. Enzyme-inducing drugs may reduce the serum level of topiramate. Common side effects include paresthesias because of inhibition of carbonic anhydrase, drowsiness, fatigue, and cognitive symptoms. The incidence of nephrolithiasis was 1.5% in clinical trials, and mild weight loss is often noted. The propensity for weight reduction in some patients has led to investigation of its potential as a weight-reducing agent.[63]

The initial dose is 50 mg at bedtime, with increases to an upper limit of 200 mg twice daily. Studies have demonstrated that pain relief begins to occur at doses of 200 mg/day. Two large trials on migraine prophylaxis with topiramate were published in 2004, and topiramate received FDA approval for this indication.[64,65] A review of multiple double-blind studies examining the efficacy of topiramate for PDN failed to show significant analgesic benefit.[44] However, a more recent 12-week, double-blind study showed that it had greater efficacy than placebo in relieving the pain sensed by patients with PDN.[66] Topiramate has also been studied for other painful conditions. In a double-blind, randomized, crossover trial, topiramate, 50 to 400 mg, was assessed in patients with chronic lumbar radicular pain; it resulted in an improved global pain relief score, but it did not reduce leg pain.[67] The study was limited by frequent side effects and a high dropout rate. The exact role of topiramate has yet to be determined, and thus it may best be reserved as an adjunct for pain management with other membrane stabilizer agents. Case reports in the literature have also highlighted the use of this agent for additional forms of NP, including PHN, intercostal neuralgia, and CRPS.

LACOSAMIDE (VIMPAT)

Lacosamide is an effective and well-tolerated antiepileptic drug that is used as adjuvant treatment of focal-onset seizures uncontrolled by other agents.[68] Although it has not been compared directly with other adjuvant treatment options, its different mechanism of action and favorable safety profile make this antiepileptic agent a valuable addition to the treatment options available. The primary action of lacosamide is enhancement of slow inactivation of voltage-gated sodium channels without any apparent interaction with fast inactivation, a mechanism that differs from that of other sodium channel–blocking membrane stabilizers. In addition to treatment of epilepsy, lacosamide has been found to be beneficial in the treatment of PDN. Evidence of the efficacy of lacosamide in patients with PDN has been found in the results of a phase II trial[69] and phase III trials.[70,71] In a later trial, the primary end point of pain reduction was not reached.[72]

GABAergic MEDICATIONS

VALPROIC ACID (DEPAKOTE)

First synthesized in 1882, valproate became available in the 1960s as an antiepileptic agent and received FDA approval in 1978 as an immediate-release formulation.[73] The drug has a broad spectrum of use for seizure disorders, including absence seizures, and is now also used extensively by psychiatrists for mood disorders. The exact molecular mechanisms responsible for its clinical effects are unknown. Catabolism of GABA is inhibited and the synaptic release of GABA is increased. There are conflicting reports in the literature regarding the efficacy of this agent for NP, although studies have demonstrated that it is effective as migraine therapy at dosages of 750 mg/day for a period of 3 months.[74] In an RCT it was found to be mildly beneficial in the treatment of PDN and had a relatively high NNT of 7.[75] Side effects include gastrointestinal upset, somnolence, and dizziness. The exact role of valproic acid in the armamentarium of the pain practitioner is yet to be elucidated.[6]

DIAZEPAM (VALIUM), LORAZEPAM (ATIVAN), CLONAZEPAM (KLONOPIN)

Benzodiazepines, such as diazepam, lorazepam, and clonazepam, facilitate the actions of GABA in the CNS as a result of their binding to the $GABA_A$ receptor. The side effects of drowsiness and ataxia and the development of tolerance to the antiseizure effect limit the usefulness of benzodiazepines for chronic use. Clonazepam is also used for chronic facial pain and has had some success in small clinical trials.[76] A randomized, double-blind trial of a benzodiazepine for pain compared lorazepam with amitriptyline for PHN, but lorazepam was found to be less effective.[77]

Although benzodiazepines are frequently prescribed for multiple pain syndromes, there is little, if any evidence of their benefit as pain therapy, and they are more commonly associated with adverse events.[78] Recently, use of the benzodiazepine diazepam was evaluated for the treatment of neuropathic radicular pain in an randomized controlled trial (RCT) and found to have no benefit beyond placebo.[79]

LOCAL ANESTHETICS

Local anesthetics are used in NP states to block the aberrant firing of abnormal nerves, although they also block normally conducting (non-nociceptive) nerves. As a group, they are effective in the treatment of PHN, TN, radiculopathies, and peripheral neuropathies.

LIDOCAINE

The typical dose of lidocaine is 1 to 5 mg/kg intravenously. Side effects include dizziness, blurred vision, and seizures, which typically occur at a plasma level of 10 mg/mL.[48] Given that lidocaine is an antiarrhythmic, bradycardia and cardiac depression (present at a 20- to 25-mg/mL plasma concentration) are potential risks with this agent; therefore, electrocardiographic studies are indicated for long-term or high-dosage use of lidocaine. This therapy is severely limited by the method of medication delivery, and its most likely utility is as a diagnostic test for a disease process (e.g., erythromelalgia) or as therapy with mexiletine.

A patch formulation of 5% lidocaine (Lidoderm) is available in a topical preparation. Approved by the FDA for PHN, it has also proved to be of benefit in patients with various other types of NP, including PDN, post-thoracotomy pain, intercostal neuralgia, and meralgia paresthetica.[80] The eutectic mixture of local anesthetics (EMLA)—composed of prilocaine and lidocaine—has also been advocated for use as a topical local anesthetic. This agent is sometimes used as an adjunct for venipuncture in the pediatric population, but care must be taken with the amount of EMLA cream given to patients to avoid toxicity. Prilocaine is readily metabolized to *O*-toluidine, which can lead to methemoglobinemia. However, if dosages of prilocaine are kept below 600 mg, clinical methemoglobinemia is less likely to develop. These topical formulations are discussed at greater length in Chapter 42.

MEXILETINE

Mexiletine is an antiarrhythmic and, for pain relief, can be considered an oral analogue of lidocaine. Pain physicians may provide intravenous lidocaine for pain management, with monitoring of dose and effect. After receiving a dose of intravenously administered drug, treatment may readily be converted to oral mexiletine. The standard starting dose is 75 to 150 mg/day with a target of 300 to 450 mg/day.

Mexiletine can be used for PDN, thalamic stroke pain, spasticity, allodynia, and myotonia, although its effects are minimal.[81,82] It has been used successfully in patients with the rare $Na_v1.7$ mutation causing erythromelalgia.[83] Common side effects, including somnolence, irritability, blurred vision, and nausea and vomiting, severely limit the utility of this medication. Patients are also at risk for the development of blood dyscrasias, and blood tests should be obtained on a regular basis.

MISCELLANEOUS

MAGNESIUM

Research has recently been performed to evaluate antagonists of the *N*-methyl-D-aspartate (NMDA) receptor, including the membrane-stabilizing effect of magnesium. In a study of seven patients with PHN, intravenous infusion of 30 mg/kg of magnesium sulfate over a 30-minute period was found to be more effective in relieving pain than an intravenous infusion of saline.[84] Significant limitations with this therapy include the method of medication delivery (intravenous) and lethargy and muscle flaccidity following its use. Further, RCTs with alternative formulations need to be conducted to establish its role in the treatment of pain.

LEVETIRACETAM (KEPPRA)

Levetiracetam is a newer anticonvulsant that was approved in 1999 as adjunctive therapy for partial seizures in adults. It appears that inhibition of voltage-gated sodium channels or T-type calcium channels is not involved in the anticonvulsant effects of levetiracetam, which does not appear to have direct $GABA_A$ receptor effects. The mechanism of action of levetiracetam thus does not involve modulation of the four main systems. The starting dose of levetiracetam is 500 mg twice daily, and it may be increased to a recommended 3000 mg/day in divided doses. Dosages of up to 5000 mg/day have been assessed for the treatment of NP.[85] Its linear pharmacokinetics results in predictable effects as the dosage is increased. Levetiracetam is not metabolized by the cytochrome P-450 system and thus does not have significant drug interactions.[86] Adverse effects include asthenia, dizziness, somnolence, and headache. The drug has a number of favorable characteristics and has therefore been investigated for adjuvant use in areas such as pain. Unfortunately, in a number of well-conducted RCTs, it was found to be ineffective in the treatment of NP secondary to spinal cord injury,[87] polyneuropathy,[88] and postmastectomy pain.[89]

CONCLUSION

There are now a wide variety of neuronal membrane-stabilizing medications available for the treatment of NP conditions. The majority of RCTs to determine the effectiveness of these agents have involved select NP conditions such as PDN and PHN, with extrapolation of these results to other neuropathic conditions. As the science of pain medicine has advanced, studies have begun to examine less common NP conditions and the efficacy of these agents. Conditions such as chemotherapy-induced neuropathy and HIV-associated neuropathy have proved to be exceptions to the common belief that all NP responds to the standard group of membrane-stabilizing agents, and this reinforces the understanding that nerve-related pain may have similar symptoms or pain qualities but may not respond to the same treatments.

KEY POINTS

- Multimodal medical management of cancer- and non–cancer-related pain can involve the use of nonopioid medications, as well as opioid medications.
- The NNT is the number of patients needed to be treated with a particular drug to obtain one patient with a defined degree of relief.
- Drugs with a low NNT/NNH ratio are superior to drugs with a high NNT/NNH ratio.
- Calcium channel modulators that are used for the treatment of neuropathic pain, such as gabapentin and pregabalin, bind to the $\alpha_2\delta$ subunit of L-type voltage-gated calcium channels and result in decreased release of glutamate, norepinephrine, and substance P.
- The combination of low doses of gabapentin with low doses of morphine or nortriptyline provides significantly greater analgesia with lower side effects than do these agents used alone.
- Recently, use of the benzodiazepine diazepam was evaluated for the treatment of neuropathic radicular pain in a randomized, controlled trial and was found to have no benefit beyond placebo.
- Levetiracetam was found to be ineffective in the treatment of neuropathic pain secondary to spinal cord injury, polyneuropathy, and mastectomy.

SUGGESTED READINGS

Backonja M, Beydoun A, Edwards K, et al. Gabapentin monotherapy for the treatment of painful neuropathy: a multicenter, double-blind, placebo-controlled trial in patients with diabetes mellitus. *JAMA.* 1998;280:1831-1836.

Backonja MM, Canafax DM, Cundy KC. Efficacy of gabapentin enacarbil vs placebo in patients with postherpetic neuralgia and a pharmacokinetic comparison with oral gabapentin. *Pain Med.* 2011;12:1098-1108.

Dworkin RH, O'Connor AB, Backonja M, et al. Pharmacologic management of neuropathic pain: evidence-based recommendations. *Pain.* 2007;132:237-251.

Gilron I, Bailey JM, Tu D, et al. Morphine, gabapentin, or their combination for neuropathic pain. *N Engl J Med.* 2005;352:1324-1334.

Gilron I, Bailey JM, Tu D, et al. Nortriptyline and gabapentin, alone and in combination for neuropathic pain: a double-blind, randomized controlled crossover trial. *Lancet.* 2009;374:1252-1261.

Nikolajsen L, Finnerup NB, Kramp S, et al. A randomized study of the effects of gabapentin on postamputation pain. *Anesthesiology.* 2006;105:1008-1015.

Rauck R, Wallace M, Leong M, et al. A randomized, double-blind, placebo-controlled study of intrathecal ziconotide in adults with severe chronic pain. *J Pain Symptom Manage.* 2006;5:393-406.

Rauck RL, Shaibani A, Biton V, et al. Lacosamide in painful diabetic peripheral neuropathy: a phase 2 double-blind placebo-controlled study. *Clin J Pain.* 2007;23:150-158.

Simpson DM, McArthur JC, Olney R, et al. Lamotrigine for HIV-associated painful sensory neuropathies: a placebo-controlled trial. *Neurology.* 2003;60:1508-1514.

Taylor C. The biology and pharmacology of calcium channel alpha2-delta proteins. *CNS Drug Rev.* 2004;10:183-188.

The references for this chapter can be found at www.expertconsult.com.

40

Nonsteroidal Anti-inflammatory Drugs, Acetaminophen, and COX-2 Inhibitors

Brian Birmingham | Asokumar Buvanendran

Nonsteroidal anti-inflammatory drugs (NSAIDs) are a diverse group of chemically unrelated compounds that are classified together based on their therapeutic property of possessing anti-inflammatory action (Fig. 40.1).[1] NSAIDs are the most widely prescribed drugs for the treatment of acute and chronic pain, and they account for about 6 to 7 billion dollars in sales worldwide.

Extracts from the bark and leaves of willow, myrtle, and other plants have therapeutic effects because of the presence of salicylic acid and were first used for the treatment of fever in 1763 by Edward Stone. In 1829, Henri Leroux in France obtained a compound of salicylic acid (known as salicin) in crystalline form and succeeded in splitting it to obtain the acid in its pure state. Professor Hermann Kolbe in Germany discovered the compound's chemical structure and succeeded in synthesizing it in 1859. Sodium salicylate was first used for the treatment of rheumatic fever in 1875. Bayer Pharmaceutical started manufacturing aspirin (acetylsalicylic acid) by 1914 and currently sells about 11 billion tablets annually. Shortly after aspirin was manufactured, other drugs with diverse chemical structures but similar antipyretic, anti-inflammatory, and analgesic properties were discovered; these drugs were grouped together as NSAIDs. John R. Vane elucidated the mechanism of NSAIDs in 1971 and shared the Nobel Prize in Physiology and Medicine with Sune Bergström and Bengt Samuelsson in 1982.

MECHANISM OF ACTION

PROSTAGLANDIN SYNTHESIS AND PHARMACOLOGY

Von Euler[2] coined the term *prostaglandin* (PG) to describe an extract from semen that contracted uterine smooth muscle. Although PGs are derived from arachidonic acid and other polyunsaturated fatty acids, the 20-carbon polyunsaturated essential fatty acid (arachidonic acid) is the major source in mammalian tissues. PGs derived from arachidonic acid (prostaglandin E_2 [PGE_2], thromboxane, and prostacyclin) contain two double bonds. Analogous compounds synthesized from eicosatrienoic (linoleic) and eicosapentaenoic acids contain one less or more double bond in the side chains (PGE_1, PGE_3, respectively).[3] The various groups of PGs, thromboxanes, hydroxy acids, and leukotrienes that retain the 20-carbon unsaturated fatty acid structure are collectively known as eicosanoids. The three fatty acid precursors (eicosapentaenoic acid) are derived directly or indirectly from dietary fat and are esterified into cell membranes.[4] Their release, usually as a result of trauma, is the major stimulus for eicosanoid production because PGs cannot be stored and are released as soon they are synthesized.[5] Disruption of the cell membrane leads to the release of phospholipid, which is converted to arachidonic acid by the action of phospholipase A_2. Arachidonic acid in turn acts as a substrate for cyclooxygenase (COX). COX-catalyzed peroxidation of arachidonic acid results in a cyclic structure, whereas peroxidation catalyzed by lipoxygenase produces straight-chain hydroxy-peroxy acids, which can then be converted to hydroxy acids (Fig. 40.2).

PGs are also involved in the pyretic response. After injection of pyrogens, there is a rise in PG levels in cerebrospinal fluid (CSF) that is prevented by pretreatment with aspirin.[6] It is of interest that acetaminophen, which is antipyretic but not anti-inflammatory, blocks brain PG synthetase.[7] Prostanoids do not generally activate nociceptors directly but sensitize them to mechanical stimuli and chemical mediators of nociception, such as bradykinin.[8] PGE_2 is the predominant eicosanoid released from the endothelial cells of small blood vessels[9] and a key mediator of both peripheral and central pain sensitization.[4] Because PGE_2 is the prostanoid most associated with inflammatory responses, the formation of PGE_2 at inflammatory sites is often considered an indicator of local COX activity, and suppression of PGE_2 is an indicator of a decreased inflammatory process.[10] Production of PGE_2 is slow in onset and of long duration in response to inflammation.[11] It is currently recognized that COX is encoded by two genes.[12] Although the isomerization of PGH_2 into PGE_2 has been well characterized biochemically and pharmacologically, the enzyme responsible, PGE synthase, has been purified and cloned only rather recently.[13] This enzyme is one of the membrane-associated proteins in the eicosanoid and glutathione metabolism superfamily, which consists of six proteins with divergent functions.[14]

COX-1 AND COX-2 SELECTIVITY

The existence of a COX isoform that is positively and negatively regulated by cytokines and glucocorticoids, respectively,

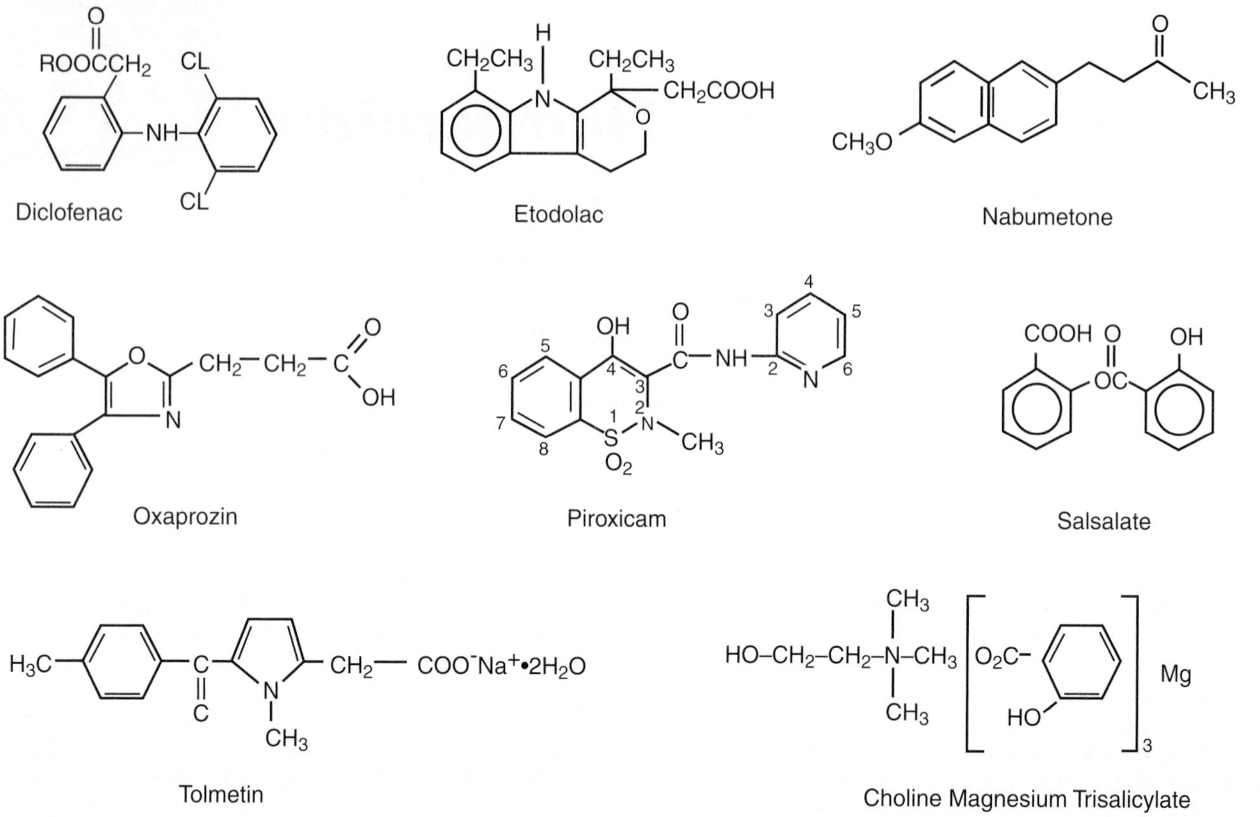

Diclofenac

Etodolac

Nabumetone

Oxaprozin

Piroxicam

Salsalate

Tolmetin

Choline Magnesium Trisalicylate

Figure 40.1 Structures of several different nonsteroidal anti-inflammatory drugs revealing the wide variation in chemical structures of the compounds that are grouped into this one therapeutic class.

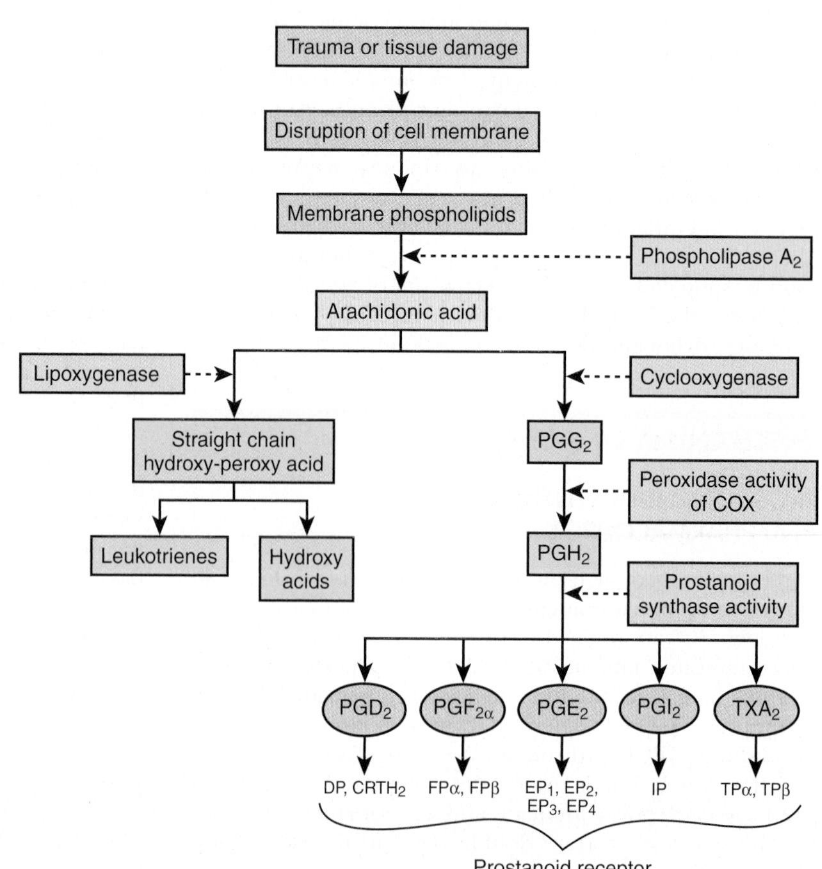

Figure 40.2 Pathway for the formation of prostaglandins. COX, cyclooxygenase; $CRTH_2$, chemoattractant receptor-homologous molecule; DP, PGD receptor; EP_1, EP_2, EP_3, EP_4, PGE receptors; FPα, PGF receptor α; FPβ, PGF receptor β; IP, PGI receptor; PG, prostaglandin; TPα, TXA_2 receptor α; TPβ, TXA_2 receptor β; TXA_2, thromboxane A_2.

was long suspected, but it was only in the early 1990s that an inducible COX isoenzyme (COX-2) was successfully cloned.[15] The identification of two COX isoforms, COX-1 and COX-2, has generated intense effort to characterize the relative contribution of each isoform to prostanoid production in specific situations. The development of isoform-specific antagonists has been extremely useful, first as experimental tools and, more recently, for clinical therapy.

Both COX-1 and COX-2 isoenzymes are composed of three independent folding units: (1) an epidermal growth factor–like domain, (2) a membrane-binding moiety, and (3) an active enzymatic domain that consists of a long hydrophobic channel.[16] Despite their remarkable structural similarity, the two COX isoforms have different gene expression profiles, distinct kinetic properties, and different interactions with phospholipase A_2 and synthases.[17] The genes for COX-1 and COX-2 are located on human chromosomes 9 and 1, respectively.[18] Whereas COX-1 represents a housekeeping gene that lacks a TATA box, the promoter of the immediate-early gene COX-2 contains a TATA box and binding sites for several transcription factors, including the nuclear factor κB (NF-κB), the nuclear factor for interleukin-6 (IL-6) expression (NF IL-6), and the cyclic adenosine monophosphate (cAMP) response element–binding protein.[19]

COX-1 is expressed constitutively and produces prostanoids that fine-tune physiologic processes requiring instantaneous or continuous regulation (e.g., hemostasis).[16] COX-2 expression is usually low but can be induced by numerous factors, including neurotransmitters, growth factors, proinflammatory cytokines, lipopolysaccharide, calcium, phorbol esters, and small-peptide hormones.[20] However, there are exceptions to the original constitutive versus inducible theory of COX expression. COX-1 expression can be induced in some stress conditions, such as nerve injury, whereas many tissues, including the central nervous system (CNS) and kidney, constitutively express COX-2.[20] In the spinal cord there are detectable basal levels of both COX-1 and COX-2, which might enable immediate reactions to release of transmitter that result in prostanoid production.[21]

It has been suggested that there is another COX enzyme formed as a splice variant of COX-1, known as COX-3.[22] Canine COX-3 expressed by transfected insect cells can be inhibited by therapeutic concentrations of analgesic or antipyretic drugs, such as acetaminophen, phenacetin, antipyrine, and dipyrone. However, it has been reported that this COX-1 variant (COX-3) is not expressed in humans,[23] rats, or mice because the corresponding additional intron 1 sequence in the mRNA transcript spans 94 (human) or 98 (rat and mouse) nucleotides, thus shifting the coding sequence out of frame.[24,25]

PERIPHERAL AND CENTRAL INDUCTION OF COX-2

The original hypothesis formulated by Vane in his Nobel Prize–winning work on the mechanism of action of NSAIDs was that these compounds inhibit prostanoid production in the periphery, thereby preventing a sensitizing action of PGE_2 on the peripheral terminals of sensory fibers.[26] More recently, peripheral inflammation has also been shown to induce a widespread increase in COX-2[27] and PGE synthase expression in the CNS. The proinflammatory cytokine IL-1β is upregulated at the site of inflammation and plays a major role in inducing COX-2 in local inflammatory cells by activating NF-κB.[28] IL-1β is also responsible for induction of COX-2 in the CNS in response to peripheral inflammation, but this is not the result of neural activity arising from sensory fibers innervating the inflamed tissue or the result of systemic IL-1β in plasma. Instead, peripheral inflammation produces some other signaling molecule that enters the circulation, crosses the blood-brain barrier, and acts to elevate IL-1β levels, which leads to COX-2 expression in neurons and non-neuronal cells in many different areas of the spinal cord.[4,29] An elevation in COX-2 also occurs at many levels in the brain and spinal cord, mainly in the endothelial cells of the brain vasculature.[30]

Thus, there appear to be two forms of input from peripheral inflamed tissue to the CNS. The first is mediated by electrical activity in sensitized nerve fibers innervating the inflamed area, which signals the location of the inflamed tissue, as well as the onset, duration, and nature of any stimuli applied to this tissue.[26] This input is sensitive to peripherally acting COX-2 inhibitors and neural blockade with local anesthetics, such as occurs with epidural anesthesia.[31] The second is a humoral signal originating from the inflamed tissue that acts to produce widespread induction of COX-2 in the CNS. This input is not affected by regional anesthesia[29,32] and can be blocked only by centrally acting COX-2 inhibitors.[29,31] This implies that patients undergoing neuraxial anesthesia for surgery also need a centrally acting COX-2 inhibitor for optimal reduction of postoperative pain and the postoperative stress response.[31]

It is therefore clear that the permeability of the blood-brain barrier to currently used NSAIDs and COX-2 inhibitors is important.[33,34] Inhibitors of COX-2 that penetrate the blood-brain barrier more effectively might represent more efficient painkillers and could also act to reduce many of the more diffuse aspects of inflammatory pain, such as generalized aches and pains, depression, and loss of appetite, which are key aspects in determining the quality-of-life response to treatment.[35] The main process whereby a drug passes from the bloodstream to the CNS is passive diffusion, for which lipophilicity and ionization are critical determinants of transfer.[36] CSF represents a convenient sampling point for drugs that enter the CNS; however, there are very few NSAIDs for which CSF pharmacokinetics has been defined. For example, the CSF-to-plasma concentration ratio of oxyphenbutazone has been determined to be 0.0074 (0.7%). This ratio is close to the free fraction of oxyphenbutazone in plasma, which is about 0.5%.[37] The high lipid solubility of indomethacin allows it to cross into CSF rapidly and equilibrate with the free plasma concentration.[38] Similar results have been noted with ketoprofen.[39]

PROSTANOID RECEPTORS: EXPRESSION, REGULATION, AND FUNCTION

The first prostanoid receptor to be isolated and cloned was the thromboxane A_2 (TXA_2) receptor,[40] a guanine (G) protein–coupled receptor with seven transmembrane domains. Homology screening of complementary DNA (cDNA) libraries has resulted in the isolation and identification of seven other prostanoid receptors that had been predicted pharmacologically: the PGD receptor (DP), four PGE receptors (EP_1, EP_2, EP_3, and EP_4), the PGF receptor (FP), and the PGI receptor (IP). Prostanoid receptors are expressed in many tissues and cell types. Among the EP receptors, EP_3 and EP_4 are the most widely distributed, whereas the distribution of EP_1 and EP_2 is restricted to the kidney, stomach, and uterus, as well as to neuronal and non-neuronal cells in the nervous system.[41] EP_1, EP_3, and EP_4 mRNA is expressed in primary sensory neurons in the dorsal root and trigeminal ganglia,[42] thus suggesting involvement in PGE_2-mediated peripheral sensitization. Inflammation affects the level of expression of many prostanoid receptor subtypes. Further studies are needed to determine which of the EP receptors are involved in analgesia and their respective antagonists.

Inhibition of PG biosynthesis may only partly explain the therapeutic effects of NSAIDs.[43] Another postulated mechanism includes interactions with the adenylate cyclase system. Indomethacin and some other NSAIDs inhibit phosphodiesterase, thereby elevating the intracellular concentration of cAMP.[44]

PHARMACOKINETICS

NSAIDs are weak acids with pK_a values typically lower than 5. Because weak acids will be 99% ionized 2 pH units above their pK_a, these anti-inflammatory agents will be present in the body mostly in the ionized form.

GENERAL FACTORS AFFECTING NSAID PHARMACOKINETICS

Although NSAIDs differ in their individual pharmacokinetic properties, some general factors affecting NSAID pharmacokinetics can enable clinicians to select among the different agents available.

ABSORPTION

Most NSAIDs are absorbed rapidly following oral administration, and peak plasma concentrations are generally reached within 2 to 3 hours after administration. Slow-release dosage forms have been developed to maintain active plasma levels for prolonged periods. Factors affecting gastric emptying may have a profound effect on the time course of the clinical effect of the NSAID administered. The extent of drug absorption from the gastrointestinal (GI) tract is more important than the rate.[45] The rectal route of administration has been used to minimize GI side effects, which are a common feature of these agents. In general, the rate and extent of NSAID absorption are comparable for the rectal and oral routes.[46]

DISTRIBUTION

All NSAIDs are lipid soluble, weakly acidic, and highly bound to plasma proteins, with the exception of aspirin. In most cases, less than 1% of the total plasma concentration is in the unbound form. Albumin is the major binding protein for NSAIDs. Disease conditions that cause hypoalbuminemia will result in an increased free fraction of NSAIDs in plasma, thus affecting the distribution and elimination of these agents.[47] Most NSAIDs have distribution volumes between 0.1 and 0.15 L/kg.

In inflammatory joint diseases, the effect of an NSAID is related to its level in the affected synovial fluid. This level correlates closely with the concentration of drug at the active site because there is simple transport of drugs across the synovial membrane.[48,49] The amount of drug in synovial fluid is dependent on the level of albumin in the joint, which is lower than in plasma.[50]

ELIMINATION

Hepatic biotransformation is the main elimination pathway for most NSAIDs.[51] Most are metabolized by cytochrome P-450–mediated oxidation, glucuronide conjugation, or both. Renal excretion of nonmetabolized drug is a minor elimination pathway for most NSAIDs and accounts for less than 10% of the administered dose. Some NSAID metabolites are also excreted to a significant extent in bile.

PATHOPHYSIOLOGIC CONDITIONS AFFECTING NSAID KINETICS

Renal failure and hepatic disease are common disorders that affect the kinetics of NSAIDs.

RENAL FAILURE

Renal failure has a variety of influences on drug kinetics, not only by reducing the renal excretion of drugs and metabolites normally excreted in urine but also by affecting the absorption, distribution, and biotransformation of drugs.

Absorption and Distribution

Absorption of NSAIDs is not impaired in patients with renal failure. However, the plasma protein binding of many acidic compounds such as the NSAIDs is impaired in those with renal failure.[52] The result is an increase in the volume of distribution of the unbound fraction of the drug in plasma.

Elimination

An increase in the unbound fraction of the drug in plasma may lead to an increase in total plasma clearance of the NSAID. The clearance of NSAIDs (e.g., diflunisal, ketoprofen, naproxen, indoprofen, benoxaprofen, tiaprofenic acid) for which the formation of acyl glucuronides is a major elimination pathway is significantly reduced in patients with renal failure.[53] The effect of renal failure on the oral clearance of several other NSAIDs (e.g., ibuprofen, fenbufen, isoxicam, piroxicam) is small.[54] Most of these compounds are metabolized by oxidative pathways. All NSAIDs are highly bound to plasma proteins, and hemodialysis will probably not result in increased elimination of these agents. No dosage adjustments are therefore necessary for patients being administered NSAIDs who are undergoing hemodialysis.[53]

HEPATIC DISEASE

Impaired liver function can affect the disposition of NSAIDs.

Absorption and Distribution

Most NSAIDs are low-clearance drugs, and liver disease should theoretically not be expected to interfere with the oral bioavailability of these agents. Because the liver is the major organ for the synthesis of albumin, the major binding protein for NSAIDs in plasma, it would be expected that hepatic dysfunction could lead to alterations in the unbound drug fraction present in plasma.

Table 40.1 Generic and Trade Names of Nonsteroidal Anti-inflammatory Drugs

Generic Name	Trade Names
Aspirin	
Diflunisal	Dolobid
Diclofenac	Voltaren, Cataflam, Arthrotec (combination with misoprostol
Indomethacin	Indocin
Sulindac	Clinoril
Tolmetin	Tolectin
Ketorolac	Toradol
Etodolac	Lodine, Lodine XL
Ibuprofen	Motrin, Advil, Vicoprofen (combination with hydrocodone), Combunox (combination with oxycodone)
Flurbiprofen	Ansaid
Naproxen	Naproxen, Aleve
Ketoprofen	Orudis
Fenoprofen	Nalfon, Nalfon 200
Oxaprozin	Daypro
Mefenamic	Ponstel
Meclofenamic	Meclomen
Phenylbutazone	Butazolidin
Piroxicam	Feldene
Nabumetone	Relafen
Acetaminophen	Tylenol
Celecoxib	Celebrex
Rofecoxib	
Valdecoxib	
Meloxicam	Mobic

Elimination

Because most NSAIDs have low total intrinsic clearance (oral clearance) relative to blood flow, hepatic clearance is essentially independent of flow and reflects drug-metabolizing capacity. Elimination of ibuprofen does not seem to be affected in patients with liver disease.[55]

SPECIFIC DRUGS

Generic and trade names of NSAIDs are listed in Table 40.1.

SALICYLATES

The major salicylates currently used are aspirin, diflunisal, choline magnesium trisalicylate, and salsalate.

ASPIRIN

Aspirin is the most studied and commonly used NSAID. Aspirin has an elimination half-life that increases from 2.5 hours at low doses to 19 hours at high doses. It is well absorbed in the stomach and small intestine, with a peak blood level attained 1 hour after an oral dose. Rapid conversion of aspirin to salicylates then takes place as a result of a high first-pass effect, which occurs in the wall of the small intestine and in the liver. The metabolic pathways follow first-order and zero-order kinetics.[56]

Aspirin inhibits the biosynthesis of PGs by irreversible acetylation and consequent inactivation of COX. This is in contrast to the action of newer NSAIDs, which are reversible inhibitors of the COX enzyme.[57] Although most cells can synthesize new COX, platelets cannot; thus, the acetylation of their microsomal enzyme lasts for the life of the platelet (10 to 14 days). The ability of aspirin to acetylate proteins may be one reason for its superiority over other salicylate derivatives as an anti-inflammatory agent. Of all the NSAIDs, only aspirin has been associated with Reye's syndrome, a combination of seizures, coma, and sometimes death related to the use of aspirin during a viral illness in children.[58]

DIFLUNISAL

Diflunisal is potentially better tolerated in the GI system because it is not metabolized to salicylic acid in plasma, based on a study comparing diflunisal, 250 and 500 mg twice daily, with aspirin, 600 mg four times daily.[59] It has a short half-life relative to aspirin and causes less inhibition of platelets than aspirin does.[60]

CHOLINE MAGNESIUM TRISALICYLATE AND SALSALATE

Both are nonacetylated salicylates that have minimal effect on platelet function and less effect on the GI mucosa than their acetylated counterparts do. They produce similar analgesia and blood levels of salicylate as those of the acetylated class.[61]

ACETAMINOPHEN

Acetaminophen is a *p*-aminophenol derivative with analgesic and antipyretic properties comparable to those of aspirin. Antipyresis probably occurs because of direct action on the hypothalamic heat-regulating centers via the inhibiting action of endogenous pyrogen.[62] Recently, it has been hypothesized that acetaminophen may be acting via the serotonergic pathway to provide analgesia.[63] Though equipotent to aspirin in inhibiting central PG synthesis, acetaminophen exhibits no significant peripheral PG synthetase inhibition. Doses of 650 mg have been shown to be more effective than doses of 300 mg, but little additional benefit is seen at doses higher than 1000 mg, thus indicating a possible ceiling effect.[64]

Acetaminophen has few side effects in the usual dosage range; no significant GI toxicity or functional changes in platelets occur. It is almost entirely metabolized in the liver, and the minor metabolites are responsible for the hepatotoxicity seen with overdose.[65] Inducers of the cytochrome P-450 enzyme system in the liver (e.g., alcohol) increase the formation of metabolites and therefore increase hepatotoxicity. In certain patients (chronic ethanol users, patients suffering from malnutrition, and fasting patients), repeating therapeutic or slightly excessive doses may precipitate hepatotoxicity. A dosage of 2600 to 3200 mg/day may represent a safer chronic daily dosage, and dosing should not exceed 4 g/day.[66] Toxic doses may be a function of baseline glutathione levels and other dose-related factors. Acetaminophen is completely and rapidly absorbed following the oral route. Peak serum concentrations are achieved within 2 hours of a therapeutic dose; therapeutic serum concentrations are 10 to 20 μg/mL.[67] About 90% of acetaminophen is hepatically metabolized to sulfate and glucuronide conjugates for renal excretion, with a small amount being secreted unchanged in urine.[68]

The bioavailability of rectally administered acetaminophen is variable. It is approximately 80% that of tablets, and the rate of absorption is slower, with the maximum plasma concentration being achieved about 2 to 3 hours after administration.[69] Doses of 40 to 60 mg/kg of rectal acetaminophen have been shown to have an opioid-sparing effect in postoperative pain models.[70] Propacetamol, an injectable prodrug of paracetamol, is completely hydrolyzed within 6 minutes of administration, and 1 g of propacetamol yields 0.5 g of paracetamol. Injectable paracetamol has been shown to reduce opioid consumption by about 35% to 45%[71] in postoperative pain studies.[72] In a study examining the analgesic serum concentrations of paracetamol, it was demonstrated that a ceiling effect of paracetamol may be present at intravenous doses of 5 mg/kg, which corresponds to a serum concentration of 14 mg/mL.[73] Recently, an intravenous form of acetaminophen has become available. One gram of injectable acetaminophen is equivalent to 2 g of propacetamol and has a lower incidence of pain at the injection site.[74] Intravenous acetaminophen has been demonstrated to be an effective adjunctive analgesic after orthopedic, ear-nose-throat, and dental surgery.[75-77] Intravenous acetaminophen also provided analgesia superior to that with oral acetaminophen after cardiac surgery.[78]

ACETIC ACID DERIVATIVES

This group of NSAIDs contains two subclasses, pyrrole acetic acids (indomethacin, sulindac, tolmetin, ketorolac, etodolac) and phenylacetic acids (diclofenac, bromfenac).

INDOMETHACIN

Indomethacin has good oral and rectal absorption, although the extent of absorption varies widely among patients. There is also large interpatient variability in its elimination half-life as a result of extensive enterohepatic recirculation of the drug. It is highly bound to albumin. Metabolism involves demethylation and deacetylation in the liver, with subsequent excretion of inactive metabolites and unchanged drug in bile and urine.[79] Its clinical application is somewhat limited by a relatively high incidence of side effects (primarily gastritis and renal dysfunction), but it is used in patients with acute gouty arthritis and osteoarthritis.

SULINDAC

Sulindac was developed as the result of a search for a drug similar to indomethacin but with lower toxicity. The GI toxicity associated with sulindac may be lower because it is an inactive prodrug that is converted after absorption by liver microsomal enzymes to sulindac disulfide, which appears to be the active metabolite.[80,81] It is eliminated from plasma, predominantly by excretion in bile, but is subject to enterohepatic circulation. Peak plasma levels of 0.1 to 0.2 mg/100 mL occur 2 to 3 hours after an oral dose of 200 mg. Steady-state plasma levels of the sulfide are reached after 4 to 5 days of therapy with 200 mg twice daily by mouth. It is available in 150- and 200-mg tablets and administered twice daily for the treatment of gouty arthritis, osteoarthritis, and various inflammatory diseases.[82]

Huskisson and Scott[82] reported that only 25% of patients have GI problems with sulindac; constipation is common. Sulindac seems to have less effect on the CNS than indomethacin does, possibly because it has an indene nucleus, rather than the indole nucleus present in indomethacin and serotonin, an important mediator in the CNS.

TOLMETIN AND ETODOLAC

Both these drugs have fewer side effects than other NSAIDs do. Tolmetin is available in 100- and 200-mg tablets and has a half-life of 60 minutes. It is excreted in urine partly unchanged, partly conjugated, and as an inactive dicarboxylic acid metabolite.[83] Tolmetin can cause edema because of sodium retention and abnormal liver function, both of which are reversible on discontinuation of this NSAID.

Etodolac is an acidic compound with a pK_a of 4.65. It is manufactured as tablets and capsules, with a normal dosage ranging from to 1 to 1.2 g daily. Clinical doses of 200 to 300 mg twice daily for the relief of low back or shoulder pain have been equated to analgesia with naproxen, 500 mg twice daily.[84] From large clinical trials it has been found that the incidence of abdominal pain and dyspepsia is similar to that with several other NSAIDs, and GI ulceration develops in less than 0.3% of patients.[85] Dyspepsia occurs in 10% of patients taking etodolac, with a somewhat lower incidence of abdominal pain.

KETOROLAC

Ketorolac is currently the most commonly used parenteral NSAID in the United States. Although indomethacin has been available as an injectable form for years, it was used only in low dosages for the treatment of patent ductus arteriosus. Ketorolac is almost entirely bound to plasma proteins (more than 99%), which results in a small apparent volume of distribution, and it is extensively metabolized by conjugation and excreted via the kidney.[86] Its analgesic effect occurs within 30 minutes, its maximum effect takes place in 1 to 2 hours, and it has a duration of analgesia of 4 to 6 hours.[87] Ketorolac has been demonstrated to be efficacious in treating postoperative pain in several studies, both as a single agent and as an adjunct to opioids.[88-90] There is evidence that ketorolac may be acting at the CNS in addition to its peripheral mode of action.[38] Dental surgery studies with ketorolac have also indicated that it acts centrally,[91] but measurement of drug levels in CSF has demonstrated poor penetration of the compound from plasma.[92]

Oral ketorolac was approved for use in the United States approximately 3 years after the parenteral form and has an efficacy similar to that of naproxen and ibuprofen.[93] However, the parenteral form can be administered at single doses of 30 mg intravenously or up to 60 mg intramuscularly. A 30-mg dose can be repeated intravenously or intramuscularly every 6 hours. The oral dose is limited to 10 to 20 mg. Ketorolac should not be used for more than 5 days because of GI toxicity. Since there have been reports of deaths caused by GI and operative site bleeding,[94] the drug's license was suspended in Germany and France. In response to these adverse events, the drug's manufacturer recommended reducing the dose of ketorolac from 150 to 120 mg/day.[87] The European Committee for Proprietary Medicinal Products has recommended a further maximal daily dose reduction to 60 mg for older patients and 90 mg for younger adults. Recent studies have examined the efficacy of this drug when administered intranasally.[95,96] The intranasal route of administration may offer the added advantage of better brain penetration via the olfactory route and might provide higher levels of the drug in the CNS and CSF, with minimal GI side effects.

DICLOFENAC

Diclofenac has a carboxylic acid functional group and is rapidly and completely absorbed after oral administration. Oral preparations include diclofenac potassium, which is rapidly absorbed in the stomach, and enteric-coated diclofenac sodium, which resists dissolution at low pH and is released in the duodenum. A parenteral form has been used in Europe, with one study showing it to be effective in reducing opioid requirements and reducing pain after thoracotomy.[97] Diclofenac sodium has also been tested in clinical trials in a gel form for relief of pain from superficial burns, with good success.[98] A Cochrane collaborative meta-analysis showed that diclofenac was effective in treating postoperative pain, with a dose-response relationship demonstrating increasing efficacy of diclofenac at 25- , 50-, and 100-mg doses.[99]

Diclofenac binds extensively to plasma albumin.[100] Substantial concentrations of the drug are attained in synovial fluid, which may be one of the sites of action of diclofenac.[101] Concentration-effect relationships have been established for total bound, unbound, and synovial fluid diclofenac concentrations.[102] Diclofenac is eliminated following biotransformation to glucuroconjugated and sulfate metabolites, which are excreted in urine, and very little drug is eliminated unchanged.

Diclofenac differs from other NSAIDs in that it has a high first-pass effect and hence lower oral bioavailability. Diclofenac may also be associated with a significantly higher incidence of hepatotoxicity than other NSAIDs. The excretion of conjugates may be related to renal function. Accumulation of conjugates occurs in patients with end-stage renal disease; however, no accumulation is apparent on comparison of younger and older adults.[103] Dosage adjustments in older adults, children, or patients with various disease states (e.g., hepatic disease, rheumatoid arthritis) may not be required. Significant drug-drug interactions have been demonstrated with aspirin, lithium, digoxin, methotrexate, cyclosporine, cholestyramine, and colestipol.[104]

PROPIONIC ACID DERIVATIVES

This class of compounds includes ibuprofen, fenoprofen, ketoprofen, flurbiprofen, and naproxen. A newer drug in this class is oxaprozin, which has received attention because of its once-daily dosage regimen, but it has no distinct advantage over other NSAIDs.[105]

IBUPROFEN

Ibuprofen is well absorbed, and peak plasma levels of 15 to 20 μg/mL are achieved about 1 to 2 hours after a single dose. Its half-life is about 3.5 hours. An intravenous form of ibuprofen has been developed, and an 800-mg intravenous dose is well tolerated and results in faster and higher peak drug levels but a similar total bioavailability and elimination profile as oral dosing.[106] The drug is metabolized mostly in the liver, with less than 10% excreted unchanged in urine and bile.[107] Ibuprofen at a dose of 1200 mg/day produces effective analgesia in arthritis patients. At the high end of the recommended dosage, 2400 mg/day, it produces GI side effects, of which nausea and dyspepsia are predominant. Renal side effects of ibuprofen appear to be dose dependent and have not been reported at the recommended over-the-counter drug dosage (0.2 to 0.8 g/day). Even at anti-inflammatory dosages (>1.6 g/day), renal side effects are almost exclusively encountered in patients with low intravascular volume and low cardiac output, particularly in older adults.[108] Ibuprofen antagonizes the irreversible platelet inhibition induced by aspirin. Therefore, treatment of patients at increased cardiovascular risk with ibuprofen may limit the cardioprotective effects of aspirin.[109]

KETOPROFEN

Ketoprofen is available in oral form and reaches its peak plasma level in 0.5 to 2 hours. Its half-life is 2.4 hours, with an analgesic duration of 4 to 6 hours.[110] The maximum recommended dosage is 300 mg/day. Pharmacokinetic data indicate that plasma levels of ketoprofen with oral administration (100 mg) are higher than when applied via a patch. Ketoprofen, 100 mg, has been tried as a patch to directly deliver the compound to the site of injury. Because the patch facilitates delivery of ketoprofen over a 24-hour period, the drug remains continually present in the tissue adjacent to the site of application. High tissue but low plasma ketoprofen concentrations mean that although tissue concentrations are high enough to exert a therapeutic effect, plasma concentrations remain low enough to minimize systemic adverse events.[111]

FENOPROFEN

The calcium derivative of fenoprofen is more commonly used; it is well absorbed and achieves a peak plasma level of 20 to 30 μg/mL 2 hours after a single oral dose, with a plasma half-life of 2 to 3 hours.[112] The drug is available as 300-mg capsules, and the recommended dosage is 2.4 g/day. Steady-state plasma levels are reached within the first 24 hours of therapy. Fenoprofen is well tolerated in comparison to aspirin and causes minimal occult GI bleeding; nevertheless, dyspepsia remains its most common side effect. Most of the drug is excreted as glucuronide in urine.

NAPROXEN

Naproxen is well absorbed in the upper GI tract and is highly bound to plasma albumin. Because of its long half-life of 13 hours, it is suitable for twice-daily administration.[113] Equilibrium is reached in about 3 days. Excretion is almost entirely in urine, mainly as an inactive glucuronide metabolite.

Naproxen is available as 250-, 375-, and 500-mg tablets and has been used for the treatment of arthritis and other inflammatory diseases, with efficacy superior to that of aspirin.[114] It causes less GI irritation than aspirin does. Naproxen increases bleeding time by inhibiting platelet aggregation. When given during pregnancy, it can cross the placenta in 20 minutes and cause neonatal jaundice.

OXAPROZIN

Oxaprozin is effective in the management of adult rheumatoid arthritis, osteoarthritis, ankylosing spondylitis, soft tissue disorders, and postoperative dental pain. It has high oral bioavailability (95%), with peak plasma concentrations being achieved 3 to 5 hours after dosing.[115] It is metabolized in the liver by oxidative and conjugative pathways and readily eliminated by the renal and fecal routes. The strong analgesic qualities of oxaprozin are particularly useful for painful musculoskeletal conditions because, for example, it inhibits COX-1 and COX-2 isoenzymes, inhibits nuclear translocation of NF-κB and metalloproteinases, and modulates the endogenous cannabinoid system.[116] In a randomized study of patients with refractory shoulder pain, oxaprozin, 1200 mg once daily, was superior to three doses per day of diclofenac (50 mg) in reducing pain and improving quality of life.[117]

Oxaprozin can diffuse easily into inflamed synovial tissue after oral administration.[118] Though discovered more than 20 years ago, it is now under intensive investigation because of its unusual pharmacodynamic properties. Other than being a nonselective COX inhibitor, the drug is capable of inhibiting both anandamide hydrolase in neurons, with consequent potent analgesic activity, and NF-κB activation in inflammatory cells.[116] Moreover, oxaprozin induces apoptosis of activated monocytes in a dose-dependent manner. Because the monocyte, macrophage, and NF-κB pathways are crucial for the synthesis of proinflammatory and histotoxic mediators in inflamed joints, oxaprozin appears to have pharmacodynamic properties exceeding those presently assumed as markers of classic NSAIDs.[119]

OXICAM DERIVATIVES

The only NSAID in this class in clinical use is piroxicam. Unlike other NSAIDs, the peak serum concentration following oral dosing is attained more slowly, with a duration of 5.5 hours. It is notable for its long elimination half-life, 48.5 hours, so up to 1 week may be needed to achieve steady-state blood concentrations, although it does also allow once-daily dosing.[120]

PYRAZOLONE DERIVATIVES

The only drug in clinical use in this class is phenylbutazone. Although phenylbutazone is a very effective anti-inflammatory and analgesic, its clinical use has been severely limited because of an association with aplastic anemia and agranulocytosis.[121]

ANTHRANILIC ACID DERIVATIVES

These NSAIDs are unique because they block PG synthesis and the tissue response to PGs. Mefenamic acid has been associated with severe pancytopenia and many other side effects. Therefore, it cannot be used for longer than 1 week.[122] Meclofenamate has a high incidence of GI toxicity and is also not a first-line drug. It is well absorbed orally; peak plasma levels are reached after 2 hours, with a half-life of about 4 to 6 hours.

NAPHTHYLALKANONES

This newer class of NSAIDs is most noted for its nonacidic chemical structure, similar to naproxen but unlike that of other clinically used NSAIDs. The only clinically available NSAID in this class is nabumetone. Studies have shown that its use results in fewer gastric lesions than occur with aspirin, naproxen, or ibuprofen.[123] Also, dosages of 1 g/day for 7 days in volunteers resulted in no changes in bleeding time. Only 35% of the drug is converted to its active form after oral administration. None of the parent drug can be measured in plasma after oral administration because of the rapid biotransformation that occurs during the first-pass effect, which makes nabumetone a prodrug.[124]

MELOXICAM

Meloxicam is a relatively new NSAID approved for the treatment of osteoarthritis in the United States. It has also been evaluated for the treatment of rheumatoid arthritis, ankylosing spondylitis, and acute rheumatic pain.[125] Meloxicam has been shown to be COX-2 preferential, particularly at its lowest therapeutic dose, and to exert an anti-inflammatory action by inhibiting prostanoid synthesis in inflammatory cells. Because it is COX-2 preferential, it would be expected to have less GI toxicity than nonselective NSAIDs do. In clinical trials of meloxicam for osteoarthritis, it was found to be as effective as piroxicam, diclofenac, and naproxen, with fewer GI symptoms and a lower incidence of perforation, obstruction, and bleeding.[126]

Meloxicam has a plasma half-life of approximately 20 hours and is convenient for once-daily administration in 7.5- and 15-mg tablets.[127] Neither moderate renal nor hepatic insufficiency has significantly altered the pharmacokinetics of meloxicam in short-term studies; however, it should not be used in patients with renal failure. Furthermore, dose adjustment is not required in older adults. Drug-drug interaction studies have demonstrated that meloxicam interacts with some medications, including cholestyramine, lithium, and some inhibitors of cytochrome P-450 2C9 and 3A4. Consequently, increased clinical vigilance should be maintained when co-prescribing some medications with meloxicam. No interactions have been observed following the concomitant administration of food, antacid, aspirin, β-acetyldigoxin, methotrexate, warfarin, or furosemide.

Concentration-dependent therapeutic and toxicologic effects have yet to be extensively elucidated for meloxicam.[127] Its pharmacokinetic profile is characterized by prolonged, almost complete absorption, and the drug is more than 99.5% bound to plasma proteins. Meloxicam is metabolized to four biologically inactive main metabolites, which are excreted in urine and feces. Steady-state plasma concentrations are achieved within 3 to 5 days. The pharmacokinetic parameters of meloxicam are linear over the dose range of 7.5 to 30 mg, and bioequivalence has been shown for a number of different formulations.

COX-2 INHIBITORS

COX-2–specific inhibitors were developed with the aim of reducing the incidence of serious GI adverse effects associated with the administration of traditional NSAIDs, the assumption being that these side effects were mediated by COX-1. Assessment of COX-1 and COX-2 selectivity in vitro in whole-blood assays (Table 40.2) of the cellular capacity to produce prostanoids has shown that selectivity is a continuous variable of COX inhibitors.

The initial COX-2 inhibitors approved by the U.S. Food and Drug Administration (FDA) were celecoxib and rofecoxib. Overall, a meta-analysis of clinical studies evaluating COX-2 inhibitors versus traditional NSAIDs for postoperative

Table 40.2 IC_{50} Ratios for Inhibition of COX-1 and COX-2 in Human Whole Blood*

Drug	IC_{50} Ratio
Lumiracoxib	700
Etoricoxib	344
Rofecoxib	272
Valdecoxib	61
Celecoxib	30
Meloxicam	18
Naproxen	0.7
Ibuprofen	1.5
Indomethacin	0.02
Aspirin	0.007

IC_{50}, concentration needed to inhibit 50% of COX-1 and COX-2.
*A higher ratio indicates greater COX-2 selectivity.

pain has shown that the analgesic efficacy of COX-2 inhibitors 0 to 6 hours postoperatively is similar to or better than that of ibuprofen.[128] The initial clinical trials using COX-2 inhibitors for the management of pain evaluated efficacy in the immediate postoperative period and demonstrated a reduction in postoperative opioid consumption. A meta-analysis examined the advantage of multimodal analgesia with acetaminophen, with NSAIDs, and when COX-2 inhibitors were added to patient-controlled analgesia with morphine.[129,130] The results suggested that all the analgesic agents provide an opioid-sparing effect (25% to 55%). The use of nonselective NSAIDs was associated with a decrease in the incidence of postoperative nausea, vomiting, and sedation. In addition, the use of COX-2 inhibitors or acetaminophen did not decrease the incidence of opioid-related adverse events when compared with placebo. Clinical trials of COX-2 inhibitors used during the preoperative period and into the postoperative period (2 weeks) for patients undergoing both major surgery[131] and minimally invasive surgery[132] have demonstrated improved clinical outcomes. Perioperative administration of COX-2 inhibitors for total joint arthroplasty has been shown to result in a reduction in perioperative pain and improvement in outcomes without the added risk of increased perioperative bleeding.[131,132]

It was recently demonstrated that preoperative administration of oral COX-2 inhibitors can reduce CSF PGE_2 levels in humans during the perioperative period, which has resulted in improved outcomes following hip replacement surgery.[31] In addition to the effect on CSF PGE_2, COX-2 inhibitors[31] were able to modulate the level of CSF IL-6. The exact mechanism responsible for the reduction in interleukin level has yet to be determined but is probably related to the PGE_2 pathway.[31]

CELECOXIB

Celecoxib was the first COX-2 inhibitor approved by the FDA (December 1998). It has now been approved for the relief of pain from osteoarthritis, rheumatoid arthritis, acute pain, dysmenorrhea, and familial adenomatous polyposis. It has good selectivity for the COX-2 enzyme (see Table 40.2). Celecoxib is available in 100-, 200-, and 400-mg capsules, with a maximum recommended dosage of 400 mg/day for chronic pain. The dose recommended for the management of acute pain is 400 mg followed by 200 mg within the first 24 hours. If celecoxib is administered with aluminum- or magnesium-containing antacids, plasma levels of celecoxib are reduced. Peak plasma levels occur 3 hours after oral administration, and the drug crosses into CSF.[33] Celecoxib is 97% protein bound, with an apparent volume of distribution of 400 L. It is metabolized via cytochrome P-450 2C9 and eliminated predominantly by the liver. It is not indicated for pediatric use and is a category C drug for pregnancy. The drug has a half-life of about 11 hours.[133] Adverse events noted in the various clinical trials include headache, edema, dyspepsia, diarrhea, nausea, and sinusitis. It is contraindicated in patients with sulfonamide allergy or known hypersensitivity to aspirin or other NSAIDs. Because celecoxib does not interfere with platelet function,[134] it can be administered perioperatively as a multimodal analgesic without increasing the risk for bleeding. The incidence of NSAID gastropathy may also be lower with celecoxib than with nonselective NSAIDs.[135]

ROFECOXIB

Rofecoxib is a selective COX-2 inhibitor indicated for use in patients with osteoarthritis, rheumatoid arthritis, dysmenorrhea, and acute pain. The drug is administered orally, its bioavailability is 93%, and 87% of the absorbed dose is bound to plasma proteins.[136] The metabolism of rofecoxib in the liver yields metabolites that have no COX-1 or COX-2 activity. Though metabolized by the liver, adjustment in dosage for patients with liver disease is not necessary. The metabolites are predominately eliminated from the body in urine. Analgesic efficacy occurs 0.7 to 1.5 hours after oral dosing and continues for more than 24 hours.[137] Steady-state plasma concentrations of rofecoxib are achieved after 4 days, a function of its 17-hour half-life. It is supplied in 12.5-, 25-, and 50-mg tablets, including a suspension (5 mL contains 12.5mg/5mL or 25mg/5mL).

When compared with other NSAIDs, rofecoxib has less effect on the GI mucosa and therefore has less likelihood of GI complications; adverse events reported with rofecoxib include dyspepsia, peripheral edema, and hypertension.[138] Because rofecoxib has no effect on platelet aggregation[139] and has minimal interaction with warfarin,[140] it has been used extensively in the perioperative arena as a preemptive analgesic for various types of surgeries.[31,131,140,141] Larger clinical trials and long-term follow-up studies undertaken to demonstrate the efficacy of this compound in the prevention of cancer have demonstrated an increased incidence of cardiovascular events,[142] which prompted voluntary withdrawal of rofecoxib by the manufacturer in 2004 (see more detailed discussion later).

VALDECOXIB AND PARECOXIB

Valdecoxib is a derivative of isoxazole and binds noncovalently to COX-2 to form a tight and relatively stable enzyme-inhibitor complex. It is a potent inhibitor of PGE_2 production in humans.[143] Valdecoxib and its metabolites are also the active moieties of a parenteral COX-2 inhibitor, parecoxib sodium.[144]

Valdecoxib has good oral bioavailability (83%) and a minimal first-pass effect. It achieves its maximal plasma concentration in 3 hours, with an elimination half-life of about 8 to

11 hours.[145] It is metabolized by the liver via the cytochrome P450 3A4 isoenzyme. About 70% of the dose is excreted in urine as metabolites. Valdecoxib has been approved for use in patients with osteoarthritis (10 mg), rheumatoid arthritis (10 mg),[146] and acute pain (up to 40 mg). Several clinical studies have demonstrated the efficacy of valdecoxib in patients undergoing oral surgery[147,148] and major orthopedic surgery at doses of 40 mg.[149] Common adverse events reported include GI[150] and renal toxicity.[151] Clinical studies in high-risk cardiac patients in which a significantly increased incidence of major cardiovascular adverse events and increased risk for serious skin reactions (e.g., toxic epidermal necrolysis, Stevens-Johnson syndrome, erythema multiforme) were demonstrated led to withdrawal of this COX-2 inhibitor from the U.S. market in 2005.

New COX-2 inhibitors that are in clinical use in Europe include etoricoxib and lumiracoxib. However, these drugs have not yet been approved by the FDA. Concerns about their cardiovascular risk profile are as yet unresolved.

ETORICOXIB

Etoricoxib (MK-663) is a dipyridinyl derivative that contains a phenyl group attached to the central ring. Etoricoxib is highly selective for COX-2 (IC_{50} ratio, 344; see Table 40.2), with substantial distribution into tissue and 92% bound to plasma.[152] It is distributed rapidly, with the peak concentration being reached within 1 to 2 hours, and has an elimination half-life of approximately 22 hours.[153] Etoricoxib is metabolized via cytochrome P-450–dependent oxidation, which results in prolonged elimination in patients with liver disease. The highest recommended daily dosage for chronic use is 60 to 90 mg; for acute pain, the dose is 120 mg.[154]

Clinical trials of etoricoxib have demonstrated its analgesic efficacy for various types of arthritis,[155] acute dental pain,[156] dysmenorrhea, and chronic pain conditions such as back pain. Adverse effects include GI, renal, and cardiovascular manifestations. There is a 40% reduction in the relative risk for GI side effects with etoricoxib in comparison to other NSAIDs.

LUMIRACOXIB

Lumiracoxib is structurally distinct from other COX-2 inhibitors; it is a phenylacetic acid derivative with a short mean plasma half-life of 4 hours, but it provides analgesic efficacy for 24 hours with a single dose.[157] It is 99% protein bound, with a volume of distribution of 13 L and a bioavailability of 74% after oral administration. Lumiracoxib has been found to bind and interact with the COX-2 enzyme via a mechanism different from that of other COX-2–selective inhibitors and carboxylate-containing nonselective COX inhibitors. The carboxylate group of lumiracoxib forms hydrogen bonds with the catalytic Tyr385 and with Ser530 on COX-2 rather than with the larger hydrophobic side pocket or with Arg120.[158] Lumiracoxib is highly selective for COX-2 (see Table 40.2). It has been shown clinically to provide analgesia for the treatment of knee osteoarthritis,[159] acute pain after dental surgery,[160] and pain after major joint replacement surgery.[161] Like other COX-2 inhibitors, lumiracoxib has been shown to have a reduced incidence of GI side effects. In a large controlled study (TARGET study) including 18,325 patients, lumiracoxib, 400 mg daily, was shown to cause fewer gastric ulcers than other NSAIDs do; no increase in cardiovascular risk was demonstrated in this study.[162]

COMBINATION DRUGS

To enhance the efficacy and safety of NSAID analgesia, drugs have been formulated in combination with NSAIDs. Formulations of ibuprofen-containing hydrocodone are available, and diclofenac has also been formulated in combination with misoprostol. Although such combinations are more convenient, there is no evidence that they are any more effective or safer than when administered separately. Caffeine, long sold in combination with acetaminophen and aspirin in over-the-counter analgesic preparations, has also been studied in combination with ibuprofen.[163,164] The effect of the added analgesia from caffeine is measurable but not substantial. The enhanced NSAID analgesia seen in combination with caffeine probably does not result from alterations in absorption or distribution of the NSAID.[165]

An oxycodone-ibuprofen combination, 5 mg/400 mg, is manufactured as Combunox. It is an oral fixed-dose combination tablet with analgesic, anti-inflammatory, and antipyretic properties. It is approved in the United States for short-term use (up to 7 days) in the management of acute, moderate, and severe pain and is the first and only fixed-dose combination of ibuprofen and oxycodone.[166] A single dose of oxycodone-ibuprofen (5 mg/400 mg) provided better analgesia than did low-dose oxycodone or ibuprofen administered alone in most trials. It is generally well tolerated after single or multiple doses, and short-term use is not expected to produce any of the serious adverse effects typically associated with the long-term use of opioids or NSAIDs.

ADVERSE EFFECTS OF NSAIDS

The clinical utility of NSAIDs has been limited greatly by concerns of adverse effects. Such concerns have included inhibition of platelet function and renal and GI effects. Recently, concerns about bone healing and cardiovascular risk have become prominent.

HEMATOLOGIC EFFECTS

Arachidonic acid is converted into the PG endoperoxides PGG_2 and PGH_2 by the action of COX (see Fig. 40.2). These endoperoxides in turn are converted to TXA_2 in platelets by the action of TXA_2 synthase, but in vascular endothelium they are converted to PGI_2 by the action of PGI_2 synthase. TXA_2 functions as a platelet activator and vasoconstrictor, whereas PGI_2 is a platelet inhibitor and vasodilator. Furthermore, activated platelets divert some of their endoperoxides to vascular cells ("endoperoxide steal") to provide more substrate for PGI_2 formation.[167] Platelet activity, therefore, is the result of a constant balance between the effects of PGI_2 in the endothelium and TXA_2 in platelets. Platelets are especially vulnerable to COX inhibition because unlike most other cells, they cannot regenerate this enzyme. Presumably, this reflects the inability of platelets to synthesize proteins independently. Thus aspirin, which irreversibly acetylates the COX enzyme, causes inhibition of platelet aggregation for the life span of the platelet, which is 7 to 10 days.[167] In contrast, nonselective NSAIDs reversibly inhibit the COX enzyme and thus cause a transient reduction in the formation of TXA_2 and inhibition of platelet activation, which resolves after most of the drug is eliminated.[167] A single dose of 300 to 900 mg of ibuprofen can inhibit platelet aggregation for 2 hours after administration, but the effect is largely dissipated by 24 hours.[167,168] Similarly, both sulindac and diclofenac also cause a short-term (<24 hours) reduction in platelet aggregation. The antiplatelet effects of long-acting NSAIDs such as piroxicam, however, can last for several days after use of the drug is discontinued.[169]

Studies have shown variable clinical effects of NSAIDs on perioperative bleeding. Most of the studies that have found an association between NSAID use and blood loss have included surgeries with relatively high unsutured tissue surfaces, such as tonsillectomy and total joint replacement. In one study of patients undergoing total hip replacement surgery, those who received NSAIDs had more intraoperative and postoperative blood loss than did those who did not.[170] A meta-analysis of clinical trials of NSAID use for tonsillectomy showed an increase in post-tonsillectomy bleeding.[171] Studies have noted more complications in patients given NSAIDs with half-lives longer than 6 hours and when NSAIDs are administered before surgical control of bleeding. Many studies of perioperative NSAIDs have not demonstrated an increased risk for bleeding. No difference was found in clinical blood loss during total hip replacement or transurethral resection of the prostate in patients taking diclofenac versus those taking placebo.[172,173] A study of ketorolac, 60 mg, administered during anorectal surgery did not find any association with intraoperative or postoperative bleeding.[174] A meta-analysis of the perioperative use of NSAIDs in patients undergoing a variety of surgical procedures revealed a slight, but statistically significant, risk for "any bleeding" (1.7 % vs. 0.2%), as well as "severe bleeding" (1.7% vs. 0%), associated with the perioperative use of nonselective NSAIDs.[175]

Finally, most NSAIDs potentiate the anticoagulant activity of warfarin by displacing the protein-bound drug or by inhibiting its metabolism by hepatic microsomal enzymes.[167] Thus, they should be used with caution in patients taking oral anticoagulants, especially older patients, who can have a significant increase in bleeding and hospitalization when the two are used in combination.[176]

CARDIOVASCULAR EFFECTS

NSAIDs and COX-2 inhibitors may cause an increased incidence of serious cardiovascular thrombotic events, myocardial infarction, and stroke.[177] This effect has been noted most markedly with COX-2 inhibitors. Unbalanced biosynthesis of PGI_2 and TXA_2 seems to play a role in atherogenesis and thrombosis. It is postulated that prolonged administration of COX-2 inhibitors, which inhibit PGI_2, may lead to several adverse effects, including a rise in blood pressure, initiation and early development of atherosclerosis, and architectural and functional responses of blood vessels to such stress. These changes may predispose individuals to an exaggerated thrombotic response on rupture of atherosclerotic plaque.[178] Aspirin and traditional NSAIDs suppress the activities of COX-1 and COX-2 and therefore reduce both TXA_2 and PGI_2 levels. In contrast, COX-2 inhibitors suppress the production of PGI_2 without affecting TXA_2 synthesis.[179] These mechanisms may be responsible for the increased incidence of acute myocardial infarction observed with prolonged use of COX-2 inhibitors.[180]

A fivefold increase in the incidence of myocardial infarction was noted in the Vioxx Gastrointestinal Outcome Research (VIGOR) study.[181] This study involved the use of rofecoxib, 50 mg daily, for a median of 9 months in a high-risk rheumatoid arthritis patient population in which the use of aspirin was precluded.[182] Similarly, the Adenomatous Polyp Prevention on Vioxx (APPROVe) study, which evaluated a 25-mg daily dose of rofecoxib in patients with a history of colorectal adenoma, demonstrated a 1.7-fold increase in the risk for myocardial infarction and cerebrovascular events associated with rofecoxib that became apparent after 18 months of therapy.[142] Epidemiologic database studies, which reflected actual drug use and included higher-risk patients, also found a correlation between normal- or high-dose rofecoxib use and adverse cardiovascular outcomes.[142,183] The drug manufacturer voluntarily withdrew rofecoxib from the world market on September 30, 2004.

Subsequently, on December 17, 2004, the Adenoma Prevention with Celecoxib (APC) trial was halted because of an increased occurrence of cardiovascular events. The APC trial compared the efficacy of celecoxib (200 or 400 mg twice daily) with that of placebo for 33 months in preventing colorectal adenoma.[183] Celecoxib was associated with a dose-related 2.3- to 3.4-fold increase in serious adverse cardiovascular events, which became apparent after 12 months of treatment. However, two other large long-term placebo-controlled studies had different results. The Prevention of Spontaneous Adenomatous Polyps (PreSAP) trial,[184] which included patients taking 400 mg of celecoxib daily or placebo for an average of 32 months, found no difference in risk for cardiovascular events. The Alzheimer's Disease Anti-Inflammatory Prevention Trial (ADAPT)[185] found no increased risk with celecoxib, 200 mg daily, but noted a statistically significant increase in cardiovascular risk with naproxen.[186]

Valdecoxib and the parenteral prodrug parecoxib have also been associated with the potential risk for adverse postoperative cardiovascular events, including an increase in cerebrovascular events (2.9% vs. 0.7%) and myocardial infarction (1.6% vs. 0.7%), after the administration of a supramaximal dose (40 mg twice daily) for 14 days following coronary artery bypass graft surgery.[187] However, no increases in cardiovascular events were observed with therapeutic dosing of parecoxib followed by valdecoxib for general and orthopedic surgery.[146,148,149]

A joint meeting of the FDA's Arthritis Advisory Committee and the Drug Safety and Risk Management Advisory Committee was convened in February 2005 to discuss the safety of COX-2 inhibitors and nonspecific NSAIDs. These committees jointly reaffirmed that COX-2 inhibitors are important treatment options for pain management and that the preponderance of data demonstrates that the cardiovascular risk associated with celecoxib is similar to that associated with commonly used older nonspecific NSAIDs.[177] The rationale behind this conclusion is that COX-2 inhibitors collectively increase cardiovascular risk when compared with placebo but not when compared with nonselective NSAIDs. It was noted that rigorous scientific studies are needed to characterize the longer-term cardiovascular risks associated with these analgesics.

Subsequently, on April 7, 2005, the FDA announced a series of changes applicable to the entire class of NSAIDs.

Table 40.3 Cardiovascular Risk with NSAIDs

Drug	Pooled RR (95% CI)
Naproxen	1.09 (1.02, 1.16)
Ibuprofen	1.18 (1.11, 1.25)
Celecoxib	1.17 (1.08, 1.27)
Rofecoxib	1.45 (1.33, 1.59)
Diclofenac	1.40 (1.27, 1.55)
Indomethacin	1.30 (1.19, 1.41)
Piroxicam	1.08 (0.91, 1.30)
Meloxicam	1.20 (1.07, 1.33)
Etodolac	1.55 (1.28, 1.87)
Etoricoxib	2.05 (1.45, 2.88)
Valdecoxib	1.05 (0.81, 1.36)

CI, confidence interval; NSAIDs, nonsteroidal anti-inflammatory drugs; RR, relative risk.

Adapted from McGettigan P, Henry D. Cardiovascular risk with NSAIDS: systematic review of population-based controlled observational studies. *PLoS Med*. 2011;8:e1001098.

These included an FDA boxed warning for the potential increased risk for cardiovascular events and GI bleeding associated with all prescription NSAIDs, including celecoxib. The manufacturers were asked to revise their labeling to include a medication guide for patients to help make them aware of the potential for cardiovascular and GI adverse events. In addition, the FDA requested that the manufacturers of all over-the-counter NSAIDs revise their labels to include more specific information about the potential cardiovascular and GI risks and include information to assist consumers in the safe use of these drugs. Finally, the FDA concluded that the overall risk-benefit profile of valdecoxib is unfavorable and requested that the manufacturer voluntarily withdraw valdecoxib from the market.

The FDA noted that all NSAIDs can lead to the new onset of hypertension or worsening of preexisting disease, which may contribute to an increased incidence of cardiovascular events.[177]

Follow-up studies have demonstrated concerns about cardiovascular safety for a wide variety of NSAIDs (Table 40.3). A systematic review of 51 observational studies involving more than 3 million patients found that several NSAIDs of various categories were associated with a significantly increased risk for cardiovascular events: rofecoxib with a 45% increase in cardiovascular events, diclofenac with a 40% risk that increased at higher doses, indomethacin with a 30% increased risk, meloxicam with a 20% increased risk, and ibuprofen with elevated risk at higher but not at lower doses. Naproxen at any dose had the least association with adverse cardiovascular events.[188,189] Furthermore, a dose-response relationship was demonstrated for many of these NSAIDs.

Similarly, a nationwide cohort study from Denmark revealed that patients with established cardiovascular disease who used NSAIDs had an odds ratio (OR) of 1.45 for recurrent myocardial infarction in comparison to those who did not take NSAIDs. This effect was apparent at the beginning of treatment and persisted throughout treatment. Diclofenac had the highest association (OR = 3.96) and naproxen the lowest.[190]

Another recent review of the cardiovascular effects of NSAIDs that included only randomized controlled trials confirmed the relatively low risk associated with naproxen and the higher risk with other NSAIDs.[191] International guidelines now discourage the use of NSAIDs in patients with established cardiovascular disease.[190,191] Additional studies are needed to further delineate the relative cardiovascular risk associated with each NSAID and enable the most appropriate selection to be made for patients with cardiovascular disease in whom NSAIDs cannot be avoided entirely.

BONE HEALING

Another concern regarding the perioperative use of NSAIDs is the possible deleterious effect on osteogenesis and spinal fusion.[192] PGs have been known for many years to have potent effects on bone metabolism, including osteoblastic and osteoclastic activity, as well as being essential for bone repair.[193] The exact mechanism by which NSAIDs impair spinal fusion has not yet been elucidated. It has been hypothesized that the effect may be mediated by inhibition of the inflammatory process with a concomitant reduction in blood flow in the early period of osteogenesis, decreased mesenchymal cell proliferation, or inhibition of calcification of the bone matrix.[194] Many investigators have recommended that NSAIDs not be used in the multimodal management of acute pain for patients undergoing spinal fusion surgery.[192-195] Although the data are conflicting, a large body of literature derived from laboratory animal studies has suggested that COX-2 inhibitors delay or inhibit bone healing.[192-194] However, in these studies COX-2 inhibitors were administered over a period of several weeks to months at doses higher than those approved for acute pain.

A recent Cochrane database study pooled the results of 11 cohort and case-control trials involving fracture, osteotomy, and spine fusion in patients with NSAID exposure and nonunion as an outcome. In the initial analysis of the pooled data of the 11 studies, the OR for nonunion with NSAID exposure was 3 (confidence interval [CI] = 1.6 to 5.6). However, when only higher-quality studies were considered, which included primarily spine fusion patients, no significant outcome was detected.[196]

Another study evaluated 9995 patients with humeral shaft fractures, including 105 with nonunion. A total of 10.3% were exposed to NSAIDs within 90 days of their index fracture. NSAID exposure within the first 90 days was significantly associated with nonunion (OR = 3.7, CI = 2.4 to 5.6). When the data for each of the three 30-day periods were placed in the same multivariate model, only the period from 61 to 90 days showed a relationship between NSAID use and nonunion. A similar relationship was demonstrated for opioids and nonunion during this period. These results suggest that painful nonhealing fractures may be the cause of NSAID use rather than the result.[197]

A small study investigating the utility of indomethacin in preventing heterotopic ossification in patients with long-bone fractures undergoing hip replacement noted a higher risk for nonunion in the indomethacin group[198] (26%) than in the radiation therapy group (7%).

Conversely, a recent study compared the efficacy and safety of etoricoxib with tramadol in patients undergoing hallux valgus repair. Etoricoxib provided superior pain relief and patient recovery scores without any effect on quality of bone or wound healing.[199]

These conflicting results indicate that large randomized prospective trials are needed to better delineate causality and determine risk. Given the relatively low incidence of nonunion, large cohorts will be needed.

TENDON AND SOFT TISSUE HEALING

Several animal investigations have raised questions regarding the effect of NSAIDs on soft tissue healing.[200,201] Lower tensile strength was noted in healing of the Achilles tendon in rats treated with indomethacin or parecoxib than in controls.[201] In another study of rodent patellar tendon healing, both traditional and COX-2–selective NSAIDs impaired healing, with the COX-2–selective medications having the most dramatic effect.[201]

In a small randomized controlled trial of marathon runners, ibuprofen was shown to decrease patellar tendon PGE_2 levels and impair load-induced adaptive collagen synthesis in the patellar tendon when compared with placebo. Further investigations delineating the clinical relevance of these findings are needed.[202]

ALLERGY, HYPERSENSITIVITY, AND ASTHMA

All NSAIDs, including acetylsalicylic acid, may induce hypersensitivity reactions, which are of two general types. Both may be related to inhibition of PG synthesis. The two types of hypersensitivity reactions are (1) the syndrome of asthmatic attacks in patients with vasomotor rhinitis, nasal polyposis, and bronchial asthma and (2) the syndrome of urticaria and angioedema. PGE_2 is a bronchodilator. It stabilizes histamine stores in mastocytes and thus helps inhibit the inflammatory response.[8,19,203] In a susceptible person, the result of inhibition of PG biosynthesis may be spontaneous degranulation of mastocytes, with release of histamine into the respiratory tract and skin leading to bronchoconstriction and asthma, as well as urticaria.

Recent data have demonstrated that acetaminophen can deplete pulmonary antioxidant levels, which can result in an increased risk for newly diagnosed asthma.[204] Previous research has demonstrated that acetaminophen may be associated with an increased risk for newly diagnosed asthma if used for 14 days or more per month. Increasing use of acetaminophen may be associated with an increased prevalence of asthma and chronic obstructive pulmonary disease.

GASTROINTESTINAL EFFECTS

The first evidence that aspirin could damage the stomach was reported in 1938 based on gastroscopic observations.[205] In the 1950s and 1960s, case-control studies indicated that melena was associated with NSAID use. NSAIDs cause hemorrhagic gastric erosions in the corpus and antrum of the stomach. The mortality rate attributed to NSAID-related GI toxic effects is 0.22% per year, with an annual relative risk of 4.21. It has been estimated that 16,500 NSAID-related deaths occur per year as a result of gastric complications, similar to the number of deaths annually from acquired immunodeficiency syndrome (16,685) and higher than the deaths caused by multiple myeloma and asthma. Some risk factors identified for the development of NSAID-induced ulcers include advanced age; history of ulcer; concomitant use of corticosteroids; higher doses of NSAIDs, including the use of more than one NSAID; concomitant administration of anticoagulants; serious systemic disorder; cigarette smoking; consumption of alcohol; and concomitant infection with *Helicobacter pylori*.

NSAIDs cause ulceration in the stomach by their topical irritant effect on the epithelium and their ability to suppress PG synthesis.[206] The ability of NSAIDs to cause gastric damage correlates with the time and dose dependency for PG suppression in the stomach.[207] Inhibition of PG synthesis leads to a reduction in the ability of the gastric mucosa to defend itself against luminal irritants; bicarbonate secretions, blood flow, and epithelial cell turnover are influenced by PGs. Another feature of NSAIDs that probably contributes to gastric bleeding from preexisting ulcers is their effect on platelet aggregation through the suppression of thromboxane synthesis.[208] Mediators in the pathway whereby decreased PG levels cause gastric irritation and damage have been extensively studied. These mediators include leukotrienes,[209] tumor necrosis factor-α (TNF-α),[210] and neutrophil adherence substances.[211]

NSAID-induced enteropathy has been documented in the small intestine and colon, although the exact mechanism is not fully understood. Various preventive strategies have been developed to reduce NSAID gastroenteropathy.[212] Enteric-coated and slow-release formulations of NSAIDs have been ineffective in preventing the gastric side effects seen with NSAID consumption. Other agents used for the prevention of ulcer formation with NSAIDs include sucralfate (controversy exists about its efficacy), histamine 2 (H_2) receptor antagonists (famotidine), proton pump inhibitors (omeprazole), and PGs (misoprostol).

NSAID gastric-induced complications led to the development of COX-2 inhibitors. These agents have shown promise in reducing NSAID-associated gastropathy. In the SUCCESS-I study, celecoxib was compared with nonspecific NSAIDs in 13,274 patients with osteoarthritis.[213] Patients were randomly assigned to either celecoxib, 100 or 200 mg twice daily, or nonselective NSAID therapy (diclofenac, 50 mg twice daily, or naproxen, 500 mg twice daily) for 12 weeks. The study revealed that both dosages of celecoxib were as effective as the nonselective NSAIDs in treating osteoarthritis. However, significantly more gastric ulcer–related complications occurred in the nonselective NSAID group of patients (0.8/100 patient-years) than in the celecoxib group (0.1/100 patient-years) (OR = 7.02, $P = 0.008$). The results of the SUCCESS-I study are different from those of the Celecoxib Long-term Arthritis Safety Study (CLASS),[135] which did not demonstrate an advantage of celecoxib in reducing the incidence of upper GI ulcer complications; this was attributed by the SUCCESS-I study authors to the low dropout rate and design of the newer study.

Preferential use of COX-2 inhibitors[214] because of their gastric enteropathy safety properties led to the increased incidence of cardiovascular effects that resulted in the withdrawal of some COX-2 inhibitors from the market. Guidelines for gastric protection when NSAIDs are needed have been suggested.[189] For all patients, nonpharmacologic methods (e.g., lifestyle changes) should be initiated first. Topical agents should be considered. Acetaminophen can be used safely for many conditions. Nevertheless, NSAID therapy may be needed. In patients who have no cardiovascular risk factors and are at low or no risk for GI complications, monotherapy with one of the traditional nonselective NSAIDs can be prescribed (Table 40.4). In patients who do not require aspirin prophylaxis and who are at risk for NSAID-induced

Table 40.4 Recommended Use of NSAID or COX-2 Inhibitor Based on Cardiovascular Risk

CV Risk Factors or Rx?	History of GI Ulcers or GI Bleeding? No	Yes
No	Nonselective NSAIDs	COX-2 with GI prophylaxis
Yes	Nonselective NSAIDs	Nonselective NSAIDs with GI prophylaxis

COX, cyclooxygenase; CV, cardiovascular; GI, gastrointestinal; NSAID, nonsteroidal anti-inflammatory drug; Rx, medical prescription.

GI complications, an initial approach would be to prescribe a COX-2 inhibitor or a traditional NSAID and proton pump inhibitor. In contrast, in patients with cardiovascular risk who require aspirin prophylaxis, COX-2 inhibitors should be avoided; in patients with no GI risk factors, traditional NSAIDs can be used; and if they are at risk for GI complications, a proton pump inhibitor must also be prescribed.[215]

RENAL TOXICITY

Aspirin and other NSAIDs cause a transient decrease in renal function. This effect may occur more often in patients with underlying renal disease.[216] The postulated mechanism is inhibition of the renal synthesis of PG, which may be important in the autoregulation of renal blood flow. Aspirin may also block the diuretic effect of spironolactone by inhibiting its binding to the tubular cell receptor. Similarly, NSAIDs may alter a patient's responses to thiazides or loop diuretics. Fluid retention and edema have been observed in some patients taking NSAIDs.

The renal profile of traditional NSAIDs and COX-2 inhibitors may be described by the following: sodium retention is mediated by COX-2 inhibition, and changes in the glomerular filtration rate are caused by inhibition of COX-1 and COX-2. All NSAIDs, including COX-2 inhibitors, are associated with hypertension and edema.[217] Most cases resolve with continuation of therapy, with resolution generally occurring over a period of 1 to 8 weeks. Risk factors for NSAID-induced renal toxicity include chronic NSAID use, multiple NSAID use, dehydration, volume depletion, congestive heart failure, vascular disease, hyperreninemia, shock, sepsis, systemic lupus erythematosus, hepatic disease, sodium depletion, nephrotic syndrome, diuresis, concomitant drug therapy (e.g., diuretics, angiotensin-converting enzyme inhibitors, β-blockers, potassium supplements), and age 60 years or older.[216]

HEPATIC TOXICITY

Aspirin is clearly hepatotoxic in certain situations, and this effect is not dose dependent. However, the effect is reversible when use of the drug is discontinued.[218]

CENTRAL NERVOUS SYSTEM EFFECTS

Direct toxic reactions are of several types. Symptoms of the ear in the form of tinnitus or deafness are usually an early warning of toxicity. Toxic manifestations are directly related to free drug levels, which vary inversely with albumin levels; the adverse event is typically reversed when the dose is reduced or discontinued. The most frequently implicated class of drugs in hypersensitivity-induced aseptic meningitis is the NSAIDs. Four NSAIDs—ibuprofen, sulindac, tolmetin, and naproxen—have been implicated in drug-induced aseptic meningitis. Patients typically complain of fever, headache, and stiff neck, which generally commence within weeks of beginning therapy.[219]

USE IN SPECIFIC POPULATIONS

PREGNANT AND LACTATING WOMEN

When administered to pregnant women, salicylates may reach substantial levels in the fetus. Birth defects have not been reported to occur in regular users; however, experimental evidence has shown that it is teratogenic in monkeys.[220] Aspirin taken at term may delay the onset of labor for 3 to 10 days, and it has been associated with increased bruising of the newborn child, particularly when instrumentation is necessary. Administration of aspirin or indomethacin at term to delay the onset of labor has been reported to cause serious pulmonary vascular disease in the newborn infant.

PEDIATRIC USE

NSAIDs are often used "off label" in pediatric populations.[221] In the United States and Canada, NSAIDs approved for children include ibuprofen, naproxen, tolmetin, aspirin, and choline magnesium salicylate. In the United Kingdom, diclofenac, indomethacin, piroxicam, and mefenamic acid are also approved for use in children. Review of the available pharmacokinetic data before use of any NSAID not approved for pediatric populations is suggested to minimize adverse effects and maximize efficacy.[222] GI toxicity from NSAIDs does occur in children, but estimates of frequency vary. In a large retrospective study of 702 children examined for gastropathy, only 5 (10 events) were documented with gastric ulcers or gastritis.[222] Other toxicities related to NSAID use in children are renal (rare) and skin reactions, which are all reversible.[223]

Oral administration of ibuprofen (15 mg/kg) every 4 to 6 hours at a fixed dose and the option of using opioid at an adjustable dose could be beneficial for the relief of pain in pediatric patients. When oral administration is not possible, rectal ibuprofen (40 mg/kg/day) or indomethacin is useful.[221] In situations in which the oral or rectal route is not optimal, intravenous ketorolac, 0.5 mg/kg, followed by repeated doses every 6 hours to a maximum of 60 mg/day, can be used.[224] Ketorolac can be of great benefit in pediatric patients with sickle cell crisis, but renal function in these patients needs to be monitored closely.

Oral acetaminophen at doses of 15 mg/kg every 4 to 6 hours is an effective analgesic for children; when the oral route is not available, acetaminophen suppositories may be used. Absorption of rectal acetaminophen is slow and sometimes erratic.[225] Studies have suggested that an initial dose of 40 mg/kg followed by 20 mg/kg every 6 hours may be needed to maintain therapeutic blood levels.[226] An intravenous formulation of acetaminophen is now available that is well tolerated and effective at a dose of 15 mg/kg.[227]

OLDER ADULTS

Absorption of NSAIDs is not affected by the diminished active transport systems in the GI tract of older adult patients because most of the absorption of these compounds occurs via passive diffusion.[228] Changes in body composition, such as a decrease in albumin levels in older adult patients, might be expected to increase the toxicity of highly protein-bound compounds; however, such compounds seldom produce clinically important effects if hepatic and renal function is normal.[229]

Piroxicam and ibuprofen have been shown to have longer plasma half-lives in older women and men, respectively.[230,231] These drugs also undergo biotransformation largely by oxidation. There is evidence that drugs undergoing biotransformation by phase II reactions are more slowly eliminated, as may be the case with naproxen and ketoprofen.[232,233] Acute renal failure may occur, especially in older adult patients, when the renin-angiotensin system is activated and a PG inhibitor is prescribed.[233]

Older patients are subject to a number of diseases for which they receive multiple medications. Drug-drug interaction is therefore a serious issue. Some important examples include the interaction of NSAIDs such as phenylbutazone or azapropazone with warfarin, which can lead to an enhanced anticoagulation effect.[234] Indomethacin nullifies the hypotensive effects of atenolol, propranolol, prazosin, captopril, and thiazide diuretics. It also blunts the diuretic response of furosemide, triamterene, and spironolactone. Phenylbutazone and oxyphenbutazone increase the rate of synthesis of the cytochrome P-450 enzyme, thereby reducing the hydroxylation activity of tolbutamide; thus, the plasma half-life of this agent is prolonged, which can result in hypoglycemia. Azapropazone also enhances the hypoglycemic action of tolbutamide. Salicylate in therapeutic doses has been shown to enhance the effects of oral hypoglycemic agents, especially chlorpropamide.

CONCLUSION

NSAIDs have been a mainstay of acute and chronic pain management for decades and will continue to play this role in the foreseeable future.[235,236] A deeper understanding of their complex effects on the PG pathways in normal and disease states will be necessary to tailor these drugs for best efficacy and safety. Their effects are widespread and encompass all organ systems in both health and disease. Further investigation of the effects of NSAIDs on this complex balance is essential. This will allow physicians to apply the risk-benefit ratio to each individual.

A greater variety of modes of administration are now available. Intranasal and intravenous forms are available for patients who cannot take oral medications. Transdermal preparations may allow drugs to be delivered directly to tissues while limiting systemic effects.

Despite recent setbacks with the withdrawal of newer, more selective NSAIDs from the market because of safety concerns, continued development of anti-inflammatory drugs that are capable of targeting specific points of the PG pathway is necessary to optimize pain management.

KEY POINTS

- Prostanoids are arachidonic acid derivatives that are essential to the central and peripheral inflammatory response. The phospholipid released as a result of disruption of cell membranes is converted by phospholipase A_2 to arachidonic acid.
- Cyclooxygenase (COX) catalyzes the conversion of arachidonic acid to prostanoids by the addition of molecular oxygen. The prostanoid most prominently associated with the inflammatory response is prostaglandin E_2.
- COX-1 and COX-2 are two different isoforms of COX that have very different functions. COX-1 is primarily expressed constitutively. It serves to maintain homeostasis, stimulate angiogenesis, regulate gastric pH, and regulate platelet reactivity, as well as other functions. COX-2 is a highly inducible enzyme importantly associated with the inflammatory response. The relative effects of anti-inflammatory drugs on COX-1 and COX-2 have important implications for the efficacy and safety of these drugs.
- Peripheral inflammation leads to induction of COX-2 and expression of prostaglandin E synthase in the central nervous system by both neural and humoral components. The humoral component can be blocked only by centrally acting COX-2 inhibitors.
- Most nonsteroidal anti-inflammatory drugs (NSAIDs) currently available can be broadly classified as salicylates (e.g., aspirin), acetaminophen, acetic acid derivatives (e.g., indomethacin), propionic acid derivatives (e.g., ibuprofen), and COX-2 inhibitors.
- Unlike other NSAIDs, acetaminophen inhibits prostaglandin synthesis in the central nervous system, but not in peripheral tissues.
- The utility of all NSAIDs is limited by concerns of adverse events, including effects on the gastric mucosa, renal function, platelet reactivity, bone and tissue healing, cardiovascular risk, and interactions with other patient medications.
- Selective COX-2 inhibitors were developed to reduce some of the adverse effects of COX-1 inhibition, such as GI ulcers and platelet inhibition. However, serious concerns have arisen about increased cardiovascular risk with these medications. This led to withdrawal of several of the newer COX-2–selective medications from the market.
- A thorough and individualized assessment of the potential benefits and adverse effects for each patient is critical to successful use of these drugs.
- Areas for future investigation include novel methods of drug delivery, drugs with specific targets on the prostaglandin pathway, central versus peripheral sites of action, epidemiologic studies on drug safety, and nonanalgesic uses, including prophylaxis for cancer, cardiovascular disease, and dementia.

SUGGESTED READINGS

Apfelbaum JL, Ashburn MA, Connis RT, et al. ASA task force on acute pain management: practice guidelines for acute pain management in the perioperative setting. *Anesthesiology.* 2012;116:248-273.

Bombardier C, Laine L, Reicin A, et al. Comparison of upper gastrointestinal toxicity of rofecoxib and naproxen in patients with rheumatoid arthritis. *N Engl J Med.* 2000;343:1520-1528.

Buvenandran A, Kroin JS, Tuman KJ, et al. Effects of peri-operative administration of a selective cyclooxygenase 2 inhibitor on pain management and recovery of function after knee replacement. *JAMA.* 2003;290:2411-2418.

Buvanendran A, Kroin JS, Berger RA, et al. Up-regulation of prostaglandin E_2 and interleukins in the central nervous system and peripheral tissue during and after surgery in humans. *Anesthesiology.* 2006;104:403-410.

Dodwell ER, Latorre JG, Parisini E. NSAID exposure and risk of nonunion: a meta-analysis of case-control and cohort studies. *Calcif Tissue Int.* 2010;87:193.

McGettigan P, Henry D. A systematic review of observational studies of selective and nonselective inhibitors of cyclooxygenase. *JAMA.* 2006;296:1633-1644.

McGettigan P, Henry D. Cardiovascular risk with non-steroidal anti-inflammatory drugs: systematic review of population-based controlled observational studies. *PLoS Med.* 2011;8:e1001098.

Rosenquist RW, Benzon HT, Connis RT, et al. ASA task force on chronic pain management: practice guidelines for chronic pain management. *Anesthesiology.* 2010;112:810-833.

Samad TA, Sapirstein A, Woolf CJ. Prostanoids and pain: unraveling mechanisms and revealing therapeutic targets. *Trends Mol Med.* 2002;8:390-396.

Schjerning Olson AM, Fosbol EL, Lindhardsen J. Duration of treatment with nonsteroidal antiinflammatory drugs and risk of myocardial infarction in patients with a prior myocardial infarction. *Circulation.* 2011;123:2226-2235.

Sinatra RS, Jahr JS, Reynolds LW. Efficacy and safety of single and repeat dose of 1 gram intravenous acetaminophen (paracetamol) for pain management after major orthopedic surgery. *Anesthesiology.* 2005;102:822-831.

U.S. Food and Drug Administration memorandum. Analysis and recommendations for agency action regarding non-steroidal anti-inflammatory drugs and cardiovascular risk; 2005. Available at www.fda.gov/cder/drug/infopage/COX2/NSAIDdecisionMemo.pdf.

The references for this chapters can be found at www.expertconsult.com.

Skeletal Muscle Relaxants

41

Kenneth C. Jackson, II | Charles E. Argoff | Andrew Dubin

The term *skeletal muscle relaxant* is often used to describe a diverse group of medications commonly used in the treatment of back pain (Table 41.1).[1-4] Medications commonly referred to as skeletal muscle relaxants include carisoprodol, chlorzoxazone, cyclobenzaprine, metaxalone, methocarbamol, and orphenadrine.[5] All these agents are labeled by the U.S. Food and Drug Administration (FDA) with an indication for the relief of discomfort associated with an acute, painful, musculoskeletal condition. Oral baclofen and tizanidine are also commonly used to treat acute musculoskeletal conditions and are considered by many clinicians as muscle relaxants, despite the lack of an FDA-approved indication in this regard. Baclofen and tizanidine do have FDA indications for the treatment of spasticity caused by upper motor neuron syndromes including multiple sclerosis, spinal cord disease, or injury. Benzodiazepines, principally diazepam, are also commonly used and indicated for adjunctive relief of skeletal muscle spasm and are often considered in discussions regarding skeletal muscle relaxants.

In discussing this broad class of medications, it becomes difficult to cull out the actual intended therapeutic outcomes. These agents are typically prescribed during the initial presentation of acute low back pain problem, often the result of a soft tissue mechanical injury. The injury normally occurs to the muscles, ligaments, or tendons, structures around the lumbar spine. The presentations may include local pain and tenderness, muscle spasm, and limited range of motion. Muscle spasm is often the most difficult to define and is the subject of controversy among some clinicians.[6] Muscle spasm can be described as a vicious pain-spasm-pain cycle that protects compromised tissues and structures. Secondary to these pain impulses, an involuntary reflex muscle contraction at the site of injury can occur, which in turn can lead to local ischemic injury. This can further facilitate the pain-spasm-pain paradigm. Muscle spasm phenomena may be considered a variation of a myofascial pain presentation.[7]

MECHANISM OF ACTION

In considering this discussion of muscle spasm pathophysiology, the problem with defining the activity of the skeletal muscle relaxants becomes manifest. The exact mechanism of action for these various agents has not been fully elucidated. It is generally accepted that skeletal muscle relaxants have the ability to depress polysynaptic reflexes within the dorsal horn via a variety of mechanisms (Box 41.1), which in turn may relax skeletal muscle tissue in an indirect manner.[1-3] In animal studies, these agents exert their muscle-relaxing effects by inhibiting interneuronal activity and blocking polysynaptic neurons in the spinal cord and descending reticular formation in the brain. Interesting to note is that sedating agents also depress polysynaptic reflexes, making it difficult to determine whether skeletal muscle relaxants produce their clinical activity via sedation or a change in the pain-spasm-pain cycle.

INDICATIONS FOR USE

Despite the common use of skeletal muscle relaxants, relatively little data exist to elucidate their role in the treatment of back pain, especially chronic back pain.[8,9] None of the agents discussed in this chapter have an indication for use in the setting of chronic back pain. In one survey of skeletal muscle relaxant use in the United States, muscle relaxants, although indicated for short-term treatment, are most often prescribed on a long-term basis.[10] In general, skeletal muscle relaxants, excluding baclofen and tizanidine, maintain FDA labeling as adjuncts for treatment of short-term acute low back pain (LBP) and are commonly used to treat muscle spasms and associated pain for periods of 1 to 3 weeks. This time frame coincides with how long many patients may expect it will take to recover from an initial acute low back insult. In this context, it may be difficult to discern the role of these agents, other than the palliative analgesic quality that they may provide for patients. Skeletal muscle relaxant selection depends on an evaluation of adverse effects, contraindications, patient tolerability, and clinical experience. This discussion will also include a brief review of the clinical use of botulinum toxin as a treatment for musculoskeletal pain.

SPECIFIC DRUGS

CARISOPRODOL (SOMA)

Carisoprodol is available as a 250-mg or 350-mg tablet and in combination with aspirin (soma compound) and with aspirin and codeine (soma compound with codeine). Carisoprodol dosing should not exceed four doses in a 24-hour period (Table 41.2). Similar to other muscle relaxants, carisoprodol has additive sedative effects when taken with alcohol or other central nervous system (CNS) depressants.

Carisoprodol is converted in the liver to meprobamate (Miltown), an intravenous (IV) controlled substance. Meprobamate is well known to produce phenomena that result in physical and psychological dependence.[11-16] Substance abuse is problematic with carisoprodol, probably as a consequence of meprobamate formation. Several states within the United States have begun listing carisoprodol as a controlled substance in their state formularies. However,

Table 41.1 Skeletal Muscle Relaxant Profiles

Drug	Onset of Action	Duration (Hr)	Side Effects	Important Drug Interactions
Carisoprodol	30 min	4-6	Drowsiness, N/V, dizziness, ataxia; withdrawal potential	Additive effects with alcohol and other CNS depressants
Chlorzoxazone	~1 hr	3-4	N/V, headache, drowsiness, dizziness	Additive effects when taken with alcohol or other CNS depressants
Cyclobenzaprine	~1 hr	12-24	Drowsiness, dizziness, dry mouth	Additive effects with barbiturates, alcohol, other CNS depressants; seizures with tramadol and MAOIs; additive effects with TCAs
Metaxalone	1 hr	4-6	Dizziness, headache, drowsiness, N/V, rash	Additive effects when taken with alcohol or other CNS depressants
Methocarbamol	30 min (PO)	4-6	Dizziness, blurred vision, with drowsiness	Additive effects when taken with alcohol or other CNS depressants
Orphenadrine	1 hr (PO)	4-6	Tachycardia, lightheadedness, anxiety	Propoxyphene (confusion, N/V, dry mouth, tremors)
Diazepam	30 min (PO)	Variable, depending on elimination	Sedation, fatigue, hypotension ataxia, respiratory depression	Potentiation of effects when taken with phenothiazines, opioids, barbiturates, MAOIs
Baclofen	3-4 days (PO) 4-6 hr (IT) 30 min (IT)	Variable (PO)	Drowsiness, slurred speech, hypotension, constipation, urinary retention	Antidepressants (short-term memory loss); additive effects with imipramine
Tizanidine	2 weeks	Variable	Drowsiness, dry mouth, dizziness, hypotension, increased spasm, or muscle tone	Additive effects with alcohol and other CNS depressants; reduced clearance with oral contraceptives

CNS, central nervous system; IT, intrathecal; MAOIs, monoamine oxidase inhibitors; N/V, nausea and vomiting; TCA, tricyclic antidepressant.

Box 41.1 Classification of Agents by Proposed Mechanism of Action

CNS Depressants

Antihistamine: orphenadrine
Sedatives: carisoprodol, chlorzoxazone, metaxalone, methocarbamol
TCA-like: cyclobenzaprine

Central α_2 Agonists

Tizanidine

GABA Agonists

Baclofen, benzodiazepines

CNS, central nervous system; GABA, gamma-aminobutyric acid; TCA, tricyclic antidepressant.

Table 41.2 Comparative Dosing of Commonly Used Muscle Relaxants

Agent	Dosage
Baclofen	5-10 mg PO tid
Carisoprodol*	250 mg PO qid
Chlorzoxazone	250-750 mg PO qid
Cyclobenzaprine	5-10 mg PO tid
Diazepam*	2-10 mg PO qid
Metaxalone	800 mg PO qid
Methocarbamol	750-1500 mg PO qid
Orphenadrine	100 mg PO bid
Tizanidine	4-8 mg PO qid

*Not recommended.

carisoprodol is not considered a controlled substance at the federal level. Because of the dependence potential, carisoprodol use should be avoided. It should also be cautiously tapered as opposed to immediately discontinued following long-term use.

CHLORZOXAZONE (PARAFLEX, PARAFON FORTE DSC)

Chlorzoxazone is available as 250- and 500-mg tablets, taken up to four times daily. It has been suggested that chlorzoxazone may be less effective than the other skeletal muscle relaxants.[8] It does not have any significant drug-drug interactions, but it does have a significant adverse effect profile that includes a rare idiosyncratic hepatocellular reaction.[17] The role of this agent is unclear, considering the potential lack of efficacy and significant toxicity profile.[18]

CYCLOBENZAPRINE (FLEXERIL)

Cyclobenzaprine is available as 5- and 10-mg tablets, with recommended dosing of up to three times daily. Cyclobenzaprine is more structurally and pharmacologically related to the tricyclic antidepressants than to the CNS depressant skeletal muscle relaxants. As with other skeletal muscle relaxants, cyclobenzaprine does not have activity directly on muscle tissue, with animal data suggesting that this agent acts primarily in the brainstem. The net result of this action is a reduction in tonic somatic motor activity.[19] Although no human evidence exists to support this mechanism, the newer 5-mg dose has yielded similar clinical efficacy with less sedation than the more sedating 10-mg dose.[20] In the future, this may prove to be an important distinction with the CNS depressant agents. In an open-label study of patients with acute neck or low back pain associated with muscle spasm who were randomized to be treated for 7 days with cyclobenzaprine 5 mg PO three times daily alone or cyclobenzaprine 5 mg PO three times daily in combination with ibuprofen, at doses of 400 mg PO three times daily or 800 mg three times daily, no significant treatment differences were found among these groups.[21]

Because of the structural relationship to tricyclic antidepressants (TCAs), clinicians must be cognizant of the anticholinergic side effects, such as dry mouth, urinary retention, dizziness, hypotension, and constipation, seen with cyclobenzaprine. Use of cyclobenzaprine is contraindicated in the setting of arrhythmias, congestive heart failure, hyperthyroidism, acute glaucoma, narrow angle glaucoma, or during the acute recovery phase of a myocardial infarction. One report suggested that coadministration with pro-serotonergic agents such as selective serotonin reuptake inhibitors (SSRIs) may predispose patients to life-threatening serotonin syndrome.[22]

Cyclobenzaprine labeling suggests that concomitant use with tramadol may place patients at higher risk for developing seizures.[19] Attendant use of cyclobenzaprine with monoamine oxidase inhibitors or use within 14 days after their discontinuation is contraindicated. It can also enhance the effects of agents with CNS depressant activity. Older adults appear to have a higher risk for CNS-related adverse reactions, such as hallucinations and confusion, when using cyclobenzaprine. Withdrawal symptoms have been noted with the discontinuation of chronic cyclobenzaprine use. Use of a medication taper may be warranted for chronic-use patients.

METAXALONE (SKELAXIN)

Metaxalone is available as a 400- and 800-mg tablet and has a recommended maximal dose of 800 mg three or four times daily. Metaxalone does not have any significant drug-drug interactions and appears to have a fairly benign side effect profile, although fatalities attributed to the use of metaxalone have been reported.[23,24] Hemolytic anemia, leukopenia, and impaired liver function have been seen with the use of metaxalone, but they are uncommon. Metaxalone is contraindicated in patients who have severe renal or hepatic impairment. It is known to cause an elevation in the cephalin flocculation test, necessitating serial liver function assessments. Metaxalone can also produce a false-positive result for Benedict's test. In this scenario, alternatives to urine glucose testing may be necessary.[25] Although FDA approved since the 1980s, there are few published placebo-controlled studies comparing metaxalone with placebo for the treatment of musculoskeletal pain.[26]

METHOCARBAMOL (ROBAXIN, ROBAXISAL)

Methocarbamol is available in oral and parenteral forms for IV or intramuscular use. However, many complications have arisen with the injectable form, including pain, sloughing of the skin, and thrombophlebitis. The injectable form should be used cautiously in patients with known latex hypersensitivity. The oral dosage form of the medication is marketed as a 500- and 750-mg tablet, with a recommended daily dosage range of 4000 to 4500 mg as three or four divided doses daily. For difficult situations, the dose for the first 24 to 48 hours can be up to 6 to 8 g/day. Methocarbamol is also combined with aspirin and marketed as Robaxisal. Similar to metaxalone, although FDA approved in the 1980s, there are few published placebo-controlled studies comparing methocarbamol with placebo for the treatment of musculoskeletal pain.[27]

ORPHENADRINE CITRATE (NORFLEX, NORGESIC, NORGESIC FORTE)

Orphenadrine is a direct descendant of diphenhydramine and thus exhibits antihistaminic and anticholinergic properties. Like methocarbamol, orphenadrine is available in a parenteral dosage formulation. There have been reports of severe adverse reactions with parenteral use (e.g., anaphylactoid reaction), making this formulation difficult to use. Orphenadrine is available as a 100-mg tablet (Norflex) and in combination with aspirin (Norgesic) and caffeine (Norgesic Forte).

Orphenadrine use with propoxyphene (removed from the U.S. market in 2011) may cause confusion, anxiety, and tremors, perhaps because of additive effects. Orphenadrine's anticholinergic actions have been noted to produce significant adverse effects at high dosages, such as tachycardia, palpitations, urinary retention, and blurred vision.[28] Given its significant anticholinergic profile, orphenadrine use is contraindicated in patients with underlying neuromuscular junction defects such as myasthenia gravis and Lambert Eaton syndrome.

DIAZEPAM (VALIUM)

This is the most commonly prescribed and referenced benzodiazepine for the treatment of muscle spasms.[29] Diazepam demonstrates hypnotic, anxiolytic, antiepileptic, and antispasmodic properties. With respect to muscle relaxation, gamma-aminobutyric acid (GABA)–mediated presynaptic inhibition at the spinal level is thought to be the main mechanism of action for diazepam. Sedation and abuse potential are the main concerns with this agent; therefore, it should not be used as a first-line muscle relaxant agent. It is important to taper this agent slowly after long-term use to avoid any withdrawal symptoms. Diazepam is available in a wide range of dosages, and each patient should be treated on an individual basis. The recommended dosage range for musculoskeletal pain is 2 to 10 mg four times daily. Coadministration of the benzodiazepine class of medications with opioids, as they are commonly prescribed, can lead to significant morbidity in the form of respiratory depression and mortality from respiratory failure.

BACLOFEN (LIORESAL)

Baclofen is chemically related to GABA and produces its effects by inhibiting monosynaptic and polysynaptic transmission along the spinal cord. This drug is mainly used for spasticity associated with CNS disorders (multiple sclerosis [MS], spinal cord lesions). Studies have shown baclofen to have superior efficacy when compared with diazepam.[2] Baclofen is unique in that it can be administered intrathecally in cases of severe spasticity and for patients who do not tolerate or have failed oral therapy. It has also found a niche in the treatment of trigeminal neuralgia because of a more favorable side effect profile. Baclofen is available in 10- and 20-mg tablets, with a therapeutic range of 40 to 80 mg daily. The medication should be started at 5 mg three times daily and tapered up to a therapeutic level of 5 mg every 3 to 5 days. It should be tapered slowly after long-term use to avoid a withdrawal reaction, rebound phenomena, and potential withdrawal seizures that can occur with sudden cessation. It should be used with caution in older patients and patients with renal impairment.

TIZANIDINE (ZANAFLEX)

Tizanidine (Zanaflex) is a short-acting inhibitor of excitatory (presynaptic) motor neurons at the spinal and supraspinal levels, producing agonistic activity at the noradrenergic α_2 receptors. This activity results in the inhibition of neurotransmitter release from spinal interneurons and the concomitant inhibition of facilitatory spinal pathways that enhance muscle movement. Tizanidine is related chemically to clonidine, but it has significantly lower antihypertensive effects.[30] The main adverse effect for most patients is sedation.[31] Currently, tizanidine is FDA approved for the management of increased muscle tone associated with spasticity resulting from CNS disorders, such as multiple sclerosis or spinal cord injury. There are published studies on the use of tizanidine in the setting of back pain or muscle spasm, either alone or in combination with ibuprofen, as well as a report of effective use for myofascial pain.[32-34] In a multicenter placebo-controlled study evaluating the efficacy and safety of tizanidine for the treatment of low back pain, tizanidine was found to provide more pain relief and less restriction of movement compared with placebo. Drowsiness was the most common side effect, but this adverse effect may actually be desired in patients with nighttime exacerbations of their pain.[32] In a separate study, 105 patients with acute low back pain were given tizanidine 4 mg PO three times daily in conjunction with ibuprofen 400 mg PO three times daily, or ibuprofen 400 mg PO three times daily with placebo. The study results suggested that the tizanidine-ibuprofen combination is more effective for the treatment of moderate or severe acute low back pain than ibuprofen only.[33] Tizanidine is available as 2- and 4-mg tablets; treatment should be instituted with a 4-mg single dose, increasing by 2- to 4-mg increments up to a therapeutic dose. The maximum daily dose should not exceed 36 mg.

Tizanidine should be used with caution in the setting of renal impairment. Tizanidine clearance decreases by 50% in patients with creatinine clearance lower than 25 mL/min. Coadministration with alcohol can increase the area under the curve (AUC) of tizanidine by approximately 20% and increase the maximum concentration (C_{max}) by approximately 15%. Use with oral contraceptives can decrease the clearance of tizanidine and place patients at higher risk for sedating adverse effects.

BOTULINUM TOXINS (BOTOX-ONABOTULINUMTOXINA, DYSPORT-ABOBOTULINUMTOXINA, XEOMIN-INCOBOTULINUMTOXINA AND MYOBLOC-RIMABOTULINUMTOXINB)

Botulinum toxin is a potent neurotoxin produced by the gram-positive anaerobic bacterium *Clostridium botulinum*. Of the seven known immunologically distinct serotypes of botulinum toxin (A to G), only types A and B have been developed for routine commercial use. Historically, the toxin's primary mechanism of action has been linked to its ability to inhibit the release of acetylcholine from cholinergic nerve terminals. However, it is now appreciated that these neurotoxins may also inhibit the release of glutamate, substance P, and calcitonin gene-related peptide. These effects may strongly contribute to the analgesic effects of these toxins.[35-37] Botulinum toxin has been studied in a number of chronic pain conditions associated with painful muscle spasm, including cervicogenic headache, temporomandibular joint disorders, craniocervical dystonia syndromes, chronic myofascial pain, and chronic low back pain.

The potential benefit of the use of botulinum toxin for the treatment of cervicogenic headache associated with "whiplash" injuries has been noted. In 1997, Hobson and Gladish reported that botulinum toxin type A (onabotulinumtoxinA) injections could be effective in reducing cervicogenic headache resulting from cervical whiplash-type injuries.[38] In a randomized, double-blind, placebo-controlled study, Freund and Schwartz found that the botulinum toxin type A–treated patients (onabotulinumtoxinA) demonstrate significant greater improvement from baseline with respect to pain reduction and cervical range of motion.[39] Mixed results have been observed in evaluating the effect of botulinum toxin injection on temporomandibular joint and other orofacial-related pain. In an open-label study completed by Freund and Schwartz,[40] patients with temporomandibular joint dysfunction believed to be related to myofascial dysfunction were treated with a total of 200 units of botulinum toxin A (onabotulinumtoxinA) (masseter and temporalis muscles injected), with most patients experiencing pain reduction as well as improvements in jaw function. Von Lindern and colleagues' study of patients with chronic facial pain associated with muscular hyperactivity also demonstrated improvement in botulinum toxin type A (onabotulinumtoxinA)–treated patients.[41] However, in a placebo-controlled crossover trial evaluating botulinum toxin type A (onabotulinumtoxinA) in patients with chronic moderate to severe orofacial pain of muscular origin, no statistically significant differences were seen between placebo and active treatment.[42]

There have been several published evaluations of the use of botulinum toxin for the treatment of myofascial pain in the cervicothoracic regions. In a small crossover trial ($N = 6$), patients whose cervical myofascial trigger points were injected with botulinum toxin type A (onabotulinumtoxinA) had an average of 30% pain reduction.[43] In a separate study, Wheeler and associates[44] completed a randomized, double-blind, prospective, placebo-controlled study in 33 patients with chronic cervical myofascial pain who were injected with either 50 or 100 units of botulinum toxin type A (onabotulinumtoxinA) or normal saline. No clear benefit was found in the botulinum toxin–treated patients. Porta,[45] in a single-blinded study, evaluated the potential difference between "conventional" lidocaine-methylprednisolone trigger point injections and botulinum toxin type A injections (onabotulinumtoxinA) for myofascial pain treatment and concluded that although each group received benefit, the duration of benefit was longer in the botulinum toxin–treated group.

Botulinum toxin injections have also been studied in the treatment of chronic low back pain. In one study, 31 patients with chronic low back pain were randomized to be treated with 200 units of botulinum toxin A (onabotulinumtoxinA) into five sites (L1-5 or L2-S1, 40 units/site) or placebo injections. Pain and disability were measured at 3 and 8 weeks following injection using the visual analog scale and the Oswestry Low Back Pain and Disability Questionnaire. At 3 and 8 weeks, the pain reduction experienced by the botulinum toxin–treated group was greater than that experienced by the placebo group, and at 8 weeks there was less disability in the botulinum toxin–treated group compared with placebo.[46] A report evaluating the use of botulinum toxin type A (abobotulinumtoxinA) for the relief of upper back myofascial pain syndrome concluded that several secondary parameters, such as physicians' global assessment and patients' global assessment, significantly favored abobotulinumtoxinA over placebo at weeks 8 and 12.[47] The precise role of botulinum toxin injection therapy in the management of conditions associated with chronic muscle spasm remains to be determined.

CONCLUSION

Available clinical data indicate that skeletal muscle relaxants are more effective than placebo with respect to relieving acute low back pain.[8] Most of this information is dated, however, with study designs and analyses that would not be acceptable if this research were conducted today. In general, no data support any one agent being more efficacious than another. Some reports have suggested that chlorzoxazone may be less effective than other agents, which puts into question the viability of using this agent.[8,48]

Most clinical guidelines list skeletal muscle relaxants as optional agents for use individually or in combination with an NSAID. The Agency for Health Care Policy and Research (AHCPR) guidelines, published in 1995, specifically noted that skeletal muscle relaxants alone or in combination with an NSAID are no more effective than using an NSAID alone.[49] This conclusion has been supported in systematic reviews by van Tulder and colleagues.[8,48] Skeletal muscle relaxants have been shown to be more effective than placebo for patients with acute LBP with respect to outcomes such as short-term pain relief, global efficacy, and improvement of physical outcomes,[50-53] but there remains no quality evidence that allows for a direct comparison of skeletal muscle relaxants with NSAIDs. Most clinicians and researchers agree that skeletal muscle relaxants may be of benefit to patients with acute low back pain by reducing the duration of their discomfort and accelerating recovery. A meta-analysis of cyclobenzaprine use in acute low back pain by Browning and associates concluded that despite limitations in the available evidence, the combination of an NSAID with cyclobenzaprine appears to be warranted.[54] It is probably best to consider the use of skeletal muscle relaxants as an adjunct or alternative to NSAIDs, especially in cases in which NSAID toxicity is a concern or when NSAID monotherapy proves suboptimal. Two Cochrane reviews concluded that that there is little evidence to support the use of muscle relaxants for the management of pain associated either with inflammatory arthritis or rheumatoid arthritis.[55,56]

Skeletal muscle relaxants have CNS depressant effects and should be used with caution, particularly for patients with concomitant use of alcohol, anxiolytics, opioid analgesics, or other sedating medications. There is strong evidence that skeletal muscle relaxants are associated with higher risks for total adverse effects, especially those related to the central nervous system.[8,9,48] The most common and consistent adverse effects noted with the central nervous system were drowsiness and dizziness.[25] The benzodiazepines-muscle relaxants such as diazepam and sedative-muscle relaxants such as carisoprodol are highly addictive and should never be used as first-line agents.

Thus, skeletal muscle relaxants remain an enigmatic collection of agents with an ill-defined role in the treatment of chronic back pain. This is partly because of the nature of their discovery and early clinical applications that predate more modern research approaches. Considering the many issues currently facing clinicians (e.g., adverse effects of NSAIDs), it will become necessary to re-evaluate the role and use of skeletal muscle relaxants in the future.

KEY POINTS

- Muscle relaxants may treat muscle spasticity in two manners. First, they can modify the stretch reflex arc, either by reducing the excitatory signals or by augmenting the inhibitory interneurons. This decreases activation of the alpha motor neuron. Second, they can disrupt the excitation-contraction coupling that produces muscle contraction.
- Cyclobenzaprine is a centrally acting skeletal muscle relaxant that is structurally related to tricyclic antidepressants; it acts primarily at the level of the brainstem.
- Baclofen, as a $GABA_b$ agonist, causes hyperpolarization and thus decreases the release of excitatory neurotransmitters in the brain and spinal cord. It causes less sedation than benzodiazepines and may reduce pain by decreasing substance P release.
- Skeletal muscle relaxants have been shown to be more effective than placebo for patients with acute LBP with respect to outcomes, such as short-term pain relief, global efficacy, and improvement of physical outcomes.
- Botulinum toxin type A (onabotulinumtoxinA) injections could be effective in reducing cervicogenic headache resulting from cervical whiplash-type injuries.
- Carisoprodol is converted in the liver to meprobamate (Miltown), an intravenous (IV) controlled substance. Meprobamate is well known to produce phenomena that result in physical and psychological dependence.

SUGGESTED READINGS

Bailey DN, Briggs JR. Carisoprodol: an unrecognized drug of abuse. *Am J Clin Pathol.* 2002;117:396-400.

Berry H, Hutchinson DR. A multicentre placebo-controlled study in general practice to evaluate the efficacy and safety of tizanidine in acute low back pain. *J Int Med Res.* 1988;16:75-82.

Borenstein DG, Korn S. Efficacy of a low-dose regimen of cyclobenzaprine hydrochloride in acute skeletal muscle spasm: results of two placebo-controlled trials. *Clin Ther.* 2003;25:1056-1073.

Reeves RR, Carter OS, Pinkofsky HB, et al. Carisoprodol (soma): abuse potential and physician unawareness. *J Addict Dis.* 1999;18:51-56.

van Tulder MW, Touray T, Furlan AD, et al. Muscle relaxants for nonspecific low back pain. *Cochrane Database Syst Rev.* 2003;(3):CD004252.

The references for this chapter can be found at www.expertconsult.com.

42 Topical Analgesics

Charles E. Argoff

In contrast to the use of a systemic analgesic, use of a topical analgesic may result in relief of pain without the requirement for notable systemic absorption. A topical analgesic is *not* a transdermal analgesic. For example, the mechanism of action of *transdermal* nitroglycerin or fentanyl and clonidine patches is systemic, which requires systemic absorption through the skin, as well as a systemic concentration of the specific drug. A *topical* analgesic requires neither systemic absorption nor a significant systemic concentration to be clinically effective. A topical analgesic is an analgesic that is applied locally and directly to the painful areas, with the primary site of action being local to the site of application. As noted previously, it is not a "transdermal analgesic," which unlike a topical analgesic, requires a systemic analgesic concentration for its analgesic action. This is not a trivial distinction; analgesics have been inappropriately considered "topical" agents even when formal pharmacologic studies to demonstrate a lack of systemic activity or systemic drug concentration (or both) had not been completed, and at other times, true topical agents have been incorrectly described as transdermal agents. As discussed in this chapter, topical analgesics have been studied and are used for acute pain, as well as for a variety of types of chronic neuropathic and non-neuropathic pain. Different topical analgesics are associated with different mechanisms of action, a point to be considered when choosing a topical analgesic for a patient with chronic pain. Of great interest is the recent observation (described in greater detail later in this chapter) that although a topical analgesic's primary mechanism of action may occur locally and within the peripheral nervous system (PNS), the effect of a topical analgesic can be detected in the central nervous system (CNS) by functional neuroimaging.

BACKGROUND

Undoubtedly, pain cannot be ultimately experienced in the absence of relevant brain activity; however, we have also appreciated for many years the importance of PNS activity, including provision of input to the CNS, in initiating and maintaining acute and some chronic painful conditions. There are specific painful conditions, such as central post-stroke pain and spinal cord injury pain, in which the pain mechanisms lie within the CNS and do not respond to topical analgesics. Many common chronic pain syndromes, including post-herpetic neuralgia (PHN), chronic low back pain (CLBP), and osteoarthritis (OA), probably result from mechanisms involving both the PNS and CNS.

If pain cannot be experienced without brain activation, how can a topical analgesic whose primary mechanism of action is largely within the PNS be helpful? A topical analgesic may interrupt, depending on the specific analgesic, certain mechanisms of pain transmission and by doing so may actually lead to a reduction in central pain mechanisms and thus pain as well. In other words, acknowledging that the experience of pain cannot occur without the brain, less pain may be experienced if use of a topical analgesic leads to reduced activation of PNS mechanisms, which if activated would facilitate transmission of pain signals to the CNS for central processing. This chapter reviews the use of topical analgesics for the treatment of various painful conditions and provides an update of previously published similar reviews.[1-3]

The potential clinical benefit of any analgesic—or for that matter any medical treatment—is diminished by its adverse effect profile, toxicities, and drug-drug interactions. When considering the use of a topical analgesic, the risk for and severity of significant adverse effects and drug-drug interactions are often less than those for the same analgesic administered systemically.[4] Consider, for example, the treatment of OA with a nonsteroidal anti-inflammatory drug (NSAID). If one can successfully treat someone with a topical NSAID versus a systemic NSAID, this may be helpful in reducing the risk for systemic side effects typically associated with NSAIDs. Rash and unpleasant skin sensations may occur with the use of a topical analgesic, but neither is typically experienced.[5] Among the topical analgesics currently approved by the Food and Drug Administration (FDA) (see Box 42.1), the 5% lidocaine patch (Lidoderm) has been studied widely. Several studies of the 5% lidocaine patch have been designed to evaluate its safety and tolerability. For example, the outcome of one study assessing the tolerability and safety of 24-hr/day use of four 5% lidocaine patches demonstrated that there were no significant systemic side effects and that plasma lidocaine levels remained below those known to be associated with cardiac abnormalities. In this study, the safety and tolerability were similar if the subject used the patch for 12 or for 24 hr/day.[6] In a multicenter open-label study, patients with a history of CLBP from a variety of causes were treated safely with four 5% lidocaine patches every 24 hours for extended periods.[5] In each of these reports, no significant dermal reactions were experienced.[6,7]

Dermal sensitivity is a potential side effect of all topical analgesics; however, other adverse effects may be experienced as a result of the use of a specific topical analgesic that may be more related to the specific medication in the specific topical analgesic. An example is capsaicin. After the topical application of capsaicin, severe burning at the site of application commonly occurs. This particular side effect may in fact not infrequently lead to reduced clinical

Box 42.1 Food and Drug Administration–Approved Topical Medications

Lidocaine
Lidocaine/prilocaine
Diclofenac
Doxepin
Capsaicin

effectiveness of this specific topical analgesic. Capsaicin, when applied topically in its currently available forms, does not result in significant systemic accumulation or in any life-threatening outcomes, and the incidence of burning may decrease with repeated use; however, frequent occurrence of this side effect may negatively affect treatment adherence and consequently the patient's ability to benefit from its use.[8] The 8% capsaicin patch (Qutenza), approved by the FDA for the treatment of PHN, was generally well tolerated in clinical trials even though burning did occur. In contrast to over-the-counter preparations of capsaicin that may need to be applied multiple times daily, the 8% capsaicin patch is applied for a single hour and may result in effective outcomes for 12 weeks or longer.

It is generally acknowledged that a patient being treated for chronic pain may also have other medical comorbid conditions that would be treated with pharmacologic therapies as well. Recognizing that drug-drug interactions are minimized with topical analgesics may be clinically relevant when managing a patient who has been prescribed systemic medications concurrently for comorbid medical conditions. Recently published guidelines regarding the pharmacologic management of persistent pain in older adults emphasize this point in their recommendations.[9] A clinical example would be a 79-year-old woman being treated for hyperlipidemia, hypertension, coronary artery disease, and type 2 diabetes mellitus and OA. She requires analgesics for the chronic pain associated with her OA and is already taking four oral systemic medications on a daily basis for the other chronic medical conditions A trial of the use of a topical medication for her may offer several advantages over a systemic medication because of reduced drug-drug interactions, assuming that she achieves adequate pain relief.[10] Since the topical analgesics available typically do not involve dose titration and many systemic agents do, this may provide an additional potential benefit for a patient.

The prescriber must recognize the difference between topical analgesics that are prescribed as commercially available, FDA-approved agents and those that are touted as "topical" agents by various compounding pharmacies but in fact have not been proved to be such following appropriate testing. Commercially available FDA-approved topical analgesics must have demonstrated to the FDA consistent manufacturing standards and quality control, in contrast to those manufactured and sold by a specialized compounding pharmacy. The reader should keep in mind that the so-called topical analgesics that may be made by a compounding pharmacy may consist of a combination of substances, such as a local anesthetic, NSAID, and antidepressant combined together in a chemical base, that are *not* commercially available, FDA-approved topical products. There is no current general requirement for compounding pharmacies to demonstrate manufacturing consistency, and this is an important point for a prescriber to recognize. Even though for many compounding pharmacies there is no documentation of quality control or preparation consistency such as would be required for an FDA-approved product, these products are commonly prescribed. In a survey of members of the American Society of Regional Anesthesia and Pain Medicine, 27% of the respondents reported prescribing such an agent, and 47% of the respondents noted a positive impression suggesting that they thought that patients responded well to the preparation.[11] Of interest is continued commercial development of new topical analgesic preparations. Recently, three topical NSAIDs and the 8% capsaicin preparation have been approved by the FDA. Topical preparations containing opioids, local anesthetics, antidepressants, glutamate receptor antagonists, α-adrenergic receptor agonists, adenosine, cannabinoids, cholinergic receptor agonists, gabapentinoids, prostanoids, bradykinin, adenosine triphosphate, biogenic amines, and nerve growth factor are each at various stages of clinical development.[12]

As one would expect for an oral systemic analgesic, the mechanism of action of a specific topical analgesic depends on the chemical entity or entities in the specific agent, and this may be considered when choosing a particular agent for a patient. The mechanism of action of the topical agent capsaicin, for example, appears to be through agonist activity at the transient receptor potential vanilloid 1 (TRPV1) on Aδ and C fibers.[13,14] As a result of this activity at the TRPV1 receptor, release of substance P and calcitonin gene-related peptide takes place, and it is hypothesized that reduced peripheral as well as central excitability with resulting less pain through reduced afferent input occurs because of the depletion of substance P in C fibers associated with the application of topical capsaicin.[8,13,15] The results of both human nerve biopsy and animal studies demonstrate nerve fiber degeneration in the skin underneath the site of capsaicin application. Such nerve fiber degeneration associated with the application of capsaicin has been suggested to be one of the mechanisms through which its use results in pain relief.[16] The mechanism of action of a topical NSAID, in contrast to capsaicin, is probably associated with inhibition of prostaglandin synthesis and the resulting anti-inflammatory effect. Keeping in mind that the extent of anti-inflammatory effect is not consistently proportional to the pain relief experienced, perhaps other mechanisms of action might be considered.[17] It may be worthwhile to consider the potential benefit of an agent with more than one mechanism of action. For example, the antinociceptive effects of topical morphine may be enhanced by a topical cannabinoid as demonstrated in a study in rats in which the radiant tail flick test was used.[18] Local anesthetic agents are known to suppress the activity of peripheral sodium channels within sensory afferents and subsequent pain transmission; however, other mechanisms of action are under investigation. It has been noted that decreased expression of mRNA for specific sodium channel subtypes may occur following local anesthetic use.[1,5] Several local anesthetic-containing topical analgesics are currently available commercially, including the 5% lidocaine patch, EMLA cream (eutectic mixture of local anesthetics, 2.5% lidocaine/2.5% prilocaine), and the Synera patch (lidocaine, 70 mg/tetracaine, 70 mg). Of these three agents, only the 5% lidocaine patch is associated with an *analgesic* effect without creating *anesthetic* skin, whereas use of EMLA cream or the FDA-approved Synera patch may create both analgesia and anesthesia. This difference among the preparations is useful to apply in specific clinical settings, such as venipuncture, lumbar puncture, intramuscular injections, and circumcision, for which creating both anesthesia and analgesia would be helpful.[5] Choosing which topical analgesic to use clearly depends on the clinical setting in which the medication is being used. At least for the 5% lidocaine patch, it has been noted that application of the patch itself, by protecting allodynic skin from being stimulated, may reduce the allodynia experienced by those afflicted by neuropathic pain states such as PHN.[1]

One novel area of topical analgesic development involves the use of tricyclic antidepressants as topical analgesics. Certain tricyclic antidepressants such as amitriptyline and doxepin have been demonstrated to block sodium channels, and the potential clinical benefit of this mechanism when such an agent is topically applied is being actively investigated at this time.[19,20] One commercially available topical antidepressant, doxepin hydrochloride (Zonalon) cream, is currently approved by the FDA for the short-term treatment of adult patients with pruritus associated with atopic dermatitis or lichen simplex chronicus. Of interest have been reports of use of this agent in an "off-label" manner as a topical analgesic.[21] Other topical agents, including topical opioids, glutamate receptor antagonists, and cannabinoids, have potential as topical analgesics as well. Certain studies of some of these agents are discussed in the following sections.

USE OF TOPICAL ANALGESICS FOR SPECIFIC CLINICAL CONDITIONS (SEE BOX 42.2)

NEUROPATHIC PAIN

The use of specific topical analgesics for the management of neuropathic pain has been established by a number of clinical trials, and more than one published review of the management of neuropathic pain has emphasized their efficacy.[22-24]

LOCAL ANESTHETICS

The first medication to receive FDA approval for the treatment of PHN was in fact the 5% lidocaine patch. The clinical trials that led to the FDA approval of this preparation for the management of PHN demonstrated that when compared with patients treated with placebo patches, patients who were treated with 5% lidocaine patches experienced statistically significantly more pain reduction in a safe and well-tolerated manner.[25,26] A phase IV open-label study involving PHN patients was completed to evaluate whether treatment of PHN with the 5% lidocaine patch affected various quality-of-life measures. A study of 332 patients with PHN used the Brief Pain Inventory (BPI), a validated pain assessment tool. During the study period, enrolled patients were able to use up to three 5% lidocaine patches 12 hours each day, and the BPI was completed daily for 4 weeks. Sixty-one percent (204/332) of the subjects enrolled noted decreased pain intensity by the end of the first week of the study. A reduction in pain intensity was noted by the second week of patch use in more than 40% of the 128 subjects who had not experienced pain relief by the end of the first week of the study. Overall, 70% of enrolled patients experienced improvement by the study's conclusion.[27] In another open-label study, treatment with the 5% lidocaine patch was compared with treatment with pregabalin (Lyrica) for PHN. The study results demonstrated that the 5% lidocaine patch was at least as effective as pregabalin for pain relief in PHN patients. Among the study's most interesting results was that for patients who had not responded to either the 5% lidocaine patch or pregabalin alone, using these agents in combination resulted in greater benefit, and the combination was well tolerated by these patients.[28] This observation is particularly important to note when managing patients with PHN.

Box 42.2 Pain Conditions Treated with Topical Analgesics

Neuropathic pain (various syndromes)
Musculoskeletal pain (acute and chronic)
Soft tissue pain (acute and chronic)
Other pain (dressing changes, cancer treatment related)

In addition to PHN, use of the 5% lidocaine patch for the management of other neuropathic pain states has been evaluated in various studies. A study conducted in Europe, a randomized, double-blind, placebo-controlled trial evaluated the analgesic efficacy of the 5% lidocaine patch for the treatment of "focal" neuropathic pain syndromes.[29] The painful conditions included in the study were mononeuropathies, intercostal neuralgia, and ilioinguinal neuralgia. The results of this study demonstrated that adding the 5% lidocaine patch to other pharmacotherapeutic regimens could reduce ongoing pain and allodynia as quickly as within the first 8 hours following application in some patients, as well as in other patients over a period of 7 days.[29] A smaller open-label study of 16 patients with various chronic neuropathic pain conditions (post-thoracotomy pain, complex regional pain syndrome, postamputation pain, painful diabetic neuropathy, meralgia paresthetica, postmastectomy pain, neuroma-related pain) demonstrated that the 5% lidocaine patch provided pain relief without significant side effects in 81% of these patients.[30] It is worthy to note that according to the study's authors, patients enrolled in this study, before use of the 5% lidocaine patch, had experienced suboptimal outcomes with numerous other agents commonly prescribed for the treatment of neuropathic pain. Several other noncontrolled studies of patients with painful diabetic neuropathy who were treated with the 5% lidocaine patch have been completed. These studies allowed patients to use as many as four 5% lidocaine patches for as long as 18 hr/day. Viewing these studies as a group, the majority of enrolled subjects reported pain reduction and good tolerability of this medication.[31-34] An additional study, a 3-week single-center, open-label study of the 5% lidocaine patch in patients with painful idiopathic sensory polyneuropathy, noted significant improvements in both pain and quality-of-life measures.[35]

In addition to measuring any changes in pain intensity or function (or both) in patients treated with the 5% lidocaine patch, changes in pain quality in patients with PHN have been studied as well. Changes in the quality of pain in patients with PHN treated with the 5% lidocaine patch versus placebo were evaluated in a multicenter, randomized, vehicle-controlled study of 150 PHN patients.[36] Reduced intensity of certain neuropathic pain qualities according to the Neuropathic Pain Scale was more likely to occur in patients treated with the 5% lidocaine patch than in those given the placebo patch (up to three patches for 12 hours each day). Also of interest was that certain types of neuropathic pain (deep, sharp, and burning) that were reduced had previously been assumed to not be related to PNS but to CNS mechanisms. In their discussion of the study's results, the authors proposed that given the localized primary PNS mechanism of action of the 5% lidocaine patch, peripheral mechanisms of neuropathic pain might also be important in the development of these neuropathic pain qualities.[36] The results of a functional brain magnetic resonance imaging study of patients with PHN treated with the 5% lidocaine patch for various lengths of time demonstrated that the brain activity occurring with the spontaneous pain of PHN appeared to be modulated in a manner related to the length of application of this medication, thus suggesting again that a peripherally acting agent may have an impact on CNS pain mechanisms.[37]

Another local anesthetic preparation that is currently commercially available is EMLA cream. Its FDA-approved indication is as a topical anesthetic for use on normal intact skin for analgesia, but it is not FDA-approved for any specific neuropathic pain disorder. Several studies of EMLA cream for the treatment of PHN have been completed, with mixed results. The results of a randomized, controlled study of PHN patients treated with EMLA cream or placebo cream did not demonstrate a significant difference in treatment outcome between the two groups.[38] The results of two uncontrolled studies were more favorable and suggested that use of EMLA cream could relieve the pain associated with PHN.[39,40]

CAPSAICIN

Even though there has been interest in using capsaicin for a number of neuropathic pain disorders such as diabetic neuropathy, painful human immunodeficiency virus (HIV)-related neuropathy, PHN, and postmastectomy pain, many of the older studies had yielded disappointing results, perhaps partly as a result of the weakness of past available strengths of capsaicin (0.025% and 0.075%), as well as poor toleration of the treatment, poor treatment adherence, and the resulting insufficient pain relief.[41] However, in contrast, the results of a higher-strength capsaicin preparation demonstrated better analgesia. In one reported study of patients with painful HIV neuropathy treated with 7.5% topical capsaicin cream, the patients experienced notable pain relief, but to be able to tolerate this medication, concurrent treatment with epidural anesthesia was required.[42] At the 2004 Annual Scientific Meeting of the American Academy of Neurology, two open-label studies, one involving patients with PHN and one involving patients with painful HIV-associated distal symmetrical polyneuropathy, reported notable pain relief in the majority of patients following the single application of a high-concentration (8%) capsaicin patch. The duration of pain relief lasted as long as 48 weeks (PHN).[15,43] A review of the published randomized trials on the use of topical capsaicin for the treatment of either neuropathic or musculoskeletal pain syndromes concluded that "although topically applied capsaicin has moderate to poor efficacy in the treatment of chronic musculoskeletal or neuropathic pain, it may be useful as an adjunct or sole therapy for a small number of patients who are unresponsive to, or intolerant of, other treatments."[44] Recently, the 8% capsaicin patch (Qutenza) received FDA approval for the treatment of PHN. In studies leading to its FDA approval, it was shown to be more effective in reducing pain intensity than was an active, lower-concentration capsaicin product that served as placebo, and it was generally well tolerated. It has also been studied for other neuropathic pain states such as painful HIV neuropathy, with a favorable outcome as well.[45-49]

The results of a novel study comparing the pain-reducing effect of a topical preparation containing 3.3% doxepin alone or a topical preparation containing 3.3% doxepin combined with 0.075% capsaicin versus placebo in patients with a variety of chronic neuropathic pain problems indicated that each treatment provided similar pain-reducing effects and that each was superior to placebo.[50]

OTHER AGENTS

Interest in the use of topical tricyclic antidepressants for the treatment of neuropathic pain has resulted in multiple clinical trials, including the trial on topical doxepin described earlier. For several such trials, the topical preparation examined was a combination of 2% amitriptyline and 1% ketamine. One of these studies, a double-blind, randomized, placebo-controlled study involving 92 patients with diabetic neuropathy, PHN, or postsurgical or post-traumatic neuropathic pain, resulted in no difference in analgesic benefit among any of the four treatment groups (placebo, 2% amitriptyline alone, 1% ketamine alone, or a combination of 2% amitriptyline and 1% ketamine).[51] The results of an open-label study completed by similar investigators involving 28 patients with neuropathic pain for 6 to 12 months treated with the combination topical analgesic 2% amitriptyline and 1% ketamine demonstrated that the average reduction in pain was 34%.[52] Another open-label study by similar investigators using the same type of preparation also demonstrated encouraging results.[53] Noncontrolled trials evaluating the use of topical ketamine, one in PHN patients and one in patients with complex regional pain syndrome type 1, each concluded that topical ketamine may be an effective topical analgesic; however, serum ketamine levels were not measured in either study, and thus it is not clear how truly "topical" the ketamine preparations were.[54] There is one report suggesting that topical application of geranium oil may provide temporary relief of PHN.[55]

SOFT TISSUE INJURIES AND OSTEOARTHRITIS

Common musculoskeletal pain conditions include soft tissue injuries and OA. Since 2007, the FDA has approved three topical NSAIDs, including 1% diclofenac sodium gel (1% Voltaren gel), the 1.3% diclofenac epolamine topical patch (Flector patch), and 1.5% diclofenac topical solution (Pennsaid). Each of these FDA-approved topical NSAIDs has different indications. Diclofenac sodium 1% gel (1% Voltaren gel) is FDA-approved for treating pain associated with OA in joints that can be managed with topical treatment, such as the knees and hands. The diclofenac epolamine topical patch (Flector patch) is FDA-approved for the topical treatment of acute pain from minor strains, sprains, and contusions. The diclofenac sodium topical solution (Pennsaid) is FDA-approved for treatment of the signs and symptoms of OA of the knee.[56]

NONSTEROIDAL ANTI-INFLAMMATORY DRUGS

The use of other topical NSAIDs has been studied most notably outside the United States. For example, a topical ketoprofen patch (100 mg) was found to be superior to placebo in reducing pain intensity following 7 days of treatment in a 2-week randomized, placebo-controlled study of 163 patients with pain from an ankle sprain.[57] In a separate study, a comparable topical ketoprofen preparation was evaluated in patients with tendinitis in a randomized, double-blind, placebo-controlled study. Subjects treated with the active medication fared better than the placebo-treated group did, and except for the skin irritation experienced by some, the treatment was otherwise well tolerated.[58] Ketoprofen gel has been reported to be helpful when used as an adjunct to physical therapy, with benefit reported in a child with Sever's disease, a not uncommon source of heel pain in growing children.[59] A randomized, controlled study of use of a diclofenac patch in 120 individuals experiencing acute pain after a "blunt" injury demonstrated that it was not only well tolerated but also reduced pain intensity greater than did placebo treatment.[60] Treatment of acute sports injury-related pain with a diclofenac patch has also been studied. Two studies, one not controlled and the other a multicenter randomized, controlled study, noted that a diclofenac patch was found to be well tolerated and effective in patients with acute sports injuries. Patients experienced an average of 60% pain relief in the open-label study.[61,62] Additional NSAIDs have also been studied, and in a noncontrolled study of patients described as experiencing "soft tissue pain," the reported results indicated that topical flurbiprofen was associated with greater pain reduction than oral diclofenac was and that fewer adverse effects occurred when the topical preparation was used.[63] This study is one of very few that actually compared a topical NSAID with an oral agent—an important study design for comparing not only efficacy but also adverse events. In another controlled study, use of topical ibuprofen cream for the management of acute ankle sprains was found to be superior to placebo in reducing pain.[64] In a controlled study of ketoprofen gel for the management of acute soft tissue pain, it was found to be more effective than placebo in providing pain relief.[65] A topical formulation of 5% ibuprofen gel was examined in a placebo-controlled study in patients with painful soft tissue injuries. Patients received either 5% ibuprofen gel or placebo gel for a maximum of 7 days. Pain intensity levels, as well as limitations in physical activity, were assessed daily. A significant reduction ($P < 0.001$) in pain intensity plus improvement in physical activities was experienced by the patients who received the 5% ibuprofen gel versus placebo.[66] A second study with similar patient types completed by the same investigators demonstrated similar results.[67] Also of interest is a recent Cochrane database review in which it was concluded that topical NSAIDs can provide good levels of pain relief without the systemic adverse effects of oral NSAIDs in the treatment of acute musculoskeletal pain.[68]

The use of topical analgesics for the treatment of OA has also been studied, and in fact, multiple reviews of this subject have recently been published.[69-72] A diclofenac patch preparation, studied in a randomized, double-blind, controlled study in patients with chronic pain secondary to knee OA, demonstrated that this patch may be safe and effective for this common condition.[73] A randomized controlled study comparing the use of a topical diclofenac solution and oral diclofenac for the treatment of OA of the knee concluded that use of the topical diclofenac solution produced relief of symptoms that was equivalent to that of oral diclofenac and resulted in a significantly reduced incidence of diclofenac-related gastrointestinal complaints.[74] A recently published long-term study with the same topical diclofenac solution confirmed its safety during the study period.[75] A study of individuals with pain in the temporomandibular joint compared treatment with diclofenac solution applied topically several times daily and treatment with oral diclofenac. Even though there was no significant difference in analgesic benefit between the two groups, significantly fewer gastrointestinal side effects were experienced by the patients receiving the diclofenac topical solution.[76] Other completed topical NSAID trials include a placebo-controlled trial that demonstrated efficacy of 1.16% topical diclofenac gel in patients with OA of the knee and a randomized controlled study demonstrating benefit from the application of a topical diclofenac solution versus placebo after 6 weeks of treatment in patients with painful OA of the knee.[77,78] One meta-analysis examining the use of topical NSAIDs for the treatment of OA found evidence suggesting that topical NSAIDs are more effective than placebo during the initial 2 weeks of treatment only.[79] The authors concluded that the evidence available indicates that topical NSAIDs are inferior to oral NSAIDs during the first week of treatment.[79] A separate meta-analysis reviewed the evidence for the use of topical NSAIDs for chronic musculoskeletal pain and concluded that topical NSAIDs are effective and safe in treating chronic musculoskeletal conditions for 2 weeks.[80] Another meta-analysis on the use of topical NSAIDs for OA suggested that of the four studies that compared a topical NSAID with placebo or vehicle in patients with OA of the knee, pain relief did occur for a longer period with the topical NSAID than with placebo but that the results were not uniform for the preparations reviewed.[81]

Health care professionals and especially prescribers must be aware of the fact that topical salicylates are used by patients in over-the-counter preparations. A meta-analysis reviewed the limited data available from trials of musculoskeletal and arthritic pain and concluded that topically applied rubefacients containing salicylates have moderate to poor efficacy in relieving acute and chronic pain. The authors emphasized that estimates of the efficacy of these rubefacients are currently unreliable because of a lack of appropriately designed clinical trials.[82] A randomized controlled study completed in Europe with the topical NSAID eltenac examined its effect in comparison to placebo in 237 patients with knee OA and concluded that use of topical eltenac for the treatment of OA of the knee versus placebo is safe and effective.[83] In an additional clinical trial, topical eltenac gel was compared with oral diclofenac and placebo in patients with knee OA. Each active treatment resulted in analgesia superior to that achieved with placebo, but as reported in the meta-analysis mentioned earlier, the incidence of gastrointestinal side effects was notably lower in the group treated with topical eltenac gel than in those treated with the oral NSAID diclofenac.[84] Additional studies have demonstrated that topical diclofenac may be effective in reducing the pain associated with various types of degenerative joint disease.[85-87]

Other topical agents have been studied for these musculoskeletal pain conditions as well. Capsaicin 0.025% cream was determined to be no better than the vehicle (not active) cream in a randomized, double-blind study of 30 patients with pain in the temporomandibular joint.[88] A randomized controlled study of a topical cream containing glucosamine sulfate, chondroitin sulfate, and camphor for OA of the knee showed a significant reduction in pain in the treatment group after 8 weeks when compared with the placebo group.[89]

Although a published case series reported the potential benefit of "topical" morphine in the management of chronic OA-related pain, this report emphasized that morphine or its metabolites, or both, were identifiable in the urine of treated patients, thus calling into question how truly "topical" this preparation was given its systemic effects.[90]

LOW BACK AND MYOFASCIAL PAIN

Regrettably, substantially fewer studies examining the use of topical analgesics for low back pain or myofascial pain, two very common conditions, have been published. A randomized, double-blind, placebo-controlled study comparing the use of topical capsaicin with placebo in 154 patients with CLBP resulted in 60.8% of capsaicin-treated patients versus 42.1% of placebo patients experiencing 30% pain relief after 3 weeks of treatment ($P < 0.02$).[91] Unfortunately, additional studies have been published in abstract form only—two are novel (one will be mentioned) because they each involve the use of a local anesthetic for conditions not typically thought of as being responsive to this form of treatment. In one, a multicenter, open-label study involving 120 patients with acute (<6 weeks), subacute (<3 months), short-term chronic (3 to 12 months), or long-term chronic (>12 months) low back pain with four 5% lidocaine patches applied to the most painful areas in the low back region demonstrated that during the 6-week study period the majority of patients experienced moderate or a greater degree of pain relief.[71]

OTHER USES OF TOPICAL ANALGESICS

It is important to note other painful conditions in which topical analgesics have been used even if the number of patients studied in each study was relatively small. Various types of topical analgesics, including opiates, may be helpful in reducing the pain associated with pressure ulcers or dressing changes.[92-98] Controlled studies have demonstrated the benefit of EMLA cream in reducing the pain associated with circumcision and venipuncture and, in addition, in reducing the pain associated with breast cancer surgery.[5,99] At least two studies have suggested that either topical ketamine or topical morphine can be used for mucositis-associated pain following chemotherapy or radiation therapy in patients with head and neck carcinoma.[100,101] Topical opiates have been reported to reduce pain in two children with epidermolysis bullosa.[102] In one report, the analgesic effect of menthol, an ingredient common in many over-the-counter analgesic preparations, is hypothesized to be the result of activation of κ-opioid receptors.[103] Burn pain has been reported to be treated effectively with a topical loperamide preparation.[104] Two randomized controlled studies—one involving postoperative pain (diclofenac patch) and the other involving wound pain treatment (capsicum plaster topically applied at acupuncture sites)—have been published as well.[105,106] Central neuropathic itch was treated successfully with the 5% lidocaine patch in a single case report.[107] The results of an enriched enrollment study in which an open-label initial study led to the randomization of responders in a placebo-controlled study of the use of either 4% amitriptyline/2% ketamine cream, 2% amitriptyline/1% ketamine cream, or placebo in patients with PHN demonstrated that after 3 weeks of treatment the average daily pain intensity was lower in patients receiving the higher-concentration combination cream than in those receiving the lower concentration combination or placebo ($P = 0.026$ for the high-concentration cream vs. placebo).[108] Plasma levels of either drug were detected in less than 10% of the patients receiving active treatment. An open-label study of the use of a 0.25% capsaicin topical agent in a lidocaine-containing vehicle in 25 patients with painful diabetic polyneuropathy and 7 patients with PHN demonstrated pain relief in the majority of patients who were studied.[109] In a noncontrolled study of 23 patients with acute migraine headache, 0.1% capsaicin gel applied topically was helpful in reducing mild or moderate pain.[110] In a randomized, double-blind study assessing 154 patients with chronic pain from lateral epicondylitis, topical glyceryl trinitrate (0.72 mg/day) was found to provide statistically significantly greater pain relief after 8 weeks when compared with placebo.[111] In a study of 52 patients with chronic pain secondary to chronic Achilles tendinopathy, patients who had been treated with topical glyceryl trinitrate for 6 months were more likely 3 years after treatment ended to have less pain and more function than those who had been treated with placebo.[112] Published reports of the use of topical phenytoin for the treatment of pain from superficial burns or chronic leg ulcers are noted as well.[113,114]

CONCLUSION

The clinician should consider the use of topical analgesics for a variety of painful conditions. Of note is that the number of FDA-approved topical agents has increased. Off-label use of the available therapies must include careful consideration of the potential risks, as well the benefits of such. Given the repeated observations that topical analgesic use is generally associated with a more desirable side effect profile than are orally, transdermally, parenterally, or intrathecally administered analgesics, this factor should be considered when developing a pain management treatment regimen for individual patients, especially when pharmacotherapy will be involved. Certainly, additional large, well-designed studies that include comparative trials with nontopical analgesics would be helpful to better understand the role of topical analgesics in the management of acute and chronic pain.

KEY POINTS

- In contrast to using a systemic analgesic, use of a topical analgesic is less likely to be associated with systemic side effects since the systemic concentration of a topical analgesic is likely to be lower than that with systemic administration.
- Topical analgesics are *not* equivalent to transdermal analgesics.
- Despite the localized, peripheral mechanism of action of a topical analgesic, there may be central nervous system effects related to the topical analgesic.
- The clinical benefit of topical analgesics for a broad range of chronic pain conditions has clearly been established.

SUGGESTED READINGS

Argoff CE. New analgesics for neuropathic pain: the lidocaine patch. *Clin J Pain.* 2000;16(suppl 2):S62-S65.

Attal N, Brasseur L, Chauvin M, et al. Effects of single and repeated applications of a eutectic mixture of local anesthetics (EMLA) cream on spontaneous and evoked pain in post-herpetic neuralgia. *Pain.* 1999;81:203-209.

Galer BS, Rowbotham MC, Perander J, et al. Topical diclofenac patch significantly reduces pain associated with minor sports injuries: results of a randomized, double-blind, placebo-controlled, multicenter study. *J Pain Symptom Manage.* 2000;19:287-294.

Galer BS, Jensen MP, Ma T, et al. The lidocaine patch 5% effectively treats all neuropathic pain qualities: results of a randomized, double-blind, vehicle-controlled, 3-week efficacy study with use of the Neuropathic Pain Scale. *Clin J Pain.* 2002;18:297-301.

Mason L, Moore RA, Derry S, et al. Systematic review of topical capsaicin for the treatment of chronic pain. *BMJ.* 2004;328:991-996.

Rowbotham MC, Davies PS, Verkempinck C, et al. Lidocaine patch: double-blind controlled study of a new treatment method for post-herpetic neuralgia. *Pain.* 1996;65:39-44.

Sawynok J, Esser MJ, Reid AR. Antidepressants as analgesics: an overview of central and peripheral mechanisms of action. *J Psychiatry Neurosci.* 2001;26:21-29.

Watson CPN. Topical capsaicin as an adjuvant analgesic. *J Pain Symptom Manage.* 1994;9:425-433.

The references for this chapter can be found at www.expertconsult.com.

43 Neuraxial Agents

Robert W. Hurley | Dustin Anderson | Steven P. Cohen

Medication delivery to the spinal cord or the dorsal nerve roots via the intrathecal or epidural route exploits the endogenous pharmacology of the neuraxis to relieve pain in patients. These methods of delivery require a certain degree of expertise and are commonly used by anesthesiologists and interventional pain management specialists. In 1885, Leonard Corning described the first neuraxial administration of a medication, first in a dog and then in a man suffering from "seminal incontinence."[1] Fourteen years later, Augustus Bier (Fig. 43.1) reported the first case whereby cocaine was administered intrathecally to provide surgical anesthesia for lower limb orthopedic procedures.[2] The first use of a neuraxial technique to treat chronic pain was in 1901 when Sicard administered a local anesthetic epidurally via the caudal route.[3] Another significant breakthrough occurred in 1942 when Manalan used a catheter to continuously administer medication for labor analgesia.[4] The epidural injection of steroids for the treatment of sciatica was first described in 1953.[5] Several years after the discovery of the endogenous opioid receptors and their respective agonists, Wang reported treating cancer pain with intrathecal morphine.[6]

This chapter focuses on the current pharmacologic agents that are administered into the epidural or intrathecal space to produce antinociception (in animals) or analgesia (in humans), as well as future potential agents. The outcomes of neuraxial anesthesia and analgesia on postsurgical morbidity, as well as long-term neuraxial analgesia either by intrathecal pump or a tunneled epidural catheter, are covered elsewhere in this text and, hence, are not addressed in this chapter.

PERIPHERAL NERVE NEUROTRANSMITTERS AND THE SPINAL CORD

A variety of mechanical, thermal, or chemical stimuli can result in the sensation of pain. Information about these painful or noxious stimuli is carried to higher brain centers by receptors and neurons that are distinct from those that carry innocuous somatic sensory information. Small-diameter A-delta and C fibers primarily transmit nociceptive information. Neurotransmission by A-delta and C fibers is accomplished via the release of numerous peptides, including substance P, calcitonin gene-related peptide, galanin, vasoactive intestinal peptide, and somatostatin into the spinal cord. The excitatory amino acid, glutamate, is also present within small-diameter primary afferents and can be released by noxious stimulation, resulting in the activation of second-order neurons in the dorsal horn of the spinal cord.[7] The presynaptic nerve terminals of primary afferents in the spinal cord are potential therapeutic targets. They possess numerous receptor systems that can enhance transmission by increasing the release of excitatory amino acids and other transmitters, activating voltage-gated calcium channels and purinergic receptors, and inhibiting pathways involved in the modulation of pain, such as alpha$_2$-adrenergic, cholinergic, serotonergic, and opioid receptors as well as gamma-aminobutyric acid (GABA) systems.[8-12]

Primary afferent neurons release neurotransmitters, activating postsynaptic receptors on second-order projection neurons in the spinal cord (Fig. 43.2).[13] Second-order neurons in the dorsal horn possess a wide variety of neurotransmitter receptors. A subset of these receptors, including those involving substance P and the excitatory amino acid glutamate (e.g., N-methyl-D-aspartate [NMDA] and α-amino-3-hydroxy-5-methylisoxazole-4-propionic acid [AMPA] kainate, mGluR), can induce depolarization of the neuron, leading to increased nociceptive transmission. Activation of other receptors such as opioid, GABA$_A$-ergic and serotoninergic incites hyperpolarization of postsynaptic neurons, thereby inhibiting the transmission of noxious stimuli. Neurotransmission by second-order neurons on bulbar or thalamic targets is primarily through glutamate, resulting in depolarization of postsynaptic AMPA and NMDA receptor-containing neurons.[14]

NEURAXIAL AGENTS

Medications approved by the Food and Drug Administration (FDA) can be used for a multitude of purposes, including not only the approved indication, but for off-label indications as well. This practice is common with systemically delivered medications. Unfortunately, it has also become common practice to use medications approved for systemic use in anatomic sites that have not been tested for safety. These sites include the intrathecal or epidural compartments that can result in actual or potential risk to the spinal cord of patients.[15] During 2007-2008, the journals–*Anesthesia & Analgesia, Anesthesiology, and Regional Anesthesiology and Pain Medicine*–revised their instructions to authors to address this concern and established the following policy:[16]

1. Is the drug approved by the FDA for this indication?
2. If the drug is not approved, is it widely used off-label (e.g., in tens of thousands of patients)? [The] editorial board concluded that if multiple textbooks indicated that the drug could be safely used in a given manner, this was a suitable surrogate demonstration that the drug was widely used for the indication.

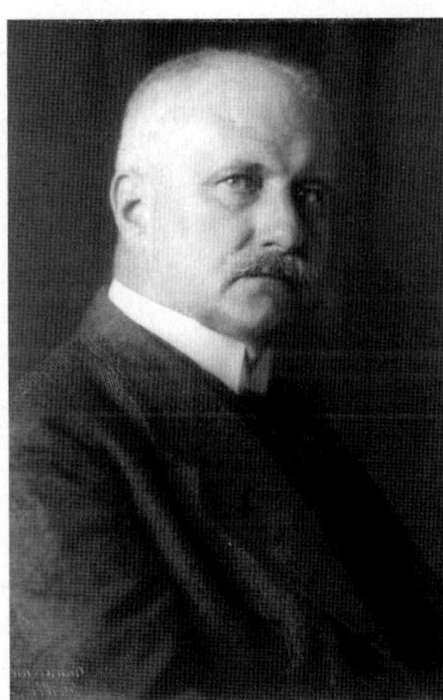

Figure 43.1 August Karl Gustav Bier (November 24, 1861–March 12, 1949) was a German surgeon and a pioneer of spinal anesthesia.

3. If neither 1 nor 2 applies, was the study performed with an "Investigator Investigational New Drug (IND)" from the FDA or an equivalent regulatory authority?

This chapter is divided into three categories: (1) medications with FDA approval for neuraxial administration; (2) medications without FDA approval but which are commonly used; and (3) experimental medications that have neither received approval nor are in common use.

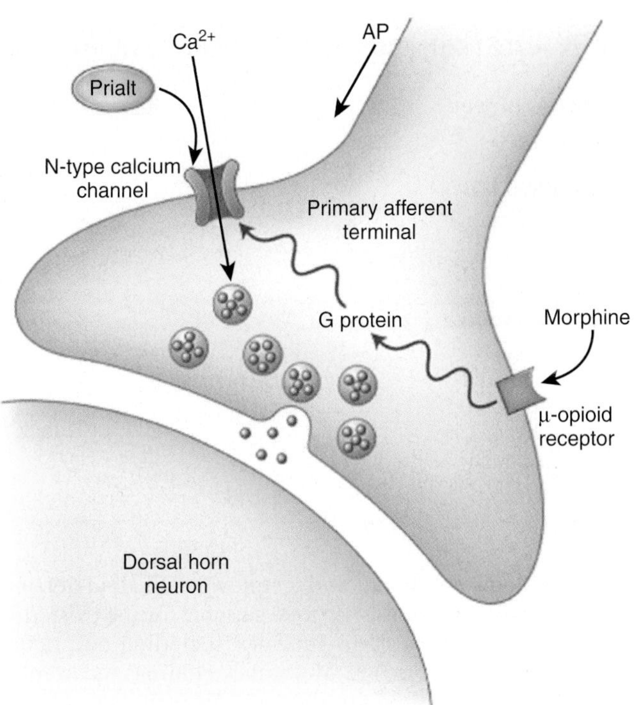

Figure 43.2 A nerve terminal of a primary afferent nociceptor is depicted, which is stimulated by noxious stimuli in peripheral tissues, such as the skin or joints. Transmitters (e.g., glutamate and substance P) released from these neurons stimulate secondary neurons in the dorsal horn of the spinal cord, which send the noxious signal to the brain. (From Lawson EF, Wallace MS. Current developments in intraspinal agents for cancer and noncancer pain. *Curr Pain Headache Rep.* 2010;14:8-16.)

LOCAL ANESTHETICS (BOX 43.1)

The most widely used drugs for neuraxial analgesia are local anesthetics, which produce a reversible conduction blockade of impulses in peripheral and central nerves. Local anesthetics have proven to be safe and reliable in interrupting nerve impulse conduction in both peripheral and central nerves. Local anesthetics are most commonly used to provide surgical anesthesia, postoperative pain relief, and relief of cancer pain. The discussion of local anesthetic agents will be brief.

Electrical impulses in the form of action potentials are conducted along nerve fibers. The propagation of electrical impulses along nerve fibers in the form of action potentials is responsible for transmitting sensory and motor information along the nerves. Action potentials are dependent on maintaining a resting membrane potential of approximately 60 to 70 mV, which requires various pumps and channels to sustain an electrochemical gradient.[17] The most important channel is the voltage-gated sodium channel, which allows the influx of sodium ions during the depolarization phase of the action potential, thus enabling an impulse to travel down the nerve fiber. These sodium channels are complex three-dimensional structures integrated into the membrane lipid bilayer of the nerve cells.[18] Local anesthetic agents act by interrupting the propagation of an impulse, thereby inhibiting the nerve conduction of a painful stimulus.[19] Local anesthetics gain access to the sodium channel from either the plasma or cytoplasmic side of the channel protein, and bind within the pore of the channel. The binding of sodium channels by local anesthetics is state dependent. The local anesthetic can bind to the channel when it is open (active), closed (inactivated), or in a resting state. However, the receptor has the highest affinity when the channel is open or closed and the lowest affinity in the resting state. These processes are not sensory specific; thus, local anesthetics are capable of blocking the transmission of all nerve fibers, not just A-delta and C fibers. Therefore, the potential for motor blockade, as well as sensory blockade, limits the use of these agents.

Box 43.1 FDA Package Insert Labeling

Intrathecal	*Epidural*
Bupivacaine with 7.5% dextrose	Lidocaine
Lidocaine with 7.5% dextrose	Bupivacaine
	Ropivacaine
	Mepivacaine
	Chloroprocaine

OPIOIDS (BOX 43.2)

Opioid analgesics exert their actions through the inhibition of target cell activity. The existence of multiple types of opioid receptors was originally proposed by Martin and colleagues.[20] Subsequent studies using both in vitro and in vivo

Box 43.2 Intrathecal Opioid Medications

FDA Approved

Morphine

Common Use

Hydromorphone
Fentanyl
Sufentanil

Investigational

Methadone
Meperidine
Levorphanol
Butorphanol
Oxymorphone
Pentazocine

pharmacologic methods, and employing alkaloid-derived and synthetic compounds, provide support for the existence of multiple opioid receptor subtypes, including mu, delta, and kappa receptors.[21-23] Molecular cloning techniques have, thus far, identified three gene families that encode for these receptors.[24-26] In addition, an "orphan" opioid receptor (ORL1), which shares substantial sequence homology but does not bind prototypic opioid receptor agonists with high affinity, has also been identified[27] and structured.[28] All of the opioid receptors belong to the GTP-binding protein superfamily of metabotropic receptors. Agonist binding to opioid receptors results in activation of inwardly rectifying potassium channels, the inhibition of N-type and L-type calcium channels, or the inhibition of adenylate cyclase activity, all processes by which neuronal excitability can be suppressed.

Whereas peripherally located opioid receptors have been identified, the predominant analgesic sites are believed to reside in the central nervous system (CNS). In the brain, these receptor sites include the brainstem, thalamus, forebrain, and mesencephalon. In the spinal cord, they include the postsynaptic receptors located on cells originating in the dorsal horn, as well as presynaptic receptors found on the spinal terminals of primary afferent fibers.[9]

The effects of opioids are determined not only by their affinity for endogenous receptors but also by their ability to reach those receptors. The onset of analgesia is similar for intrathecal and epidural narcotics, suggesting that the penetration of neural tissue—and not the meninges—is the rate-limiting step. Intrathecal opioids exert their analgesic properties by presynaptically inhibiting the release of glutamate, substance P, and calcitonin gene-related peptide, molecules believed to be responsible for transmitting nociceptive signals across synapses. Epidurally administered opioids may operate via an additional mechanism. The systemic absorption of an epidural bolus of lipophilic opioids (e.g., fentanyl and sufentanil) is similar to that which follows an intramuscular injection and may play a role in the analgesic effects.[29,30] The conflicting theories regarding how epidural lipophilic opioids exert their pain-relieving properties may be partially explained by the differing modes of administration. For example, a bolus of epidural fentanyl appears to produce analgesia mostly via

Table 43.1 Dosing of Intrathecal Opioid Agents

Maximum 24-Hour Dose	Maximum Concentration
Morphine	20 mg/mL
15 mg/day	
Hydromorphone	10 mg/mL
4 mg/day	
Fentanyl	2 mg/mL
—No known upper limit	
Sufentanil	50 μg/mL
—No known upper limit	

spinal mechanisms, whereas uptake into the systemic circulation plays a major role in the analgesic effects produced by continuous epidural infusion. In contrast, hydrophilic opioids as morphine are more likely to diffuse across dural membranes where their primary analgesic effect is exerted through receptors in the dorsal horn.[31,32]

Lipid solubility determines, in part, several other important characteristics of intrathecal opioids, including the spread of analgesia and side effects. Opioids that are highly water soluble, such as morphine, exhibit a greater degree of rostral spread when injected into the subarachnoid or epidural space than lipid-soluble compounds, so that in pain conditions requiring higher spinal levels or more extensive coverage, the degree of analgesia they confer may be superior. Conversely, because many of the adverse effects of spinal opioids, such as nausea, vomiting, and delayed respiratory depression, are the result of interaction with opioid receptors in the brain, the more water-soluble compounds are associated with a higher incidence of these problems.

Whereas the earliest studies evaluating the chronic use of intrathecal opioids were conducted in patients suffering from cancer pain, other studies have found intrathecal and epidural narcotics to be effective in nonmalignant pain as well.[33-35] These conditions include not only nociceptive pain but also neuropathic pain, a heterogeneous group of disorders originally believed to be resistant to narcotics. Certain aspects of neuropathic pain, such as tactile allodynia, may be less responsive to the effects of spinal opiates. Therefore, many neuropathic conditions require adding nonopioid adjuvants to spinal opioids for successful pain relief.[36-39] The caveat with the treatment of nonmalignant pain via intrathecal opioids is that these patients have a higher likelihood of complications resulting from the opioid therapy because of their normal life expectancy compared to those with cancer. Aside from the common intrathecal opioid side effects such as tolerance, constipation, sweating, nausea, and urinary retention, these patients are at risk for the development of intrathecal granulomas.[40] Factors that are positively associated with the development of catheter tip granuloma include drug dosage, drug concentration, and the duration of intrathecal opioid therapy. In 2008, Deer and associates[41] published recommendations for the maximum daily dose and maximum concentration of intrathecal medications (Table 43.1).

When opioids are administered directly into the cerebrospinal fluid, only a fraction of the systemic dose is required, as there are no anatomic barriers to be crossed, and vascular reuptake is slow. Not all side effects of intrathecal opioids are

Box 43.3 Intrathecal Calcium Channel Medications

FDA Approved

Ziconotide

Common Use

None

Investigational

Gabapentin
Verapamil

dose related, but in many instances, the drastic reduction in dosage translates into reduced side effects. In fact, one of the primary indications for a trial with intrathecal or epidural narcotics is a good analgesic response to systemic opioids coupled with intractable side effects. Among the adverse opioid effects reduced by switching from oral formulations to spinal administration are sedation and constipation. Effects that may be increased include pruritus, urinary retention, and edema. The mechanisms contributing to the various adverse effects of opioids are incompletely understood but probably multifactorial and include those that are mediated via interaction with specific opioid receptors and those that are not. Undesirable effects not mediated by opioid receptors, such as CNS excitation and hyperalgesia, cannot be reversed with naloxone. The incidence of various opioid-induced side effects depends on a number of different factors including the opioid infused, route of administration and dosage, extent of disease, concurrent drug (e.g., oral opioids, adjuvants), age, concomitant medical problems, and prior exposure to opioids. The most frequent side effects of intrathecal morphine are constipation, sweating, urinary retention, nausea and vomiting, and disturbances of the libido.[42-45]

CALCIUM CHANNEL ANTAGONISTS (BOX 43.3)

Voltage-dependent calcium channel (VDCC) conduction plays an integral role in pain transmission. Diversity among these voltage-gated calcium channels was originally described through differences in the biophysical properties of calcium currents recorded from individual neurons. Multiple distinct voltage-gated calcium currents were observed, including the L-type responsive to dihydropyridines, the T-type responsive to ethosuximide, and the N-type and P/Q-type responsive to conotoxins. Molecular cloning has led to the identification of multiple genes encoding the calcium channels that correspond to the biophysical and pharmacologic profiles of the receptor subtypes. VDCCs are located in the plasma membrane of all excitable cells, including the neurons of the peripheral and central nervous system. These calcium channels are found in high concentrations in the dorsal horn of the spinal cord and dorsal root ganglia.[46]

The neuraxial administration of some VDCC modulators has been shown to produce antinociception, antiallodynia, and antihyperalgesia in animals. High threshold VDCCs, including N- and P/Q channels, are primarily found at synaptic sites involved in the release of transmitters; L-type channels are mainly observed at cell bodies and dendrites.[47,48] Several VDCCs have been found to co-localize in the same neuron; therefore, antagonists to a given channel type usually block only a fraction of the VDCCs present and hence may have additive effects when combined. Finally, the relative importance of the various channel types depends on the functional status of the neuron. For instance, in acute models of nociception in uninjured naïve animals, there is a large body of evidence implicating N types, limited evidence for L types, and no evidence for P/Q types in producing antinociception. However, under conditions of persistent nociception induced in animals by chemical, inflammatory, or neuropathic stimuli, all three of these subtypes have been found to have anti-allodynic or anti-hyperalgesic properties.[49,50] Although the physiologic and pharmacologic properties of VDCCs are largely determined by the molecular identity of the $\alpha 1$ subunit, the auxiliary subunits, including a_2d_1, also play a substantial role in the receptors' characteristics. Gabapentin and pregabalin are two medications originally designed as structural analogs of GABA; however, neither drug acts as an agonist at $GABA_A$ or $GABA_B$ receptors, and neither drug acutely alters GABA uptake. It is likely that their analgesic effects are mediated at the a_2d_1 subunits of VDCCs, for which both have a substantial affinity.[51,52] Intrathecal gabapentin has no effect on an animal's nociceptive threshold in the uninjured state, but it does possess antihyperalgesic and anti-allodynic properties in animal models of chronic pain.[53,54] A substantial portion of the effects exerted by gabapentin are mediated by the N-type VDCC.[53,54]

Ziconotide is a synthetic form of the peptide, ω-conotoxin MVIIA, which is isolated from the venom of the marine cone snail, *Conus magus*.[55] It potently blocks N-type VDCCs in vitro and inhibits wind-up. The process of wind-up involves the activation of spinal NMDA receptors after injury, which induces a state of facilitated processing from repetitive small afferent fiber stimulation. This in turn leads to an increased response to high and low threshold stimulation and enhanced receptor field size. Ziconotide is the first member in the new drug class of selective N-type voltage-sensitive calcium channel blockers. It has been approved by the U.S. Food and Drug Administration and the European Medicines Agency for intrathecal treatment of patients with severe chronic pain that is refractory to other treatment modalities.[56] Ziconotide blocks N-type calcium channels in the spinal cord and inhibits release of pain neurotransmitters from the central terminals of primary afferent neurons. By way of this mechanism, ziconotide has been found to effectively reduce pain. In a multicenter, double-blind, placebo-controlled study evaluating intrathecal ziconotide for the treatment of refractory pain in 111 patients with cancer and acquired immunodeficiency syndrome (AIDS), Staats and colleagues[57] found that the treatment group obtained significantly enhanced pain relief compared to the control group (53% versus 18% improvement). The observation that there was no loss of efficacy for ziconotide in the maintenance phase is consistent with animal studies showing the absence of tolerance with calcium channel blockers. The most common side effects noted in this study were confusion, somnolence, and urinary retention; however, 97% of patients receiving ziconotide experience side effects, and 30% had serious adverse events. All side effects were reversible, with their incidence decreasing after the initial dosing period.

Table 43.2 Intrathecal Calcium Channel Agents: Dosing

Maximum 24-Hour Dose	Maximum Concentration
Ziconotide 19.2 mg/day	100 μg/mL

In a randomized, double-blind, placebo-controlled trial, Wallace and colleagues demonstrated that intrathecal (IT) ziconotide provides relief in patients suffering from severe chronic nonmalignant pain who are unresponsive to conventional therapy.[58] Patients were treated over a 6-day period and were found to respond to dosing of 0.1 μg/hr to 2.4 μg/hr. The original starting dose of 0.4 μg/hr was decreased due to a high incidence of side effects. The mean reduction in pain score from baseline was 31.2% in the treatment group compared to 6.0% in the placebo group. Patients in the treatment group reported suffering more side effects, including abnormal gait, amblyopia, dizziness, nausea, nystagmus, pain, urinary retention, and vomiting. However, Rauck and associates[59] demonstrated that slow titration can provide comparable pain relief while minimizing the side effects experienced by patients. Wallace and colleagues[60] showed that ziconotide could be safely given for long-term treatment of refractory pain. More than 644 patients with severe chronic pain participated in this open-label, multicenter longer-term trial. Thirty-two percent of patients receiving ziconotide for over 360 days, with a dose range between 0.048 μg/day and 240 μg/day, experienced greater than or equal to 32.7% improvement in pain scores. Although only FDA approved as single therapy (Table 43.2), emerging evidence suggests that ziconotide can be safely combined when administered intrathecally with baclofen, morphine, sufentanil, and bupivacaine.[61-63] Webster and colleagues added morphine to stable IT ziconotide therapy in 25 patients, which resulted in a mean 26.3% reduction in pain and a 49.1% reduction in opioid consumption at week 4 of treatment. This study suggests a synergism between morphine and ziconotide.[64] When IT ziconotide is combined with other drugs such as opioids and baclofen, the stability declines, which may necessitate more frequent refills.[65]

More recently, ziconotide has been anecdotally reported to successfully treat neuropathic pain and trigeminal neuralgia.[66] The main limitations regarding the use of IT ziconotide are its steep cost and the high incidence (> 80% in many studies) of side effects, which can include the neurologic, psychiatric, cardiovascular, gastrointestinal, and genitourinary systems. Although in some guidelines ziconotide is now considered to be a first-line treatment for chronic pain,[33,67] this therapy has an extremely narrow therapeutic window with substantial side effects and should be reserved for patients for whom other agents and therapies have been exhausted.

The epidural administration of VDCC modulators has also been examined. In a double-blind study conducted in healthy cohorts, adding a low dose (5 mg) of the L-type calcium channel blocker, verapamil, to epidural bupivacaine both pre- and postsurgical incision was found to reduce postoperative analgesic requirements in patients undergoing abdominal surgery.[68] In a case report, Filos and collaborators[69] described a modest and short-lived analgesic benefit for epidural nimodipine in two terminal cancer patients. The authors reported significant discomfort upon administration, but with no increased incidence of sedation, mood disturbances, or hypotension.

Box 43.4 Intrathecal GABAergic Medications

FDA Approved

Baclofen

Common Use

None

Investigational

Muscimol
Midazolam

GAMMA-AMINOBUTYRIC ACID AGONISTS (BOX 43.4)

Three types of GABA receptor are currently recognized: $GABA_A$, $GABA_B$, and $GABA_C$. Only $GABA_A$ and $GABA_B$ receptors are present in significant quantities within the CNS. The $GABA_A$ receptor is a ligand-gated ion channel. Activation of this receptor by GABA results in an influx of chloride ions and stabilization of the membrane potential, which decreases neuronal excitability. The receptor possesses two binding sites for GABA, as well as sites at which barbiturates, inhalational anesthetics, neurosteroids, and benzodiazepines bind to modulate the action of GABA. The receptor itself is a pentameric arrangement of different subunits. In contrast, the $GABA_B$ receptor is a metabotropic receptor. Activation of the $GABA_B$ receptor by GABA results in activation of inwardly rectifying potassium channels, inhibition of calcium channels, or inhibition of adenylate cyclase activity, all of which suppress neuronal excitability.

In laboratory animals, $GABA_A$ agonists including muscimol, isoguvacine, and midazolam have anti-allodynic and antihyperalgesic effects in chronic pain models, whereas the $GABA_A$ antagonists, bicuculline and picrotoxin, induce allodynia and hyperalgesia in naïve rats. However, $GABA_A$ receptors are also closely linked to large-diameter afferents and, thus, are likely involved in modulating innocuous sensations as well. Similar to $GABA_A$ receptors, $GABA_B$ receptors are found in greatest abundance in the superficial dorsal horn of the spinal cord. Within the GABAergic system, nociceptive transmission is primarily regulated primarily by $GABA_B$ receptor activity. The $GABA_B$ receptor agonist, baclofen, blocks the activity of peripheral C and A-delta nociceptive fibers. Further, in the spinal cord, $GABA_B$ receptors are found on interneurons as well as on terminals from primary afferent neurons. $GABA_B$ receptor agonists administered via the intrathecal or epidural route produce pre- and postsynaptic inhibition, and therefore block the release of glutamate, substance P, and calcitonin gene-related peptide (CGRP) from primary afferents, and GABA from interneurons.

In naïve animals, the intrathecal administration of antagonists to either receptor increases pain behaviors, suggesting that tonic release of GABA in the spinal cord prevents innocuous stimuli from being perceived as noxious. In animal models of acute and persistent nociception, $GABA_B$ agonists such as baclofen produce antinociception and anti-allodynia, respectively, at doses in which no motor impairment is observed.[70,71] In contrast, the highly selective $GABA_A$ agonist, muscimol, was found to be effective only in animal models of persistent nociception.[72] Interestingly, in the same study, midazolam, the only $GABA_A$ agonist presently available for human use, was ineffective in either acute or persistent pain models at doses that did not produce substantial motor impairment. In summary, the results from animal studies suggest that both $GABA_A$ and $GABA_B$ receptor agonists could be used to treat chronic pain.

In human studies, both $GABA_A$ and $GABA_B$ agonists have been shown to contain analgesic effects when injected into the intrathecal or epidural space. The literature shows that the neuraxial administration of $GABA_A$ agonists in combination with local anesthetics increases the duration of motor and sensory block, increases the time to first analgesic request, and decreases postoperative analgesic requirements. The administration of the $GABA_A$ agonist, midazolam, via either the intrathecal or the epidural route in combination with a mixture of other analgesics, including local anesthetics and opioids, was found to reduce opioid requirements and enhance postoperative analgesia for a variety of different surgical procedures.[73-77] Ghai and associates[78] found that adding 20 µg/kg/hr of midazolam to a continuous postoperative epidural of 0.125% bupivacaine reduced the requirement for rescue analgesia in children following upper abdominal and flank surgery. In a meta-analysis of 13 randomized controlled trials involving 672 patients, Ho and Ismail[75] found that adding midazolam to other spinal medications delayed the time to request for rescue analgesia and reduced the incident of nausea and vomiting. A prospective, randomized, double-blind study by Shadangi and associates[77] involving patients undergoing elective lower abdominal, lower limb, and gynecologic procedures found that adding midazolam to bupivacaine significantly improved analgesia. One hundred patients were randomized to receive a combination of either 0.4 mL (2 mg) midazolam with 3 mL of 0.5% bupivacaine or 0.4 mL normal saline with 3 mL of 0.5% bupivacaine. The duration of sensory blockade was prolonged in the group receiving midazolam by over 25 minutes without increasing motor blockade. In a double-blind study evaluating the effects of adding intrathecal midazolam to bupivacaine in patients undergoing hemorrhoidectomy, the addition of midazolam was found to expedite the onset of spinal analgesia in a dose-dependent manner.[79] Other studies have found intrathecal midazolam to be effective in treating chronic mechanical low back pain, musculoskeletal pain, and neurogenic pain.[80] In an open-label study, Prochazka and colleagues[81] demonstrated the effectiveness of midazolam in the treatment of chronic low back pain and failed back surgery syndrome. Midazolam 2 to 5 mg was administered 500 times in 126 patients from 1995 to 2010. The analgesic effect lasted 9.7 weeks, with 65% of patients experiencing relief lasting 4 weeks or longer. The administration of subarachnoid midazolam was shown to be effective in treating pain associated with chronic, nonmalignant pain.[80]

The safety of neuraxial administration of midazolam is controversial. Numerous animal studies have shown evidence of neurotoxicity with intrathecal midazolam. Svensson and associates[82] found histologic evidence of neuronal death in the spinal cords of rats after 20 consecutive days of 100 µg intrathecal injections of midazolam. Unfortunately, the relative doses and concentrations of midazolam used in these animal studies were many times higher than those used in human studies. Malinovsky and colleagues[83] reported that midazolam (1 mg/mL) produced histologic pathology that was greater than that of lidocaine or saline controls. Similar results were obtained by Erdine and colleagues,[84] who found that rabbits infused with both preservative-containing and preservative-free intrathecal midazolam (300 µg daily, 1 mg/mL) over 5 days displayed vascular and other histologic spinal cord lesions on microscopic examination. Part of the controversy revolves around the pH of the medications administered. In an attempt to resolve this controversy, Bozkurt and colleagues[85] administered normal saline, midazolam, and a saline vehicle control with the same acidic pH as midazolam epidurally in newborn rabbits. During electron microscopy examination on days 2 and 7, both the acidic midazolam and saline groups displayed significant pathologic spinal cord changes, such as degeneration of vacuoles, cytoplasm, and neurofilaments, disruption of myelin sheaths, lysis of cell membranes, perivascular edema, and pyknosis of nuclei. In contrast, the normal pH saline group displayed normal histology on spinal cord sectioning. More recent literature evaluating multiple doses of commercially available concentrations of midazolam in two species of animals found no histopathologic or behavior differences compared with saline controls.[86] At present, the use of midazolam as a spinal analgesic is not FDA approved due to safety concerns. However, in clinical studies, there have been no reported adverse cardiovascular (hypotension or bradycardia), urologic (urinary hesitance or incontinence), or gastrointestinal (nausea or vomiting) side effects when compared to administering the local anesthetic alone.[13] Prochazka and associates[81] injected doses of 0.02 to 0.06 mg/kg into 14 patients with 10 administrations or more and reported that none of them displayed any clinical signs of neurotoxicity, such as bladder or bowel dysfunction, motor or sensory deficits, or new neuropathic pain. Canavero and colleagues[87] reported successful intrathecal treatment of neuropathic pain with midazolam in a 60-year-old woman. They reported that intrathecal midazolam ranging from 2 to 4.6 mg successfully controlled neuropathic pain for over 6½ years. In one human study involving 1100 patients who were either administered intrathecal local anesthetic or local anesthetic and midazolam 2 mg for surgery, the authors reported no increased incidence of postoperative neurologic signs or symptoms or any other difference in complication rates between the two groups.[88] Midazolam is currently considered a fifth-line neuraxial treatment for chronic pain.[89]

Numerous studies support the use of neuraxial baclofen for spasticity in humans. There are multiple uncontrolled studies showing intrathecal baclofen to be effective for a variety of central pain conditions as well, including stroke, phantom limb pain, spinal cord injury, cerebral palsy, amyotrophic lateral sclerosis, and multiple sclerosis.[90-93] Intrathecal baclofen has also been found to be an effective treatment for peripheral neuropathic pain conditions, such complex regional pain syndrome.[94-96] In a small study by Lind and

Table 43.3 Intrathecal GABAergic Agents: Dosing

Maximum 24-Hour Dose	Maximum Concentration
Baclofen 2 mg/day	4 mg/mL

coworkers,[97] the authors found that the addition of intrathecal baclofen in patients being treated with spinal cord stimulation for neuropathic pain improved pain scores to a greater degree than concomitant treatment with oral baclofen. The beneficial effect of intrathecal baclofen was dose dependent, peaking at 50 μg. Furthermore, at follow-up Lind and colleagues[98] found that patients who were treated for a mean of 67 months enjoyed the same degree of pain relief, requiring only a modest (30%) dose increase. More recently, van Rijn and associates[99] found that intrathecal baclofen provides substantial improvement in patients suffering from dystonia and in those with complex regional pain syndrome (CRPS). Thirty-six patients received a pump for continuous intrathecal baclofen for 12 months. Patients experienced a decrease in pain and disability as well as an improved quality of life. However, patients did experience a high complication rate, most often associated with pump or catheter system defects. Intrathecal baclofen administration as a therapeutic modality remains promising and would benefit from more research.[100] Neuraxial baclofen has also been found to be beneficial in the treatment of musculoskeletal pain. Loubser and Akman found that intrathecal baclofen reduced musculoskeletal, but not neurogenic, pain in 12 patients with chronic spinal cord injury–related pain.[101] Based on the results of this study and the temporal disparity regarding its analgesic effects on central pain and muscle spasm, it is likely that different pain-relieving mechanisms exist for these two conditions.

At therapeutic doses, baclofen is associated with numerous adverse effects, including drowsiness, flaccidity, headache, confusion, hypotension, weight gain, constipation, nausea, urinary frequency, and sexual dysfunction.[102,103] Intrathecal baclofen overdose can lead to respiratory depression, seizures, obtundation, and, if not adequately treated, death. Withdrawal from abrupt cessation of intrathecal baclofen treatment can last days to weeks, or possibly longer,[104,105] and can also be life threatening. There is growing evidence to suggest that replacement with oral baclofen may not always be adequate to control the symptoms, possibly because oral baclofen does not reach the central concentrations near the range achieved with intrathecal administration.[104,106] Some studies suggest that tizanidine may represent a viable option for patients with spasticity and blood pressure lability, specifically with hypertension. Currently, there is animal model evidence to support intrathecal tizanidine for neuropathic pain, but it is not approved for use in humans. Baclofen is currently considered a fourth-line treatment for chronic pain (Table 43.3).[89]

ADRENERGIC AGONISTS (BOX 43.5)

Adrenergic agonists have analgesic effects when applied for the management of chronic pain. Alpha-adrenergic receptors are widely distributed throughout the body and consist of two clinically significant classes: $alpha_1$ and $alpha_2$. $Alpha_1$ receptors are found in the smooth muscle cells of the peripheral vasculature and play an essential role in the regulation of systemic vascular resistance;[107] they have no known significant role in analgesia. $Alpha_2$ receptors however, are present throughout the peripheral and central nervous system and play a substantial role in modulating pain signals. There are several known subunits of the alpha-receptor: 2a, 2b, and 2c. Clonidine binds to pre- and post-synaptic α2 receptors in the dorsal horn. Activation of these receptors depresses presynaptive C-fiber transmitter release and hyperpolarizes the postsynaptic membrane through the Gi-coupled potassium channel.[107,108] A different physiologic effect transpires, depending on the particular alpha subunit involved. The neuronal responses can be either inhibitory or excitatory.[109] For example, the 2b subtype produces hemodynamic responses (primarily hypotension), whereas the 2a receptor is responsible for analgesia.[109,110] The mechanism of action of neuraxial $alpha_2$ agonists is similar to that for opioids[110] in that they can exert effects on presynaptic and postsynaptic neurons. On the presynaptic neuron, they bind to $alpha_2$ receptors of primary afferent neurons, resulting in hyperpolarization and depressed release of neurotransmitters involved in pain transmission. On postsynaptic neurons, $alpha_2$ agonists hyperpolarize the cell by increasing the transmission of potassium through G_i-coupled potassium channels.[108] Among the alpha-adrenergic agonists used for analgesia, clonidine remains the prototypical nonselective $alpha_2$ agonist, partly because it has been the most studied (Table 43.4). Clonidine is a nonselective agonist that produces antinociception via interaction with the alpha 2a receptor. However, it also produces substantial hemodynamic side effects due to its interaction with the 2b receptor. A newer agent, dexmedetomidine, is a selective $alpha_{2a}$ receptor agonist that contains analgesic and sedative properties, with less respiratory depression and fewer cardiovascular effects.[111-114] Dexmedetomidine demonstrates increased selectivity of the alpha 2a subunit than previous alpha-adrenergic agonists.[112,115] Alpha-adrenergic agonists have also been shown to activate spinal cholinergic neurons,

Box 43.5 Intrathecal Adrenergic Medications

FDA Approved
None

Common Use
Clonidine

Investigational
Dexmedetomidine

Table 43.4 Intrathecal Adrenergic Agents: Dosing

Maximum 24-Hour Dose	Maximum Concentration
Clonidine 1 mg/day	2 mg/mL

which may contribute to their analgesic effects. In addition to their antinociceptive properties, $alpha_2$ agonists can produce dose-dependent sedation, presumably by inhibitory mechanisms involving the brainstem.[116,117]

$Alpha_2$ agonists have been administered intrathecally in humans since 1985. The antihypertensive medication, clonidine, is the most studied $alpha_2$ agonist for neuraxial use. Although it is FDA approved for epidural use only in cancer pain, clinical reports have shown it to be effective intrathecally and epidurally for nonmalignant pain as well.[118,119] Intrathecal clonidine has been reported to provide significant analgesia in combination with opioids for neuropathic pain and cancer pain, and it has been used in the pediatric population for these reasons.[119] Clonidine has not consistently been shown to be effective as a single agent, but studies have shown it to prolong and enhance the effects of spinal and epidural anesthesia when coadministered with local anesthetics.[120-122] When added to opioids, clonidine can extend the duration of pain relief for labor analgesia and postoperative pain.[123-125] However, for acute pain, the evidence that adding clonidine to an epidural or intrathecal opioid is more effective than either analgesic alone is weak and inconsistent. Neuraxial clonidine has shown efficacy in treating central pain and spasticity after spinal cord injury.[126] Studies show that dexmedetomidine prolongs local anesthetic motor and sensory blockade when compared to opioids.[125,126] $Alpha_2$ receptor agonists may also be suitable for patients suffering from neuropathic pain. In a randomized, placebo-controlled trial evaluating epidural clonidine in refractory reflex sympathetic dystrophy, Rauck and colleagues[127] found that 300 µg of clonidine was equally effective but associated with less side effects than 700 µg.

Wu and collaborators[128] compared preoperative epidural clonidine followed by patient-controlled epidural analgesia (PCEA) with clonidine, morphine, and ropivacaine to a control group who received preoperative epidural saline followed by PCEA with morphine and ropivacaine in 40 patients scheduled for elective colorectal surgery. Patients in the clonidine group exhibited longer PCEA trigger times, lower pain scores at rest and while coughing, less morphine consumption, and a faster return of bowel function throughout the 72-hour postoperative period compared with patients in the control group. Interestingly, the concentration of certain proinflammatory cytokines was also decreased in the clonidine group 12 and 24 hours following surgery. The most common side effects of neuraxial clonidine are sedation, hypotension, nausea and vomiting, and bradycardia. Hypotension and bradycardia are likely the result of $alpha_2$ effects on preganglionic fibers in the thoracic spinal cord. Sedation results from their action exerted at supraspinal sites.

The interest in dexmedetomidine has grown in recent years because of its decreased cardiovascular and respiratory effects. Kanazi and colleagues[122] showed, in a prospective, double-blind study, that 60 patients undergoing transurethral resection of prostate or bladder tumor under spinal anesthesia experienced a prolonged duration of motor and sensory blockade, with no increase in adverse hemodynamic effects or level of sedation. Patients were randomized to three groups receiving either dexmedetomidine (3 µg) or clonidine (30 µg) added to bupivacaine or bupivacaine alone. These results suggest that low-dose dexmedetomidine has similar analgesic efficacy to clonidine.

Box 43.6 Intrathecal Glutamatergic Medications

FDA Approved

None

Common Use

None

Investigational

Ketamine

Clonidine has been studied extensively in animals and has produced no evidence of neurotoxicity.[129] The number of studies involving human exposure continues to grow, and these studies have not revealed any clinical evidence of neurotoxicity. Clonidine, therefore, appears to be a drug that can be administered safely in humans via the spinal route.

GLUTAMATERGIC RECEPTOR ANTAGONISTS (BOX 43.6)

Similar to GABAergic and cholinergic receptors, glutamatergic receptors are divided into the G-protein-coupled (metabotropic) receptors (mGluR) and ion channel (ionotropic) receptors, which include NMDA, AMPA, and kainite receptors. The NMDA receptors contain ion channels permeable to calcium, sodium, and potassium. The NMDA ion channel is somewhat unique in that ambient concentrations of magnesium block NMDA responses in a use- and voltage-dependent manner.[130] In addition to the glutamate binding site, the NMDA receptor has binding sites for glycine, which functions as an obligatory co-agonist, phencyclidine-like compounds, and endogenous protons and polyamines. Endogenous protons inhibit NMDA receptors via their interactions with an extracellular proton sensor on one of the receptor's subunits. Endogenous polyamines such as spermine and spermidine bind at a separate site but shield this proton receptor, thereby potentiating NMDA receptor activity.[130,131] The AMPA and kainate receptors function as ion channels that are permeable to sodium and potassium. Activation of the ionotropic receptors results in depolarization and neuronal excitation. Metabotropic glutamate receptors are divided into three groups. Group I receptors are positively coupled to phosphatidylinositol hydrolysis, and activation of these receptors ultimately increases intracellular calcium levels. The second and third groups of mGluRs are similar to opioid receptors in that they are negatively coupled to adenylate cyclase; hence, activation of these receptors results in neuronal inhibition.

In animal studies, intrathecally applied, selective agonists at the NMDA, AMPA, kainite, and group I mGlu receptors produce spontaneous pain behavior in naïve animals, and allodynia and hyperalgesia in neuropathic and inflammatory models of persistent pain. Antagonists to these receptors can reverse these nociceptive responses.

For humans, there are no AMPA, kainate, or mGluR agonists or antagonists available for clinical use. As such, the most studied glutamate modulators are the NMDA receptor antagonists. Perhaps the most studied NMDA antagonist for neuraxial use is ketamine, a noncompetitive NMDA antagonist that has been administered both epidurally and intrathecally in humans for acute and chronic pain relief. Following tissue injury, the activation of spinal NMDA receptors induces a state of facilitated processing from repetitive small afferent fiber stimulation, leading to an increased response to high and low threshold stimulation and enhanced receptor field size. This process, known as "wind-up," is thought to be responsible for phenomena such as allodynia and hyperalgesia.[132]

In a case report by Kristensen and colleagues,[133] the spinal administration of CPP (3-[2-carboxypoperazin-4-yl]propyl-1-phosphonic acid), a competitive NMDA antagonist, was noted to suppress wind-up, but not spontaneous pain or allodynia in a patient with a peripheral nerve injury. Four hours after the last injection of CPP, psychomimetic side effects developed that were attributed to the rostral spread of medication. In combination with intrathecal morphine or other analgesic agents in patients suffering from cancer pain, the addition of intrathecal ketamine was shown to enhance the analgesic effects of opioids and other drugs while reducing the development of tolerance.[134] In two case studies, Selda and colleagues[135] found that adding low doses of epidural ketamine to morphine and bupivacaine improved analgesia while minimizing the side effects in patient suffering from terminal cancer with neuropathic components of pain. Bion[136] reported that hyperbaric intrathecal ketamine mixed with epinephrine provided adequate short-term anesthesia in young soldiers undergoing field surgery. More recently, Murali Krishna and coworkers[76] demonstrated that a combination of low doses of intrathecal ketamine and midazolam with bupivacaine improved postoperative analgesia in patients undergoing orthopaedic surgery. However, an open-label study by Hawksworth and Serpell[137] conducted in 10 male patients undergoing prostate surgery found that the high frequency of psychomimetic disturbances, the short duration of action, and the high incidence of incomplete anesthesia precluded its use as a sole anesthetic agent. Similar findings were reported by Kathirvel and colleagues[138] in a prospective study involving 30 healthy women undergoing a brachytherapy application for cervical cancer. The authors found that although the addition of 25 mg of ketamine had local anesthetic-sparing effects, it neither extended postoperative analgesia nor reduced the postoperative analgesic requirements. Compared to the patients who received bupivacaine alone, those who received bupivacaine and ketamine experienced an increased incidence of nausea, vomiting, sedation, dizziness, and "strange feelings." In an interesting case report, the long-term intrathecal administration of the S(+)-ketamine enantiomer was found to be effective in a patient with severe neuropathic cancer pain refractory to conventional therapy.[139] This study reported no adverse side effects and found low plasma concentrations of ketamine after the third week of treatment.

Epidurally administered ketamine has been found to be a clinically more viable treatment than intrathecal delivery, with a lower incidence of dysphoric and other adverse effects. In a randomized clinical study performed by Sethi and coworkers,[140] low-dose ketamine was added to the epidural mixture patients undergoing major upper abdominal surgery. Ketamine added to bupivacaine in postoperative PCEA was found to provide better pain control with less opioid use. In addition, patients experienced significantly less nausea, vomiting, and pruritus. More recently, Amr demonstrated in a large randomized, double-blind, controlled trial that ketamine administered epidurally with steroids and a local anesthetic provided superior pain relief in 200 patients suffering from lumbar radiculopathy from disk herniation than steroids and a local anesthetic alone. Patients receiving ketamine by injections reported significantly decreased pain scores lasting up to 12 months postinjection, though six patients in the ketamine group experienced short-lasting delusions immediately after injection.[141] In a study involving patients undergoing hepatic resection, the combination of epidural ketamine and morphine was found to provide superior pain relief compared to morphine alone. In elderly patients, the epidural ketamine dose was reduced by 33% (20 mg versus 30 mg).[142] There were no reports of psychomimetic effects, neurologic findings, or any other complications in this study. In a study by Himmelseher and colleagues[143] assessing the impact of adding S(+) ketamine to epidural anesthesia with ropivacaine in patients undergoing knee arthroplasty, the combination group experienced significantly longer pain relief than patients receiving the local anesthetic alone. A review of 13 randomized controlled studies involving 584 children reported that patients receiving 0.25 to 0.5 mg/kg ketamine via caudal administration extended the time needed for rescue medication by about 5 hours. Furthermore, these findings held true irrespective of the local anesthetic dose.[144] One of the theoretic advantages of ketamine for chronic pain is that it is not associated with tolerance.

Not all studies have found epidural ketamine to be beneficial. Lauretti and colleagues[145] found no benefit to adding epidural ketamine to clonidine in 56 patients undergoing orthopedic surgical procedures. The 24-hour postoperative pain scores, time to first rescue medication, and quality of analgesia were similar in the clonidine, ketamine, and ketamine-clonidine combination groups. In a double-blind study by Weir and associates,[146] the authors found that adding ketamine to epidural bupivacaine for knee replacement surgery failed to prolong postoperative analgesia or reduce analgesic requirements, but it did result in significantly more side effects. The majority of the existing literature demonstrates that epidural ketamine in doses ranging from 0.5 to 1 mg/kg is well tolerated in patients of all age groups and is most effective when combined with opioids or local anesthetics.

The potential neurotoxicity of intrathecal ketamine remains a subject of controversy. In most countries, racemic formulations (50% S(+) and 50% R(−)-ketamine) are available either preservative-free or with preservatives, such as benzethonium chloride and chlorobutanol. Compared to the racemic mixture, the S(+) enantiomer has a fourfold greater affinity for NMDA receptor, and consequently possesses 2 to 3 times the analgesic potency. Karpinski and colleagues[147] reported that a terminal cancer patient who received a 3-week intrathecal infusion of racemic ketamine was found to have subpial vacuolar myelopathy on autopsy; a similar finding was reported by Stotz and coworkers.[148] On postmortem examination of a terminal cancer patient who received a 7-day trial of intrathecal ketamine, focal

Box 43.7 Intrathecal COX Medications

FDA Approved

None

Common Use

None

Investigational

Ketorolac
Aspirin

Box 43.8 Intrathecal Cholinergic Medications

FDA Approved

None

Common Use

None

Investigational

Neostigmine

lymphocytic vasculitis close to the catheter injection site was noted. Subarachnoid S(+)-ketamine is a matter of much debate, as the results regarding its toxicity are contradictory. Although no human studies of preservative-free racemic or pure S(+)-ketamine have examined the histopathologic effects in humans, preservative-free racemic ketamine has been shown to be without apparent neurotoxic effects after repeated administration in pigs.[149] However, S(+) ketamine without preservative injected into dogs resulted in significant histologic abnormalities, including gliosis, axonal edema, central chromatolysis, lymphocyte infiltration, and fibrous thickening of the dura mater. Similar findings have been reported in rat models and rabbits.[150,151] At present, ketamine is not FDA approved for neuraxial use in the United States and is considered experimental or only for use in palliative care.

CYCLOOXYGENASE INHIBITORS (BOX 43.7)

Research was conducted with animal models that implicate the cyclooxygenase isoenzymes, COX-1 and COX-2, as playing a role in the development and maintenance of spinal neuropathic pain.[152] In the spinal cord, prostaglandin E2 (PGE_2) acts presynaptically to increase the release of glutamate from primary afferent C fibers and postsynaptically to directly excite dorsal horn neurons by activation of nonselective cation currents.[153-155] Both effects promote the development and maintenance of central sensitization and enhanced pain states. The intrathecal administration of nonsteroidal anti-inflammatory drugs (NSAIDs) prevents the development of hyperalgesia and inhibits the release of PGE_2.[153,156] In an animal experiment using a peripheral nerve injury model, the nonselective COX inhibitor ketorolac provided significantly longer antinociception than the COX-2 selective NSAID, NS-398 (6 days versus 2 hours).[157] These findings are consistent with recent experiments showing potent antinociceptive effects without neurotoxicity following intrathecal ketorolac administration.[158] In a study by Parris and colleagues[159] investigating intrathecal ketorolac and morphine in an animal model of neuropathic pain, the authors demonstrated that both drugs possess antinociceptive properties, with morphine being more potent than ketorolac for all outcome measures except cold allodynia, in which the effects of the two drugs were found to be similar.

Despite the promising evidence produced in animal studies, several well-designed studies have failed to demonstrate the efficacy of intrathecal ketorolac in clinical or experimental pain. Eisenach and associates[160] tested the efficacy of intrathecal ketorolac in a randomized controlled, chronic pain study involving patients suffering primarily low back and lower extremity pain with a combination of somatic and neuropathic components. This study failed to demonstrate a difference between patients receiving ketorolac intrathecally compared with saline. In a second clinical study, Eisenach and collaborators[161] found that 2 mg of intrathecal ketorolac combined with 15 mg bupivacaine failed to prolong postoperative analgesia when compared with normal saline. These results are disappointing and imply that intrathecal ketorolac are of limited utility for alleviating pain in humans. However, these studies included a small number of subjects, and more studies involving larger numbers of subjects are needed before conclusions can be made about the effectiveness of intrathecal ketorolac. Two studies examined the analgesic effects of intrathecal aspirin in patients with chronic refractory pain.[162,163] In a large study conducted in 60 cancer patients with intractable pain, a single intrathecal dose of isobaric lysine acetylsalicylate (doses ranged from 120 to 720 mg) resulted in excellent pain relief in 78% of cases, with the duration of analgesia lasting from 3 weeks to 1 month on average. Neuraxial ketorolac is not FDA approved and is considered investigational or only for use in palliative care.

CHOLINERGIC AGONISTS (BOX 43.8)

Cholinergic receptors are divided into the G-protein-coupled (metabotropic) receptors (i.e., the muscarinic subtype) and ion channel (ionotropic) receptors (i.e., the nicotinic subtype). Pharmacologic molecular cloning studies have led to the classification of muscarinic acetylcholine receptors (mAChRs) in central and peripheral tissues into five distinct subtypes: M1, M2, M3, M4, and M5. Studies of radioligand binding and analysis of mRNA have demonstrated the existence of M1, M2, M3, and M4 receptors in the spinal cord. Neuronal nicotinic acetylcholine receptors (nAChRs) are pentameric ligand-gated ion channels, and molecular cloning has identified nine alpha and three beta subunits. These subunits assemble to form functional receptors in heteromeric combinations or as homopentamers. Receptor subunit composition underlies the differences in functional properties, and there is considerable variation in subunit expression throughout the spinal cord.

In animal models, the spinal administration of muscarinic cholinergic agonists results in antinociception, an effect that is reversed by muscarinic antagonists.[164,165] In contrast, the intrathecal administration of nicotinic agonists results in a decrease in nociceptive threshold (hyperalgesia) or increase in spontaneous pain behaviors[164,165] in most studies, but antinociception in others.[166,167] The increase in pain-related behaviors after the intrathecal administration of nicotonic agonists may be the result of an associated increase in excitatory transmitter release. This hyperalgesia is reversed by the administration of intrathecal nicotinic or glutamate receptor antagonists.[166,168,169] The diversity of nAChR subunits likely contributes to the seemingly paradoxical analgesic and hyperalgesic effects of nicotinic agonists. However, the predominant analgesic effects of neuraxial cholinergic drugs are thought to be mediated by muscarinic M1 and M3 receptors found in the dorsal root ganglia and superficial laminae of the dorsal horn, with a more modest contribution by nicotonic receptors.[170,171] Cholinesterase inhibitors, including neostigmine and physostigmine, increase the amount of available acetylcholine by inhibiting its metabolism. These drugs have been found in numerous animal studies to produce antinociception, anti-allodynia, and antihyperalgesia after neuraxial administration.[169,172,173]

Because of the lack of available selective muscarinic agonists and the paradoxical and unpredictable effects of neuraxially administered nicotinic agonists, human research has focused on the administration of cholinesterase inhibitors, primarily neostigmine. Despite promising data from animal studies, the administration of intrathecal neostigmine alone in humans has been somewhat disappointing. After preclinical toxicity screening, neostigmine was introduced into clinical trials for intrathecal administration. Spinal administration was found to produce analgesia to experimental pain stimuli in naïve volunteers and patients suffering from cancer and postoperative pain.[174-176] Unfortunately, the pain relief was accompanied by severe and debilitating nausea. Thus, the use of intrathecal neostigmine as a sole analgesic is not currently recommended. However, the addition of neostigmine to intrathecal opioids and local anesthetics has been found to prolong and enhance analgesia, with only a modest increase in the incidence of nausea and vomiting.[176-178] The most recent literature has focused on using neostigmine in combination with other neuraxial agents and has helped to better define the use of neostigmine in neuraxial analgesia. One finding is that neostigmine, when used in combination with an alpha-adrenergic agonist such as clonidine, might provide superior labor analgesia while reducing the risk of side effects when compared with either of these two drugs given alone.[178]

Roelants and coworkers[176] compared a single epidural dose of clonidine (150 μg) together with a single dose of neostigmine (750 μg) to three combinations of clonidine (75 μg) and neostigmine (250, 500, and 750 μg). The study found that only the combinations of 75 μg clonidine with 500 or 750 μg neostigmine provided visual analog scale (VAS) pain scores significantly lower than baseline, and that the effect was significantly longer than in the three other groups. Furthermore, the combination of these two drugs did not result in any increase in maternal adverse outcomes, such as nausea, hypotension, or sedation, or any neonatal adverse outcome. In another study, Van de Velde and colleagues[123] found that a combination of clonidine 75 μg and neostigmine 500 μg, administered epidurally as part of a combined spinal-epidural anesthetic (CSE) technique with ropivacaine and sufentanil, did not result in maternal adverse effects.[123] The authors found that the combination prolonged the initial analgesic effect of the spinal component of the CSE and decreased the requirement for local anesthesia. Furthermore, the investigators were able to demonstrate that this combination prolonged the initial analgesic effect of the spinal component of the CSE and provided a subsequent local anesthetic-sparing effect.

Neostigmine has also been coadministered for caudal analgesia in children with bupivacaine[179-181] or ropivacaine,[182] where it was reported to provide prolonged analgesia without any adverse effects. This benefit was demonstrated in a double-blind, randomized, prospective study by Karaaslan and coworkers,[183] whereby 60 male patients between the ages of 5 months and 5 years undergoing genitourinary surgery were allocated randomly to one of three groups. One group received caudal 0.25% levobupivacaine (1 mL/kg) alone (note that levobupivacaine is no longer available in the United States). The next two groups of patients received neostigmine (2 and 4 μg/kg, respectively) together with levobupivacaine. Both groups receiving intrathecal neostigmine combined with levobupivacaine showed decreased pain scores postoperatively, a longer duration of analgesia, and lower analgesic consumption compared with the group administered levobupivacaine alone. There was no difference in analgesic efficacy between groups receiving different doses of neostigmine, nor were the adverse effects different among the three groups.[183] The benefit of combining neostigmine with local anesthetics is not limited to levobupivacaine. Batra and colleagues[184] demonstrated that combining neostigmine at a dose of 0.75 μg/kg with bupivacaine significantly extends spinal anesthesia duration, reduces postoperative pain scores, and decreases the need for rescue analgesia in infants undergoing lower abdominal and urogenital procedures. The study showed no benefit by increasing the dose to 1 μg/kg. Animal studies have shown that the coadministration of neostigmine does not decrease the neurotoxicity of lidocaine.[185]

The combination of neostigmine with morphine via the epidural route has been shown to decrease the incidence of postoperative urine retention and prolong analgesia.[186] The synergistic effect of combining neuraxial neostigmine with local anesthetics was confirmed in a randomized double-blind study by Kumar and colleagues,[179] which assessed the addition of neostigmine, ketamine, and midazolam to bupivacaine in 80 children administered a single-shot caudal injection for inguinal hernia repair. The duration of complete analgesia was significantly longer in the neostigmine-bupivacaine group than in patients who received midazolam-bupivacaine, ketamine-bupivacaine, and bupivacaine alone. In addition to enhancing sensory blockade, combining neostigmine with an assortment of other intrathecal medications may also prolong muscle weakness and increase sedation.[187] The most commonly encountered side effects of intrathecal neostigmine are nausea, vomiting, and, at doses exceeding 150 μg, sedation and leg weakness. At low doses, neostigmine is devoid of significant hemodynamic effects, but at higher doses (750 μg), increases in blood pressure, heart rate, respiratory rate, and anxiety may occur.

The epidural administration of neostigmine alone, or in combination with local anesthetics or opioids, has been found to effectively decrease postoperative pain. In contrast to intrathecally administered neostigmine, neostigmine administered via the epidural route enhances opioid and local anesthetic analgesia without increasing the incidence of nausea. In a prospective, randomized, double-blind study, Caliskan and collaborators[188] demonstrated that patients who received 1 μg/kg of neostigmine in addition to 20 mL of bupivacaine experienced faster restoration of bowel sounds and a shortened duration of postoperative ileus after abdominal aortic surgery compared to patients receiving 20 mL of bupivacaine and an equal volume of normal saline. In the first of a two-phase randomized controlled study evaluating bolus (40 and 80 mcg) epidural neostigmine in women scheduled for elective cesarean section, Ross and colleagues[189] found that epidural neostigmine boluses did not alter baseline fetal heart rate, induce contractions, or produce nausea. In the second, randomized phase comparing patient controlled epidural analgesia with either bupivacaine alone (1.25 mg/mL) or bupivacaine combined with neostigmine (4 mcg/mL), those who received the combination treatment had a 19% decrease in bupivacaine requirements. In parturients receiving treatment for longer than 4 hours, the decrease was 25%. Similar to a previous study, those patients who received combination did experience a slight increase in sedation.

Unfortunately, there are few studies evaluating the long-term use of neuraxial neostigmine for chronic pain. Lauretti and coworkers[190] found that the epidural administration of a low dose of neostigmine (100 μg) in combination with morphine was associated with improved analgesia when compared to opioid treatment alone in terminal cancer patients followed for 20 days. This improvement was not associated with an increased incidence of adverse effects. Neostigmine is considered investigational or only for use in palliative care of terminal patients without further options and full consent of the patient.

OTHER EXPERIMENTAL NEURAXIAL AGENTS

ADENOSINE AGONISTS

Extracellular adenosine and adenosine tri-phosphate (ATP) have been proposed as neurotransmitters. Adenosine is thought to modulate the transmission of nociceptive information by its action at peripheral, spinal, and supraspinal receptor sites. These receptors are divided into two groups: purinergic 1 (P_1) and purinergic 2 (P_2) receptors at which adenosine and ATP act, respectively. These receptors can be further subdivided into adenosine A_1, A_{2a}, A_{2b}, and A_3 receptors, all of which are metabotropic, and ATP P_{2X} and P_{2Y} receptors, which are ionotropic and metabotropic, respectively.

Numerous studies in animals have demonstrated that the spinal or systemic administration of adenosine and adenosine analogs inhibit pain behavior in response to noxious stimuli in acute and chronic models of nociception. Neuraxially administered A_1 receptor agonists produce antinociceptive properties in a number of acute, inflammatory, and neuropathic pain models.[191,192] In contrast, the spinal administration of ATP results in pronociceptive behaviors and a decrease in nociceptive thresholds[193] through the activation of the P_{2X} receptor. Activation of spinal P_{2Y} receptors results in antinociception,[193,194] although this effect is subordinate to the pronociceptive properties of the P_{2X} receptor.

In a phase I clinical safety study published in 1998 by Rane and colleagues,[195] intrathecal injection of adenosine in 12 healthy volunteers reduced areas of secondary allodynia after skin inflammation and decreased forearm ischemic tourniquet pain, but it had no effect on the cold-pressor test. No adverse side effects were noted, although one patient who received a 2000 μg injection (ranges tested were from 500 μg to 2000 μg) experienced transient low back pain. In a case report on a patient with neuropathic leg pain and tactile allodynia, a single intrathecal injection of the A_1 agonist, R-phenylisopropyl adenosine (R-PIA), provided relief of the patient's stimulus-dependent pain.[196] However, in a randomized study evaluating 1000 μg of intrathecal adenosine given before and after hysterectomy, the treatment produced no significant impact on postoperative analgesic requirements or visual analog scale (VAS) pain scores compared to placebo.[197] In a randomized, double-blind study conducted in 25 healthy parturients, Rane and colleagues[198] found no clinically or statistically significant benefit when a one-time dose of adenosine 500 μg was added to intrathecal sufentanil for labor pain. In an assessment using a different formulation of adenosine currently marketed in the United States, Eisenach and coworkers[199] found that intrathecal adenosine reduced hyperalgesia and allodynia associated with intradermal capsaicin injection, but it had no effect on acute noxious chemical or thermal stimulation. A follow-up study by the same group of investigators showed that intrathecal adenosine reduced areas of allodynia by 25% in volunteers given subdermal capsaicin.[200] These findings are consistent with those of Rane and colleagues and indicate that adenosine may be more effective for neuropathic pain than it is for acute pain. The only side effects noted in the initial safety studies were headache and back pain.

There are no published studies investigating the long-term infusion of intrathecal adenosine in patients with chronic pain. To date, all human studies assessing neuraxial adenosine have been in either the perioperative setting or experimental pain models. Although adenosine shows promise as a treatment for chronic pain, it is premature to comment on its safety or efficacy.[13] At present, adenosine is considered investigational or only for use in palliative care of terminal patients without further options and full consent of the patient.

SOMATOSTATIN AGONISTS

There is extensive literature on the use of neuraxial somatostatin for pain relief. To date, at least six somatostatin receptors have been identified, which are dispersed throughout the periaqueductal gray matter, ventral horn, primary afferent neurons, and substantia gelatinosa. The antinociceptive effects of somatostatin result from presynaptic inhibition. Stimulation of the somatostatin receptors results in hyperpolarization of the cell via a G-protein-coupled inwardly rectifying potassium current. This serves to block coupled calcium channels, reduce transmitter release, and decrease the synthesis of cyclic adenosine monophosphate (cAMP).

Epidural somatostatin has been demonstrated in several studies to provide postoperative pain relief for patients undergoing major surgical procedures.[201-203] In an open-label study assessing the effect of 250 μg of epidural somatostatin on postoperative pain after abdominal surgery, complete pain relief (no other analgesics required) was obtained in all eight patients.[202] In two patients, an epidural somatostatin infusion also provided adequate intraoperative analgesia. There were no reported side effects in this pilot study.

There are also reports of intrathecal and epidural somatostatin being used in cancer pain. In a study performed by Mollenholt and associates[204] examining the efficacy of continuous intrathecal and epidural infusions of somatostatin in eight patients with intractable cancer pain unresponsive to opioids, the authors described demyelination of spinal nerve roots and dorsal columns in two of their eight patients at autopsy. None demonstrated any clinical signs of neurologic deficits during their treatment. As the patients were receiving other treatments for cancer, including chemotherapy and radiation treatment, the pathologic changes could not definitively be attributed to somatostatin. All patients in this investigation required rapid dose escalation over a relatively short time period, perhaps indicating the development of tolerance. Analgesia was rated as either "good" or "excellent" in six of the eight patients. One patient experienced nausea, headache, and vertigo during the last 5 days of somatostatin treatment, and another became agitated and tremulous during the first night of therapy.

Research efforts have now turned to octreotide, a synthetic analog of somatostatin with a longer half-life. In preclinical studies involving rats with chronic constriction injury of the sciatic nerve, octreotide has been shown to reduce the behavioral effects of thermal hyperalgesia.[205] In a dog model, IT octreotide infusions of 40 µg per hour were not found to be neurotoxic.[13] Human use, although limited, has also not revealed any neurotoxicity. Deer and colleagues[206] conducted a randomized, double-blind study comparing the safety and adverse effects with normal saline. Twenty patients received intrathecal doses of octreotide as high as 405 to 650 µg per day and showed no neurotoxicity or adverse effects. Intrathecal octreotide was found to provide long-term pain relief in two patients, one of who was suffering from refractory central pain secondary to multiple sclerosis. In this patient, a double-blind "N of 1" trial with saline resulted in a sharp increase in pain during the 2-week placebo period, necessitating an increase in supplemental opioids. The patient continued on the intrathecal somatostatin therapy for 5 years with no adverse side effects. The increase in somatostatin required during this period was modest, from 20 µg/hr to 29 µg/hr.

Not all studies examining spinal somatostatin or octreotide for pain relief have found the drug to be of benefit.[207] In a randomized controlled trial assessing epidural diamorphine and somatostatin in 24 patients undergoing cholecystectomy, only patients who received intraoperative diamorphine required less postoperative analgesics.[208] The neuraxial use of somatostatin was associated with minimal side effects. However, neuraxial somatostatin and its analogs have been reported to produce substantial neurotoxicity in animals,[209,210] and there have been no recent clinical trials assessing neuraxial somatostatin as an analgesic. Octreotide is considered experimental or only for use in palliative care of terminal patients without further options and full consent of the patient.

DOPAMINE AGONISTS

The mechanism by which neuraxial droperidol, a butyrophenone, exerts its antinociceptive effects is not fully understood, but appears to involve D1 and D2 receptors in descending dopaminergic tracts in the dorsal horn of the spinal cord.[211,212] When administered parenterally, neuroleptic drugs have been demonstrated to have analgesic, as well as sedative and anti-emetic, effects in humans.[213] The use of epidural droperidol has been shown to enhance analgesia in several studies. In several clinical trials including two randomized controlled trials, droperidol was shown to potentiate epidural analgesia with opioids.[214-216] Naji and colleagues[216] reported significantly enhanced analgesia with lower morphine usage in patients undergoing hip replacement surgery. Wilder-Smith and collaborators[217] followed up with a double-blind, placebo-controlled study demonstrating that a combination of epidural droperidol and intravenous sufentanil significantly reduced both the duration of analgesia and adverse effects compared with intravenous (IV) sufentanil alone. Several studies have reported that epidurally administered droperidol with opioids provides better analgesia with less nausea than epidural opioids alone.[218,219] Furthermore, two prospective, randomized studies have demonstrated that epidural droperidol enhances analgesia when combined with tramadol, a combination analgesic that possesses weak µ-opioid, noradrenergic, and serotoninergic effects.[220,221] Gurses and colleagues[221] demonstrated that a one-time bolus of epidural droperidol in combination with epidural tramadol increased the quality and duration of analgesia over tramadol alone in the immediate postoperative period in 90 patients undergoing abdominal surgery. Finally, Bach and associates[215] conducted a retrospective study assessing the effect of adding epidural droperidol to epidural opioids in 20 patients with chronic pain, 17 of whom suffered from a malignancy. The authors found that adding droperidol to epidural morphine resulted in significantly reduced opioid requirements and improved pain relief (80% of patients reported decreased pain), with seven patients reporting reversible side effects.

The potential benefits of combining epidural droperidol with opioids include a reduction in opioid-related side effects, including nausea, vomiting, pruritus, urinary retention, and hypotension.[213] Side effects of epidural droperidol include sedation, respiratory depression, and Parkinsonian sequelae.

There are no studies to date on the long-term intrathecal use of neuroleptics. The literature that does exist on neuraxial neuroleptics primarily deals with either the intrathecal effects of droperidol in animals or epidural droperidol in the perioperative setting.

PRECLINICAL AGENTS

Xen2174 is a structural analog of Mr1A, a chi-conopeptide recently isolated from the venom of the marine cone snail, *Conus marmoreus*.[222] Its mechanism, similar to tricyclic antidepressants, is effected by inhibiting the norepinephrine transporter. However, chi-conopeptides are highly selective for the norepinephrine transporter and are less likely to cause the side effects associated with tricyclic antidepressants. Nielsen and colleagues[223] compared intrathecal bolus doses of Xen2174 with tricyclic antidepressants and clonidine. They found that IT Xen2174 reduced allodynia in rats with either a chronic constriction injury of the sciatic nerve or an L5/L6 spinal nerve injury.[223] It is hypothesized that the anti-allodynic, antihyperalgesic, and antinociceptive effects of IT Xen2174 are due to upregulation of descending noradrenergic inhibition in the dorsal horn.[222]

CGX-1160 is a conopeptide-based drug that produces analgesia through activation of the neurotensin receptor type 1 (NTR1).[222] It has been shown to produce significant analgesia in dogs,[224] but has not been tested in humans. Resiniferatoxin is an investigational drug that desensitizes primary dorsal root ganglion neurons.[225] It is extracted from a cactus-like plant and is a potent capsaicin analog that has been found to produce analgesia in animal studies.[225] P-Saporin is a neurotoxin that selectively destroys cells containing neurokinin-1 receptor neurons.[226] Animal studies have demonstrated reduction in pain-related behaviors without long-lasting toxicity or adverse effects.[226-228] P-Saporin is currently being evaluated for IT use in cancer patients with chronic intractable pain.[228]

CONCLUSIONS

The use of neuraxial analgesics to modulate pain has generated intense interest. Despite this interest and need for alternatives in pain care of patients in dire need, there is a saddening lack of effective analgesic agents that are already FDA approved. Compared to the oral and intravenous routes of administration, the intrathecal and epidural administration of analgesics is associated with a reduced incidence of most, but not all, side effects. To date, most of the literature regarding spinal analgesics has been conducted in surgical and cancer patients, in whom the development of cumulative side effects, tolerance, and system malfunction is less of a concern than it is for chronic, nonmalignant pain patients. In these patients, treatment with neuraxial analgesics is more controversial, and long-term safety and efficacy studies are surprisingly scarce. One area that demonstrates particular promise is combining various neuraxial analgesics to enhance efficacy and reduce side effects and tolerance. In addition to the agents mentioned in this chapter, other substances that show promise for future study include nitric oxide inhibitors, dynorphins, calcitonin, neurotensin, antidepressants, β-blockers, and cannabinoids. Clearly, more research is needed to determine the best candidates for neuraxial therapy and which drug combinations have the best efficacy and side effect profiles.

KEY POINTS

- The FDA has approved only morphine, baclofen, and ziconotide for intrathecal use.
- The FDA has not approved the use of hydromorphone, fentanyl, sufentanil, clonidine, or bupivacaine for intrathecal use, but these agents have historically found common off-label use.

KEY POINTS—cont'd

- The FDA has labeling for intrathecal bupivacaine and lidocaine when used in combination with dextrose.
- Intrathecal granulomas have been reported to form at the tip of the intrathecal catheter when infusing morphine, hydromorphone, and baclofen.
- Intrathecal fentanyl has not been associated with granuloma development; however, with its lipophilic properties it remains in the intrathecal space a very short time and requires catheter placement at the spinal level associated with the patient's pain.
- Intrathecal medication pumps with opioid and nonopioid adjuvants can be extremely helpful in patients with cancer-related pain who are unable to be controlled or have significant side effects with standard parenteral therapies.
- Intrathecal ziconotide has efficacy in some neuropathic pain conditions but is often associated with severe side effects.
- Intrathecal therapy is much less effective in the treatment of non-cancer-related pain.
- The future of intrathecal therapy lies in the development of targeted, non-neurotoxic medications.

SUGGESTED READINGS

Deer TR, Smith HS, Cousins M, et al. Consensus guidelines for the selection and implantation of patients with noncancer pain for intrathecal drug delivery. *Pain Physician.* 2010;13:E175-E213.

Deer TR, Smith HS, Burton AW, et al. Comprehensive consensus based guidelines on intrathecal drug delivery systems in the treatment of pain caused by cancer pain. *Pain Physician.* 2011;14:E283-E312.

Eisenach JC, Curry R, Rauck R, et al. Role of spinal cyclooxygenase in human postoperative and chronic pain. *Anesthesiology.* 2010;112:1225-1233.

Errando CL, Sifre C, Moliner S, et al. Subarachnoid ketamine in swine—pathological findings after repeated doses: acute toxicity study. *Reg Anesth Pain Med.* 1999;24:146-152.

Hood DD, Eisenach JC, Tuttle R. Phase I safety assessment of intrathecal neostigmine methylsulfate in humans. *Anesthesiology.* 1995;82:331-343.

Kamibayashi T, Maze M. Clinical uses of alpha2-adrenergic agonists. *Anesthesiology.* 2000;93:1345-1349.

McClelland S III, Bethoux FA, Boulis NM, et al. Intrathecal baclofen for spasticity-related pain in amyotrophic lateral sclerosis: efficacy and factors associated with pain relief. *Muscle & Nerve.* 2008;37:396-398.

Schmidtko A, Lotsch J, Freynhagen R, et al. Ziconotide for treatment of severe chronic pain. *Lancet.* 2010;375:1569-1577.

Shafer SL. Anesthesia & Analgesia's policy on off-label drug administration in clinical trials. *Anesth Analg.* 2007;105:13-15.

Stotz M, Oehen HP, Gerber H. Histological findings after long-term infusion of intrathecal ketamine for chronic pain: a case report. *J Pain Symptom Manage.* 1999;18:223-228.

Zuniga RE, Perera S, Abram SE. Intrathecal baclofen: a useful agent in the treatment of well-established complex regional pain syndrome. *Reg Anesth Pain Med.* 2002;27:90-93.

The references for this chapter can be found at www.expertconsult.com.

44 Pharmacology for the Interventional Pain Physician

Magdalena Anitescu | Honorio T. Benzon | Renata Variakojis

This chapter reviews the clinical pharmacology, pharmacokinetics, therapeutic mechanisms, and side effects of corticosteroids and botulinum toxins. Radiocontrast agents are reviewed in greater detail elsewhere in this text. All of these drugs have the potential to produce physiologic toxicity and therefore should be administered appropriately and in the smallest dose that will reliably produce the desired effect; an increase in total dose or volume should not be used to compensate for inadequate injection technique. In addition, this chapter reviews the main characteristics of the available injectable bone cements, their use, and their handling as an effective treatment in vertebral compression fractures. Novel techniques involving gene therapy in the treatment of chronic, unrelenting pain syndromes are also explored.

CORTICOSTEROIDS

Corticosteroids (CSs) are key mediators in the maintenance of normal physiology and in the complex adaptive mechanisms that protect an organism in the setting of internal or external stressors.[1] CSs maintain the function and integrity of many important physiologic and biochemical processes, including the regulation of protein, carbohydrate, and lipid metabolism.[2,3] Naturally occurring corticosteroids are classified into three functional groups: mineralocorticoids, glucocorticoids, and adrenal androgens.[4]

Mineralocorticoids maintain normal fluid and electrolyte balance. Glucocorticoids (GCs) act primarily to enhance the production of high-energy fuel, glucose, and reduce other metabolic activity.[2,5] Injections of glucocorticoids for the relief of vertebrogenic, arthritic, and radiculopathic pain are widely accepted.[6]

GENERAL EFFECTS OF THE ENDOGENOUS CORTICOSTEROIDS

PHYSIOLOGIC EFFECTS OF CORTICOSTEROIDS

GCs stimulate hepatic gluconeogenesis, increase hepatic glycogen content, and inhibit insulin-mediated peripheral blood glucose uptake.[2] They modulate protein metabolism by decreasing peripheral protein synthesis (by inhibiting amino acid incorporation) and stimulating protein catabolism while stimulating protein and enzyme synthesis in the liver.[2] CSs regulate lipid metabolism largely by potentiating catecholamine-enhanced activation of cellular lipase, resulting in lipolysis.[3]

GC actions on protein and lipid tissues vary in different parts of the body. Whereas cortisol can deplete the protein matrix of the vertebral column (trabecular bone), there may be minimal effect on long bones (compact bone).[2] For adipose tissue, the subcutaneous lipid cell mass of the arms and legs decreases while that of the abdomen and interscapular area increases.

Cortisol maintains vascular responsiveness to circulating vasoconstrictors and, in high doses, may restore circulatory function in shock (hemorrhage, endotoxin, anaphylaxis, and trauma). Hemodynamically, GCs modulate α-adrenergic receptor synthesis and cell density,[7] prevent α-adrenergic receptor desensitization and uncoupling,[8] and inhibit nitric oxide synthase.[9]

Cortisol maintains the microcirculation in the setting of acute inflammation by reducing capillary endothelial permeability and preventing edema formation. GCs modulate the immune response at many levels.[2] They cause leukocytosis by enhancing the release of mature leukocytes from the bone marrow as well as inhibiting their egress from the circulation.

STEROID SYNTHESIS

All CSs are produced in the cortex of the adrenal gland, which is composed of three distinct zones.[4,10] The outer zone, the zona glomerulosa, produces mineralocorticoids, specifically aldosterone, which is synthesized in response to stimulation by the renin-angiotensin-aldosterone system or hyperkalemia. The middle zone, the zona fasciculata, comprising more than 70% of the cortex, is the site of glucocorticoid production. Cortisol is the primary glucocorticoid and represents about 80% of GC production.[10] The inner zone, the zona reticularis, produces GCs and in some species small amounts of androgens.

Adrenocortical cells contain large stores of lipid used for steroidogenesis. Adrenocorticotropic hormone (ACTH) induces physiologic, molecular, and morphologic changes in the adrenal cortex.[11,12] In addition to releasing GCs, the adrenal gland undergoes upregulation of steroidogenic cytochrome P-450 mRNAs, as well as hypervascularization and cellular hypertrophy and hyperplasia.

Circulating plasma lipoproteins provide most of the cholesterol for steroid synthesis. Cholesterol uptake by the adrenal cortex is mediated by the low-density-lipoprotein (LDL) receptor, whose quantities increase with ACTH stimulation. The first and rate-limiting step in steroid

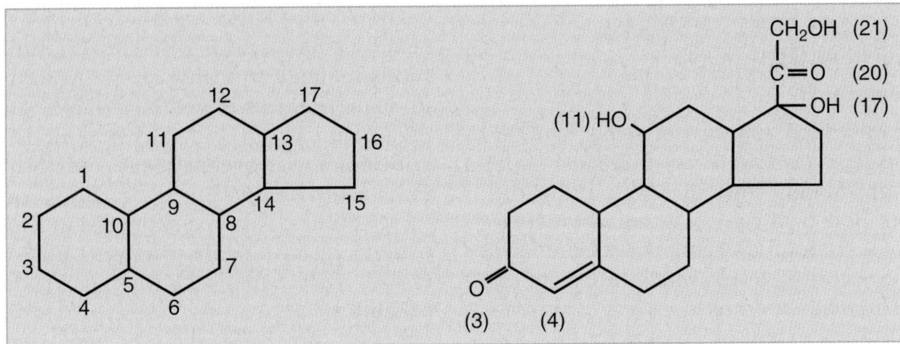

Figure 44.1 Cyclopentanoperhydrophenanthrene ring.

biosynthesis is the conversion of cholesterol to pregnenolone under the control of ACTH and by the cytochrome P-450 enzymes in the mitochondria and smooth endoplasmic reticulum.[10] Corticosterone is the immediate precursor to cortisol, and it is the principal glucocorticoid in certain animal species.[10]

Adrenal steroids share a common carbon skeleton, the cyclopentanoperhydrophenanthrene ring, composed of three cyclohexane rings and one cyclopentane ring (Fig. 44.1). Variation among naturally occurring steroid compounds is related to the manner in which hydrogen, hydroxyl, and oxygen radicals and carbon atoms are attached to the basic steroid nucleus.[4] Cortisol and other anti-inflammatory steroids contain a two-carbon chain attached to position 17, and are termed C21 steroids. Even the commonly administered steroid cortisone must be converted in vivo to hydrocortisone (cortisol) by the liver before it is biologically active.

STEROID SECRETION

Cortisol secretion is under the control of the hypothalamic-pituitary-adrenal (HPA) axis. Cortisol synthesis depends on three factors: negative feedback by serum cortisol levels, normal circadian cycle, and responses to central nervous system (CNS) activation by physical and emotional stress. During nonstress periods, cortisol production is under the influence of CNS activation by baroreceptor, chemoreceptor, nociceptor, and emotional afferent signals.

Negative Feedback

Cortisol exerts a negative feedback inhibition of corticotropin-releasing hormone (CRH) secretion by binding to specific steroid receptors in the CNS.[13] It also inhibits both ACTH secretion and proopiomelanocortin (POMC) gene transcription. Systemic hypoperfusion, with decreased adrenal blood flow and certain drugs, may also inhibit cortisol synthesis.

Circadian Pattern of Secretion

It is estimated that human cortisol production is approximately 5 to 10 mg/m^2 per day.[14,15] This amount is the equivalent of about 20 to 30 mg/day of hydrocortisone or 5 to 7 mg/day of oral prednisone.[14] The range of the circadian pattern of cortisol production varies more than threefold. Peak levels of ACTH and cortisol secretion occur between 4 and 8 a.m. There is minimal production of cortisol during the evening, and the lowest levels are observed between 8 p.m. and 12 a.m.[4] In abnormal sleep-wake cycles, this diurnal pattern will adjust, so that peak cortisol levels occur just prior to awakening.

CNS Control of Secretion

Baroreceptor and chemoreceptor afferent inputs to the medulla are transmitted via the pons to the hypothalamus. Nociceptive afferent signals activate both the medulla and thalamus, which independently activate the hypothalamus via the paleocortex limbic system.[13] Emotional triggers also activate the hypothalamus through the paleocortex limbic system.[13]The arrival of afferent input into the hypothalamic paraventricular nucleus stimulates the synthesis of CRH, which is secreted into the hypophyseal portal system to the anterior pituitary, causing ACTH release.[13] In addition to afferent signals, other substances can stimulate the hypothalamus to secrete CRH and cause ACTH release. These include the proinflammatory cytokines IL-1β, IL-6, and tumor necrosis factor α (TNF-α).[13,16] Other substances that influence CRH and ACTH secretion include vasopressin, angiotensin II, norepinephrine (NE), prostaglandin $F_{2\alpha}$ ($PGF_{2\alpha}$), and thromboxane A_2 (TXA_2). Cortisol synthesis can increase 5- to 10-fold during severe stress, to a maximal level of approximately 100 mg/m^2 per day.[4,17]

PHARMACOKINETICS AND PHARMACODYNAMICS OF THE STEROIDS

Cortisol circulates in the blood in three forms: free cortisol (5%), protein-bound cortisol, and cortisol metabolites.[2] It is this unbound (free) portion that is the physiologically active hormone. Approximately 90% of cortisol is bound to cortisol-binding globulin (CBG), also known as transcortin, and albumin. CBG has a high affinity for cortisol but is present in small amounts. The second serum-binding protein, albumin, binds cortisol with less affinity but is abundantly present. During stress, there is a characteristic increase in total cortisol blood levels, including an increase in the unbound percentage.[13] The level of CBG is increased in high-estrogen states, in pregnancy, and during administration of contraceptives.[2] Most synthetic glucocorticoids have less affinity for CBG (approximately 70% binding), and this may account for their propensity to produce cushingoid symptoms at low doses. Cortisol primarily is metabolized in the liver, with subsequent renal excretion of the metabolites.

CORTICOSTEROID LEVELS IN STRESS RESPONSE AND IN VARIOUS CLINICAL SITUATIONS

Endogenous Corticosteroids

Cortisol levels increase within minutes of stress, whether physical (trauma, surgery, exercise), psychological (anxiety, depression), or physiologic (hypoglycemia, infection). Pain, fever, and hypovolemia all cause a sustained increase in ACTH and cortisol secretion.[17] Surgery is associated with elevations in ACTH and cortisol levels, which usually persist for 24 to 48 hours. The magnitude of the stress response is directly proportional to the extent of surgical trauma. Less extensive procedures such as surgery on the joints, breasts, or neck produce a 36% increase in cortisol levels, whereas laparotomy is associated with an 84% increase in the serum cortisol level for 2 days postoperatively. Adult adrenal glands produce about 50 mg of cortisol/24 hours during minor surgery and 75 to 150 mg/24 hours during major surgery.[18]

Elevated levels of circulating cytokines, which appear within minutes of trauma, stimulate the HPA axis to increase production of cortisol. Increased tissue corticosteroid levels are an important protective and life-sustaining response in these settings. Corticosteroids improve survival in stress by reducing the duration of shock, decreasing the severity of inflammation, improving vessel contractility and hemodynamics, and preventing inflammatory cell recruitment, proliferation, and release of proinflammatory mediators.[19] Corticosteroids also improve outcome by modulating α-receptor responsiveness to catecholamines. GCs both increase the number of α receptors and prevent uncoupling of the α receptor from adenylate cyclase.[7,8]

Exogenous Corticosteroids

The introduction of cortisone, a purified glucocorticoid preparation, revolutionized the treatment of a number of medical diseases and provided physiologic replacement in patients with adrenal insufficiency.[4] Shortly thereafter, a number of case reports and studies appeared describing the catastrophic effects of inadequate corticosteroid supplementation in glucocorticoid-treated patients with medical or surgical stresses. Glucocorticoid therapy is the most common cause of secondary adrenal insufficiency.[4] Initially, glucocorticoid administration suppresses CRH and ACTH stimulation. Over time, tertiary iatrogenic adrenal insufficiency develops as the adrenal gland atrophies. Adrenal atrophy may persist for months, following even short courses of corticosteroid therapy.[20]

The dose and duration of corticosteroid administration are only fair predictors of the extent of adrenal suppression, because ACTH and cortisol production vary greatly among individuals. The time to recovery from HPA suppression is highly variable, ranging from 2 to 5 days to 9 to 12 months.[21] The hypothalamus is the first to be suppressed by steroid dosing but the first to recover (normalizing ACTH in several months), whereas the adrenal glands are the last to be suppressed and the slowest to recover, a process that may take 6 to 12 months. Data regarding corticosteroid-induced adrenal suppression are varied. Suppression of the HPA axis should be anticipated in any patient who has been receiving more than 30 mg/day of hydrocortisone (or 7.5 mg of prednisolone or 0.75 mg of dexamethasone) for more than 3 weeks.[22]

Given the large variation in cortisol production in healthy patients, it is difficult to predict the need for GC supplementation during stress. Also, the adrenal response to acute medical illness is variable. An intact HPA axis is paramount to survival during periods of major stress and critical illness. Adrenal insufficiency with decreased GC levels is associated with a significantly increased mortality in these settings. Adrenal suppression should be suspected in patients receiving corticosteroids, and these patients should receive replacement GCs when facing major surgery or critical illness.[22]

Expert recommendations have suggested lower doses and shorter duration of glucocorticoid administration (Table 44.1). Patients undergoing minor procedures such as routine dental work, skin biopsy, inguinal repair, or minor orthopaedic surgery only require their normal daily dose of replacement, and not a supplemental dose.[17] Some clinicians have advocated using hydrocortisone continuous infusions to limit the rapid clearance and peaks and nadirs of bolus therapy.[4,17,20] Others have suggested using longer-acting glucocorticoid agents, such as methylprednisolone or dexamethasone.[4,17,20]

CORTICOSTEROIDS USED IN CLINICAL PRACTICE

Cortisol has a half-life of 70 to 90 minutes, whereas all synthetic analogues of cortisol have longer half-lives, based on slower rates of metabolism.[3] The half-life does not reflect duration of action, which is best represented by the duration of ACTH suppression. Short-acting synthetic GCs have durations of action of 8 to 12 hours; these include the active agent hydrocortisone and the inactive cortisone (converted by the liver to the biologically active cortisol). The intermediate-acting GCs prednisone, prednisolone, methylprednisolone, and triamcinolone have durations of action of 24 to 36 hours. Prednisone is an inactive agent, which is metabolized to the active agent prednisolone by the liver. The longest acting GCs, dexamethasone and betamethasone, have durations of action longer than 48 hours (Table 44.2).

Short-acting GCs are advantageous when a rapid clinical effect is desired such as in allergic reactions. Long-acting agents are of interest for their prolonged anti-inflammatory effects and are well suited for disorders requiring inhibition of ACTH secretion. Because all GCs have some mineralocorticoid effect, their administration can have profound consequences for patients with impaired cardiovascular function. The shorter-acting GCs have the highest mineralocorticoid potency, and the long-acting agents have the weakest.

THERAPEUTIC EFFECTS OF CORTICOSTEROIDS

Corticosteroids are predominantly used in interventional pain management because of their proven anti-inflammatory effects with subsequent temporary relief of symptoms. They are the most potent and effective agents in controlling inflammation through numerous mechanisms, including effects on cytokines, inflammatory mediators, inflammatory cells, nitric oxide synthase, and adhesion molecules.

Effects on Cytokines

Cytokines are important mediators of inflammation, and the pattern of their expression largely determines the magnitude and persistence of the inflammatory response.[23]

Table 44.1 Guidelines for Adrenal Supplementation Therapy

Surgical Stress	Glucocorticoid Dosage	Medical Stress	Glucocorticoid Dosage
Minimal			
<1 hr under local anesthesia (e.g., dental work, skin biopsy)	Usual replacement dose, 15-30 mg hydrocortisone/day	Nonfebrile cough or upper respiratory tract infection	Usual replacement dose, 15-30 mg hydrocortisone/day
Minor			
Inguinal hernia repair Colonoscopy	Intravenous hydrocortisone 25 mg equivalent at start of the procedure 5 mg of methylprednisolone IV on day of procedure only; usual replacement dose after procedure	Viral illness Bronchitis Uncomplicated urinary tract infection Uncomplicated cellulitis	Double or triple the usual dose of glucocorticoid until recovery (e.g., 40-60 mg oral hydrocortisone daily in divided doses)
Dental procedure requiring > 1 hr under local anesthesia (multiple extractions)	Double the daily dose of glucocorticoid on day of procedure; usual replacement dose next day		
Moderate			
Open cholecystectomy Segmental colon resection Lower limb revascularization Total joint replacement Abdominal hysterectomy	Intravenous hydrocortisone 75 mg/day (25 mg every 8 hr) or 10-15 mg of methylprednisolone on day of procedure; taper over the next 1-2 days to usual replacement doses in uncomplicated cases	Gastroenteritis Pneumonia Pyelonephritis	Intravenous hydrocortisone 25 mg every 8 hr until recovery
Severe			
Cardiothoracic surgery Whipple procedure Esophagogastrectomy Total proctocolectomy Liver resection Pituitary adenomectomy Dental procedures under general anesthesia	Intravenous hydrocortisone 150 mg/day (50 mg every 8 hr) or 20-30 mg of methylprednisolone; taper over the next 2-3 days to usual replacement dose in uncomplicated cases	Pancreatitis Myocardial infarction Labor	Intravenous hydrocortisone 150 mg/day; taper once clinical condition is stable
Critical Illness/Intensive Care			
Major trauma Life-threatening complications	Maximum 200 mg/day intravenous hydrocortisone (50 mg every 6 hr or by continuous infusion)	Septic shock	Maximum 200 mg /day intravenous hydrocortisone (50 mg every 6 hr or by continuous infusion 0.18 mg/kg/hr + 50 mcg/day of fludrocortisone until shock is resolved); may take several days to a week or more; gradually taper, following vital signs and serum sodium level determination

Data are based on extrapolation from the literature, expert opinion, and clinical experience. Patients receiving 5 mg/day or less of prednisone should receive their normal daily replacement but do not require supplementation. Patients who receive more than 5 mg/day of prednisone should receive the above therapy in addition to their maintenance therapy.

Reproduced from Jung C, Inder WJ. Management of adrenal insufficiency during stress of medical illness and surgery. *Med J Australia.* 2008;188:409-413.

Steroids have potent inhibitory effects on cytokine transcription and synthesis, especially the ones relevant in chronic inflammation (IL-1, IL-3, IL-4, IL-5, IL-6, IL-8, TNF-α, and granulocyte-macrophage colony-stimulating factor).[24,25] Steroids interfere with cytokine synthesis by blocking their synthesis.[25] They inhibit the synthesis of the IL-2 receptor and oppose the induction of IL-2 and T-lymphocyte activation and proliferation.

Effects on Inflammatory Mediators

The activation of phospholipase A_2 leads to the hydrolysis of arachidonic acid from membrane phospholipids and the

Table 44.2 Properties of Synthetic Cortisol Analogues

Steroid	Half-Life (hours)	Relative Glucocorticoid Activity	Relative Mineralocorticoid Activity	Glucocorticoid Dose Equivalency (mg)	Relative Anti-inflammatory Activity
Short Term					
Cortisone	8-12	1	1	25	NAE
Hydrocortisone	8-12	0.8	0.6	20	1
Intermediate Acting					
Prednisone	8-36	4	0.8	5	NAE
Prednisolone	8-36	4	0.8	5	3
Methylprednisolone	18-36	5	0.5	4	6.2
Triamcinolone	18-36	5	0	4	5
Long Acting					
Dexamethasone	36-54	20-30	0	0.75	26
Betamethasone	36-54	20-30	0	0.6	NAE

NAE, no available equivalency.
Reproduced from Deer T, Ranson M, Kapural L. Guidelines for the proper use of epidural steroid injections for the chronic pain patient. *Tech Reg Anesth Pain Manag.* 2009;13:288-295. Adapted from Harris E. *Kelley's Textbook of Rheumatology.* 7th ed. Philadelphia: Saunders; 2005.

production of arachidonic acid metabolites. Arachidonic acid metabolism via the cyclooxygenase pathway produces prostaglandins and thromboxanes, and through the lipoxygenase pathway it produces leukotrienes. Steroids increase the synthesis of lipocortin (annexin) 1, a phospholipase A_2 inhibitor, and thus decrease the production of inflammatory mediators such as leukotrienes, prostaglandins, and platelet-activating factor.[25,26] GCs also upregulate the transcription of other anti-inflammatory genes such as neutral endopeptidase and inhibitors of plasminogen activator.[27]

The primary anti-inflammatory effect of steroids appears to be the suppression of transcription of genes involved in inflammation such as collagenase, elastase, plasminogen activator, cyclooxygenase (COX)-2, and most chemokines.[27] Steroids directly inhibit the transcription of a cytosolic form of phospholipase A_2 induced by cytokines, and they inhibit the gene expression of cytokine-induced COX-2 in monocytes.[28] Cortisol, 6-methylprednisolone, and dexamethasone suppress lipopolysaccharide-induced synthesis of PGE_2 and cyclooxygenase-2 expression and activity in human monocytes.[29] In addition, steroids inhibit the synthesis of early genes c-fos and c-jun triggered by increased levels of mediators of inflammation such as leukotriene B_4 and platelet-activating factor.[30]

Effects on Inflammatory Cells

GCs interfere with macrophage activity by impairing phagocytosis, intracellular digestion of antigens, and macrophage release of IL-1 and TNF-α.[2] By inhibiting the expression of chemokines, GCs prevent the activation and recruitment of inflammatory cells, including eosinophils, basophils, and lymphocytes.[27] Steroids also markedly decrease the survival of certain inflammatory cells, such as eosinophils. Eosinophil activity is dependent on the presence of cytokines IL-3, IL-5, granulocyte-macrophage colony-stimulating factor (GM-CSF), and interferon-γ. The presence of these cytokines promotes prolonged eosinophil survival, increased adhesion molecule expression, potentiated eosinophil degranulation, and movement of eosinophils across an endothelial barrier. Steroid administration blocks these cytokine effects, leading to programmed cell death, or apoptosis. GCs cause an expansion in the number of circulating neutrophils secondary to decreased adherence to vascular endothelium (demargination) and stimulation of bone marrow production.[31] GCs interfere with T-cell mediated immunity. They inhibit the production of T lymphocytes by downregulating T-cell growth factors IL-1β and IL-2, and they inhibit the release of various T-lymphocyte cytokines.[2]

Effects on Nitric Oxide Synthase

Various cytokines induce nitric oxide synthase (NOS), resulting in increased nitric oxide production. Nitric oxide increases plasma exudation in inflammatory sites. Steroids potently inhibit the inducible form of NOS in macrophages, and steroid pretreatment prevents the induction of NOS expression by endotoxin.[25]

Effects on Adhesion Molecules

Adhesion molecules facilitate the trafficking of inflammatory cells to sites of inflammation. The expression of the adhesion molecules E-selectin, P-selectin, and intracellular adhesion molecule-1 on the surface of endothelial cells is induced by the cytokines IL-1β and TNF-α.[25] These adhesion molecules enable the endothelium to recruit leukocytes actively and nonselectively, including neutrophils, eosinophils, mononuclear cells, and basophils from the circulation.[27] GCs are effective and potent inhibitors of TNF-α and IL-1 release from macrophages, monocytes, and other infiltrating cells. There is a second class of cytokines that selectively activate the endothelium—IL-4 and IL-13, two cytokines associated with allergic diseases. Their release causes the endothelial expression of vascular cell adhesion molecule-1 only. Consequently, only circulating basophils, eosinophils, monocytes, and lymphocytes, but not neutrophils, can bind to the endothelial surface.[27]

Other Anti-inflammatory Effects

Steroids inhibit plasma exudation from postcapillary venules at inflammatory sites. This effect is delayed, suggesting that gene transcription and protein synthesis are involved.[25] It appears that the antipermeability effect is linked to the synthesis of vasocortin. In addition to nuclear anti-inflammatory effects, GCs also have direct effects on cells and cell membranes. Cortisol stabilizes lysosomal membranes, thus inhibiting lysosomal enzyme release. GCs prevent the sequestration of water intracellularly and the swelling and destruction of cells.[3] GCs inhibit leukocyte accumulation and complement-induced polymorphonuclear neutrophil (PMN) aggregation and decrease PMN chemotaxis, T-cell and B-cell proliferation, and the differentiation and function of macrophages.

Other Mechanisms of Pain Relief

Following peripheral nerve injury, a number of morphologic and biochemical changes occur at the injury site including the formation of neuromas, which leads to increased electrical excitability. Ectopic discharge from the injury site leads to a persistent afferent barrage, which maintains neuralgic pain and paresthesias. GCs have been demonstrated to suppress spontaneous ectopic neural discharge originating in experimental neuromas and prevent the later development of ectopic impulse discharge in freshly cut nerves.[32] The topical application of methylprednisolone was noted to block transmission of C-fibers but not the A-β fibers.[33]

SIDE EFFECTS OF CORTICOSTEROIDS

Short courses of GC therapy (less than 2 to 3 weeks) are usually safe. Side effects from short-term therapy are rare but may include fluid retention, hyperglycemia, elevated blood pressure, mood changes, menstrual irregularities, gastritis, Cushing's syndrome, increased appetite, weight gain, increased infections, delayed wound healing, and acneiform eruptions. Long-term GC therapy with near-physiologic GC doses is relatively safe. With long-term supraphysiologic doses of steroids, more serious side effects may occur.

Cushing's Syndrome

Cushing's syndrome is characterized by sudden weight gain, hypertension, glucose intolerance, oligomenorrhea, decreased libido, and spontaneous ecchymoses. There is centripetal weight gain, involving thickening of the facial fat that rounds the facial contour (moon facies), enlargement of the dorsocervical fat pad (buffalo hump), and truncal obesity. The development of multiple striae wider than 1 cm on the abdomen or proximal extremities is almost unique to Cushing's syndrome. Mild hirsutism, acne, personality changes, depression, insomnia, and edema also occur. Despite the external signs of excess GC production, patients receiving GCs develop adrenal atrophy and are at risk for adrenal crisis in the setting of stress.[34] Laboratory tests reveal low blood ACTH and cortisol and low urinary cortisol levels.

Skeletal Effects

Osteoporosis, aseptic necrosis, and growth retardation are all potential complications of long-term GC therapy. Osteoporosis occurs in as many as 50% of patients treated with long-term supraphysiologic doses of prednisone. Trabecular bone, found in the axial skeleton (vertebrae and ribs), is more susceptible to demineralization due to high metabolic turnover rate (eight times more) when compared with that of cortical bone. Corticosteroid-induced osteoporosis (CIOP) has a multifactorial cause–impaired intestinal absorption of calcium coupled with its increased renal excretion, increased osteoclast activity with resultant bone resorption, inhibition of osteoblast activity with decreased bone synthesis, and secondary hyperparathyroidism. The incidence of fractures in patients receiving GCs has been reported to be between 10% and 20%.[35] Patients at greatest risk for corticosteroid-induced osteoporosis are postmenopausal women, children, immobilized patients, and patients with rheumatoid arthritis. Agents such as activated vitamin D products, hormone replacement therapy, fluoride, calcitonin, and bisphosphonates have been shown to maintain or improve bone mineral density in corticosteroid-induced osteoporosis.[36]

Aseptic necrosis is a severe musculoskeletal complication of GC therapy. It occurs with greater incidence in alcoholics, patients with systemic lupus erythematosus, patients with fatty degeneration of the liver, patients with altered lipid metabolism, and renal transplantation patients. The mechanism is related to deposits of fat in terminal arterioles of certain sites of bone. The femoral head is the site most commonly affected, although the humeral head or knee may also be involved. Bone pain is almost always the first symptom and precedes radiologic signs of osteonecrosis by up to 6 months.[35,36]

Muscle Effects

The incidence of myopathy secondary to high-dose GC therapy has been reported to vary from 7% to 60%.[37] There is no consistent relationship between the dose and duration of steroid administration and the occurrence of myopathy, but the condition develops more often with the use of potent fluorinated steroids such as triamcinolone, dexamethasone, and betamethasone. Symptoms include skeletal muscle weakness, tenderness, and pain with proximal or pelvic muscles typically affected.[37] Recovery may take months to 1 year; treatment includes a reduction in the GC dose and physical therapy with a rehabilitation exercise program.

Ophthalmologic Effects

Cataracts and glaucoma may occur with chronic GC therapy. Steroid-induced cataracts occur in the posterior subcapsular region of the lens and may be asymptomatic until well formed. Children are at greatest risk for this complication. Glaucoma is caused by swelling of collagen strands at the angle of the anterior chamber of the eye, with resistance to the outflow of aqueous humor. The process is usually reversible after GC therapy is discontinued.

Gastrointestinal Effects

Nausea and vomiting are not uncommon with oral steroid therapy. Peptic ulcer disease is slightly increased with GC therapy and is more likely to be gastric than duodenal. GCs cause a decrease in mucus production and mucosal cell renewal. Concomitant use of aspirin and nonsteroidal anti-inflammatory drugs increase this risk and should be avoided, along with tobacco and alcohol, which also are ulcerogenic.[38]

Metabolic Effects

Hyperglycemia results from GC effects of increased hepatic glucose synthesis and increased gluconeogenesis. GCs also antagonize peripheral insulin effects and can occasionally produce insulin resistance. Exacerbation of glucose intolerance is common, but the development of new cases of diabetes mellitus is not, and ketoacidosis is rare. Weight gain is a common side effect of GC therapy and may be the result of increased appetite or fluid retention. Facial edema and fat are estimated to occur in 10% to 25% of patients on steroid therapy for 2 months.

Hyperlipidemia is another metabolic consequence of GC therapy and is likely secondary to relative insulin resistance. Increased plasma triglyceride levels are more common than increased cholesterol levels. Patients with previous lipid level elevations are at higher risk for this side effect. Electrolyte abnormalities such as hypokalemic alkalosis may also occur, usually with GCs possessing strong mineralocorticoid properties.

Cardiovascular Effects

Hypertension, edema, and atherosclerosis may occur with GC therapy. Elevations in blood pressure occur because of increased sodium retention and vasoconstriction. GCs cause vasoconstriction by potentiating the effect of norepinephrine and opposing the effect of endogenous vasodilators such as histamine. This side effect occurs more frequently in patients with preexisting hypertension, older adults, GCs with high mineralocorticoid potency, and high-dose or prolonged (longer than 2 weeks) glucocorticoid treatment courses. Edema occurs from fluid retention secondary to sodium retention. With initial GC dosing, there is a paradoxical diuresis caused by an early blockade of antidiuretic hormone release.

Hematologic Effects

Blood cell effects, immunosuppression, and impaired fibroplasia occur with steroid therapy. Immunosuppression is produced by GCs at many levels. GCs increase the release of granulocytes from bone marrow, thus increasing the number of circulating leukocytes.[39] Lymphopenia occurs, with predominant depression of T-cell production and decreased eosinophil counts with enhanced eosinophil destruction. Tissue inflammation is reduced by inhibition of cytokine production and by impaired chemotaxis of macrophages, neutrophils, basophils, and eosinophils. There is inhibition of the metabolism of arachidonic acid into prostaglandin and leukotriene mediators, as well as a direct inhibition of COX-2. Steroid therapy increases susceptibility to many bacterial, fungal, viral, and parasitic infections. Wound healing is delayed by GC inhibition of fibroblasts, collagen production, and suppression of wound reepithelialization.[40]

Nervous System Effects

Mood changes, nervousness, euphoria, insomnia, and headache are common side effects of GC therapy and are dose related.[41] Psychosis is an uncommon side effect and is seen more commonly in patients with previous psychiatric disorders.

Cutaneous Effects

Skin changes typical of the hyperadrenal state may occur; these include purpura, telangiectasia, atrophy, striae, pseudo-scars, and facial plethora.[42] The skin becomes thin and fragile. Hair growth changes include transient scalp hair loss and hirsutism on other parts of the body. Hyperpigmentation or hypopigmentation may occur, as well as acneiform eruptions. Steroid acne commonly presents on the back and chest as fine, uniform papulopustules.

Pregnancy and Lactation

There appears to be no teratogenic contraindication to corticosteroid therapy in pregnancy. However, intrauterine growth retardation has been reported, and steroid use late in pregnancy may cause adrenal suppression in the fetus. Corticosteroids are secreted in small amounts into breast milk, thus exposing the infant to the risk of adrenal suppression.[35]

INJECTABLE STEROIDS IN INTERVENTIONAL PAIN MANAGEMENT

The most commonly used synthetic CSs for interventional pain procedures are derivatives of prednisolone (analog of cortisol) either by methylation (methylprednisolone) or fluorination (triamcinolone, betamethasone, and dexamethasone). As most corticosteroid solutions contain water-insoluble CS esters, they appear as microcrystalline suspensions in commercial preparations. Dexamethasone preparations are free of ester CSs and appear clear and nonparticulate. In the commonly used particulate CS preparations, the biologically active moiety is released by the action of cellular local esterases (hydrolysis) and therefore has the potential of lasting longer at the level of placement (joint, nerve root, intra-articular facets, etc.).[43] On the other hand, the water-soluble CS solutions are taken up quickly by the cells and have a quicker onset of effect, but with a possible reduced duration of action. Many in vitro studies have demonstrated that for the ester CSs, in addition to variations in particle size, there are also differences in propensity of different CS crystals to aggregate into larger particles.[44] Concentration of crystals also varies to compensate for different potencies and to allow equivalent doses between different CSs (Table 44.3).[45-47]

The duration of action of injectable CSs depends on their biologic and pharmacologic half-lives as well as the duration of clinical benefits. Although the length of pain relief in response to a CS injection may be the most practical assessment, it is also a subjective variable on which literature data vary widely. Despite the assumption that heavy particulate formulations are expected to have a longer-lasting effect because they depend on the patient's own hydrolytic enzymes (esterases) to release the active moiety, CS knee injection in rheumatoid arthritis provided pain relief for 14 to 66 days after triamcinolone[48,49] and 8 to 56 days after methylprednisolone.[50,51] Other studies comparing an ester CS with dexamethasone for major joint injections have shown no statistically significant difference between their onset, duration, or efficacy.[52]

When used in neuraxial techniques such as interlaminar or transforaminal epidural injections, the steroid injection has shown both short (less than 6 weeks) and long (more than 6 weeks) pain relief.[53] Studies of steroid doses have found no difference in outcome between low-dose (40 mg) and high-dose (80 mg) methylprednisolone.[54] Some authors have suggested that the depot formulation of steroids (Depo-Medrol) provided better pain control at 4 weeks than the aqueous preparation of betamethasone.[55] In addition,

Table 44.3 Properties of Commonly Used Injectable Corticosteroids

Steroid	Commercial Name	Equivalent Potency (mg)	Relative GC Potency	Solubility	Maximum Particle Size (microns)	Particles > 10 Microns (%)	Particle Aggregates
Methylprednisolone acetate	Depo-medrol, Solu-medrol	4	5	0.001	> 500	45	Extensive
Triamcinolone acetonide	Kenalog	4	5	0.0002	> 500	45	Extensive
Betamethasone acetate, betamethasone sodium phosphate	Celestone Soluspan, Betaject	0.75	33	Acetate form, "practically insoluble" Sodium phosphate form, freely soluble	500	35	Some
Dexamethasone sodium phosphate	Decadron phosphate, Adrenocort, Decaject	0.75	27	Freely soluble	0.5	0	None

Reproduced and adapted from MacMahon PJ, Eustace SJ, Kavanagh EC. Injectable corticosteroids and local anaesthetic preparations: a review for radiologists. *Radiology.* 2009;252:647-681; and Benzon HT, Chew TL, McCarthy RJ, et al. Comparison of the particle sizes of different steroids and the effect of dilution. *Anesthesiology.* 2007;106:331-338.
GC, glucocorticoids.

evidence from the literature supports minimizing the steroid used either by adding clonidine or by increasing the volume of injectate, as evidence suggests that a larger volume may provide the added benefit of adhesiolysis.[56]

COMPLICATIONS OF STEROID INJECTIONS

Although some patients experience no changes in fasting blood glucose or lipid levels after a single epidural injection of dexamethasone,[57] other patients may experience a host of side effects. The depot steroid preparations used for epidural injections may produce ACTH suppression and cushingoid symptoms that can last up to a few weeks.[58] Cushing's syndrome has occurred following a single epidural injection of 60 mg of methylprednisolone[34] or triamcinolone,[59] and it has been reported in several patients following repeated epidural steroid injections when 200 mg of methylprednisolone was exceeded.[60]

Steroid myopathy involving the proximal muscles of the lower extremity has been reported following a single epidural triamcinolone injection. The progressive weakness developed over 2 to 4 weeks and did not resolve for 12 to 16 weeks.[59] Lumbar epidural injection of triamcinolone, 80 mg, caused profound HPA axis suppression for 3 weeks, although steroid was undetectable in the plasma during this time. This suggests that GCs act directly on central GC receptors, presumably via CSF absorption.[61] Comparable studies of patients who have received intra-articular steroid injections have shown detectable levels in the circulation and HPA axis suppression for up to 4 weeks.[62]

Epidural injection of triamcinolone, 80 mg, caused a marked reduction in insulin sensitivity in patients with normal glucose tolerance and caused fasting hyperglycemia in patients with a preexisting degree of insulin resistance.[63] In this study, insulin sensitivity and fasting glucose levels were normal 1 week after injection. Because patients with diabetes commonly experience increased insulin requirements for several days following injection, it is suggested that they be given specific advice on the management of their condition following epidural GC injection.

Sterile meningitis and arachnoiditis have been reported following intrathecal injection of methylprednisolone but may have been related to the polyethylene preservative.[64] Rare anaphylactoid reactions have occurred following intravenous, intramuscular, and soft tissue injections of the succinate salts of methylprednisolone and hydrocortisone.[65-67] Most of these patients were chronically atopic, and in two cases the patients had aspirin sensitivity.[65,68] Signs and symptoms of anaphylaxis reported with the use of various hydrocortisone preparations include bronchospasm, shock, urticaria, and angioedema.[66] Any type of anaphylactic reaction warrants prompt and aggressive life support therapy, including resuscitation of airway, breathing, and circulation, with oxygen support and cardiac life support when indicated.

CENTRAL NERVOUS SYSTEM EVENTS AFTER TRANSFORAMINAL EPIDURAL STEROID INJECTIONS

The overall safety of fluoroscopically guided epidural steroid injections has been confirmed in a retrospective study.[69] However, there have been several reported cases of central nervous system injuries after transforaminal epidural steroid injections (Table 44.4).[70-78]

These injuries occurred after injection not only of the steroid but also of the local anesthetics and contrast. In addition, they have also been reported not only after fluoroscopy but also after computed tomography. These injuries involve the spinal cord in the form of paraplegia or the brain as embolic cerebrovascular accidents. The mechanisms of the spinal cord injuries have been ascribed to injury or spasm of the blood vessels supplying branches to the spinal cord (segmental artery, deep cervical, or ascending cervical arteries),

Table 44.4 Adverse Central Nervous System Events after Transforaminal Epidural Steroid Injections

Study	Site	Injectate	Needle	Event*
Brouwers et al.[70]	C6-7	Triamcinolone, 0.5 mL + 0.5% bupivacaine, 0.5 mL	22 G	C3 quadriplegia (spinal cord infarct)
Rozin et al.[74]	C7	Methylprednisolone, 80 mg + 0.75% bupivacaine (3 mL total)	25 G Quincke	Death (brainstem hemorrhage)
Tiso et al.[75]	C5-6	Triamcinolone 80 mg + 0.25% bupivacaine, 2 mL	25 G, Quincke	Cerebellar infarct
Karasek and Bogduk[77]	C6-7	2% lidocaine, 0.8 mL	needle size not specified	Paralysis of all four extremities for 20 min
McMillan and Crompton[73]	C5-6	Iopamidol, 2 mL	22 G	Cortical blindness for 3 wk (edema of occipital cortex)
Houten and Errico[71]	L3-4, L4-5	Betamethasone, 12 mg + 0.25% bupivacaine (3 mL total)	25 G spinal	L1 paraplegia (spinal cord edema)
	L3-4	Methylprednisolone, 40 mg + 1% lidocaine, 1 mL + iodine (Isovue 300), 0.2 mL	20 G spinal	Low thoracic paraplegia (spinal cord edema)
	S1	Methylprednisolone, 40 mg + 1% lidocaine, 1 mL	22 G spinal	T10 paraplegia
Huntoon and Martin[76]	L1	Triamcinolone 40 mg + 0.12% bupivacaine, 5 mL	25 G; 22 G, Quincke	T10 paraplegia (spinal cord infarct)
Somayaji et al.[78]	L2-3	Triamcinolone, 40 mg + 0.5% bupivacaine, 1 mL	21 G, spinal	L2 paraplegia (spinal cord infarct)

*The MRI findings in the "Event" column are in parentheses. The cases of Huntoon, Houten, and colleagues had lumbar spine surgeries. The case of Somayaji and associates was performed under computed tomographic guidance.

C, cervical; G, gauge; L, lumbar; S, sacral; T, thoracic.

Reprinted with permission from Benzon HT, Chew TL, McCarthy R, et al. Comparison of the particle sizes of different steroids and the effect of dilution: a review of the relative neurotoxicities of the steroids. *Anesthesiology.* 2007;106:331-338.

proximal intraneural spread of the injectate, or embolization of the particulate steroid through these vessels.[79-81] Injury to these vessels is possible. Huntoon has shown in cadaver studies that the entry of the ascending cervical and deep cervical vessels in the posterior portion of the cervical intervertebral foramen is within a few millimeters of the path of the needle placed for transforaminal epidural steroid injections,[82] and these findings were confirmed by Hoeft and colleagues.[83] Spasm of the blood vessels occurs after trauma by the needle or after injection of the dye. Another mechanism is embolization of the particulate steroid through these blood vessels, resulting in segmental infarct of the spinal cord or embolization through the vertebral or an end cerebral artery, resulting in cerebral or cerebellar infarct.

Tiso and colleagues,[75] Benzon and associates,[44] and Derby and colleagues [81] examined the sizes of the particles in the steroid preparations. They found that methylprednisolone has a significantly higher percentage of large particles (Fig. 44.2) and that the particles are large enough to occlude the vessels. One type of available betamethasone (Celestone Soluspan) had the smallest particle sizes, followed by triamcinolone acetonide (Figs. 44.3 and 44.4).

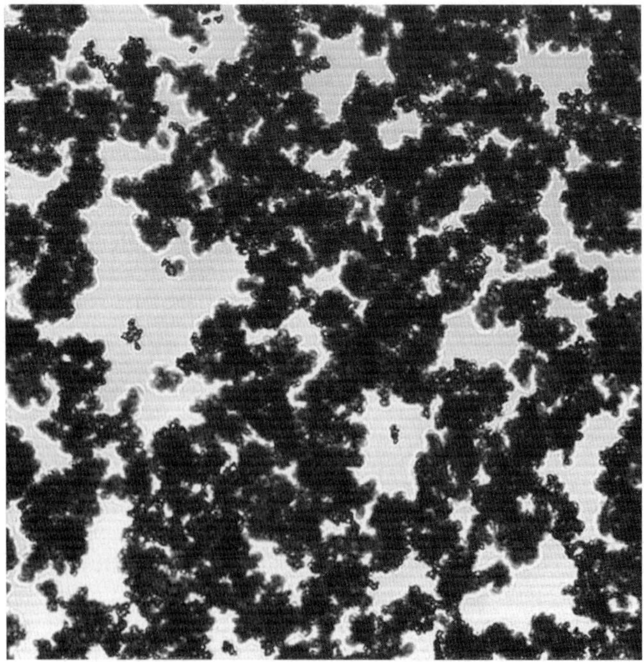

Figure 44.2 Particle size in methylprednisolone.

A compounded form of betamethasone, which can be ordered from compounding companies, does not appear to offer an advantage over triamcinolone, because the sizes of their particles appear to be the same.[44,81] Whereas Tiso and coworkers noted small particles in dexamethasone and betamethasone sodium phosphate,[75] the short-acting component in the commercial type of betamethasone, Benzon and colleagues noted that the two steroids are pure liquid, with no identifiable particles.[44] It should be noted that the commercially available betamethasone preparation (Celestone Soluspan) contains 3 mg/mL of betamethasone sodium phosphate and 3 mg/mL of betamethasone acetate.

An outbreak of fungal infections *(Exserohilum rostratum)* from epidural injections of contaminated methylprednisolone

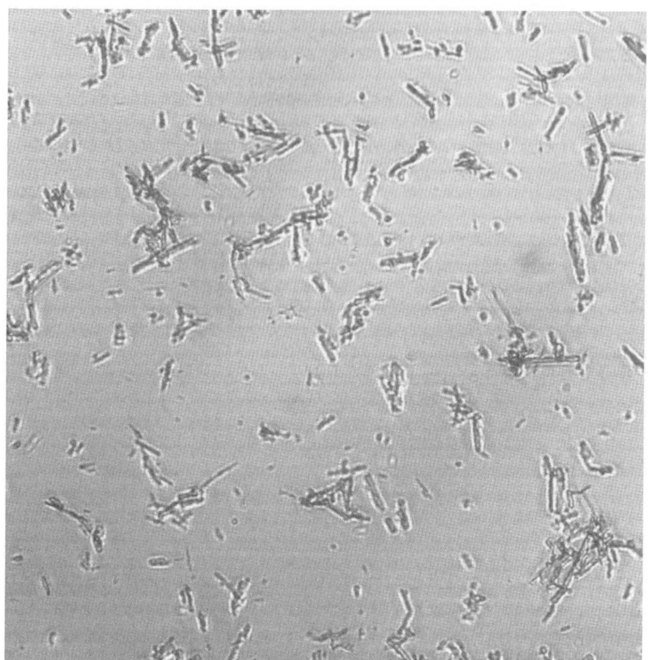

Figure 44.3 Particle size in betamethasone.

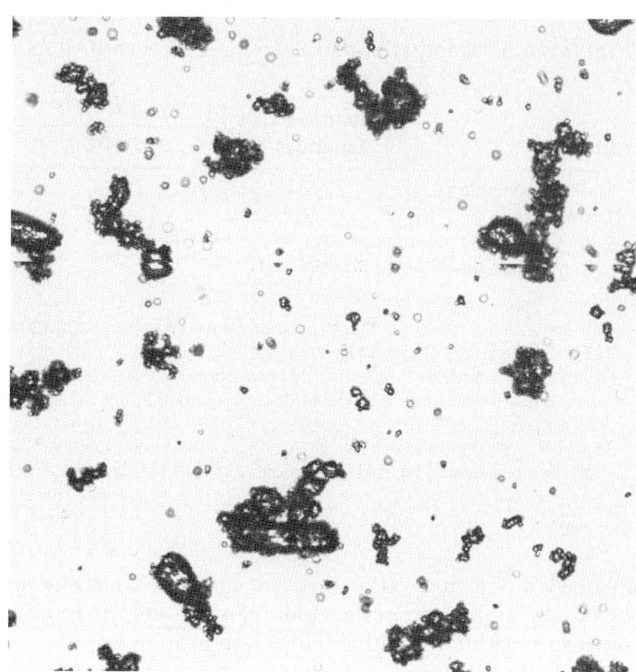

Figure 44.4 Particle size in triamcinolone.

occurred in September 2012; the contaminated steroid was manufactured by the New England Compounding Company in Framingham, Massachusetts. The infections were initially noted in Tennessee, where the initial 66 cases presented with either meningitis, cauda equine syndrome or focal infection, or posterior cerebral artery distribution such as basilar stroke with or without meningitis.[84] The risk of infection was noted to increase with the older vials, higher doses, multiple procedures, and translaminar approaches. Voriconazole was used to treat most of the patients, whereas the other patients were treated with liposomal amphotericin B.[84] At least 4300 patients have been infected, and more are expected because approximately 14,000 patients had injections from the contaminated lots.[85-87] Some of the spinal infections progressed into abscesses.

Compounding companies fall into a gray area between federal and state oversight. These companies are not registered with the U.S. Food and Drug Administration (FDA) as drug manufacturers, and adverse events do not have to be reported to the FDA.[86] The authority of the FDA is limited to investigating problems once the problem is obvious.[86] The lack of clear oversight on the safe and sterile practices of compounding companies led to calls for stronger oversight by the FDA on compounding companies.[88]

For economic reasons or because of the lack of availability (e.g., high concentration bupivacaine), drugs will continue to be compounded. Between 1% and 3% of all prescriptions are compounded.[87] These include drugs used in pain management such as oral ketamine and intrathecal drugs. Standards for compounding of drugs are written under United States Pharmacopeia, chapter 797 (USP 797), and include the particulate matter in the room air where the drug is compounded and the colony forming units per cubic meter of air per plate.[89] There are approximately 7500 compounding companies in the United States; only 2% participate in the industry's voluntary accreditation program.[87] The pain medicine physician can ensure sterility of the compounded drug that he or she is using by getting the drug from a company accredited by the Pharmacy Compounding Accreditation Board (www.pcab.org).

In a laboratory study, the injection of the particulate steroid methylprednisolone into the carotid artery resulted in cerebral hemorrhage in 8 of 11 rats.[90] This is compared to the lack of such injury when dexamethasone or saline was injected. Interestingly, the nonparticulate carrier of methylprednisolone caused the same injury in half of the rats. Another study of methylprednisolone injection into the vertebral artery of pigs resulted in brainstem edema, hypoxic and ischemic brain damage, ventilatory support, and inability to regain consciousness.[91] In comparison, there was full recovery with dexamethasone and prednisolone.

Dexamethasone is a nonparticulate steroid, is long-acting, and has minimal or no mineralocorticoid activity. It has increased GC activity, theoretically resulting in a greater elevation of the blood glucose level. A dose ranging study compared transforaminal epidural dexamethasone, 4 mg versus 12 mg.[92] The authors noted a reduction in radicular pain by 42%, 34%, and 27% at 4, 8, and 12 weeks, respectively, whereas the Oswestry Disability ratings improved from "moderate" at baseline to "minimal" at 12 weeks. There was no difference between the two doses. Studies comparing dexamethasone with a particulate steroid are few. One clinical study on dexamethasone showed it to be slightly less efficacious than triamcinolone.[93] Another study compared 10 mg dexamethasone with 40 mg triamcinolone for cervical transforaminal epidural steroid injection and showed no difference in efficacy.[94] However, the study was not randomized; dexamethasone was used between 2006 and 2007, whereas triamcinolone was employed between 2007 and 2008. Also, the follow-up was short (1 month). Triamcinolone was slightly more effective (80% versus 69%) but did not reach statistical significance. It therefore appears that dexamethasone is slightly less effective than triamcinolone for transforaminal injections. However, clinical studies of better quality

Table 44.5 Comparison of Steroids in Terms of Glucocorticoid Potency, Component Vehicles, and Preservatives

Steroid	Relative GC Potency*	Vehicle	Preservatives		
		PEG	Benzyl Alcohol	Methylparaben	Sodium Bisulfite
Methylprednisolone	5	+	+	–	–
Triamcinolone	5	+/–†	+	–	–
Betamethasone	33	–	–	–	–
Dexamethasone	27	–	–	+	+

All the steroids in Table 44.5 have minimal mineralocorticoid activity.
*Relative milligram potency to hydrocortisone.
†Triamcinolone acetonide does not contain polyethylene glycol (PEG), whereas triamcinolone diacetate does; both contain benzyl alcohol. Triamcinolone diacetate has been recently discontinued in the United States.
GC, glucocorticoid.
Reprinted with permission from Benzon HT, Chew TL, McCarthy R, et al. Comparison of the particle sizes of different steroids and the effect of dilution: a review of the relative neurotoxicities of the steroids. *Anesthesiology*. 2007;106:331-338.

are needed. The theoretical disadvantages of dexamethasone are its easy washout from the epidural space and the reports of convulsions after intrathecal injection in animals.[58,44]

The better efficacy of the transforaminal approach over the interlaminar approach has not been completely established; one study showed the two approaches to be similar in efficacy in terms of pain relief and functional capacity.[95] If cervical transforaminal epidural steroid injection is to be given, dexamethasone should be used; particulate steroid should not be injected in the cervical levels. For lumbar transforaminal injections, dexamethasone should preferably be tried first. If the relief is short, then a steroid with smaller particles (i.e., commercial betamethasone or triamcinolone) is then tried. The CNS events have not been reported after interlaminar injections, so any of the available steroids can be used. Digital subtraction angiography should be employed for cervical and upper lumbar transforaminal injections to detect intravascular injections.

The question of neurotoxicity and possible allergic reactions to steroids arises from the vehicle and preservatives of the commercially available steroids (Table 44.5).

Dexamethasone contains methylparaben and sodium bisulfite, compounds that have been implicated in allergic reactions to local anesthetics.[44] Polyethylene glycol, the vehicle used in methylprednisolone and triamcinolone, can decrease the compound action potential of the A, B, and C fibers.[96] However, these changes are reversible, and concentrations above 20% are required for this effect (methylprednisolone and triamcinolone contain only 3% polyethylene glycol [PEG]). In addition, the concentration of PEG in the vial can be significantly decreased by inverting the vial for 1 to 2 hours and aspirating and using the steroid component.[97] Interestingly, the intrathecal injection of the vehicle in dogs showed minimal histologic changes, whereas methylprednisolone resulted in a dose-dependent intrathecal inflammatory reaction.[98]

BOTULINUM TOXIN THERAPY

HISTORY

Botulinum toxins are produced by the gram-negative anaerobic bacterium *Clostridium botulinum*. They produce flaccid paralysis by preventing the presynaptic release of acetylcholine (Ach) at the neuromuscular junction. There are eight botulinum toxin (BTX) subtypes: A, B, C_1, C_2, D, E, F, and G.[99] Types A, B, E, and F have been described to cause botulism, a syndrome of generalized muscle weakness following the ingestion of botulinum-contaminated food. The FDA approved the use of onabotulinum toxin A for the treatment of strabismus, blepharospasm, and hemifacial spasm. In 2000, the FDA approved botulinum toxin B for treating cervical dystonia, and 10 years later the agency approved the use of onabotulinum toxin (Botox or Botox Cosmetic) for chronic migraine treatment.

PHARMACOLOGY OF BOTULINUM TOXIN

TOXIN STRUCTURE AND QUANTIFICATION

Botulinum toxin is synthesized as a single-chain polypeptide, consisting of a heavy chain (H chain; molecular weight [MW], 100,000) and a light (L) chain (MW, 50,000). The H chain is responsible for binding to presynaptic cholinergic nerve terminals at the neuromuscular junction, whereas the L chain is the neurotoxic component. The H and L chains are bound together by disulfide bonds, and the toxin is activated by proteolytic enzymes in a cleaving process. BTX is quantified in mouse units (MU); 1 MU is the dose required to kill 50% of a batch of 18- to 20-g female Swiss-Webster mice (LD_{50}). It is estimated that the human lethal dose of botulinum toxin A (BTX-A) is about 2800 to 3500 units for a 70-kg adult. The lethal dose of BTX-B in humans is estimated at 144,000 units. The type A subtypes appear to be the most potent and have the longest duration of action.

PREPARATION AND DOSING

Two botulinum neurotoxins, types A and B, are used in clinical practice. There are three commercially available type A preparations: Botox, Dysport, and Xeomin. Each vial of Botox (Allergan, Inc., Irvine, California) contains 100 units of onabotulinum toxin A as a sterile, vacuum-dried form without preservative (the toxin is redissolved prior to drying in a solution containing saline and albumin and sterile filtered through a 0.2 µm filter) that can be reconstituted with sterile nonpreserved saline prior to injection. Dysport (abobotulinum toxin A) (Ipsen, Ltd., Berkshire,

United Kingdom) is marketed in the form of 500-MU vials. Data from patients treated for cervical dystonia suggest that 1 MU of Botox equals 3 to 5 MU of Dysport. Xeomin (Merz Pharmaceutical, Greensboro, NC) is marketed as 100 units of incobotulinum toxin A powder, reconstituted upon use in normal saline. Myobloc (Solstice Neurosciences, Inc.) is marketed as a sterile liquid formulation of a purified botulinum toxin B (rimabotulinum toxin B). Each 3.5 ml glass vial of Myobloc contains 5000 units of B toxin per milliliter in 0.05% human serum albumin, 0.01 M sodium succinate, and 0.1 M sodium chloride at approximate pH 5.6.

BTX-A in the Botox formulation, the commercially available product in the United States, is inactivated by heat, shaking, excessive dilution, and surface tension from bubbles during reconstitution. Boiling dissolves the disulfide bonds between the heavy and light chains of BTX-A, thus rendering the toxin inactive, because neither chain can exert neurotoxicity independently. BTX-A must be reconstituted with normal saline without a preservative. Dilution of a 100-MU vial may be performed with 1, 2, 5, or 10 mL of 0.9% sodium chloride. This will yield a concentration of 10, 5, 2, or 1 MU/0.1 mL, respectively. The higher concentrations are appropriate for larger muscles—for example, hip flexors or piriformis muscles. Lower concentrations are used for facial injections, such as for the glabella, temporalis, and frontalis muscles. Tuberculin syringes are used to dilute and draw up the toxin, and new 30-gauge needles are used to give the injections so as to reduce discomfort, local trauma, and bleeding. BTX-A should be used within 4 hours of preparation and stored at 2° to 8° C during this time. It has been shown that there is no loss of activity 6 hours after reconstitution at room temperature; however, a 44% loss of activity is observed at 12 hours.[100] Refreezing the toxin after reconstitution causes a 70% reduction in bioactivity at 1 to 2 weeks.

MECHANISMS OF ACTION

Botulinum toxins act by blocking the presynaptic release of ACh from cholinergic terminals of motor and autonomic nerves. BTX neurotoxicity occurs in three stages: binding, internalization, and proteolysis.[101] Following activation by proteolytic cleavage, the BTX heavy chain binds irreversibly to the presynaptic terminals of cholinergic neurons. The C-terminal region of the heavy chain binds in a serotype-specific manner to receptors on the motor end plates and at autonomic cholinergic ganglia.

In addition to the pain relief associated with its paralytic effect, BTX-A has been studied in relation to its effect on noncholinergic neurons to reduce peripheral sensitization. By acting as an inhibitor for the release of glutamate, BTX-A subsequently decreases the amount of substance P, the neuropeptide essentially involved in pain perception, vasodilation, and neurogenic inflammation. This mechanism is modulated by the synaptosomal-associated protein 25 (SNAP-25). In addition to substance P, other mediators have been involved in response to the BTX-A. Those neuropeptides, calcitonin gene-related peptide and neurokinin A, play a major role in neurogenic inflammation and are released from dense-core vesicles at sites away from the synaptic active zone, as part of the nonadrenergic, noncholinergic (NANC) transmitter system.

The effects of BTX-A on inhibiting central sensitization stem from studies suggesting the transport of BTX-A by axons to the CNS after intramuscular injections. Because many neurotransmitters released in vesicles by exocytosis mechanisms are dependent on **s**oluble *N*-ethylmaleimide **s**ensitive **f**actor **a**ttachment protein **r**eceptor (SNARE) proteins, the target of botulinum toxins, it appears that BTX-A may be implicated in nervous pathways whose transmitters extend beyond acetylcholine-dependent mechanisms. Therefore, BTX-A may play an important role in central nervous system "neuroplasticity" that involves pain transmission and modulation.[102-105]

CLINICAL EFFECTS

Botulinum neurotoxins irreversibly inhibit the release of Ach from cholinergic terminals of motor neurons, preganglionic sympathetic fibers, and pre- and postganglionic parasympathetic fibers. The BTX molecule cannot cross the blood-brain barrier and therefore does not have any direct CNS effects.[102] At the neuromuscular junction, BTXs cause a chemical denervation, thereby inhibiting skeletal muscle contraction. Experiments on mouse phrenic nerve have revealed that binding of BTX to nerve terminals takes about 32 to 64 minutes. In humans, clinical effects typically appear after 2 to 3 days, but peak effects are observed at 2 to 6 weeks. The primary muscle relaxant effect is on α motor neuron function, but it may also affect the γ motor neurons in the muscle spindles, resulting in lower resting muscle tone.[103] In both animal and human muscle biopsy studies, muscle atrophy occurs within 2 weeks of injections. Atrophy continues for about 4 weeks and then stabilizes. Muscle mass has been estimated to return to about 70% to 80% of original size after 3 months.[104]

BTX may also have other mechanisms of analgesia in addition to those related to the relief of muscle spasm. Specifically, there is evidence to suggest that BTX-A may block the release of glutamate, substance P, calcitonin g-related peptide, and neurokinin A.[105] The subcutaneous injection of BTX-A into the paws of rats exposed to the formalin experimental pain model, although causing no motor effects, results in reduced pain behaviors, decreased release of glutamate, and inhibition of c-fos expression in the dorsal spinal cord.[106]

RECOVERY

BTX-induced chemical denervation is permanent, so skeletal muscle remains paralyzed until new axons and synapses have formed to reestablish the neuromuscular junction. Functional recovery takes place by neurogenesis in the form of axonal sprouting, reinnervation and enlargement of some end plates, and the formation of new smaller end plates.[104] The number of muscle fibers innervated per axon also increases. Sprouting begins within 10 days of BTX exposure. Functional denervation is apparent for 6 weeks up to 6 months following injection, but it typically lasts for 3 to 4 months. Recovery is complete after allowing sufficient time for reinnervation, and neuromuscular function returns essentially to normal, even after multiple cycles of injection and recovery.

THERAPEUTIC USES IN PAIN MANAGEMENT

CERVICAL DYSTONIA

Cervical dystonia is characterized by involuntary head and neck movements, in the form of either sustained muscle contraction or intermittent jerking motions. Both types may coexist and cause significant disability. Neck pain with or without headaches is a complaint in 70% of patients. Treatment with oral medications may yield inconsistent and unsatisfactory results. Surgical treatments, including thalamotomy, myelectomy, neurotomy, and selective peripheral denervation of neck muscles, may produce limited benefits. It is estimated that treatment with BTX-A is effective in over 80% of cases, with an average duration of benefit of 3 to 4 months. A survey of 19 studies in which BTX-A was used to treat cervical dystonia revealed a mean weighted percentage of 76% (range, 50% to 100%) of patients reporting pain relief, from 16 studies that reported pain results.[107] Injections into the superficial neck muscles, such as the sternocleidomastoid, splenius capitis, levator scapulae, and trapezius, may be done without electromyelographic guidance. The dose of BTX-A per muscle ranged from 50 to 100 MU. It has been suggested to divide the dose into 25-MU quanta and inject these in an even distribution throughout the length of the muscle. A study of patients with cervical dystonia treated with BTX-A has revealed that pain relief occurs long before any reduction in muscle spasm can be detected.[108]

MIGRAINE HEADACHE

Since 2010, onabotulinum toxin A (Botox, Allergan, Inc., Irvine, California) has been FDA approved for the treatment of patients with chronic migraine headaches. The diagnosis of chronic migraine can be made for individuals who experience 15 or more headache days each month, at least 8 of which would be consistent with migraine, for at least 4 hours per day for at least 4 months. Multiple studies led to the Phase REsearch Evaluating Migraine Prophylaxis Therapy (PREEMPT) trials, which ultimately led to the FDA approval of onabotulinum toxin A for chronic migraine.

In a multicenter, open-label study on the efficacy of Botox (BTX-A) for the acute and prophylactic management of migraine, BTX-A was injected into the glabellar, temporal, frontal, or suboccipital muscles of the head and neck.[109] In 77 true migraine patients treated prophylactically with a mean dose of 31 units (range, 5 to 110 units), 51% reported complete response with a mean duration of relief of 4.1 months, and 38% reported a partial response with a mean duration of relief of 2.7 months. In the acute treatment group, 70% of 10 true migraine patients treated with a mean dose of 31 units reported complete response at 1 to 2 hours after treatment. A double-blind, vehicle-controlled study was done on 123 migraineurs in which the patients were randomized to receive the vehicle or BTX-A 25- or 75-unit injections at one visit into symmetric points in the frontalis, temporalis, and glabellar muscles.[110] BTX-A, 25 units, was significantly superior to vehicle in reducing migraine frequency and severity, the use of acute migraine medication, and migraine-associated vomiting. The beneficial effects of BTX-A were observed at 2 and 3 months. The 75-unit dose of BTX-A had a higher incidence of side effects, including blepharoptosis, diplopia, and injection site weakness. BTX-B (Myobloc) has been evaluated for treating transformed migraine headaches.[111] Forty-seven patients received injections of 5000 units of BTX-B into three or more muscles. Of these, 64% reported improvement in headache intensity and severity, and all patients experienced a decrease in migraine frequency over 4 weeks.

Two large randomized, controlled, multicenter clinical trials, PREEMPT I and II,[112,113] reported their results in 2010. Each study enrolled approximately 700 patients with a comparable number in toxin treatment and placebo administration groups in a 24-week blinded arm followed by a 32-week open arm. In the treatment group, patients received 155 U of onabotulinum toxin A divided in 31 injections sited across 7 head and neck muscles using a fixed-site fixed-dose (FSFD) paradigm (Table 44.6). Each injection was performed with 5 U in 0.1 ml, obtained by reconstituting the toxin powder in 2 ml of normal saline.[114]

The primary outcomes and a number of secondary outcomes were evaluated at 24 weeks for both studies. PREEMPT II met its primary and secondary outcomes at all time points, whereas PREEMPT I met only its secondary outcomes and not the primary ones.[115] However, the number of headache days (the reached primary outcome for PREEMPT I) was considered the better outcome measure than the headache episodes (not the reached primary outcome for PREEMPT II) for the study of chronic migraine (headache with a frequency of 15 or more headache days per month for more than 3 months). Therefore based on those studies, Botox or Botox Cosmetic (manufactured by Allergan) was approved in October 2010 to be used for the treatment of chronic migraine.

Overall, the use of onabotulinum toxin A for chronic migraine significantly improves headache symptoms and demonstrates improved patient functioning, vitality, psychological distress, and overall quality of life.[116]

TENSION HEADACHE

Tension-type headache (TH) is characterized as a dull, aching, pressure-like or squeezing feeling; the International Headache Society (IHS) has characterized the pain as pressing or tightening.[117] A population study of 1000 adult patients revealed a lifetime prevalence of TH of 78%, with 87% of chronic headache sufferers demonstrating pericranial muscle tenderness and pain threshold abnormalities. Onabotulinum toxin A has shown some efficacy in the treatment

Table 44.6 Onabotulinum Toxin A Dosing for Chronic Migraine by Muscle Using the PREEMPT Injection Paradigm

Head/Neck Area	Recommended Dose: Total Dosage (number of sites*)
Frontalis†	20 units (in four sites)
Corrugators†	10 units (in two sites)
Procerus	5 units (in one site)
Occipitalis†	30 units (in six sites), rebreak up to 40 units in 8 sites
Temporalis†	40 units (in eight sites), rebreak up to 50 units in 10 sites
Trapezius†	30 units (in six sites), rebreak up to 50 units in 10 sites
Cervical paraspinal muscle†	20 units (in five sites)

*Each intramuscular injection site = 0.1 ml = 5 U onabotulinum toxin A.
†Dose distributed bilaterally for the minimum 155 U dose.
Total dose range: 155 units to 195 units.

of TH. In one retrospective study, 21 patients with chronic TH were injected with onabotulinum toxin A, 100 units, divided evenly over five injection sites representing the most tender muscle points in the scalp and upper neck.[118] There was a 50% reduction in headache frequency in 18 of the 21 patients and a 50% reduction in tenderness to palpation in 20 patients. In another study, the efficacy of onabotulinum toxin A was assessed in a randomized, double-blind, placebo-controlled trial in 37 patients.[119] Patients received onabotulinum toxin A, 100 units, or placebo, divided among six injection sites—two in the temporal muscles and four in the cervical muscles. The actively treated group experienced decreased headache severity and more headache-free days over 3 months following injection.[119]

WHIPLASH INJURY

Whiplash-associated disorders (WADs) include a number of clinical features, including neck pain, nonspecific headache, and temporomandibular joint pain. Clinical findings in WADs include myofascial tenderness, trigger points in the affected musculature, increased pain with function, and cervical muscle spasm.[120] Onabotulinum toxin A has been studied in small trials of WADs and has been found to relieve pain and increase range of motion. A randomized, double-blind, placebo-controlled study has examined the effects of onabotulinum toxin A in patients with motor vehicle accident (MVA)-associated WADs of longer than 6 months' duration. Half of the patients received onabotulinum toxin A, 100 units, into five trigger points, and the other 50% received normal saline injections. The muscles treated bilaterally included the splenius capitis, rectus capitis, semispinalis capitis, and trapezius. At 4 weeks postinjection, the onabotulinum toxin A treatment group demonstrated improvement in range of motion (ROM) and subjective pain. Another randomized, placebo-controlled study evaluated the potential benefits of relaxing selected neck muscles with onabotulinum toxin A.[121] Twenty-eight patients with chronic grade 2 WADs received injections of onabotulinum toxin A, 100 units, or saline placebo. Each patient received five injections into the five most tender cervical muscular points. At 2 weeks, the onabotulinum toxin A group showed a trend of improvement in ROM and pain reduction. At 4 weeks postinjection, this group was significantly improved from preinjection levels.

Botulinum toxin B has also been studied in WADs. An open-label study evaluated botulinum toxin-B for the treatment of 31 patients with chronic headaches following injury. Botulinum toxin B, 5000 units, was injected in divided doses into the suboccipital muscles (rectus capitis posterior major and minor, oblique capitis inferior and superior). Of these, 71% experienced a decrease in headache pain and frequency.[122]

HEMIFACIAL SPASM

Hemifacial spasm is usually caused by irritation or compression of the root of the facial nerve by an anomalous blood vessel. This is a slowly progressive syndrome characterized by intermittent tonic or clonic contractions of the muscles supplied by the facial nerve. Treatment with anticonvulsants such as carbamazepine may provide relief initially but becomes less effective with long-term use. Surgical microvascular decompression of the facial nerve may be highly successful in relieving this condition, but serious potential complications, such as facial paralysis, hearing loss, and stroke, deter many patients from this procedure. Onabotulinum toxin A injections into the facial muscles have now become the treatment of choice for hemifacial spasm.[123,124] It is recommended that for the first treatment only the orbicularis oculi be injected, with a starting dose of 12.5 units of onabotulinum toxin A.[104] Other commonly injected muscles include the frontalis (5 to 10 MU), risorius (2.5 to 5 MU), depressor anguli oris (5 MU), platysma (2.5 MU per strand of muscle), and zygomatic major (2.5 MU). The dose for botulinum toxin B is 125 to 250 units per muscle site (total dose, 750 to 5000 units).

LOW BACK PAIN

The efficacy of botulinum toxins for the relief of chronic low back pain was investigated in a randomized, double-blind study of 31 patients who had nonradiating back pain for at least 6 months.[125] Fifteen patients received 200 units of onabotulinum toxin A, 40 units per site at five lumbar paravertebral levels on the side of maximum discomfort, and 16 patients received normal saline. At 3 weeks, 86% of patients in the onabotulinum toxin A group and 31% of patients in the saline group reported some degree of pain relief, with 73% in the onabotulinum toxin A group reporting more than 50% relief. At 8 weeks, 60% in the botulinum toxin group versus 12.5% in the saline group reported pain relief exceeding 50%. Onabotulinum toxin A was not associated with any increase in low back pain or worsening in functioning.

MYOFASCIAL PAIN

Botulinum toxin injections may be used for cases refractory to a series of trigger point injections with local anesthetics and steroids. Onabotulinum toxin A was evaluated for the treatment of chronic myofascial pain in a randomized, double-blind, placebo-controlled study of six patients with myofascial pain involving cervical paraspinal and shoulder girdle muscles.[126] Patients were injected with 50 units of onabotulinum toxin A or normal saline on two occasions. Four of the 6 patients experienced more than a 30% reduction in pain and muscle spasm following botulinum toxin injections. The onset of the response occurred within the first week, and the mean duration of response was 5 to 6 weeks.

Studies have shown the lack of efficacy of botulinum toxin injections for myofascial pain syndrome. In a randomized, double-blind crossover study, onabotulinum toxin A (25 units per trigger point) was found to provide the same degree and duration of pain relief compared with 0.5% bupivacaine.[127] Another study has shown no difference in results between onabotulinum toxin A, at 5 units per trigger point, and saline.[128] Finally, a study that compared different doses of onabotulinum toxin A (5, 10, 25, or 50 units per trigger point) with saline showed no differences in the pain scores, pain threshold as measured by pressure algometry, and number of rescue medications.[129] It appears, therefore, that onabotulinum toxin A does not offer any advantage over bupivacaine or saline, regardless of the dose.

PIRIFORMIS SYNDROME

Initial treatment of piriformis syndrome is conservative and includes physical therapy combined with anti-inflammatory drugs, analgesics, and muscle relaxants to reduce inflammation, spasm, and pain.[130] When conservative therapy fails, patients may benefit from local anesthetics, steroid injections, or both into the piriformis muscle; caudal epidural steroid injections;[131] botulinum toxin injections; or surgery. A randomized, double-blind study of 72 cases of piriformis syndrome has examined the effect of onabotulinum toxin A, 200 units, compared with lidocaine and triamcinolone or placebo. Onabotulinum toxin A therapy resulted in a 50% pain reduction in 65% of patients as compared with a 32% response in the triamcinolone and lidocaine group and 6% in the placebo group.[132]

ANTIBODY FORMATION AND ADVERSE REACTIONS

Repeated injections of onabotulinum toxin A have been associated with antibody formation, which renders subsequent onabotulinum toxin A injections ineffective. A study of 32 patients with spasmodic torticollis treated with repeated onabotulinum toxin A injections has revealed that 4 patients (12.5%) produced antibodies after 2 to 9 months of treatment.[133] The larger doses used likely explain this relatively high incidence. The data from numerous studies have suggested that the incidence of antibody formation with onabotulinum toxin A for the treatment of cervical dystonia is probably less than 5%.[101] Because onabotulinum toxin A and botulinum toxin B are structurally different, it has been thought that neutralizing antibodies to onabotulinum toxin A would not cross-react with botulinum toxin B. It appears that higher toxin doses and frequent injections are the leading factors in the development of neutralizing antibodies.[134] The reported complications of botulinum toxin injection include brachial plexopathy, polyradiculoneuritis, and local psoriasiform dermatitis. Muscle weakness occurs if more than 50 units of onabotulinum toxin A are injected into a muscle.[129]

SUMMARY OF CLINICAL EVIDENCE FOR USE OF BOTULINUM TOXIN IN HUMAN SUBJECTS

Jabbari and Machado,[115] in an evidence-based review, used American Academy of Neurology (AAN) methodology as stated by the guidelines of the society's Therapeutics and Assessment Subcommittee to rate the scientific evidence for the use of BTXs in clinical practice. They found four levels of clinical evidence (Table 44.7). Although evidence supports using this treatment in several specific conditions such as cervical dystonia and chronic migraine, clinical studies for other chronic pain conditions have produced contradictory results.[135,136]

OTHER AGENTS USED IN INTERVENTIONAL PAIN MANAGEMENT

INJECTABLE BONE CEMENT

Vertebroplasty and kyphoplasty are minimally invasive interventions routinely used to treat vertebral body compression fractures of multiple etiologies (osteoporosis, malignancy, metastasis). By injecting bone cement into the fractured vertebral body, the procedure aims to stabilize the fracture and, it is hoped, prevent further collapse. It is reported to be highly effective, with an immediate and lasting pain relief seen in 80% to 90% of cases.[137,138]

The most common injectable bone cement used in clinical practice is polymethylmethacrylate (PMMA). Its main effect is to reinforce the fragile or broken vertebral bodies, thus leading to extensive bone stiffening. However, its handling differs between vertebroplasty and balloon kyphoplasty.[139] More fluid PMMA with a longer liquid phase working time and a very short set time is necessary in vertebroplasty procedures where the cement is injected directly into the bone

Table 44.7 Summary of Levels of Evidence for Use of Botulinum Toxins in Various Painful Clinical Conditions

Level of Evidence	Recommendations	Clinical Condition
A	Established and recommended	Cervical dystonia Chronic migraine Chronic lateral epicondylitis
B	Probably effective; should be considered for treatment	Post-herpetic neuralgia Post-traumatic neuralgia Plantar fasciitis Pyriformis syndrome Total knee arthroplasty
C	Possibly effective; can be used at the discretion of the physician	Allodynia in diabetic neuropathy Chronic low back pain Knee osteoarthritis Anterior knee pain with vastus lateralis imbalance Pelvic pain Postoperative pain in children with cerebral palsy Postoperative pain after mastectomy Sphincter spasm and pain after hemorrhoidectomy
U	Insufficient evidence due to contradictory results	Myofascial pain syndrome Chronic daily headaches

Reproduced from Jabbari B, Machado D. Treatment of refractory pain with botulinum toxins: an evidence-based review. *Pain Med.* 2011;12:1594-1606.

through the introducer with relatively higher pressure. Kyphoplasty involves the introduction of an inflatable bone tamp into the compressed vertebrae with creation of a cavity, which is subsequently filled with partially cured PMMA with a short liquid phase and a longer "doughy" phase working time.

PMMA is a bio-inert material considered an ideal substrate for use in vertebral augmentation procedures, specifically because of its ease of handling, strength, and cost-effectiveness. It has a number of disadvantages, including its lack of biologic potential to remodel or integrate into the surrounding bone; it has an excessive inherent stiffness, a high polymerization temperature, and potential monomer toxicity. Several studies have demonstrated temperatures as high as 70° C in the center of the vertebrae during setting.[140-142] Accidental release of the component monomer can be associated with cytotoxic effects such as tissue irritation, inflammation, or systemic effects on lungs, kidneys, and liver resulting from circulatory uptake. Although PMMA's main indication is for vertebral fracture stabilization, with increased strength, it may excessively increase the stiffness of the augmented vertebrae, sometimes up to 174% when compared to the intact osteoporotic bone.[143] This overly rigid reinforcement of the broken vertebrae may enhance the risk of an additional fracture in adjacent levels.

PMMA consists of several components: a polymer powder and a monomer liquid whose admixture renders an exothermic reaction with in vitro temperatures as high as 113° C and in vivo temperatures of 40° to 56°.[144-146] *N,N*-dimethyl-p-toluidine acts as an accelerator while the traces of hydroquinone stabilize the monomer, preventing premature polymerization. The major characteristics of PMMA that affect its use in vertebral augmentation are polymerization time and opacification. The polymerization time, or curing rate, varies among the different products, and the preparation material may be suited for injection in as little as 5 minutes to close to 20 minutes. The polymerization time of any PMMA can be prolonged by refrigerating its components prior to their use or by wrapping syringes filled with the acrylic in a sterile glove filled with ice. For acrylics with a longer curing time, the powdered polymer component needs to dissolve completely in the liquid monomer before injecting. Some manufacturers recommend the addition of a "rest period" of approximately 1 minute after mixing and before injection.

The amount of barium sulphate within the products, the quality of the imaging chain, the size of the patient, and the location of the targeted vertebral body influence visualization of the bone cement. The common materials present in the currently used commercial preparations for vertebral augmentation are listed in Table 44.8.

The most feared complication of PMMA is leakage of the filler material in the adjacent structures with devastating nerve root impingement and cord compression. In addition, during liquid phase PMMA injection, fatal complications have been reported due to pulmonary cement embolism via venous sinuses. This risk seems to be slightly decreased with the use of partially cured cement that is injected under low pressure in kyphoplasty.

The cement monomer is arrhythmogenic and cardiotoxic at the volumes used in total hip arthroplasties, with an estimated risk of 1 in 3000 to 5000 surgeries.[147,148] Assuming the same risk for vertebral augmentation procedures at a mean of 6 cc of cement injected per vertebral body, it might be prudent to limit the kyphoplasty/vertebroplasty levels treated to 2 (12 cc of PMMA total) per surgical intervention. In addition, a potentially higher incidence of cement leak and embolization may occur in vertebroplasty, where liquid PMMA with a higher concentration of "free" toxic monomer (available to enter the systemic circulation) is forcibly injected within the vertebra body.

BIOLOGIC AGENTS IN CHRONIC PAIN THERAPY

Advances in the understanding of chronic pain mechanisms allowed the emerging of new treatment strategies involving the delivery of short-lived potent bioactive molecules with therapeutic properties to sensory nerves, spinal cord, and meninges[149] for the treatment of refractory pain. Building on a number of preclinical studies, researchers focused on the use of nonviral or viral vector-based gene transfer for the treatment of chronic pain.[150] When comparing those two systems, the viral agents seemed to be more efficient in delivering exogenous genes to target cells and inducing long-term gene expression than their nonviral counterparts and are currently viewed as the preferred target delivery system in chronic pain. Table 44.9 summarizes preclinical data on various animal pain models that use viral system loaded genes targeting specific structures implicated in chronic pain states.

The use of viral vectors loaded with genes targeting specific structures for the treatment of chronic pain involves genetically engineering the viral genome to create a nucleic acid sequence that encodes a promoter to drive both the gene expression and the analgesic transgene. This delivering system exploits the properties of the virus to enter a normal cell and alter its transduction. Targeted vector delivery also evades the side effects of systemic administration. The ideal viral system needs to be safe and well tolerated, should not elicit any immune response, and should also be replication incompetent, and thus unable to produce an infection.[165] In addition, it should be able to infect multiple cell types and express large and small transgenes. Its mode of delivery should be varied depending on the targeted cell: either directly via neuro-axial administration (injected in the sensory nerves, intrathecal, meninges) or indirectly via distal, subcutaneous injection of a virus with engineered increased tropism for dorsal root ganglia.

The first human trial of gene therapy for chronic pain started enrolling patients with chronic cancer pain in 2008,[166] and it is currently in phase II. The product, named NP2, is a replication-defective herpes simplex virus (HSV)–based vector expressing human preproenkephalin (PENK). Injected subcutaneously in a dermatomal distribution of focal pain in individuals with moderate to severe cancer pain requiring more than 200 mg morphine equivalents daily, it proved to decrease pain scores in escalating doses.[166] Another vector expressing glutamic acid decarboxylase, potentially beneficial in neuropathic pain, is currently being studied by the same research group.

Gene therapy is an exciting new development in treating chronic refractory pain. Perfecting the genetically engineered viral vectors as well as correctly identifying delivery modes is possible due to our increased understanding of pain generation, transmission, and maintenance. Other therapies, such as the regulation of neurotropic factors and cell transplantation, currently still in preclinical trials may emerge as effective pain treatments for chronic unrelenting pain.[165]

Table 44.8 Injectable Bone Cements

Injectable Bone Cement	Manufacturer	Materials (description, feature)
Polymethylmethacrylate (PMMA)		
Simplex P	Stryker Orthopedics Mahwah, NJ, United States	**(Powder)** 75% w/w methylmethacrylate–styrene–copolymer, 10% w/w barium sulfate, 15% w/w polymethyl methacrylate **(Liquid)** 97.4% v/v methylmethacrylate **(Monomer)** 2.6% v/v *N,N*-dimethyl-p-toluidine, 75±15 ppm hydroquinone
HV-R	Medtronic, Kyphon Northridge, CA, United States	**(Powder)** 68% w/w methylmethacrylate–styrene–copolymer, 30% w/w barium sulfate, 2% w/w benzoyl peroxide **(Liquid)** 99.1% v/v methylmethacrylate **(Monomer)** 0.9% v/v *N,N*-dimethyl-p-toluidine, 75 ppm hydroquinone
Palacos R	Biomet Orthopedics, Inc. Warsaw, IN, United States	**(Powder)** 81.8% w/w methyl acrylate, methylmethacrylate, 14.9% w/w zirconium dioxide, 0.78% w/w benzoyl peroxide, 2.4% chlorophyll **(Liquid)** 96% v/v methyl methacrylate **(Monomer)** 2.0% v/v *N,N*-dimethyl-p-toluidine, 0.40 mg chlorophyll
DePuy 1	DePuy Orthopedics Inc. Warsaw, IN, United States	**(Powder)** 88.85% w/w polymethyl methylmethacrylate, 9.1% w/w barium sulfate, 2.05% w/w benzoyl peroxide **(Liquid)** 98.18% v/v methylmethacrylate **(Monomer)** 0.82% v/v *N,N*-dimethyl-p-toluidine, 25 mg hydroquinone
Osteobond	Zimmer Inc. Warsaw, IN, United States	**(Powder)** 88.75% w/w polymethyl methylmethacrylate–styrene, 10% w/w barium sulfate, 0.0125% w/w benzoyl peroxide **(Liquid)** 97.3% v/v methylmethacrylate **(Monomer)** 2.7% v/v *N,N*-dimethyl-p-toluidine, 80 ppm hydroquinone
Composite Materials		
Cortoss	Orthovita Inc. Malvern, PA, United States	**(Resin components)** 2,2-bis-4-(2-hydroxy-3-methacryloxy-propoxy) phenylpropane, (2,2-bis-4-(2-methacryloxy-ethoxy) phenylpropane, triethylene glycol dimethacrylate, 2,2′-(4-methylphenyl) imino bis-ethanol, benzoyl peroxide 98%, 2-hydroxy-4-methoxy-benzophenone, 2,6-di-tert-butyl-p-cresol **(Reinforcing components)** silane treated combeite glass-ceramic (Na_2O-CaO-P_2O5-SiO_2), silane treated baria-boroa lumino-silicate glass (Bao-B_2O_3-Al_2O_3-SiO_2), silane treated amorphous silicon dioxide (SiO_2), methacryloxypropyltrimethoxysilane
Calcium Phosphate Cement		
Bone source	Stryker Orthopedics Malvern, PA, United States	**(Powder)** 72.3% w/w tetracalcium phosphate, 27.7% w/w dicalcium phosphate anhydrous **(Fluid)** 0.25 mol/L phosphate solution and distilled water-(Ca9.970 (HPO_4)0.080(PO_4) 5.892(CO_3)0.080(OH)1.944)
Biopex	Mitsubishi Materials Tokyo, Japan	**(Powder)** α-tricalcium phosphate, tetracalcium phosphate, dicalcium phosphate, and hydroxyapatite **(Liquid)** chondroitin sodium sulfate, sodium succinate, and water
Calcium Sulphate Cement		
BonePlast	Interpore Cross International Irvine, CA, United States	**(Powder)** calcium sulphate **(Liquid)** saline

Reproduced from Lieberman I, Togawa D, Kayanja MM. Vertebroplasty and kyphoplasty: filler materials. *Spine J.* 2005;5(6 suppl):305S-316S.
v/v, percent volume in volume; w/w, percent weight.

Table 44.9 Preclinical Data for Development of Viral Vectors for Gene Therapy for Chronic Pain

Pain Models	Gene Products	Inoculation	References
HSV Vectors			
Acute pain	Preproenkephalin	Skin of dorsal hind paw	Wilson[151]
Inflammatory pain	Preproenkephalin A, Endomorphine 2	Infected or scarred footpad, subcutaneous	Braz, Hao[152,153]
Neuropathic pain	Proenkephalin A, Endomorphine 2, IL-4,	Unilateral peripheral inoculation, subcutaneous	Meunier, Wolfe, Hao [154-156]
Cancer pain	Proenkephalin	Subcutaneous	Goss [157]
Adeno-Associated Viral Vectors			
Neuropathic pain	IL-10, Prepro-β-endorphin	Intrathecal	Milligan, Storek [158,159]
Inflammatory pain	μ opioid receptor	Into the DRG	Xu[160]
Neuropathic pain	BDNF	Into the dorsal horn	Eaton[161]
Adenovirus Vectors			
Pathologic pain	IL-10	Intrathecal	Milligan[158]
Inflammatory pain	β-endorphin	Intrathecal	Finegold[162]
Neuropathic pain	Interleukin 2	Intrathecal	Yao[163]
Lentivirus			
Neuropathic pain	GDNF	Intrathecal	Nagano[159]
Human Foamy Virus			
Mechanical allodynia	GAD	Into the dorsal root ganglia	Liu[164]

DRG, dorsal root ganglia; BDNF, brain-derived neurotropic factor; its overexpression reduces allodynia and hyperalgesia in chronic constriction injury model; GDNF, glial cell line-derived neurotrophic factor; in neuropathic pain it is decreased; increased, its expression may be effective in treatment of neuropathic pain; GAD, glutamic acid decarboxylase; its expression can decrease mechanical allodynia and thermal hyperalgesia in spinal cord injury model; HSV, herpes simplex virus.

Reproduced from Huang Y, Liu X, Dong L, et al. Development of viral vectors for gene therapy of chronic pain. *Pain Res Treat.* 2011;2011:968218.

KEY POINTS

- There are theoretical advantages for the use of the transforaminal technique, but the reports of central nervous system injuries make its continued use in the cervical area inadvisable. These events have been described with all the steroids, local anesthetics, and contrast. The use of computed tomography does not prevent the occurrence of these injuries.
- Recommended precautions for preventing CNS events include aspiration before injection, the use of blunt needles, flexible extension tubing, and digital subtraction imaging.
- Steroids with larger particles, such as methylprednisolone, should not be used in transforaminal epidural steroid injections. The commercial form of betamethasone, with its small particles, may be the ideal particulate steroid for transforaminal injections.
- Soluble steroids such as dexamethasone have no particles, are long acting, and have minimal mineralocorticoid properties. However, they have increased glucocorticoid activity, similar to betamethasone, and are easily washed out from the epidural space. Definitive prospective, randomized, controlled studies on the efficacy of these steroids are lacking.
- CNS injuries have not been described with the interlaminar epidural technique. Any of the steroids can be used with this technique.
- The outbreak of fungal *(Exserohilum rostratum)* meningitis in September 2012 was associated with contaminated methylprednisolone from a compounding company. The pain medicine physician can ensure sterility of the compounded drug that he or she is using by obtaining the drug from a company accredited by the Pharmacy Compounding Accreditation Board.
- Botulinum toxins are effective drugs when used for their FDA-approved indications. Studies have shown inconsistent efficacy for patients with myofascial pain syndromes.
- New indications for the botulinum toxin are emerging. When used for chronic migraine, onabotulinum toxin A significantly improved headache symptoms and demonstrated improved patient functioning, vitality, psychological distress, and overall quality of life.

KEY POINTS—cont'd

- Injectable bone cements are widely used in vertebral augmentation procedures. In vertebroplasty, the currently preferred product, polymethylmethacrylate, can be injected into the vertebral body under high pressure and in liquid form. An alternate technique, kyphoplasty, involves injecting the vertebral body with semisoft, partially cured acrylic paste under low pressure, possibly allowing for better control for the dispersed substance. Several other agents are under investigation as injectable bone cements.
- Gene therapy is an emerging technique to treat chronic unrelenting pain. Genetically engineered herpes simplex virus type 1 (HSV 1) vector has been used to treat cancer pain in a phase I study with favorable results. Other methods of vector delivery are under investigation for the treatment of neuropathic pain.

SUGGESTED READINGS

Ahadian FM, McGreevy K, Schulties G. Lumbar transforaminal epidural dexamethasone: a prospective, randomized, double-blind, dose response trial. *Reg Anesth Pain Med.* 2011;36:572-578.

Aurora SK, Dodick DW, Turkel CC, et al. Onabotulinum toxin A for the treatment of chronic migraine: results from the double blind, randomized placebo-controlled phase of the PREEMPT 1 trial. *Cephalalgia.* 2010;30:793-803.

Belkoff SM, Molloy S. Temperature measurement during polymerization of polymethyl-methacrylate cement used for vertebroplasty. *Spine.* 2003;28:1555-1559.

Benzon HT, Gissen AJ, Strichartz GR, et al. The effect of polyethylene glycol on mammalian nerve impulses. *Anesth Analg.* 1987;66:553-559.

Benzon HT, Chew TL, McCarthy RJ, Benzon HA. Comparison of the particle sizes of different steroids and the effect of dilution: a review of the relative neurotoxicity of the steroids. *Anesthesiology.* 2007;106:331-338.

Deer T, Ranson M, Kapural L, Diwan SA. Guidelines for the proper use of epidural steroid injections for the chronic pain patient. *Tech Reg Anesth Pain Manag.* 2009;13:288-295.

Derby R, Lee SH, Date ES, et al. Size and aggregation of corticosteroids used for epidural injections. *Pain Med.* 2008;9:227-234.

Diener HC, Dodick, Aurora SK, et al. Onabotulinum toxin A for treatment of chronic migraine: results from the double-blind, randomized, placebo controlled phase of the PREEMPT 2 trial. *Cephalalgia.* 2010;30:804-814.

Drazen JM, Curfman GD, Baden LR, Morrissey S. Compounding errors. *N Engl J Med.* 2012;367:2436-2437.

Friedrich MJ. Research yields new insights into mechanisms and treatment of pain. *J Am Med Assoc.* 2012;307:239-240.

Grady D. Dangerous abscesses add to tainted drug's threat. *New York Times.* December 22, 2012;pA3.

Huang Y, Liu X, dong L, et al. Development of viral vectors for gene therapy of chronic pain. *Pain Res Treat.* 2011;2011:968218.

Jung C, Inder WJ. Management of adrenal insufficiency during the stress of medical illness and surgery. *MJA.* 2008;188:409-413.

Kainer MA, Reagan DR, Nguyen DB, et al. Fungal infections associated with contaminated methylprednisolone in Tennessee. *N Engl J Med.* 2012;367:2194-2203.

Lieberman IH, Togawa D, Kayanja MM. Vertebroplasty and kyphoplasty: filler materials. *Spine J.* 2005;5:305S-316S.

MacMahon PJ, Eustace SJ, Kavanagh EC. Injectable corticosteroids and local anesthetic preparations: a review for radiologists. *Radiology.* 2009;252:647-661.

McGrath JM, Schaefer MP, Malkamaki DM. Incidence and characteristics of complications from epidural steroid injections. *Pain Med.* 2011;12:726-731.

Outterson K. Regulating compounding pharmacies after NECC. *N Engl J Med.* 2012;367:1969-1972.

Owczarek J, Jasinska M, Orszulak-Michalak D. Drug-induced myopathies: an overview of the possible mechanisms. *Pharmacolog Rep.* 2005;57:23-34.

Sitzman T, Chen Y, Rallo-Clemans R, et al. Drugs for the interventional pain physician. In: Benzon HT, Raja S, Molloy RE, et al, eds. *Essentials of Pain Medicine and Regional Anesthesia.* New York: Elsevier Churchill Livingstone; 2005:166-180.

US Pharmacopeia, 27th revision, The National Formulary. 22nd ed. Rockville, Md: The US Pharmacopeia Convention; 2004:2350-2370.

Wilson LE, Blythe D, Sharfstein JM. Fungal meningitis from injection of contaminated steroids. *JAMA.* 2012;308:2461-2462.

The references for this chapter can be found at www.expertconsult.com.

Psychological Interventions

45

Dennis C. Turk

A number of psychological interventions have been developed for patients with chronic pain, with a large body of research supporting their efficacy. Before reviewing the approaches with the greatest empirical support, it is important to consider the plight of a person with chronic pain, the role of psychological factors, and the mechanisms involved in the experience of chronic pain because these factors serve as the basis for the development of treatment modalities. The various psychological models and conceptualizations of chronic pain will then be outlined and the most commonly used treatment interventions described.

Note that the term *patient* will be used to designate individuals when they are in the health care provider's office, clinic, or hospital and the term *person* to designate those with chronic pain when they are outside the confines of health care facilities. This is an important distinction because chronic pain is by definition not curable and can persist over extended periods, for years and even decades. Persons with a chronic pain syndrome must learn how to adapt and self-manage their pain, associated symptoms, and lives. Chronic pain might be viewed as analogous to diabetes; in the physician's office a person with diabetes is a diabetic patient but, at all other times, is someone who has to learn how to live with diabetes. This involves carrying out all the necessary activities—routinely testing glucose levels (if insulin dependent), taking medication orally or injecting with insulin, maintaining an appropriate diet, modulating exercise patterns, and monitoring skin for infections. All these activities occur outside the formal health care system. Similar behavior is required of those with various types of chronic pain. In the absence of cure, self-management becomes critical.

PLIGHT OF THE PERSON WITH CHRONIC PAIN

People with chronic and recurrent acute pain (e.g., migraine, trigeminal neuralgia, sickle cell episodes) often feel rejected by the very elements of society that exist to serve them. They lose faith and may become frustrated and irritated when the health care system that initially might have created expectations for cure turns its back when treatments prove ineffective. They feel victimized and traumatized by repeated and invasive medical procedures; they become disillusioned and feel disbelief when it seems as though medical professionals expect them to find the cause of the pain on their own and when they have to convince skeptical providers to take their symptoms seriously.

Although patients with acute pain can often obtain relief from primary health care providers, people with persistent pain become enmeshed in the medical system as they shuttle from physician to laboratory test to imaging procedure to medical specialist in a frustrating quest to have their pain diagnosed and successfully treated, if not eliminated completely. Thus, at the same time that returning to work and earning an income become less possible, medical bills for unsuccessful treatments accumulate. This experience of "medical limbo"—the presence of a painful condition that in the absence of acceptable pathology might have psychiatric causation, suggests malingering, or perhaps might even be an undiagnosed but potentially progressive disease—is itself a source of significant and persistent stress that can initiate emotional distress or aggravate a premorbid psychiatric condition.

People with chronic pain reside in a complex and costly world that is also populated by their significant others, health care providers, employers, and third-party payers. Family members feel increasingly hopeless and distressed as medical costs, disability, and emotional suffering mount while income and available treatment options decline. Health care providers grow increasingly frustrated and feel defeated and ineffective as available treatment options are exhausted while the pain condition remains a mystery and may worsen. Employers, who are already resentful of growing workers' compensation benefits, pay higher costs while productivity suffers because the employee frequently calls in sick or cannot perform at the usual level ("presenteeism"). Third-party payers watch as health care expenditures soar with repeated diagnostic tests and treatments, often with inconclusive results. Over time, the legitimacy of the individual's report of pain may be questioned because often a medical reason fails to substantiate the cause of the symptoms.

People with chronic pain may begin to feel that their health care providers, employers, and even family members are blaming them when their condition does not respond to treatment as expected. Some may suggest that the individual is complaining excessively to receive attention, avoid undesirable activities, or be relieved from onerous obligations (e.g., gainful employment, household responsibilities). Others may suggest that the pain reported is not real, people reporting unremitting pain are feigning or exaggerating their symptoms, and it is all in their heads, "psychogenic." Third-party payers may even suggest that the individual is intentionally exaggerating the pain to obtain financial gain, whereas others may attribute the reported symptoms to the desire to obtain mood-altering medications. In this way, people reporting pain may come to be regarded as wimps, crocks, or fakes.

As a result of these attitudes and the absence of cure or even substantial relief, those with chronic pain may withdraw from society, lose their jobs, alienate family and friends, and become more and more isolated, despondent, depressed, and in general *demoralized.* Their bodies, the health care system, and their significant others have let them down. They may even believe that they have failed themselves as they relinquish their usual activities and responsibilities because of symptoms that are intractable but frequently almost invisible when not validated by objective pathologic findings. This emotional distress, however, can be exacerbated by other factors, including fear, inadequate or maladaptive support systems, inadequate personal and material coping resources, treatment-induced (iatrogenic) complications, overuse of potent drugs, inability to work, financial difficulties, prolonged litigation, disruption of usual activities, and sleep disturbance.

Fear of pain or movement and injury or reinjury is an important contributor to the disability associated with several chronic pain disorders, including back pain and fibromyalgia syndrome.[1] People with chronic pain often anticipate that certain activities will increase their pain or induce further injury. These fears may contribute to avoidance of activity and subsequently greater physical deconditioning, emotional distress, and ultimately, greater disability. Their failure to engage in activities prevents them from obtaining any corrective feedback about the association between activity and pain and injury.

In addition to fear of movement, people with persistent pain may be anxious about the meaning of their symptoms for the future—will their pain increase, will their physical capacity diminish, will they have progressive disability and ultimately end up in a wheelchair or become bedridden? In addition to these anxieties, people in pain may fear that others will not believe that they are suffering or will tell them that they are beyond help and will just have to "learn to live with it." Such fears can contribute to additional emotional distress and increased physiologic arousal, which may directly exacerbate and maintain the pain. Living with persistent pain conditions requires considerable emotional resilience. It tends to deplete people's emotional reserves and taxes not only the individual but also the capability of family, friends, coworkers, and employers to provide support.

Chronic pain is estimated to be present in up to 30% of the adult U.S. population.[2] If we assume that most people do not live alone but in a social context with significant others, more than the majority of the population may be affected directly or indirectly. Pain is expensive; health care and indirect costs associated with disability compensation, lost tax revenues, retraining, less than optimal performance on the job, and legal fees exceed $550 billion each year.[2] To put it bluntly, pain hurts—it hurts the person with the symptoms, it hurts significant others, and it hurts society.

Despite advances in knowledge of the neurophysiology of pain and the development of new pharmacologic agents with analgesic properties, sophisticated surgical interventions, and advanced technologies (e.g., spinal cord stimulation, implantable drug delivery systems), cure of pain has eluded the best efforts of health care providers. Regardless of the treatment, the amount of pain reduction averages only about 35%; less than 50% of persons treated with these interventions obtain even this result, and the extent of improvement in emotional, physical, and social functioning is often below this level.[3]

As noted, chronic pain is by definition incurable. People with chronic pain continually confront noxious sensations and other aversive symptoms that affect every aspect of their lives—social, emotional, interpersonal, and economic, as well as physical. Thus, those with chronic pain are faced with managing their symptoms on their own. Faced with this task, the common response is, "How?"

It is well to recall Bonica's[4] comment in the preface to the first edition (1954) of his seminal work *The Management of Pain* (and repeated in the third edition almost 50 years later):

> *The crucial role of psychological and environmental factors in causing pain in a significant number of patients only recently received attention. As a consequence, there has emerged a sketch plan of pain apparatus with its receptors, conducting fibers, and its standard function which* [sic] *is to be applicable to all circumstances. But…in so doing, medicine has overlooked the fact that the activity of this apparatus is subject to a constantly changing influence of the mind.*

Based on the overview provided, two conclusions should be obvious: (1) psychological factors play a significant role in the experience, maintenance, and exacerbation, if not the cause, of pain, and (2) because there are no cures for chronic pain and some level of pain will persist in most people with chronic pain regardless of treatment, psychological approaches may be useful complements to more traditional medical and surgical approaches.

PSYCHOLOGICAL FORMULATIONS OF CHRONIC PAIN

A number of different psychological perspectives on chronic pain have evolved over time. It is important to consider these initially because psychological treatments are based on different, and at times competing, psychological principles.

PSYCHOGENIC VIEW

As is frequently the case in medicine, when physical explanations seem inadequate or when the results of treatment are inconsistent, reports of pain are attributed to a psychological cause (i.e., psychogenic). Although psychogenic views of pain have been discussed since the formulation of psychodynamic theory, a psychodynamic perspective on chronic pain was first described systematically in the 1960s, when people with pain were viewed as having compulsive and masochistic tendencies, inhibited aggressive needs, and feelings of guilt—"pain-prone personalities."[5] It was commonly believed that people with pain had childhood histories fraught with emotional abuse, family dysfunction (e.g., parental quarrels, divorce), illness or death of a parent, early responsibilities, and high motivation toward achievement.[6] Some studies reported associations between chronic pain and childhood trauma, although the findings are not consistent.[7,8]

Based on the psychogenic perspective, assessment of those with chronic pain is directed toward identifying the psychopathologic tendencies that instigate and maintain pain. Although evidence to support this model is scarce, the American Psychiatric Association[9] has created a psychiatric diagnosis, somatoform pain disorder. Diagnosis of a pain disorder requires that the person's report of pain be inconsistent with the anatomic distribution of the nervous system or, if it mimics a known disease entity, cannot be adequately accounted for by organic pathology after extensive diagnostic evaluation. Even in the presence of a medical condition that may cause pain, psychological factors may be implicated, and thus the person may receive a psychiatric diagnosis of "pain disorder associated with *both* psychological factors and a general medical condition."[9]

It is assumed that reports of pain will cease once the psychogenic mechanisms have been resolved. Treatment is geared toward helping patients gain insight into the underlying maladaptive psychological contributors.[10,11]

Empirical evidence supporting the psychogenic view is scarce. A number of people with chronic pain do not exhibit significant psychopathology. Furthermore, insight-oriented psychotherapy has not been shown to be effective in reducing symptoms in most patients with chronic pain. Studies have suggested that the emotional distress observed in patients with chronic pain more typically occurs in response to the persistence of pain and is not a causal agent[12,13] and may resolve once the pain is treated adequately.[14] The psychogenic model has thus come under scrutiny and may be flawed in its view of chronic pain.[15]

BEHAVIORAL FORMULATIONS

According to the classical or respondent conditioning model, if a painful stimulus is repeatedly paired with a neutral stimulus, the neutral stimulus will by itself come to elicit a pain response. For example, a person who experienced pain after performing a treadmill exercise may become conditioned to experience a negative emotional response to the presence of the treadmill and to any stimulus associated with it (e.g., physical therapist, gym). The negative emotional reaction might instigate tensing of muscle in anticipation, thereby exacerbating the pain and further reinforcing the association between the stimulus and pain. Based on this conditioned correlation, people with chronic pain may avoid activities previously associated with onset or exacerbation of the pain.

In 1976, Fordyce[16] extended operant conditioning to chronic pain. This view proposes that acute pain behavior (e.g., avoidance of activity for fear of pain) may come under the control of external contingencies of reinforcement (i.e., responses increase or decrease as a function of their reinforcing consequences) and thus develop into a persistent pain problem. Fordyce underscored that because there is no objective means of measuring pain, the only way that we can know of other people's pain is by their behavior, expressed verbally or nonverbally. Overt pain behavior includes verbal reports, paralinguistic vocalizations (e.g., sighs, moans), motor activity, facial expressions, body postures and gesturing (limping, rubbing a painful body part, grimacing), functional limitations (e.g., reclining for extensive periods, inactivity), and behavior designed to reduce pain (e.g., taking medication, use of the health care system).

The central features of pain behavior are that behavior is (1) a source of communication and (2) observable. Observable behavior is capable of eliciting a response, and the consequences of the behavior will influence subsequent behavior. Through a learning process, behaviors that receive positive consequences will more likely be maintained, whereas types of behavior that fail to achieve positive consequences or that receive negative consequences will be less likely to occur (i.e., extinguished). Pain behavior may be positively reinforced directly, such as by attention from a spouse or health care provider, monetary compensation, or avoidance of undesirable activity.[17] It may also be maintained by escape from noxious stimulation through the use of drugs or rest or by avoidance of undesirable activities such as work. In addition, "well behavior" (e.g., activity, working) may not be positively reinforcing and the more rewarding pain behavior may therefore be maintained.

The operant conditioning model does not concern itself with the initial cause of pain. Rather, it considers pain an internal subjective experience that can be directly assessed and may be maintained even after an initial physical basis of the pain has resolved. The pain behavior originally elicited by organic factors as a result of injury or disease may come to occur, totally or in part, in response to reinforcing environmental events.

It is important, however, not to make the mistake of viewing pain behavior as synonymous with malingering. Malingering involves consciously and purposely faking a symptom such as pain for some gain, usually financial. Contrary to the beliefs of many third-party payers, there is little support for the contention that outright faking of pain for financial gain is prevalent.

The social learning model emphasizes that behavior can be learned not only by actual reinforcement of behavior but also by observation of what happens to others. This is a particularly powerful way of learning when the others being observed are judged to be similar to the observer. For example, a middle-aged man might learn what to expect by observing how other middle-aged men with similar medical problems are treated, as opposed to observing young women with a very different pain disorder. Thus, the development and maintenance of pain behavior may occur by observational learning and modeling processes. Specifically, people can acquire responses that were not previously in their behavioral repertoire by the observation of others performing these activities. Expectations and actual behavioral responses to nociceptive stimulation are based, at least partially, on people's prior learning histories.[18]

Children develop attitudes about health and health care and about the perception and interpretation of symptoms and physiologic processes from their relatives and others whom they confront in their social environment. They learn how others respond to injury and disease and thus may ignore or over-respond to symptoms that they experience based on the behavior modeled in childhood. For example, children of chronic pain patients have been shown to exhibit more pain-related responses during stressful times or exhibit more illness behavior (e.g., complaining, days absent, visit to the school nurse) than children of healthy parents based on what they have observed and learned at home.[19]

Expectations and actual behavioral responses to nociceptive stimulation are based partially on prior social learning history. Models can influence the expression, localization, and methods of coping with pain. Even physiologic responses may be conditioned during observation of others in pain.[20]

A central construct of the social learning perspective is self-efficacy.[21] This is a personal expectation that is particularly important for patients with chronic pain. A self-efficacy expectation is defined as a personal conviction that a course of action (e.g., performing the required behavior) can successfully be executed to produce a desired outcome in a given situation.[21] Given sufficient motivation to engage in a behavior, it is a person's self-efficacy beliefs that determine the choice of activities that the person will initiate, the amount of effort that will be expended, and how long the individual will persist in the face of obstacles and aversive experiences. In this way, self-efficacy plays an important role in therapeutic change.[22]

Efficacy judgments are based on four sources of information regarding one's capabilities, listed in descending order of effect[16]: (1) one's own past performance at the task or similar tasks; (2) the performance accomplishments of others who are perceived to be similar to oneself; (3) verbal persuasion by others that one is capable; and (4) perception of one's own state of physiologic arousal, which in turn is partly determined by previous estimation of efficacy. Performance mastery can then be achieved by encouraging people to undertake subtasks that are initially attainable but become increasingly difficult and to subsequently approach the desired level of performance. It is important to remember that coping behavior is influenced by a person's beliefs that the demands of a situation do not exceed her or his coping resources.

How people interpret, respond to, and cope with illness is determined by cultural norms and perceptions of self-efficacy. These two sets of factors contribute to the marked variability in response to objectively similar degrees of physical pathology noted by health care providers.

GATE CONTROL MODEL

Though not a psychological formulation itself, the gate control model[23] was the first to popularize the importance of central psychological factors in perception of pain. Perhaps the most important contribution of the gate control theory is the way in which it changed thinking about pain perception. Melzack and Casey[24] differentiated three systems related to the processing of nociceptive stimulation, all thought to contribute to the subjective experience of pain—sensory-discriminative, motivational-affective, and cognitive-evaluative. Thus, the gate control theory specifically includes psychological factors as an integral aspect of the pain experience. It emphasizes central nervous system mechanisms and provides a physiologic basis for the role of psychological factors in chronic pain.

The gate control model contradicts the notion that pain is either somatic *or* psychogenic. Instead, it postulates that both factors have potentiating and moderating effects. According to this model, both the central and peripheral nervous systems interact to contribute to the experience of pain. It is not only these physical factors that guide the brain's interpretation of painful stimuli that are at the center of this model; psychological factors (e.g., thoughts, beliefs, emotions) are also actively involved.

Before formulation of the gate control theory by Melzack and Wall,[23] psychological processes were largely dismissed as reactions to pain. Although the physiologic details of the gate control model have been challenged,[25] it has had a substantial impact on basic research and can be credited as a source of inspiration for diverse clinical applications to control or manage pain, including neurophysiologically based procedures (e.g., neural stimulation techniques involving peripheral nerves and collateral processes in the dorsal columns of the spinal cord), pharmacologic advances, behavioral treatments, and interventions that target modification of the attentional and perceptual processes involved in the pain experience.

COGNITIVE-BEHAVIORAL PERSPECTIVE

The cognitive-behavioral (CB) model, perhaps the most commonly accepted model for the psychological treatment of individuals with chronic pain,[26,27] incorporates many of the psychological variables previously described—anticipation, avoidance, and contingencies of reinforcement—but suggests that cognitive factors rather than conditioning factors are of central importance. The model proposes that conditioned reactions are largely self-activated on the basis of learned expectations rather than being automatically evoked. The model suggests that behavior and emotions are influenced by interpretations of events, and emphasis is placed on how people's beliefs and attitudes interact with physical, affective, and behavioral factors. In other words, it is the individual's information processing that results in anticipatory anxiety and avoidance. The critical factor, therefore, is that people learn to anticipate and predict events and to express appropriate reactions.[28]

In the CB model, people with pain are viewed as having negative expectations about their own ability to control certain motor skills without pain. Moreover, people with chronic pain tend to believe that they have limited control over their pain. Such negative maladaptive appraisals about the situation and personal efficacy may reinforce the experience of demoralization, inactivity, and over-reaction to nociceptive stimulation. These appraisals and expectations are postulated to have an effect on behavior by leading to reduced effort and activity, which may contribute to increased psychological distress (helplessness) and subsequent physical limitations. If one accepts that pain is a complex subjective phenomenon that is uniquely experienced by each person, knowledge about idiosyncratic beliefs, appraisals, and coping ability becomes critical for optimal treatment planning and for evaluating treatment outcome accurately.

Several important factors may facilitate or disrupt people's sense of control: their beliefs and appraisals, their expectations about pain, their ability to cope, their social supports, their disorder, the medicolegal and health care systems, and their employers. These factors also influence patients' investment in treatment, acceptance of responsibility, perceptions of disability, adherence to treatment recommendations, support from significant others, expectations for treatment, and acceptance of treatment rationale.

Cognitive interpretations also affect how people experiencing pain present their symptoms to others, including health care providers. Overt communication of pain, suffering, and distress will enlist responses that may reinforce the pain behavior and impressions about the seriousness, severity, and uncontrollability of the pain. That is, complaints of pain may induce physicians to prescribe more potent medications, order additional diagnostic tests, and in some cases, perform surgery. Significant others may express sympathy, excuse the person with chronic pain from responsibilities, and encourage passivity, thereby fostering further physical deconditioning.

People with persistent pain often have negative expectations about their own ability and responsibility to exert any control over their pain and frequently view themselves as helpless. Such negative maladaptive appraisals about their condition, situation, and personal efficacy in controlling their pain and problems associated with the pain reinforce their experience of demoralization, inactivity, and overreaction to nociceptive stimulation. These cognitive appraisals are posited to have an effect on behavior by leading to reduced effort, less perseverance in the face of difficulty, lowered activity level, and increased psychological distress. It should be obvious that the CB perspective integrates the operant conditioning emphasis on external reinforcement with the respondent view of conditioned avoidance within the framework of information processing.

The CB perspective on pain management focuses on providing patients techniques to gain a sense of control over the effects of pain on their lives, as well as on actually modifying the affective, behavioral, cognitive, and sensory facets of the experience. Behavioral experiences help show persons with pain that they are capable of more than they assumed, thereby increasing their sense of personal competence. Cognitive techniques (e.g., self-monitoring to identify the relationships among thoughts, mood, and behavior; distraction using imagery; and problem solving, described below) help place affective, behavioral, cognitive, and sensory responses under the person's control.

The assumption is that long-term maintenance of behavioral changes will occur only if the person with pain has learned to attribute success to his or her own efforts. It has been suggested that such treatments can result in changes in beliefs about pain, coping style, and reported pain severity, as well as in direct behavioral changes. Treatment that results in increases in perceived control over pain and decreased catastrophizing also results in decreases in pain severity and functional disability. When successful rehabilitation occurs, there is a major shift from beliefs about helplessness and passivity to resourcefulness and ability to function regardless of pain, as well as a shift from an illness conviction to a rehabilitation conviction.

A number of studies have supported the contribution of cognitive factors to pain and disability.[22,29] These studies have consistently demonstrated that individuals' attitudes, beliefs, and expectations about their plight, themselves, personal coping strategies, and the health care system affect reports of pain, activity, disability, and response to treatment. For example, people respond to medical conditions in part based on their subjective ideas about their illness and symptoms. When pain is interpreted as signifying ongoing tissue damage or a progressive disease, it is likely to produce considerably more suffering and behavioral dysfunction than if it is viewed as being the result of a stable problem that is expected to improve.

Once beliefs and expectations are formed, they become stable, rigid, and relatively impervious to modification. Individuals with chronic pain tend to avoid experiences (e.g., physical activity) that could invalidate their beliefs (disconfirmations) and guide their behavior in accordance with these beliefs, even in situations in which these beliefs are no longer valid. It is thus essential for people with chronic pain to develop adaptive beliefs about the relationships among impairment, pain, suffering, and disability and to de-emphasize the role of experienced pain in their regulation of functioning.

Distorted thinking can also contribute to the maintenance and exacerbation of pain. A particularly potent and pernicious thinking style that has been observed in people with chronic pain is catastrophizing—holding negative thoughts about one's situation and interpreting even minor problems as major catastrophes.[30] Research has indicated that people who spontaneously use more catastrophizing thoughts report more pain than do those who do not catastrophize.[30]

Coping strategies, or a person's specific ways of adjusting to or minimizing pain and distress, act to alter both the perception of pain intensity and the ability to manage or tolerate pain and continue daily activities. Overt behavioral coping strategies include rest, medication, and the use of relaxation. Covert coping strategies include various means of distracting oneself from pain, reassuring oneself that the pain will diminish, seeking information, and problem solving.

Active coping strategies, such as efforts to function despite pain or distracting oneself from pain, tend to be associated with adaptive functioning, and passive coping strategies, such as depending on others for help with pain control, avoiding activities because of fear of pain or injury, self-medication, and alcohol, tend to be related to greater pain and depression.[29] Regardless of the type of coping strategy, if people with chronic pain are instructed in the use of adaptive coping strategies, their rating of the intensity of the pain decreases and their tolerance of the pain increases.[29] Thus, the perspective on how people function and the emphasis on facilitating self-management are more important than any specific cognitive or behavioral techniques used to bring about changes in thinking and behavior.

BIOPSYCHOSOCIAL MODEL

Although the gate control theory introduced the role of psychological factors in the maintenance of pain symptoms, it focused primarily on the basic anatomy and neurophysiology of pain. The biopsychosocial model, which expands the CB model of pain, views illness as a dynamic and reciprocal interaction between biologic, psychological, and sociocultural variables that shape the experience and the response to pain.[22,29] What is unique about this model is that it takes into consideration the influence of higher-order cognition, including perception and appraisal. It accepts that people are active processors of information and that behavior, emotions, and even physiology are influenced by interpretation of events rather than solely by physiologic factors.[28,29] People with chronic pain may therefore have negative expectations about their own ability and responsibility to exert any control over their pain. Moreover, those with pain behavior elicit responses from significant others that can reinforce adaptive and maladaptive modes of thinking, feeling, and behaving.

The biopsychosocial model presumes some form of physical pathology or at least physical changes in muscles, joints, or nerves that generate nociceptive input to the brain. At the periphery, nociceptive fibers transmit sensations that may or may not be interpreted as pain. Such sensation is not pain until subjected to higher-order psychological and mental processing that involves perception, appraisal, and behavior. Perception entails the interpretation of nociceptive input and identifies the type of pain (e.g., sharp, burning, punishing). Appraisal involves the meaning attributed to the pain and influences subsequent behavior. A person may choose to ignore the pain and continue working, walking, socializing, and engaging in previous levels of activity or may choose to leave work, refrain from activities, and assume the sick role. In turn, this interpersonal role is shaped by responses from significant others that may promote the healthy response or the sick role. The biopsychosocial model has been instrumental in the development of CB treatment approaches for chronic pain, including assessment and intervention (described later in this chapter).[28,29]

FAMILY SYSTEMS PERSPECTIVE

In family systems—and this could be expanded to significant others, not only to traditional concepts of nuclear families—the individual and his or her behavior are placed within a social unit. The family is viewed as an interactional unit, and family members (significant others) have a profound impact on each other's emotions, thoughts, and behavior. Thus, the functioning of family members is interdependent, and family relationships are important for not only psychological but also physical health.[31,32]

Increasing evidence supports the concept that family members contribute to behavioral risk factors such as smoking, lack of exercise, and poor diet, which can influence the development of numerous chronic illnesses, as well as compliance or noncompliance with treatment regimens.[33] Additionally, families influence the development of chronic pain via operant theory. As noted, expressions of acute pain (e.g., reporting pain, grimacing, avoidance of activity, use of pain medication), because they are overt and observable, may be reinforced through expressions of concern from family members. Furthermore, in support of this idea, a number of investigators[34-36] have found that spousal attentiveness to expressions of pain is positively correlated with higher levels of reported pain, pain behavior frequency, and disability.

The experience of chronic stress within the family has also been hypothesized to contribute to the development of chronic illness.[37] Specifically, chronic stress may play an important role in the sympathetic nervous system and endocrine dysregulation often found in chronic pain patients.

As noted, pain does not take place in isolation but in a social context. Pain does not occur solely in people's bodies, nor does it occur solely in their brains, but rather it occurs in their lives. The emphasis on the role of significant others is important. It reminds us that treating a chronic pain patient successfully requires that we not only assess and treat the patient but also target significant others, who can be supportive but can also be impediments to rehabilitation when they are overly punitive or solicitous.[35,37]

INTERFACES OF PSYCHOLOGY, PHYSIOLOGY, AND NEUROCHEMISTRY

Pain is a biopsychosocial phenomenon, with the implication being that psychological, social, and biologic factors contribute to the experience. Moreover, these factors interact: psychological and social factors are reflected in bodily processes and have physiologic consequences, and psychological and social variables are influenced by an individual's unique biology. Advances in research and technology are permitting increased understanding of the intricate associations between biology and behavior.[28,29]

Psychoneuroendocrinology is a specialized field of research that studies the interactions between behavior and the brain, nervous system, and endocrine system. The primary emphasis of this area is on the hypothalamic-pituitary-adrenal (HPA) axis. The HPA axis is believed to be the primary part of the neuroendocrine system that responds to stress.[38-40]

Several investigators have proposed that chronic or extensive activation of the HPA axis can lead to deleterious effects on somatic and psychological well-being.[38-41] The long-term effects of altered secretion of glucocorticoids have adverse effects on various health outcomes, and dysregulation of the HPA axis has been associated with many chronic pain conditions. There have been discrepant findings in research regarding enhanced versus attenuated HPA axis activity.[38] Although the dysregulation cannot be accounted for entirely by psychosocial distress and somatization,[40] release of hormones by the HPA axis in the face of psychosocial stress has been established, and dysregulation of the HPA axis does appear to contribute significantly to the maintenance and severity of chronic pain conditions.[39,41,42]

Psychophysiology is the science of understanding the link between psychology and physiology. Psychophysiology examines how psychological activities (e.g., stressful events or emotions) produce a physiologic response. Thus, in individuals with chronic pain, psychophysiology examines how exposure to a stressful situation or strong emotions produces a result expressed as the pain experience.[28] Commonly used measures of psychophysiology include measures of brain activity event-related potentials, functional magnetic resonance imaging (fMRI), skin temperature, skin conductance (also known as the galvanic skin response), cardiac measures (heart rate, heart rhythm, heart rate variability), and muscle responses (electromyogram, muscle tension, and myofascial trigger points).[28,43,44]

Autonomic dysregulation is the main component of psychophysiology that has been investigated.[44,45] Although autonomic dysregulation has not been confirmed as a causative factor in chronic pain, dysregulation with evidence of sympathetic tone has been demonstrated to be a significant mediator in the long-term maintenance and subjective severity of the pain experience in many chronic pain conditions.[45,46] The results of studies examining psychoneuroimmunology and psychophysiology, along with more recent studies using brain imaging, are not only beginning to confirm the interrelationships between physiologic and psychological factors in chronic pain but are also demonstrating the mechanisms involved in such interactions[47] (see Chapter 12).

ASSESSMENT AND EVALUATION

To understand and appropriately treat a person whose primary symptom is pain, one must begin with a comprehensive history and physical examination. Physical examination procedures and sophisticated laboratory and imaging techniques are readily available for use in detecting organic pathology. Physical and laboratory abnormalities, however, correlate only modestly with subjective reports of pain, and it is often not possible to make any precise pathologic diagnosis or even to identify an adequate anatomic origin of the pain. Thus, adequate pain assessment also requires the use of clinical interviews, observation, and assessment tools to help evaluate the myriad psychosocial and behavioral factors that influence the subjective report.[48]

There is no "pain thermometer" that can provide an objective quantification of the amount or severity of pain experienced; it can be assessed only indirectly based on a patient's description, verbally and behaviorally. Patients are usually asked to describe the characteristics (e.g., stabbing, burning), location, and severity of their pain. However, even this can make pain assessment difficult because, as outlined, pain is a complex, subjective phenomenon composed of a range of factors and is uniquely experienced by each person. Wide variability in pain severity, quality, and impact may be noted in reports of people with pain as they attempt to describe what appear to be objectively identical phenomena. Their pain descriptions are also colored by cultural and sociologic influences, as well as by previous experiences.

INTERVIEW

A list of topics that can be covered in an assessment interview is presented in Box 45.1.[48] A functional assessment of the pain can also be made by asking the person about the current level of pain or pain over the past week or month, or a diary or journal can be maintained to indicate pain intensity, with ratings recorded several times daily for several days or weeks. Merely inquiring about the characteristics of the pain, though necessary, is not sufficient. Diaries or journals can provide more information than just the varying pain intensity. A clinician can use information about the pain obtained during the interview and from a patient's writings to identify patterns in behavior, including potential antecedents and consequences of exacerbation of the pain, and treatment decisions can be facilitated by the availability of such data.

Box 45.1 Areas Covered in Clinical Interviews

- Patient's perception about the cause of the pain
- Patient's experience of the pain (how often and when it occurs) and related symptoms
- Treatments received and currently receiving
- Impact of pain on daily activities
- Impact of pain on interpersonal relationships
- Level and nature of emotional distress
- Current stressors and areas of conflict
- Methods used to cope with symptoms
- Alcohol and substance abuse history and current use
- Behavior used to let others know pain is present
- Responses by significant others
- Social history
- Education and vocational history
- Receiving or seeking compensation and involvement in litigation
- Concerns and expectations

The beliefs of people with pain about the cause and trajectory of their symptoms and the availability of beneficial treatments will have important influences on coping with the pain and adhering to therapeutic interventions. Thus, when conducting an interview with a person chronically in pain, focus should be on the specific thoughts, types of behavior, emotions, and physiologic responses that precede, accompany, and follow the pain episodes or exacerbations, including environmental and temporal conditions and the consequences associated with the patient's responses (e.g., cognitive, emotional, and behavioral, including frequency, specificity, and generality). It is important to note any patterns of maladaptive thoughts because they may contribute to a sense of hopelessness, dysphoria, and unwillingness (e.g., fears) about engaging in specific activities.

It is also important to determine expectations and goals of treatment for patients and their significant others. For example, an expectation that pain will be eliminated completely may be unrealistic and should be addressed to prevent discouragement if it does not occur. Additionally, formulating treatment goals (e.g., reduction in symptoms; reduced emotional distress; improved physical, social, and vocational functioning; reduction of inappropriate use of the health care system) is helpful in returning individuals to optimal functioning given their age, sex, education, and presence of physical impairments.

BEHAVIORAL OBSERVATION

A number of different observational procedures have been developed to quantify pain behavior.[49] Behavioral checklists can identify the frequency and type of pain behavior exhibited by a person with pain. Such checklists can be self-reports or reports by others—for example, behavioral observation scales can be used by significant others, and health care providers can use observational methods to quantify various types of pain behavior systematically (e.g., observing the person in the waiting room, while being interviewed, during a structured series of physical tasks, in the presence of a significant other). Noting the type and frequency of pain behavior can provide detailed information about when someone performs pain behavior, around whom the behavior is elicited, and the responses of others to the pain behavior. It is not surprising to find that people with chronic pain tend to carry out more pain behavior around others who give them positive reinforcement of the pain behavior (e.g., providing soothing statements, physical intimacy, assistance in performing tasks). Obtaining details about factors that increase and decrease behavior (e.g., patterns) can be useful when developing treatment goals.

SELF-REPORT QUESTIONNAIRES

A number of assessment instruments designed to evaluate people's attitudes, beliefs, and expectations about themselves, their symptoms, and the health care system have been developed (some common assessment instruments have been described by Turk and Melzack[50]). There are many advantages to the use of standardized instruments—they are easy to administer, require minimal time, assess a wide range of behavior, and obtain information about behavior that may be private (sexual relations) or unobservable (thoughts, emotional arousal), and most importantly, they can be submitted to analyses that permit determination of their reliability and validity. These instruments should not be viewed as alternatives to interviews; rather, they may suggest issues to be addressed in more depth during an interview or to be investigated with other measures. Additionally, they allow comparison among groups of people with pain and provide valuable information about the functional status of individuals in relation to others with the same condition. Questionnaires have been developed to assess reports of engaging in a range of functional activities, such as the ability to walk up stairs, sit for specific periods, lift specific weights, and perform activities of daily living, as well as the severity of the pain experienced when performing these activities.[49,50]

Measures of psychosocial functioning have been developed for use specifically in people with pain to assess psychological distress, impact of pain on their lives, feeling of control, coping behavior, and attitudes about disease, pain, and health care providers and the person's plight.[49,50] However, these responses to pain may be distorted as a function of the disease or as a result of medications taken. For example, common measures of depression ask people about their appetites, sleep patterns, and fatigue. Because disease status and medication can affect the responses to such questions, scores may be elevated and thus distort the validity of the responses. Therefore, it is always best to corroborate information gathered from these instruments with other sources, such as personal interview, report by significant others, and chart review.

REFERRAL FOR PSYCHOLOGICAL INTERVENTION

The health care provider should be alert for red flags that may serve as an impetus for more thorough evaluation by a psychologist who specializes in the treatment of pain. Box 45.2 lists questions worth considering for persons who report persistent or recurring pain. Positive responses to these questions should not be viewed as sufficient to make a referral for more extensive evaluation, but when more than six or seven of them are positive, referral should be considered. These questions need not be regarded as an interview or questionnaire but should be routinely included when interacting with chronic pain patients during the course of the history and physical examination if appropriate. By the end of the evaluation, the health care provider should have elicited enough information to make a decision whether a psychological evaluation is warranted.

Box 45.2 Screening Questions*

1. Has the patient's pain persisted for 3 months or longer despite appropriate interventions and in the absence of progressive disease? [Yes]
2. Does the patient repeatedly and excessively use the health care system, persist in seeking invasive investigations or treatments after being informed that these are inappropriate, or use opioid or sedative-hypnotic medications or alcohol in a pattern of concern to the patient's physician (e.g., escalating use)? [Yes]
3. Does the patient come in requesting specific opioid medication (e.g., hydromorphone [Dilaudid], oxycodone [OxyContin])? [Yes]
4. Does the patient have unrealistic expectations of the health care provider or the treatment offered ("total elimination of pain and related symptoms")? [Yes]
5. Does the patient have a history of substance abuse or is he or she currently abusing mind-altering substances? [Yes]
   - Patients can be asked, "Have you ever found yourself taking more medication than was prescribed or have you used alcohol because your pain was so bad?" *or* "Is anyone in your family concerned about the amount of medication you take?" [Yes]
6. Does the patient display a large number of types of pain behavior that appear to be exaggerated (e.g., grimacing, rigid or guarded posture)? [Yes]
7. Does the patient have litigation pending? [Yes]
8. Is the patient seeking or receiving disability compensation? [Yes]
9. Does the patient have any other family members who have had or currently suffer from chronic pain conditions? [Yes]
10. Does the patient demonstrate excessive depression or anxiety? [Yes]
    - Straightforward questions such as "Have you been feeling down?" or "What effect does your pain have on your mood?" can clarify whether this area is in need of more detailed evaluation.
11. Can the patient identify one significant or several stressful life events before symptom onset or exacerbation? [Yes]
12. If married or living with a partner, does the patient indicate a high degree of interpersonal conflict? [Yes]
13. Has the patient given up many activities (e.g., recreational, social, familial, in addition to occupational and work activities) because of pain? [Yes]
14. Does the patient have any plans for renewed or increased activities if the pain is reduced? [No]
15. Was the patient employed before the onset of pain? [No] If yes, does he or she wish to return to that job or any job? [No]
16. Does the patient believe that he or she will ever be able to resume normal life and normal functioning? [No]

*If there is a combination of more than six "yes" answers to questions 1 to 13 and "no" answers to questions 14 to 16 or if there are general concerns in any one area, consider referral for psychological assessment.

THERAPEUTIC INTERVENTIONS

A number of different clinical approaches to the treatment of chronic pain have been developed based on the models and variables described, including insight-oriented approaches, behavioral approaches, cognitive-behavioral therapy (CBT), family systems perspective, and biobehavioral interfaces. In addition, several specific techniques based on these models have been used successfully (e.g., motivational interviewing, biofeedback, relaxation, guided imagery, hypnosis, meditation) on their own or as part of more comprehensive treatment regimens. Each of these will be described briefly. Perhaps the most commonly used approach, however, is CBT, which incorporates and integrates many techniques from other approaches.[3,26-28,51] Thus, more attention will be given to this general approach to patients and treatment.

INSIGHT-ORIENTED THERAPIES

Therapy based on the psychodynamic view and insight-oriented approaches are primarily focused on early relationship experiences, which are reconstructed within the context of the therapeutic relationship. The therapeutic relationship is meant to "correct" the person's previous maladaptive experience by reintegrating emotions into symbolic and available mental processes to achieve improved emotional regulation.[6] It is important for the person with pain and the therapist to have a supportive and trusting relationship. Although insight-oriented psychotherapy may be useful in selected individuals,[11] this approach has rarely been shown to be effective in reducing symptoms in most persons with chronic pain. No well-designed, randomized controlled trials have been published that demonstrate the efficacy of insight-oriented psychotherapy for those with chronic pain problems.[52]

BEHAVIORAL APPROACHES

RESPONDENT CONDITIONING

If a nociceptive stimulus is repeatedly paired with a neutral stimulus in close temporal proximity, the neutral stimulus will come to elicit a pain response. This is referred to as classical, respondent, or pavlovian conditioning. In chronic pain, many activities that were neutral or even pleasurable may come to elicit or exacerbate pain and are thus experienced as aversive and actively avoided. Over time, a growing number of stimuli (e.g., activities and exercises) may be expected to elicit or exacerbate pain and will be avoided, a process termed *stimulus generalization*. The anticipatory fear of pain and restriction of activity—and not just the actual nociception—may contribute to disability. Anticipatory fear can also elicit a physiologic reaction that may aggravate the pain. Thus, conditioning may directly increase nociceptive stimulation and pain.

As long as avoidance of activity succeeds in preventing initiation or exacerbation of the pain, the conviction of pain sufferers that they must remain inactive is difficult to modify. Treatment of pain via the classical conditioning model involves repeated exposure to feared or avoided activities that result in less pain than the patient may have predicted (i.e., corrective feedback). In this way patients' anticipatory fear of the activity is reduced or extinguished.[53,54] Such transformations add support to the importance of quota-based physical exercise programs, with participants progressively increasing their activity levels despite fear of injury and discomfort associated with the use of deconditioned muscles.

OPERANT APPROACH

Operant approaches focus on extinction of pain behavior by withdrawal of positive attention from pain behavior and increasing well behavior by positive reinforcement. As noted, the operant learning paradigm does not seek to uncover the cause of the pain but focuses primarily on maintenance of the pain behavior and deficiency of well behavior. Target pain behavior is identified, as are its controlling antecedents and consequent reinforcers or punishments,[50] such as overly solicitous, distracting, or ignoring behavior by a spouse.[34]

Removal of the contingent relationship between overt pain behavior and its positive or negative consequences, along with positive and negative reinforcement, is used to increase and maintain the desired behavior and decrease pain-compatible behavior (e.g., with operant behavioral treatment) because patients are expected to be active in setting treatment goals and following through with recommendations.[50] The efficacy of operant treatment has been demonstrated in several studies of persons with chronic pain disorders, including low back pain[35] and fibromyalgia syndrome.[55]

Box 45.3 Assumptions of the Cognitive-Behavioral Perspective

- People are active processors of information and not passive reactors.
- Thoughts (e.g., appraisals, expectations, beliefs) can elicit and influence mood, affect physiologic processes, have social consequences, and also serve as an impetus for behavior; conversely, mood, physiology, environmental factors, and behavior can influence the nature and content of thought processes.
- Behavior is reciprocally determined by individual *and* environmental factors.
- People can learn more adaptive ways of thinking, feeling, and behaving.
- People should be active collaborative agents in changing their thoughts, feelings, behavior, and physiology.

COGNITIVE-BEHAVIORAL THERAPY

As noted, it is important to make a distinction between the CB perspective and cognitive and behavioral techniques.[22,29] The CB perspective is based on the idea that people believe that they cannot function because of their pain and that they are helpless to improve their situation (Box 45.3). Treatment goals thus focus on helping patients with pain realize that they can manage problems and on providing the skills to respond in more adaptive ways that can be maintained after the treatment has ended. These techniques include those described earlier and more specific interventions, as noted here.

The CBT approach combines cognitive and behavioral techniques, including assertiveness, stress management, relaxation training, goal setting, guided imagery, and pacing of activities.[22,29] Biofeedback, meditation, and hypnosis can all be incorporated within the framework of CBT. Therapists assist patients with concerns about the future, returning to work, and physical limitations; they help people build their communication skills, gain a sense of control over their pain, and cope with fear of pain and reinjury and with frustration resulting from the responses of others (e.g., physicians, insurance companies, employers, family, significant others) to the patient's pain reports or behavior. Individuals are educated in developing positive coping strategies and are encouraged to increase their activities in a graded fashion. It is expected that they will gain mastery over their pain, which will then result in improved mood and foster self-confidence.[22,29,55]

Four key components of CBT have been described[22,29]—education, skills acquisition, skills consolidation, and generalization and maintenance. The education component consists of helping the patient challenge negative perceptions regarding his or her ability to manage pain through a process termed *cognitive restructuring* by making the person aware of the role of thoughts and emotions in potentiating and maintaining stress and physical symptoms. Steps in cognitive restructuring include identifying maladaptive thoughts during problematic situations (e.g., during pain exacerbations, stressful events), introduction and practice of coping thoughts, shifting from self-defeating to coping thoughts, introduction and practice of positive or reinforcing thoughts, and finally home practice and follow-up. Using these steps, the therapist encourages patients to test the adaptiveness (not the so-called rationality) of thoughts, beliefs, expectations, and predictions. The crucial element in successful treatment is bringing about a shift from well-established, habitual, and automatic but ineffective responses to systematic problem solving and planning, control of affect, behavioral persistence, and disengagement, when appropriate.[22,29]

The goal of skills acquisition and consolidation is to help patients learn skills for new pain management behavior and cognition, including training in relaxation, problem solving, distraction, activity pacing, and communication. Using role-playing techniques and homework assignments, patients can practice emerging skill sets and evaluate their usefulness for the management of their pain.

Finally, generalization and maintenance are aimed at solidifying skills and preventing relapse. Problems that arise throughout treatment are viewed as opportunities to assist patients in learning how to handle any setbacks and lapses that may occur following treatment. During this phase they can learn how to anticipate future problems and high-risk situations so that they can think about and practice the behavioral responses that may be necessary for successful coping. The goal of this phase is to enable patients to develop a problem-solving perspective in which they believe that they have the skills and competency to respond appropriately to problems as they arise. In this manner, attempts are made to help the patient learn to anticipate future difficulties, develop plans for adaptive responding, and adjust behavior accordingly.

Recently, some variations in CBT have been proposed. Acceptance-based approaches use a series of exercises to teach patients to be more mindful and less judgmental about their experience and to focus on achieving valued goals.[56,57] However, the specific techniques used and mediating variables targeted by CBT interventions may turn out to be less important than the overall objective of helping patients change their view of themselves as being helpless, passive, and dependent to a view of themselves as active agents who are resourceful and capable of self-managing their symptoms and their lives.[29]

The efficacy of CBT has been demonstrated in a large number of studies of chronic pain disorders and has been reviewed extensively.[26,58-60] Evidence suggests that individual and group CBT can help restore function and mood, as well as reduce pain and disability-related behavior.[26,54] Despite the fact that CBT is undoubtedly the intervention used most often for those with chronic pain, it has limitations. For example, although CBT has been found to be helpful for a number of individuals, there are some for whom CBT is not beneficial. Researchers are just beginning to explore different aspects of CBT to answer the question, "what works for whom?"[61-63]

Some specific techniques can be incorporated into CBT when treating chronic pain patients. The specific details involved in these techniques may be less important than the primary objective. Each technique described is designed to help patients feel a sense of control; a common feature is their ability to combat the feelings of helplessness and demoralization experienced by many of those with chronic pain.[22]

MOTIVATIONAL INTERVIEWING

Most people with chronic pain adhere to a biomedical model; for example, the nature of their symptoms is closely aligned with physical pathology. As the pain persists, some people may become aware of the role of factors such as emotional stress in their experience of pain. They may begin to consider that they can learn and use self-management techniques to help them adapt to life with a chronic pain condition. Others with chronic pain, however, have difficulty with this expanded perspective. The stage of acceptance of self-management is important because those who are not ready for the use of psychological techniques will tend to avoid and dismiss such methods. Thus, the clinician needs to be aware of an individual's readiness to accept and undertake the steps necessary to achieve self-management. The assessment process described earlier should help the health care provider determine the patient's readiness for the use of nonphysical approaches.

Motivational interviewing as a treatment intervention was initially developed for those with substance abuse disorders,[55] although it has been used increasingly for chronic pain patients.[64] Specific stages of change have been postulated, and interventional techniques are tailored to each stage.

In the precontemplation stage, patients with chronic pain have not yet begun to consider changing from a purely somatic view of pain and have adopted a passive role as they wait for the health care provider to identify and provide appropriate treatment. The clinician attempts to assist the person by fostering acknowledgment of risks and problems resulting from inactivity, such as increased pain and physical deconditioning.[65]

Once patients with chronic pain take responsibility for their prior inactivity, they enter the next of the proposed stages, the contemplation stage. Here, the clinical goal is to encourage the patient to conclude that the risks associated with inactivity outweigh the perceived benefits. When they are ready to become more active (the preparation stage), the clinician helps outline appropriate structured physical activities in which the patient is willing to participate. Finally, in the action stage, the clinician helps the patient increase activity levels. This is followed by maintenance geared toward the individual's ongoing motivation and commitment.[65]

It is important for physicians to be tolerant as patients move through these stages. Clinicians can encourage transition to different stages by providing motivational statements, listening with empathy, asking open-ended questions, providing feedback and affirmation, and handling resistance.[55,65] Because motivational interviewing has been applied to chronic pain only rather recently,[63] the efficacy of this intervention in different chronic pain populations is not yet well documented. Motivational interviewing is a general framework for preparing persons for treatment and for adherence to the CB perspective and can be readily used with CBT.

BIOFEEDBACK

Developed in the 1960s, biofeedback is a self-regulation technique that has been used successfully to treat a number of chronic pain states, such as headache, back pain, chronic myofascial pain, and irritable bowel syndrome.[66,67] The objective of biofeedback is to teach people to exert control over their physiologic processes. During biofeedback, the patient is connected by electrodes to equipment linked to a computer that records physiologic responses. These processes may include skin conductance, respiration, heart rate, heart rate variability, skin temperature, brain wave activity, and muscle tension. The recording equipment amplifies and converts the readings into visual or auditory signals on a monitor that the patient can observe. In this way, the information recorded is "fed back" to the person, which potentially helps the individual learn to change physiologic responses by manipulating the auditory or visual signals.

Important forms of biofeedback therapy include electromyographic biofeedback, in which patients (e.g., those with tension headaches) are provided with information fed back to them from the physiologic recordings and taught to manipulate the tension in their frontalis muscle. Patients with migraine are provided with thermal feedback. They are instructed to warm the temperature of their hands by using visual or auditory cues.[29] Alternatively, patients may be given biofeedback associated with heart rate variability, which has been shown to be associated with pain perception.[68,69]

Real-time fMRI has been used as a sophisticated source of biofeedback to help train participants to control activation in the rostral anterior cingulate cortex (rACC) and has shown promising results. This brain region is reputedly involved in pain perception and regulation. When the participants deliberately induced changes in the rACC, there was a corresponding change in their perception of the pain.[70]

With practice, most people can learn to control voluntarily important physiologic functions that may be associated directly with pain and stress.[71] Biofeedback generates a state of general relaxation. Typically, patients being treated with biofeedback will be instructed to practice using the methods that have been successful in altering physiologic parameters in the clinic.

The actual mechanisms involved in the success of biofeedback are still unknown. However, the assumption of biofeedback treatment is that the level of pain is maintained or exacerbated by dysregulation of the autonomic nervous system, which is believed to be associated with the production of nociceptive stimulation (e.g., muscle tension in a person with low back pain). In addition to the physiologic changes accompanying biofeedback, patients are provided with a sense of control over their bodies. Given the high levels of helplessness observed in those with chronic pain problems, the perception of control may be as important as the actual physiologic changes observed. A general sense of relaxation is also an important feature of biofeedback. Again, it is not clear whether the alterations in specific physiologic parameters putatively associated with pain are the most important component of biofeedback or whether it is the broader relaxation and self-control created.

There are many relaxation techniques that have been used in combination with biofeedback and on their own. However, reports are mixed about whether biofeedback is any more effective than relaxation. The pain condition being treated may differ in regard to the greatest contribution of a possible component (relaxation, sense of control, general relaxation). Moreover, the components may not be mutually exclusive and may even be synergistic.

MEDITATION

Meditation is a 2500-year-old practice that has become a popular mental exercise. It is defined as the "intentional self-regulation of attention," a systematic inner focus on particular aspects of inner and outer experience.[72,73] Unlike many approaches in behavioral medicine, such as biofeedback, meditation was developed in a religious or spiritual context. It is regarded as the ultimate goal of spiritual growth in that it can end suffering, enable personal transformation, and provide a transcendental experience.[74] However, as a health care intervention, it has been taught effectively, regardless of the individual's cultural or religious background.[75,76]

Many forms of meditation are practiced worldwide. Here, two general approaches are described that have been researched extensively: transcendental meditation and Zen or mindfulness meditation.[77] Transcendental meditation is concentrative in that it involves focus on one of the senses, like a zoom lens focusing on a specific object. For example, the individual repeats a silent word or phrase (mantra) with the goal of transcending the ordinary stream of mental discourse.[74,78] Mindfulness meditation is the opposite of transcendental meditation in that its goal is awareness of the whole perceptual field, like a wide-angle lens. Thus, it incorporates focused attention and whole-field awareness in the present moment. For example, the individual simply observes without judgment, thoughts, emotions, sensations, and perceptions as they arise moment by moment.[75,79] Bonadonna[80] has proposed that those with chronic illness have an altered ability to concentrate; therefore, transcendental meditation may be less useful than mindfulness meditation.

Mindfulness meditation reframes the experience of discomfort such that physical pain, malaise, or suffering becomes the object of meditation. The attention and awareness of discomfort or suffering are another part of human experience; rather than being avoided, which is the most common reaction, it is to be investigated, experienced, and explored.[80] This form of meditation was incorporated into behavioral medicine in the 1980s[75] and has been used successfully as an adjunctive intervention for health conditions such as fibromyalgia, psoriasis, and cancer pain. Studies have found that mindfulness-based interventions decrease pain symptoms, increase healing speed, improve mood, reduce stress, contain health care costs, and decrease visits to primary care facilities.[73,74,81]

Meditation has captured the attention of medicine, behavioral medicine, psychology, and neurocognitive science, partly because experienced meditators demonstrate calmer responses to daily stress and perform better at tasks that require focused attention. Many believe that meditation can confer health benefits.[82,83] Lazar and associates[82] found that long-term meditation by Western practitioners who were not monks results in increased cortical thickness in areas related to somatosensory, auditory, visual, and interoceptive processing. They found thickening in the right Brodmann areas 9 and 10, which have been shown to be involved in the integration of cognition and emotion. A hypothesis based on this structural change is that by becoming increasingly aware of sensory stimuli during practice, the practitioner is gradually able to use self-awareness to navigate potentially stressful encounters more successfully. This may be useful for those experiencing chronic pain because of the reciprocal relationship between stress and pain symptoms.

Additionally, Lutz and coworkers[83] observed that Buddhist practitioners at baseline and while in a state of unconditional loving kindness and compassion while meditating have higher self-induced gamma-wave synchrony than do controls. Gamma-wave activity is the synchrony of areas of the brain communicating with each other. This also suggests how meditation may be beneficial for people with chronic pain because of dysregulation within the HPA axis and autonomic nervous system. Furthermore, meditators have demonstrated changes in electroencephalographic activity; specifically, they have higher alpha brain wave activity. This has been found to have beneficial health effects and to promote a general sense of well-being.[84-86]

GUIDED IMAGERY

Guided imagery can be useful for helping people with pain relax, achieve a sense of control, and distract themselves from pain and the accompanying symptoms. This modality involves the generation of mental images by oneself or the practitioner. Thus, it overlaps with the available relaxation techniques and hypnosis. Although guided imagery has been advocated as a stand-alone intervention to reduce presurgical anxiety and postsurgical pain and accelerate healing,[87] it is most often used in conjunction with other treatment interventions, such as CBT or relaxation.[22,28]

With guided imagery using visualization or imagination, patients are asked to evoke specific images that they find pleasant and engaging. In this way, a detailed representation tailored to the individual can then be created. When the person with chronic pain is feeling pain or is experiencing an exacerbation of pain, he or she can use imagery to help redirect attention away from the pain and achieve a psychophysiologic state of relaxation.

Images can be sensory or affective; however, the most successful images tend to be those that involve all the senses (vision, sound, touch, smell, and taste). People with chronic pain are thus encouraged to use images that evoke these senses. Some patients, however, may have difficulty generating a particularly vivid visual image and may find it helpful to listen to a taped description or look at a poster on which they can focus their attention as a way of assisting their imagination.

HYPNOSIS

Hypnosis has been defined as a "natural state of aroused attentive focal concentration coupled with a relative suspension of peripheral awareness." There are three central components of a hypnotic trance: (1) absorption, or intense involvement in the central object of concentration; (2) dissociation, in which experiences that would commonly be felt consciously occur outside of conscious awareness (i.e., the converse of meditation); and (3) suggestibility, in which persons are more likely to accept outside input without cognitive censorship or criticism.[88]

Hypnosis has been used as a treatment intervention for pain control since at least the 1850s. It has been shown to be beneficial in relieving pain in people with headache, burn injury, arthritis, cancer, and chronic back pain.[89-91] As with imagery, relaxation, and biofeedback, hypnosis is infrequently used alone for chronic pain; although it has been used as a psychological model with some success in cancer patients,[92] it is often used concurrently with other treatment interventions. Hypnotic suggestions have been used to instill positive attitudes in people, facilitate compliance with treatment, foster distraction from negative thoughts or stimuli, alleviate anxiety related to medical procedures, reduce reliance on medication, and promote relaxation and rehearsal of adaptive behavior.[91,93]

A meta-analysis[91] has suggested an overall benefit of the addition of hypnosis to nonhypnotic pain management strategies, although this may be affected by the level of hypnotic suggestibility. Furthermore, there are discrepancies in the literature with regard to the methods used to induce hypnosis, thus making it difficult to evaluate the efficacy of this intervention accurately.[92] Finally, based on systematic reviews, Patterson and Jensen[89,90] suggested that hypnosis has more usefulness for the treatment of acute pain than chronic pain. Thus, the degree to which hypnosis is helpful beyond the effectiveness of other interventions and for which populations it is useful remain to be elucidated.

I have only briefly described the range of psychological approaches and techniques that have been used in chronic pain patients. Some illustrative studies have been highlighted and reference made to systematic reviews and meta-analyses; the reader may wish to consult these sources to learn more about these approaches. These methods can readily be integrated into more comprehensive rehabilitation programs. They can be useful complements to physical therapy, medication management, and vocational rehabilitation by helping patients become active participants in their own care when pain flares up, as well as being a routine part of a self-management program. Using these techniques, the patient may feel more hopeful rather than helpless and dependent.

INTERDISCIPLINARY PAIN REHABILITATION PROGRAMS

Psychological approaches and techniques have found strong support in the literature when used on their own. However, interdisciplinary pain rehabilitation programs (IPRPs) are also efficacious because the CB perspective and cognitive and behavioral techniques are often important components of these programs[26,58-60] and have been recommended for use in combination.[3,28] The premise underlying the development of IPRPs is that patients with complex pain problems are best served by the collaborative efforts of a team of specialists, which often includes physicians, nurses, physical therapists, occupational therapists, vocational counselors, and psychologists. IPRPs operate under the assumption that pain is not just the result of body damage but also has psychological and environmental origins. In other words, IPRPs treat more than pain—they treat the whole person.[94]

The primary goal of IPRPs is to improve physical performance and coping skills and to transfer the responsibility for pain management from the health care provider to the individual. The treatment plan is rehabilitative rather than curative and encourages people to take a more active role in the management of their pain.

IPRPs adopt the biopsychosocial model of chronic pain, which assumes that all human behavior, including the report of pain, reflects a combination of the events occurring within the person's body, recognition and appraisal of these events, affective responses to these events, and the influence of the environment.[3,94] Comprehensive and concurrent treatment interventions may include drug detoxification, psychological treatment (e.g., relaxation training, problem solving), physical conditioning, acquisition of coping and vocational skills, and education about pain and how the body functions.

A large number of published studies and several meta-analyses have supported the clinical effectiveness of IPRPs.[26,95] In general, when compared with pharmacologic, medical, and surgical alternatives, IPRPs appear to be equally effective in reducing pain and significantly more effective in reducing health care consumption and can lead to closure of disability claims, increased functional activities, and a higher rate of return to work.[3,51] Even at long-term follow-up, people who are treated in IPRPs appear to maintain their reductions in pain and emotional distress.[96,97] An additional benefit of IPRPs is that they cost substantially less per person annually than medications and surgery do, thus rendering treatment more cost-effective. However, somewhat paradoxically, the availability of these types of programs is limited and appears to be shrinking.[51]

CONCLUSION

A person experiencing chronic pain is continually in quest of relief that often remains elusive, which leads to feelings of helplessness, hopelessness, demoralization, and outright depression. Emotional distress may be attributed to various factors, including inadequate or maladaptive coping resources, iatrogenic complications, overuse of medication, disability, financial difficulties, litigation, disruption of usual activities, inadequate social support, and sleep disturbances. Thus, chronic pain represents a demoralizing situation; the individual with pain not only faces the stress created by the pain but also experiences a cascade of ongoing stressors that compromise all aspects of life. Living with chronic pain requires considerable emotional resilience, tends to deplete emotional reserve, and taxes not only the pain sufferer but also the capability of family members and significant others to provide support.

A large body of evidence demonstrates that psychological factors can interfere with or hinder a person's ability to cope with the pain experience. As a result, psychological intervention in the assessment and treatment of chronic pain is becoming standard practice. Psychological treatment can focus on the emotional distress that accompanies chronic pain and provide education and training in the use of cognitive and behavioral techniques, which may reduce perceptions of pain and related disability. Psychologists and psychological principles have played a major role in understanding and treating people with pain, and psychologists have an important function in IPRPs as clinicians and researchers.

None of the treatments described are successful in eliminating pain completely; the same statement can be made in reference to the most commonly used pharmacologic, medical, and surgical interventions.[51] Consequently, most people have to adapt to the presence of chronic pain and learn self-management in the face of persistent pain and accompanying symptoms. The psychological interventions described in this chapter provide a general overview of various treatment strategies. By far, however, treatment with CBT alone or within the context of an IPRP holds the greatest empirical evidence for success. There is a substantial and overwhelming body of research supporting the effectiveness of various psychological approaches. It therefore seems prudent to consider the use of psychological treatment in conjunction with traditional medical interventions.

Currently, few data are available that consistently identify the characteristics of those who would most likely benefit from the pain treatment methods described in this chapter, although some studies have suggested that individualized treatment is associated with more relief of symptoms than standard treatment is.[61,98-100] Further studies are needed to determine which treatments—and how they should be delivered—are most effective for patients with certain characteristics and result in the fewest iatrogenic complications and adverse events.[28,55] Positive results will permit more clinically effective and cost-effective ways to treat the difficult population of patients with chronic pain.

KEY POINTS

- Pain is a complex, subjective experience with psychosocial and behavioral as well as biologic contributors.
- The biologic treatments currently available are inadequate, and significant levels of pain persist despite the most advanced pharmaceutical, anesthetic, and surgical treatments.
- Persistent pain has an impact on all aspects of individuals' lives.
- People with chronic pain are demoralized because their bodies and the health care system have let them down.
- The presence of chronic pain affects not only patients but also their significant others, health care providers, employers, and third-party payers.
- There is wide individual variation in the experience of chronic pain, styles of coping and adaptation, and response to treatment.

Continued

KEY POINTS—cont'd

- Environmental factors (e.g., attention by significant others, including health care providers) can reinforce behavioral responses by patients.
- Patients' beliefs, attitudes, and expectations influence the experience of pain, disability, and treatment response.
- A comprehensive approach to assessment of patients with chronic pain that addresses the medical, psychological, and environmental contributors is necessary to develop an optimal treatment plan.
- The cognitive-behavioral perspective makes several assumptions about patients: (1) they are active processors of information and not passive responders; (2) thoughts, mood, behavior, and physiology are interdependent and interactive; (3) patient behavior is influenced by both personal and environmental factors; (4) patients can learn more adaptive ways of thinking, feeling, and behaving in response to persistent pain; and (5) patients should be actively involved as agents in changing their thoughts, feelings, and behavior, and this may in turn have an impact on the physiologic factors associated with persistence and magnitude of the pain.
- Since there is no cure for chronic pain, patients need to learn to accept their own role in self-management of their pain and their lives.
- A number of behavioral (e.g., relaxation, biofeedback) and cognitive (e.g., problem solving, meditation) modalities that may be helpful to patients can be taught and learned as complements to traditional medical treatments.
- Interdisciplinary pain rehabilitation programs that integrate psychological and physical treatments have been demonstrated to provide benefits to patients with recalcitrant chronic pain.
- Research is needed to identify the best treatment combination for patients with different physical and psychosocial characteristics.

ACKNOWLEDGMENT

Support for preparation of this chapter was provided by grants from the National Institutes of Health/National Institute of Arthritis and Musculoskeletal and Skin Diseases (AR 59102).

SUGGESTED READINGS

Committee on Advancing Pain Research, Care, and Education, Institute of Medicine. *Relieving Pain in America: Blueprint for Transforming Prevention, Care, Education, and Research.* Washington, DC: National Academies Press; 2011.

Flor H, Turk DC. *Chronic Pain: An Integrated Biobehavioral Approach.* Seattle: IASP Press; 2011.

Fordyce WE. *Behavioral Methods for Chronic Pain and Illness.* St. Louis: Mosby; 1976.

Gatchel RJ, Peng YB, Peters ML, et al. The biopsychosocial approach to chronic pain: scientific advances and future directions. *Psychol Bull.* 2007;133:581-624.

Henschke N, Ostelo RW, van Tulder MW, et al. Behavioural treatment for chronic low-back pain. *Cochrane Database Syst Rev.* 2010;7:CD002014.

Hoffman BM, Papas RK, Chatkoff DK, et al. Meta-analysis of psychological interventions for chronic low back pain. *Health Psychol.* 2007;26:1-9.

Okifuji A, Turk DC, Sherman JJ. Evaluation of the relationship between depression and fibromyalgia syndrome: why aren't all patients depressed? *J Rheumatol.* 2000;27:212-219.

Rusu A, Boersma K, Turk DC. Subgroups of pain patients—the potential of customizing treatments. In: Hasenbring M, Rusu A, Turk DC, eds. *From Acute to Chronic Back Pain: Risk Factors, Mechanisms, and Clinical Implications.* London: Oxford University Press; 2012:485-511.

Skinner MS, Wilson HD, Turk DC. Cognitive-behavioral perspective and cognitive-behavioral therapy for people with chronic pain—distinctions, outcomes, and innovations. *J Cogn Psychother.* 2012;26:93-113.

Turk DC, Swanson K, Tunks E. Psychological approaches in the treatment of chronic pain patients—when pills, scalpels, and needles are not enough. *Can J Psychiatry.* 2008;53:23-33.

Turk DC, Melzack R, eds. *Handbook of Pain Assessment.* 3rd ed. New York: Guilford Press; 2011.

Turk DC, Robinson JP. Assessment of patients with chronic pain—a comprehensive approach. In: Turk DC, Melzack R, eds. *Handbook of Pain Assessment.* 3rd ed. New York: Guilford Press; 2011:188-210.

Turk DC, Wilson HD, Cahana A. Treatment of chronic noncancer pain. *Lancet.* 2011;377:2226-2235.

Vlaeyen JWS, Morley S. Cognitive-behavioral treatments for chronic pain: what works for whom? *Clin J Pain.* 2005;21:1-8.

The references for this chapter can be found at www.expertconsult.com.

46

Physical Medicine Techniques in Pain Management

Benoy Benny | Martin Grabois | Kwai-Tung Chan

This chapter focuses on the physical medicine techniques used to treat patients in pain. At the conclusion of reading this chapter the reader will have a thorough understanding of physical medicine techniques and how they fit into the multidisciplinary comprehensive treatment of patients with pain. Although the physical medicine approach can help decrease pain and increase function, if combined with medication, behavioral modification, cognitive modification, and sometimes interventions, the results can be much more dramatic.

In the third edition of this text, Linchitz and Sorell[1] defined physical medicine and rehabilitation and the role of the physiatrist. They noted that "Physical medicine and rehabilitation have traditionally been the medical specialty that oversees and prescribes the application of physical modalities to treat disease and disorders, including the rehabilitation of patients with pain. The physiatrist, whose primary perspective is typically one of the functions, is an expert on the musculoskeletal and locomotor systems and is knowledgeable about how to use physical agents and how to coordinate the rehabilitation team. As part of the multidisciplinary medical team, the physiatrist participates in the evaluation and treatment of those individuals with pain."[1]

However, there are not enough physiatrists to treat all patients with pain. Therefore, all physicians need to understand the rationale, indications, contraindications, and prescription of physical medicine techniques and their appropriate use. Many of these techniques can be used for acute, subacute, and chronic pain. However, with progression to more chronic pain, techniques should be more active and less passive and more behavioral and cognitive in nature. Although many of these techniques will help decrease pain, the long-term goal should be to increase function despite the presence of the pain syndrome.

APPROACH TO TREATMENT

Patients with pain can be evaluated and treated by individual physicians and therapists. This type of approach is more often used and successful in patients with acute or subacute pain. However, as the pain becomes more chronic and includes psychosocial and vocational issues, a multidisciplinary or interdisciplinary approach is recommended.

Although the terms *multidisciplinary* and *interdisciplinary* are often used interchangeably, multidisciplinary more formally refers to collaboration among members of different disciplines (including various medical specialists and therapists), managed by a leader who directs a range of ancillary services.[2] Interdisciplinary describes a deeper level of consensus-based collaboration in which the entire process (i.e., evaluation, goal setting, and delivery of treatment) is orchestrated by the team, facilitated by regular face-to-face meetings, and primarily delivered at a single facility.[2] The interdisciplinary team is commonly led by a pain specialist and includes physical and occupational therapists; pain psychologists; relaxation training experts; vocational, rehabilitation, and therapeutic recreational specialists; social workers; and nurse educators.[3] The role of these team members is discussed later in this chapter.

It should be noted that comprehensive reviews of the cost-effectiveness and efficacy of interdisciplinary programs have demonstrated significant improvements in return to work, increased function, reduced health care use, and closure of disability claims.[4] These comprehensive programs have also shown clear benefits over conventional management with regard to decreasing pain behavior and improving mood.[4,5] The interdisciplinary model provides ongoing communication among all members of the treatment team, which helps facilitate patients' care while they progress to behavioral, cognitive, and active therapy.[6]

ROLE OF THE THERAPY TEAM

Ideally, a pain program should be comprehensive and interdisciplinary. Typically, the team is led by a physician and consists of physical therapists, occupational therapists, and often recreational therapists, dieticians, and psychologists.[7] Combined assessment by these professionals is used to devise a comprehensive approach to allow the patient to benefit maximally, reintegrate fully into life, and have as few restrictions as possible.

It is important that realistic goals be set before therapy begins. Such goals include but should not be limited to decreasing muscle tightness, increasing strength in areas of muscle weakness, increasing general aerobic conditioning, and improving ease in performance of activities of daily living. In general, one wants to first restore flexibility and then increase strength and develop endurance. Completely removing the pain may not be a realistic goal of therapy, but increased function should be. Box 46.1 lists the goals of therapy to be accomplished.

Sometimes, the distinction between physical and occupational therapists is lost. Physical therapists focus on the strength, flexibility, and coordination of large muscle groups. They assess and help in developing strength and flexibility of the legs, pelvic girdle, and trunk and address mobility by ambulation. They also train patients in back and body mechanics.[8] Occupational therapists focus on fine and gross motor strength, flexibility and coordination of the hands, and activities of daily living. For pain patients, they are also good in teaching conservation techniques. They can help patients in their work by instructing them in ergonomics, work simplification, and energy conservation.[9] Another important aspect that they address is proper posture, which can result in a significant reduction in pain if put into practice daily. The roles of physical and occupational therapists are presented in Box 46.2.

Recreational therapists assist in providing pleasurable outlets to help maintain physical conditioning. Instead of prescribing a boring set of home exercises, incorporating pleasurable activities that are also distracting often increases the patient's interest and cooperation. The psychologist's role is to identify factors that may be complicating the pain experience and help the patient deal with the process in a better way. There are many useful tools and tests to help the psychologist determine other confounding factors so that the patient's functioning can be increased maximally. These include the Minnesota Multiphasic Personality Inventory, Beck Depression Inventory, Oswestry scale, Symptom Checklist 90, and McGill Pain Questionnaire.[10] The psychologist, working alone or with the team, can encourage pain reduction by teaching the patient stress management, relaxation, and self-monitoring techniques. Stress reduction can be achieved through cognitive-behavioral therapy.[11]

The physician's role is mainly to lead the team in complete management of the patient. This includes making sure that there is no disease process that might be causing the pain and, if present, that there is no other treatment or intervention that should be pursued before initiating therapies. It also includes monitoring safe participation in physical rehabilitation while optimizing medication management. If it is thought that the patient could benefit from interventions, it is easier if this is done before initiating a comprehensive rehabilitation program.[10]

Physical conditioning programs use a cognitive-behavioral approach plus intensive physical training that includes aerobic capacity, muscle strength and endurance, and coordination. These approaches can be work related, given and supervised by a physiotherapist or multidisciplinary team, and seem to be effective in reducing the number of sick days for some with chronic back pain when compared with usual care.[12]

Box 46.1 Goals of Therapy

Restore biomechanical dysfunction.
Improve strength.
Improve posture.
Improve gait symmetry.
Improve general aerobic conditioning.
Improve efficiency of activities of daily living.
Decrease edema.
Instruct patients to monitor pain response and to pace activity.
Use back or joint conservation techniques.

Box 46.2 Role of Physical Therapists and Occupational Therapists

Physical Therapists

Loss of flexibility
Strength and weakness of trunk and limb muscles
Core strengthening
General aerobic conditioning
Balance and coordination
Contractures
Assisted mobility

Occupational Therapists

Joint conservation techniques
Work simplification techniques
Back conservation
Posture
Energy conservation techniques
Activities of daily living and self-care
Edema control

BASIC MANAGEMENT CONSIDERATIONS

CLINICAL EVALUATION

Patients with acute or chronic pain may be referred for physical medicine evaluation and treatment as a component of a multidisciplinary management approach or for certain specific treatments. Before initiating treatment, it is important to perform a history and physical examination (Chapter 13), review the medical records to identify factors contributing to the patient's complaints, and assess the impact of pain on the patient's functioning. Contraindications to physical medicine treatments and precautions for treatment should be identified. A careful and thorough history and physical examination also help establish trust between the clinician and patient and facilitate consensus with treatment recommendations.

HISTORY

A detailed history is obtained by interviewing the patient and reviewing questionnaires and medical records. It is important to obtain information about the time course, intensity, and location of the pain, as well as relieving and exacerbating factors. The functional state of the patient before onset of the problem and the current functional level should be determined to establish a baseline and guide expectations for improvement. The patient's experiences and responses to previous diagnostic and therapeutic interventions should be noted because they may predict responses to future treatment. Medical conditions that can affect or be affected by physical medicine treatments should be identified. It is also important to obtain information on medications, coexisting psychological and psychiatric disorders, substance abuse or addiction, and involvement in litigation because these factors can affect the patient's response to treatment.

PHYSICAL EXAMINATION

A complete physical examination with a focus on the neurologic and musculoskeletal systems should be performed. Active and passive joint range of motion (ROM), muscle bulk, strength, and sensation should be assessed and documented. Findings in the involved area should be compared with those on the asymptomatic side when possible. Patterns of pain and sensory loss can provide clues to the site of nervous system pathology or dysfunction. Signs of vasomotor instability, such as changes in skin temperature and alterations in hair, nails, or perspiration, may indicate autonomic dysfunction. Pain may limit testing of ROM, strength, and sensation; if this is the case, it should be noted. Reflex testing can be particularly helpful because it is one of the more objective parts of the examination. Abnormal or asymmetrical reflex responses may indicate dysfunction or pathology of the nervous system. Evidence of previous surgery or injury should be noted.

A patient's gait, posture, and movement can provide diagnostic clues to the source and severity of the pain. It is helpful to observe the patient and form a general impression before carrying out the formal physical examination. Inconsistencies between the patient's complaints and behavior should be noted.

FUNCTIONAL EVALUATION

A functional evaluation should be performed on pain patients before, during, and after completion of any treatment or functional restoration program.[7] Functional evaluation may range from direct observation of function by the clinician to formal functional capacity evaluation (FCE) performed by trained health care personnel.

Functional assessment can provide additional useful information because tests of pain perception, psychological distress, and self-perception of abilities and limitations do not accurately assess a person's physical capacity for work.[13] Physicians and patients often have great difficulty estimating functional limitation and physical ability.[14]

FCEs have existed in one form or another since the 1940s, although their use and application have changed over time. They are primarily used in industrial medicine and in legal and disability settings.[15] Reasons for ordering an FCE include making disability determinations, setting goals and planning treatment for industrial rehabilitation, monitoring progress through industrial rehabilitation, determining a person's readiness to return to work after injury, performing pre-employment evaluation, and determining case closure.[16]

Most FCE protocols include some or most of the following components: an interview, record review, self-administered questionnaire, psychological test battery, musculoskeletal evaluation, functional testing, validation of sincerity of effort, and comparisons to specific job requirements.[7,16] Functional testing may include material handling, specific tasks, holding static postures, and repetitive task performance.[7,16] A job analysis should be done before administration of an FCE because measurement of work capacity is specific to the demands posed by a job.[15]

There are scientific and practical limitations associated with FCEs with regard to standardization, validity, and reliability.[15,16] They have not necessarily been shown to predict return to work. However, they may be helpful in charting changes in function, comparing functional disparities with job demands, identifying nonmedical factors influencing the ability to work, and serving as a tool to guide work restrictions for patients returning to work or for initial therapy prescriptions for patients beginning a rehabilitation program.[7,16]

PSYCHOLOGICAL EVALUATION

A psychological evaluation should be considered when the pain is resulting in significant impairment in psychological, vocational, or social functioning. Such evaluations can determine the emotional, cognitive, behavioral, social, or vocational factors that could be affecting the patient's perception of pain.[7]

It is important that the psychological evaluation of a patient in chronic pain be conducted by a clinician who is sensitive to and knowledgeable about the psychological aspects of chronic pain. It should be appreciated that many chronic pain patients may be defensive about a psychological referral and are more likely to be evaluated if they are provided with an appropriate rationale and explanation for the referral. This topic is discussed further in Chapter 16.

ELECTRODIAGNOSTIC TESTING

Electrodiagnostic testing encompasses nerve conduction studies (NCSs) and electromyography (EMG), which provide information about the peripheral nerves and muscles, and evoked potentials, which are used mainly to assess the central nervous system (Fig. 46.1). Chapter 14 presents a more detailed discussion of the role of electrodiagnostic testing.

Electrodiagnosis can play an important role in identifying an underlying problem in a patient with a pain disorder. It helps not only in diagnosis but also in determining the

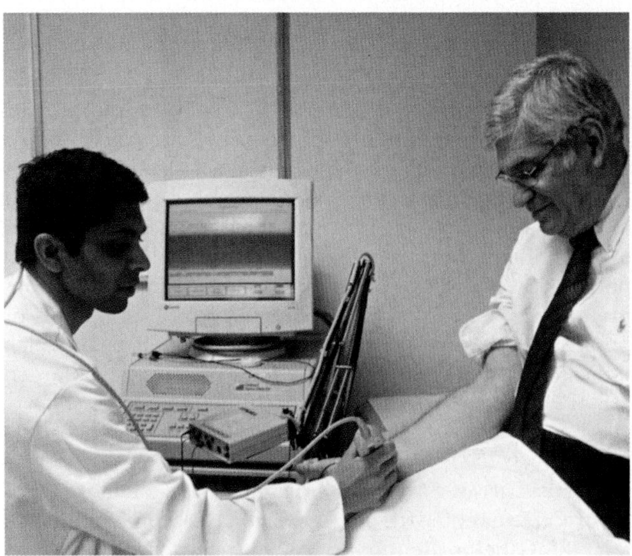

Figure 46.1 Performing electrodiagnostic testing.

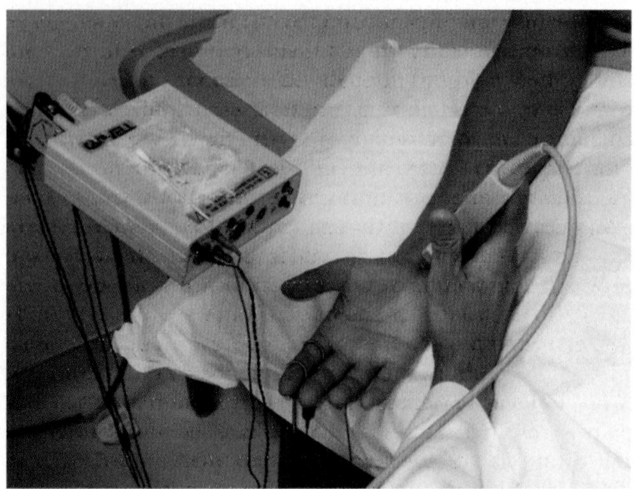

Figure 46.2 Performing nerve conduction studies.

chronicity and severity of the condition and can even assist in prognosis. Electrodiagnostic testing has another advantage when dealing with a pain patient who has signs of radiculopathy. Because disk bulges seen with magnetic resonance imaging (MRI) may be found routinely at many levels, EMG can help determine whether one of these disk bulges is actually producing nerve damage.[17] In addition, this test may be helpful in patients who have radiculitis with no structural disk herniation and often normal results on MRI. EMG has also been shown to help in making the diagnosis of spinal stenosis but does not predict future pain.[18] However, it has also been shown that the findings on EMG do not necessarily correlate with severity of the pain.[19]

Most physicians will perform NCSs and EMG together in the same session. The NCSs usually involve testing of sensory and motor nerves and sometimes reflex studies. Common nerves studied in the lower extremity include the sural, tibial, and deep peroneal and, in the upper extremity, the median, ulnar, and radial nerves. The facial and trigeminal nerves are tested less often.

When performing a motor NCS, the active electrode is placed over the muscle belly, the reference electrode is placed over the tendon insertion, and the nerve is stimulated at a fixed distance from the muscle. F-wave responses can also be recorded during motor studies; they can indicate the integrity of the entire motor nerve.

When performing a sensory NCS (usually done antidromically), the active and reference electrodes are placed over a distal nerve segment and the nerve is stimulated proximally (Fig. 46.2). The EMG study can be done with concentric or monopolar needles. There are two parts of EMG—evaluation of spontaneous activity and evaluation of motor unit action potentials (MUAPs). Typically, in neurogenic conditions the electromyographer will notice fibrillation potentials or positive sharp waves (PSWs) with spontaneous activity, which indicates instability of the muscle fiber membrane, enlarged MUAPs, and decreased MUAP recruitment.

RADICULOPATHY

The sensitivity of EMG in the diagnosis of radiculopathy is lower than that of MRI, but its specificity is significantly better.[17] EMG helps identify not only which nerve is involved but also the severity and chronicity of the lesion. It is important to remember that in radiculopathy, sensory NCS findings are normal because compression of the nerve root usually occurs proximal to the dorsal root ganglion, which therefore spares it. In S1 radiculopathy, the H-reflex is often prolonged.

Diagnosis of radiculopathy relies primarily on the electromyogram. With subacute, single–nerve root involvement, one should find denervation (fibrillation potentials, PSWs, or both) in two or more muscles of that myotome, involvement of the paraspinal muscles at the same level, and no denervation in other myotomes. It usually takes about 3 to 4 weeks for denervation to appear in the extremity muscles, but there may be earlier signs, such as decreased recruitment of motor units in muscles innervated by the involved root or signs of denervation in the paraspinal muscles. A more detailed discussion is presented in Chapter 14, so Table 46.1 summarizes abnormalities in some common disorders found by only NCSs and EMG.

REFLEX SYMPATHETIC DYSTROPHY

Despite the involvement of sympathetic nerves, electrophysiologic studies do not reveal specific abnormalities unless there is an associated nerve injury. One study has suggested relative reductions in the amplitude of the sympathetic nerve fiber function in the affected area as compared with the affected extremity.[20]

TREATMENT GOALS

The etiology of the pain syndrome should be determined from a medical and psychosocial point of view, and if possible, the location of the "pain generator" should be identified.[20] Attempts to decrease or eliminate pain generators are important and should be carried out first, followed by consideration of other treatment options.[7]

The goals of treatment center on moderating pain, increasing function, decreasing psychosocial issues, and reducing health care use.[21] These objectives can be achieved by modifying pain medication and pain behavior, decreasing reliance on medical care, increasing activity through exercise, and dealing with psychological and vocational issues.[6]

The Fordyce model of behavioral modification is useful in the treatment of patients with chronic pain syndromes.[22] The goal in these patients is not to cure the pain but to interrupt the pain behavior reinforcement cycle by rewarding healthy behavior and setting appropriate goals for the patient. Such goals include a reduction in the use of medications, modulation of the pain response, increased activity, and reduction in pain behavior.[23]

ROLE OF MEDICATIONS

Pain commonly limits participation in a physical therapy or rehabilitation program. Adequate pain management is an important component of rehabilitation. Many patients may be free of pain at rest and have incident pain provoked by activity or movement. Analgesic medications that are not timed to the patient's pain may lead to overdosing at rest and underdosing during pain or activity. Simple measures such as taking oral analgesic medications 30 to 60 minutes before the onset of therapy or other activity that incites pain

Table 46.1 Summary of Abnormalities on NCSs and EMG in Some Common Disorders

Disorder	Motor Study	Sensory Study	EMG	F and H Waves
Radiculopathy	Usually normal; if severe, may have a reduction in amplitude	Normal	Fibs and PSWs in muscles supplied by that root	Mild to moderate prolongation of H and F response latencies
Axonal polyneuropathy	Reduced amplitude in distal muscles	Reduced amplitude of distal nerves	Fibs and PSWs in distal muscles	Mild to moderate prolongation of H and F response latencies
Demyelinating polyneuropathy	Slowing of CV, prolongation of distal latency	Reduced amplitude and CV	Fibs, PSWs, variable reinnervation; reduced recruitment of motor units	Severe prolongation, absence of F and H responses
Compression neuropathy	Focal slowing of CV across the affected segment if mild, reduction in amplitude if severe	Slowing of CV across the affected segment, reduction in amplitude if severe	Fibs and PSWs in muscles supplied by that nerve	Mild prolongation in F responses
Plexopathy	Reduced amplitude in muscles supplied by affected fibers	Reduced amplitude in sensory nerves traversing the affected part of the plexus	Fibs and PSWs in muscles supplied by affected fibers	Mild to moderate prolongation of F and H latency
Mononeuropathy multiplex	Focal "axonal" lesions of multiple nerves with markedly decreased amplitude	Reduced or absent responses in affected nerves	Marked abnormalities in muscles supplied by the affected nerve	Mild prolongation or absence of H and F responses

CV, conduction velocity; EMG, electromyography; Fibs, fibrillation potentials; NCSs, nerve conduction studies; PSWs, positive sharp waves.

can provide satisfactory pain relief and increase the success of therapy.

In the postoperative setting, patients may benefit from multimodal analgesic techniques, including the use of combinations of analgesic medications and regional-peripheral nerve blocks.[24] Parenterally administered analgesic medications are more effective for treating severe, acute, or rapidly changing pain because of their rapid onset of action and ease of dose titration.[25] Patient-controlled analgesia allows self-titration of analgesic medication to an individual's pain and activity level.[26]

Patients with different types of pain—neuropathic, musculoskeletal, inflammatory—will benefit from medications that address the different causes of pain. Some patients have comorbid conditions that can increase the experience of pain, such as soft tissue inflammation, muscle spasms, or depression.[27] The concurrent use of medications to treat these coexisting symptoms may help reduce the degree of pain experienced.

ROLE OF PHYSICAL MODALITIES

Physical modalities are physical agents and techniques used to produce a therapeutic response. There is a long history of use of physical modalities to treat pain that dates back to ancient human prehistory and civilizations. Physical modalities and techniques commonly used to relieve pain include therapeutic heat and cold, hydrotherapy, ultrasound, electricity, and traction. Evidence-based guidelines regarding the use of physical modalities for acute and musculoskeletal pain have been published.[28,29]

It is important to realize that physical modalities do not eliminate pain by themselves and generally should not be prescribed as stand-alone treatments. Rather, they are best used as adjunctive treatments to an active exercise program. Modalities that the patient can safely use at home, such as hot and ice packs and transcutaneous electrical nerve stimulation (TENS), are more useful for chronic pain management. Modalities that require health care personnel to administer are best reserved for those with acute pain syndromes or intermittent exacerbations of chronic pain.

Before prescribing or administering a physical modality, an accurate diagnosis needs to be established and the goals of treatment determined. It is important to be aware of contraindications to the use of a specific modality. Precautions that need to be taken should be specified in the prescription.

PHYSICAL MODALITIES

THERAPEUTIC HEAT

Heat is one of the oldest physical modalities used to relieve and reduce pain. In addition to relief of pain, heat elicits other physiologic responses in local tissues that may be therapeutic, including increased blood flow, increased connective tissue extensibility, decreased muscle spasm, decreased joint stiffness, and reduced edema.[30] Heat may also have a modulating effect on pain at the spinal and supraspinal levels.[31] There is evidence that heat wrap therapy provides a short-term reduction in acute or subacute low back pain.[28,29]

Clinicians considering the use of therapeutic heat should first decide whether superficial or deep heat is required and then choose the appropriate heating modality. Superficial modalities include hot packs, heating pads, heat lamps, paraffin and whirlpool baths, and fluidotherapy. Deep heating agents include ultrasound, short wave, and microwave.

Contraindications to therapeutic heat are listed in Box 46.3. The risk for burns from external heat sources is real, and physicians should always write precautions to monitor for burns when heat is prescribed.

Superficial heat is delivered primarily by conduction, convection, and conversion. Modalities that transfer heat by conduction include hot packs (hydrocollator packs), heating pads, and paraffin baths. These heating modalities generally penetrate to depths of less than 2 cm from the skin. Skin and subcutaneous tissue temperatures are increased by 5° C to 6° C after 6 minutes and maintained for up to 30 minutes after application.[32]

A heating duration of 15 to 30 minutes may be necessary to increase muscle temperature by 1° C at depths of up to 3 cm.[33] A 1.2° C increase in knee intra-articular temperature has been demonstrated after superficial heat application.[33]

Hydrocollator packs are hot packs that contain a silicate gel product encased in canvas. These packs are heated and stored in thermostatically controlled water baths. Before application, the packs should be wrapped in several layers of towels and excess water allowed to drain off. To minimize the risk for burns, hot packs should be placed on the patient rather than under the patient because body weight and pressure impair circulation and dissipation of heat from the heated area.

Heat lamps provide superficial heating through conversion. Heat is generated in tissue through induction of molecular vibration by infrared waves emitted by the lamps. The degree of heating is a function of lamp wattage, angle of application, and distance to the body part. Radiant heat from lamps may be preferred when heating a diffuse area is required or when direct contact of a heating pad with the skin is not desirable.

Paraffin baths are a superficial heat modality commonly used for the treatment of distal extremity pain and stiffness from rheumatoid arthritis, osteoarthritis, and other connective tissue diseases. The two primary methods of application are dip and wrap and dip and immerse.[32] The former is more popular; it consists of dipping and removing the body part from the paraffin bath 8 to 10 times, followed by wrapping to assist in retention of heat. The paraffin–mineral oil mixture used should be heated in a bath with a thermostatically controlled heater.

Hydrotherapy is the use of water for medical purposes; it includes treatments as diverse as aquatic therapy and wound care. Patients with painful musculoskeletal conditions can often exercise more easily in water because of reduced weight bearing and additional support. Warm water also provides heat transferred by convection to immersed body areas. A whirlpool or agitation device can be used to maintain a constant water temperature around the treated areas and provide gentle mechanical stimulation to the immersed body parts.

Fluidotherapy uses glass beads, pulverized corncobs, or other finely pulverized substances with low heat affinity that are heated by hot air to form a warm medium with liquid-like properties. The body part or extremity to be treated is immersed in a cabinet containing this dry and warm medium for treatment.[32] Fluidotherapy is particularly useful for treating limbs affected by complex regional pain syndrome because it provides gentle tactile desensitization through stimulation of thermoreceptors and mechanoreceptors. Unlike hot packs and paraffin baths, there is no loss of heat over time. Stretching and exercise can also be performed during application of the heat.

When deep heating is required, ultrasound, short wave, and microwave diathermy can be used. These modalities deliver heat to deep tissues via conversion of physical energy to heat.

Ultrasound uses high-frequency sound waves to deliver energy to the target tissue. The sound waves produce thermal and nonthermal therapeutic effects.[34] Ultrasound waves pass through, are absorbed, or are reflected, depending on the type of tissue encountered. Higher temperatures are generated when the ultrasound energy is absorbed. Energy is absorbed more effectively at muscle-bone interfaces, which results in higher tissue temperatures in these areas. Ultrasound is also more effective in heating tendons and ligaments than in heating muscle, which absorbs ultrasound relatively poorly.

Ultrasound is used clinically to treat subacute and chronic inflammatory soft tissue disorders such as tendinitis and bursitis. There is evidence that therapeutic ultrasound may improve acute shoulder pain in patients with calcific tendinitis.[28,29] It can also be used for deep heating to facilitate stretching of contractures and shortened soft tissue structures. Low-intensity pulsed ultrasound has been shown to facilitate tissue repair and healing.[34,35] Contraindications to the use of ultrasound are listed in Box 46.4.

Short wave diathermy uses electromagnetic radio waves to deliver heat down to 3 to 5 cm below the skin without overheating the skin and subcutaneous tissue. Indications for short wave diathermy are similar to those for ultrasound. Contraindications include the presence of metal, implanted pacemakers, spinal cord stimulators, surgical implants, and copper-containing intrauterine devices, because of the risk for excessive heating.

Box 46.3 Contraindications to Therapeutic Heat

Insensate skin
Atrophic skin
Inability to communicate or respond to pain
Acute inflammation
Malignancy
Ischemia
Growth plates
Peripheral vascular disease
Demyelinating disease

Box 46.4 Contraindications to Ultrasound

Contraindications to therapeutic heat
Laminectomy sites
Over a pregnant uterus
Over the heart or carotid sinus
Over an implanted pacemaker

Microwave diathermy uses electromagnetic radio waves with frequencies of 915 and 2456 MHz. It is rarely used in current clinical practice. Protective eyewear must be worn during its application to minimize the risk for cataract formation. Because of its more rapid heating of tissues with high water content, it should not be used in patients with edema, blisters, or hyperhidrosis.

Short wave and microwave diathermy is not commonly used in clinical practice, partly because there are more contraindications (Box 46.5) than with other heat agents and partly because of the availability and ease of use of other therapeutic heating options.

THERAPEUTIC COLD

Therapeutic cold is another time-tested modality used for pain relief and reduction of edema and muscle spasm. Other effects of cold include reduction of metabolic activity, muscle tone, and spasticity.[32] Evidence that local cooling postoperatively reduces pain is mixed, with reports of a significant reduction in pain scores and opioid use after certain types of orthopedic surgery, but such results have not been demonstrated in other studies. There is no good-quality evidence that local cooling is effective in the treatment of low back pain.[28] The rationale for using cold is similar to that for using therapeutic heat—as an adjunctive treatment to physical therapy and exercise.

Therapeutic cold can be delivered by means such as ice packs and slushes, iced whirlpools, ice rubs, chemical ice packs, and evaporative cooling sprays. The same general precautions for therapeutic heat should be used during therapeutic cold treatments to avoid thermal injury. Contraindications to therapeutic cold are listed in Box 46.6.

CONTRAST BATHS

Contrast baths are a combination of therapeutic heat and cold and are generally used for the treatment of complex regional pain syndrome and sympathetically mediated pain syndromes. One method is to immerse the limb or body part in a warm bath at a temperature of 38° C to 43° C for about 6 minutes, transfer the limb to a cold bath at 13° C to 18° C for about 4 minutes, and then transfer the body part back to the warm bath. This cycle is then repeated several times.[36]

Box 46.5 Contraindications to Short Wave and Microwave Diathermy

- Contraindications to therapeutic heat
- Near metallic implants
- Over a pregnant uterus
- Implanted pacemaker

Box 46.6 Contraindications to Therapeutic Cold

- Insensate skin
- Ischemia
- Peripheral vascular diseases
- Raynaud's phenomenon
- Cold insensitivity
- Cold urticaria
- Cryoglobulinemia
- Paroxysmal cold hemoglobinuria

TRANSCUTANEOUS ELECTRICAL NERVE STIMULATION

TENS involves the application of electrical stimulation across the skin to the peripheral nerves. Many acute and chronic pain syndromes have been treated with TENS because of its ease of use and relatively low side effects.[28,37-39] There is evidence that high-intensity TENS can reduce postoperative analgesic requirements and improve pain relief after inguinal herniorrhaphy, laparoscopic tubal ligation, and thoracotomy, and it has been found to be of value in the treatment of primary dysmenorrhea.[28] However, there is insufficient evidence to support the use of TENS for various musculoskeletal conditions such as acute shoulder pain, acute neck pain, and low back pain.[29] Based on the gate theory of pain, TENS is thought to block or modulate pain transmission in C fibers through stimulation of large myelinated A fibers. Research has indicated that there are probably more complex mechanisms to explain its clinical effect.[40]

Currently, many different types of TENS units are available, which allows a variety of settings and modes of application. The different TENS modes include conventional narrow pulse duration, high pulse rate, low frequency, burst, modulation, and hyperstimulation.[37] Use of conventional TENS results in a comfortable electrical paresthesia, whereas low-frequency modes result in rhythmic muscle contractions. There are many different protocols for the placement of electrodes and TENS settings. The efficacy of TENS can be optimized by an individualized approach to parameter settings and electrode placement. When the unit and electrodes are used appropriately, side effects are minimal. Contraindications to the use of TENS are listed in Box 46.7.

IONTOPHORESIS

Iontophoresis is the use of direct electrical current to drive electrically charged molecules actively, such as those in medications, across the skin and into the underlying tissue. It functions more as a drug delivery system than as a therapeutic modality. The most popular agents transported are local anesthetics such as lidocaine, steroids, and nonsteroidal anti-inflammatory drugs. Iontophoresis is generally well tolerated, and few complications have been reported.

Box 46.7 Contraindications to Transcutaneous Electrical Nerve Stimulation

- Demand-type cardiac pacemakers
- Pregnancy
- Over the carotid sinus or eyes
- Across the chest

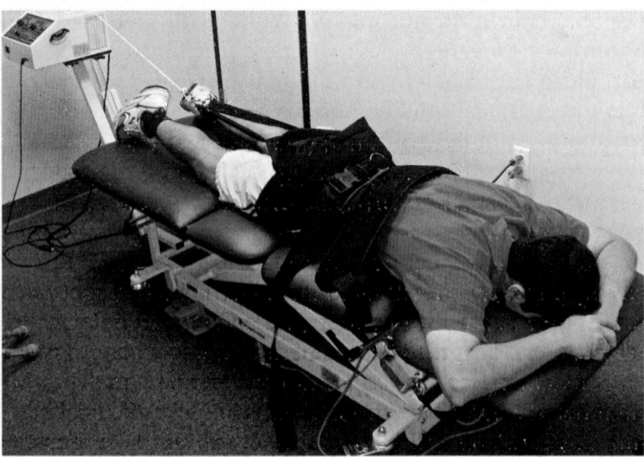

Figure 46.3 Lumbar traction.

Box 46.8 Contraindications to Traction

General Traction

Osteomyelitis or diskitis
Osteoporosis
Spinal cord compression
Malignancy
Unstable fracture
Uncontrolled hypertension
Severe cardiovascular disease

Cervical Traction

Central disk herniation
Hypermobility
Rheumatoid arthritis
Carotid or vertebral artery disease
Temporomandibular joint dysfunction (with a chin strap)

Lumbar Traction

Pregnancy
Hemorrhoids and intra-abdominal conditions that may be affected by increased intra-abdominal pressure
Cauda equina syndrome

TRACTION

Traction is the application of forces in direct opposition to each other to produce a separation of two body parts or stretching of soft tissues. In the area of spine care, traction is commonly used to treat cervical and lumbar pain. Despite a seemingly endless variety of traction techniques and treatment protocols, most types of traction are applied by a therapist (manual traction), by machine (mechanical traction), or by weight (gravitational traction) in a sustained or intermittent manner.[41]

Traction has been prescribed to treat various spinal disorders, including radiculopathy, disk herniation, disk degeneration, foraminal stenosis, and nonspecific low back pain (Fig. 46.3). Research in this area has been confounded by the multiple types of traction techniques and treatment protocols and by methodologic flaws.[41-46] The benefits of traction for neck and back pain may be mediated through anatomic changes such as diminution of disk protrusion, reduction of disk pressure, widening of disk spaces and intervertebral foramina, reduction of pressure on exiting nerve roots, stretching or separation of joints and ligaments, and relaxation of muscle spasm.[47]

Contraindications to the use of traction are listed in Box 46.8. Cervical traction should be avoided in patients with rheumatoid arthritis and significant vertebral or carotid artery disease. Lumbar traction should be done cautiously, if at all, in patients who are pregnant or have abdominal conditions that may be worsened by increased intra-abdominal pressure. Inversion lumbar traction can increase systolic and diastolic blood pressure and increase oxygen uptake; it should be avoided in patients with cardiac or pulmonary insufficiency.[48] Despite controversy about its physical and physiologic effects and benefits, it continues to be part of the treatment armamentarium for spinal pain.

MANUAL TECHNIQUES

Manual medicine refers to hands-on therapy and includes gentle joint stretching or mobilization to improve joint mobility and muscle dysfunction in the spine or adjacent structures based on the concept that joint restriction contributes to pain.[49] Integral to the skills of ancient surgeons and physicians from Greece to China, manipulation and mobilization are still practiced after thousands of years, not just by chiropractors and medically trained practitioners but as part of folk practice in many parts of the world. Hippocrates (460-355 BC) was the first in recorded history to describe and illustrate joint manipulation and traction techniques.[50]

There is debate on the long-lasting effects of manual techniques, but few can argue that there is at least subjective short-term relief of neck and low back symptoms. Guidelines of the Agency for Health Care Policy and Research include manipulation as an effective strategy for the initial treatment of acute low back pain.[51] Studies by Bronfort and Van Tulder and colleagues[52,53] have suggested that manual therapy is effective for the treatment of acute and chronic musculoskeletal pain. A randomized controlled trial comparing spinal manipulative therapy with exercise therapy (16 treatments delivered over a 2-month period) found that spinal manipulation significantly decreased pain and increased functioning and return to work at 12 months when compared with exercise therapy.[54] Geisser and associates[55] have shown that patients with chronic low back pain benefit from manual therapy with specific adjuvant exercise.

Many theories have been proposed to explain how manual therapy actually reduces pain. Skyba and coworkers[56] have shown that joint manipulation produces a nonopioid form of analgesia mediated by spinal serotonergic and noradrenergic receptors. DiGiovanna[57] theorized that manual therapy increases circulation via local effects or sympathetic reflex and increases venous and lymphatic drainage, which leads to decreased local swelling and edema. Vernon and colleagues[58] have shown that manual therapy causes a change in the pain threshold secondary to an increase in serum endorphin levels.

Modern manipulative therapy can range from slow oscillating glides to high-velocity, low-amplitude (HVLA) techniques.[59] It has been shown that spinal manipulative therapy reduces pain over the short term (<6 weeks) and long term (>6 weeks) when compared with sham manipulation and improves function over the short term.[60]

TYPES OF MANUAL THERAPY

Biomechanical Model (Osteopathic Approach)

This model can be used in several ways. Using muscle energy, manual medical treatment involves voluntary contraction of the patient's muscle in a precisely controlled direction against a counterforce applied by the operator.[61] Use of strain-counterstrain can help relieve spinal pain by passively placing the joint in its position of greatest comfort.[62]

Manipulation

This is similar to the biomechanical model and is also used by osteopaths and chiropractors. Manipulation refers to a modality in which the practitioner passively, often forcefully, moves (or "thrusts") a bone through its physiologic barrier in an attempt to improve ROM or alignment of a joint. The goal is to improve function and decrease pain. The thrust is an HVLA movement. Use of this HVLA technique is what differentiates manipulation from mobilization.[50] The ROM of a joint during HVLA movement depends on where the restriction lies in the joint's normal ROM.

When performed appropriately and by a trained person, manipulation can usually result in immediate relief of pain. This is thought to be due to a decrease in muscle spasm while increasing ROM and the level of serum endorphins.[57] Contraindications to manipulation include osteoporosis, acute inflammation, infection, vertebral-basilar insufficiency, fracture, or any other cause of structural instability.

Norwegian Approach (Kaltenborn)

The range (hypomobility, hypermobility, or normal mobility) and quality of movement are evaluated by using translatory movement in addition to rotational movement.[63] During treatment, translatory traction and gliding movements rather than rotational movements are preferred to avoid compressing a joint that is already strained by pathology.[64]

Maitland (Australian) Approach

With this approach there is continual (ongoing) assessment and reassessment of the patient and consideration of the pathology and anatomy in relation to the signs and symptoms manifested by the patient. The accessory and physiologic joint movements are tested. Treatment strategies involve the use of mobilization, manipulation, adverse neural tissue mobilization, traction, and exercise based on this continual assessment.[47]

McKenzie Approach

This is a popular approach to patients with back pain that uses pain centralization and decentralization methods to diagnose and treat spinal pathology. The key concept here is that during movements of the spine there is a change in position of the nucleus pulposus and that a flexed lifestyle generally leads to a more posterior position of the nucleus. The treatment involves having the patient use repeated movements to treat the spinal pathology (Fig. 46.4).

Myofascial Release

This type of soft tissue treatment stretches the fascial structures of the body along its planes.

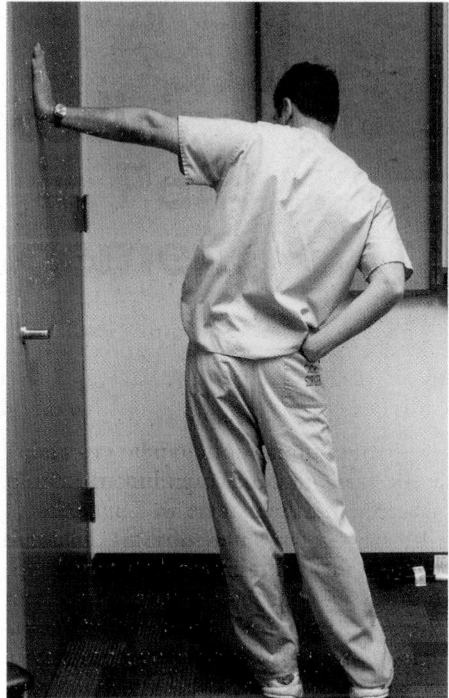

Figure 46.4 McKenzie approach.

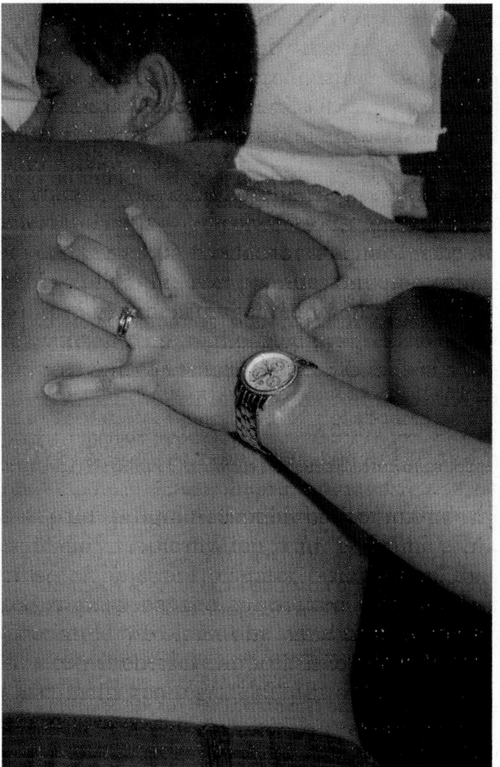

Figure 46.5 Massage.

MASSAGE

Massage is a general term that refers to application of the hands to soft tissues (e.g., skin, muscles, ligaments, tendons) to produce a therapeutic effect (Fig. 46.5). Even though preferred and appreciated by many, massage has little objective research to support its long-term benefit.[65] Massage can be subcategorized as classic massage, sports massage, reflexology, shiatsu, and acupuncture. There are many forms of classic massage, including the following:

1. *Stroking or effleurage.* This is light movement, either superficial or deep, over the skin in a slow, rhythmic fashion.[49]
2. *Kneading and pétrissage.* Pétrissage is the application of firm but gentle pressure in a rhythmic fashion while gently grasping the underlying tissues and lifting and squeezing them. Movement is accomplished by gliding of the hands in a centripetal pattern. Kneading lifts, squeezes, and moves larger amounts of tissue than pétrissage does.[65]
3. *Friction massage.* This is carried out by applying pressure in a slow circular pattern with the fingers or ball of the thumb. It is used primarily to loosen scars or adhesions.
4. *Tapotement.* This technique involves applying light "chops" or "cups" in series as percussive methods.

Sports massage is massage therapy for athletes that focuses on the muscles. A literature review by Callaghan[65] showed subjective reports of benefit, but little agreement on the efficacy of massage has been documented.

Reflexology is a massage system based on a series of points in the hands and feet that are believed to correspond to a reflex pattern in all areas of the body. Treatment consists of compression of the hands or feet by firm pressure applied by the thumbs of the practitioner.[65]

Shiatsu and acupressure are massage techniques that use pressure applied by the practitioner's fingers over predetermined points. These are the same points and meridians used for acupuncture. Shiatsu, on the other hand, is derived from traditional Japanese massage, called *anma*, and has a more anatomic and physiologic basis.[66]

The indications for massage are muscle cramps, stress and tension, contracture of joints, strains and sprains, tendinitis or tenosynovitis, and edema and lymphedema. Contraindications to massage include local malignancy, local infection, calcification of soft tissues, inflammatory arthritis (gout, infective), bursitis, open wounds, bleeding disorders, and entrapment neuropathy.

The theoretical mechanical effects of massage include improved circulation, breakdown of soft tissue adhesions, and activation of the peripheral nervous system. Arterial flow, venous flow, and lymphatic flow are all theoretically improved with massage.[67] Benefits on the peripheral circulation include improvement in local nutrition and removal of waste products.[65] This helps decrease aches in muscles and facilitate healing. Activation of the peripheral nervous system is thought to be beneficial via the gate control theory of Melzack and Wall[68,69] and inhibition of overactive proprioceptors.

ROLE OF EXERCISE

In physiology, we learn that regular exercise may increase strength, muscle bulk, and stamina. Physiologically, exercise does not directly reduce pain, although reports have indicated that the performance of exercise modulates pain by a physiologic mechanism that has not yet been fully elucidated.[70] Reports on the efficacy or benefit of therapies are mixed, but most physicians agree that being more active rather than less active is more beneficial for most pain patients. A recent Cochrane review has shown that performance of strengthening exercises, trunk stabilization, and advice to stay active had more beneficial results than placebo did.[71]

Exercise has systemic and local effects on the body. Systemically, it increases blood flow and cardiac output; locally, it helps increase flexibility of the muscles and mobilize joints. In addition, it also strengthens weak muscles, builds endurance and speed, and establishes balance and coordination.[18] Therapeutic exercise should include not only flexibility and strengthening exercises but also exercises for redeveloping the normal patterns of movement of specific muscle groups.[18]

Physical inactivity, if helpful at all, is helpful only during the acute inflammatory phase of an injury, and activities should be resumed rapidly, unless an obvious risk for structural damage is present.[72]

With sprains and strains of joints and ligaments, the acronym RICE is used—*r*est, *i*ce, *c*ompression, and *e*levation. Kellett[73] has explained that the duration of rest and icing should be 48 to 72 hours, so progressive mobilization within the limits of pain is prescribed. Acute soft tissue injuries should be rested, supported, and iced, and nonpainful early mobilization is probably beneficial.

EXERCISE FOR PATIENTS WITH LOW BACK PAIN

Regarding low back pain, the benefit of rest is debatable, with the current trend being toward shorter periods of rest or none at all. Thirty years ago it was believed that there does need to be a period of rest, ranging from days to longer than a month. Deyo and colleagues[72] noted that there is no advantage to bed rest and that those who do not have complete bed rest have fewer missed days of work and better disability scores. Hagen and associates,[74] in a literature search of musculoskeletal controlled trials, deduced that "bed rest compared to advice to stay active will, at best, have small effects, and at worst might have harmful effects on acute low back pain."

In patients with back pain it has been shown that both stretching and strengthening exercises are important. Khalil and colleagues[75] studied patients with myofascial low back pain and noted that stretching plus a multimodality rehabilitation program versus only a rehabilitation program improves measures of muscle function and significantly decreases pain in 2 weeks. Takemasa and associates[76] have shown that strengthening exercises not only improve strength but also reduce pain. Several studies have shown that exercises, whether flexion based (Fig. 46.6) or extension

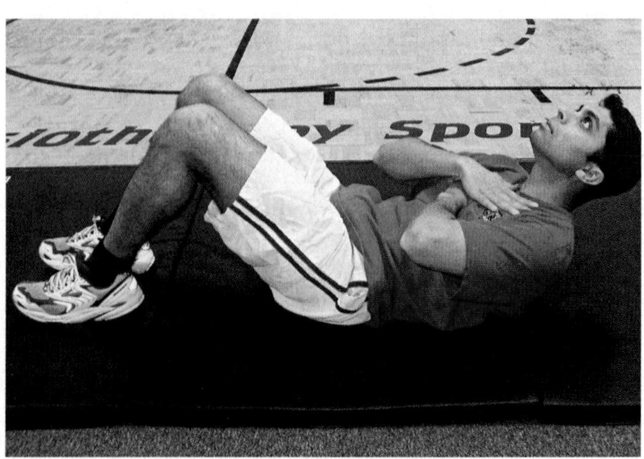

Figure 46.6 Abdominal curls.

based (Fig. 46.7), improve back pain more than treatment with only modalities does.[77,78]

It is important to understand that in chronic pain patients, physical therapy alone will not completely eradicate the pain. Physical therapy and exercise, however, can decrease the musculoskeletal sequelae of chronic pain. Exercise can improve the patient's tolerance of functional activity by increasing flexibility, strengthening weaker muscles, and improving aerobic endurance.

TYPES OF EXERCISES

There are three main types of therapeutic exercises—stretching, strengthening, and endurance activities. Strengthening exercises involve the application of weights or resistance to a muscle group during several repetitions at maximal effort to increase the force of the muscle. Stretching involves sustained static lengthening of a muscle to increase the flexibility of that specific muscle. Figure 46.8 demonstrates stretching exercises. Endurance exercises involve the application of repeated movements with low resistance to large locomotive muscle groups to increase cardiopulmonary stamina.

There are three types of strengthening exercises. Isometric exercises involve exertion of force against a fixed object or a muscle contraction that holds an object in one position. Isotonic exercises involve exertion of force against weight that moves it through a specific ROM (e.g., handheld weights). Isokinetic exercises entail exertion of force against an object that moves it at a fixed velocity. Table 46.2 lists the indications and precautions for these types of exercises.[8] Table 46.3 summarizes some useful exercises and assistive devices for various painful medical and surgical diagnoses.[9]

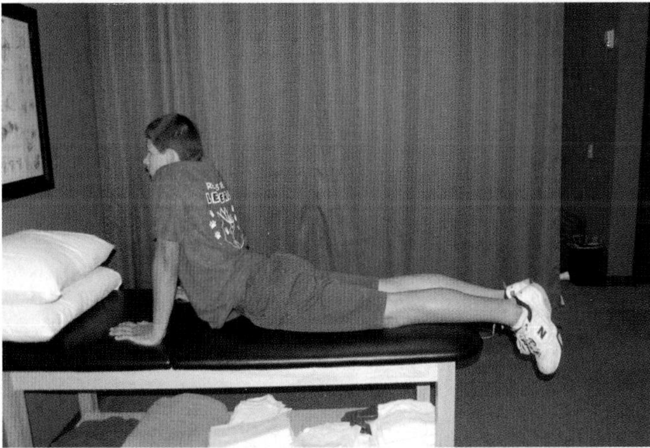

Figure 46.7 Prone press-ups.

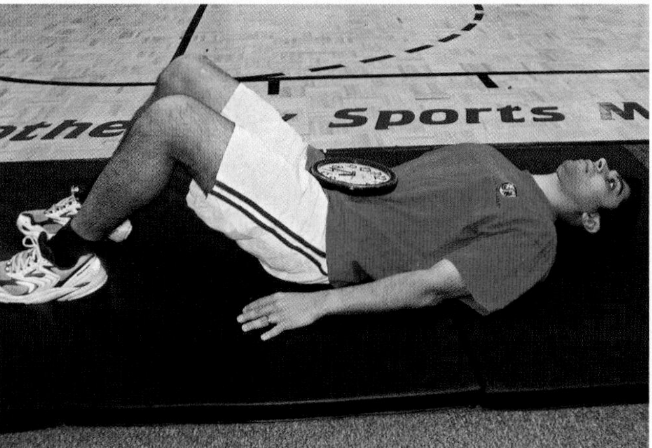

Figure 46.8 Pelvic rock.

PRECAUTIONS AND CONTRAINDICATIONS

Patients with unstable medical and surgical conditions, including unhealed fractures, unstable angina, and uncompensated

Table 46.2 Indications and Precautions for Different Types of Exercise

Exercise	Indication	Precautions
Isometric	Range of motion over a joint not desired because of fracture or painful arthritis	Evaluation of blood pressure with sustained contraction; strengthens muscle only at that length
Isotonic	Low-weight strengthening, intense weight training for competitive body building	Weak person may incur tendon injury; only to be done with a spotter because may cause severe injury if done improperly
Isokinetic	Strengthening with the arc and velocity of motion controlled; more suitable for a noncompetitive weight trainer	May raise systolic blood pressure mostly at maximal torque; requires access to a facility with machines

Table 46.3 Useful Exercises and Assistive Devices for Different Disease Entities

Diagnosis	Exercises to Consider
Reflex sympathetic dystrophy	Edema control Gentle desensitization Assisted range of motion Prevention of secondary contracture
Facet arthropathy	Sustained hamstring stretches Pelvic tilts (abdominal and gluteal strengthening) Lumbar stabilization Posture monitoring Back conservation techniques
Hip arthritis	Cane to unweight the limb Hip extension and abduction
Knee arthritis	Cane use Joint conservation techniques (e.g., straight-leg raises and short-range quadriceps contractions)
Spondylolisthesis	Core strengthening Bracing in flexion
Osteoporosis	Cane use in extension Cane use with extreme pain Thoracic extension exercises Low-impact weight-bearing activity

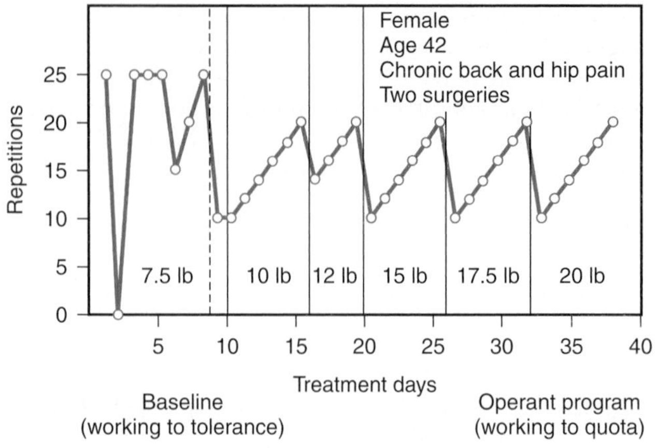

Figure 46.9 Behavior modification approach to exercise.

cardiac, pulmonary, hypertensive, and thrombotic disorders, should not participate in strengthening, endurance, or flexibility exercises.

Precautions for resistive exercises include cardiovascular factors, overwork, osteoporosis, and immediate muscle soreness associated with exercise. A specific complication of isometric exercise is the potential for a significant increase in blood pressure.[79]

BEHAVIORAL MODIFICATION APPROACH TO EXERCISE

We suggest that physical medicine techniques performed in conjunction or along with a behavioral modification approach should produce a better outcome, especially in patients with chronic pain. Figure 46.9 graphically depicts the use of exercise within a behavioral concept.[9]

Appropriate exercises specific for the painful area and general conditioning exercises such as bicycling, walking, or swimming are usually indicated. Fordyce[80] has noted that appropriate exercise in a behavior modification program must be relevant to the patient's pain and limitations, as well as being quantifiable, visible, and accessible. The patient's baseline exercise level is determined by asking the patient to exercise to tolerance (until pain, weakness, or fatigue necessitates stopping) over a few days.[9] Once the patient's baseline has been established, the initial goal of exercise is set within the patient's tolerance and then gradually increased, with new goals being set every few days.[9] Rewards and reinforcement are given when established goals are accomplished without demonstration of pain behavior.[81] In some patients, however, it is necessary to reduce excessive activity levels by teaching them to pace themselves more appropriately.[9]

This concept makes sense because among the treatment goals of pain management are a decrease in illness behavior (reduced drug use and visits to physicians) and an increase in well behavior (increased physical activities and mobility and return to gainful employment).[82] This may be accomplished by blocking noxious sensory input, decreasing tension and depression, rearranging reinforcement contingencies, or assisting in the learning of new behavior.[83] Biofeedback, cognitive-behavioral modification, operant approaches, hypnosis, operant pain hypnosis, and relaxation techniques can assist in the treatment of chronic pain behavior.[84-87]

CONCLUSION

In this chapter we discussed the physical medicine techniques used for treating pain. We presented the concept that although there are a number of approaches to the treatment of patients with pain, a multidisciplinary or interdisciplinary approach is recommended as the symptom becomes more chronic. Additionally, the treatment modalities used should be more successful if carried out within a behavioral modification approach.

Before treatment is undertaken, a comprehensive evaluation is necessary, including assessment of function and setting of treatment goals that need to be delineated and agreed on by all involved in the treatment program. Physical modalities, manual techniques, and exercise can modify pain symptoms but will probably not cure them, especially in patients with chronic pain. The appropriate use of medications, injections, and psychosocial intervention, in conjunction with physical medicine techniques, is often required to achieve the maximum outcome.

KEY POINTS

- All physicians need to understand the rationale, indications, contraindications, and prescription of physical medicine techniques and their appropriate use. Many of these techniques can be used for acute, subacute, and chronic pain. However, with progression to more chronic pain, techniques should be more active and less passive and more behavioral and cognitive in nature. Although many of these techniques will help decrease pain, the long-term goal should be to increase function despite the presence of the pain syndrome.
- Patients with pain can be evaluated and treated by individual physicians and therapists. This type of approach is more often used and successful in patients with acute or subacute pain. However, as the pain becomes more chronic, a multidisciplinary or interdisciplinary approach is recommended.
- The role of the therapy team in a pain program should be comprehensive and interdisciplinary. Typically, the team is led by a physician and consists of physical therapists, occupational therapists, and often recreational therapists, dieticians, and psychologists.[7] Combined assessment by these professionals is used to devise a comprehensive approach to allow the patient to benefit maximally, reintegrate fully into life, and have as few restrictions as possible.
- Patients with acute or chronic pain may be referred for physical medicine evaluation and treatment as a component of a multidisciplinary management approach or for certain specific treatments.
- Electrodiagnostic testing encompasses nerve conduction studies and electromyography, which provide information about the peripheral nerves and muscles, and evoked potentials, which is used mainly to assess the central nervous system. Electrodiagnosis can play an important role in identifying an underlying problem

KEY POINTS—cont'd

in a patient with a pain disorder. Electrodiagnostic testing helps not only in diagnosis but also in determining the chronicity and severity of the condition and can even assist in prognosis.

- Pain commonly limits participation in a physical therapy or rehabilitation program. Adequate pain management is an important component of rehabilitation.
- Physical modalities and techniques commonly used to relieve pain include therapeutic heat and cold, hydrotherapy, ultrasound, electricity, and traction. They are best used as adjunctive treatments to an active exercise program.
- Manual medicine refers to hands-on therapy and includes gentle joint stretching or mobilization to improve joint mobility and muscle dysfunction in the spine or adjacent structures based on the concept that joint restriction contributes to pain.
- Various types of manual therapy exist: the biomechanical model, manipulation, the Norwegian approach, the Maitland approach, the McKenzie approach, and myofascial release.
- Massage is a general term that refers to application of the hands to soft tissues (e.g., skin, muscles, ligaments, tendons) to produce a therapeutic effect. Massage can be subcategorized as classic massage, sports massage, reflexology, shiatsu, and acupuncture.
- In physiology, we learn that regular exercise may increase strength, muscle bulk, and stamina. Reports on the efficacy or benefit of therapies are mixed, but most physicians agree that being more active rather than less active is more beneficial for most pain patients.
- There are three main types of therapeutic exercises—stretching, strengthening, and endurance activities. Strengthening exercises involve the application of weights or resistance to a muscle group during several repetitions at maximal effort to increase the force of the muscle. Stretching involves sustained static lengthening of a muscle to increase the flexibility of that specific muscle.
- We suggest that physical medicine techniques performed in conjunction or along with a behavioral modification approach should produce a better outcome, especially in patients with chronic pain.

SUGGESTED READINGS

Aure OF, Nilsen JH, Vasseljen O. Manual therapy and exercise therapy in patients with chronic low back pain: a randomised, controlled trial with 1-year follow-up. *Spine.* 2003;28:525-532.

Australian Acute Musculoskeletal Pain Guidelines Group. *Evidence-Based Management of Acute Musculoskeletal Pain.* Brisbane: NHMRC Australian Academic Press; 2003.

Bloodworth D, Calvillo O, Smith K, et al. Chronic pain syndromes: evaluation and treatment. In: Braddom RL, ed. *Physical Medicine and Rehabilitation.* 2nd ed. Philadelphia: Saunders; 2000:913-933.

Callaghan MJ. The role of massage in the management of the athlete: a review. *Br J Sports Med.* 1993;27:28-33.

Clarke J, van Tulder M, Blomberg S, et al. Traction for low back pain with or without sciatica: an updated systematic review within the framework of the Cochrane collaboration. *Spine.* 2006;31:1591-1599.

Gatchel RJ, Turk DC. *Psychological Approaches to Pain Management: A Practitioner's Guide.* New York: Guilford Press; 1998.

Geisser M, Wiggert E, Haig A, et al. A randomized, controlled trial of manual therapy and specific adjuvant exercise for chronic low back pain. *Clin J Pain.* 2005;21:463-470.

Grabois M. Comprehensive evaluation and management of patients with chronic pain. *Cardiovasc Res Center Bull.* 1981;19:113-117.

Greenman PE. *Principles of Manual Medicine.* 2nd ed. Baltimore: Williams & Wilkins; 1996.

Hagen KB, Hilde G, Jamtvedt G, et al. Bed rest for acute low back pain and sciatica. *Cochrane Database Syst Rev.* 2000;2:CD001254.

Haig AJ, Tong HC, Yamakawa KS, et al. Predictors of pain and function in persons with spinal stenosis, low back pain, and no back pain. *Spine.* 2006;31:2950-2957.

Haldeman S. Manipulation and massage for the relief of pain. In: Melzack R, Wall PD, eds. *Textbook of Pain.* 2nd ed. New York: Churchill Livingstone; 1989:942-951.

Linchitz RM, Sorell PJ. Physical methods of pain management. In: Raj PP, ed. *Practical Management of Pain.* 3rd ed. St. Louis: Mosby; 2000:529-543.

Melzack R. The gate control theory 25 years later: new perspectives in phantom limb pain. In: Bond MR, Charlton JE, Woolf CJ, eds. *Proceedings of the Sixth World Congress on Pain.* Amsterdam: Elsevier; 1991:9-21.

Nussbaum EL, Behrens BJ. Therapeutic ultrasound. In: Behrens BJ, Michlovitz SL, eds. *Physical Agents: Theory and Practice.* 2nd ed. Philadelphia: Davis; 2006:57-79.

Pransky GS, Dempsey PG. Practical aspects of functional capacity evaluations. *J Occup Rehabil.* 2004;14:217-229.

Rutkove SB, Lichtensteni SH. Role of electrodiagnostics in pain assessment. In: Warfield CA, Bajwa ZH, eds. *Principles and Practice of Pain Medicine.* Philadelphia: McGraw-Hill; 2004:112-120.

Schonstein E, Kenny DT, Keating J, et al. Work conditioning, work hardening and functional restoration for workers with back and neck pain. *Cochrane Database Syst Rev.* 2003;3:CD001822.

Sluka KA, Walsh D. Transcutaneous electrical nerve stimulation: basic science mechanisms and clinical effectiveness. *J Pain.* 2003;4:109-121.

Stanos SP, Tyburski MD, Harden RN. Management of chronic pain. In: Braddom RL, ed. *Physical Medicine and Rehabilitation.* 3rd ed. Philadelphia: Saunders; 2006:951-988.

The references for this chapter can be found at www.expertconsult.com

47 Physical Rehabilitation for Patients with Chronic Pain

Harriët Wittink | Jeanine A. Verbunt

Ideally, patients with pain-related disability resulting from chronic pain are treated by a team of health professionals, commonly consisting of physicians, psychologists, physical and occupational therapists, social workers and nurses, to address the biopsychosocial nature of pain. Within the interdisciplinary team, the physical therapist is responsible for a comprehensive assessment with emphasis on the musculoskeletal system, including assessment of impairments, limitations in activities, restrictions in participation, environmental and personal factors that may influence physical functioning, as well as the management of the physical rehabilitation process. Physical therapists are thus intimately involved in pain management and, where possible, pain treatment.

Patients come to our clinics with certain expectations of evaluation and treatment. One study investigated the expectations of patients with chronic pain of their first outpatient visit to a pain management program.[1] In that study, most patients expected an explanation or an improved understanding of their pain problem. The most common satisfying outcome was relief or control of pain and the most common disappointing outcome was being told nothing could be done. The majority of patients expected further medical investigations and changes to the prescribed medication. There was no mention of patients expecting a referral for pain management, and only a small percentage of patients wanted advice on coping with pain, or self-management of pain. Although this study needs to be duplicated in other centers, it has a great deal of face validity. Many patients with chronic pain resist referral to physical rehabilitation. Part of the difficulty lies in the history of treatment failures with which patients often present. A number of factors may be responsible for past treatment failures, including persistent failure of physical therapists to recognize and treat the differences between acute and chronic pain states, past treatment that did not address the emotional and cognitive aspects of chronic pain, and an inability of the patient to recognize anything less than total pain relief as success.[2] It is therefore important to identify patient expectations at the initial visit to prevent disappointment with referrals to physical rehabilitation for pain management.

PHYSICAL THERAPY EVALUATION

In evidence-based practice, clinical decisions must include consideration of, first, the patient's clinical and physical circumstances to establish what is "wrong" and what treatment options are available to address this problem. Second, the latter need to be tempered by research evidence concerning the efficacy, effectiveness, and efficiency of the treatment options. Third, given the likely consequences associated with each option, the clinician must consider the patient's preferences and likely actions (in terms of what interventions she or he is ready and able to accept). Clinical expertise is needed to bring these considerations together and recommend a treatment that the patient agrees to accept.[3] Accordingly, the purposes of a physical therapy evaluation are to establish a baseline from which to plan and begin interventions, assist in the selection of appropriate interventions, and evaluate the efficacy of interventions.

As described in the biopsychosocial model of pain introduced by Fordyce, contributing factors to disability can be biologic, psychological, as well as social.[4] Essential in this model is the idea that factors maintaining the pain problem are not necessarily the same as those initiating pain. To establish a baseline, therefore, a thorough inventory of all factors contributing to a patient's perceived level of disability is important. The International Classification of Functioning, Disability and Health (ICF) provides a biopsychosocial model that identifies three concepts described from the perspective of body systems, the individual, and society. Within the context of health, the ICF defined *bodily functions and structures* as physiologic functions of body systems or anatomic elements, such as organs, limbs, and their components. *Activity* is defined as the execution of specific tasks or actions by an individual, whereas *participation* is envisioned as encompassing involvement in a life situation. In the ICF, *functioning* refers to all body functions, activities, and participation. *Disability* is the ICF umbrella term for impairment, activity limitation, and participation restrictions. Contextual factors are provided within the ICF framework (Fig. 47.1), consisting of external environmental factors (such as significant others, employers, medications, and health care providers) and personal factors (such as age, education, income, worry that activity will exacerbate pain or injury resulting in avoidance of activity to prevent anticipated negative consequences).

Qualifiers for the Activities and Participation classification make it possible to clearly separate the patient's inherent capacity to perform actions within a domain and performance in his or her actual environmental context.[5] *Capacity* refers to the environmentally adjusted inherent ability of the individual or, in other words, the highest probable functioning of a person in a given domain at a given point in time, in a standardized environment. Capacity can be measured by physical tests or by questionnaires that ask, "Can you?" Performance describes what a person actually does in her or his current environment and thus describes

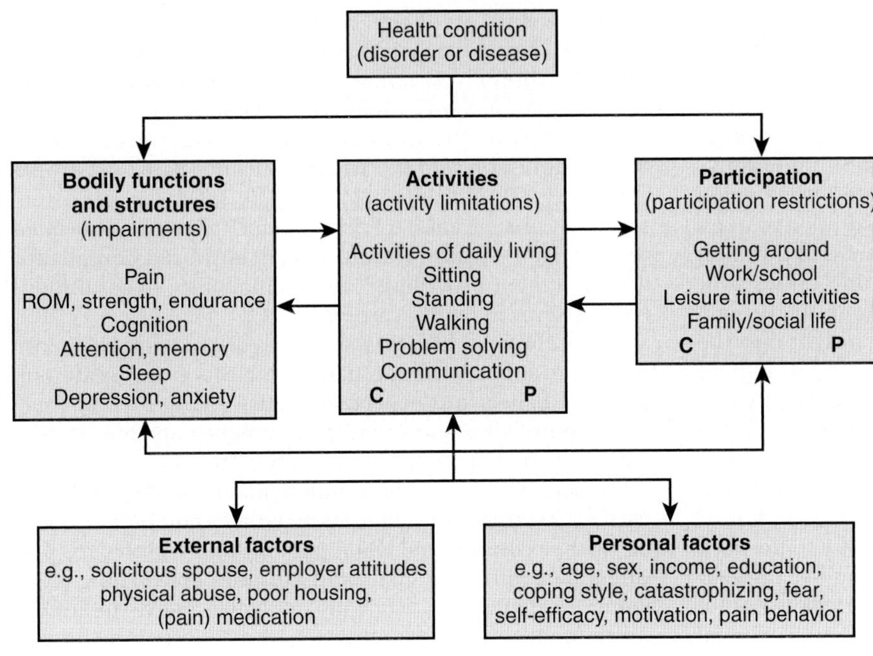

Figure 47.1 Example of International Classification of Functioning, Disability, and Health (ICF) framework. C, capacity; P, performance; ROM, range of motion. (Adapted from Ustun TB, Chatterji S, Bickenbach J, et al: The International Classification of Functioning, Disability and Health: a new tool for understanding disability and health. *Disabil Rehabil.* 2003;25:565-571.)

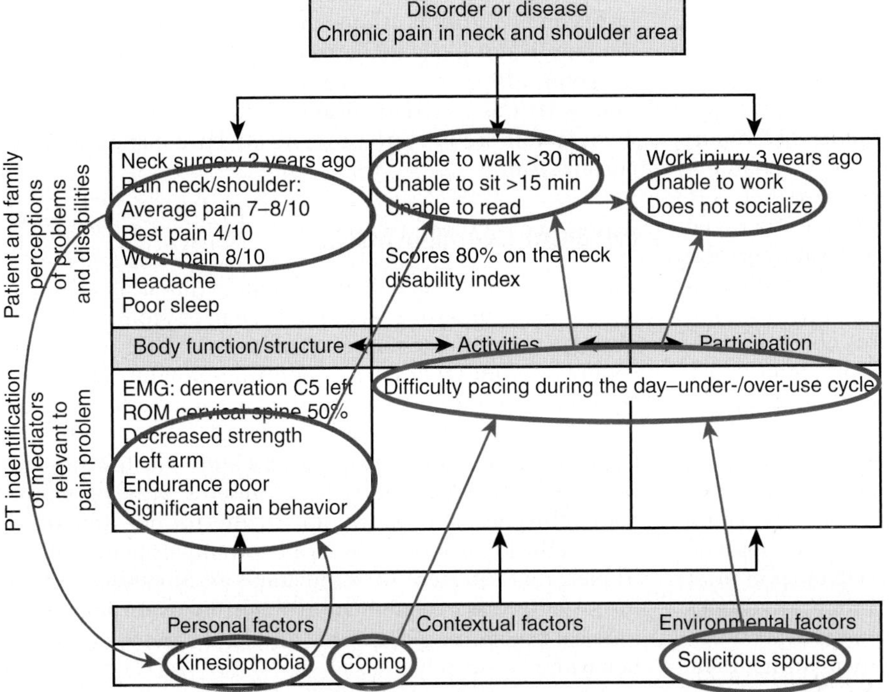

Figure 47.2 Rehabilitation Problem-Solving (RPS) form used for a patient with chronic neck and shoulder pain. EMG, electromyelogram; PT, physical therapist; ROM, range of motion. (Adapted from Steiner WA, Ryser L, Huber E, et al: Use of the ICF model as a clinical problem-solving tool in physical therapy and rehabilitation medicine. *Phys Ther.* 2002;82:1098-1107.)

the person's functioning as observed or reported in the person's real-life environment with the existing facilitators and barriers.[6] Performance can be measured by direct observation. As this is often highly impractical, self-report measures can be substituted that ask, "Do you?"

The Rehabilitation Problem Solving (RPS) form is based on the ICF[7] and is a practical tool to use to visualize the patient's state of functioning and disability. The form is used to specify precise and relevant target problems, discern factors that cause or contribute to these problems, and plan the most appropriate intervention. In addition, the form was designed as a tool to facilitate both intra- and interprofessional communications and improve the communication between health care professionals and their patients.[7] The form is divided into three parts: (1) the header provides basic information, (2) the upper part is used to describe the patient's perspective, and (3) the lower part is used for the analysis of the health care professionals.

The form can visualize the current understanding of the patient's state of activities and participation, his or her target problems, and how the health care team relates them to hypothetical mediators and contextual factors (Fig. 47.2).

From the information obtained through carefully selected questionnaires, an interview, the physical examination, and physical tests, most of the information needed to develop an appropriate treatment plan should be obtained.

PATIENT INTERVIEW

The Joint Commission on Accreditation of Health Care Organizations requires that all patients have the right to an adequate pain assessment, including documentation of pain location, intensity, quality, onset/duration/variations/rhythms, manner of expressing pain, pain relief, what makes it worse, effects of pain, and a pain plan. In addition to questions about the location, intensity, frequency, and duration of pain, questions such as "What do you think causes your pain?" and "What is the worst thing you think might happen to you because of your pain?" will give insight into the patient's belief system—especially important if the patient comes from a different culture—and the presence of catastrophizing. In addition, physical therapists focus on determining how much the pain interferes with activities and participation: activities of daily living such as housework, grocery shopping, and getting around in the community; recreational and social activities; and the ability to do work and sleep. The number of hours lying down and changes in the level of activity because of pain during a day is noted. Patients are further asked about significant others, partners, parents, and children; do they help out, ignore the patient, or prevent the patient from doing things as they fear the patient might "harm" him- or herself.

Unfortunately there are no perfect measures of physical activity or activity limitations. Comparison measures include both "subjective" measures (based on self-report) and "objective" measures (based on direct measurement). Self-report measures can be self-administered or interviewer administered, both in person or on the telephone. However, self-report of physical activity can reflect a difference between how active patients really are and how active they perceive they are, resulting in a difference between self-reported physical activity level and the actually observed active behavior.[9] Studies including both self-report and objective measures on activity and activity-related disability indicated a gap between self-report and objective measurement.[10]

In rehabilitation practice, there is a tendency to use objective as well as self-report measures to assess physical activity. Objective measures include functional capacity tasks, markers of movement (accelerometers or activity monitors), and observed or videotaped activity (direct observation).[11] Self-reported status often involves outcomes of most relevance and importance to patients and their loved ones because they capture patient experience and perspective.[12] Therapists should be aware of these differences during their assessment. In addition to assessing a patient's level of activity, labeling a patient's activity-related behavior style seems of additional value when choosing the most appropriate ingredients for treatment: Will this patient avoid activities because of pain (avoider), or will he or she persist in the performance of activities regardless of pain (persister)?[13]

Psychosocial factors have been found to have a significant impact on perceived disability, particularly among persons with chronic pain. The physical therapist's observations of a patient's behavior during the interview or functional testing as a part of a screening procedure can deliver valuable information and should be communicated clearly to the rest of the team, which can then direct appropriate psychological and psychiatric treatment. Psychological screening by means of history taking has been shown to have low sensitivity and predictive value for identifying distressed patients. Thus, formal screening of some sort, such as with a questionnaire, is recommended.[14] Psychosocial factors contributing to a patient's disability level that can be assessed by a questionnaire are, for instance, fear of movement (Tampa Scale of Kinesiophobia),[15] catastrophizing (Pain Catastrophizing Scale),[16] and depression (the Beck Depression Inventory).[17] Consideration of the patient's views is associated with greater satisfaction with care,[18] improved compliance with treatment programs,[19] and maintenance of continuous relationships in health care.[20]

As previously mentioned, particularly important are questions about what the patient expects from treatment. Patients' beliefs and expectations play a large role in treatment compliance and eventual treatment outcome. Studies have shown that high patient expectations may positively influence clinical outcome independent of the treatment itself.[21] Treatment of chronic pain is often complex and may be further complicated when patients and health care providers have differing goals and attitudes concerning treatment. Difficulties in engaging in collaborative treatment decision making may result. A negative expectation on treatment outcome can influence treatment compliance. For instance, a patient, who is looking for pain relief only and insists on medication management as the sole treatment for the pain is not likely going to comply with a rehabilitation program. Efforts to enhance patient-provider communication as well as to systematically examine nonspecific treatment factors are likely to promote effective management of chronic pain.[22]

PHYSICAL EXAMINATION

The traditional rehabilitation-oriented physical examination assesses impairments in joint range of motion (ROM), strength, neurologic integrity, and gait. Diagnostic procedures should focus on identifying potentially serious "red flag" conditions that require prompt medical evaluation. The main objective is to determine whether there is a relationship between pain reports and objective physical findings or whether the patient presents with intractable pain (chronic pain syndrome). In the former, rehabilitation might focus more specifically on impairments related to pain that interfere with the ability to function, whereas in the latter case rehabilitation might focus on improving physical functioning in general and have a more significant behavioral approach.

Patient anxiety may complicate the physical examination. Catastrophic cognitions, behavioral displays of pain, and somatic sensations measured during examination have been shown to uniquely predict anxiety experienced during examination.[23] Muscle guarding and pain behaviors are often displayed during physical examination and include moaning, sighing, rubbing, reluctance to perform any active movement (ROM), and the presence of giveaway weakness and nonphysiologic signs. Waddell's[24] nonphysiologic or behavioral signs in patients with back pain can be assessed through palpation and simulation tests including axial loading (pressure applied to the top of the patient's head), simulated rotation (moving shoulders and hips together so that no rotation occurs in the trunk), inconsistency between the straight leg raise in a sitting versus supine position, giveaway weakness with resisted muscle testing, and regional sensory change. One study examined the cross-sectional construct validity of the Waddell score and found evidence that it measures a combination of pain intensity, illness behavior, physical dysfunction, and psychological functioning. However, the associations with the different domains were, in general, weak, which underscores the complexity of illness behavior as measured with the Waddell score.[25]

Recognizing that studies in patients with chronic pain have identified discrepancies between self-report of physical activity and actual level of physical activity, capacity testing is performed in addition to traditional impairment examination. This involves direct observation of patient performance on specific tasks and assessment of whether the patient is willing to move or fears performing specific tasks. Baseline functional ability assessment can provide objectively verifiable information about a patient's quality of life and ability to participate in normal life activities.

Functional tests can be used to focus on performance in basic daily life activities, such as walking, stair climbing, and lifting. Various specific tasks or sets of tests that intend to represent daily functioning are available for this purpose. Simple tasks such as 5-minute walking, 50-foot walking, sit-to-stand, 1 minute stair climbing, loaded forward reach, or various lifting tasks are available to test a patient's capacity during one specific activity. However, the ability of the tests to reflect the level of functioning in patients with pain have to be taken with caution. The test-retest reliability[26] and responsiveness[27] appeared to be only moderate for most of the tests. In addition to single tests, test batteries have been introduced to represent functioning in patients with pain. For example, the Back Performance Scale is a condition-specific performance measure of activity limitation in patients with back pain and includes five tests of daily activities requiring mobility of the trunk: sock test, pickup test, rollup test, fingertip-to-floor test, and lift test. The psychometric properties of this test battery have been demonstrated.[28,29] A second example of a test battery is a generic test battery that includes nine physical performance tests: the time taken to complete various tasks (e.g., picking up coins, tying a belt, reaching up, putting on a sock, standing from sitting, a 50-foot fast walk, a 50-foot walk at preferred speed), the distance walked in 6 minutes, and the distance reached forward while standing. The reliability and discriminant ability of this battery have been confirmed.[30]

In the assessment of work-related performance, a functional capacity evaluation (FCE) is often used.[31] An FCE is an evaluation of capacity of activities that is used to make recommendations for participation in work while considering the person's body functions and structures, environmental factors, personal factors, and health status.[32] The purpose of an FCE is to test a person's physical abilities to the maximum in order to produce objective documentation regarding work and activities of daily life. The FCE has become part of the accepted practice in work injury prevention and rehabilitation.[33] During an FCE, the patient has to complete a standard protocol of physical tasks while a trained observer records the capacity and limitations. Assessment includes ability to lift weights from floor to waist and from waist to overhead, carry, crawl, squat, sit, stand, walk, climb stairs, and push and pull weights. Aerobic capacity may be determined from a maximal bicycle or treadmill test. Additional specific tests may be performed, such as those used to evaluate fine motor skills for the hands and handgrip strength. Practical data on the use of FCEs to determine an individual's physical capacities have been available since the early 2000s and normative data have now been established.[34] Biopsychosocial factors may influence FCE test results, although it is not quite clear to what extent and which factors are important. A systematic review concluded that there is conflicting evidence for the influence of psychological factors and absence of evidence for the influence of social and biologic/physiologic factors in patients with nonspecific chronic low back pain (CLBP) that influence capacity test results.[35] Interpretation of FCE test results is therefore not fully objective because the observer has to decide if a patient performed maximally or submaximally during the test.

A number of studies have shown that self-report and performance and capacity tests, although related, appear to tap into different aspects of the physical functioning domain.[36] For instance, patients with CLBP showed considerable differences in limitations when comparing self-report, clinical examination, and functional testing for assessing work-related limitations. Professional health care workers should be aware of these differences when using them in daily practice.[37,38]

THERAPY FOR CHRONIC PAIN

An important difference between patients with acute pain and those with chronic pain is the variation in relationships between pain, activity limitations, and participation restrictions. For patients with acute pain, nociception, perceived pain, activity limitations, and participation restrictions often have a close relationship. Therefore, treatment in the acute phase focuses on eliminating the causal factor of the pain, resulting in a reduction of activity limitations and the prevention of disability. For patients with chronic pain, however, this treatment strategy is often insufficient. Patients with chronic pain may never return to work even when the only impairment identified is pain. Treatments that address chronic pain as a warning of tissue damage do not alter the illness and disability behavior of patients with chronic pain, nor will they improve their health-related quality of life. The focus of therapy should be to help these patients regain control over their lives by active participation in their pain management program and learning to cope with pain. To achieve this goal, an active partnership is needed between the patient and the therapist. Like other patients, patients with chronic pain want a confidence-based association that includes understanding, listening, respect, and being included in decision making.[39]

Patients with chronic pain are not a homogeneous group and there is no magic bullet that fits all. Because each patient has a unique set of circumstances, psychosocial issues, and physical findings, treatment is individualized and based on the comprehensive assessment of the patient and the patient's individual goals.

In general, chronic pain management should include the following, as noted by Von Korff and colleagues:[40]

- Collaboration between physical therapist and the patient
- A personalized rehabilitation plan

- Tailored education of the patient on the nature of the problem
- Resolution of treatable barriers related to functional goal attainment
- Tailored instruction in independent management of pain
- Instruction in methods to prevent future problems
- Monitoring of outcome (achievement of patient goals)
- Monitoring of adherence to treatment
- Planned follow-up

COLLABORATION BETWEEN PHYSICAL THERAPIST AND PATIENT

Implementing patient-centered approaches in caring for individuals with chronic pain and using principles drawn from the chronic disease management model to improve care systems may improve both patient and provider satisfaction with chronic pain care.[41] For instance, significant positive associations were found between a positive therapeutic alliance and the patient's global perceived effect of treatment, change in pain, physical function, patient satisfaction with treatment, depression; and general health status in patients with chronic musculoskeletal pain in physical rehabilitation.[42] Contributing to a positive therapeutic alliance are (1) therapist-patient agreement on goals of treatment, (2) therapist-patient agreement on intervention, and (3) the affective bond between patient and therapist.[43]

Coming to mutual agreement on goals and intervention can be a challenge. To decrease the negative impact of chronic pain on functioning and health-related quality of life, patients must adopt self-management skills. In order to do so, patients have to be ready to stop focusing on further medical diagnostics in order to find a definite medical solution for pain and change to an active orientation regarding self-management. Not all patients are ready for this. For a good collaboration between the physical therapist and the patient, the patient must at least be planning to take an active orientation toward self-management, and the therapist should support and encourage this goal. Motivational interviewing (MI) techniques can be applied to support patients in enhancing behavioral change and finding an active orientation toward self-management. MI, originally developed in the field of addiction, has recently been introduced in various health care domains, including the care for patients with chronic pain. In the treatment of patients with chronic low back pain, an MI-adapted intervention added to physical therapy effectively enhanced motivation and exercise compliance compared to physiotherapy alone.[44] Patients with chronic musculoskeletal pain who followed an exercise program containing an additional motivation program were more likely to attend the exercise classes.[45] Further research is, however, needed to study whether these positive effects on motivation and adherence will eventually improve treatment outcomes.

Not only do patients bring expectations about treatment but the provider does as well. Treatment decisions are often heavily influenced by personal beliefs of the provider. Results of several studies indicate that the personal attitudes and beliefs regarding pain of physiotherapists and other health care providers are associated with their advice to patients regarding regaining activities and return to work. Practitioners with a more biomedical orientation are more likely to use a pain-contingent treatment approach and focus on "curing" impairments, whereas practitioners with a more biopsychosocial orientation will more likely use a time-contingent treatment approach and focus on increasing activities. Linton and associates investigated the level of fear-avoidance beliefs in practicing general practitioners and physical therapists.[46] Compared to providers with low fear avoidance, providers with high levels of fear-avoidance belief had an increased risk for believing sick leave to be a good treatment, not providing good information about activities, and being uncertain about identifying patients at risk for developing persistent pain problems. The combination of a high fear avoidant provider with a high fear avoidant patient seems a recipe for disaster in chronic pain management and should at all cost be avoided.

Different assessment tools are currently available to measure practitioners' beliefs toward pain, such as the Attitudes to Back Pain scale for musculoskeletal practitioners (ABS .mp), the Health Care Providers' Pain and Impairment Relationship Scale (HC-PAIRS), and the Pain Attitudes and Beliefs Scale for Physiotherapists (PABS.PT).[47]

It can be concluded that for optimal interaction with his or her patient, a physical therapist should have (1) a dynamic, multidimensional knowledge base that is patient centered, (2) a clinical reasoning process that is embedded in a collaborative, problem-solving venture with the patient, (3) a central focus on movement assessment linked to patient function, and (4) consistent virtues seen in caring and commitment to patients as has been shown to be central to expert physical therapy care.[48]

PERSONALIZED REHABILITATION PLAN

To win the collaboration of patients and their families, physical therapists need to negotiate and agree on a definition of the problem they are working on with each patient. They must then agree on the targets and goals for management and develop an individualized collaborative self-management plan.[49] The patient and physical therapist need to agree on the goals of treatment to prevent confusion and disappointment on both sides and to establish a collaborative relationship. Adopting a shared decision-making approach to goal and treatment setting may be useful. Training and support for both health professionals and patients may facilitate a shared decision-making approach.[22] Establishing specific but attainable goals can facilitate task performance. In contrast, unrealistic goals can lead to decreased motivation and a sense of failure. Self-efficacy facilitates goal setting. People with high self-efficacy choose to perform more challenging tasks.[49] They set themselves higher goals and stick to them. Self-efficacy can be understood as the confidence one has in one's ability to deal with certain life stressors. High self-efficacy is related to better treatment outcomes, such as higher levels of physical functioning and the use of pain coping strategies related to better adjustment to chronic pain.

Goals must be measurable so that treatment can be time limited and have an observable end point. Return to a pain-free state is a good example of an unrealistic goal. Common (realistic) goals are associated with a reduction of the impact of pain on the patient's life (i.e., increased level of activities and participation), independent pain management, and the attainment of functional goals. Examples of functional goals are being able to walk for an hour, sitting through a meal or a movie, being able to carry and lift a certain amount of weight, playing with the kids, going out with the family, and being able to perform essential job components. Return to work or vocational rehabilitation should be part of the treatment plan when appropriate. Goals must be realistic and attainable within a reasonable time. A gauge such as the Canadian Occupational Performance Measure (COPM) can be helpful during the process of goal setting and goal attainment during treatment.[50] It is helpful to determine the number of treatments per week and the number of weeks of treatment before initiating treatment (i.e., treatment will occur 3 times per week for 6 weeks). Having a definite end point increases patient adherence and provides a framework to the patient and the treatment team in which to achieve goals. A treatment contract that includes goals, the intensity and frequency of treatment, and expected compliance with treatment can be helpful.

During treatment, the use of goal-setting charts is recommended. Patients set a target for activities each week, record their achievements on the chart, note the nature of any difficulties and how these will be tackled next time, and make other comments. Patients may comment on their performance or on the appropriateness of the goals they had set. In this manner they can monitor their progress and improve their accuracy in goal setting.

EDUCATION ON THE NATURE OF THE PROBLEM

A number of studies have shown that most patients expect an explanation or an improved understanding of their pain problem, a clear diagnosis of the cause of their pain, information, and instructions. They expect confirmation from the health care provider that their pain is real.[52,53] For patients attending pain clinics, the explanation of their pain problem is rated as important as the cure or relief of their pain.[51] Education on the neurophysiology of pain seems therefore quite important and may be considered a precondition for pain management success.

The sensitization model can be used to explain pain as a physical cause related to changes in the nervous system and to explain how chronic pain exists without tissue damage. This explanation may improve the patient's motivation to discuss the importance of psychosocial factors that contribute to the maintenance of chronic pain.[52] Unfortunately, the underestimation of patients' ability to understand currently accurate information about the neurophysiology of pain represents a barrier to reconceptualization of the problem in chronic pain within the clinical and lay arenas.[53] Most patients are quite capable of understanding the complexities of pain if explained well. The textbook *Explain Pain* can help to guide educational sessions with patients.[54] For chronic musculoskeletal pain disorders, there is compelling evidence that an educational strategy addressing the neurophysiology and neurobiology of pain can have a positive effect on pain, disability, catastrophization, and physical performance.[55] The main goals of education are reassurance and empowerment for further treatment. When treating patients in a group, education comes from other patients as well. They may share solutions to functional problems, ways to better pace their activities, or independent pain management techniques they have found helpful.

RESOLUTION OF TREATABLE BARRIERS RELATED TO FUNCTIONAL GOAL ATTAINMENT

Barriers related to the attainment of functional goals in patients with chronic pain are usually due to a combination of physical factors and patient beliefs and cognitions. Physical conditioning programs that include a cognitive-behavioral approach plus intensive physical training (specific to the job or not) that includes aerobic capacity, muscle strength, endurance, and coordination; are in some way work related; and are given and supervised by a physical therapist or a multidisciplinary team seem to reduce the number of sick days for some workers with chronic back pain, when compared to usual care.[56] Ideally, exercise therapy is combined with a cognitive-behavioral approach in a chronic pain rehabilitation program.

EXERCISE THERAPY

The "deconditioning syndrome"[57,58] was postulated in the mid-1980s as a factor contributing to the intolerance to physical activities and subsequent (further) loss of function and disability in patients with chronic pain. Physical disuse has been presented as one factor that perpetuates chronic pain in theoretical pain research models. Although current evidence does not support the disabling influence of a deconditioning syndrome in chronic pain syndromes,[59] reconditioning is still used as a fundament for various pain rehabilitation programs. Enhancing physical activity and fitness can, however, indeed have a beneficial effect in patients with chronic pain. For example, meta-analyses have demonstrated strong evidence for the efficacy of muscle conditioning and aerobic exercise to lessen symptoms in persons with arthritis, other rheumatic diseases,[60] and shoulder pain.[61] There is evidence (although the studies have been classified as low quality) for the effectiveness of exercise therapy compared to usual care in patients with back pain.[62]

Exercise therapy encompasses a heterogeneous group of interventions, and a number of studies have found beneficial effects of exercise on pain and function; however, there continues to be uncertainty about the most effective exercise approach. Most studies had insufficient data to provide useful guidelines on optimal exercise type or dosage, although some evidence exists that "sicker" patients may benefit from more intensive treatment. Haldorsen and associates,[63] for instance, showed that patients with a poor return-to-work prognosis returned to work at significantly higher rates when they completed a more intense multidisciplinary treatment program, whereas patients with a good return-to-work prognosis benefited equally from ordinary treatment and multidisciplinary treatment. Patients thus do not all benefit from the same exercise program. Exercise programs therefore need to be designed and tailored to the individual needs of the patient. In addition, the mechanisms by which physical treatment supports improvement in patients with chronic pain may not only be based on changes in muscle strength or fitness. In a study of Smeets and coworkers, it appeared that pain catastrophizing mediated results in both cognitive-behavioral treatment and in physical treatment.[26] Changes in the level of catastrophizing, instead of changes in physical fitness, were associated with changes in disability during treatment.

There is little evidence that supports the use of passive modalities in the treatment of patients with chronic pain.

High-quality evidence suggests that there is no clinically relevant difference between spinal manipulative therapy and other interventions for reducing pain and improving function in patients with chronic low-back pain.[64] There is currently insufficient evidence to draw a firm conclusion on the clinical effect of low-level laser therapy, massage, traction, superficial heat/cold, and lumbar supports for patients with chronic low-back pain.[62]

Published literature on transcutaneous electrical nerve stimulation (TENS) lacks the methodological rigor or robust reporting needed to make confident assessments of the role of TENS in chronic pain management.[65] Passive modalities (TENS, ultrasound, massage, corsets, traction, acupuncture) should be limited and used only in combination with an active exercise program.

COGNITIVE-BEHAVIORAL APPROACH

Cognitive-behavior therapy (CBT) is a combination of cognitive and behavioral therapy. Behavioral therapy addresses the connections between situations and patients' habitual reactions to them (i.e., walking with a limp because it gets positive attention from the spouse). Cognitive therapy addresses patients' thoughts or beliefs that cause them to feel and act the way they do ("If I use my back I will become paraplegic, so the safest thing to do for me is to lie on the couch and do nothing"). Therefore, if patients exhibit unwanted behaviors, it is important to identify the beliefs that cause the behaviors and to teach patients how to replace or modify the beliefs so that more desirable behavior might ensue.

Cognitive-behavior modification can be accomplished in a number of ways: by talking about beliefs, by gaining exposure to avoided activities, by increasing the number and duration of usual activities, by participating in a "reward system" in which healthy behavior is rewarded and encouraged and nonhealthy behavior is ignored, and by listening to feedback from other patients on their behavior.

Pain-related fear has been consistently associated with initiation and maintenance of chronic pain disability.[66] For patients with high levels of pain and activity-related fear who avoid activities, behavioral methods such as graded activity and graded exposure treatment have both been shown to be effective in reducing disability.[67] Repeated exposure to avoided activities decreases anxiety and fear about them. In graded exposure, patients are challenged to actually perform the specific physical activities that they believe will harm them. Most of the time exposure treatment is performed in combined therapy with a physical therapist and a behavioral therapist.

Although multidisciplinary programs have shown effectiveness in patients with chronic pain,[62] it is still unclear which component is most effective. In a study in which the effectiveness of three rehabilitation interventions (an active physical, a cognitive-behavioral, and a combined treatment) for patients with chronic low back pain was compared with that for a waiting list control group, it appeared that all three active treatments were effective in comparison to no treatment, but no clinically relevant differences between the combined and the single-component treatments were found.[21] A new approach in CBT, or the third-wave CBT, has been introduced in pain treatment. An example of a third-wave CBT approach is acceptance commitment therapy (ACT). ACT differs from traditional CBT in that instead of trying to teach people to better control their thoughts, feelings, and sensations, ACT teaches them to "just notice," accept, and embrace personal life events. ACT aims to help individuals clarify their personal values and take action on them in order to bring more meaning to their lives.

SELF-MANAGEMENT TECHNIQUES

Self-management ensures active patient participation in managing pain and achieving reasonable goals of functional restoration. Self-management ensures active patient participation and includes the following:

- The use of pain-control modalities (e.g., ice, heat, self-massage, relaxation, cognitive- behavioral techniques)
- A graded, gradually progressive exercise program to encourage overall fitness, activity, and a healthy lifestyle

There is emerging evidence that interactive online self-management programs are helpful in reducing pain intensity, psychological distress, and disability.[68,69]

INSTRUCTION IN METHODS TO PREVENT FUTURE PROBLEMS

It is almost inevitable that a patient with chronic pain will experience an exacerbation of the pain problem at some time. Relapse may be due to an individual physical event or it may result from cumulative physical and psychological stresses that challenge patients' coping resources. The physical therapist can help to identify situations that are challenging and develop strategies to cope with them. Strategies may include setting criteria to visit health professionals, using pain medication, or briefly resting and relaxing. Plans for resuming activity following an exacerbation are critical.[70] Technological applications, such as the online self-management programs described previously, or telephone-based interventions may help patients maintain the skills they learned in their pain management programs and prevent relapse.

If returning a patient to work is an important goal, a job description with as much detail as possible provides important ergonomic information. Patients can then practice components of the job description with the physical therapist and at home.

The goal of ergonomics is to ensure that the workplace is designed to prevent work-induced injuries. Non-neutral postures, forceful exertions, constrained or static postures, repetitive work, use of pinch grip, work over shoulder height, prolonged periods of time with the trunk inclined forward, heavy lifting, twisting while lifting, and whole body and vibration are all risk factors for work-related musculoskeletal disorders. A common type of ergonomic instruction during physical therapy is educating the patient on manual handling and lifting, optimal seated postures and activities, and the relationship of the seat to the workbench or desk. The patient is taught to take "stretch breaks" during work or to alternate job components.

At the end of treatment, a vocational assessment is advised, which preferably includes an FCE assessment. Then the FCE is matched with the job description. Recommendations for return to work are based on this evaluation. Changes in the job that would enable the patient to return to work may be suggested. If possible, a worksite analysis also should be performed to help identify risks to the patient and to suggest changes to the work environment to accommodate the patient.

For return to work, a "light duty" job or a gradual increase in the hours worked per day is usually recommended. Some therapists offer a "work hardening" program in which a pain patient gradually "works" up to a simulated 8-hour workday. In workers with chronic back pain, pooled results of five physical conditioning studies showed a small effect on sickness absence at long-term follow-up. The addition of cognitive behavioral therapy to physical conditioning programs was not more effective than the physical conditioning alone. Workplace involvement might improve the outcome.[71] After discharge from these programs, full-time return to work is appropriate.

MONITORING OF OUTCOME (ACHIEVEMENT OF PATIENT GOALS)

Generic and disease-specific measurement tools have been developed. Recommendations based on the Initiative on Methods, Measurement, and Pain Assessment in Clinical Trials (IMMPACT) can be helpful for designing sets for routine assessments in order to monitor treatment progress.[72] Important domains to consider for assessment as advised by IMMPACT are pain, fatigue, disturbed sleep, physical functioning, emotional functioning, patient global ratings of satisfaction, and health-related quality of life. In addition, patients' treatment goals can serve as outcome measures to determine treatment efficacy. A simple visual analog scale (VAS) can visualize progress, for instance:

In the past week were you able to walk a mile?

Completely unable_______________Completely able

MONITORING OF ADHERENCE TO TREATMENT

As early as 1991, Turk and colleagues reported that nonadherence with therapeutic recommendations during treatment and subsequent to treatment termination are neglected topics in the treatment of patients with chronic pain.[73] The topic remains under-researched.

Besides outcome domains as mentioned earlier, IMMPACT focuses also on participant disposition (e.g., adherence to the treatment regimen and reasons for premature withdrawal from the trial). Adherence to pain management treatment recommendations and the number of "no shows" should be monitored in clinical practice as well. Physical therapists need to offer an appropriate behavioral framework by maintaining a clear structure, consistent rules, and rewards for positive patient response during treatment. When a patient is persistently nonadherent, the problem should be addressed and the reasons for nonadherence explored. Reasons for nonadherence can include poor satisfaction with treatment results or a patient-provider relationship that does not work well.

PLANNED FOLLOW-UP

There is a paucity of literature on planned follow-up after multidisciplinary treatment. Planned follow-up can be done on an individual basis or in group settings and serves to prevent crisis management. It can also serve as an external motivator (they are going to know I did not do my exercise/self-management techniques). To date, there is no evidence as to the optimal frequency or duration of follow-up visits.

CONCLUSION

Generally, the evaluation and treatment of chronic pain patients are difficult tasks that are best performed in an interdisciplinary team setting, because both biomedical and psychosocial aspects related to the pain problem have to be addressed. The role of the physical therapist is to form a close partnership with patients, help patients set and attain individual goals at activities and participation level, and teach patients self-management skills. Ultimately, patients should become experts on managing their own chronic pain in order for them to enjoy the best health-related quality of life possible.

KEY POINTS

- Multidisciplinary care of patients with chronic pain has proven to be of significant value.
- A collaborative relationship between patient and therapist is essential to enhance successful outcomes.
- The pain management treatment plan must be tailored to the individual patient.
- Establishing treatment goals, patient education, therapeutic exercise and behavioral techniques are at the core of physical therapy pain management.
- Active involvement of patients and treatment adherence are necessary.

SUGGESTED READINGS

Apeldoorn AT, Ostelo RW, Fritz JM, van der PT, et al. The cross-sectional construct validity of the Waddell score. *Clin J Pain.* 2012;28:309-317.

Bishop A, Thomas E, Foster NE. Health care practitioners' attitudes and beliefs about low back pain: a systematic search and critical review of available measurement tools. *Pain.* 2007;132:91-101.

Huijnen IP, Verbunt JA, Peters ML, et al. Do depression and pain intensity interfere with physical activity in daily life in patients with chronic low back pain? *Pain.* 2010;150:161-166.

Jordan JL, Holden MA, Mason EE, Foster NE. Interventions to improve adherence to exercise for chronic musculoskeletal pain in adults. *Cochrane Database Syst Rev.* 2010:CD005956.

Lin CW, McAuley JH, Macedo L, et al. Relationship between physical activity and disability in low back pain: a systematic review and meta-analysis. *Pain.* 2011;152:607-613.

Macedo LG, Smeets RJ, Maher CG, et al. Graded activity and graded exposure for persistent nonspecific low back pain: a systematic review. *Phys Ther.* 2010;90:860-879.

Schaafsma F, Schonstein E, Whelan KM, et al. Physical conditioning programs for improving work outcomes in workers with back pain. *Cochrane Database Syst Rev.* 2010:CD001822.

Smeets RJ, Hijdra HJ, Kester AD, et al. The usability of six physical performance tasks in a rehabilitation population with chronic low back pain. *Clin Rehabil.* 2006;20:989-997.

Ustun TB, Chatterji S, Bickenbach J, et al. The International Classification of Functioning, Disability and Health: a new tool for understanding disability and health. *Disabil Rehabil.* 2003;25:565-571.

van Middelkoop M, Rubinstein SM, Kuijpers T, et al. A systematic review on the effectiveness of physical and rehabilitation interventions for chronic non-specific low back pain. *Eur Spine J.* 2011;20:19-39.

Verbeek J, Sengers MJ, Riemens L, Haafkens J. Patient expectations of treatment for back pain: a systematic review of qualitative and quantitative studies. *Spine.* 2004;29:2309-2318.

The references for this chapter can be found at www.expertconsult.com.

48 Acupuncture

Yuan-Chi Lin

Acupuncture is an ancient medical modality of traditional Chinese medicine. It was described in the *Huang Di Nei Jing* (*Yellow Emperor's Internal Classic*) in 100 BC. Called *jin jiao*, acupuncture generally consists of the practices of needling and moxibustion. Moxibustion is a warming sensation produced by placing smouldering moxa (*Artemisia vulgaris*) over the acupuncture points. The practice of acupuncture also includes electroacupuncture, laser acupuncture, cupping, Chinese tui na massage, Gua Sha, and acupressure. With the advances in biochemical and biophysical technology, the mechanisms of acupuncture analgesia have been elucidated as being a consequence of peripheral acupuncture point stimulation, mobilization of central neural peptides, and triggering of the central inhibitory pathway for modulation of pain sensation.

THEORIES OF ACUPUNCTURE

The concept of yin and yang is one of the essential theories of traditional Chinese medicine. The principle is simple, but its implication is philosophical. It was first mentioned in *The Book of Changes and Simplicity* (*Yi Jing*), a text from about 700 BC. Yin and yang are natural phenomena that exist within the body. They are interdependent and can be transformed into each other. They exist in a constant state of dynamic balance. Yang is related to bright, hot, activity, light, above, outward, increase, dry, and male. Yin is present in the qualities of dark, cold, rest, passivity, below, inward, decrease, wet, and female. Yin and yang define aspects of a whole and are therefore dependent on each other. For example, "bright" is difficult to define without "dark." "Above" is meaningless without "below." Yin-yang interdependence is the relationship between structure and function. Optimal physical condition requires a balance of yin and yang within the body. Disease is associated with a disharmony or imbalance between yin and yang. Acupuncture can be used to balance and promote yin and yang energy within the body.

There are more than 365 identifiable acupuncture points in the human body. There are also pathways, called meridians, connecting acupuncture points to each other. Qi (pronounced "chee") is the energy flow through these meridians. Difficult to define, qi represents power and movement, similar to energy. Qi is a functional, dynamic force that resides in living creatures. It is a result of the interaction between heaven and earth, an energy that is manifested concurrently in the physical and spiritual levels of human existence. Qi flows throughout the meridians of the body to maintain life and health. These meridians are not defined by physical structures such as blood or lymphatic vessels, but by their function. The body is viewed as a dynamic system of organs connected by the flow of qi through the meridians.

When there is stagnation or inadequate flow of qi through the meridians, pain or illness may result. The flow of qi may be restored by the insertion of very fine needles into a combination of appropriate acupuncture points along the meridians. Manual twirling of these needles produces a sore, heavy, or numb sensation known as "de qi" (obtaining qi). Acupuncture practitioners have observed that stimulating specific acupuncture points results in predictable responses in patients with a given pattern of signs and symptoms. Practitioners of acupuncture routinely request the patient's detailed history of the present illness in pursuing the diagnosis. Physical attention is also focused on disposition of the pulse and appearance of the tongue. In traditional Chinese medicine, there are six pathologic factors that cause disease—wind, cold, heat, dampness, dryness, and fire. The goal of the history and physical examination is to assess the patient's balance of yin and yang and to gain insight into other symptoms.

There are eight principal classifications of symptoms, which include yin or yang, external or internal, cold or hot, and deficient or excess. The aim of acupuncture therapy is to restore deficiencies or correct excesses in qi, thus restoring health. It is frequently used for preventive care, as well as for therapeutic purposes.

A Treatise on Acupuncturation, written by James Morss Churchill in 1823, was the first text about acupuncture published in English. Dr. Churchill described his success in using acupuncture for rheumatic conditions, sciatica, and back pain. Sir William Osler's *Principles and Practice of Medicine*, first published in 1892, recommended the use of acupuncture for the treatment of sciatica and lumbago. Public awareness and use of acupuncture increased in the United States following *New York Times* writer James Reston's account of his emergency appendectomy in a Chinese hospital. His article described how physicians eased his postsurgical abdominal pain with acupuncture.[1]

ACUPUNCTURE POINTS

Acupuncture points are generally located in the deep depressions of muscles, joints, or bones and are often sensitive to pressure. The unit of measurement used to determine the locations of acupuncture points on the body is called a *tsun*, and measurement of a tsun is relative to the patient's own body. One tsun (approximately 1 inch) is equal to the space

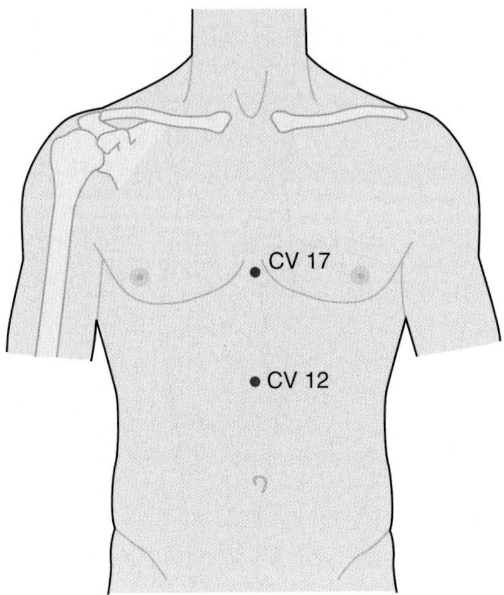

Figure 48.1 Acupuncture points CV 12 and CV 17.

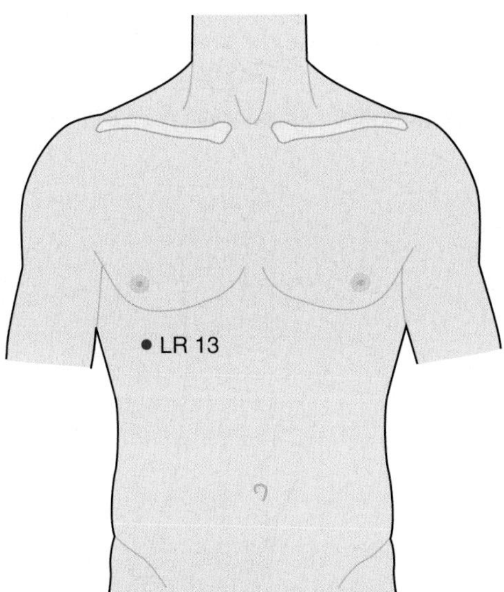

Figure 48.2 Acupuncture point LR 13.

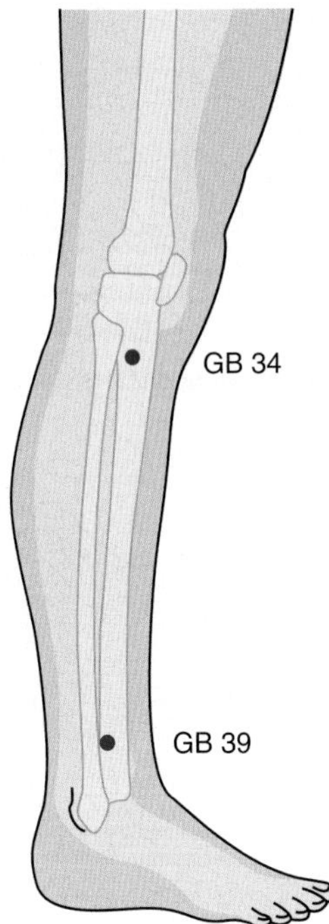

Figure 48.3 Acupuncture points GB 34 and GB 39.

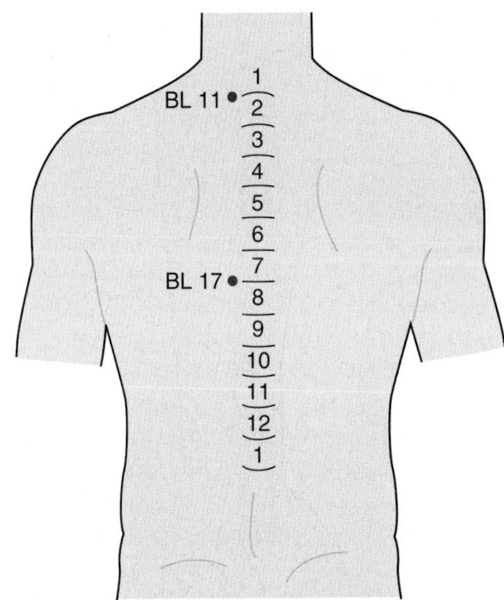

Figure 48.4 Acupuncture points BL 11 and BL 17.

between the distal interphalangeal joint and the proximal interphalangeal joint on the middle finger.

- CV 12 (zhong guan; "central venter")—located in the midline, 4 tsun above the umbilicus (Fig. 48.1)
- CV 17 (tan chung; "chest center")—located in the midline of the sternum, between the nipples, at the level of the fourth intercostal space (Fig. 48.1)
- LR 13 (zhang men; "camphor wood gate")—located on the lateral side of the abdomen, below the free end of the 11th rib, 2 tsun above the navel and 6 tsun on either side of the midline (Fig. 48.2)
- GB 34 (yang ling quan; "young mound spring")—located in the deep depression 1 tsun anterior and 1 tsun inferior to the head of the fibula (Fig. 48.3)
- GB 39 (xuan zhong or jue gu; "suspended bell or severed bone")—located 3 tsun directly above the tip of the lateral malleolus in the depression between the posterior border of the fibula and the tendons of the peroneus longus and brevis (see Fig. 48.3)
- BL 11 (da zhu; "great shuttle")—located 1.5 tsun lateral to the lower border of the spinous process of the first thoracic vertebra (Fig. 48.4)
- BL 17 (ge shu; "diaphragm shu")—located 1.5 tsun lateral to the lower border of the spinous process of the seventh vertebra (Fig. 48.4)
- LU 9 (tai yuan; "great abyss")—located at the transverse crease of the wrist in the depression on the lateral side of the radial artery (Fig. 48.5)

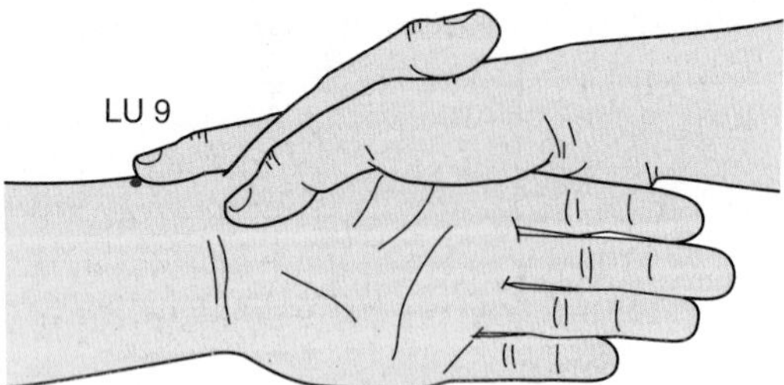

Figure 48.5 Acupuncture point LU 9.

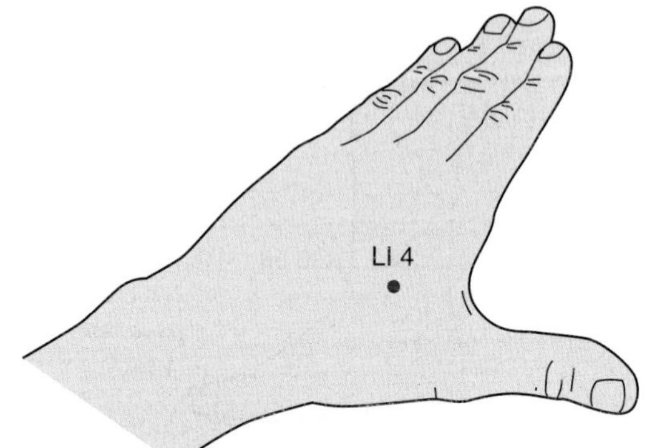

Figure 48.6 Acupuncture point LI 4.

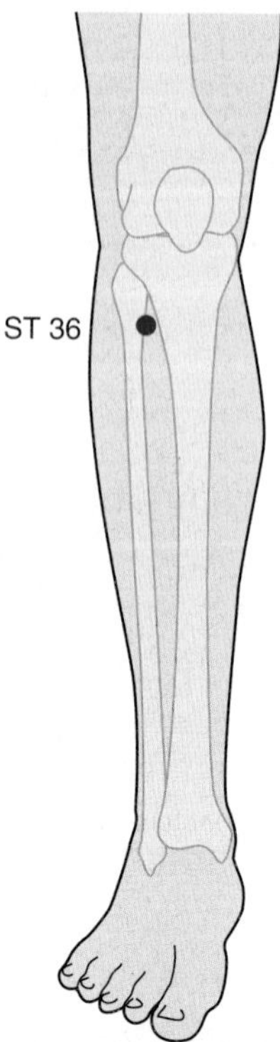

Figure 48.8 Acupuncture point ST 36.

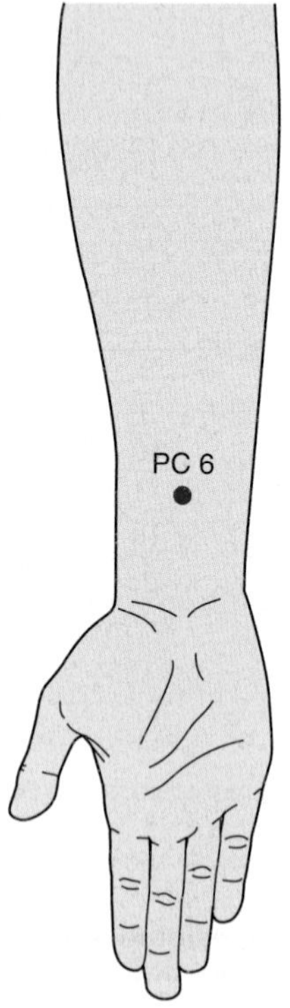

Figure 48.7 Acupuncture point PC 6.

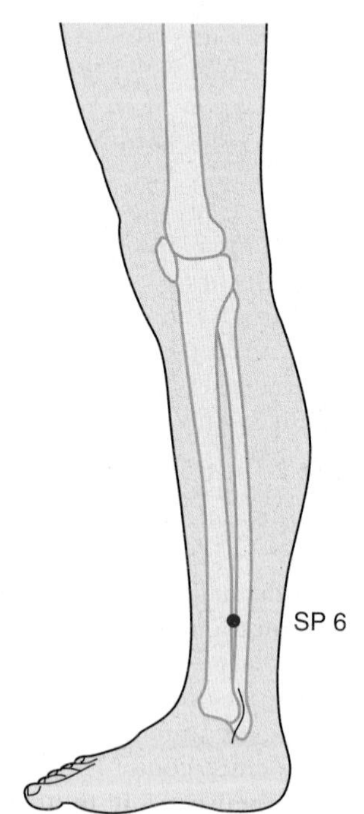

Figure 48.9 Acupuncture point SP 6.

- LI 4 (he gu; "union valley")—located between the first and second metacarpal bones in the deep depression of the web space (Fig. 48.6)
- PC 6 (nei guan; "internal gate")—located 2 to 3 tsun above the transverse crease of the wrist, a deep depression between the tendons of the long palmar muscle and the radial flexor muscle of the wrist (Fig. 48.7)
- ST 36 (zu san li; "leg three miles")—located 3 tsun below the patella and 1 tsun lateral to the crest of the tibia (Fig. 48.8)
- SP 6 (san yin jiao; "three yin intersection")—located 3 tsun above the tip of the medial malleolus on the posterior border of the tibia (Fig. 48.9)

BASIC RESEARCH

Numerous reports confirm that acupuncture has reproducible neurobiologic effects. Acupuncture inhibits the transmission of pain according to the gate control theory.[2] It may act by stimulating sensory Aβ fibers and directly inhibiting the spinal transmission of pain by smaller Aδ and C fibers.[3] Researchers have also been paying attention to the relationship between acupuncture and the production of endogenous opioid peptides, such as the endorphins and enkephalins, and stimulation of the endogenous descending inhibitory pathways. In an analysis of human cerebrospinal fluid, Sjolund and colleagues[4] determined that endorphin levels in subjects become elevated following electroacupuncture. Acupuncture analgesia is caused mainly by activation of the endogenous antinociceptive system to modulate transmission of pain and the pain response.[5]

Electroacupuncture at 2 Hz accelerates the release of enkephalin, β-endorphin, and endomorphin, whereas at 100 Hz it selectively increases the release of dynorphin. A combination of the two frequencies produces simultaneous release of all four opioid peptides, thereby resulting in a maximal therapeutic effect.[6] Peripheral stimulation of the skin or deeper structures activates various brain structures, the spinal cord, or a combination via specific neural pathways.[7] A human study by Mayer and associates indicated that acupuncture analgesia can be reversed by naloxone.[8] Several serotonin antagonists inhibit the effects of electroacupuncture. Electroacupuncture attenuates behavioral hyperalgesia and stress-induced colonic motor dysfunction in rats.[9] It also attenuates behavioral hyperalgesia and stress-induced colonic motor dysfunction in rats via serotonergic pathways.

Neuronal correlation to acupuncture stimulation in the human brain has been investigated with functional magnetic resonance imaging (fMRI). Acupuncture needle manipulation on the LI 4 (he gu) point modulates the fMRI activity of the limbic system and subcortical structure.[10] Acupuncture stimulation at analgesic points involving the pain-related neuromatrix have been studied. Acupuncture stimulation at the GB 34 (yang ling quan) acupuncture point has elicited significantly higher activation than has sham acupuncture over the hypothalamus and primary somatosensory motor cortex and deactivation over the rostral segment of the anterior cingulated cortex.[11]

SIDE EFFECTS

The use of disposable sterile acupuncture needles avoids the risk of cross-contamination. Occasionally, the patient may experience bruising at the acupuncture site. Mild transient drowsiness may also occur. Pneumothorax is the most frequently reported serious complication related to acupuncture.[12,13] In a study of the cases of 78 acupuncturists involving 31,822 acupuncture treatments in the United Kingdom, the most common adverse events reported were bleeding (310/10,000 consultations) and needling pain (110/10,000 consultations).[14] The York acupuncture safety study surveyed 34,000 treatments by traditional acupuncturists. Aggravation of symptoms occurred in 96 of 10,000 cases, but none of these events were serious. There was subsequent improvement in the main complaint in 70% of cases.[15] Major adverse consequences of acupuncture appear to be extremely rare.[16] Acupuncture can be considered safe when performed by a competent and experienced acupuncturist,[17] including appropriately trained practitioners in the pediatric population.[18]

CLINICAL USE OF ACUPUNCTURE

Acupuncture as a therapeutic intervention is currently practiced widely in the United States. In 1997, the National Institutes of Health[19] concluded that there are promising results supporting its efficacy for adult postoperative and chemotherapy-related nausea and vomiting and for postoperative dental pain. There are reasonable studies concluding that the use of acupuncture results in satisfactory treatment of addiction, stroke rehabilitation, headache, menstrual cramps, tennis elbow, fibromyalgia, myofascial pain, osteoarthritis, low back pain, carpal tunnel syndrome, and asthma. Depending on the situation, acupuncture may be used as an adjunctive treatment or acceptable alternative therapy or be integrated into a comprehensive management program.

Clinical research on the use of acupuncture for the treatment of pain has consisted primarily of uncontrolled trials. Although beneficial results have frequently been demonstrated, the flawed design of many of the studies places limited value on the outcomes. Systematic reviews of randomized controlled trials (RCTs) have provided the best evidence and the least bias in assessing the efficacy of any medical intervention. Several difficulties are inherent in designing valid, blinded RCTs of acupuncture.[20,21] An appropriate placebo for the acupuncture control group is difficult to determine. Various studies have used placement of needles at nonmeridian sites, called "sham" acupuncture, to model acupuncture in control group patients.

Thirty percent of study subjects may respond positively to placebo. There are very few criteria in the current literature for the use of placebo in acupuncture research. Sham acupuncture is frequently used as the control treatment in research trials involving acupuncture; however, it presents a unique problem as a placebo. The well-outlined energy channels of the acupuncture meridian systems cover the entire body and link wei-qi (defense qi), rong-qi (growth and development qi), and yuan-qi (the original qi inherited at birth). Because the meridian systems affect the entire body, sham acupuncture still does provide some acupuncture effect and therefore cannot be considered to produce a true placebo effect. In an attempt to address this problem, a placebo acupuncture needle that retracts back into the handle of the acupuncture needle and does not penetrate the skin has been developed.[22]

Richardson and Vincent[23] reviewed 27 controlled studies of acupuncture for the treatment of acute and chronic pain, as well as several large uncontrolled studies. In 50% to 80% of the patients studied, they noted that it was difficult to assess the long-term effectiveness of acupuncture based on the collected data. In a meta-analysis of 14 RCTs of acupuncture for chronic pain in adults, Patel and coworkers[24] found that although few of the individual trials demonstrated statistically significant benefit from acupuncture, the pool-

results for several subgroups did, in fact, attain statistical significance in favor of acupuncture.

POSTOPERATIVE PAIN

Acupuncture may be most useful in predictable situations involving acute pain, such as dental procedures and postoperative pain, or in the setting of medical conditions characterized by recurrent episodes of acute pain, such as sickle cell crisis and recurrent abdominal pain. Although effective treatment is available in many cases (e.g., local anesthetics for dental procedures, opioids for severe postoperative pain), side effects such as respiratory depression may occur. Taub and colleagues[25] used acupuncture for the treatment of dental pain in a single-blind RCT in which 39 adult patients underwent dental restoration for cavities. Patients were randomized between real and sham acupuncture groups. Seventy percent of the experimental group and 53% of the control group reported good or excellent pain reduction. The results for the two groups showed no statistical significance. A systematic review has suggested that acupuncture is effective in relieving dental pain.[26] Also, a study of the effect of acupuncture for pain after lower abdominal surgery revealed that preoperative treatment with low- or high-frequency electroacupuncture reduced postoperative analgesic requirements and decreased the side effects of systemic opioids.[27]

Acupuncture has been shown to reduce postoperative opioid dose requirements in patients and to decrease discomfort. In a randomized, controlled, double-blind study of patients scheduled for elective upper and lower abdominal surgery, acupuncture was found to reduce postoperative pain. Consumption of supplemental intravenous morphine was reduced 50%, and the incidence of postoperative nausea was reduced 20% to 30%. Plasma cortisol and epinephrine concentrations were reduced 30% to 50% in the acupuncture group.[28] In an RCT of electroacupuncture in 100 women undergoing lower abdominal surgery, the incidence of nausea and dizziness during the first 24 hours after surgery was significantly reduced in the electroacupuncture group when compared with the control and sham groups. Preoperative treatment with low- and high-frequency electroacupuncture reduced postoperative analgesic requirements and associated side effects.[29] A study of 27 patients with operable non–small cell lung carcinoma who underwent either electroacupuncture or sham acupuncture for control of post-thoracotomy pain revealed that electroacupuncture may reduce narcotic analgesic use in the early postoperative period.[30] In a study of 36 patients undergoing thoracotomy, epidural and intradermal insertion of acupuncture needles was well tolerated by the patients and did not interfere with standard preoperative care.[31]

In a study of pediatric patients undergoing bilateral myringotomy tube placement, acupuncture treatment provided a significant benefit in alleviating pain and reducing agitation. The median time until the first postoperative administration of an analgesic, acetaminophen, was significantly shorter in the control group. The number of patients who required analgesia was considerably smaller in the acupuncture group than in the control as well. No adverse effects related to the acupuncture treatment were observed.[32] A systematic review was performed to quantitatively evaluate the [illegible] of acupuncture and related techniques as adjunctive analgesics for the management of acute postoperative pain. Fifteen RCTs compared acupuncture with sham control for the management of acute postoperative pain. The acupuncture treatment group had a lower incidence of opioid-related side effects, such as nausea, dizziness, sedation, pruritus, and urinary retention. Perioperative acupuncture may thus be a useful adjunct for acute postoperative pain management.[33]

NAUSEA AND VOMITING

Acupuncture performed with acupuncture needles, an electrical apparatus, pressure, or magnets is commonly used for the management of nausea and vomiting after surgery or chemotherapy. Stimulation of the PC 6 (nei guan) acupuncture point is also used to treat nausea and vomiting caused by sea sickness or pregnancy and to treat side effects from surgery or chemotherapy. A systematic review revealed that beneficial results were achieved in 27 of 33 RCTs of acupuncture, acupressure, or both for the treatment of nausea and vomiting.[34] An RCT of pediatric patients undergoing tonsillectomy in whom electroacupuncture was used for control of nausea showed a significant reduction in the occurrence of nausea when compared with the sham and control groups. This study demonstrated that the efficacy of acupuncture for prevention of postoperative nausea and vomiting is similar to that achieved with commonly used pharmacotherapies.[35] These results have been most consistent with its use for postoperative nausea and vomiting. In 26 trials studying the care of more than 3000 patients, stimulation of the PC 6 acupuncture point was superior to sham acupuncture for the treatment of nausea and vomiting in both adults and children.[36]

LOW BACK PAIN

In a meta-analysis of 12 RCTs, acupuncture was found to be superior to various control interventions for the management of low back pain.[37] An RCT of acupuncture versus transcutaneous electrical nerve stimulation for chronic low back pain in the elderly revealed that both were equally effective, with acupuncture improving spinal flexion.[38] An RCT of 50 patients with low back pain showed a significant decrease in pain intensity at 1 and 3 months in the acupuncture groups in comparison to the placebo group. Acupuncture treatment significantly shortened the time that patients were out of work, improved their quality of sleep, and decreased analgesic intake.[39] An RCT revealed significant improvement in chronic low back pain with traditional acupuncture versus physiotherapy, but not versus sham acupuncture. Benefits included decreases in pain intensity, pain disability, and psychological distress at the end of 12 weeks of treatment. At the 9-month follow-up, the superiority of acupuncture over the control group had lessened.[40] An RCT of 298 patients with low back pain revealed that acupuncture was more effective than no acupuncture treatment in improving pain, but there were no significant differences between acupuncture and minimal acupuncture.[41]

A meta-analysis of 33 RCTs of acupuncture for low back pain indicated that acupuncture effectively relieves chronic low back pain.[42] An RCT of 241 patients with low back pain revealed that a short course of treatment by a qualified traditional acupuncturist is a safe and acceptable method of pain management.[43] Additionally, acupuncture care for low back pain is a cost-effective therapy in the long term.[44]

HEADACHE

Several studies have shown acupuncture therapy to be efficacious for migraine headache.[45,46] In an RCT of 168 women with migraine, acupuncture was found to be adequate for migraine prophylaxis. When compared with flunarizine therapy, acupuncture treatment exhibited greater effectiveness in the first months of therapy and superior tolerability.[47] A prospective, randomized, double-blind study has shown the efficacy of acupuncture for migraine prophylaxis. The reduction of migraine days in patients receiving acupuncture treatment was statistically significant in comparison to baseline. Treatment outcomes for migraine do not differ between patients treated with acupuncture or standard therapy.[48] A systematic review of 22 trials involving a total of 1042 patients concluded that acupuncture has a role in the treatment of recurrent headaches.[49] In an RCT of 179 patients with acute migraine, acupuncture and sumatriptan were more effective than placebo injection for the early treatment of an acute migraine attack.[50] An RCT of 114 patients with migraine compared acupuncture with the use of metoprolol and determined that acupuncture might be an effective and safe treatment option for patients unwilling or unable to use drug prophylaxis.[51]

Supplementing medical management with acupuncture can result in improvement in health-related quality of life, as well as the perception by patients that they suffer less from their headaches.[52] A Cochrane Database Systematic Review of acupuncture for migraine prophylaxis involved 22 trials with 4419 participants. The available studies suggested that acupuncture is at least as effective as or possibly more effective than prophylactic drug treatment and has fewer adverse effects. Acupuncture should be considered as a treatment option for patients with migraine headaches.[53] A Cochrane Database Systematic Review of 11 trials with 2317 participants also indicated that acupuncture can result in at least a 50% reduction in headache frequency, headache days, pain intensity, and analgesic use. Acupuncture could be a valuable nonpharmacologic tool for patients with frequent episodic or chronic tension-type headaches.[54]

TEMPOROMANDIBULAR JOINT DYSFUNCTION

Three RCTs of acupuncture treatment involving 205 patients with temporomandibular joint dysfunction revealed positive results. Acupuncture appears to be an effective treatment of painful dysfunction of the temporomandibular joint, but the results still require confirmation from more rigorous trial methods.[55,56]

NECK PAIN

Several clinical reports have suggested that acupuncture can be useful for the treatment of patients with neck pain. However, 14 RCTs involving 724 subjects with various causes of neck pain did not provide significant evidence in support of acupuncture for the treatment of neck pain.[57] There have been too few studies of sufficient quality and homogeneity to be able to draw conclusions about its effectiveness as treatment. A scoring system to gauge the effects of acupuncture on neck pain has been proposed, but there are problems with its use.[58] In an RCT of 177 individuals with chronic neck pain, patients were randomly assigned to treatment with acupuncture (56 patients), massage (60 patients), or "sham" laser acupuncture (61 patients) over a period of 3 weeks. The patients received five acupuncture treatments during this 3-week period, and acupuncture was found to be an effective short-term treatment.[59] An RCT of acupuncture in 123 patients with chronic neck pain revealed that at 6 months of follow-up, acupuncture was more effective than placebo treatment. Acupuncture treatment improved the patient's quality of life from a physical aspect, improved active neck mobility, and reduced the need for rescue medication.[60] There is some evidence that acupuncture relieves neck pain more effectively than sham treatment or no treatment does.[61]

MYOFASCIAL PAIN SYNDROME

Myofascial pain syndrome is one of the most common causes of chronic musculoskeletal pain. Melzack and colleagues reported a 71% correlation between acupuncture points and trigger points used for the treatment of myofascial pain.[62] In an uncontrolled study, Lewit reported immediate relief in 87% of cases and long-term benefit in at least 92 of 288 patients.[63]

KNEE PAIN AND OSTEOARTHRITIS

Osteoarthritis of the knee is a common joint disorder, especially in women older than 50 years. In a randomized controlled trial of 570 patients with osteoarthritis of the knee, patients underwent 23 weeks of acupuncture treatment. Acupuncture seemed to provide improvement in function and pain relief as an adjunctive therapy when compared with sham acupuncture and education control groups.[64] A systematic review and meta-analysis of 13 RCTs of acupuncture for knee pain revealed acupuncture to be significantly superior to sham acupuncture in both pain control and regaining function. The differences were still significant at long-term follow-up.[65]

LOW BACK PAIN

Low back pain limits daily activities and is a common reason for physician visits. Acupuncture is widely used by patients with low back pain. A meta-analysis of 33 RCTs of acupuncture for low back pain indicated that acupuncture is significantly more effective than sham treatment and no treatment.[42] A study of 298 patients with chronic low back pain compared acupuncture, minimal acupuncture (superficial needling at nonacupuncture points), and a waiting list group as the control. Low back pain was shown to improve after acupuncture treatment for at least 6 months. The effectiveness of acupuncture, either verum or sham, was almost twice that of conventional therapy.[66]

CARPAL TUNNEL SYNDROME

Carpal tunnel syndrome is a common entrapment neuropathy of the median nerve. Eleven patients with mild to moderate carpal tunnel syndrome were randomized into groups receiving real or sham laser acupuncture treatment.

Significant decreases in the McGill Pain Questionnaire score, median nerve sensory latency, and Phalen's and Tinel's signs after the actual laser acupuncture treatment series were observed, but not in the placebo group.[67] A study of fMRI in patients with carpal tunnel syndrome revealed that hyperactivity in the contralateral sensorimotor cortex diminishes after acupuncture treatment.[68]

NEUROPATHIC PAIN

The efficacy of acupuncture in patients with peripheral neuropathy is unclear. Peripheral neuropathy is common in patients infected with human immunodeficiency virus (HIV). Neither acupuncture nor amitriptyline was found to be more effective than placebo in relieving pain caused by HIV-related peripheral neuropathy.[69] Reports are available on the benefits of traditional acupuncture therapy and auricular therapy in treating complex regional pain syndrome, formerly known as reflex sympathetic dystrophy.[70,71] However, each of these reports involved only one to five patients in uncontrolled studies.

REFERRING PATIENTS FOR ACUPUNCTURE TREATMENT

Differentiating between disease and illness is important. A disease is what physicians diagnose, whereas an illness is what the patient feels or suffers. There are many diseases for which there is no cure, but acupuncture can be used as a complementary intervention for the associated illnesses or for the side effects related to conventional medical therapies. Licensing guidelines for the practice of acupuncture are determined by each state. The National Commission for the Certification of Acupuncturists has developed standards for training and certification of licensed acupuncturists, and the American Board of Medical Acupuncture has established guidelines and qualification requirements for physicians to practice medical acupuncture.

Over the past several years the use of traditional Chinese medicine has become more common and accepted in the United States. Some health maintenance organization insurance plans have begun to cover acupuncture treatments for their patients. Some workers' compensation boards and personal injury insurance policies will also cover acupuncture. If there is an increase in the number of insurers willing to reimburse acupuncture therapy, patients will be more likely to seek acupuncture treatment in the future.[72]

How can we best advise patients with pain-related disorders who are interested in acupuncture? The pain service practitioner should discuss with patients what their treatment preferences and expectations of outcome are. It is also essential to review the safety and efficacy of the therapy thoroughly with patients. Patients should be referred to qualified acupuncture providers, and follow-up appointments should also be scheduled to monitor response to treatment.

Acupuncture is steadily becoming an integral part of the health care delivery system. Research on acupuncture has allowed its integration into conventional Western medical practice. More prospective, randomized, and controlled studies on acupuncture are needed to better understand its mechanisms, efficacy, and side effects.

KEY POINTS

- Acupuncture is part of traditional Chinese medicine. The practice of acupuncture includes electroacupuncture, laser acupuncture, moxibustion, cupping, Chinese tui na massage, Gua Sha, and acupressure.
- The theory of yin and yang is essential in traditional Chinese medicine. Yin and yang are natural phenomena that exist within the body. They are interdependent and can be transformed into each other. They exist in a constant state of dynamic balance.
- Optimal physical condition requires a balance of yin and yang within the body. Disease is associated with a disharmony or imbalance between yin and yang.
- There are approximately 365 identifiable acupuncture points in the human body. The pathways connecting the acupuncture points are called meridians. Qi is the energy flow through these meridians. Qi is a functional, dynamic force that resides in living creatures. It is the result of the interaction between heaven and earth, an energy that is manifested concurrently in the physical and spiritual levels of human existence.
- Side effects of acupuncture are extremely rare. The use of disposable sterile acupuncture needles avoids the risk of cross-contamination. Occasionally, patients may experience bruising at the acupuncture site. Mild transient drowsiness may also occur. Pneumothorax is the most frequently reported serious complication related to acupuncture. Acupuncture can be considered safe when performed by competent and experienced licensed providers.
- Acupuncture as a therapeutic intervention is widely practiced in the United States. There are promising results supporting its efficacy for adult postoperative and chemotherapy-related nausea and vomiting and for postoperative dental pain. There are reasonable studies that conclude that the use of acupuncture results in satisfactory treatment of addiction, stroke rehabilitation, headache, menstrual cramps, tennis elbow, fibromyalgia, myofascial pain, osteoarthritis, low back pain, carpal tunnel syndrome, and asthma.
- Acupuncture may be used as a complementary treatment or acceptable alternative therapy or be integrated into a comprehensive management program.
- The LI 4, he gu, acupuncture point is located between the first and second metacarpal bones in the deep depression of the web space.
- The PC 6, nei guan, acupuncture point is located three fingerbreadth proximal to the transverse crease of the wrist, a deep depression between the tendons of the long palmar muscle and the radial flexor muscle of the wrist.

SUGGESTED READINGS

Acupuncture. NIH Consensus Statement. *JAMA.* 1997;15:1-34.

Han JS. Acupuncture and endorphins. *Neurosci Lett.* 2004;361:258-261.

Lin YC. Perioperative usage of acupuncture. *Paediatr Anaesth.* 2006;16:231-235.

Lin YC, Tassone RF, Jahng S, et al. Acupuncture management of pain and emergence agitation in children after bilateral myringotomy and tympanostomy tube insertion. *Paediatr Anaesth.* 2009;19:1096-1101.

Linde K, Allais G, Brinkhaus B, et al. Acupuncture for migraine prophylaxis. *Cochrane Database Syst Rev.* 2009;1:CD001218.

Linde K, Allais G, Brinkhaus B, et al. Acupuncture for tension-type headache. *Cochrane Database Syst Rev.* 2009;1:CD007587.

Manheimer E, White A, Berman B, et al. Meta-analysis: acupuncture for low back pain. *Ann Intern Med.* 2005;142:651-663.

Sun Y, Gan TJ, Dubose JW, et al. Acupuncture and related techniques for postoperative pain: a systematic review of randomized controlled trials. *Br J Anaesth.* 2008;101:151-160.

Thomas KJ, Macpherson H, Thorpe L, et al. Randomised controlled trial of a short course of traditional acupuncture compared with usual care for persistent non-specific low back pain. *BMJ.* 2006;333:623.

The references for this chapter can be found at www.expertconsult.com.

49 Integrative Approaches to Pain Management

Delia Chiaramonte | Chris D'Adamo | Brian Morrison

INTEGRATIVE MEDICINE: OVERVIEW

Integrative medicine is a philosophy of care that integrates conventional allopathic medical therapies with modalities not typically included in conventional care and addresses the physical, emotional, and spiritual needs of the patient. This field of medicine is sometimes referred to as complementary medicine or complementary and alternative medicine (CAM). However, these terms refer more precisely to modalities such as acupuncture, meditation, nutritional supplements, and massage, all of which may be included in the integrative medicine "tool box." In 2005 the Consortium of Academic Health Centers for Integrative Medicine defined integrative medicine as follows:

The practice of medicine that reaffirms the importance of the relationship between practitioner and patient, focuses on the whole person, is informed by evidence, and makes use of all appropriate therapeutic approaches, health-care professionals and disciplines to achieve optimal health and healing.

The use of complementary medicine modalities in the United States is increasing. One study found that 62% of adults had used some form of complementary therapy in the previous 12 months.[1] The most commonly used CAM therapies were prayer for the improvement of health, natural products, deep-breathing exercises, meditation, chiropractic care, yoga, massage, and diet-based therapies. It is estimated that in 1997, between $36 and $47 billion was spent on CAM therapies in the United States.[2]

Pain syndromes, such as chronic back pain, appear to be increasing and are associated with significant health care costs.[3] Unresolved pain has a wide-reaching impact in that it affects physical, emotional, and spiritual wellness and has a negative impact on social and occupational functioning. Integrative medicine, which adopts a mind-body approach to the treatment of pain and uses multiple effective CAM modalities, is well suited to address chronic pain syndromes. In 2002, 6% of the U.S. population used complementary medicine modalities for the treatment of back pain and 60% of respondents who used CAM for back pain perceived a "great deal" of benefit.[4]

MULTIDIMENSIONAL PERCEPTION OF PAIN

Perception of pain is multifactorial and involves a complex interplay between the peripheral and central nervous systems. As pain signals reach the brain from the periphery, the brain can modify these signals by activating inhibitory pathways and releasing substances such as endorphins and neurotransmitters. Alternatively, the brain can magnify nociceptive signals if they are perceived to be threatening, thus increasing the perception of pain. Connections between the cerebral cortex and the limbic system allow the brain to give meaning to the pain experience. It is this connection between emotions and pain perception that forms the basis of the mind-body approach to pain. Psychological factors such as the tendency to catastrophize have been associated with chronic pain,[5] and the literature suggests a clear link between psychological variables and neck and back pain.[6] Life stress in childhood[7] or adulthood[8] can be associated with adult pain syndromes, and anxiety and chronic pain often coexist.[9] Depression and pain are related, with each negatively affecting the other,[10] and negative emotional states of any kind can increase the severity of pain. Even brief interventions designed to address the emotional components of pain have been effective in decreasing its severity.[11]

Using real-time functional magnetic resonance imaging (fMRI) to guide training, subjects were able to learn to control regions of the brain involved in pain perception and regulation, specifically, the rostral anterior cingulate cortex (rACC).[12] When activation of the rACC was intentionally increased or decreased, there was a simultaneous change in the perception of pain from an experimentally induced pain. Subjects who trained with sham real-time fMRI did not show a similar change in pain perception. In addition, chronic pain patients who were trained to control activation of the rACC reported decreased levels of chronic pain after training. This experiment illustrates that patients can learn to control specific regions of the brain that are involved in pain perception, thus learning to exert control over their own pain. This is a form of biofeedback and contributes to scientific understanding of the mind-body connection.

Neuroimaging studies have shown that social pain and physical pain are reflected similarly in the brain. In one study, subjects played a virtual game that elicited feelings of being excluded. The rACC showed an increase in activity during exclusion—physiologic changes that are similar to those seen with physical pain.[13] In addition, hypnotic suggestion of pain has been shown to create changes on fMRI in the rACC, thalamus, insula, prefrontal cortex, and parietal cortex, which are also influenced by pain originating in peripheral tissues.[14] This suggests that pain initiated by the brain has significant similarity to pain originating in the periphery. This concept highlights the mind-body connection and is important for understanding and treating patients with acute and chronic pain.

INTEGRATIVE MEDICINE MODALITIES AND PAIN

Varied complementary medicine techniques have shown benefit in the treatment of pain. Domains such as traditional Chinese medicine (TCM), mind-body medicine, manual medicine, and others have an increasing body of evidence supporting their use for management of pain. The most commonly used and well-supported modalities are discussed in the following sections.

ACUPUNCTURE AND TRADITIONAL CHINESE MEDICINE

TCM is an inclusive medical system based on 3000-year-old ancient texts. It incorporates varied treatment modalities, including acupuncture, acupressure, Chinese herbal medicine, meditative movement such as tai chi and qi gong, moxibustion, cupping, and specialized massage techniques referred to as tui na.

Acupuncture and TCM are based on the theory that health is determined by the balance of vital energy flow, called qi (pronounced "chi"), which is thought to be present in all living creatures. TCM uses concepts such as yin and yang and dampness and wind, which have no equivalents in conventional medicine and are therefore difficult to explain in standard medical terms. "Yin" represents the concept of cold, slow, and passive, whereas "yang" represents energy that is hot, fast, and active. Health is believed to be based on a balance of these and other opposing forces, such as dampness and dryness, and to require free flow of qi. Disease is thought to arise from an imbalance in these forces. Imbalance leads to blockage of qi (vital energy) along specified pathways. In all organisms, qi is believed to flow through particular channels called meridians, and TCM therapies are used to unblock the flow of qi. Unlike conventional medicine, treatment plans are highly individualized and based on an individual's constitution, as assessed by the TCM provider, as well as on the individual's symptoms. Thus, two patients with identical complaints might receive entirely unique treatment plans based on their baseline characteristics.

Acupuncture points are located along the recognized meridians, and the process of acupuncture involves the insertion of thin needles into these points. Although meridians cannot be visualized anatomically, acupuncture points often correspond to depressions in muscles, bones, or neural foramina and may have their own neurovascular bundle that distinguishes the acupuncture point from surrounding tissue.[15] They are often palpable and may be tender to palpation.

The mechanism of action of acupuncture, from a conventional medicine point of view, has not been unequivocally determined. Theories on the efficacy of acupuncture include release of endorphins and neurotransmitters, enhanced local immune response, enhanced circulation and smooth muscle relaxation, stimulation of tissue growth and repair, and spinal and peripheral nerve stimulation. Substantial evidence supports the theory that acupuncture creates physiologic change at the site of needle insertion, in the cerebral cortex, and in the release of hormones and endorphins.[15] Endorphin levels in cerebrospinal fluid have been shown to rise after acupuncture treatment.[16]

Despite abundant evidence supporting the use of acupuncture for varied medical conditions, there are particular challenges in conducting research on acupuncture that may affect the results. Acupuncture has no true placebo control, and sham acupuncture has sometimes been shown to be as effective as true acupuncture.[17] Inserting needles in "sham" acupuncture points might elicit physiologic changes, and even sham acupuncture needles that press but do not puncture the skin may approximate the effects of acupressure if they are used at specified acupuncture points. In addition, standardized acupuncture treatments are often used in research in an effort to provide a standardized and replicable approach. That is, all patients with back pain would receive acupuncture at the same acupuncture points. However, this does not replicate the individualized treatment approach to acupuncture used in practice, thus creating a research environment that does not reflect real-life conditions.

Acupuncture is used for a wide variety of health conditions and is also used by those without specific symptoms to maintain optimal health. It is most commonly used for relief of musculoskeletal pain. A 2001 review on acupuncture safety found that minor adverse events were common but serious adverse events were rare. The most commonly reported adverse events were needle pain (1% to 45%), tiredness (2% to 41%), nausea or vomiting (0.01% to 0.2%), and slight bleeding or bruising (0.03% to 38%). Feeling faint was very rare (0% to 0.3%), and pneumothorax was extremely rare—occurring only twice in nearly a quarter of a million treatments.[18]

Laws concerning the practice of acupuncture are defined by each state. Practitioners may include licensed acupuncturists who have completed more than 1000 hours of training at a college of Oriental medicine or masters-level program, chiropractors who may receive some training within their professional course of study and may choose to pursue additional postgraduate training, and physicians and dentists who pursue acupuncture training after completing their professional programs. Most programs targeted to physicians, chiropractors, and dentists include approximately 200 to 400 hours of training. Board certification is available to physicians through the American Board of Medical Acupuncture. Acupuncture styles differ and can include traditional Chinese acupuncture, five-element acupuncture, Korean or Japanese acupuncture, and auricular acupuncture. Evidence of superiority of one form over the others is not available.

A Cochrane review on acupuncture for pain found that it was effective for migraines, neck disorders, tension-type headaches, and peripheral joint osteoarthritis.[19] One well-designed randomized controlled trial of acupuncture for the treatment of knee osteoarthritis involved 507 patients recruited from two university outpatient clinics. The patients were randomized into one of three groups: true acupuncture, sham acupuncture, or education control. The primary outcomes measured were changes in the Western Ontario and McMaster Universities Osteoarthritis Index (WOMAC) pain and function scores at 8 and 26 weeks. Secondary outcomes were patient global assessment, 6-minute walk distance, and physical health scores on the 36-Item Short-Form Health Survey (SF-36). Participants in the true acupuncture group experienced significantly greater improvement in the WOMAC function score than did both the sham acupuncture and education groups at 8 weeks, but not in the WOMAC pain score or patient global assessment. At 26 weeks, the true acupuncture group experienced significantly greater improvement than did the sham and education groups in the WOMAC function score, WOMAC pain score, and patient global assessment. The authors concluded that acupuncture can be used as adjunctive therapy for the treatment of knee osteoarthritis.[20] Another randomized controlled trial in which acupuncture was added to advice and exercise in patients with osteoarthritis showed only small improvements in pain and no superiority of true acupuncture over sham acupuncture.[21]

A recent Cochrane review of acupuncture revealed that sham-controlled trials show statistically significant benefits; however, these benefits are small and may be due partly to placebo effects from incomplete blinding.[22] Acupuncture has been shown to improve chronic low back pain symptoms in some studies,[23] but not in others.[24] However, another Cochrane review of acupuncture for the treatment of chronic tension-type headache suggested that acupuncture could be a valuable nonpharmacologic tool for patients with frequent episodic or chronic tension-type headache.[25] A recent meta-analysis using individual patient data evaluated the efficacy of acupuncture for the treatment of chronic pain. Data from 29 studies of back and neck pain, osteoarthritis, chronic headache, and shoulder pain were evaluated, and true acupuncture was found to be more effective than either sham acupuncture or nonacupuncture control in decreasing pain.[26]

Thus, although the evidence is suggestive that acupuncture is beneficial for the treatment of varied pain syndromes, the picture is not entirely clear. Expectation of benefit, possible physiologic action of supposed sham controls, different styles of acupuncture, and acupuncture research protocols that may not match the "real-life" practice of acupuncture all create some uncertainty regarding the effectiveness of acupuncture for the treatment of pain. On the other hand, a mounting body of evidence suggests acupuncture to be beneficial when added to conventional care, with clear evidence of safety.

MIND-BODY MEDICINE

The term *mind-body medicine* does not refer to a specific treatment modality; rather, it refers to a group of modalities that are unified by the underlying concept of an intricate connection between the mind and the body. The physical, emotional, spiritual, and social aspects of our lives have an impact on health and well-being, and dysfunction in one domain can lead to dysfunction in another. Mind-body medicine asserts that the mind can positively affect the body in the pursuit of health and wellness. Our daily experience makes it clear that the mind can affect physiology. Blushing from social embarrassment results from increased blood flow to the face, frightening movies can increase cardiovascular vital signs, and sexually stimulating visual material can increase blood flow to the penis. Similarly, psychological stress can lead to clear physiologic changes, most of which are potentially harmful. Chronically elevated blood pressure, muscular tension leading to headaches or neck pain, and the increased incidence of chronic pain syndromes may all be associated with stress. Pain and stress are interconnected, and a vicious cycle is often generated in which pain causes stress and subsequently stress causes more pain. Mind-body techniques can provide an improved ability to cope with pain, decreased perception of pain, and an increased sense of well-being and relaxation. The psychological tendency to catastrophize has been associated with increased pain perception,[27] and mind-body techniques can help temper this anxious state.

The relaxation response is a physical state or reaction that counteracts the physiologic and emotional responses to stress and is essentially the opposite of the fight-or-flight response. It was first described by Herbert Benson and colleagues at Harvard Medical School in the 1970s.[28] Just as eliciting the stress response can generate unhelpful physiologic changes, eliciting the relaxation response can result in health-inducing physiologic effects. The relaxation response is different from simply relaxing with a book or in front of the television. Although these activities may be considered "relaxing," they do not generate the physiologic changes associated with the relaxation response. The relaxation response is elicited by focusing the mind on a particular word, phrase, breath, image, or action and adopting a passive attitude toward one's thoughts. Modulation of cardiovascular parameters, muscular relaxation, and normalization of stress hormones such as cortisol, epinephrine, and norepinephrine are all associated with the relaxation response.

Mind-body techniques are varied and become easier to do with practice. Techniques include abdominal breathing, meditation, guided imagery, biofeedback, yoga, tai chi, qi gong, therapeutic arts, and even prayer. No mind-body technique is intrinsically more effective than another, and all can be used to decrease stress and elicit the relaxation response. Some involve movement and stretching, whereas others are practiced in seated or recumbent positions. They can be performed in groups, with an individual instructor, or alone. Patients may choose to try different mind-body techniques to find one, or several, that they prefer. Mind-body techniques have been shown to be helpful for varied conditions such as osteoarthritis, rheumatoid arthritis, headaches, procedural pain, and stress management.[29] Specific mind-body techniques are described in the ensuing paragraphs.

PROGRESSIVE MUSCLE RELAXATION

Progressive muscle relaxation is a technique commonly used for eliciting the relaxation response and relieving muscular tension. It is easy to learn and is accessible even to people who may not be familiar with or interested in meditation. It involves sequentially relaxing various muscle groups, often starting at the head and moving down the body to the feet. Participants may tense a muscle before relaxing it (for example, clenching the jaw and then releasing it) or simply bring their attention to a muscle group and intentionally relax it. A sample progressive muscle relaxation script is provided in Appendix A.

MEDITATION

The term *meditation* refers to a broad variety of practices that are similar in form but may be quite distinct in intention. Depending on the culture and tradition of the meditator, meditation may be used to induce relaxation, increase vital energy ("qi" or "prana"), attain closeness to God, or induce a state of contemplation or ultimate consciousness. Many religious faiths, both Western and Eastern, include meditative practices within their traditions, and in the past 40+ years, more secular versions of meditation have gained popularity. These forms of meditation are generally considered relaxation techniques, and they involve an intentional focus on the act of breathing, a sound, an object, a phrase, or a movement. The goal of these forms of meditation is generally to increase awareness of the present moment, elicit the relaxation response, reduce stress, and enhance personal growth.

Two common forms of meditation used in the West are mindfulness meditation and concentrative meditation. In mindfulness meditation, participants direct their full attention to their breathing by focusing on each inhalation and exhalation. When thoughts, feelings, or sensations arise, the meditator simply notices and accepts them nonjudgmentally and brings attention back to the breath. In concentrative meditation, attention is focused intently on one thing such as an object (a candle) or a sound or on a word or phrase, which is repeated silently with each breath cycle. Common words and phrases might include "peace" with inhalation and "love" with exhalation or "all will/be well."

Practicing focused attention in the present moment and nonjudgmental acceptance of experiences or thoughts decreases the mind's tendency to worry about the future or ruminate about the past. It has also been found to be useful in pain conditions. In one interesting study of experimental pain, subjects were taught mindfulness meditation, which they practiced 20 minutes daily for 3 days. The investigators measured pain sensitivity before and after meditation training and found decreased sensitivity after 3 days of meditation. The authors believed that the increased ability to tolerate pain was related to decreased anxiety and an increased ability to focus on the present moment.[30]

Mindfulness meditation has also been used successfully in older adults with chronic low back pain. Patients were randomized to an 8-week mindfulness meditation group or a wait-list control. The meditators had statistically significant improvements in pain acceptance, activity engagement, and physical functioning.[31] Qualitative assessment of the same subjects revealed that meditation was beneficial for pain, sleep, attention, and well-being.[32] It has also been shown to decrease the severity of bowel symptoms in women with irritable bowel syndrome, with benefits lasting for at least 3 months after mindfulness training.[33]

GUIDED IMAGERY

Guided imagery is the generation of specific mental images to evoke a state of relaxation or physiologic change. It takes advantage of the communication links between the mind and the body and uses the imagination to generate intentional physiologic states, such as relaxation or relief of pain. It can be performed with a therapist and patient in person or by a patient alone listening to a recording.

One study of fibromyalgia patients randomized subjects to either 6 weeks of daily guided imagery audiotapes or usual care. People in the guided imagery group had statistically significant improvements in their ability to cope with fibromyalgia, with a decrease in the Fibromyalgia Impact Questionnaire (FIQ) score and increased self-efficacy in managing pain.[34] Interestingly, the imagery dose was not significantly associated with outcome. This lack of dose-response relationship suggests that even using guided imagery infrequently might be beneficial. Guided imagery has also been shown to be beneficial for tension-type headache,[35] recurrent abdominal pain in children,[36] and musculoskeletal pain,[37] although large, higher-quality studies are needed to confirm these results.

There is suggestive evidence that guided imagery is helpful in the perioperative period. It has been shown to reduce length of hospital stay and pharmacy costs[38] and to decrease postoperative pain.[39] A study of patients undergoing colorectal surgery showed that guided imagery significantly reduced postoperative pain, anxiety, and narcotic requirements while increasing patient satisfaction.[40]

HYPNOSIS

Hypnosis involves leading the patient into a focused, trance-like state. By concentrating attention intensely on one specific thought, memory, feeling, or sensation and blocking out all distractions, patients become calm, relaxed, and open to hypnotic suggestion. Health-inducing suggestions can be offered, including a decrease in anxiety or pain. Patients' free will remains intact during hypnosis, and they cannot be led against their will to actions that are dangerous to themselves or others.

There is evidence supporting the use of hypnosis for various pain syndromes such as chronic pain, cancer, osteoarthritis, sickle cell disease, temporomandibular disorder, fibromyalgia, non–cardiac-related chest pain, and disability-related chronic pain.[41] In a review of hypnosis for procedure-related pain in children, hypnosis was consistently found to be more effective than control conditions in alleviating the discomfort of bone marrow aspiration, lumbar puncture, voiding cystourethrography, the Nuss procedure, and postsurgical pain.[42] Hypnosis decreased anxiety and depressed mood in patients about to undergo excisional breast biopsy.[43]

YOGA

Yoga originated in India but is now widely practiced throughout the world and is generally used to improve relaxation, strength, and flexibility. Yoga's combined focus on mindfulness, breathing, and physical movements is health inducing for the mind and the body. Several styles of yoga are commonly practiced in the United States, including Hatha, Vinyasa, Ashtanga, Iyengar, Anusara, and Bikram, and each has unique intentions and techniques. Hatha yoga may be more appropriate for beginners, whereas Ashtanga yoga tends to be more physically demanding. "Power yoga" classes are appropriate for people seeking aerobic exercise, and they are often modifications of the Ashtanga style. Bikram yoga, often referred to as "hot yoga," is practiced in a room heated to between 95° F and 100° F, and Iyengar yoga is particularly concerned with bodily alignment.

Yoga is often used as a relaxation practice, but it has also been shown to be helpful for pain conditions. In one study, yoga was found to be more effective than a self-care book but equal to a stretching regimen in relieving chronic low back pain. The benefits lasted for several months.[44] Iyengar yoga was also found to reduce pain intensity, functional disability, and depression, and patients with chronic low back pain showed a trend toward decreased use of pain medication when compared with controls.[45] Six months after the intervention, the yoga group still showed decreased functional disability, pain intensity, and depression when compared with the control group.

In a systematic review of yoga interventions, 9 of 10 randomized controlled trials suggested that yoga leads to a significantly greater reduction in pain than do the various control interventions, such as standard care, self-care, therapeutic exercises, touch and manipulation, or no intervention. The authors noted, however, that study quality was less than ideal and definitive judgment was not possible.[46]

TAI CHI AND QI GONG

Tai chi and qi gong are ancient meditative movement techniques that combine standardized physical movements with meditation and relaxation breathing techniques. They have been used for thousands of years in China and as part of TCM theory and are thought to unblock and balance vital energy ("qi"). In the United States, tai chi and qi gong are often used to relieve stress, improve balance, and reduce pain. These techniques use conscious, often slow movements and focus on goals different from those of conventional Western exercise, such as developing consciousness within the body and enhancing the smooth flow of energy.

One study found that tai chi improves immunity and resistance to the virus that causes shingles in older adults,[47] and several have shown benefits in alleviating osteoarthritis symptoms.[48-50] A Cochrane review of the medical literature showed that tai chi may be helpful in rheumatoid arthritis patients by increasing range of motion of the ankle, hip, and knee. Patients enjoyed the exercise and reported subjective improvement.[51]

Practice of qi gong has been shown to decrease weight, waist circumference, and insulin resistance and to increase leg strength.[52] It might therefore be useful for patients with weight- and deconditioning-related painful conditions such as knee osteoarthritis, although in a meta-analysis of internal qi gong it was not shown to improve chronic pain syndromes.[53] Very few high-quality studies of qi gong for pain have been published, and thus more evidence is needed to evaluate the utility of qi gong for pain conditions.

A recent review of the medical literature found significant beneficial health effects of tai chi and qi gong. The authors reviewed 77 articles reporting the results of 66 randomized controlled trials of the health effects of tai chi or qi gong in more than 6000 patients. Control groups included nonexercise controls, exercise controls, or both. The most convincing evidence of health benefits in this review was for bone density, cardiopulmonary fitness, prevention of falls, balance, quality of life, and self-efficacy.[54]

Tai chi has also been shown to benefit patients with fibromyalgia. A single-blind, randomized trial of tai chi versus an attention control was recently published in the *New England Journal of Medicine*.[55] The intervention group received tai chi instruction and practiced twice per week for 12 weeks, whereas the control group received an equivalent amount of wellness education and stretching. Subjects who practiced tai chi had highly statistically significant decreases in FIQ scores, and the benefit was maintained at 24 weeks. No adverse events were noted.

THERAPEUTIC ART AND MUSIC

Creative arts can be used in the therapeutic environment to relieve stress, anxiety, and pain in patients and caregivers.[56,57] Art therapy has been used to stimulate relaxation in the palliative care setting,[58] as distraction from the negative side effects of bone marrow transplantation[59] and to increase patient empowerment.[60]

Music therapy was more effective in decreasing anxiety in ventilated patients in the intensive care unit than was an uninterrupted period of rest,[61] and it was more effective than treatment as usual or scheduled rest in decreasing anxiety, pain, and pain-related distress in patients after open heart surgery.[62] Patients randomly assigned to music during colposcopy had decreased pain and lower anxiety than did a non–music therapy group.[63]

A Cochrane review of music therapy in people with cancer assessed 30 trials with a total of 1891 participants. They used music from multiple sources, including recorded music and music provided by trained music therapists, and found that music interventions may have beneficial effects on pain, anxiety, mood, and quality of life in people with cancer.[64]

ENERGY MEDICINE

Energy medicine modalities, sometimes called biofield therapies, are based on the idea that all living creatures have energy that can be manipulated in the pursuit of health by a trained practitioner.

A recent 3-year study of 118 chemotherapy patients investigated the role of Reiki in the management of anxiety, pain, and global wellness in cancer patients. Pain and anxiety were evaluated with a visual analog scale (VAS). In patients who received the full treatment course (four Reiki sessions), mean VAS anxiety scores decreased from 6.77 to 2.28, which was a highly significant result. Mean VAS pain scores also decreased from 4.4 to 2.32, but this did not reach statistical significance.[65] Another small study of the use of Reiki in community-dwelling older adults found significant improvements in pain, depression, and anxiety in patients who received Reiki,[66] whereas another found a highly significant reduction in pain of varied causes after Reiki treatment.[67]

A Cochrane review of touch therapies for pain evaluated the evidence for the efficacy of therapeutic touch, healing touch, and Reiki. Randomized controlled trials or controlled clinical trials evaluating the effect of touch on any type of pain were included. Twenty-four studies involving 1153 participants met the inclusion criteria, and only studies using a sham placebo or a "no treatment" control were included. Small, but statistically significant effects were found in patients receiving touch therapy. Interestingly, experienced practitioners of Reiki appeared to be slightly more effective. Two of the five studies evaluating analgesic use suggested that touch therapies minimized analgesic use.[68]

Despite the presence of evidence suggesting that Reiki and related therapies are effective in controlling pain, the evidence is contradictory. Distant Reiki was not found to be effective in controlling pain in women after cesarean section.[69] A review of the Reiki literature found that most trials suffered from methodologic flaws such as small sample size, inadequate study design, and poor reporting. The authors concluded that the evidence is insufficient to suggest that Reiki is an effective treatment of any condition.[70] In another systematic review, 9 of the 12 trials detected a significant therapeutic effect of the Reiki intervention. However, using the Jadad quality score, 11 of the 12 studies were ranked "poor."[71] Thus, although Reiki is probably safe and may be effective in relieving pain and anxiety, higher-quality studies are needed to clarify its clinical indications.

MANUAL THERAPIES

The term *manual therapy* is nonspecific and refers to techniques that use the hands to diagnose and treat disorders of the musculoskeletal system. It is often used to treat a variety of painful musculoskeletal conditions, and several studies have demonstrated its effectiveness.[72-77] Many studies show a significant effect on pain and improvement in outcome measures, although in some cases the effect size is small.[72,75,78] Manual therapy may be performed by physical therapists, chiropractors, massage therapists, osteopathic physicians, and others and may include techniques such as craniosacral therapy and osteopathic manipulative techniques (OMTs).

Practitioners of manual therapy generally believe that musculoskeletal problems arise from abnormal movement patterns or postures, which lead to asymmetrical musculoskeletal forces and subsequent pain. Examples of musculoskeletal asymmetry that can lead to painful conditions include chronic elevation of one shoulder when carrying a heavy purse, abnormalities in tissue texture after prolonged immobilization, and forward head carriage associated with desk work, computer use, and prolonged sitting causing intervertebral disk deformation.

Several models attempt to explain the mechanisms by which manipulation or manual therapy modulates pain. There are three primary models:

Structural model: Misaligned structures impinge on nerves and stress soft tissues, thereby stimulating nociceptors. Common terminology includes "subluxation," "pelvic obliquity," "leg length inequality," and "torsion." It is believed that correction of these misalignments via manual methods eliminates pain.

Functional model: Muscular imbalance leads to abnormal joint loading, which in turn causes loss of joint function at the level of accessory motion. Terminology includes "somatic dysfunction," "biomechanical lesion," "blockage," "muscular inhibition/facilitation," and "instability/stabilization." Syndromes include upper and lower crossed syndromes,[79,80] each characterized by specific patterns of muscular facilitation (tightness) and inhibition (weakness). For example, upper crossed syndrome is characterized by facilitation or "tightness" of the upper trapezius, levator, sternocleidomastoid, and pectoralis muscles, whereas the deep cervical flexors, lower trapezius, and serratus anterior muscles are inhibited and weak. Practitioners use rehabilitative exercise and manipulation with the intention of correcting the imbalance and reducing nociceptive input. This is the current model presented in most chiropractic, physical therapy, and osteopathic programs.

Neurophysiologic model: This model is consistent with the emerging concept that the pain experience is a central nervous system output that is modulated by multiple factors such as stress, anxiety, fear avoidance, experience, and context in the brain's "neuromatrix."[80] Wellens proposed that manual therapy introduces a novel stimulation into the central nervous system that may help the brain downregulate the perceived threat of nociceptive stimuli, thereby decreasing the pain by descending inhibition and other peripheral and central mechanisms. This in turn may stimulate a change in the maladaptive motor responses produced by the brain in response to pain. Other reflexive reactions at the spinal cord level may affect temporal summation and downregulate the value (threat) of the nociceptive input even more.[81] Even though this model is hypothetical, there is an impressive emerging body of supportive literature.[82-85]

It is likely that manual therapy provides pain relief through an interplay of all three models. Future research may help determine each model's relative contribution.

Myofascial pain syndrome is a chronic musculoskeletal pain condition with a poorly defined and somewhat controversial pathophysiology. It may emerge after tissue injury, chronic stress-related muscular contraction, or excessive strain on a muscle, tendon, or ligament. Tender regions of hyperirritable, contracted muscle fibers, called trigger points, may form in the affected muscle group and cause local and referred pain. Myofascial trigger points are palpable, tender nodules within skeletal muscle that have characteristic referred pain patterns and physiologic activity that are different from those in normal muscle tissue.[86] Trigger points may be treated with physical therapy, massage, transcutaneous electrical stimulation, selective voluntary contraction of antagonist muscles or muscle groups,[87] injection of saline or local anesthetic medications, dry needling, or application of coolant spray combined with focused muscular stretching. Botulinum toxin has also been used.[88]

MASSAGE

Massage refers to the application of varied techniques to the muscles, ligaments, tendons, and related structures in the pursuit of health and wellness. Massage may be performed with the hands, elbows, forearms, or feet, as well as with appliances such as warmed stones. There are many types of massage, each with unique techniques and goals, such as Swedish massage, trigger point massage, reflexology, and lymphatic drainage.

Massage is often used to address pain syndromes such as back pain, neck pain, and sports injuries, as well as to aid in stress reduction and generation of the relaxation response. It has been found to improve symptoms of osteoarthritis of the knee[89] and chronic low back pain, decrease medication use and medical costs,[24,90,91] and decrease perception of cancer pain.[92]

It is not clear whether some forms of massage are superior to others or whether all are equally effective. One recent study randomized 401 patients with nonspecific low back pain to relaxation massage, structural massage, or usual care and assessed their symptoms with the Roland Disability Score and the Symptom Bothersome Score. Participants were blinded to the type of massage but not to massage versus usual care. At 10 weeks, both massage groups had statistically significant improvements in both outcome measures when compared with those receiving usual care.[93]

Although massage is generally safe for healthy populations, it can be dangerous in certain circumstances.

Contraindications include, but are not limited to metastatic lesions, severe osteoporosis, thrombosis, infections or wounds, active inflammatory conditions, and bleeding disorders.

CHIROPRACTIC

Doctors of chiropractic focus primarily on the interaction between the structure and the function of the body, with particular attention paid to the spine. Historically, the primary goal was to correct musculoskeletal misalignments (subluxations) to relieve nerve pressure and thus alleviate pain and improve the body's innate self-healing capability. The primary modality of chiropractic manipulative therapy is high-velocity, low-amplitude (HVLA) thrust manipulation (spinal adjustment). Adjustments generally involve use of the hands or a device to apply an intentional, controlled, rapid force to a joint or body segment thought to have impaired alignment or restricted motion. Restored intersegmental motion or joint position is believed to improve both function and general health. There are multiple chiropractic techniques, each with its own unique set of diagnostic and treatment protocols. Some use very little force, whereas others can be quite aggressive. The most common technique encountered is termed "diversified" and encompasses HVLA maneuvers for all joints of the spine and extremities. In addition to manual therapies, chiropractors may incorporate relaxation techniques, dietary guidance, nutritional supplements, physical therapy modalities, and rehabilitative exercise into their treatment plans. The combination of HVLA manipulation and rehabilitative exercise appears to provide the best outcomes.[94]

Most patients who choose chiropractic care do so because of back and neck problems. Patients are generally satisfied with their chiropractic care.[95] Although some have expressed concern that chiropractic treatment of the neck increases the risk for stroke, a large study that included more than 100 million person-years showed that these concerns are unfounded.[96] Debate on this topic persists.[97,98]

A systematic review of randomized clinical trials of manual therapies evaluated the evidence for spinal manipulation or mobilization in treating several different conditions, including 13 musculoskeletal conditions and headaches. The authors reviewed 49 systematic reviews, 16 evidence-based clinical guidelines, and an additional 46 randomized clinical trials not yet included in systematic reviews and guidelines. They found spinal manipulation to be effective in adults for acute, subacute, and chronic back pain, migraine and cervicogenic headache, and cervicogenic dizziness, and thoracic manipulation or mobilization was determined to be effective for acute and subacute neck pain.[77]

Research is inconsistent regarding the efficacy of spinal manipulation or mobilization for the treatment of neck pain. One study found spinal manipulation or mobilization to be effective in improving neck pain symptoms when combined with exercise but not when used alone,[99] but a literature review found chiropractic spinal manipulation to be ineffective for neck pain.[100] A more recent Cochrane review detected a suggested benefit but also noted the need for higher-quality studies to confirm the result.[75] A 2011 study provided evidence suggesting that HVLA manipulation of the cervicothoracic and upper cervical segments is superior to mobilization techniques for the relief of neck pain.[101]

OSTEOPATHIC MANIPULATION

Doctors of osteopathy earn their DO degree from 1 of 26 osteopathic medical schools in the United States and are approved for the unlimited practice of medicine in all 50 states, the District of Columbia, and U.S. territories. Their scope of practice includes the ability to prescribe medications and perform surgery. Osteopathic medical education is similar to that found in allopathic medical schools, with the added focus on a holistic and preventive approach to medicine. In addition, osteopathic physicians learn OMT, which is not included in the allopathic medical school curriculum. OMT is a hands-on practice that attempts to restore normal movement and function and decrease pain.

Osteopathic physicians may choose any specialty and can earn board certification from both osteopathic and allopathic medical boards. Some osteopathic physicians complete allopathic residencies and practice indistinguishably from allopathic physicians, whereas others remain committed to osteopathic principles and practices.

Osteopathic principles include working in partnership with patients to facilitate wellness and prevent disease and the concept that structure influences function. That is, a structural problem in one part of the body may affect function in that region and possibly others. Osteopaths generally believe that the body has an innate ability for self-healing, and OMT techniques are thought to support this process.

OMT procedures are directed at increasing mobility in restricted areas of musculoskeletal function and reducing pain. Some practitioners focus on pain relief, whereas others are more interested in the influence of increased mobility within the system. The stated goal of OMT is to restore maximal, pain-free movement of the musculoskeletal system in postural balance.[102] Techniques include a muscle energy technique, mobilization with and without impulses, indirect technique, myofascial release, and integrated neuromusculoskeletal technique.[102]

OMT has been demonstrated to be effective for neck pain[103] and migraine headache symptoms, with pain intensity, functional disturbance, and days of disability all showing improvement when compared with control.[104] A systematic review and meta-analysis of OMT for low back pain concluded that OMT significantly reduces low back pain symptoms, with the effect lasting at least 3 months.[105]

Orthopedic manual therapy is the name given to manual therapy as practiced by physical therapists. Manual therapy has only recently been introduced as part of the core physical therapy curriculum, with most practitioners gaining knowledge and skills through continuing education or fellowships. Physical therapists trained in manual therapy use techniques such as stretching, mobilization, manipulation, and muscle energy–related techniques to increase range of motion, improve function, modulate pain, decrease tissue inflammation, and facilitate tissue repair.

Practitioners of manual medicine may be trained as physical therapists, osteopathic physicians, chiropractors, and to some extent, massage therapists, and strict distinction between practice styles and techniques is lacking. A standardized knowledge base with certification available to all relevant practitioners would be valuable. It is not clear whether one profession will eventually "own" manual medicine or whether a new specialty will emerge. One suggested model is to offer fellowships in manual medicine with board certification that would be available to physical therapists, chiropractors, osteopathic physicians, allopathic physicians, and massage therapists.

HOMEOPATHY

The field of homeopathy was developed by the German physician Samuel Hahnemann at the end of the 18th century in an effort to find a way to trigger the body's natural ability to heal disease. Homeopathic medicines, called "remedies," are made at homeopathic pharmacies by using a specialized process of dilution and shaking, called succussion. Remedies, which are often in tablet form, are individualized, and patients with the same symptom may be given very different remedies. Homeopathy is based on two principles that may be challenging for conventional health practitioners to accept: the "law of similars" and the "law of minimum dose." The "law of similars" suggests that the substance that is most helpful for a disease or symptom is one that causes these same symptoms in a healthy person. For example, if a substance causes sleeplessness when taken at full strength, it might be used to treat insomnia homeopathically.

The "law of minimum dose" is based on the principle that the efficacy of a remedy increases as the dose is decreased. Homeopathic remedies are serially diluted, often until the remedy no longer contains any molecules of the original medication. The diluent, frequently water, is thought by homeopaths to be "imprinted" by the original substance, thus imparting therapeutic efficacy.

Most rigorous clinical trials and systematic analyses of the research on homeopathy have concluded that there is little evidence to support homeopathy as effective treatment of any specific condition.[106] However, some reviews have found suggestions of positive results,[107] and a randomized, controlled study of homeopathic treatment of fibromyalgia showed significant decreases in tender points in the treatment group.[108] One randomized, double-blind controlled trial of homeopathy for rheumatoid arthritis showed that it was the homeopathic consultation rather than the remedy itself that led to positive outcomes.[109] Anecdotal claims of the efficacy of homeopathic treatments are common from both practitioners and users of homeopathy, and the remedies tend to be safe. Large, well-designed studies are needed to clarify the effectiveness of homeopathy for varied health conditions.

BIOLOGICALLY BASED PRODUCTS: HERBS, NUTRACEUTICALS, AND NUTRITIONAL SUPPLEMENTS

A large body of clinical evidence supports the use of biologically based natural products for the alleviation of pain. This supportive evidence for pain reduction spans a wide variety of herbs, nutraceuticals, nutritional supplements, and food-derived topical products. Although the majority of the evidence assessed the effects of these products on osteoarthritis pain, there is also evidence from well-designed clinical trials supporting the use of natural products for rheumatoid arthritis, neuropathy, persistent neck and back pain, dysmenorrhea, and inflammatory bowel disease. The following products have the strongest evidence supporting their use for the reduction of pain.

CAPSAICIN

Capsaicin is derived from chili peppers of the genus *Capsicum,* which includes the cayenne pepper commonly used in cooking. Topical application of gel ranging from a 2.5% to 8% concentration of capsaicin is used to provide pain relief. The primary mechanism through which capsaicin is believed to reduce pain is depletion of substance P, a neuropeptide involved in the transmission of pain signals from nerve endings to the brain, as well as the activation of inflammatory cytokines in joints.

Many high-quality, randomized, double-blind placebo-controlled trials have found that topical application of capsaicin is an effective treatment of osteoarthritis pain. A meta-analysis found that topical capsaicin in concentrations between 2.5% and 7.5% was four times as effective as placebo in reducing osteoarthritis pain.[110] No serious side effects were noted in these trials, although a burning sensation following topical application of capsaicin at these concentrations is common. Motivated by the relatively common sensation of burning experienced at these concentrations, a recent trial assessed topical application of capsaicin at a concentration of 1.25% in 100 patients with osteoarthritis of the knee.[111] Capsaicin at this lower concentration was effective in improving pain. Even though a mild burning sensation was common, no participants dropped out of the study for this reason. Consequently, lower concentrations of topically applied capsaicin appear to be an effective treatment option for mild to moderate osteoarthritis pain.

Although most capsaicin research to date has focused on osteoarthritis pain, several recent studies have assessed its efficacy for neuropathic pain.[112-114] Transient application of a dermal patch containing 8% capsaicin has been shown to be an effective option for reducing neuropathic pain. The patch was applied for between 30 and 90 minutes in these studies and repeated, as required, every 90 days. The capsaicin patch was generally well tolerated in these studies. However, as has been the case in studies using capsaicin gel, irritation localized to the site of application was the most common adverse event.

BOSWELLIA SERRATA

Extracts of the *B. serrata* plant have been used as an important component of Ayurvedic medicine for thousands of years. Western science has validated the traditional use of *B. serrata* for pain inasmuch as its extracts elicit powerful anti-inflammatory activity through its inhibition of the 5-lipoxygenase (5-LOX) enzyme. Several forms of *B. serrata* have been studied and used clinically, including traditional 60% to 70% extracts of *B. serrata* gum resin, as well as the commercial preparations Aflapin and 5-Loxin.

Five randomized controlled trials have been conducted to assess the effects of *B. serrata* on the pain associated with osteoarthritis of the knee.[115-119] All these trials found statistically and clinically significant reductions in pain. Symptoms improved as early as 5 days after treatment commenced. In one trial, the reduction in pain persisted 1 month after the conclusion of treatment. The lasting reduction in pain is a unique benefit of *B. serrata* when compared with traditional pharmacologic therapies for pain. Daily dosages used in these studies were 333 mg of 65% standardized *B. serrata* extract, 100 mg of Aflapin, and 250 mg of 5-Loxin. *B. serrata* was well tolerated in all trials, and very few side effects were noted aside from minor gastrointestinal distress in some participants.

GLUCOSAMINE AND CHONDROITIN

Numerous meta-analyses have determined that glucosamine, either combined with chondroitin or alone, is an effective treatment of osteoarthritis pain.[120-122] A meta-analysis of 16 randomized, double-blind studies found glucosamine to be significantly more effective than placebo and more effective than or equal to nonsteroidal anti-inflammatory drugs (NSAIDs) with minimal adverse effects. Another review of randomized trials of both glucosamine and chondroitin found moderate to large effect sizes (0.44 and 0.78, respectively). A large randomized controlled trial ($N = 212$) published since the aforementioned reviews[75] found that patients taking 1500 mg of oral glucosamine sulfate daily for 3 years experienced no significant joint space loss and minimum joint space narrowing when compared with patients taking placebo.[123]

Despite the abundance of positive evidence for glucosamine and chondroitin, the large Glucosamine/chondroitin Arthritis Intervention Trial (GAIT) found mixed results, which are often misinterpreted.[124] This five-arm trial compared glucosamine alone, chondroitin sulfate alone, glucosamine/chondroitin sulfate, and celecoxib with placebo. Participants in the glucosamine/chondroitin group did not demonstrate a statistically significant improvement over placebo in the primary outcome (20% improvement in the WOMAC pain score) of the overall study sample of patients with osteoarthritis of the knee (mild [$n = 1229$] vs. moderate to severe [$n = 354$]). However, 67% of the overall study sample in the glucosamine/chondroitin group experienced at least a 20% improvement in pain with a trend toward statistical significance ($P = 0.09$). The lack of statistical significance at the $P = 0.05$ level was thought to be due to the unexpectedly high improvement in the placebo group (60.1%). Furthermore, among the 354 participants with moderate to severe osteoarthritis of the knee, 79% of those in the glucosamine/chondroitin combination group experienced at least a 20% improvement in the WOMAC pain score, which was statistically significant when compared with placebo ($P = 0.002$). Interestingly, participants with moderate to severe arthritis pain in the celecoxib group did not demonstrate statistically significant improvement when compared with placebo, a finding that is rarely reported. Although a statistical comparison between the glucosamine/chondroitin and celecoxib groups was not reported in the paper, glucosamine/chondroitin was shown to be more effective than celecoxib in patients with moderate to severe osteoarthritis.

Even though the findings from the more than 50 randomized controlled trials of glucosamine/chondroitin for osteoarthritis pain have not been universally positive, consideration of the body of evidence suggests that glucosamine/chondroitin is a safe and at least moderately effective treatment of osteoarthritis pain. A daily dose of 1500 mg glucosamine and 1200 mg chondroitin has been studied most frequently and is the typical recommended dosage.

S-ADENOSYLMETHIONINE

The reduction in joint pain provided by *S*-adenosylmethionine (SAM-e) was first observed as side effects in clinical trials for depression. Produced from L-methionine and adenosine triphosphate, SAM-e is a methyl donor involved in a wide variety of metabolic processes. Although its mechanism of action is not completely understood, SAM-e has been shown to possess anti-inflammatory and analgesic effects without causing gastrointestinal damage in animal models. SAM-e has also demonstrated chondroprotective effects through stimulation of chondrocytes and a subsequent increase in cartilage production.

A meta-analysis of 13 clinical trials revealed that SAM-e is comparable to ibuprofen and superior to placebo in reducing osteoarthritis pain.[125] A large randomized controlled trial published subsequent to this review compared the efficacy of SAM-e with that of celecoxib in patients with osteoarthritis pain.[126] This study found that SAM-e was as effective as celecoxib in relieving pain after 16 weeks of treatment. The onset of pain relief is slower than with some pharmacologic pain relievers, but SAM-e has no known side effects. Most clinical trials to date have used a daily dosage of between 400 and 1600 mg.

ω-3 FATTY ACIDS

Dietary ω-3 fatty acids, including α-linolenic acid (ALA), eicosapentaenoic acid (EPA), and docosahexaenoic acid (DHA), can interrupt the production of inflammatory compounds such as prostaglandin E_2, leukotriene B_4, interleukin-1β, and tumor necrosis factor-α. ω-3 Fatty acids also inhibit the platelet-activating factor synthesis pathway, the cyclooxygenase pathway, and the 5-lipoxygenase pathway. Accordingly, ω-3 fatty acids are known to play an important role in modulating the inflammatory cascade and the pathophysiology of autoimmune conditions. Chief among the conditions affected by ω-3 fatty acids is rheumatoid arthritis.

ω-3 Fatty acids have been shown in numerous systematic reviews to reduce the pain and joint tenderness of rheumatoid arthritis.[127-130] Multiple studies have also found that ω-3 supplementation can reduce dependence on NSAIDs and antirheumatic drugs.[131-134] In addition to reduction of the pain associated with rheumatoid arthritis, ω-3 fatty acids have also been determined to be effective in reducing neck and back pain,[135] neuropathic pain,[136] and the pain from inflammatory bowel disease and dysmenorrhea.[137] No significant toxicities have been associated with the use of ω-3 fatty acids, although patients taking anticoagulant medications should be mindful of the potential for interaction.

The ω-3 fatty acids EPH, DHA, and ALA are not produced endogenously in human beings and must be obtained through the diet. Dietary sources of ω-3 fatty acids include salmon, sardines, and other cold-water fish, fish and krill oil, and plant oil from flaxseed or walnuts. Although all forms of ω-3 fatty acids are important, EPA and DHA have direct anti-inflammatory effects and are more easily used by the body.[138] Conversion from ALA to EPA and DHA is poor, particularly in men.[139] Consequently, the optimal forms of ω-3 fatty acids taken for therapeutic purposes to relieve painful conditions are EPA and DHA. Therefore, most studies to date have investigated the effects of fish oil because of its high concentration of EPA and DHA. These studies show that a minimum daily dosage of 3 g of EPA and DHA is required for clinical efficacy in pain conditions. Benefits in alleviating pain generally become apparent after a period of at least several weeks.

SUMMARY

An integrative approach to the treatment of pain that incorporates complementary medicine approaches into the care plan can provide clinical benefit with minimal additional risk. An understanding of the mind-body connection and its relevance to pain perception and treatment is important for the care of patients with both acute and, especially, chronic pain. Biologically active products, mind-body therapies, and manipulative and body-based treatments can all benefit patients with pain. Energy medicine and homeopathy have some evidence of benefit, although more research is needed. Large, well-designed studies of diverse complementary medicine modalities are needed to confirm which modalities are best suited to which conditions.

KEY POINTS

- The integrative approach to pain management takes into account the biopsychosocial etiology of pain and provides effective tools not conventionally used by allopathic physicians.
- Patients' level of anxiety, psychological characteristics such as the tendency to catastrophize, and the meaning assigned to the pain experience can significantly affect the perception of pain.
- Acupuncture has shown efficacy in relieving migraines, neck disorders, tension-type headaches, and osteoarthritis and may improve chronic low back pain.
- The term "mind-body medicine" refers to a group of modalities, such as guided imagery, qi gong, and meditation, that are unified by the belief that the mind and body can positively affect each other in the pursuit of health and wellness.
- Mind-body techniques have been shown to be helpful in varied conditions such as osteoarthritis, rheumatoid arthritis, headache, procedural pain, and stress management.
- Guided imagery may be particularly helpful in the perioperative period to decrease pain, opioid use, and length of hospital stay.
- Manual therapy may be helpful in varied pain syndromes and may be performed by osteopathic physicians, appropriately trained allopathic physicians, chiropractors, physical therapists, and to some extent, massage therapists.
- Osteopathic manipulative treatment has been shown to be helpful for neck pain, migraine headaches, and low back pain.
- Biofield therapies and homeopathy have evidence suggesting benefit in patients with pain syndromes, but more robust studies are needed.
- Capsaicin, *Boswellia serrata*, glucosamine/chondroitin, S-adenosylmethionine, and ω-3 fatty acids are the biologically based products with the strongest evidence supporting their use for the treatment of pain.

SUGGESTED READINGS

Astin JA. Mind-body therapies for the management of pain. *Clin J Pain.* 2004;20:27-32.

Clegg DO, Reda DJ, Harris CL, et al. Glucosamine, chondroitin sulfate, and the two in combination for painful knee osteoarthritis. *N Engl J Med.* 2006;354:795-808.

Halpin LS, Speir AM, CapoBianco P, et al. Guided imagery in cardiac surgery. *Outcomes Manag.* 2002;6:132-137.

Kanodia AK, Legedza AT, Davis RB, et al. Perceived benefit of complementary and alternative medicine (CAM) for back pain: a national survey. *J Am Board Fam Med.* 2010;23:354-362.

Karels CH, Bierma-Zeinstra SM, Burdorf A, et al. Social and psychological factors influenced the course of arm, neck and shoulder complaints. *J Clin Epidemiol.* 2007;60:839-848.

Lee MS, Chin EE. Acupuncture for pain: an overview of Cochrane reviews. *J Integr Med.* 2011;17:187-189.

Licciardone JC, Brimhall AK, King LN. Osteopathic manipulative treatment for low back pain: a systematic review and meta-analysis of randomized controlled trials. *BMC Musculoskelet Disord.* 2005;6:43.

Rakel D. *Integrative Medicine.* 3rd ed. St. Louis: Elsevier; 2012.

Reginster JY, Deroisy R, Rovati LC, ed. et al. Long-term effects of glucosamine sulphate on osteoarthritis progression: a randomised, placebo-controlled clinical trial. *Lancet.* 2001;357:251-256.

Sikdar S, Ortiz R, Gebreab T, et al. Understanding the vascular environment of myofascial trigger points using ultrasonic imaging and computational modeling. *Conf Proc IEEE Eng Med Biol Soc.* 2010;2010:5302-5305.

United Kingdom back pain exercise and manipulation (UK BEAM) randomized trial: effectiveness of physical treatments for back pain in primary care. UK BEAM Trial Team. *BMJ.* 2004;329:1377.

Williams KA, Petronis J, Smith D, et al. Effect of Iyengar yoga therapy for chronic low back pain. *Pain.* 2005;115:107-117.

Zeidan F, Gordon NS, Merchant J, et al. The effects of brief mindfulness meditation training on experimentally induced pain. *J Pain.* 2010;11:199-209.

The references for this chapter can be found at www.expertconsult.com.

A Appendix

Find a comfortable position where you won't be interrupted. You may sit up or lie down, however you are most comfortable.

You will be focusing your attention on your body for the next few minutes. If your mind wanders, simply bring your attention back to your body.

Take a deep breath into your abdomen while trying to push your belly button out as you breathe in. Hold your breath for a few seconds, and then slowly breathe out. Take another deep breath while trying to push out your belly button as you take in a healing breath.…Hold for a few seconds…then slowly release your breath.

As you exhale, imagine the tension in your body being released and flowing out of your body. And again inhale… hold…and exhale. Feel your body beginning to relax.

Now tighten the muscles in your forehead by raising your eyebrows as high as you can. Hold for about 5 seconds. And abruptly release and feel that tension fall away.

Pause for about 10 seconds. Now smile widely and feel your mouth and cheeks tense. Hold for about 5 seconds, and release; noticing the softness in your face. Now just breathe slowly for about 10 seconds while feeling your face relax more and more with each breath.

Next, tighten your eye muscles by squinting your eyelids tightly shut. Hold for about 5 seconds and release.

Pause for about 10 seconds while breathing slow, relaxing breaths.

Now lift your shoulders up as though they could touch your ears. Hold for about 5 seconds and release quickly while feeling their heaviness. Pause for about 10 seconds; feel your arms getting heavy and warm as you continue to breathe slow, relaxing breaths.

Tense your upper back by pulling your shoulders back while trying to make your shoulder blades touch. Hold for about 5 seconds and release.

Pause for about 10 seconds while breathing slow, relaxing breaths.

Tighten your chest by taking a deep breath in, hold it for about 5 seconds, and exhale to blow out all the tension.

Breath in…and out. In…and out. Let go of all the stress. In…and out.

Now, tightly but without straining, clench your fists. Hold for about 5 seconds and release.

Pause for about 10 seconds. Now, flex your biceps. Feel that buildup of tension. You may even visualize that muscle tightening. Hold for about 5 seconds, release, and enjoy that feeling of limpness. Breath slowly in…and out.

Now tighten your triceps by extending your arms out and locking your elbows. Hold for about 5 seconds and release. Pause for about 10 seconds while imagining that all your stress and tension are leaving your body through your fingertips.

Now tighten the muscles in your abdomen by sucking your abdomen in. Hold for about 5 seconds and release. Pause for about 10 seconds while breathing slowly deep into your abdomen and notice your belly button moving away from your body with each inhalation.

Gently arch your lower back. Hold for about 5 seconds and relax. Pause for about 10 seconds.

Feel the limpness in your upper body letting go of the tension and stress, hold for about 5 seconds, and relax. Your arms are heavy and warm…the tension is leaving your body through your fingertips.

Tighten your buttocks. Hold for about 5 seconds…, release, and imagine your hips falling loose. Pause for about 10 seconds while breathing slow, relaxing breaths.

Tighten your thighs by pressing your knees together. Hold for about 5 seconds…and release.

Pause for about 10 seconds. Now flex your feet, pull your toes toward you, and feel the tension in your calves. Hold for about 5 seconds and relax; feel the weight of your legs sinking down. Pause for about 10 seconds.

Curl your toes and tense your feet. Hold for about 5 seconds and release. Pause for about 10 seconds.

Now imagine a wave of relaxation slowly spreading through your body beginning at your head and going all the way down to your feet.

Breathe in…and out…in…out…in…out.

Adapted from Bourne EJ. *The Anxiety and Phobia Workbook.* Oakland, New Harbinger Publications Inc., 2005.

50

Pain and Addictive Disorders: Challenge and Opportunity

Edward C. Covington | John A. Bailey

It is essential that pain specialists have an understanding of addiction since patients with both conditions are increasingly being encountered in pain clinics and are among the most challenging that we see. Addiction not only alters the experience of pain[1] but also changes the reporting of it. Trough levels of opioids in addicts may create hyperalgesia,[2] and reinforcing drugs may increase "pain behavior" (see Treisman and Clark[3]). Addiction impairs function and thereby directly antagonizes efforts to promote functional restoration in pain management. Pain is also likely to be augmented by the dysphoria associated with addiction.[4,5] The risk for trauma and medical complications of addiction have an impact on pain treatment and may worsen outcomes. Finally and perhaps of greatest concern to pain specialists, addiction carries the risk that misuse will cause our treatments to become harmful to patients.

The actual prevalence of addiction in those with chronic pain is unknown, and reports vary from 1% to 40%. Reasons for this variability include differences in time frame (past 30 days vs. lifetime, for example), different definitions, failure to obtain full information, and different patient populations, among others.[6] It is clear that many patients with chronic noncancer pain (CNCP) have comorbid substance use disorders (SUDs),[7] especially those receiving chronic opioid therapy (COT) for pain.[8] In a recent comparison of *Diagnostic and Statistical Manual of Mental Disorders*, Fourth Edition (DSM-IV), and proposed DSM-V criteria for addiction, Boscarino and coworkers found that 35% of patients receiving COT for pain had an opioid use disorder.[9] Similarly, addiction treatment facilities have found that an increasing proportion of their admitted patients, up to 61%, suffer from chronic pain.[10-12] Clearly, the extent of pain and addiction comorbidity requires that pain specialists be able to competently treat patients with both.

The presence of comorbid addiction complicates the treatment of pain in numerous ways. Patients can be argumentative and unpleasant, and providers unprepared to deal with them may either give in to unreasonable demands or inappropriately refuse to provide care. The former error not only leads to patient harm but also leaves the provider vulnerable to sanctions.[13]

Addiction also complicates pain management because of the fact that individuals with previous addictions are the ones most likely to have problems when prescribed therapeutic opioids. The pain clinician has an obligation to screen for this risk before prescribing opioids and to be skillful in directing the patient to appropriate care if addictive behavior develops during treatment.

THE EPIDEMIC OF PRESCRIPTION OPIOID ABUSE AND ADDICTION

Media attention has created general awareness that there has been a "dark" side to the liberalization of opioid prescribing, which began in the late 1980s. The epidemic of prescription analgesic abuse now exceeds the use of cocaine and heroin combined.[14] As opioid sales have increased, there has been a parallel increase both in admissions to addiction treatment facilities and in overdose deaths.[15] Fatal poisonings involving opioids more than tripled between 1999 and 2006, from approximately 4000 to 13,800.[16]

The relationship between opioid addiction and opioid treatment of pain is a complex one. A review by Minozzi and colleagues found that it is rare for pain treatment to result in opioid addiction,[17] and the majority of abused prescription drugs are obtained from illicit sources rather than from a single, legitimate prescriber.[18] However, in a sample of patients entering treatment for opioid dependence, Cicero and coworkers found that more than 80% had been exposed via a therapeutic prescription, which they then abused. Most had a previous SUD during their early or late teens and had received multiple treatments of substance use.[19] Weisner and associates studied 4 million customers of two large insurance companies and found that those with an identified SUD were more likely to receive schedule II opioid prescriptions, received opioids in higher doses for longer periods, and were more likely to receive concomitant sedative-hypnotics than were those without an SUD.[20]

These studies sound much more contradictory than they in fact are. Together, they portray a situation in which therapeutic opioids do not usually lead to addiction; however, they are commonly prescribed to people who have or have had an SUD. Furthermore, prescription recipients contribute heavily, intentionally or inadvertently, to drugs that are abused in society, often with disastrous results.

Thus, this epidemic is of concern to pain specialists for three reasons: (1) a large percentage of patients being prescribed COT suffer from comorbid addiction (often unknown to the prescriber) and are therefore at increased risk for harm; (2) the abused drugs are frequently diverted from legitimate prescriptions, thereby creating an obligation for the prescriber to be vigilant for signs of diversion, to be responsible in performing and responding to toxicology screens, and to educate patients regarding the necessity for secure handling and storage of prescription medications; and (3) patients with previous SUDs are at high risk for "transferring" their addiction to prescribed opioids.

DEFINITIONS

There is disagreement concerning the optimal definition of addiction. The American Psychiatric Association and the World Health Organization both wished to avoid stigmatizing patients with the label "addict" and therefore substituted the word *dependence*. Unfortunately, this had the effect of creating ambiguity. The problem is the inevitable confusion between the terms *dependent* and *physically dependent* (which refers to the normal development of the potential for a withdrawal syndrome in nearly all continuous users of dependence-producing drugs). This chapter uses the terms "addict" and "addiction" for the sake of clarity and brevity. We recognize addiction as a disease that arose not because the patient intended it, but despite efforts to avoid it. The individual is thus the victim of the disease, not a perpetrator, and the term is not used disparagingly.

ADDICTION AND SUBSTANCE DEPENDENCE

In an effort to use a common taxonomy, the American Society of Addiction Medicine, the American Pain Society, and the American Academy of Pain Medicine formed a consensus panel to define tolerance, physical dependence, and addiction. They adopted the following definition[21]:

Addiction is a primary, chronic, neurobiologic disease, with genetic, psychosocial, and environmental factors influencing its development and manifestations. It is characterized by behaviors that include one or more of the following: impaired control over drug use, compulsive use, continued use despite harm, and craving.

Since the biologic changes that are the essence of addiction are not clinically detectable, the diagnosis must be based on behavioral abnormalities and patient reports. The current standard criteria for substance dependence are those of the DSM-IV[22]; however, these criteria will be obviated by the publication of DSM-V, scheduled for May 2013. The DSM-IV term *substance dependence disorder* closely approximates what is generally considered to be addiction; nonetheless, accurate diagnosis is contingent on attention to the paragraph preceding the bulleted criteria, which requires "a maladaptive pattern of substance use" that leads to "clinically important distress or impairment." Without this, many nonaddicted patients receiving COT would meet the criteria for a substance use diagnosis. These and other criteria not only risk diagnosing addiction in its absence but can also contribute to failure to diagnose the condition when present because the detrimental effects of drug use on lifestyle and psychosocial functioning may be less evident in pain patients and, when they do occur, are likely to be ascribed to pain rather than to drug use.

The proposed DSM-V criteria for "opioid use disorder" will require a maladaptive pattern of use leading to significant impairment or distress, as manifested by at least two of the following occurring within a 12-month period (the criteria have been abbreviated)[23]:

1. The opioid is often taken in larger amounts or over a longer period than intended.
2. There is a persistent desire or unsuccessful efforts to cut down or control use.
3. A great deal of time is spent on activities necessary to obtain, use, or recover from the effects of the opioid.
4. Recurrent use results in failure to fulfill major role obligations.
5. Use is continued despite persistent or recurrent social or interpersonal problems caused or exacerbated by the substance.
6. Important social, occupational, or recreational activities are reduced because of use.
7. Use occurs in situations in which it is physically hazardous.
8. Use is continued despite knowledge of a persistent or recurrent physical or psychological problem likely to have been caused or exacerbated by the opioid.
9. Tolerance is present (not counted for those taking medications under medical supervision).
10. Withdrawal occurs (not counted for those taking medications under medical supervision).
11. There is craving or a strong desire or urge to use the opioid.

There are many idiosyncratic definitions created by governmental and health-related organizations. For example, the Controlled Substances Act defines an "addict" as a person who "habitually uses any narcotic drug so as to endanger the public morals, health, safety, or who is so far addicted to the use of narcotic drugs as to have lost power of self-control with reference to his addiction."[24]

PHYSICAL DEPENDENCE

It must be emphasized that "drug dependence" is not synonymous with "physical dependence," which is normal and to be expected with prolonged use of opioids and does not indicate the presence of any disorder. In fact, physical dependence, as manifested by withdrawal on administration of naloxone, can be elicited in normal subjects following a single dose of morphine,[25] which confirms that this phenomenon is not useful as a diagnostic criterion in patients taking prescribed opioids.

Physical dependence is neither necessary nor sufficient for the diagnosis of SUD. It commonly occurs with substances that lack addictive potential and is universal in those taking significant doses of prescribed opioids or benzodiazepines on a continuous basis. It is said to be present if a withdrawal syndrome occurs on cessation of use, dose reduction, or administration of an antagonist.[26,27] Physical dependence can be a major issue in addiction to opioids and alcohol, is minimal with cocaine and amphetamines,[28-30] and is absent in addiction to hallucinogens and inhalants. It can be a major problem with discontinuation of such nonreinforcing substances as paroxetine, venlafaxine, some antiepileptics, clonidine, and baclofen.

TOLERANCE

Tolerance is a state of adaptation in which exposure to a substance induces physiologic changes that diminish its effects.

It develops more rapidly in some individuals than in others. It develops with effects such as sedation from antiepileptics, nausea from serotonin-norepinephrine reuptake inhibitors, and hypotension from clonidine. Tolerance usually develops rapidly to opioid-induced sedation, itching, and nausea and more slowly to analgesia and may not develop at all to constipation. Because of tolerance, patients who take a stable dose of opioids on a scheduled basis can usually safely return to work and drive.[31,32]

Analgesic tolerance is one of the reasons that opioids are more effective for acute than for chronic pain.[33-37] Clinically, patients who have severe pain despite high doses of opioids often report that low to moderate doses of opioids initially produced satisfactory analgesia. It is important to explain tolerance to patients. They should understand that efforts to regain initial analgesia through repeated dose escalation can lead to falls, fractures, and fatalities, as well as side effects such as low testosterone and opioid-induced hyperalgesia. Strategies for reducing tolerance include opioid rotation and the addition of adjunctive medications that are opioid sparing.

PSEUDOADDICTION

Pseudoaddiction describes a state in which inadequate analgesia leads to behavior that mimics addictive behavior. This drug-seeking behavior improves when the pain is controlled. Although the concept is simple, in practice, both undermedicated patients in pain and patients with actual addiction may be drug seeking, and both cease drug seeking, at least transiently, when their needs are met. So the distinction is often made with difficulty and usually in retrospect (i.e., when the patient's behavior normalizes for an extended period after adequate pain control is provided).[38,39]

DRUG MISUSE

Drug abuse and misuse are defined in various ways that have in common the fact that the drugs either were not prescribed or were used in a manner different than instructed. They differ from addiction in that those who abuse drugs can choose to quit in the event of adverse consequences. The term *chemical coping* has been used to describe persons who use opioids to ameliorate uncomfortable emotion. For example, opioids may reduce fear of cancer. They temporarily decrease depression, anxiety, anger, and symptoms of post-traumatic stress disorder (PTSD). In fact, there is some evidence that PTSD may share a common neurobiology with addiction, which in part accounts for their high comorbidity[40] (for review, see Logrip and colleagues[41]).

NEUROBIOLOGY OF ADDICTION

Increased understanding of the neurobiology of addiction has had both medical and cultural benefits as the traditional views of addicts as people who were immoral or lacking in willpower have become untenable.[42] It is established that neural mechanisms evolved that link behavior necessary to survival (e.g., acquisition of food, sex, and nurture) to dopaminergic (DA) activity in the ventral tegmental area and the nucleus accumbens. These areas are involved in salience, reward, expectation of reward, and habit.[43] In other words, important or pleasurable activities increase midbrain dopamine. Importantly, all rewarding drugs also act in the ventral tegmental area and nucleus accumbens to increase DA function, a remarkable fact given that some are sedatives, others stimulants, and others analgesics. Since reinforcing drugs increase dopamine even more than natural rewards do, our brains are hardwired to experience pleasure from and attach importance to these drugs. Thus, recreational drug use in essence hijacks neurologic systems that are essential for survival. Evidence that release of dopamine with opioid use is attenuated in animals that have chronic inflammatory or neuropathic pain may explain the observation that people are less likely to become addicted after opioid use for pain than after use for euphoria.

Imaging also implicates dysfunctional activity in the prefrontal cortex (PFC) in addiction. This functionally heterogeneous structure plays a crucial role in regulating limbic reward regions and higher-order executive functions, including self-control, judgment, salience attribution, and awareness. In addiction, PFC dysfunction is thought to impair impulse control. PFC dysfunction could also explain patients' lack of awareness of their addiction in the face of overwhelming evidence.[44] This decreased awareness, or "denial," is a hallmark of addiction and a barrier to treatment acceptance.

It has become clear that addictive behavior has other driving forces. For example, negative reinforcement results from both withdrawal anhedonia and the anxiety driven by sympathetic rebound.[4] Important insights have been provided by study of what have been called opponent processes.[45] Many drugs elicit homeostatic mechanisms that antagonize some or all of their effects; in fact, withdrawal symptoms typically consist of processes that oppose a drug that is no longer present. Thus, sedative withdrawal is characterized by stimulation, stimulant withdrawal is associated with lethargy, withdrawal of constipating drugs causes diarrhea, and stopping anticonvulsants (e.g., benzodiazepines) can produce seizures.

It has been shown that processes are engendered by euphorigenic drugs that oppose euphoria and create dysphoria. As drug use continues, euphoria diminishes, whereas dysphoria increases, can be intense, and is relieved only by the substance of abuse. Thus, the transition from drug use to addiction involves stages. Recreational users are initially motivated by positive reinforcement (i.e., substance use generates a pleasurable state). However, after the transition to addiction, negative reinforcement is increasingly determinative; people use substances not so much to feel good as to avoid feeling bad. With continued use, release of dopamine in response to dosing is reduced, whereas release of corticotropin-releasing factor (a "stress hormone"), adrenocorticotropic hormone, corticosterone, norepinephrine, and neuropeptide Y during periods of abstinence is increased. It is believed that the decrease in reward function combined with the recruitment of antireward systems provides a powerful negative reinforcement that contributes to compulsive drug seeking and addiction.[46,47] Furthermore, the transition from controlled use to compulsive drug seeking seems to be associated with the migration of control neural circuitry to the more dorsal areas of the striatum that are involved in habit and compulsion.[48]

Heroin addicts often report that they have spent years trying without success to recapture the highs that they experienced when they initiated use or, more commonly, that they no longer use heroin to get high but only to stop feeling bad. In this way, recreational addicts are similar to those with chronic pain—their use is motivated primarily by a desire to end suffering, not to achieve euphoria. The brain changes result in an increase in the perceived importance of drug-related issues, a reduction in the perceived importance of other things, and diminished impulse control over use.

It is well known that marked physical and emotional distress can result from abrupt drug discontinuation; however, it is less commonly appreciated that subsequent to the resolution of obvious symptoms, during the so-called post-acute withdrawal period, there may be persistent anhedonia and depression. The endogenous opioid systems may take months to normalize, during which time patients may experience insomnia, anxiety, depression, inability to concentrate, clumsiness, and disturbing dreams.[49-51] Recent studies suggest that a specific set of genetic transcriptional regulations may underlie protracted abstinence symptoms from compounds as disparate as nicotine, alcohol, tetrahydrocannabinol (THC), and morphine.[52] This could in part explain the vulnerability of abstinent addicts to the development of addiction to an unrelated substance.

Some of the neuroplastic changes associated with addiction are thought to be permanent,[53] which may explain why addiction is associated with a lifelong vulnerability to relapse. Fortunately, the likelihood of relapse decreases with time, as well as with continued participation in an ongoing recovery program.

DEVELOPMENT OF ADDICTION

Addictive behavior is heavily influenced by genetic factors. Selective breeding easily produces animals that have a strong baseline propensity to self-administer rewarding drugs and other animals that require high doses and prolonged exposure to develop evidence of "drug liking."[54,55] These studies, as well as twin studies and family hereditary patterns, support the belief that vulnerability to addiction is partially genetic. Animal and human imaging suggests that those more vulnerable to addiction have decreased baseline DA activity and may therefore attach even more importance to dopamine-elevating drugs.[56] Vulnerability to addiction is also influenced by life events. Childhood physical, sexual, and emotional trauma, as well as major adult stress,[57] is important in this regard.

Previous exposure to a rewarding substance can increase consumption of subsequent substances,[58,59] and previous drug abuse or addiction increases the likelihood of future SUDs; for example, those who have smoked tobacco or marijuana may have increased vulnerability to other SUDs.[60]

Factors that promote *addiction* should be distinguished from those that trigger *relapse* in individuals with prior addiction. Common triggers include drug exposure, environmental stimuli (people, places, and things associated with drug use), and stress.[61]

Many people incorrectly attribute addictive behavior to psychiatric comorbidity and believe that if the underlying psychiatric disorder is corrected, the addiction will go away. In fact, although patients may believe that their substance use would cease if they were relieved of their anxiety, depression, panic, or stress, experience shows that such is rarely the case.

CROSS-ADDICTION

A tenant of most addiction treatment and education is the concept that a person addicted to one reinforcing substance is at high risk for addiction to all such substances and should therefore abstain even from substances that have never been problematic. This caution is based on two considerations: (1) a person who takes an intoxicant is less able to resist other temptations (e.g., a person working on nicotine abstinence is more likely to relapse after a few drinks), and (2) the neurologic changes that occur with addiction appear to be common to most substances (i.e., the changes in people with alcohol dependence and those with opioid dependence are similar). Thus, it makes sense to caution those attempting to recover from opioid dependence to avoid alcohol, benzodiazepines, carisoprodol, and illicit substances. Unfortunately, there are few data to confirm these beliefs other than the high prevalence of polysubstance abuse or dependence, which shows that people who develop one SUD often develop several (see Compton and colleagues[62]).

IATROGENIC ADDICTION

Although COT can cause physical dependence, trigger relapse in those recovering from addiction, and elicit addiction in some, it is clear that preexisting vulnerability plays a critical role in this process. Early in the last century it was often believed that anyone who used opioids chronically became addicted.[63] However, the distinction between physical dependence and addiction was not appreciated and therefore addiction rates were probably exaggerated.[42]

Until recently, many believed that addiction was *rare* in those who took long-term opioids to treat pain, unlike those who sought euphoria or relief from emotional distress. Now, concern is being raised that opioid therapy is causing a wave of addiction. Probably much of the uncertainty and disagreement relate to the distinction between those who *have* an addiction and are treated with COT versus those who have an addiction *because* they were treated with COT. The ambiguity surrounding triggering addiction versus triggering relapse is also a confounder.

Even though most pain specialists believe that iatrogenic addiction is uncommon, there are few data to determine its exact incidence.[17] Extant studies are largely poorly done and brief. Accurate data are frequently difficult to obtain, and there is often ambiguity not only about the presence of addiction but also about the time of its onset. It is widely believed that the risk for inducing an addictive disorder with *short-term* opioid therapy is extremely low, around 3 per 1000. However, there seems to be no data on this question beyond two very old studies, both widely cited and widely criticized on methodologic grounds.[64,65] Nonetheless, clinical experience supports their findings in that it is quite rare to see patients in whom iatrogenic addiction has developed as a result of brief treatment. Unfortunately, these early studies addressing *acute* opioid therapy have been cited as evidence of the safety of *chronic* opioid therapy, which they did not address.

IATROGENIC RELAPSE

Several studies suggest that the vast majority of patients who manifested addiction while being treated long-term with opioids had preexisting drug or alcohol disorders. For example, in a retrospective study of 48 patients hospitalized for addiction to oxycodone (OxyContin), Potter and associates[66] found that 77.1% reported previous nonopioid substance use problems (including alcohol) and 48% had prior problems with other opioids. Similarly, an older study of 200 patients with chronic low back pain found that substance abuse preceded the pain in 94% of those with both conditions.[67] In a highly selected group of patients undergoing pain rehabilitation, our group found that of those with an addictive disorder, medical exposure was responsible in 33%, recreational use in 64%, and undetermined causes in 3%.[68] Needless to say, the proportion of patients in a pain clinic who became addicted medically would be much higher than the proportion in the community.

It seems that most patients thought to have iatrogenic addiction instead had a recreationally induced addiction that transformed into prescription use or were abstinent addicts who relapsed on re-exposure to opioids. The latter is predictable given that animal[69] and human[70] studies have demonstrated that one of the most powerful stimuli for eliciting resumption of dormant drug-seeking behavior is re-exposure to the drug of choice. A recovering heroin addict came to our attention who had maintained sobriety for longer than 1 year until exposed to intravenous midazolam for procedural sedation. He experienced an immediate onset of drug craving, subsequently obtained and injected heroin, to which he was no longer tolerant, and died. Studies are lacking to clarify the risk for relapse if, for example, a patient who has been sober from alcoholism for a number of years is exposed to COT. However, based on animal studies and observation, most addiction specialists believe that ingestion of alcohol or any reinforcing drug may increase craving for the addict's drug of choice and other reinforcing drugs.

The brain changes that underlie addiction are multifactorial, and it appears that the development of addiction is a function of the molecule involved, dose administered, duration of use, genetic and personal vulnerability, and perhaps route and rate of administration. Thus, in a patient with no predisposition, COT would be unlikely to trigger addiction, whereas in those with high vulnerability, addiction might develop easily and early.[71] Such patients would be likely to have a history of nicotine dependence or overuse of alcohol or other substances.

In addition to vulnerability and length of exposure, the substance itself plays a role. For example, drugs that rapidly and markedly increase dopamine (e.g., crack cocaine) often produce addictive behavior quickly. Other drugs, such as alcohol, seem to take much longer for most. Furthermore, the delivery system plays a role, with slow-onset preparations such as chewed tobacco or coca leaves producing addiction more slowly than cigarettes or smoked cocaine. This suggests that opioids that rapidly enter the central nervous system (CNS), such as fentanyl given by the intravenous or transmucosal route, may be more likely to trigger addiction or relapse than the same molecule administered transdermally.[72,73]

DETECTING AND PREDICTING ABUSE AND ADDICTION

SCREENING AND UNIVERSAL PRECAUTIONS

Appropriate screening takes considerable time, which can lead providers to neglect it. A self-report questionnaire can facilitate this task and help ensure adequate information to guide the prescriber. If the state has an electronic prescription-monitoring program (42 of 50 do so as of this writing[74]), this should be reviewed and compared with the patient's information. One of the most valuable ways to detect addiction is by interviewing the patient's relatives or significant others. They may be both more honest in revealing signs of addiction and more aware than the patient of such issues as drug-induced sedation, cognitive impairment, and changes in personality.

Legitimate patients (as opposed to scammers) generally understand that prescription opioids are a public health concern and that prescribers have a responsibility to mitigate societal risk. Patients should be informed of clinic rules and philosophies before the initial prescription. Some find it helpful to frame the first appointment as a screening and compatibility visit and to make it clear that controlled medications will not be prescribed on the first visit.

Gourlay and colleagues developed guidelines for opioid prescribing that they liken to the universal precautions used for infection control.[75] The rationale is that providing the same standard of care to all patients minimizes risk to both the patient and provider. The guidelines recommend that such things as thorough assessment, documentation, testing, and follow-up standards be applied to all who are prescribed COT, regardless of perceived risk for aberrant behavior (Box 50.1).

SCREENING FOR LIABILITY TO ADDICTION

Instruments have been devised to alert the clinician to the likelihood that a patient has or is at risk for drug-related difficulties (Box 50.2). Positive screening does not necessarily exclude patients from opioid therapy; rather, it identifies

Box 50.1 The Ten Steps of Universal Precautions in Pain Medicine

1. Diagnosis with appropriate differential
2. Psychological assessment, including risk for addictive disorders
3. Informed consent
4. Treatment agreement
5. Preintervention/postintervention assessment of pain level and function
6. Appropriate trial of opioid therapy with or without adjunctive medication
7. Reassessment of pain score and level of function
8. Regular assessment of the "four A's" of pain medicine (analgesia, activity level, adverse effects, and aberrant behavior)
9. Periodic review of diagnosis and comorbid conditions, including addictive disorders
10. Documentation

Box 50.2 CAGE* Questions Adapted to Include Drugs (CAGE-AID)

1. Have you felt that you ought to cut down on your drinking or drug use?
2. Have people annoyed you by criticizing your drinking or drug use?
3. Have you felt bad or guilty about your drinking or drug use?
4. Have you ever had a drink or used drugs the first thing in the morning to steady your nerves or to get rid of a hangover (eye opener)?

*C, cut down; A, annoyed; G, guilty; E, eye opener.
Modified from Brown RL, Rounds LA. Conjoint screening questionnaires for alcohol and drug abuse. *Wisc Med J.* 1995;94:135-140.

those who have a lower than usual benefit-to-harm ratio and who therefore require more thorough assessment, closer monitoring and accountability, and possibly referral for addiction treatment. Simple questioning may fail to reveal SUDs because of concealment, unawareness, or forgetfulness on the part of patients.[76] In a study of 109 patients with CNCP, Berndt and associates[77] found that 32% of the toxicology results were discordant with patients' reports and that 21% concealed drug use.

The Screener and Opioid Assessment for Patients with Pain (SOAPP) comes in 5-, 14-, and 24-question versions, in addition to the Revised SOAPP (SOAPP-R). These questionnaires assess the risk for prescription opioid abuse. The test may be used in conjunction with other information to help assess patient suitability for COT, as well as to identify the need for more intense monitoring. The drug abuse screening test (DAST), though not developed for patients taking prescribed drugs, does contain several items that screen for drug use problems.[78,79] The SOAPP-R[80] and the Opioid Risk Tool (ORT)[81] are widely used to help assess the risk for aberrant opioid use behavior in patients being considered for a trial of COT. The ORT is a questionnaire that asks yes or no questions about risk factors such as family and personal substance abuse history, age, preadolescent sexual abuse, and psychological comorbidity. Though brief and easy, the questions are not disguised and stand out as screening questions and thus may invite dishonesty if the patient is seeking to obtain controlled medications.

Unlike these self-report instruments, the Diagnosis, Intractability, Risk, Efficacy (DIRE) score is a tool for use by clinicians to aid in determining the risks and benefits likely to accrue from COT.[82] A comparison of these screens suggests that all have value and are most useful when supplemented by clinical interview.[83]

RED FLAGS

The dividing line between characteristics that predict substance use and those that ascertain its presence is somewhat arbitrary. All the signs are clinically important.[84-90]

AT RISK FOR ADDICTION

- Young age
- Novelty-seeking/thrill-seeking personality
- Smoker
- History of substance abuse
- Family history of addiction, especially first-degree relatives
- History of physical, emotional, or sexual abuse
- History of "process addiction": sex, gambling, food, shopping

LIKELIHOOD OF EXISTING ADDICTION

- Previous drug-related treatment, arrests, driving under the influence
- Anger, arguing, bargaining
- Numerous emergency room visits for opioids
- Requesting highly abused medications, such as carisoprodol, barbiturates, stimulants
- Requesting rapid-onset opioids or those with easily defeated delivery systems
- Failure to bring requested medication bottles or amounts or dates that do not "add up"
- Statements such as "I have a high tolerance"
- Multisourcing/doctor shopping
- Wrong or no contact information
- Focus on opioids/disinterest in other treatment
- Extensive knowledge about abusable medications
- Previous noncompliance with other pain treatment programs
- Vernacular such as "oxy's," "roxy's," "bars," "xanny bars," "eating" versus "taking" pills
- Traveling long distances to the pain clinic
- Failure to produce medical records
- Obtaining medications from nonmedical sources
- Numerous allergies or intolerances to less reinforcing medications
- Positive, diluted, contaminated, or wrong temperature urine drug screen
- Failure to produce urine for drug testing
- Liver dysfunction, hepatitis B or C, or human immunodeficiency virus infection
- Physical findings: drug-related tattoos, track marks, needle bruising, "seed burns," signs of withdrawal or intoxication
- Appearance discordant with professed dysfunction—muscular, tanned

TOXICOLOGIC STUDIES

It is necessary to verify that patients are taking prescribed medications and not using illicit drugs. Urine drug testing (UDT) and hair testing can help provide this information and assist the patient in maintaining compliance by providing accountability. Additionally, UDT results can be of value to patients who need to document treatment adherence for reasons that range from child custody to probation. An excellent primer of UDT is available in a monograph prepared for the California Academy of Family Physicians that is available online.[91] It is important to understand the limitations of the testing used, and most companies have experts available to assist in interpretation.

In clinical practice, UDT is the mainstay because it is relatively inexpensive and noninvasive and provides a reasonable window of detection. The initial office screening test is usually an immunoassay. These "dipsticks" are economical and consist of antibodies that react with the drug or its metabolite. A positive test can be confirmed with gas chromatography–mass spectrometry or equivalent testing.[92] Standard tests, such as the Substance Abuse and Mental Health Services Administration's standard workplace drug panel (SAMHSA 5), are often insufficient in the pain clinic setting[93] because of limited detection capability. The SAMHSA 5 detects only marijuana, cocaine, morphine, phencyclidine, and amphetamines. Heroin and codeine are metabolized to morphine and are therefore detected; however, synthetic and semisynthetic opioids are not. Other screening tests are available that may include methadone, propoxyphene, benzodiazepines, barbiturates, and EDDP (2-ethylidene-1,5-dimethyl-3,3-diphenylpyrrolidine)—a methadone metabolite.

UDT can lead to erroneous conclusions for several reasons. Immunoassays are vulnerable to cross-reactivity; for instance, decongestants may test as amphetamines. Misleading results can occur when a prescribed substance is converted to another nonprescribed substance (e.g., hydrocodone and morphine can be converted to hydromorphone[92]). Spurious results can also occur from the consumption of legal substances; for example, poppy seeds contain morphine and some nasal inhalers contain l-methamphetamine.

In contrast, a finding of cocaine or THC is reliable and, in the case of THC, cannot be caused by being in a room in which a great deal of marijuana is being smoked. A urine screen that fails to contain a prescribed opioid may indicate diversion, but it can also mean that the patient exhausted the supply of medication several days before the test or that the patient used someone else's urine to conceal the use of illicit drugs.

It is helpful to have a breathalyzer available since alcohol is often not detected by urine drug testing. Ethyl glucuronide testing is widely available and can detect alcohol consumption for the previous 3 days; however, the test is so sensitive that exposure to alcohol from mouthwash or hand cleaner can produce a positive result. If levels exceed 500 ng/mL, deliberate alcohol ingestion is probable.

Drug testing should be performed before initiation of COT and randomly during treatment. Importantly, testing should not be limited to patients suspected of abuse because this strategy is open to bias (e.g., disproportionate testing of minorities) and has been shown to miss 50% of those using nonprescribed or illicit drugs.[94]

Even though there are safeguards, urine drug screens can be defeated. "Clean" urine may be obtained via the Internet or from friends and delivered by ingenious worn devices that are difficult to detect even with direct observation. These devices can even maintain urine at an appropriate temperature, typically, 90° F to 100° F within 4 minutes of voiding.

The most common strategy for avoiding detection is to dilute the urine through aggressive fluid ingestion or by adding tap water. Therefore, reasonable care should be taken that the sample is not obtained in a room with access to water for dilution and that the color and temperature are appropriate. Urine creatinine, specific gravity, and pH should be determined.[95]

Hair and saliva testing is now available. Hair testing is extremely accurate and virtually impossible to defeat and can detect use in the past 2 or more months since hair grows about half an inch per month. Recent use will be missed because it takes about 1 week for hair to grow from the follicle to a length at which it can be collected. THC levels are relatively low in hair follicles in comparison to most other drugs, and occasional use can be missed. Hair testing cannot be defeated by coloring or bleach since the chemicals tested are at the core. If scalp hair is absent, body hair may be used.[96,97] The cost of hair testing is no longer prohibitive, and its use in monitoring is increasing. For example, the Florida Physicians Health Program has used hair testing to monitor recovering physicians since 2006.[98]

It is reasonable for the clinician, without getting into a dispute about patients' rights to use substances or the benefits of "medical marijuana," to make access to opioid therapy contingent on the patient's willingness to produce urine that is free of illicit substances. This can be presented in a nonjudgmental manner as a way to ensure the patient's access to treatment and the provider's continued ability to prescribe. If the person is *unwilling* to relinquish recreational use, it suggests that the pain problem does not warrant COT. If the patient is *unable* to relinquish the drugs, addiction treatment is indicated.

TREATING PAIN IN PATIENTS WITH ADDICTION

A number of authors in the past emphasized the importance of distinguishing pain patients from addicts (e.g., Ling and colleagues[99]). The rub, obviously, is that the conditions are not mutually exclusive and, in fact, co-occur more frequently than would be expected by chance given that chemically dependent persons are at increased risk for trauma and painful illnesses and that pain patients have some finite risk for iatrogenic addiction.

Numerous authorities and professional organizations agree that it is unethical to withhold opioid analgesia from addicts. For example, the American Society for Pain Management Nursing has upheld this principle and described strategies for dealing with patients at different stages of the addictive disease process.[100] The policy of the American Academy of Addiction Psychiatry is cautionary regarding COT in general.[101] However, no one believes that patients should receive ineffective or harmful treatment, and all agree that opioids are not helpful in every case of chronic pain. Thus, there will be some patients with pain complaints who seek opioids and should be denied. Even though there are almost no data clarifying the risks and benefits of chronic opioid analgesia in addicts, it is clear that such therapy has hazards exceeding those of opioid therapy in nonaddicts given the potential for overuse and loss of control.

A patient's former drug of choice will have the most power to elicit cravings and relapse, which may explain the clinical impression (and pilot data[102]) that COT in recovering alcoholics is often more successful than COT in recovering opioid addicts. Nevertheless, the concept of cross-addiction suggests that a patient with any prior addiction, including alcohol dependence, is at elevated risk for new addiction, even to unrelated substances.[103,104] Thus, a chronic marijuana user may be at special risk for the development of an opioid use disorder. It is therefore essential that the clinician identify preexisting problems with all rewarding/reinforcing substances.

Treating pain in a person with an active SUD is complicated by several factors. Such patients are likely to believe that they are entitled to pain relief (regardless of whether this goal is attainable), and the prescriber is likely to suspect that some portion of the pain complaint represents drug seeking. Thus, the stage is set for conflict, which is further promoted by the previously mentioned adverse childhood experiences that predispose to both addiction and somatization. These experiences additionally engender mistrust, anger, and resentment of authority figures, who may be seen as betraying and withholding.

A distinction must be made between acute pain and chronic nonmalignant pain and between a patient who is actively engaging in substance abuse and a patient in recovery.

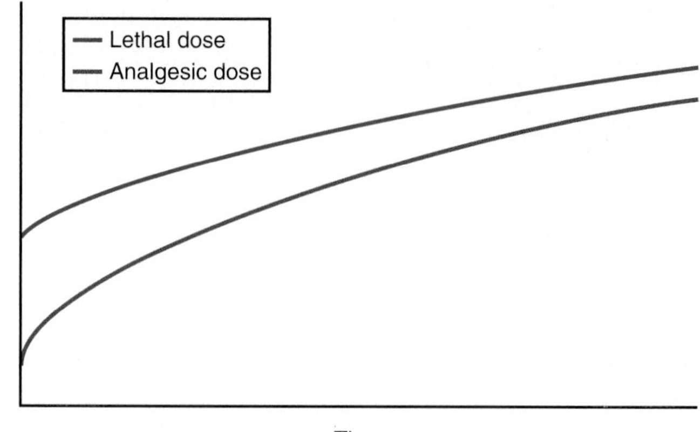

Figure 50.1 Hypothetical graph of progressive diminution of the therapeutic window as opioid tolerance develops.

ACUTE PAIN

Substance abuse not only leads to trauma[105] but also probably increases the pain associated with trauma based on the observations that addiction often leads to lower pain thresholds and tolerance[106] and that patients taking preoperative opioids have substantially greater postoperative pain and opioid requirements than do those not taking opioids.[107,108]

Therefore, acute injuries in addicts, even in those with sustained recovery, frequently require more aggressive analgesia than in patients with no addiction history because of the presence of tolerance. (It is commonly observed that a period of abstinence eliminates apparent drug tolerance; however, on resumption of use, tolerance is rapidly re-established in the previously tolerant person or animal.) The need of opioid-tolerant patients for more analgesia than expected can collide with staff desires to limit opioids in those with an addictive disorder. The result is likely to be a dissatisfied and uncomfortable patient—perhaps a vociferous one—and an unpleasant experience for staff. Management is facilitated by recognizing that a patient who is loudly demanding analgesia is unlikely to be overly medicated. It may be helpful to rotate opioids to identify a medication with incomplete cross-tolerance with the patient's drug of choice. Methadone and buprenorphine may provide satisfactory analgesia in these conditions.[109,110]

Difficulties arise in the treatment of acute (including perioperative) pain in a patient who is tolerant and physically dependent on opioids because of licit or illicit use. Not only may these patients require substantial doses of opioids simply to prevent withdrawal, but in addition they may require considerably more acute opioids for analgesia than a nontolerant patient.

PATIENTS RECEIVING PHARMACOTHERAPY FOR ADDICTION

Patients whose addiction is under treatment with opioid agonists (methadone, buprenorphine) require special consideration when they experience trauma or acute painful illness.[111] Their maintenance dose of methadone will not provide analgesia but must be continued to prevent withdrawal. Doverty and coworkers found that blood levels of morphine typically adequate for relief of postoperative pain had minimal analgesic effect in patients maintained on stable doses of methadone.[112] Thus, higher than usual doses of μ-opioid agonists may be required for acute pain. Administration of buprenorphine, a partial μ-agonist, to a patient taking full μ-agonists may produce an abstinence syndrome; however, the cautious addition of full agonists to a baseline dose of buprenorphine is effective.

Alcohol and opioid addiction may be treated with naltrexone, a long-acting μ-antagonist, as a relapse prevention strategy. When such patients require acute opioid therapy, much higher than usual doses are required. Close observation is necessary because these doses may become toxic as the naltrexone level decreases over time.

It seems counterintuitive, but acute analgesia with opioids may be more hazardous in tolerant than in nontolerant patients. Figure 50.1 is hypothetical but conveys the idea of what seems to happen clinically—as tolerance develops differentially to the analgesic versus the sedating and respiratory depressant effects of the drugs, the therapeutic window narrows, and the therapeutic dose begins to approach the lethal dose. (A part of this phenomenon may result from opioid-induced hyperalgesia since this would create the appearance of a high degree of analgesic tolerance without inducing tolerance to toxic drug effects.)

Rapp and colleagues compared the results of patient-controlled analgesia in tolerant and nontolerant patients, and although the former reported less nausea, vomiting, and pruritus than did opioid-naïve controls, the incidence of moderate or severe sedation was 50.3% as compared with 19.0% in controls.[108] We have seen postoperative patients who were highly opioid tolerant before surgery and in whom there seemed to be virtually no therapeutic window—careful bedside titration of intravenous opioids failed to reduce pain below a level of 9 to 10 out of 10 before the development of an unacceptable degree of sedation or respiratory depression.

Mehta and Langford reviewed recommendations for the treatment of acute or postoperative pain in patients maintained on opioid agonists.[113] These recommendations included continuing maintenance opioids and supplementing them with additional analgesia, multimodal when possible, including short-acting opioids, local anesthetics, and adjuvant nonsteroidal anti-inflammatory drugs. They also recommended patient-controlled analgesia with higher than usual bolus doses and shorter than usual lock-out intervals. Transdermal opioids and implantable pumps were noted as alternatives. A review by Huxtable and associates supported recommendations for multimodal analgesia.[114]

A special problem is created by the emergency department (ED) "frequent flyer"—a patient who is known to the staff of several local EDs and habitually shows up, often at night and on weekends, demanding opioids for a chronic (e.g., back pain), recurrent (migraine, sickle cell disease), or idiopathic pain condition. Fragmented care, as the person engages different shifts at different hospitals, presents a severe challenge to the development of a rational treatment plan; however, such a plan is mandatory. It is useful to establish liaison with a nonemergency provider in the relevant field of medicine and to arrange for consultation so that a plan of management for pain and addiction can be developed. Assessment for an addictive disorder should also be arranged. It is useful to recall that unrewarded behavior is not long repeated, so patients who resist daytime consultation should be limited, when possible, to noneuphorigenic medications in the ED (e.g., parenteral phenothiazines for migraine, ketorolac for other types of pain). ED guidelines on the administration and dispensing of opioids are essential so that house staff and faculty will have a consistent approach to provision of opioids for chronic pain. States and hospitals have developed guidelines that typically emphasize avoiding provision of opioids for chronic pain in the emergency setting, refusing to provide long-acting opioids or to refill lost or stolen prescriptions, avoiding parenteral opioids, using non-opioid–containing medications whenever possible, and creating a care plan for frequent patients that provides continuity of care with a nonemergency clinician (for examples, see the websites provided[115,116]).

PATIENTS IN RECOVERY

Patients recovering from an addictive disorder may face elective surgery with trepidation because they fear having to choose between unrelieved pain and relapse of their addiction. Some even refuse analgesia in an effort to preserve their hard-won sobriety. Experience suggests that this is unnecessary. They should be encouraged to advise the surgeon or anesthesiologist in advance of elective procedures that they are in recovery, will probably require higher than average doses of analgesics, but wish to preserve their sobriety by avoiding their previous drug of choice, transitioning to long-acting oral agents as soon as possible, and making arrangements for the safe use of opioids after discharge. The patients should increase their recovery work (12-step meetings, office sessions with an addiction counselor) and should notify their treating professionals and sponsor of their pending surgery so that support is in place. It is advisable to have a spouse, friend, or sponsor safeguard any home-going opioids and provide the patient a supply each day so that the patient is protected from the temptation of a bottle of opioids within easy reach.

CHRONIC PAIN

SAMHSA recently published a "treatment improvement protocol" that addresses the treatment of chronic pain in patients who have active or recovering SUDs (download available).[117] Recommendations include avoidance of chronic opioid analgesic therapy in active addiction unless and until the person commits to a treatment/recovery program. Further recommendations include implementation of nonopioid therapies when effective (both pharmacological and nonpharmacological), avoidance of other reinforcing drugs (e.g., benzodiazepines, benzodiazepine receptor agonists, carisoprodol), and aggressive treatment of psychiatric comorbidity.

Optimal treatment of comorbid pain and addiction nonetheless remains controversial, and there are few data on which to base therapy.[118] Current practice is largely guided by recommendations from clinicians in the field; however, we must recall how often "clinical wisdom" has been proved wrong when data became available. Among the most notable were the recommendations 50 years ago to minimize opioids for terminal cancer pain because of the risk for addiction.[119]

OPIOID-BASED TREATMENT

In a 1991 survey, Joranson and colleagues found that 58% of state medical board members considered it a probable violation of federal or state laws and regulations to prescribe COT to a person with a history of opioid abuse.[120] A subsequent survey demonstrated marked liberalization of this attitude[121]; however, many continue to doubt the wisdom of prescribing COT to those with SUDs, in part because of the paucity of data on the outcomes of such treatment. The lack of data may reflect a sense that the practice is hazardous. In fact, the use of chronic, home-going opioids in a person with an untreated addiction seems to be an invitation to abuse (altered routes of administration), diversion (exchanging therapeutic opioids for a different drug of choice), and death as a result of overdose and combinations of abused substances. Ironically, those with the least evidence of benefit from COT (most opioid studies excluded this population) and the most evidence of harm may be the ones most likely to receive it, as noted earlier.[20]

Studies of opioid analgesia in addiction are sparse. Dunbar and Katz treated 20 such patients with COT for longer than 1 year and found that those who abused treatment did so early. Those who did not were likely to be active in Alcoholics Anonymous, to have stable support systems, and not to be recent polysubstance abusers.[102] Unsurprisingly, those who did not abuse opioid treatment were more likely to benefit from it. Kennedy and Crowley used methadone and weekly psychotherapy to treat four patients with chronic pain and comorbid SUDs.[122] Three patients remained in treatment (19 to 21 months), stopped needle use or markedly decreased substance abuse, and demonstrated functional improvement. All three had significant psychopathology requiring psychotropics. Currie and coworkers treated 44 patients with comorbid chronic pain and addiction in cognitive-behavioral groups with an emphasis on substance abuse education and relapse prevention.[123] Some chose to discontinue opioids. Those who continued opioids were transitioned to longer-acting medications (excluding methadone). "As-needed" opioids were prohibited, and once titrated to the optimal dosage, patients could not obtain additional medication. There were significant improvements in pain, emotional functioning, and medication reliance. At the 12-month follow-up, half the patients were opioid free and the remainder had reduced their use from 17 to 12 days per month. There was no significant difference in outcomes in opioid and nonopioid users, although those who continued to take opioids appeared to function better overall. It was suggested that long-acting opioids may provide both analgesia and reduction of cravings in this population.

From these studies, as well as clinical reports, it is reasonable to conclude that chronic opioid analgesic therapy will help some patients despite comorbid addiction if managed optimally. Ensuring concomitant addiction treatment is often key to management. For readers with interest in the treatment of addiction, the *Textbook of Substance Abuse Treatment*[124] provides detailed descriptions of psychosocial treatments, including psychodynamic, network, cognitive-behavioral, motivational, individual, group, and family psychotherapy, as well as 12-step–based approaches.

Several authors and publications have developed recommendations for opioid therapy in patients with SUDs. Most of these are not strictly data based; however, they are a reasonable guide given that patient management cannot be deferred until we have certainty. There is considerable overlap in recommendations; that is, experts tend to be in general agreement. This list is largely based on the sources listed.[118,125-127]

Opioid Treatment of Patients with Substance Use Disorder

1. Wean opioids and avoid COT if acceptable comfort and function can be maintained with nonopioid medications, behavioral methods, physical therapy, neuroaugmentation, or other therapies. Non-opioid–based treatments may be effective in this population.[128]
2. If a patient weaned from opioids continues to have craving and preoccupation, sublingual buprenorphine should be offered.
3. Require that the patient sign an agreement that constitutes informed consent (i.e., provides information regarding the risks and probable benefits of COT) and establishes the expected behavior of the patient and provider for continued management.
4. Make it clear that initiation of COT is always an "*N* of 1 experiment" and that it will be continued only if there is objective evidence of improved quality of life. "Taking the edge off" is not successful therapy.
5. Present COT as only one component of the treatment of chronic pain, which optimally includes education, fitness, and relaxation and coping skills training.
6. Ensure that the patient and family members understand that zero pain is not achievable with current technology and will not be pursued. Chasing this goal leads to indefinite dose escalation.
7. Frequent visits are necessary during dose finding (perhaps weekly) and initial treatment (at least monthly). Those who demonstrate the ability to use the medications appropriately may be seen less frequently and given multiple prescriptions with "do not fill until ___" instructions.
8. Avoid highly reinforcing opioids, primarily those with rapid onset and short action. Consider abuse-deterrent formulations that may impede crushing, injecting, and nasal insufflation.
9. A patient unable to maintain control of opioid use may respond to treatment with transdermal agents and an agreement that refills are contingent on return of used patches. This is also an option if the patient cohabits with a person who abuses substances.
10. Make it clear, in writing, at the onset that lost or stolen opioids or prescriptions will be treated like lost or stolen cash—it is not the prescriber's role to replace them. It is clearly toxic to society to replace lost opioids since they lead to abuse and death, especially in young people.
11. Maintain accountability for medications with strategies such as pill counts.
12. Require permission to communicate with cohabitants, sponsors, pharmacies, and other providers.
13. Closely monitor the "four A's"—analgesia, activity level, adverse effects, and aberrant behavior. In the event of poor outcomes, there is no defense for having continued an obviously ineffective treatment.
14. Obtain toxicologic verification that the patient is not taking unauthorized substances and is taking the prescribed opioid.
15. Do not combine opioids in this population with benzodiazepines, benzodiazepine receptor agonists, or carisoprodol. Instead, treat anxiety and insomnia with sedating antidepressants or antiepileptic drugs (AEDs).
16. If COT fails because of noncompliance, do not dismiss the patient; rather, dismiss the opioids and provide non-addicting treatments.

Opioid Selection

The goals in selecting an opioid are optimal analgesia with minimal risk for addictive relapse. Pharmacokinetic factors that promote inappropriate self-administration include rapid absorption and high bioavailability, rapid delivery to the CNS, low protein and peripheral tissue binding, small volume of distribution, short half-life, and high free drug clearance[129] (see also Quinn and colleagues[130]). Thus, drugs that are "fast in" with a bolus into the neuron and "fast out," other things being equal, will be most subject to abuse. This is consistent with observations that delivery systems developed for euphorigenic effects are almost invariably in the direction predicted by these factors; for example, smoked cocaine is profoundly more rewarding than chewed coca leaves, and transdermal nicotine has little appeal to smokers.

Mironer and associates compared patients dismissed from treatment because of opioid misuse with those continuing to receive opioids.[131] They compared the frequency of prescription of various opioids with their frequency of abuse to generate a relative risk for misuse. The results, from highest to lowest risk for abuse, are as follows: butorphanol (4.4), propoxyphene (2.5), hydrocodone (1.61), codeine with acetaminophen (1.45), oxycodone immediate release (1.35), oxycodone delayed release (0.73), morphine 12 hour (0.66), transdermal fentanyl (0.23), and methadone (0.08). The conclusions are tentative given that patients were not randomly assigned to medications; however, they tend to support the clinical impression that patients are more likely to experience difficulty with some drugs than with others. Unfortunately, the study did not include many commonly prescribed opioids, and we lack good empirical data to guide opioid selection.

Brookoff asked prescription drug abusers to estimate the street price of various opioids. Of subjects who had tried controlled-release preparations, 60% found them to be of little use and estimated their street value to be lower than that of other opioids.[132] Reformulated OxyContin has a lower street price than the older, easy-to-crush formulation.[133] It seems reasonable to conclude that when abuse is a concern, there should be a preference for opioids with delayed and prolonged action and avoidance of rapid-onset drugs and those that can be inhaled or injected.

Abuse-Deterrent Drugs

People abuse drugs in different ways—the most common is simple overuse of oral medications in an effort to become "high." However, other methods to intensify the drug experience include crushing, grinding or chewing, dissolving, solvent extraction, nasal insufflation, and injection. Most strategies represent efforts to minimize T_{max} and achieve immediate neuronal entry of the substance.

In response, manufacturers have used a number of strategies to render drugs less abusable. Early "abuse-deterrent" formulations included Lomotil, which contains a subtherapeutic amount of atropine to discourage overuse, and Talwin-NX, in which naloxone was added to pentazocine in response to widespread abuse in the 1970s. The low dose of oral naloxone has no pharmacological activity; however, if injected, it antagonizes the action of pentazocine.

Currently, manufacturers are investigating a variety of techniques to impede rapid-onset preparations or routes (nasal, intravenous, smoked) or to limit the attractiveness of large doses:

- Physical barriers
  - Impede crushing, dissolving, chemical manipulation
  - Gel forming (difficult to inject, use by nasal insufflation)
- Antagonist-agonist combinations
  - Typically release an antagonist if crushed or dissolved or contain an inactive oral dose of antagonist that is active if injected
- Prodrugs
  - Minimal effect until metabolized and thus little effect if injected or snorted
  - Lengthening of T_{max}
- Aversive stimulus
  - Niacin (induces flushing with overdose)
  - Capsaicin (painful nasally)
  - Sodium lauryl sulfate (irritates the nasal mucosa)
- Depot drugs/implants
  - Slow release rendering the drug inaccessible for manipulation

Although it seems that strategies that impede opioid abuse without reducing therapeutic use offer great promise, there are a number of barriers, including the difficulties associated with prescribing a proprietary abuse-deterrent drug when a cheaper generic is equally effective, the hurdle of convincing the Food and Drug Administration (FDA) that a new drug warrants an "abuse-deterrent" designation, and the fact that the benefit of the costly formulation will accrue more to society than to the recipient (purchaser) of the prescription.

Intrathecal analgesia has been used as a strategy for providing opioid therapy to patients who have difficulty controlling their use. Although this route impedes abuse, patients have withdrawn opioid from the pump and injected it intravenously, as well as injected illicit drugs into the port.[134-136]

Buprenorphine

The synthetic opioid buprenorphine is a partial μ-opioid agonist with unusually high affinity for the μ receptor.[137] Because it is a partial agonist, there is a ceiling on both its analgesic and respiratory depressant effects, which may provide a considerable margin of safety in a population at risk for losing control of impulses to overuse.[138] A sublingual form is available with naloxone that has little effect sublingually, but it antagonizes the opioid with parenteral use.[139] Sublingual buprenorphine is approved only for use in the treatment of opioid addiction, but it is also an excellent analgesic and can be used to treat both conditions.[138,140]

The Drug Addiction Treatment Act of 2000 permits physicians to obtain a waiver that authorizes the prescription of approved medications (only sublingual buprenorphine at this point) for the treatment of opioid addiction. It is otherwise unlawful to prescribe opioids for the treatment of addiction except in a licensed methadone treatment program. The waiver is available from the Drug Enforcement Administration for physicians who have completed a small amount of training and meet other qualifications (details available online[141]).

Sublingual buprenorphine represents an appealing choice for patients with coexisting pain and addiction given its demonstrated benefit in both conditions and the reduced abuse liability of the naloxone-containing product. Transdermal buprenorphine is approved only for the treatment of pain. The packaging carries the warning of possible QT prolongation at dosages higher than 20 μg/hr, and hepatic impairment may increase this risk. The FDA has mandated studies to determine whether sublingual forms also carry this risk since the dosages are higher.[142]

Because buprenorphine is only a partial agonist and has high receptor affinity, it can precipitate withdrawal in a patient taking a full μ-agonist since the full agonist is displaced from the receptor by the partial agonist. If a patient maintained on COT is allowed to go into mild withdrawal and is then given buprenorphine, it relieves withdrawal symptoms.

Though used for the treatment of addiction, buprenorphine is also a drug of abuse. In Finland it has been the most misused opioid in recent years,[143] and its illicit use has been increasing in the United States.[144] The buprenorphine/naloxone combination is considerably less abusable as an intravenous preparation.[143,145] Despite the relative safety of buprenorphine, it may be lethal when combined with benzodiazepines or other sedatives.[146]

Methadone

Methadone warrants special mention.[147] It is approved for addiction treatment (by specially licensed facilities), is inexpensive and long acting, and seems less likely than other μ-opioid agonists to promote dose escalation,[148] possibly because of *N*-methyl-D-aspartate (NMDA) receptor blockade by the *d*-isomer.[149] However, it has many interactions with drugs and other substances[150] (e.g., grapefruit, nicotine, antiretrovirals), has unpredictable kinetics leading to overdose fatalities, and prolongs the QT interval, which leads to a risk for torsades de pointes.[151] Data from the American Association of Poison Control Centers demonstrated that the fatality rate per 100 exposures to methadone was several times that of other commonly prescribed analgesics.[152] Therefore, it is best prescribed by those with expertise in its use.[153]

Additional Reinforcing Medications

The presence of comorbid psychiatric illness is typical in both individuals with disabling chronic pain and those with addictive disorders. Thus, a preponderance of these patients will have psychiatric symptoms, most commonly anxiety or depression, which accounts for the frequent prescription of benzodiazepine anxiolytics in this population. Even though primary addiction to benzodiazepines is uncommon, its prevalence is increasing, and they are commonly abused by patients with other SUDs.[154] There seems to be little justification for prescribing controlled substances for anxiety, muscle spasm, and insomnia given the availability of non-addicting alternatives. Most antidepressants have anxiolytic properties and are not subject to abuse.[155-158] This is also true of many AEDs commonly used for pain treatment.[159-161] When needed, drugs from both categories (antidepressants and AEDs) that have sedative properties can be selected to minimize polypharmacy and unnecessary exposure of vulnerable patients to addicting substances.[162] Chronic pain is also strongly associated with sleep disorders,[163,164] which amplify the pain and should be addressed; however, the potentially habituating benzodiazepine receptor agonists are best avoided in those with addiction and tend to be of only transient benefit in any case.[165,166] Most so-called muscle relaxants are not habituating, with the exception of carisoprodol, which should therefore be avoided in addicted patients.

NON-OPIOID–BASED TREATMENTS OF PAIN

It has been well demonstrated that some patients with chronic pain are more comfortable and functional without opioids, and there are a number of pharmacological and nonpharmacological options to opioids, as detailed in Chapters 38 to 43 and 45 to 49.

The role of fitness training and physical therapy is increasingly being recognized not only for improving pain and function in persons with CNCP[167] but also for improving comorbid psychological distress.[168,169] Cognitive-behavioral therapy[170,171] and behavioral modification[172] have well-demonstrated efficacy as well. Interdisciplinary pain rehabilitation programs that combine reconditioning, cognitive-behavioral therapies, and (usually non-opioid–based) pharmacotherapy have been shown to produce marked and lasting benefit in pain, mood, and function.[173,174]

Since we lack accurate predictors of which patients will do well with opioids, we are essentially limited to a therapeutic trial to ascertain who will show improved pain, function, and mood and to assess side effects and aberrant behavior. It is likely that patients with addiction will be overly represented in the group who are better without opioids since their risks are clearly increased. It is noteworthy that most of the patients who improve with opioid elimination had believed that they were being helped by the drugs. We have compared treatment outcomes of CNCP patients who had comorbid addiction with those of nonaddicted patients and found that with nonopioid management of both conditions, outcomes were equally good.[175]

Since studies that extend beyond 18 months rarely show more than a 33% reduction in pain with COT (and a >50% dropout rate), it is apparent that even when opioids are necessary, they are rarely sufficient in patients with CNCP, and this is even more the case in those with comorbid addiction. Fitness, psychological counseling, and use of adjuvant analgesics are essential for most patients.

PROTECTING THE CLINICIAN

A medical text should properly be concerned primarily with the well-being of patients, which is the goal of health care. However, one impediment to such care is providers' appropriate concern for their own protection and the protection of their livelihood. This concern has an impact on patient access to care.

Prescribers may face sanctions for treating addicts with opioids, and addicts may seek compensation from providers whom they claim caused their addiction.[176] In a study of malpractice claims against anesthesiologists by patients with chronic pain, Fitzgibbon and colleagues found that medication management was responsible for 17% of the claims. Of the patients involved, 94% were prescribed opioids, which were combined with additional psychoactive medications in 58%. Eighty percent had at least one factor commonly associated with medication misuse, and 24% had three or more factors. Most claims involved patients who did not cooperate in their care (69%). Death was the most common outcome (57%), although iatrogenic addiction was the complaint in 24%.

The fact that addiction is much more likely to have arisen from recreational drug use does not alter the fact that iatrogenic addiction does occur and may constitute a compensable injury. A greater risk, however, is that a patient who had a preexisting addiction may falsely believe or claim that the prescriber caused it. Personal knowledge of physicians who have been sanctioned or sued for issues related to opioid prescribing suggests that the problems are most likely to occur during treatment of people with an addictive disorder. Although it is critical to recognize that addiction is a disease that no one chooses to have, it is associated with the emergence of antisocial behavior, to which the prescriber must not become vulnerable. Thus patients must be held accountable. Addicts making a sincere effort to recover will appreciate this because it helps reduce the likelihood of relapse (like being "weighed in" at Weight Watchers).

Protection of the provider's interests is promoted by diligent documentation and diagnosis of any preexisting addictive disorder. Some states require that COT in those with a previous addiction be initiated only after consultation with an addictionologist. It is equally critical that the provider meticulously document treatment response (perhaps with spousal confirmation)—or the lack thereof—and terminate opioid therapy unless it is clearly beneficial.

Prescribers may assume that patients will accept a small risk for the development of addiction to have a substantial likelihood of pain relief. This should not be assumed because that decision belongs to the patient. It should be clearly documented that the patient understood the risk for potential addiction and opted for COT before its institution.

CONCLUSION

The pain/addiction interface is quite complex. It poses special challenges and requires special techniques. Accurate diagnosis is critical and often difficult. A guiding principle is that even though patients with addictive disorders are entitled to aggressive pain treatment, they are not all entitled to opioids, which may be more of a liability than an asset. There is the potential for an excellent outcome in these cases since most patients with an addictive disorder and chronic pain can be restored to good function and comfort, sometimes with and sometimes without opioids. Such an outcome is unlikely unless the clinician exercises due diligence in identifying preexisting SUDs. A particular challenge is the apparent fact that excellent pain treatment or excellent addiction treatment will be of little value to these patients unless they have both. The pain specialist is in a unique position to ensure that this occurs.

Although addiction is generally described as a chronic relapsing illness, many sufferers are restored to fully normal and productive lives for prolonged periods, and some never relapse. In fact, it may be that those with iatrogenic opioid addiction have a better long-term prognosis than those who acquired the disease through recreational use. Thus, it is essential that pain specialists be able to understand patients who manifest addictive behavior as people with a bad disease rather than as bad people. By diagnosing addiction and facilitating treatment, pain specialists are in a position not only to decrease suffering but also to save lives.

KEY POINTS

- Addiction is a primary, chronic, neurobiologic disease with genetic, psychosocial, and environmental factors influencing its development and manifestations. It is characterized by behavior that includes one or more of the following: impaired control over drug use, compulsive use, continued use despite harm, and craving.
- Physical dependence is normal and is expected after prolonged use of opioids; it does not indicate the presence of any disorder.
- Tolerance is a state of adaptation in which exposure to a substance induces physiologic changes that diminish its effects. Analgesic tolerance is one of the reasons that opioids are more effective for acute than for chronic pain.
- Pseudoaddiction describes a state in which inadequate analgesia leads to behavior that mimics addictive behavior.
- Heroin addicts often report that they have spent years trying without success to recapture the highs that they experienced when they initiated use or that they no longer use heroin to get high but only to stop feeling bad.
- A tenant of most addiction treatment and education is the concept that a person addicted to one reinforcing substance is at high risk for addiction to all such substances and should therefore abstain even from substances that have never been problematic.
- Although chronic opioid therapy can cause physical dependence, trigger relapse in those recovering from addiction, and elicit addiction in some, it is clear that preexisting vulnerability plays a critical role in this process.
- Several studies suggest that the vast majority of patients who manifested addiction while being treated with chronic opioids had preexisting drug or alcohol disorders.

KEY POINTS—cont'd

- The development of addiction is a function of the molecule involved, dose administered, duration of use, genetic and personal vulnerability, and perhaps the route and rate of administration.
- Drugs that rapidly and markedly increase dopamine, such as crack cocaine, often produce addictive behavior quickly.
- A positive screening test does not necessarily exclude patients from opioid therapy. Rather, it identifies those who have a lower than usual benefit-to-harm ratio and therefore require more thorough assessment, closer monitoring and accountability, and possibly referral for addiction treatment.
- Urine drug testing can lead to erroneous conclusions for several reasons. Immunoassays are vulnerable to cross-reactivity, misleading results can occur when a prescribed substance is converted to another nonprescribed substance, and spurious results can occur from the consumption of legal substances.
- Hair and saliva testing is now available. Hair testing is extremely accurate and virtually impossible to defeat and can detect use in the past 3 or more months. Recent use will be missed because it takes about 1 week for hair to grow from the follicle to a length where it can be collected.
- It has been shown that blood levels of morphine typically adequate for relief of postoperative pain had minimal analgesic effect in patients maintained on stable doses of methadone.
- Buprenorphine is a partial agonist with a ceiling on its analgesic and respiratory depressant effects, and this may provide a considerable margin of safety in a population at risk for losing control of impulses to overuse. Sublingual buprenorphine is approved only for use in the treatment of opioid addiction.
- Primary addiction to benzodiazepines is uncommon, but its prevalence is increasing. It is commonly abused by patients with other substance use disorders. There is little justification for prescribing controlled substances for anxiety, muscle spasm, and insomnia to patients with comorbid addiction given the availability of nonaddicting alternatives.
- The role of fitness training and physical therapy is increasingly being recognized not only for improving pain and function in persons with chronic non-cancer–related pain but also for improving comorbid psychological distress.
- Reports of physicians who have been sanctioned or sued for issues related to opioid prescribing suggest that problems are most likely to occur during treatment of people with an addictive disorder. Protection of the provider's interests is promoted by diligent documentation and diagnosis of any preexisting addictive disorder. Some states require that chronic opioid therapy in those with a previous addiction be initiated only after consultation with an addictionologist.

SUGGESTED READINGS

Center for Substance Abuse Treatment. *Managing Chronic Pain in Adults With or in Recovery From Substance Use Disorders.* Rockville, Md: U.S. Substance Abuse and Mental Health Services Administration; 2012.

Chapman CR, Davis J, Donaldson GW, et al. Postoperative pain trajectories in chronic pain patients undergoing surgery: the effects of chronic opioid pharmacotherapy on acute pain. *J Pain.* 2011;12: 1240-1246.

Davis MP. Twelve reasons for considering buprenorphine as a frontline analgesic in the management of pain. *J Support Oncol.* 2012;10:209-219.

Fishbain DA, Cutler RB, Rosomoff HL, et al. Are opioid-dependent/tolerant patients impaired in driving-related skills? A structured evidence-based review. *J Pain Symptom Manage.* 2003;25:559-577.

Gardner E. The neurobiology and genetics of addiction: implications of the reward deficiency syndrome for therapeutic strategies in chemical dependency. In: Elster J, ed. *Addiction: Entries and Exits.* New York: Russell Sage Foundation; 1999:57-120.

Gatchel RJ, Okifuji AJ. Evidence-based scientific data documenting the treatment and cost-effectiveness of comprehensive pain programs for chronic nonmalignant pain. *J Pain.* 2006;7:779-793.

Gourlay DL, Heit HA, Almahrezi A. Universal precautions in pain medicine: a rational approach to the treatment of chronic pain. *Pain Med.* 2005;6:107-112.

Gourlay DL, Heit HA, Caplan YH. *Urine Drug Testing in Clinical Practice.* 4th ed. California Academy of Family Physicians. Available at http://www.familydocs.org/files/UDTMonograph_for_web.pdf. Accessed May 30, 2010.

Koob G, Le Moal M. Plasticity of reward neurocircuitry and the "dark side" of addiction. *Nat Neurosci.* 2005;8:1442-1444.

Koob G, Le Moal M. Addiction and the brain antireward system. *Annu Rev Psychol.* 2008;59:29-53.

Minozzi S, Amato L, Davoli M. Development of dependence following treatment with opioid analgesics for pain relief: a systematic review. *Addiction.* 2013;108:688-698.

Turk D, Swanson K, Gatchel R. Predicting opioid misuse by chronic pain patients: a systematic review and literature synthesis. *Clin J Pain.* 2008;24:497-508.

Weisner CM, Campbell CI, Ray GT, et al. Trends in prescribed opioid therapy for non-cancer pain for individuals with prior substance use disorders. *Pain.* 2009;145:287-293.

Yaksh TL, Onofrio BM. Retrospective consideration of the doses of morphine given intrathecally by chronic infusion in 163 patients by 19 physicians. *Pain.* 1987;31:211-223.

The references for this chapter can be found at www.expertconsult.com.

51

Issues Associated with Opioid Use

Mohammed Issa | James Celestin | Ajay D. Wasan

Chronic pain is a widespread, costly condition that influences every aspect of normal functioning[1-4]; collectively, pain imposes a greater economic burden than any other disease, with estimates of annual cost near $300 billion.[4-7] Opioids have been used to relieve pain for thousands of years, and prescription opioid medications continue to be a very common treatment modality for chronic non–cancer-related pain. Simultaneously, prescription opioid medications used for nonmedical purposes have rapidly become common drugs of abuse and the most likely cause of unintentional overdose.[8-10] As a result, the relationship between pain and addiction is a complicated one that poses several challenges for both patients and physicians.

A large percentage of patients with chronic pain disorders have preexisting comorbid addiction disorders or such disorders develop after receiving treatment for pain.[11] Studies have found rates as high as 15% to 28% for current substance disorders and 2% to 54% for lifetime prevalence in chronic pain patients,[11-14] both rates significantly higher than in the general population. In one study of 200 patients with low back pain it was found that substance use and anxiety disorders seem to precede the onset of chronic pain.[11] In the primary care setting it has been shown that substance use disorders precede the onset of chronic pain in 77% of patients who are actively using illicit substances and in 63% of patients with lifetime substance use disorders.[15] Even though a significant proportion of patients seeking treatment of their pain may have a comorbid addiction problem, addiction problems can make it difficult to diagnose and treat pain.[11] Chronic pain is more likely to develop in those with a preexisting history of substance abuse, and comorbid substance use disorders are more likely to develop in those with chronic pain and no history of substance abuse than in those without pain. It behooves the pain physician to have a good understanding of how pain and addiction are intertwined to skillfully manage these problems in an attempt to prevent worse outcomes.

Patients with chronic pain often have other psychiatric comorbid conditions (such as major depression or a generalized anxiety disorder), which may increase the risk for substance abuse and thereby create a more complex diagnostic and treatment conundrum for treating these patients' pain.[16] Some data suggest connections between chronic pain, mood disorders, and substance abuse.[17] Moreover, it has been shown that patients who have chronic pain are not only at a higher risk for opioid abuse but also have higher rates of mood disorders.[17,18] This constellation of diagnoses and problems compounds the difficulty that a physician will face when attempting to treat pain in patients who fall into this category.

This chapter covers the scope of these issues, from the neurobiology of addiction, to characterizing those at risk for opioid misuse and distinguishing opioid misuse without major negative consequences from prescription opioid addiction, to treatment considerations in patients with pain and substance use comorbidity. The topics are discussed primarily from the perspective of treatment of non–cancer-related pain with opioids. Even though those with cancer-associated pain are also at risk for substance use disorders, this phenomenon has not been well described.

NEUROBIOLOGY OF ADDICTION TO OPIOIDS

Any drug addiction is now understood to be a disease that is very much brain based. This phenomenon is a consequence of repeated exposure to the addictive drugs that leads to behavior characterized by loss of control over the use of such drugs. The behavioral abnormalities are connected to physiologic underpinnings, which mutually reinforce each other, and substance use disorders can be thought of as disorders of motivated behavior. Effective treatment involves simultaneously changing behavior and addressing the underlying physiologic drives sustaining the aberrant behavior. Addiction can be conceptualized as a chronic neurobiologic disease and a model of the relationship between the brain and behavior.[18]

There remains a great deal of uncertainty regarding the exact neural correlates of addiction. Nonetheless, it is believed that key brain regions constituting the brain networks for addiction are found within the mesocorticolimbic dopamine systems, which start in the ventral tegmental area and connect to the amygdala, prefrontal cortex, and nucleus accumbens (Fig. 51.1).

This pathway has been called the "dopamine reward pathway," and all addictive drugs ultimately act through different mechanisms to potentiate euphoria or other positive reward symptoms that subsequently reinforce behavior for ongoing use of the drug. Opioids, in particular, work by inducing the release of dopamine in the ventral tegmental area[19-21] and by binding to receptors in the nucleus accumbens.[22,23] It has been postulated that the experience of withdrawal uses this same pathway to create the negative reinforcement that contributes to compulsive behavior and cravings.[21,24]

Moreover, some of the biologic correlates connecting negative affect, increased pain, and opioid use have been described. These include the spinolimbic pathway, also known as the "medial pain system." This pathway travels parallel to

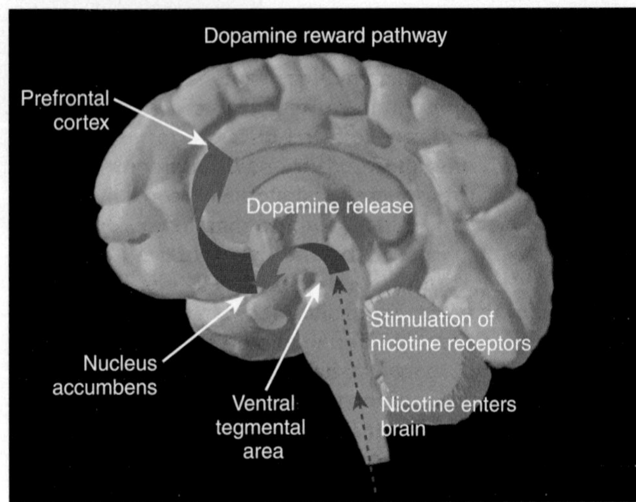

Figure 51.1 Dopamine reward pathway. (This slide is made available to the public through the National Institute on Drug Abuse Web page at www.nida.nih.gov/Teaching/largegifs/slide-9.gif.)

the spinothalamic tracts in the spinal cord and receives direct input from the dorsal horn of the spinal cord.[25] This pathway will lead to regions in the brain, such as the anterior cingulate cortex, insula, and prefrontal cortex, that not only process both pain and affect but are also regions with a very high concentration of opioid receptors.[26,27]

Vulnerability to the development of addiction is very much linked to genetic factors, as shown by genetic epidemiologic studies using twin, family, and adoption designs. Heritability can range from 0.3 to 0.5, depending on the drug of use.[28-32] Although a specific "addiction gene" has not been identified, these studies point to a very strong biologic influence of addiction, whose assessment must be incorporated into the everyday clinical practice of addiction medicine and pain medicine. Thus, taking a detailed family history, including a family history of substance abuse, is valuable in providing data for comprehensive pain assessment. The different terminology used in the context of chronic pain with addiction and opioid misuse or abuse is summarized in Box 51.1.

Box 51.1 Definition of Terms Used in Opioid Addiction

Pain is an unpleasant sensory and emotional experience associated with actual or potential tissue damage or described in terms of such damage.[33]

Addiction is a chronic, relapsing brain disease characterized by compulsive drug behavior and use despite harmful consequences.[34]

Pseudo-addiction is a condition in which patients taking opioids seek additional opioid medications because of inadequate dosing. These patients may exhibit behavior suggestive of addiction, but it resolves with an increase in opioid dose to provide adequate analgesia.[35]

Iatrogenic addiction is a condition in which patients without a genetic predisposition for abuse are overly prescribed opioids, thereby leading to addiction.[36]

Physical dependence is a state of adaptation that causes a drug class–specific withdrawal syndrome because of abrupt drug cessation, rapid reduction, or use of an antagonist.[37,38]

Tolerance is an adaptation state that develops over time to a drug that requires increased doses to create the same drug effect or a reduction in one or more of a drug's effect over time.[39]

Misuse is the use of medications other than as directed whether willfully or unintentionally and regardless of whether harm results.

Abuse is the use of illicit or licit substances intentionally for nonmedical purposes.

Diversion is the intentional removal of a drug from legitimate distribution and dispensing channels. Much of the opioid medications "sold on the street" have come from pharmacies.[10,40,41]

Aberrant behavior is a breach of mutually established medical boundaries by the patient.

NOSOLOGY OF PRESCRIPTION OPIOID MISUSE, ABUSE, AND ADDICTION

Many terms are used to describe substance use disorders in patients with chronic non–cancer-related pain, and clarification of the terminology is important. The American Academy of Pain Medicine (AAPM), the American Pain Society, and the American Society of Addiction Medicine (ASAM) define *prescription opioid addiction* in patients with pain as "a primary, chronic, neurobiologic disease that is characterized by behaviors that include one or more of the following: impaired control over drug use, compulsive use, continued use despite harm, and craving."[42] As noted, the behavioral characteristics of prescription opioid addiction may be perpetuated by a physiologic drive that comes with using prescription opioids[18]; in this case the mesolimbic motivational circuits are "hijacked" to perpetuate a disorder of motivated behavior.[43,44]

For many pain medicine and addiction specialists, this definition of addiction is preferred in patients prescribed opioids for pain over the *Diagnostic and Statistical Manual of Mental Disorders*, Fourth Edition (DSM-IV), definition of substance dependence because physical dependence in these patients, as evidenced by tolerance and withdrawal, is normal. Although the DSM-IV definition does not require tolerance or withdrawal to make the diagnosis of substance dependence, these conditions do fulfill two of three major criteria required to make the diagnosis (Table 51.1). Thus, there are phenomenologic quandaries in applying the DSM-IV criteria for evaluation of substance dependence in patients prescribed opioids for pain. Given these issues, the AAPM and ASAM refer to *substance misuse* in this patient group as the use of any drug in a manner other than how it is indicated or prescribed.[42] *Substance abuse* is defined as the use of any substance when such use is unlawful or detrimental to the user or others.

Hence, opioid misuse may indicate a treatment compliance issue or may signal a more serious addiction problem if accompanied by a lack of control over use despite negative consequences. These distinctions are somewhat blurry, and in a clinical pain medicine practice it is often unclear whether a patient is simply noncompliant with the medication or is truly dependent. The presence of craving is central to this distinction in applying the AAPM and

Table 51.1 Substance Abuse and Dependence Symptoms in the DSM-IV

Brief Symptom Descriptor	Abstracted DSM-IV Definition
Abuse Symptoms	
Role impairment	Frequent intoxication leading to failure to fulfill major role obligations
Hazardous use	Recurrent use when it is physically hazardous (e.g., drunk driving)
Legal problems	Recurrent substance-related legal problems
Social problems	Continued use despite social or interpersonal problems caused or exacerbated by use
Dependence Symptoms	
Tolerance	Need to consume more to achieve the same effect; decreased effect with the same amount
Withdrawal	Signs of withdrawal syndrome; use to avoid withdrawal
Larger/longer	Often using more or for a longer period than intended
Quit/cut down	Persistent desire or unsuccessful attempts to quit or cut down substance use
Much time spent using	Lots of time spent using, obtaining, or being affected by a substance
Reduced activities	Important social activities given up or reduced because of substance use
Psychological/physical causes	Continued use despite psychological or physical problems or problems exacerbated by use

Note: Abuse is diagnosed when at least one of the four abuse criteria are present, and dependence is diagnosed when at least three of the seven dependence criteria occur within the same year.
DSM-IV, *Diagnostic and Statistical Manual of Mental Disorders*. Fourth Edition. American Psychiatric Association; 1994.)

ASAM criteria for prescription opioid addiction. Moreover, DSM-V will add craving to the diagnostic criteria for opioid addiction and is changing the terminology from *opioid dependence* to *opioid addiction*.[45] However, it remains unclear to what extent craving is indicative of prescription opioid dependence or addiction since those without opioid dependence who are taking prescription opioids have appropriately also reported some craving. Furthermore, across many different substances, reporting craving is significantly associated with a substance use disorder.[46,47] A few studies have examined craving in patients with pain who have been prescribed opioids, and craving is significantly associated with an elevated risk for opioid misuse.[48,49]

SIGNS OF PROBLEMATIC OPIOID USE

One major concern for the long-term use of opioids in patients with chronic non–cancer-related pain is their potential for misuse and abuse. Multiple cross-sectional studies in clinic populations have indicated that treatment of noncancer pain with opioids is associated with a 40% prevalence of opioid misuse.[50,51] Clinicians have reported several types of aberrant drug-related behavior (ADRB) that may be indicative of opioid misuse.[52-54] Although such behavior is problematic and indicative of nonadherence to opioid therapy at the very least, many have not been empirically tested to distinguish opioid misuse without negative consequences from prescription opioid addiction. Of course, certain types of extreme behaviors, such as injecting oral formulations or compulsive, uncontrolled use of medication, have face validity suggestive of addiction. According to Portenoy,[53,55] there are three major types of ADRBs: loss of control over the drug, compulsive drug use, and continued use despite harm. He suggested the following sets of drug-related behavior that may cause suspicion about problematic use in opioid-treated pain patients:

ADRB more predictive of addiction

- Prescription forgery
- Stealing or "borrowing" drugs from others
- Injecting oral formulations
- Obtaining prescription drugs from nonmedical sources
- Concurrent abuse of alcohol or illicit drugs
- Multiple dose escalation or other noncompliance with therapy despite warnings
- Multiple episodes of prescription "loss"
- Repeatedly seeking prescriptions from other clinicians or from emergency departments (EDs) without informing the prescriber or after a warning to desist
- Evidence of deterioration in the ability to function at work, in the family, or socially that appears to be related to use of the drug
- Repeated resistance to changes in therapy despite clear evidence of adverse physical or psychological effects from the drug
- Selling prescription drugs (which is termed *diversion* and is not indicative of a substance use disorder per se but does signify a major ADRB)

ADRB less predictive of addiction (may be more indicative of poorly controlled pain or misuse without significant negative consequences)

- Aggressive complaining about the need for more drug
- Drug hoarding during periods of reduced symptoms
- Requesting specific drugs
- Openly acquiring similar drugs from other medical sources
- Unsanctioned dose escalation or other noncompliance with therapy on one or two occasions
- Unapproved use of the drug to treat another symptom
- Reporting psychic effects not intended by the clinician
- Resistance to change in therapy associated with "tolerable" adverse effects with expressions of anxiety related to the return of severe symptoms

Savage in 2002[56] also formulated a short list of patterns that may suggest addiction ("look for the four C's"):

*Adverse **C**onsequences/harm as a result of use*

- Intoxicated, somnolent, sedated
- Declining activity
- Irritable, anxious, labile mood
- Increasing sleep disturbances
- Increasing pain complaints
- Increasing relationship dysfunction

Impaired ***Control*** *over use/****Compulsive*** *use*

- Reports lost or stolen prescriptions or medication
- Frequent early renewal requests
- Urgent calls or unscheduled visits
- Abusing other drugs or alcohol
- Cannot produce medication on request
- Withdrawal noted at clinic visits
- Observers reporting overuse or sporadic use

Preoccupation with use because of ***Craving***

- Frequently missed appointment unless opioid renewal expected
- Does not try nonopioid treatments
- Cannot tolerate most medications
- Requests medication with high reward
- No relief with anything else except opioids

It is important to remember that many of the types of behaviors listed may occur occasionally in isolation in patients using opioids appropriately, for the most part in the treatment of their chronic pain. However, a pattern of such behavior in the context of titrated pain therapy may suggest the need for further evaluation to determine the presence of prescription opioid addiction. It is still unclear exactly which constellations of symptoms or behaviors accurately distinguish misuse from abuse and addiction. These are thought to exist on a continuum, with the most severe form of nonadherence—addiction—characterized by the four "C's."

Early and proper identification, as well as careful monitoring for signs of problematic opioid use and ADRB, is warranted. Once identified, several measures may be taken by the prescribing physician to control for such aberrant behavior and reduce risk for the subsequent development of an addiction problem, including the following:

- Writing an opioid pain treatment agreement, if one is not available, in which expectations and conditions for termination of opioid prescription are clearly outlined
- Increasing the number of office visits and more frequent monitoring
- Decreasing the number of medication dispensed per visit
- Performing random pill counts on visits
- Recommending the use of only one pharmacy
- Using prescription drug–monitoring programs (PDMPs) to determine whether the patient has been getting prescriptions from multiple providers, EDs, or both
- Avoiding early prescriptions and excluding any replacement of lost or stolen prescriptions
- Requiring police reports for stolen medications
- Performing random urine drug screens and considering consultation with an addiction specialist if true addiction to the opioid medication is suspected

Careful assessment is essential to determine the underlying cause and co-occurring physical and mental comorbid conditions that may contribute to such behavior.[51,57-60] Reliance on patient self-reports of medication use to determine inappropriate behavior has been shown to be notoriously unreliable and inaccurate since patients tend to underestimate their medication use.[61-66] Cook and colleagues[65] found that when patients' self-reports were compared with urine toxicology screens, the actual prevalence rate of drug use was approximately 50% higher than the estimate produced by self-reports. Berndt and coauthors[62] also reported that 32% of patients' self-reports of their use of medication did not match with their urine tests.

In addition, "gut feelings" by some prescribers who are confident that they can identify vulnerable individuals should be avoided since empirical evidence has shown them to be ineffective.[16,51] Wasan and associates[16] found that even though prescribers had judged only 14% of their chronic pain patients to have ADRB, approximately 50% were found to have positive urine drug screens for illicit drugs and 8.7% had no evidence of any opioids in their urine.

In an attempt to decrease the risk for opioid misuse and iatrogenic addiction to prescribed opioid medications, Gourlay and coworkers[67] recommended establishing a policy of "universal precautions" when prescribing opioid analgesics:

1. Making a diagnosis with appropriate differential
2. Psychological assessment, including risk for addictive disorders
3. Informed consent
4. Treatment agreement (previously called an "opioid contract")
5. Preintervention and postintervention assessment of pain level and function
6. Appropriate trial of opioid therapy with or without adjunctive medication
7. Reassessment of pain score and level of function
8. Regular assessment of the "four A's" of pain medicine (analgesia, activity, adverse effects, and aberrant behavior)
9. Periodic review of the pain diagnosis and comorbid conditions
10. Proper documentation

SCREENING/RISK TOOLS FOR SUBSTANCE ABUSE

Screening for risk for addiction should be performed before chronic opioid therapy is initiated to provide the treating physician with clues about the necessity for increased monitoring in susceptible individuals and to assist in making the decision of whether to prescribe opioids at all. If opioid treatment results in good pain control, a better level of functioning, and improved overall quality of life, opioid treatment could reasonably be continued even in patients susceptible to addiction. However, the important point is that patients thought to be at greater risk for opioid misuse will require special attention with a focus on compliance and with proper communication about the potential risks and consequences if opioid treatment is getting out of control.

The ideal screening tool for medication misuse or abuse in patients with chronic pain should be easy to administer, reliable, and well validated.[68] An outline of such different screening tools is summarized in Box 51.2.

Though conceptually distinct from instruments designed to detect existing addictive disorders, measures whose purpose is to predict aberrant prescription opioid–related behavior in pain patients are closely related, with identification of similar risk factors. As a whole, this body of research is remarkably consistent in identifying the most significant risk factors for predicting prescription opioid misuse: current reports of misuse, past or current history

Box 51.2 Screening Tools for Opioid Misuse or Abuse

Well Validated Tools

Pain Medicine Questionnaire: high validity and reliability; patients answering the questionnaire may not feel opposed to or prejudiced against the questions since opioids are not specifically mentioned.[69]

Current Opioid Misuse Measure (COMM): can identify aberrant drug-related behavior in patients who are currently taking opioids.[70]

Screener and Opioid Assessment for Patients with Pain—Revised (SOAPP-R): consists of 24 items and a cut-off score of 14 or higher for classifying those at greater risk for opioid misuse.[71]

Less Validated Tools

CAGE questionnaire (CAGE-AID): primarily used for brief screening for alcohol abuse but has been adapted to include drugs.[72]

Short Michigan Alcoholism Screening Test (SMAST-AID): also adapted to include drugs.[72]

Prescription Opioid Abuse Checklist: based on DSM-III-R parameters.[54]

Prescription Drug Use Questionnaire (PDUQ): developed by Miotto and colleagues and includes 42 items to be administered by trained clinicians.[73]

Substance Use Questionnaire: capable of differentiating between chronic pain patients and heroin street abusers.[58]

Opioid Risk Tool (ORT): categorizes patients into low (score of 3 or lower), moderate (score of 4 to 7), or high (score of 8 or higher) risk for aberrant drug-related behavior.[74]

Screening Tool for Addiction Risk (STAR) questionnaire: developed by specialists in both pain and addiction medicine. History of treatment in a drug or alcohol rehabilitation facility is a significant predictor of ongoing addiction with a positive predictive value of 93% and a negative predictive value of 5.9%.[75]

DSM-III-R, *Diagnostic and Statistical Manual of Mental Disorders*, Third Edition, Revised.

of an addiction disorder to any substance (except perhaps for alcohol dependence in remission for several years), concurrent negative affective disorder (such as major depression or an anxiety disorder), previous or current history of sexual or physical abuse, family history of substance use disorders, and a history of illegal activities. Remarkably, ongoing pain levels have *not* been shown to be strong, consistent predictors of opioid misuse, albeit some misuse behavior may purely be a consequence of underdosing of opioids (pseudo-addiction).

URINE TOXICOLOGY SCREENING

Urine toxicology screens continue to be the most widely used and possibly the "gold standard" for detecting illicit substance use in chronic pain patients treated with opioids. Patients should be screened at baseline before starting opioids and then periodically throughout the course of treatment. However, the results of baseline screening should be interpreted with caution and not considered indicative of future aberrant behavior. Katz and Fanciullo[60] found that 72% of patients with positive baseline screens (i.e., inappropriate results) did not have evidence of any aberrant behavior after initiation of treatment. Conversely, patients with an initial negative toxicology screen may later demonstrate behavior indicative of problematic drug use. Many types of urine toxicology screens and many testing technologies are available, so it is important to choose the type of screening that most closely and accurately identifies the substances of interest.

OPIOID THERAPY AGREEMENTS

As noted, it is important for clinicians to discuss their management plan regarding chronic opioid therapy with their patients before initiating treatment and on an ongoing basis during therapy.[76] The management plan should include the goals of therapy, how opioids will be prescribed and taken, alternatives to opioid therapy, expectations for follow-up, monitoring, and use of concomitant therapies, as well as potential reasons for terminating opioid therapy, which may include failure to meet the therapeutic goals, serious side effects, or repeated ADRB.

Although evidence of the most effective methods to convey this management plan is lacking, written documentation through an opioid therapy agreement signed by both the patient and clinician may be an appealing tool for managing many of the potential difficulties related to chronic non–cancer-related opioid therapy.[77] Despite the widespread use of therapy agreements and some evidence of their effectiveness, their efficacy has not yet been proved (i.e., compared with a control condition in a prospective study). Nevertheless, multiple opioid therapy treatment guidelines appropriately emphasize the benefits of such an agreement in all patients prescribed opioids for noncancer pain. They can be particularly helpful for patients at higher risk for opioid misuse, to reinforce expectations about the appropriate and safe use of opioids, and to convey the consequences of violating such terms. The contents of signed opioid agreements may vary,[78] and there is still insufficient evidence to guide specific recommendations on which provisions to include. Some common provisions include

- Obtaining opioids from one prescriber
- Filling opioid prescriptions at one designated pharmacy
- Random urine drug screens
- Office visits at a specified minimum interval
- Use of pill counts
- Limited prescriptions (in weekly or biweekly instead of monthly amounts)
- Description of behavior that may lead to discontinuation of chronic opioid therapy

Although the opioid agreement may be helpful in some ways, it may not be entirely benign for either the patient or clinician. There is always the potential of carrying some degree of stigma or even the appearance of punishment with such agreement forms, particularly in those with a history of addiction.[79] It may also inappropriately reassure clinicians that patients are completely adherent to the treatment plan, which then results in less stringent monitoring of opioid use and treatment efficacy. Opioid agreements are still considered binding contracts and thus carry with them an increased risk for liability should the clinician violate their terms or place patients at risk for reduced autonomy.[80] Careful consideration should be given to restrictions placed on patients, such as limitations on driving or prohibiting pregnancy, since the literature is still inconclusive on these subjects.

PRESCRIPTION DRUG-MONITORING PROGRAMS

PDMPs are statewide electronic databases that collect data on controlled substances dispensed in the state. They are housed by specified statewide regulatory, administrative, or law enforcement agencies (most commonly state boards of pharmacy). Information is stored in a central database and can be accessed by authorized users, including prescribers, dispensers, law enforcement for drug investigations, licensing and regulatory boards, Medicaid programs, medical examiners, and research organizations. Their main goal is to identify and prevent drug abuse and diversion, as well as to facilitate the identification of, intervention in, and treatment of persons addicted to prescription drugs. The data collected can help provide information for public health initiatives about the use and abuse trends of different substances statewide, including prescription opioids. PDMPs also ensure patient privacy since law enforcement personnel cannot access patient-specific PDMP data unless an active investigation is ongoing and health care providers can access only the PDMP data relevant to their patients.

Several studies have shown that PDMPs are effective when fully used. A 2010 study found that when PDMP data were used in an ED, 41% of cases had altered prescribing after the clinician reviewed PDMP data: 61% of the patients received no or fewer opioid pain medications than had been originally planned by the physician before reviewing the PDMP data, and 39% received more opioid medication than previously planned because the physician was able to confirm that the patient did not have a recent history of controlled substance use.[81] Another 2010 independent evaluation of Kentucky's PDMP, KASPER, found that 90% of those surveyed believed that KASPER was effective in preventing drug abuse, diversion, and doctor shopping.[82]

RISK EVALUATION AND MITIGATION STRATEGIES

In response to disturbing rises in prescription opioid abuse, the Food and Drug Administration proposed the implementation of aggressive risk evaluation and mitigation strategies (REMSs) that will require prescribers to obtain mandatory education, provide mandatory patient education, register patients into registries, and other measures before prescribing certain opioids. The first opioid to be subject to the new REMSs was the fentanyl buccal soluble film (Onsolis), and it has now been extended to include multiple opioids, including extended-release and long-acting forms. The applicability, usefulness, and acceptance of REMSs by prescribers remain controversial. A recent survey by Slevin and Ashburn[83] found that 50% of surveyed primary care physicians reported being unwilling to prescribe opioids controlled by the new REMSs, which could have the unintended effect of decreasing access to these medications for legitimate medical purposes.

FACTORS PREDICTIVE OF OPIOID MISUSE OR ABUSE

As noted, the risk for addiction in the context of chronic non–cancer-related pain is believed to be due to a combination of factors, including genetic predisposition,[84] brain reward mechanisms, psychosocial factors, and drug exposure. The most consistent risk factor in the context of opioid therapy as identified by several studies[50,85-88] is a personal or family history of addiction, more so with multiple substances rather than a sole history of alcohol dependence. Turk and coworkers[85] also identified other possible predictive factors, including a history of psychiatric comorbid conditions, especially unipolar depression, and a history of legal problems such as driving under the influence, previous motor vehicle collisions, or drug convictions. Dunbar and Katz[89] identified not being members of a 12-step group such as Alcoholics Anonymous (for those with a past history of alcohol dependence) and having poor social support as additional risk factors. Michna and colleagues[87] found that the presence of two or more risk factors, including a personal or family history of substance abuse or legal problems related to substance abuse, was significantly associated with clinical evidence of opioid misuse. Schieffer and associates[88] also found that patients with a history of drug and alcohol abuse and patients with a prior psychiatric diagnosis (such as depression or an anxiety disorder) showed greater risk for medication misuse than did those without such a history. The results for other variables such as age, gender, and marital status are mixed.[85]

TREATMENT OF PAIN IN HIGH-RISK PATIENTS AND THOSE WITH KNOWN ADDICTION

A number of authors have emphasized the importance of differentiating pain patients from addicts. However, realistically, the two conditions are not mutually exclusive and occur concurrently more frequently than would be expected by chance. Jamison and colleagues[90] interviewed 248 patients at methadone maintenance centers and found that 61.3% reported chronic pain as a primary medical condition. Rosenblum and coworkers[91] found that severe chronic pain was present in 37% of 390 methadone maintenance treatment patients and in 24% of 531 chemically dependent inpatients. On the other hand, reports regarding the prevalence of current substance use disorders in patients receiving opioids for chronic pain range from 3% to 43%, with a lifetime prevalence as high as 54%.[12,15,92] Thus, documentation of the prevalence of pain in addicts and the prevalence of addiction in those with pain makes it clear that it is often necessary to treat persons with both conditions.

Pain, as well as pain management, in high-risk patients and those with substance dependence is a complex topic that sometimes leads to uncertainty or conflict between the patient and practitioner. It is important to remember that pain is more commonly undertreated in individuals perceived to have an addictive disorder secondary to fear of causing or exacerbating their addiction. However, this may increase the distress over and anxiety and craving for pain-relieving medications and thus potentially create more potent factors for relapse. Treating physicians should inform patients with addictive disease that they are aware of their addiction and reassure them early that this will not be an obstacle to relief of their pain. Addiction counseling should be offered any time during treatment as long as the pain is adequately controlled. It is unclear to what extent this subgroup of patients can be adequately managed in a medical setting, such as a pain medicine clinic, or under what conditions these patients should have opioids prescribed only by an addiction medicine specialist.

CROSS-ADDICTION OF NONOPIOIDS

It is a truism in addiction medicine that a patient's former drug of choice will have the most power to elicit cravings and relapse, which probably explains the clinical impression that opioid therapy in recovering alcoholics is often more successful and less likely to lead to adverse outcomes than such therapy in recovering opioid addicts. Nevertheless, the concept of cross-addiction suggests that a patient with *any* previous addiction is at heightened risk for new addiction, even to unrelated substances. Thus, a chronic marijuana user may be at special risk for the development of opioid addiction, even though the substances are unrelated. It is therefore essential that the clinician identify preexisting problems not only with opioid abuse but also with all rewarding or reinforcing substances. A distinction must be made between acute pain and chronic nonmalignant pain and between a patient who is actively engaging in substance abuse and one in recovery.

ACUTE PAIN

OPIOID ADDICTS

Acute injuries in addicts, even those with sustained recovery, often require higher doses of analgesia (about three times on average) than needed in patients with no addiction history because of higher tolerance levels to opioids. Research has shown that tolerance is rapidly re-established in a previously tolerant person or animal once opioid use is resumed. Care should be taken to educate the supporting staff well regarding tolerance and the higher analgesia requirements of such patients with a history of addiction to avoid possible collisions between the patient and staff.

Management of acute and postoperative pain in patients with addiction should include continuing the patients' maintenance opioids, if any, to meet their baseline opioid requirements and supplementing them with additional analgesia, multimodal when possible, such as adjuvant nonsteroidal anti-inflammatory drugs (NSAIDs), neuropathic medications, local anesthetics, or short-acting opioids if needed. However, if opioids are to be used, they should be given on a scheduled or continuous basis rather than as-needed dosing. Giving the patient specific times for drug administration is also helpful. Intermittent, nonscheduled medications are appropriate when the individual has pain that is related only to specific activities or to help adjust the dosing schedule. If the individual has difficulty controlling medication use, a trusted other may help dispense the medications. The patient should always be included in the decision-making process regarding dosing and scheduling since this helps alleviate anxiety and may also give the physician valuable insight in designing an effective treatment regimen.

The use of patient-controlled analgesia (PCA) in individuals with addictive disease has been recommended by some[93] to help provide more uniform pain relief at a lower total dose of medications and to eliminate the need for the patient to request opioids, thus avoiding conflicts between the staff and patient. However, others worry that because PCA requires self-administration, this may create ambivalence in recovering addicts who have difficulty limiting their administration of opioids to levels that provide analgesia without intoxication. It may also reinforce pain through pairing of pain with self-administration of opioids. Thus, as with all pain control measures, use of PCA should be considered on a case-by-case basis. If used, higher than usual bolus doses and shorter than usual lock-out intervals are generally recommended.[93]

Transdermal opioids and implantable devices (discussed later in detail) have also been noted as alternatives. Other promising adjuvant analgesics that have been gaining more interest in controlling postoperative pain in patients taking long-acting opioids are ketamine and α_2-agonists such as dexmedetomidine. Such agents may reduce opioid tolerance and attenuate opioid-induced hyperalgesia and have proven analgesic properties of their own. A recent meta-analysis of 37 trials that included more than 2200 patients by Bell and associates[94] indicated that ketamine probably reduces postoperative opioid requirements, at least during the first 24 hours. In addition, Loftus and coauthors reported almost a 30% reduction in morphine consumption over the first 48 hours and a 25% reduction in visual analog pain scores in the postoperative care unit with the intraoperative administration of ketamine.[95]

As a general rule, when there is doubt regarding whether a patient is in pain or is requesting drugs because of addiction, it is always more appropriate to err on the side of giving adequate pain relief, preferably with "nonopioid" interventions. In addition, associated symptoms such as sleep disturbance, anxiety, depression, or secondary physical problems should be identified and treated properly. Once the acute pain has completely resolved, the addiction problem can be addressed through detoxification, rehabilitation, therapy, or medications as deemed appropriate.

PATIENTS RECEIVING OPIOID AGONIST THERAPY

Both pain and addiction treatment issues should be addressed concurrently in patients with acute pain who are receiving opioid agonist therapy (such as methadone or buprenorphine).

First, in regard to their pain, it is crucial to relieve patients' anxiety by discussing the plan with them in a nonjudgmental manner. Opioid tolerance and pain sensitization will often necessitate higher opioid analgesic doses administered at shorter intervals. Conventional analgesics, including opioids, should be used aggressively to treat the painful condition and should be given via continuous or scheduled dosing rather than as-needed dosing and for only a limited period. Mixed agonist-antagonist opioids such as pentazocine and nalbuphine should be avoided since they will displace the maintenance opioid from the μ-opioid receptor and precipitate acute opioid withdrawal. If the patient is receiving methadone maintenance treatment, methadone can be continued and its dose titrated slowly in 5- to 10-mg increments at least every 5 to 7 days to achieve proper analgesia. Short-acting opioid analgesics can be used for breakthrough pain if needed. If the patient is receiving buprenorphine maintenance therapy and requires opioid analgesics, different options may be available:

1. Discontinue buprenorphine and titrate the opioid analgesics to effect to avoid withdrawal first and then to achieve analgesia.
2. Divide the buprenorphine dose to every 6 to 8 hours (although this by itself is usually insufficient to provide proper analgesia).
3. Convert buprenorphine to methadone at 30 to 40 mg daily (methadone binds less tightly to the μ-opioid receptor, and thus response to additional opioids will be as expected).
4. Buprenorphine can be continued and a short-acting opioid added and titrated to effect.

However, since dissociation of buprenorphine from the μ-opioid receptor is highly variable and high doses of opioids are usually required to over-ride buprenorphine secondary to its high receptor affinity, naloxone should be readily available at the bedside and the patient's level of consciousness and respiration monitored closely.

Second, regarding their addiction issues, patients have to be reassured that their addiction history will not in any way prevent adequate pain management. The opioid agonist medication should be continued at the usual or equivalent dosing after being verified by the methadone maintenance clinic or prescribing physician. The addiction treatment program or prescribing physician should be notified regarding the patient's admission and discharge from the hospital, and the time and amount of the last maintenance opioid dose have to be confirmed. Proper communication with the addiction treatment maintenance program or prescribing physician regarding any opioids or benzodiazepines given to the patient during hospitalization should be maintained since they may show up on routine urine drug screening.

NONOPIOID ADDICTS

Management of acute pain in patients with nonopioid addiction should entail providing effective analgesia with interventions that do not involve medication initially, such as local anesthetic blocks, thermal treatment, or transcutaneous electrical nerve stimulation. If ineffective, nonopioid analgesics as NSAIDs and neuropathic medications should be tried before opioids are used. Again, it is important to avoid as-needed dosing in such patients, and the opioid medication has to be tapered off immediately as the acute pain resolves. Sometimes withdrawal symptoms are misidentified by the patient and staff as reflecting pain, which may lead to increasing the opioid dose, often without relief of the symptoms. Thus, withdrawal symptoms should be properly identified and treated promptly to avoid such confusion. The underlying addiction should also be evaluated and treated.

EMERGENCY DEPARTMENT PATIENTS ("FREQUENT FLYERS")

Approximately 11% of patients seeking treatment in the ED have chronic pain as their complaint,[96] and a significant number of them are receiving opioids for non–cancer-related pain. A "frequent flyer" is a patient who is known to all the ED staff in the area and habitually shows up, usually on nights and weekends, demanding opioids for some chronic (e.g., pancreatitis) or recurrent (e.g., migraine, sickle cell disease) condition. Since the patient engages different shifts at different hospitals, the lack of continuity of care presents a severe challenge to the development of a rational treatment plan. However, such a plan is mandatory.

It is useful to establish a liaison with specialists in the relevant fields and to arrange for consultation so that a plan of management for both pain and addiction can be developed. It is useful to recall that unrewarded behavior is not repeated for long, so patients who resist daytime consultation should be limited, when possible, to noneuphorigenic medications in the ED (e.g., parenteral phenothiazines for migraine, ketorolac for other types of pain) until they accept appropriate consultation. Use of nationwide PDMPs can be very helpful in identifying frequent flyers.

PERSISTENT (SUBACUTE) PAIN

If pain persists beyond the expected time of healing, physical causes should initially be explored such as delayed healing, undetected trauma or abscess, disuse phenomena (muscle spasm, contractures), neuropathic pain (neuritis, neuroma, deafferentation), or sympathetic pain (complex regional pain syndrome). If no physical cause can be identified, possible pain-sustaining factors such as sleep disturbance, anxiety, depression, and secondary gain must be considered. Physical dependence on the opioid medication has to be ruled out. If this is the case, a slow taper of the current opioid or an equianalgesic dose of a long-acting opioid would be appropriate. Taper is preferably performed at a scheduled time contingent rather than at symptom contingent intervals, and associated withdrawal symptoms should be treated symptomatically if present. If addiction is suspected, consider obtaining an evaluation by an addiction specialist and referral to a recovery program if needed. Pain can be managed as a chronic problem at this time.

CHRONIC PAIN

Appropriate treatment of comorbid chronic pain and addiction remains controversial, and data on which to base therapy are still limited. However, it is important to remember that the goals of treatment of chronic pain in patients with and without an addiction history would be identical and should include reduction of pain, restoration of function, improved coping with pain, and improvement in associated symptoms such as sleep disturbance, depression, and anxiety if present. Both addiction and the physical components of pain have to be addressed concurrently through detoxification or substitution with a long-acting opioid if detoxification is not possible early in treatment. For pain management, non–medication-based approaches and the use of non–dependence-producing analgesics should take priority. Physical, social, and productive activity should be strongly encouraged to help improve the patient's overall functional status. Chronic pain control in general in patients with addiction revolves mainly around opioid- and non–opioid-based therapies.

OPIOID-BASED TREATMENT

Use of chronic opioid therapy in patients with suspected ADRB or a history of substance abuse is challenging because such patients are more vulnerable to prescription drug misuse and abuse. In some patients, such as those actively using illicit drugs, the potential benefits from chronic opioid therapy are outweighed by the potential risks, and opioids should not be prescribed outside highly controlled and specialized settings such as an opioid treatment program with directly observed therapy. However, in other patients with no active substance use disorder, the potential benefits may outweigh the risks. Although evidence is still lacking on the best way to manage these patients, potential risks may be minimized by some of the measures mentioned previously, such as more frequent monitoring and scheduled visits, limiting the amount of dispensed medication, and clear communication with the patient regarding expectations and conditions for termination of opioid therapy. It is still unclear what degree of monitoring is needed and how effective these measures may be. However, as discussed below, some studies suggest that these measures are quite helpful and can readily be undertaken in a medical setting, such as a pain clinic.

Multiple guidelines for the treatment of chronic non–cancer-related pain have been developed, with some variability in their recommendations in regard to concurrent addictive disorder. Portenoy,[97] among others, considered a history of alcohol abuse to be a relative contraindication to opioid therapy, whereas Kalso and coworkers[98] considered it an absolute contraindication. Most guidelines emphasize the need for special attention in patients with a history of drug or alcohol abuse and recommend that such patients be referred to a multidisciplinary pain clinic[99,100] or a specialized drug unit.[97,101] All but one guideline[101] recommend that opioid therapy be considered after all other reasonable attempts have failed or have been considered. Some guidelines recommend that a second opinion be sought at a multidisciplinary pain clinic before long-term opioid treatment is initiated.[97-102] Another publication recommended that the final decision for initiating opioid treatment be made by a team of two or more practitioners.[102] However, most guidelines recommend that only one physician should be responsible for the opioid prescribing. Sustained-release opioids taken by mouth and by the clock are recommended by all guidelines,[97-102] and some consider transdermal fentanyl patches a useful alternative for patients with morphine intolerance who are at risk for inappropriate self-medication with oral opioid formulations.[100,101] Again, all guidelines recommend close monitoring of patients to include adequate pain relief, adverse effects, functional capacity, and quality of life.

With such guidelines in place, many prescribers are still reluctant to prescribe opioids for patients with concurrent chronic pain problem and substance use disorder. A survey of physician attitudes across the United States[103] found generalized reluctance regarding the prescription of opioids for chronic noncancer pain. Concerns about addiction, tolerance, and dependence were the most important cited, followed by regulatory pressure and finally side effects. Another survey by Joranson and colleagues[104] found that 58% of surveyed state medical board members considered prescribing opioids for patients with a history of opioid abuse a probable violation of federal or state laws. Two subsequent follow-up surveys[105,106] revealed some liberalization of this attitude in light of increased emphasis on pain management and educational programs for state medical boards; however, many still believe that federal and state law enforcement agencies have increased criminal investigations and prosecutions of physicians. It is important to remember that federal law prohibits the prescription of opioids to maintain addiction or prevent withdrawal but does not prohibit long-term prescription of opioids to persons with addictive disorders for the relief of pain.

Data on the outcome of opioid therapy in patients with chronic pain and addiction are very limited, and most studies conducted thus far have been small. In 20 patients with chronic non–cancer-related pain and a comorbid history of substance abuse who were treated for more than 1 year, Dunbar and Katz[89] found that those who abused opioids did so early in treatment and those who did not were more likely to be active in 12-step meetings, to have stable support systems, and to be less likely to be recent polysubstance abusers. Those who did not abuse were more likely to benefit from the opioids. Currie and associates[107] used cognitive-behavioral therapy with an emphasis on substance abuse education and relapse prevention to treat 44 patients with comorbid chronic pain and addiction who were receiving chronic opioid therapy. Some chose to discontinue opioids because they felt unable to control their use. Those who continued opioids were transitioned to longer-acting medications (excluding methadone). As-needed opioids were prohibited, and once titrated to the optimal dosage, patients could not obtain additional medication. There were significant improvements in pain, emotional functioning, and medication reliance. At the 12-month follow-up, 50% of the patients were opioid free and the remainder had reduced their use from 17 to 12 days/mo. There was no significant difference in outcomes for opioid and nonopioid users, although those who continued to take opioids appeared to function better overall. The authors suggested that long-acting opioids may provide both analgesia and reduction of cravings in this population. Jamison and colleagues[108] conducted a 6-month-long randomized trial of opioid adherence strategies in 60 subjects with chronic non–cancer-related pain who were at high risk for opioid misuse but had no active substance use disorder. They found that an intervention consisting of monthly physician visits, urine toxicology screening every 3 months, and a monthly session with a psychologist conducting motivational interviewing for opioid adherence reduced opioid misuse from a 75% rate in the control group receiving usual care to 25% in the intervention group.

From these studies, as well as clinical reports, it is reasonable to conclude that chronic opioid therapy may be indicated in selected patients with concurrent chronic non–cancer-related pain and addictive disorder (or in those at risk for misuse but no active substance use disorder) when no other realistic treatment option is available. Long-term opioids may be considered in such cases if they provide subjective pain relief and improved level of function and do not result in adverse consequences, such as signs of loss of control over medication use or return to addictive drugs. The issue of ensuring that addiction is being adequately treated is often key to the management of these patients. A team approach consisting of a pain specialist, an addiction specialist, and the patient's primary care physician in a highly structured program setting is strongly recommended. A team physician should meet regularly with the patient to assess efficacy of the medication and monitor for any evidence of misuse or abuse of the prescribed medication. In addition, an exit strategy should be planned ahead and communicated appropriately with the patient and should include discontinuation of opioid therapy in case of lack of improvement in pain or function, failure to comply with the treatment plan, unexpected findings in urine drug screens, or documented misuse of the prescription in any form. Patients should clearly understand that if a decision is made to discontinue opioid therapy, this would not in any way affect their pain management treatment or support by the treating physician.

NON–OPIOID-BASED TREATMENT

A number of pharmacological and nonpharmacological interventions have proved useful for chronic pain and are effective in addition to or in lieu of opioids. It has been compellingly demonstrated over the course of several decades that there is a group of patients with chronic pain who are more comfortable and more functional without opioids. To date, we still lack accurate predictors of patients who will do well with opioids and are essentially limited to a therapeutic trial to ascertain patients who will show improved function, mood, and relief of pain and to assess side effects and aberrant behavior. It is likely that patients with addiction will be over-represented in the group who are better served without opioids because their risks are clearly increased. No randomized trials so far have directly evaluated the efficacy of behavioral therapy, psychiatric treatment, multidisciplinary rehabilitation, or functional restoration versus or in addition to chronic opioid therapy in patients with chronic pain.

INTRATHECAL DRUG DELIVERY

The appropriateness of intrathecal (IT) drug delivery in chronic pain patients with current or a past history of addiction remains a controversial topic. Although some may consider addiction an absolute contraindication to IT delivery, others would recommend it as an option, provided that the patient is treated appropriately for the addictive disorder. According to one recent consensus panel,[109] selected patients with addiction may be reasonable candidates for IT opioid therapy since eliminating oral opioids and using only IT opioids shift the control of medication administration from the patient to the pump as prescribed by the physician. However, it is often quite difficult to eliminate the need for oral opioids to control pain in the treatment of cancer- or non–cancer-related chronic pain with an IT pump, and thus these risks of misuse and addiction are most often unchanged with IT therapy. The panel also recognized the potential risks and problems associated with IT opioid delivery in this population secondary to the higher incidence of associated personality problems since such patients can be demanding, manipulative, passive-aggressive, and generally noncompliant. Moreover, there is no assurance that these patients will not turn to other substances such as alcohol, benzodiazepines, or illicit drugs following resolution of the pain problem. There have been a few case reports of patients who attempted to penetrate their pump or catheter to gain access to the drug. Burton and coauthors[110] reported a case of self-administration of phencyclidine, methamphetamine, and propoxyphene via an IT pump by an incarcerated patient. Thus, it is strongly recommended that if IT therapy is to be used, patients have to be monitored closely and treated appropriately for their addiction. Non–opioid-based IT therapy may also be a reasonable alternative for patients with serious abuse problems or an active addiction.

SPINAL CORD STIMULATION

Data on the outcomes of spinal cord stimulation (SCS) in patients with addiction and chronic pain are lacking, possibly because addiction is still considered an exclusion criterion for a trial of SCS by many physicians. Pain specialists are still unclear about the role of drug addiction and psychiatric comorbid conditions on SCS outcomes. Some would recommend treatment of the drug addiction before undergoing an SCS trial,[111,112] whereas others have strongly related a history of drug addiction with poor outcomes regardless of current addiction status. Most authors, however, still consider an active alcohol or drug dependency that assumes an over-riding importance in the patient's behavior or in whom there is obviously excessive drug-seeking behavior or uncontrolled escalation of prescribed or nonprescribed substances to be a contraindication to a trial of SCS. Such patients must first demonstrate an ability to conform to a reasonable medication regimen before implantation for SCS is attempted or else they are unlikely to do so afterward. However, patients may be reconsidered for SCS candidacy if they are able to demonstrate a minimum of 3 months of appropriate control of substance use.[113]

SPECIALIZED PAIN SERVICES VERSUS PRIMARY CARE SETTING

Pain practitioners often find themselves in a difficult situation in which the current reimbursement system favors procedures and brief visits for medication management. However, this bias neglects a longitudinal management approach that integrates medical, physical, and psychological therapies, which is essential to address the biopsychosocial factors causing and perpetuating chronic pain. Thus, in this current practice environment, many practitioners tend to rely on opioids alone to help relieve their patients' pain, although it may not be the most beneficial for them. The pain medicine and primary care community rehabilitation model emphasizes training primary care providers to use evidence-based clinical algorithms to manage different chronic pain conditions. Ideally, a multidisciplinary pain medicine team should be readily accessible to support primary care providers when algorithms are not effective in controlling pain and its consequences in a timely fashion. Referral to addiction specialists and rehabilitation facilities should also be made readily available if needed.

PHYSICIAN CONCERNS

As clinicians who are dedicated to the treatment of patients, the priority in the doctor-patient relationship is always focused on the well-being of the patient. However, the practice of medicine often requires a balance between physicians' responsibilities to care for their patients and the appropriate concern of physicians to protect themselves from a medical-legal standpoint. Most often, these concerns are aligned; good patient care is also safe care, with the risks well articulated to the patient. However, maintaining this balance may have an impact on access to care and how care is ultimately delivered. One could argue that treating pain in the context of addiction disorders provides an excellent example of the difficulties involved in striking this balance.

Pain physicians who prescribe opioids to patients with addiction disorders may be at elevated medical-legal risk if patients suffer significant negative consequences of their care. For instance, physicians are at risk for medical malpractice suits from patients who may claim to be victims of iatrogenic addiction as a result of a physician's prescribing. Ultimately, protection of the physician is best achieved through meticulous and diligent documentation, diagnosis of a preexisting addictive disorder or a genetic predisposition for one, and a treatment plan accounting for these risks in the treatment of pain. Just as important is the responsibility of the clinician to document treatment response or lack thereof. In addition, clinicians who prescribe opioids on a regular basis should have access and the ability to seek consultation from an addiction specialist when needed.

As noted previously in this chapter, use of an opioid therapy agreement in both the acute and chronic settings is key not only for documentation purposes but also for establishing a clear agreement with the patient and the expectations regarding the guidelines and boundaries of opioid prescribing.[78] Important points in such a contract would be keeping all appointments, even those with other professionals (psychiatry, physical therapy, marriage counselor, and others). One would also want to see progress toward goals of improving function and life satisfaction. In addition, the agreement should include patient consent to the use of appropriate screening tools, such as random urine toxicology screens.

KEY POINTS

- The powerful analgesic benefit of opioids comes with its own risk for addiction.
- Physicians should be aware of this complex challenge when they decide to prescribe opioids.
- Treatment plans for chronic pain should not always include opioids.
- If necessary, opioid therapy should always be considered a trial and be ended if there is poor evidence of significant improvement in pain or function.
- Improvements in pain and function and adherence to therapy must be demonstrated by the patient for continued opioid prescription.

KEY POINTS—cont'd

- When taking opioids, careful monitoring is necessary.
- Clinicians should identify any aberrant behavior early and respond appropriately to decrease the risk for subsequent addiction.
- Stringent measures of monitoring should be applied in such circumstances.
- Opioid therapy agreements are recommended but should be used with caution.
- Good communication with the patient during each step is crucial for success of treatment. Physicians must also have access to and know when to seek consultation with addiction specialists.

SELECTED READINGS

Ballantyne JC, Laforge KS. Opioid dependence and addiction during opioid treatment of chronic pain. *Pain.* 2007;129:235-255.

Brown RL, Patterson JJ, Rounds LA, et al. Substance abuse among patients with chronic back pain. *J Fam Pract.* 1996;43:152-160.

Chabal C, Erjavec MK, Jacobson L, et al. Prescription opioid abuse in chronic pain patients: clinical criteria, incidence, and predictors. *Clin J Pain.* 1997;13:150-155.

Fishman SM, Bandman TB, Edwards A, et al. The opioid contract in the management of chronic pain. *J Pain Symptom Manage.* 1999;18:27-37.

Gourlay DL, Heit HA, Almahrezi A. Universal precautions in pain medicine: a rational approach to the treatment of chronic pain. *Pain Med.* 2005;6:107-112.

Ives TJ, Chelminski PR, Hammett-Stabler CA, et al. Predictors of opioid misuse in patients with chronic pain: a prospective cohort study. *BMC Health Serv Res.* 2006;6:46.

Jamison RN, Ross EL, Michna E, et al. Substance misuse treatment for high-risk chronic pain patients on opioid therapy: a randomized trial. *Pain.* 2010;150:390-400.

Michna E, Jamison RN, Pham LD, et al. Urine toxicology screening among chronic pain patients on opioid therapy: frequency and predictability of abnormal findings. *Clin J Pain.* 2007;23:173-179.

Nestler EJ. Under siege: the brain on opiates. *Neuron.* 1996;16:897-900.

Portenoy RK. Chronic opioid therapy in non-malignant pain. *J Pain Symptom Manage.* 1990;5:S46-S62.

Savage SR, Joranson DE, Covington EC, et al. Definitions related to the medical use of opioids: evolution towards universal agreement. *J Pain Symptom Manage.* 2003;26:656-666.

Turk DC, Swanson KS, Gatchel RJ. Predicting opioid misuse by chronic pain patients: a systematic review and literature synthesis. *Clin J Pain.* 2008;24:497-508.

Wasan AD, Butler SF, Budman SH, et al. Psychiatric history and psychological adjustment as risk factors for aberrant drug-related behavior among patients with chronic pain. *Clin J Pain.* 2007;23:307-315.

The references for this chapter can be found at www.expertconsult.com.

PART 6

NERVE BLOCK TECHNIQUES

HONORIO T. BENZON, EDITOR

PART OUTLINE

52 Nerve Blocks of the Head and Neck

Kenneth D. Candido | Miles Day

The primary indication for nerve blocks of the head and neck is for diagnostic and therapeutic purposes in cases of head and neck pain. Some of the more common indications are discussed in detail in this chapter, including the rationale for selecting regional nerve blocking techniques in the care and management of these patients.

HEADACHES

Differentiating the etiology for headaches is a vexing task, often requiring the skill and experience of multiple clinicians from diverse specialties. The pain practitioner and skilled regional block specialist are well suited to the task by virtue of their respective experiences in performing conduction blockade of the greater and lesser occipital nerves (occipital headache), the cervical medial branches of the facet joints (cervicogenic headache), the cervical epidural nerve block (nonspecific headache), and the atlanto-axial joint (suboccipital headache). Therefore, it is by use of the various modalities of regional block that a diagnostic/therapeutic block of the respective structures implicated in a given patient's pain may be discernible. The anatomic method is a more scientific method of pursuing the source of a headache than that of solely relying on historical information presented by the patient.

ATLANTO-AXIAL JOINT BLOCK

The primary indication for performing atlanto-axial (A-A) nerve block is for the diagnostic and therapeutic evaluation of suboccipital pain that occasionally radiates into the temporomandibular joint (TMJ) area that is exacerbated by head rotation. Whiplash injuries and cervicogenic headaches are two of the more common indications for this block. The A-A joint (Figs. 52.1 and 52.2) lacks posterior articulations and therefore is neither a bona fide facet joint nor a true zygapophyseal joint. Also, there is no intervertebral disk between the atlas (C1) and the axis (C2), nor is there an intervertebral foramen at that level to accommodate an exiting nerve root. At the A-A joint, the head flexes, extends, and rotates in a horizontal plane, up to 60 degrees, giving the joint significant responsibility for both the stability and the mobility of the head and neck. The joint can be injured by seemingly trivial insults and trauma. The resulting pain syndrome can be significant, manifesting as dull, continual and achy pain in the posterior neck and suboccipital region. More severe injuries, such as those caused by motor vehicle accidents, might subject the joint to acceleration-deceleration type injuries, with sequelae exceeding pain and dysfunction. Indeed, paralysis and even death could result from ligamentous disruption, analogous to an odontoid fracture. The fibers of the respective spinal nerves C1 and particularly C2 contribute to the formation of the occipital nerves (greater and lesser), which are frequent targets for the practicing pain physician. An extremely important anatomic concept involves the relationship of the vertebral artery to the A-A joint; whereas the artery is medial to the atlanto-occipital (A-O) joint,[1] it is found lateral to the A-A joint. Therefore, needles directed at the joint during nerve block need to be oriented slightly more medially, cognizant of the danger of aiming toward the interlaminar space, or even toward the foramen magnum.

TECHNIQUE OF ATLANTO-AXIAL NERVE BLOCK (SEE FIGS. 52.3 AND 52.4)

Blockade of the A-A joint requires fluoroscopic assistance to ascertain that the advancing needle does not encroach on the critical anatomic structures such as the vertebral artery and the spinal cord. Patients are placed prone, after obtaining the appropriate medical history, performing a targeted physical examination, and establishing that there are no bleeding problems or infectious issues related to the target for intended needle placement. Baseline vital signs are obtained and recorded. It is recommended that an intravenous access be established for prophylactic purposes. Bolsters are typically placed beneath the chest to elevate the shoulders off the procedure table, permitting the patient to flex the neck and rest the forehead on a neurosurgical donut or pillow. After performing a sterile skin preparation and draping, the fluoroscopic unit is oriented in an anterior-posterior direction to identify the atlas and the foramen magnum, implementing a moderate craniad tilt of the unit until all structures are clearly visualized. The A-A joint is located lateral and inferior to both the foramen magnum and the atlas (see Fig. 52.2). A local anesthetic skin wheal is made over the intended injection site using a small gauge, 1.5-inch needle. Next, an 18-gauge skin core is made using a sharp cutting needle to permit the passage of a blunt, 22-gauge, styletted Whitacre type subarachnoid needle. A curve is made at the distal tip of the needle to allow better steering once it has been advanced through the skin and subcutaneous tissues. The needle is advanced under continued fluoroscopic guidance, rotating the beam of the unit until the needle appears in tunnel or "gun barrel" view, which is represented as a dot advancing toward the posterolateral

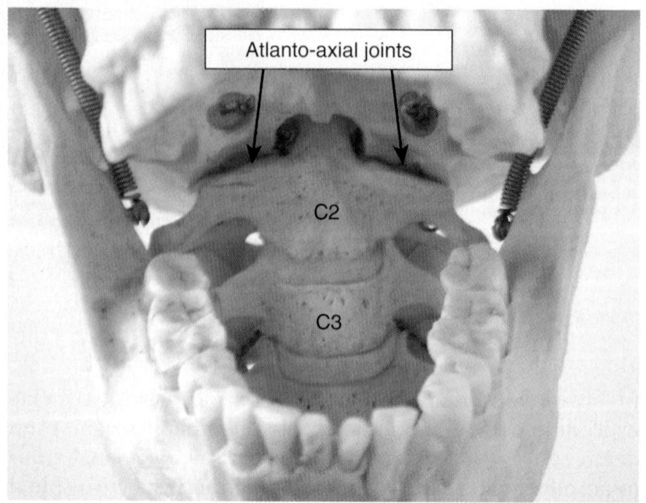

Figure 52.1 Demonstration of the mouth open view to reveal the anterior atlanto-axial (C1-C2) joint. (Photo courtesy of Kenneth D. Candido, M.D.)

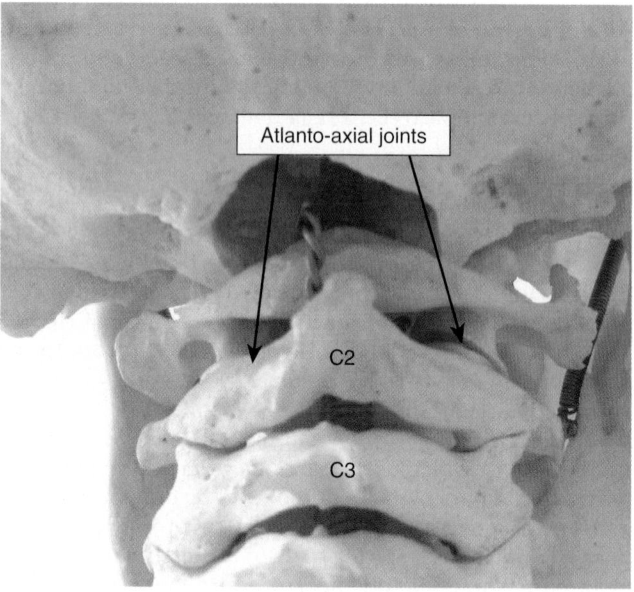

Figure 52.2 Posterior view of the atlanto-axial (C1-C2) joint. (Photo courtesy of Kenneth D. Candido, M.D.)

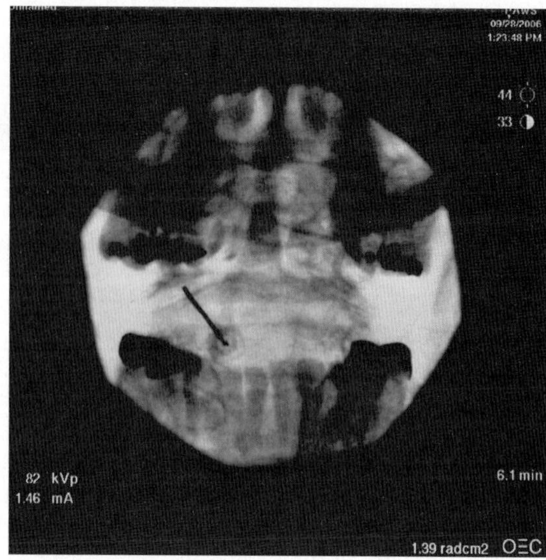

Figure 52.3 Posterior-anterior radiograph demonstrating correct needle placement using a posterior approach to the left atlanto-axial joint. (Photo courtesy of Kenneth D. Candido, M.D.)

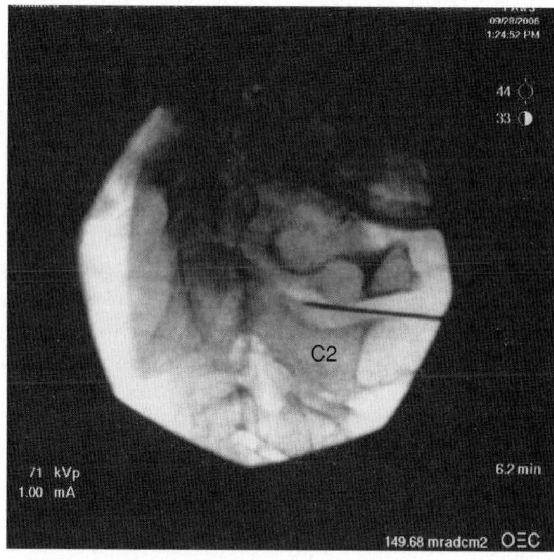

Figure 52.4 Lateral fluoroscopy demonstrating appropriate needle placement for an atlanto-axial joint injection. (Photo courtesy of Kenneth D. Candido, M.D.)

aspect of the A-A joint. The needle should be directed slightly medially to avoid the vertebral artery, which is situated laterally, but not too medially, as this would potentially engage the spinal cord. Occasionally, but not always, a "popping" sensation will be appreciated as the needle traverses the joint and enters it from posterior to anterior (see Fig. 52.3). The fluoroscopic unit must then be rotated laterally (see Fig. 52.4) to confirm the needle placement at the appropriate depth between the atlas and axis. Once placement has been verified, gentle aspiration of the needle is undertaken to assess for the presence of cerebrospinal fluid (CSF) or blood. If none is present, a small (i.e., 1-mL) volume of radiocontrast media may be incrementally injected under real-time fluoroscopy. If the needle is situated within the confines of the joint, a bilateral concavity will be demonstrated, indicative of an intact joint capsule. If the joint capsule has been ruptured, then the dye may be seen as spreading into the peridural space, and care should be taken not to inject long-acting local anesthetic (bupivacaine, ropivacaine) through the needle. Rapid runoff of the dye may signify vascular injection and is to be guarded against, particularly if it is suspected that the needle may have entered the laterally situated vertebral artery. If this occurs, the needle should be redirected medially, re-aspiration of the needle in four quadrants undertaken, and re-injection of contrast material prior to considering injecting local anesthetics or adjuvants. Even without directly injecting into the vertebral artery (even miniscule volumes of dilute local anesthetics injected here can lead to grand mal seizures), ataxia following A-A block is not uncommon[2] and is likely due to vascular uptake of local anesthetics in this extremely vascular region.

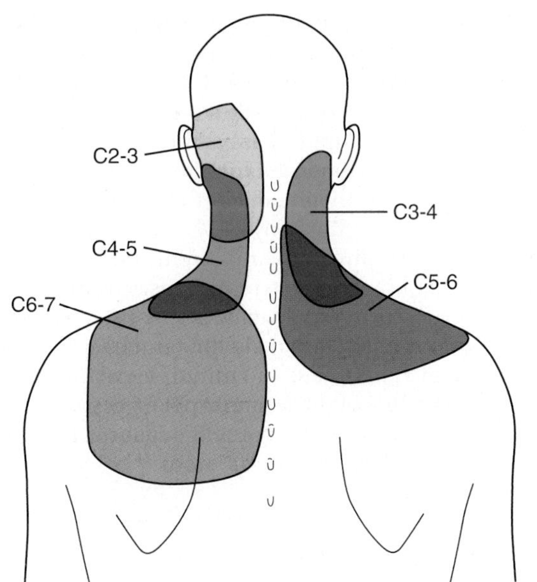

Figure 52.5 Map of areas invested by the sensory nerves of the cervical medial branches. (From Cooper G, Bailey B, Bogduk N. Cervical zygapophysial joint pain maps. *Pain Med*. 2007;8:344-353.)

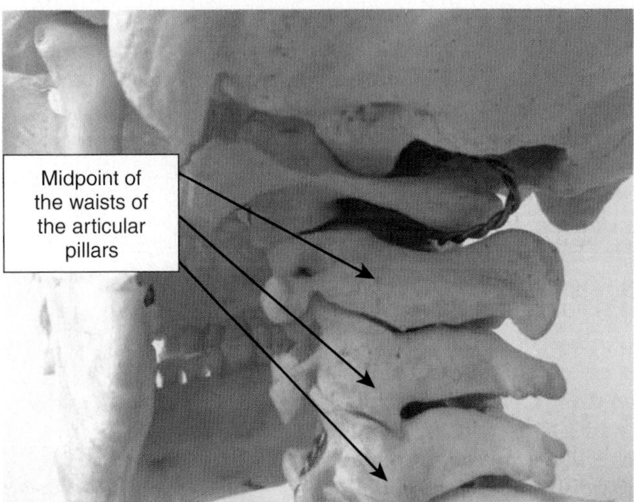

Figure 52.6 Lateral oblique view demonstrating close-up of the needle insertion points for medial branch blocks and radiofrequency ablation techniques of cervical facet joint denervation. (Photo courtesy of Kenneth D. Candido, M.D.)

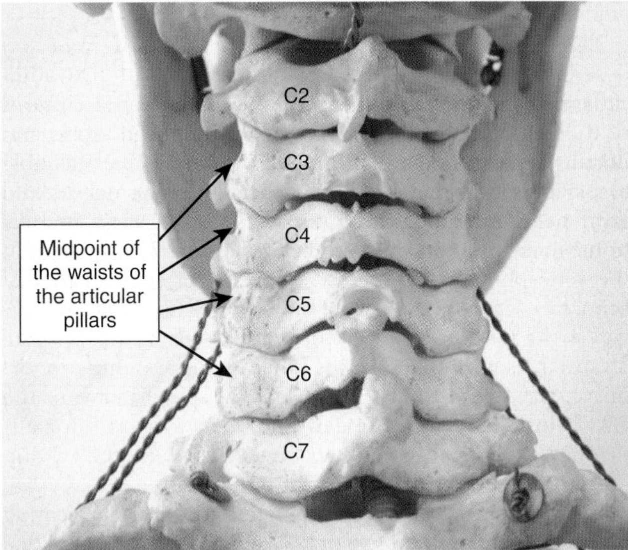

Figure 52.7 Posterior view of the scalloped areas representing the waists of the cervical articular pillars, the site of needle placement for both local anesthetic medial branch facet joint block, as well as for RFA procedures and pulsed-RF techniques of denervating or neuromodulating the cervical facet joint nerves. The C7-T1 interlaminar opening is more capacious than more proximal levels and is the site frequently chosen for cervical epidural needle placement. (Photo courtesy of Kenneth D. Candido, M.D.)

THIRD OCCIPITAL NERVE BLOCK

Diverse pain syndromes result from disorders of the cervical intervertebral disks, the facet joints (zygapophyseal, or Z joints), or both. When confronted by individuals with headache and neck or shoulder pain, the clinician is compelled to seek a diagnosis based largely on history and physical examination. The physical examination is complicated by the finding of significant variability and overlap in the innervation patterns related to the sensory distribution of the cervical medial branch nerves (Fig. 52.5). The third occipital nerve has been implicated in chronic headache pain, primarily as attributed to cervicogenic headache. Syndromes related to dysfunction of the medial branches of the upper cervical spine have at times been misdiagnosed as being due to tension-type and other forms of headache. Patients, having been misdiagnosed as such, have ultimately failed to derive analgesic benefit from medication administration and other conservative treatment measures that were misguided.

The third occipital nerve (TON) is the superficial branch of the C-3 dorsal ramus. It is the only medial branch that innervates the facet joint at C2-C3 (Figs. 52.6 through 52.8). Therefore, successful blockade of the TON, and the resultant block of the facet joint at C2-C3, has been associated with relief of headache pain in individuals suffering from "third occipital headache."

ANATOMIC CONSIDERATIONS

The C2-C3 joint is the first joint of the cervical spine possessing a true joint capsule and synovium, and this level is the first wherein an intervertebral disk exists and wherein a foramen exists to accommodate the exiting C3 nerve root. In this regard, the C2-C3 joint is distinct from the atlanto-occipital (A-O) (C0-C1) and atlanto-axial (A-A) (C1-C2) joints superior to it. This level, then, represents a sort of transitional zone between the rotational joint of the neck (AA) and the lower cervical facet joints, which function not in neck and head rotation but in neck flexion and extension.

Facet joints contain free and encapsulated nerve endings. In addition, nerves in the zygapophyseal joint (Z joint) contain substance P and calcitonin gene-related peptide (CGRP). The capsule of the Z joint contains low-threshold mechanoreceptors, mechanically sensitive nociceptors, and silent nociceptors. Each of these may respond to noxious stimulation, including moderate to severe levels of osteoarthritis, with the result being a nociceptive stimulation perceived as headache or neck pain.

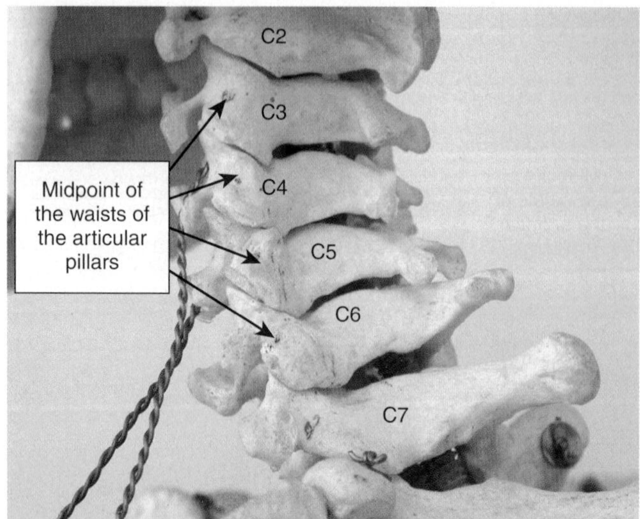

Figure 52.8 Lateral oblique view demonstrating the waists of the articular pillars in consideration of medial branch blocks of the cervical facet joints. Also demonstrated is the interlaminar space at C7-T1 for cervical epidural block needle placement. (Photo courtesy of Kenneth D. Candido, M.D.)

The clinical anatomy of the cervical dorsal rami was described by Bogduk, following dissections of five adult cadavers.[2] He pointed out that classic textbook descriptions of the cervical dorsal rami had been limited in scope and detail. While dissecting the medial branches, he was able to place wires superficially and parallel to the nerves and then perform radiographic analyses of the wires in relationship to the cervical vertebral skeleton. He noted that the semispinalis capitis muscle covers the cervical medial branches, whereas the lateral branches of C3-C7 lie superficial to the tendons of origin of that muscle. The TON penetrates the semispinalis capitis. The C3 dorsal ramus, a short nerve, was noted to arise from the C3 spinal nerve in the C2-C3 intervertebral foramen and then to curve dorsally through the intertransverse space. At this point, the C3 dorsal ramus was noted to divide into major branches: the two medial branches, the lateral branch, and a communicating branch. In three out of five of his specimens, the two medial branches of C3 were noted to arise from a common stem, and in the other two specimens they had their own respective origins. The third occipital nerve (TON) was the principal and constant medial branch of the C3 dorsal ramus.[2] After arising from the C3 dorsal ramus, the TON was found to curve dorsally and medially around the superior articular pillar of the C3 vertebral body, crossing the C2-C3 Z joint either just below the joint itself or at the joint level. The TON runs transversally medially through the fibro-adipose tissue below the obliquus inferior and dorsal to the lamina of the C2 vertebra.

A branch of the TON supplies the semispinalis capitis, which lies superficial to it. A communicating branch to the greater occipital nerve (GON) is also given off. This branch arises just above the level of the C2 spinous process. The TON then passes dorsally and pierces the semispinalis capitis and the splenius capitis, turning rostrally to pierce the trapezius, which lies over it. The more medial terminal branch supplies the skin of the rostral neck and the occiput below the external occipital protuberance. More lateral branches travel toward the mastoid process, communicating with the cutaneous rami of the GON and lesser occipital nerves (LONs). Because of the transverse direction of the GON and the TON, these two nerves may be injured by parasagittal incisions made in the upper part of the neck.

The target branch for nerve block, the TON, wraps dorsally and medially around the middle of the waist of the articular pillar of C3 (center of the bony trapezoid). As it moves more medially, the TON invests the multifidus muscle. There is a communicating branch that typically arises from the C3 dorsal ramus, running rostromedially across the posterior part of the C2-C3 Z joint.[2] The anatomic target for locating the nerve percutaneously, then, is to utilize lateral fluoroscopy to identify the waistline of the articular pillars of C2 and C3 and to advance a needle or radiofrequency cannula toward the Z joint at C2-C3. As Bogduk stated,

> *[N]eedles or electrodes introduced obliquely, ventromedially onto the dorsolateral aspect of the articular pillar, will rest on the medial branch. The relationship of the nerve to bone at this site is constant, because the medial branches are bound to the periosteum by an investing fascia and are held against the articular pillar by tendons of the semispinalis capitis.*[2]

This target is removed from any major arterial (vertebral artery) or other vascular structure, as well as from the exiting spinal nerve and spinal cord; it is therefore an appropriate target in terms of affording access to the medial branches as well as one that provides for an approach likely to minimize unwanted trespass into nontargeted tissues.

THE THIRD OCCIPITAL NERVE AND HEADACHE PAIN

Osteoarthritis of the C2-C3 Z joint and trauma related to motor vehicle accidents are causes of persistent occipital or suboccipital headache pain. As there is no clear-cut clinical evaluative technique or diagnostic tool for determining who is suffering from headache due to disease of this joint or from neck trauma (or that mediated by the TON), it is somewhat intuitive and logical that blockade of the TON should be performed in cases of persistent headache that are unresponsive to conventional medication management.[3]

Bogduk and Marsland conducted fluoroscopically guided TON blocks in 10 consecutive patients presenting with occipital or suboccipital headache. They elected to place their needles at the lower half of the silhouette of the C2-C3 Z joint, recognizing the landmark on x-ray as a convexity arising upward from the concavity of the C3 articular pillar, lying horizontally opposite the level of the C2 spinous process and C2-C3 disk space (Figs. 52.9 through 52.11). All procedures were performed with patients in the prone position and with a bolster beneath the upper chest and shoulders to permit head flexion forward toward the procedure table. A solution of 0.5 mL of 0.5% bupivacaine was injected at three distinct sites: in the middle of the Z joint at C2-C3, at the lower end of the joint, and between the first two needle placements (for bilateral blocks the total volume was therefore 3 mL; 1.5 mL per side). Seventy percent of patients manifest total pain relief lasting the duration of the bupivacaine, following unilateral blocks.[3] The 30% failures did not have positive responses to the bilateral blocks performed on their behalf.[3] Bogduk stated that blockade of the medial

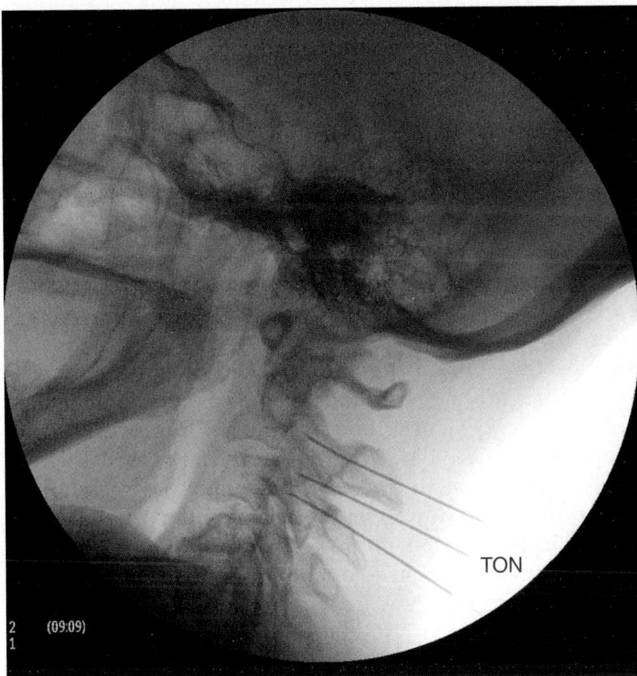

Figure 52.9 Three needles in place, lateral fluoroscopic view, for C2, C3, and third occipital nerve (TON) block, right side. (Figure courtesy of Kenneth D. Candido, M.D.)

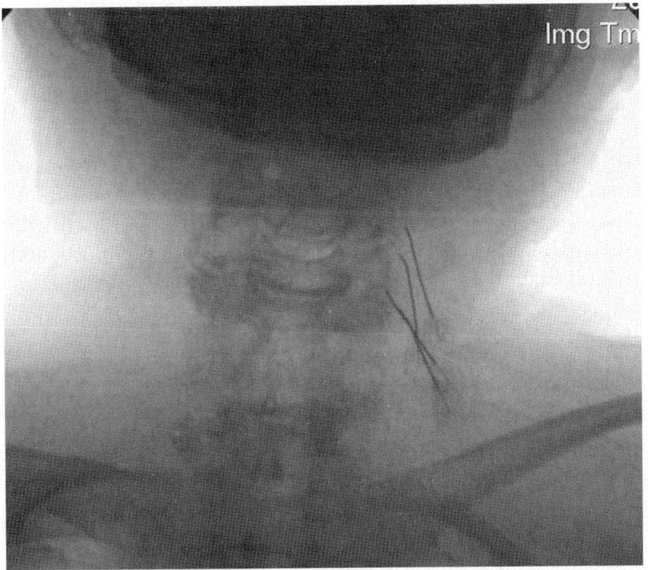

Figure 52.10 Three needles in place, Anterior-posterior fluoroscopic view; right-sided C2, C3, and third occipital nerve block (TON). (Photo courtesy of Kenneth D. Candido, M.D.)

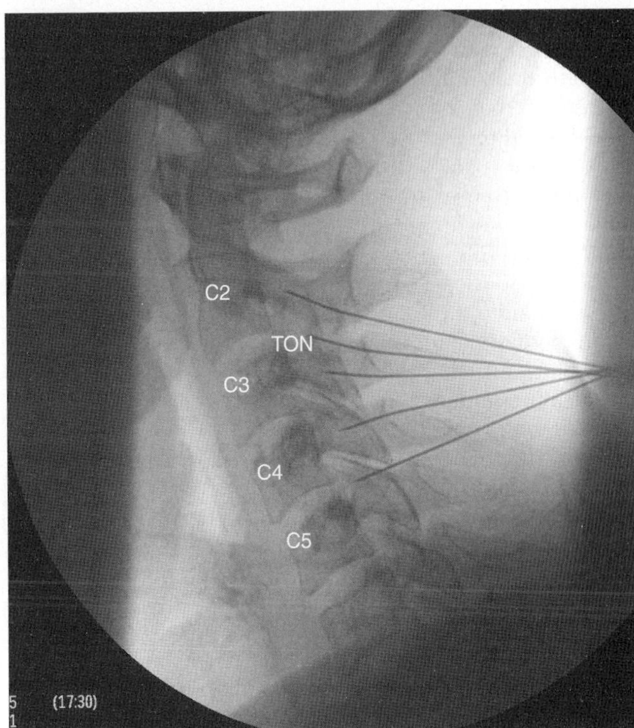

Figure 52.11 Lateral fluoroscopic image demonstrates placement of 22-gauge, 3.5 inch Whitacre subarachnoid needles at the middle of the waist of the articular pillars for C2, third occipital nerve (TON), C3, C4, and C5 blocks of the medial branches. A single skin wheal has been used for entry of all five needles, minimizing patient discomfort for the performance of the procedure. (Photo courtesy of Kenneth D. Candido, M.D.)

branch nerves, particularly the TON, are easier for patients to tolerate than intraarticular injections because they are more easily performed and are associated with less pain during their performance than are the articular injections. Furthermore, it is apparent that local anesthetic injected into a joint may not actually stay within the joint space, potentially limiting any diagnostic information that might otherwise be derived from the procedure. Finally, markedly degenerated joints might not readily accommodate an advancing needle tip, rendering the choice of this articular approach potentially useless overall.[2] If the ventral margin of the joint space is penetrated, there is also a distinct possibility that entrance into the epidural or subarachnoid spaces may occur, with potentially devastating consequences.

Although no one knows for certain how likely it is that pain in the occipital and suboccipital area emanates from the C2-C3 Z joint and although various studies show greatly disparate findings, several compelling attempts at determining the incidence (a measure of the risk of developing some new condition within a specified period of time) or prevalence (the total number of cases in the population, divided by the number of individuals in the population) need to be reviewed.

A study involved 24 consecutive patients presenting with undiagnosed neck pain who were evaluated using controlled diagnostic blocks incorporating low-volume local anesthetic injections.[4] For individuals with occipital or suboccipital headache and neck pain, the lower half of the lateral margin of the C2-C3 Z joint was selected as the injection site. Complete pain relief was considered to occur if the patients, having received the bupivacaine blocks and then going home to perform their activities of daily living, noted at least 2 hours of total analgesia. Failure to derive pain relief resulted in patients undergoing additional cervical medial branch blocks at contiguous levels. Nineteen out of 24 patients had positive results, with 9 of these ultimately having pain isolated to the C2-C3 level. Therefore, in 47% of patients who had diagnostic block-proven cervical Z joint pain, the TON was the nerve responsible for mediating the pain. Although this study has not been replicated, it is tempting to use the information as a general rule of thumb when approaching individuals with neck pain resulting from degenerative disease of the cervical spine and when planning nerve blocks based on the correlation of symptoms with joint pain maps.[5,6] If it is known that in half of cases the level responsible for a given pain problem is at the C2-C3 joint, then it might save time, expense, and patient discomfort to rapidly move toward ruling in or ruling out that level, and the TON, at the outset as part of the diagnostic workup. However, as discussed later, these figures may be overreaching in terms of the actual prevalence of C2-C3–related pain. Although TON block may be performed easily and typically is without significant complications, side effects do occur commonly. Indeed, any patient presenting for this type of procedure must be duly appraised that successful blockade of the TON (or GON) will likely result in the temporary development of ataxia and some gait unsteadiness. For this reason, bilateral blocks at these levels should likely be staggered, or else the benefit-risk ratio must be significant enough that performing bilateral blocks is clearly warranted.

The subject of joint pain maps merits special mention, as noted previously (see Fig. 52.5). Multiple attempts have been made at delineating the specific cutaneous area of sensation, and hence pain, invested by each respective facet joint and medial branch.[5-9] In the report by Fukui and associates,[8] the site of Z joint intraarticular injection and electrical stimulation (selected cases) was chosen based on any focal paraspinal tenderness. They observed that with injections performed at C2-C3 (n = 14), symptoms were referable to the upper posterior cervical region (64%), the occipital region (50%), or the upper posterolateral cervical region (50%).[8] Windsor and colleagues[9] electrically stimulated the cervical medial branches, including the TON in 9 patients suffering from chronic neck pain. They used the lateral midpoint of the C2-C3 Z joint to indicate the location of the TON. Relatively reproducible referral patterns were identified for the TON nerve distribution as well as for the other medial branch nerves studied.[9]

When reviewing these studies, however, considerable overlap in the areas served by each of the respective segments is noted, much more so than that observed with attempts at mapping spinal nerve dermatome distributions. This produces a diagnostic conundrum, as it is entirely conceivable when approaching cervical spine pain that even perfectly performed techniques, using standardized and accepted anatomic landmarks, may result in failures to derive antinociception with the resultant confusion on behalf of the patient and treating physician.

Because both the intervertebral disk and facet joint are fairly equivalently represented as sources of neck pain (approximately 40% each as sources of neck pain, according to two separate studies), a missed diagnosis might lead a pain physician in the wrong direction when seeking to provide pain relief to a given individual.[10,11] Mapping studies may help to pinpoint discrete areas of pain referral sources that are then amenable to local anesthetic blockade or radiofrequency lesioning techniques. In one such study, joint maps were created by distending the respective joint capsules at segments from C2-C3 to C6-C7. This was done by sequential injections of contrast media, which could be subsequently identified using fluoroscopy. Each joint was noted to produce a characteristic, distinguishable pain pattern from which pain charts could be constructed (see Fig. 52.5).[6] Although only four subjects were evaluated, that number is not too disparate from the original small group of subjects selected to develop the original dermatome charts in neurologically impaired individuals; such charts have been mostly unchallenged since the 1950s.[12] In 10 subjects who received injections based on maps such as those derived and described earlier, 90% had complete concordance of the predicted level of pain and the positive response to the blocks.[7] The C3-C4, C4-C5, and C5-C6 levels were most commonly affected, with only 10% (1 of 10) patients having pain that was documented to result from processes occurring at the C2-C3 (TON) level. These percentages are therefore less indicative of the possibility of the C2-C3 level being primarily involved in head and neck pain than they are of alternative levels lower in the cervical spine. However, a study by Barnsley and Bogduk demonstrated that, following cervical medial branch injections performed in 16 patients suffering from chronic neck pain, 33% (3 of 9) patients who had complete pain relief were patients for whom the TON was treated.[13] It remains unclear how likely the TON is to be implicated in individuals suffering from chronic head and neck pain. The closest studies performed to identify the prevalence of TON-induced headache and neck pain may have been those performed by Lord and Barnsley and colleagues.[14,15] In the first study, 100 consecutive patients underwent double-blind, controlled diagnostic blocks of the TON. On two separate occasions the nerve was blocked using either lidocaine or bupivacaine. The diagnosis of TON nerve involvement was only made if the double diagnostic blocks both relieved the symptoms, with the bupivacaine injection-induced pain relief outlasting that provided by the lidocaine. The prevalence of TON headache among whiplash patients was 27% and among those with dominant headache was 53%.[14]

In the second study, 50 consecutive patients with chronic neck pain and whiplash injury underwent double-blind, controlled diagnostic medial branch blocks using either 0.5-mL lidocaine (2%) or bupivacaine (0.5%) in a random fashion. In 12 of 27 patients (44%), the source of symptoms was identified as being isolated primarily to the C2-C3 Z joint.[15]

These findings corroborated the impression that although there may be substantial overlap in cutaneous innervations of the central and peripheral nervous systems, these joint maps are essential tools in assessing the appropriate approach to a given pain process in any individual. They also demonstrated variability in determining the relative incidence and prevalence of C2-C3 Z joint pain, depending on technique of assessment and provocation maneuvers to assess the joint and the medial branch nerve (TON).

RATIONALE FOR BLOCKING THE TON

The TON block is useful in the diagnostic and therapeutic phases of treating cervicogenic headache. Evidence of efficacy for both local anesthetic blocks as well as for radiofrequency ablation of the cervical medial branches has accrued. However, only recently has the use of medial branch blocks and radiofrequency ablation techniques received scientific support in the literature. Indeed, two separate attempts at meta-analysis have shown somewhat disparate results. The first paper, published in 2001, suggested that radiofrequency neurotomy used for treating pain from the cervical Z joints after flexion-extension injury was only supported by limited scientific data.[16] However, a mere six total studies satisfied the authors' criteria for inclusion, and so it is entirely possible that the data suffer lack of suitable cohort studies to make a true assessment of its validity. The second review performed in 2007 liberalized the inclusion criteria somewhat and found that the support for medial branch cervical block was moderate (level III) as was the support for cervical medial branch neurotomy.[17] Here the authors relied on the criteria established by the Agency for Healthcare Research and Quality (AHRQ), which included some nonrandomized trials. They also incorporated studies from the Cochrane Musculoskeletal Review Group, which were randomized trials. One of the important points noted was that the evidence for performing cervical intra-articular facet joint injections was limited both for short-term as well as for long-term analgesia efficacy. This corroborates Dr. Bogduk's earlier assertions that not only are medial branch techniques more likely to target the real source of pain associated with cervical degenerative facet conditions, but also that articular procedures have an inherently high failure rate because there is no guarantee that injected local anesthetic will remain in the confines of the joint.

The rationale for blocking the TON is twofold:

1. To provide a diagnostic evaluation of the C2-C3 facet joint as being the source of pain in the occipital and suboccipital area
2. To provide an indication as to whether or not neuroablative techniques applied over that nerve might be fruitful in treating pain on a long-term basis

We suggest performing double-diagnostic blocks using 0.5 mL of local anesthetic solutions, typically 0.5% ropivacaine plain, before undertaking neurotomy of the TON. Ropivacaine is used for two major reasons. It has intrinsic vasoconstrictor properties, and epinephrine does not have to be added to it. It also has a cardiovascular safety profile that is superior to that for bupivacaine. Unintentional injection into vascular structures, including the vertebral artery, is less likely to result in serious morbidity when ropivacaine is used, in contradistinction to bupivacaine. The further rationale for using ropivacaine is to provide duration of analgesia that exceeds that provided by shorter-acting agents such as lidocaine or mepivacaine. In terms of assessing efficacy, it is likely that longer-acting local anesthetics may provide greater information than shorter-acting drugs, as the effect of the short-acting drugs may be so fleeting as to provide confusing or inexact clinical information.

Double-diagnostic blocks have been described for assessing the efficacy of cervical medial branch blocks.[18] Barnsley and associates compared single to double-diagnostic blocks in 55 adult patients who had been having neck pain for longer than 3 months. They used 0.5 mL of either 0.5% bupivacaine or 2% lidocaine, randomly selected. The duration of analgesia was assessed in a double-blind fashion. They found that the false-positive rate (a test that shows evidence of a disease when it not present) of single blocks was 27% (16/60).[18] They also found that the most common positive levels were at C2-C3 and C5-C6.[18] Lord and colleagues found that comparative blocks of the medial branches using lidocaine, bupivacaine, or normal saline in a randomized, double-blind, placebo-controlled fashion in 50 patients had a specificity (the statistical probability that an individual who does not have the particular disease being tested for will be correctly identified as negative, expressed as the proportion of true negative results to the total of true negative and false positive results) (TN/TN + FP) of 88%, but only marginal sensitivity (the proportion of individuals in a population that is correctly identified when administered a test designed to detect a particular disease, calculated as the number of true positive results divided by the number of true positive and false negative results) (TP/TP + FN) (54%).[19] Hence, some 46% of patients who are not placebo responders would incorrectly be labeled as placebo responders if diagnoses were based solely on comparative blocks.[19]

Slipman and colleagues retrospectively reviewed 18 patients with chronic persistent daily headaches lasting a mean of 34 months following whiplash injury who underwent intraarticular C2-C3 facet joint injections.[20] They noted that in 61% of cases, headache frequency diminished from daily to less than three headaches per week. Although this work is retrospective, the results are nevertheless supportive for targeting the TON in chronic headache conditions refractory to conventional conservative management. Furthermore, because the injections were articular and not at the medial branch (TON), the information gleaned from this report may not be useful in determining candidacy for radiofrequency neurotomy.

TECHNIQUE FOR TON BLOCK

We perform C2-C3 medial branch (TON) procedures with the patient in the prone position using continual live fluoroscopic guidance throughout the injection phase (see Figs. 52.9 through 52.11).[21] A bolster is placed beneath the shoulders and chest to elevate the thorax off of the table and to permit gentle head and neck flexion forward. An intravenous cannula is placed for purposes of administering resuscitative medications in the unlikely event that it is necessary to treat vasovagal syncope or for supportive medication administration in cases of unintentional vascular injection. Vital signs are monitored using standard American Society of Anesthesiologists (ASA) basic monitors including pulse oximetry and noninvasive blood pressure assessment. After performing a sterile skin preparation, scout films are obtained of the neck in an effort to identify the scalloped margins of the lateral vertebral bodies. Then, skin wheals are raised over the intended target(s) using a hypodermic needle and 1 to 3 mL of lidocaine solution with epinephrine, 1:200,000 (5 mcg/mL). Using short-beveled, 22-gauge, 2.5- to 3.5-inch needles, the targeted lateral scalloped margins of the vertebral bodies are advanced upon until bony contact is made. At this point the fluoroscopy unit is rotated laterally to assess the relationship of the advancing needle tip to the TON target, in the center of the C2-C3 Z joint (discussed previously). The needle tip must be recessed posteriorly away from the C2-C3 intervertebral foramen as well as from the known location of the vertebral artery. If bone has not been contacted and 2 cm of the needle has been inserted into the skin, then a reassessment of the approach and direction is undertaken while still in the A-P fluoroscopy mode. Once the needle is appropriately seated on bone at the target site (Fig. 5.4), the A-P view is once again undertaken to verify that the needle(s) is in the correct position vis-à-vis the lateral vertebral body margin.

Ultrasound-guided approaches are rapidly gaining popularity for all forms of interventional pain procedures, but in our experience they have not yet reached the level of sophistication to supplant fluoroscopy use for this particular procedure. At this point, aspiration tests are performed to verify the absence of blood or cerebrospinal fluid, and the patient is queried to ascertain that no paresthesias have been elicited. If there are none and vital signs remain stable and close to baseline values, 0.5 mL of 0.5% ropivacaine is injected. No glucocorticoid is added to the solution, as Manchikanti and associates, have demonstrated that there is little value, if any, of adding steroid to the blocks.[22] Still, many clinicians continue to add a steroid in their practice. If the risk-benefit ratio favors using steroids in an individual suspected of having an inflammatory component to his or her pain, then there may be little harm in adding a nonparticulate steroid in judicious doses. After injection, the needle(s) is cleared and withdrawn, and a sterile dressing is applied over the injection site. The patient should be observed for at least 30 minutes, as it is common for patients to become ataxic or have unsteady gait following successfully performed procedures. Discharge instructions should be clear and precisely instruct patients to seek emergency medical care if they develop any delayed-onset side effects or complications from the procedure.

RADIOFREQUENCY NEUROTOMY

In selected patients, radiofrequency (RF) of the TON may be considered for long-term therapeutic benefit. In a study published in 1995, Lord and colleagues demonstrated the efficacy of performing radiofrequency ablation (RFA) of the TON in only 40% of patients (4 of 10), with only three having long-lasting pain relief.[23] They used 10-cm needles with either 4-mm or 6-mm exposed tips. No stimulation test was performed to assure concordance of needle placement with the nerve; instead, the authors relied solely on fluoroscopic anatomic cannula placement. The mean duration of the C2-C3 neurotomy procedure was stated to have been 1.5 hours.[23] The rather meager success rate was in sharp contrast to the 70% success that they noted for lower cervical medial branch procedures. The authors stated that radiofrequency of the cervical medial branches "carries a high rate of technical failure.[23]" In 1996,[24] Lord and associates noted that RFA of the cervical medial branches, performed in 24 patients with a median duration of pain of 34 months following motor vehicle accidents, provided a median duration of analgesia persisting 263 days. This contrasted sharply to the median analgesia of 8 days in a control group of patients. However, they excluded individuals with C2-C3 Z joint pain based on their rather dismal results from the previous study noted earlier. In a subsequent study published by the same group of investigators, complete pain relief was found in 71% of 28 patients following a single RF procedure, persisting a mean duration of 219 days. When failures were excluded from consideration, the mean duration extended out to 422 days (60 weeks).[25] Again, excluded from study were individuals suffering from TON-mediated C2-C3 pain. In 2003, Govind and associates[26] used three large-gauge electrodes to perform RFA procedures of the TON. Following controlled diagnostic blocks, 51 nerves in 40 patients were treated with RFA. Eighty-eight percent (43 of 49) achieved successful outcomes using this approach, with a median duration of 297 days (42 weeks). Side effects included slight ataxia, numbness, and temporary dysesthesias.[26] Their improved success was attributed to use of three needles, as well as use of Ray electrodes instead of SMK electrodes (smaller), as well as the assurance that each of the three lesions was made at a distance no greater than one electrode width from an adjacent lesion.[26]

Cohen found that the only factor predicting the success of RFA, defined as at least 50% pain reduction lasting at least 6 months, was paraspinal tenderness.[27] Although the authors stated that C2-C3 pain was included in this analysis, they never indicated how many individuals were thusly treated or what the success rate was for TON RFA.

CERVICAL FACET BLOCK; MEDIAL BRANCH BLOCK (FIGS. 52.6 THROUGH 52.12)

The cervical facet joints and medial branches are commonly implicated in the etiology of cervicogenic headache. C2 and C3 blocks are undertaken to effectively disrupt neural

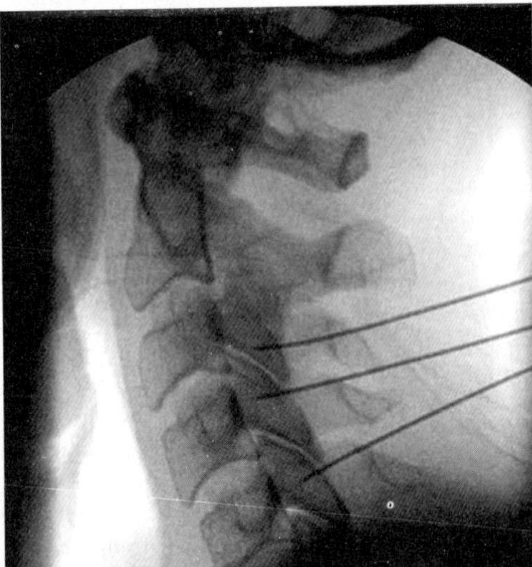

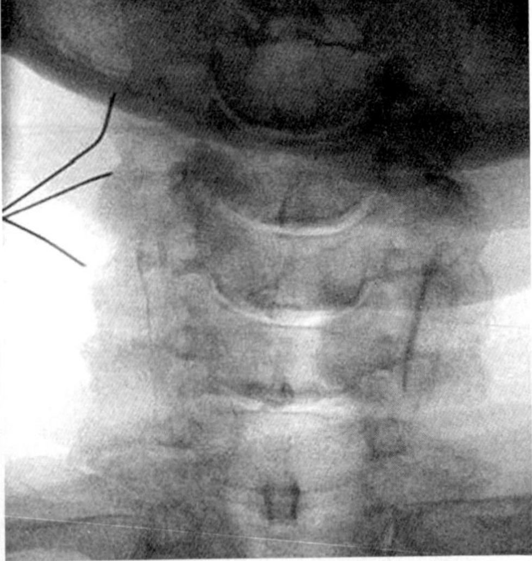

Figure 52.12 Lateral and posterior-anterior fluoroscopic images using cephalad tilt of the fluoroscopy unit, with patient in prone position demonstrating needles appropriately placed for blockade of C3, C4, C5 medial branch nerves, left sided. (Photos courtesy of Kenneth D. Candido, M.D.

pathways giving rise to greater and lesser occipital nerve dysfunction. Blockade of the joints via the medial branches is typically undertaken for such headaches as well as for the treatment of nonspecific neck pain, degenerative arthropathies of the cervical spine, degenerative disk disease, cervical sprain, and trauma-related pain. Pain may be localized to the neck or may radiate in a capelike fashion from the neck over the shoulders, with extension to the suboccipital area and the supraclavicular area (see Fig. 52.5). The cervical facet joints are present from C2 toC3 caudally, as the atlanto-occipital (A-O) and atlanto-axial (A-A) joints are not true zygapophyseal joints, as described previously. From C2 to C3 caudally, the joints are lined by synovium and possess a true joint capsule, which is generously innervated and which may be a source of neck pain and headache pain in certain individuals. The joints themselves may be injured in acceleration-deceleration types of injuries or may be affected by chronic degenerative arthritic changes. Pain results from synovial joint inflammation caused by irritation from repetitive motion at an injured segment. The cervical facet joints, like the thoracic and lumbar facet joints, receive innervation from two adjacent spinal levels. The dorsal ramus from the level above the joint as well as from the level at the joint provides fibers that invest the joint. This forms the foundation for blocking both the affected level and superior levels to completely denervate the facet joint. Each dorsal ramus innervates two facet joints, and each facet joint receives its innervation from two separate nerves. The medial branch, which wraps around the waist of the articular pillars of the vertebral bodies (see Figs. 52.6 through 52.8), is the site for peripheral nerve block as well as for neuromodulation techniques of radiofrequency at the joint. These nerves are held against the bone by a fascial envelope and are anchored there by tendons of the semispinalis capitis. The medial branch is consistently found at this anatomic location between C4 and C7, making needle placement for these levels a relatively simple task to accomplish. For example, at the C4-C5 facet joint, the medial branches of C4 and C5 are blocked at their respective articular pillars to anesthetize the joint. At C2-C3, the joint receives innervation from the third occipital nerve (one of two median branches of the C3 dorsal ramus, as discussed previously), and also somewhat by the C2 dorsal ramus. The medial branch of the C2 dorsal ramus is the greater occipital nerve (discussed later). C2-C3 facet joint innervation is a complex anatomic scheme, and for practical purposes, our technique of blocking the third occipital nerve at the C3 articular process waist is sufficient for denervating or anesthetizing this joint.

TECHNIQUE OF BLOCKING THE MEDIAL BRANCHES FOR CERVICAL FACET JOINT PAIN (SEE FIGS. 52.9 THROUGH 52.11)

Our technique of blocking the medial branches requires the use of fluoroscopic guidance, although there are increasingly more advocates of performing an ultrasound-guided technique.[28-30] We believe this is essential to minimize the likelihood of advancing our needles too far ventrally with the patient in the prone position. Advancing too far ventrally could cause injury or irritation to the exiting cervical spinal nerve roots or to the more ventrally situated vertebral artery. Also, if strict adherence to maintaining needle-to-bone contact is not maintained, it could be possible for advancing needles to stray too far medially toward the interlaminar or transforaminal spaces, or too far laterally with a resultant failure of accessing the medial branches, which are secured to the waists of the articular pillars by a fascial sheath and the semispinalis capitis tendons. Appropriately screened candidates (i.e., no coagulation problems, no infection at the intended insertion site, etc.) are placed in the prone position, with a bolster placed under the chest to permit flexion of the head on the neck. The forehead is supported using a ring neurosurgical donut or pillow, with unrestricted breathing and with minimal to no sedation utilized. Vital signs are monitored using standard ASA monitors, and an intravenous cannula is placed in a distal extremity for purposes of administering resuscitative medications or adjuvants, as indicated. A careful sterile skin prep and drape is performed using a generic antiseptic solution. The fluoroscope is oriented anterior to posterior with a moderate-steep cephalad orientation. This is an essential step that if not undertaken inhibits or impairs the ability to visualize the periarticular osseous structures because of the obstruction imposed by the thick mandible. Scout films are obtained using sterile needles placed over the skin of the intended needle entry sites, and local anesthetic skin wheals are raised using a 27-gauge, short (1.5-inch) needle with a short acting local anesthetic agent (i.e., lidocaine 1% without epinephrine), in doses of 2 to 3 mL per site. Next, a 22-gauge, 3.5-inch blunt (i.e., Whitacre type or equivalent) subarachnoid or block needle is advanced completely perpendicular to the skin toward the lateral-most edge of the vertebral body on the side selected. In this position, it may not be practical to gauge the exact site (i.e., C3 versus C4) where the needle is being directed. When 2 cm of needle have been introduced, it is essential to switch to a straight lateral view to observe the depth of needle advancement, as well as to ascertain which anatomic segment is being addressed. This is usually of little concern, as two levels (the level at the joint and the level cephalad to the joint) are being blocked to anesthetize a single level. So even if C4 was chosen, and the needle is seen as advancing toward the trapezoid body articular pillar at C3, the second needle may merely need to be placed caudad to the first to block both medial branches. Once the needle is seated at the appropriate depth, as seen on lateral fluoroscopy (see Fig. 52.9) and is seen not to be encroaching on either the visible neural foramen, or too far ventral, toward the anatomic site of the vertebral artery, the needle is checked to ascertain that the tip is touching bone. Using a curve tipped needle helps to realign the needle in cases where the depth appears appropriate, but the needle tip is laterally directed away from bone. In such cases, a mere twisting of the needle hub will usually suffice to turn and steer the tip toward, and subsequently against, the bone where the medial branches are situated in their respective fascial planes and are anchored by the semispinalis capitis tendons. When all needles are in the appropriate anatomic position for a given individual, they should be aligned like a picket fence. The lateral fluoroscopic image should demonstrate almost perfect parallel lines derived from the needles. An alternative technique is to place the patient prone and advance the needle from lateral to medial toward the bone under fluoroscopic guidance. This technique is clearly fraught with greater danger of striking the vertebral artery or an exiting cervical spinal nerve root than the technique described previously as a result of the direction of the needle toward the central neuraxis. Additionally, and potentially more than a mere nuisance, the clinician who subsequently determines that the patient might derive benefit from a radiofrequency or a neurodestructive procedure of the cervical medial branches is then faced with the prospect of performing the procedure with the active tip of any RF needle making minimal and insignificant contact with the target area/nerve of interest. Contrast this with the approach described earlier, where the RF needle's active tip will be hugging the bone through its entire length, making the likelihood of success inherently much greater. Additionally, there is less muscle in the pathway of the advancing needle using the lateral approach. This increases the likelihood that needles with not be firmly seated against the target and will be easily displaced once the second and possibly third or fourth needles are inserted at a given level.

Whichever technique is chosen, once the needles are situated, and once there has been no paresthesia or blood from the needle during aspiration, a small (typically 0.5 mL to 1 mL) volume of radiocontrast media may be injected merely to verify that no arterial cannulation has occurred. The incidence of intravascular injection following this procedure in the cervical spine is about 3.9%.[31] If this injection proves negative for such a cannulation, the same volume of a short-acting (i.e., lidocaine, mepivacaine) local anesthetic with or without corticosteroid may be added. We prefer to use the nonparticulate steroid dexamethasone acetate for this purpose, in doses of 2 mg per medial branch (up to 12 mg total), because the particulate agents such as methylprednisolone acetate tend to flocculate or clump, with the potential for neurologic compromise if such a phenomenon occurs in an end artery. When assessing response to local anesthetic (LA) blocks, it may be prudent to query patients on more than one occasion to minimize a perception bias associated with single time frame, snapshot data capture.[32]

If RF procedures are anticipated to ameliorate recalcitrant symptoms, we typically perform double-diagnostic blocks as a prelude to RF, accepting an arbitrary 60% or better response prior to doing the actual RF. In the future, pulsed RF techniques may replace conventional RFA lesioning in the neck for the most part. These are performed by applying 42° to 45° C temperatures for 120 seconds to each nerve in question. Success rates of RFA in carefully selected patients may be found in up to 74% of patients for up to 20 months.[33] If performed following cervical spine surgery in patients with ongoing neck pain, success may be found in 59.4% for up to 15 months.[34] However, when data from eight cervical RFA studies were summarized in a systematic review, the average duration of analgesia was found to be more modest, at about 7 to 9 months.[35] Even pulsed RF techniques of the cervical dorsal root ganglia may provide significant analgesia in patients with radicular pain, lasting up to 12 months.[36] Using ultrasound guidance in the performance of the procedure has been associated with similar rates of success for RFA of the medial branches as that identified for fluoroscopic techniques.[37]

OCCIPITAL NERVE BLOCK (FIGS. 52.13 AND 52.14)

The greater occipital nerve (GON) arises from the dorsal primary rami of C2, with occasional contributions from C3. The nerve penetrates the fascia inferior to the superior nuchal crest, where it runs alongside the occipital artery for a variable distance. The sensory area innervated by the nerve includes the medial portion of the posterior scalp, with radiation ventrally up to the vertex. The lesser occipital nerve (LON) arises from the ventral primary rami of C2 and C3 and passes superiorly and laterally from the occiput to the lateral edge of the sternocleidomastoid muscle. Here the nerve divides into cutaneous branches that innervate the lateral portion of the posterior scalp and the cephalad surface of the ear pinna. Along with the great auricular nerve, the GON and LON provide the majority of sensory afferent information for the occipital area and are responsible for transmitting information derived from C2-C3 facet joint derangements to the referral area described.

Occipital nerve block has have become an increasingly popular method of managing headaches of diverse

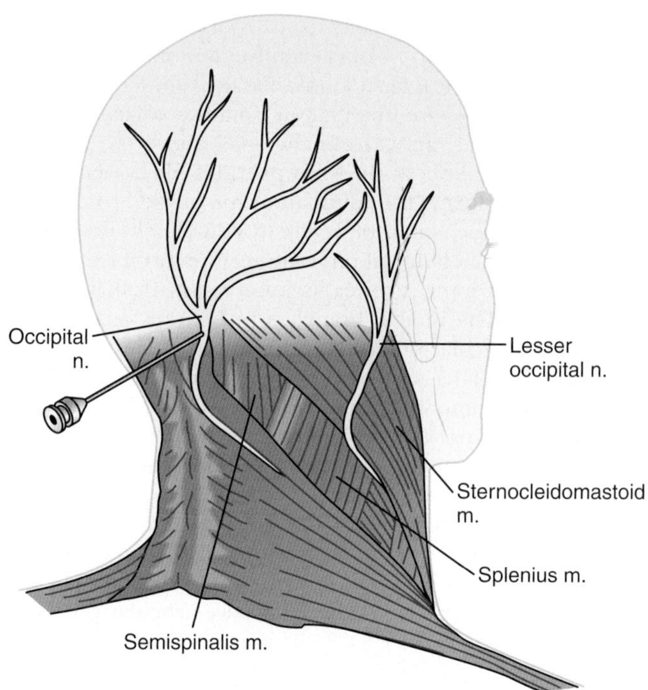

Figure 52.13 The anatomy and site of nerve blocking for the greater occipital nerve.

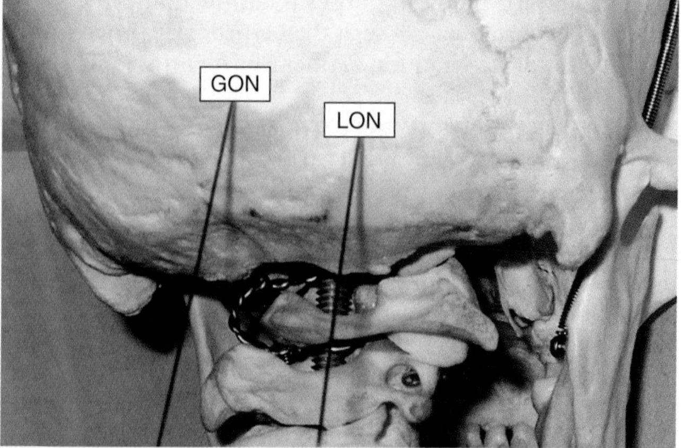

Figure 52.14 Needles inserted for right-sided greater occipital nerve (GON) and lesser occipital nerve (LON) blocks. (Photo courtesy of Kenneth D. Candido, M.D.)

etiologies, even though the scientific support for doing so is limited. GON blocks have been shown to be ineffective for chronic tension type headache when prilocaine and dexamethasone were used in a group of 15 patients.[38] They have been used with various degrees of success for postconcussive headaches[39] (80% successful in then patients), atypical orofacial pain,[40] and especially for migraine headaches, when they are often combined with trigger point injections[41] or supraorbital nerve blocks,[42] in both cases affording a very high degree of success for ameliorating pain and brush allodynia. A novel use of GON block has been in the successful treatment of patients with abnormal head movements who also suffered from tinnitus and dizziness associated with a previous history of trauma.[43] Although oftentimes the diagnosis of headache due to occipital neuralgia is not too difficult to make,[44] there are cases of refractory headache that require advanced evaluation techniques. Some suggest performing computed tomography (CT)–guided C2-C3 nerve blocks as a prelude to considering patients who may be candidates for percutaneous rhizotomy[45]; in our experience, fluoroscopically guided techniques of C2-C3 nerve block have been extremely useful and have precluded the requirement to seek more advanced imaging for guidance (see Figs. 52.8 and 52.9).

TECHNIQUE OF BLOCKING THE GREATER AND LESSER OCCIPITAL NERVES

Occipital nerve blocks have been erroneously described by some to be merely a field block of local anesthetic and steroid layered somewhere in the posterior part of the occiput, without regard to anatomic landmarks or consequences of errantly placed medications. Indeed, there are cases of sudden unconsciousness reported following LON block, some resulting from occipital artery injection and at least one the result of unintentionally injecting local anesthetic into a previous bone defect from a craniotomy.[46] Also, it is possible that unconsciousness might occur after GON block has been made too far inferiorly toward the foramen magnum. Additionally, if practitioners are not careful and discriminating in their choices of frequency of GON block, and use judicious doses of agents including corticosteroids, additional complications like the development of Cushing syndrome may result.[47] Our technique of blockade of the occipital nerves is to perform the procedure with the patient in the sitting position, with the forehead forward, resting on either a Mayo stand, the edge of a padded table, or on a gurney. If possible, the occipital artery is palpated at the superior nuchal ridge. Using ultrasound guidance may help to identify the artery, which is often not robust or bounding and, subsequently, not always readily discernible as a distinct structure. As it is virtually impossible to completely disinfect the scalp injection site, we utilize alcohol wipes or a Betadine-soaked pledget to soak the area with disinfectant prior to inserting the needle, without expectations of complete asepsis. Next, we insert a fine-gauge (25-gauge, 1.5-inch) cutting needle immediately medial to the artery and advance it perpendicular to the skin until the needle tip touches periosteum. Once the occipital bone has been thusly contacted, the needle is retracted about 1 mm and is redirected slightly cephalad. After gently aspirating, 5 mL of local anesthetic (0.5% bupivacaine or ropivacaine) with 4 mg of dexamethasone or 6 mg of betamethasone is injected in a fanlike manner, taking care not to direct the needle too far medially toward the foramen magnum. The lesser occipital nerve may be blocked, as can the greater auricular nerve, by removing the needle and placing it into the skin about 3 to 4 cm lateral to the entry point for GON block, while also directing it inferiorly instead of superiorly as for GON block. After gentle aspiration, 5 mL of the same combination of local anesthetic with or without corticosteroid as noted previously may be injected, again in a fanlike distribution, to block the nerve. After completing GON and LON blocks, it is important to gently massage the tissues of the scalp to assist in the spread of the agents while maintaining pressure over the injection site(s). This will minimize ecchymosis or hematoma formation from this highly vascular area. Often, an ice pack is applied for 20 to 30 minutes post-procedure to further minimize swelling and inhibit vascular absorption of the local anesthetic agents, particularly if bilaterally blocks have been performed.

FACIAL PAIN

SUPRAORBITAL, INFRAORBITAL, MENTAL NERVE BLOCKS (FIGS. 52.15 AND 52.16)

Peripheral branches of the trigeminal system may be readily accessible through percutaneous needle techniques.

Supraorbital nerve block is useful in the treatment of painful conditions of the frontal nerve, a branch of cranial nerve V1. The nerve leaves the superior orbital fissure to enter the orbit, passing ventrally under the periosteum of the roof of

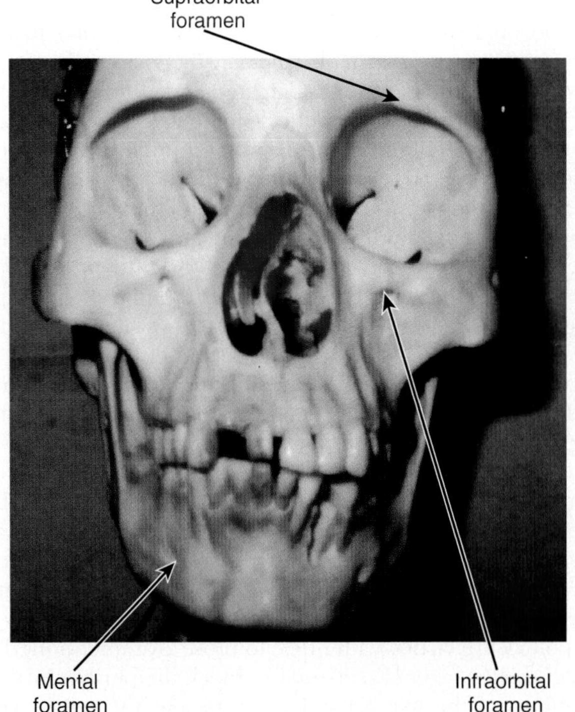

Figure 52.15 Anterior view of the facial skeleton revealing three foramina; supraorbital, infraorbital, and mental, for needle placement. (Photo courtesy of Kenneth D. Candido, M.D.)

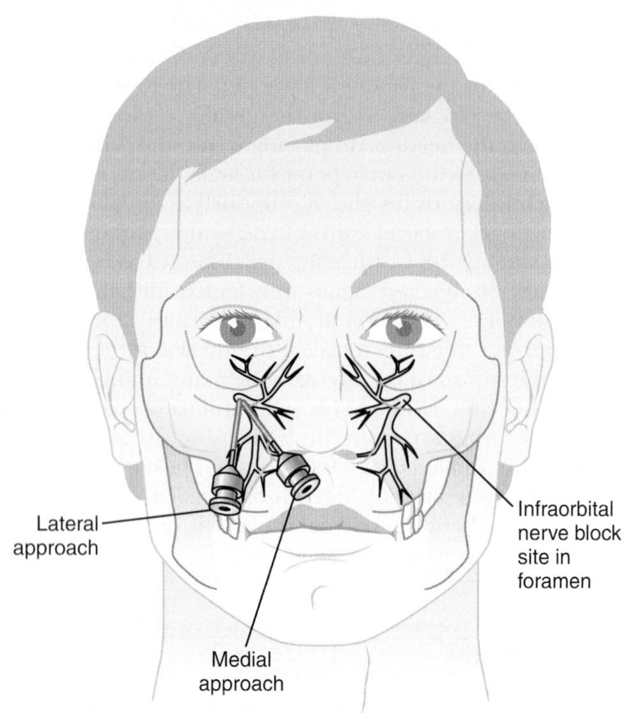

Figure 52.16 Anatomy of the infraorbital nerve block; lateral and medial approach.

the orbit. The frontal nerve gives off two corollary branches: the supraorbital and the supratrochlear nerves. The supraorbital nerve is larger and more laterally situated than the supratrochlear nerve, and it supplies sensory fibers to the forehead, upper eyelid, and anterior scalp. The nerve is typically blocked by injecting a small volume of dilute local anesthetic, with or without corticosteroid added, into the supraorbital foramen. A 22- to 25-gauge, 1.5-inch needle is typically employed for the block, which is readily accomplished once the foramen is palpated and after a sterile skin prep is performed. The goal of needle insertion is to avoid placing the needle tip through the foramen, which would assuredly elicit a paresthesia of the supraorbital nerve as it pins the nerve against the periosteum. It is more desirable to guide the needle toward the foramen, and, once periosteum is contacted, the needle should be slid slightly medially so that its tip is abutting the rim of the foramen. Following a negative aspiration, 3 to 4 mL of local anesthetic with 2 mg of dexamethasone or 6 mg of betamethasone may be incrementally injected. The needle should be flushed and withdrawn, and a dressing is applied over the injection site. Supraorbital nerve block has been successfully employed in the treatment of hemicrania continua.[48] Supratrochlear nerve block may be performed at a point slightly medial to the insertion site described earlier for supraorbital nerve block, using the same needle types and volumes and concentrations of local anesthetics and adjuvants. The indications, contraindications, complications, and side effects of this block are virtually identical to those aforementioned.

Infraorbital nerve block is used to block the peripheral contribution of the maxillary nerve, typically affected by conditions of chronic facial pain such as those resulting from complex regional pain syndrome and occasionally herpes zoster. The infraorbital nerve enters the orbit via the infraorbital fissure and passes along the floor of that structure in the infraorbital groove. It exits the skull through the infraorbital foramen, innervating the lower eyelid, lateral nose, and part of the superior lip. A branch of the nerve, the superior alveolar nerve, innervates the upper incisors, canine, and contiguous soft tissue.

Infraorbital block is performed with the patient in the supine position and with the head maintained in a neutral position. The infraorbital foramen is palpated, and a mark is placed over it using a marking pen. A sterile skin prep is performed, after which a fine-gauge (25- or 27-gauge), 1.5 inch needle is advanced into the foramen, while maintaining a slight medial direction of the advancing needle tip. This maneuver minimizes the pinning of the infraorbital nerve against bone and potentially traumatizing the nerve. Even taking such precautions, the nerve may be stimulated, resulting in a paresthesia to the teeth or lateral naris. After aspirating for the presence of blood, a small volume (3 mL) of local anesthetic, with or without a nonparticulate corticosteroid, is incrementally injected. After clearing the needle, it is withdrawn, and a small bandage is applied over the injection site. The patient should be observed for 20 minutes and examined for an expanding hematoma of the face, which, if present, is usually readily treated with pressure and occasionally with an ice pack.

INFERIOR ALVEOLAR (MENTAL) NERVE BLOCK

The inferior alveolar nerve is a distal branch of the mandibular nerve. The nerve exits the mental foramen at the level of the second molar tooth, having divided into an incisor branch and a mental branch. After exiting the foramen, the nerve sends a ramus superiorly, innervating the lower lip, inferior oral mucosa, and the chin (mental branch). This nerve block has been used in the treatment of mental neuralgia, facial herpes zoster, and cases of trigeminal neuralgia (TGN) of the V3, where the nerve is readily accessible for cryolesioning.[49] As in the infraorbital nerve block technique, there is both an extraoral and an intraoral technique of mental nerve block. The intraoral technique is less painful for patients and provides a similar degree of successful block compared to the latter agent.[50] When evaluated in 123 patients using a standardized alveolar nerve block method, the block provided analgesia/anesthesia to the first molar (92%), first premolar (55.3%), and canine (38.2%) teeth of the lower jaw.[51] Additionally, levobupivacaine 0.5% with epinephrine 1:200,000 (5 μg/mL) was shown to be equipotent and equi-effective to the same concentration and dose of bupivacaine when used for inferior alveolar nerve block. Because of its inherent reduced systemic and cardiac toxicity, levobupivacaine may replace the latter agent for peripheral nerve blocks of the trigeminal system.[52]

Inferior alveolar nerve block is performed with the patient in the supine position and the head maintained in a neutral position. After palpating the mental foramen and performing a sterile skin prep, a small (25- or 27-gauge), 1.5-inch needle is advanced toward the foramen using a slight medial approach, as noted earlier for infraorbital nerve block, to minimize the likelihood of pinning the exiting nerve against periosteum. A paresthesia may nevertheless be obtained while performing the needle insertion, and patients need to be appraised of this possibility. After a negative aspiration test, 3 mL of local anesthetic with or without a nonparticulate corticosteroid are incrementally injected. The needle is cleared and withdrawn, and a small bandage is applied over the injection site. The patient should be observed for approximately 20 minutes to guard against the development of a hematoma, which is typically amenable to compression or the application of an ice pack.

TRIGEMINAL NERVE BLOCK AND GASSERIAN GANGLION BLOCK

Gasserian ganglion block is an underutilized technique for managing chronic face pain resulting from trigeminal neuralgia (TGN) and for persistent pain resulting from conditions such as recalcitrant herpes zoster ophthalmicus and postherpetic neuralgia. It has also been utilized for diagnostic purposes to differentiate pain originating from somatic structures from those mediated by sympathetic mechanisms. By far the most common indication, however, remains pain caused by malignancy with invasion of neural structures of the head and face. In these cases, local anesthetic nerve blocks may be accomplished as prognostic blocks, prior to subjecting patients to alcohol or phenol blocks, or to radiofrequency (conventional or pulsed) or cryo-neurolysis of the gasserian ganglion. Some of the more common malignancies involving the respective structures innervated by the trigeminal nerve include tumors of the orbit, maxillary sinus, and mandible. At times, gasserian ganglion block may be undertaken in cases where neurosurgical management (i.e., Janetta's procedure) is not feasible or practical. Occasional uses of the block and of neurodestruction of the ganglion include intractable cluster[53-57] and migraine headache (reflecting the second author's experience) and ocular pain due to glaucoma. Idiopathic TGN is due to vascular contact at the proximal portion of the preganglionic segment of the trigeminal nerve with preganglionic deformity and is observed in up to 97% of individuals so affected,[58] with the remedy often being gasserian ganglion block. For individuals suffering from isolated dysfunction of either the maxillary (V2) or mandibular (V3) division of the trigeminal nerve, it is often more feasible to perform single nerve injections on these structures, as the success rate of performing blocks at the foramen rotundum (maxillary) and foramen ovale (mandibular) have been shown to be 84% and 92%, respectively, for chronic facial pain.[59] When compared to peripheral nerve procedures, however, ganglion level procedures (radiofrequency thermocoagulation, balloon compression, glycerolysis) are more effective overall and should probably be attempted by skilled interventionalists if long-term success is sought.[60] The median pain-free interval that may be expected after percutaneous retrogasserian glycerol injection is 32 months, although the complication rate (hypesthesias, dysesthesias, anesthesia dolorosa) may approach 50% or more using this technique.[61] In another study using the same technique, the success rate, as defined by complete pain relief at 3.5 years, was 71.4%, with a 32% rate of mild hypesthesias, a 19% rate of paresthesias, and a 3% rate of dysesthesias.[62] The choice of whether to perform percutaneous neurodestructive ganglion procedures using fluoroscopic guidance or CT scan guidance is operator dependent. The largest case series to date have included more than 2000 percutaneous ethanol or RFA blocks over a 13-year period using fluoroscopy with excellent success.[63] On the other hand, the foramen ovale is often difficult to visualize using fluoroscopy alone. In recent times, CT-guided or CT-fluoroscopy-guided gasserian ganglion thermolysis procedures have become increasingly popular because of the ability to more readily identify osseous structures (Fig. 52.17).[64] In the evolving practice of using CT scanning for head and neck nerve blocks, determinations are being made for the most appropriate skull-rotation angles in which the foramen ovale is best visualized, the relationship between the virtual puncture point and anatomic landmarks, and the distance between the virtual puncture point and the foramen.[65]

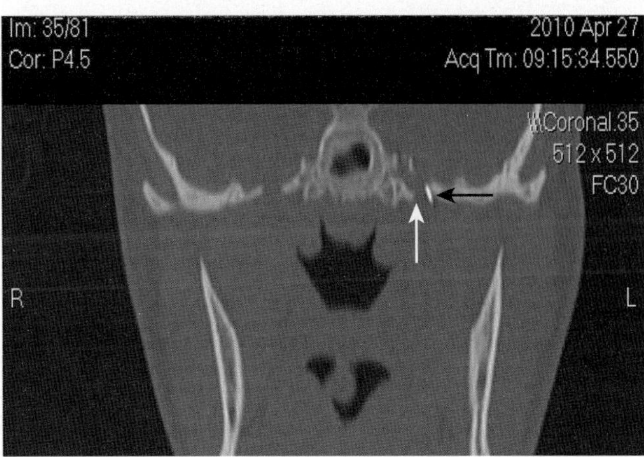

Figure 52.17 CT-guided trigeminal ganglion block. The vertical, white arrow indicates the foramen ovale. The horizontal, black arrow indicates the needle through the foramen.

TECHNIQUE OF BLOCKING THE TRIGEMINAL NERVE VIA THE GASSERIAN GANGLION

The gasserian ganglion resides in the middle cranial fossa.[66-68] It is situated in a fold of dura mater that forms an invagination around the posterior two thirds of the ganglion. This region is referred to as Meckel's cavity and contains cerebrospinal fluid. The ganglion is bound medially by the cavernous sinus and optic and trochlear nerves, superiorly by the inferior surface of the temporal lobe of the brain, and posteriorly by the brainstem. The ganglion is formed by the fusion of a series of cell bodies that originate at the midpontine level of the brainstem.

The ganglion has three major divisions: ophthalmic (V1), maxillary (V2), and mandibular (V3). The ophthalmic division is located dorsally, the maxillary branch intermediate, and the mandibular branch ventrally. The ophthalmic division leaves the ganglion and passes into the orbit through the superior orbital fissure. It further divides into the supraorbital, supratrochlear, and nasociliary nerves, which innervate the forehead and the nose.[63] The maxillary division exits the middle cranial fossa via foramen rotundum, crosses the pterygopalatine fossa, and enters the orbit through the inferior orbital fissure. Branches include the infraorbital, superior alveolar, palatine, and zygomatic nerves, which carry sensory information from the maxilla and overlying skin, the nasal cavity, palate, nasopharynx, and meninges of the anterior and middle cranial fossa.[68] The mandibular division exits through the foramen ovale and divides into the buccal, lingual, inferior alveolar, and auriculotemporal nerves. These nerves carry sensory input from the buccal region, the side of the head and scalp, and the lower jaw including teeth, gums, anterior two thirds of the tongue, chin, and lower lip.[68] The motor component of V3 innervates the several muscles including the masseter, temporal, and medial and lateral pterygoids. The ganglion interfaces with the autonomic nervous system via the ciliary, sphenopalatine, otic, and submaxillary ganglia. It also communicates with the oculomotor, facial, and glossopharyngeal nerves.[69]

All patients considered candidates for either diagnostic or therapeutic block, or for neurolysis procedures, need to be evaluated to rule out the presence of coagulation disorders or the historical use of medications that might impair platelet aggregation and adhesiveness. The practitioner should also inquire about homeopathic medications, which patients tend to forget to include on intake questionnaires. All procedures are performed using radiologic assistance, either CT scan or fluoroscopy. After securing intravenous access and placing patients supine, a full complement of noninvasive hemodynamic monitors is applied, and baseline vital signs are obtained and recorded. Oxygen is typically administered via a nasal cannula. Modest amounts of sedative-hypnotic medication may be used to allay fears and limit apprehension in appropriate individuals.

The head of the patient is kept in a neutral position, and a site 2 to 3 cm lateral to the corner of the mouth on the ipsilateral side is chosen as the needle entry point. The needle direction is toward the ipsilateral, midline pupil, with a slight mesiad direction taken beneath the zygoma. The fluoroscope should be used to obtain anterior-posterior images. The beam should be oriented in a steep cephalad direction to attempt to visualize the foramen ovale. Even using this, or the submental view, does not guarantee that the foramen will be visualized. In the submental view, the orbital line and petrous ridge are visualized through the orbits using an A-P image. Then, the C-arm is moved slightly laterally and obliquely. The foramen ovale should appear medial to the medial edge of the mandible. Once the anatomic boundaries have been identified, the skin of the lateral area of the cheek is prepped and draped. A skin wheal is raised at the point chosen, using 1% lidocaine plain. Next, a 22-gauge, blunt nerve block or Whitacre subarachnoid needle is advanced toward the foramen ovale as described previously. If using a blunt needle, an 18-gauge introducer needle should be inserted first. Usually a paresthesia in the distribution of the mandibular nerve is obtained once the foramen is entered. Once the needle appears to be in proximity of the foramen, the C arm is switched to lateral to show the needle approximating the angle made by the clivus and petrous ridge of the temporal bone (Fig. 52.18). This is an area close to the pituitary fossa and sphenoid sinus, as well as the external auditory canal, so obviously every effort must be made to ascertain that the needle is situated where intended. If the needle tip has entered Meckel's cavity, it is not unusual for the dura to be punctured and for cerebrospinal fluid (CSF) to be aspirated through the needle. Theoretically, CSF should not be obtained when using a blunt block needle. Nevertheless, the next step in the block sequence is to inject 0.1 to 0.5 mL of nonionic, water-soluble contrast media into the space to verify that no vascular structure has been entered and that the

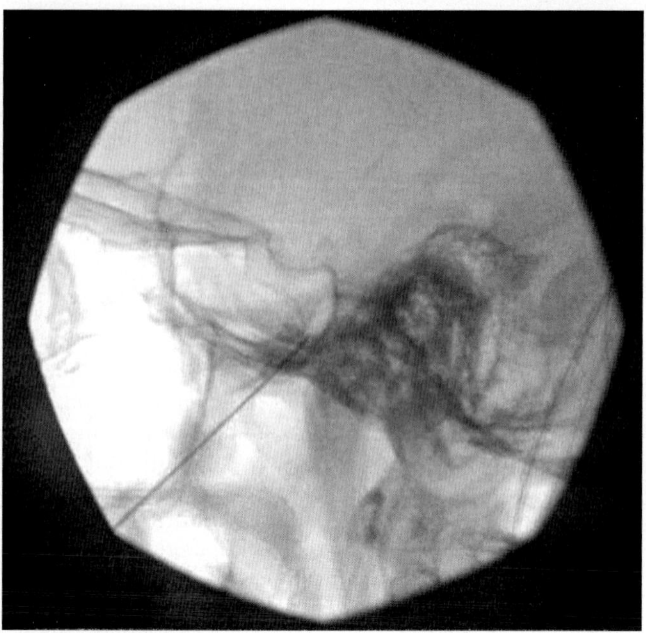

Figure 52.18 Lateral fluoroscopic image of a 22-gauge, curved, blunt block needle through the foramen ovale.

needle is still not in the subarachnoid space. If a diagnostic block is being performed, then 0.1 mL of 1% lidocaine without epinephrine, 0.2% ropivacaine, or 0.25% bupivacaine can be incrementally injected using a tuberculin syringe, to a total volume of about 0.5 mL, with continual intermittent aspiration. If neurolysis is desired, the same volume of 6.5% phenol in glycerin or absolute alcohol may be incrementally injected using a tuberculin syringe in the manner described previously for local anesthetic injection. For using hyperbaric phenol solutions, the patient should be placed in the sitting position with the chin aiming toward the chest prior to injecting the agent; this will help maximize the likelihood that the phenol will spread preferentially to V2 and V3 and avoid the ophthalmic division of the TGN. For absolute alcohol, the patient should be left in the supine position.

The same approach to gasserian ganglion block can be undertaken for radiofrequency (conventional or pulsed), cryolesioning, balloon compression, or even for placing stimulating electrode leads for subsequent attachment to an implanted pulse generator. For conventional radiofrequency lesioning, a 3- to 5-mm active-tip needle is placed. The target depth of the needle tip depends on the division of the trigeminal nerve that needs to be lesioned. The mandibular division is rostral and lateral, the maxillary division is intermediate, and the ophthalmic division is mostly cephalad and medial. Location of the needle tip on the appropriate division(s) is determined by the response to sensory and motor stimulation (50 Hz, 1 volt and 2 Hz, 2 volts, respectively) of the ganglion. Paresthesia should be perceived at less than 0.3 volt, with little to no muscle contraction of the masseter muscle at 0.6 to 1 volt.[69] If no contraction is observed, then the tip of the needle is on the ophthalmic or maxillary divisions. Once the patient senses paresthesia in the painful area, inject 0.5 mL of 0.25% bupivacaine or 0.2% ropivacaine with steroid. Wait 30 to 60 seconds and begin lesioning at 60° C for 90 seconds. If the patient cannot tolerate the lesioning, stop and wait an additional 30 seconds, then try again or add another 0.5 mL of local anesthetic prior to resuming lesioning. If more than one branch of the trigeminal nerve is affected, perform several lesions of the ganglion. Reposition the needle and repeat the stimulation test to get paresthesia in the desired site. For lesioning of the ophthalmic division, assess the corneal reflex during and after each lesion. Lesioning is typically started at temperatures of 55° to 65° C to preserve this reflex. One or two lesions are recommended. If the corneal reflex diminishes, lesioning should be stopped. Pulsed radiofrequency is not a temperature-dependent technique. It is a nondestructive method of providing long-term pain relief.[70] After proper positioning of the needle tip, perform two to four pulsed radiofrequency cycles for 120 seconds each at 45 to 60 volts. The temperature of the needle tip rarely exceeds 42° C, thus local anesthetic is not required. If significant masseter contraction is noted during pulsing, inject 1 to 2 mL of local anesthetic to diminish this effect, or hold the patient's mouth closed with your hand while the cycles complete.

MAXILLARY AND MANDIBULAR NERVE BLOCKS

The trigeminal nerve branches may also be blocked using a coronoid approach. The benefit of accessing the V2 and V3 nerves using this approach is the facility in doing so, the ease of reproducibility, and the possibility, albeit not recommended, of doing the procedure absent the requirement for radiologic guidance. The coronoid approach is a useful technique of accessing V2 as it leaves the foramen rotundum. From a technical ease standpoint, coronoid trigeminal block far surpasses the classical technique of gasserian ganglion block, so it is probably our technique of choice in all situations where a V1 block is not essential for diagnosis or management of facial pain (as noted by the first author).

With the patient in the supine position, the head is turned to the side opposite of the intended block. The coronoid notch is easily identified by asking patients to open and close their mouths and with palpation anterior and inferior to the external auditory meatus. Once the landmarks are identified, the patient is asked to maintain the mouth in a neutral position, while a 22-gauge, 3.5-inch Whitacre or other blunt-tipped block needle is advanced perpendicular to the skin of the side of the face, just below the zygomatic arch directly in the center of the coronoid arch. Once the lateral pterygoid plate is contacted (at about 4 to 5 cm from the skin), the needle is withdrawn about 22 mm. Withdrawing the needle slightly as such improves the likelihood of successfully blocking the mandibular nerve (V3) in addition to V2. A total of 5 to 10 mL of local anesthetic, with or without corticosteroid, is used for diagnostic/therapeutic block, whereas the same volume of alcohol may be carefully injected using the same approach if neurolysis is desired. The mandibular (V3) branch may be separately blocked here, or it may be blocked in tandem with V2 as described previously. If the nerve is to be blocked as noted previously for the V2 block, the simplest and likeliest chance for success is via the coronoid approach. If one desires to block the nerve separately, then, once the needle contacts the lateral pterygoid plate, it should be redirected posteriorly and inferiorly until it passes the inferior aspect of the plate. At a point corresponding to approximately 1 cm deeper than the contact point of the lateral pterygoid plate, there will typically be a V3 paresthesia elicited. A usual dose of local anesthetic, or of neurolytic agent, is 3 to 5 mL using continual intermittent aspiration tests because of the high degree of vascularity in the area. Because the mandibular nerve (V3) has motor branches, it is not inconceivable that a well-performed local anesthetic or neurolytic procedure might result in paresis or weakness of the muscles of mastication and also some facial asymmetry resulting from muscle weakness. This may be more than a nuisance and should be clearly described during the informed consent process with the patient.

Mandibular and maxillary nerve blocks are typically used for ameliorating pain related to TGN, but indications for surgical analgesia, including using mandibular block as an adjunct for cervical plexus block (CPB) for carotid endarterectomy surgery, have been described.[71] Although most clinicians continue to use fluoroscopic guidance in most instances of mandibular nerve block, the technique of CT-guided block has been described and may be a suitable alternative if this modality is considered necessary to delineate the relevant anatomy.[72] Continuous catheter techniques of mandibular block have also been described both for cancer pain management[73] and for analgesia after mandibular fracture repair.[74] Neural complications after mandibular nerve injury are not uncommon and involve the lingual nerve more commonly than the inferior alveolar nerve, oftentimes lasting much longer than other common peripheral nerve injuries such as neuropraxias.[75] These injuries may represent neurotoxicity as a central etiology, according to one recent review undertaken in 52 patients who had received these blocks.[75] Otherwise, intravascular injection, hematoma, dizziness, and ataxia occur with some frequency after these procedures and should be discussed with patients during the informed consent process.[76]

For maxillary nerve block using the coronoid approach, it is important to not advance the block needle more than 0.25 cm once the pterygoid plate has been contacted in order to minimize the chance of causing neural injury.[77] And as for mandibular nerve block described earlier, a CT-guided technique and a continuous catheter technique of maxillary nerve block have both been described, the former to increase the likelihood of success[78] and the latter to extend the duration of analgesia in a group of patients undergoing radical maxillary sinusotomy.[79]

GLOSSOPHARYNGEAL NERVE BLOCK AND RADIOFREQUENCY

The glossopharyngeal nerve (GPN) (cranial nerve IX) is infrequently implicated in painful conditions of the face and neck. Nevertheless, because of the lack of familiarity of many pain practitioners with the anatomy and implications of glossopharyngeal nerve dysfunction, it is an important entity to consider in cases of recalcitrant pain particularly of the tongue, mouth, and pharynx. GPN block may be suitable for conditions such as glossopharyngeal neuralgia and pain from malignancy. The nerve may be affected by tumors of the tongue, hypopharynx, and palatine tonsils. The block is also used during the anatomic evaluation method of differential nerve block. The GPN is a mixed cranial nerve carrying both motor and sensory fibers. The nerve is attached by three or four filaments to the medulla oblongata in a groove between the olive and inferior peduncle.

Motor fibers, from cells of the nucleus ambiguus, innervate the stylopharyngeus muscle, while the sensory branches, from cells of the superior and petrous ganglia, innervate the tongue (the posterior third), palatine tonsil, fauces, and mucous membranes of the mouth and pharynx. A branch of the GPN, the carotid sinus nerve, is important in the regulation of blood pressure, pulse, and respiration, as this branch innervates the carotid body and carotid sinus. Sympathetic efferent fibers from the nucleus ambiguus are both preganglionic motor fibers and preganglionic secretory fibers of the sympathetic system. Parasympathetic fibers pass to the otic ganglion, and postganglionic fibers innervate the parotid gland. In conjunction with the vagus and spinal accessory nerves (cranial nerves X and XI), the GPN exits the jugular foramen near the internal jugular vein. All three cranial nerves as well as the hypoglossal nerve (cranial nerve XII) lie between the internal jugular vein and the internal carotid artery. The styloid process of the temporal bone is a major landmark for successfully blocking the GPN. GPN block is performed with the patient in the supine position and the head turned slightly opposite to the affected side.

Our practice includes the use of fluoroscopic imaging to help delineate and define the ipsilateral mastoid and the ipsilateral angle of the mandible, as the styloid process is typically found equidistant between those two respective structures. Fluoroscopy also permits real-time imaging of the pattern of injection of contrast media, so that in cases where the needle tip has penetrated either the carotid or jugular systems, this activity should be observable and intravascular injection subsequently preventable. Once baseline scout films have been obtained, intravenous access assured, and baseline vital signs documented, the skin overlying the styloid process should be prepped and draped in sterile fashion. A small skin wheal may be made over the styloid process using a 25-gauge 1.5-inch needle and 1% plain lidocaine, 3 to 4 mL. Next, a 22-gauge, 1.5- to 2-inch blunt tipped block needle may be advanced perpendicular to the skin toward the process, aiming for its posterior aspect. The usual depth of contact of the styloid varies from about 1.5 cm to 4 cm. Once the needle tip has slipped posteriorly off of the process, 1 mL of iodinated contrast media should be incrementally injected under live continuous fluoroscopy (Fig. 52.19). Then, barring any intravascular spread, a short-acting (lidocaine, mepivacaine) and dilute (1% concentration) local anesthetic with epinephrine 1:200,000 (5 μg/mL) in a volume of 5 to 8 mL should be incrementally injected in divided doses. If indicated, a modest dose of nonparticulate corticosteroid (dexamethasone, betamethasone) may be added to the injectate. Patients need to be monitored for a minimum of 30 minutes following the block to verify that there has been no systemic response to the injected local anesthetic solution. Even taking these precautions and using fluoroscopic guidance does not completely eliminate the possibility of local anesthetic spillover onto the vagus nerve (with resultant ipsilateral vocal cord paralysis, or bradycardia, asystole, reflex tachycardia, and syncope) or onto the spinal accessory nerve (weakness of the trapezius muscle).

There is also an intraoral approach that can be utilized when there is an anatomic distortion externally by previous surgery or tumor. The patient is placed in a supine position with the mouth wide open and the tongue is retracted

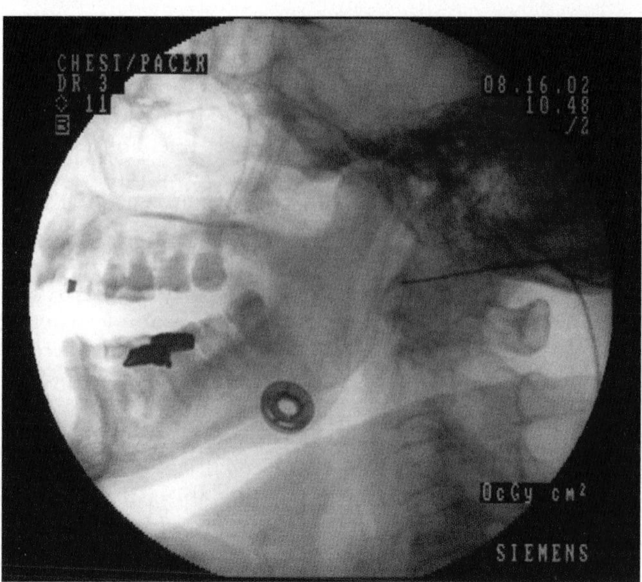

Figure 52.19 Lateral fluoroscopic image for a glossopharyngeal nerve block. Note the tip of the needle is at the base of the styloid process.

downward and medially using a tongue depressor or a laryngoscope blade. The nerve will be located at the inferior portion of the tonsillar pillar and is accessed via the palatoglossal fold. Once the fold is identified, a topical local anesthetic spray or pledget with 1 mL of saline with epinephrine is applied for hemostasis. A 22- or 25-gauge needle with a slight distal bend (25 degrees) is advanced to depth no more than 0.5 cm into the mucosa. After negative aspiration, 2 mL to 3 mL of local anesthetic (0.2% ropivacaine) with or without steroid is injected. With the intraoral approach, there is a potential of vessel trauma and neurotoxicity but much less than might occur with the extraoral approach.

SPHENOPALATINE GANGLION BLOCK AND RADIOFREQUENCY

The sphenopalatine ganglion (SPG) block is useful for treating acute migraine headaches, acute and chronic cluster headache,[80] post-traumatic headache,[81] and facial neuralgias including Sluder's, Vail's, and Gardner's syndromes.[82] Some have suggested that SPG block using 4% viscous lidocaine is not superior to placebo in the analgesic management of patients suffering from myofascial pain of the head.[83] Others have found that RF of the SPG relieved the symptoms of episodic cluster headache in 60.7% of 56 patients and in 30% of 10 patients with chronic cluster headache. An infrazygomatic approach was used, and complications were transient in all cases.[84] The ganglion resides in the pterygopalatine fossa. The fossa is bordered anteriorly by the maxillary sinus, posteriorly by the medial pterygoid plate, medially by the palatine bone, and superiorly by the sphenoid sinus. The pterygomaxillary fissure allows passage of a needle into the fossa, whereas the pterygopalatine foramen is located medial to the ganglion and is just posterior to the middle turbinate. The fossa is approximately 1 cm wide and 2 cm high and resembles a V-shaped vase on a lateral fluoroscopic image. The SPG is covered by a 1- to 1.5-mm thick layer of connective tissue and mucous membrane and is approximately 5 mm in size and triangular in shape. A large venous plexus overlies the fossa. Foramen rotundum and the pterygoid canal are located on the superolateral and inferomedial aspect of the fossa, respectively. The maxillary artery resides in the fossa. The ganglion is "suspended" from the maxillary nerve by the pterygopalatine nerves and is medial to the maxillary nerve. Posteriorly the ganglion is connected to the vidian nerve, which is formed by the deep petrosal (sympathetic from the upper thoracic spinal cord) and greater petrosal (parasympathetic from the superior salivatory nucleus) nerves. The ganglion has efferent branches and forms the superior posterior lateral nasal and pharyngeal nerves. Caudally, the greater and lesser palatine nerves exit the ganglion. Sensory fibers arise from the maxillary nerve, pass through the SPG, and innervate the upper teeth, nasal membranes, soft palate, and some parts of the pharynx. A small number of motor nerves are believed to travel with the sensory trunks.

There are several techniques to block the SPG, one of which is to block the ganglion using the topical application approach. With the patient in the supine position and the head maximally extended, as in the sniffing position, the practitioner applies 3 mL of 4% viscous lidocaine absorbed onto cotton-tipped pledgets. The pledgets are advanced slowly and deliberately, to minimize the chance of causing epistaxis, in a direction that is directly perpendicular to the floor. The path taken with the pledgets is along the superior border of the middle turbinate of each nostril until the tip contacts the mucosa overlying the SPG. The pledgets are left in place for 30 minutes while the patient's vital signs are monitored, and then they are removed and discarded. Side effects are typically related to iatrogenic epistaxis, as local anesthetic toxicity is exceedingly rare using this approach.

Another technique is the infrazygomatic approach to SPG blockade, which can be technically challenging. It can be performed without fluoroscopy, but fluoroscopic guidance is highly recommended, as this will anecdotally improve the success of the block and the speed at which it is performed, and will decrease potential complications. Noninvasive monitors should be used to record vital signs. Place the patient in the supine position. Sterilely prep and drape the appropriate side of the face. Obtain a lateral fluoroscopic image. Palpate the mandibular notch and anesthetize the skin. If the notch is not palpable, identify the notch on a lateral fluoroscopic view. Identify the pterygopalatine fossa (which appears as a "V") on the lateral image and superimpose the right and left fossae. This is accomplished by manipulating the C arm or the head. The block can be performed with a 3.5-inch, 22-gauge, short-bevel needle with the distal tip bent at a 30-degree angle or with a curved, blunt, 10-cm, 20- or 22-gauge needle. The technique described reflects the use of a blunt needle. Anesthetize the skin and insert a 1.25-inch, 16-gauge angiocatheter through the skin and advance until it is just medial to the ramus of the mandible. This can be checked on an A-P image. Pass the block needle through the angiocatheter and advance it medial, anterior, and slightly cephalad. Obtain a lateral image to check the direction of the needle. Your target is the midportion of the pterygopalatine fossa (Fig. 52.20). Get an A-P view and advance the needle toward the middle turbinate, stopping when the tip is adjacent to the palatine bone (Fig. 52.21). If resistance is encountered at any point, withdraw and redirect the needle. Given the small size of the fossa, frequent A-P and lateral images are may be required to redirect the needle. Once in the fossa, inject 0.5 to 1 mL of nonionic, water-soluble contrast and observe for intravascular spread or intranasal placement of the needle. Once correct placement has been confirmed, inject 1 to 2 cc of local anesthetic, with or without steroids.

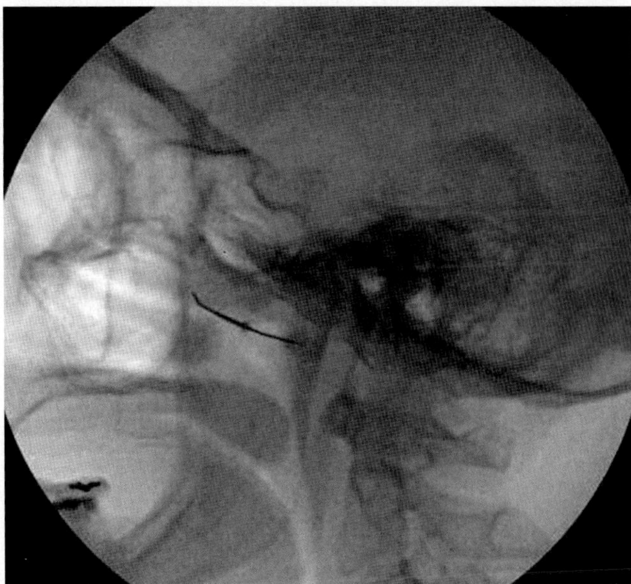

Figure 52.20 Lateral fluoroscopic image of a 22-gauge, curved, blunt block needle in the pterygopalatine fossa.

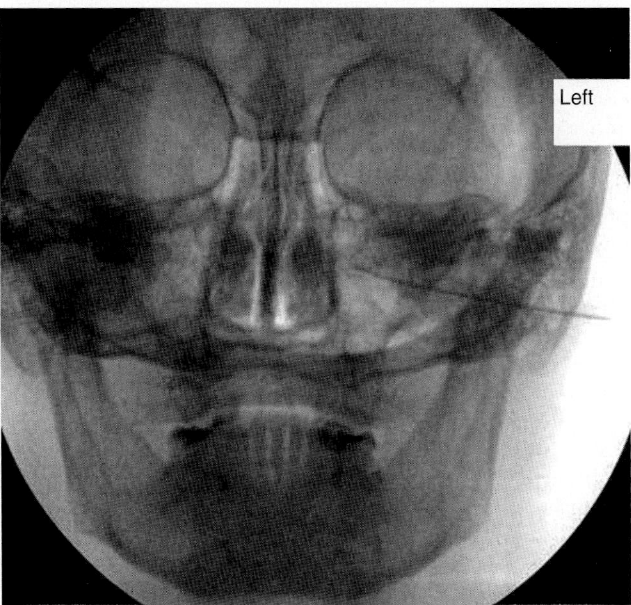

Figure 52.21 Posteroanterior fluoroscopic image of a 22-gauge, curved, blunt block needle just lateral to the middle turbinate. Sensory stimulation confirmed the tip of the needle is on the sphenopalatine ganglion.

After a successful diagnostic block, two therapeutic choices are available: conventional radiofrequency lesioning (RFTC) and pulsed radiofrequency (PRF). An insulated RF needle with a 3- to 5-mm active tip is placed using the infrazygomatic approach. Once in place, sensory stimulation is performed at 50 Hz up to 1 volt. If the tip of the needle is adjacent to the SPG, the patient should perceive a paresthesia at the root of the nose at less than 0.3 volt. If the paresthesia is felt in the hard palate, the needle should be redirected cephalad and medial. A paresthesia in the upper teeth indicates stimulation of the maxillary nerve, and the needle should be more caudal and medial. Motor stimulation is not necessary. After appropriate sensory stimulation, RFTC can be performed at 67° C for 90 seconds times two cycles. Before lesioning, 2 to 3 mL of local anesthetic should be injected. To avoid inadvertent lesioning of other nerves around the SPG, a 3-mm active tip is a better choice. For pulsed RF, the size of the active tip is not important as the electromagnetic field is projected from the tip of the needle and not from the shaft. With pulsed RF, two to four 120-second cycles are performed at 45 volts. Local anesthetic is not required for pulsed RF. The choice of whether to do a conventional or a pulsed RF lesion after a successful block is up to the discretion of the pain practitioner. Bradycardia ("Konen" reflex) has been noted during both conventional and pulsed RF lesioning and can be prevented with pretreatment with atropine or glycopyrolate.[85]

SUMMARY

Facial, head, and neck pain remains a diagnostic and therapeutic challenge for many pain practitioners. Knowledge of relevant anatomy is crucial to avoid complications and to increase the success of the therapeutic procedure. Appropriate patient selection, monitoring, proper injection technique, and knowledge of the pharmacokinetics and pharmacodynamics of the agents used are mandatory. The possible drug-drug interactions, increasing use of anticoagulant agents by individuals at high risk, and anatomic variation found in clinical practice serve to confound the picture even further. With proper education and training, pain management interventionalists can add these techniques to their everyday skills and open an avenue to patients suffering from these maladies.

One of the most daunting challenges in contemporary pain medicine is that presented by the patient complaining of head or neck pain. The complexities of the anatomy and the overlapping zones of innervation of somatic and sympathetic nerve pathways and ganglia leads commonly to implementation of incomplete treatment strategies and resultant partial remedies. The astute pain practitioner is well served to approach the chronic head and neck pain sufferer using an algorithmic approach that relies on a comprehensive appreciation of anatomy, physiology, and pharmacology but that progresses in an orderly fashion from simpler to more complex. For example, in the chronic headache patient who complains of symptoms in the posterior head and cervical spine following a motor vehicle accident, and following a comprehensive diagnostic workup, simpler attempts at analgesia using occipital nerve blocks should precede attempts at cervical medial branch neurotomy. Similarly, for someone complaining of supraorbital type pain, a supraorbital or supratrochlear nerve block should be considered before doing a CT scan–guided V-1 nerve block at the foramen ovale. A modicum of conservatism, coupled with a multimodal systematic evaluation and implementation approach, is the most prudent way of dealing with these difficult cases.

KEY POINTS

- Detailed knowledge of the anatomy of the facial structures will improve the success of trigeminal ganglion, sphenopalatine ganglion, and glossopharyngeal nerve blocks.
- Expected side effects (e.g., numbness in the distribution of the targeted nerve) versus complications of trigeminal ganglion rhizotomy should be fully explained to and comprehended by the patient before proceeding.
- The use of pulsed radiofrequency for trigeminal-mediated pain syndromes should be considered prior to using thermal radiofrequency after a successful diagnostic block.
- The practitioner should be prepared to treat bradycardia, which is commonly seen with trigeminal and sphenopalatine ganglion procedures.
- Given the complexity of the facial pain syndromes, the sphenopalatine ganglion block should be considered for diagnostic and therapeutic purposes.

SUGGESTED READINGS

Antonaci F, Pareja JA, Caminero AB, Sjaastad O. Chronic paroxysmal hemicrania and hemicrania continua: anaesthetic blockades of pericranial nerves. *Funct Neurol.* 1997;12:11-15.

Barnsley L, Bogduk N. Medial branch blocks are specific for the diagnosis of cervical zygapophyseal joint pain. *Reg Anesth.* 1993;18:343-350.

Barnsley L, Lord S, Wallis BJ, et al. The prevalence of chronic cervical zygapophyseal joint pain after whiplash. *Spine.* 1995;20:20-26.

Bogduk N, Aprill C. On the nature of neck pain, discography and cervical zygapophyseal joint blocks. *Pain.* 1993;54:213-217.

Bogduk N, Marsland A. The cervical zygapophyseal joints as a source of neck pain. *Spine.* 1988;13:610-617.

Boswell M, Colson J, Sehgal N, et al. A systematic review of therapeutic facet joint interventions in chronic spinal pain. *Pain Physician.* 2007;10:229-253.

Choi G, Ahn S, Cho Y, Lee D. Long-term effect of pulsed radiofrequency on chronic cervical radicular pain refractory to repeated transforaminal epidural steroid injections. *Pain Med.* 2012;13:368-375.

Cohen S, Bajwa Z, Kraemer J, et al. Factors predicting success and failure for cervical facet radiofrequency denervation: a multi-center analysis. *Reg Anesth Pain Med.* 2007;32:495-503.

Cooper G, Bailey B, Bogduk N. Cervical zygapophyseal joint pain maps. *Pain Med.* 2007;8:344-353.

Konen A. Unexpected effects due to radiofrequency thermocoagulation of the sphenopalatine ganglion: two case reports. *Curr Rev Pain.* 2000;10:30-33.

Lord SM, Barnsley L, Bogduk N. The utility of comparative local anesthetic blocks versus placebo-controlled blocks for the diagnosis of cervical zygapophyseal joint pain. *Clin J Pain.* 1995;11:208-213.

Lord SM, Barnsley L, Bogduk N. Percutaneous radiofrequency neurotomy in the treatment of cervical zygapophyseal joint pain: a caution. *Neurosurgery.* 1995;36:732-739.

Manchikanti L, Damron K, Cash K, et al. Therapeutic cervical medial branch blocks in managing chronic neck pain: a preliminary report of a randomized, double-blind, controlled trial. *Pain Physician.* 2006;9:333-346.

McDonald G, Lord S, Bogduk N. Long-term follow-up of patients treated with cervical radiofrequency neurotomy for chronic neck pain. *Neurosurgery.* 1999;45:61-68.

Narouze S, Kapural L, Casanova J, Mekhail N. Sphenopalatine ganglion radiofrequency ablation for the management of chronic cluster headaches. *Headache.* 2009;49:571-577.

Ruiz-Lopez R, Erdine S. Treatment of cranio-facial pain with radiofrequency procedures. *Pain Practice.* 2002:206-213.

Sanders M, Zuurmond WW. Efficacy of sphenopalatine ganglion blockade in 66 patients suffering from cluster headache: a 12- to 70-month follow-up evaluation. *J Neurosurg.* 1997;87:876-880.

Siegenthaler A, Schliessbach J, Curatolo M, Eichenberger U. Ultrasound anatomy of the nerves supplying the cervical zygapophyseal joints: an exploratory study. *Reg Anes Pain Med.* 2011;36:606-610.

Sluijter M, van Kleef M. Characteristics and mode action of radiofrequency lesioning. *Curr Rev Pain.* 1998:143-150.

Smuck M, Crisostomo R, Trivedi K, Agrawal D. Success of initial and repeated medial branch neurotomy for zygapophyseal joint pain: a systematic review. *PM & R.* 2012;4:686-692.

The references for this chapter can be found at www.expertconsult.com.

53 Upper Extremity Blocks

Joseph M. Neal | Edward R. Mariano | Francis V. Salinas

Regional anesthetic approaches to the brachial plexus are a mainstay of surgical anesthesia practice and play an increasingly important role in postoperative analgesia. Well-designed outcome studies have confirmed the benefits of regional anesthesia in patients undergoing upper extremity surgery. When compared with traditional opioid-based postoperative analgesia for outpatient shoulder, arm, or hand surgery, single-injection regional anesthesia techniques provide superior analgesia, reduce opioid-related side effects, improve patient satisfaction, and reduce the number of unplanned admissions. Although these benefits are generally limited to the day of surgery, they nevertheless represent a valuable alternative to general anesthetic and postoperative opioid techniques.[1-4] Furthermore, limited comparative studies have shown that an interscalene or suprascapular block provides better analgesia than does an intra-articular injection or infusion of local anesthetic[5,6] and without any risk for chondrolysis. Continuous perineural catheter techniques provide superior analgesia for total shoulder arthroplasty and various ambulatory shoulder surgeries. Similar to single-injection techniques, the prolonged analgesia afforded by continuous perineural catheters is associated with fewer opioid-related side effects and higher patient satisfaction. What remains unclear is whether these techniques substantially improve economic outcomes such as faster rehabilitation or return to work.[7-9] This chapter offers a brief review of brachial plexus anatomy and pertinent pharmacology, with a primary focus on the techniques and complications of upper extremity blocks.

BRACHIAL PLEXUS ANATOMY

The brachial plexus is composed of the ventral primary rami of cervical nerves C5 to C8 and thoracic nerve T1, with occasional contributions from C4 and T2 (Fig. 53.1). Understanding the complex interdigitations that define the brachial plexus is important for two reasons. First, brachial plexus approaches are directed toward its various anatomic divisions. For example, the interscalene approach is directed toward the level of the distal roots and proximal trunks, whereas the infraclavicular approach is directed toward the level of the cords. This anatomic subarchitecture, in turn, determines the expected motor response to peripheral nerve stimulation and the distribution of anesthetic resulting from the particular approach. Second, supplemental procedures are often necessary to anesthetize nerves that are distinct from the brachial plexus or are intermediary branches. For example, the intercostobrachial nerve is primarily derived from T2, which is not part of the brachial plexus and must therefore be blocked separately if anesthesia of the medial aspect of the upper part of the arm is desired. Therefore, basic knowledge of brachial plexus anatomy is crucial for understanding the advantages and limitations of the various approaches to upper extremity regional anesthesia.

The functional neuroanatomy of the upper extremity is critically important for determining selection of the block and assessment. Motor function is generally well correlated with an observed motor response after electrical stimulation of a specific terminal nerve; for example, distal stimulation of the radial nerve consistently elicits wrist and finger extension. In contrast, as one moves proximally along the brachial plexus, stimulation yields muscle movements of a mixed nature. As an example of this concept, electrical stimulation of the superior trunk during the interscalene approach results in mixed muscle stimulation that produces shoulder elevation (Table 53.1).

Sensory innervation of the upper extremity is inconsistent and widely overlapping (Fig. 53.2). Certain areas of the arm, such as the distal palmar aspect of the forearm, have overlapping sensory innervation from the medial and lateral antebrachial cutaneous nerves, plus occasional contributions from the median nerve. A practical implication of this neuroanatomic overlap is that most areas of the upper extremity require anesthesia of two or more terminal nerves, which supports the effectiveness of plexus-based regional anesthesia over multiple selective nerve blocks at the elbow or wrist. Furthermore, overlapping cutaneous sensory fields and motor function can be problematic for assessing anesthesia, which is best accomplished by testing end functions that can be attributed only to a single nerve. The "four P's"[11] is an example of such a tool (Table 53.2).

PHARMACOLOGIC CONSIDERATIONS

Selection of a local anesthetic for brachial plexus anesthesia is based on the expected duration of surgery and the optimal duration of postoperative analgesia. When considering block duration, anesthesiologists should be cognizant of the expected degree of postoperative pain. For mildly painful procedures, some patients may interpret prolonged arm numbness as bothersome, whereas dense analgesia may mask early signs of impaired circulation in crush injuries or surgeries with potential for the development of compartment syndrome.[12] Thus, selection of a local anesthetic for an upper extremity block is best individualized to achieve specific therapeutic goals.

Potency studies of long-acting local anesthetics applied to the brachial plexus suggest that 0.5% bupivacaine is

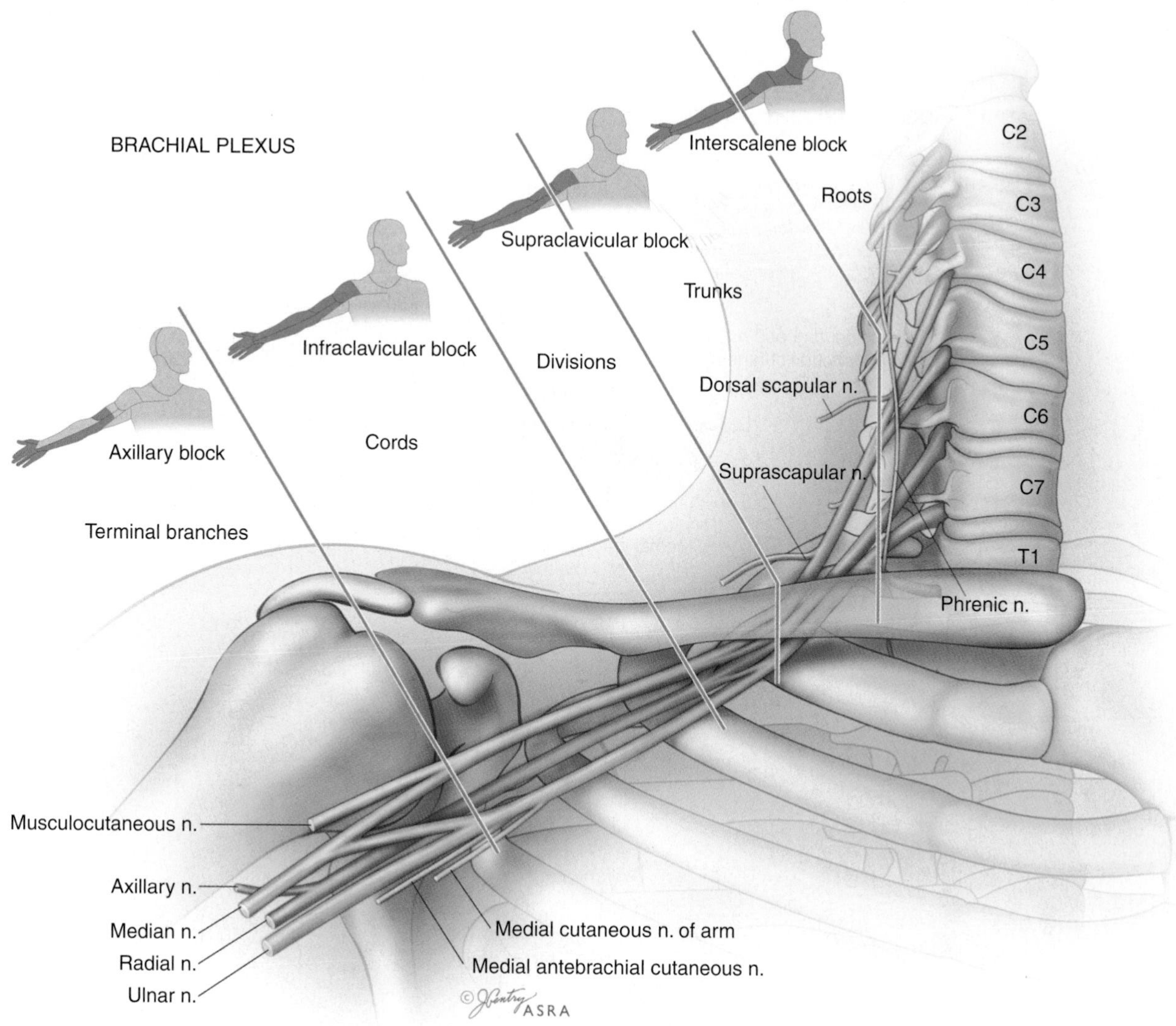

Figure 53.1 Anatomic architecture of the brachial plexus. The illustration shows the various portions of the brachial plexus. Note how different approaches to upper extremity regional anesthesia result in different distributions of anesthetic. (©American Society of Regional Anesthesia and Pain Medicine and Jennifer Gentry. Used with permission. All rights reserved.[10])

Table 53.1 Brachial Plexus Stimulation: Expected Motor Response

Approach	Stimulated Portion of the Brachial Plexus	Expected Motor Response
Interscalene	Superior trunk	Shoulder abduction, elbow flexion
Supraclavicular	Middle and inferior trunk	Hand movement
Infraclavicular	Lateral cord	Forearm flexion, hand pronation (the little finger moves laterally)
	Posterior cord	Wrist extension (the little finger moves posteriorly)
	Medial cord	Finger flexion, thumb opposition (the little finger moves medially)
Axillary	Musculocutaneous nerve	Forearm flexion, hand supination
	Median nerve	Forearm pronation, wrist flexion
	Ulnar nerve	Finger flexion, thumb opposition
	Radial nerve	Wrist extension

Modified from Rathmell JP, Neal JM, Viscomi CM. *Regional Anesthesia. The Requisites in Anesthesiology*. Philadelphia: Elsevier Mosby; 2004.

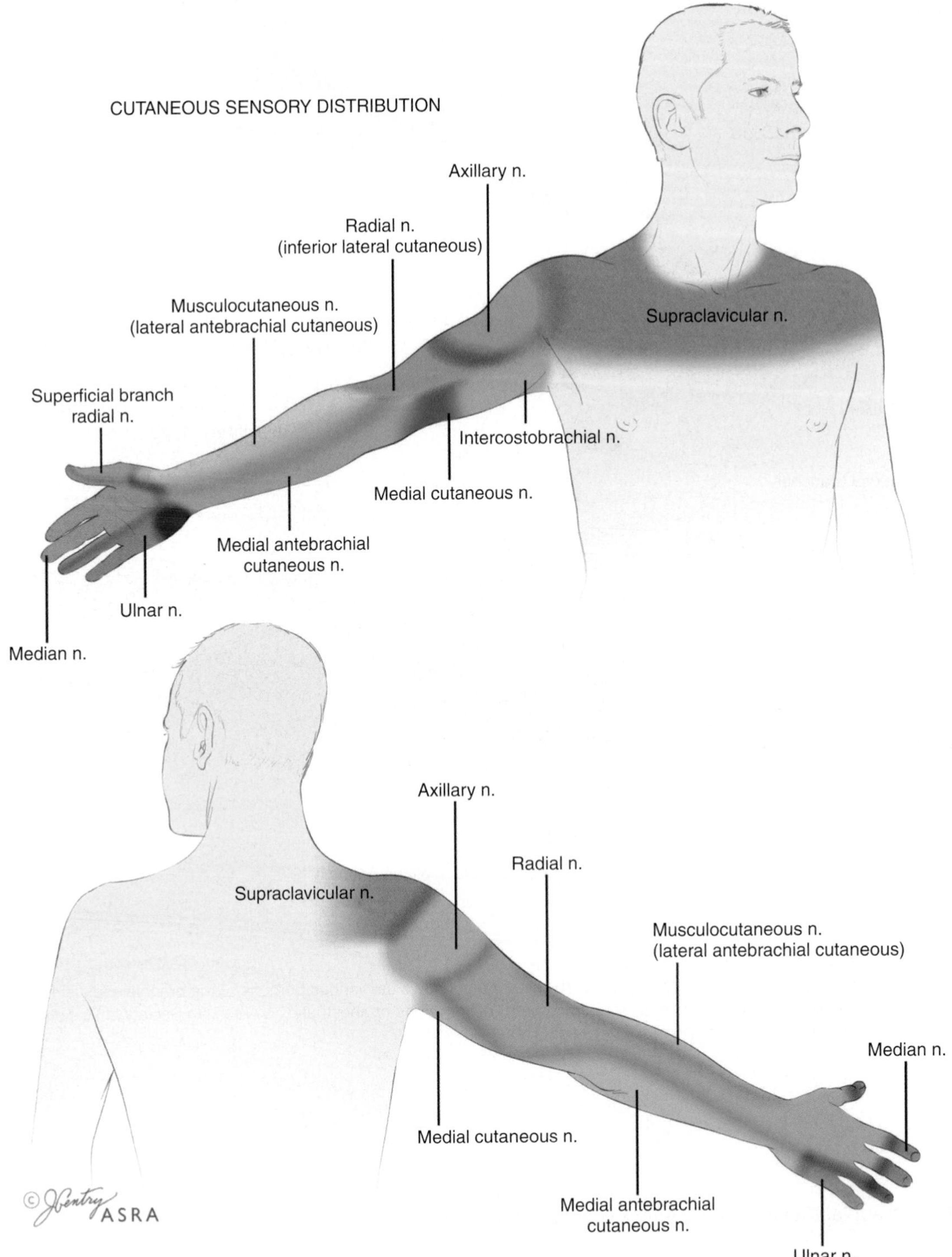

Figure 53.2 Cutaneous innervation of the upper extremity. In practice, cutaneous sensory zones are not distinct but, instead, are widely overlapping. The blending of colors demonstrates this overlap. (©American Society of Regional Anesthesia and Pain Medicine and Jennifer Gentry. Used with permission. All rights reserved.[10])

equipotent to 0.75% ropivacaine.[13,14] This equivalence is important because a tendency to use more ropivacaine to attain the same effect as bupivacaine will probably negate the lower cardiotoxicity properties of ropivacaine. When considering the total mass (dose) of a local anesthetic, decisions are best skewed toward using a lower volume, concentration, and dose. Although it may appear counterintuitive, the work of Vester-Andersen and colleagues,[15-17] along with other confirmatory investigations,[18-20] clearly demonstrates that block onset, quality, and duration are not improved by using larger volumes or concentrations of local anesthetic. Indeed, doing so risks local anesthetic

Table 53.2 Assessing Upper Extremity Nerve Block: The Four P's

P	Action	Nerve Assessed
Push	Extend the forearm against resistance	Radial
Pull	Flex the forearm against resistance	Musculocutaneous
Pinch	Pinch the palmar base of the index finger	Median
Pinch	Pinch the palmar base of the little finger	Ulnar

concentration-dependent neurotoxicity and dose-dependent systemic toxicity. Therefore, traditional local anesthetic volumes for an upper extremity plexus block are generally between 20 and 40 mL, depending on the approach chosen, and concentrations to produce surgical anesthesia should be 1.5% or less for lidocaine or mepivacaine, 0.75% or less for ropivacaine, and 0.5% or less for bupivacaine.[10] Conversely, if one seeks only postoperative analgesia, ultrasound guidance facilitates the use of much lower volumes of local anesthetic for an interscalene block.[19,21] However, further evidence suggests that ultrasound-guided regional anesthesia (UGRA) with low-volume blocks may indeed result in a shorter duration of analgesia.[22-24]

Four local anesthetic additives have proven value when applied to the brachial plexus. Epinephrine, 2.5 μg/mL (1:400,000), prolongs the duration, acts as a marker of intravascular injection, and decreases systemic uptake of local anesthetic.[10] The ability of epinephrine to prolong a local anesthetic block is a consequence of reduced clearance from the injection site,[25] and it is unlikely to involve a significant α_2-adrenergic agonist effect.[26] Epinephrine is unique among local anesthetic additives in that its associated tachycardia can serve as a marker of intravascular injection. Clonidine, 0.5 μg/kg, prolongs anesthesia and analgesia by 50% without systemic side effects such as hypotension or sedation.[27,28] Clonidine does not improve block quality during continuous perineural catheter techniques.[29] The effect of epinephrine and clonidine on intermediate-acting local anesthetics is clinically significant, but they do not reliably prolong the duration of long-acting local anesthetics.[30-32] Buprenorphine, 0.3 mg, also prolongs anesthesia and analgesia, but at the expense of nausea and vomiting.[33] Dexamethasone can also prolong intermediate-acting agents to a degree similar to epinephrine, but the optimal dose and any potential long-term effects of dexamethasone remain uncertain.[34,35] The beneficial effects of these additives, as well as their potential neurotoxicity, alone and in combination, are currently still under investigation.[35,36] Other opioids, neostigmine, calcium channel blockers, hyaluronidase, and tramadol either do not improve local anesthetic blocks or have unresolved neurotoxicity issues.[10]

Alkalinization of intermediate-acting local anesthetics facilitates faster onset of the block during epidural anesthesia but does not have the same effect at the brachial plexus. Onset is not hastened by adding sodium bicarbonate to plain local anesthetic or to local anesthetic freshly mixed with epinephrine.[10] Indeed, animal models have shown that alkalinization of local anesthetic reduces block intensity and duration.[37]

BLOCK TECHNIQUES FOR MAJOR APPROACHES TO THE BRACHIAL PLEXUS

A number of techniques involving various nerve localization modalities may be used for successful brachial plexus blocks, but only a sample can reasonably be presented in one chapter. When using ultrasound, target nerves can theoretically be imaged in short or long axis; target imaging is then combined with the needle guidance technique, in plane or out of plane, to fully describe the approach, for instance, short axis in plane or short axis out of plane. Since long-axis imaging for nerve blocks is limited to lower extremity techniques to date[38] and in-plane needle guidance permits visualization of the tip of the needle, this chapter will cover only short-axis in-plane techniques using ultrasound.

CONTINUOUS PERIPHERAL CATHETERS

Prolonged analgesia of the upper extremity can be accomplished with continuous perineural catheter techniques. Surgeries expected to cause prolonged, moderate to severe pain are appropriate for catheter placement. Such surgeries include total shoulder arthroplasty, rotator cuff repair, and major reconstructive operations on the elbow, wrist, or hand. Accumulated evidence suggests that perineural catheters can be managed efficiently in the ambulatory setting with a high degree of patient acceptance.[39,40] Key to successful management is establishing clear lines of contact with the physician and patient.[8] Even major surgeries such as total shoulder arthroplasty can be managed on an outpatient basis when perineural catheters are used to control pain and facilitate rehabilitation.[9] Recent data indicate that ultrasound guidance can decrease the time needed to successfully place upper extremity perineural catheters in comparison to traditional nerve stimulation techniques.[41,42] For infraclavicular perineural catheter insertion, ultrasound may reduce the incidence of unintentional vascular puncture when compared with nerve stimulation techniques.[41] Limited data suggest that patient-controlled perineural analgesia techniques are superior to continuous infusion techniques.[40,43] However, in the ambulatory setting, perineural infusion regimens that combine patient-controlled boluses with a continuous infusion rate are preferred.[44]

INTERSCALENE BLOCK

INDICATIONS

For an interscalene block, the brachial plexus is approached at the level of its distal roots/proximal trunks. The most consistent local anesthetic distribution resulting from this approach involves the shoulder and upper part of the arm (Fig. 53.3). The inferior trunk (C8, T1) is unaffected by local anesthetic in approximately 50% of cases,[45] so an interscalene block is not recommended for surgeries involving the medial aspect of the upper part of the arm, the forearm, and the hand. Ultrasound-guided approaches are also likely to spare the lower trunk distribution, although some investigators describe targeting these nerves.[46]

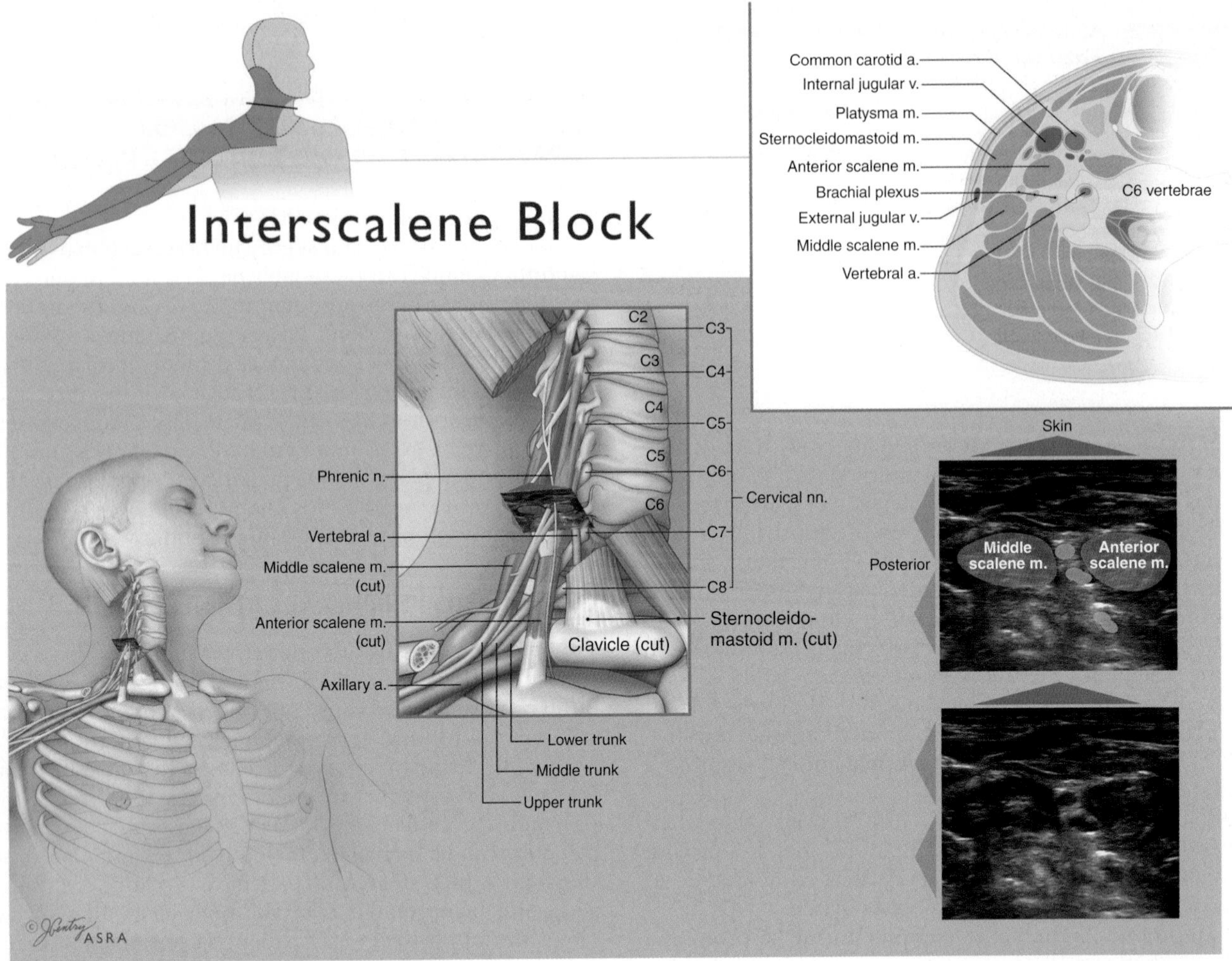

Figure 53.3 Interscalene block. The upper right inset notes the proximity of the brachial plexus to the neuraxis and major vascular structures. The upper left inset illustrates the expected anesthetic distribution of an interscalene block. Note how the spinal roots begin to form the three trunks as the brachial plexus passes through the interscalene groove. The sonogram most likely reveals the C5-C7 nerve roots or the upper/middle trunk. (©American Society of Regional Anesthesia and Pain Medicine and Jennifer Gentry. Used with permission. All rights reserved.[10])

TECHNIQUES

Traditional Techniques

The brachial plexus traverses the interscalene groove, which is bordered by the anterior and middle scalene muscles. In the classic Winnie[47] technique, the patient's head is turned 30 degrees to the contralateral side, and then a 50-mm or shorter needle is inserted into the interscalene groove at the level of the sixth cervical vertebra. The needle is oriented perpendicular to all planes of the skin and then advanced with a slightly caudad angulation, which lessens the risk of entering the intervertebral foramen and encountering spinal nerves or the vertebral artery (Fig. 53.4). The end point for advancement of the needle is either paresthesia or an evoked motor response (from peripheral nerve stimulation) in the arm or anterior aspect of the shoulder.[48,49] Movement of the posterior portion of the shoulder indicates that the needle is too posterior and is stimulating the dorsal scapular nerve (C5), whereas a diaphragmatic motor response indicates placement of the needle too far anterior with resultant stimulation of the phrenic nerve. Once paresthesia or a motor response at approximately 0.5 mA is obtained, a 1-mL local anesthetic test dose is injected to rule out intravascular injection, followed by incremental injection of 20 to 30 mL of local anesthetic.

Borgeat and colleagues'[50] modified lateral interscalene approach has reportedly facilitated perineural catheter placement by reducing the angle that a catheter must take as it exits the block needle and enters the perineural area. Because the lateral approach directs the needle away from the vertebral column, this approach theoretically reduces the risk for injection of the vertebral artery or contact of the needle with the spinal cord or perispinal neural elements.

Ultrasound-Guided Technique

With the patient positioned as just mentioned, a high-frequency linear-array transducer should be placed at the level of the cricoid cartilage along the posterior border of the sternocleidomastoid (SCM) muscle (Fig. 53.5). After identifying the SCM, the scalene muscles are reliably located deep to the SCM fascia posterior to the internal jugular vein and carotid artery. If the fascial plane between the anterior and middle scalene muscles (interscalene groove) is not easily visualized, slide the transducer caudad toward the clavicle while keeping the scalene muscles in the center of the screen

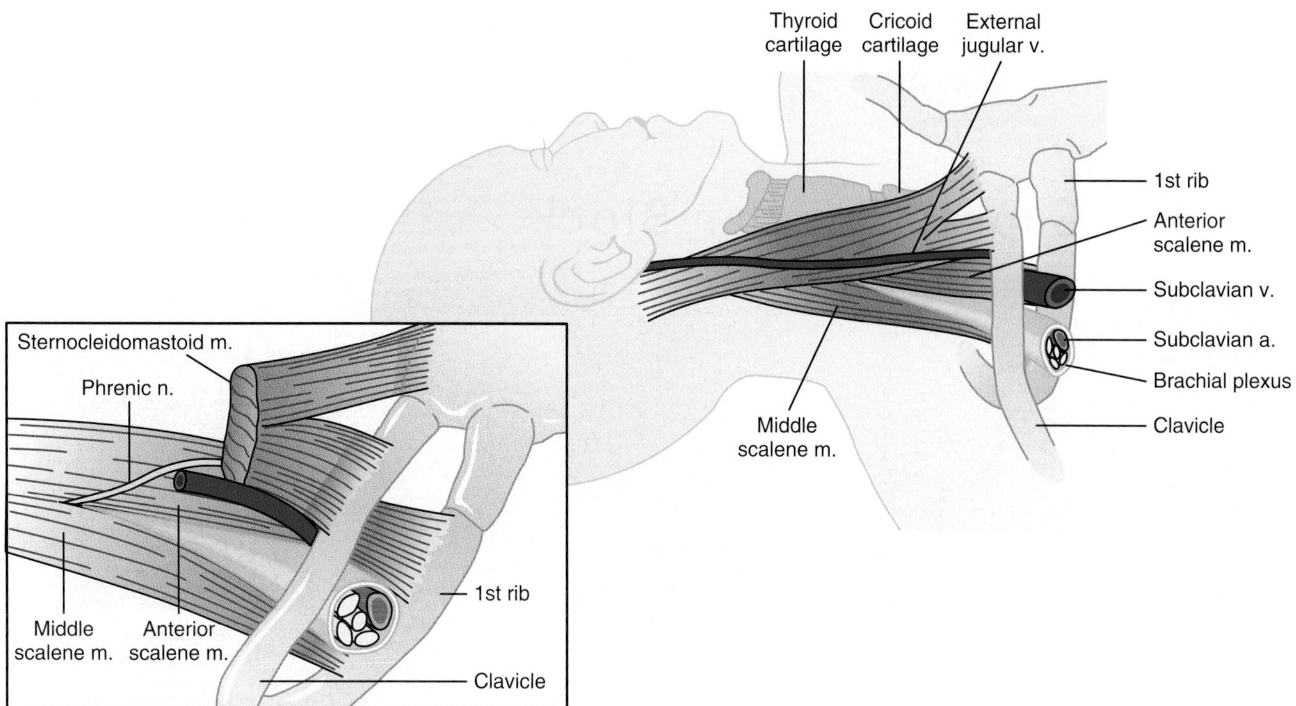

Figure 53.4 Interscalene approach of Winnie. The brachial plexus traverses through the interscalene groove, where a needle can approach it at the C6 level. Note that the phrenic nerve lies on the anterior scalene muscle, which exposes it to unintended stimulation. a., artery; m., muscle; n., nerve; v., vein. (Adapted from Rathmell JP, Neal JM, Viscomi CM. *Regional Anesthesia. The Requisites in Anesthesiology*. Philadelphia: Elsevier Mosby; 2004:63.)

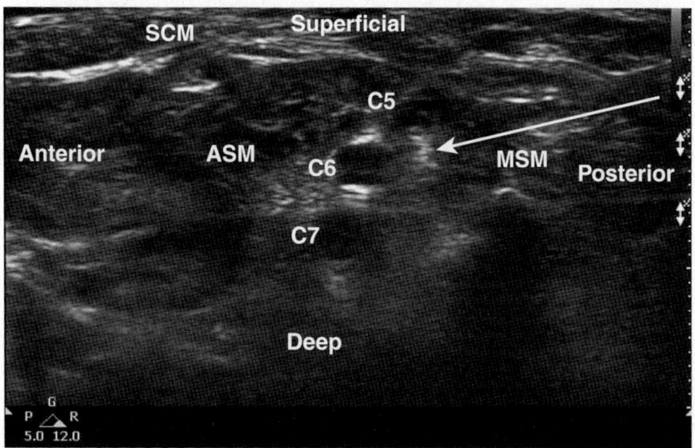

Figure 53.5 Ultrasound-guided interscalene block—short-axis view of the brachial plexus located in the interscalene groove. The roots (C5, C6, and C7) or trunks (upper and middle) appear as hypoechoic (dark), monofascicular to oligofascicular structures located in between the fascial compartment between the anterior scalene muscle (ASM) and middle scalene muscles (MSMs). The interscalene groove is typically located posterior to the sternocleidomastoid muscle (SCM). The arrow illustrates the typical "in-plane" needle path in the anterior direction through the MSM toward the brachial plexus.

until the interscalene groove widens to reveal the brachial plexus. Following infiltration of the skin and subcutaneous tissue with local anesthetic posterior to the transducer, advance the block needle in an anteromedial trajectory in plane through the middle scalene muscle and into the interscalene groove.[51,52] Proceed with incremental injection of local anesthetic solution as described previously. In this region, successful interscalene blocks with injectate volumes of less than 5 mL have been reported.[21,53] For perineural catheter insertion, placing the patient in the lateral decubitus position with the operative side up may facilitate this posterior approach when using ultrasound guidance.[52,54]

SUPRACLAVICULAR BLOCK

INDICATIONS

The supraclavicular approach aims to encounter the brachial plexus at the juncture of the distal trunks and divisions as the brachial plexus courses under the clavicle and across the superior surface of the first rib (Fig. 53.6). This area represents the most compact architecture of the brachial plexus, which has been postulated (but never proved) to explain the propensity of supraclavicular blocks for rapid onset and nearly complete anesthesia of the upper extremity. This block is indicated for any surgery on the arm (see Fig. 53.1), although shoulder surgery may require supplemental blockade of the supraclavicular nerve (C3-4) to ensure anesthesia of the cape area around the shoulder. A supraclavicular block is successful in approximately 95% of patients, including those who are obese.[55]

TECHNIQUES

Traditional Techniques

A variety of techniques have been described for performing a supraclavicular block.[56-58] With the patient in the supine position, the plumb bob technique places the needle just above the clavicle at the lateral border of the SCM muscle. The original description by Brown and associates[56] involved directing the needle straight downward, similar to a brick

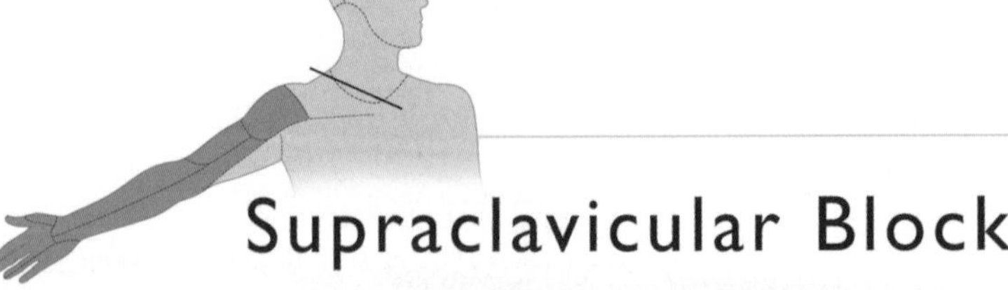

Supraclavicular Block

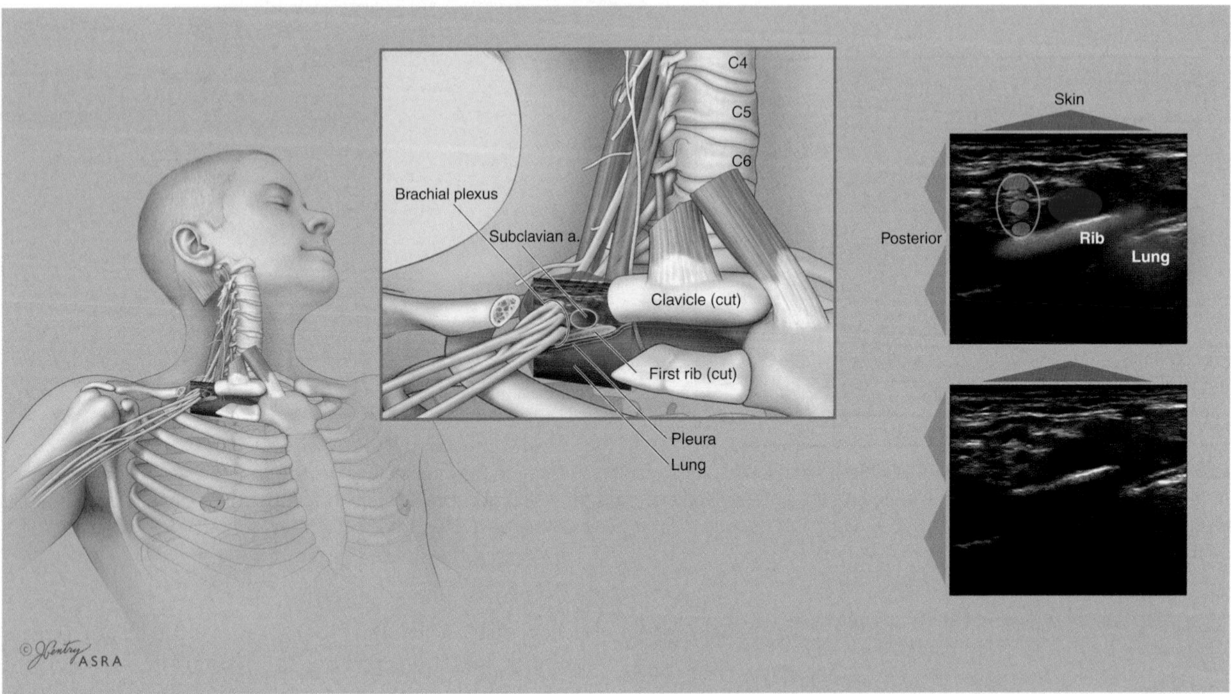

Figure 53.6 Supraclavicular block. The upper inset illustrates the expected distribution of anesthetic with a supraclavicular block. Note how the three trunks begin to form the anterior and posterior divisions as the brachial plexus passes under the clavicle and over the first rib. The sonogram shows the plexus lateral to the subclavian artery. Note the shimmering of the pleura and the acoustic shadowing caused by the first rib. (©American Society of Regional Anesthesia and Pain Medicine and Jennifer Gentry. Used with permission. All rights reserved.[10])

mason's plumb bob. If a motor response or paresthesia is not elicited, the needle is incrementally fanned 20 degrees cephalad and then 20 degrees caudad in the parasagittal plane until the desired motor response is obtained. In a modification of this technique, the initial needle pass is made 45 degrees cephalad, followed by incremental caudad angulation until a suitable paresthesia or motor response is obtained. The logic of this modification is that it reduces the risk for contact with the lung copula in tall individuals.[59] If during the course of a supraclavicular block the needle encounters the subclavian artery, the needle should be redirected posteriorly and laterally to identify the brachial plexus. Injecting 20 to 30 mL of local anesthetic after a single paresthesia or motor response into the arm or shoulder at less than 0.5 to 0.9 mA[60] completes the block procedure.

Ultrasound-Guided Technique

Using the same surface anatomic landmarks as presented for the traditional techniques, a high-frequency linear-array transducer is placed with its midpoint centered posterior to the clavicle and along the posterior border of the SCM (Fig. 53.7). The subclavian artery is the most important sonographic anatomic landmark and helps localize the divisions of the brachial plexus, which is reliably superficial and

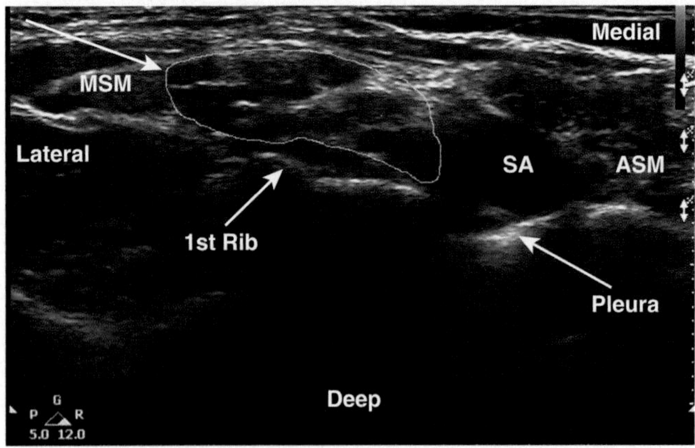

Figure 53.7 Ultrasound-guided supraclavicular block—short-axis view of the brachial plexus with the supraclavicular approach. The brachial plexus elements (trunks, divisions) appear as hyperechoic, polyfascicular structures typically located posterosuperior to the subclavian artery (SA) lying on the superior aspect of the first rib. Note that the first rib appears hyperechoic with posterior acoustic dropout. The pleura also appears hyperechoic but has a shimmering appearance. The arrow *(top left)* illustrates the typical "in-plane" needle approach in an anterior direction toward the brachial plexus. ASM, anteriior subclavian muscle; MSM, middle subclavian muscle.

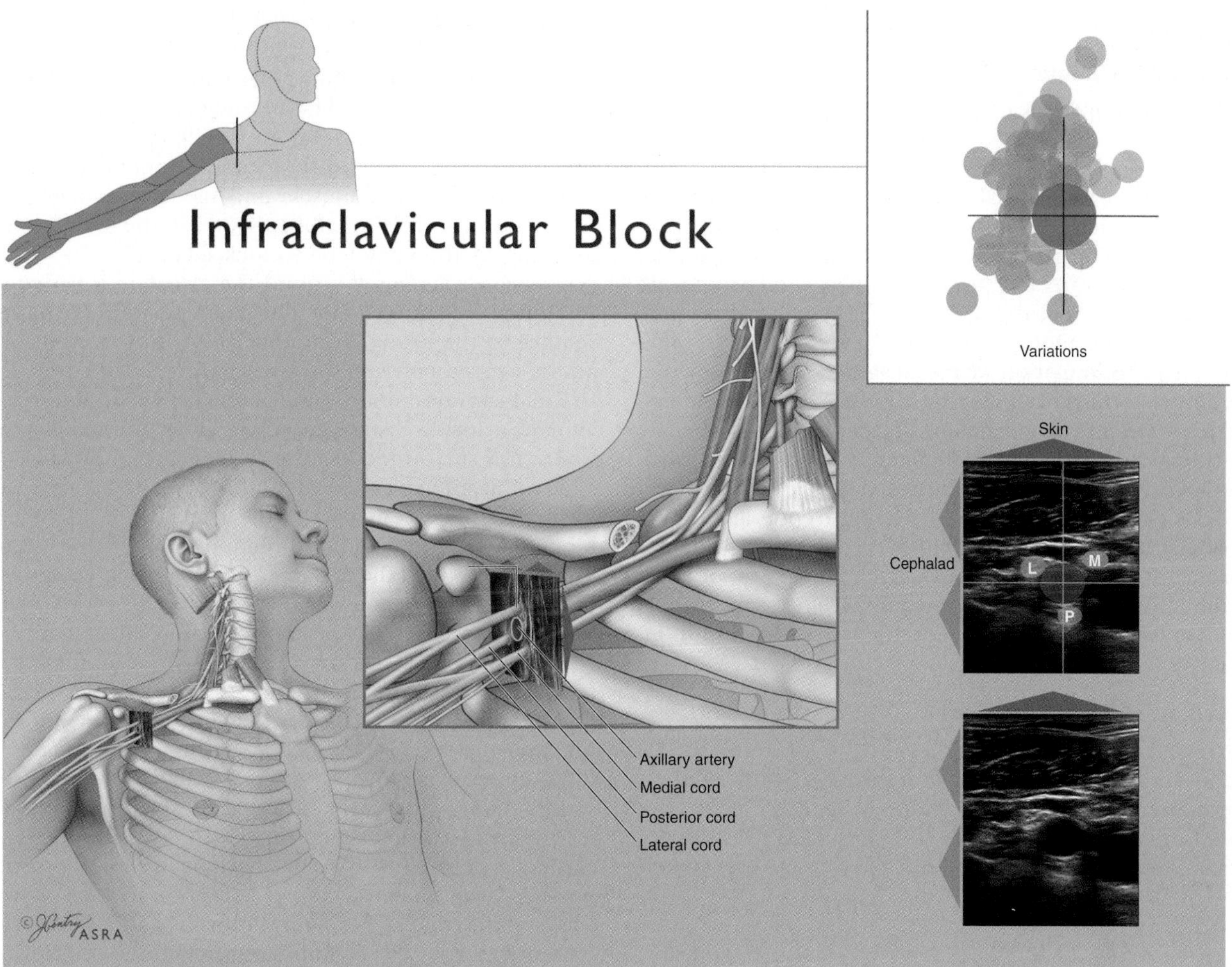

Figure 53.8 Infraclavicular block. The upper left inset illustrates the expected distribution of anesthetic with an infraclavicular block. Note how the three cords are arranged around the second part of the axillary artery in positions roughly equivalent to their name. However, as shown in the upper right inset, the cords manifest considerable positional overlap (lateral cord = green, medial cord = blue, posterior cord = orange). The medial cord frequently lies between the axillary artery and vein. (©American Society of Regional Anesthesia and Pain Medicine and Jennifer Gentry. Used with permission. All rights reserved.[10])

posterior to the artery. With the transducer in this position, tilt the plane of the ultrasound beam more laterally to visualize the subclavian artery over the first rib. At this location the divisions of the inferior trunk, composed of C8 and T1, should be visualized in the "corner pocket" posterior to the subclavian artery and superficial to the first rib.[61,62] The subclavian artery and brachial plexus at this level are still within the interscalene groove. After infiltration of the skin and subcutaneous tissue with local anesthetic posterior to the transducer, advance the block needle in an anteromedial trajectory in plane through the middle scalene muscle and into the interscalene groove.[58,61] Ultrasound-guided supraclavicular perineural catheter insertion has been described with this approach, although there may be an analgesic advantage to using the infraclavicular technique for the postoperative management of patients undergoing distal upper extremity surgery.[63] Alternatively, when using ultrasound guidance, the block needle may be directed in a posterolateral direction.[64] Inject the local anesthetic solution incrementally and visually confirm spread of the injectate in the vicinity of the target nerves. Unlike an interscalene block, an ultrasound-guided supraclavicular block requires a volume of injectate similar to that used with the traditional techniques.[65,66]

INFRACLAVICULAR BLOCK

INDICATIONS

The infraclavicular block, which is indicated for surgery on the arm distal to the shoulder, approaches the brachial plexus at the level of the cords (Fig. 53.8). This block anesthetizes the axillary and musculocutaneous nerves more reliably than does the axillary approach.[67,68] Infraclavicular block techniques have the advantage of not requiring a specific arm position during placement, which is useful for patients with limited arm motion because of pain, casts, or dressings.[69] The infraclavicular approach is frequently used for continuous perineural catheter placement because the catheters reliably remain in place during use. There have been reports of successful use of continuous infraclavicular perineural infusion for the treatment of complex regional pain syndrome of the upper extremity[70] and for upper extremity limb salvage.[71]

TECHNIQUES

Traditional Techniques

Similar to the supraclavicular approach, several techniques have been described for an infraclavicular block; none are inherently superior. The coracoid approach[72] begins with identification of the lateral aspect of the coracoid process in a supine patient. From this point, an entry point 2 cm caudad and 2 cm medial is marked (Fig. 53.9). A stimulating needle is directed posteriorly, perpendicular to all planes. Stimulation of the various cords can be ascertained by their resulting motor response—"at the cords, the pinkie towards." Stimulation of the posterior cord causes the little finger to move posteriorly, stimulation of the medial cord results in medial movement, and stimulation of the lateral cord results in lateral movement.[73] The posterior cord occupies the middle position and is the deepest of the three cords. Block success is maximized when two cords are identified and subsequently bathed with local anesthetic[74]; identification and subsequent injection around the posterior cord are the most important determinants of block success.[75,76] A total of 30 to 40 mL of local anesthetic is sufficient for an infraclavicular block.

Ultrasound-Guided Technique

With the arm abducted 90 degrees and the coracoid process used as a surface landmark, the transducer is oriented in the parasagittal plane with its midpoint slightly medial and caudad to the coracoid process[77,78] (Fig. 53.10). Although a small-footprint, lower-frequency curvilinear transducer may have advantages because of this region's limited space and the expected steep angle of the block needle,[78,79] a high-frequency linear transducer may also be used in most nonobese patients.[80,81] The optimal short-axis ultrasound image should demonstrate the axillary artery and the brachial plexus cords to be located immediately deep to the pectoralis minor muscle and its accompanying clavipectoral fascia. It is helpful to visualize the axillary artery as being in the center of a clock face, with the brachial plexus cords arranged around the artery in a parasagittal topographic arrangement. The exact position of the cords relative to the artery is variable, but the posterior cord is always located between the lateral and medial cords. Deep to the pectoralis minor muscle and clavipectoral fascia, the axillary artery is visualized cephalad to the axillary vein, where it is surrounded by the three brachial plexus cords. After infiltration of the skin and subcutaneous tissue with local anesthetic cephalad to the transducer, advance the block needle in a caudad direction through the pectoralis muscles toward the axillary artery. Local anesthetic may be deposited separately around each cord[78] or via a single injection incrementally posterior to the axillary artery with comparable block efficacy.[80,81] Similar to a supraclavicular block, injectate volume when using ultrasound guidance for an infraclavicular block does not seem to differ significantly from that used with traditional techniques.[66] For distal upper extremity postoperative analgesia, many ultrasound-guided infraclavicular perineural catheter insertion techniques have been described.[79,82,83] Continuous infraclavicular perineural infusions have been shown to provide postoperative analgesia that is superior to that achieved with supraclavicular perineural infusions after distal upper extremity surgery.[63] A combination of continuous infusion and patient-controlled boluses optimizes analgesia when compared with either a basal-only or a bolus-only dosing regimen.[44]

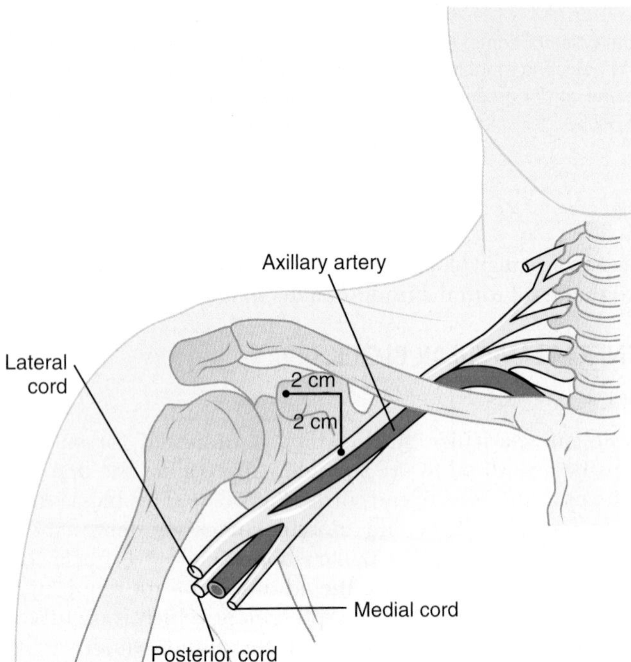

Figure 53.9 The infraclavicular approach. The entry point is marked after identifying the lateral edge of the coracoid process and then moving 2 cm medial and 2 cm caudad. A needle is then directed posteriorly toward the three cords of the brachial plexus and the axillary artery, which is approximately 4 ± 1.5 cm from the skin. (Adapted from Rathmell JP, Neal JM, Viscomi CM. *Regional Anesthesia. The Requisites in Anesthesiology*. Philadelphia: Elsevier Mosby; 2004:67.)

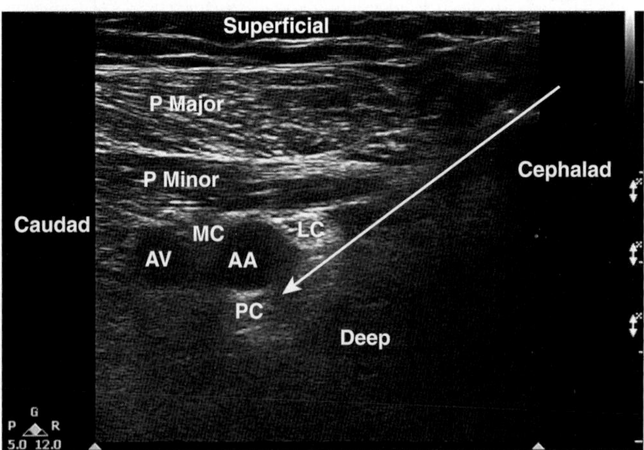

Figure 53.10 Ultrasound-guided infraclavicular block—short-axis view of the infraclavicular approach. The neurovascular structures are located deep to the pectoralis major and pectoralis minor. The axillary artery (AA) is located cephalad to the axillary vein (AV), where it is surround by the lateral cord (LC), posterior cord (PC), and medial cord (MC) of the brachial plexus. The optimal location for injection of local anesthetic is typically located closest to the PC and just deep to the AA. The arrow illustrates the typical needle path needed to place the tip of the needle in close proximity to the PC.

AXILLARY BLOCK

INDICATIONS

The axillary block anesthetizes the brachial plexus at the level of the four terminal nerves: the radial, ulnar, median, and musculocutaneous nerves (Fig. 53.11). It is indicated for surgeries distal to and including the elbow[84] (see Fig. 53.1). With the exception of very proximal approaches high in the axilla, the axillary block is not as ideally suited for continuous catheter techniques as are the infraclavicular approach and approaches above the clavicle.

TECHNIQUES

Traditional Techniques

The patient lies supine with the arm abducted approximately 90 degrees and externally rotated such that the dorsum of the hand lies flat while supported by one or two pillows. Classic descriptions of the axillary neurovascular bundle place the radial nerve nearly posterior to and slightly inferior to the artery, the ulnar nerve more superficial but also inferior to the artery, the median nerve superficial and superior to the artery, and the musculocutaneous nerve superior to the artery and residing deeper within the fascial plane between the coracobrachialis and biceps muscles or within the belly of the coracobrachialis muscle (Fig. 53.12). However, anatomic variation is frequently present, especially with regard to nerve position relative to the axillary artery.[85] These inherent variations may partially explain why the various techniques for axillary block have similar success rates.

The transarterial technique generally achieves higher success rates with two 10- to 20-mL local anesthetic injections anterior and posterior to the axillary artery.[86] Success rates are similar with the paresthesia and peripheral nerve stimulation techniques.[10,87] Either technique's success is enhanced by identifying and subsequently injecting local anesthetic near three or four terminal nerves rather than using a single injection. Four injections may increase performance time without appreciably affecting success rates.[10,88,89] The motor responses expected for each nerve are listed in Table 53.1. Further technical refinement suggests that success is most dependent on identifying and

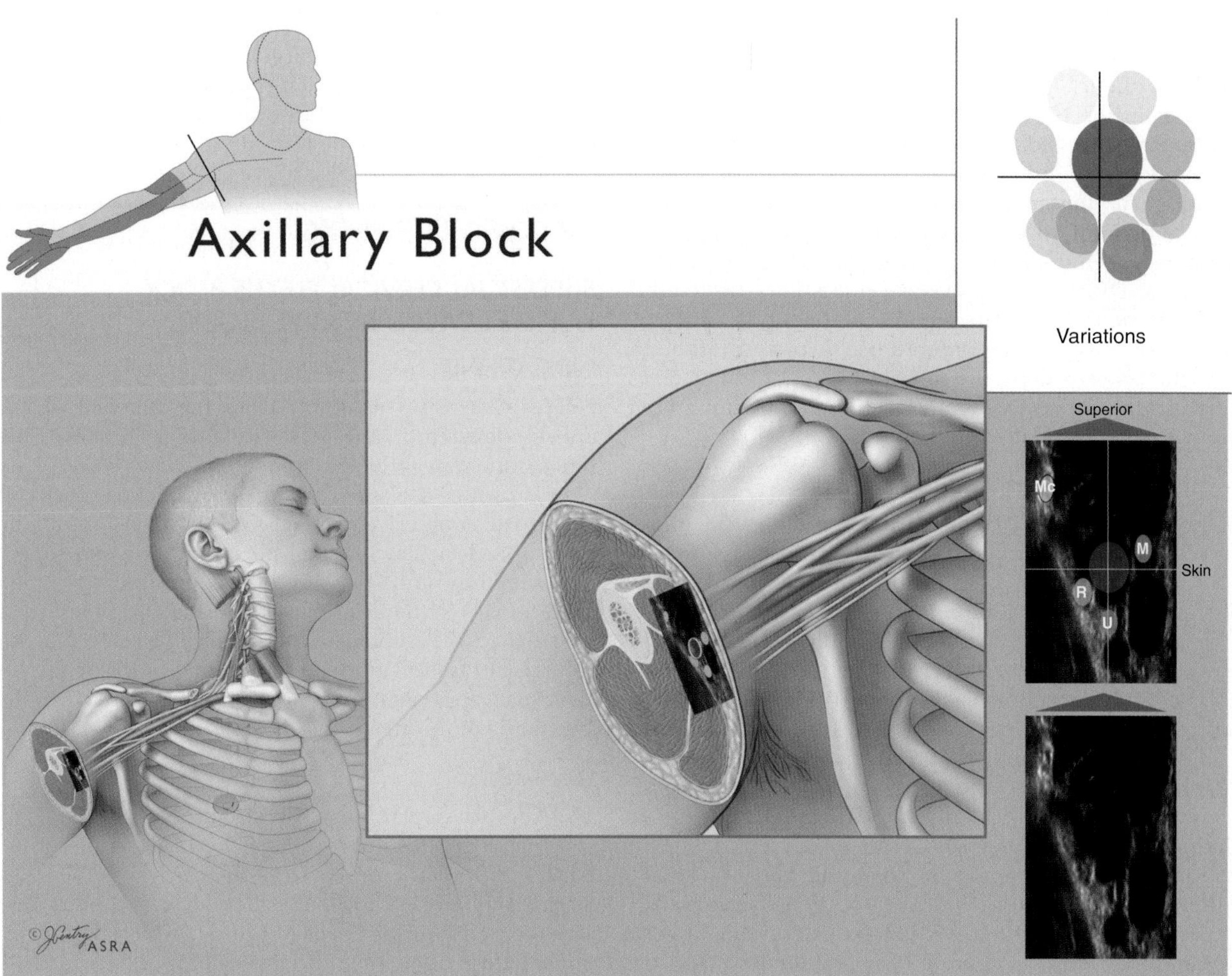

Figure 53.11 Axillary block. The upper left inset illustrates the expected distribution of anesthetic with an axillary block. The musculocutaneous nerve (MC) is superior to the axillary artery and typically within the fascial plane between the coracobrachialis and biceps muscles. Note how the other three terminal nerves are arranged around the axillary artery. As shown in the upper right inset (which is rotated 90 degrees clockwise from its normal patient-oriented view), the terminal manifests considerable positional overlap (median nerve = green, ulnar nerve = blue, radial nerve = orange). The medial cord frequently lies between the axillary artery and vein. (©American Society of Regional Anesthesia and Pain Medicine and Jennifer Gentry. Used with permission. All rights reserved.[10])

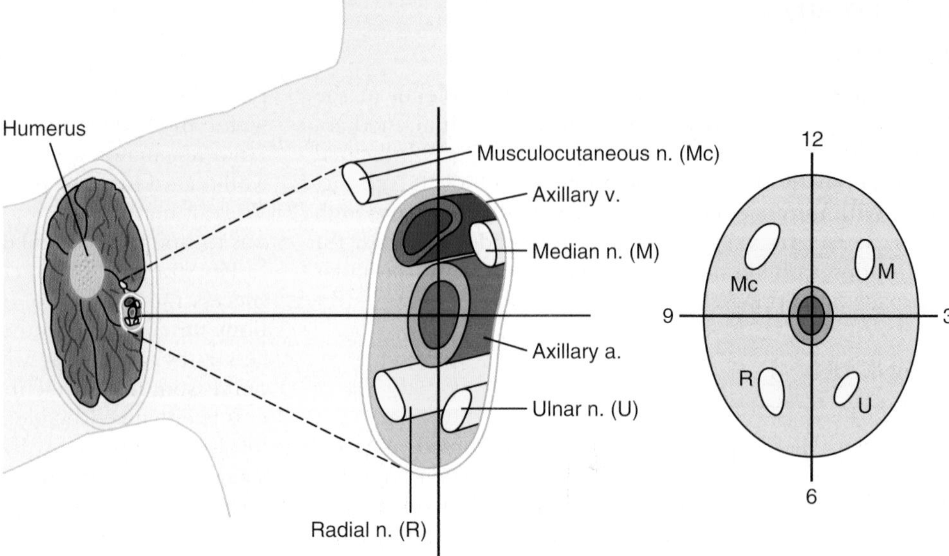

Figure 53.12 Axillary block. At the level of the axilla, the four terminal nerves of the brachial plexus maintain a quadrant-like relationship to the axillary artery. Although there is substantial variation between patients, the radial and ulnar nerves are typically inferior (6-o'clock position) to the artery, with the radial artery being deeper. The median nerve is typically superficial and superior (12-o'clock position) to the artery. The musculocutaneous nerve requires a separate anesthetizing procedure. (Adapted from Rathmell JP, Neal JM, Viscomi CM. *Regional Anesthesia. The Requisites in Anesthesiology*. Philadelphia: Elsevier Mosby; 2004:67.)

subsequently injecting local anesthetic near the radial and median nerves and least dependent on injection around the ulnar nerve.[89,90] Clinical trials suggest that traditional axillary block techniques should require less than 40 mL of local anesthetic.[17] Because the musculocutaneous nerve diverges from the plexus at the level of the axilla, it may remain unanesthetized during transarterial or single-injection techniques. If not localized by ultrasound or nerve stimulation, the musculocutaneous nerve is easily blocked by infiltrating 5 mL of local anesthetic into the belly of the coracobrachialis muscle. The perivascular infiltration technique[91] uses a continuously moving needle to fan 10 to 15 mL of local anesthetic next to the superior border of the axillary artery in three progressively outward needle passes and then repeats the process along the inferior aspect of the artery. Because of this outwardly fanning technique, the musculocutaneous nerve is usually anesthetized.

Ultrasound-Guided Technique

With the arm abducted 90 degrees at the shoulder, the midpoint of a high-frequency linear-array transducer is placed over the axillary artery pulse in the proximal part of the axilla. Such placement and orientation will provide a short-axis view of the axillary artery, the terminal nerves, and the surrounding perineural musculature (conjoint tendon and biceps and coracobrachialis muscles) (Fig. 53.13). The artery and other blood vessels may be clearly identified with the aid of color flow Doppler. The locations of the terminal branch nerves relative to the artery, especially the musculocutaneous nerve,[92] are highly variable, and ultrasound-guided axillary blocks may still result in nerve sparing.[93] Therefore, it may be advantageous to identify the individual peripheral nerves more distally and trace them back toward the axilla. After visualizing the axillary artery and target nerves and following injection of local anesthetic lateral to the transducer, the block needle is advanced in a medial direction toward the axillary artery and local anesthetic is injected so that each target nerve is surrounded.[94,95] With an ultrasound-guided multiple-injection technique, the volumes of local anesthetic required may be drastically reduced as compared with the traditional techniques.[93,96] However, recent prospective randomized controlled studies indicate that when using traditional volumes of local anesthetic (35 to 40 mL), an ultrasound-guided double-injection (with one injection specifically targeting the musculocutaneous nerve) perivascular approach results in success comparable to that achieved with an ultrasound-guided quadruple-injection perineural technique but with fewer needle passes.[97,98]

ACCESSORY BLOCKS

SUPERFICIAL CERVICAL PLEXUS BLOCK (SUPRACLAVICULAR NERVE BLOCK)

INDICATIONS

Nerves that arise separately from the brachial plexus or are inconsistently anesthetized with a brachial plexus block innervate selected upper extremity sensory fields. Also known as the superficial cervical plexus block, blockade of the supraclavicular nerve (C3-4) is a useful adjunct to a supraclavicular brachial plexus block when surgery is performed around the cape of the shoulder (Fig. 53.14). Traditional techniques for the interscalene block typically anesthetize the supraclavicular nerve. However, a lower-volume ultrasound-guided interscalene block or the supraclavicular approach may be associated with insufficient anesthesia of this nerve.[10]

TECHNIQUES

The supraclavicular nerve is anesthetized by injecting a subcutaneous wheal of local anesthetic along the posterior border of the SCM muscle from the clavicle to the mastoid. Several milliliters of local anesthetic can also be infiltrated into the midpoint of the SCM muscle, which the nerve traverses before branching into three components.

SUPRASCAPULAR NERVE BLOCK

INDICATIONS

The suprascapular nerve (C5-6) branches from the superior trunk of the brachial plexus to supply the posterior

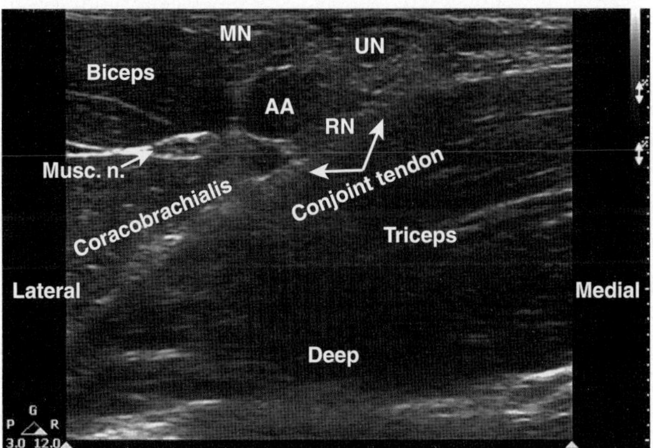

Figure 53.13 Ultrasound-guided axillary block—short-axis view of the axillary brachial plexus. The terminal nerves of the brachial plexus (median nerve [MN], ulnar nerve [UN], and radial nerve [RN]) appear as hyperechoic, polyfascicular structures *("honeycomb" appearance)* that surround the axillary artery (AA). The axillary neurovascular structures are located in the bicipital groove (between the biceps and triceps muscles) and lay directly superficial to the conjoint tendon (of the teres major and latissimus dorsi muscles). The musculocutaneous nerve (Musc. n.) typically lies either within the body of the coracobrachialis muscle or less commonly in between the fascial plane of the coracobrachialis and biceps muscles.

two thirds of the shoulder joint and the acromioclavicular joint. Blocking this nerve prolongs analgesia after shoulder arthroscopy performed under general anesthesia[4] but adds no value to an interscalene block for open, anterior shoulder surgery.[99] A suprascapular block with local anesthetic and steroid also provides prolonged relief of acute painful conditions and the chronic degenerative shoulder conditions commonly encountered in pain medicine practice.[100] The block can also be used for diagnostic purposes.

TECHNIQUES

A suprascapular nerve block is accomplished by depositing local anesthetic near the suprascapular notch. Drawing a line along the scapular spine and bisecting it with a second line drawn parallel to the vertebral spine outlines the surface landmarks. The resultant upper outer quadrant is then entered with a needle traveling cephalad to caudad and directed toward the scapular spine. This approach, rather than posterior to anterior, avoids entry into the suprascapular notch and the possibility of pneumothorax (Fig. 53.15). Once contact is made, 10 mL of local anesthetic is injected in a fanning manner.

An ultrasound-guided approach involves placing the transducer in a coronal plane over the suprascapular fossa. The suprascapular nerve and artery can usually be visualized along the floor of the suprascapular fossa between the suprascapular and spinoglenoid notches (Fig. 53.16).

SELECTIVE NERVE BLOCKS AT THE TERMINAL BRANCHES

There are few indications for selective nerve blocks of the upper extremity because innervation of the forearm and hand is typified by extensive crossover of the cutaneous sensory distribution; therefore, single-nerve blockade is rarely adequate. Selective blocks at the elbow or wrist as a sole anesthetic are also problematic if prolonged use of a pneumatic tourniquet is required. One indication for a selective block is use of a median nerve block at the wrist for carpal tunnel release,[101] although supplemental local anesthesia may still be required.

Ultrasound may be used to identify the distal peripheral nerves of the upper extremity,[102] and ultrasound-guided blocks of these nerves in the forearm may be performed.[103] The use of ultrasound-guided pulsed radiofrequency ablation of the median nerve has been reported for recurrent carpal tunnel syndrome following surgical intervention.[104]

COMPLICATIONS OF UPPER EXTREMITY BLOCK

NERVE INJURY

Permanent nerve injury after an upper extremity block is extremely rare and probably occurs in 0 to 16 per 10,000 patients (95% confidence interval [CI]).[105] Nerve dysfunction, particularly persistent paresthesia or numbness, is relatively common (up to 19%) immediately after surgery, but the vast majority of these symptoms resolve within 4 weeks.[10,106] Warning signs that an injury may be particularly worrisome include complete absence of nerve function immediately after surgery (probably indicative of nerve transection or ischemia), motor deficit, worsening symptoms over time, or failure to show early signs of resolution. Particularly in these cases, early neurologic consultation is recommended to rule out reversible causes, establish bilateral baseline function, and coordinate further diagnostic workup and rehabilitation.[107]

Whether brachial plexus blocks should be attempted in anesthetized or heavily sedated patients is controversial. Especially with interscalene blocks, a series of case reports[108,109] clearly point to the risk for intramedullary injection with devastating consequences. As the approach moves away from the neck, the risk for spinal cord injury probably lessens, but the chance of unrecognized intraneural (specifically, intrafascicular) injection remains poorly quantified. Some peripheral nerve injuries have occurred in nonanesthetized patients without a preceding warning such as pain on injection or severe paresthesia, whereas other patients have noted these warnings and have still sustained injury. Yet another subset of patients has experienced pain on injection but no subsequent injury.[105,110,111] Until our understanding of peripheral nerve injury and premonitory symptoms becomes clearer, the American Society of Regional Anesthesia (ASRA) recommends that patients be given every opportunity to recognize potential injury by not routinely placing brachial plexus blocks in anesthetized patients.[112]

Clinicians must recognize that neither peripheral nerve stimulation nor ultrasound guidance consistently protects against nerve injury.[113] Peripheral nerve stimulation is neither sensitive nor specific for detecting subepineurial needle placement.[114-116] Indeed, with the supraclavicular approach, stimulation thresholds between 0.2 and 0.5 mA may indicate either extraneural or subepineurial needle placement.[114] There is no evidence that UGRA reduces the incidence of neural injury,[113,117,118] and there are reports of injury despite its use.[119-121]

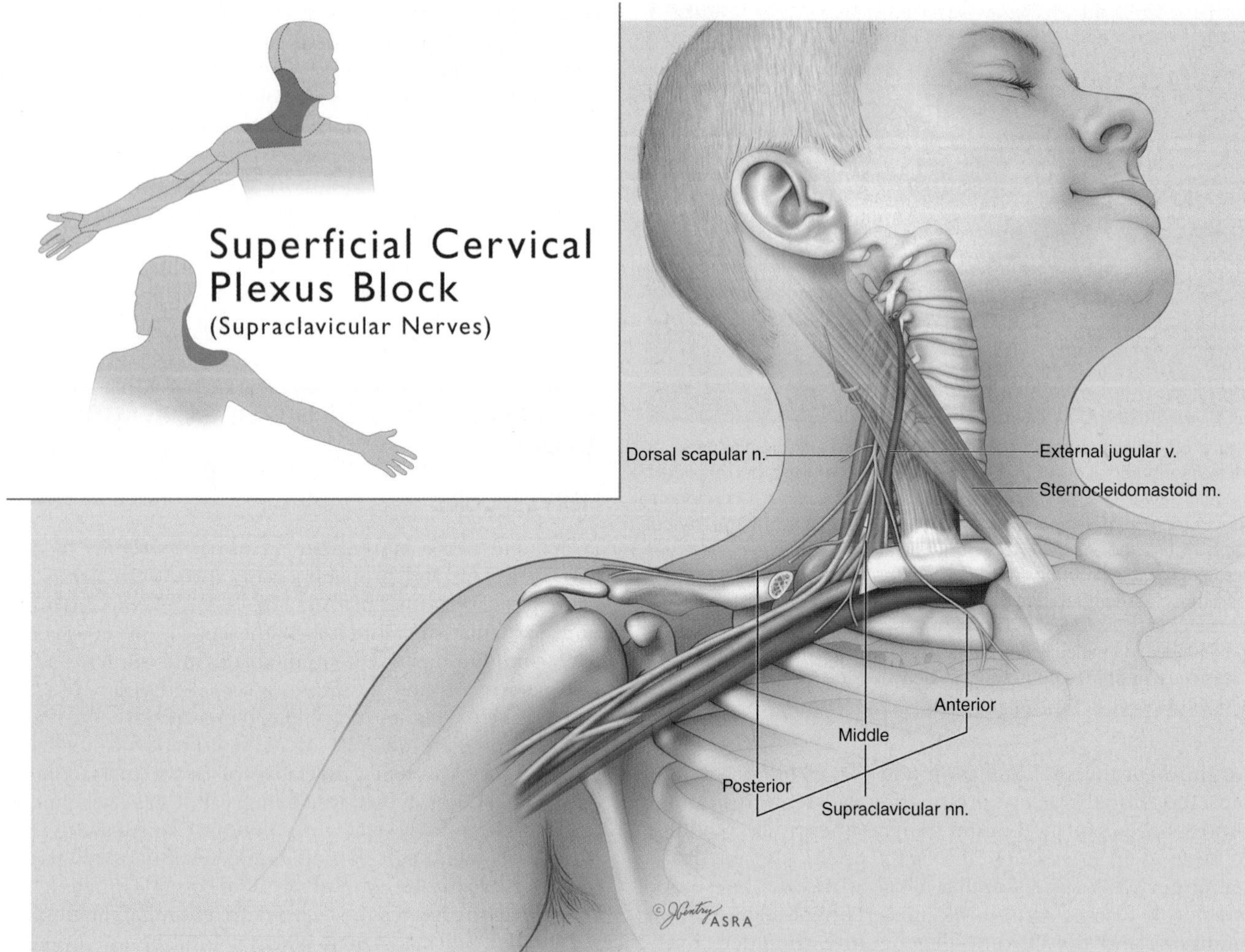

Figure 53.14 Superficial cervical plexus block. The inset illustrates the expected distribution of anesthetic with a superficial cervical plexus (supraclavicular nerve) block. The supraclavicular nerve supplies the cutaneous innervation to the cape of the shoulder. (©American Society of Regional Anesthesia and Pain Medicine and Jennifer Gentry. Used with permission. All rights reserved.[10])

Whether a brachial plexus block is contraindicated in patients with preexisting nerve injury is unclear. Patients who underwent ulnar nerve transposition were no more likely to sustain a postoperative exacerbation or new symptoms regardless of whether they received general anesthesia or a brachial plexus block.[122] In contrast to these reassuring data, postoperative dysfunction has developed in patients with preexisting nerve dysfunction, even of a subclinical nature.[123]

INTRAVASCULAR INJECTION

Brachial plexus blocks have a relatively low risk for delayed local anesthetic systemic toxicity (LAST) when compared with epidural or intercostal blocks, but there are no reliable data on which to base the maximum recommended doses of local anesthetic.[124] Furthermore, the risk for seizure secondary to intravascular injection is five times higher with peripheral nerve blocks than with epidural blocks.[105] This risk is particularly relevant to brachial plexus regional anesthesia because of the proximity of the vertebral, carotid, and subclavian (via retrograde flow) arteries to direct injection during placement of an interscalene or supraclavicular block.[125] Because upper extremity regional anesthesia typically uses volumes of local anesthetic that are capable of inducing severe systemic toxicity, it is recommended that practitioners be familiar with and have readily available the ASRA checklist for managing LAST.[126,127]

UNINTENDED DESTINATIONS OF LOCAL ANESTHETICS

Because the neck contains so many vital structures, it is common for local anesthetics intended for the brachial plexus to affect other structures. Most serious is when local anesthetic is unintentionally placed near the neuraxis and causes epidural or spinal anesthesia during attempted interscalene anesthesia. The C6 foramen is only 23 mm from the skin in the average patient,[128] so it is easy to conceive how excessively deep needle placement could result in this complication. Neuraxial injection of local anesthetic is manifested by the rapid (total spinal anesthesia) or delayed (massive epidural anesthesia) appearance of a bilateral upper and lower extremity block, which is often associated with hypotension, bradycardia, and apnea. This complication must be diagnosed and treated rapidly with airway control, volume

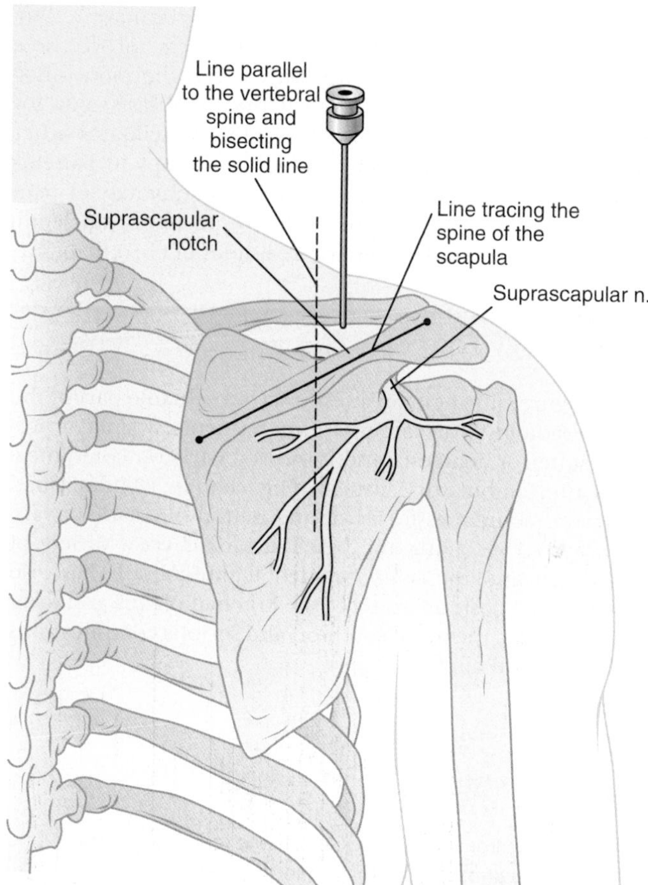

Figure 53.15 Suprascapular nerve block. A line is drawn along the scapular spine and then bisected by a second line parallel to the vertebral spine. The entry point is 2 to 3 cm into the upper outer quadrant. The needle is directed from the top to avoid entry deep into the suprascapular notch, which could pose a risk for pneumothorax. (Adapted from Rathmell JP, Neal JM, Viscomi CM. *Regional Anesthesia. The Requisites in Anesthesiology*. Philadelphia: Elsevier Mosby; 2004:69.)

expansion, and early provision of exogenous epinephrine to counteract blockade of the cardioaccelerator fibers and absent vascular tone.[10] An ultrasound-guided interscalene block and the modified lateral interscalene block use a more superficial approach to the brachial plexus. Though not proved in randomized trials, these approaches are theoretically less likely to result in neuraxial deposition of local anesthetic than the classic Winnie approach is.

Local anesthetics intended for the brachial plexus during blocks above the clavicle and infraclavicular blocks can also spread to the cervical sympathetic chain, where they cause Horner's syndrome. Another unintended effect is anesthesia of the recurrent laryngeal nerve, which results in hoarseness or difficulty swallowing. Both these nuisance side effects resolve in unison with resolution of the anesthetic block.[10]

HEMIDIAPHRAGMATIC PARESIS

Impairment of diaphragmatic function is common during above-the-clavicle approaches. Hemidiaphragmatic paresis (HDP) occurs in all patients who undergo an interscalene block via the traditional techniques, and about one in four of these patients will have a 25% to 32% reduction in spirometric measures of pulmonary function.[129] Ultrasound-guided interscalene blocks that use low volumes of local anesthetic (5 to 10 mL) result in a reduced incidence and severity of HDP, but the side effect still occurs unpredictably.[19,21,130,131] The incidence of HDP is less (95% CI = 14% to 86%) in patients undergoing a supraclavicular block. Although healthy volunteers experienced no diminution in pulmonary function during the supraclavicular approach, this may not hold true for patients with underlying pulmonary disease.[99] A low-volume supraclavicular block performed under ultrasound guidance reduces the incidence of HDP to almost 0.[132] Nevertheless, it is recommended that any patient unable to withstand a 25% or greater reduction in pulmonary function not be given an

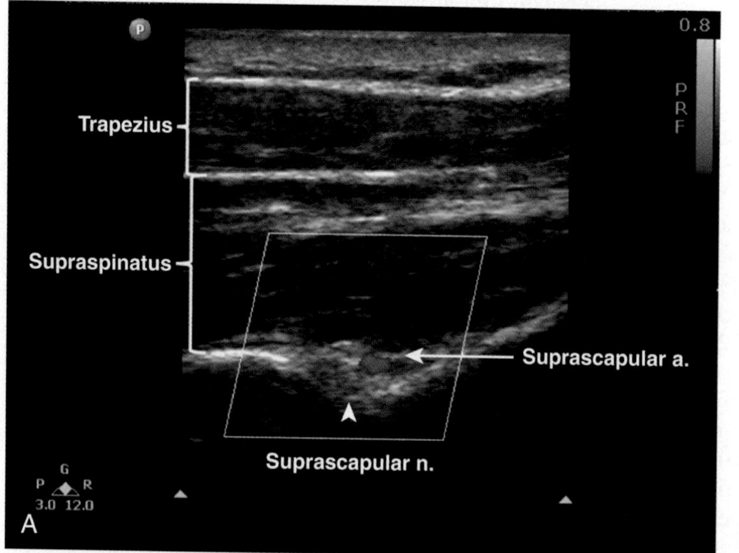

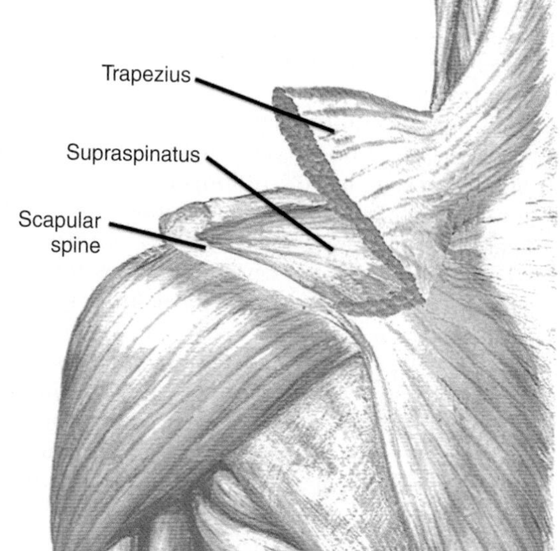

Figure 53.16 Ultrasound-guided suprascapular nerve block. **A,** The suprascapular nerve resides between the suprascapular notch and the spinoglenoid notch on the floor of the scapular fossa. The arrowhead indicates the suprascapular nerve and the arrow indicates the artery. **B,** Proper transducer position, which is in the short axis to a line that joins the coracoid process and the acromion. (Reproduced with permission from *Ultrasound for Regional Anesthesia*. Available at www.usra.ca).

above-the-clavicle brachial plexus block, even when using ultrasound guidance.

The incidence of HDP is lower with infraclavicular approaches and may be specific to the approach. For instance, in 26% of patients given a vertical infraclavicular block, reduced or paradoxical hemidiaphragmatic function developed along with an approximate 30% diminution in spirometric values.[133] Conversely, no ventilatory dysfunction was observed with the more distal coracoid approach.[134] HDP during continuous perineural infusion appears to lessen over time. In a study of patient-controlled perineural interscalene catheter analgesia with 0.2% ropivacaine, diaphragmatic function and spirometric values were no different from those observed in patients randomized to receive opioid patient-controlled analgesia.[135]

PNEUMOTHORAX

The incidence of pneumothorax associated with a supraclavicular block has probably decreased with the advent of techniques such as the plumb bob and ultrasound-guided approaches, which avoid needle contact with the pleural dome. Nevertheless, there remains a small (<1%) but poorly defined risk for pneumothorax with the supraclavicular and inter-SCM approaches. Even though extremely rare, pneumothorax has been reported with the interscalene and coracoid infraclavicular approaches. There are reports of pneumothorax despite the use of ultrasound guidance.[136,137] Clinicians should recognize that the symptoms of pneumothorax are typically delayed 6 to 12 hours after initial needle puncture and are more likely to consist of pleuritic chest pain than dyspnea.[10]

PERIPHERAL NERVE BLOCKS FOR CHRONIC PAIN MANAGEMENT

Peripheral nerve blocks are usually performed for diagnostic, prognostic, and therapeutic reasons in chronic pain management. A block may help in confirming the etiology and pathway of the patient's pain, for example, a suprascapular nerve block for relief of frozen shoulder. Prognostically, it may predict the efficacy of more definitive procedures, such as pulsed radiofrequency ablation of the nerve. Interestingly, the duration of pain relief may outlast the duration of nerve blockade by 50% or longer.[138]

In a review of the published literature by Vlassakov and colleagues, single-injection peripheral nerve blocks with local anesthetic alone at certain locations resulted in pain relief durations of longer than 1 week. In fact, some patients experienced relief for 1 to 3 weeks, 7 to 13 months, and 2 to 4 years.[138] In pain practice, a series of blocks are usually performed every 1 to 3 weeks. It is common for the pain physician to add steroid to the local anesthetic solution (4 mg dexamethasone or 40 mg methylprednisolone/triamcinolone per 30 mL local anesthetic) to reduce inflammation in the nerve. Topical application of steroid on a peripheral nerve has also been shown to suppress nociceptive impulses by blocking the motor and sensory fibers.[139] The lasting effect of local anesthetic blocks has been attributed to "interruption of the vicious cycle of pain." Another explanation is elimination of maintenance of central sensitization in neuropathic pain conditions (most neuralgias have a neuropathic pain component).[140] It is difficult to prove these theories despite the frequency with which the pain physician sees these responses. Even if the relief lasts only for the duration of the block, such numbness facilitates other therapeutic modalities such as physical therapy in patients with complex regional pain syndrome or myofascial pain syndrome. Nerve blocks are therefore an important component of the multidisciplinary treatment of chronic pain.

SUMMARY

Upper extremity regional anesthesia is a valuable part of the anesthesiologist's armamentarium, particularly since it provides superior analgesia and improved early outcome measures after ambulatory surgery. This chapter has described common techniques for achieving neural blockade at various approaches along the brachial plexus via a variety of traditional and ultrasound-guided techniques. It has also reviewed the basic anatomy of the brachial plexus and drug selection, plus the more common and serious complications of these useful blocks.

KEY POINTS

- Upper extremity regional anesthetic techniques can improve analgesia in the immediate postoperative period, reduce opioid-related side effects, improve patient satisfaction, and reduce unplanned hospital admissions. Single-injection brachial plexus blockade does not affect outcome measures beyond the first 24 hours.
- The functional anatomy of the upper extremity is variable. Relying on a single cutaneous distribution to plan which nerve requires blockade or to assess the adequacy of anesthesia is unreliable.
- The primary determinant in selecting a local anesthetic for an upper extremity block is anesthetic or analgesic duration. Epinephrine, clonidine, dexamethasone, and buprenorphine extend the duration of intermediate-acting local anesthetics, but not long-acting ones.
- As one proceeds distally along the brachial plexus when using traditional techniques, multiple-injection techniques improve block success. Ultrasound-guided blocks tend to involve multiple injections. There is no evidence that any regional anesthetic technique—paresthesia, peripheral nerve stimulation, perivascular, ultrasound, or transarterial—is inherently more effective or safer than another.
- Shoulder surgery is best accomplished with an interscalene block; arm or hand surgery is amenable to an infraclavicular block; and arm surgery, including the elbow and areas distal, is a classic indication for an axillary block. A supraclavicular block is most likely to anesthetize the entire upper extremity, although it will occasionally not anesthetize the supraclavicular or ulnar nerves.

KEY POINTS—cont'd

- Accessory blocks are valuable for surgeries that involve a cutaneous sensory distribution outside the brachial plexus. A supraclavicular (superficial cervical plexus) nerve block anesthetizes the cape distribution around the shoulder, and a suprascapular block adds value to general anesthesia for shoulder arthroscopy or for pain management indications.
- Continuous perineural catheter techniques provide analgesia superior to that achieved with placebo or opioid techniques. Data are as yet insufficient to show meaningful improvement in other outcomes such as rehabilitation or earlier return to work.
- Permanent anesthesia-related nerve injury after a brachial plexus block is distinctly rare. Particularly when using the interscalene approach, it is recommended that placing these blocks in anesthetized or heavily sedated patients be avoided.
- Local anesthetic systemic toxicity is relatively common with brachial plexus regional anesthesia, at least in part because of unintentional injection into arteries that directly supply the brain.
- Anesthesiologists must be vigilant for the rare complication of neuraxial anesthesia during the course of an interscalene brachial plexus block. Signs and symptoms of high spinal or massive epidural anesthesia require prompt airway control and aggressive treatment of hypotension and bradycardia with potent α-adrenergic agonists such as epinephrine.
- Above-the-clavicle blocks are not recommended in patients who are unable to withstand a 25% to 30% reduction in pulmonary function.
- Selected upper extremity blocks have a diagnostic, therapeutic, and prognostic role in chronic pain management.

SUGGESTED READINGS

Bigeleisen PE, Moayeri N, Groen GJ. Extraneural versus intraneural stimulation thresholds during ultrasound-guided supraclavicular block. *Anesthesiology*. 2009;110:1235-1243.

Chan VW, Perlas A, Rawson R, et al. Ultrasound-guided supraclavicular brachial plexus block. *Anesth Analg*. 2003;97:1514-1517.

Handoll HHG, Koscielniak-Nielsen ZJ. Single, double or multiple injection techniques for axillary brachial plexus block for hand, wrist or forearm surgery. *Cochrane Database Syst Rev*. 2006;1:CD003842.

Ilfeld BM. Continuous peripheral nerve blocks in the hospital and at home. *Anesthesiol Clin*. 2011;29:193-211.

Mariano ER, Sandu NS, Loland VJ, et al. A randomized comparison of infraclavicular and supraclavicular continuous peripheral nerve blocks for postoperative analgesia. *Reg Anesth Pain Med*. 2011;36:26-31.

McCartney CJ, Xu D, Constantinescu C, et al. Ultrasound examination of peripheral nerves in the forearm. *Reg Anesth Pain Med*. 2007;32:434-439.

Neal JM, Gerancher JC, Hebl JR, et al. Upper extremity regional anesthesia: essentials of our current understanding, 2008. *Reg Anesth Pain Med*. 2009;34:134-170.

Neal JM, Bernards CM, Butterworth JF, et al. ASRA practice advisory on local anesthetic systemic toxicity. *Reg Anesth Pain Med*. 2010;35:152-161.

Renes SH, Rettig HC, Gielen MJ, et al. Ultrasound-guided low-dose interscalene brachial plexus block reduces the incidence of hemidiaphragmatic paresis. *Reg Anesth Pain Med*. 2009;34:498-502.

Tran de QH, Bertini P, Zaouter C, et al. A prospective, randomized comparison between single- and double-injection ultrasound-guided infraclavicular brachial plexus block. *Reg Anesth Pain Med*. 2010;35:16-21.

Tran de QH, Dugani S, Correa JA, et al. Minimum effective volume of lidocaine for ultrasound-guided supraclavicular block. *Reg Anesth Pain Med*. 2011;36:466-469.

Tran de QH, Pham K, Dugani S, et al. A prospective, randomized comparison between double-, triple-, and quadruple-injection ultrasound-guided axillary brachial plexus block. *Reg Anesth Pain Med*. 2012;37:248-253.

The references for this chapter can be found at www.expertconsult.com.

54 Lower Extremity Nerve Blocks

Uma Shastri | Kwesi Kwofie | Emine Aysu Salviz | Daquan Xu | Admir Hadzic

INTRODUCTION

Lower extremity blocks (LEBs) are common techniques for surgical anesthesia and postoperative analgesia. They are being used more frequently in the setting of outpatient surgery worldwide because of their favorable recovery and side effect profile when compared with general and neuraxial anesthesia.[1-3] LEBs may decrease the incidence of postoperative pain syndromes, including chronic postamputation phantom limb pain.[4,5] In addition to surgical applications, LEBs have also been reported to be beneficial in patients with complex regional pain syndrome, chronic cancer pain, peripheral vascular diseases (ischemia, Reynaud's disease, peripheral embolism), intractable phantom limb pain, and spasticity.[6-9] Continuous LEBs with perineural catheters can also provide analgesia for an extended period.[6,10] Moreover, neurolysis of lower extremity peripheral nerves can also be performed with techniques analogous to peripheral nerve blockade.[11,12]

Ultrasound-guided techniques are becoming more prevalent methods of performing LEBs in many centers. Several reports have suggested that ultrasound guidance results in more precise needle and catheter placement during LEBs than do blocks performed with nerve stimulator or landmark techniques only or with both.[13]

This chapter provides an overview of the relevant anatomy of the lower extremity, technical aspects of performing LEBs, and common indications for their use in clinical practice.

ANATOMY

Innervation of the lower extremity is derived from both the lumbar plexus and the sacral plexus, sometimes referred as the lumbosacral plexus.

LUMBAR PLEXUS

The lumbar plexus is made up of the L1 through L5 spinal nerve roots. As the L2, L3, and L4 roots of the lumbar plexus depart from their spinal nerves and emerge from the intervertebral foramen, they enter the posterior third of the psoas muscle.[14] Once in the muscle, these roots then become organized into anterior and posterior divisions. The divisions reunite to form the iliohypogastric, ilioinguinal, genitofemoral, lateral femoral cutaneous, femoral, and obturator nerves[15] (Fig. 54.1). The most significant nerves in the lower extremity are the femoral, lateral femoral cutaneous, and obturator nerves.

The *femoral nerve* is formed by the posterior divisions of L2-4. The nerve descends from the plexus lateral to the psoas muscle. The femoral nerve innervates the rectus femoris, vastus medialis, vastus intermedius, and vastus lateralis muscles. It also provides cutaneous sensory innervation to much of the anterior and medial aspects of the thigh, as well as the medial part of the leg distal to the knee (Fig. 54.2).

The *lateral femoral cutaneous nerve* is formed from the L2 and L3 nerve roots and, as its name indicates, is a cutaneous, sensory nerve. It provides sensation to the lateral aspect of the thigh (see Fig. 54.2).

The *obturator nerve* (L2-4) provides sensory innervation to a variable portion of the leg proximal to the knee, as well as motor innervation to the adductor muscles (see Fig. 54.2).

The *iliohypogastric* and *ilioinguinal nerves* are primarily sensory nerves that arise from L1 and supply innervation to the skin of the suprapubic and inguinal regions.

The *genitofemoral nerve* arises from the L1 and L2 roots and supplies motor innervation to the cremasteric muscle and additional sensory innervation to the inguinal area.

SACRAL PLEXUS

The sacral plexus is formed from the L4-S3 nerve roots (Fig. 54.3). It is shaped like a triangle pointing toward the sciatic notch, with its base spanning across the anterior sacral foramina. The roots of the sacral plexus lie on the anterior surface of the lateral sacrum and form the sciatic nerve on the ventral surface of the piriformis muscle.[16] The sacral plexus gives rise to one major nerve and six collateral nerve branches. The sciatic nerve exits the pelvis through the greater sciatic notch and then descends between the greater trochanter of the femur and the ischial tuberosity. It runs along the posterior part of the thigh to the lower third of the femur, where it diverges into two divisions: the tibial and common peroneal. The sciatic nerve provides motor and sensory innervation to the hamstring muscles and the entire leg below the knee with the exception of the cutaneous region medially, which is innervated by the saphenous nerve (see Fig. 54.2). The posterior cutaneous nerve of the thigh exits the pelvis with the sciatic nerve but then diverges posteriorly to become a cutaneous nerve that is the major sensory nerve from the sacral plexus within the thigh.[17]

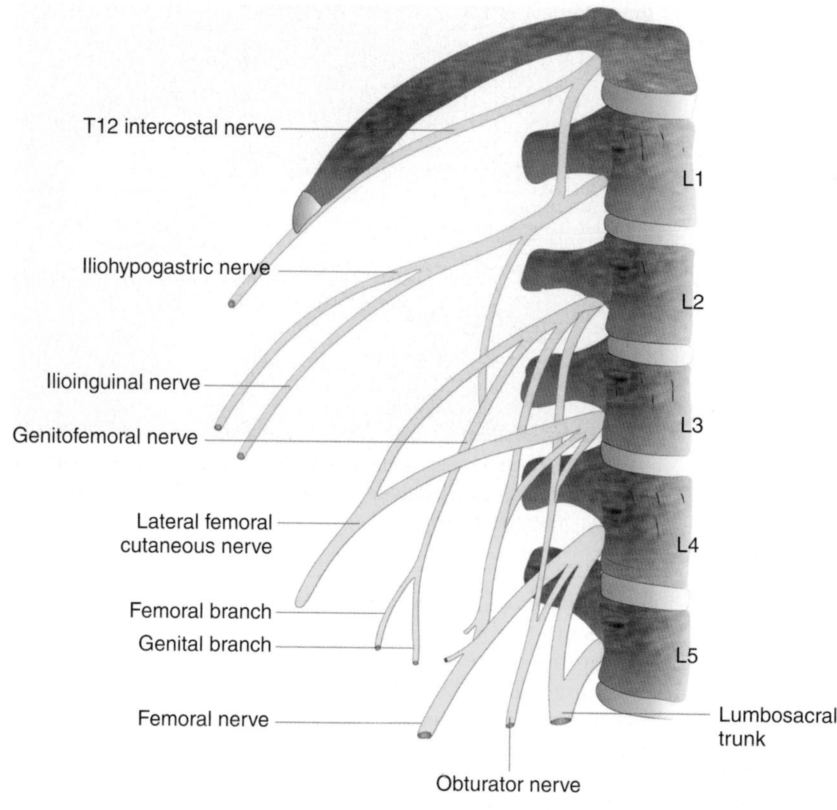

Figure 54.1 Schematic representation of the lumbar plexus and its branches. (From Hadzic A, ed. *Hadzic's Peripheral Nerve Blocks and Anatomy for Ultrasound-Guided Regional Anesthesia*. 2nd ed. New York: McGraw-Hill: 2012. Used by permission.)

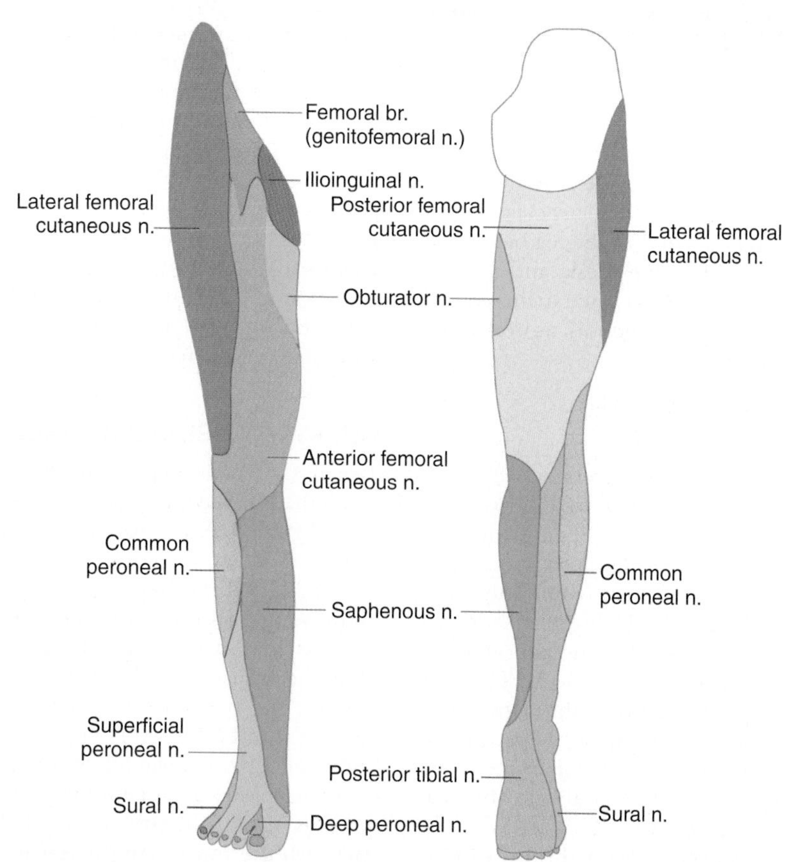

Figure 54.2 Schematic representation of the sensory distribution in the lower extremity.

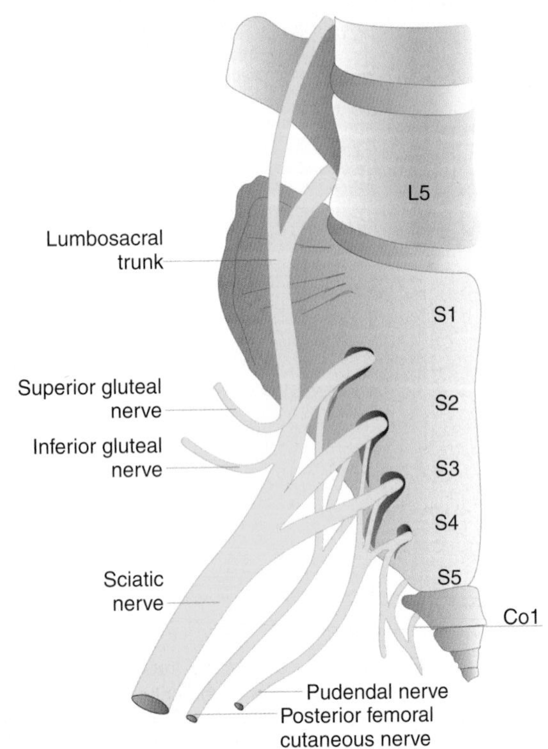

Figure 54.3 Schematic representation of the sacral plexus and its branches. (From Hadzic A, ed. *Hadzic's Peripheral Nerve Blocks and Anatomy for Ultrasound-Guided Regional Anesthesia*. 2nd ed. New York: McGraw-Hill: 2012. Used by permission.)

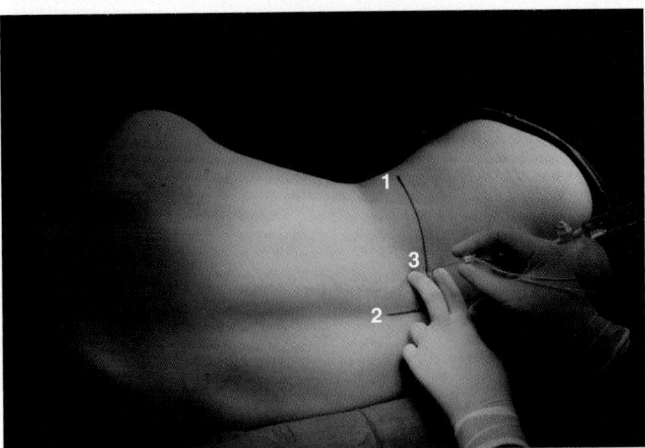

Figure 54.4 Anatomic landmarks with the needle insertion site for a lumbar plexus block include (1) the iliac crest, (2) the midline, and (3) 4 cm from the midline.

NERVE BLOCK TECHNIQUES

LUMBAR PLEXUS BLOCK

CLINICAL APPLICATIONS

A lumbar plexus block (LPB) can provide anesthesia or analgesia to the anterolateral and medial aspects of the thigh, the knee, and the medial portion of the leg below the knee. Common indications include anesthesia and analgesia following total hip arthroplasty, total knee arthroplasty, and anterior cruciate ligament reconstruction, as well as for treatment of chronic hip pain.[18-23]

NERVE STIMULATOR– AND SURFACE-BASED TECHNIQUES

An LPB is a deep block and the needle traverses several layers of structures, including (from posterior to anterior) the posterior lumbar fascia, paraspinous muscle, anterior lumbar fascia, quadratus lumborum muscle, and psoas muscle.[17]

Nerve stimulation is probably the most commonly used method to localize the lumbar plexus during blockade. To perform the block, the patient is placed in the lateral decubitus position with the operative side up (Fig. 54.4). The foot on the side to be blocked is positioned over the dependent leg so that the motor response of the quadriceps muscle can easily be seen. The two surface anatomic landmarks for determining the insertion point for the needle are the iliac crest and the midline spinous processes.

The top of the iliac crest correlates with the L3-4 interspace in most patients.[24] The point 3 to 3.5 cm lateral to the intersection of the iliac crest and the midline spinous processes marks the needle insertion site (see Fig. 54.4). After setting the nerve stimulator to an initial current of 1.5 mA (0.1 msec, 2 Hz) and skin preparation, a 4-inch insulated needle is advanced in a posterior-to-anterior manner. As the needle is advanced, local contractions of the paravertebral muscles are commonly elicited and indicate that placement of the needle is too shallow. The needle is advanced further until the transverse process is encountered. Contact with the transverse process is not routinely sought, but when present, it provides a consistent landmark. After contact with the transverse process, the needle is redirected cephalad or caudad and advanced approximately 2 cm beyond the transverse process. Starting from the level of the skin, the lumbar plexus is located between 6.1 and 10.1 cm in men and 5.7 and 9.3 cm in women.[25]

Once a quadriceps muscle–evoked response is obtained between 0.5 and 1.0 mA, 20 to 35 mL of local anesthetic is injected slowly, with frequent aspiration between injection aliquots. Unintentional deep placement of the needle carries a risk for injury to internal organs, such as renal hematoma.[26] Epidural spread of local anesthetic has been reported to occur in as many as 16% to 27% of blocks.[17] Limiting the force of injection decreases the risk for epidural spead.[27]

ULTRASOUND-GUIDED TECHNIQUES

Because of the deep location of the plexus, ultrasound-guided LPBs have not become as rapidly adopted as ultrasound-guided blocks of more peripheral sites. To obtain adequate views, a low-frequency (4 to 8 MHz) curvilinear probe is used. Perhaps the most common approach is an ultrasound-assisted technique in which the scanning is performed in the parasagittal axis. After preparation of the skin and transducer, the transverse processes are identified first on the parasagittal axis (Fig. 54.5). Starting from the sacrum, the L5 transverse process is identified. Continuing the scan cephalad will allow visualization of the other transverse processes in ascending order.[28] Once the transverse process of L3 is identified, the needle is inserted until contact with the transverse process and then "walked off" until contractions of the quadriceps muscle are elicited. The rest

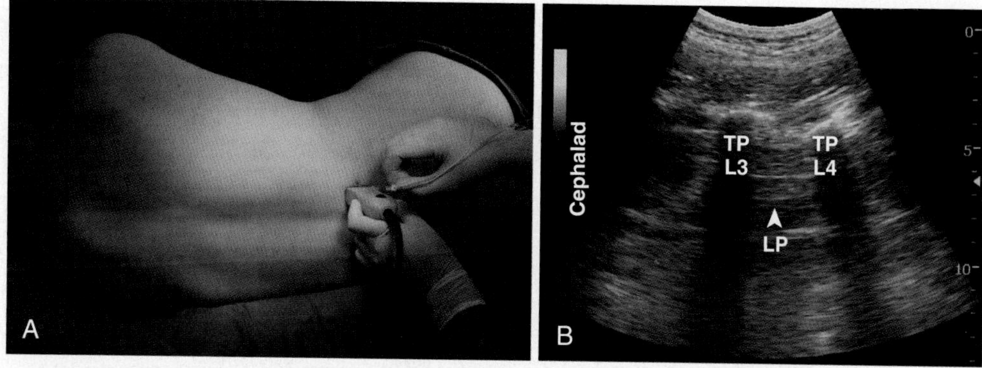

Figure 54.5 **A,** Ultrasound-guided lumbar plexus block with parasagittal transducer placement and an out-of-plane needle approach. **B,** Ultrasonography is used to guide the needle between the transverse processes (TP) and advanced to a point 1 to 2 cm deep to the level of the transverse processes to elicit stimulation of the lumbar plexus (LP).

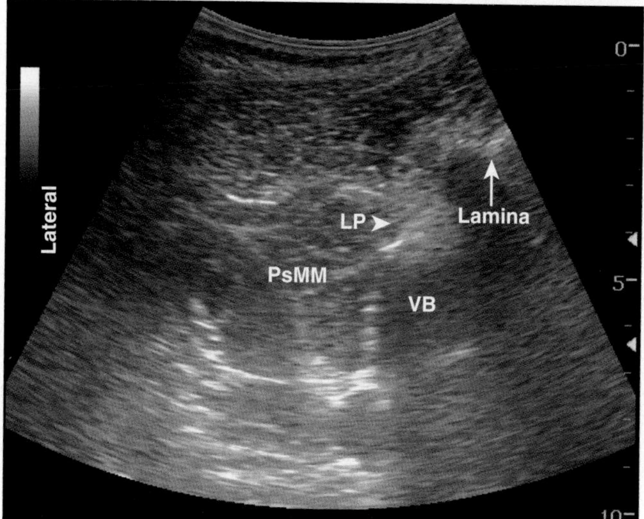

Figure 54.6 Ultrasound image with a transverse oblique view of the lumbar plexus (LP) within the posterior third of the psoas major muscle (PsMM). The vertebral body (VB) and vertebral lamina are medial to the plexus. Ultrasound is used to guide the needle to the LP in an in-plane approach.

of the injection procedure is similar to the nerve stimulator–guided technique.

More recently, a transverse oblique technique has been suggested in which the stimulating needle is directed into the posteromedial aspect of the psoas muscle.[29] With this technique the roots of the lumbar plexus may be seen exiting through the intervertebral foramen (Fig. 54.6).[30-32] The needle is advanced in plane, and its position is routinely monitored by nerve stimulation.

COMPLICATIONS

Complications associated with LPB fall into one of three categories: (1) systemic toxicity of local anesthetics, (2) neuraxial spread, and (3) needle misadventures.[33,34] Epidural spread of the local anesthetic, total spinal anesthesia, and circulatory collapse have been reported.[35-37] Care should be taken to avoid major vascular structures and the lower pole of the kidney because cases of subcapsular renal hematoma have been reported.[26,38-41] The reported cases of delayed retroperitoneal hematoma after LPB in the absence of anticoagulation underscore the need for caution in patients treated with anticoagulants. Although there are no clear guidelines on the safety of LPB in the presence of anticoagulation,[42-44] it is prudent to consider alternative anesthetic plans for patients with known coagulopathy.

LATERAL FEMORAL CUTANEOUS NERVE BLOCK

CLINICAL APPLICATIONS

Blockade of lateral femoral cutaneous nerve (LFCN) is indicated for anesthesia or analgesia of the anterolateral aspect of the thigh, as well as for the diagnosis and treatment of meralgia paresthetica.[45-47]

ANATOMY

The LFCN is typically blocked 1 to 2 cm medial and inferior to the anterior superior iliac spine (ASIS). At this location the nerve lies beneath the fascia iliaca, just lateral to the sartorius muscle and medial to the tensor fasciae latae muscle (TFLM).

NERVE STIMULATOR– AND SURFACE-BASED TECHNIQUES

Surface-based techniques yield variable success rates because of the anatomic variability of the LFCN.[48] Electrical nerve stimulation can be used to elicit paresthesia in the sensory distribution of the nerve to increase the chance of success. With either technique, the needle is inserted 1 to 2 cm medial and inferior to the ASIS and advanced until loss of resistance is felt as the needle penetrates the fascia iliaca.[49] When the technique is aided by nerve stimulation, current intensity is set to 1.0 to 2.0 mA with a pulse duration of 1.0 msec for greater sensitivity.

ULTRASOUND-GUIDED TECHNIQUE

After preparation of the skin and transducer, a high-frequency linear probe is placed inferior to the ASIS, parallel to the inguinal ligament, to identify the sartorius and TFLM first.[50] The LFCN is visualized as a small oval hypoechoic structure beneath the fascia iliaca, just lateral to the sartorius muscle, and medial to the TFLM (Fig. 54.7). A 2-inch, 22-gauge needle is used to approach the nerve, typically in an in-plane technique, and 5 to 10 mL of the local anesthetic of choice is injected.

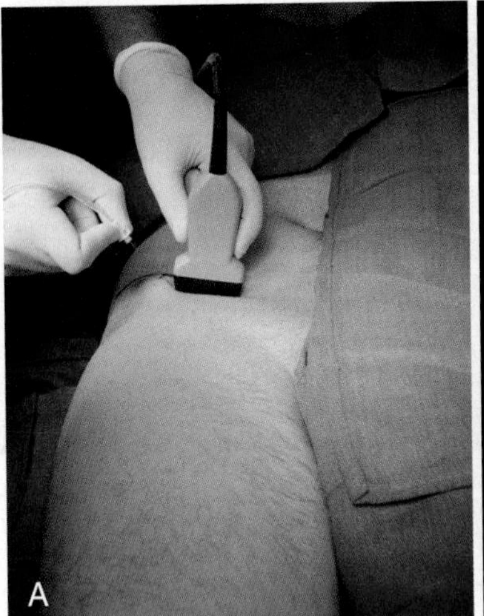

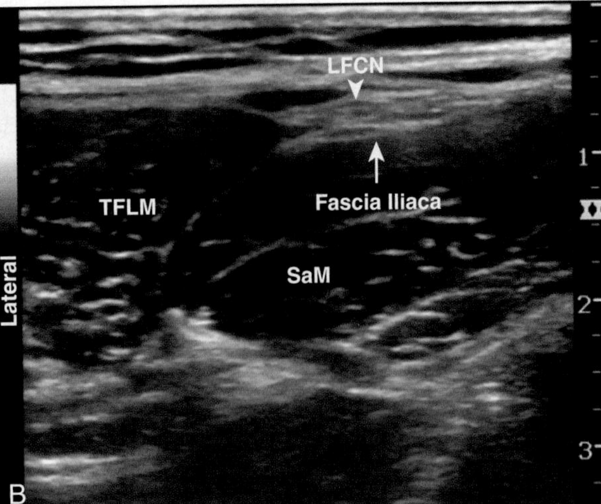

Figure 54.7 **A,** Position of the transducer and needle insertion for a lateral femoral cutaneous nerve (LFCN) block. **B,** Ultrasound image demonstrating the LFCN, tensor fasciae latae muscle (TFLM), sartorius muscle (SaM), and fascia iliaca.

COMPLICATIONS

Because no large vascular structures or other organs are nearby, an LFCN block is associated with a low risk for complications.

FEMORAL NERVE BLOCK

CLINICAL APPLICATIONS

A femoral block is one of the most commonly used peripheral nerve block techniques in clinical practice. It is often used for anesthesia or postoperative analgesia (or both) in patients undergoing surgery on the anterior aspect of the thigh and the knee, quadriceps tendon repair, and femoral surgery. A continuous femoral nerve block has become a mainstay analgesic technique in patients after knee arthroplasty.[51] It has also been reported to be used for palliative care, and in such cases an indwelling catheter can be left in situ for up to several weeks.[10]

ANATOMY

The femoral nerve arises from the L2-4 roots of the lumbar plexus. The nerve travels through the psoas muscle and ends on the anterior surface of the iliopsoas as it passes under the inguinal ligament. At this level the nerve lies beneath the fascia iliaca and lateral to the femoral artery (Fig. 54.8). A femoral nerve block provides sensory anesthesia to the anterior aspect of the thigh, the knee, and the medial portion of the calf and ankle.

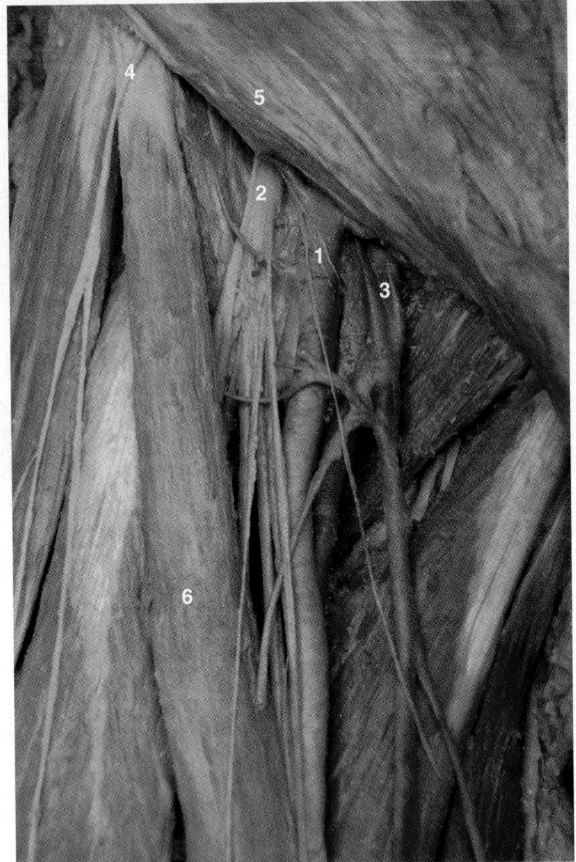

Figure 54.8 Cadaveric dissection at the inguinal crease. 1, Femoral artery; 2, femoral nerve; 3, femoral vein; 4, lateral femoral cutaneous nerve; 5, inguinal ligament; 6, sartorius muscle.

TECHNIQUE

Nerve Stimulator– and Surface-Based Techniques

After skin preparation, the needle is introduced in a sagittal, slightly cephalad plane immediately lateral to the femoral artery at the femoral crease to obtain a femoral nerve response (quadriceps twitch). If a sartorius muscle twitch is obtained first (twitch of the medial aspect of the thigh with no patellar movement), the needle is advanced deeper and more lateral to ensure that the needle is positioned closer to the main trunk of the femoral nerve.[52] A recent report suggests that injection of local anesthetic after obtaining a sartorius motor response results in a successful femoral nerve block.[53] However, a sartorius response can also take place when a sartorius branch is stimulated remotely from the main trunk of the femoral nerve, particularly in patients with less than ideal anatomy (e.g., obese). Once a quadriceps muscle twitch at a current of 0.2 to 0.5 mA is elicited, 10 to 15 mL of local anesthetic is injected to accomplish the block.

Ultrasound-Guided Techniques

A high-frequency linear transducer (8 to 14 MHz) is used in most patients. After preparation of the skin and transducer,

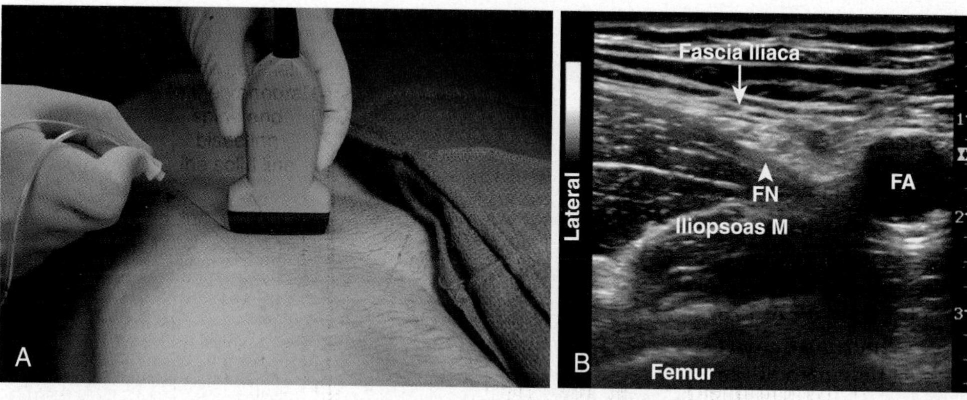

Figure 54.9 Ultrasound-guided femoral nerve block. **A,** The ultrasound probe is placed about the inguinal ligament. An in-plane needle approach (as shown) or out-of-plane approach can be used. **B,** Within the ultrasound view the femoral artery (FA), fascia iliaca, and femoral nerve (FN) are identified.

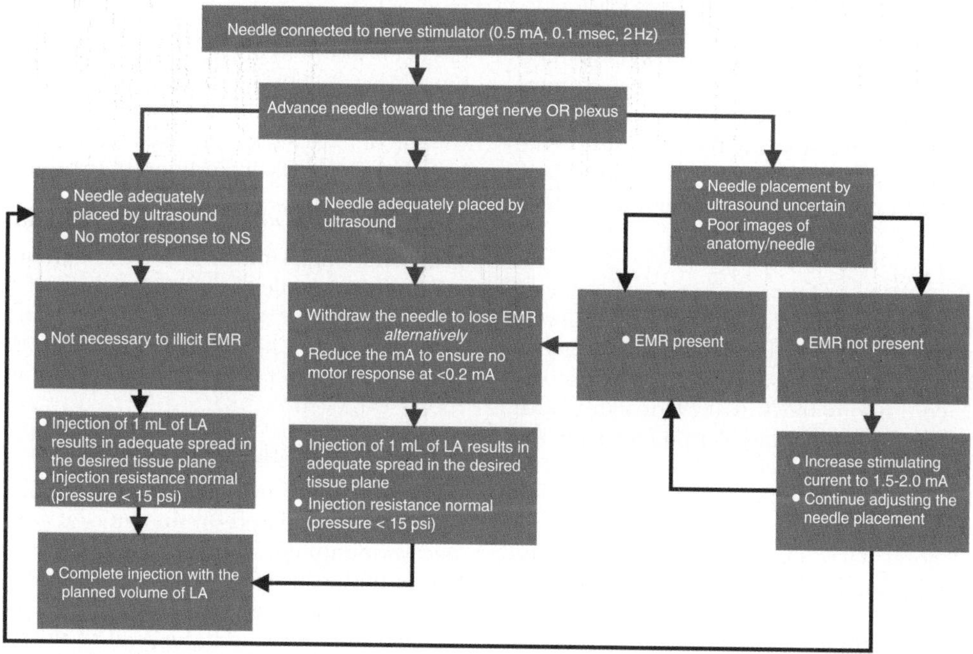

Figure 54.10 Algorithm for combining monitoring modalities during ultrasound-guided femoral nerve block.

the transducer is placed parallel to the inguinal crease to identify the femoral artery and vein. The nerve is imaged just lateral to the femoral artery on the surface of the iliacus muscle, underneath iliacus fascia (Fig. 54.9). A 4-inch nerve block needle can be inserted in an in-plane or out-of-plane fashion, the former being favored by many clinicians. The needle is advanced underneath the iliacus fascia to allow spread of the local anesthetic around the femoral nerve. When adequate needle-nerve imaging is present, it is not necessary to elicit a motor response. However, when a motor response is elicited, the current is reduced to ensure that the response is not present below 0.2 mA because a motor response to a very low current intensity may indicate intraneural placement of the needle. Injection underneath the fascia iliaca (perineural) should not result in significant resistance to the injection. A monitoring algorithm combining nerve stimulation with ultrasound guidance for a femoral nerve block, as well as most other peripheral major nerve blocks, is outlined in Figure 54.10.

CONTINUOUS FEMORAL NERVE BLOCK

A continuous femoral nerve block is similar to the single-shot technique except that a larger-gauge needle is used to allow insertion of the catheter.[54,55] Once the tip of the needle is deemed to be in the correct position, the catheter is inserted through the needle approximately 3 cm beyond the tip. After an initial bolus of local anesthetic, a continuous infusion is started at a rate of 5 mL/hr, typically with a patient-controlled bolus of 5 mL/hr. Ultrasound imaging can be used to confirm proper spread of local anesthetic underneath the fascia iliaca in the vicinity of the femoral nerve.

A continuous femoral nerve block is used to provide postoperative analgesia after knee surgery, and catheters may be left in situ for several days.[51] Perineural infusion for up to several weeks has also been reported to be useful in palliative care.[10]

THREE-IN-ONE BLOCK

A 3-in-1 block refers to a modification of the standard femoral block in which a larger volume of local anesthetic is

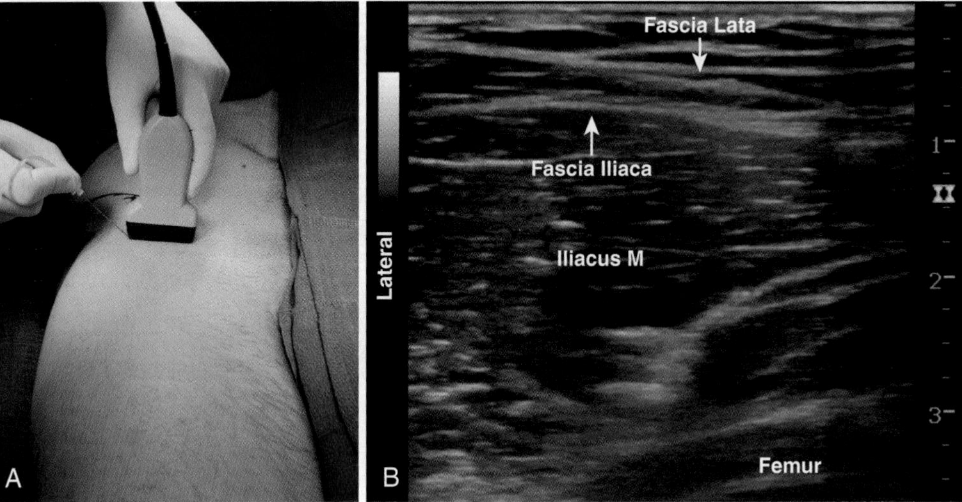

Figure 54.11 A, Ultrasound-guided fascia iliaca block with probe placement and in-plane needle approach. **B,** Ultrasound image demonstrating the fascia iliaca between the fascia lata and the iliacus muscle.

injected, with pressure being held distal to the needle injection site. Although this technique is still used in clinical practice, several studies have failed to document reliable spread of the local anesthetic.[56] Usually, the obturator nerve is not blocked with this technique. Technically, a 3-in-1 block is essentially the same as a large-volume femoral block or fascia iliaca block.

COMPLICATIONS

Complications of a femoral nerve block include injury to the nerve itself, vascular injury, and loss of muscle strength. The incidence of transient adverse neurologic symptoms associated with a continuous block is 0.4% to 0.5% with femoral catheters.[51,57] The rate of vascular puncture during placement of a femoral nerve block has been reported to be as high as 5.6%, but this rate may be decreased with the use of ultrasound.[58] Femoral neuropathy secondary to compression of the femoral nerve by a retroperitoneal hematoma has also been documented.[57] Quadriceps weakness in patients with femoral nerve blocks may lead to falls, which can cause significant morbidity. The frequency of falls in these patients may have been underreported.[59,60]

The incidence of bacterial colonization associated with continuous femoral nerve blocks was evaluated in 208 patients.[58] Fifty-seven percent were found to have positive bacterial colonization of the catheter 48 hours postoperatively. Three patients had transient symptoms of bacteremia that resolved with removal of the catheter, but there was no report of long-term infectious complications.[61] Two case reports of a psoas abscess requiring drainage and intravenous antibiotic therapy after a continuous femoral nerve block have been described,[62,63] but there are no case reports of infection after a femoral nerve block performed with a single injection.

FASCIA ILIACA BLOCK

A fascia iliaca block is an alternative approach to a femoral nerve block in which local anesthetic is injected underneath the fascia iliaca at a distance from the femoral nerve. The rationale is that because the femoral nerve and LFCN both lie deep to the iliacus fascia, a sufficient volume of local anesthetic deposited beneath the fascia iliaca will spread underneath the fascia and reach these nerves. Ultrasound has been shown to improve the success rate of a fascia iliaca block over the landmark-only approach.[64] Functionally, the technique is similar to a femoral block except that the large volume of local anesthetic used has a greater chance of also blocking the LFCN in addition to the femoral nerve.

SURFACE ANATOMY–BASED TECHNIQUE

The traditional landmark-based technique involves placement of the needle at the lateral third of the distance from the ASIS and the pubic tubercle by using a "double-pop" technique as the needle passes through the fascia lata and fascia iliaca. Block success can be sporadic because false "pops" can occur.

ULTRASOUND-GUIDED TECHNIQUE

With the patient in the supine position, a high-frequency linear probe is placed on the femoral crease and the fascia iliaca is identified. The probe is then moved to the medial border of the sartorius muscle (Fig. 54.11). At this position a 4-inch 22-gauge needle is inserted in an in-plane approach, the fascia is pierced, and the local anesthetic is placed below the fascia iliaca, above the iliopsoas muscle (see Fig. 54.11). If infiltration is observed within the muscle, the needle should be withdrawn slightly. Proper injection will result in separation of the fascia iliaca from the muscle in a medial-to-lateral direction.

SAPHENOUS NERVE BLOCK

Techniques for saphenous nerve blockade include the perifemoral, trans-sartorial, below-the-knee field block, and above-the-medial-malleolus approaches.[65] The perifemoral approach may be associated with weakness of the quadriceps muscles. The trans-sartorial approach may be most effective in blocking the saphenous nerve. However, use of the landmark-based technique for the trans-sartorial approach may result in inconsistent results because deposition of local anesthetic into the trans-sartorial canal cannot be monitored with ultrasound.

ULTRASOUND-GUIDED SAPHENOUS NERVE BLOCK

Several different approaches to ultrasound-guided saphenous nerve block have been described.[66] Most techniques involve placement of the transducer proximal to the knee joint. Typically, the sartorius muscle is visualized in relation to the vastus medialis and gracilis muscles, and local anesthetic is injected anterolateral to the femoral artery. Five to 10 mL of local anesthetic is injected. An advantage of the subsartorial technique is that blockade of the motor branches for the entire quadriceps muscle may be avoided.

SCIATIC NERVE BLOCK

CLINICAL APPLICATIONS

The primary indications for sciatic nerve blockade are for foot and ankle surgery. A sciatic nerve block can also be combined with a femoral nerve block to provide analgesia after knee surgery, amputation, or tibial osteotomy. Along with a lumbar plexus block or a femoral block, a sciatic block can also provide anesthesia of the entire lower extremity.[67,68]

A continuous sciatic nerve block has been used for analgesia and sympatholysis in patients with severe ischemia-induced pain.[69] A single or continuous femoral block may also be used with a sciatic nerve block for chronic pain and treatment of pressure ulcers, which need multiple surgeries and have a high recurrence rate.[70,71] Sciatic nerve injections with alcohol neuroablation were helpful in the treatment of a patient with knee and hip flexor spasticity and related right trochanteric and ischial pressure ulcers.[70]

If blockade of the posterior femoral cutaneous nerve of the thigh is desired (such as for surgical anesthesia for above-knee amputation), a block of the sciatic nerve at the subgluteal level or above is indicated. However, the frequency of posterior femoral cutaneous nerve block with different approaches to blockade of the sciatic nerve has not been well established by clinical trials.[17]

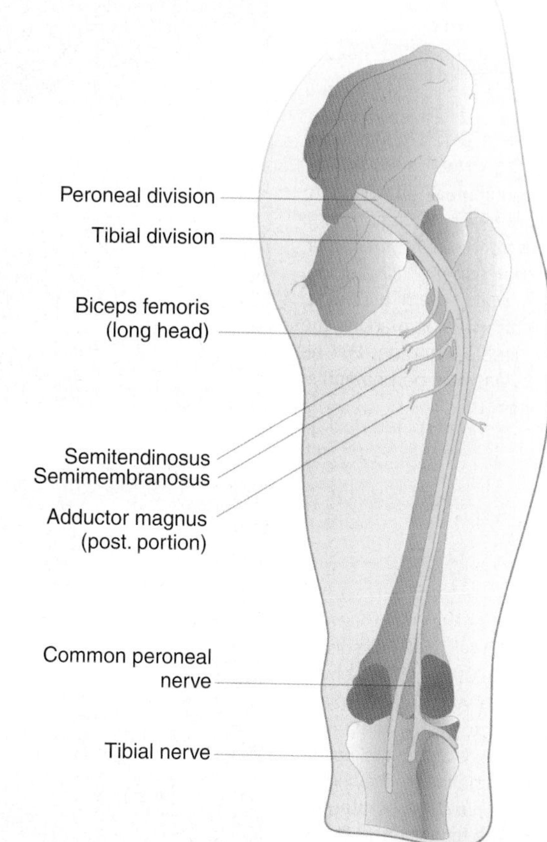

Figure 54.12 Schematic representation of the branches and course of the sciatic nerve. (From Hadzic A, ed. *Hadzic's Peripheral Nerve Blocks and Anatomy for Ultrasound-Guided Regional Anesthesia*. 2nd ed. New York: McGraw-Hill: 2012. Used by permission.)

ANATOMY

The sciatic nerve is the largest nerve of the sacral plexus, and it innervates almost the entire leg below the knee. The sciatic nerve passes from the pelvis through the sacrosciatic foramen between the ischial tuberosity and greater trochanter of the femur. It lies anterior to the gluteus maximus muscle and runs with the sciatic artery. It courses down the posterior aspect of the thigh to the popliteal fossa, where it diverges into the tibial nerve (TN) and the common peroneal nerve (CPN) (Fig. 54.12). Sensation to the posterior aspect of the thigh is provided by the posterior femoral cutaneous nerve, which also originates from the sacral plexus, follows a similar course as the sciatic nerve in the thigh, but is not formally part of the sciatic nerve (see Fig. 54.2).

TECHNIQUE

There are several approaches to block the sciatic nerve. The level at which it should be blocked depends on the surgical site.

Nerve Stimulator– and Surface-Based Techniques

Transgluteal Approach. This approach is based on the geometric relationship of the posterior superior iliac spine (PSIS) and greater trochanter to the sciatic nerve with the patient in a modified Sims position. Winnie modified the original description by adding another landmark, the sacral hiatus, to account more precisely for the variability in body habitus.[72,73]

A line is drawn from the PSIS to the greater trochanter. A second line is drawn perpendicular to the midpoint of the first line drawn and extended 4 cm. This point is the site of needle insertion (Fig. 54.13). After skin preparation, the needle is introduced perpendicular to all planes until the appropriate motor response below the knee (dorsiflexion or plantar flexion) is elicited. Once a twitch is obtained, 10 to 20 mL of local anesthetic is injected to accomplish the blockade. Regardless of the technique, the motor response and local anesthetic dose are similar.

Anterior Approach. A line is drawn over the femoral crease. The femoral artery is palpated, and a second line is drawn perpendicular to the first line originating at the femoral pulse. The line is extended 2 to 4 cm from the femoral crease. The greater trochanter is palpated and a line is extended from its tuberosity medially across the anterior surface of the thigh, parallel to the inguinal ligament. The point of intersection of this line and the perpendicular line from the inguinal crease marks the entry site for the needle.[74]

After skin preparation, a 6-inch needle is inserted perpendicular to the skin. Once bone is contacted, the needle is withdrawn and redirected medially to pass 5 cm beyond the femur, where it should be resting slightly posterior and medial to the femur to elicit a motor response in the calf or foot. Slight internal rotation of the leg can greatly facilitate

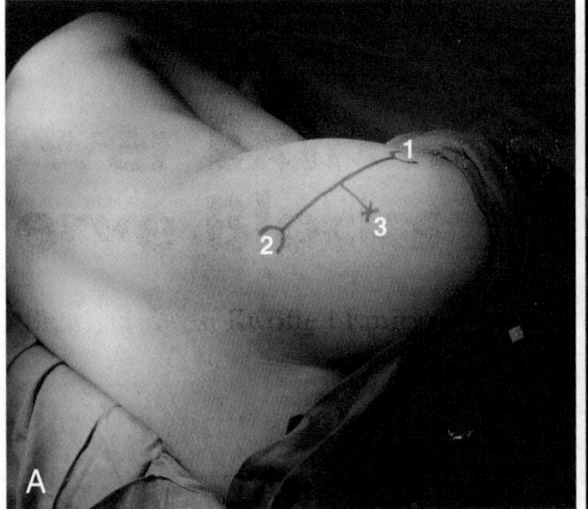

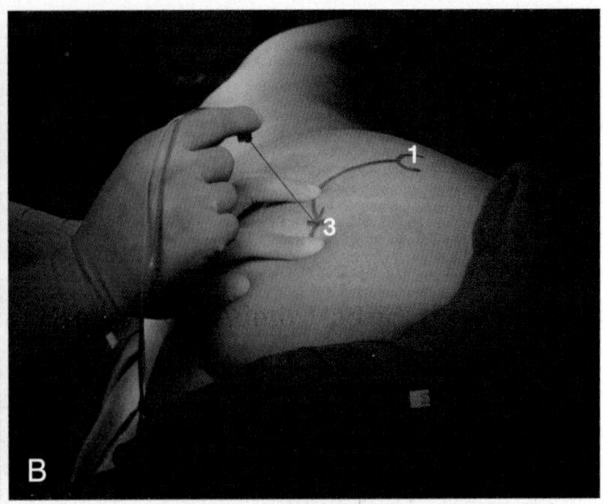

Figure 54.13 Nerve stimulation–guided transgluteal approach to the sciatic nerve. **A,** landmarks: (1) greater trochanter of the femur, (2) posterior superior iliac spine, and (3) a point 4 cm caudal to the point of bisection marking the spot for needle insertion. **B,** The needle is inserted perpendicular to all planes.

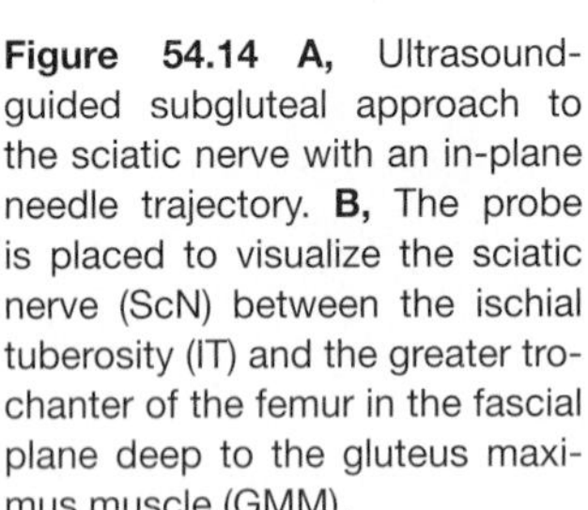

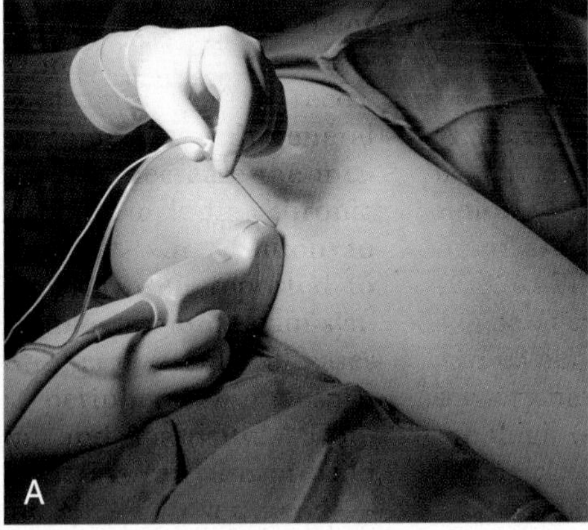

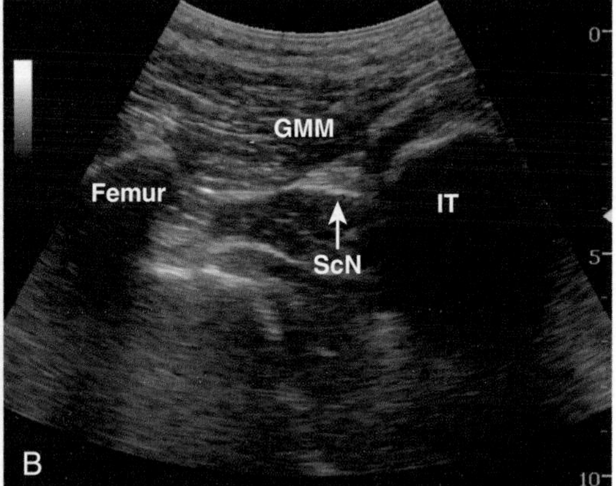

Figure 54.14 **A,** Ultrasound-guided subgluteal approach to the sciatic nerve with an in-plane needle trajectory. **B,** The probe is placed to visualize the sciatic nerve (ScN) between the ischial tuberosity (IT) and the greater trochanter of the femur in the fascial plane deep to the gluteus maximus muscle (GMM).

finding the sciatic nerve because it swings the lesser trochanter away from the path of the needle.[75]

Ultrasound-Guided Techniques

Depending on the level at which the sciatic block is performed, either a low-frequency transducer (transgluteal approach) or a high-frequency transducer (subgluteal approach) can be used. We limit description in this section to the subgluteal technique because it is probably the most common method. However, once the reader is familiarized with the ultrasound anatomy of the sciatic nerve at the subgluteal location, the block can be accomplished at any desired level.

Subgluteal Approach

The patient is placed in a modified Sims position and the ischial bone is located. The sciatic nerve is lateral to the ischial bone and medial to the greater trochanter. It lies anterior to the gluteus maximus muscle (Fig. 54.14*A*).

A 5-MHz low-frequency curvilinear probe is used. The transducer is placed in a transverse plane. The sciatic nerve is seen as a hyperechoic structure between the greater trochanter and ischial tuberosity, laterally and medially, respectively (Fig. 54.14*B*). In addition, it also lies in the plane with the fascia of the surrounding muscles; this appears as a hyperechoic line extending from the nerve in the same plane. A 4-inch nerve-stimulating needle is used in either an in-plane or out-of-plane approach. If a combined nerve stimulator– and ultrasound-guided technique is used, the appropriate evoked motor response should be observed. Once satisfactory ultrasound images and nerve stimulation are obtained, 20 to 30 mL of local anesthetic can be injected.

POPLITEAL BLOCK

Popliteal approaches to a sciatic nerve block are performed from the lateral or posterior aspect of the leg. The lateral approach offers the benefit of maintaining the patient in the supine position, and the posterior approach offers the benefit of easily identifiable landmarks and ease of performance. The level in the thigh at which the sciatic nerve branches into the TN and CPN varies greatly; to block both components, a more proximal needle insertion site should be chosen. Alternatively, an injection can be made between the TN and the CPN in the common epineurial sheath. With an ultrasound-guided technique, the block can be performed in either position by using the same end point—injection of local anesthetic within the epineurial sheath to encircle the sciatic nerve and its two divisions.

TECHNIQUE

Nerve Stimulator– and Surface-Based Techniques

Lateral Approach. The landmarks for the lateral approach to a popliteal block are 7 cm above the popliteal fossa crease, the posterolateral border of the vastus lateralis muscle, and the superior lateral border of the biceps femoris muscle (Fig. 54.15). After skin preparation, the needle insertion site is 7 cm cephalad to the popliteal fossa crease, between

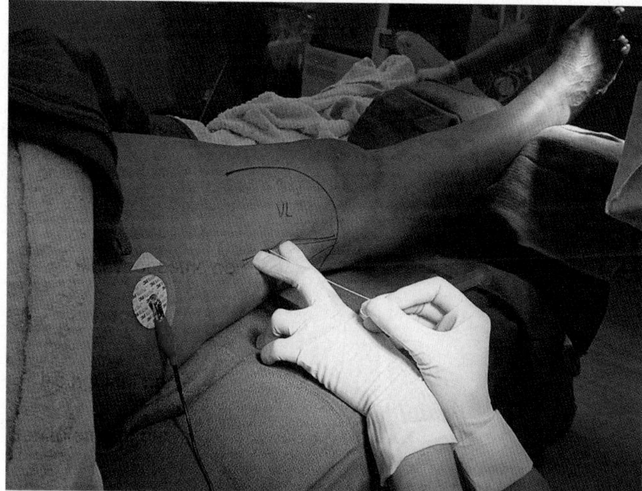

Figure 54.15 Lateral nerve stimulator–guided approach to the sciatic nerve. The needle is placed between the vastus lateralis and the biceps femoris.

the two muscles. The needle is inserted perpendicular to the skin and advanced until it touches the femur. The depth is marked and the needle is withdrawn to the skin and advanced at a 30-degree angle posterior to the angle that produced contact with the femur initially.[76,77] The needle is advanced 2 cm past the skin-femoral distance to reach the sciatic nerve. A double-injection technique with a slightly caudal needle orientation that requires stimulation of both the TN and CPN components of the sciatic nerve has also been described.[78]

Posterior Approach. Originally, the needle insertion site for a sciatic nerve block was described to be at a level 5 cm above the popliteal fossa (classic approach).[79] However, the sciatic nerve diverges into the CPN and TN more proximally in the thigh (7 to 12 cm). The tendons of the biceps femoris (laterally) and the semitendinosus and semimembranosus muscles (medially) provide consistent landmarks for identifying the needle insertion site.[80]

Once the popliteal crease and the tendons of the hamstring muscles are identified and after skin preparation, the needle insertion site is labeled 7 cm proximal to the popliteal crease at the midpoint between the two tendons (Fig. 54.16). Twitches of the foot or toes should be visible with a current of between 0.2 and 0.5 mA, and 20 to 30 mL of local anesthetic is injected incrementally. Inversion is associated with the highest success rate since this evoked motor response implies stimulation of both the TN and CPN.[81]

Ultrasound-Guided Techniques

A high-frequency linear transducer (8 to 12 MHz) is used for most patients. The transducer should be placed at the level of the popliteal crease and the popliteal artery located at this level. The sciatic nerve can then be located as a hyperechoic round or oval structure lateral and superficial to the artery. Frequently, the TN is identified first. The TN is traced to where it joins the CPN. The sciatic nerve is reimaged both distally to observe its divergence into the CPN and TN components and proximally to see the nerves form a single sciatic nerve. This is to confirm that what is seen is indeed

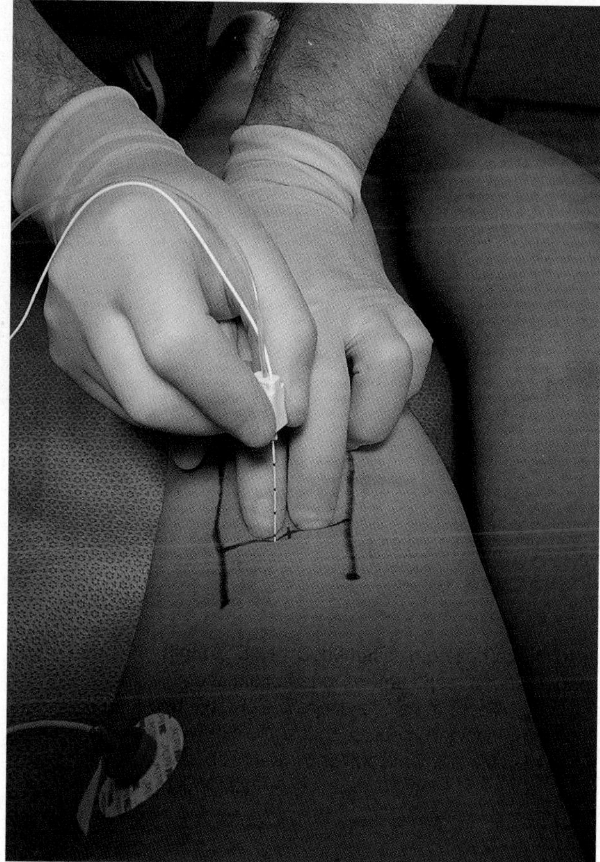

Figure 54.16 Posterior nerve stimulator–guided popliteal block with the patient in the prone position. The needle is placed 7 cm proximal to the popliteal crease at the midpoint between the tendons of the biceps femoris and the semimembranosus/semitendinosus muscles.

the sciatic nerve rather than muscles or their tendons. Once adequate views are observed, the nerve should be blocked before or at its division. The nerve can be approached in either an in-plane or out-of-plane technique (Fig. 54.17). The injection is made between the TN and CPN.[82]

COMPLICATIONS

The incidence of transient adverse neurologic symptoms associated with a continuous block is 0% to 1.0% for sciatic catheters.[83,84]

Persistent paresthesia after use of a popliteal sciatic catheter and pressure ulcers have been described in some patients receiving peripheral nerve blocks because of lack of sensation in the foot.[85,86] The risk for pressure ulcers can be decreased by padding the pressure points and improved teaching of the nursing staff caring for these patients.

Footdrop is a complication of total knee surgery and is usually surgically induced. To avoid confusion with regard to its cause, a selective TN block instead of a sciatic nerve block has been recommended. Such individual block of the TN, in conjunction with a femoral nerve block, has been shown to be as effective as a sciatic nerve block at the popliteal fossa (and femoral nerve block) in terms of postoperative pain control.[87] Preservation of peroneal nerve integrity (i.e., no footdrop after the nerve block and before surgery) allows easy determination of the cause of the footdrop.

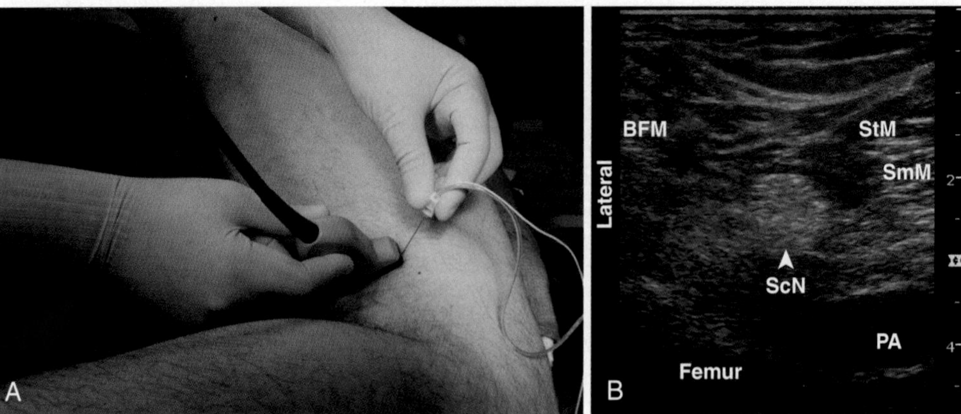

Figure 54.17 A, Transducer placement and needle insertion for an in-plane popliteal nerve block with the patient in the oblique position. **B,** Ultrasound image of the sciatic nerve in the popliteal fossa. BFM, biceps femoris muscle; PA, popliteal artery; ScN, sciatic nerve; SmM, semimembranosus muscle; StM, semitendinosus muscle.

ANKLE BLOCK

All terminal nerves to the foot are branches of the sciatic nerve (deep peroneal, superficial peroneal, posterior tibial, sural) except the saphenous nerve, a branch of the femoral nerve. Because of variations in the distribution of sensory innervation provided by each nerve, some have recommended blocking all five nerves for any procedure on the foot. An ankle block is typically used for surgery on the distal end of the foot. For more proximal or extensive surgery involving the calcaneus or ankle joint (or both), a popliteal block may result in a longer duration of analgesia and better patient satisfaction.[88] These are all important considerations when deciding between ankle and popliteal blocks.

CLINICAL APPLICATIONS

An ankle block is useful for a wide variety of procedures on the feet and toes. Some examples of common procedures include midfoot and toe amputations, toe deformities, forefoot reconstruction, arthroplasty, metatarsal osteotomy, bunionectomy, hallux valgus, neuromas, cysts, tumors, fractures, soft tissue injury, gouty arthritis, and incision, drainage, and débridement procedures.[89-94]

TECHNIQUE

Surface-Based Techniques

Deep Peroneal Nerve. The needle insertion site is immediately lateral to the dorsalis pedis artery, lateral to the tendon of the extensor hallucis longus muscle. After skin preparation the needle is advanced through the skin until bone is contacted. The needle is then withdrawn back 1 to 2 mm, and 2 to 3 mL of local anesthetic is injected. A fan technique is then used in which the needle is redirected 30 degrees medially and laterally, and additional injections of 2 to 3 mL of local anesthetic are made in both directions (Fig. 54.18).

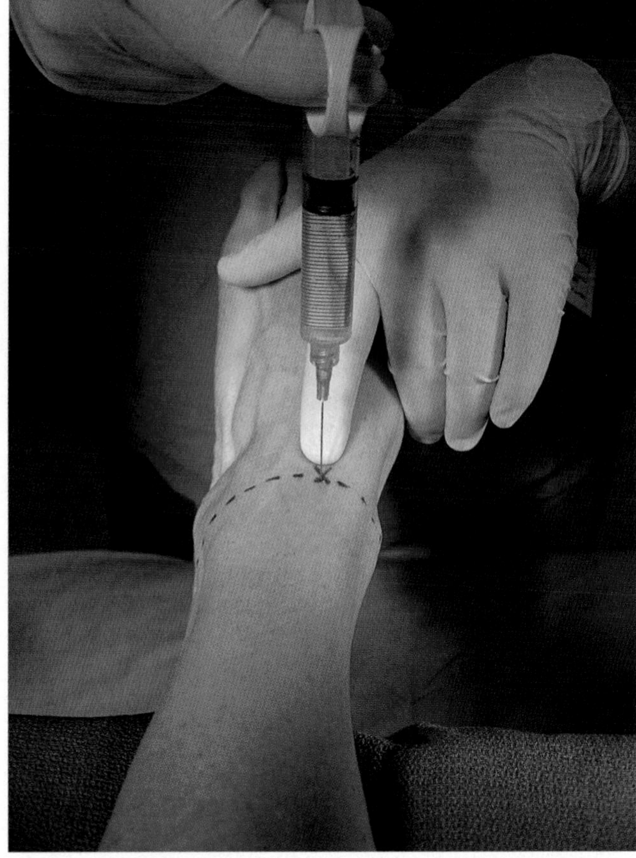

Figure 54.18 Deep peroneal nerve block. The needle is inserted lateral to the tendons of the extensor hallucis longus medially and the extensor digitorum longus.

Posterior Tibial Nerve. The TN is anesthetized by injecting local anesthetic just behind the medial malleolus, followed by a fan technique similar to that described for the deep peroneal nerve (Fig. 54.19).

Superficial Peroneal, Sural, and Saphenous Nerves. The superficial peroneal and sural nerves are superficial cutaneous extensions of the sciatic nerve, and the saphenous nerve is a superficial cutaneous extension of the femoral nerve. Blockade of all three nerves is accomplished by using a simple circumferential injection of local anesthetic subcutaneously at the level of the medial and lateral malleoli (Fig. 54.20).

Ultrasound-Guided Techniques

Ultrasound guidance can be used to perform the two deep blocks of the ankle, the posterior tibial and deep peroneal

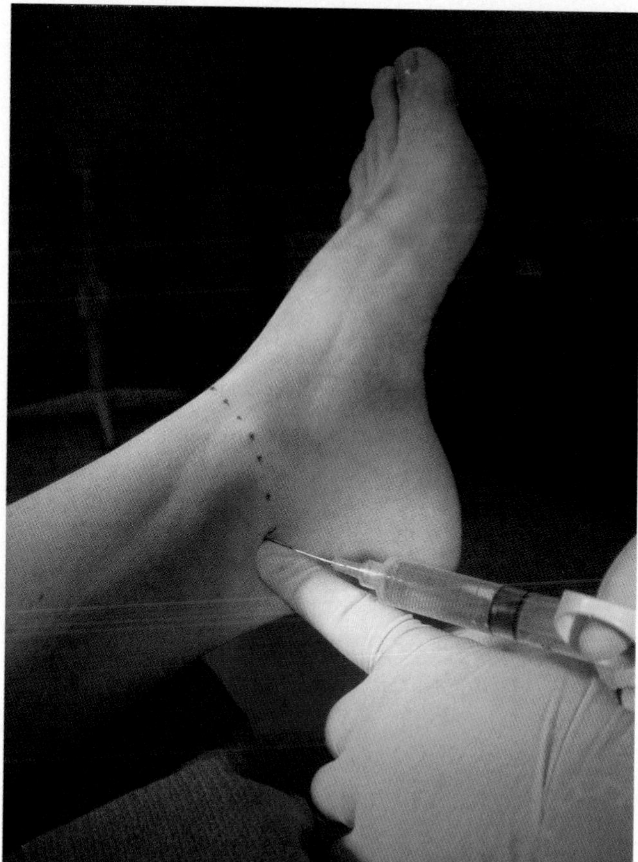

Figure 54.19 Posterior tibial nerve block at the ankle. The needle is inserted posterior to the medial malleolus.

nerves. To avoid compressing the artery, the lighter ultrasound probe should be used.

Posterior Tibial Nerve. A high-frequency transducer is placed in a transverse view, just above the medial malleolus. At this position the pulsatile posterior tibial artery can be observed, and the TN is the hyperechoic oval structure just posterior to the artery (Fig. 54.21). The nerve can be approached in an in-plane or out-of-plane technique.[95,96]

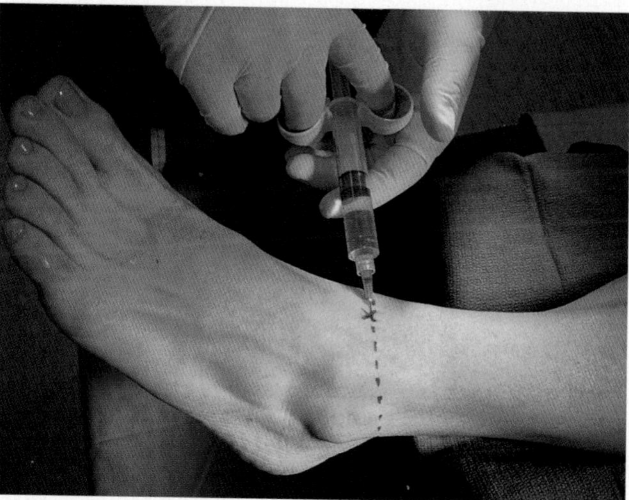

Figure 54.20 Block of the cutaneous nerves at the ankle. A superficial peroneal nerve block is shown. The sural and saphenous nerves are blocked with a subcutaneous injection of local anesthetic.

Deep Peroneal Nerve. The transducer is positioned on the dorsum of the foot at the intermalleolar line in a transverse view. The dorsalis pedis artery should be seen at this level. The nerve can be viewed as a hypoechoic structure just lateral to the dorsalis pedis artery.[97] Two to 3 mL of local anesthetic can be injected on either side of the nerve. If the nerve cannot be viewed, 2 to 3 mL of local anesthetic can be injected on either side of the artery (Fig. 54.22).

CONCLUSION

LEBs are safe, reliable methods of anesthesia and analgesia and good alternatives for patients who may not tolerate general anesthesia or large doses of opioids. LEBs can also be very useful in austere environments.[98] The introduction of ultrasound guidance has allowed more widespread use of LEBs in the modern practice of anesthesia and pain medicine.

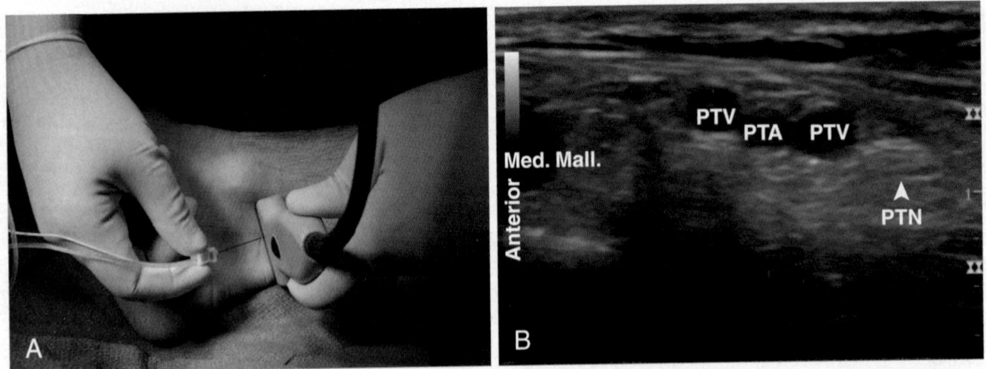

Figure 54.21 **A,** Ultrasound-guided posterior tibial nerve block. The transducer is placed behind the medial malleolus. The needle is shown inserted in an out-of-plane approach. **B,** Ultrasound image of the posterior tibial nerve. Med. Mall., medial malleolus; PTA, posterior tibial artery; PTN, posterior tibial nerve; PTV, posterior tibial veins.

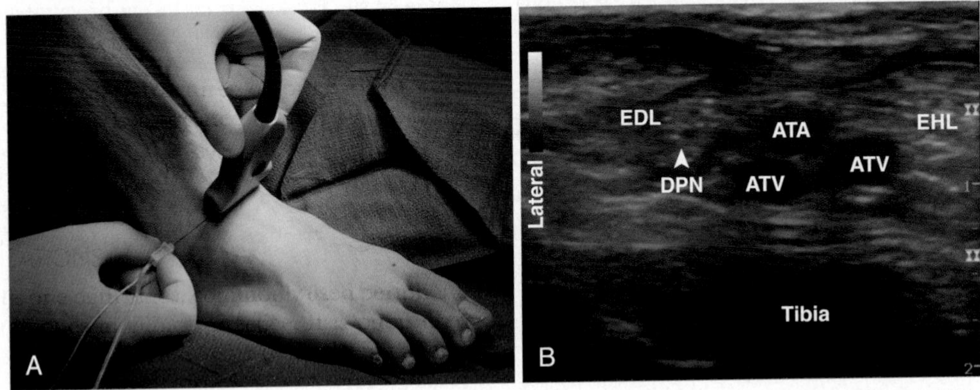

Figure 54.22 **A,** Ultrasound-guided deep peroneal block. The transducer is placed over the dorsalis pedis pulse. **B,** Ultrasound image. ATA, anterior tibial artery; ATV, anterior tibial veins; DPN, deep peroneal nerve; EDL, extensor digitorum longus tendon; EHL, extensor hallucis longus tendon.

SUGGESTED READINGS

Allen JG, Denny NM, Oakman N. Postoperative analgesia following total knee arthroplasty: a study comparing spinal anesthesia and combined sciatic femoral 3-in-1 block. *Reg Anesth Pain Med.* 1998;23:142-146.

Capdevila X, Macaire P, Dadure C, et al. Continuous psoas compartment block for postoperative analgesia after total hip arthroplasty: new landmarks, technical guidelines, and clinical evaluation. *Anesth Analg.* 2002;94:1606-1613.

Capdevila X, Pirat P, Bringuier S, et al, for the French Study Group on Continuous Peripheral Nerve Blocks. Continuous peripheral nerve blocks in hospital wards after orthopedic surgery: a multicenter prospective analysis of the quality of postoperative analgesia and complications in 1,416 patients. *Anesthesiology.* 2005;103:1035-1045.

Dadure C, Motais F, Ricard C, et al. Continuous peripheral nerve blocks at home for treatment of recurrent complex regional pain syndrome I in children. *Anesthesiology.* 2005;102:387-391.

Enneking FK, Chan V, Greger J, et al. Lower-extremity peripheral nerve blockade: essentials of our current understanding. *Reg Anesth Pain Med.* 2005;30:4-35.

Gadsden JC, Lindenmuth DM, Hadzic A, et al. Lumbar plexus block using high-pressure injection leads to contralateral and epidural spread. *Anesthesiology.* 2008;109:683-688.

Gold BS, Kitz DS, Lecky JH, et al. Unanticipated admission to the hospital following ambulatory surgery. *JAMA.* 1989;262:3008-3010.

Karmakar MK, Ho AM, Li X, et al. Ultrasound-guided lumbar plexus block through the acoustic window of the lumbar ultrasound trident. *Br J Anaesth.* 2008;100:533-537.

Ng I, Vaghadia H, Choi PT, et al. Ultrasound imaging accurately identifies the lateral femoral cutaneous nerve. *Anesth Analg.* 2008;107:1070-1074.

Salinas FV. Ultrasound and review of evidence for lower extremity peripheral nerve blocks. *Reg Anesth Pain Med.* 2010;35(suppl 2):S16-S25.

Stevens RD, Van Gessel E, Flory N, et al. Lumbar plexus block reduces pain and blood loss associated with total hip arthroplasty. *Anesthesiology.* 2000;93:115-121.

Tran de QH, Clemente A, Finlayson RJ. A review of approaches and techniques for lower extremity nerve blocks. *Can J Anaesth.* 2007;54:922-934.

Vloka JD, Hadzic A, April E, et al. The division of the sciatic nerve in the popliteal fossa: anatomical implications for popliteal nerve blockade. *Anesth Analg.* 2001;92:215-217.

Weller RS, Gerancher JC, Crews JC, et al. Extensive retroperitoneal hematoma without neurologic deficit in two patients who underwent lumbar plexus block and were later anticoagulated. *Anesthesiology.* 2003;98:581-585.

Wiegel M, Gottschaldt U, Hennebach R, et al. Complications and adverse effects associated with continuous peripheral nerve blocks in orthopedic patients. *Anesth Analg.* 2007;104:1578-1582.

The references for this chapter can be found at www.expertconsult.com.

Truncal Blocks

55

Patrick Narchi | François Singelyn | Xavier Paqueron | Barry Nicholls

Similar to peripheral nerve blocks of the upper or lower limb, truncal blocks provide excellent postoperative pain relief, avoid the risk for major complications associated with central nerve blockade such as epidural hematoma or abscess, and can be used as a sole anesthetic technique for some types of surgery. However, their use in daily practice has remained limited until recently. Because of the many advantages that they offer, truncal blocks should have a place in the armamentarium of every anesthesiologist involved in the management of postoperative analgesia, particularly in the outpatient setting. In this chapter, the following truncal blocks are discussed: paravertebral, intercostal, ilioinguinal, iliohypogastric, genitofemoral, transverse abdominal plane, and rectus sheath blocks.

PARAVERTEBRAL NERVE BLOCKADE

The renewed interest in paravertebral nerve blockade is related to many factors: the involvement of anesthesiologists in postoperative pain control, the development of ambulatory surgery, and the need to apply simpler and more reliable techniques to reduce postoperative stay in the intensive care unit. Paravertebral blockade consists of injecting local anesthetic close to the vertebra at the level where the spinal nerves exit the intervertebral foramina. Such injection induces an ipsilateral somatic and sympathetic blockade that extends, most of the time, longitudinally above and below the injected vertebral level. It is indicated for acute as well as unilateral chronic pain syndromes. Such blockade is associated with no major cardiovascular or respiratory effects.

ANATOMY

The paravertebral space is triangular shaped. It is limited by the superior costotransverse ligament posteriorly, by the parietal pleura anterolaterally, and by the head and neck of the adjacent ribs superiorly and inferiorly. It is in continuity with the epidural space through the intervertebral foramen, with the intercostal space, and with the contralateral paravertebral space anteriorly. It contains the dorsal and ventral rami and the sympathetic chain. Hence, injection of local anesthetic into the area results in unilateral sensory, motor, and sympathetic blockade (Fig. 55.1).

In the paravertebral space, the endothoracic fascia is firmly applied to the ribs and fuses medially on the vertebral body.[1] It thus divides the paravertebral space into two compartments: the extrapleural space anteriorly and the subendothoracic space posteriorly. Naja and coworkers[2] claim that longitudinal spread of local anesthetic is better when the injection is performed ventral to the endothoracic fascia whereas a dorsal injection results in localized spread. However, another author[3] has questioned the significance of the endothoracic fascia.

Whether local anesthetic injected into the low paravertebral thoracic segments spreads to the lumbar levels remains controversial. Some authors question the anatomic barrier created by the psoas muscle. Others stress that local anesthetic can spread through the posterior insertion of the diaphragm when the solution is injected deeper to the endothoracic fascia[4] or along the lateral border of the psoas muscle.

TECHNIQUE

As for any regional technique, standard monitoring includes electrocardiography, pulse oximetry, and noninvasive blood pressure monitoring.

POSITIONING

The sitting position is usually preferred since it facilitates palpation of the landmarks. The lateral decubitus position is an alternative.

APPROACHES

Several approaches have been suggested for locating the paravertebral space.

Blind Approach

Once the transverse process is contacted (usually at a maximum distance of 4 to 5 cm from the skin), the needle is withdrawn to subcutaneous tissue, reoriented caudally (but sometimes cephalad when caudal insertion is impossible because of contact with bone), and advanced 1 to 1.5 cm deeper to the transverse process.

Loss-of-Resistance Approach

Loss of resistance (a syringe filled with saline, air, or both is connected to the needle) is felt once the paravertebral space is entered. This approach may be associated with the blind approach.

Nerve Stimulator Approach

Clinical studies have shown that use of a peripheral nerve stimulator may improve the position of the needle with respect to the nerve.[3,5]

Effective intravenous sedation and local anesthetic infiltration of the puncture sites are mandatory. Indeed, needle insertion through the different muscular structures and bone contact are painful.

Single Injection Technique. The needle entry site is located 2.5 to 3 cm lateral to the cephalad border of each spinous

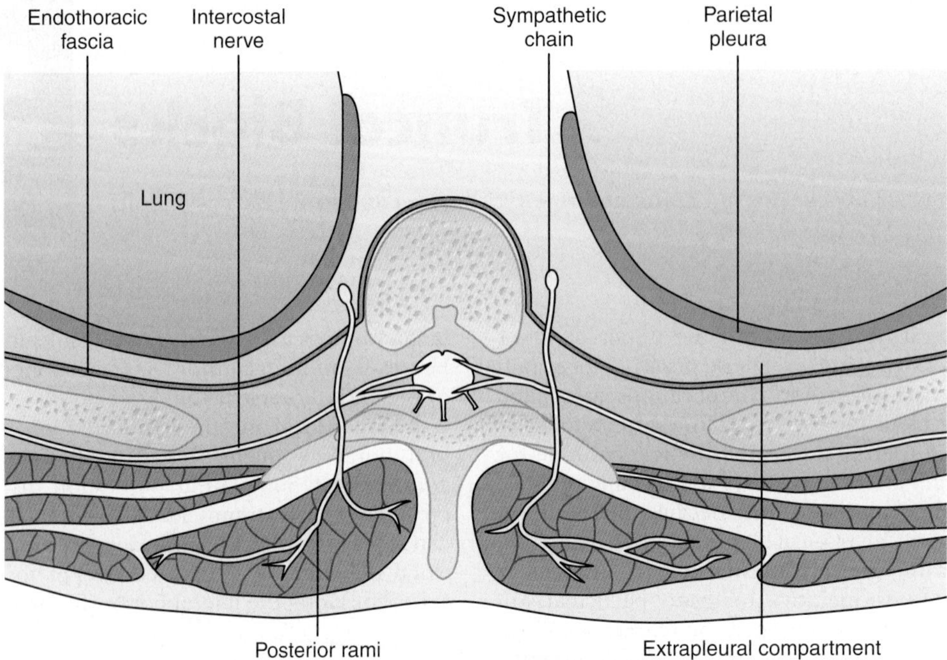

Figure 55.1 Cross section of the paravertebral space at the thoracic level.

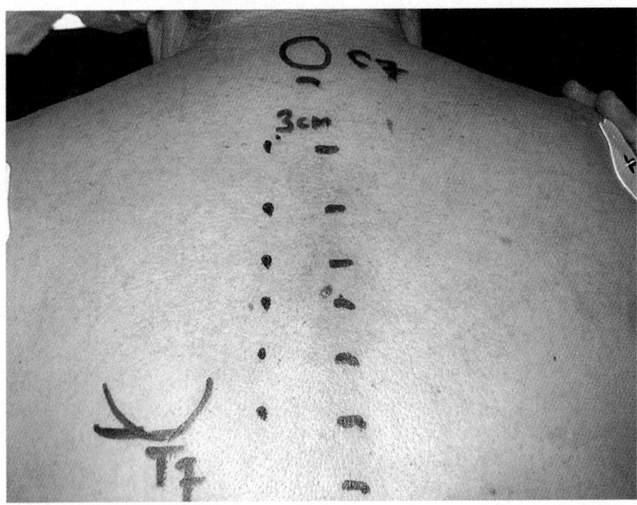

Figure 55.2 Landmarks for a high thoracic paravertebral block.

process ipsilateral to the side to be operated on (Fig. 55.2). The needle, attached via extension tubing to a syringe, is advanced anteriorly in the parasagittal plane until it contacts the transverse process. It is then withdrawn and reoriented caudally so that it can be walked off the caudad edge of the transverse process. The needle is then advanced anteriorly approximately 1 to 1.5 cm deeper to the transverse process. Note that Naja and colleagues[6] have shown that the distance from the skin to the paravertebral space is greater at the upper and lower thoracic levels than at the midthoracic levels (T4-8). Their median needle insertion depth was 55 mm. They also determined that body mass index influences the depth at the upper and lower thoracic levels but not at the midthoracic ones. After negative aspiration, 4 to 5 mL of a long-acting local anesthetic (e.g., 0.5% ropivacaine or levobupivacaine) is injected at each level, with the total volume not to exceed 0.3 mL/kg. The onset of sensory loss and surgical anesthesia typically occurs 10 minutes and 20 to 30 minutes, respectively, after injection.

Some studies[7] suggest that a single-injection technique is as effective as a multiple-injection one (average of five dermatomes blocked) as long as the total volume of 0.3 mL/kg is used. These results were confirmed in a thermographic study by Cheema and coworkers.[8] However, it seems preferable to use a "multiple-injection" technique when extensive spread of local anesthetic is required[9] because of the risk for bilateral or epidural spread associated with a single large-volume injection.

Catheter Technique. Once the paravertebral space has been identified, the catheter is threaded 2 to 3 cm through the needle. A bolus dose of 20 mL of long-acting local anesthetic is injected for surgery (an average of six to eight segments are blocked), followed by continuous infusion of a dilute solution (e.g., 0.125% levobupivacaine or 0.2% ropivacaine) at a rate of 5 to 10 mL/hr. The catheter technique has the advantage of providing surgical anesthesia and prolonged postoperative analgesia.[10] Bilateral paravertebral block catheters have been shown to be effective after bilateral thoracotomy in children, after major abdominal vascular surgery, and in outpatient bilateral reduction mammaplasty.[11]

Ultrasound Approach

Initially, ultrasound was used to visualize landmarks such as the transverse process and to measure the distance from the skin before inserting the needle. Pusch and coauthors[12] reported good correlation between the depth of needle insertion, from the skin to the transverse process, and such distance when measured by the ultrasound machine. Presently, anesthesiologists are using ultrasound guidance to perform paravertebral blocks because it allows reliable identification of critical anatomic structures such as the pleura.

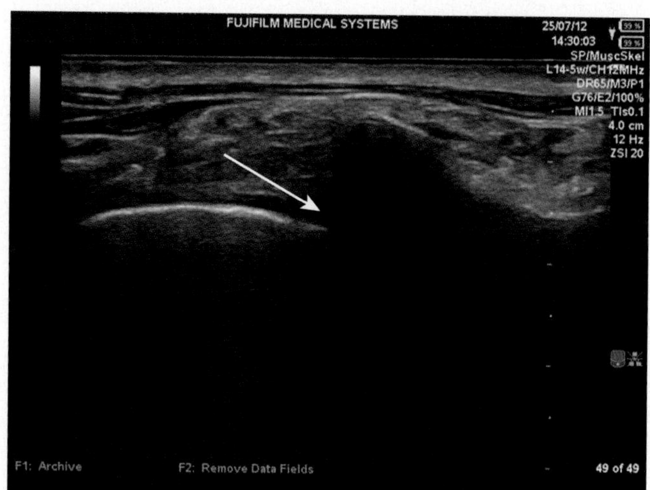

Figure 55.3 Sonographic anatomy of the paravertebral space (arrow) via a transverse scan.

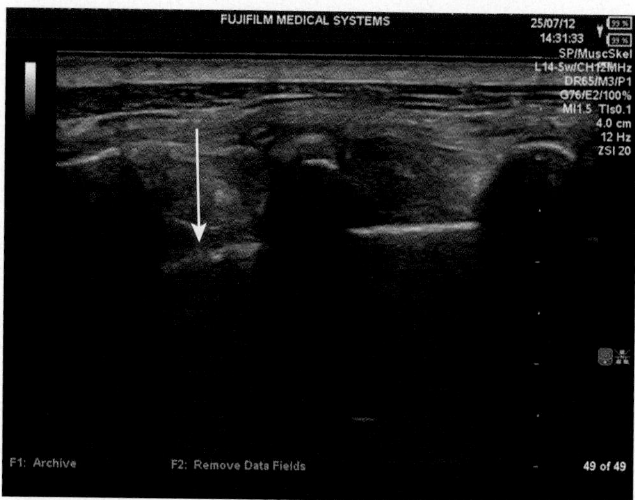

Figure 55.4 Sonographic anatomy of the paravertebral space (arrow) via a parasagittal scan.

Being able to preview the paravertebral anatomy and determine the depth of the transverse process and pleura helps in reducing the incidence of pleural puncture. Moreover, ultrasound guidance allows visualization of the spread of local anesthetic.

The thoracic paravertebral space can be scanned in two different anatomic planes:

- Transverse scan (Fig. 55.3). Performed with a high-frequency probe, a transverse scan allows identification of the apex of the paravertebral space as a triangular hypoechoic area limited by the hyperechoic parietal pleura anteriorly and the internal intercostal membrane posteriorly.
- Sagittal paramedian scan (Fig. 55.4). This scan allows identification of the transverse processes, the intertransverse and costotransverse ligaments, and the hyperechoic pleura.

Under ultrasound guidance, the needle approach can be either in plane or out of plane. Thus, four different techniques to approach the thoracic paravertebral space are described.

- Transverse scan with an "in-plane" approach.[13-15] The transverse process is identified as an acoustic shadow hiding the visibility of the paravertebral space. The block needle is inserted in the plane of the ultrasound beam in a lateral-to-medial direction. Note that as the needle is advanced medially in the direction of the intervertebral foramen, there is a risk for central spread of local anesthetic or catheter placement. Moreover, such an approach seems to be less comfortable for the patient because the needle path is long and a 100-mm needle is usually required to reach the paravertebral space.
- Transverse scan with an "out-of-plane" approach.[16] When compared with the previous one, this approach has the advantage of significantly reducing the distance between the skin and the paravertebral space, thus making it more comfortable for the patient. In addition, because the direction of the needle remains in the paramedian plane, the risk for central spread of the local anesthetic solution should be lower than with the previous approach.
- Sagittal scan with an "out-of-plane" approach.[17] Once the pleura has been carefully identified between two adjacent transverse processes, the needle is advanced until it crosses the costotransverse ligament. Two to 3 mL of local anesthetic is injected into the paravertebral space. Such injection displaces the parietal pleura anteriorly. This approach appears to be the easiest one for the single-shot technique because the path of the needle is very short (3 to 4 cm) and the pleura is easily visible.
- Sagittal scan with an "in-plane" approach.[18] With this approach it is often difficult to visualize the complete path of the needle because the angle of needle insertion is very steep. Nevertheless, it is the authors' preferred approach for catheter insertion.

With all these approaches, hydrolocation with very small amounts of either local anesthetic or saline during needle insertion is helpful to accurately check the location of the needle tip. As soon as the paravertebral space is entered and injected, the parietal pleura is displaced anteriorly by the injected solution.

EQUIPMENT

An 8- to 10-cm needle is required to perform this block. It can be a 22-gauge spinal, a 19-gauge Tuohy epidural, or an insulated stimulating needle.

PUNCTURE SITE

The puncture site is determined by the type of surgery. At the thoracic level, breast surgery requires blockade of the T1-6 dermatomes, whereas thoracotomy requires lower dermatomal blockade (T4-10). At the lumbar level, an extensive block (T10-L2) is required.

DRUGS AND ADDITIVES

A bolus dose of 2 mg/kg of ropivacaine can be used safely as demonstrated in a recent pharmacokinetic study.[19] The authors recommended the addition of epinephrine (1:200,000) to ropivacaine to decrease C_{max} and delay T_{max} and the rapid absorption phase. The measured venous plasma ropivacaine concentration (2.83 ± 1.31 μg/mL) did

Box 55.1 Indications for Paravertebral Blockade

Major breast surgery
Thoracic surgery
Laparoscopic cholecystectomy
Inguinal hernia repair
Renal surgery
Percutaneous transhepatic biliary drainage
Labor pain, first stage
Rib fractures
Intercostal neuralgia
Pleuritic pain
Coronary syndromes

not exceed the toxic threshold when a continuous infusion rate of 0.1 mL/kg/hr of a 0.5% solution was used.

INDICATIONS

A paravertebral block is associated with excellent analgesia after many types of chest surgery and a reduction in the incidence and severity of chronic pain syndromes[20] (Box 55.1).

MAJOR BREAST SURGERY

In addition to postoperative pain, a high incidence of nausea and vomiting has been reported after general anesthesia during the first 24 hours following breast cancer surgery. Paravertebral blockade results in effective anesthesia for operative procedures on the breast and axilla, reduces postoperative nausea and vomiting, and provides prolonged postoperative analgesia, thereby minimizing narcotic requirements. When compared with the standard analgesic regimen, which usually requires an overnight hospital stay, a paravertebral block allows discharge of the patient on the same day, for a total cost savings of up to 22%.[21]

When performed as a multiple-injection technique, paravertebral blockade has been shown to be effective for breast surgery. Moreover, the unilateral sympathetic blockade that it induces improves oxygenation of the flap tissue after breast reconstruction with the latissimus dorsi,[22] thus potentially improving healing of the flap.

Breast surgery may result in a "postmastectomy pain syndrome." Its incidence varies between 20% and 50%.[23,24] Risk factors include the severity of postoperative pain, anxiety, and young age. Interestingly, preincisional paravertebral blockade has been shown to reduce the prevalence of motion-related and chronic pain 1 year after such surgery.[25,26] It should be kept in mind that because of potential complications such as pneumothorax or epidural spread, the risk-benefit ratio does not favor its use for minor breast surgery. Moreover, the relatively low pain scores and the very low incidence of postoperative nausea and vomiting after minor breast surgery do not warrant the use of a paravertebral block in these situations.[27]

THORACIC SURGERY

Although thoracic epidural analgesia is still considered the "gold standard" for postoperative analgesia after thoracic surgery, continuous paravertebral analgesia has been shown to be as effective as epidural analgesia.[28] Such efficacy occurs whether the catheter is inserted blindly by the anesthesiologist or under direct vision by the surgeon before wound closure. Moreover, a paravertebral catheter avoids the potential risks observed with epidural analgesia, including epidural hematoma, infection, and spinal cord injury. Chronic pain after thoracotomy occurs in 20% to 50% of patients.[29] The occurrence of this syndrome is significantly reduced when early and effective postoperative pain treatment (e.g., epidural analgesia, paravertebral block) is provided.[30]

CARDIAC SURGERY

A unilateral continuous paravertebral block has been shown to be effective in managing pain after major unilateral thoracic surgery, such as minimally invasive coronary artery bypass surgery.[31]

INGUINAL HERNIA REPAIR[32,33]

The effectiveness of a paravertebral block in providing adequate and long-lasting postoperative relief of pain after herniorrhaphy is well documented in the literature. In this setting, a paravertebral block should be performed between the T10 and L2 levels. In pediatric surgery, a paravertebral block with a mixture of 2% lidocaine, epinephrine, and clonidine provided better postoperative analgesia during the first 48 hours than did standard general anesthesia. In adults, Hadzic and associates[32] showed that a paravertebral block (T9-L1) using 20 mL of 0.75% ropivacaine was more effective than the combination of general anesthesia and wound infiltration. This was supported by more patients bypassing the postanesthesia care unit, less need for supplemental analgesics, and earlier discharge home.

MULTIPLE RIB FRACTURES

A paravertebral block provides effective pain relief after multiple rib fractures.[34] It can be performed either as a single shot (bolus of 15 to 20 mL of a long-acting local anesthetic) or as a continuous technique. It has been shown to improve both ventilatory and arterial blood gas parameters.

NEURALGIA AND PLEURITIC PAIN

Paravertebral blocks have been used to treat chronic pain after thoracotomy or mastectomy.[35]

CONTRAINDICATIONS

Contraindications to paravertebral blockade include infection (local, empyema), allergy to local anesthetics, major chest deformity, previous ipsilateral thoracic surgery, and coagulation abnormalities.

FAILURE RATE

A paravertebral block is an easy technique to learn. Even in inexperienced hands, it rapidly provides a high success rate. Indeed, it has been shown that the success rate is significantly improved after a cutoff of 15 blind paravertebral blocks. The failure rate with the blind technique varies between 6% and 15%, depending on the experience of the operator.[36] Recently, ultrasound assistance has made this block much easier and more popular than in the past.

Box 55.2 Complications from Paravertebral Blocks

Pneumothorax (0.5% to 1.5%)
Hypotension
Vascular puncture (6%)
Intrathecal spread (1%)
Toxic seizures
Horner's syndrome
Epidural spread

COMPLICATIONS

The incidence of complications after paravertebral blocks varies between 2% and 5% (Box 55.2). The incidence of hypotension requiring a low dose of vasopressors (e.g., ephedrine) is 4%. The hypotension may be due to either sympathetic blockade (unilateral or bilateral) or a vasovagal event during the procedure. Horner's syndrome is due to cephalad spread of the local anesthetic after a high thoracic paravertebral block. With regard to epidural spread, dye injection studies have shown the incidence of unilateral epidural spread to be up to 70% when using the blind approach. However, its clinical effects are negligible because of the small amount of local anesthetic injected.[37]

INTERCOSTAL NERVE BLOCKADE

ANATOMY

The intercostal nerves are the anterior divisions of the thoracic spinal nerve from T1 to T11. They are distributed mainly to the thoracic pleura and abdominal peritoneum. The first two nerves supply fibers to the upper limb in addition to their thoracic branches, the next four are limited in their distribution to the parietal pleura of the thorax, and the lower five supply the parietal pleura of the thorax and abdomen. The 7th intercostal nerve terminates at the xiphoid process, the 10th intercostal nerve terminates at the umbilicus, and the 12th (subcostal) thoracic nerve is distributed to the abdominal wall and the groin.

TECHNIQUE AND DRUGS

An intercostal block (ICB) is usually performed at the level of the posterior axillary line (Fig. 55.5). The needle is inserted until it contacts the rib. It is then partially withdrawn, reoriented caudally, and advanced less than 0.5 cm deeper than the bone contact. Use of a stimulating needle connected to a peripheral nerve stimulator may be helpful. Elicitation of intercostal muscle contractions indicates adequate needle location. It is preferable to block the two proximal and two distal adjacent nerves from the selected level to cover all the areas affected by the surgical incision.

During thoracotomy, the block may be performed by the surgeon under direct vision either at the beginning or at the end of the operation before skin closure.

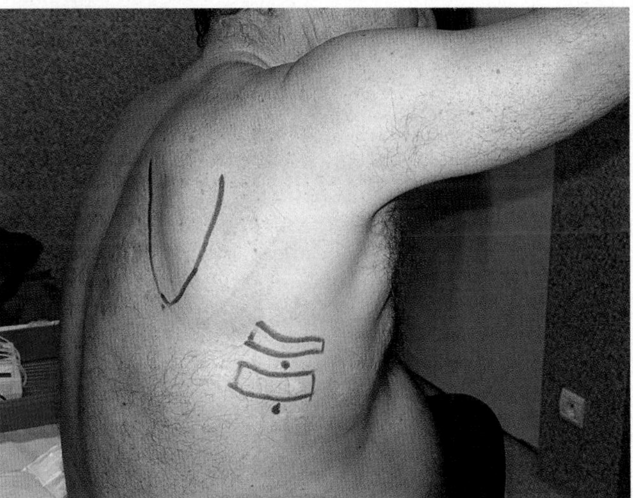

Figure 55.5 Landmarks for an intercostal nerve block.

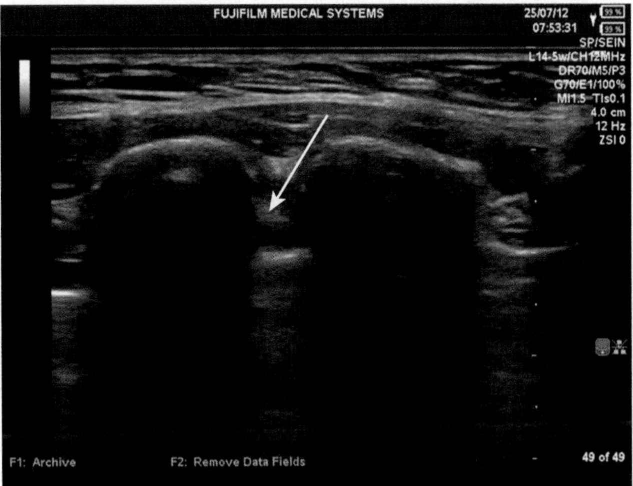

Figure 55.6 Sonographic anatomy of the intercostal space (arrow).

ULTRASOUND-GUIDED TECHNIQUE[38]

With direct visualization of the ribs and pleura (Fig. 55.6), ultrasound guidance allows the anesthesiologist to perform an ICB proximal to the scapula, where the intercostal nerve can be blocked before its division to ensure adequate anesthesia of the pleura. In addition, ultrasound guidance allows visualization of injection of the local anesthetic into the intercostal space, thereby enabling the provider to adjust the trajectory and depth of the needle to ensure adequate spread of anesthetic and avoid pleural puncture. The patient is positioned prone, and the spinous processes of the thoracic vertebra are identified by palpation. The chest wall is best imaged in a parasagittal plane. The intercostal space is visualized with a high-frequency linear probe. The ribs appear as an oval structure with a bright surface (periosteum). A dark shadow is seen deep to the rib secondary to echo shadowing. The pleura and lungs are visualized deep to the intercostal space between the echo shadows. The needle target is the internal intercostal muscle.

After subcutaneous infiltration of local anesthetic, a 22-gauge needle is inserted either in plane or out of plane toward the plane just deep to the internal intercostal muscle. Then, 3 mL of a long-acting local anesthetic with epinephrine is injected into the intercostal space.

With continuous techniques, the infusion rate is 5 to 7 mL/hr for an average-sized adult. Many studies have shown that C_{max} occurs rapidly within 3 to 20 minutes after the block.[39] Administration of 16 mL of either 0.5% plain bupivacaine or 1.5% lidocaine with epinephrine results in an acceptable range of local anesthetic plasma concentrations (1.44 ± 0.2 μg/mL for bupivacaine and 2.78 ± 0.2 μg/mL for lidocaine).

INDICATIONS

Indications for ICB include relief of postoperative pain after breast surgery, thoracotomy, video-assisted thoracic surgery, and coronary artery bypass surgery. It has been used for the relief of pain after rib fractures and with chronic pain syndromes involving the chest.

For minor breast surgery, multiple ICBs (T3-6) result in a significantly better quality and duration of postoperative analgesia than afforded by general anesthesia alone.

Many studies have confirmed the effectiveness of ICB in relieving pain after thoracic surgery.[40] It has been noted that when performed at five levels, ICB results in effective analgesia during the first 6 hours after thoracotomy, similar to thoracic epidural analgesia. In contrast, interpleural analgesia was ineffective in providing adequate pain relief.[40]

Video-assisted thoracic surgery is less invasive than open thoracotomy but is still followed by postoperative pain and impairment of lung function.[41] Bilateral ICB of the second, third, and fourth intercostal nerves, under direct vision during surgery, has been shown to be safe and effective in reducing postoperative pain and analgesic requirements.[42] However, another study[41] was unable to show any difference between ICB, intrapleural analgesia, and opioid analgesia.

The efficacy of ICB in relieving pain and improving ventilatory parameters after multiple rib fractures has clearly been demonstrated.[43-45]

For minimally invasive coronary bypass surgery, it has been shown that when compared with opioid analgesia, ICB (four levels, 5 mL of 0.1% ropivacaine per level) provides better pain relief in the early postoperative period and allows earlier patient discharge to the intermediate care ward.[46]

CONTRAINDICATIONS AND COMPLICATIONS

Contraindications to ICB include local infection and contralateral pneumothorax. Its major complication is pneumothorax, the incidence of which is estimated to be 1.4% for each intercostal nerve blocked.[47]

ILIOINGUINAL, ILIOHYPOGASTRIC, AND GENITOFEMORAL NERVE BLOCKADES

ANATOMY

The ilioinguinal (II) and iliohypogastric (IH) nerves originate from the T12 and L1 nerve roots of the lumbar plexus. Both nerves pass through the fascia lumborum at the lateral border of the quadratus lumborum muscle and then extend to the area between the obliquus internus abdominis and transversus abdominis muscles. The IH nerve is located superior and medial to the II nerve. In the area of the anterior superior iliac spine, it bifurcates into the lateral and medial cutaneous rami as its two terminal branches. The lateral cutaneous ramus passes through the obliquus internus abdominis and externus abdominis muscles and provides sensory innervation to the skin in the region of the anterior aspect of the buttock. The medial cutaneous ramus passes through both the obliquus internus abdominis muscle and the aponeurosis of the obliquus externus abdominis muscle and supplies the skin of the abdominal wall region above the symphysis. The II nerve supplies the skin region of the superomedial aspect of the thigh, as well as the anterior region of the scrotum in males or the mons pubis and labia majora in females.

The genitofemoral (GF) nerve is mainly a sensory nerve. It is formed from L1-2 in the substance of the psoas major muscle. At the L3-4 level, it emerges on the ventral surface of the muscle along its medial border. It runs downward on the muscular surface and divides into genital and femoral branches above the inguinal ligament. The genital branch enters the inguinal canal through the deep inguinal ring. It supplies motor fibers to the cremasteric muscle and sensory fibers to the skin over the scrotum in men and the mons pubis and labia majora in women. The femoral branch accompanies the external iliac artery and, below the inguinal ligament, remains enveloped by the femoral vascular sheath lateral to the femoral artery. It supplies the skin over the femoral triangle.

INDICATIONS

ILIOHYPOGASTRIC AND ILIOINGUINAL NERVE BLOCKS

In conjunction with GF nerve blockade, these blocks are indicated as anesthetic and analgesic techniques for inguinal herniorrhaphy, orchidopexy, and hydrocelectomy. Combined IH and II nerve blocks significantly reduce pain scores and supplemental analgesia after discharge following inguinal herniorrhaphy.[48] When compared with spinal anesthesia, these blocks are associated with a shorter time to discharge home, lower pain scores at discharge, higher satisfaction scores at 24-hour follow-up, and lower cost.[49] These blocks have been suggested as an alternative anesthetic technique for repair of strangulated hernias in high-risk patients who are not suitable candidates for general or neuraxial anesthesia.[50] In children, the effectiveness of the blocks appear to be similar to that of caudal blocks.[51]

The amount of postoperative intravenous morphine needed during the first 24 hours after cesarean section was significantly reduced by bilateral II nerve blocks.[52] However, no difference in the incidence of opioid-related adverse effects was noted.[53]

II nerve blocks have been recommended in patients with persistent pain and paresthesia after inguinal herniorrhaphy, appendectomy, cesarean section, and hysterectomy. Successful pain relief after a diagnostic II nerve block may indicate II nerve entrapment.

GENITOFEMORAL NERVE BLOCK

In conjunction with II and IH nerve blocks, a GF block is indicated for inguinal herniorrhaphy, orchidopexy, and

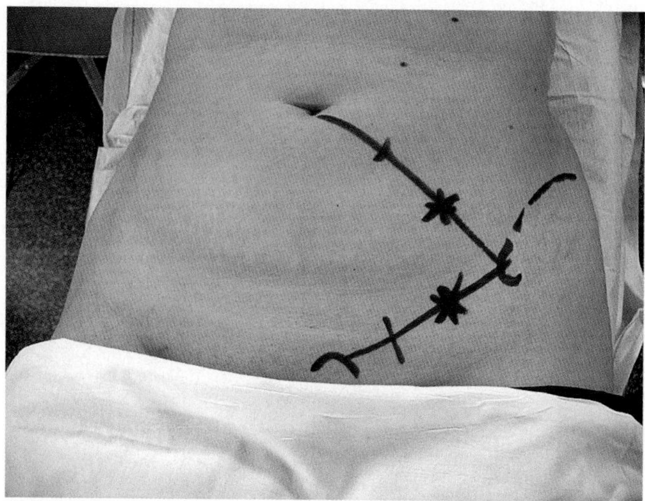

Figure 55.7 Landmarks for ilioinguinal and iliohypogastric nerve blocks.

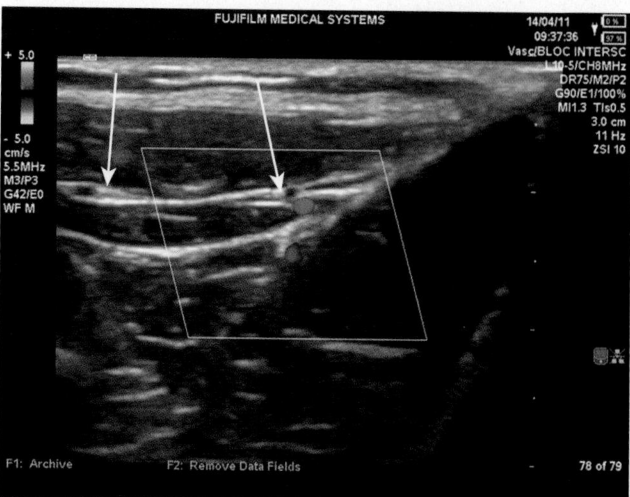

Figure 55.8 Sonographic anatomy of the ilioinguinal and iliohypogastric nerves (arrows).

hydrocelectomy. However, when compared with combined II and IH nerve blocks during inguinal herniorrhaphy, its benefit is limited to pain related to traction on the hernia sac, and it has no additional postoperative analgesic effect.

In addition to a femoral nerve block, it is an effective anesthetic and analgesic technique for stripping of the long saphenous vein.[54]

CONTRAINDICATIONS AND DRUGS

Local infection and previous II, IH, or GF nerve injury are the only contraindications.

Bupivacaine has been the most commonly used local anesthetic. However, it is more rapidly absorbed from the injection site and thus results in higher plasma concentrations than ropivacaine does.[55] At the present time, 0.5% ropivacaine or levobupivacaine appears to be the more appropriate local anesthetic solution to perform the blocks. Both drugs combine rapid onset of anesthesia and prolonged (i.e., up to 12 hours) postoperative analgesia.[56] The addition of clonidine[57] offers no advantage over plain local anesthetic solution.

TECHNIQUE

ILIOINGUINAL AND ILIOHYPOGASTRIC NERVE BLOCKADE

Classic Approach

The patient lies supine. The landmarks are the umbilicus, the ipsilateral anterior superior iliac spine, and the pubic tubercle (Fig. 55.7). A line is drawn between the anterior superior iliac spine and the umbilicus, and another line is drawn between the anterior superior iliac spine and the pubic tubercle; both lines are divided into three equal segments. On each line, the site of puncture is located at the junction of the lateral and middle thirds. At both puncture sites, a short-beveled needle is inserted at a 50- to 70-degree angle to the skin in an anteroposterior and caudal direction. It is advanced until loss of resistance is felt, which occurs as the aponeurosis of the external oblique muscle is pierced. After negative aspiration, 5 mL of local anesthetic is injected. The needle is then advanced deeper to pierce the internal oblique muscle aponeurosis, and a similar amount of local anesthetic is administered.

Ultrasound-guided Technique

The classic approach can be inaccurate. A failure rate as high as 20% to 30% has been reported. The safety and effectiveness of these blocks can be greatly improved by direct visualization with ultrasonography.[58,59] The ultrasound examination should be performed with a high-frequency linear probe (Fig. 55.8). The II nerve is best visualized immediately medial to the anterior superior iliac spine. It is located at a mean distance of 6 mm from this bony landmark. The IH nerve is close (<1 cm) to the II nerve, and both nerves are located close to the peritoneum. With an out-of-plane approach, the needle is inserted between the obliquus internus abdominis and transversus abdominis muscles. The volume of local anesthetic required to anesthetize both nerves is 0.075 mL/kg in children and 0.2 mL/kg in adults,[59] doses much smaller than those recommended with the "blind" technique. The ultrasound-guided technique resulted in a 96% success rate[58,59] and significantly reduced the risk for complications such as intestinal puncture.

GENITOFEMORAL NERVE BLOCKADE

With the patient in the supine position, the following landmarks are identified: the pubic tubercle, inguinal ligament, inguinal crease, and femoral artery. The femoral branch of the nerve is blocked by inserting the needle at the lateral border of the femoral artery in the inguinal crease. A fan-like infiltration of the subcutaneous tissue with 10 to 15 mL of local anesthetic solution is performed in a medial, caudal, and cephalad direction. The genital branch of the nerve is blocked by infiltration of 10 mL of local anesthetic just lateral to the pubic tubercle, below the inguinal ligament.

COMPLICATIONS

Transient femoral nerve palsy,[60,61] pelvic[62] or bowel[63] hematoma, and small bowel[64] or colonic puncture have been described mainly with the blind techniques. These complications can be avoided when an ultrasound-guided technique is performed. However, additional large-scales studies are required to confirm the safety of such techniques.

RECTUS SHEATH BLOCKADE

ANATOMY

The umbilical area is innervated by the 10th right and left intercostal nerves. Each nerve passes between the transverse abdominal and internal oblique muscles. It runs between the sheath and the posterior wall of the rectus abdominis muscle and ends as the anterior cutaneous branch supplying the skin of the umbilical area. The rectus abdominis muscles extend between the xiphoid and the pubic tubercle. The nerves are enclosed in the rectus sheath, which is formed by the aponeurosis of the external and internal oblique and the transverse muscles.

INDICATIONS, CONTRAINDICATIONS, AND DRUGS

The limited area of anesthesia and analgesia that rectus sheath blockade provides (midline to the linea semilunaris) makes it inadequate as the sole technique for surgery. It is generally used in combination with general anesthesia for surgery around the umbilicus (umbilical hernia) and for upper abdominal midline incisions. More recently, it has been used for midline incisions above and below the umbilicus and for postoperative analgesia as part of an enhanced postoperative recovery technique consisting of the use of indwelling local anaesthetic catheters.[65] Because of crossover innervation, bilateral blocks need to be performed in all patients. However, unilateral injections may be performed as part of management of chronic pain syndromes in adults and children.

A rectus sheath block is indicated as an analgesic technique after umbilical or epigastric hernia repair.[66] It has been noted to decrease pain after laparoscopy and midline laparotomy.[67] Local infection is a specific contraindication.

Bupivacaine has been the most commonly used local anesthetic. Less cardiotoxic drugs such as 0.5% ropivacaine or levobupivacaine are effective alternatives, particularly when high doses are used.

TECHNIQUE

CLASSIC APPROACH

The aim of the block is to inject the local anesthetic solution between the muscle and the posterior aspect of the rectus sheath. The needle is inserted 0.5 cm medial to the linea semilunaris in a perpendicular plane, just above or below the umbilicus (Fig. 55.9). The anterior rectus sheath is identified by moving the needle in a back-and-forth motion until a "pop" is felt. The rectus sheath and the belly of the muscle are entered. The needle is then advanced further up to the posterior aspect of the rectus sheath. After a negative aspiration test for blood, 10 to 15 mL of local anesthetic is injected on each side.

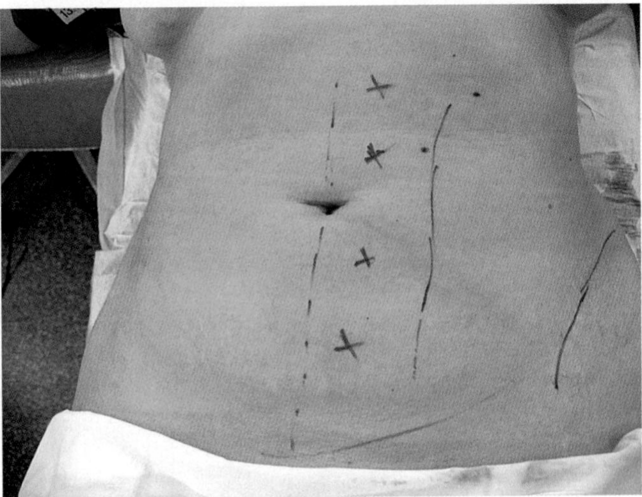

Figure 55.9 Landmarks for a rectus sheath block.

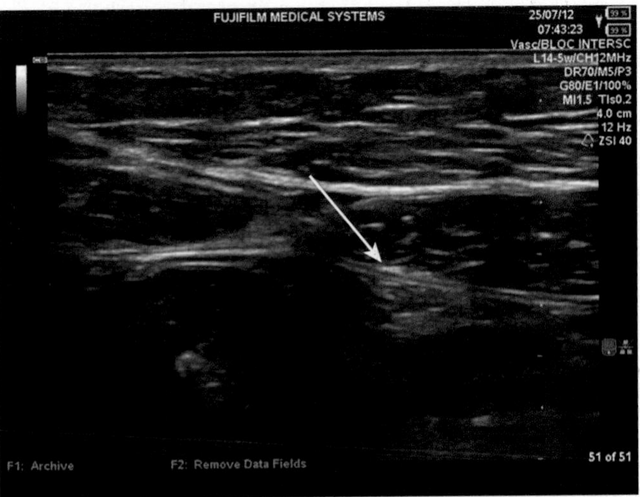

Figure 55.10 Sonographic anatomy for a rectus sheath block (arrow).

ULTRASOUND GUIDED TECHNIQUE

An ultrasound-guided technique has recently been described (Fig. 55.10) and appears to be beneficial, especially in children, in whom the depth of the posterior rectus sheath is unpredictable. It provides a high success rate with few complications. Dolan and colleagues[68] reported that the incidence of accidental intraperitoneal injection of local anesthetic during a blind rectus sheath block is as high as 20.9%, as opposed to 0% with an ultrasound-guided approach.

COMPLICATIONS

Intravascular injection is a potential complication. A case of retroperitoneal hematoma has recently been reported.[69]

TRANSVERSE ABDOMINAL PLANE BLOCK

This technique allows placement of local anesthetic in the abdominal neurovascular plane at the level of the lumbar triangle. The inferior lumbar triangle of Petit is a triangular area located at the posteroinferior part of the lower abdominal wall. It is limited anteriorly by the posterior border of the external oblique muscle and posteriorly by the lateral border of the latissimus dorsi muscle, with the internal oblique and transversus abdominis muscles as the floor. Deep to the transversus abdominis muscle is the parietal peritoneum. It separates the floor of the triangle from the peritoneal cavity. The transverse abdominal plane block was first described in 2001 by Rafi[70] as an abdominal field block performed with the use of superficial landmarks and a loss-of-resistance technique.

INDICATIONS

This block has been used as postoperative analgesia for most abdominal surgical procedures, bilaterally for midline surgery or unilaterally for unilateral surgery. A catheter technique has recently been advocated for prolonged postoperative analgesia after cesarean section,[71] colectomy, open prostatectomy, or abdominal hysterectomy.[72]

TECHNIQUE

BLIND TECHNIQUE

The triangle of Petit is identified by palpation. While standing opposite the operated site, the crest of the ileum is identified at the midaxillary line. The finger is moved posteriorly and a gap is felt in the musculature of the lateral abdominal wall. A 22- or 24-gauge, 50-mm blunt needle is inserted perpendicular to the skin, approximately 1 to 2 cm above the iliac crest, toward the apex of the triangle. Two distinct pops (loss of resistance) are felt. After negative aspiration, 15 to 20 mL of local anesthetic is injected.

ULTRASOUND-GUIDED TECHNIQUE

Ultrasound allows direct visualization of the external oblique, internal oblique, and transverse abdominal muscles, thus allowing accurate placement of the local anesthetic solution within the relevant plane (i.e., between the internal oblique and transverse abdominal muscles). Two ultrasound approaches have been described.

Midaxillary Approach[73]

A high-frequency linear probe (small adults and children) or a low-frequency curvilinear probe (large adults, obesity) is placed transversely on the abdomen at the midline just below the umbilicus. The rectus abdominis muscle is then identified. Moving the probe laterally, the three abdominal muscles (external and internal obliques and transverse abdominal) are identified in a superficial-to-deep direction (Fig. 55.11). The probe is positioned posterior to the midaxillary line midway between the rib cage and the iliac crest, a point where the three muscle layers can easily be delineated. Using either an in-plane or an out-of-plane approach, a 22-gauge, 50- to 100-mm needle is inserted. The tip of the needle is placed between the internal oblique and transverse abdominal muscles, and its position is confirmed by hydrolocation. Fifteen to 20 mL of the local anesthetic solution is injected; separation of the two muscular layers confirms correct placement of the tip of the needle.

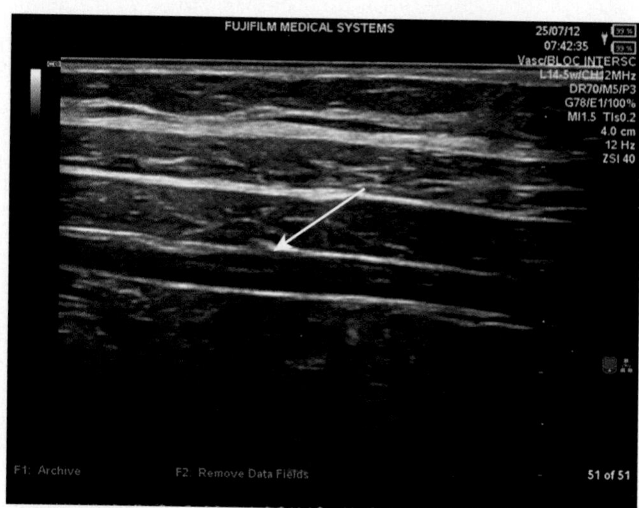

Figure 55.11 Sonographic anatomy for a transversus abdominis plane block (arrow).

Subcostal Approach[74]

The probe is placed transversely in the midline just below the sternum and moved laterally along the lower border of the ribs. The rectus muscle and then the three abdominal muscles (external and internal obliques and transverse abdominal) are identified. A 50- to 100-mm needle is inserted in a medial-to-lateral direction in an in-plane approach. This technique is specifically used for upper abdominal and subcostal incisions.

KEY POINTS

- A paravertebral block provides excellent pain relief after thoracotomy and major breast surgery. A continuous catheter technique could be used in this setting. The incidence of side effects and complications remain low when compared with thoracic epidural analgesia.
- Intercostal blocks are effective in relieving pain after unilateral thoracic or abdominal surgery. However, the need to block multiple intercostal nerves limits their wider use in clinical practice.
- Minor blocks such as ilioinguinal, iliohypogastric, and rectus sheath blocks are very helpful in managing postoperative pain after ambulatory procedures, such as inguinal or umbilical hernia repair. These blocks have a low incidence of complications and side effects.
- A transversus abdominis plane block is considered an effective alternative to epidural analgesia after major abdominal surgery. It is easy to perform under ultrasound guidance, is very effective, and has a better safety profile than epidural analgesia does.

SUGGESTED READINGS

Boezaart AP, Raw RM. Continuous thoracic paravertebral block for major breast surgery. *Reg Anesth Pain Med.* 2006;31:470-476.

Davies RG, Myles PS, Graham JM. A comparison of the analgesic efficacy and side-effects of paravertebral vs epidural blockade for thoracotomy—a systematic review and meta-analysis of randomized trials. *Br J Anaesth.* 2006;96:418-426.

Dolan J, Lucie P, Geary T, et al. The rectus sheath block: accuracy of local anesthetic placement by trainee anesthesiologists using the loss of resistance or ultrasound guidance. *Reg Anesth Pain Med.* 2009;34:247-250.

Eichenberger U, Greher M, Kirchmair L, et al. Ultrasound guided blocks of the ilioinguinal and iliohypogastric nerve: accuracy of a selective new technique confirmed by anatomical dissection. *Br J Anaesth.* 2006;97:238-243.

Karmakar MK, Chung DC. Variability of a thoracic paravertebral block: are we ignoring the endothoracic fascia? *Reg Anesth Pain Med.* 2000;25:325-327.

Luyet C, Eichenberger U, Greif R, et al. Ultrasound-guided paravertebral puncture and placement of catheters in human cadavers: an imaging study. *Br J Anaesth.* 2009;102:534-539.

McDonnell JG, O'Donnell BD, Curley G, et al. The analgesic efficacy of transversus abdominus plane block after abdominal surgery: a prospective randomized controlled trial. *Anesth Analg.* 2007;104:193-197.

Naja MZ, Ziade MF, El Rajab M, et al. Varying anatomical injection points within the thoracic paravertebral space: effect on spread of solution and nerve blockade. *Anaesthesia.* 2004;59:459-463.

Naja MZ, Gustafsson AC, Ziade MF, et al. Distance between the skin and the thoracic paravertebral space. *Anaesthesia.* 2005;60:680-684.

O'Riain SC, Donnell BO, Cuffe T, et al. Thoracic paravertebral block using real-time ultrasound guidance. *Anesth Analg.* 2010;110:248-251.

Willschke H, Marhofer P, Bösenberg A, et al. Ultrasonography for ilioinguinal/iliohypogastric nerve blocks in children. *Br J Anaesth.* 2005;95:226-230.

The references for this chapter can be found at www.expertconsult.com.

56

Peripheral and Visceral Sympathetic Blocks

Michael Gofeld | Hariharan Shankar

CERVICAL SYMPATHETIC (STELLATE GANGLION) BLOCK

Stellate ganglion block (SGB) was originally introduced by René Leriche for the treatment of angina pectoris. Findley and Patzer eventually modified the technique, which has remained largely unchanged since then and was named the anterior approach.[1] This method is the most popular technique in North America. In addition, lateral, superolateral, and posterior approaches were introduced in the first half of the 20th century.[1] All techniques are based on bony landmarks, such as the transverse process of C6, the spinous process of C7, and the first rib. Eventually, these techniques were empirically validated with fluoroscopy and computed tomography (CT) and later with ultrasonography.

CLINICALLY RELEVANT ANATOMY

The stellate ganglion, also known as the cervicothoracic ganglion, represents a fusion of the inferior cervical and first thoracic ganglia of the sympathetic trunk. It can be found in about 80% of the population. The anatomy and position of the stellate ganglion have been investigated by dissection, magnetic resonance imaging (MRI), and CT.[2-6] It is usually situated at the lateral border of the longus colli muscle (LCM) anterior to the neck of the first rib (Fig. 56.1). It lies posterior to the vertebral vessels and is separated from the cervical pleura by the suprapleural membrane inferiorly. The stellate ganglion measures 1 to 2.5 cm in length, is about 1 cm wide and 0.5 cm thick, and may be fusiform, triangular, or globular in shape.[5]

INDICATIONS

SGB is commonly used for the diagnosis and management of sympathetically mediated pain and vascular insufficiency of the upper extremity. In addition, more esoteric indications that have been advocated include the treatment of a variety of medical conditions, such as phantom pain, post-herpetic neuralgia, cancer pain, cardiac arrhythmias, orofacial pain, and vascular headache.[7] Recently, cervical sympathetic blockade has been suggested as an effective method for prevention and treatment of cerebral vasospasm, hot facial flushes, and post-traumatic stress disorder.[8-10]

EVIDENCE FOR STELLATE GANGLION BLOCK

Clinical effectiveness of SGB can be defined as undetermined. The majority of publications are case reports and case series. Neurolytic SGB is currently rarely practiced because the evidence is anecdotal. Malmqvist and colleagues assessed 54 SGBs performed blindly with bupivacaine. Their criteria for effective sympathetic blockade included Horner's syndrome in combination with increased skin temperature, increased skin blood flow, and a completely abolished skin resistance response on both the radial and ulnar sides of the blocked hand. Only 15 of 54 blocks met four of the five criteria for an effective block.[11] Another study examined the efficacy of SGB in patients with complex regional pain syndrome (CRPS) type 1. Pain relief and improved skin perfusion were observed in 40% of patients who had CRPS symptoms for 12 or fewer weeks, but no improvement occurred in the group with more protracted disease (35.8 ± 27 weeks).[12] Two small pilot studies suggested that SGB can provide relief from hot flushes and sleep dysfunction with few or no side effects in survivors of breast cancer and post-traumatic stress disorder.[9,10]

No clinical studies have compared a "blind" with fluoroscopy-guided SGB or fluoroscopy-guided with ultrasound-guided SGB. According to a study that evaluated the oblique and anterior paratracheal fluoroscopic approaches, both techniques were equally effective. However, improved safety and better satisfaction were reported with the former approach.[13] Comparison of an ultrasound-guided with a surface landmark–based technique showed that less volume of local anesthetic was used with ultrasound-guided injection (5 vs. 8 mL). Hematoma did not develop in the ultrasound group, but it did develop after the procedure in three patients in the blind injection group. Ultrasound guidance resulted in more rapid onset of Horner's syndrome.[14]

AVAILABLE TECHNIQUES

Although a C7 approach to the stellate ganglion has been described,[13] SGB is still routinely performed at the C6 level by using the following anatomic landmarks: prominent anterior tubercle of the transverse process (Chassaignac's tubercle) and cricoid cartilage, both of which facilitate identification of the level and finally the location of the carotid artery.[2] Given that only traversing sympathetic fibers or middle cervical ganglia can be found at the C6 level,[15] the procedure should more accurately be called a cervical sympathetic block. The middle cervical ganglion or traversing sympathetic fibers are located anterolateral to the belly of the LCM.[15] Conceivably, such a "convenient" location makes it easy to access the sympathetic chain for either diagnostic or therapeutic blockade.

Cervical sympathetic block is traditionally performed as a "blind" injection via the anterior approach. It is accomplished

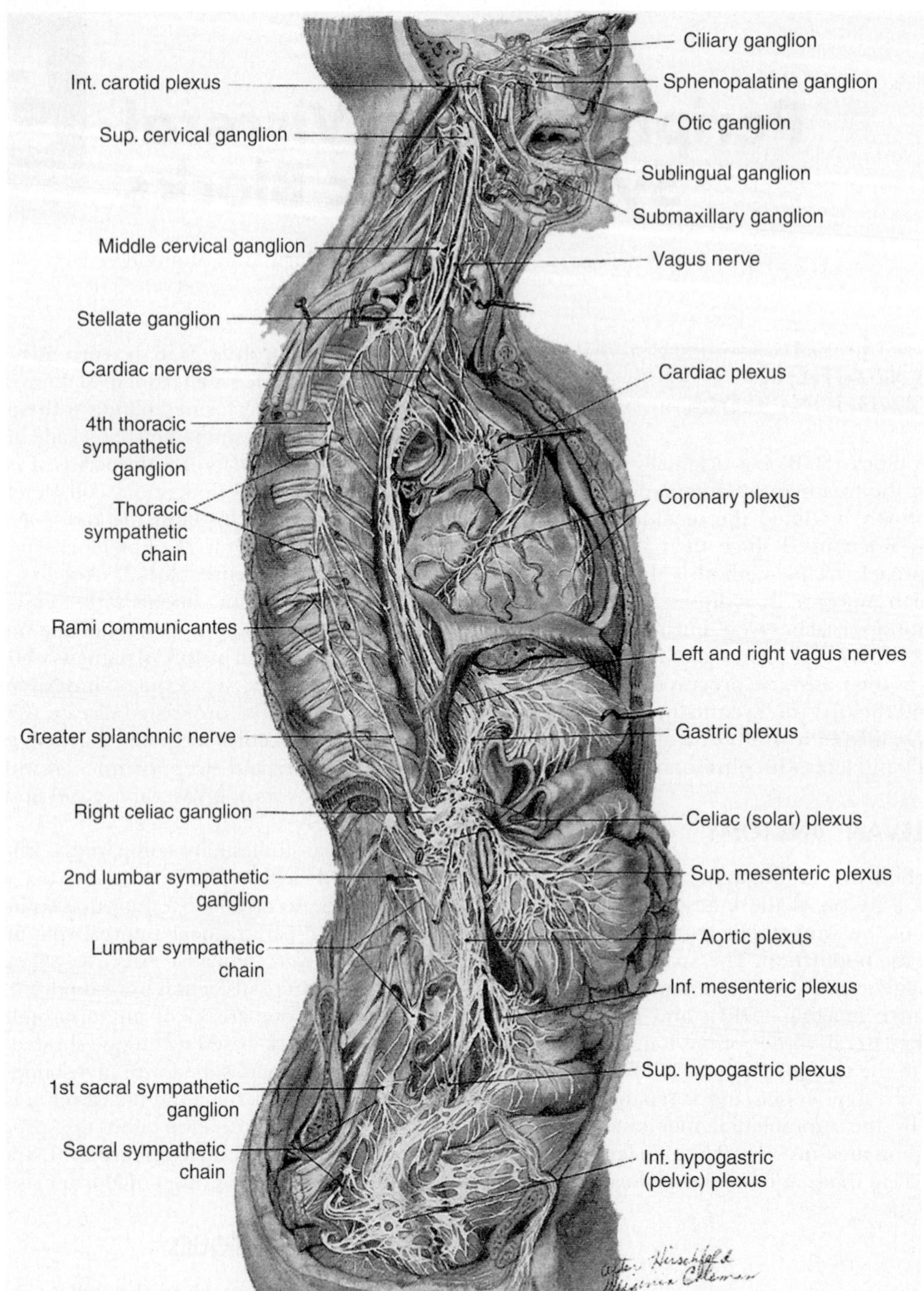

Figure 56.1 The peripheral autonomic nervous system. (From Bonica JJ. *The Management of Pain*. Philadelphia: Lea & Febiger; 1953.)

by positioning the patient supine with the head rotated to the opposite side. Following palpation of the anterior tubercle of the C6 transverse process (Chassaignac's tubercle), the carotid artery is gently retracted laterally. The needle is then inserted paratracheally until it contacts bone, presumably the lateral part of the vertebral body (Fig. 56.2). The needle is then withdrawn 1 to 5 mm, and the medication is injected. This maneuver was presumed to be sufficient to position the needle outside the LCM, where the sympathetic ganglion is likely to be situated.

Fluoroscopic guidance reduces the overall risks associated with the "blind" technique. It has the advantage of identifying the bony anatomy, although the anatomic position of the cervical sympathetic trunk (CST) is confined to the soft tissues (LCM, thyroid, and esophagus) rather than to the cervical vertebrae. Injection of a contrast dye helps to confirm the procedural accuracy, although it may show aberrant and inconsistent spread. Such injection will, however, significantly decrease, if not eliminate the risk for intravascular injection. Typically, fluoroscopically guided SGB is performed similar to the blind technique just described. A coaxial anteroposterior view is used to direct the block needle toward the anterior base of either the C6 or C7 transverse process. Alternatively, the injection can be

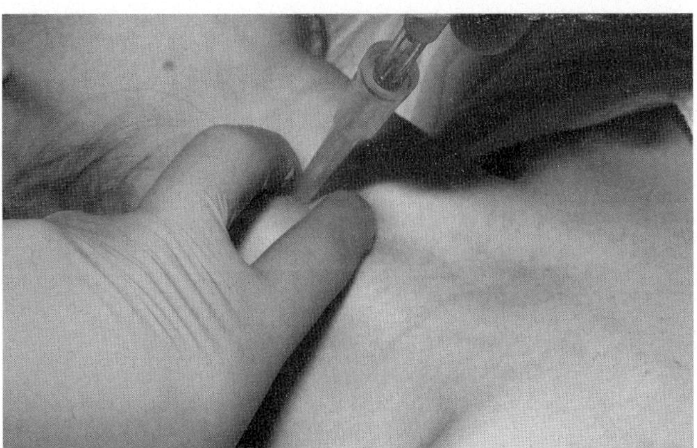

Figure 56.2 Two fingers are placed lateral to the cricoid cartilage to gently displace the carotid artery laterally and palpate Chassaignac's tubercle. The needle is inserted between the fingers and directed to the tubercle.

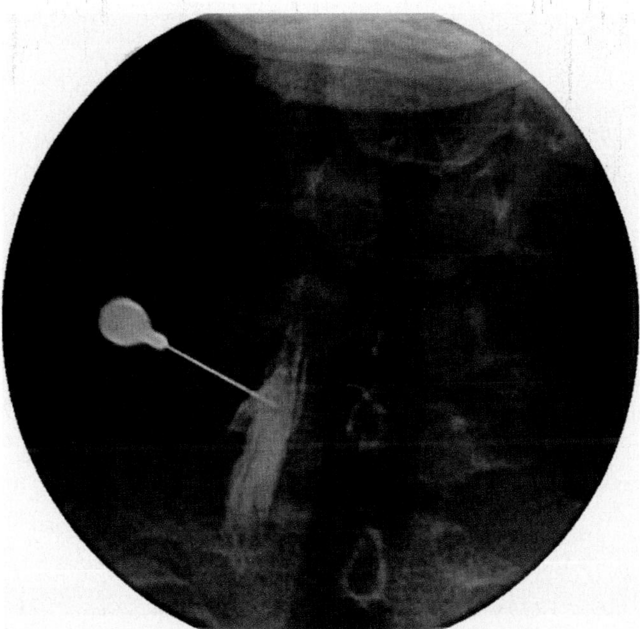

Figure 56.3 Anteroposterior fluoroscopy shows a block needle placed at the anterior base of the C6 transverse process. Injected contrast material is seen within the longus colli muscle.

performed via an oblique fluoroscopic view (Fig. 56.3).[13] Most likely, neither "blind" nor fluoroscopically guided injection can ensure reliable results. Since the ultimate thickness of the LCM remains unknown, the contrast dye and subsequently the local anesthetic are injected into the muscle and then reach the sympathetic trunk by overflow or diffusion.

Several clinical and cadaver trials have been conducted in an attempt to elucidate the pattern of spread when solutions are injected at the C6 level.[6,16-19] The results of these studies have been conflicting, probably because of differences in study design: cadavers or live subjects, low or high volume of injectant, and CT or fluoroscopy control. The results of one cadaver study suggested that deposition of a solution only into the prevertebral "interlaminar space" provides reliable spread to the stellate ganglion.[18] The cervical prevertebral fascia is attached to the base of the skull and extends over the prevertebral muscles (longus capitis, rectus capitis, and longus colli) to the T4 vertebra, just beyond the LCM. This positioning of the fascia forms a plane along which the injected fluid can flow.

Although some anatomic and imaging studies indicate a subfascial position,[15,19] textbooks allocate the path of the CST to the suprafascial plane.[3,20] Two recently published studies have hopefully resolved this issue. The first used cadaver dissection and human MRI and showed a subfascial position of the stellate ganglion. This study found the thickness of the LCM to be highly variable, which may lead to negative block results.[21] The second study was designed as a step-by-step methodology to validate a new ultrasound-guided approach (described below); a subfascial position of the sympathetic trunk was detected by three-dimensional ultrasonography and confirmed by cadaver dissection. In addition, this study measured the thickness of the LCM at the C6 level and proved that the muscle is 2 to 10 times thicker than was previously suggested in the regional anesthesia literature. Accordingly, routine injection by the traditional method would have resulted in an intramuscular injection, and the CST would be anesthetized only by overflow or diffusion of the injectant.[22]

Ultrasound guidance is a logical solution to ensure accurate injection when soft tissues are involved. Clear imaging of the muscles, fasciae, blood vessels, viscera, and bone surface makes ultrasonography superior to fluoroscopy for image-guided CST blockade. In 1995 Kapral and coworkers[14] described an ultrasound-guided anterior technique and published the results of a case series.

The patient is placed in the supine position. A pillow can be placed under the lower part of the neck to achieve some extension. The head may be rotated slightly contralateral to the injection side to increase the distance between the carotid artery and the trachea and improve the sonographic view. Ultrasonography of the anterior part of the neck is performed by initially placing the transducer at the level of the cricoid cartilage, anterior to the sternocleidomastoid muscle. Short-axis ultrasonography reveals the typical appearance of the C6 transverse process: a prominent anterior tubercle, a short posterior tubercle, and the exiting C6 nerve root (Fig. 56.4). Scanning caudally and dorsally brings the C7 transverse process into view. The C7 transverse process has no anterior tubercle. The C7 nerve root is situated just anterior to the posterior tubercle (Fig. 56.5). At the C6 level, the LCM is seen as an oval structure adjacent to the base of the transverse process and vertebral body. Sometimes the caudal portion of the longus capitis muscle can be seen as well. The CST is visualized as a spindle-shaped structure (the midcervical ganglion) and is typically situated on the posterolateral surface of the LCM. If the CST cannot be identified, some widening of the tissue plane below the prevertebral fascia can usually be seen. Once the correct level for injection is localized, the surrounding anatomic structures should be identified and the feasibility of the "anterior" approach determined. Frequently, the distance between the carotid artery and the trachea is wide enough, and therefore only thyroid tissue and superficial neck muscles are seen between the needle entry point and the surface of the LCM. Gentle pressure may actually decrease the skin-to-target distance and further separate the carotid artery from the trachea. Additional scanning should be performed to confirm

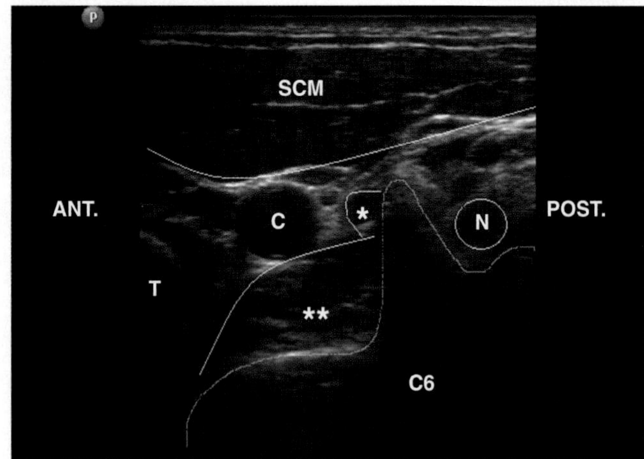

Figure 56.4 Short-axis view at the C6 level. Asterisk, longus capitis muscle; two asterisks, longus colli muscle; C, carotid artery; C6, sixth cervical vertebra with a prominent anterior tubercle. N, C6 nerve root; SCM, sternocleidomastoid muscle; T, trachea.

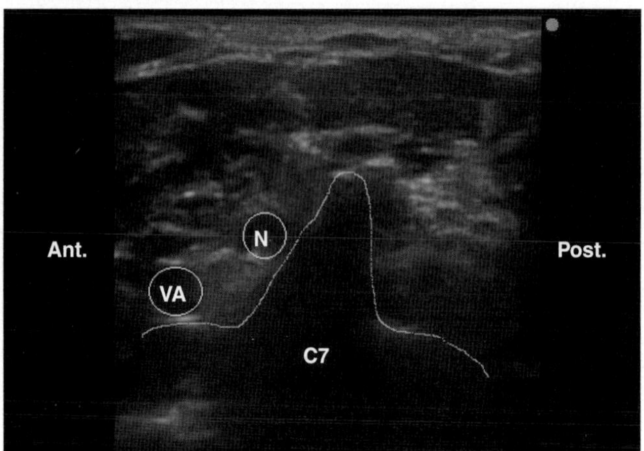

Figure 56.5 Short-axis view at the C7 level. C7, seventh cervical vertebra with only one tubercle; N, C7 nerve root; VA, vertebral artery.

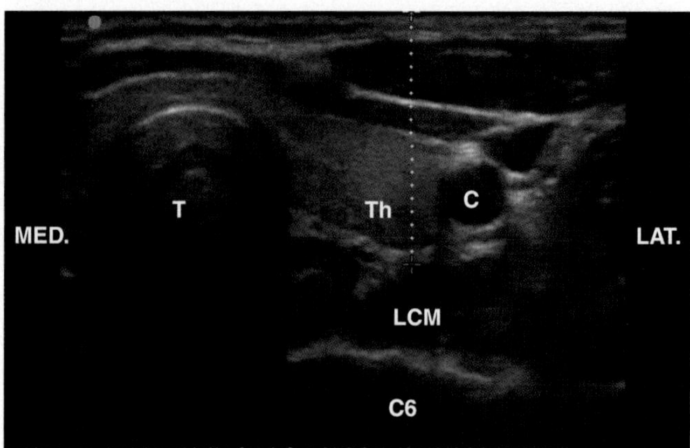

Figure 56.6 Anterior ultrasound-guided approach. The dotted line represents the needle trajectory; it is trespassing through the thyroid (Th). C, carotid artery; C6, sixth cervical vertebra; LCM, longus colli muscle; T, trachea.

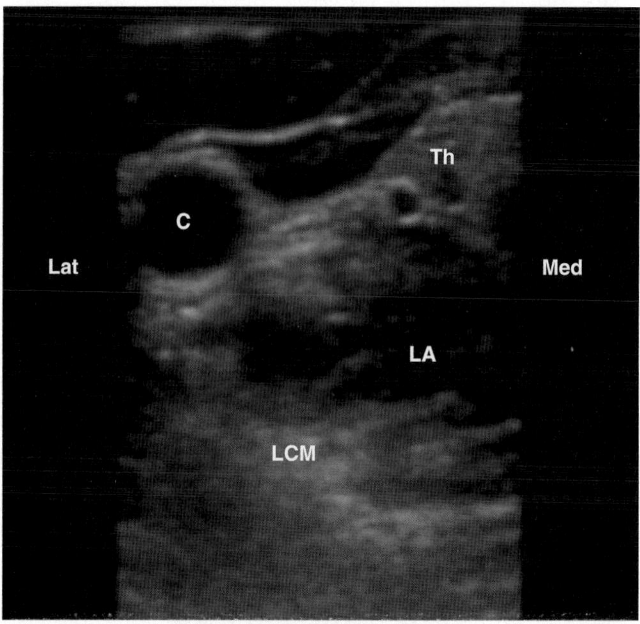

Figure 56.7 Injection of local anesthetic (LA) produced an anechoic signal. After injection, the longus colli muscle (LCM) appears hyperechoic. C, carotid artery; Th, thyroid.

that the inferior thyroid artery is not seen immediately caudad. The injection is performed in a short-axis, out-of-plane approach (Fig. 56.6). The skin is anesthetized immediately caudad or cephalad to the transducer. The injection is performed with a spinal needle (22 to 25 gauge and 2 to 3.5 inches long), three-way stopcock, and extension tubing connecting two syringes, one with 0.9% NaCl and the other with local anesthetic. The needle is inserted under continuous ultrasound guidance and directed to the anterior surface of the LCM via a short-axis, out-of-plane approach. When the tip of the needle is visualized, either directly or indirectly (tissue movement) as the target is approached, 1 to 2 mL of saline is injected to confirm placement of the needle under the prevertebral fascia and facilitate clear separation of the tissue planes (Fig. 56.7). If the injectant is observed above the fascia or within the muscle, the needle must be carefully repositioned. If the spread is appropriate, 5 mL of local anesthetic is injected and the needle is withdrawn.

A lateral approach has recently been described and validated.[22] The patient is placed in the lateral decubitus position with the side to be treated uppermost. Preparation and ultrasonography are performed as described previously. The ultrasound transducer is centered on the C6 transverse process and not the anterior aspect of the neck. With the transducer placed as shown in Figure 56.6, only the anterior tubercle of the C6 transverse process is visible adjacent to the projected entry point of the needle, and no visceral or neural elements are present between the entry site and the anterolateral surface of the LCM. The needle track should be entirely intramuscular and pass through the sternocleidomastoid muscle, the anterior scalene muscle, or both. Occasionally, the internal jugular vein is seen within the projected needle track, but it can readily be collapsed by placing light pressure on the transducer.

Skin anesthesia is performed immediately posterior to the ultrasound transducer. Under continuous ultrasound guidance, the needle is inserted via a short-axis, in-plane technique (Fig. 56.8). The advantage of the lateral approach, in addition to avoiding trespassing through the thyroid, is

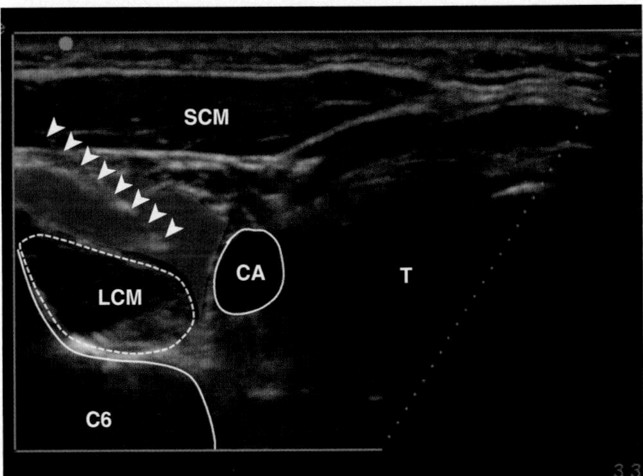

Figure 56.8 Lateral ultrasound-guided approach. The needle (arrowheads) is placed under the prevertebral fascia. Local anesthetic (semitransparent figure) spread superficially to the longus colli muscle (LCM) and posteriorly to the carotid artery (CA). C6, sixth cervical vertebra; SCM, sternocleidomastoid muscle; T, trachea.

totally controllable, visible progression of the needle from the skin entry point to the target. Verification of needle position and performance of the rest of the procedure are the same as for the anterior approach.

Injection of 5 mL of a local anesthetic typically results in C3-T1 prevertebral spread and complete blockade of the CST and stellate ganglion. If anesthetic blockade of the upper cervical ganglion is not desirable, it would be prudent to limit the volume of injectant to 3 mL.

COMPLICATIONS

Blind paratracheal injection produces unreliable results and is associated with a variety of side effects and complications, such as intravascular injection, formation of hematomas, temporary paralysis of the recurrent laryngeal nerve, diskitis, and esophageal injury.[7,14,23-26] Narouze and associates further emphasized the risks inherent with a blind approach[25] by pointing out that blind injection at the C6 level on the left side may cause inadvertent esophageal puncture or may traverse the thyroid. Hematoma formation is probably related to damage to the inferior thyroid artery.

Fluoroscopic guidance may prevent adverse outcomes related to intravascular, nerve root, or neuraxial injection. However, visualization of the soft tissue, vessels, and cervical sympathetic ganglia makes guidance with ultrasound superior to fluoroscopic guidance. Subfascial injection of 5 mL of an injectant reliably produces cervical sympathetic blockade. Ultrasound guidance may prevent the complications and adverse outcomes associated with either blind or fluoroscopically guided techniques.

CELIAC PLEXUS BLOCK

Max Kappis has frequently been cited as the person who developed the technique of celiac plexus block (CPB).[27] However, he never described this technique. Kappis showed that pain from the upper abdominal organs is conducted via the splanchnic nerves and that experimental abdominal pain can be relieved by infiltration of the splanchnic nerves with procaine from the back. Theoretically, this was not a CPB but a splanchnic nerve block. Perhaps it was John Bonica who described the technique that is currently named percutaneous transcrural CPB.[28] Both surface landmark–based and fluoroscopically guided approaches were described in this seminal work. He also advocated the use of neurolytic celiac plexus block (NCPB) with alcohol for palliation of pain related to abdominal malignancies, although it was Bridenbaugh and associates who published their experience in the peer-reviewed literature.[29]

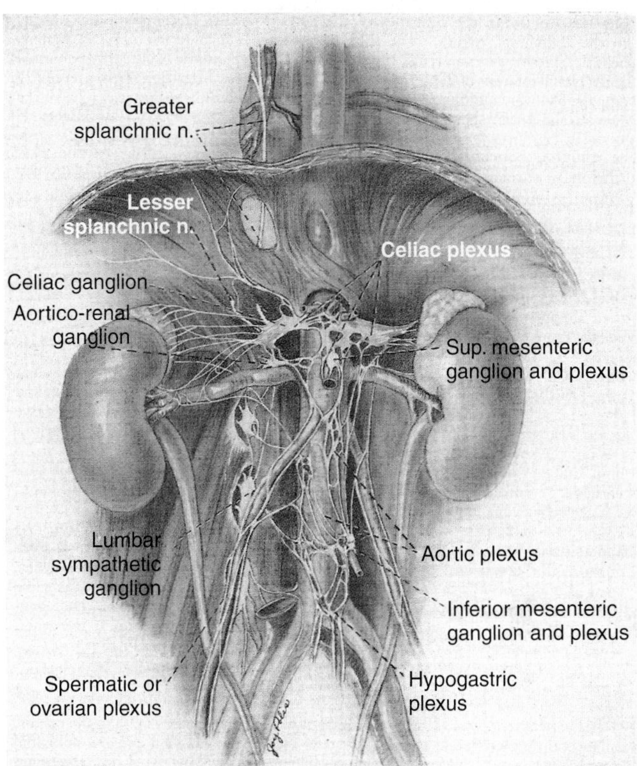

Figure 56.9 Celiac plexus anatomy (From Bonica JJ. *The Management of Pain*. Philadelphia: Lea & Febiger; 1953.)

CLINICALLY RELEVANT ANATOMY

Innervation of the viscera originates from the T5 to T11 spinal segments, with occasional contribution of the T4 and T12 preganglionic fibers. They do not synapse in the sympathetic chain but rather pass through the chain to synapse at distal locations (i.e., the celiac, renal, and superior mesenteric ganglia). The T5 to T9 preganglionic fibers coalesce to form the greater splanchnic nerve; T10 and T11 constitute the lesser and T12 the least splanchnic nerves.[30]

Efferent fibers of the splanchnic nerves end up in the celiac plexus. Located approximately at the level of T12 or L1, or both, the celiac plexus is composed of several celiac ganglia that surround the celiac trunk and the superior mesenteric artery at its root.[31] It is located in front of the aorta and the crus of the diaphragm and posterior to the stomach and omental bursa (Fig. 56.9). The plexus in turn supplies the various upper abdominal viscera through multiple smaller plexuses and nerve fibers. These viscera include the diaphragm, liver, stomach, spleen, suprarenal glands, kidneys, ovaries and testes, small intestine, and colon up to the splenic flexure. The celiac plexus also sends branches to the superior and inferior mesenteric plexuses. In addition, the plexus receives parasympathetic supply from the vagus. The sensory (afferent) fibers do not synapse in the plexus but rather traverse it and ascend to spinal levels through the splanchnic nerves.

EVIDENCE FOR CELIAC PLEXUS BLOCK

Multiple clinical studies have demonstrated level I efficacy of NCPB as a minimally invasive modality for managing cancer-related pain. Bridenbaugh and colleagues performed 41 CPBs in which 50 mL of a 50% alcohol solution was used. It was effective in 40 patients and had no significant side effects.[29] Ischia and coworkers compared three common techniques in a randomized controlled fashion and found that all approaches were equally effective and abolished cancer pain in 70% to 80% of patients immediately after the block and in 60% to 75% until death.[32] Several large-scale randomized controlled trials were published and unequivocally demonstrated superiority of CPB over oral opioid therapy.[33-35] In addition, one demonstrated improved survival.[34] Finally a meta-analysis suggested that (1) NCPB produces long-lasting benefit in 70% to 90% of patients with pancreatic and other intra-abdominal cancers regardless of the technique used, (2) adverse effects are common but transient and mild, and (3) severe adverse effects are uncommon.[36] CPB was somewhat efficacious in managing nonmalignant pain, such as chronic pancreatitis.[37,38] A recent randomized, controlled study showed that in patients with critical illness, CPB was effective in treating feeding intolerance when intravenous drug therapy had failed to improve gastrointestinal dysfunction.[39]

INDICATIONS

Major causes of visceral pain include functional gastrointestinal disorders, abdominal malignancies, and chronic pancreatitis. NCPB is indicated for the management of pain related to cancer of the pancreas, stomach, duodenum, and proximal part of the small bowel. In addition, metastatic tumors in the lymph nodes may cause similar pain and might be amenable to NCPB. In the case of benign conditions, analgesic prognostic CPB is performed and may be repeated as needed. Alternatively, if the reduction in pain was significant but lasted only short-term, NCPB may be attempted.

AVAILABLE TECHNIQUES

Surface landmark–based techniques for CPB were introduced in the beginning of the 20th century. Later, fluoroscopic guidance was strongly advocated. Other high-quality and accurate images of fluoroscopically controlled transcrural CPB are presented in Bonica's pivotal book *The Management of Pain*. With the overwhelming recommendation for mandatory use of imaging guidance, such as fluoroscopy, CT, and ultrasonography, these aids became standard features, although only a few studies have directly compared different imaging modalities.[32,37,40,41] A variety of techniques and approaches are described in the literature, including the retrocrural, antecrural, transcrural, transdiscal, and transaortic approaches and splanchnicectomy. Both single-needle and two-needle techniques have been advocated.[42-49] Each technique has its proponents and opponents claiming advantages and disadvantages. The spread of cancer, as seen on CT, may sometimes dictate the approach.[49]

NCPB is usually performed with either 6% to 10% phenol or 50% to 100% alcohol after a diagnostic local anesthetic injection despite a low negative predictive value of the diagnostic block.[32,50]

Anterior and posterior approaches to the plexus have been described.[51] The anterior approach is used intraoperatively or percutaneously with ultrasound guidance. Fluoroscopic- and landmark-based injections approach the plexus posteriorly. CT-guided CPB may be performed through an anterior or posterior approach, although the posterior approach is commonly preferred. CT may provide finer details about the plexus, celiac artery, and neighboring structures, which can facilitate improved safety and better targeting. Fluoroscopy is based solely on skeletal imaging and requires additional aids, such as a loss-of-resistance device and injection of a contrast dye. Open MRI guidance has been reported to result in a 57% success rate for CPB, but this method is definitely time-consuming and costly.[52]

Endoscopic ultrasound–guided CPB has been performed safely with clear visualization of the ganglia, but it frequently relies on a second imaging aid (e.g., radiography). Endoscopic CPB may be more cost-effective than CT-guided CPB.[38] Ultrasound-guided percutaneous CPB may have several benefits when compared with other modalities. It may be performed at the bedside and has no radiation hazards. In addition, the supine position is more comfortable for patients. It allows real-time visualization of spread of the injectant. Its disadvantages include poor visualization of deeper structures, including the pancreas, and interference by air in the intestinal loops. Similar to anterior CT guidance, it may be associated with perforation of the stomach, intestine, pancreas, or liver.

POSTERIOR TRANSCRURAL (CLASSIC) FLUOROSCOPICALLY GUIDED APPROACH

The patient is positioned prone on the fluoroscopic table. Bolsters usually have to be placed under the chest and pelvis to alleviate pressure on the abdomen, which may not be tolerated by patients. Standard monitoring and supplemental oxygen are applied. To prevent a sudden decrease in blood pressure related to visceral vasodilation, 500 mL of an isotonic intravenous fluid is administered. After the usual sterile preparation, thoracolumbar spine fluoroscopy is performed and the L1 vertebra is placed at the center of the scout image. Next, the image intensifier is rotated to an oblique position. The degree of obliquity is usually judged by observing contralateral movement of the spinous process. It has to be aligned with the contralateral facet joint. In addition, a cephalad or caudad tilt is used to "eliminate" the L1 transverse process from view. The radiologic target is the middle of the L1 vertebral body. Local anesthesia is performed and a 20- or 21-gauge Chiba-type needle is inserted and advanced via a coaxial view (Fig. 56.10*A*). The needle has to contact the L1 vertebral body just 1 to 2 mm medial to the lateral bony shadow, or further advancement will be difficult. Some practitioners manually bend

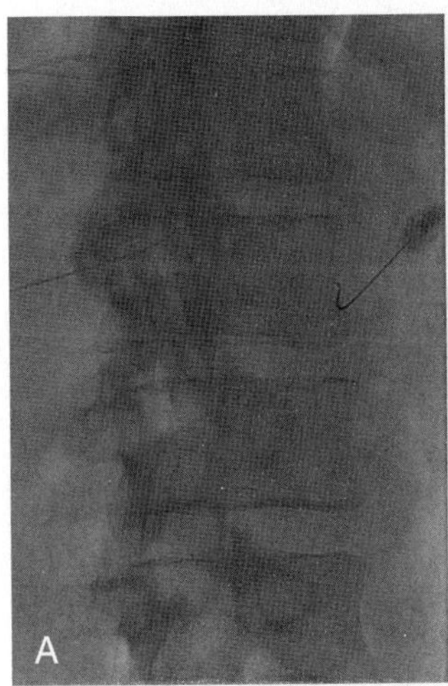

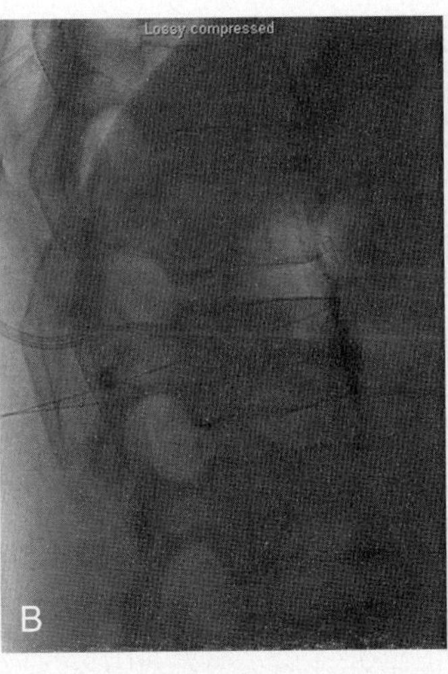

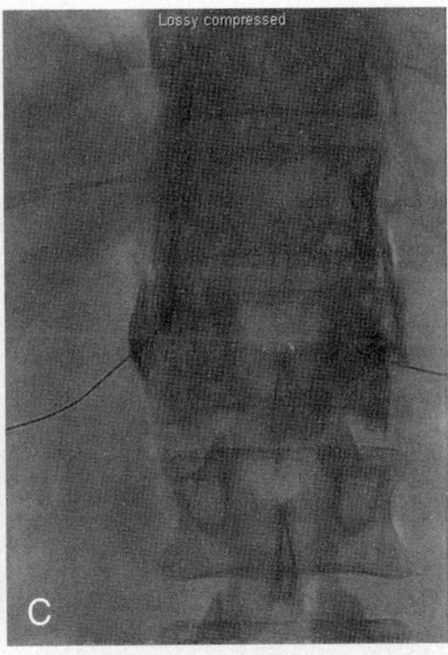

Figure 56.10 Fluoroscopy-guided celiac plexus block. **A,** Chiba needle inserted via the coaxial view on the right. Radiopaque contrast material was injected on the left. **B,** Lateral view showing longitudinal prevertebral spread of contrast agent. **C,** "Honeycomb" appearance of the contrast agent on the anteroposterior view.

the tip of the needle 10 to 15 degrees to improve steering. After the bone has been contacted, the image intensifier is rotated into the lateral position and further needle progress is monitored with this view. It is also advisable to remove the stylet and use a loss-of-resistance devise filled with either 0.9% NaCl or diluted radiopaque contrast dye. Typically, once the needle is advanced about 1 cm past the anterior bony shadow, the resistance drastically decreases and prevertebral/preaortic longitudinal spread of the contrast dye is observed (Fig. 56.10*B*). On the anteroposterior view, a "honeycomb" contrast shadow is seen (Fig. 56.10*C*). The procedure is performed in the same fashion on the contralateral side. If arterial blood is obtained or the injected contrast dye produces an aortogram, the procedure may be converted to a transaortic single-needle technique. In this case, the needle is advanced through the anterior aortic wall and additional contrast dye is injected. Its spread should be confined to the retroperitoneal compartment. Once the needle's position is verified, 5 to 10 mL of a local anesthetic mixed with contrast dye is injected and the patient is closely monitored for signs of intravascular injection or neuraxial blockade. After 3 to 5 minutes, 20 to 40 mL of 50% to 80% alcohol or 6% phenol is injected slowly. Alcohol can be mixed with the contrast dye to further ensure accurate injection.

POSTERIOR TRANSCRURAL (CLASSIC) COMPUTED TOMOGRAPHY–GUIDED APPROACH

Patient position and preparation are similar to the fluoroscopically guided approach.

CT guidance can be facilitated by using a standard planning grid or a three-dimensional reconstruction and cone beam guidance. With the former, CT planning is performed while paying attention to direction and depth. The patient is removed from the scanner and the needle is inserted; a second CT scan is obtained to confirm final needle position. If the placement is satisfactory, either contrast dye is injected and further confirmation with CT or ancillary fluoroscopy is performed or a neurolytic solution is injected slowly (Fig. 56.11). If needle placement is inaccurate, the process is repeated. This method is definitely time-consuming and associated with significant radiation exposure.

A novel cone beam CT procedure uses 50% to 70% less radiation than conventional CT scanners do and combines

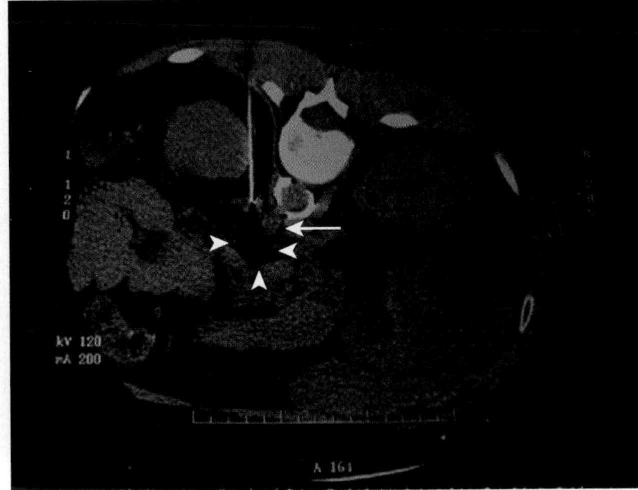

Figure 56.11 Computed tomography–guided celiac plexus block. The needle is positioned adjacent to the aorta and alcohol is injected (the arrowheads are pointing to the black shadow). The arrow indicates the celiac trunk.

the capabilities of CT scanning and fluoroscopy. The procedure is planned with specialized software showing the entry point, direction, and depth of the needle (Fig. 56.12). Next, the procedure is performed with live fluoroscopic guidance overlaid on the CT image. This radiologic method may effectively reduce radiation exposure and minimize procedure time without sacrificing technical accuracy (Fig. 56.13).

TECHNIQUE OF PERCUTANEOUS ULTRASOUND-GUIDED CELIAC PLEXUS BLOCK

With the patient positioned supine, standard monitoring and preparation are performed. Patients may be instructed to control their respiration during the procedure. A low-frequency, curved-array, 3- to 5-MHz transducer is used. The ultrasound scan is performed by starting from the epigastrium and moving caudad to visualize the aorta, vertebral body, and the liver in a transverse view (Fig. 56.14). Once the celiac trunk is localized, color Doppler flow is turned on to verify the vessels. Next, the transducer is turned longitudinally to visualize the celiac trunk and superior mesenteric artery (Fig. 56.15). Color flow Doppler is used to verify the

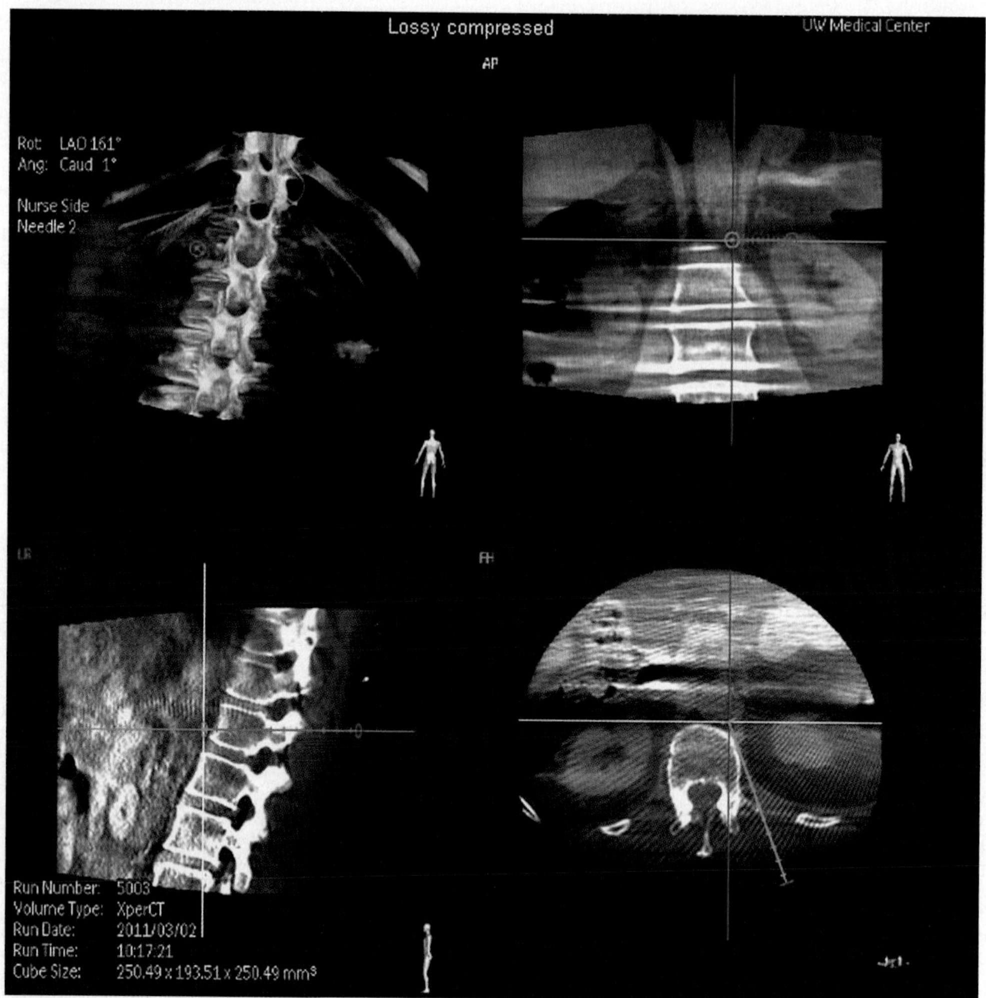

Figure 56.12 Procedural planning with cone beam computed tomography.

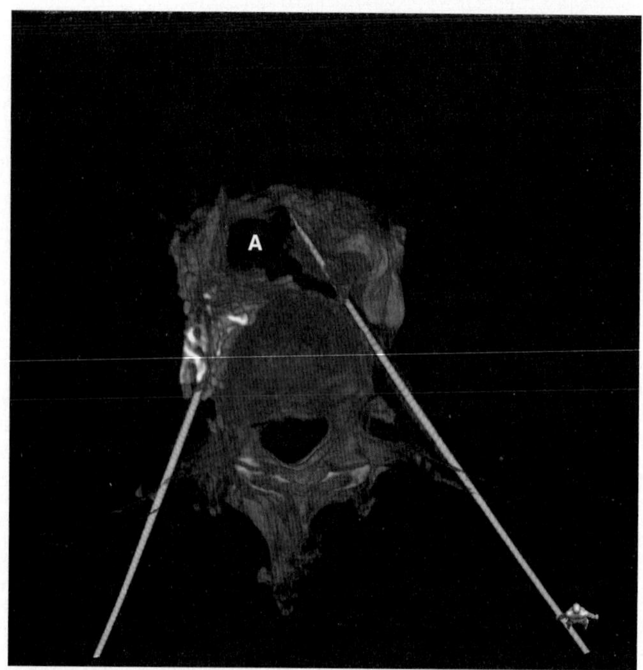

Figure 56.13 Three-dimensional axial reconstruction. A contrast dye encircles the aorta (A).

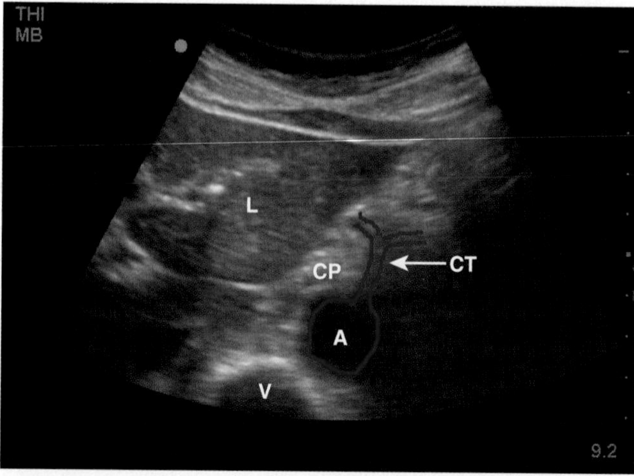

Figure 56.14 Short-axis ultrasound view. A, aorta; CP, celiac plexus; CT, celiac trunk; L, liver; V, L1 vertebral body.

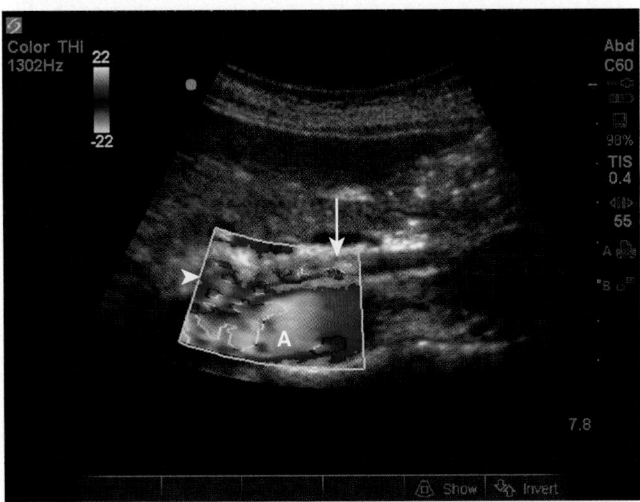

Figure 56.15 Long-axis ultrasound view. A, aorta; arrow, superior mesenteric artery; arrowhead, celiac trunk.

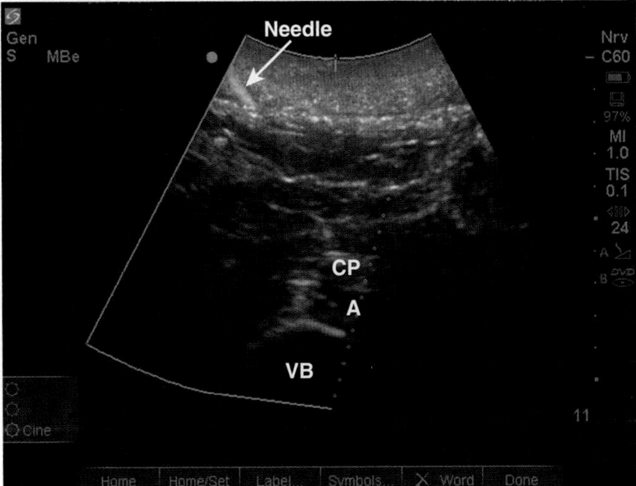

Figure 56.16 Needle inserted in plane in a short-axis view and placed onto the celiac plexus (CP). A, aorta; VB, vertebral body.

vessels. The target is the space between the celiac trunk and the superior mesenteric artery. The tip of the needle may be also positioned cephalad to the celiac trunk to ensure better spread of the neurolytic agent.[53] Deviations in local anatomy related to the malignancy or previous surgery may influence spread of the injectant more than the position of the needle does.

A 22-gauge, 10- to 15-cm Chiba-type needle is advanced to the space between the celiac trunk and the superior mesenteric artery in a longitudinal view. The needle may be advanced in plane or out of plane, depending on the size of the needle, the safest path to the target area, and personal preference of the physician (Fig. 56.16). After negative aspiration, a test dose of 3 mL of 1% lidocaine with epinephrine is injected in real time to rule out any intravascular uptake. Subsequently, real-time injection of the neurolytic agent in 5-mL increments is done. The typical volume of injectant used varies from 10 to 50 mL. The concentrations of alcohol used vary from 50% to 100%. With phenol, the concentration ranges from 6% to 10%. The needle is flushed with 1 mL of local anesthetic at the end of the procedure to flush the needle track of any neurolytic agent remaining.

An alternative two-needle technique has also been described in which the celiac trunk is visualized in a transverse view and the needles are introduced from the lateral sides of the transducer. The authors claim better visualization of the injectant with this approach.[54]

COMPLICATIONS

Side effects such as orthostatic hypotension and transient diarrhea are known to occur in approximately 38% and 44% of patients, respectively. A frequently reported complication is postprocedural pain, which occurs in about 90% of patients. The original abdominal pain may be aggravated, or new pain may appear in the back or shoulder. The pain usually subsides in 24 to 48 hours. Other rare complications are retroperitoneal hematoma, pneumothorax, renal and intestinal injury, and paraplegia secondary to neurolytic injection into the epidural or spinal canal or secondary to accidental injection of neurolytic agent into the artery of Adamkiewicz, all of which are reported in less than 1% of patients.[55] Superior mesenteric vein thrombosis has been reported with alcohol NCPB.[56] Intravascular injection of the neurolytic agent is a potential complication and can cause tremors and convulsions with phenol.[57]

CONCLUSION

CPB is a century-old interventional technique that has the most rigorous evidence-based assessment of its efficacy. It is generally safe and accurate and compares favorably with conservative analgesic methods. Newer approaches, such as bedside ultrasound guidance and cone beam CT, are promising.

SUPERIOR HYPOGASTRIC PLEXUS BLOCK

A variety of visceral and somatic causes can lead to pelvic pain. Such conditions may include endometriosis, inflammatory disease, postoperative adhesions, and cancer. Frequently, the pain is diffuse and vague, a condition called visceral pain, and may be interrupted with a targeted sympathetic blockade. The original technique of percutaneous superior hypogastric plexus neurolytic blockade for pelvic pain was developed by Plancarte in 1990 following reports of pain relief after cordotomy.[58] This spurred investigation for alternative techniques to perform a superior hypogastric plexus block (SHPB), including the use of image guidance.

CLINICALLY RELEVANT ANATOMY

The superior hypogastric plexus (SHP) is a bilateral continuation of the paravertebral sympathetic chain with contribution from aortic plexus nerve fibers. It is a retroperitoneal midline structure that is usually located anterior to the lower third of the fifth lumbar vertebral body and extends caudally to the upper third of the first sacral body (see Fig. 56.1). The plexus lies anteromedial to the psoas muscle and caudal to the bifurcation of the iliac vessel. The SHP sends out multiple branches to various smaller plexuses supplying sympathetic innervation to all the pelvic viscera except the ovaries and fallopian tubes. It extends distally as the hypogastric nerves, which form the inferior hypogastric plexus.

INDICATIONS

Blockade of the SHP provides relief of pain originating from pelvic viscera secondary to various types of cancer and endometriosis. SHGB has also been reported to provide relief from postprostatectomy penile pain, urethral pain, and post–uterine artery embolization pain.[59-62]

EVIDENCE FOR SUPERIOR HYPOGASTRIC BLOCK

Using a bilateral posterior paravertebral needle insertion technique under fluoroscopic guidance, SPHB provided greater than a 70% reduction in pain in 28 patients with cancer pain. This was replicated in another 26 patients with similar results and no major complications.[63] A subsequent 3-year review of 115 neurolytic blocks from two centers showed similar success with decreased opioid consumption.[64] A volume of 8 mL on each side provided successful pain relief in 72% of patients. The spread of tumor may hinder adequate distribution and thus require higher volumes with limited pain relief. The transdiscal approach offers similar pain relief with decreased procedure time, although infectious diskitis has been reported. There is still a potential for vascular and ureteral injury, but it may not have any long-term implications.[65]

AVAILABLE TECHNIQUES

The original description outlined a posterior approach under fluoroscopic guidance for placement of needles on either side of the anterolateral part of the fifth lumbar vertebral bodies. Neurolytic blocks are performed after diagnostic local anesthetic injections have confirmed spread of the contrast dye. The main disadvantage of this approach is the necessity for multiple redirections secondary to encountering the transverse process or the nerve roots. A modification of this technique is the simpler fluoroscopically guided anterior approach[66] or the posterior transdiscal approach.[65] CT guidance has been used for both the posterior and anterior approaches. Anterior placement may be advantageous when a patient is unable to lie prone, and contact of the needle with the lumbar nerve roots is avoided. Antibiotic prophylaxis is recommended with the anterior and transdiscal approaches because of the potential for bowel perforation and diskitis, respectively. A single-needle technique may be possible when spread of the tumor is not extensive.[67,68] Single-needle and two-needle techniques with the target being inferior to the aortic bifurcation and just anterior to the iliac vessels have been used.[68-70] Fluoroscopy- and CT-guided transdiscal approaches have also been used with no complications reported.[71-73] With the patient prone, an oblique fluoroscopic image is centered on the lateral part of the L5/S1 intervertebral disk such that about 1 cm of it is seen lateral to the S1 superior articular process. A 22-gauge Chiba-type needle is directed via the coaxial view through the disk and placed just anteriorly. Following injection of contrast dye and real-time visualization for appropriate spread, a local anesthetic or neurolytic solution is injected (Fig. 56.17). Injectants containing steroids have also reported to provide

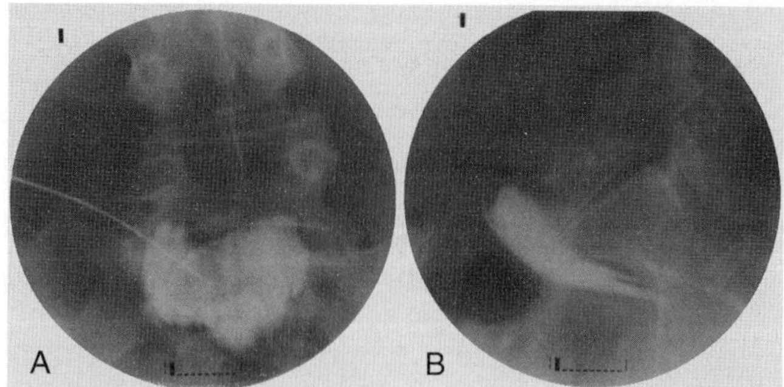

Figure 56.17 Transdiscal superior hypogastric plexus block. **A,** A single needle placed through the disk. Contrast dye was injected. **B,** Retroperitoneal spread of contrast material has a typical radiographic appearance and shape.

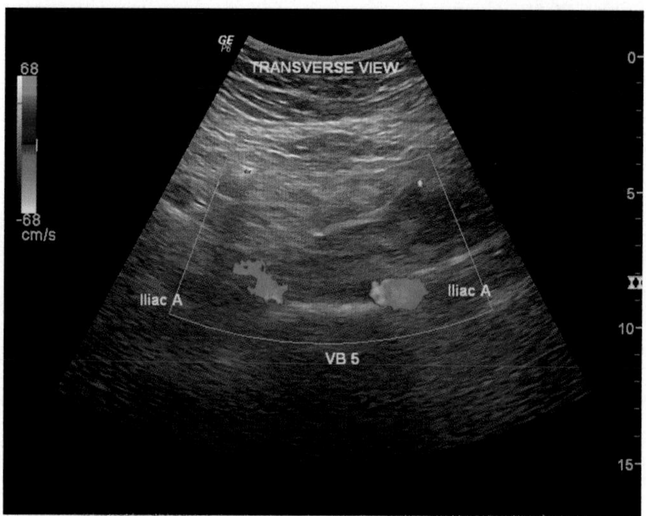

Figure 56.18 Transverse sonographic view in Doppler mode showing the bifurcation of the aorta into the iliac vessels.

lasting pain relief.[59] Despite better visualization of soft tissue and vascular structures, CT guidance carries the risk of an increased radiation dose. More recently, an ultrasound-guided anterior approach was described that permits visualization of the iliac vessels and vertebral body.[73] It may be prudent to confirm spread of contrast dye with fluoroscopy, especially before instillation of neurolytic solutions, when the needle was placed under ultrasound guidance.

With a curved-array transducer and the patient supine, the aorta is traced caudally until it bifurcates into the iliac arteries (Fig. 56.18). Use of color Doppler facilitates proper identification. Medial and posterior to the bifurcation, the fifth lumbar vertebral body may be visualized. The target is over the anterior and most caudal portion of the fifth lumbar vertebral body. Planning of the trajectory is based on the location of the vessels (Fig. 56.19). The area over the possible needle entry point is prepared and draped. Using sterile technique, a 22-gauge spinal needle is advanced either out of plane or in plane to the anterolateral border of the vertebral body. Following placement it may be prudent to confirm accuracy with digital subtraction angiography before injection of local anesthetic. The typical volume used is approximately 10 mL on each side. Neurolytic agents may be

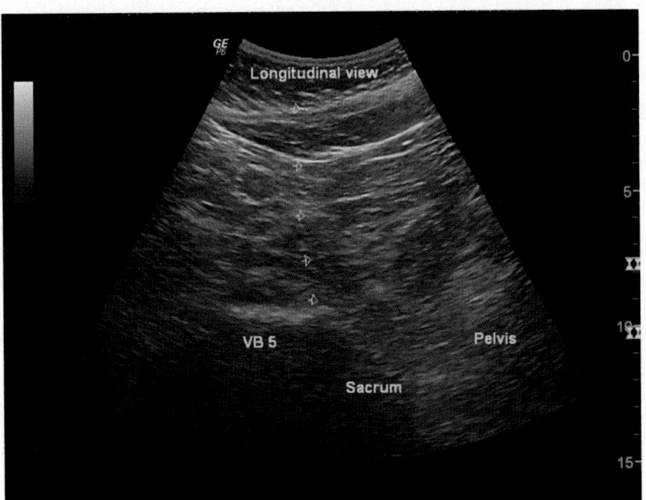

Figure 56.19 Transverse sonographic view showing the fifth lumbar vertebral body. The line marks the trajectory for the needle.

used after confirmation of pain relief with local anesthetic. Administration of antibiotic beforehand is recommended.

COMPLICATIONS

Intravascular injection, inadequate spread, incomplete pain relief, and prolonged sensory and motor deficits have all been reported.[63,74] Other potential complications include diskitis with the transdiscal approach, dislodgment of atheromatous plaque from major vessels, retroperitoneal hematoma, and perforation of the bowel or urinary bladder with the anterior approach.

CONCLUSION

SHPB may be performed for relief of pelvic pain under imaging guidance through either an anterior or posterior approach. The major advantage of an anterior approach is patient comfort. Although CT- and fluoroscopy-guided approaches have been described, they have the disadvantage of excessive radiation exposure. An ultrasound-guided anterior approach may be used for needle placement with subsequent fluoroscopic contrast confirmation. The safety, reproducibility, and efficacy of this technique still need to be established.

ULTRASOUND-GUIDED GANGLION IMPAR BLOCK

The bilateral paravertebral sympathetic chain terminates anteriorly as the midline single fused ganglion impar (the ganglion of Walther), which supplies sympathetic innervation to the perineum. Relief of perineal pain with a ganglion impar block (GIB) was originally reported by Plancarte and coauthors in 1990.[75] Their original description of a landmark-based injection fell into disfavor because of a potential for rectal perforation and a higher failure rate. Interest in this block has since been regained with the increasing use of image guidance.

CLINICALLY RELEVANT ANATOMY

The ganglion impar is an irregularly shaped terminal ganglion of the sympathetic chain that is usually located close to the midline. The variably shaped ganglion is approximately 4 mm long. It may be located anywhere from the anterior surface of the sacrococcygeal junction to the lower coccygeal vertebral bodies. The exact location follows a gaussian distribution centered on the first to second coccygeal vertebrae.[76] The rectum is situated anterior to the ganglion. Fibers from the ganglion travel to the sacral spinal nerves along the gray rami communicantes.

INDICATIONS

GIB is indicated for sympathetically mediated pain in the region of the anus, distal part of the rectum, urethra, and vagina. Coccygodynia following trauma, infection, degenerative changes, and subluxation has also been relieved temporarily with this block.[77-85]

EVIDENCE FOR THE USE OF GANGLION IMPAR BLOCK

Anecdotal evidence has demonstrated the usefulness of GIB and different techniques. Greater than 50% relief of pain from a variety of painful perineal disorders was obtained following GIB under fluoroscopic guidance via a transsacrococcygeal approach.[85,86] Retrospective reviews of CT-guided GIB have shown greater than a 75% decrease in pain scores for up to 6 months.[78,80] No adverse events have been reported. More recently, ultrasound-guided, fluoroscopy-confirmed GIB has also been found to be successful.[81,87]

AVAILABLE TECHNIQUES AND APPROACHES

The initial description of GIB outlined a method based on insertion of a bent needle through the anococcygeal ligament with a finger in the rectum to detect perforation.[75] Imaging guidance markedly increased technical success rates. Fluoroscopy facilitated further development, including the transcoccygeal, transarticular, transdiscal, intracoccygeal, and paracoccygeal approaches.[77,79,83,85,86,88-90] When combined with the use of contrast agents to visualize the spread of injectant, these techniques were associated with a modicum of safety. However, bowel gas shadow, tumor infiltrates, and osteoporosis may hinder proper visualization. Other limitations include an inability to visualize adjacent soft tissues and radiation exposure. CT-guided techniques from a lateral approach provide visualization of the ganglion and soft tissues.[78,80] Ultrasound-guided techniques provide the advantage of real-time visualization and avoidance of radiation. To enhance safety, most practitioners using ultrasound guidance recommend fluoroscopic confirmation of the spread of contrast dye before injection of neurolytic agents.[81,86] Several modifications in needle design, including arc and double-bent needles, were claimed to improve the safety of the procedure.[91] However, cryotherapy or radiofrequency ablation cannulas cannot be customized. In addition, such modifications make it more difficult to extract the stylet after proper positioning of the needle. A needle-in-needle technique may avoid trauma to the disk and coccyx, in addition

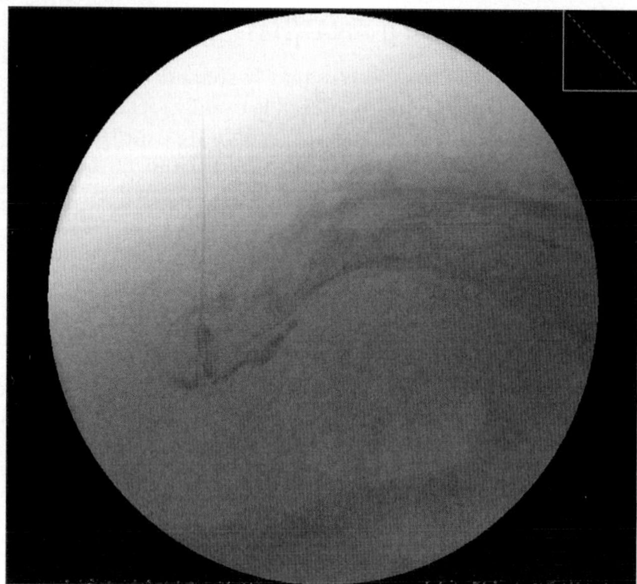

Figure 56.20 Fluoroscopic transverse image of the sacrum and coccyx with the needle in a transcoccygeal approach showing spread of contrast dye along the anterior surface of the coccyx.

to decreasing needle breakage during the transcoccygeal approach (Fig. 56.20).[92] It may also decrease the incidence of infection. Following diagnostic local anesthetic injection, either neurolytic injection, cryoablation, or radiofrequency ablation of the ganglion may be performed.[84,92,93]

TECHNIQUE OF ULTRASOUND-GUIDED GANGLION IMPAR BLOCK

The patient is positioned prone with a pillow underneath the pelvis and the hips externally rotated to provide exposure of the perineum. The skin is prepared with a suitable antiseptic solution and draped in a sterile manner. A preliminary scout scan is performed in the transverse and longitudinal views with a linear-array transducer in a sterile sleeve to visualize the sacrum and coccyx. The coccyx is then brought to the middle of the field in a longitudinal view and a suitable trajectory is planned (Figs. 56.21 and 56.22). While keeping the coccyx in the longitudinal view, a skin wheal is raised with 1% lidocaine at the point of needle entry just caudal to the transducer. A Quincke-type spinal needle is then directed from the caudad to the anterior part of the first coccygeal vertebral body via an in-plane technique with real-time visualization of the needle (Fig. 56.23). The tip of the needle may not be visualized clearly beneath the coccyx because of the acoustic shadow. Alternative methods are to use an out-of-plane technique for the trans-sacrococcygeal or paracoccygeal approaches. This provides a smaller trajectory, but needle visualization is poorer.

Further confirmation is provided by a lateral fluoroscopic view, which should show the needle to be suitably positioned just anterior to the coccyx and posterior to the rectum. Under fluoroscopic guidance, 0.5 to 1 mL of contrast agent is injected to confirm proper spread of the dye, which appears as a "comma sign," before injecting a local anesthetic, steroid, or neurolytic substance (see Fig. 56.20). Injection of a local anesthetic first to confirm pain

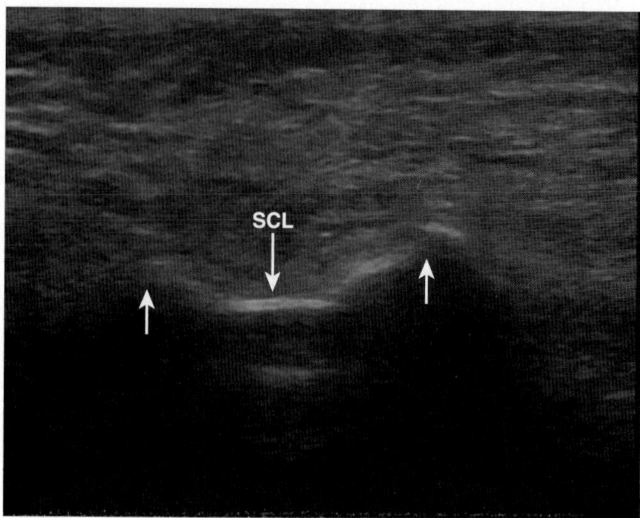

Figure 56.21 Transverse sonographic view of the sacral hiatus. The arrows point to the cornu of the sacral hiatus. SCL, sacrococcygeal ligament.

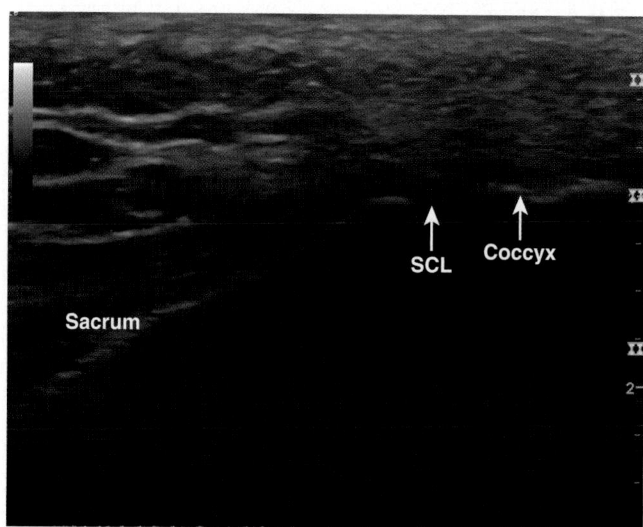

Figure 56.22 Longitudinal sonographic view of the sacrum and coccyx. SCL, sacrococcygeal ligament.

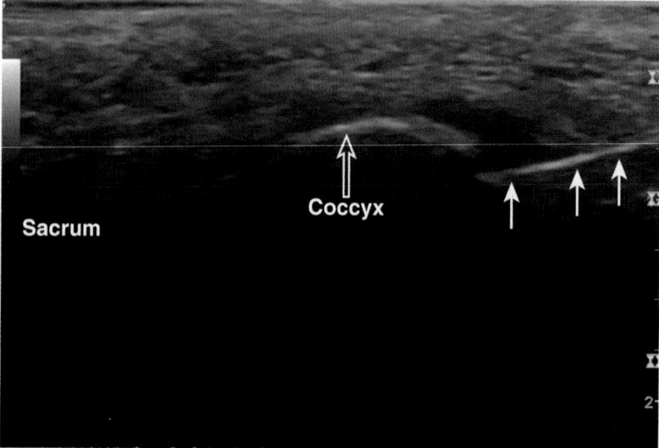

Figure 56.23 Longitudinal sonographic view of the sacrum, coccyx, and needle (arrows) placed in an in-plane approach through the anococcygeal ligament.

reduction before steroid injection or neurolytic intervention may be recommended. The total volume required is usually about 2 to 4 mL.

COMPLICATIONS

The potential for perforation of the rectum may lead to infection. In addition, because of its proximity to the perineum, there is an additional risk for infection. Damage to the sacrococcygeal nerves is possible with the lateral approach.

CONCLUSION

Despite limited evidence, GIB is a commonly implemented technique for the management of visceral pain. Imaging guidance provides better accuracy and safety.

KEY POINTS

Stellate Ganglion Block

- A stellate ganglion block has historically been used to treat numerous pain-related and unrelated conditions.
- Evidence of its efficacy is limited.
- Blind injections are inaccurate and risky.
- Ultrasound guidance is the preferred method to ensure accuracy and safety.

Celiac Plexus Block

- The celiac plexus is supplied by the greater, lesser, and least splanchnic nerves originating from T5 to T12.
- Sensory visceral nerve fibers traverse the celiac plexus and ascend to spinal centers.
- Neurolytic celiac plexus blockade is an established evidence-based method to alleviate severe abdominal pain related to inoperable malignancies.
- An analgesic or neurolytic celiac plexus block is less effective in managing nonmalignant abdominal pain.
- Bedside ultrasound guidance is particularly valuable in a palliative care setting.
- Newer cone beam computed tomography guidance is a promising technique that ensures superior procedural accuracy, limits radiation exposure, and saves time.

Superior Hypogastric Plexus Block

- The superior hypogastric plexus is a midline sympathetic center located in the retroperitoneum anterior to the fifth lumbar and first sacral vertebral bodies.
- A superior hypogastric block is an interventional technique for the management of pelvic pain.
- Fluoroscopy, computed tomography, and ultrasound have been used to guide access to the plexus.
- No formal clinical studies of ultrasound guidance for performance of this block are presently available to attest to its safety and efficacy.

KEY POINTS—cont'd

Ganglion Impar Block

- The ganglion impar is the terminal midline sympathetic ganglion.
- The ganglion impar is commonly found over the first coccygeal vertebral body and the sacrococcygeal junction.
- A ganglion impar block provides relief of coccygodynia and pain involving the lower part of the rectum, anus, urethra, and vagina.
- Imaging guidance for performance of this block is provided by fluoroscopy, computed tomography, and ultrasound, each with its own inherent advantages and disadvantages.

SUGGESTED READINGS

Ateş Y, Asik I, Ozgencil E, et al. Evaluation of the longus colli muscle in relation to stellate ganglion block. *Reg Anesth Pain Med.* 2009;34:219-223.

Bhatnagar S, Gupta D, Mishra S, et al. Bedside ultrasound-guided celiac plexus neurolysis with bilateral paramedian needle entry technique can be an effective pain control technique in advanced upper abdominal cancer pain. *J Palliat Med.* 2008;11:1195-1199.

de Leon-Casasola OA, Kent E, Lema MJ. Neurolytic superior hypogastric plexus block for chronic pelvic pain associated with cancer. *Pain.* 1993;54:145-151.

Eisenberg E, Carr DB, Chalmers TC. Neurolytic celiac plexus block for treatment of cancer pain: a meta-analysis. *Anesth Analg.* 1995;80:290-295.

Gamal G, Helaly M, Labib YM. Superior hypogastric block: transdiscal versus classic posterior approach in pelvic cancer pain. *Clin J Pain.* 2006;22:544-547.

Gofeld M, Bhatia A, Abbas S, et al. Development and validation of a new technique for ultrasound-guided stellate ganglion block. *Reg Anesth Pain Med.* 2009;34:475-479.

Ina H, Kitoh T, Kobayashi M, et al. New technique for the neurolytic celiac plexus block: the transintervertebral disc approach. *Anesthesiology.* 1996;85:212-217.

Ischia S, Luzzani A, Ischia A, et al. A new approach to the neurolytic block of the coeliac plexus: the transaortic technique. *Pain.* 1983;16:333-341.

Ischia S, Polati E, Finco G, et al. 1998 Labat lecture: the role of the neurolytic celiac plexus block in pancreatic cancer pain management: do we have the answers? *Reg Anesth Pain Med.* 1998;23:611-614.

Kapral S, Krafft P, Gosch M, et al. Ultrasound imaging for stellate ganglion block: direct visualization of puncture site and local anesthetic spread: a pilot study. *Reg Anesth.* 1995;20:323-328.

Kiray A, Arman C, Naderi S, et al. Surgical anatomy of the cervical sympathetic trunk. *Clin Anat.* 2005;18:179-185.

Michalek P, Dutka J. Computed tomography–guided anterior approach to the superior hypogastric plexus for noncancer pelvic pain: a report of two cases. *Clin J Pain.* 2005;21:553-556.

Narouze S, Vydyanathan A, Patel N. Ultrasound-guided stellate ganglion block successfully prevented esophageal puncture. *Pain Physician.* 2007;10:747-752.

Plancarte R, Amescua C, Patt RB, et al. Superior hypogastric plexus block for pelvic cancer pain. *Anesthesiology.* 1990;73:236-239.

Wong GY, Schroeder DR, Carns PE, et al. Effect of neurolytic celiac plexus block on pain relief, quality of life, and survival in patients with unresectable pancreatic cancer: a randomized controlled trial. *JAMA.* 2004;291:1092-1099.

The refrences for this chapter can be found at www.expertconsult.com.

57 Intraarticular Analgesia

Anil Gupta

INTRODUCTION

An ideal analgesic should provide pain relief locally at the site of trauma without any systemic or local side effects, preferably as long as the pain persists. Scientists have searched for this ideal analgesic for several centuries, but as yet, no such drug exists. Local anesthetics (LAs) provide excellent analgesia with minimal toxicity when they are used in safe doses. In addition, they have anti-inflammatory and antithrombotic effects. However, LAs have a short duration of effect,[1] which limits their usefulness to the immediate postoperative period unless injected intermittently or continuously into traumatized tissues. Therefore, the search for LA enclosed in microspheres or administered through catheters to prolong the duration of their effect continues.[2] Opiates are efficacious, specifically following major surgery, but have several disadvantages, including nausea and vomiting, pruritus, constipation, and rarely, respiratory depression, when administered systemically. Following the discovery and isolation of opioid receptors on peripheral nerves and joints in the late 1980s,[3] intensive investigation into the use of opiates peripherally to obtain pain relief without significant side effects ensued. Thus, analgesia with intra-articular (IA) morphine for the relief of postoperative pain following arthroscopy and arthroscopic knee surgery has been the focus of more than 60 publications involving humans during the last 20 years, when the first reports described the clinically beneficial effects of morphine. Recently, there has been increasing focus on the use of large-volume LA injections, with or without other adjuvants, into periarticular tissue during surgery to achieve sustained analgesia following knee and hip arthroplasty.[4,5] Although this method has been reported in several publications, consensus on its applicability has not yet been attained.

Most authors have used the knee joint as a model for research. However, morphine and other drugs have also been injected into other joints, including the ankle, shoulder, and elbow, for assessment of clinical effects. Among the drugs and drug combinations that have been studied, the following are the most common: LAs, opioids, nonsteroidal anti-inflammatory drugs (NSAIDs), α_2-adrenergic agonists, anticholinesterase drugs, steroids, and ketamine (Table 57.1). Despite the relatively large number of publications on these issues, a well-designed study recruiting a sufficient number of patients and asking the relevant questions has yet to be performed. This review of the literature summarizes the findings of some of the studies published and focuses on the drawbacks, limitations, and problems that surround this complex but interesting question of the efficacy of IA analgesics in the clinical setting.

VARIATIONS IN PAIN INTENSITY AND METHODS OF MEASUREMENT

INTENSITY OF POSTOPERATIVE PAIN

Studying the efficacy of analgesics following procedures associated with only mild pain is likely to either be unsuccessful (i.e., not show analgesic efficacy) or require forbiddingly large numbers of patients to achieve statistical significance. In addition, even when statistical difference is seen, it may not be clinically meaningful since minor differences in pain intensity are questionable. Although a difference in pain intensity of 30% and higher is thought to be relevant, a 30% reduction in pain from 1.5 to 1.0 cm on a visual analog scale (VAS) is not necessarily of clinical importance. Therefore, when assessing the efficacy of drugs injected intra-articularly, it is likely to be more meaningful to study either patients *or* procedures associated with moderate to severe postoperative pain. In this way it is estimated that 20% to 30% fewer patients may need to be studied, as well as to provide meaningful assessment of drug efficacy.[6] Because of the variation in pain intensity between operative procedures, international experts have suggested evidence-based guidelines for procedure-specific pain management, which are frequently updated with new evidence (www.postoppain.org).

BIOLOGIC VARIATIONS IN PAIN INTENSITY

Recent evidence suggests that women have more pain following arthroscopic surgery than men do, which is important when managing postoperative pain after arthroscopic procedures.[7-9] In one study, Taenzer and colleagues studied 736 patients undergoing arthroscopic anterior cruciate ligament reconstruction (ACLR) and found that women experience greater pain intensity, which is associated with a worsened functional outcome.[10] They concluded that these differences might result from variations in either response to analgesics or neuron processing. In another study, Rosseland and Stubhaug showed that gender might account for the differences in analgesia experienced by women after arthroscopic knee surgery, with women experiencing more pain than men do.[11] Cepeda and Carr found that women have more intense pain and require 30% more morphine to achieve a similar degree of analgesia than do men.[12] In addition to sex differences, variation in pain intensity during the menstrual cycle should also be considered in studies on analgesic efficacy since analgesic consumption is greater in women during the luteal phase of the menstrual cycle.[13] There is also a clinically significant reduction in the intensity of pain perception or symptoms with increasing age,[14] which could be related to the decrease in Aδ- and C-fiber nociceptive function, delay in central sensitization, or an increase in pain thresholds.[15-17]

ASSESSMENT OF PAIN

Pain is a subjective sensation and varies between individuals. Several methods to measure pain have been described in the literature. Although the VAS and numeric rating scale (NRS) are well described and validated in the literature,[18] other scales have also been used. When presenting the results, it is important to specify whether pain has been assessed at rest (static pain) or during provocation (dynamic pain) since mobilization often aggravates the intensity of pain. Dynamic pain can be measured as "pain on coughing," "pain on movement," or pain during "knee flexion" or "leg elevation" and should be described appropriately. Measuring pain intensity at fixed time intervals after the operation may sometimes give inaccurate results, depending on the last intake of analgesics, as well as the time of the day that the pain is being measured. Thus, both pain intensity and total analgesic consumption are important when drawing conclusions. Sometimes, the "area under the curve" for pain intensity may be more relevant than the pain intensity at fixed time points. Finally, in studies on postoperative pain and analgesic consumption, it may be equally important to measure pain relief as pain intensity. However, the former is more difficult to measure since VASs or NRSs may not correctly describe pain relief, as they do for pain intensity.

PLACEBO IN CLINICAL STUDIES

In a randomized controlled trial, Rosseland and colleagues showed that pain after knee arthroscopy is modest and short-lived and can be treated successfully with IA saline (placebo).[19] They also showed that the addition of 2 mg of morphine to 10 mL of saline does not reduce pain following arthroscopic knee surgery in patients with moderate to severe pain.[20] IA saline may produce analgesia by cooling (cryoanalgesia) or by diluting IA algogenic substances. Indeed, this may represent a true therapeutic effect of saline attributable to the removal or dilution of pain-mediating substances (histamine, potassium, or vasoactive polypeptides) in the wound.[21,22] Alford and Fadale also found that IA saline infusions provide similar pain relief as bupivacaine infusion following anterior cruciate ligament repair,[23] thus suggesting that local pain mediators may be washed away by the infusion of saline. The placebo effect is well defined in the literature in studies on analgesics, and therefore it is important to include this group in randomized, double-blind trials, specifically when studying new analgesics or techniques. However, the use of placebo groups in pain trials is controversial, and this has been highlighted in the updated Helsinki declaration of 2001.

DRUGS USED INTRA-ARTICULARLY

LOCAL ANESTHETICS

Single doses of LAs administered intra-articularly are used frequently. LAs have been used successfully as the sole anesthetic for minor arthroscopic procedures (Fig. 57.1) and, when used in this way, provide adequate analgesia of short duration. In the only systematic review published in the literature on the efficacy of LA injected intra-articularly, Møiniche and associates evaluated randomized, double-blind controlled, controlled trials comparing LA with placebo or no treatment for the relief of postoperative pain following arthroscopic knee surgery.[1] They found a significant prolongation of pain relief lasting between 30 and 50 minutes in only 2 of 6 studies; in addition, these authors also found that in 9 (of 20) studies, consumption of supplementary analgesics was reduced by 10% to 50% during observation periods of up to 4 hours (Fig. 57.2). However, in most cases, the

Table 57.1 Intra-articular Analgesics

Drug	Doses Used	Number of Studies Published	Number of Systematic Reviews Published
Local anesthetics		>20	1
Opioids			4
Morphine*	0.5, 1, 2, 3, 4, 5, 10 mg	>50	
Pethidine	10, 50, 100, 200 mg	5	
Fentanyl	10, 50 µg	<5	
Sufentanil	5, 10 µg	<5	
NSAIDs			0
Ketorolac	5, 30, 60 mg	5-10	
Tenoxicam	20 mg	5-10	
α_2-Agonists			0
Clonidine	150, 1 µg/kg	5-10	
Others			0
Neostigmine	500 µg	<5	
Ketamine	0.5 mg/kg		
Oxycodone	5 mg	1	
Diamorphine	5 mg	1	

*For studies on intra-articular morphine, the reader is referred to already published systematic reviews with extensive reference lists.[6-9]
NSAIDs, nonsteroidal anti-inflammatory drugs.

analgesic requirements were small to moderate, thus suggesting mild pain intensity in these studies. They concluded that the pain relief obtained with LA injected intra-articularly is mild to moderate and of short duration. This may, however, be of clinical significance in day-case surgery. In another recent systematic review and meta-analysis of the literature, the efficacy of LA injection via catheters was assessed following non–orthopedic-related surgery.[24] The authors found very little benefit of this technique, except for short-lasting effects in patients undergoing obstetric surgery. LAs have been administered via catheters as intermittent injections or as continuous infusions into the knee joint intra-articularly,[25] subacromially,[22] intra-abdominally following hysterectomy,[26] and subcutaneously following cesarean section,[27] as well as during peripheral nerve blocks,[28] with variable success.

MAJOR KNEE SURGERY

A summary of the articles published and the conclusions drawn by the authors during knee surgery is presented in Table 57.2.[29-33] The anterior synovium, infrapatellar fat pad, and joint capsule are very sensitive to pain stimuli.[34] Chew and coworkers tested the analgesic efficacy of 0.25% or 0.5% bupivacaine administered into the intrapatellar fat pad via a catheter after ACLR.[29] A self-administered infusion pump (50 mL) allowed the patients to administer 4-mL doses of bupivacaine. The authors found no significant difference between 0.5% and 0.25% bupivacaine, thus suggesting absence of correlation between the dose of bupivacaine and pain intensity. It is likely that there is no direct relationship between the concentration and volume of LAs injected intra-articularly.[35] Continuous catheter techniques were used for pain relief after knee replacement in three studies. In one study, DeWeese and associates compared continuous infusion of 0.5% bupivacaine at 2 mL/hr intra-articularly with a historical group in which patients were given controlled epidural analgesia with 0.125% bupivacaine plus fentanyl, 2 μg/mL.[30] The IA infusion was less efficient, and higher analgesic consumption was registered during the 24-hour test period. In a double-blind study, 0.25% bupivacaine, 5 mL/hr, was compared with saline during a 48-hour IA infusion. The authors noted a significant reduction in opioid consumption, which resulted in less nausea, fatigue, and malaise and even enhanced rehabilitation and increased satisfaction.[31] In another study, Hoenecke and colleagues found that patients undergoing knee surgery and receiving an LA infusion postoperatively experience less pain and require fewer doses of narcotic.[32] They also found that the disposable pump allows administration of the medication on an outpatient basis. The site of LA injection (IA vs. intracapsular) was studied.[36] In this study no differences were found between the groups, and the authors concluded that intracapsular LA has similar analgesic efficacy as IA LA after total knee arthroplasty. Warming of lidocaine appears to improve intraoperative anesthetic and postoperative analgesic conditions.[33] Several published studies have focused on a new technique of high-volume LA (with or without adjuvants) infiltration periarticularly, often called local infiltration analgesia, for relief of postoperative pain.[4,5,36] Although the majority of these studies appear to be promising, some have not been equally positive. It is possible that a combination of drugs rather than simply LAs injected during surgery will offer better analgesia without significant side effects. Further studies on short- and long-term outcomes following this technique are awaited.

In summary, IA injection of LA after total knee replacement, specifically, the recently used technique of local infiltration analgesia, offers an efficacious and inexpensive method for achieving good pain relief following total knee arthroplasty.

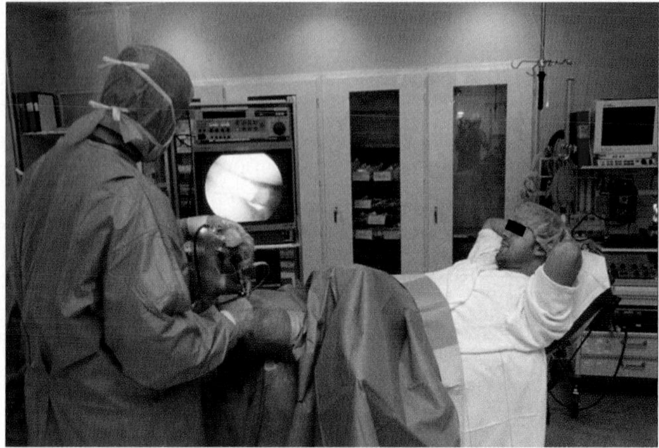

Figure 57.1 Arthroscopy is now commonly performed under local anesthesia.

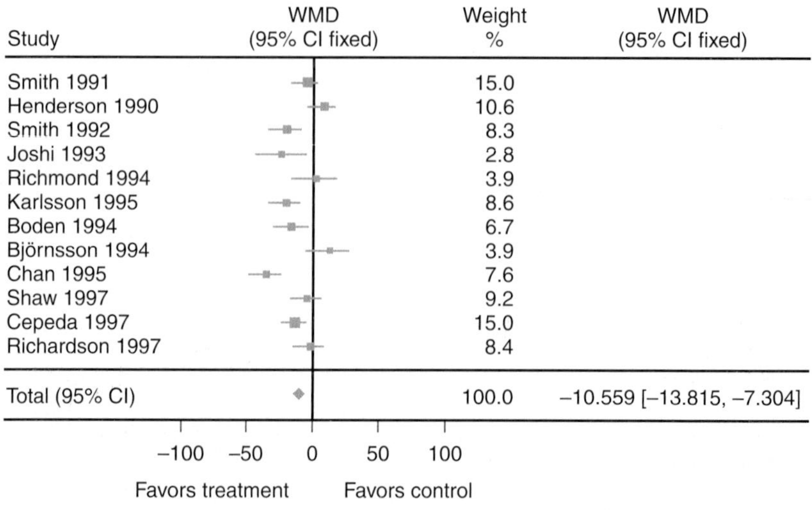

Figure 57.2 Meta-analysis of studies using a single dose of local anesthetic injected intra-articularly. The weighted mean difference (WMD) with 95% confidence intervals (95% CI, horizontal lines) in visual analog scale (VAS) pain scores early postoperatively (1 to 4 hours) is shown in the intra-articular local anesthetic and control groups. (Data from Møiniche S, Mikkelsen S, Wetterslev J. A systematic review of intraarticular local anesthesia for postoperative pain relief after arthroscopic knee surgery. *Reg Anesth Pain Med.* 1999;24:430-437.)

TOTAL HIP ARTHROPLASTY

Several studies have assessed the analgesic effects of LAs, with or without adjuvants, following IA and periarticular infiltration during surgery. A majority of these studies have shown better analgesia, a shorter duration of hospital stay, and improved mobilization,[37,38] with some exceptions.[39,40] Ropivacaine combined with ketorolac and adrenaline and infiltrated periarticularly reduced rescue analgesic consumption and decreased postoperative hospital stay when compared with epidural analgesia.[37] Busch and colleagues found a reduction in pain during rest and on mobilization with LA infiltration and multimodal pain management in comparison to saline.[39] In another study, no benefit of continuous infusion of 0.5% bupivacaine was noted when compared with saline for relief of pain after arthroplasty.[40] Prolonging analgesia with postoperative infusion of drugs following hip arthroplasty does not seem to reduce pain intensity.[40] Finally, adding LA infiltration to a multimodal pain management protocol involving the use of several analgesics does not add to the pain relief already achieved with these drugs.[41] In summary, local infiltration analgesia using a combination of drugs is probably beneficial, but not the use of LAs alone. When using multimodal analgesia, adding LA infiltration does not add to the analgesia, and postoperative infusion of LA is not recommended for pain relief following total hip arthroplasty.

SHOULDER SURGERY

A summary of articles published on continuous LA infusion during shoulder surgery and the conclusions drawn by the authors is presented in Table 57.3. To treat postoperative

Table 57.2 Local Anesthetics for Knee Surgery

Drug/Concentration	Method of Drug Delivery	Type of Surgery	Type of Study	Effect (VAS or Analgesic Intake)	Reference
Bupivacaine, 0.25% and 0.5%	Intermittent injection via catheter	ACLR	Open	No difference between 0.25% and 0.5%	29
Bupivacaine, 0.5%	Continuous infusion	TKR	Open	Epidural better than IA LA	30
Bupivacaine, 0.25%	Continuous infusion	TKR	Double blind	Lower morphine requirement in IA LA group	31
Bupivacaine, 0.25%	Continuous infusion	ACLR	Double blind	Lower VAS and analgesic needs	32
Bupivacaine, 0.25%	Continuous infusion	TKR	Double blind	No difference between saline and LA	33

ACLR, anterior cruciate ligament repair; IA, intra-articular; LA, local anesthetic; TKR, total knee replacement; VAS, visual analog scale.

Table 57.3 Local Anesthetics for Shoulder Surgery*

Drug/Concentration	Method of Drug Delivery	Type of Surgery	Type of Study	Effect (VAS or Analgesic Intake)	Reference
0.25% bupivacaine, 2 mL/hr	Continuous infusion	Subacromial decompression	Double blind	Lower VAS scores and analgesic consumption	42
0.5% ropivacaine, 2 mL/hr	Continuous infusion	Unilateral shoulder arthroscopy	Double blind	Lower VAS scores at rest and with movement	43
0.2% and 0.375% ropivacaine	Continuous infusion	Cuff repair	Double blind	Lower VAS scores and analgesic consumption	44
0.5% bupivacaine, 2 mL/hr	Continuous infusion	Rotator cuff repair	Double blind	Lower VAS scores	45
0.25% bupivacaine, 2 mL/hr	Continuous infusion	Subacromial surgery	Double blind	Mild analgesic effect	46
Ropivacaine, 6 mL/hr	Continuous infusion	Acromioplasty	Double blind	No benefit	47
0.2% ropivacaine	Continuous infusion and bolus	Rotator cuff repair	Open	Interscalene block better than IA infusion of LA	48
0.5% ropivacaine	Intermittent injection	Subacromial decompression	Double blind	Lower VAS score and analgesic consumption	22
0.125% bupivacaine, 2.5-10 mL/hr	Intermittent injection	Subacromial decompression	Open	Good analgesia	49
2% lidocaine, 2 mL/hr, plus bolus	Continuous infusion plus intermittent injection	Subacromial decompression	Open	Better pain relief than with placebo	50
0.2% ropivacaine plus bolus	Continuous infusion plus intermittent injection	Subacromial decompression	Double blind	Lower VAS score by 44%	51

*Effect of IA LA on postoperative pain following shoulder surgery. The list of studies shown is not exhaustive.
IA, intra-articular; LA, local anesthetic; VAS, visual analog scale.

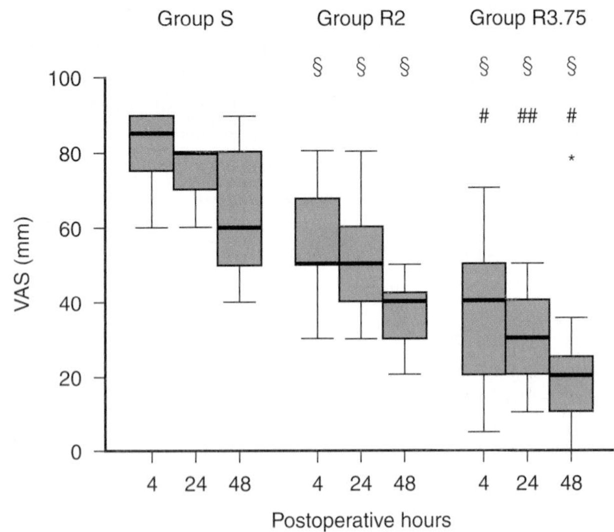

Figure 57.3 Comparison of 0.2% and 0.375% ropivacaine with saline infusion for 48 hours postoperatively. VAS, visual analog scale. *Greater than 3 times the quartile range; #$P < 0.05$ versus group R2; §$P < 0.005$ versus group S. (Data from Gottschalk A, Burmeister M-A, Radtke P, et al. Continuous wound infiltration with ropivacaine reduces pain and analgesic requirement after shoulder surgery. *Anesth Analg*. 2003;97:1086-1091.)

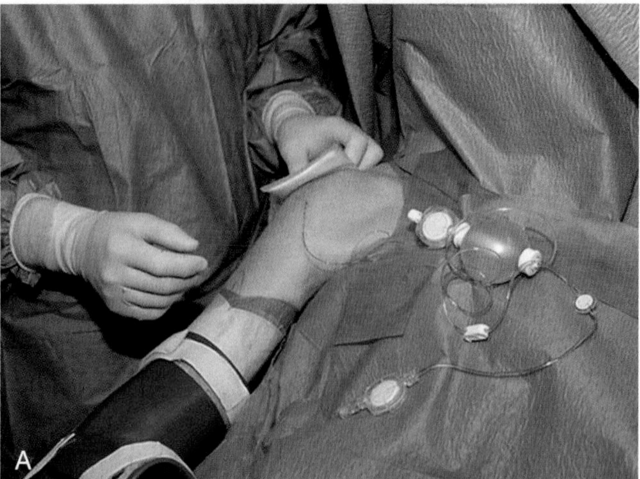

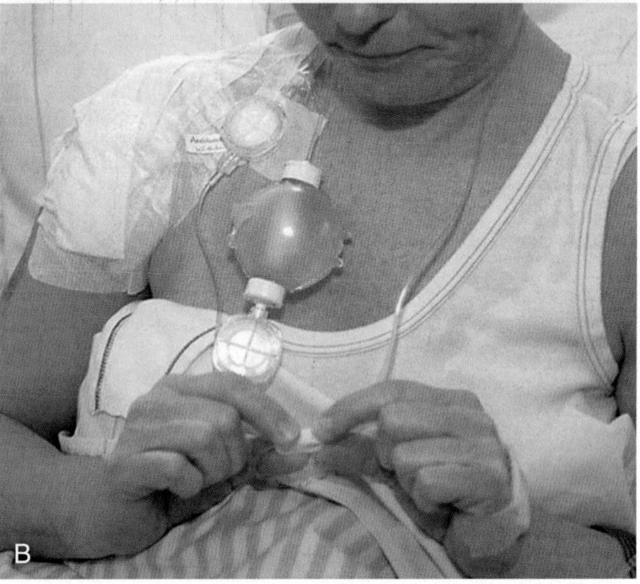

Figure 57.4 Postoperative pain management using an elastometric pump (**A**) and patient-controlled regional analgesia (PCRA) following subacromial decompression (**B**).

pain after acromioplasty, LA administered subacromially has recently been found to be effective. In seven studies,[42-48] continuous infusion was used, and in four studies, patient-controlled regional analgesia (PCRA) was used.[22,49-51] Savoie and colleagues[42] found that 0.25% bupivacaine infused at a rate of 2 mL/hr decreases not only VAS scores during 48 hours of LA administration but also analgesic consumption during the first 5 postoperative days. Others reported significantly decreased VAS scores in comparison to saline when 0.5% bupivacaine was administered at an infusion rate of 2 mL/hr.[45] In contrast to studies following knee surgery, the analgesic effect was dose dependent when 0.2% and 0.375% concentrations of ropivacaine were compared[44] (Fig. 57.3). In two other studies, however, continuous IA bupivacaine infusion resulted in only minor analgesic effects.[46,47] The use of chilled compressive dressings and NSAID medication may have contributed to the small difference seen between the test drug and placebo.[46]

Klein and coworkers[43] evaluated postoperative pain relief when a long-acting preoperative interscalene block (0.5% ropivacaine) was compared with continuous IA infusion of 0.5% ropivacaine, 2 mL/hr for 24 hours. IA ropivacaine resulted in lower VAS scores both at rest and during movement. Delaunay and associates compared interscalene block with subacromial LA infusion following arthroscopic rotator cuff repair.[48] A continuous interscalene block provides better analgesia than does continuous subacromial infusion, but with an increased incidence of minor side effects. In an open study, Mallon and Thomas[50] described a patient-controlled catheter technique based on both continuous subacromial infusion of 2% lidocaine at 2 mL/hr and self-administration of 1-mL lidocaine boluses at 15-minute intervals as needed. During the 72-hour infusion, pain *relief* was significantly increased in the lidocaine relative to the placebo group. In another PCRA study, 0.2% ropivacaine infused at 5 mL/hr was combined with 2-mL boluses of 0.2% ropivacaine with a 15-minute lockout time.[51] The authors reported a significant 44% decrease in VAS scores during 48 hours. We have tested the combined analgesic effect of LA administered both into the subacromial bursa and intra-articularly via a PCRA technique[22] (Fig. 57.4). Patients given LAs both in the bursa and subacromially had significantly lower VAS scores early postoperatively and lower morphine consumption than did those administered saline.

PITFALLS IN STUDIES ON INTRA-ARTICULAR LOCAL ANESTHETICS

Intermittent versus Continuous Techniques

Intermittent injection of drugs offers an advantage in that it prevents “overdosing” since pain is not continuous but exacerbated during certain maneuvers, such as movement, and can be either prevented or treated by the self-injection of fixed amounts of drugs intra-articularly through a catheter and an infusion pump. This technique, called PCRA and originally described by Rawal and colleagues,[49] has now been used effectively in several studies for postoperative analgesia following shoulder surgery,[22] hand surgery,[52] laparoscopic cholecystectomy,[53] and cesarean section.[27] In contrast, continuous infusion of LA or other analgesic combinations has an advantage in that the patient may be pain free during an unplanned movement, but at the cost of drug overdose. This method also has the disadvantage that pain relief may be inadequate during maximal pain intensity. Perhaps a combination of low-dose infusion and intermittent injections as needed may be best.[51]

Site of Injection of Local Anesthetic

Injections of LA at portal sites may reduce postoperative pain for short periods in a similar way as has been shown for IA injections. However, the anterior synovium, infrapatellar fat pad, and joint capsule are very sensitive to pain stimuli,[34] and injections into these areas may provide better pain relief. Subacromial injections of LA have been found to provide good pain relief in comparison to placebo following shoulder surgery.[22,51,54] No differences were seen in one study in which the authors injected LA intracapsularly versus extracapsularly. However, the study was small in size, and this issue has not been resolved to date.

Use of Adrenaline

Although adrenaline has been known to have analgesic efficacy for more than 100 years and recent evidence suggests that its pharmacodynamic effect is exerted via α_2 adrenoceptors in the substantia gelatinosa in the dorsal horn of the spinal cord,[55] controlled studies on the use of adrenaline intra-articularly as an analgesic are lacking. Certainly, epidurally administered LA with fentanyl added to adrenaline provides better pain relief than do LA and fentanyl alone.[56] Whether adrenaline has a preventive, pharmacologic (α_2 adrenoceptors), or physiologic effect (decrease in blood flow) remains uncertain. More studies on this important subject are warranted.

Volume and Dose of Local Anesthetic Injected Intra-articularly

Both the volume and the dose (milligrams) of LA injected intra-articularly may play a role in the analgesic efficacy of LA postoperatively. Small volumes of LA injected intra-articularly may theoretically leak out of the IA space, thus limiting its usefulness. It is difficult to fill the entire joint with LA because of the sensitive joint capsule. Similarly, small doses of LA may not have the desired effects. In one study, Gottschalk and coworkers found a reduction in pain intensity postoperatively at some time points in patients receiving 3.75 mg/mL versus 2 mg/mL ropivacaine[44] (see Fig. 57.3). In a systemic analysis of the effect of IA LA on postoperative pain by Møiniche and colleagues, a mean dose of 90 mg bupivacaine was recommended with an injection volume of between 20 and 40 mL.[1] Recent studies have found no relationship between the volume, concentration, or dose of LA and postoperative pain, except perhaps following shoulder surgery.

MORPHINE

The presence of peripheral morphine receptors has been noted.[3] The first clinical study on the efficacy of morphine injected intra-articularly by Stein in 1991 found a reduction in pain intensity during the first 6 postoperative hours following minor arthroscopic surgery.[3] This analgesic effect could be confirmed due to morphine via peripheral receptors since IA injection of naloxone reversed the analgesic effect.[3] Since then, interest in the IA effects of morphine has grown by leaps and bounds, with more than 50 published studies assessing the efficacy of morphine injected intra-articularly into the knee joint. The results and conclusions have, however, been contradictory in these studies. In a systematic review of the literature in 1997, Kalso and coauthors concluded that "intra-articular morphine may have some effect in reducing postoperative pain intensity and consumption of analgesics."[7] Gupta and colleagues evaluated 45 studies in a meta-analysis of the literature and found "a definite but mild analgesic effect, which could be dose-dependent" (Fig. 57.5). However, these authors could not completely exclude a systemic effect of IA morphine.[8] Another systematic review by Kalso and coworkers found that 5 mg of morphine injected intra-articularly into the knee joint provides relief of postoperative pain for up to 24 hours.[9] They also concluded that when there is "no pain, there is no gain," thus suggesting that pain intensity must be at least moderate to detect any significant analgesic effects of morphine administered intra-articularly. Rosseland and colleagues confirmed that a postoperative analgesic effect of IA morphine is found only in a subgroup of patients with greater pain intensity in the immediate postoperative period.[57] They also found that women perceive greater pain than men do, and therefore it is important to consider sex differences in studies on pain, thus adding another dimension to this complex problem. In one published systematic review, the authors showed that when only high-quality studies were considered in which pain intensity was moderate to severe, 5 mg IA morphine provided no significant analgesia postoperatively.[4] This was in contrast to the findings of Kalso and associates presented earlier.[9]

PITFALLS IN STUDIES ON INTRA-ARTICULAR MORPHINE

Use of Systemic Opioids Intraoperatively

A substantial number of studies have used intraoperative analgesics such as fentanyl, which complicates the issue since analgesic efficacy (when seen) could be due to the preemptive or pharmacologic effect of these opiates in the early postoperative period. Studies in which only LAs are used intraoperatively without general anesthesia or in which general anesthesia is given without opioids may be more important to exclude this possibility. In two studies, the authors assessed postoperative pain following arthroscopy performed under LA without intraoperative opioids. In one study, Gupta and colleagues found no benefit of morphine, 3 mg intra-articularly, over saline.[58] In another published study, Ng and coworkers found improved analgesia when morphine and ketorolac are combined with ropivacaine versus ropivacaine or bupivacaine alone.[59] Whether this effect was due to ketorolac alone or its combination with morphine remains unclear.

Method of Injection of Drugs Intra-articularly

Variations in techniques of injection of drugs intra-articularly may account for some of the differences seen between studies. For instance, drugs have been injected via the arthroscope

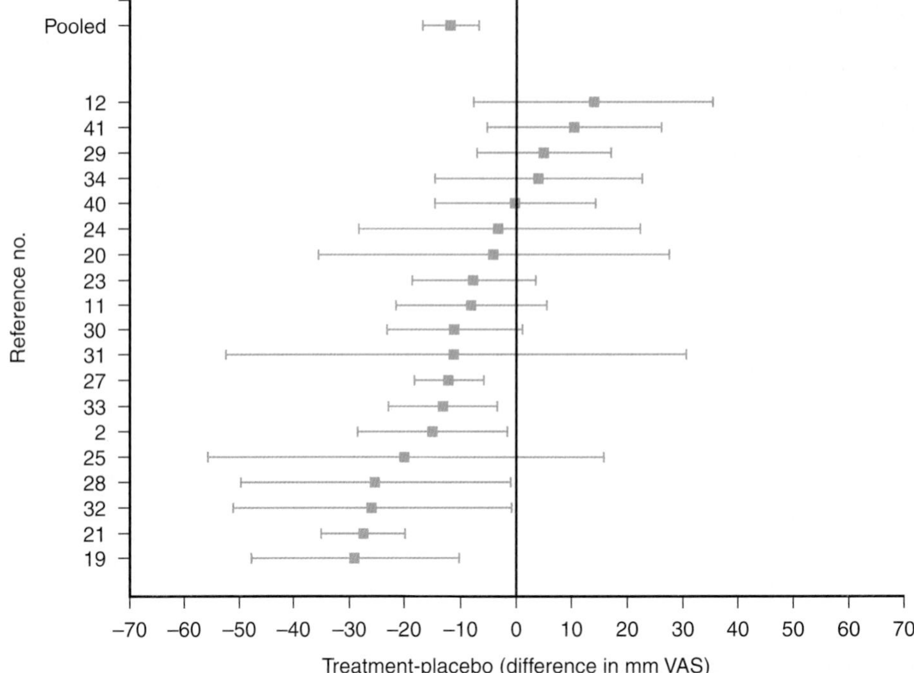

Figure 57.5 Early (0 to 2 hours) postoperative pain following intra-articular morphine. VAS, visual analog scale. (Data from Gupta A, Bodin L, Holmstrom B, et al. A systematic review of the peripheral analgesics effects of intraarticular morphine. *Anesth Analg*. 2001;93:761-770.)

under direct vision or at the end of surgery intra-articularly via a needle. Injection of drugs through the arthroscope before it is removed may result in some of the drug either "running out" from the site of injection into tissue planes or, in the worst scenario, exiting through the incision sites. This depends naturally on the volume of the injectant and the meticulousness of the operator. A small volume of injectant that leaks out of the sore would not have any meaningful effect, whereas large volumes may not remain in the limited IA space. Similarly, a quick injection through the arthroscope and immediate removal may not ensure that the drugs remain where they are intended to be. Thus, the volume of drug remaining in the IA space may vary and account for some of these differences. Injections of drugs postoperatively through a catheter placed intra-articularly via an arthroscope may enable the entire volume of the drug to remain intra-articularly, but very few studies have used this simple but effective method. Finally, intermittent or continuous infusion of drugs via a catheter may prolong the analgesic effects and has been used recently in many studies. This technique, as opposed to a single injection of the drug via the arthroscope or a needle, needs to be further evaluated.

Systemic Effect of Intra-articular Morphine

It remains unclear whether the analgesic effects of IA morphine are due to its systemic absorption. Therefore, a similar dose of morphine was injected by the intramuscular (IM), intravenous (IV), and IA routes in several studies.[3,60-64] The results were equivocal, with some studies documenting an equianalgesic effect[61,62,64] and others documenting better analgesia with IA morphine.[3,33,60] No clear relationship appears to exist between the dose of morphine and analgesia when comparing IA with IM/IV morphine. Plasma concentrations of morphine were measured after IA injection of 1 and 5 mg morphine in one study[60] and after IV and IA injection (5 mg) in another study.[63] In the first study, two patients had spuriously large concentrations and two others had undetectable levels (<1 ng/mL).[60] In the remaining 6 of 10 patients, the authors found lower concentrations of morphine than usually described after parenteral morphine administration. In the second study, the plasma concentration measured 2 hours after IA morphine administration was approximately 50% of the concentration achieved after the same dose administered by the IV route.[63] In a third study, although the maximum plasma concentration following IA injection was lower than after IV injection, the area under the curve during hours 0 to 6 was similar, thus suggesting that substantial amounts of morphine are absorbed into the systemic circulation over time.[65] In conclusion, whether there is a systemic effect of morphine following IA injection remains unclear.

Dose-Response Effect

The effects of increasing IA doses of morphine on postoperative analgesia have also been studied.[66,67] Better postoperative analgesia was obtained with 5 mg than with lower doses. Denti and coworkers found that 2 mg of morphine is adequate for minor arthroscopic procedures but 5 mg is necessary for anterior cruciate ligament surgery, thus suggesting that the dose of IA morphine is dependent on pain intensity.[67] Although low doses of IA morphine (<1 mg) should theoretically produce a high concentration of IA morphine,[7] a dose-response effect was demonstrated by Likar and associates[66] with IA doses of 1 to 4 mg. Kalso and colleagues also demonstrated in their systematic review of the literature that all studies in which 5 mg of morphine was injected intra-articularly showed a positive result at all time periods.[9] Thus, clinical data seem to suggest that larger IA doses of morphine result in better pain relief.

Use of a Tourniquet

Use of a tourniquet on the thigh has been proposed to reduce pain intensity and may account for the differences in results. The mechanism for this effect is unclear, and

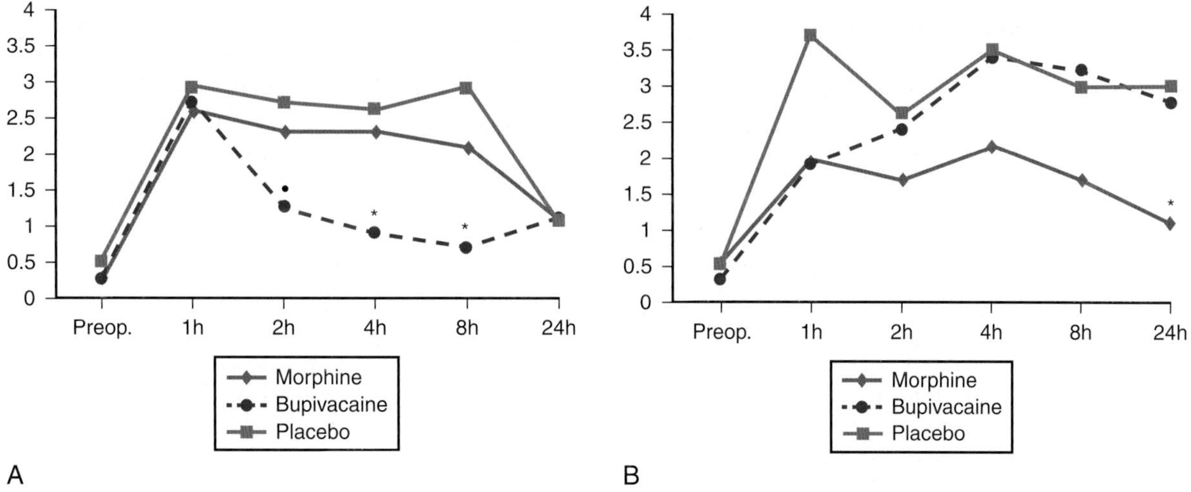

Figure 57.6 Effect of intra-articular morphine in patients with low and high inflammation. **A,** Postoperative pain in the low-inflammatory group. Mean visual analog scale (VAS) values were obtained at different intervals. $^{*}P < 0.05$; $\bullet P = 0.06$ (not significant). **B,** Postoperative pain in the high-inflammatory group. Mean VAS values were obtained at different intervals. $^{*}P < 0.05$. (Data from Marchal JM, Delgado-Martinez AD, Poncela M, et al. Does the type of arthroscopic surgery modify the analgesic effect of intraarticular morphine and bupivacaine? A preliminary study. *Clin J Pain.* 2003;19:240-246.)

therefore the role of the tourniquet remains controversial. Whitford and coauthors suggested that retaining the tourniquet for 10 minutes after the injection of morphine postoperatively provides better pain relief than if it is released immediately,[68] a finding that has not been confirmed by others.[69] Many surgeons do not use a tourniquet while performing arthroscopic procedures on the knee, and some joints are not accessible to a tourniquet, so this method may not always be applicable.

Role of Inflammation

Marchal and colleagues classified procedures a priori into low inflammatory (diagnostic arthroscopy, partial meniscectomy) or high inflammatory (synovial plicae removal, patellar shaving, anterior cruciate ligament repair) and found that operative procedures associated with low-inflammatory states respond best to bupivacaine whereas those associated with high-inflammatory states respond better to IA morphine, thus supporting the theory that inflammation is a prerequisite for the peripheral analgesic effect of opioids[70] (Fig. 57.6). Others have also suggested that upgrading of morphine receptors during states of inflammation may account for its improved efficacy, a phenomenon that has been well documented in a rat model.[71] However, this was not found in one study in which the authors concluded that the dose-response relationship of IA morphine analgesia is not shifted by enhanced inflammation in synovial tissue.[66] Further clinical studies in this area are urgently needed.

PETHIDINE

In addition to being an opioid, pethidine is unique in having LA effects and has been used as the sole anesthetic during spinal anesthesia and analgesia.[72] Therefore, the analgesia following IA injection of pethidine may have an effect as an LA, as well as via peripheral morphine receptors. IA administration of 5% pethidine with adrenaline was found to be comparable to 5% lidocaine with adrenaline during arthroscopy of the ankle. However, lower pain scores at rest were found postoperatively than with IA prilocaine.[73] In another study, 1 mg morphine, 10 mg pethidine, or 10 μg fentanyl resulted in similar pain intensity and analgesic consumption regardless of whether the drugs were administered intra-articularly or systemically.[74] The authors concluded that the analgesia seen following IA pethidine may be identical to that following its systemic administration. Lyons and coworkers compared the effects of morphine, pethidine, and placebo and concluded that the LA effect of pethidine may be responsible for the improved early analgesia but that its duration of action was shorter than that of morphine.[75] Finally, Ekblom and colleagues found that pethidine, 200 mg intra-articularly, provides the best analgesia and that the effect is not potentiated by the addition of adrenaline and prilocaine.[76] However, in the dose range of 50 to 200 mg of pethidine intra-articularly, analgesia is due to both peripheral and central mechanisms.[77] A summary of the studies on IA administration of pethidine is presented in Table 57.4.

FENTANYL

Studies published on IA fentanyl are summarized in Table 57.5. Fentanyl, like pethidine, has been shown to have some LA effect.[83] In a randomized double-blind study, IA fentanyl, 50 μg, was compared with IA bupivacaine after knee arthroscopy.[78] During the first 2 postoperative hours, patients receiving 0.25% IA bupivacaine had superior analgesia in comparison to IA fentanyl. However, VAS pain scores during the next 18 hours were similar between IA bupivacaine and fentanyl. In another study, 50 μg fentanyl was compared with placebo. Pain scores were lower during 8 hours in the IA fentanyl group than in the placebo group.[79] Thus, fentanyl at a dose of 50 μg does produce analgesia that is better than placebo but similar to that with bupivacaine. However, more studies are warranted, specifically to compare IV with IA fentanyl. Plasma concentrations of fentanyl have not been measured following IA injection to exclude a possible systemic effect.

Table 57.4 Intra-articular Pethidine

Drug/Concentration	Comparator Drug	Type of Surgery	Type of Study	Effect (VAS or Analgesic Intake)	Reference
Pethidine, 5%	Local anesthesia	Ankle surgery	Double blind	Lower pain scores in the pethidine than in the LA group	73
Pethidine, 10 mg	Fentanyl, morphine, saline injected IA or systemically	Arthroscopic knee joint surgery	Double blind	Similar analgesia as with morphine or fentanyl and similar to systemic drug	74
Pethidine, 50 mg	Morphine or saline	Arthroscopic knee joint surgery	Double blind	Early, short-lasting analgesia (0.5-2 hr) with pethidine	75
Pethidine, 200 mg	LA (prilocaine plus adrenaline)	Arthroscopic knee joint surgery	Double blind	Good analgesia with pethidine IA during 1-4 hr	76
Pethidine, 50, 100, 200 mg	LA (prilocaine plus adrenaline)	Arthroscopic knee joint surgery	Double blind	Pethidine, 100-200 mg, provided good postoperative analgesia	77

IA, intra-articularly; LA, local anesthetic; VAS, visual analog scale.

Table 57.5 Intra-articular Fentanyl and Sufentanil

Drug/Concentration	Method of Drug Delivery	Type of Surgery	Type of Study	Effect (VAS or Analgesic Intake)	Reference
Fentanyl	Bupivacaine	Knee arthroscopy	Double blind	IA bupivacaine better during 0-2 hr	78
Fentanyl, 50 μg	Morphine or saline	Arthroscopic knee surgery	Double blind	Fentanyl better than morphine, 3 mg	79
Sufentanil, 5 or 10 μg	Sufentanil, 5 or 10 μg IV	Arthroscopic procedures	Double blind	Lower VAS scores in the sufentanil groups vs. sufentanil IV	80
Sufentanil, 10 μg	Methylprednisolone plus sufentanil or saline	Arthroscopic knee surgery	Double blind	Lower pain scores and analgesic consumption in the combined group	81
Sufentanil, 2.5 μg/hr	Epidural, femoral nerve block	ACLR	Not blinded	Epidural or femoral nerve block better than IA sufentanil for ACLR	82

ACLR, anterior cruciate ligament repair; IA, intra-articular; IV, intravenously; LA, local anesthetic; VAS, visual analog scale.

SUFENTANIL

Studies published on IA sufentanil are summarized in Table 57.5. Sufentanil is very fat soluble and can therefore easily cross the synovial membrane. When 10 μg of IA or 5 μg of IV sufentanil was compared with placebo after arthroscopic knee surgery, it was found that VAS scores at rest and during movement are significantly lower in the sufentanil groups than in the control group postoperatively and at day 1.[80] In addition, analgesic consumption was significantly lower and time until discharge home from the postanesthesia care unit was significantly shorter in the sufentanil groups. However, there was no significant difference between IA and IV sufentanil. Therefore, a systemic effect of IA sufentanil could not be ruled out. In another study, Kizilkaya and colleagues injected sufentanil, 10 μg intra-articularly, and found better postoperative analgesia and less analgesic consumption than with saline following knee arthroscopy.[81] In yet another study, a continuous 5-mL/hr infusion of ropivacaine, 2 mg/mL, plus sufentanil, 0.2 mg/mL, combined with patient-controlled analgesia boluses of 5 mL, each with a lock-out period of 2 hours, was administered intra-articularly and compared with epidural analgesia or continuous femoral blockade with the same infusion regimen postoperatively.[82] In one study, the authors did not find improved analgesia when IA sufentanil was added to a multimodal analgesic regimen following anterior cruciate ligament repair.[84] The analgesic effect of the IA infusion was insufficient when pain scores were higher.

STEROIDAL AND NONSTEROIDAL ANTI-INFLAMMATORY DRUGS

Several studies published in the literature have assessed the effects of NSAIDs, specifically, ketorolac and tenoxicam injected intra-articularly, on postoperative pain following arthroscopic surgery (Table 57.6).[85-93] Studies on IA methylprednisolone are few and involve mostly chronic pain states, which does not allow any definite conclusions to be drawn. In one study on acute pain, the authors injected methylprednisolone combined with LA and morphine into the ankle joint and compared it with placebo.[94] This combination reduced pain, joint swelling, time of immobilization, duration of sick leave, and return to sports after the arthroscopic procedure. However, 1 of 18 patients had transitory purulent arthritis requiring antibiotics and arthroscopic synovectomy. In another study, sufentanil was compared with sufentanil and methylprednisolone during arthroscopic meniscectomy. The combined use of IA

Table 57.6 Intra-articular Nonsteroidal Anti-inflammatory Drugs

Drug/Concentration	Comparator Drug	Type of Surgery	Type of Study	Effect (VAS or Analgesic Intake)	Reference
Ketorolac, 60 mg	Morphine, and combination	Arthroscopic meniscus repair	Double blind	Ketorolac or morphine equally good; combination not better	85
Ketorolac, 60 mg	Bupivacaine, and combination	Arthroscopic surgery	Double blind	Combination of bupivacaine and ketorolac was best	86
Ketorolac, 30 and 60 mg	Morphine, placebo	Arthroscopic surgery	Double blind	Ketorolac, 60 mg, better than 30 mg and placebo	58
Ketorolac, 60 mg	Bupivacaine, morphine, saline	Arthroscopic meniscectomy	Double blind	Ketorolac better than bupivacaine or morphine	87
Ketorolac, 5 mg	Ketorolac, 10 mg IV	Arthroscopy of the knee	Double blind	Ketorolac IA better than IV	88
Tenoxicam, 20 mg	Tenoxicam, 20 mg IV	Arthroscopy of the knee	Double blind	Tenoxicam IA provided better analgesia	89
Tenoxicam, 20 mg IA	Tenoxicam, 20 mg IV	Arthroscopy of the knee	Double blind	Tenoxicam IA provided better analgesia	90
Tenoxicam, 20 mg	Morphine or saline	ACLR	Double blind	Tenoxicam IA provided better analgesia	91
Tenoxicam, 20 mg	Bupivacaine or combination	Arthroscopic knee surgery	Double blind	Combination of tenoxicam and bupivacaine provided best analgesia	92
Tenoxicam, 20 mg	Bupivacaine or saline	Arthroscopy of the knee	Double blind	Lower analgesic requirements but no difference in pain intensity	93

ACLR, anterior cruciate ligament repair; IA, intra-articularly; IV, intravenously; LA, local anesthetic; VAS, visual analog scale.

sufentanil (10 μg) and methylprednisolone (40 mg) during surgery reduced both postoperative pain scores and the use of additional analgesics.[81] Use of steroids intra-articularly following arthroscopy can lead to a 2% incidence of postoperative infections.[95] In this study, the initial phase of the outbreak of infection correlated with the use of intraoperative IA corticosteroids.

KETOROLAC

In a study on the effects of ketorolac and bupivacaine, it was noted that the group that received a combination of IA bupivacaine and IA ketorolac had decreased postoperative pain, decreased need for postoperative analgesics, and increased analgesic duration.[86] Some studies using IA ketorolac for postoperative pain management have been withdrawn from the literature since the previous edition of this book and are therefore excluded from this review. Gupta and colleagues found a dose-dependent reduction in pain intensity following ketorolac injected intra-articularly, with the maximal effect occurring with 60 mg.[58] Calmet and coworkers found that 60 mg ketorolac provides a better analgesic effect than does 10 mL of 0.25% bupivacaine or 1 mg of morphine when injected intra-articularly.[87] In another study, Convery and associates showed that 5 mg IA ketorolac provides similar analgesia as 10 mg IV ketorolac following knee arthroscopy.[88] It is possible that the large doses of ketorolac administered intra-articularly by Gupta and colleagues[58] and Calmet and coworkers[87] may exert their effects via systemic absorption of the drug injected intra-articularly. However, as in the case of morphine, it is not known whether therapeutic plasma concentrations of IA ketorolac can be achieved, which may suggest a systemic as well as a peripheral effect.

TENOXICAM

Colbert and associates showed that IA tenoxicam results in superior postoperative analgesia and reduces postoperative analgesic requirements when compared with IV tenoxicam in patients undergoing day-case knee arthroscopy.[89] Elhakim and coworkers showed that IA tenoxicam, 20 mg, provides better analgesia and decreases the requirement for postoperative analgesics when compared with IV tenoxicam, 20 mg.[90] Guler and colleagues found that better analgesia is attained with IA tenoxicam than with saline.[91] Talu and associates found that IA injection of tenoxicam, 20 mg, and bupivacaine is a simple, safe, and effective method of analgesia after arthroscopic meniscectomy with high patient satisfaction.[92] Cook and coworkers showed that the use of IA tenoxicam, 20 mg, at the end of arthroscopy reduces oral analgesic requirements during the first day after the operation but does not alter the patient's perception of pain.[93] Finally, in a systematic review of the literature, Rømsing and associates found four studies comparing IA NSAIDs with systemic administration (Fig. 57.7). The results showed a statistically significant effect in favor of IA NSAIDs. The authors concluded that there is evidence for a clinically relevant peripheral analgesic action of IA NSAIDs.[96]

In summary, when comparing ketorolac or tenoxicam with placebo injected intra-articularly, all studies found a better analgesic effect of these drugs. The duration of postoperative analgesia varied in these studies. Several studies reported better pain relief following IA than following IV

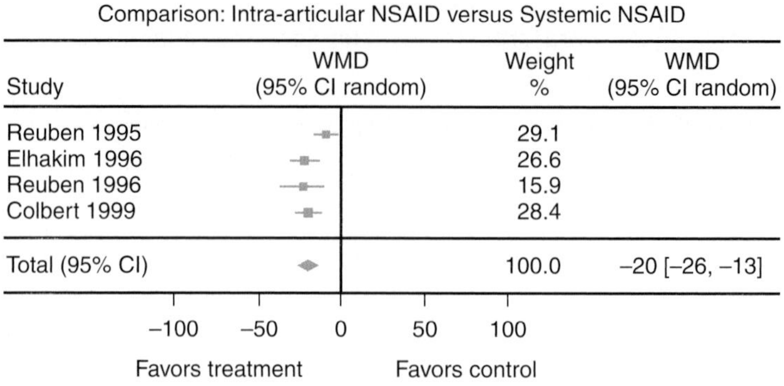

Comparison: Intra-articular NSAID versus Systemic NSAID

Study	WMD (95% CI random)	Weight %	WMD (95% CI random)
Reuben 1995		29.1	
Elhakim 1996		26.6	
Reuben 1996		15.9	
Colbert 1999		28.4	
Total (95% CI)		100.0	−20 [−26, −13]

−100 −50 0 50 100

Favors treatment Favors control

Figure 57.7 Pooled data on the efficacy of intra-articular nonsteroidal anti-inflammatory drug (NSAID) on postoperative pain following arthroscopic surgery. CI, confidence interval; WMD, weighted mean difference. (Data from Romsing J, Møiniche S, Ostergaard D, et al. Local infiltration with NSAIDs for postoperative analgesia: evidence for a peripheral analgesic action. *Acta Anaesthesiol Scand*. 2000;44:672-683.)

Table 57.7 Intra-articular Clonidine*

Drug/Concentration	Method of Drug Delivery	Type of Surgery	Type of Study	Effect (VAS or Analgesic Intake)	Reference
Clonidine, 150 μg	Clonidine, 150 μg subcutaneously, saline, or morphine	Arthroscopic knee surgery	Not blinded	Clonidine IA provided better analgesia	97
Clonidine, 150 μg	Morphine, 2 mg, combination	Arthroscopy of the knee	Double blind	Similar analgesia	98
Clonidine, 150 μg	Morphine, combination or saline	Arthroscopic knee surgery	Double blind	Combination of clonidine and opiate best	99
Clonidine, 150 μg	Morphine, 5 mg, or saline	Arthroscopic knee surgery	Double blind	Clonidine IA provided better analgesia	100
Clonidine, 1 μg/kg	Bupivacaine, morphine, 3 mg, combination	Arthroscopic meniscus repair	Double blind	Combination of clonidine and morphine was best	101
Clonidine, 1 μg/kg	Bupivacaine, combination, clonidine subcutaneously	Arthroscopic knee surgery	Not blinded	Combination of clonidine and bupivacaine was best	102
Clonidine, 1 μg/kg	Morphine, neostigmine, tenoxicam, bupivacaine	Arthroscopic knee surgery	Double blind	Clonidine or neostigmine provided best analgesia	103

*The list of studies is not exhaustive.
IA, intra-articularly; VAS, visual analog scale.

tenoxicam, which would suggest that analgesia is mediated via peripheral IA receptors.

CLONIDINE

α_2-Adrenergic agonists have been shown to have a central effect via the dorsal horn of the spinal cord and even supratentorially, as well as via peripheral analgesic receptors. All studies using IA clonidine have universally found improved analgesia when injected alone or in combination with other drugs (Table 57.7). Gentili and colleagues found that 150 μg clonidine administered intra-articularly provides analgesia unrelated to vascular uptake of the drug since subcutaneous administration of a similar dose is not equally effective.[97] In a second study comparing the effects of 150 μg clonidine with 2 mg morphine, Gentili and associates found a similar analgesic effect of both drugs.[98] In another study, peripheral codelivery of an opioid and an α_2-agonist resulted in improved postoperative pain relief when compared with each single agent given alone.[99] IA administration of 150 μg clonidine was also found to have longer-lasting pain relief postoperatively than was 5 mg of preservative-free morphine.[100] The combination of morphine (3 mg) and clonidine (1 μg/kg) resulted in decreased postoperative pain and analgesic use, as well as an increased analgesic duration when compared with either drug alone in patients undergoing knee arthroscopy[101] (Fig. 57.8). There was also a significant benefit from the individual IA administration of both clonidine and morphine versus placebo. A significant improvement in analgesia was found when clonidine was administered intra-articularly along with bupivacaine as opposed to either drug alone.[102] Furthermore, there was an increased time to first analgesic request and a decreased need for postoperative analgesics. Finally, in a comparative study of several different IA analgesics, the authors found that clonidine or neostigmine provides the best analgesia.[103]

In summary, clonidine produces analgesia when injected intra-articularly, and the effects are probably comparable to that of morphine or neostigmine alone. Clonidine combined with morphine appears to increase analgesia but not combinations with neostigmine. However, hypotension can be a problem when 150 μg clonidine is administered intra-articularly.

KETAMINE

In an animal study, Zhou and colleagues found that peripheral injections of ketamine and other *N*-methyl-D-aspartate (NMDA) receptor antagonists reduce glutamate-induced

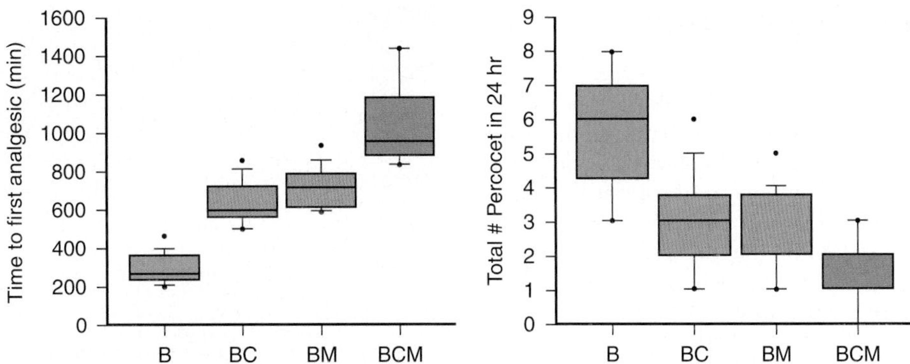

Figure 57.8 Effect of combining bupivacaine, clonidine, and morphine versus individual drugs. B, bupivacaine; BC, bupivacaine and clonidine; BCM, bupivacaine, clonidine, and morphine; BM, bupivacaine and morphine. (Data from Joshi W, Reuben SS, Kilaru PR, et al. Postoperative analgesia for outpatient arthroscopic knee surgery with intraarticular clonidine and/or morphine. *Anesth Analg*. 2000;90:1102-1106.)

pain.[104] Long-lasting analgesia was found in humans following IA ketamine, which was comparable to IA neostigmine but less effective than IA bupivacaine.[105] Rosseland and coworkers[106] studied patients with moderate to severe pain after IA arthroscopy. In this study, IA ketamine, 10 mg, had no analgesic effect on pain after arthroscopy when compared with IA injection of saline, 10 mL. IM ketamine, however, showed significantly better early pain relief than IA administration did, thus suggesting a systemic effect. In another study, no differences were found when ketamine, 0.5 mg/kg, was injected intra-articularly versus saline injected intra-articularly.[107] Batra and colleagues found that the combination of bupivacaine-ketamine appears to provide better pain relief than IA ketamine alone after day-case arthroscopic knee surgery.[108] In conclusion, the efficacy of IA ketamine, if any, is limited, and therefore it cannot be recommended today for postoperative pain management following arthroscopic surgery.

TRAMADOL

Tramadol is a weak µ-agonist and serotonin antagonist. In three studies, IA tramadol has been found to be equianalgesic to fentanyl or morphine administered intra-articularly. In a dose-response study, 20, 50, and 100 mg of IA tramadol was compared with IV tramadol in the same doses. It was found that IA administration of tramadol prolongs the duration of analgesia, which was longest when 100 mg was administered.[109] However, nausea and vomiting were most frequent when using this dose. In another study, IA tramadol, 1.5 mg/kg, resulted in pain relief comparable to that with IA fentanyl, 1.5 µg/kg.[110] It has been reported that 50 mg IA tramadol provides analgesia equivalent to that with 5 mg IA morphine.[111] The combination of IA tramadol plus periarticular bupivacaine has also been shown to give better pain relief with less analgesic requirement following arthroscopic outpatient partial meniscectomy.[112] However, the pain relief was better only during minutes 0 to 30. In another study, the authors found that an IA admixture of 100 mg tramadol with 0.25% bupivacaine provides a pronounced prolongation of analgesia when compared with either drug alone.[113] In summary, mild analgesic effects of tramadol comparable to those of IA morphine have been demonstrated, but side effects, including postoperative nausea and vomiting, dominate when the dose is 100 mg or higher.

NEOSTIGMINE

Cholinergic agonists and cholinesterase inhibitors administered systemically display a dose-dependent analgesic effect mediated through the activation of ascending and descending cerebral cholinergic pathways.[114,115] These effects are even more profound when the drugs are administered spinally.[116] Although Gentili and colleagues found that neostigmine, 500 µg, is equianalgesic to clonidine, 150 µg, but better than placebo,[117] others have not found any analgesic effect of IA neostigmine over placebo but an excellent effect when injected epidurally.[118] In another study, IA neostigmine was found to be equianalgesic to ketamine.[105] Alagol and associates compared the analgesic efficacy of neostigmine with that of clonidine, tenoxicam, bupivacaine, morphine, and placebo and reported that the best analgesia is produced by neostigmine or clonidine.[103] In a dose-response study it was found that neostigmine, 500 µg, produces moderate but significant analgesia.[119] Shafer argued that release of acetylcholine does not occur at the nerve endings within the IA space and, therefore, neostigmine cannot have an effect via anticholinesterase activity.[120] However, other mechanisms such as hyperpolarization of neurons, reduction in the release of pronociceptive neurotransmitters, or activation of the nitric oxide–cyclic guanosine monophosphate pathway might mediate this peripheral cholinergic antinociception by elevating endogenous acetylcholine levels.[119]

In summary, it is difficult to draw any definite conclusions on the effects of neostigmine injected intra-articularly because of opposing results in the literature. Although some studies have found it to be efficacious, a theoretical explanation for its analgesic effect is currently lacking.

DRUG COMBINATIONS

Many drugs have been used in combination to potentiate the effects of single agents. Combining analgesics with different mechanisms of action has the advantage of reducing the side effects of individual drugs. However, few studies have compared these combination of drugs administered by the IV or IA route to exclude a systemic effect.

INTRA-ARTICULAR INJECTIONS WITHOUT CATHETERS

Ketorolac has been combined with morphine and ropivacaine and shown to reduce pain after arthroscopic knee surgery.[121] In a recent study, Ng and colleagues compared the analgesic efficacy of a combination of ropivacaine, morphine, and ketorolac with that of ropivacaine administered alone intra-articularly and found that morphine and ketorolac enhance the analgesia produced by LA alone, reduce postdischarge analgesic consumption, and improve activities of daily living without increasing side effects after ambulatory arthroscopic knee surgery.[59] Ketorolac has also been combined with LAs and, when compared with ketorolac alone, was found to reduce pain intensity.[86] Similarly, clonidine has been combined with morphine,[98,101] as well as with LAs,[102] and was demonstrated to improve analgesia. When comparing the analgesic effects of clonidine with those of neostigmine, it was shown that IA administration of 150 µg clonidine, 500 µg neostigmine, or both produces postoperative analgesia and that their combination is not more effective.[117] However, a significantly greater number of patients who had received clonidine had at least one episode of hypotension or bradycardia. The combination of lidocaine, pethidine, and tenoxicam given intra-articularly resulted in superior analgesia and reduced oral analgesic requirement during the first day after arthroscopy when compared with lidocaine and pethidine alone.[122] It has also been shown that soft tissue and IA injection of a long-acting LA with epinephrine and morphine provides better pain control in the immediate postoperative period, decreases blood loss, and decreases the need for rescue narcotics and reversal agents.[123] As mentioned earlier, several studies have been performed in the last few years in which the authors used a combination of LA, NSAID, and epinephrine periarticularly and intra-articularly in large volumes via the local infiltration analgesia technique during knee and hip arthroplasty, and most studies have shown positive effects on pain intensity, rescue analgesic requirements, duration of hospital stay, and pain satisfaction.

INTRA-ARTICULAR INJECTIONS VIA CATHETERS

In contrast to single injections, intermittent injections or infusions of analgesics have been used intra-articularly to prolong analgesia. Thus, in one study, 0.2% ropivacaine was combined with sufentanil, 0.2 µg/mL, as an infusion (5 mL/hr) during arthroscopic ACLR.[82] The authors concluded that either an epidural or continuous femoral nerve block results in adequate pain relief in patients undergoing ACLR. However, IA analgesia seemed to be insufficient for pain management. In contrast, Rasmussen and Kehlet used a continuous infusion of a combination of ropivacaine and morphine following total knee replacement in a nonrandomized nonblinded study and found that it reduces pain and enhances rehabilitation.[94] Morphine administered intra-articularly may reduce postoperative pain when combined with other drugs. In one study, morphine combined with ketorolac for IA pain relief following minor arthroscopic procedures resulted in a synergistic effect.[58] When using PCRA, the combination of IA ropivacaine, morphine, and ketorolac has also been demonstrated to be superior to saline or a combination of ropivacaine and morphine administered intra-articularly following repair of the anterior cruciate ligament.[121] A continuous infusion of morphine and bupivacaine has been used for pain relief after subacromial arthroscopy.[54] These authors studied the analgesic effect of a continuous subacromial infusion of bupivacaine and morphine and found that pain scores at rest and supplemental analgesic requirements were lower postoperatively than in patients receiving saline infusion.

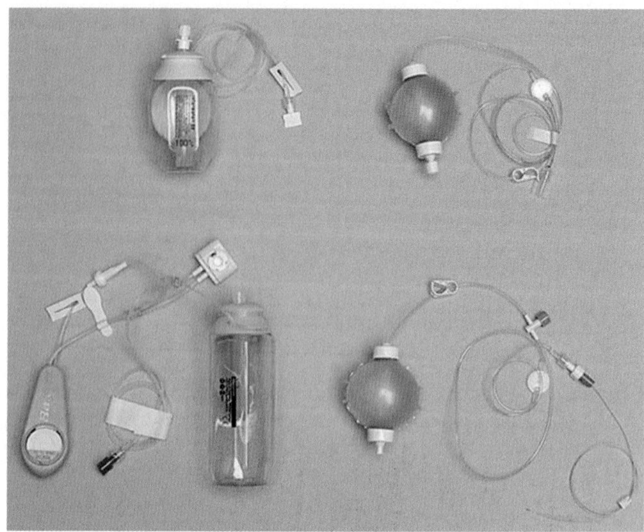

Figure 57.9 Different elastometric pumps available for the delivery of local anesthetic into the wound or intra-articularly.

In summary, combinations of drugs may be used for pain relief postoperatively after knee surgery with the following results: ketorolac combined with morphine, LA, or both results in better pain relief than either drug alone. Clonidine combined with morphine or LA offers better pain relief in some studies but not all. Morphine and LA combined together have mild benefits and are not as efficacious as when they are combined with NSAIDs.

SAFETY OF INTRA-ARTICULAR ANALGESICS

SAFETY OF DELIVERY SYSTEMS

For ambulatory practice, the IA catheters are connected to either disposable elastomeric pumps (Homepump, I-Flow Corp; Infusor, Baxter) (Fig. 57.9) or electronic pumps (Graseby PCA, Microject Sorensen Medical). The IA analgesic techniques are based on continuous, patient-controlled, or both continuous and patient-controlled infusions. When the continuous-infusion technique with elastomeric pumps is used, the rate of flow is controlled by the lumen of the catheter. By using simple techniques (i.e., opening a clamp [Homepump] or pressing a button [Infusor or Homepump]), the patient may self-administer analgesics using the concept of patient-controlled regional analgesia (PCRA). Ilfeld and colleagues[124] tested different pumps for continuous regional analgesia and found that accuracy differed significantly among the pumps, with variations in flow rate of ±15%. An increase in temperature also affected flow rates to varying degrees, with infusion rates increasing from

Table 57.8 Risk for Infection

Control/Local Anesthetic	Surgery	Positive Culture	Growth	Clinical Wound Infection	Reference
Saline	Subacromial decompression	30%	Coagulase-negative staphylococci	Negative	22
Bupivacaine plus fentanyl	Knee replacement	0.6%	*Streptococcus pneumoniae*	Positive	30
Ropivacaine plus morphine	Knee replacement	1%	?	Deep infection	25
Ropivacaine plus morphine	Anterior cruciate ligament repair	7.8%	*Staphylococcus epidermidis*	Negative	121

Table 57.9 Systemic Toxicity of Local Anesthetic

Local Anesthetic*	Dose	Surgery	Total Concentration (mg/mL)	Free Concentration (mg/mL)	Reference
Ropivacaine	225 mg	Shoulder	1.42	0.08	127
Ropivacaine	500 mg (1 hr)	Subacromial compression	2.23	0.12	22
Ropivacaine	225 mg plus 900 mg/48 hr	Shoulder/rotator cuff	—	<0.6	44
Lidocaine-adrenaline	400 mg	Knee arthroscopy	0.8	0.2	59
Ropivacaine	150 mg	Knee arthroscopy	1.2	0.06	59
Ropivacaine	200 mg	Knee arthroscopy	1.29	0.047	128

*The systemic toxicity of local anesthetics is shown with different drugs injected at different sites. Mild toxic symptoms occurred at a free concentration 0.6 mg/mL.[131]

0% to 25% for different models. Capdevila and associates[125] compared an elastomeric pump (Infusor) and electronic pumps (Graseby and Microject) and found that the elastomeric pump is as effective as the electronic pump and that the elastomeric pump is less expensive, has fewer technical problems, and gives better patient satisfaction.

TECHNICAL PROBLEMS WITH CATHETERS

In some studies it has been reported that the catheter can be dislodged,[22] disconnected,[126] or partially blocked at the outlet.[29] Better methods need to be explored to retain the catheter firmly in position while allowing easy removal. With the older elastomeric balloon pump technique there was a risk that the patient would fail to close the clamp, thereby resulting in the contents of the pump emptying within 1 hour. However, no case of systemic LA toxicity has been reported in the literature. The risk for systemic toxicity is low because absorption of LA from the joint structure is slow, which results in low plasma concentrations of LA[22,44,59,127] (see below for further details). Also, newer and safer elastometric pumps allow delivery of LA only if the patient presses a button, thus reducing the risk for accidental delivery of large volumes of LA. Long-acting LAs with low systemic toxicity, such as ropivacaine and levobupivacaine, are therefore recommended rather than bupivacaine.

LOCAL AND SYSTEMIC INFECTIONS

Infections at the site of drug injection or systemic infections are a major concern, but the reported incidence is very low. A summary of studies published in the literature in which culture specimens were taken from the catheter tip following IA placement is presented in Table 57.8. In two studies, positive isolated bacterial cultures from the catheter tip were reported in a few patients without any sign of clinical infection.[22,121] In one of these studies,[123] despite an increase in body temperature and higher level of C-reactive protein, the patient responded well to antibiotics and wound healing was considered to be normal. However, in two other studies,[30,94] two patients were reported to have deep infection that required long antibiotic therapy. Thus, proper catheter technique using bacterial filters, sterile preparation and injection of drugs, and aseptic catheter placement during surgery is vital, particularly during orthopedic surgery.

LOCAL ANESTHETIC TOXICITY

Plasma concentrations of LAs have been measured following IA injection in several studies (Table 57.9). It was found that free and total plasma concentrations are much lower than known toxic plasma concentrations in humans despite sufficiently high doses of LA.[22,59,127,128] Single injections of up to 500 mg ropivacaine subacromially have not produced toxic symptoms in humans.[22] In the only study published on continuous infusion of ropivacaine following shoulder surgery, a dose higher than 1000 mg resulted in a free plasma concentration of less than 0.6 μg/mL, which is far below known toxic concentrations in humans.[129] Therefore, the likelihood of any significant LA toxicity when the drugs are used in these doses appears to be small.

SIDE EFFECTS AND COMPLICATIONS

Before a new technique is used in daily clinical practice, it is important to show efficacy, as well as a low incidence of side effects and complications, in relation to existing techniques. Although the IA technique has been used extensively, reports of side effects and complications have been few. This could be because authors have not adequately documented side effects or because the incidence of side effects with this technique is truly low. Among the side effects of IA morphine that have been reported, itching is probably the most frequent but the least worrisome. Other side effects have included nausea and vomiting and redness at the injection site when catheters have been used. There has also been a serious concern with the IA use of NSAIDs and their effect on bone healing. Though shown to be true in animal studies, there is a lack of evidence in human studies, particularly during single-dose administration. A single dose of ketorolac injected intra-articularly in rats was found to result in significantly more inflammation than occurred with saline on histologic examination after 5 days that was not attributable to the alcohol in the injectant.[130] Morphine and ketorolac have both been found to produce mild histopathologic changes in rabbit knee joints, with morphine causing more changes than ketorolac.[131] However, the authors concluded that both these drugs can be used intra-articularly with safety. In another study by the same group, IA bupivacaine and neostigmine were also found to cause histopathologic changes in rabbit knee joints, with neostigmine having a greater effect than bupivacaine.[132] More studies, however, are needed on this important question. Operative site bleeding following the administration of NSAIDs is a real risk when these drugs are administered systemically. Nonetheless, apart from spontaneous IA bleeding following the use of clopidogrel or aspirin,[133] no significant bleeding complications have been reported following IA injection of NSAIDs. Finally, evidence seems to suggest that chondrotoxicity may be a rare but serious complication of injecting LA intra-articularly. This has been specifically documented when using bupivacaine in higher concentrations and over a longer period.[134] Therefore, we are currently using 0.2% ropivacaine without additives intra-articularly, and although our patients have been monitored for up to 6 months after surgery, no such complication has been described after more than 10 years of clinical practice. Other minor side effects do not appear to be significantly different between patients given IA neostigmine, morphine, tenoxicam, clonidine, or bupivacaine.[109]

FUTURE STUDIES

Despite the large volume of information available, as well the enormous number of studies published on the subject, the impact of individual drugs on postoperative pain management remains unclear. Combinations of drugs have been shown to produce maximum benefit with the lowest risk, and optimal selection of the different combinations of drugs and doses needs to be established through well-designed studies that include a sufficiently large number of patients. The question of the analgesic efficacy of morphine following IA surgery is still unclear because of deficiencies in study design and choice of the patient population. The ideal opioid for pain relief intra-articularly needs to be identified and perhaps more specific drugs effective on peripheral receptors developed. Prolonging the effects of LAs, opioids, and other IA analgesics through the use of IA catheters needs further documentation. In view of the huge costs involved in the development and marketing of pumps for use with the catheter techniques, both the safety and cost-effectiveness of these techniques need to be further analyzed. The risk for infection in joints has been one of the concerns of orthopedic surgeons when LAs are injected via catheters intra-articularly. Therefore, considering that insertion of a catheter at the end of the operation is a simple procedure, it would be important to exclude any significant risk for infection when using IA catheters. Specifically, IA analgesia should be assessed during procedures associated with moderate to severe pain, such as anterior cruciate ligament repair and total knee replacement, with assessment of not only the efficacy of this technique but also its side effects and complications, such as postoperative infections. The answer to all questions cannot be provided by retrospective analysis of data or by systematic reviews but by well-designed large prospective studies that take into consideration some of the problems highlighted earlier. Safety is only in numbers, and authors should therefore be asked to report not only efficacy variables but also any and all adverse effects. Analysis of the side effects of drugs injected intra-articularly should be obligatory in future studies on IA analgesia to confirm that they indeed have advantages that overweigh their disadvantages. Issues relating to the cost of drugs and equipment in relation to the benefits offered should also be documented.

CONCLUSION

IA analgesics have been used for more than a decade with variable results. In studies in which postoperative analgesia was provided with IA morphine, the effects have been mild, and it has been difficult to exclude systemic effects. In contrast, NSAIDs (ketorolac and tenoxicam) have consistently shown efficacy. However, the important question on the effect of NSAIDs on bone healing has not been answered. Combinations of several drugs, including LA, ketorolac, adrenaline, and even morphine, have shown efficacy in several studies, but the exact combination of drugs and doses needs to be elucidated. It is difficult to draw any conclusions on drugs such as clonidine, neostigmine, ketamine, fentanyl, and pethidine because of the limited number of studies published in a varying patient population. The use of catheters intra-articularly has the advantage of prolonging analgesia when LA or a combination of drugs is used, and this method needs to be developed further. Local infiltration analgesia using large volumes of diluted LA combined with an NSAID may provide such good analgesia of sufficiently long duration that the catheter technique may become obsolete in the future.

KEY POINTS

- Several analgesics have been injected alone or in combination intra-articularly, primarily into the knee and shoulder joints, to achieve relief of postoperative pain. Drugs that have been tested in clinical studies include local anesthetics, opiates (morphine, pethidine, fentanyl, and sufentanil), nonsteroidal anti-inflammatory drugs (NSAIDs—ketorolac, tenoxicam), clonidine, ketamine, corticosteroids, and neostigmine.
- Local anesthetics provide good pain relief but of short duration. Some concern exists about the risk for chondrolysis when higher concentrations of bupivacaine are injected into the shoulder joint, specifically over longer periods of time.
- Although evidence of the existence of peripheral opiate receptors exists, clinical studies have been equivocal. The analgesic effect, if any, is mild but relatively long lasting.
- NSAIDs appear to be efficacious in most studies, but some concern remains from animal studies regarding delay in bone healing.
- Clonidine is also efficacious when used in low doses intra-articularly. However, it remains unclear whether this effect is local or occurs via systemic absorption.
- The results of studies using ketamine, neostigmine, and corticosteroids are equivocal, or very few studies have been performed to be able to draw any definite conclusions.
- Combinations of drugs, specifically NSAIDs and local anesthetics, have produced added effects, and possibly even a synergistic effect of certain combinations has been described but not confirmed.
- Recently, high volumes of local anesthetics combined with NSAIDs have been used periarticularly during surgery (local infiltration analgesia) to produce analgesia of long duration. Most studies have shown good results, but the technique is under continuous development.
- The major advantage of intra-articular analgesia appears to be its efficacy combined with a low risk for side effects. The main uncertainty remains whether the effect is indeed local or occurs via systemic absorption of components of the analgesic mixture of drugs.

SUGGESTED READINGS

Andersen KV, Pfeiffer-Jensen M, Haraldsted V, et al. Reduced hospital stay and narcotic consumption, and improved mobilization with local and intraarticular infiltration after hip arthroplasty: a randomized clinical trial of an intraarticular technique versus epidural infusion in 80 patients. *Acta Orthop.* 2007;78:180-186.

Gupta A, Bodin L, Holmstrom B, et al. A systematic review of the peripheral analgesics effects of intraarticular morphine. *Anesth Analg.* 2001;93:761-770.

Gupta A, Favaios S, Perniola A, et al. A meta-analysis of the efficacy of wound catheters for post-operative pain management. *Acta Anaesthesiol Scand.* 2011;55:785-796.

Kalso E, Kramer M, Carroll D, et al. Pain relief from intra-articular morphine after knee surgery: a qualitative systematic review. *Pain.* 1997;71:642-651.

Kalso E, Smith L, McQuay HJ, et al. No pain, no gain: clinical excellence and scientific rigour—lessons learned from IA morphine. *Pain.* 2002; 98:269-275.

Likar R, Mousa SA, Philippitsch G, et al. Increased numbers of opioid expressing inflammatory cells do not affect intra-articular morphine analgesia. *Br J Anaesth.* 2004;93:375-380.

Rosseland LA, Stubhaug A, Sandberg L, et al. Intra-articular (IA) catheter administration of postoperative analgesics: a new trial design allows evaluation of baseline pain, demonstrates large variations in need of analgesics, and finds no analgesic effect of IA ketamine compared with IA saline. *Pain.* 2003;104:25-34.

Rosseland LA, Stubhaug A. Gender is a confounding factor in pain trials: women report more pain than men after arthroscopic surgery. *Pain.* 2004;112:248-253.

The references for this chapter can be found at www.expertconsult.com.

58 Chemical Neurolytic Blocks

Meredith C.B. Adams | Honorio T. Benzon | Robert W. Hurley

Neurolytic therapy remains a therapy of last resort. However, for the appropriate patient, it can result in significant improvement of quality of life and possibly improved function. Few other interventional pain therapies have such extreme risk/benefit profiles requiring targeted patient selection and meticulous procedural technique. Evaluating neurolysis as a therapeutic option is usually reserved for end-stage therapy, primarily patients with refractory cancer pain resulting from the significant possibility of severe side effects. For instance, neuraxial neurolysis can provide profound pain relief for patients with pain related to invasive tumors involving the pelvis, but this approach often also leads to loss of bowel or bladder function and may well also produce weakness in the lower extremities. It should also be emphasized that relief from neurolytic blocks is usually not complete, as most patients with cancer pain have multiple sources of their pain. Although this therapeutic modality is no longer novel in development or application, neuraxial neurolysis is an important treatment modality for patients *in extremis.* Neurolytic agents available in the United States for common use in the neuraxis include ethanol and phenol. The five criteria for neurolysis[1] are (1) the presence of severe pain, (2) the failure of less invasive techniques to relieve the pain, (3) the presence of well-localized pain, (4) the relief of pain with diagnostic local anesthetic blocks, and (5) the absence of undesirable effects after diagnostic blocks (Box 58.1).

Neurolytic blocks can be peripheral, neuraxial, or visceral. Of the three, visceral blocks are most commonly performed (this subject will be covered in Chapter 60), whereas neuraxial and peripheral neurolytic blocks are performed less frequently for many reasons. In the case of peripheral neurolytic nerve blocks, blocking mixed motor and sensory nerves can cause motor deficit leading to loss of functionality for the patient. In addition, peripheral neuritis and deafferentation pain are potential painful consequences, whereas the block itself is not predictably permanent.[1] Finally, the patient may also be dissatisfied with the subsequent numbness of the area and complain of symptoms of *anesthesia dolorosa.* Neuraxial neurolytic blocks, including both intrathecal and epidural alcohol or phenol neurolytic blocks, are rarely used today because neuraxial analgesics including opioids, local anesthetics, and clonidine can effectively and safely be used to treat cancer pain. Where an intrathecal drug delivery system can provide widespread pain relief that can be adjusted to accommodate many scenarios, a successful neurolytic block may have to be repeated with changes in pain pathology, such as the presence of new metastatic lesions. In such cases, it is impractical to perform subsequent subarachnoid neurolytic injections because of their attendant risks, whereas an indwelling intrathecal (and occasionally epidural) drug delivery system will cover new areas of pain and continue to be useful. This chapter reviews the technical approaches and pharmacological agents used for neurolytic blocks.

NEUROLYTIC AGENTS (Table 58.1)

ALCOHOL

Ethyl alcohol (ethanol) is the classic neurolytic agent first reported by Dogliotti in 1931 for intrathecal injection.[2] Anhydrous ethanol is commercially available undiluted (100% concentration) but will absorb a small amount of water from the air upon exposure to the atmosphere. Although neurolytic blocks have been shown to require a concentration of 33% or greater to effect neurolysis,[3] the most common concentrations used are ≥80% when diluted with contrast medium or local anesthetic. The neurolytic action of alcohol is produced by the extraction of neural cholesterol, phospholipids, and cerebrosides, and the precipitation of mucopeptides.[4] These actions result in sclerosis of the nerve fibers and myelin sheath, leading to demyelination.[5] The basal lamina of the Schwann cell sheath remains intact, allowing for new Schwann cell growth, thereby providing the framework for subsequent nerve fiber growth. This framework encourages the regeneration of axons, but only if the cell bodies of these nerves are not completely destroyed.[6] The pathway of degeneration is nonselective and can be observed in peripheral nerves and spinal nerve roots following intrathecal injection. Areas of demyelination can be seen in posterior columns, Lissauer's tract, and the dorsal root, followed by Wallerian degeneration to the dorsal horn.[7] Intrathecal alcohol injection results in rapid uptake of alcohol and variable injury to the surface of the spinal cord.

Ethanol is quickly absorbed from the cerebrospinal fluid (CSF) so that only 10% of the initial dose remains in the CSF after 10 minutes and only 4% after 30 minutes.[8] The rapid spread from the injection site means larger volumes are required than for phenol, which in turn may result in local tissue damage.[9] In the case of celiac plexus blocks, alcohol is rapidly absorbed into the bloodstream. It has been shown that serum ethanol levels up to 54 mg/dL can occur after a celiac plexus block.[10] However, following the intrathecal administration of alcohol, it is unlikely that there will be significant vascular uptake. Ethanol has a specific gravity of less than 0.8, and CSF has a specific gravity of slightly greater than 1. Within the CSF, alcohol is hypobaric and will move against gravity, "floating" upward. Therefore, positioning

Box 58.1 Criteria for Use of Neurolytic Blockade

- Pain is severe and unremitting
- Pain is unresponsive to medical management
- Pain is relieved with diagnostic blocks using local anesthetic
- No undesirable effects appear during local anesthetic blocks
- Pain is well localized
- Pain affects the patient's function
- Patient is not a candidate for neuraxial medication delivery systems
- Patient has failed neuraxial medication delivery
- The patient is able perform informed consent or has appropriate advance directive

Table 58.1 Characteristics of Chemical Neurolytic Agents

	Alcohol	Phenol
Physical properties	Low water solubility	Absorbs water on air exposure
Stability at room temperature	Unstable	Stable
Concentration	100%	4%-8%
Diluent	None	Glycerin
Relative to CSF	Hypobaric	Hyperbaric
Injection sensation	Burning pain	Painless, warm feeling
Onset of neurolysis	Immediate	Delayed (15 min)
CSF uptake ends	30 minutes	15 minutes
Full effect of neurolysis	3-5 days	1 day

of the patient is an extremely important factor to consider when planning the procedure.

The use of ethanol as a neurolytic agent has been associated with a disulfram-like effect, acetaldehyde syndrome. Case reports include patients taking moxalactam, a beta lactam antibiotic that inhibits aldehyde dehydrogenase, documented disulfram-like effects, and another taking 1-hexyl carbamoyl-5-fluorouracil, an anticancer drug, experienced similar symptoms.[11] The patients experienced flushing, hypotension, tachycardia, and diaphoresis within 15 minutes of alcohol administration. The symptoms resolved 4 to 6 hours later, and efforts were undertaken to stabilize hemodynamics. Both cases occurred after celiac plexus blocks. It is important for the pain practitioner to recognize medications that may cause disulfram-like effects, such as chloramphenicol, beta-lactams, metronidazole, tolbutamide, chlorpropamide, and disulfram, after peripheral neurolytic blocks with alcohol.[12]

Perineural administration of ethanol is associated with burning dysesthesias in the distribution of the nerve. This sensation is often extremely unpleasant for the patient and can last from a few minutes to a few weeks. To alleviate this outcome, local anesthetic is administered prior to the use of ethyl alcohol. The use of this initial dose of local anesthetic can also provide diagnostic guidance on the correct location for the neurolytic that has enormous importance. The administration of ethanol for the purpose of neurolysis can have catastrophic consequences. It has been associated with both transient and permanent paraplegia in both celiac plexus and intrathecal blocks. It has been postulated that these effects are secondary to vasospasm of the spinal arteries by the direct action of alcohol or direct damage to the spinal motor nerves.[9]

PHENOL

Phenol is a benzene ring with one hydroxyl group substituted for a hydrogen atom. It is usually prepared by the hospital pharmacy because it is not commercially available in premixed liquid form. Phenol is poorly soluble in water and, at room temperature, forms only a 6.7% aqueous solution. It has a shelf life of approximately 1 year if refrigerated and shielded from light exposure. When phenol is exposed to room air, it oxidizes and turns a reddish color. Phenol is frequently prepared with contrast and sterile water, sterile saline, or glycerin. When it is prepared with glycerin, it has limited anatomic spread, and, hence, injections are well localized. In rats, the aqueous solution of phenol has greater ability to penetrate the perineurium and produce greater endoneurial damage than glycerin preparations, but there is no difference in results following intraneural injection.[13] Unlike alcohol, phenol injection has an initial local anesthetic effect. It is not associated with localized burning but instead creates a sensation of warmth for a short time after injection. The distribution of this sensation can help the practitioner verify proper needle placement similar to a diagnostic local anesthetic injection. Concentrations of 4% to 10% are typically used for neurolysis. When phenol is prepared in glycerin, it has a specific gravity of 1.25, making it hyperbaric. Preparations of phenol in glycerin are highly viscous, which may make administration through a small (22 or 25 gauge) spinal needle difficult.

Putnam and Hampton first used phenol as a neurolytic agent in 1936. Mandl used it for a sympathetic ganglion block in animals in 1947.[14] Phenol was first used as a medication in an intrathecal injection in humans in 1955.[15] It was once believed that phenol's neurolytic effects might be due to local ischemia because of its greater affinity for vascular tissue compared to neural tissue.[16,17] Racz found that unlike epidural injection, tissue destruction resulted after intrathecal injection even though the vasculature was intact in the areas of spinal cord destruction.[18] This finding points toward direct neurotoxic effects rather than effects secondary to local ischemia. Phenol's effects may be a combination of direct neurotoxic and ischemic effects.[19] Originally, it was surmised that phenol had a selective effect on small-diameter, unmyelinated nerve fibers, such as C-fiber afferents and lightly myelinated A-δ afferents. Subsequent studies have shown that phenol concentrations determine the type and extent of nerve disruption. Dilute intrathecal phenol can produce a transient local anesthetic blockade, whereas increased concentrations can produce significant neural damage.[20] At concentrations less than 5%, phenol results in protein denaturation of axons and surrounding blood vessels. At concentrations >5%, phenol can produce protein coagulation and nonselective segmental demyelination.[9] Nathan confirmed the nonselective effects of phenol using histologic studies combined with evidence of electrophysiologic changes to Aα and Aβ fibers.[21] Smith showed that intrathecal phenol injections in cats and humans primarily destroyed axons in dorsal rootlets and in the dorsal columns of the spinal cord. It was also noted to exert some effects on the ventral root axons.[22] Maher and Mehta noted that motor blocks by phenol were possible at concentrations greater than 5%, whereas intrathecal injections of less than 5% produced mostly sensory blocks.[23] At higher concentrations, the extent of damage can increase significantly, with the potential of axonal nerve root damage and spinal cord infarcts. Injections of high-concentration phenol have also been associated with arachnoiditis and meningitis.[24]

Systemic doses of phenol in excess of 8.5% are associated with toxic side effects. These effects initially are convulsions, followed by central nervous system depression, and, finally, cardiovascular collapse. Chronic long-term exposure may be associated with renal toxicity, skin lesions, and gastrointestinal effects. However, phenol is not classically used in long-term settings, and the customary doses of less than 100 mg are unlikely to produce any systemic effects.[5]

When compared to alcohol, phenol seems to facilitate axonal regeneration in a shorter period of time. Electrophysiologic studies comparing peripheral nerve destruction in cats showed that those injected with phenol had returned to normal by 2 months, whereas at the end of the same time period, those injected with alcohol still demonstrated depression of compound action potentials.[25]

GLYCEROL

Glycerol is a colorless, odorless, viscous, liquid, polyol compound. It has three hydroxyl groups that result in high water solubility and it is hygroscopic in nature. The glycerol backbone is central to all lipids known as triglycerides. When placed on nervous tissue, myelin disintegration and axonolysis occur in both myelinated and unmyelinated fibers. In the uninjured nerve, the c-fiber and lightly myelinated fibers are the most sensitive to neurolysis, requiring higher concentrations to destroy the heavily myelinated fibers. However, this order is altered in the injured nerve; the heavily myelinated fibers become very sensitive to the neurolytic properties of glycerol. In 1981, Hakanson was the first to use glycerol for neurolysis of the trigeminal ganglion.[26] The success is most likely related to a combination of the viscous nature of glycerol and resultant lack of spread into other sensitive structures, the low concentration required to destroy the abnormally firing myelinated fibers while preserving the uninjured sensory afferents. The use of glycerol for neurolysis is now primarily restricted to the neurolysis of the Gasserian ganglion.

NEUROLYTIC BLOCKS

Neurolytic agents can be injected surrounding peripheral nerves, along the neuraxis within the intrathecal or epidural spaces, or adjacent to visceral sympathetic nerves. Each of these sites of injection is associated with specific benefits, risks, and complications. Peripheral neurolysis can include injection into the trigeminal ganglion, truncal, upper, and lower extremities.[1]

Head and Neck

Gasserian Ganglion Neurolysis. Peripheral nerves in the head and neck are destroyed for a variety of reasons. These include blockade of the trigeminal ganglion for trigeminal neuralgia that is not responsive to medical management and for relief of cancer pain secondary to invasive tumors of the orbit, maxillary sinus, and mandible; and blockade of individual peripheral nerves in the head.

The gasserian ganglion is formed from two trigeminal roots that exit the ventral surface of the brainstem at the midpontine level.[27] The roots pass forward and in a lateral direction, in the posterior fossa of the cranium, across the border of the petrous temporal bone. It then enters the Meckel's cave in the middle cranial fossa. The gasserian ganglion contains the ophthalmic, maxillary, and mandibular divisions. A smaller motor root joins the mandibular division as it exits the foramen ovale. It should be noted that a dural pouch, the trigeminal cistern, lies behind the trigeminal ganglion. In gasserian ganglion block, the needle is inserted approximately 2.5 cm lateral to the side of the mouth and advanced, perpendicular to the middle of the eye (with the eye in the midposition), in a cephalad direction toward the auditory meatus.[28] When contact is made with the base of the skull, the needle is withdrawn and "walked" posteriorly toward the foramen ovale (Fig. 58.1). A free flow of CSF is usually noted, and fluoroscopy is then used to confirm correct needle placement. Very small amounts (i.e., 0.1-mL increments) of local anesthetic or neurolytic agent (commonly glycerol) are injected to a total of 0.4 to 0.5 mL. Because of their different baricity, the patient remains supine if alcohol is used but placed in a sitting position with the chin on the chest prior to the injection of phenol. This maneuver localizes the phenol around the maxillary and mandibular divisions of the trigeminal nerve, avoiding the ophthalmic division and the risk of keratitis from loss of the conjunctival reflex. If glycerol is used, the patient is kept in a "seated"/head-up position. The pterygopalatine space is highly vascular, and significant hematoma of the face and subscleral hematoma of the eye can occur. Veins in the subtemporal region can be punctured, causing hemorrhage in the temporal fossa. Local anesthetic injection can lead to spinal anesthesia because the ganglion lies within the cerebrospinal fluid. Blockade of the motor fibers of the trigeminal nerve can interfere with mastication.[29] Oculomotor palsy, which results in diplopia and strabismus, is usually temporary. Abducens palsy is also temporary, although cases of permanent lateral rectus palsy have been reported.[30] Spread of the neurolytic agent into the facial nerve results in paralysis of the facial muscles and inability of the eyelid to close, resulting in keratitis or corneal ulceration. Blockade of the greater superficial petrosal nerve may result in lack of tear formation and conjunctivitis. Blockade of the acoustic nerve may result in deafness or dizziness. The delayed effects of gasserian ganglion neurolytic block include trophic problems such as keratitis, ulcerations in the nose, and erosions in the mouth. These disturbances usually occur after trauma to the area. Another delayed complication is anesthesia dolorosa seen more commonly with alcohol and phenol neurolysis. Because the neurolytic block of the gasserian ganglion is associated with myriad devastating complications, many neurosurgeons and pain medicine physicians choose to perform radiofrequency rhizotomy of the ganglion instead.[30] The technical difficulty and complications associated with gasserian ganglion block led some investigators to perform peripheral branch (supraorbital, infraorbital, and mandibular nerves) injections with 10% phenol to relieve the pain of tic douloureux.[31]

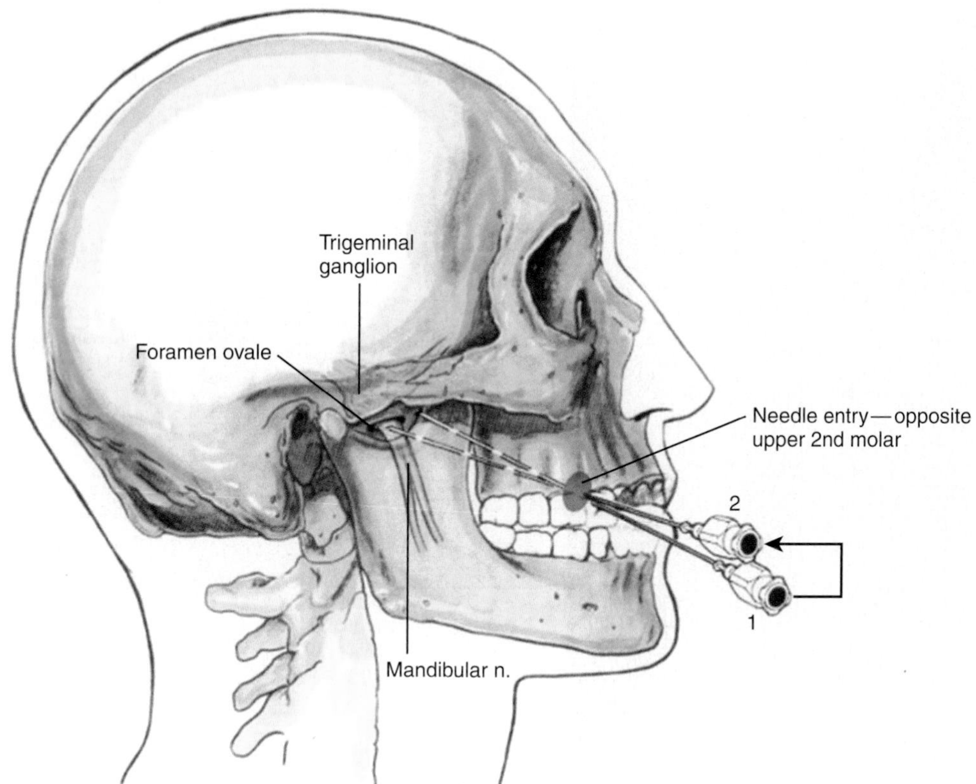

Figure 58.1 Trigeminal ganglion block: anatomy and technique. (Reprinted with permission from Brown D. *Atlas of Regional Anesthesia*. 3rd ed. Philadelphia: Saunders, an Imprint of Elsevier; 2006, Figure 20-5.)

Other Neurolytic Blocks of the Head and Neck. Neurolytic blocks of individual cranial nerves and their branches have also been performed, and complications are related to nerve location and the tissues it innervates. Neurolytic block of the maxillary nerve at the foramen rotundum or of the infraorbital nerve may cause ulceration and sloughing of the alar of the nose and the cheek, ischemic necrosis of the palate, or sloughing of the posterior portion of the superior ridge of the maxilla.[30] Blockade of the mandibular nerve at the foramen ovale may result in weakness of the muscles of mastication in the blocked side, whereas blockade of the facial nerve causes weakness or paralysis of the facial muscles. Blockade of the glossopharyngeal nerve is rarely performed because of the proximity of the nerve to the vagus, spinal accessory, and hypoglossal nerves. The close location of the other nerves led investigators to recommend blockade of the glossopharyngeal nerve under fluoroscopic control[32] or to use radiofrequency rhizotomy.[33] The sensory area of innervation of the glossopharyngeal nerve includes the nasopharynx, eustachian tube, uvula, tonsil, soft palate, base of the tongue, and part of the external auditory canal.[1] Paralysis of the pharyngeal muscles is a consequence of blockade of the glossopharyngeal nerve. The authors do not recommend any of these neurolytic procedures for use by pain physicians.

PARAVERTEBRAL SYMPATHETIC NEUROLYSIS

STELLATE GANGLION NEUROLYSIS

The cervical sympathetic trunk contains the superior, middle, and inferior cervical ganglia. In 80% of the population, the lowest cervical ganglion is fused with the first thoracic ganglion, forming the cervicothoracic (stellate) ganglion. The cervical sympathetic chain lies anterior to the prevertebral fascia, which encloses the prevertebral muscle. The sympathetic chain is enclosed within the alar fascia, a thin fascia that separates the cervical sympathetic chain from the retropharyngeal space. The carotid sheath is connected to the alar fascia by a mesothelium-like fascia. The fascial plane that encloses the sympathetic chain may be in direct communication with several spaces and structures, including the brachial plexus, vertebral artery, endothoracic fascia, and the thoracic wall muscle at T1-T2. At the C6 level, the cervical sympathetic trunk is located posterolaterally to the prevertebral fascia on the surface of the longus colli muscle.[34] The carotid vessels are anterior, whereas the nerve roots that contribute to the inferior portion of the brachial plexus are lateral to the ganglion. The vertebral artery passes over the ganglion and enters the vertebral foramen posterior to the anterior tubercle of C6. The communications of the fascia covering the stellate ganglion with several structures, as noted previously, and the proximity of the stellate ganglion to the vertebral and carotid vessels, phrenic nerve, and the recurrent laryngeal nerve explain some of the potential complications of the stellate ganglion block (Fig. 58.2).[35]

Several techniques of stellate ganglion block have been described. These include insertion of the needle at the level of C6, placement of the needle at C7, and the posterior thoracic approach.[35] With C6 placement, the needle is placed in contact with either the C6 tubercle or the junction between the C6 vertebral body and the tubercle. The needle is withdrawn 1 to 2 mm and an initial test dose of 0.5 to 1 mL

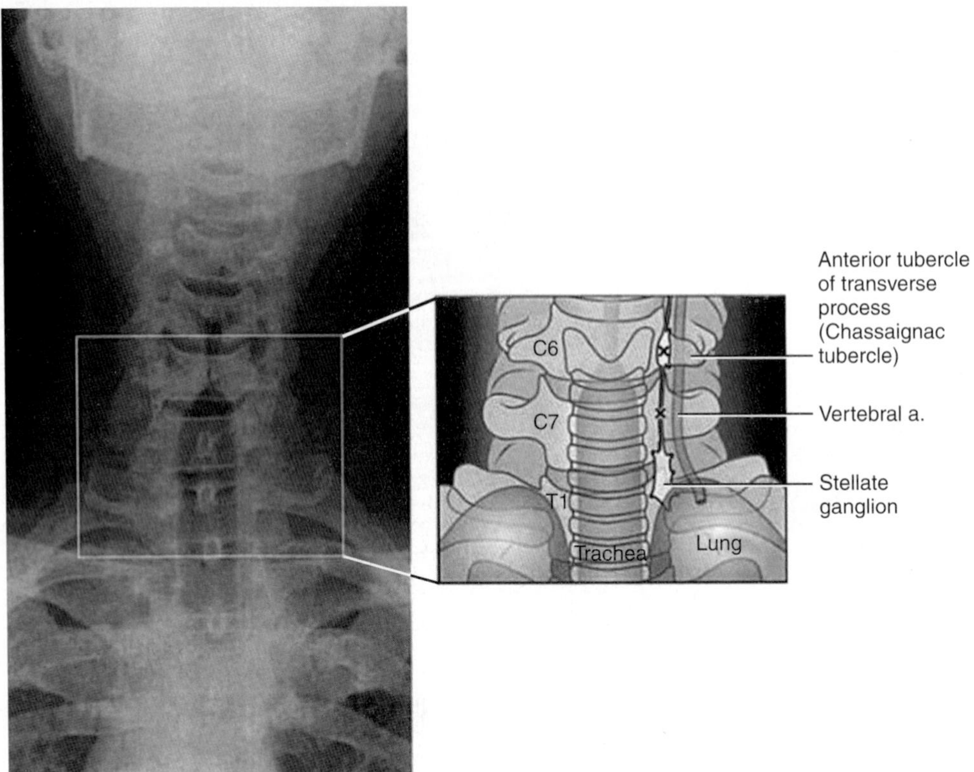

Figure 58.2 Stellate ganglion anatomy. Relative position of the stellate ganglion, the vertebral artery, and the inferior cervical vertebrae. The relative positions of the C6, C7, T1 vertebral bodies of the Chassaignac tubercle (anterior tubercle of C6 transverse process), and the vertebral artery are illustrated. The vertebral artery traverses within the bony foramen at the C6 level, but the presence of a bony foramen at C7 is variable, and here the artery often courses unprotected anterior to the C7 transverse process. (Adapted from Janik IE, Hoeft MA, Rathmell J. Anatomic variation of Chassaignac tubercle measured by computed tomography: implications for stellate ganglion block. Presented at the annual fall meeting of the American Society of Regional Anesthesia and Pain Medicine; November 7-10, 2002, Phoenix, AZ; and Rathmell JP. *Atlas of Image-Guided Intervention in Regional Anesthesia and Pain,* 2005, Figure 10-2.)

is injected, or volumes of 5 to 10 mL can be injected. If the patient is positioned in reverse Trendelenburg, the injectate travels caudad and reaches the stellate ganglion and the upper thoracic sympathetic ganglia.[36] A smaller volume of drug is adequate when the needle is placed at the level of C7. However, there is increased incidence of vertebral artery injection with this approach because the artery lies anterior to the C7 transverse process. There is also an increased risk of pneumothorax because the dome of the lung is closer to the injection site. These risks are reduced when an oblique approach aiming at the uncinate process of C7 is taken.[37,38] The posterior thoracic approach requires fluoroscopic guidance to identify the lamina of T1 or T2, and dye injection is recommended to document the spread of the drug. In this approach, the needle contacts the lamina of T1 or T2, is moved laterally off the lamina, and is advanced to pass the costotransverse ligament at a depth of 2 cm beyond the lamina. Either loss of resistance is used or dye is injected to confirm proper needle placement.

Kapral developed a technique, involving the use of ultrasound, to visualize the stellate ganglion.[39] Since the initial technique was developed, many modifications have been made to increase the safety, efficacy, and speed of the block.[34,40] The patient is positioned supine with the neck slightly hyperextended, and an ultrasound probe is placed at the level of C6, providing a cross section of the anatomy at this level. Visible are the trachea, esophagus, thyroid gland, carotid artery, jugular vein, longus colli muscle, and transverse process of C6. A 22G × 2-inch needle can be advanced in plane with the ultrasound probe paratracheally toward the longus colli muscle, while avoiding the other structures, and stopping once the tip reaches the prevertebral fascia. At this point, 5 to 10 mL of local anesthetic is deposited under direct visualization and can be seen spreading along the prevertebral fascia.[41]

The complications of an intravascular injection of local anesthetic are well known. These include loss of consciousness, apnea, hypotension, and seizures. Local anesthetic blocks of the stellate ganglion have been performed for complex regional pain syndrome, vascular insufficiency of the upper extremities, and hyperhidrosis of the face and upper extremities. Neurolytic blockade of the stellate ganglion has been performed for complex regional pain syndrome when there is consistent relief after diagnostic block with local anesthetic and without prolongation of the duration of pain relief. The overall incidence of complications is 0.17%.[42] The exact incidence of pneumothorax is not known. Aside from Horner's syndrome, hoarseness, blockade of the brachial plexus, subarachnoid and epidural spread, and cord infarction have been reported.[43] Brachial plexus block is secondary to the needle being inserted too lateral or from the spread of the drug along the prevertebral fascia. Ptosis can be corrected by suspension operation of the upper eyelid. Additionally, retropharyngeal hematomas have been reported, ranging from minimal patient discomfort to complete loss of airway.[44,45] An unusual reported complication is transient locked-in syndrome, in which the patient is paralyzed and cannot breathe or speak, but can only move his or her eyes due to accidental intravascular anesthetic injection.[46] These complications led other investigators to use alternative techniques to cervicothoracic sympathectomy, including radiofrequency rhizotomy and thoracoscopic sympathectomy.

LUMBAR SYMPATHETIC NEUROLYSIS

Paravertebral sympathetic blocks are performed for the treatment of complex regional pain syndromes, vascular insufficiencies of the lower extremities, phantom limb pain, and other conditions such as hyperhidrosis. Percutaneous thoracic paravertebral sympathetic neurolysis is rarely performed because of the high incidence of pneumothorax. A thoracic surgeon who does a surgical sympathectomy under direct vision usually performs treatment of this region. Lumbar paravertebral sympathetic neurolysis can be more safely performed. In this technique, the needles are placed in the anterolateral surface of L2 or L3. Fluoroscopy is used to confirm vertebral level of placement, correct position of the needle tip, and adequate spread of the dye along the anterolateral aspect of the vertebral bodies. Although a single needle technique can be used, two needles (one at L2 and the other at L3) are recommended for chemical neurolysis so that a smaller volume can be injected per needle. One to 2 mL of local anesthetic is injected, and if it is followed by a temperature increase, 3 to 4 mL of 6% to 10% phenol is injected per needle. The reported complications of the block include subarachnoid injection secondary to injection near the dural cuff at the intervertebral foramen, sensory and motor block resulting from nerve root injury, paresthesias, and backache. The ureter can be injured from the needle or from phenol-induced thrombosis of the branch of the ovarian artery supplying the ureter. Genitofemoral neuralgia occurs in 7% to 20% of patients and may last 4 to 5 weeks.[47] Postsympathectomy dysesthesias result in numbness and pain in the thigh and may last several months. The use of guidance (fluoroscopy, computed tomography [CT], or ultrasound) is mandatory when neurolytic block of the sympathetic chain is performed. Alternate nonchemical neurolytic techniques, including radiofrequency rhizotomy of the lumbar sympathetic nerves, have been employed to avoid the complications from spillage of the neurolytic agent; however, this technique did not result in long-term relief,[48] although other studies have found benefit.[49,50] Compared with phenol neurolysis, incomplete neurolysis appears to be more common with radiofrequency rhizotomy,[51] but the incidence of postsympathectomy neuralgia was higher in the phenol group (33% versus 11%).

NEUROLYTIC BLOCKS OF THE TRUNK AND EXTREMITIES

INTERCOSTAL NEUROLYSIS

Peripheral neurolysis is a controversial subject. Although some argue that it has no real use in pain management, it has found a role in intercostal neurolytic blocks for the management of malignant chest wall pain. The use of peripheral neurolysis follows successful diagnostic blocks using local anesthetics. Peripheral neurolytic blocks are frequently associated with neuritis and deafferentation pain, in addition to postinjection dysesthesias (Box 58.2). Although these complications are unpleasant, they may be preferable to the patient's current pain, or the patient may succumb to his or her primary disease before these complications fully manifest themselves.[52] Intercostal blocks are used in the treatment of thoracic or abdominal wall pain and as adjunct in surgery.[53,54] Complications include pneumothorax, intravascular injection, intrapulmonary injection with consequent bronchospasm, and neuraxial spread (Table 58.2). The incidence of pneumothorax detected by radiograph is 0.082 to 2%.[55] Clinically significant pneumothorax occurs at a low rate and chest tube insertion is rarely required. Another reported complication is total spinal anesthesia after intraoperative intrathoracic injection.[56] The intrathoracic injection at a medial location resulted in the injection of the local anesthetic into a dural cuff or into the nerve itself, with proximal spread of the drug. Bronchospasm from intrapulmonary injection of phenol has been reported.[57] Persistent paraplegia from intercostal block with 7.5% phenol has additionally been reported, with the authors suspecting the damage occurred via spread of phenol through the intervertebral foramen and subsequent destruction of motor and sensory nerve roots.[58] Similar to the advantages of its use in other peripheral nerve blocks, ultrasound has made intercostal nerve block a safer technique in that the pleura is visualized, preventing its puncture and avoiding pneumothorax.[59]

Box 58.2 Limitations of Peripheral Neurolytic Blocks

- Motor deficits are likely when mixed sensory-motor nerves are blocked.
- Neuritis/deafferentation pain may occur and can be more severe than preexisting pain.
- Neurolytic blocks are not permanent.
- Sensory loss following peripheral neurolysis can in some cases become more distressing than the original pain.

Table 58.2 Complications after Truncal Blocks

Block	Complications
Intercostal	Pneumothorax
	Intravascular injection
	Bronchospasm (intrapulmonary injection)
	Neuraxial block
Somatic	Hypotension
	Urinary retention
Lumbar	Subarachnoid injection

ILIOINGUINAL AND ILIOHYPOGASTRIC NEUROLYSIS

Ilioinguinal and iliohypogastric nerve blocks are used in the perioperative management of pain after inguinal herniorrhaphy. Preoperative wound infiltration can decrease pain scores and analgesic requirements after inguinal herniorrhaphy. The preemptive analgesic effect of the preincisional infiltration of local anesthetic before herniorrhaphy has not been firmly established. In the pain clinic, ilioinguinal and iliohypogastric nerve blocks are performed in the diagnosis and treatment of inguinal and suprapubic pain after lower abdominal surgery or inguinal hernia repair. Complications of the block include unintentional blocks of the lateral femoral cutaneous and femoral nerves. The incidences of these complications are not known. Neurolytic blocks of these nerves are presently being supplanted by pulsed radiofrequency treatment (this is not a neurolytic procedure) and radiofrequency rhizotomy.[60] The advantage of radiofrequency techniques includes the ability to first stimulate the nerves to provide exact localization in a manner similar to sensory and motor testing of medial branch nerves in facet joint denervation. Diagnostic blocks are recommended before neurolytic (chemical or thermal) procedures are performed.

NEUROLYSIS OF OTHER PERIPHERAL NERVES

Neurolytic injections have been reported to be useful in patients with palpable painful neuromas (0.2 to 0.5 mL of 5% phenol),[61] patients with poststernotomy pain secondary to scar neuroma (2 to 3 mL of 6% phenol),[62] and patients with painful surgical scars (1 mL of absolute alcohol).[63] Neuritis has not been reported after these peripheral neurolyses.

Nerve root destruction in the extremities is rarely performed because of the attendant paralysis of the extremity. Mullin reported neurolytic blockade of the brachial plexus with 10 mL of 10% phenol in a patient with a painful arm secondary to Pancoast tumor.[64] The patient had short-term pain relief with minimal motor blockade. The complications from neurolysis of peripheral nerves include painful dysesthesias and sensory and motor blockade. The exact incidences of these complications are not known but are high enough that this treatment is not recommended.

NEUROLYSIS FOR MYOFASCIAL PAIN AND SPASTICITY

Neurolytic blocks of peripheral nerves are useful in patients with acquired spasticity in order to facilitate rehabilitation and restore normal position of the limb for maintenance of hygiene. Examples of these blocks include obturator block to relieve hip adduction, musculocutaneous nerve block for elbow flexion, and posterior tibial nerve block for plantar flexion.[65] Peripheral nerve blocks with phenol have been performed in patients with spasticity to improve their gait and balance and to assist in their rehabilitation. In this technique, the motor or mixed nerves are targeted preferentially. A nerve stimulator is used for nerve identification. Injections of small volumes of 3% to 5% phenol are effective in relieving the hypertonicity of affected muscles, and relaxation of the muscle usually lasts 2 months. During this time, extensive physical therapy is employed for functional training of the limb. It appears that ethanol treatment can extend the therapeutic benefit. In a randomized controlled trial (RCT) of 20 patients evaluating phenol (5%) versus ethanol (50%) in neurolysis of tibial motor branches for gastrocnemius spasm after stroke, ethanol maintained its effect for 6 months in 9 of the 10 patients, whereas phenol lasted the same amount of time in 7 of the 10 patients.[66] The reported complications include focal motor weakness in 15% of patients and dysesthesias in 10% of patients, but there were no differences between those that received ethanol and those that received phenol. The motor weakness usually lasts 1 week, whereas the dysesthesias last several days to weeks. Others have reported a rare complication of arterial occlusion of the patient's upper limb after phenol block of the brachioradialis and musculocutaneous nerves.[67] Of note, the development and widespread use of botulinum toxin has made neurolysis a therapy of last resort for this condition.

NEURAXIAL NEUROLYSIS

Intrathecal Alcohol

A neurolytic intrathecal procedure should be performed at the level where the targeted dorsal root leaves the spinal cord and not at the level where it passes through the intervertebral foramen. The latter is not recommended due to mismatch of the spinal cord level and vertebral bone level (especially as one progresses from thoracic spinal cord to lower lumbar). An accurate determination of the level to be blocked should be evaluated according to dermatome and sclerotome charts, as well as selective local anesthetic intrathecal blockade.[68] The patient should be positioned laterally so that the rootlets (dorsal root entry zone [DREZ]) are above the injection site.[69] This positioning is necessary given that alcohol will float in the CSF due to its hypobaric nature.[70] The patient should also be turned 45 degrees toward the prone position (Fig. 58.3). This will raise the targeted area (DREZ) horizontally so it will be superior to the ventral nerve rootlets, and it makes contact with the neurolytic.[69] After proper patient positioning, a short beveled (e.g., small Touhy, 22 gauge) needle is placed into the predetermined level slowly until arriving at the epidural space. This is best confirmed using loss of resistance to air and guided by fluoroscopy. After ascertaining that the epidural space has been reached, the needle should be advanced slowly while aspirating continuously until it reaches the intrathecal space and contrast dye administration (Fig. 58.4). The physician should then inject a low volume/high concentration of rapidly acting local anesthetic to provide anesthesia and clinical feedback of needle location. The lack of pretreatment with local anesthetic will result in significant discomfort and the possibility of patient movement. Using a 1-mL syringe, the alcohol is injected in 0.1-mL increments, with at least 60 to 90 seconds between repeat administrations. The maximum dose per nerve is usually 0.3 mL and the total alcohol volume should not exceed 0.5 to 0.7 mL when several nerve roots are neurolyzed.[71] After injection, the patient should remain in the same position for 15 to 30 minutes. This immobilization allows the alcohol to exert its maximal effect at the desired location, with minimal spread to adjacent levels. After the 30-minute time period, a neurologic exam should be performed. Three to 5 days after the alcohol injection, the patient's pain should be reassessed to determine the effectiveness of the procedure.

Intrathecal Phenol

The same considerations that occur prior to the injection of alcohol also apply to that of phenol. The pain location should be determined with dermatome and sclerotome mapping and isolated with a diagnostic injection of local anesthetic or contrast dye under fluoroscopy. There are two fundamental differences between alcohol and phenol administration. When using phenol, the patient's targeted anatomy must be facing down, the patient must be leaned 45 degrees supine, and the spinal needle diameter must be larger because of the increased viscosity of phenol. The hyperbaric nature of phenol in glycerin requires positioning so that the phenol sinks to targeted DREZ and rootlets. A short, 20-gauge needle should allow the thick phenol

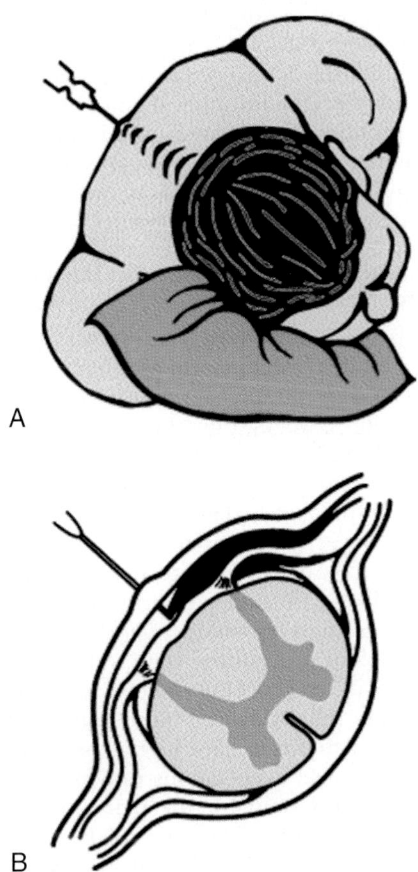

Figure 58.3 **A,** Proper positioning of a patient with left-sided pain for intrathecal alcohol injection. Note the 45-degree anterior tilt, intended to bathe the dorsal (sensory) nerve roots with hypobaric alcohol while sparing the ventral (motor) roots. **B,** Cross-sectional diagrammatic depiction of the above. (Reprinted with permission from Candido K, Stevens RA. Intrathecal neurolytic blocks for the relief of cancer pain. *Best Pract Res Clin Anaesthesiol.* 2003;17:407-428, Figure 4.)

solution to be injected in most situations. However, if this proves difficult, warming the injectate in a warm water bath before drawing may ease the flow of the injection.

Although positioning can be challenging, a common technique involves elevating the head of the bed slightly, with the bed under the target flexed, and the patient turned 45 degrees supine (Fig. 58.5). Using supporting devices such as pillows, towels, and foam and a judicious amount of intravenous sedation can facilitate a reasonable level of comfort to prevent failure of the technique resulting from patient movement. Unlike alcohol, phenol does not require pretreatment with local anesthetic to provide analgesia of the site; however, the diagnostic value (needle localization) of the local anesthetic is still imperative. Similar to alcohol neurolysis, phenol is injected in 0.1-mL increments, with 60 to 90 seconds between subsequent injections. Phenol is injected up to a total dose of 0.5 to 0.7 mL. The feeling of warmth from the phenol is fleeting and may provide some pain relief. Although there is less diffusion with phenol compared to alcohol, the patient should be maintained in position for 30 minutes after phenol administration. The full effect of phenol manifests over approximately 24 hours.

Epidural Neurolytic Block

Epidural neurolysis is used for abdominal cancer pain of both visceral and mixed somatic and visceral origin. Epidural neurolysis remains popular in comparison to intrathecal neurolysis, not only because of its increased safety index and the ease for repeated injections but also for its greater efficacy on thoracic and cervicothoracic junction pain. However, it often provides less complete anesthesia of the patient's painful areas when compared with intrathecal administration. Although the traditional technique is described in this chapter, one study demonstrated that the use of a transforaminal approach when necessary provided excellent results.[72] Selecting the appropriate size needle depends on the agent used, as discussed previously. If alcohol is used, the physician may use an epidural catheter for delivery. An epidural catheter approach provides advantages of repeated injections and can be performed without accessing the epidural space multiple independent times; however, the indwelling catheter can be an entry site for epidural infection. The most appropriate catheter to use is a soft-tipped styletted catheter that can be maneuvered with

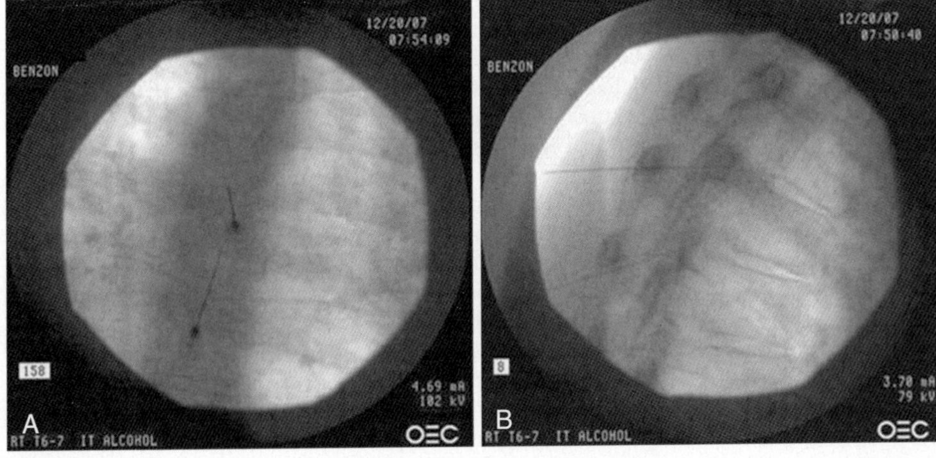

Figure 58.4 **Intrathecal neurolysis.** **A,** Anterior-posterior fluoroscopic view. **B,** Lateral fluoroscopic view. (Reprinted with permission from Benzon H, Raja S, Fishman S, et al, eds. *Essentials of Pain Medicine.* 3rd ed. Philadelphia: Elsevier; 2011, Figure 72-3.)

precision and allows confirmation of position with the injection of a small amount of contrast and local anesthetic.

Unlike the intrathecal administration of neurolytic agents, needle or catheter tip location should be chosen near the vertebral bone that corresponds to the dermatomal levels manifesting in the patient's pain area in order to deposit the medication over the appropriate nerve roots. The injections should be performed under sterile conditions. It has been recommended that injections be repeated over the course of several days to improve efficacy and outcome. Once needle and patient positioning have been established, contrast-enhanced fluoroscopic imaging and a local anesthetic test dose can be performed to confirm proper needle depth and location. The appropriate volume of injectate depends on the level of the neurolysis being performed. Doses ranging from 2 to 5 mL are usually adequate, with doses increasing as location moves more caudally. Racz and colleagues endorse daily injections until noticeable changes in pain levels no longer occur or the patient is pain-free after 24 hours. For up to 3 days after the initial placement of an epidural catheter 3 to 5 cm into the epidural space, ethanol can be injected daily. Before each daily administration, the researchers reconfirmed placement with a local anesthetic test dose.[73] Using 0.2-mL increments, they administered 3 to 5 mL of alcohol over a period of 20 to 30 minutes. Although initial relief was achieved in all cancer patients, results are less significant in patients with chronic nonmalignant pain.[74] In four studies, the results of thoracic epidural neurolysis revealed a significant improvement of cancer pain.[6] Pain relief, ranging from 65% to 100%, was achieved in 80% of patients. Pain relief varied among populations and reflected the severity of disease; nonetheless, many patients were pain-free until the time of their death. In the patients who survived, the duration of pain relief varied from less than 1 month to in excess of 3 months.

Neuraxial neurolytic procedures for cancer pain are rarely used now because intrathecal opioid pumps have supplanted it. Intrathecal medication infusion pumps have the advantage of managing pain from progression of the disease or future sites of painful metastases, which are common occurrences in a patient with malignancy.

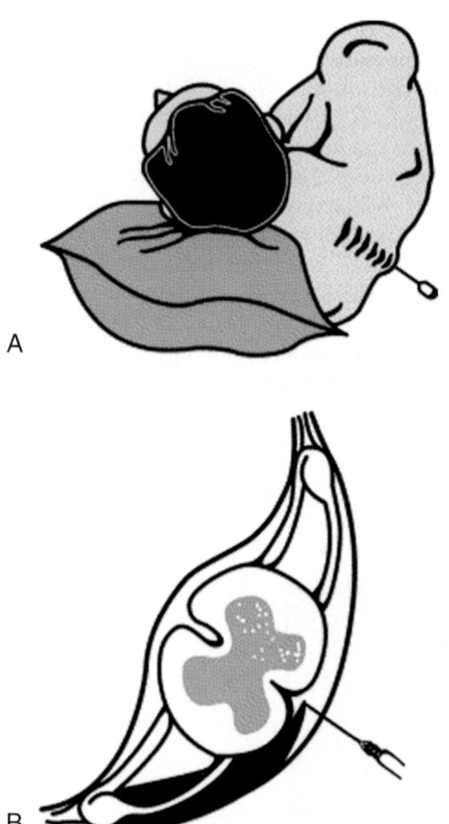

Figure 58.5 **A,** Proper positioning of a patient with left-sided pain for intrathecal phenol in glycerin. Note the 45-degree posterior tilt, intended to bathe the dorsal (sensory) nerve roots with hyperbaric phenol, while sparing the ventral (motor) roots. **B,** Cross-sectional diagrammatic depiction of the above. (Reprinted with permission from Candido K, Stevens RA. Intrathecal neurolytic blocks for the relief of cancer pain. *Best Pract Res Clin Anaesthesiol.* 2003;17:407-428, Figure 5.)

Other Complications Associated with Intrathecal and Epidural Neurolysis

Although ease of administration is a factor, there does not appear to be an increased margin of safety of epidural neurolysis compared to intrathecal neurolysis. A study done by Katz showed that 2 weeks after the lumbar epidural injection of phenol in a group of primates, predominant posterior nerve root damage was noted, in addition to anterior nerve root and spinal cord damage. These test subjects also demonstrated lower extremity motor weakness on physical examination.[75] Complications with neurolysis range in frequency from 1% to 14%, and in severity between incomplete block to limb weakness or bladder/rectal paresis.[5] Like most interventional pain procedures, the most common complication is failure of the procedure to provide significant pain relief. Poor pain relief can have numerous etiologies. It is not unusual for patients to have high expectations for pain relief and have those expectations not met by neurolysis. Therefore, it is important for the pain physician to have clear communication and discuss rational expectations with the patient prior to the procedure to prevent these disappointments. Another cause of inadequate pain relief may be as simple as an incomplete block that can be remedied with a repeat dose. If tumor growth is extensive or crosses several dermatomes, neurolysis may be less effective. Unfortunately, there is always the possibility that the block works well but that local spread of the neurolytic agent may have produced peripheral damage.

There are complications due to entry into the anatomic space where these medications are administered. They include postdural puncture headache, meningitis, arachnoiditis, and neural damage from trauma. Postdural headaches usually resolve quickly, within 1 to 5 days. Complications related to neurolytic agents include loss of motor function due to neurolysis of the ventral rootlets, loss of touch and proprioception, and loss of sphincter tone. Of these potential complications, loss of bowel or bladder sphincter tone is relatively common. The complications resulting from the neurolytic agents are usually transient. According to Gerbershagen, who observed the duration required for resolution of neurolytic complications, 28% resolved within 3 days, 23% within 1 week, 21% within 1 month, 9% within 4 months, and 18% longer than 4 months.[76] Complication rates appear to be similar between alcohol and phenol as shown by Swerdlow, who analyzed complications in a series of 145 patients.[77]

Complications can be specific to location along the spine where the neurolysis is performed. At the cervical level, damage can occur to the brachial plexus, most often manifesting as limb paresthesias. Complications at the thoracic level are the least common relative to the cervical and lumbar level. Below the L1 spinal level, injections may travel into the cauda equina, where anterior and posterior roots are not separated. This factor may make the degree of motor or sensory effect difficult to predict.

Changes in opioid use may occur after a neurolytic block. Patients who have typically been on high doses of opioids for long periods of time will have reduced requirements for pain control with a successful neurolysis. Rapid discontinuation of opioids will cause withdrawal side effects; without pain as a stimulus, preneurolysis opioid doses may produce excessive sedation and respiratory depression. Careful observation of the patient in the hours to days post successful neurolysis can circumvent these problems.

KEY POINTS

- Chemical neurolytic therapy should only be considered after other pain modalities have been exhausted. These therapies are usually reserved for patients with terminal disease. Very clear therapeutic goals and limitations need to be communicated between patient and practitioner.
- Chemical neurolytics can offer patients the ability to decrease their systemic pain medications that can improve their quality of life and allow them the opportunity to clearly communicate with loved ones during difficult times.
- Alcohol and phenol are the primary agents used in intrathecal and epidural chemical neurolysis. Alcohol is associated with burning upon injection, so it is preceded by local anesthetic injection. Phenol injection is relatively painless and is associated with a feeling of warmth. Glycerol is used or trigeminal neurolysis.

KEY POINTS—cont'd

- Pain location should be pinpointed with sclerotome, dermatome mapping, and radiologic survey. For neuraxial injections, the patient's positioning for injection is determined by patient comfort and by which agent is to be injected. Alcohol is hypobaric and "floats" in CSF, whereas phenol is hyperbaric and "sinks" in CSF.
- The most common complication is poor pain relief. Proper location is paramount. Often, pain relief may require several injections. Other complications related to intrathecal or epidural neurolytics are loss of motor function, loss of touch or proprioception, and loss of bowel or bladder sphincter tone.

SUGGESTED READINGS

Abdi S, Zhou Y, Patel N, et al. A new and easy technique to block the stellate ganglion. *Pain Physician.* 2004;7:327-331.

Candido KD, Philip CN, Ghaly RF, et al. Transforaminal 5% phenol neurolysis for the treatment of intractable cancer pain. *Anesth Analg.* 2010;110:216-219.

Gofeld M, Bhatia A, Abbas S, et al. Development and validation of a new technique for ultrasound-guided stellate ganglion block. *Reg Anesth Pain Med.* 2009;34:475-479.

Hakanson S. Trigeminal neuralgia treated by the injection of glycerol into the trigeminal cistern. *Neurosurgery.* 1981;9:638-646.

Nabil Abbas D, Abd El Ghafar EM, Ibrahim WA, et al. Fluoroscopic stellate ganglion block for postmastectomy pain: a comparison of the classic anterior approach and the oblique approach. *Clin J Pain.* 2011;27:207-213.

Racz GB, Noe C. Do neurolytic blocks have a role in chronic nonmalignant pain? *Curr Rev Pain.* 1998;2:181-186.

Totoki T, Kato T, Nomoto Y, et al. Anterior spinal artery syndrome: a complication of cervical intrathecal phenol injection. *Pain.* 1979;6:99-104.

Wilkinson HA. Trigeminal nerve peripheral branch phenol/glycerol injections for tic douloureux. *J Neurosurg.* 1999;90:828-832.

The references for this chapter can be found at www.expertconsult.com.

59 Neurolysis of the Sympathetic Axis for Cancer Pain Management

Matthew J.P. LoDico | Oscar de Leon-Casasola

INTRODUCTION

Neurolytic blocks of the sympathetic axis were procedures that were widely used in the past for control of chronic upper abdominal pain or pelvic pain in patients with cancer. However, recent studies suggest that these blocks are not effective in treating pain that is not visceral in origin. Consequently, when there is evidence of disease outside the viscera, for example, lymphadenopathy, the success rate decreases significantly. Moreover, a controlled randomized study has shown that even in the best-case scenario, the duration of full pain control is 2 months. Thus we should reconsider the indications for these procedures, and when indicated, they should be performed early in the course of the disease.

Stretching, compressing, invading, or distending visceral structures can result in poorly localized, noxious visceral pain. Patients experiencing visceral pain often describe the pain as vague, deep, squeezing, crampy, or colicky. Other signs and symptoms include referred pain (e.g., shoulder pain that appears when the diaphragm is invaded by tumor) and nausea and vomiting as a result of vagal irritation.

Visceral pain associated with cancer may be relieved by oral pharmacologic therapy, which classically includes combinations of nonsteroidal anti-inflammatory drugs (NSAIDs), opioids, and co-adjuvant therapy. NSAIDs have begun to fall out of favor with some clinicians for the treatment of chronic pain because they have been implicated in thrombotic events. In addition to pharmacologic therapy, neurolytic blocks of the sympathetic axis are also effective in controlling visceral cancer pain and should be considered as important adjuncts to pharmacologic therapy for relief of severe visceral pain. These blocks rarely eliminate cancer pain because patients frequently experience somatic and neuropathic pain as well. Therefore, oral pharmacologic therapy must be continued in the majority of patients with advanced stages of their disease. The goals of performing a neurolytic block of the sympathetic axis are to maximize the analgesic effects of opioid or nonopioid analgesics and reduce the dosage of these agents to alleviate side effects.

Since neurolytic techniques have a narrow risk-to-benefit ratio, undesirable side effects and complications from neurolytic blocks can be minimized by sound clinical judgment and by assessment of the potential therapeutic effect of the technique on each patient. This chapter discusses pertinent information regarding neurolytic block of the celiac plexus, superior hypogastric plexus, and ganglion impar.

CELIAC PLEXUS BLOCK

The celiac plexus is situated retroperitoneally in the upper part of the abdomen. It is at the level of the T12 and L1 vertebrae, anterior to the crura of the diaphragm. The celiac plexus surrounds the abdominal aorta and the celiac and superior mesenteric arteries. The plexus is composed of a network of nerve fibers from both the sympathetic and parasympathetic systems. It contains two large ganglia that receive sympathetic fibers from the three splanchnic nerves (greater, lesser, and least). The plexus also receives parasympathetic fibers from the vagus nerve. Autonomic nerves supplying the liver, pancreas, gallbladder, stomach, spleen, kidneys, intestines, and adrenal glands, as well as blood vessels, arise from the celiac plexus.

Neurolytic block of the celiac plexus has been used for malignant and chronic nonmalignant pain. In patients with acute or chronic pancreatitis, celiac plexus block has been used with variable success.[1] Likewise, patients with upper abdominal cancer who have a significant visceral pain component have responded well to this block.[2]

The Cochrane collaboration performed a systematic review of all randomized controlled studies investigating the effectiveness of celiac plexus block in the management of pancreatic cancer pain. They concluded that despite only a small amount of evidence for an increase in pain relief, the improved side effect profile as a result of the reduced need for opiates is desirable.[3] It must be considered that many of the studies comparing the various interventional procedures with oral pharmacotherapy included NSAIDs. If more protocols in the future exclude NSAIDs, there may become a bigger statistical difference between the interventional and pharmacotherapy groups.

Three approaches to block nociceptive impulses from viscera in the upper abdominal region include the retrocrural (or classic) approach, the anterocrural approach, and neurolysis of the splanchnic nerves.[4-7] Regardless of the approach, the needle or needles are inserted at the level of the first lumbar vertebra, 5 to 7 cm from the midline. Then the tip of the needle is directed toward the upper third of the body of L1 for the retrocrural and toward the lower third of the body of L1 for the anterocrural technique (Fig. 59.1). In the case of the retrocrural approach, the tip of the needle is advanced no more than 0.5 cm anterior to the anterior border of L1, and with the anterocrural approach (see Fig. 59.1), the tip of the needle is advanced

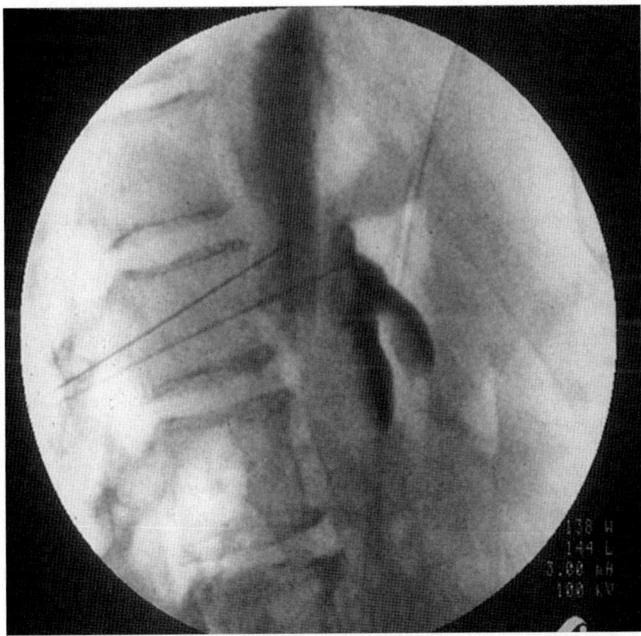

Figure 59.1 Neurolysis of the celiac plexus, retrocrural versus anterocrural positions of the tip of the needle on the lateral view. Note that for a retrocrural technique, the tip of the needle is in the upper third of L1 and about 1 cm beyond its anterior border. Moreover, the spread of contrast medium is cephalad. In contrast, the tip of the needle is in the lower third of L1 and about 3 cm beyond its anterior border for an anterocrural technique. In this case, the spread of contrast medium occurs caudad.

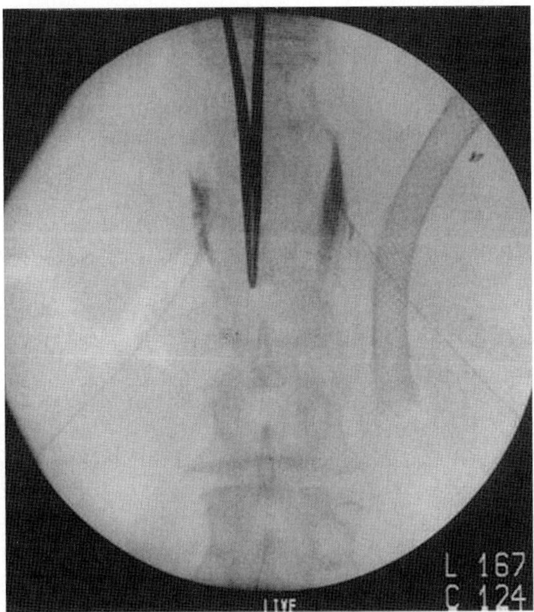

Figure 59.2 Neurolysis of the splanchnic nerves with needle position on the anteroposterior view. Note that the spread of contrast medium is limited to the lateral portion of T12.

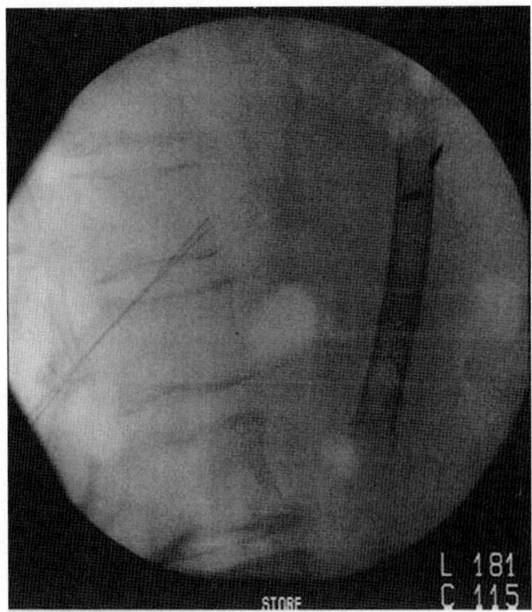

Figure 59.3 Neurolysis of the splanchnic nerves with needle position on the lateral view. Note that the tip of the needle is advanced until it is at the same level of the anterior border of T12 to avoid potential puncture of the pleura.

through the aorta on the left side until no more blood flow is noted through the needle. This is why the anterocrural approach is also known as transaortic approach. In the case of a splanchnic nerve block, the needle is directed toward the body of T12 (Fig. 59.2). Perfect needle positioning in this case is achieved when the tip of the needle is at the anterior portion of the T12 vertebral body on the lateral view (Fig. 59.3).

More recently, computed tomography (CT) and ultrasound techniques have allowed pain specialists to perform neurolysis of the celiac plexus via a transabdominal approach. This approach is frequently used when patients are unable to tolerate either the prone or lateral decubitus position or when their liver is so enlarged that a posterior approach is not feasible. Moreover, CT guidance allows an anterocrural technique to be performed without piercing the aorta, thus adding an element of safety in this case (see the section "Complications").

DRUGS AND DOSING

For neurolytic blocks performed via the retrocrural or anterocrural approaches, 50% to 100% alcohol is used. Injected by itself, alcohol can produce severe pain. Thus, it is recommended that 5 to 10 mL of 0.25% bupivacaine first be injected 3 to 5 minutes before injection of the alcohol or at the time of the injection by diluting 100% alcohol to a 50% concentration with the same amount of local anesthetic (0.25% bupivacaine). Phenol in a 6% to 10% final concentration may also be used; it has the advantage of being painless on injection, and both agents seem to have the same clinical efficacy. The dose of alcohol or phenol administered varies with the approach to be used. For the retrocrural approach, 20 to 25 mL of alcohol is injected on each side. Consequently, the need to inject this high volume precludes the use of phenol in the retrocrural approach. For the anterocrural approach, 8 to 10 mL of either neurolytic agent is used per side. For splanchnic nerve blocks, 6 to 8 mL of phenol per side is recommended.

COMPLICATIONS

The incidence of complications from neurolytic celiac plexus blocks (NCPBs) was evaluated by Davis[8] in 2730 patients who had blocks performed from 1986 to 1990. The overall incidence of major complications (e.g., paraplegia, bladder and bowel dysfunction) was 1 in 683 procedures. However, the report does not describe which approach or approaches were used to perform the blocks.

Complications associated with celiac plexus block appear to be related to the technique used: retrocrural,[5] transcrural,[6] or transaortic.[7] In a prospective, randomized study of 61 patients with cancer of the pancreas, Ischia and colleagues[4] compared the efficacy and incidence of complications associated with these three approaches with those of celiac plexus neurolysis. Orthostatic hypotension occurred more often when the retrocrural (50%) or splanchnic (52%) technique was used, thus suggesting associated neurolysis of the sympathetic chain. In contrast, the anterocrural approach produced a 10% incidence of hypotension. Conversely, transient diarrhea was more frequent with the anterocrural approach (65%) than with the splanchnic nerve block technique (5%) or the retrocrural approach (25%). The incidence of dysesthesia, interscapular back pain, reactive pleurisy, hiccups, or hematuria was not statistically different among the three groups.

The following paragraphs discuss several aspects involved in the diagnosis and management of specific complications.

Malposition of the needle is avoided with radiologic imaging before injection of a neurolytic agent inasmuch as the tip of the needle may be intravascular, in the peritoneal cavity, or in a viscus. Imaging guidance techniques currently used include biplanar fluoroscopy, CT, and ultrasound. However, no study has evaluated the superiority of one technique over the others. Wong and Brown[9] suggested that the use of radiologic imaging does not alter the quality of the block or the incidence of complications based on a retrospective study of 136 patients with pancreatic cancer pain treated with a celiac plexus block with or without radiologic control of the position of the tip of the needle. However, it is not clear how many of these patients underwent radiologic imaging. Assuming that half the patients did not, the upper 95% confidence limit for complications would be 5%.[10]

Orthostatic hypotension may occur up to 5 days after the block. Treatment includes bed rest, avoidance of sudden changes in position, and replacement of fluids. Once the compensatory vascular reflexes are fully activated, this side effect disappears. Wrapping the lower extremities from the toes to the upper part of the thighs with elastic bandages has been successful in patients in whom orthostatic hypotension developed and thus enabled them to walk during the first week after the block.

Backache may result from local trauma during needle placement and subsequent retroperitoneal hematoma or from irritation of retroperitoneal structures by alcohol. Patients with a backache should have at least two hematocrit measurements at a 1-hour interval. If there is a decrease in the hematocrit, radiologic imaging is indicated to rule out a retroperitoneal hematoma. Urinalysis positive for red blood cells suggests renal injury.

Retroperitoneal hemorrhage is rare; however, in patients with orthostatic hypotension, the possibility of hemorrhage must be ruled out before assuming that it is a physiologic response to the block. Patients in whom backache and orthostatic hypotension develop after a celiac plexus block should be admitted to the hospital for serial hematocrit monitoring. If the hematocrit level is low or decreasing, patients should undergo radiologic evaluation to rule out injury to the kidneys, the aorta, or other vascular structures. Surgical consultation should be obtained as soon as feasible.

Diarrhea may occur as a result of sympathetic block of the bowel. Treatment includes hydration and antidiarrheal agents. Oral loperamide is a good choice, although any anticholinergic agent may be used. Matson and colleagues[11] reported nearly fatal dehydration from diarrhea following this block. In debilitated patients, diarrhea must be treated aggressively.

Abdominal aortic dissection has also been reported.[12,13] The mechanism of aortic injury is direct damage with the needle during performance of the block. As expected, the anterocrural approach is more frequently associated with this complication. Thus, this approach should be avoided in patients with atherosclerotic disease of the abdominal aorta.

Paraplegia and *transient motor paralysis* have occurred after celiac plexus block.[14-20] These neurologic complications may be due to spasm of the lumbar segmental arteries that perfuse the spinal cord.[21] In fact, canine lumbar arteries undergo contraction when exposed to both low and high concentrations of alcohol.[21] Thus, these data suggest that alcohol should not be used if there is evidence of significant atherosclerotic disease of the aorta because the circulation to the spinal cord may also be impaired and be dependent only on lumbar artery flow. However, there is also a report of paraplegia after the use of phenol,[14] which suggests that other factors (e.g., direct vascular or neurologic injury or retrograde spread to the spinal cord) may come into play. These complications further support the need for radiologic imaging when performing these blocks.

EFFICACY

To date, only three randomized, controlled trials[4,22,23] and one prospective study[24] have evaluated the efficacy of celiac plexus neurolysis in relieving pain caused by upper abdominal cancer. In a prospective, randomized study, Ischia and coworkers[4] evaluated the efficacy of three different approaches to celiac plexus neurolysis for pancreatic cancer. Of 61 patients with pancreatic cancer pain, 29 (48%) experienced *complete* relief of pain after the neurolytic block. The remaining 32 patients (52%) required further therapy for residual visceral pain secondary to technical failure in 15 patients and neuropathic or somatic pain in 17 patients. The second trial,[22] which compared the procedure with oral pharmacologic therapy in 20 patients, concluded that celiac plexus neurolysis results in an equal reduction in visual analog scale (VAS) pain score as does therapy with a combination of NSAIDs and opioids. However, opioid consumption was significantly lower in the group of patients who underwent neurolysis than in the group receiving oral pharmacologic therapy during the 7 weeks of the study. Moreover, the incidence of side effects was greater in patients who received oral pharmacologic therapy than in those who underwent neurolytic block. Regarding the third randomized controlled study, Wong and collaborators[23] are to be congratulated for designing and completing this study. Their results are welcome in light of a lack of properly designed comparative studies between neurolytic techniques and comprehensive medical management (CMM). However, several issues in the design and results of this study need to be highlighted:

1. Patients enrolled in the study did not have severe pain at study entry. Mean pain scores at baseline were 4.4 ± 1.7 in the NCPB group and 4.1 ± 1.8 in the CMM group. This is a surprising finding in patients with this type of malignancy and may reflect ethnic and racial differences in pain perception and reporting by the population enrolled in the study.
2. Although the authors reported a significant statistical reduction in pain scores 1 week after therapy when comparing the NCPB group with the CMM group, the difference between the two groups may not be clinically important. Patients assigned to the NCPB group reported mean pain scores of 2.1 ± 1.4, whereas those randomized to the CMM group reported pain scores of 2.7 ± 2.1 at that time interval. Moreover, statistical difference was found only when the percent reduction from baseline in the NCPB and the CMM group was analyzed separately (53% reduction from baseline in the NCPG group, $P = 0.05$, versus a 27% reduction observed in the CMM group, $P = 0.01$).
3. In analyzing these results it is critically important to note that most patients (93%) took opiates during the first week of therapy, with similar amounts of opiates being administered to the two treatment groups. In fact, opiate consumption increased with time with no differences between groups at the different time intervals during the study. Furthermore, the incidence of side effects was not different between the two treatment groups at any point in time.
4. Likewise, quality-of-life measurements and the physical and functional well-being subscales of the Functional Assessment of Cancer Therapy for Prostate Cancer did not differ between the two groups at any evaluation point.

Two important questions stem from these results:

1. Can the authors truly conclude that the major finding of the study was that NCPB significantly improves relief of pain in patients with advanced pancreatic cancer when compared with those who received optimized CMM?
2. Based on these results, are we justified to submit a patient with advanced pancreatic cancer to NCPB in view of the potential side effects and complications associated with this procedure?

We do not believe that the authors can conclude that NCPB significantly improves pain relief in patients with *advanced pancreatic cancer*. This is partly because the levels of analgesia achieved by the patients assigned to either group after 1 week of therapy can be considered clinically acceptable. Additionally, statistical difference was found only when the authors analyzed the percent reduction in pain from baseline in each of the treatment groups.

Likewise, based on these results we do not believe that we would recommend NCPB to a patient with *advanced pancreatic cancer* because in this not so perfect world, complications do occur, as has been addressed earlier.

Given these reservations, does this mean that we should not perform NCPB in patients with pancreatic malignancy? As with every clinical study, the results of Wong and associates apply only to the population studied and under the conditions of the study protocol design. The critical issue is that *all* patients had nonresectable disease, which suggests that the patients were likely to have other pain components such as somatic or neuropathic, which are not responsive to NCPB.[4] This is because neurolytic blocks of the sympathetic axis are effective in treating visceral pain only. Moreover, previous studies have suggested that in patients with evidence of disease outside the pancreas, such as celiac or portal adenopathy, the success rate of this block decreases significantly.[24] In the study by De Cicco and collaborators, long-lasting pain relief was described in 9 of 9 patients (95% confidence interval of 60 to 100) when contrast medium spread into the four quadrants and in 10 of 21 patients (95% confidence interval of 26 to 70) when contrast medium spread into three quadrants. None of the 75 patients with spread of contrast agent into two or one quadrant experienced long-lasting pain relief.[24] Thus, the presence of adenopathy secondary to metastasis is a poor prognostic factor for success of the block. This decrease in effectiveness is not due to a mechanical factor such as big lymph nodes blocking spread of the neurolytic agent; rather, it is simply a marker of more extensive disease that often includes nonvisceral pain components and is therefore less amenable to NCPB. The results of the study by Wong and collaborators further support the notion that NCPB should *not* be performed in patients with advanced unresectable carcinoma of the pancreas. This block should be reserved for patients without evidence of disease outside the viscera so that one is guaranteed that the patient has a visceral pain component only.

A prospective, nonrandomized study[25] compared 41 patients treated according to the World Health Organization guidelines for relief of cancer pain with 21 patients treated by NCPB. The authors concluded that this technique can play an important role in managing pancreatic cancer pain.

Since one of the three randomized, controlled studies compared different approaches to the celiac plexus and had no control group[4] and the other study compared the procedure with an analgesic drug,[22] it is not possible to estimate the success rate of this technique. In contrast, the results of a meta-analysis that evaluated the findings of 21 *retrospective* studies with a total of 1145 patients concluded that adequate to excellent pain relief can be achieved in 89% of patients during the first 2 weeks following the block.[26] Partial to complete pain relief continued in approximately 90% of the patients who were alive at the 3-month interval and in 70% to 90% of patients during the 3-month interval before death. Moreover, its efficacy was similar in patients with pancreatic cancer as in those with other upper intra-abdominal malignancies. However, these results are based on *retrospective* evaluation, which may not yield reliable information or may be subject to publication bias. In addition, the statistical techniques used for the analysis must account for the heterogeneity produced by patient selection criteria, technical differences in performance of the blocks, choice of neurolytic agents and doses used, diversity in the tools for evaluation of pain, goals of therapy, and other factors. Thus, the meta-analysis must be interpreted with caution because the report may be overly enthusiastic.

As discussed previously, oral pharmacologic therapy with opioids, NSAIDs, and co-adjuvants is used frequently for the treatment of cancer pain. However, the evidence suggests that chronic use of high doses of opioids may have a negative effect on immunity.[27] Thus, analgesic techniques that lower opioid consumption may have a positive effect on patient outcomes. Lillemoe and colleagues[28] showed in a prospective, randomized trial that patients with nonresectable cancer of the pancreas who underwent splanchnic neurolysis lived longer than did those who did not undergo neurolysis. These findings may be the result of lower opioid use in the neurolysis patients, who not only had better-preserved immune function but also experienced fewer side effects (e.g., nausea and vomiting), thus allowing them to eat better. Although the study by Wong and colleagues[23] did not show that patients randomized to the neurolytic arm of the study lived longer, this may be explained by their high intake of opioids during the study period, which negated the effect of the blocks. Consequently, the effects of this procedure on long-term survival will need further experimental investigation.

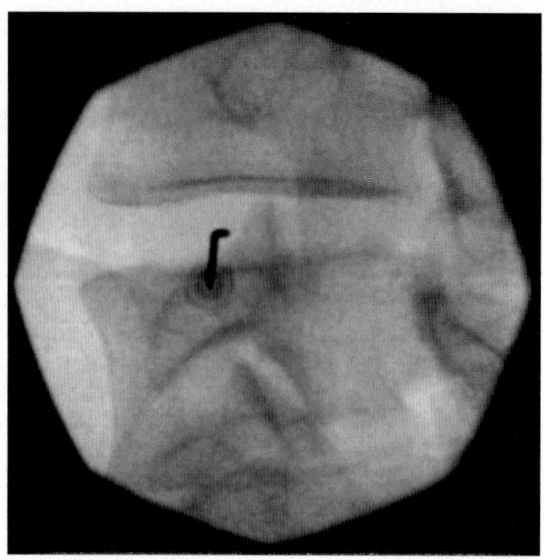

Figure 59.4 Transdiscal positioning of the needle at L5-S1 for a superior hypogastric plexus block on an oblique view.

SUPERIOR HYPOGASTRIC PLEXUS BLOCK

Cancer patients with extension of tumor into the pelvis may experience severe pain that is unresponsive to oral or parenteral opioids. In addition, excessive sedation or other side effects may limit the acceptability and usefulness of oral opioid therapy. Therefore, a more invasive approach is needed to control pain and improve the quality of life of these patients.

Pelvic pain associated with cancer and chronic nonmalignant conditions may be alleviated by blocking the superior hypogastric plexus.[29-32] Analgesia of the organs in the pelvis is possible because the afferent fibers innervating these structures travel in the sympathetic nerves, trunks, ganglia, and rami. Thus, sympathectomy for visceral pain is analogous to peripheral neurectomy or dorsal rhizotomy for somatic pain. One study[32] has suggested that visceral pain is an important component of the cancer pain syndrome experienced by patients with cancer of the pelvis, even in advanced stages. Thus, percutaneous neurolytic blocks of the superior hypogastric plexus should be considered more often for patients with advanced stages of pelvic cancer.

A Japanese study group investigated 35 patients with abdominal or pelvic pain (or both) that had a large visceral component. They performed three blocks at one time on all the patients: celiac plexus, inferior mesenteric, and superior hypogastric. They reported a 100% immediate success rate, with all patients' VAS pain scores dropping to zero. The statistically significant decrease in pain scores following the procedures persisted for 3 months. They also found a significant decrease in opiate use following the intervention that persisted for the first month.[30] This again underscores the need for selecting patients with visceral pain for neurolysis.

The superior hypogastric plexus is situated in the retroperitoneum; it extends bilaterally from the lower third of the fifth lumbar vertebral body to the upper third of the first sacral vertebral body. The technique for the blockade has been described elsewhere.[29,32,33] The patient is placed in the prone position with a pillow under the pelvis to flatten the lumbar lordosis. Two 7-cm needles are inserted with the bevel directed 45 degrees medially and 30 degrees caudad so that the tips lay anterolateral to the L5-S1 intervertebral disk space. Aspiration is important to avoid injection into the iliac vessels. If blood is aspirated, a transvascular approach can be used (see the section "Complications"). Accurate placement of needle is verified by biplanar fluoroscopy. Anteroposterior (AP) views should reveal the tip of the needle to be at the level of the junction of the L5 and S1 vertebral bodies. This is an important safety step to avoid potential spread of the neurolytic agent toward the L5 roots (see "Complications"). Lateral views will confirm placement of the needle's tip just beyond the vertebral body's anterolateral margin. Injection of 3 to 5 mL of water-soluble contrast medium is used to verify accurate needle placement and to rule out intravascular injection. In the AP view, spread of contrast material should be confined to the midline region. In the lateral view, a smooth posterior contour corresponding to the anterior psoas fascia indicates that the needle is at the appropriate depth. For a prognostic hypogastric plexus block or for patients with non–cancer-related pain, local anesthetic alone is used. For therapeutic purposes in patients with cancer-related pain, phenol is typically used as the neurolytic solution.

Mastering this technique is not easy because the transverse process of L5 makes it difficult to access the anterior portion of the L5-S1 region. Consequently, a transdiscal approach has been suggested (Figs. 59.4 to 59.6). However, this approach may be associated with the inherent risk of puncturing the intervertebral disk.[31]

COMPLICATIONS

The combined experience of more than 200 cases from the Mexican Institute of Cancer, Roswell Park Cancer Institute, and M.D. Anderson Cancer Center indicates that neurologic complications have not occurred as a result of this block.[33] However, extreme care should be exercised because placing the tip of the needle in the upper middle portion

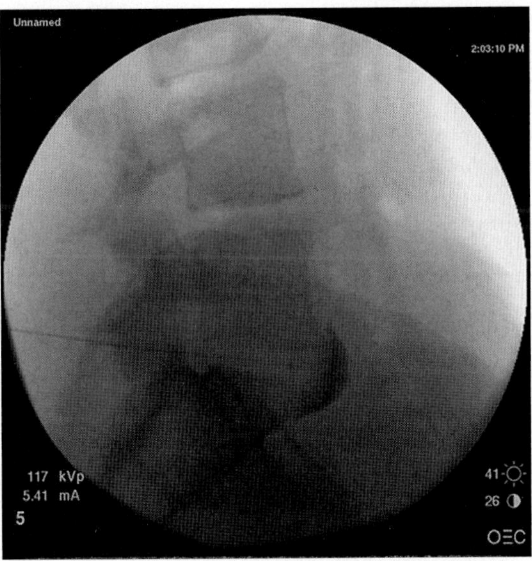

Figure 59.5 Transdiscal positioning of the needle at L5-S1 for a superior hypogastric plexus block on a lateral view.

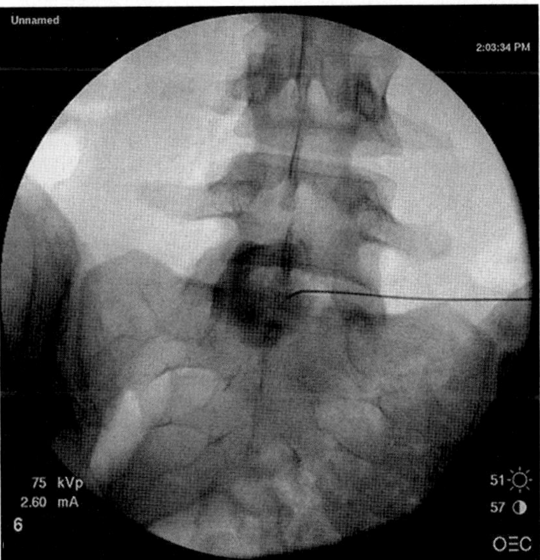

Figure 59.6 Transdiscal positioning of the needle at L5-S1 for a superior hypogastric plexus block on an anteroposterior view.

of L5 may be associated with retrograde spread to the nerve roots. If such spread is not recognized, injection of the neurolytic agent could result in predictable neurologic deficits (Figs. 59.7 and 59.8).

EFFICACY

Effectiveness of the superior hypogastric plexus block was originally demonstrated by a significant decrease in pain via VAS pain scores. In their study, Plancarte and colleagues[29] showed that the block was effective in reducing VAS pain scores in 70% of patients with pelvic pain associated with cancer. The majority of the patients enrolled had cervical cancer. In a subsequent study,[32] 69% of the patients experienced a decrease in VAS pain scores. Moreover, a mean daily reduction in opioid use of 67% was seen in the success group (736 ± 633 reduced to 251 ± 191 mg/day) and 45% in the failure group (1443 ± 703 reduced to 800 ± 345 mg/day).[32] In a later

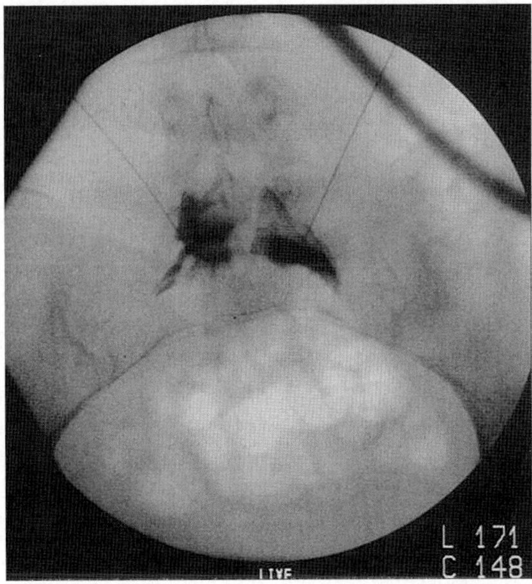

Figure 59.7 Improper needle placement for intended superior hypogastric neurolysis. Note the spread of contrast medium to the L5 nerve root.

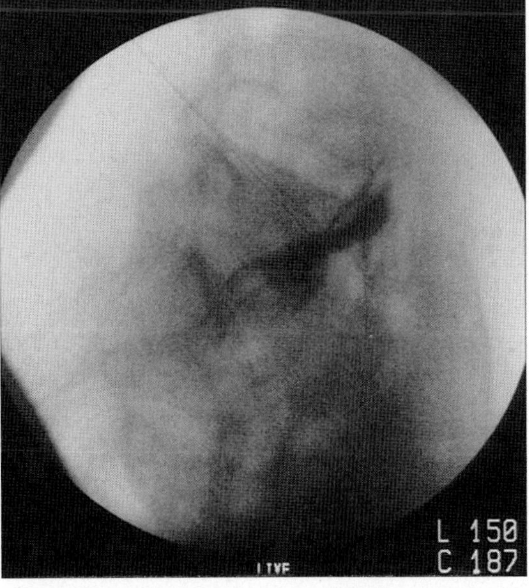

Figure 59.8 Lateral view of the same patient as in Figure 59.7.

multicenter study,[33] 159 patients with pelvic pain associated with cancer were evaluated. Overall, 115 patients (72%) had satisfactory pain relief after one or two neurolytic procedures. Mean opioid use decreased by 40% from 58 ± 43 to 35 ± 18 mg/day of morphine equivalents 3 weeks after treatment in all the patients studied. This decrease in opioid consumption was significant in both the success group (56 ± 32 reduced to 32 ± 16 mg/day) and the failure group (65 ± 28 reduced to 48 ± 21 mg/day).[33] Success was defined in the two studies as the ability to reduce opioid consumption by at least 50% in the 3 weeks following the block and a decrease in VAS pain scores to below 4 of 10.[21,32]

In a case report, Rosenberg and colleagues[34] reported on the efficacy of superior hypogastric plexus block in a patient with severe chronic nonmalignant penile pain after transurethral resection of the prostate. Although the patient did not receive a neurolytic agent, a diagnostic block performed with 0.25% bupivacaine and 20 mg methylprednisolone acetate was effective in relieving the pain for more than 6 months. The usefulness of this block for chronic benign pain conditions has not been adequately documented.

GANGLION IMPAR BLOCK

The ganglion impar is a solitary retroperitoneal structure located at the level of the sacrococcygeal junction. This unpaired ganglion marks the end of the two sympathetic chains. Visceral pain in the perineal area associated with malignancy may be treated effectively by neurolysis of the ganglion impar (Walther's).[35] Patients who will benefit from this block frequently have vague, poorly localized pain that is frequently accompanied by sensations of burning and urgency. However, the clinical value of this block is not clear because the published experience is limited.

ANATOMY

The ganglion impar has gray nerve fiber communication from the ganglion to the spinal nerve but appears to lack white nerve fibers, which communicate pulses from the spinal nerves to the ganglion in the thoracic and upper lumbar regions.[35] Visceral afferents innervating the perineum, distal part of the rectum, anus, distal end of the urethra, vulva, and distal third of vagina converge at the ganglion impar. The original technique was described by Plancarte and collaborators.[35] The technique calls for the patient to be placed in the lateral decubitus position with the hips fully flexed. A standard 22-gauge, 3.5-inch spinal needle is bent 1 inch from its hub to form a 30-degree angle. The needle is then introduced under local anesthesia through the anococcygeal ligament with its concavity oriented posteriorly, and under fluoroscopic guidance it is directed along the midline at or near the sacrococcygeal junction while placing a finger in the rectum to avoid puncturing this structure. Retroperitoneal location is verified by observation of the spread of 2 mL of water-soluble contrast medium. An alternative needle geometry, in which the needle is bent to the shape of an arc, has been proposed by Nebab and Florence.[36]

An easier technique is the trans-sacrococcygeal approach,[37] in which the tip of the needle is placed directly into the retroperitoneal space by inserting a 20-gauge, 1.5-inch needle through the sacrococcygeal ligament under fluoroscopic guidance so that the tip of the needle is just anterior to the anterior portion of the sacrum. This technique avoids invasion of more caudal structures (rectum) by the needle and the need to insert a finger in the rectal lumen.

For diagnostic blocks, local anesthetic alone is used. For neurolytic blocks, 6% phenol is recommended. Cryoablation of the ganglion impar has also been described for repeated procedures via a trans-sacrococcygeal approach in a patient with chronic benign pain after abdominoperineal resection.[38]

EFFICACY

Three studies evaluated the efficacy of ganglion impar blocks in a prospective, nonrandomized, noncontrolled fashion. Plancarte and colleagues[35] evaluated 16 patients with advanced cancer (cervix, 9; colon, 2; bladder, 2; rectum, 1; endometrium, 2) and persistent pain despite treatment (pharmacologic management resulted in a 30% global reduction in pain). Localized perineal pain was present in all cases and was characterized as burning and urgent in eight patients and of mixed character in the other eight. Pain was referred to the rectum (seven patients), perineum (six patients), or vagina (three patients). After a neurolytic block via a transanococcygeal approach, eight patients reported complete pain relief, whereas the remainder experienced a significant reduction in pain (60% to 90%). Blocks were repeated in two patients, and follow-up was carried out for 14 to 120 days, depending on survival.

Swofford and Ratzman[39] reported on the efficacy of the trans-sacrococcygeal approach. Twenty patients with perineal pain unresponsive to previous intervention were studied, 18 with a bupivacaine/steroid block and 2 with a neurolytic block. In the bupivacaine/steroid group, 5 patients reported complete (100%) pain relief, 10 reported greater than a 75% reduction in pain, and 3 reported greater than a 50% reduction in pain. Both neurolytic blocks resulted in complete pain relief. Duration of the pain relief varied from 4 weeks to long-term.

Vranken and colleagues[40] studied the effect of a ganglion impar block for long-lasting, treatment-resistant coccydynia. Twenty patients, 17 women and 3 men, with a diagnosis of coccydynia (spontaneous, 7; fracture, 3; injury, 10) received a 5-mL injection of 0.25% bupivacaine. There was no reduction in pain or increase in quality of life associated with the procedure. Thus, based on this study, it would appear that this block is not effective for the treatment of coccydynia.

COMPLICATIONS

Although there is always a risk of damaging structures adjacent to the ganglion impar, no complications have been reported with this technique. Plancarte and coauthors[41] reported one case in which epidural spread of contrast medium within the caudal canal was observed. In this case, repositioning the needle resolved the problem. Although published experience is limited and criteria for predicting success or failure are not available, patients with poorly localized perineal pain with a burning character are considered candidates for a ganglion impar block. The procedure is safe and no complications have been reported.

SUMMARY

Neurolysis of the celiac plexus/splanchnic nerves, superior hypogastric plexus, or ganglion impar may be used in patients with visceral pain of the upper part of the abdomen, pelvis, and perineal region, respectively. Use of this technique in patients who do not have a significant visceral pain component is not warranted. The presence of disease in the corresponding lymph nodes is a poor prognostic marker for these blocks. The incidence of reported complications is low. However, they may occur and have significant implications on the quality of life of the patient. Thus, strict adherence to the technique is important to prevent potential problems.

KEY POINTS

- Neurolytic blocks of the sympathetic axis are used for the control of chronic upper abdominal and pelvic pain in patients with cancer.
- A study has shown that even in the best-case scenario, the duration of full pain control with a neurolytic block is 2 months.
- Visceral pain associated with cancer may be relieved by oral pharmacologic therapy.
- The goals of a neurolytic block are to maximize the analgesic effect of pharmacotherapy and reduce the dosage of these agents to alleviate side effects.
- The celiac plexus is situated retroperitoneally in the upper part of the abdomen at the level of the T12 and L1 vertebrae, anterior to the crura of the diaphragm.
- Patients with upper abdominal cancer who have a significant visceral pain component have responded well to celiac plexus blocks.
- Three approaches to block the celiac plexus include the retrocrural (or classic) approach, the anterocrural approach, and neurolysis of the splanchnic nerves.
- Studies have suggested that when there is evidence of disease outside the pancreas (including adenopathy), the success rate of a celiac plexus block decreases significantly.
- The superior hypogastric plexus is situated in the retroperitoneum and bilaterally extends from the lower third of the fifth lumbar vertebral body to the upper third of the first sacral vertebral body.
- Pelvic pain associated with cancer and chronic nonmalignant conditions may be alleviated by blocking the superior hypogastric plexus.
- The ganglion impar is a solitary retroperitoneal structure located at the level of the sacrococcygeal junction.
- Visceral pain in the perineal area associated with malignancy may be treated effectively by neurolysis of the ganglion impar.
- Use of this neurolytic technique in patients who do not have a significant visceral pain component is not warranted.

SUGGESTED READINGS

Arcidiacono PG, Calori G, Carrara S, et al. Celiac plexus block for pancreatic cancer pain in adults. *Cochrane Database Syst Rev.* 2011;3: CD007519.

De Cicco M, Matovic M, Bortolussi R, et al. Celiac plexus block: injectate spread and pain relief in patients with regional anatomic distortions. *Anesthesiology.* 2001;94:561-565.

de Leon-Casasola OA, Kent E, Lema MJ. Neurolytic superior hypogastric plexus block for chronic pelvic pain associated with cancer. *Pain.* 1993;54:145-151.

Ischia S, Ischia A, Polati E, et al. Three posterior percutaneous celiac plexus block techniques: a prospective randomized study in 61 patients with pancreatic cancer pain. *Anesthesiology.* 1992;76:534-540.

Kitoh T, Tanaka S, Ono K, et al. Combined neurolytic block of celiac, inferior mesenteric, and superior hypogastric plexuses for incapacitating abdominal and/or pelvic cancer pain. *J Anesth.* 2005;19:328-332.

Mercadante S. Celiac plexus block versus analgesics in pancreatic cancer pain. *Pain.* 1993;52:187-192.

Plancarte R, Amescua C, Patt RB, et al. Superior hypogastric plexus block for pelvic cancer pain. *Anesthesiology.* 1990;73:236-239.

Plancarte R, Velazquez R, Patt RB. Neurolytic blocks of the sympathetic axis. In: Patt RB, ed. *Cancer Pain.* Philadelphia: Lippincott-Raven; 1993:419.

Plancarte R, de Leon-Casasola OA, El-Helaly M, et al. Neurolytic superior hypogastric plexus block for chronic pelvic pain associated with cancer. *Reg Anesth.* 1997;22:562-568.

Regional anesthetic techniques for the management of cancer pain. In: Urmey W, ed. *Techniques in Regional Anesthetic and Pain Management.* Vol. 1. No 1. Philadelphia: Saunders; 1997;18-31.

Turker G, Basagan-Mogol E, Gurbet A, et al. A new technique for superior hypogastric plexus block: the posteromedian transdiscal approach. *Tohoku J Exp Med.* 2005;206:277-281.

Wong GY, Brown DL. Celiac plexus block for cancer pain. In: Urmey W, ed. *Techniques in Regional Anesthetic and Pain Management.* Vol. 1. No 1. Philadelphia: Saunders; 1997.

Wong G, Schoeder DR, Carns PE, et al. Effect of neurolytic celiac plexus block on pain relief, quality of life, and survival in patients with unresectable pancreatic cancer. *JAMA.* 2004;291:1092-1099.

The references for this chapter can be found at www.expertconsult.com.

PART 7

INTERVENTIONAL TECHNIQUES

ROBERT W. HURLEY | JAMES P. RATHMELL, EDITORS

PART OUTLINE

60

Interlaminar and Transforaminal Therapeutic Epidural Injections

Meenal Patil | Marc A. Huntoon

The Institute of Medicine's report on chronic pain in America estimated that more than 100 million citizens are living with chronic pain.[1] Of this group, chronic low back and often associated radicular pain is the most prevalent type of pain and results in significant health care expenditure and adverse social, emotional, and financial consequences in the populace.[2] Radiculopathy is a syndrome of neurologic conductive loss (sensory or motor) arising from any compressive force (e.g., impingement of a disk on the foraminal spinal nerve, spondylosis, vertebral subluxation, ligamentum flavum cyst, infection).[3] Experimentally, displacement of the spinal nerve with a silk loop can mimic the effects of lumbar disk protrusion and produce deficits in sensory and motor conduction.[4] Radiculopathy is not uniformly associated with radicular pain. Radicular pain, or pain in the distribution of a spinal nerve, probably requires both pathologic compression of the nerve and inflammation. The resulting radiculitis is largely driven by glial production of cytokines.

Surgical treatment of acute radiculopathy is widely accepted by patients, but very few studies comparing surgery with comprehensive nonsurgical care have been reported.[5-7] The efficacy of surgical procedures for many spinal conditions has come under greater scrutiny, though, because of disparate geographic practice patterns and inconsistent outcomes.[8] Previous studies suggested that radicular pain can be treated effectively by diskectomy.[5,6] These studies also demonstrated a favorable natural history of lumbar radicular pain syndromes,[5,6] which compares well with the previous epidemiologic study of cervical radicular pain.[9] Recent data from the Spine Pain Outcomes Research Trial (SPORT) regarding nonsurgical versus surgical care of lumbar disk herniation,[7] however, demonstrated no statistically significant superiority of surgical diskectomy over conservative care for primary study outcomes, and thus conservative treatments such as injections for radicular pain will probably continue to increase (Fig. 60.1*A* to *C*). In addition, SPORT agreed with previous trials[5,6] that the natural history of discogenic radicular pain consists of slow improvement over time. Recent 5-year follow-up data from an earlier controlled trial of transforaminal epidural steroid injections suggest that conservative care may be effective in decreasing the need for disk surgery over time, with potentially lower morbidity.[10]

During the period 1993 to 1999, the number of injections billed to the U.S. Medicare system steadily increased to 680,000 epidural steroid procedures per year, with a large number of other spinal injections increasing as well. Cervical and thoracic epidural procedures increased the most, from 10,105 to 48,210 procedures (377%).[11] Because large studies suggest that the natural history of radiculopathy secondary to disk herniation is favorable,[5-8] the challenge of successful treatment of radicular pain is to achieve a reduction in pain and restoration of function while minimizing risk or harm to the patient. The uncertainty regarding nonsurgical best practice with a seemingly increasing number of serious complications[12] poses a significant challenge to interventional pain physicians.

HISTORY

Mixter and Barr were the first to suggest that intervertebral disk herniation might be responsible for radicular pain via mechanical compression on the exiting spinal nerve root.[13] Four years before the idea that the disk was somehow involved, Evans had proposed treating the syndrome of primary or idiopathic sciatica with injections of 120 mL of 2% procaine (Novocaine) via the trans-sacral canal.[14] Kelly[15] later suggested that inflammatory changes on the nerve might be the cause of the pathophysiologic injury. Building on these ideas, Lindahl and Rexed[15] demonstrated that inflammation, as evidenced by lymphocyte infiltration and edema, could be seen on histologic section of dorsal root nerve biopsy specimens in 7 of their 10 patients at the time of surgical diskectomy. Kelly[16] later suggested that inflammatory changes on the nerve might be the cause of the pathophysiologic injury.

Early work on injectable corticosteroids by Hench, Kendall, and colleagues was a Nobel Prize–winning effort that culminated in synthesis of the drug hydrocortisone.[17] Soon thereafter, corticosteroids were used in injections, initially reported as a series of knee joint injections by Hollander and associates.[18] Theorizing that inflammation might be amenable to injection in the epidural space, the first injection of epidural corticosteroids took place in Europe in 1952 by Robecchi and Capra.[19] Then in 1953, Li'evre and associates described their results in 20 patients in whom hydrocortisone was injected into the epidural space.[20]

In 1961, Goebert and colleagues discussed their results of 121 injections in 113 patients over the preceding 5-year period. Of the total, all but 27 of these injections were caudal and only 3 were cervical. The injections consisted of a mixture of 1% procaine in 30-mL volumes with 125 mg hydrocortisone acetate, usually on 3 consecutive days.[21] Between 1960 and the late 1980s, interlaminar and caudal approaches to the epidural space predominated, largely via non–image-guided

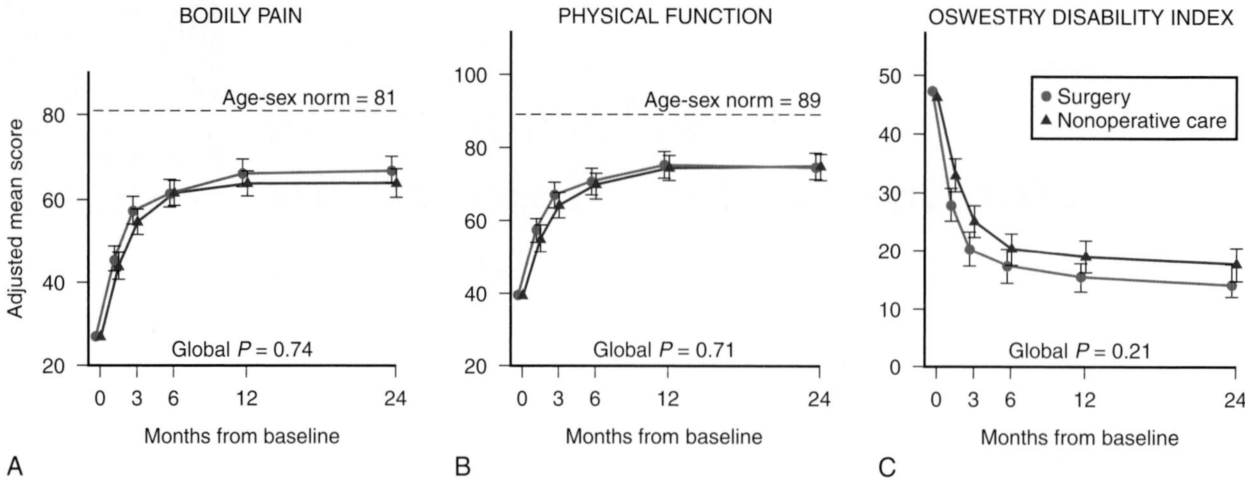

Figure 60.1 Data from the Spine Pain Outcomes Research Trial demonstrate no significant difference between bodily pain scores (**A**), physical function (**B**), and Oswestry Disability Index (**C**) over a 2-month study period in which surgery was compared with conservative care of patients with radicular pain. (From Weinstein JN, Tosteson TD, Lurie JD, et al. Surgical vs nonoperative treatment for lumbar disk herniation: the Spine Patient Outcomes Research Trial [SPORT]: a randomized trial. *JAMA*. 2006;296:2441-2450.)

techniques using surface landmarks and "loss-of-resistance" techniques. In 1988, el-Khoury and coworkers[22] published a study suggesting that a large percentage of these "blind" epidural injections were not placed appropriately, either not being in the epidural space or not properly communicating with the target area of the injection. In a subsequent large review, Johnson and colleagues described their experience with 5489 consecutive injections that resulted in only four complications. They proposed that use of a epidurogram allowed one to provide accurate localization within the epidural space while also demonstrating that the injectant reached the target area. Furthermore, only 10 patients in the entire series required sedation, thus suggesting that the procedure was exceedingly safe on an outpatient basis.[23]

Epidural steroid injections are now most widely used for radicular pain caused by herniated disk material. Guidelines from organizations such as the International Spinal Intervention Society, which are based on evidence, have become accepted by some practices.[24]

PATHOPHYSIOLOGY

Inflammation of the spinal nerve root caused by proinflammatory mediators such as prostaglandins and cytokines and by mechanical compression are now thought to be key inciting events of radicular symptoms.[25] Corticosteroids, through their anti-inflammatory effects, may reduce these inflammatory changes in or around the nerve[26] and thereby decrease pain and improve function.

Until recently the pathophysiology of nociceptive pain emanating from the disk has been poorly understood. Nociceptive neural structures have been demonstrated in the outer third of the annulus fibrosus with modern immunohistochemistry techniques. The nociceptive neural fibers are small unmyelinated C fibers that are activated by peptidergic neurotransmitters such as calcitonin gene–related peptide or substance P. In diskography-proven pathologic disks, nerve ingrowth into the disk may extend farther into the disk matrix, usually accompanied by neovascularization and further degradation of the disk matrix.[27] These nerves appear to be originating from the vertebral end-plate region, which may be the progenitor of the pathologic pain attributed to the disk itself.[28] The disk is relatively avascular, and homeostatic attempts to improve disk nutrition may explain why new blood vessels (and associated nerve fibers) invade the disk from the vertebral end-plate region. Blood flow is predominantly via passive diffusion. Circulation in the end plate is probably controlled by local neurotransmitters, which suggests that neural fibers are present as well.

The processes that lead to disk degeneration and disease may ultimately lead to herniation of the disk. Herniated nucleus pulposus results in local release of cytokines and other inflammatory mediators that cause a chemical radiculitis. Burke and associates[29] found increased levels of the inflammatory cytokines interleukin-6 (IL-6) and IL-8 in disk material taken from patients with known disk disease. Olmarker and coworkers[30] found that the application of disk material onto spinal nerve roots induced functional and morphologic changes in these nerves. In addition, disk cells express tumor necrosis factor-α (TNF-α), which when applied to spinal nerve roots, causes similar changes as those seen after the application of disk material,[31] and selective inhibition of TNF-α may reduce the intraneural edema seen in this context.[32]

CORTICOSTEROID ALTERNATIVES

Because corticosteroids have specific dose limitations and side effects, many researchers are interested in finding alternative agents for therapeutic injection in and around the epidural space and dorsal root ganglion. Systemic delivery of specific anti-inflammatory agents for the treatment of radicular syndromes in humans has shown early promise. Korhonen and colleagues[33] used intravenous infliximab, a TNF-α inhibitor, to treat patients with disk herniation and radicular pain and found that pain scores were reduced at the 1-year follow-up when compared with controls. Etanercept, another TNF-α inhibitor, has also shown promising but preliminary efficacy as systemic treatment of lumbosacral radicular syndromes.[34] Cohen and associates[35] performed a novel double-blind trial involving varying doses of etanercept in patients with subacute lumbosacral radiculopathy. The results revealed significant improvement in pain scores at 1 month when compared with saline. Unfortunately, in a follow-up, randomized, controlled, parallel-group design of epidural etanercept, saline, or steroid in which the patients and investigators were blinded, no significant difference was found between the groups.[36] Potential shortcomings of this study were that the doses of corticosteroid were somewhat lower than in previous studies and that all patients received a small dose of bupivacaine before injection of the study drug. Previously, both human and animal data have suggested that local anesthetics may not be inferior to corticosteroids in their effects.[37-39] Manchikanti and colleagues[37] performed a prospective, randomized, double-blind trial comparing local anesthetic only with local anesthetic mixed with steroid (nonparticulate betamethasone) in fluoroscopically guided cervical interlaminar epidural injections. The study group included 60 patients with central cervical spinal stenosis and upper extremity pain. Thirty patients were randomized to each group. Multiple outcome measures were studied, including the numeric rating scale (NRS), Neck Disability Index, employment status, and opioid intake at 3, 6, and 12 months after treatment. Significant pain relief was noted in 73% in group 1 (local anesthetic only) and 70% in group 2 (local anesthetic with betamethasone); however, the preliminary results showed no significant difference in pain relief or functional status whether patients received injections with or without steroid. One of the significant limitations of the study was the small sample size ($N = 60$).

Ohtori and colleagues conducted a more recent trial to test the effect of epidural etanercept on lumbar radicular pain in patients with spinal stenosis and found that etanercept was more effective than dexamethasone for leg and low back symptoms without any adverse events noted.[40]

In another study evaluating the use of alternatives to corticosteroids, Burgher and coworkers[41] studied the difference between clonidine and corticosteroid (triamcinolone) in transforaminal epidural injections for the indication of acute lumbosacral radiculopathy. Thirty-three patients were screened and randomized; ultimately, 26 patients were divided into two groups, clonidine (11) and steroid (15). Although no difference was seen between the groups in the primary outcome (11-point pain intensity NRS at 1 month), both groups showed significant improvement in pain scores at 2 weeks and 1 month when compared with baseline ($P < 0.05$). The corticosteroid group showed additional functional improvement at 1 month in comparison to clonidine ($P = 0.022$). Even though adverse effects did occur, none resulted in serious complications.

Prolonged continuous delivery of anticytokine agents to the site of inflammation has not yet been studied.

EVIDENCE-BASED THERAPY

Many reviews of trials of epidural steroid injections suggested that the early studies either were not well controlled or had methodologic deficiencies.[42-44] The effect of epidural corticosteroid injections in treating radicular pain syndromes overall appears to be a transient improvement.[45] There are multiple examples of controlled trials of procedural therapies that demonstrate little significant clinical benefit when previous noncontrolled observational studies and case series had suggested benefit.[46-48] Furthermore, "epidural" describes an anatomic space that can be accessed by injection via different approaches to reach the epidural space: interlaminar, transforaminal, and caudal. The different technical approaches to the epidural space additionally complicate the study because different approaches may have different efficacy and risks. Further complicating the clinical scenario is whether the pathology is cervical, thoracic, or lumbar, given the significant pathologic differences between different areas of the spine.[12]

Several well-designed studies have corroborated a short-term benefit with epidural steroid injections. These short-term benefits must be recognized when selecting a technique for the injection, as discussed further in the section "Complications." Given the favorable natural history of the majority of patients with radicular pain syndromes, especially those related to disk protrusion, a thorough understanding of benefits and risks associated with epidural steroid injections for radicular pain syndromes is needed. A selection of these studies with respect to interlaminar, transforaminal, and caudal epidural steroid injections is reviewed in this section.

Carette and colleagues[45] performed a randomized, placebo-controlled trial to investigate the efficacy of lumbar interlaminar epidural steroid injections (up to three) for sciatica (Table 60.1). The study group included 158 patients with unilateral or bilateral lower extremity pain, signs of nerve root irritation or compression, and computed tomography (CT) evidence of nerve root compression at the appropriate levels. A total of 78 patients were allocated to the methylprednisolone group (80 mg) and 80 to the placebo group (saline). The primary outcome was patient function as measured by the Oswestry Disability Index. The epidural injections were not fluoroscopically guided, which may have led to a significant frequency of misplaced injections.[22] The treatment group received 80 mg of methylprednisolone acetate mixed with 8 mL of isotonic saline or 1 mL of isotonic saline in the epidural space. The study did not show a statistically significant change in functional improvement as assessed by Oswestry scores, but it did find a reduction in leg pain as assessed by the visual analog scale (VAS) at 6 weeks in the corticosteroid treatment group (difference of −0.11 in mean change; 95% confidence interval, −21.1 to −0.9; $P = 0.03$); however, this improvement was no longer significant at 3 months.

Arden and colleagues[46] performed a randomized, placebo-controlled trial to examine the efficacy of lumbar interlaminar epidural steroid injections (up to three) for sciatica as well. The study group included 228 patients with unilateral lower extremity pain and signs of nerve root irritation. A total of 120 patients were allocated to the triamcinolone group (80 mg) and 108 allocated to the placebo (saline) group. The primary outcome was patient function as measured by the Oswestry Disability Questionnaire (ODQ). A number of secondary outcomes were studied, including a 100-mm VAS for leg and back pain. The epidural injections were not fluoroscopically guided. The treatment group received 80 mg of triamcinolone and 10 mL of 0.25% bupivacaine at weeks 0, 3, and 6. The placebo group received injections of 2 mL of normal saline into the interspinous ligament. The treatment

Table 60.1 Selected Studies—Interlaminar Epidural Steroid Injections

Authors	Patients	Design/Technique	Outcome Measure	Conclusion
Arden et al.[46]	C = 108 T = 120	RA, DB, PC No fluoroscopic guidance	1—Oswestry 2—VAS, others	Improvement at 3 wk with ESI but not thereafter
Wilson-MacDonald et al.[47]	C = 48 T = 44	RA, DB, PC No fluoroscopic guidance	1—Oswestry 2—Oxford pain chart	Improvement at 35 days with ESI but not thereafter
Carette et al.[45]	C = 80 T = 78	RA, DB, PC No fluoroscopic guidance	1—Oswestry 2—VAS, others	Improvement in leg pain at 6 wk but not thereafter
Cuckler et al.[48]	C = 31 T = 42	RA, DB, PC No fluoroscopic guidance	1—subjective improvement >75%	No significant improvement

C, cervical; DB, double-blind; ESI, epidural steroid injection; PC, prospective controlled; RA, randomized; T, thoracic; VAS, visual analog scale.

Table 60.2 Selected Studies—Transforaminal Epidural Steroid Injections

Authors	Patients	Design/Technique	Outcome Measure	Conclusion
Karppinen et al.[49]	C = 80 T = 80	RA, DB, PC Fluoroscopic guidance, 1 injection	1—VAS 2—Oswestry, others	Improved leg pain at 2 wk, no difference at 4 wk Increased back and leg pain at 6 mo in the steroid group
Riew et al. (both RCT and 5-yr follow-up data)[10,50]	C = 27 T = 28	RA, DB, PC Fluoroscopic guidance, up to 4 injections	1—rate of operative intervention	Reduced surgical rates in the group receiving corticosteroid plus LA
Ng et al.[51]	C = 43 T = 43	RA, DB, PC Fluoroscopic guidance, 1 injection	1—Oswestry 2—VAS	No significant difference between groups

C, cervical; DB, double-blind; LA, local anesthetic; PC, prospective controlled; RA, randomized; RCT, randomized controlled trial; T, thoracic; VAS, visual analog scale.

group reported a statistically significant improvement in self-reported function as compared with placebo at 3 weeks (improvement in the ODQ adjusted for baseline, 10.3 [14.8] vs. 6.6 [15.6]; $P = 0.017$). The number of patients achieving a 75% improvement in the ODQ was greater in the active group than in the placebo group (15 [12.5%] vs. 4 [3.7%]; $P = 0.016$). At 3 weeks the number needed to treat to achieve a 75% improvement in the ODQ over and beyond placebo injection was 11.4. There were no statistically significant differences between the groups at 6 weeks or beyond on any outcome measure.

In response to the review of Koes and coworkers,[43] Karppinen and colleagues[49] hypothesized that the poor efficacy reported may be a result of insufficient penetration of corticosteroid into the locus of nerve root irritation when administered via an interlaminar approach (Table 60.2). They conducted a randomized, double-blind trial to test the efficacy of periradicular corticosteroid injection for sciatica. The study group included 163 patients with unilateral lower extremity pain. Magnetic resonance imaging (MRI) was performed, but nerve root compression was not part of the inclusion criteria. Eighty patients were randomized to a single injection of methylprednisolone-bupivacaine and 80 were allocated to a saline injection, for a total of 160 patients. Three patients were not randomized because of an inability to produce a neurogram with fluoroscopic guidance. The primary outcome measure was back and leg pain on a 100-mm VAS. Transforaminal epidural injections were performed under fluoroscopic guidance, with injection of contrast dye to produce a neurogram. The injectant consisted of 2 to 3 mL, depending on the level, of either methylprednisolone (40 mg/mL) plus bupivacaine (5 mg/mL) or isotonic (0.9%) saline. The results showed that the effect of treatment on leg pain was significantly better in the steroid-bupivacaine group at 2 weeks, with a 45% reduction in pain versus 24% for placebo ($P < 0.01$), but not thereafter. Back pain was better in the steroid group at 3 months. Back and leg pain was better in the saline group than in the steroid group at 6 months (difference of −16.2 [−26.8 to −5.6], $P = 0.003$ for leg pain). No difference in groups was noted at 1 year. However, only one injection was used in the study. Interestingly, they noted that a single transforaminal corticosteroid injection seemed to be associated with a rebound phenomenon at 3 and 6 months.

Ng and colleagues[51] performed a randomized, double-blind controlled trial of transforaminal epidural steroid injections for sciatica as well. The study group included 88 patients with unilateral leg pain. Symptoms had to be consistent with the MRI diagnosis of nerve root compression secondary to either lumbar disk herniation or foraminal stenosis. Two patients were withdrawn because of blinding

Table 60.3 Selected Studies—Caudal Epidural Steroid Injections

Authors	Patients	Design/Technique	Outcome Measure	Conclusion
Bush and Hillier[52]	C = 11 T = 12	RA, DB, PC No fluoroscopic guidance	1—VAS 2—Grogono and Woodgate Symptomatology Questionnaire	Improved leg pain and lifestyle at 4 wk, no significant difference at 1 yr
Dashfield et al.[53]	Caudal = 33 Endoscopy = 27	RA, DB Caudal ESI versus targeted endoscopic delivery of steroid Fluoroscopy used	1—McGill Pain Questionnaire 2—Hospital Anxiety and Depression Scale 3—VAS	Reduction in pain intensity and anxiety in the caudal group at 6 wk, 3 mo, and 6 mo

C, cervical; DB, double-blind; ESI, epidural steroid injection; PC, prospective controlled; RA, randomized; T, thoracic; VAS, visual analog scale.

failure. A total of 43 patients were allocated to treatment with a transforaminal injection of 40 mg methylprednisolone and bupivacaine, along with 43 patients allocated to the placebo group (local anesthetic injection only). The primary outcome was a 10% change in the Oswestry Disability Index. Secondary outcomes assessed included the VAS (100 mm, with a 20% change being regarded as significant), change in walking distance, and the patient's level of satisfaction. The study demonstrated no statistically significant difference in outcome measures between the groups assessed at 3 months.

Riew and colleagues[50] published a prospective randomized trial of lumbar transforaminal epidural steroid injection versus local anesthetic injection in which lumbar spine surgery was used as a primary outcome. The study group included 55 patients with lower extremity pain and MRI- or CT-confirmed disk herniation or spinal stenosis. A total of 28 patients were allocated to a bupivacaine-betamethasone injection and 27 to a transforaminal bupivacaine injection only. Injections were performed under fluoroscopic guidance. They found a significant reduction in the frequency of lumbar spine surgery in patients treated with up to four transforaminal epidural steroid injections. Recently, Riew and colleagues[10] reported 5-year follow-up data on the patients who avoided operative treatment in their 2000 randomized trial. The majority of these patients still had not undergone operative treatment. There was no statistically significant difference in the number of patients in the bupivacaine versus bupivacaine-betamethasone groups with regard to lumbar spine surgery in the interval period since the original trial.

Bush and Hillier[52] studied caudal epidural corticosteroid injections in patients with intractable sciatica in a double-blind, placebo-controlled fashion (Table 60.3). Patients with lower extremity pain and a positive straight-leg raise test were included in the study. Patients with suspected cauda equina syndrome or symptoms of less than 4 weeks' duration were excluded. The study group included 23 patients with lower extremity pain and signs of lumbar nerve root irritation. A total of 12 patients were allocated to the steroid group and 11 to the placebo group. The caudal epidural injection was performed without fluoroscopic guidance, with 25 mL of injectant being administered, including 80 mg triamcinolone and 0.5% procaine hydrochloride. The placebo group received 25 mL of saline. Outcome measures studied included a symptomatology questionnaire and a VAS. The treatment group showed statistically significant improvement in lifestyle and reduction of pain at 4 weeks (VAS score of 16 vs. 45, $P = 0.02$). At 1 year, both groups showed statistically significant resolution of their symptoms. No major side effects were reported.

Dashfield and colleagues[53] performed a prospective, randomized, double-blind trial comparing caudal steroid injection with targeted steroid placement during spinal endoscopy for chronic sciatica. The study group included 60 patients with lower extremity pain in the distribution of a lumbar nerve root. A total of 30 patients were allocated to the caudal injection group and 30 to the endoscopy-guided targeted injection group. Spinal endoscopy could not be performed in three patients, who were then assigned to the caudal injection group. Injections were not fluoroscopically confirmed. The caudal injection group received 10 mL of 1% lidocaine with 40 mg triamcinolone. The endoscopy group had 10 mL of 1% lidocaine and 40 mg triamcinolone injected at the painful nerve root. The primary outcome measure was the VAS score. Additional outcome measures included the Short-Form McGill Pain Questionnaire and anxiety and depression using the Hospital Anxiety and Depression Scale. The results showed no significant difference between the groups. A significant reduction in pain as recorded by VAS was reported at 6 weeks ($P = 0.034$), 3 months ($P = 0.026$), and 6 months ($P = 0.01$) in the caudal injection group. Postprocedure adverse events included nonpersistent low back discomfort in both groups that was insufficient to require hospitalization. Otherwise, no serious complications were reported.

Few randomized, placebo-controlled studies of cervical epidural steroid injections, interlaminar or transforaminal, have been conducted to date.[54] Retrospective studies have suggested clinical improvement in radicular symptoms with interlaminar epidural steroid injections.[55,56] A number of prospective cohort studies and retrospective analyses have demonstrated benefit with transforaminal cervical epidural steroid injection.[57-59] No direct studies comparing cervical interlaminar with transforaminal administration of corticosteroid exist.[56]

In summary, the evidence seems to support the use of interlaminar, caudal, and transforaminal corticosteroid injections for radicular pain secondary to spinal stenosis or disk pathology for short-term analgesia. Most studies suggest modest benefit for variable periods of 2 weeks to perhaps 3 months. The short-term benefit from epidural injections and the natural history of radicular pain may complement each other with respect to clinical improvement. The impact of other aggressive conservative therapies such as medications, exercise, physical therapy, and cognitive-behavioral strategies combined with epidural corticosteroids has not been studied. Significant complications of epidural steroid administration can occur (see "Complications"). Certain safety measures may reduce these complications, but their effect is unclear and difficult to study given the relative rarity of these serious complications. Head-to-head studies are necessary to compare interlaminar, transforaminal, and caudal approaches to the epidural space, which may be relevant given the unique risks to the patient with each approach.

SELECTED EPIDURAL INJECTION TECHNIQUES

CERVICAL TRANSFORAMINAL

For cervical transforaminal injections, the patient is positioned supine and the head is elevated and turned slightly opposite the side being targeted. Great care is taken to mark the great vessels of the neck to avoid placement of needles through these areas. The skin is prepared with chlorhexidine solution and draped in sterile fashion. A subcutaneous skin wheal is raised, and a 25- or 22-gauge bent-tipped needle is selected for a coaxial fluoroscopic technique. An oblique lateral radiograph is adjusted to maximize the optimal transverse view of the intervertebral foramen. The superior articular process (SAP) is seen at the posterior aspect of the foramen and is optimally seen as a straight line. The needle is introduced laterally into the neck toward the SAP in the posterior foramen when the foramen is viewed in maximal breadth. From the SAP, the needle is "walked" into the posterior aspect of the foramen at its midpoint while making sure that an anteroposterior (AP) projection does not show the tip of the needle extending beyond the midsagittal plane of the cervical articular pillar.[54] Once the needle is in position, various safety measures are used, as discussed in the section "Complications," including local anesthetic test dosing, real-time fluoroscopic contrast dye injections, and digital subtraction techniques.

As noted previously in dissections of the cervical transforaminal space,[60] "critical arteries are located in the posterior aspect of the intervertebral foramen," and anastomoses between the vertebral and cervical arteries are variable. Given the risk of introducing steroid into the cervical circulation, nonparticulate steroids should be considered.

TRANSFORAMINAL LUMBAR EPIDURAL

The patient is placed prone on the fluoroscopy table, and an oblique view is obtained with the SAP at the desired injection level. The target point, the lateral surface of the SAP, is marked along a line that bisects the sagittal plane of the pedicle. The target is thus at approximately the 6-o'clock position of the pedicle at the same level[47] (Fig. 60.2). A chlorhexidine-based solution is spread over the skin in circular fashion and sterile drapes applied. A skin wheal is raised and deeper subcutaneous infiltration is provided, usually with 1% lidocaine, and the needle is usually gently bent at the tip to allow greater steerability. Either a Quincke-type

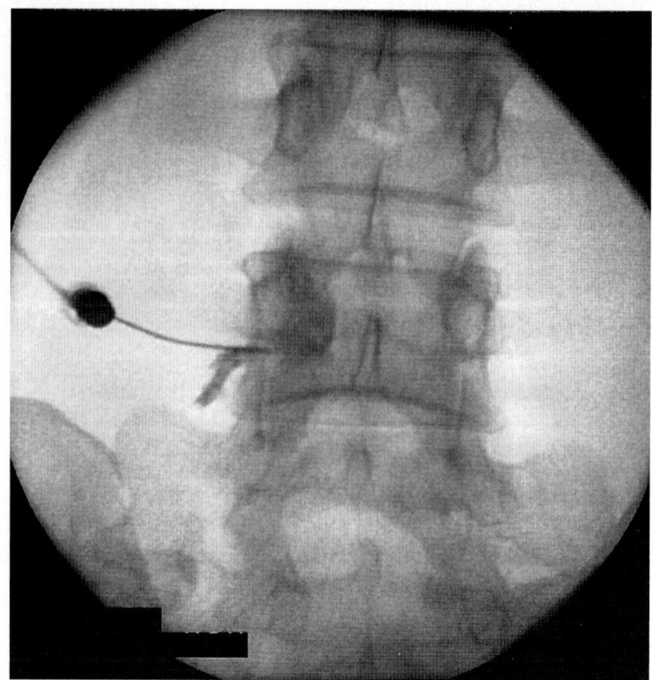

Figure 60.2 Needle placement for a left L4 transforaminal epidural block. The needle has been "walked off" the lateral edge of the superior articular process and is at approximately the midsagittal plane relative to the pedicle above.

needle or a blunt needle with a side port opening may be used, depending on preference, with some authors contending that a blunt needle may be less apt to enter blood vessels.[61] The needle is advanced with incremental fluoroscopic images until the tip approaches the appropriate depth. AP and lateral images are obtained to verify that the needle is either within the "safe triangle area" as proposed by Bogduk and Cherry[62] or is dorsal to the dorsal root ganglion (Fig. 60.3). Murthy and colleagues performed 113 angiograms to determine the most likely position of the artery of Adamkiewicz.[63] Their studies revealed that the artery was in the upper half of the foramen 97% of the time (110/113) and was never seen in the most inferior fifth of the foramen. Injection of 0.2 to 1.0 mL of nonionic contrast medium should demonstrate a neurogram, as well as epidural spread medially and outlining the pedicle (Fig. 60.4). Digital subtraction imaging is useful to substantiate absent vascular uptake (Fig. 60.5). Local anesthetic test dosing with 1 mL of 1% to 2% lidocaine is also useful to prevent accidental administration of particulate corticosteroid into a spinal segmental medullary artery. Once safe needle location is confirmed, injection of corticosteroid or other agent can commence.

Kim and coworkers studied 182 patients who received cervical and lumbar transforaminal injections to evaluate the incidence of intravascular injections.[64] Fifty-six patients (30.8%) showed intravascular spreading patterns with real-time fluoroscopic visualization. Forty-five of them occurred during cervical injection, significantly higher than the 11 that occurred during lumbar injection ($P < 0.001$). One suggestion that came about was to inject a proper volume of contrast agent (deemed to be 3 mL) to detect vascular flow given the relatively high incidence in this study.

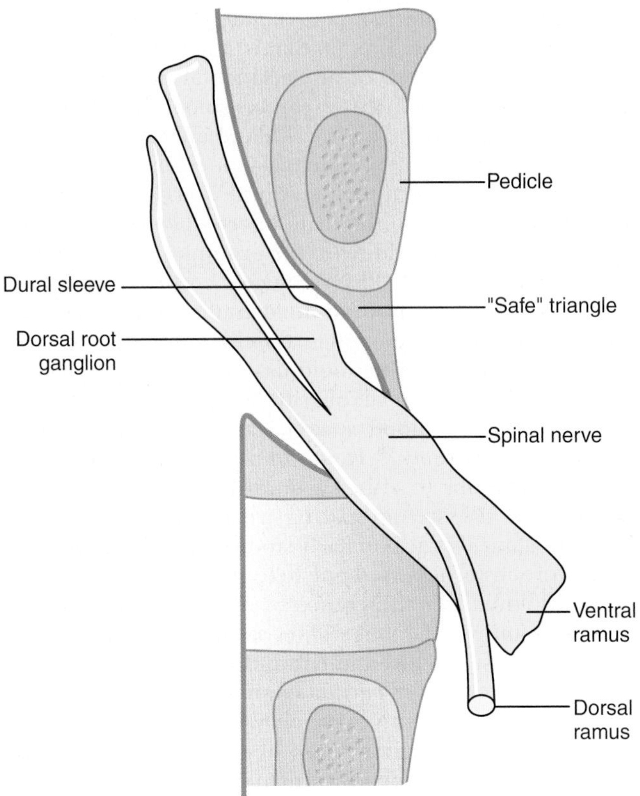

Figure 60.3 The "safe" triangle depicts the confines of the classic transforaminal epidural technique. The needle is safely placed inferior to the pedicle's inferior border, superior to the tangentially exiting spinal nerve, and lateral to the dural sleeve.

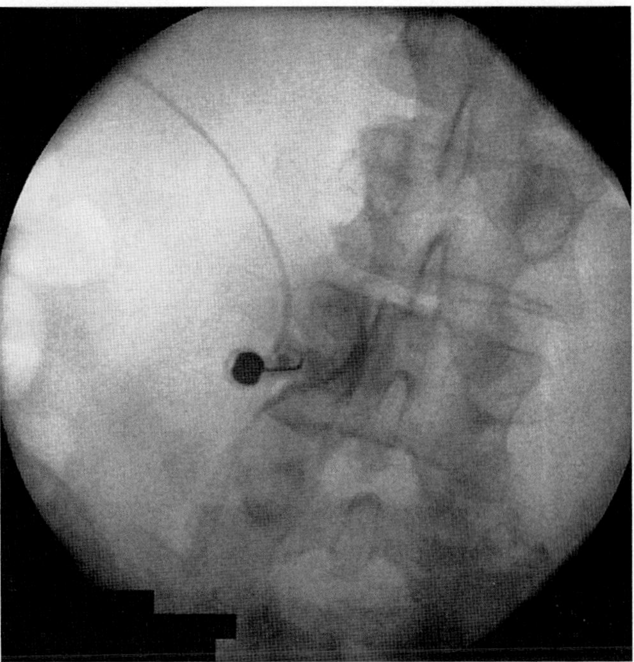

Figure 60.4 Spread of contrast dye is seen along the medial border of the pedicle and outlining the exiting spinal nerve.

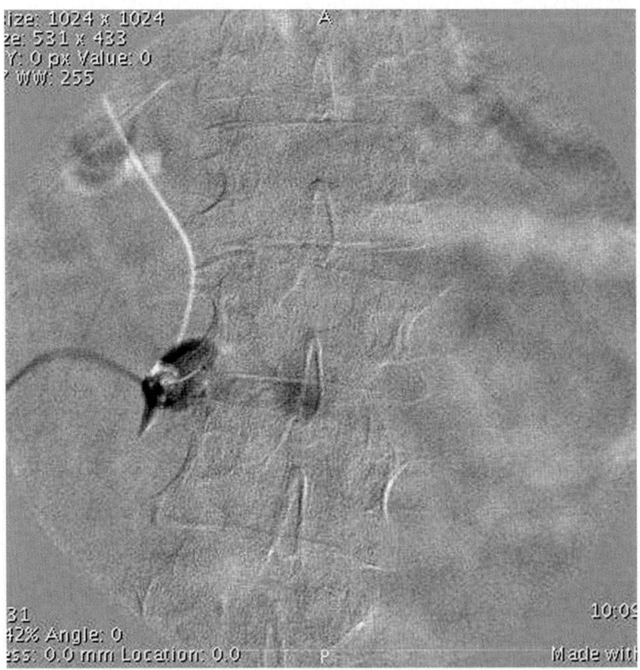

Figure 60.5 Digital subtraction sequence of a left L2 transforaminal epidural injection. The contrast dye outlines the exiting spinal nerve and displays no vascular uptake despite the high likelihood of proximity to the great segmental medullary artery of Adamkiewicz (see Fig. 60.9).

CERVICAL INTERLAMINAR EPIDURAL

Generally, the cervical interlaminar approach is most safely performed at the C7-T1 or T1-2 levels. The epidural space is widest at these levels and may be 1.5 to 2 mm. There are occasionally discontinuous areas of the cervical epidural space,[65,66] and often the width is drastically narrowed by underlying disease such as spinal stenosis or intervertebral disk herniation, which can produce significant compression of the posterior epidural space.[67] It is almost always advisable to have MRI available before performing any cervical epidural injections. Once the safety of the potential interlaminar approach is verified, chlorhexidine-alcohol preparation is performed and sterile drapes placed. The interlaminar opening is viewed in maximal diameter, usually with a caudocephalad angulation of the image intensifier. The lamina immediately inferior to the interlaminar opening target is marked. An epidural needle is chosen, generally a Tuohy or otherwise blunt-tipped needle. A skin wheal is raised and subcutaneous infiltration is performed with 1% lidocaine. The epidural needle is advanced slowly down to the inferior laminar bone via intermittent fluoroscopic guidance. Once the inferior laminar bone is contacted, the needle is gradually walked superiorly and medially into the center of the interlaminar opening until it just slips superiorly past the lamina.

At this point, a glass or plastic syringe containing 3 mL or less of saline is attached, and a lateral fluoroscopic view is obtained. The needle is then advanced slowly while the operator is correlating the tactile loss-of-resistance technique with the lateral fluoroscopic view until the anterior extent of the spinous processes is reached. A subtle loss of resistance will be detected as the needle enters the epidural space. Paresthesia or a cerebrospinal fluid aspirate should prompt abandonment of the procedure. Once the needle is in position, injection of 0.5 mL of nonionic contrast dye will

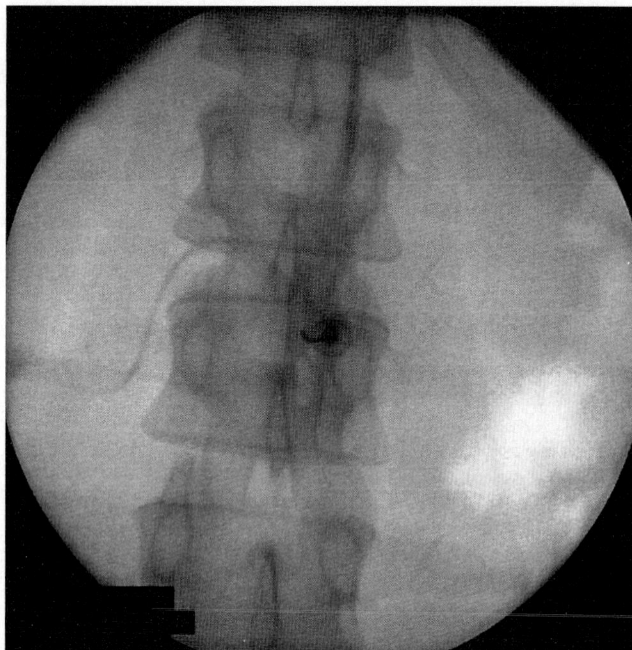

Figure 60.6 An interlaminar epidural procedure demonstrates one-sided spread at the same level and cephalad to the injection.

demonstrate cervical epidural spread of the dye. The corticosteroid or other agent can then be injected. An alternative to the direct injection technique uses a curved needle and a 20-gauge catheter that can be threaded cephalad through the needle. A very flat 45-degree or less epidural needle angle directed in a paramedian trajectory toward the targeted site can aid in threading the catheter without paresthesia.[68]

INTERLAMINAR LUMBAR EPIDURAL

After informed consent is obtained, the patient should be positioned prone on the fluoroscopic table. With the use of fluoroscopic guidance, the interlaminar space of interest is identified and marked. Our practice is to favor the side of pathology given the relative frequency of unilateral spread of contrast dye with epidurography (Fig. 60.6). A skin wheal is raised with local anesthetic after sterile preparation and draping of the injection site. An epidural needle, typically a Hustead or Tuohy, is advanced via a coaxial fluoroscopic technique. The epidural space is typically identified by loss of resistance to fluid or air, and one may choose to traverse the ligamentum flavum and enter the epidural space guided by the lateral fluoroscopic view to ensure appropriate placement. Contrast dye approved for intrathecal use is injected to confirm epidural placement with characteristic spread of the dye. Both AP and lateral fluoroscopic views provide additional support for correct needle placement. Once proper location is verified, the injectant can consist of 2 to 4 mL in total volume, including corticosteroid, preservative-free normal saline, or local anesthetic.

COMPLICATIONS

Complications from epidural steroid injections can generally be categorized as being (1) specifically related to the technique used (interlaminar, caudal, or transforaminal); (2) related to needle trauma, that is, whether a direct neural injury has occurred or any accidental puncture of the dura (post–dural puncture cerebrospinal hypotension); (3) vasospastic or ischemic (accidental injection into a vascular structure causing ischemia—anterior spinal artery syndrome); (4) infectious (epidural abscess, meningitis, diskitis); (5) related to the drug injected; or (6) related to the drug diluent or additives, for example, benzyl alcohol or polyethylene glycol (PEG). Injected corticosteroids have been associated with multiple complications, including osteoporosis and osteopenia, avascular necrosis, steroid-induced myopathy, arachnoiditis, cushingoid signs and symptoms (stria, truncal obesity, weight gain, hirsutism, edema, increased blood sugar), cataracts, risk for infection, and many others.[69] To minimize these adverse effects, recommendations to either arbitrarily limit corticosteroid exposure or use steroid-sparing treatments have become common clinical practice. Early studies of epidural or intrathecal corticosteroids used one to four doses of 80 mg methylprednisolone over the course of days to weeks until the symptoms improved.[70] It is still recommended that no more than three doses be given in 6 months.[71] Many studies have evaluated the effects of certain commercial preparations of corticosteroids. PEG can cause nerve damage; only concentrations of 20% or higher did so in isolated nerve preparations, but they responded within an hour to washout of the PEG.[72] Several studies have examined the effects of various preparations containing 0.9% benzyl alcohol, but none of these animal models demonstrated irreparable harm to tissues.[72-74] It is becoming more common for various compounding pharmacies to make steroid solutions to the specifications of client physicians, which may lessen issues of unwanted substances added as preservatives but raise the specter of infectious agents or errors in compounding to the surface. Therefore, alternative interventions with reproducible beneficial effects in the treatment of radicular pain that lack significant systemic toxicity with repeated administration would potentially represent a significant therapeutic advance over corticosteroids.

A large review of the literature from 1960 to 1994 of complications that occurred with cervical and lumbar epidural steroid injections documented 6947 cases of patients receiving one or more epidural steroid injections. Overall, the incidence of complications was very low.[75] Another large study of 1214 patients receiving predominantly lumbar interlaminar epidural injections at two university pain clinics demonstrated no major complications resulting in neurologic damage and an incidence of post–dural puncture headache of just 0.8%.[76] Other authors have proposed that the transforaminal technique may be safer because they believe that dural puncture is less likely. For example, Botwin and colleagues[77] studied 322 patients and noted no dural punctures but, instead, a 3.1% incidence of transient, non–position-related headache. Cervical interlaminar epidural injections with or without fluoroscopic guidance were similarly successful in treating radicular symptoms in approximately two thirds of patients with no major neurologic complications in past studies.[54] Case reports of spinal cord injury[78,79] have illustrated the potential for catastrophic neural injury as a result of spinal cord puncture in sedated or anesthetized patients, and also that fluoroscopic imaging is not necessarily protective. In an examination of the American Society of Anesthesiology closed claims reports during the years 1970 to 1999, 5475 total claims were noted, and it was found that injuries reported as a result of procedures for chronic pain were increasing. Epidural steroids made up most of the total number (83%) of all injections but accounted for 40% of the claims. Thirty percent of the chronic pain claims leading to payment were associated with a disabling injury and increased from the previous 2 decades by 17%.[80]

The American Society of Anesthesiologists closed claims reports from 2005 to 2008 were studied by Rathmell and colleagues to determine the injury and liability associated with cervical procedures for chronic pain.[81] Of 1627 total claims during this period, there were 294 (18%) for chronic pain management. Of those, 64 were related to cervical procedures (22% of the 294). Most (74%) of the claims cited events from 2000 or later. Overall, patients undergoing cervical procedure were healthier ($P < 0.001$) and more often women ($P = 0.011$). Of the cervical procedures, 59% of the patients experienced spinal cord damage, with direct needle trauma being the predominant cause (31%). General anesthesia or sedation was also more prevalent in cervical claims associated with spinal cord injuries. In fact, 25% of those who had spinal cord injuries were nonresponsive during the procedure as compared with 5% of those who did not sustain spinal cord injuries ($P < 0.05$, $\kappa = 0.52$).

Regarding dosages, a recent study by Ahadian and colleagues[82] investigated the potential differences between using 4-, 8-, and 12-mg doses of dexamethasone in lumbar transforaminal epidural injections. Although improvement in radicular pain was noted 12 weeks after injection in all groups ($P < 0.05$), no significant differences were found between each group.

A contradictory study was performed by Park and associates[83] in which particulate and nonparticulate steroids were compared in lumbar transforaminal epidural injections. Dexamethasone, 7.5 mg, was compared with triamcinolone acetate, 40 mg; the triamcinolone group showed a statistically significant improvement in VAS scores when compared with the dexamethasone group ($P = 0.001$).

INFECTIOUS COMPLICATIONS

Until recently, many of the cases of epidural abscess and meningitis in the literature were reported in the context of perioperative epidural catheter infusions, which is not necessarily similar to the incidence after a single corticosteroid injection. Gaul and associates[84] reviewed every patient admitted to their neurologic unit with meningitis during the years 1992 to 2000. This review yielded 128 patients, 8 of whom had previously received corticosteroid spinal injections. Review of the cases reported in the literature[85] yielded a total of 11 abscesses and 3 abscesses plus meningitis after spinal injections of corticosteroid. The cases of abscess and meningitis associated with injections appeared to overwhelmingly be caused by the *Staphylococcus* species, with 8 of 14 infections occurring in immunocompromised patients (mostly patients with diabetes and metastatic cancer). The patients were usually seen within the first 2 weeks after injection, with back pain being the most prominent symptom. A high clinical index of suspicion and laboratory findings (erythrocyte sedimentation rate and C-reactive protein) may be more helpful than the white blood cell count in screening. Ultimately, MRI is necessary to make the diagnosis (Fig. 60.7).

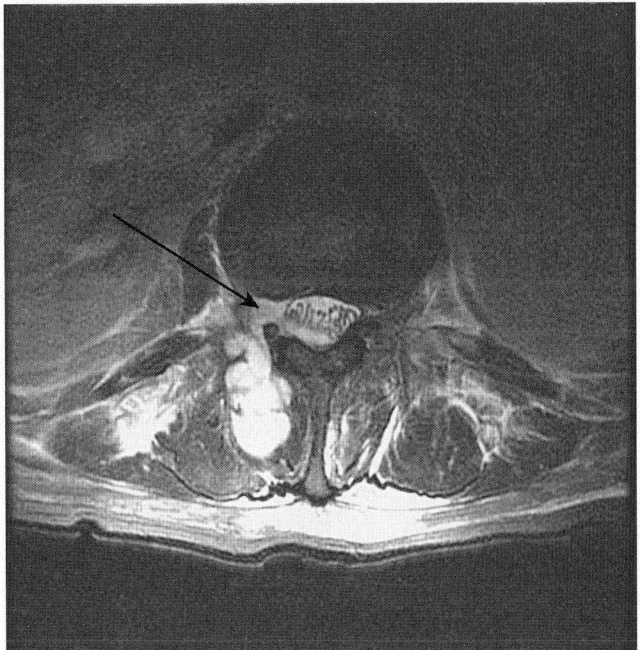

Figure 60.7 An accumulation of abscess material (arrow) is seen tracking epidurally and into the perispinal soft tissues. (From Hooten WM, Kinney MO, Huntoon MA. Epidural abscess and meningitis after epidural corticosteroid injection. *Mayo Clin Proc*. 2004;79:682-686.)

ISCHEMIC INJURY (ANTERIOR SPINAL ARTERY SYNDROME)

Carette and Fehlings have called for further studies on cervical epidural steroid injections because of increasing performance of these techniques, which have less evidence of efficacy than lumbar procedures do but a substantial number of complications.[12] Several recent reports of anterior spinal artery syndrome during cervical transforaminal epidural steroid injections have raised concerns of safety.[54,60,83-89] Anatomic studies have demonstrated that the segmental medullary arteries that supply the anterior spinal artery may be vulnerable. These arteries could be branches of the vertebral artery, ascending cervical artery, or deep cervical arteries.[60] Branches entering the posterior aspect of the cervical intervertebral foramen (Figs. 60.8 and 60.9) or anastomosing with the vertebral artery may explain some complications.[60] Likewise, a lumbar safe zone may not protect one from catastrophic injection into a tributary of the artery of Adamciewicz.[90]

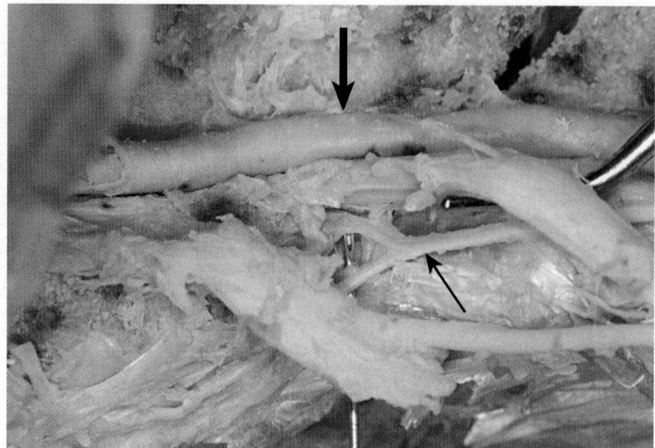

Figure 60.8 Anatomic cadaver dissection demonstrating the vertebral artery (pink, large arrow) and the exiting left C5 spinal nerve lifted by the probe. The tip of the needle is pushing on a spinal branch of the ascending cervical artery (small arrow) at the outer aspect of the C4-5 intervertebral foramen.

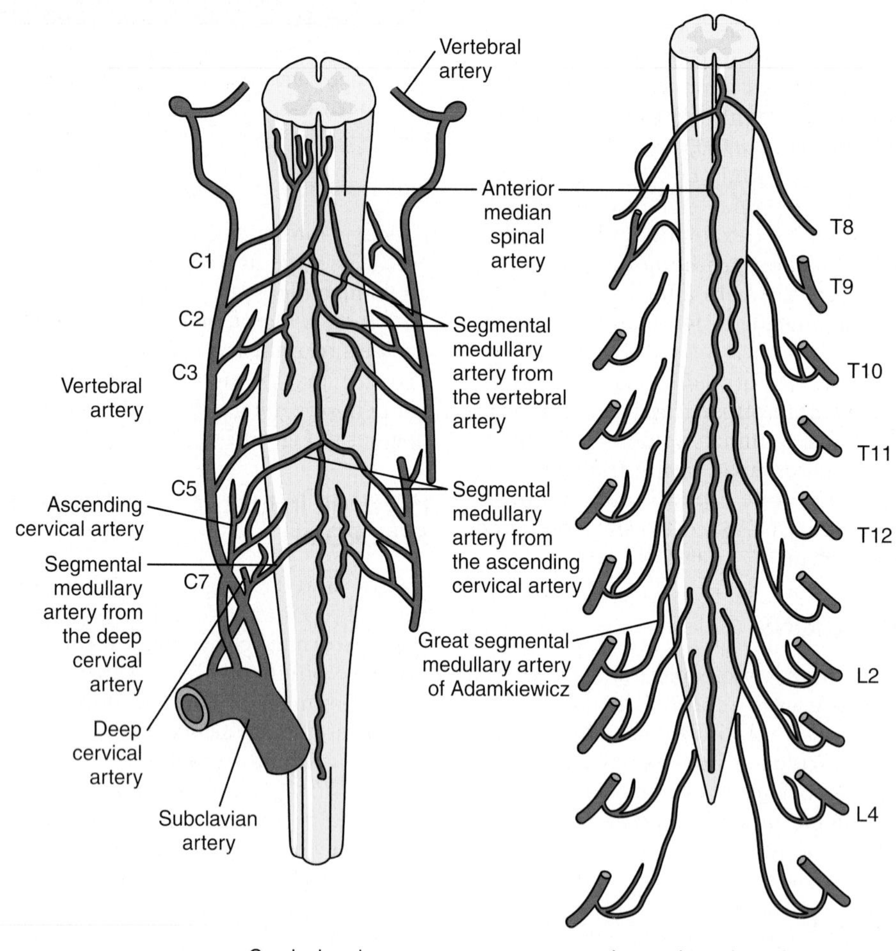

Figure 60.9 Artist's adaptation of an earlier drawing from Gillilan. Left panel, contributions of several segmental medullary vessels to the anterior median spinal artery; right panel, great segmental medullary artery of Adamkiewicz entering at the L2 intervertebral foramen on the left side. (From Gillilan LA. The arterial blood supply of the human spinal cord. *J Comp Neurol*. 1958;110:75-103.)

KEY POINTS

- The natural history of discogenic radicular pain is favorable for conservative management.
- Randomized, placebo-controlled trials show short-term benefit with epidural steroid injection via multiple techniques.
- The best practice for nonsurgical radicular pain syndromes is yet to be defined. Few comparative, nonsurgical trials have been conducted.
- Devastating complications of epidural steroid injection have occurred, especially in the cervical spine.
- Because of the rare, but catastrophic nature of some of these complications and the favorable natural history of discogenic radicular pain, safety should be of primary concern.
- Future directions in research may look at alternative pharmacologic agents or techniques to address the pathophysiology of radicular pain syndromes. Use of these agents via continuous or prolonged delivery is of interest.

SUGGESTED READINGS

Atlas SJ, Keller RB, Wu YA, et al. Long-term outcomes of surgical and nonsurgical management of sciatica secondary to a lumbar disc herniation: 10 year results from the Maine Lumbar Spine Study. *Spine.* 2005;30:927-935.

Baker R, Dreyfuss P, Mercer S, et al. Cervical transforaminal injection of corticosteroids into a radicular artery: a possible mechanism for spinal cord injury. *Pain.* 2003;103:211-215.

Brouwers PJ, Kottink EJ, Simon MA, et al. A cervical anterior spinal artery syndrome after diagnostic blockade of the right C6-nerve root. *Pain.* 2001;91:397-399.

Bush K, Hillier S. Outcome of cervical radiculopathy treated with periradicular/epidural corticosteroid injections: a prospective study with independent clinical review. *Eur Spine J.* 1996;5:319-325.

Cohen SP, White RL, Kurihara C, et al. Epidural steroids, etanercept, or saline in subacute sciatica: a multicenter, randomized trial. *Ann Intern Med.* 2012;156:551-559.

Dashfield AK, Taylor MB, Cleaver JS, et al. Comparison of caudal steroid epidural with targeted steroid placement during spinal endoscopy for chronic sciatica: a prospective, randomized, double-blind trial. *Br J Anaesth.* 2005;94:514-519.

Fitzgibbon DR, Posner KL, Domino KB, et al. Chronic pain management: American Society of Anesthesiologists Closed Claims Project. *Anesthesiology.* 2004;100:98-105.

Horlocker TT, Bajwa ZH, Ashraf Z, et al. Risk assessment of hemorrhagic complications associated with nonsteroidal antiinflammatory medications in ambulatory pain clinic patients undergoing epidural steroid injection. *Anesth Analg.* 2002;95:1691-1697.

Huntoon MA. Anatomy of the cervical intervertebral foramina: vulnerable arteries and ischemic neurologic injuries after transforaminal epidural injections. *Pain.* 2005;117:104-111.

Huntoon MA. Steroid complications. In: Neal J, Rathmell JP, eds. *Complication in Regional Anesthesia and Pain Medicine.* New York: Elsevier; 2006:331-339.

Murthy NS, Maus TP, Behrns CL. Intraforaminal location of the great anterior radiculomedullary artery (artery of Adamkiewicz): a retrospective review. *Pain Med.* 2010;11:1756-1764.

Ng L, Chaudhary N, Sell P. The efficacy of corticosteroids in periradicular infiltration for chronic radicular pain: a randomized, double-blind, controlled trial. *Spine.* 2005;30:857-862.

Olmarker K, Myers RR. Pathogenesis of sciatic pain: role of herniated nucleus pulposus and deformation of spinal nerve root and dorsal root ganglion. *Pain.* 1998;78:99-105.

Park CH, Lee SH, Kim BI. Comparison of the effectiveness of lumbar transforaminal epidural injection with particulate and nonparticulate corticosteroids in lumbar radiating pain. *Pain Med.* 2010;11:1654-1658.

Rathmell JP, Michna E, Fitzgibbon DR, et al. Injury and liability associated with cervical procedures for chronic pain. *Anesthesiology.* 2011;114:918-926.

Riew KD, Park JB, Cho YS, et al. Nerve root blocks in the treatment of lumbar radicular pain: a minimum five-year follow-up. *J Bone Joint Surg Am.* 2006;88:1722-1725.

Weinstein JN, Tosteson TD, Lurie JD, et al. Surgical vs nonoperative treatment for lumbar disk herniation: the Spine Patient Outcomes Research Trial (SPORT): a randomized trial. *JAMA.* 2006;296:2441-2450.

The references for this chapter can be found at www.expertconsult.com.

61 Pathogenesis, Diagnosis, and Treatment of Zygapophyseal (Facet) Joint Pain

Chad M. Brummett | Steven P. Cohen

Low back pain (LBP) and neck pain represent an epidemic throughout the industrialized world. More than 75% of patients reporting spine pain are between 18 and 65 years old, thereby adding cost through lost productivity and wages.[1] Although the prevalence of LBP varies greatly throughout the literature, some lifetime estimates are as high as 84% to 90%,[2,3] and the 5-year recurrence rate of LBP may be as high as 69%.[4] The lifetime prevalence of neck pain has been estimated to be about 67%.[5] The estimated cost of treatment and lost wages for spine pain in the United States each year is estimated to be more than $140 billion.[1,4] As the population ages, the impact of LBP and neck pain will continue to grow.

The zygapophyseal (facet) joint (z-joint) is a potential source of neck, shoulder, midback, low back, and leg pain. In addition, cervical facet disease can cause headaches. Interventions on the z-joints are second only to epidural steroid injections as the most common type of procedure performed in pain management centers in the United States.[6] Despite a great deal of research on the diagnosis and treatment of facet pain, the issue still remains controversial. This chapter discusses the relevant anatomy, mechanisms of injury, prevalence, pain referral patterns, diagnosis, and treatment of facet arthropathy.

ANATOMY AND FUNCTION

The spine is normally composed of 7 cervical, 12 thoracic, and 5 lumbar vertebrae (see Fig. 61.1). The z-joints are paired structures situated posterolateral to the vertebral body. In conjunction with the intervertebral disk, they make up what is commonly known as "the three-joint complex." Together, these joints function to support and stabilize the spine and prevent injury by limiting motion in all planes of movement. The lumbar z-joints are true synovial joints formed from the superior articular process of one vertebra and the inferior articular process of the vertebra above. The volume capacity of these joints is approximately 1 to 1.5 mL in the lumbar region and 0.5 to 1.0 mL in the cervical region.[7] The articular surfaces are covered by hyaline cartilage and contain a fibrous capsule. The fibrous capsule is about 1 mm thick and is formed mostly of collagenous tissue arranged in a transverse fashion to provide resistance to forward flexion.[8,9] The superior and inferior joint borders are formed by the fibrous capsule. In the lumbar spine, the multifidus muscle serves as the posterior joint border, and the ligamentum flavum replaces the fibrous capsule at the anterior border.[10] The position of the joint relative to the sagittal and coronal planes helps determine the role that the joint plays in protecting the spine against excessive motion. Joints oriented parallel to the sagittal plane provide little resistance to backward and forward shearing forces but allow a greater degree of rotation, flexion, and extension. Joints oriented closer to the coronal plane will allow less rotation, flexion, and extension but serve as excellent protection against shearing forces. The cervical z-joints are inclined at roughly 45 degrees from the horizontal plane and angled 85 degrees from the sagittal plane. This alignment functions to prevent excessive anterior translation and to assist the disks in weight bearing.[11]

The medial branch of the posterior rami supplies sensory innervation to the facet joint. Each exiting spinal nerve splits into an anterior and posterior primary ramus (Fig. 61.2). The anterior ramus is the largest of the two branches and the main source of motor and sensory fibers. The posterior ramus divides into lateral, intermediate, and medial branches. In the lumbar region, the lateral branch provides innervation to the paraspinous muscles, thoracolumbar fascia, and sacroiliac joint and variable sensory fibers to the skin overlying the spinous processes. The small intermediate branch supplies the longissimus muscle. The medial branch is the largest branch of the posterior primary ramus and innervates not only the lumbar z-joint but also the multifidus muscle, interspinal muscle and ligament, and periosteum of the neural arch. To block sensory input from one facet joint, two adjacent medial branches must be anesthetized. In some people, facet joint innervation may be derived from other sources.

Facet joints are imbued with a rich innervation containing encapsulated (Ruffini-type endings, pacinian corpuscles), unencapsulated, and free nerve endings.[12] In addition to being a potential pain generator, the z-joint capsule is thought to serve in a proprioceptive capacity as well, as evidenced by the presence of low-threshold, rapidly adapting mechanosensitive neurons. Kallakuri and colleagues used immunocytochemistry to characterize the presence of substance P and calcitonin gene–related peptide–reactive nerve fibers in the cervical facets of 12 human cadavers.[13] In addition to substance P and calcitonin gene–related peptide, a

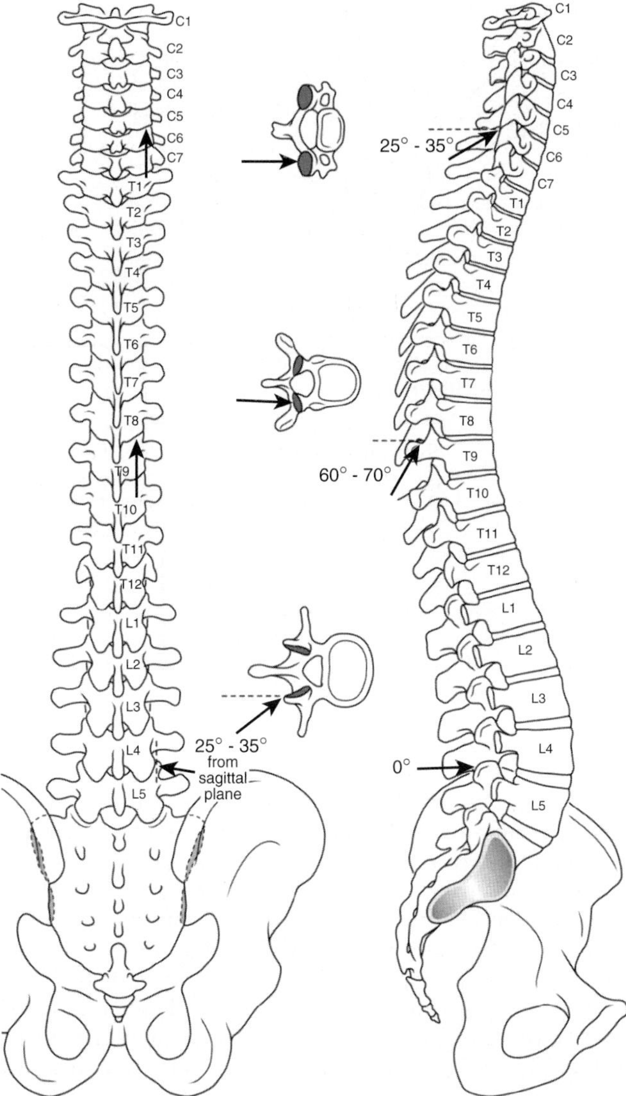

Figure 61.1 Anatomy of the facet joints. The plane of orientation of the facet joints varies significantly among the cervical, thoracic, and lumbar levels. The axis of the joints and the plane of entry for intra-articular injection are shown for the typical cervical, thoracic, and lumbar facet joints. (Reproduced with permission from Rathmell JP. *Atlas of Image-Guided Intervention in Regional Anesthesia and Pain Medicine*. Philadelphia: Lippincott; 2006:67.)

substantial percentage of nerve endings in the facet capsules contain neuropeptide Y, which is indicative of the presence of sympathetic efferent fibers.[14,15] Nerve fibers have been found in subchondral bone and intra-articular inclusions of facet joints, thus signifying that facet-mediated pain may originate in structures besides the joint capsule.[16,17] Inflammatory mediators such as prostaglandins[18] and the inflammatory cytokines interleukin-6 and tumor necrosis factor-α[19] have been found in facet joint cartilage and synovial tissue in degenerative lumbar spinal disorders.

LUMBAR FACET JOINTS

The lumbar facet joints are aligned lateral to the sagittal plane and vary in angle (Fig. 61.3). The inferior articular process faces anterolaterally, and the superior articular process faces posteromedially.[10,20] In an anatomic study published in 1940 by Horwitz and Smith,[21] the authors found that the L4-5 z-joints tended to be more coronally positioned (almost 70 degrees with respect to the sagittal plane), whereas the L2-3 and L3-4 joints were likely to be oriented more parallel (<40 degrees) to the sagittal plane. In more recent studies by Masharawi and coworkers[11] and Punjabi and associates,[22] the investigators found that the upper lumbar facet joints (T12-L2) were oriented closer to the midsagittal plane of the vertebral body (mean range, 26 to 34 degrees), whereas the lower facet joints tended to be oriented away from that plane (40 to 56 degrees). In the upper lumbar spine, approximately 80% of the facet joints are curved and 20% are flat. In the lower lumbar spine, these numbers are reversed.[21] Studies by Grobler and colleagues[23] and Boden and associates[24] found a positive association between degenerative spondylolisthesis and more sagittally oriented lower lumbar facet joints. The inferior articular processes of L5 combine with the superior articular processes of the sacrum to form the L5-S1 facet joints. The dip in the sacrum immediately lateral to the superior articular process is termed the sacral ala.

Sensory innervation of the facet joints is derived from the medial branches arising from the posterior primary rami at the same level and the level above the facet joint.[10,25] For example, the L4-5 medial branch receives its innervation from the L3 and L4 medial branch nerves. The medial branches of L1 to L4 run across their respective transverse processes one level below the named spinal nerve (e.g., L4 crosses the transverse process of L5) and traverse the dorsal leaf of the intertransverse ligament at the base of the transverse process. The nerve then proceeds along the junction of the superior articular process and the transverse process, courses underneath the mamilloaccessory ligament, and splits into multiple branches as it crosses the vertebral lamina (Fig. 61.4). Calcification of the mamilloaccessory ligament can be a source of nerve entrapment.[26] This is most common at L5 (20%) but also occurs at L4 (10%) and L3 (4%). The nerve at L5 that is amenable to blockade is actually the dorsal ramus itself, which runs along the junction of the superior articular process of the sacrum and the sacral ala.[27,28] Some authors have claimed that a branch from the S1 nerve root can run cephalad to supply a portion of the L5-S1 facet joint, although this point remains controversial.[29,30]

THORACIC FACET JOINTS

The thoracic facets are the most vertically oriented joints, as noted in Figure 61.1, with the anterior portion of the joint located more cephalad.[11,31,32] The frontal orientation permits more lateral flexion at the expense of axial rotation. In the low thoracic spine, the angle transitions from a predominantly frontal orientation to the characteristic sagittal orientation of the lumbar facets. This transition varies but generally occurs between T11-12[11] and T12-L1.[22] Unlike the lumbar facet joints, where tropism is unusual,[10,33] asymmetry is the rule rather than the exception in the thoracic spine, with the right side generally oriented more vertically and frontally than the left.[11]

Sensory innervation of the thoracic facets is comparable to that in the lumbar spine. At most levels, innervation is

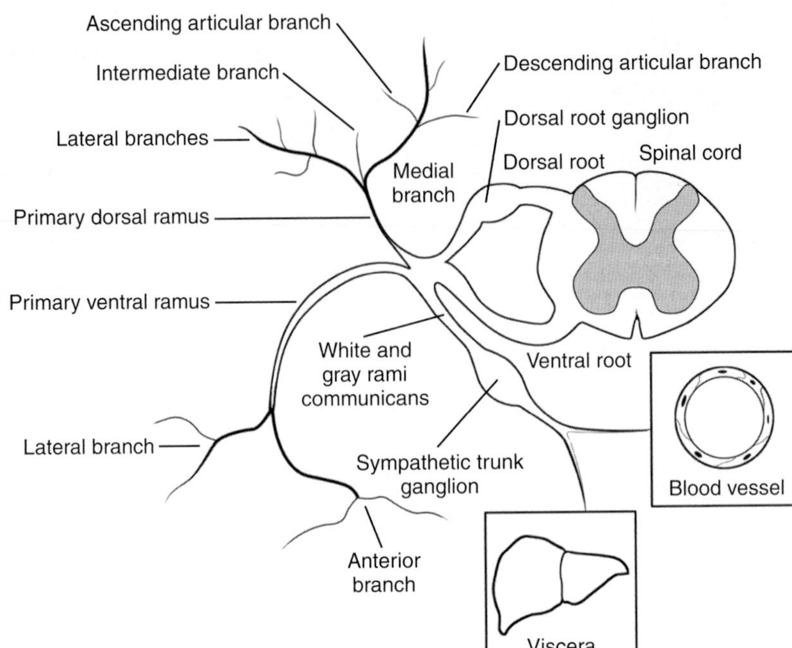

Figure 61.2 Schematic drawing of the spinal cord and segmental spinal innervation. (From Cohen SP, Raja SN. Pathogenesis, diagnosis, and treatment of lumbar zygapophysial [facet] joint pain. *Anesthesiology*. 2007;106:591-614.)

derived from the medial branch from the same level and the level above. Exceptions to this rule sometimes occur at the uppermost thoracic z-joints, where the medial branches from C7 and C8 may travel caudad to levels as low as T3.[34] In a cadaveric study by Chua and Bogduk,[35] the authors showed that the thoracic medial branches assume different courses depending on the level. In the midthoracic levels, they do not run on bone but instead are suspended in the intertransverse space. Because the thoracic medial branches also swing laterally to circumvent the multifidus muscle, motor stimulation of the multifidus muscle cannot be used reliably to confirm needle placement during radiofrequency (RF) treatment as it can be in the lumbar spine. In none of the 84 medial branch dissections did authors find the nerve crossing the junction between the superior articular process and the transverse process, as occurs in the lumbar spine. Instead, the superolateral corner of the transverse process was noted to be a more accurate target point for diagnostic blockade and denervation (Figs. 61.5 and 61.6). A recent study suggests that the posterior rami in the thoracic spine may send a branch, termed the "descending branch," to the facet joint before the bifurcations of the medial and lateral branches.[36]

CERVICAL FACET JOINTS

To facilitate the complex motions of the neck, the position and shape of the cervical z-joints change greatly from the base of the occiput to the cervicothoracic junction.[22,37,38] The occiput sits on the C1 articular processes in an orientation nearly parallel to the axial plane. The superior articular process at C3 faces posteromedially, with a 70-degree angle in the sagittal plane and a 45-degree angle in the transverse plane. The relative position of the C2-3 facet inhibits rotation and serves to anchor the C2 vertebra as a rotational pivot for the atlantoaxial joint (C1-2). Between the C3-4 and C7-T1 facet joints, the orientation transitions to the consistent posterolateral position of the C7 superior articular process. The most frequent site of this transition is at the C5-6 joint. The position of the z-joints at this level allows flexion, extension, rotation, and lateral bending. Because of the enhanced mobility of this segment, the C5-6 level is also the most prone to facet dislocations and spondylosis. The C7 superior articular processes are oriented approximately 93 degrees to the sagittal plane and 65 degrees to the transverse plane. In addition, the shapes of the facet joints between C3 and C6 tend to be round and almost flat, whereas the C6-T1 z-joints are elliptical with a more concave surface. The combination of shape and orientation at the cervicothoracic junction is designed to maximize stability.

The innervation patterns of the cervical z-joints are slightly more complicated and varied than the lumbar and thoracic levels (Fig. 61.7). There are eight cervical nerve roots, the first seven of which exit the intervertebral foramen above the vertebral body of the same number. Similar to the lumbar and thoracic z-joints, the C3-4 to C7-T1 facet joints receive dual innervation from the medial branches of the posterior rami from the same level and one level above.[39] The nerves curve around the waist of the articular pillars at their respective levels and then branch out to supply two joints. Tight fascia and the tendons of the semispinalis capitis muscle ensure that the medial branches cling closely to the periosteum, thereby making their position more predictable. On a lateral projection, the medial branches tend to lie in the center of the articular pillars.[40-42]

The cervical facet joints above the C3-4 level are slightly more complicated. The C2-3 facet joint receives the majority of its innervation from the C3 dorsal ramus. The C3 dorsal ramus normally divides into two separate medial branches. The larger superior branch is better known as the third occipital nerve, and the inferior branch is conventionally termed the deep median branch. Some innervation of the C2-3 level is also derived from the C2 dorsal rami, which may form five distinct branches, the largest of which is the

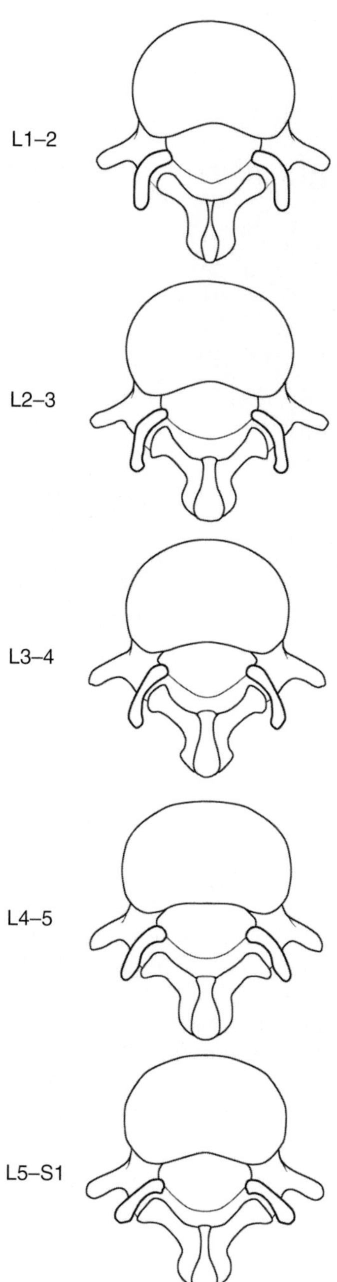

Figure 61.3 Segmental variation in lumbar zygapophyseal joint orientation in the transverse plane. (From Cohen SP, Raja SN. Pathogenesis, diagnosis, and treatment of lumbar zygapophysial [facet] joint pain. *Anesthesiology*. 2007;106:591-614.)

greater occipital nerve.[42,43] Along with the upper cervical z-joints themselves, the dorsal rami and its branches can also be a source of cervicogenic headache.[44,45]

MECHANISMS OF INJURY

In the vast majority of cases, facet joint arthropathy is the product of years of repetitive strain, low-grade trauma, and stress from intervertebral disk degeneration. This is best demonstrated by the strong association between facet arthropathy and increasing age.[46-51] Studies have demonstrated that intervertebral disk degeneration virtually always precedes facet changes in the lumbar spine.[51] At the L4-5 and L5-S1 levels, some patients have facet degeneration without disk changes. In some cases an inciting event or pathology can be identified. This is especially true in trauma patients with whiplash injuries.[41,45,52] In most patients, whiplash leads to chronic neck and shoulder pain. However, in some cases, rear impact injuries can result in radiculopathy from cervical facet dislocations or fractures or in spinal cord injury.[53-61] In addition, high-impact trauma such as motor vehicle accidents (MVAs) or sports injuries may result in z-joint pain secondary to hyperflexion,[62] rotation, and distraction injuries.[63]

CADAVERIC AND LABORATORY STUDIES

Cadaveric studies have shed some light on the mechanisms of z-joint movement and displacement. Ianuzzi and coworkers found that the joint moments occurring with any given motion are directly correlated with the magnitude of joint displacement and tend to be greatest at the L4-5 and L5-S1 joints.[64] At the three most caudad joints (L3-S1), contralateral bending is associated with greater capsular strain than ipsilateral bending is (i.e., the left facet joints are most strained during right lateral flexion). In contrast, the L1-2 and L2-3 joints undergo greater strain during ipsilateral flexion. For the upper three facet joints, the maximum joint displacement and greatest strain are associated with lateral bending, usually to the right. For the two lowest joints, the greatest degree of strain occurs during forward flexion (Table 61.1).

Later work has provided evidence that fusion of two vertebrae can lead to accelerated degeneration at adjacent levels.[65-69] Little and associates fixated human lumbar spine specimens with a single anterior thoracolumbar plate at L4-5 and measured capsular displacement and strain during a wide range of physiologic motions.[69] Motion was increased at the level of fixation and at both adjacent levels. Fusion also increased intervertebral angulation at L3-4 and L5-S1, with decreased motion at L4-5. Although fusion relieved the anterior (ipsilateral) strain at L4-5, there was greater posterior strain at L4-5 and anterior and posterior strain at both adjacent levels.

The z-joints may respond to repetitive strain and inflammation by filling with fluid and distending, thereby stretching the capsule and causing pain.[70] The pain from capsular inflammation can spread beyond the joint area due to compression of the exiting nerve root in the neural foramen or spinal canal, especially with foramina that are already narrowed by facet joint hypertrophy, osteophytes, or herniated intervertebral disks.[71-74] Inflammatory cytokines released from facet joint tissue may also contribute to the radicular symptoms in patients with spinal stenosis.[75] Facet joint pain can therefore be manifested in a radicular pattern. Irritation of the capsule may also cause reflex spasm of the erector spinae, multifidus, and other paraspinous muscles.[71,76,77]

The pathophysiologic basis for persistent lumbar facet pain was established in a series of elegant experiments conducted by Cavanaugh and colleagues,[78] Yamashita and colleagues,[79,80] and Ozaktay and colleagues[81] on New Zealand white rabbits. These studies showed that injection

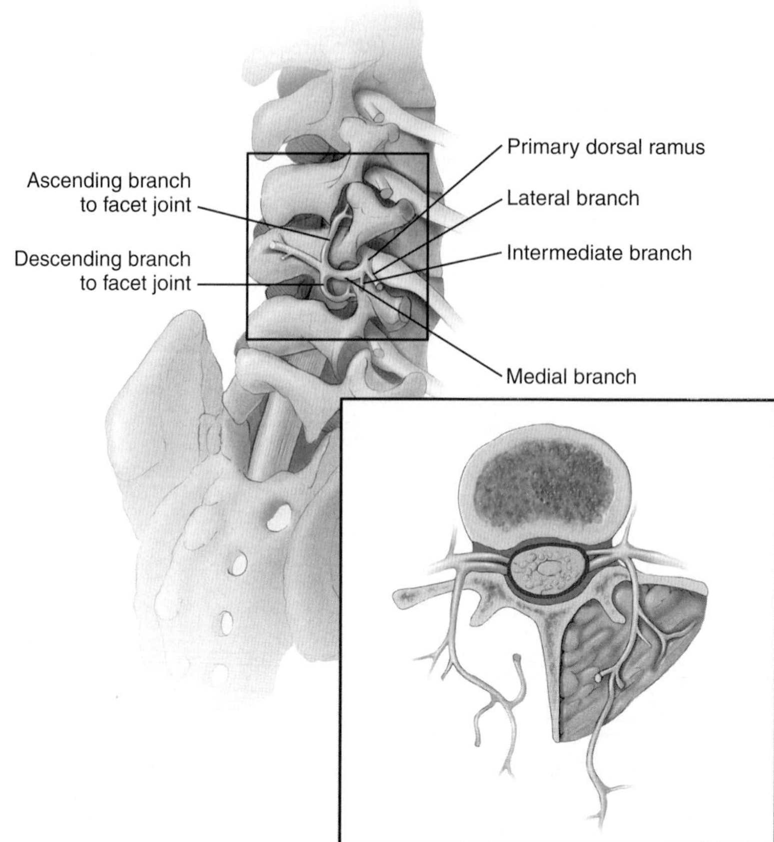

Figure 61.4 Right lateral oblique view of the lumbar vertebral bodies and the dorsal rami medial branches. (From Cohen SP, Raja SN. Pathogenesis, diagnosis, and treatment of lumbar zygapophysial [facet] joint pain. *Anesthesiology*. 2007;106:591-614.)

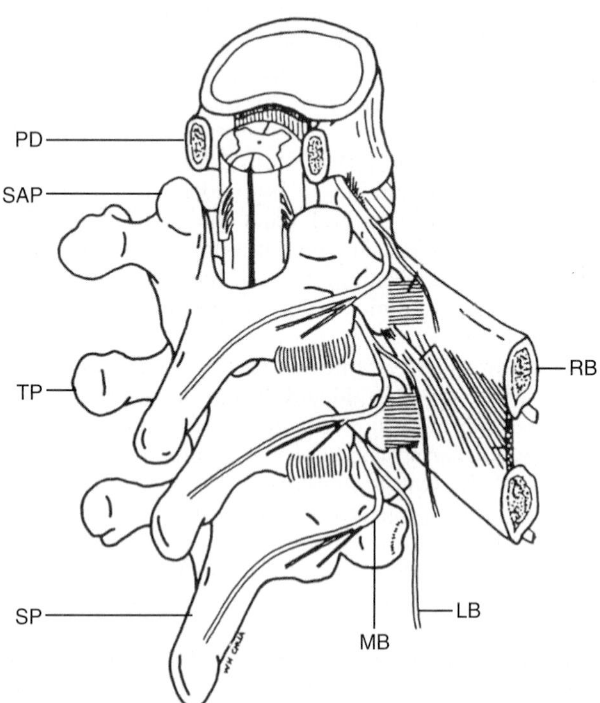

Figure 61.5 Sketch of the typical course of the thoracic medial branch from a right superior oblique view showing the target point of the superolateral corner of the transverse process. LB, lateral branch; MB, medial branch; PD, pedicle; RB, rib; SAP, superior articular process; SP, spinous process; TP, transverse process. (From Chua WH, Bogduk N. The surgical anatomy of thoracic facet denervation. *Acta Neurochir [Wien]*. 1995;136:140-144.)

of proinflammatory and algesic mediators into facet joints resulted in inflammatory changes, including vasodilation, venous congestion, and the accumulation of polymorphonuclear leukocytes. The associated inflammatory response led to sensitization and reduced the firing thresholds of both nociceptors and proprioceptive nerve fibers. The result was an increase in the discharge rate and recruitment of previously silent units.[78-81] Persistent nociception is known to cause peripheral sensitization with the potential for subsequent central sensitization and neuroplasticity.[82] Later work by Chen and colleagues showed the presence of C and Aδ fibers in the cervical facet joint capsules of goats.[83] C fibers were more prevalent in the dorsolateral aspect of the z-joint capsule, where tendons and muscles attach. Even though animal research has played a critical role in improving our understanding of the pathophysiology of facet pain, there is a wide array of anatomic and functional differences between animals and humans.[84] Rat models of facet pain have involved injection of monosodium iodoacetate into the facet joint; however, this led to mechanical hyperalgesia in the hind paw, which would not be expected in a model of axial spine pain.[85] Therefore, caution should be exercised when extrapolating the results of animal studies to humans.

These preclinical data do indicate that chronic facet pain is likely to occur with repetitive chronic strain or, less commonly, following any acute event that stretches the joint beyond its physiologic limits. Clinical studies indicating a higher prevalence of facet arthropathy in the elderly[49,86,87] and case reports of facet pain following high-energy trauma[45,63] support these preclinical findings.

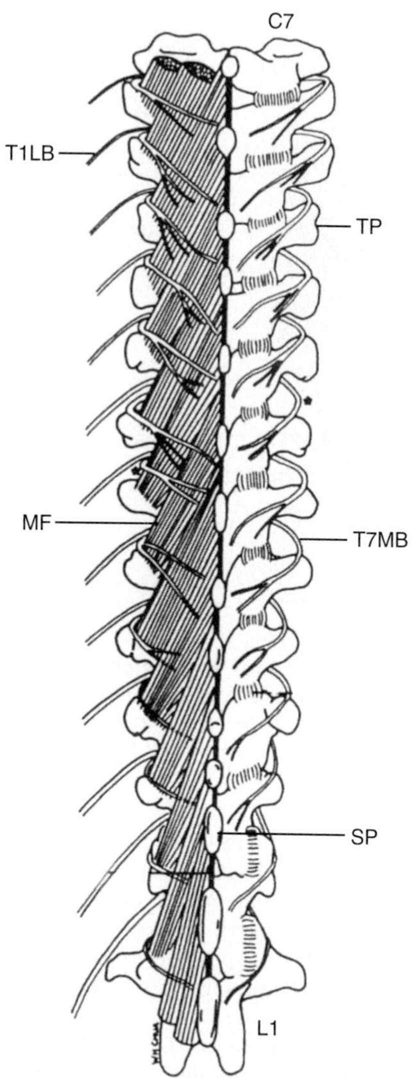

Figure 61.6 Posterior view of the course of the thoracic medial branches again showing the target points of the superolateral corners of the transverse processes. The multifidus and lateral branches are not shown on the right side. C, cervical vertebra; L, lumbar vertebra; LB, lateral branch; MB, medial branch; MF, multifidus; SP, spinous process; T, thoracic vertebra; TP, transverse process. (From Chua WH, Bogduk N. The surgical anatomy of thoracic facet denervation. *Acta Neurochir [Wien]*. 1995;136:140-144.)

HUMAN STUDIES

In clinical studies, chronic facet pain has been associated with several conditions. In patients with LBP and asymptomatic individuals, sagittally oriented facet joints were associated with degenerative spondylolisthesis.[23,24] In these patients, recurrent rotational strain results in a myriad of changes in the disks and paired facet joints, including loss of disk height, osteophyte formation, and degenerative joint hypertrophy.[88,89]

The intervertebral disk and paired facet joints work in concert. Therefore, changes in any part of the three-joint unit will alter the motion and function of the others. Degenerative disk disease (DDD) has been shown to result in concomitant changes in the facet joints.[90-92] In the reverse scenario, degeneration and motion abnormalities of the facet joints can induce and accelerate intervertebral disk degeneration.[93-95] Multiple studies have examined the relationship between DDD and facet joint osteoarthritis (OA) and concluded that DDD generally precedes facet arthritis.[51,96] In addition, facet arthropathy tends to be most pronounced at spinal levels with advanced DDD. DDD affects rotation and movement at the level of degeneration and neighboring levels.[97] However, a clinical study investigating the relationship between injection-confirmed discogenic LBP and facet joint arthropathy yielded conflicting findings.[98] Among 92 patients with axial LBP, 39% had at least one positive diskogram with a negative control disk, and 9% experienced concordant pain relief following a series of diagnostic facet blocks. Yet only 3% of patients had both positive diskography and diagnostic facet blocks.

A number of other conditions besides OA may affect the facet joint, including inflammatory arthritides such as rheumatoid arthritis, ankylosing spondylitis, and reactive arthritis.[99-102] In addition, synovial impingement, meniscoid entrapment, chondromalacia facetae, pseudogout, synovial inflammation, villonodular synovitis, and acute and chronic infection may cause facetogenic pain.[102-107] Synovial pseudocysts within the facets can result in distention and pressure on adjacent structures and thereby lead to calcification and asymmetrical facet hypertrophy.[108-113] Pseudocysts typically induce axial pain and radiculopathy but can also cause motor weakness, myelopathy, and cauda equina syndrome.[112,113] A retrospective review of magnetic resonance imaging (MRI) findings in 303 consecutive patients with LBP found that 9.5% of the patients had z-joint synovial cysts, with the majority being located posteriorly.[114]

There are a number of reported cases of lumbar facetogenic pain secondary to traumatic dislocation from rapid deceleration injuries, mostly at L5-S1.[62,63,115-119] The purported mechanism of injury in these cases was hyperflexion, rotation, and distraction. By itself, hyperextension rarely leads to facet fractures.[62] Twomey and colleagues dissected the lumbar spines of 31 subjects who died of trauma (mostly MVAs).[120] They found occult bony fractures in the superior articular process or subchondral bone plate in 35% of subjects and facet capsular or articular cartilage damage (or both) in 77% of cases. These findings indicate that occult bony and soft tissue injuries to the facet joints may be a source of LBP after trauma.

For chronic post-traumatic neck pain, the cervical z-joints have been estimated to account for upward of 60% of cases.[39,121] However, trauma is responsible for only a small percentage of chronic neck pain. An epidemiologic study conducted in patients with chronic cervical pain found trauma to be the precipitating event in only 13% of cases.[122] In patients with positive cervical facet blocks, the percentage of cases attributed to trauma varies significantly. In a small, controlled study evaluating RF denervation for cervicogenic headache, 5 of 12 patients reported a previous inciting event.[123] However, in the largest cervical facet denervation outcome study, Cohen and colleagues[124] found that only 23% of the 92 subjects with a positive response to diagnostic z-joint blocks cited trauma as the principal cause. In rare instances, tumors may also cause facet joint pain.[125,126]

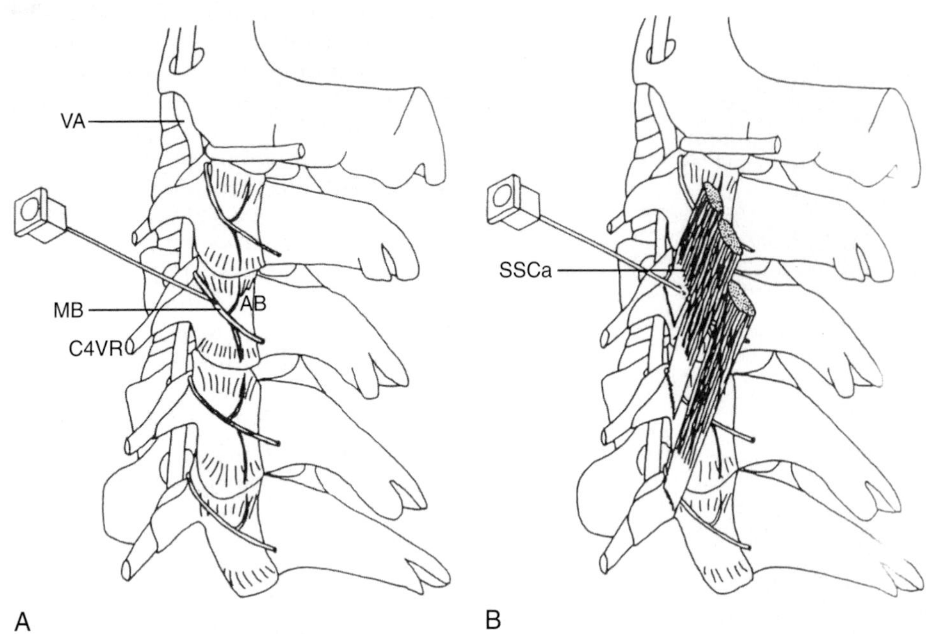

Figure 61.7 Sketches of left posterolateral views of the cervical articular pillars. **A,** The cervical medial branches course across the waist of the articular pillars. A needle inserted from a lateral approach anesthetizes the medial branch proximal to the origin of its articular branches. **B,** The articular branches lie deep to the tendinous origin of the semispinalis capitis, which acts to hold the anesthetic in place against the medial branch. AB, articular branches; C, cervical vertebra; MB, medial branch; SSCa, semispinalis capitis; VA, vertebral artery. (From Barnsley L, Bogduk N. Medial branch blocks are specific for the diagnosis of cervical zygapophysial joint pain. *Reg Anesth*. 1993;18:343-350.)

Table 61.1 Motions Associated with the Largest Intervertebral Angulation and Strain for the Lumbar Facet Joints

Facet Joint Level	Movement Associated with Maximal IVA	Largest Strain
L1-2	Right bending	Right bending
L2-3	Left bending	Right bending
L3-4	Right bending	Right bending
L4-5	Forward flexion	Forward flexion
L5-S1	Extension	Forward flexion

IVA, intervertebral angle.
Modified from Ianuzzi A, Little JS, Chiu JB, et al. Human lumbar facet joint capsule strains: I. During physiological motions. *Spine J*. 2004;4:141-152.

PREVALENCE

The prevalence of facet joint pain varies greatly throughout the literature. The lumbar facets are most commonly affected, followed in descending order by cervical and thoracic facet arthropathy.

PREVALENCE OF LUMBAR FACET ARTHROPATHY

The cited prevalence rate of lumbar z-joint pain ranges from 5% to upward of 90% in the literature.[127-134] Many of the studies investigating prevalence, however, have been flawed. Numerous reviews have found that diagnosis of facet joint pain via the history, physical examination, and radiologic findings is unreliable; the most reliable method to diagnose a painful z-joint is by image-guided medial branch blocks (MBBs) or intra-articular injections of local anesthetic (LA).[135-137] Diagnostic facet blocks without controls have been associated with false-positive rates ranging from 25% to 41%.[50,138-140] Although some consider positive MBBs to be "diagnostic," given their high false-positive rates, it is probably more appropriate to consider them as being prognostic of long-lasting treatments, such as RF ablation of the medial branch.

This high false-positive rate has led some experts to advocate controlled or comparative blocks as the only reliable method for diagnosing lumbar facetogenic pain.[141] The reported prevalence of facet pain with single LA blocks has ranged from 8% to 94%.[86,133] The addition of placebo-controlled LA blocks decreases prevalence rates significantly to between 9% and 42% (Table 61.2).[50,87,98,138-140,142-144] Not surprisingly, the estimated prevalence rates tend to increase with age.[46-51,87]

Larger epidemiologic studies by primary care physicians and spine surgeons have found much lower rates of lumbar facet pain. Newton and associates[145] studied all cases of acute and chronic LBP in a large health maintenance organization population over a 9-month period and found a 6% prevalence of facet-mediated pain. In a comprehensive epidemiologic study by Long and coworkers, spine surgeons from eight academic medical centers in the United States collected demographic and clinical information on more than 4000 patients with LBP over a 5-year period.[131] Final diagnoses were based on the history and physical examination, radiologic and other diagnostic studies, and response to treatment or diagnostic injections (or both). The diagnosis of "facet joint arthritis" was made in 4.8% of the 2374 patients who completed the study.

Table 61.2 Results of Lumbar Facet Joint Pain Prevalence Studies Conducted with Either Placebo-Controlled or Comparative Local Anesthetic Blocks

Author, Year	Patients	Interventions	Results	False-Positive Rate and Comments
Schwarzer et al.,[98] 1994	92 pts with chronic LBP without neurologic deficits or previous surgery. All pts underwent comparative facet blocks and provocative diskography.	Pts rec'd either intra-articular injection (0.5 mL) or MBB (0.5 mL) with 2% lidocaine at the 3 lowest facet levels. In pts who obtained ≥50% relief, blocks were repeated with 0.5% bupivacaine. A (+) response was pain relief sustained for ≥3 hr.	39% (n = 36) of pts achieved definite pain relief after lidocaine blocks. 25% of pts who underwent confirmatory blocks with bupivacaine obtained a (+) response, for a 9% prevalence rate.	26% rate of FP blocks. 39% of pts had (+) diskography. Only 3 pts had both (+) diskography and (+) response to facet blocks. Median age, 37 yr. Male-female ratio, 2:1.
Schwarzer et al.,[140] 1994	176 pts with chronic LBP without neurologic deficits or previous surgery.	Pts rec'd either intra-articular injection or MBB (0.5 mL) with 2% lidocaine at the 3 lowest levels. In pts who obtained ≥50% pain relief, blocks were repeated with 0.5% bupivacaine. A (+) response was pain relief sustained for ≥3 hr.	47% (n = 83) of pts reported a definite or greater response after lidocaine, with 26 of 71 pts who underwent confirmatory blocks obtaining concordant relief, for a prevalence rate of 15%.	FP rate, 38%. Median age, 38 yr.
Schwarzer et al.,[50] 1995	63 pts with chronic LBP without neurologic deficits or previous surgery.	Pts rec'd placebo injections followed by single-level intra-articular facet injections (with up to 1.5 mL of 0.5% bupivacaine) at the 3 lowest levels on separate occasions. A (+) response was pain relief sustained for ≥3 hr with only bupivacaine.	40% obtained >50% pain relief with bupivacaine but not with placebo. 37% had >90% pain relief.	32% of pts obtained >50% pain relief for ≥3 hr after placebo. 18 of 23 obtained relief at only 1 level. Median age, 59 yr. Female-male ratio, 3:1.
Revel et al.,[87] 1998	80 pts with chronic LBP not caused by sciatica without previous surgery.	Pts rec'd either placebo or 1 mL of lidocaine injected into the 2 most caudal facet joints. A (+) response was >75% pain relief.	31% of the lidocaine group obtained significant pain relief after the injection.	18% of pts receiving intra-articular saline obtained significant pain relief. Mean age, 58 yr. 2:1 female-male ratio.
Manchikanti et al.,[138] 1999	120 pts with chronic LBP without neurologic deficits.	Pts rec'd MBB with 0.4-0.6 mL of 1% lidocaine and/or 0.25% bupivacaine. In all pts a (+) response was ≥75% relief lasting longer with bupivacaine than with lidocaine.	81 (67.5%) pts reported a definite response to lidocaine MBB. 54 of them reported definite pain relief after the bupivacaine block, for a prevalence rate of 45%.	FP rate, 41%. Pts who had previous surgery were less likely to have lumbar zygapophyseal joint pain. Trauma was implicated as a cause of pain in 53% of pts. Mean age, 47 yr.
Manchikanti et al.,[139] 2000	180 pts with chronic LBP without neurologic deficits.	Pts rec'd double MBB from L1 to L5 with 0.5 mL of lidocaine and bupivacaine, LA with Sarapin, or LA with Sarapin and steroid. A (+) response was ≥75% relief lasting longer with bupivacaine than with lidocaine.	74% (n = 133) of pts obtained a (+) response to the lidocaine blocks, but only 65 reported definite pain relief after bupivacaine blocks, for a 36% prevalence rate.	25% FP rate. Mean age, 48 yr.
Dreyfuss et al.,[142] 2000	41 carefully chosen pts out of 138 screened by telephone interview with chronic LBP, no neurologic deficits, and absence of psychiatric or severe concomitant spinal pathology.	Pts rec'd MBB with 2% lidocaine at maximally tender areas. Pts who obtained ≥80% pain relief underwent confirmatory blocks with bupivacaine. A (+) response was definite pain relief lasting >2 hr.	22 pts obtained significant pain relief after lidocaine MBB, with 15 obtaining ≥80% after bupivacaine blocks, for a 37% prevalence rate.	FP rate, 17%. Mean age, 55 yr in 15 responders. Pts carefully chosen to evaluate outcomes for radiofrequency denervation.
Manchikanti et al.,[144] 2000	200 pts with chronic LBP without neurologic deficits.	Pts rec'd MBB with 1% lidocaine. All pts who obtained ≥75% pain relief underwent confirmatory blocks with 0.25% bupivacaine. A (+) response was ≥75% relief lasting longer with bupivacaine.	64% (n = 127) reported a (+) response to lidocaine blocks, with 84 obtaining definite pain relief after bupivacaine blocks, for a 42% prevalence rate.	37% FP rate. Mean age, 47 yr.
Manchikanti et al.,[143] 2004	397 pts with chronic LBP without neurologic deficits.	Pts rec'd MBB with 1% lidocaine. All pts who obtained ≥75% pain relief underwent confirmatory blocks with 0.25% bupivacaine. A (+) response was ≥80% relief lasting longer with bupivacaine.	198 (50%) of pts obtained a (+) response to lidocaine blocks, with 124 reporting definite pain relief with bupivacaine, for a 31% prevalence rate.	FP rate, 27%. Mean age, 47 yr.

The false-positive (FP) rate, if not mentioned, was determined by dividing the number of patients who obtained pain relief with the lidocaine screening block but not with the confirmatory block by the total number of blocks.
LA, local anesthetic; LBP, low back pain; MBB, medial branch block; pts, patients; rec'd, received.

The more cephalad lumbar facet joints are infrequently found to be the main source of axial LBP. In descending order, the most frequently implicated painful facet joints are L5-S1, L4-5, and L3-4.[50,98,140] The upper lumbar facet joints are far less likely to be the source of LBP independent of disease in the lower joints.

A number of factors make prevalence studies difficult to interpret. Most studies excluded patients with focal neurologic signs or symptoms, yet foraminal narrowing secondary to facet hypertrophy is a well-described cause of radiculopathy.[71,72,74] A second confounding factor is that the best studies investigating the prevalence of facet hypertrophy used comparative MBBs.[138] Although the medial branch is the largest branch of the primary dorsal ramus, the other two branches are the intermediate branch, which innervates the longissimus muscle, and the lateral branch, which supplies the iliocostalis muscle, thoracolumbar fascia, skin over the lower back and buttock region, and sacroiliac joint.[27,146-148] The medial branches above L5 are most easily blocked at the superomedial border of the transverse process at its junction with the superior articular process. In these areas, LA will almost invariably block all three primary dorsal rami branches because of their close proximity. Although it is difficult to infer the precise prevalence of lumbar facet joint pain, based on the available literature the best estimate is that it affects approximately 10% to 15% of patients with LBP.

PREVALENCE OF CERVICAL AND THORACIC FACET ARTHROPATHY

Less is known about the prevalence of cervical and thoracic facet arthropathy, although a few prospective trials have been conducted. In one of the earliest cervical z-joint prevalence studies, Aprill and Bogduk performed provocative diskography, intra-articular facet injections, or both in 318 patients with chronic nonradicular neck pain following injury. Based on concordant pain provocation to both sets of blocks, the authors estimated the prevalence of cervical z-joint pain to be 26%.[121] In addition to not using the analgesic response to facet blocks as their primary diagnostic criteria, another flaw in this study is that only 52 of the 318 patients underwent diagnostic cervical facet blocks. In an observational study by Barnsley and colleagues involving 50 patients with chronic neck pain following whiplash injury, the authors found a prevalence rate of 54% based on double-blind, comparative LA MBBs.[149]

In a prospective study of 500 patients with nonradicular neck pain (n = 255) and midback pain (n = 72) or LBP, Manchikanti and coworkers[143] used a concordant response to LA MBBs done with 1% lidocaine and 0.25% bupivacaine to diagnose a painful thoracic or cervical facet joint. The authors found the prevalence of cervical facetogenic pain in patients with neck pain to be 55%, whereas patients with midback and upper back pain had a 42% prevalence of thoracic facet pain. The latter finding is consistent with a previous study done by the same group in which a 48% prevalence of thoracic facet pain was found in patients with midback and upper back pain.[150] Bilateral involvement was present in 69% of the patients in the cervical spine, in 64% in the thoracic spine, and in 72% in the lumbar spine.[143]

Based on studies using comparative blocks, the prevalence of cervical facetogenic pain in patients with chronic neck pain has been estimated to be between 27% and 63% (Table 61-3).[41,45,143,149,151,152] The C2-3 and C5-6 levels were found to be the most prevalent levels in two studies of patients with chronic neck pain.[45,149] The C2-3 facet joint was also found to have the highest rate of degenerative disease in a study of 196 excavated human skeletons from the sixth to eighth centuries AD from Germanic row graves in southwestern Germany.[153]

The majority of well-designed cervical facet prevalence studies have been conducted in patients with whiplash injuries after MVAs, which makes it difficult to estimate the prevalence in patients with neck pain and no history of trauma. It is well known that cervical facetogenic pain accounts for a large percentage of cases of persistent whiplash injury. Based on the available literature, the prevalence of cervical facet pain is probably around 50% in patients with chronic neck pain. The prevalence of thoracic facet pain in patients with chronic axial midback pain is between 42% and 48%[143,150] (see Table 61.3).

DIAGNOSIS

Despite years of research aimed at identifying clinical factors that can be used to predict responsiveness to facet interventions, there are essentially no elements of the history or physical examination, biomarkers, or radiologic findings that are sensitive or specific for responsiveness to facet interventions. A detailed history and physical examination can help exclude other potential pain generators and may build an overall clinical picture consistent with facet pain.

HISTORY

Some patient factors are associated with possible facet pain. The majority of investigations have focused on the lumbar z-joints, although some data are available for cervical and thoracic z-joint pain. With the exception of patients with a history of whiplash or trauma (including spine surgery),[45,149,154] facet pain is often associated with older age.[46-51,87] The direct association with age is consistent with the concept that facet pain is a chronic degenerative disorder that generally coexists with DDD[51] rather than an acute inflammatory process. No self-reported patient complaints or activities, such as sitting, walking, standing, bending, twisting, or coughing, have consistently been found to be associated with responsiveness to facet interventions. Some studies have found that opioid use and previous spine surgery may be associated with poor outcomes after RF treatment,[124,155] but lack of responsiveness to RF does not rule out facet pain.

PAIN REFERRAL PATTERNS

The distribution and radiation of pain from the facet joints have been derived from patient self-report of relief with LA blocks, direct pressurization of the facet joints, and direct stimulation of the medial branches innervating the specific joints. The majority of these studies have failed to demonstrate any reliable pain referral patterns.[156,157]

Table 61.3 Results of Cervical and Thoracic Zygapophyseal Joint Pain Prevalence Studies Conducted with Either Placebo-Controlled or Comparative Local Anesthetic Blocks

Author, Year	Patients	Interventions	Results	False-Positive Rate and Comments
Barnsley et al.,[41] 1993	47 pts with chronic neck pain >3 mo after MVA.	Pts rec'd cervical MBB with 0.5 mL of either 2% lidocaine or 0.5% bupivacaine. Pts with positive block rec'd other agent. A (+) response required longer pain relief with bupivacaine.	27 pts had longer relief with bupivacaine than with lidocaine, for a 60% prevalence rate.	13 pts (27%) had a (+) response to both LAs but in excess of the expected duration. Average age, 41 yr. Female-male ratio, 1:1. All but 3 pts involved in litigation.
Barnsley et al.,[149] 1995	50 pts with chronic neck pain of >3-mo duration after whiplash injury from MVA.	Pts rec'd cervical MBB with 0.5 mL of either 2% lidocaine or 0.5% bupivacaine at random. Pts with a (+) block rec'd the complementary anesthetic. A (+) response required longer pain relief with bupivacaine.	27 pts who completed the study met the criteria for a (+) painful joint, for a 54% prevalence rate.	10 pts (20%) had longer pain relief with lidocaine than with bupivacaine or no pain relief with repeated block. Average age, 41 yr. Female-male ratio, 1.5:1. C2-3 and C5-6 most frequently affected levels.
Lord et al.,[45] 1996	68 pts with chronic neck pain of >3-mo duration after whiplash injury from MVA.	Pts rec'd diagnostic C2-3 blocks to rule out those with 3rd occipital headache. Placebo-controlled cervical facet blocks below C2-3 done with 0.5 mL of either 2% lidocaine or 0.5% bupivacaine. If (–), other levels were then attempted. If (+), pts rec'd either NS or other LA at random and then had a third block with the remaining agent.	31 of 52 pts (60%) who completed the study had cervical facet pain at C2-3 or below, for a 60% prevalence rate. Among pts with HA as the dominant Sx, 50% prevalence of C2-3 facet joint pain. In pts without C2-3 facet pain, the prevalence of lower cervical facet pain was 49%.	Average age, 41 yr. Female-male ratio, 2:1. C2-3 and C5-6 most commonly affected levels.
Manchikanti et al.,[150] 2002	46 pts with chronic thoracic pain (>6 mo) without neurologic Sxs.	Pts rec'd MBB with 1% lidocaine followed by confirmatory blocks with 0.5% bupivacaine. A (+) response was >80% concordant pain relief.	22 of 36 pts with (+) lidocaine blocks had longer relief with confirmatory bupivacaine blocks, for a 48% prevalence rate.	FP rate, 58%. Average age, 46 yr.
Manchikanti et al.,[151] 2002	106 pts with chronic neck pain with or without HA or upper extremity pain.	Pts rec'd diagnostic blocks with 0.5 mL of 1% lidocaine followed by 0.5 mL of 0.25% bupivacaine 2 wk apart.	64 of 81 pts with (+) lidocaine blocks had longer relief with confirmatory bupivacaine blocks, for a 60% prevalence rate.	40% FP rate. Mean age, 43 yr. Female-male ratio, 2:1. 15% of pts had previous neck surgery.
Manchikanti et al.,[143] 2004	500 pts with chronic neck, thoracic, and/or low back pain without neurologic Sxs. 255 pts had cervical Sxs and 72 pts had thoracic Sxs.	Pts rec'd MBB with 1% lidocaine followed by confirmatory blocks with 0.25% bupivacaine. A (+) response was ≥80% relief lasting longer with bupivacaine. Minimum of 2 levels blocked based on pain patterns.	55% prevalence rate of cervical facet joints in pts with cervical spine pain. 42% prevalence rate of thoracic facet joints in pts with thoracic pain.	FP rate of 63% for cervical and 55% for thoracic MBB. Average age, 47 yr. Female-male ratio, 2:1 for both cervical and thoracic.

FP, false-positive; HA, headache; LA, local anesthetic; MBB, medial branch block; MVA, motor vehicle accident; NS, normal saline; pts, patients; Sx, symptom.

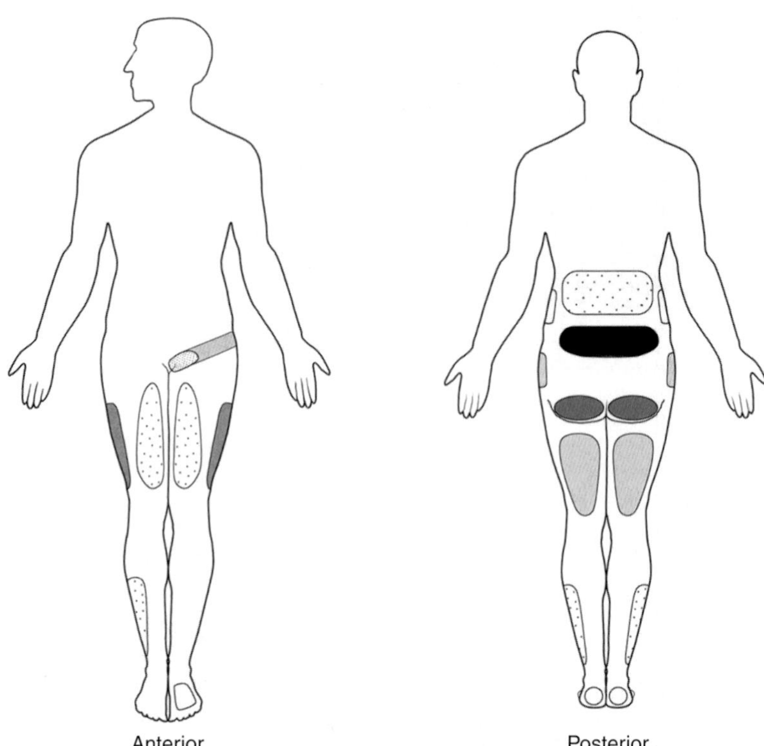

Figure 61.8 Pain referral patterns from the lumbar facet joints. In descending order, the most common referral patterns extend from the *darkest* (low back) to the *lightest* regions (flank and foot). The following key is listed in order of affected frequency (i.e., low back to foot). The *facet levels* next to each location represent the zygapophyseal joints associated with pain in each region. Low back: L5-S1, L4-5, L3-4; buttock: L5-S1, L4-5, L3-4; lateral thigh area: L5-S1, L4-5, L3-4, L2-3; posterior thigh area: L5-S1, L4-5, L3-4; greater trochanter: L5-S1, L4-5, L3-4, L2-3; groin: L5-S1, L4-5, L3-4, L2-3, L1-2; anterior thigh area: L5-S1, L4-5, L3-4; lateral lower leg area: L5-S1, L4-5, L3-4; upper back area: L3-4, L2-3, L1-2; flank: L1-2, L2-3; foot: L5-S1, L4-5. (From Cohen SP, Raja SN. Pathogenesis, diagnosis, and treatment of lumbar zygapophysial [facet] joint pain. *Anesthesiology*. 2007;106:591-614.)

These discrepancies between pain provocation patterns and pain mapping/historical findings are consistent with previous studies using sacroiliac joint and selective nerve root blocks.[158,159] Since facet pain is a usually a chronic, degenerative process, attempting to simulate this pain with maneuvers that result in acute capsular pressurization may not result in accurate findings.

When the existing data are synthesized, however, certain pain patterns do emerge (Fig. 61.8). The joint capsule appears to be more likely than the synovium or articular cartilage to generate pain. A great deal of overlap between neighboring facet joints exists. All lumbar levels are capable of producing groin pain, although it is most common in the lower levels (Table 61.4).[34,86,138,144,157,160-171] Pain from the upper lumbar facets tends to extend into the flank, hip, and upper lateral aspect of the thigh, whereas pain from the lower lumbar levels is likely to penetrate deeper into the thigh, usually in the lateral and posterior aspects. Infrequently, the L4-5 and L5-S1 facet joints can provoke pain in the lateral part of the calf and rarely in the foot. Patients with osteophytes, synovial cysts, or facet hypertrophy may also have radicular symptoms. Unilateral pain or pain in the paraspinal distribution is more likely to be associated with pain from the facet or sacroiliac joints than with discogenic or other causes of LBP.[172] In addition, pain in the low back region and thigh, especially with increasing age, was found to be more predictive of facet pain than was pain emanating from the sacroiliac joint, intervertebral disks, and other sources based on a retrospective study of patients undergoing evaluation with structured diagnostic blocks.[46]

Clinical studies have been conducted in both normal volunteers and patients with suspected cervical facet pain to determine pain referral patterns from the joints.[173-175] The results of these experiments are strikingly consistent. From C2-3, the pain pattern generally extends rostrally to the upper cervical region and suboccipital area. Infrequently, symptoms will extend toward the ear or further up the scalp. From C3-4, pain is referred to the upper and middle posterior aspect of the neck, with occasional radiation to the lower occiput. From C4-5, the most common referral pattern is to the lower posterior cervical region, although in a significant percentage of people it extends to the middle posterior aspect of the neck and suprascapular region. Pain from C5-6 is typically distributed to either the suprascapular region or lower part of the neck but can sometimes extend to the shoulder joint or midposterior neck region. From C6-7, pain is usually referred to the upper scapula or lower neck area. Pain from the C7-T1 z-joint most frequently extends further down into the midscapular area. Later work by Windsor and colleagues[176] indicated that the pain referral patterns elicited by cervical medial branch stimulation tend to be more contained and slightly different from those elicited by articular z-joint distention (Fig. 61.9).

Similar work has been done for the thoracic z-joints. Dreyfuss and coworkers[177] mapped thoracic facet pain patterns based on intra-articular injections of contrast material into the T3-4 to T10-11 z-joints in nine asymptomatic volunteers (Fig. 61.10). Fukui and associates[34] later investigated pain referral patterns during intra-articular injection of the upper- and lower-most thoracic z-joints. The resultant pain referral patterns were as follows: pain from the C7-T1 and T1-T2 z-joints typically radiates into the suprascapular region and superior angle of the scapula. Pain extending into the midscapular region may come from either C7-T1, T1-2, or T2-3, and pain from the T11-12 z-joint generally extends into the paravertebral region around the site of injection out to around the iliac crest area.

Table 61.4 Results of Studies Examining Pain Referral Patterns for Lumbar Zygapophyseal Joint Pain

Author, Year	Patients and Interventions	Results
Hirsch et al.,[160] 1963	Number of pts and characteristics not mentioned. Injected <0.3 mL of 11% hypertonic NS into 1 of the lower facet joints.	Pain distributed to the SI joint and gluteal areas, then out to the greater trochanter. Pain identical to typical LBP.
Mooney and Robertson,[161] 1976	5 controls and 15 pts with chronic LBP. Injected 1-3 mL of 5% hypertonic NS into L3-4 through the L5-S1 facet joints and S1-2 in pts with lumbarization of the sacrum.	L3-4 produced pain radiating down the lateral aspect of the leg. L4-5 and L5-S1 produced pain radiating posteriorly down the leg, often below the knee in pts with LBP. If present, S1-2 produced pain radiating under the buttock. Increasing volume increased the amount of radiation. Pts with LBP had greater radiation than did pts without back pain.
McCall et al.,[162] 1979	Intracapsular and pericapsular injection of 0.4 mL of 6% hypertonic saline into the L1-2 and L4-5 facet joints of 6 asymptomatic male volunteers.	There was little difference in pain distribution between intracapsular and pericapsular injections. Pain from L4-5 radiated to the flank, buttock, iliac crest, upper and lower groin areas, and thigh above the knee. Pain from L1-2 radiated to the flank, iliac crest, upper groin region, and occasionally the abdomen. Pain never radiated contralaterally.
Fairbank et al.,[163] 1981	25 pts with acute back and/or leg pain underwent lumbar z-joint injections at the area of maximal tenderness and 1 additional randomly chosen joint with 0.5 mL bupivacaine.	Responders had pain in the back and thigh, whereas nonresponders had pain in the back and lower part of the leg. Symptomatic pain reproduction occurred in only 6 pts.
Lippitt,[164] 1984	Retrospective review of 99 pts with LBP of varying duration who underwent lumbar z-joint injections with 1 mL of lidocaine and steroid.	No pattern of pain was noted to be more common in responders. Included pts with unilateral or bilateral hip pain, buttock pain, or pain localized to the low back area.
Lynch and Taylor,[165] 1986	50 pts with chronic LBP diagnosed by physical examination and radiographs as having facet pain underwent intra-articular steroid injections in 1 or 2 lower facet joints.	39 pts reported total (n = 11) or partial (n = 28) relief of pain after 2 wk. Over 90% of pts reported LBP during injection, with half reporting pain radiating to the ipsilateral thigh and buttock. No pts reported pain below the knee.
Helbig and Lee,[166] 1988	Retrospective review of 22 pts with chronic LBP and leg pain. Injected lumbar z-joint(s) with LA and steroid. Divided pts into (–) response (no relief), temporary response (relief lasted more than a few hr but <6 mo), and prolonged response (>6 mo relief).	80% of pts with groin or thigh pain had a prolonged response. No pts with groin pain and only 1 with thigh pain had a (–) response. Pts with pain below the knee had 37% (–) responses and only 25% prolonged responses.
Jackson et al.,[86] 1988	390 pts with LBP and no neurologic signs underwent L4-5 and L5-S1 z-joint injections with steroid and 1 mL of bupivacaine.	Postinjection pain relief was more likely to occur in patients without leg pain.
Marks,[167] 1989	138 pts with chronic LBP underwent lumbar facet blocks and MBB at the same levels. Blocks done with 1.0 mL of lidocaine, except at L5-S1, where 1.5 mL was used.	The pain produced at all levels was mostly local. The L4-5 and L5-S1 joints were also likely to radiate to the buttock, greater trochanter, and all aspects of the thigh. About 5% of the time pain extended below the knee. Pain from L2-5 sometimes extended to the groin. Stimulation of nerves was more likely to produce distally referred pain than was intra-articular provocation.

Continued on following page

Table 61.7 Results of Studies Examining Pain Referral Patterns for Lumbar Zygapophyseal Joint Pain (Continued)

Author, Year	Patients and Interventions	Results
Kuslich et al.,[168] 1991	193 pts underwent decompression surgery under local anesthesia. Stimulated a variety of tissue, including lumbar z-joints, by mechanical force or unipolar cautery.	Facet capsule stimulation produced pain in 30% of pts, but "significant pain" only 2.5% of time. Pain radiated to the back and buttock, but never the leg.
Marks et al.,[169] 1992	86 pts with chronic LBP rec'd either lumbar z-joint blocks or MBB with steroid and 1.0 or 1.5 (at L5-S1 or the L5 dorsal ramus mL of LA).	No pattern of pain predicted response to injection. Pts were included who had axial pain and pain radiating to the leg.
Schwarzer et al.,[157] 1994	90 pts with chronic LBP underwent lumbar z-joint blocks with 0.8 mL of contrast agent and lidocaine at 3 levels.	Based on analgesic response to a single block, there was a significant association between concordant pain provocation and pain relief. However, based on the concordant analgesic response to serial lidocaine and bupivacaine blocks, there was no association between pain provocation and pain relief.
Fukui et al.,[34] 1997	48 pts with chronic LBP underwent lumbar z-joint blocks with contrast material until pain was provoked, then rec'd 0.5-1.0 mL of LA. Pts who obtained excellent but temporary relief proceeded to RF denervation, with electrical stimulation being used to locate the target nerve.	Intra-articular contrast injection always reproduced the pain. Pain from the L1-2 joint always produced lumbar pain. In descending order, the L2-3 joint produced pain in the lumbar region, hip, and buttock or the lateral aspect of the thigh. L3-4 produced pain mostly in the lumbar region, buttock, or lateral or posterior aspect of the thigh. L4-5 elicited pain in the lumbar region, buttock, or lateral thigh region. L5-S1 elicited pain in the lumbar region, buttock, or lateral or posterior aspect of the thigh. Pain relief from stimulation of the medial branches was similar to that with lumbar z-joint blocks.
Kaplan et al.,[170] 1998	15 asymptomatic pts underwent painful facet capsular distention with up to 2.5 mL of contrast agent.	All subjects experienced a well-circumscribed area of pain without radiation to the inferior part of the buttock or extremity.
Manchikanti et al.,[138] 1999	120 pts with chronic LBP and no neurologic deficits underwent confirmatory MBB with 0.4-0.6 mL of lidocaine and bupivacaine.	No pattern of pain predicted response to injection. Pts were included who had axial pain only, thigh pain, groin pain, and/or leg pain.
Manchikanti et al.,[144] 2000	200 pts with chronic LBP without neurologic deficits underwent confirmatory MBB with 0.4-0.6 mL of lidocaine and bupivacaine.	No pattern of pain predicted response to injection. Pts were included who had axial pain only, thigh pain, groin pain, and/or leg pain.
Young et al.,[171] 2003	23 pts with chronic LBP and no neurologic deficits underwent lumbar z-joint injections with <1.5 mL of LA. A (+) response was designated as both concordant pain provocation and relief with LA.	The location of pain (radiating toward or away from the spinal column) was not associated with a (+) response.

LA, local anesthetic; LBP, low back pain; MBB, medial branch block; NS, normal saline; pts, patients; rec'd, received; RF, radiofrequency; SI, sacroiliac; z-joint, zygapophyseal (facet) joint.

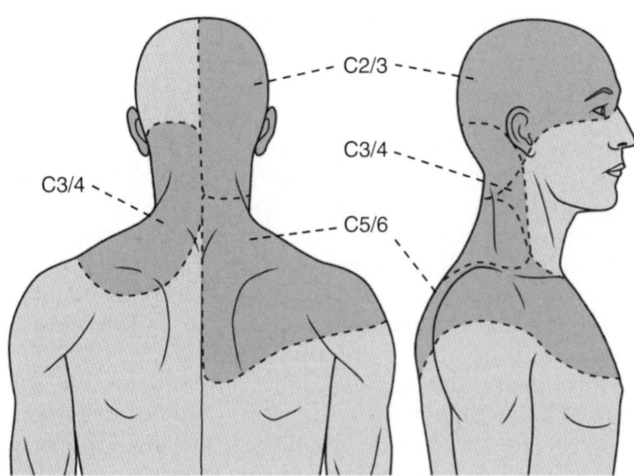

Figure 61.9 Pain referral patterns from the cervical facet joints. (From Bogduk N, Marsland A. The cervical zygapophysial joints as a source of neck pain. *Spine*. 1988;13:615.)

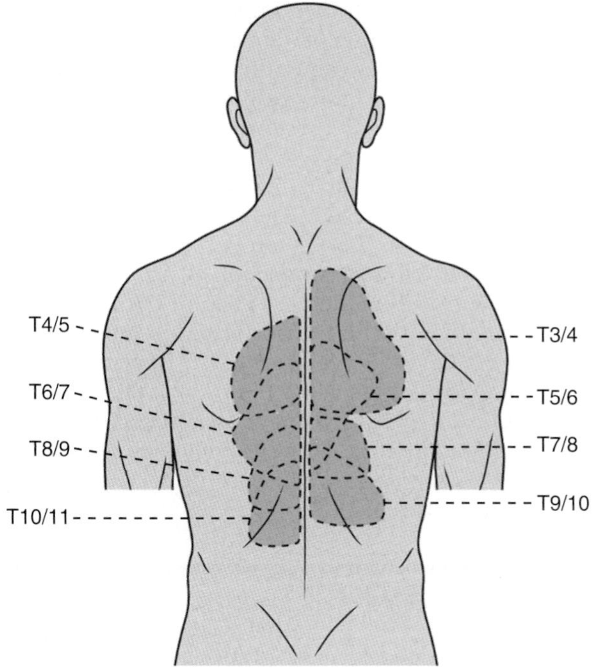

Figure 61.10 Pain referral patterns from the thoracic facet joints. (From Dreyfuss P, Tibiletti C, Dreyer SJ. Thoracic zygapophysial joint pain patterns. A study in normal volunteers. *Spine*. 1994;19:809.)

PHYSICAL EXAMINATION

As with the history and pain referral patterns, physical examination has limited value in diagnosing facet pain and is more valuable in ruling out other common causes of similar pain complaints. Of the available physical examination findings, *paraspinous muscle tenderness* is probably the only one indicative of facetogenic pain.[124,155] This finding is consistent with the self-reported patient complaints of paraspinous pain noted in the history section above.

Despite the limited value of physical examination in diagnosing facet pain, many research studies and clinicians still rely on provocative maneuvers to select patients for facet interventions. Early descriptions of physical examination findings thought to be consistent with facet pain came from retrospective studies. In a study by Fairbank and coworkers, low-volume, intra-articular bupivacaine facet blocks done on 41 patients with LBP with or without leg pain resulted in at least temporary pain relief in 14 of the 25 patients who completed the study.[163] When compared with nonresponders, subjects who responded positively to the blocks tended to have pain localized to the back and thigh and worsening pain with forward flexion. The term "lumbar facet syndrome" was coined by Helbig and Lee in 1988 based on a retrospective study of 22 patients.[166] Patients who responded to intra-articular injections were more likely to have back pain associated with groin or thigh pain, paraspinal tenderness, and reproduction of pain with extension-rotation maneuvers. Pain radiating below the knee was found to be a negative predictor.

Larger and more methodologically sound studies have failed to validate "lumbar facet syndrome" or the provocative maneuver commonly known as "facet loading." Prospective studies of 390 and 176 patients with chronic LBP were unable to correlate any historical or physical findings associated with a positive response to facet injections.[86,178] In both studies, only a small percentage (10% and 15%, respectively) of the patients responded to diagnostic blocks. A randomized, placebo-controlled study of 80 patients with chronic LBP by Revel and colleagues found seven factors to be associated with response to facet joint anesthesia: age older than 65 years and pain not exacerbated by coughing, not worsened by hyperextension, not worsened by forward flexion, not worsened when rising from forward flexion, not worsened by extension-rotation maneuvers, and well relieved by recumbency.[87] Yet subsequent investigations also failed to corroborate these findings.

Very few studies have investigated the history and physical findings most consistent with cervical and thoracic facet pain. As noted in the last section, the prevalence of facet involvement in patients with chronic neck and thoracic pain is higher than that in patients with LBP. Therefore, prognostic factors may be somewhat less important. One study found that a blinded therapist specializing in manipulation was able to diagnose symptomatic cervical facet joint pain correctly in patients with positive diagnostic cervical MBBs by means of perceived passive displacement of the joint and its resistance to displacement.[179] However, a subsequent study conducted using controlled blocks as the "gold standard" for cervical z-joint pain found that although manual examination had a sensitivity of 88%, low specificity (39%) precluded its use as a valid diagnostic tool.[180] Lord and coworkers found that patients with chronic neck pain who had a positive response to diagnostic cervical facet blocks were more likely to be female, to be victims of a rear-end collision, and to have restricted neck movement, although the findings were not statistically significant.[45] Another study showed a 94% correlation between lumbar and cervical facet pain in patients with confirmed lumbar facet pain who have concomitant neck pain.[181] The majority of cervical facet prevalence studies have been conducted on whiplash victims, thereby making it difficult to draw conclusions on the association between neck pain in nontrauma patients and cervical facet disease.

RADIOLOGIC FINDINGS

The prevalence of facet joint disease as observed with radiologic imaging is dependent on the age of patients, presence

Table 61.5 Levels of Degeneration of Facet Joints Based on Magnetic Resonance Imaging

Grade	Radiologic Findings
0	Normal zygapophyseal joints (2-4 mm in width)
1	Joint space narrowing, mild osteophyte formation, and/or mild hypertrophy of the articular process
2	Narrowing of the joint space with sclerosis or moderate osteophyte formation, moderate hypertrophy of the articular process, and/or mild subarticular bone erosions
3	Narrowing of the joint space with marked osteophyte formation, severe hypertrophy of the articular process, severe subarticular bone erosions, and/or subchondral cysts

Adapted from Weishaupt D, Zanetti M, Boos N, et al. MR imaging and CT in osteoarthritis of the lumbar facet joints. *Skeletal Radiol.* 1999;28:215-219.

of symptoms, imaging modality used, and threshold used for designating an examination as "abnormal." In LBP patients, the incidence of degenerative facet disease noted on computed tomography (CT) ranges from about 40% in some studies[127,182] to upward of 85% in others.[133] Some studies found MRI to be less sensitive than CT in detecting degenerative facet changes,[133,183,184] whereas other studies involving LBP patients revealed MRI to be more than 90% sensitive and specific when compared with CT (Table 61.5).[96,185] In a study of 14 patients with DDD, those younger than 40 years showed minimal osteoarthritic changes of the lumbar facets.[96] The prevalence of facet pathology increases significantly in patients older than 60 years; however, facet degeneration is not universal. In asymptomatic volunteers, the incidence of lumbar facet degeneration ranges from 8% to 14%.[184,186,187] In a study involving 60 asymptomatic individuals aged 20 to 50 years, MRI was used to evaluate for degenerative disk changes, end-plate abnormalities, and facet OA by two independent radiologists. Although disk bulge (62%) and protrusion (67%) were frequently present, neither radiologist noted severe facet OA.[184]

The use of radiologic imaging as a predictor of the response to diagnostic facet blocks has been conflicting at best. Even though some studies have found a positive association between CT, MRI, and other imaging and response to facet blocks,[127,130,166,182,188] an equal number have not.[49,86,133,158,163,189] In a study by Carrera and Williams, the response to high-volume (2 to 4 mL) diagnostic blocks was found to correlate with CT evidence of lumbar facet disease in 93 patients with LBP.[182] However, a larger study by Jackson and associates involving 390 patients found no relationship between x-ray findings and response to lumbar z-joint blocks.[86] Schwarzer and colleagues found no relationship between a concordant analgesic response to placebo-controlled intra-articular facet blocks and CT findings of z-joint OA in 63 patients with chronic axial LBP.[158] In a recent multicenter study by Cohen and coworkers involving 192 patients who underwent lumbar RF denervation based on a positive response to a single MBB, the authors found no association between MRI evidence of facet hypertrophy or degeneration and 6-month outcomes.[155] Finally, Kawaguchi and colleagues found no significant relationship between the degree of radiographic lumbar facet and LBP symptoms in a study of 106 patients with rheumatoid arthritis.[190] In the cervical and thoracic regions, there is a paucity of data evaluating the ability of radiologic imaging studies to predict response to diagnostic facet blocks. In the largest cervical facet denervation study ever conducted in 92 patients who underwent RF lesioning based on a positive response to a single diagnostic MBB, Cohen and coworkers found no association between 6-month outcomes and MRI evidence of facet arthritis at three different hospitals.[124]

In summary, the literature does not support the routine use of radiologic imaging as a means of diagnosing facet arthropathy. As with the history and physical examination, imaging is better used to rule out other disorders, such as corresponding neuroforaminal narrowing, spinal stenosis, vertebral fractures, and tumors. The lack of association between the degree of degeneration or damage in facet arthropathy and pain complaints and responsiveness to intervention has been used as proof against their use by those critical of facet interventions; however, the lack of an association between imaging findings and facet joint pain is consistent with virtually every pain disorder in which investigators have attempted to correlate radiologic findings with pain. The most robust example of this point lies in analyses of the most common cause of disability in the world, painful arthritis, especially knee OA. Despite well-defined grading systems for knee OA, there is no correlation between the severity of knee OA and complaints of pain, with 30% to 50% of patients with moderate to severe OA reporting no symptoms and 10% of patients with severe knee pain having normal radiographic findings.[191,192] Psychological variables account for only a small proportion of this variance.[193] Yet knee OA is a widely accepted pain diagnosis, and it is estimated that more than 1 million combined primary total knee arthroplasties and revisions are performed each year in the United States alone.[194]

DIAGNOSTIC BLOCKS

The poor correlation between historical and physical examination findings and zygapophyseal pain has led to widespread acceptance of the use of diagnostic blocks to confirm the facet joint as a primary pain generator. Even though MBB and intra-articular injections are widely touted to be equally effective diagnostic tools,[104,135,137,141] the evidence for this claim is based on two studies, neither of which used a crossover design or controlled blocks or prescreened patients for z-joint pain.[169,195] Several factors undermine the diagnostic validity of MBB. In a cadaveric study done in the 1930s, Kellegren showed that injection of 0.5 mL of fluid spread into an area encompassing 6 cm^2 of tissue.[196] Cohen and colleagues demonstrated that a reduction in LA volume in cervical MBBs from 0.5 to 0.25 mL decreased aberrant distribution, including spread to the intervertebral foramen.[197] Therefore, injection of low-volume LA is likely to block the lateral and intermediate branches in addition to the medial branch. Since these nerves supply afferent innervation to multiple potential pain-generating structures, including the paraspinal muscles, ligaments, sacroiliac joints, and skin, MBB can relieve pain even in the presence of normal facet joints. False-positive rates have been found to be as high as 63% in the cervical region, 53% in the thoracic region, and 27% in the lumbar facet region.[143] False-negative responses are also a concern and can be due to intravascular uptake of the LA or failure of patients to distinguish between procedure-related pain and their baseline pain. Given the low sensitivity of aspiration and intermittent fluoroscopy, some experts advocate using "real-time" fluoroscopy to detect intravascular uptake during MBB.[198]

Although intra-articular facet injections may inherently be more accurate in diagnosing facet pain, these blocks can be technically challenging and are fraught with limitations. Injection of 1 to 2 mL of fluid will probably rupture the joint capsule and lead to extravasation of LA onto other pain-generating structures. Depending on the point of rupture, these structures may include the epidural space, intervertebral foramen, ligamentum flavum, and paraspinal musculature.[70,132,134,169]

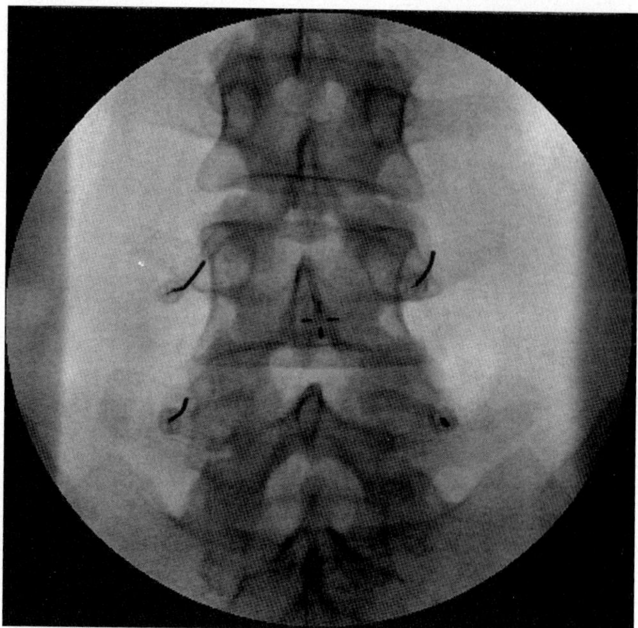

Figure 61.11 Anteroposterior fluoroscopic image demonstrating bilateral L3 and L4 medial branch blocks.

MEDIAL BRANCH BLOCK VERSUS INTRA-ARTICULAR INJECTION

Only three studies have compared MBB with intra-articular facet injections. In a prospective, randomized study by Nash, 67 patients with LBP were randomized in pairs to undergo either MBB with 2 mL of LA or intra-articular injections with 1.5 mL of LA and steroid.[195] In the 26 pairs who completed the study, 12 reported MBB to be more beneficial at their 1-month follow-up, 11 reported intra-articular injection to be better, and 3 reported no difference between the two. Marks and coworkers randomized 86 patients with LBP to receive either intra-articular injections or MBB with 2 mL of LA and steroid.[169] Although no immediate postprocedural difference was noted, patients in the intra-articular group experienced better pain relief at 1 month. At 3 months, however, no difference was noted. In the most recent study, Ackerman and Ahmad randomized 46 patients with axial LBP and a positive single-photon emission computed tomography (SPECT) scan to receive either intra-articular injections or MBB using 0.7 mL of LA and steroid. Twelve weeks after treatment, 61% of the intra-articular injection group experienced a positive outcome, which compared favorably with 26% in the MBB group.[199]

It is difficult to draw conclusions based on these comparative studies because of the multitude of design flaws, with the most prominent ones being the lack of a definitive diagnosis in the study populations and the fact that only one study[195] evaluated immediate postprocedure pain relief. Studies investigating the prevalence and false-positive rates in chronic LBP patients (see Table 61.2) found comparable diagnostic value for MBB and intra-articular injection. Only one of three placebo-controlled studies evaluating the outcome of lumbar RF denervation after intra-articular injections to "confirm" the presence of facetogenic pain demonstrated positive outcomes,[200-202] and the only study that screened patients with lumbar MBB showed a positive outcome.[203] In a prospective, randomized study comparing lumbar facet cryodenervation success rates between patients who underwent medial branch and pericapsular lumbar facet screening blocks, Birkenmaier and associates[204] found superior outcomes up to 6 months after the procedure in the MBB group. However, the excessive volumes used during both diagnostic procedures, the absence of controlled blocks, and the lack of proven validity for pericapsular injections all detract from the authors' conclusions.

Intra-articular injections can be technically more challenging, especially in the steep, frontally oriented thoracic facet joints. In addition, MBB involves anesthetization of the nerves to be lesioned and hence may serve as a "dry run" before definitive treatment. Given the lack of evidence for intra-articular injections as a superior diagnostic tool and the technical ease of performing MBB, it seems logical to use MBB as a prognostic tool for subsequent denervation (Figs. 61.11 and 61.12).

FALSE-POSITIVE BLOCKS

Numerous studies have found a high false-positive rate for diagnostic facet blocks that appears to be unaffected by the type of block used (i.e., intra-articular or MBB). Rates have ranged from 25% to 40% in the lumbar spine,[136,139,140,143] 58% in the thoracic spine,[150] and 27% to 63% in the cervical spine.[41,143,151,181,205,206] Lord and colleagues conducted a randomized, double-blind study in which 50 patients with chronic neck pain following an MVA were evaluated with serial cervical MBBs using normal saline, lidocaine, and bupivacaine in random order.[206] The authors found that the use of serial blocks with lidocaine and bupivacaine had a high degree of specificity (88%) but only marginal sensitivity (54%). Although high specificity will result in a low false-positive rate, the low sensitivity predisposes patients to false-negative diagnoses.

Reasons for false-positive facet blocks are multifactorial and include a placebo response (18% to 32%) to diagnostic interventions, use of sedation, liberal use of superficial LA, and spread of injectate to other pain-generating structures.[207] Although some investigators have disputed this assertion,[208-210] it is our belief that not only opioids but also sedatives such as midazolam can lead to false-positive blocks by interfering with interpretation of the analgesic response (i.e., preventing patients from engaging in normal activities) and by virtue of their muscle relaxant properties.[211] If sedation is used, stricter standards for a positive block should be applied. Manchikanti and coworkers[210] showed that administration of midazolam or fentanyl for the diagnosis of cervical facet joint pain using a double-block paradigm could be a confounding factor when 50% or greater pain relief is used as the cutoff for a positive response. However, when 80% or greater pain relief was used as the threshold for a positive response, the effect of sedation on validity was low. A large multicenter study by Cohen and colleagues found no difference in outcomes of lumbar facet denervation between patients who obtained 50% or greater and those who obtained 80% or greater pain relief after a single diagnostic MBB.[212] In a recent survey of 500 patients scheduled for facet blocks or epidurals at an outpatient spine center, Cucuzzella and associates found that only 17% requested sedation.[213]

Even in patients with symptomatology consistent with unambiguous pathology, diagnostic blocks may lack specificity. North and colleagues conducted a prospective study of 33 patients with L5 or S1 radiculopathy and radiologic evidence of ongoing nerve root compression.[214] All patients underwent a battery of LA blocks that included selective nerve root block, sciatic nerve block, MBB, and subcutaneous control injections. The authors found that approximately 90% of patients obtained almost complete pain relief following selective nerve root block, 70% experienced almost complete relief after sciatic block, and a majority obtained at least 50% pain relief after MBB. In contrast, the median degree of pain relief after subcutaneous injection was around 30%. The authors concluded that uncontrolled LA blocks lack specificity in the diagnostic evaluation of referred pain syndromes.

Dreyfuss and associates used postprocedural CT scans following 120 fluoroscopically guided lumbar MBBs to assess specificity and spread of contrast material.[28] Two target points were chosen, one at the superomedial border of the transverse process and a second lower site midway between the upper border of the transverse process and the mamilloaccessory ligament. In 16% of injections, contrast material was noted to spread into the intervertebral foramen or epidural space, more commonly occurring at the cephalad lumbar levels. When the lower target point was used, spread into the adjacent neural structures occurred only when the needle was inadvertently placed too high. In all cases, distal spread into the cleavage plane between the multifidus and longissimus muscles was noted. The injectate volume of 0.5 mL bathed the target in every case. The authors concluded that lower volumes may be adequate for MBB and that using a more caudad target point may increase the specificity of lumbar MBB.

Following up on the Dreyfuss study, Cohen and colleagues[215] sought to determine whether spread into the epidural space or intervertebral foramina could account for false-positive MBBs by examining the relationship between clinical signs of radiculopathy, diskographic findings, and RF outcomes in 78 patients with positive MBBs who eventually failed RF denervation. The authors found a negative correlation between discogenic pain and failed RF denervation and no association between radicular pain and RF treatment outcomes. In contrast, a trend was noted in which patients with failed back surgery syndrome experienced worse outcomes after facet denervation. The authors concluded that myofascial pain might be a significant cause of false-positive MBBs.

In a study of 24 patients undergoing cervical MBB, Cohen and associates investigated the spread of 0.5 versus 0.25 mL of LA mixed with contrast agent.[197] MBBs were performed in either the prone (posterior) or lateral position. CT scans were conducted following the MBBs to assess for aberrant spread. Blocks performed in the 0.25-mL group resulted in aberrant spread to untargeted adjacent levels and into the intervertebral foramina less than half as often as those done with 0.5 mL (16% vs. 38%). There were a total of

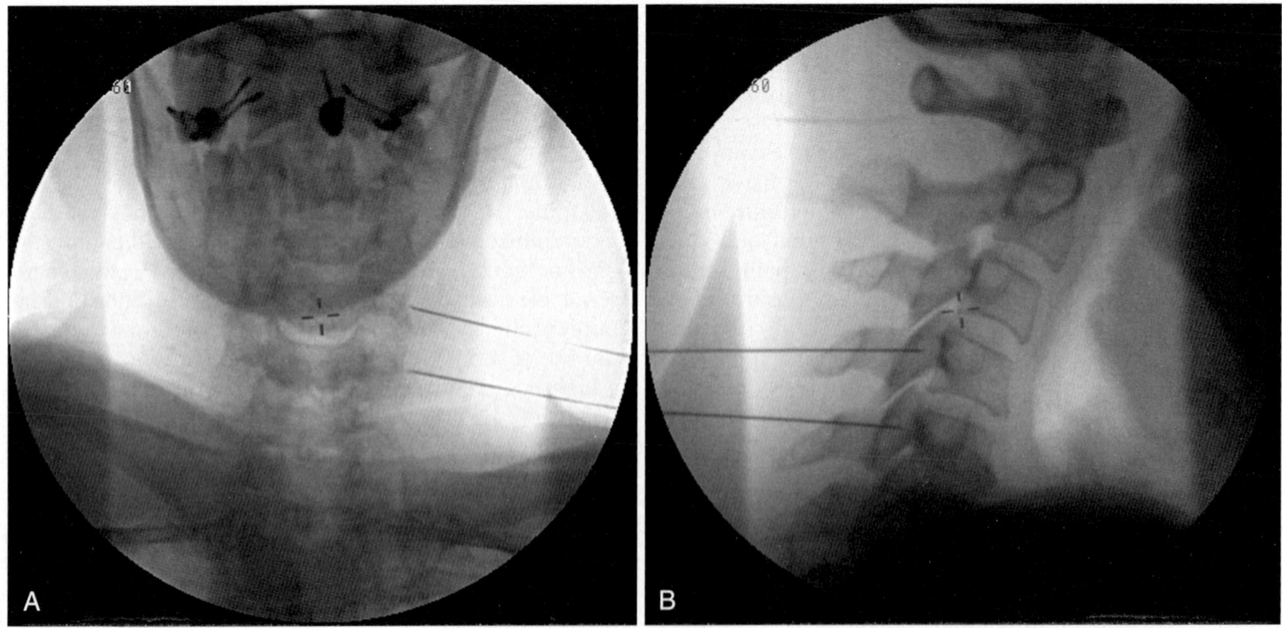

Figure 61.12 Anteroposterior (**A**) and lateral (**B**) fluoroscopic images demonstrating right-sided C4 and C5 medial branch blocks.

six "missed" medial branches in the 86 blocks performed, which were evenly distributed between the groups. These findings indicate that lower volumes may enhance specificity without negatively affecting sensitivity.

The evidence that inadvertent treatment of myofascial pain may be a significant cause of false-positive MBBs is circumstantial but multifaceted. In a large, multicenter epidemiologic study involving more than 2000 patients, Long and coworkers found myofascial pain to be the second most common cause of chronic LBP after herniated disks.[131] Controlled studies conducted in chronic LBP patients have shown both muscle relaxants and low-volume botulinum toxin injections to be efficacious, as well as electromyographic evidence of increased paraspinal muscle activity when compared with matched controls.[216-219] Finally, Ackerman and colleagues tested the hypothesis of whether myofascial pain could account for the high rate of false-positive facet blocks in a double-blind study conducted in 75 men with chronic LBP.[220] Subjects received either intra-articular facet injections or MBB via two techniques: one in which LA was used to provide superficial anesthesia down to the target point and a second in which saline was injected as the needle was advanced. The authors found that the incidence of postprocedural pain relief was significantly higher in patients who had LA injected into their musculature than in those who received saline injected superficially, thus suggesting a higher false-positive rate. Injection of LA into the skin and soft tissues may also reduce LBP by means other than the inadvertent treatment of myofascial pain. In studies by Woolf and McMahon[221] and Woolf and Wiesenfeld-Hallin,[222] the authors found that the superficial injection of even small amounts of lidocaine reduced nociceptive behavior in animal models of neuropathic pain, a finding attributed to systemic absorption of the sodium channel blocker (Box 61.1).[221,222]

In an effort to reduce the amount of superficial anesthetic used for MBB, Stojanovic and colleagues introduced a single-needle technique whereby multiple medial branches are blocked via a single skin entry point.[223] In a prospective crossover study comparing the single-needle and conventional multiple-needle techniques, the authors found that the single-needle technique required significantly less superficial LA, resulted in less procedure-related pain, and was quicker to perform than the multiple-needle approach (Fig. 61.13).[224] With regard to final needle position, spread of contrast material, and postprocedural pain relief, no differences were noted between the two techniques.

Box 61.1 Interventions That May Reduce the Incidence of False-Positive Lumbar Facet Blocks

1. Perform placebo-controlled blocks or, if not possible, comparative local anesthetic blocks.
2. Aim for a lower target point on the transverse process.
3. Reduce the injectate volume to 0.5 mL or less.
4. Be judicious with the use of superficial anesthesia.
5. Consider a single-needle approach.
6. Consider using guidance with computed tomography when doing intra-articular injections in patients with severe spondylosis.
7. Avoid the use of sedation or intravenous opioids.

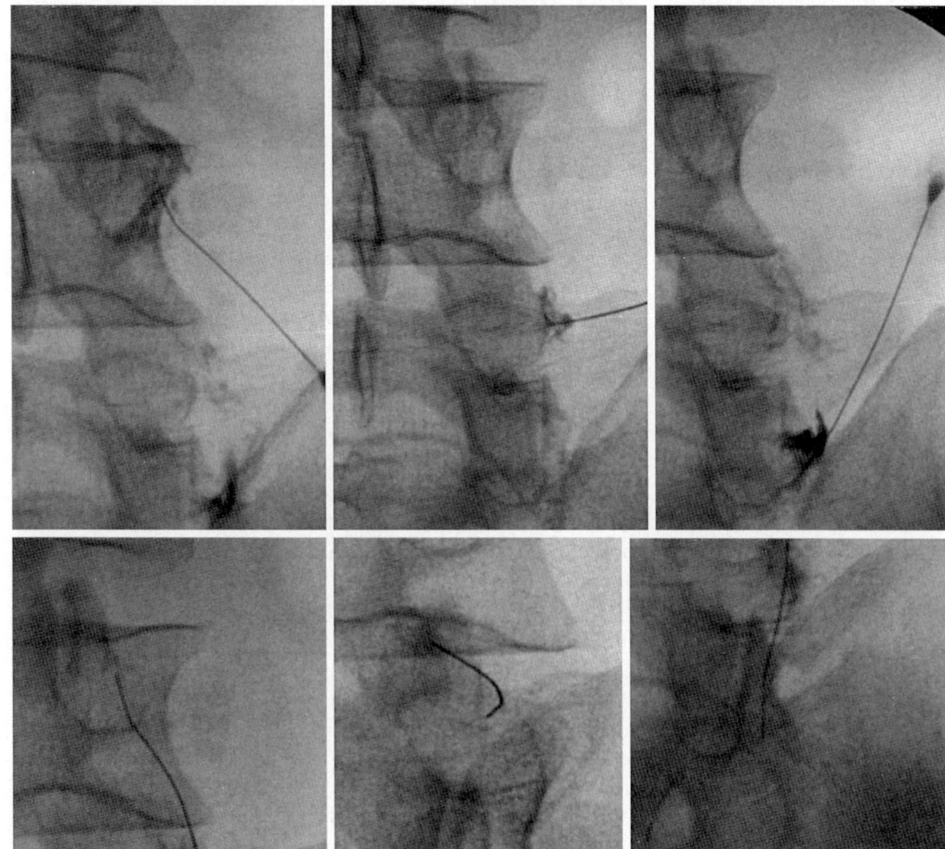

Figure 61.13 Anteroposterior fluoroscopic images showing spread of contrast material for L3 (left), L4 (middle), and L5 (right) medial branch blocks using the single-needle technique. The bottom figures show needle placement in an oblique fluoroscopic view for the same blocks.

FALSE-NEGATIVE BLOCKS

Similar to false-positive blocks, false-negative blocks may result from a multitude of factors. One study estimated the incidence of false-negative lumbar MBBs to be approximately 11%.[170] However, this study attempted to elicit pain by facet capsular distention following LA and control blocks in asymptomatic volunteers and hence would be unlikely to have significant clinical implications in patients. It suggests that some individuals may contain aberrant innervation from nerves other than the medial branches.

Venous uptake of LA was reported to occur in 8% of lumbar facet blocks in one study[28] and 33% in another.[170] In one of the studies, even after the needle was repositioned once venous uptake was detected, injection of LA failed to prevent pain from capsular distention in 50% of subjects.[170] Therefore, some experts suggest that if aspiration is positive during diagnostic MBB, it is better to abort the procedure and repeat it later rather than risk a false-negative result.[170] In a study of more than 1400 lumbar MBBs in 456 patients, Lee and coworkers found a 6.1% rate of uptake of LA, which was detected in 34% of the patients by aspiration and in 59% by spot fluoroscopy.[198] Consequently, the authors recommended the use of continuous fluoroscopy during MBBs. One of the biggest causes of false-negative blocks is the failure of patients to properly distinguish procedure-related pain from their index pain, which underscores the need for proper education regarding the use of pain diaries.

HOW MANY BLOCKS SHOULD BE DONE BEFORE RADIOFREQUENCY DENERVATION?

Many experts and organizations advocate performing multiple diagnostic blocks to reduce the high false-positive rate.[141,152,225,226] There are two problems with this argument. First, reducing the false-positive rate is important when trying to establish "efficacy" but may be counterproductive when one's objective is "effectiveness," which seeks to maximize outcomes under real-life conditions. To illustrate this point, many controlled studies evaluating RF denervation have screened hundreds of patients to enroll several dozen subjects. Although the results of the enrolled patients who received treatment are cited time and again in systematic reviews and book chapters, the ultimate outcomes of the hundreds of patients excluded from participation remain unknown. Second, many of these "false-positive" blocks may actually include "false-negatives," which can result from failure to discount procedure-related pain and discordant responses to either saline or LA, findings previously reported in clinical trials.[169,227-229] Even though performing multiple blocks will invariably reduce the false-positive rate, it will inexorably increase the false-negative rate, which translates to a safe and effective treatment being withheld from some individuals who will benefit. Undoubtedly, many of these patients eventually undergo surgery. Eliminating placebo responders may be not only impossible but also impractical since the benefits experienced by a "sham" intervention (e.g., pain relief, functional improvement) are indistinguishable from those experienced with a "true" intervention.[230]

In an attempt to determine the ideal number of diagnostic blocks under "real-life" circumstances, Cohen and colleagues performed a randomized, comparative cost-effectiveness study in which 151 patients were allocated in an equal ratio to receive lumbar facet RF denervation without MBB, after a positive response to one MBB done with bupivacaine, or only after a concordant response to comparative blocks done in random order with lidocaine and bupivacaine.[231] Predictably, a higher RF success rate was found in the double-block group, which is consistent with using this treatment paradigm in clinical trials that seek to determine efficacy. However, the overall number of patients who experienced a successful outcome at 3 months was significantly higher in the zero-block group (n = 17) than in the single- (n = 8) and double-block (n = 11) groups. Moreover, the cost per effective treatment in the zero-block group was less than half that in the other two groups. The results of this study are bolstered by theoretical computations that have determined "double blocks" not to be cost-effective at current reimbursement rates.[232] Similar comparative effectiveness studies have not been done for cervical facet joint pain; however, because the relative reimbursement rates between diagnostic blocks and RF denervation are comparable in the neck and because facetogenic pain accounts for a higher proportion of chronic neck pain than chronic LBP, it is likely that these results can be reliably extrapolated to cervical facet joint RF denervation. Currently, we believe that there is little basis for using double blocks, and the decision regarding whether to perform a single block or proceed straight to RF denervation should be made on a case-by-case basis (i.e., the risks of performing a diagnostic block might outweigh the benefits in a patient taking warfarin).

TREATMENT

CONSERVATIVE TREATMENT AND PHARMACOTHERAPY

A multimodal approach to the treatment of facetogenic pain is essential. Although many patients seen in interventional pain medicine clinics will receive a procedural approach to therapy, there is value in conservative therapy, medical management, and, when indicated, psychotherapy. Pharmacotherapy and noninterventional treatments of spinal pain have been investigated, but no study has evaluated these alternatives specifically in patients with facet pain. Tailored exercise programs and yoga have been shown to reduce pain and prevent relapses in patients with chronic LBP.[233-236] Osteopathic manipulation has produced mixed results, with two studies indicating moderate relief of LBP[237,238] and another showing no difference between true and sham manipulations.[239] For subacute neck and back pain, a randomized study comparing conservative care (i.e., physical and pharmaceutical therapy) alone with conservative care and osteopathic manipulation three to four times per week found improved outcomes in the combined therapy group at 2 months but not at 6 months after the intervention.[240] In addition, some randomized trials have found significant benefit with acupuncture and acupressure in patients with chronic LBP and neck pain.[241-245] Similar to manipulation, however, one of the largest and most methodologically sound studies found no difference between true and sham acupuncture.[246]

Nonsteroidal anti-inflammatory drugs and acetaminophen are widely considered first-line drugs for the treatment of LBP, with nonsteroidal anti-inflammatory drugs being slightly more efficacious than acetaminophen, which is devoid of anti-inflammatory properties.[247-249] A comprehensive review of published clinical trials evaluating pharmacotherapy for LBP by Schnitzer and colleagues[250] found evidence for the use of antidepressants for chronic LBP and muscle relaxants for acute LBP. However, more recent reviews have failed to find a significant benefit with antidepressants.[251] In addition to LBP, skeletal muscle relaxants have also shown efficacy in controlled trials for neck pain.[252] There is little doubt that untreated psychopathology can adversely affect back and neck pain treatment outcomes.[253,254] In a study by Polatin and coworkers[255] conducted in 200 chronic LBP patients, the authors found that 77% met the lifetime criteria and 59% demonstrated current symptoms for at least one psychiatric diagnosis, with the most common being depression, substance abuse, and anxiety disorders.[253] Reviews demonstrate that neck and back pain are associated with depression and anxiety; however, this explains only a portion of the variance and cannot be considered the primary cause of the patient's symptoms.[256] Lilius and associates[257] found a strong correlation between a negative response to intra-articular and periarticular LA and steroid injections and inappropriate signs and symptoms. Wasan and colleagues[258] found that depression and anxiety symptoms were associated with a negative response to intra-articular lumbar facet steroid injections. Some authors have postulated that depression and anxiety may be part of a broader phenotype of centralized pain, which may further explain the variance in outcomes described.[259]

Optimal management of facet joint pain should encompass both noninterventional and interventional treatment, although clinicians are encouraged to exercise caution when extrapolating the results of studies conducted in patients with nonspecific back and neck pain to those with clear-cut z-joint pathology.

INTRA-ARTICULAR STEROID INJECTIONS

There is some controversy regarding the use of intra-articular LA and steroid injections for the diagnosis and treatment of facet pain. In uncontrolled studies, success rates in individuals undergoing intra-articular steroid injections range from 18% to 63%, with most of these studies being conducted in patients who did not undergo diagnostic screening blocks.[128,130,131,133,134,164,182] Other studies have reported intermediate-term pain relief after intra-articular LA alone[163] and with hyaluronic acid.[260]

The results of controlled trials have been mixed at best (Table 61.6).[165,169,195,260-265] In a large study, Lilius and colleagues[261] found no significant differences in the outcomes of 109 patients who received large-volume (8 mm) LA and steroid injected into two joints, the same mixture administered around the joints, or physiologic saline. In another study comparing intra-articular steroid and saline in 97 patients with chronic LBP, Carette and coworkers found a statistically significant benefit only at the 6-month mark in the steroid group.[262] Although this was a large and methodologically sound study whereby patients were prescreened with diagnostic intra-articular LA blocks, the control group received intra-articular normal saline. Normal saline has been shown on multiple occasions to provide better pain relief than a true placebo for a variety of invasive procedures.[266-268] Barnsley and associates randomized 41 patients with chronic neck pain following an MVA to receive 1 mL of either intra-articular bupivacaine or betamethasone under double-blind conditions.[263] The median time to return of 50% of the patient's preinjection pain was 3 days in the steroid group and 3.5 days in the LA group, with less than half the patients reporting pain relief lasting longer than 1 week. All patients in this study were prescreened for cervical z-joint pain via comparative MBB. Wasan and colleagues found that psychopathology was associated with a negative response to intra-articular steroid lumbar facet injections in the 86 patients assessed.[258] Even though responses were better in patients in the low- and moderate-psychopathology groups, the changes in average daily pain were only 23% and 6.1% 1 month after the block, respectively, and there were no improvements in pain interference, anxiety, or depression in any of the groups.

In six recent review articles, the authors have been evenly split on the efficacy of intra-articular steroids.[136,269-273] Given basic science studies demonstrating inflammatory mediators around degenerated facet joints,[18,19] we believe that intra-articular steroid injections may provide intermediate-term relief to a small subset of patients with an actively inflamed z-joint. Evidence to support this assertion is bolstered by several recent prospective and observational studies that evaluated low- to intermediate-volume (1 to 3 mL) LA and steroid intra-articular lumbar facet joint injections performed in more than 160 patients with axial LBP.[188,264,274] In these studies, patients with positive SPECT findings experienced dramatically better pain relief (>75% success rate) than did those with negative or no SPECT findings (<40% success rate) up to 3 months after injection. In the two studies that monitored patients for 6 months after injection, the beneficial effect wore off after the 3-month evaluation.[188,264] These findings are supported by Ackerman and Ahmad, who randomized 46 patients with a positive scan and paraspinal tenderness to receive intra-articular injections or MBB with LA and steroids.[199] Three months after the injection, the patients in the intra-articular injection group experienced better pain relief than did those who received MBB. Radionuclide bone scintigraphy is capable of depicting synovial changes caused by inflammation, degenerative changes associated with bone remodeling, and increased metabolic function. In addition to radiologic evidence of joint inflammation and degeneration, intra-articular steroid injections may be more effective in patients who obtain definitive pain relief following a diagnostic screening block and when LA is added to the injectate.

THERAPEUTIC MEDIAL BRANCH BLOCKS

In a series of prospective, randomized evaluations of repeated therapeutic MBB with LA, LA plus Sarapin, LA plus steroid, and LA plus steroid and Sarapin, Manchikanti and coauthors reported significant relief of lumbar,[228,275] thoracic,[229,276] and cervical facet pain[227,277] in more than 85% of individuals in all groups for up to 2 years. Patients were screened with comparative LA blocks, but the studies lacked a placebo or sham group. No differences were

Table 61.6 Prospective Clinical Trials Evaluating Intra-articular Steroid Injections for Lumbar and Cervical Facet Joint Pain

Authors, Year, Methodology Score	Patients and Interventions	Results	Comments
Lynch and Taylor,[165] 1986; MQ score = 0	50 pts with underwent attempted intra-articular steroid injections at the 2 most caudal lumbar z-joints. Failed "extra-articular" injections were designated as the "control" group.	Relief of pain at 2 wk and 6 mo was better in pts who had 2 intra-articular injections than in the other groups. Pts who had 1 intra-articular injection had better relief than did those who had no successful injections.	Flaws include lack of randomization, poor outcome assessment, failure to identify pts based on diagnostic injections, and failure to blind the examining physician.
Lilius et al.,[261] 1989; MQ score = 1	109 pts with unilateral chronic LBP rec'd 8 mL of LA and steroid injected into 2 lumbar z-joints (n = 28) or around 2 joints (n = 39) or rec'd 8 mL of NS into 2 joints (n = 42).	All 3 groups demonstrated significant improvement in pain scores (at 3 mo), disability scores, clinical examination findings, and return to work at 6 wk after injection. No differences were noted on any variable between groups.	Lumbar z-joint pain was not diagnosed before injection. The large volumes used rendered injections nonspecific. Large standards of deviation were found for the variables measured. Other flaws include suboptimal outcomes measures and lack of a blinded observer. Pain scores measured at 3 mo by questionnaire.
Nash,[195] 1990; MQ score = 2	67 pts with chronic LBP were randomized by pairs to receive either 1.5 mL of intra-articular LA and steroid or MBB with 2 mL of LA.	At 1-mo follow-up, 12 pairs reported MBB to be more beneficial, 11 reported intra-articular injection to be better, and 3 reported no difference.	11 pts lost to follow-up. Flaws include not using lumbar z-joint blocks for diagnosis, lack of a blinded observer, poor outcome measures, and no true control group.
Carette et al.,[262] 1991; MQ score = 5	97 pts with chronic LBP who reported immediate relief after LA facet injections were injected with 2 mL of steroid and saline (n = 49) or saline (n = 48) into the L4-5 and L5-S1 lumbar z-joints.	42% of pts who received steroid and 33% who rec'd placebo reported marked improvement for up to 3 mo (not significant). At 6 mo the steroid group reported less pain and disability. Only 22% of pts in the steroid group and 10% in the placebo group had sustained improvement through 6 mo.	Differences between groups at 6 mo reduced when co-interventions taken into account. Although this is the only study that identified study pts from diagnostic injections, these injections were not "controlled." NS is known to provide pain relief greater than that expected from placebo.
Marks et al.,[169] 1992; MQ score = 3	86 pts with chronic LBP were randomized to receive either 1.5 mL of steroid and LA MBB or intra-articular injections (2 mL at the lowest level).	Pts who rec'd facet joint injections had better pain relief than did those who underwent MBB at all follow-ups, but this was significant only at the 1-mo review.	Flaws include no true control group, failure to identify pts based on diagnostic injections, no monitoring of co-interventions, lack of a blinded observer, and poor outcomes assessments.
Barnsley et al.,[263] 1994; MQ score = 5	41 pts with chronic neck pain following MVA were randomized to injection of either 1 mL of 0.5% bupivacaine or 5.7 mg of betamethasone into painful cervical z-joints diagnosed by comparative LA MBB.	Less than half the pts reported relief for more than 1 wk, and fewer than 1 in 5 reported relief for more than 1 mo, irrespective of the treatment group. Median time to return of 50% of the pre-procedure pain was 3 days in the steroid group and 3.5 days in the LA group (not significant).	All pts with neck pain following whiplash injury. May be different from chronic neck pain of other causes. Some pts with long-lasting benefit in both groups.
Fuchs et al.,[260] 2005; MQ score = 1	60 pts with chronic LBP were randomized to either 1 mL of HA or steroid into the 3 lowest facet joints at weekly intervals for 6 wk.	Pts who rec'd HA injections experienced a 40% decrease in pain scores vs. a 56% reduction in those who rec'd steroid (not significant). Greatest pain reduction observed 3 mo after treatment in the HA group and 1 wk after treatment in the steroid group.	Inclusion criteria included at least moderate facet degeneration on radiologic imaging. Flaws include lack of a control group, failure to identify pts based on diagnostic injections, no monitoring of co-interventions, and multiple injections.
Pneumaticos et al.,[264] 2006; MQ score = 3	47 pts with chronic LBP and radiologic evidence of lumbar z-joint abnormalities were randomized in a 2:1 ratio to undergo intra-articular LA and steroid injections (3 mL) based on SPECT scans or physical examination.	1 mo after injection, 87% of pts with (+) SPECT had significant pain improvement vs. 12.5% of pts with (–) SPECT and 31% of pts who underwent injections based on physical examination.	Differences remained significant at 3 mo but not 6 mo after injection. Pain scores obtained by mailed questionnaire. No functional assessment done. Use of SPECT was cost-effective.

The methodologic quality (MQ) score was based on the 5-point Jadad scale.[265] A score of 3 or higher indicates high methodologic quality.
HA, hyaluronic acid; LA, local anesthesia; LBP, low back pain; MBB, medial branch block; MVA, motor vehicle accident; NS, normal saline; pts, patients; rec'd, received; SPECT, single-photon emission computed tomography; z-joint, zygapophyseal (facet) joint.

found with the addition of either steroid or Sarapin to the LA. Even though some patients may derive long-term benefit from diagnostic MBB, either from a placebo response, from "breaking the cycle of pain," or in rare instances from the anti-inflammatory effects of steroids on a medial branch trapped beneath the mamilloaccessory ligament, most studies have failed to corroborate these findings.[169,195,278] The concept that blocking the medial branch with or without steroid would lead to sustained improvement in pain is analogous to the idea that serial blockade of the femoral nerve can successfully treat painful knee OA. Despite multiple publications reporting effectiveness by the same group of investigators, there is little supporting evidence for a prolonged benefit from MBB in most patients. Nevertheless, there is probably a small subset of patients who will experience sustained benefit following LA MBB.

PULSED RADIOFREQUENCY OF THE MEDIAL BRANCH

Pulsed radiofrequency (pRF) is a nonablative technique that has been used for the treatment of several chronic pain conditions. The conceptual appeal of pRF is that because it acts via the creation of an electrical field and enhancement of descending modulatory systems, it results in minimal nerve damage. Consequently, unlike conventional RF, which severs nerves that subsequently develop into neuromas, it is frequently used as a treatment of neuropathic pain, in which nerve damage is the underlying cause of the pain. The condition for which pRF is currently used most is chronic, refractory radiculopathy, and the dorsal root ganglion (DRG) is the target.[279-281] Although pRF of the DRG may be efficacious, its efficacy for nociceptive pain conditions (e.g., facet joint pain) and its application to peripheral nerves, such as the medial branch, have not been demonstrated. In a retrospective study involving 118 patients who responded to diagnostic MBB, only 68 derived benefit from pRF, which lasted on average less than 4 months.[282]

Two clinical trials compared conventional RF with pRF. Kroll and colleagues[283] randomized 50 patients who obtained greater than 50% relief after two MBBs to continuous RF or pRF. Almost 50% of the patients were lost to follow-up. Although no significant differences between groups were found at the 3-month follow-up, a comparison of within-group differences revealed greater improvements in pain and disability in conventional RF patients. This study was underpowered to detect between-group differences.

In the second study, Tekin and coworkers[278] randomized 60 patients with a positive response to a single MBB to either sham RF (LA only), pRF, or continuous RF. All groups, including the LA-only group, described improvements in pain and disability. However, the magnitude of improvement and the duration of benefit were significantly greater in the continuous RF group. In summary, the current state of evidence does not support the use of pRF of the medial branch for the treatment of facet pain.

RADIOFREQUENCY DENERVATION

The first description of percutaneous rhizotomy for the treatment of "intervertebral disk syndrome" was by Rees in 1971.[284] Notwithstanding his greater than 99% reported success rate, it remains a subject of controversy whether his technique actually achieved "facet rhizolysis" since the instrument that he used may not have been long enough to accomplish anything more than a myofasciotomy.[285] The technique of percutaneous RF lesioning is generally credited to Shealy, who was motivated by what he perceived to be an unacceptably high incidence of local hemorrhagic complications with the Rees technique.[286,287] Subsequently, it has been used to treat different forms of spinal pain, including whiplash,[154] sacroiliac joint pain,[147,288] discogenic pain,[289] and intractable sciatica.[290] Many uncontrolled trials have touted the benefits of RF denervation for facet pain.[290] For lumbar facet RF denervation, most studies report sustained relief in 50% to 80% of patients without previous back surgery,[155,291-297] whereas 35% to 50% of subjects with failed back surgery syndrome obtain prolonged relief.[155,298-300] In the only study comparing outcomes of cervical z-joint denervation in operated and nonoperated spines, Cohen and colleagues found no difference in success rates between patients with failed neck surgery syndrome and those who had never undergone surgery.[124]

Seven placebo-controlled studies have evaluated RF denervation for lumbar z-joint pain (Table 61.7; Fig. 61.14).[123,154,200-203,277,284,301,302] In the first study, King and Lagger randomized 60 patients with LBP and leg pain to receive empirical (without stimulation) RF denervation of the dorsal rami, an RF lesion made in the muscle, or a sham lesion after electrical stimulation.[285] At their 6-month follow-up, 27% of patients in the facet denervation group experienced satisfactory pain relief versus 53% in the myotomy group and 0% in the sham group. The main criticisms of this study are that no diagnostic blocks were performed to screen people for lumbar z-joint pain and electrode placement was suboptimal based on subsequent anatomic studies.[302] Almost 25 years later, Gallagher and coworkers randomized 41 patients to either sham or true denervation based on their response to diagnostic intra-articular blocks (equivocal or definitive response).[200] A statistically significant difference in outcomes was observed at 1 month only between sham and true RF denervation in patients who obtained a "definitive" response to diagnostic blocks. This difference persisted for the duration of the 6-month follow-up period. In one of the most methodologically sound controlled trials, van Kleef and colleagues found a 46% reduction in pain in the RF lesion group versus an 8% reduction in the placebo group.[203] At the 12-month follow-up, 7 of 15 patients in the treatment group continued to have a successful outcome versus only 2 of 16 in the sham group. In the only truly negative study, Leclaire and coworkers conducted a placebo-controlled study in 70 patients with a putative diagnosis of facet arthropathy.[201] At their 4-week follow-up, the only outcome variable that favored the treatment group was an improvement in the mean Roland-Morris disability score. At 12 weeks, no difference in pain levels or any measure of functional capacity was noted between groups. The key flaws in this study are that the authors used "significant pain relief lasting > 24 h" after an intra-articular injection of LA and steroid as their main inclusion criterion, they failed to place the electrodes parallel to the nerves, and they screened only 76 patients to enroll their 70 study participants. In addition to being ambiguous, the 24-hour threshold is inconsistent with the

Table 61.7 Outcomes of Randomized, Controlled Studies Assessing Medial Branch Radiofrequency Denervation for Lumbar and Cervical Facet Joint Pain

Study, Year	Number and Type of Patients	Follow-up Period and Methodologic Scores	Results	Comments
King and Lagger,[285] 1976	60 pts with chronic LBP, leg pain, and paraspinal tenderness were randomized to 3 groups. Group I underwent RF denervation of the primary posterior ramus, group II had RF performed with a 1.25-inch needle inserted within the area of maximum tenderness (assumed to be a myotomy), and group III rec'd stimulation but no coagulation (control).	6 mo MQ = 2 CR= 5	In group I, 27% had ≥50% relief at 6 mo vs. 53% in group II and 0% in group III.	Did not use diagnostic blocks before randomization. Probably included many pts with sciatica. In some pts, 1.25 in may be sufficient to reach the medial branch. Used a 120-sec lesion; 3 lesions were empirically made without electrical stimulation.
Gallagher et al.,[200] 1994	Subjects were 41 pts with chronic LBP who obtained "clear-cut or equivocal" relief from single intra-articular facet joint injections with LA and steroid. 18 pts with a good response and 6 pts with an equivocal response underwent RF denervation. 12 pts with a good response and 5 with an equivocal response underwent sham denervation.	6 mo MQ = 2 CR = 6	Significant differences in pain scores noted only between patients with a good response to LA blocks who underwent true RF denervation (n = 18) and those with a good response who underwent sham treatment (n = 12). Differences were noted 1 and 6 mo after procedures.	Did not define "good" or "equivocal" response to diagnostic injections. Anatomic landmarks not well described. Observer not blinded. Electrode not placed parallel to the nerve. In "Methods," stated that only LA used, but in abstract stated that LA and steroid were used. Used 90-sec lesions.
Lord et al.,[154] 1996	24 pts (12 per group) with neck pain lasting longer than 3 mo after MVA and failed conservative treatment. Included pts with a (+) response to placebo-controlled diagnostic blocks. Randomized to undergo true RF at 80°C for 90 sec or 37°C (placebo treatment) between C3 and C7 according to their response to diagnostic blocks.	3 mo (12 mo in pts with persistent relief) MQ = 5 CR = 8	Mean time to return of 50% of preoperative pain was 263 days in the RF group and 8 days in the placebo group (P = 0.04). At 27 wk, 7 pts in the RF group and 1 in the control group remained pain free.	Excluded pts with solely C2-3 facet pain. 5 pts in the RF group with numbness in the territory of the treated nerves.
van Kleef et al.,[203] 1999	Subjects were 31 pts with chronic LBP who obtained ≥50% pain relief after a single MBB (1 dropout). Compared true denervation with sham.	12 mo MQ = 5 CR = 8	After 3 mo, 9 of 15 pts in the lesion group vs. 4 of 16 in the sham group had ≥50% pain relief. At 1-yr f/u, 7 of 15 in the lesion group and 2 of 16 in the sham group had ≥50% relief.	Used 0.75 mL of injectate for diagnostic blocks. Electrode not placed perpendicular to the target nerve. Used multifidus rather than sensory stimulation to identify the medial branch. Used 60-sec lesions.
Sanders and Zuurmond,[301] 1999	Subjects were 34 pts with chronic LBP who obtained ≥50% relief after a single intra-articular injection of lidocaine. Half the pts rec'd medial branch RF denervation and half rec'd intra-articular denervation.	3 mo MQ = 1 CR = 6	Both groups improved at 3 mo, but the intra-articular denervation group improved more than the medial branch RF group.	Used 1 mL for diagnostic blocks. Medial branch lesions done at the inferolateral aspect of the facet capsule and the upper border of the transverse process. 3 intra-articular facet lesions done. Used 60-sec lesions.

Leclaire et al.,[201] 2001	Subjects were 70 pts with chronic LBP who obtained “significant” pain relief lasting >24 hr after a single intra-articular facet injection of lidocaine and steroid (4 dropouts). Compared true denervation with sham.	12 wk MQ = 4 CR = 8	At 4 wk there were modest improvements in Roland-Morris (P = 0.05) and VAS (P = NS) pain scores, but not the Oswestry score. No difference in any outcome measure at 12 wk.	Did not define “significant pain relief” with diagnostic injection. Inclusion criteria of >24-hr pain relief is inconsistent with the pharmacology of lidocaine. Performed 2 lesions, each for 90 sec. Anatomic landmarks not noted. Electrode not placed parallel to the nerve.
Stovner et al.,[123] 2004	12 pts with unilateral cervicogenic HA received comparative LA blocks and a greater occipital nerve block. Randomized to cervical facet RF or sham procedure.	24 mo MQ = 4 CR = 7	At 3 mo, 4 of 6 RF pts had a meaningful clinical response (≥30% improvement), as did 2 of the 6 in the sham group. 6 mo after the procedure, no differences noted between groups. Concluded that cervical facet denervation is not effective for cervicogenic HA.	The RF group had better response to diagnostic blocks. Able to recruit only 12 pts in 2.9 yr. Excluded pts with ongoing litigation.
Van Wijk et al.,[202] 2005	81 pts with chronic LBP who obtained ≥50% pain relief after 2-level intra-articular facet injection of LA (no dropouts). Compared true denervation with sham.	12 mo MQ = 5 CR = 7	Combined outcome measure (pain score, physical activity, and analgesic intake) showed no differences between groups at 3 mo. VAS pain score improved in both groups at 3 mo. Global perceived effect was greater in the treatment group than in the sham group at 3 mo.	Blinding ended at 3 mo in >70% of pts. Improvement in pain scores persisted throughout the 12-mo f/u. Used 60-sec lesions.
Tekin et al.,[278] 2007	60 chronic LBP pts with ≥50% relief from a single MBB at either L1-3 or L3-5 received either sham, pulsed RF, or RF denervation.	12 mo MQ =4 CR = 8	Continuous RF better than pulsed RF and sham for pain. No significant difference between sham and pulsed RF. Regarding improvement in disability, continuous RF and pulsed RF better than sham.	Used 0.3-mL diagnostic MBBs. Proper technique used for MBB and RF. Study not powered to detect between-group treatment differences.
Nath et al.,[302] 2008	40 pts with chronic LBP with >80% relief from 3 LA facet blocks.	6 mo MQ =4 CR = 6	RF group better than control group in all outcome measures, although benefits were modest.	40 of the 376 screened were randomized. Created 6 empirical lesions without stimulation.

The methodologic quality (MQ) score was based on the 5-point Jadad scale.[265] A score of 3 or greater indicates high methodologic quality. The clinical relevance (CR) score was based on patient selection parameters and description of the RF technique (0 to 9 scale) as described by Geurts and colleagues.[339]

f/u, follow-up; HA, headache; LA, local anesthetic; LBP, low back pain; MBB, medial branch block; MVA, motor vehicle accident; NS, not significant; pts, patients; rec’d, received; RF, radiofrequency; VAS, visual analog scale.

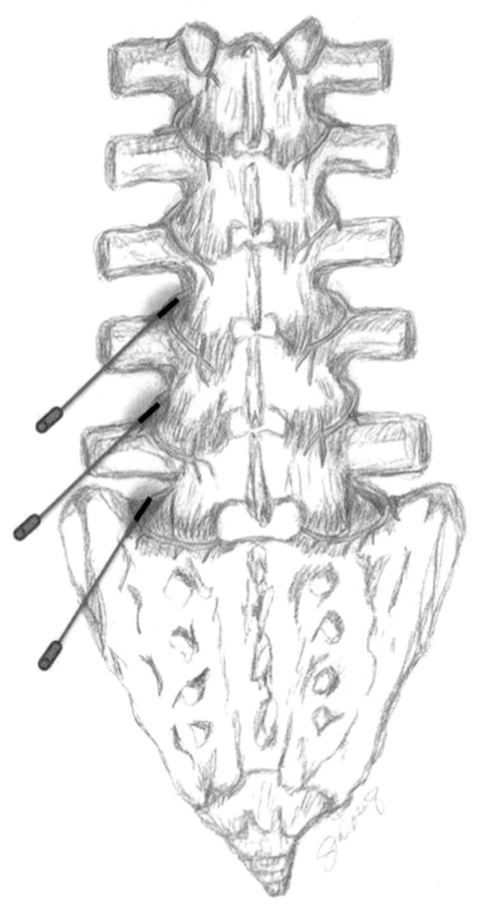

Figure 61.14 Lumbar medial branch radiofrequency denervation: posterior view of radiofrequency denervation of the medial branches of L3 and L4 and the dorsal primary ramus of L5. (Illustration courtesy of Julie HY Huang, MD, MBA.)

pharmacodynamics of lidocaine. In the largest controlled study evaluating RF denervation, van Wijk and associates[202] found that the only difference between the treatment and control groups at 3 months was that more RF patients reported a 50% or greater diminution in back pain than the sham patients did (62% vs. 39%). For the primary combined outcome measure, mean reduction in visual analog scale pain scores, change in analgesic intake, and functional assessments, no differences were noted between groups. As described earlier in the pRF section, Tekin and associates found that patients randomized to continuous RF reported greater pain relief and used less analgesics at 6 and 12 months after treatment than did those undergoing pRF or a sham procedure (LA only after placing an RF probe).[278] All groups had significant improvements in function as measured by the Oswestry Disability Index (ODI) without differences between the three groups. In the most recent controlled study, Nath and colleagues screened 376 patients with LBP by using MBBs consisting of 1 mL of 0.5% bupivacaine, with 115 excluded for a negative response to MBB.[302] The remaining 276 patients underwent comparative LA MBB, from which 221 were excluded for various reasons, including a negative response to MBB ($n = 45$), a prolonged analgesic response to MBB ($n = 105$), practical reasons, and refusal to participate. The remaining 40 patients were randomized to either sham or continuous RF with six empirical lesions. RF patients described higher self-reported improvement and significant improvements in back and leg pain, generalized pain, quality of life, and analgesic requirements when compared with the sham group.

A key flaw in many of these studies is the failure to select patients based on placebo-controlled or comparative LA blocks, which are now acknowledged to be inferior to placebo controls. Although double blocks are often impractical and will inevitably result in a lower overall success rate with higher total cost, elimination of "false-positive" responders is ideal for studies that seek to establish efficacy. In addition, electrode positioning was suboptimal in several studies, including the Leclaire and van Wijk trials.[201,202] One final point that should be considered when screening patients is that all negative[192,193] and equivocal[200] studies used intra-articular injection rather than MBB to screen patients.

In an uncontrolled study designed to determine efficacy under ideal conditions, Dreyfuss and coworkers[142] evaluated outcomes in 15 patients who underwent lumbar facet RF denervation. Their strict inclusion criteria and treatment parameters included 80% or greater relief with comparative MBB, elimination of patients with concomitant pain generators (e.g., discogenic pain), and the use of large-bore 16-gauge electrodes. They reported that 87% of 15 patients obtained at least 60% relief 12 months after RF denervation, with 60% of patients achieving at least 90% relief. Similar to the trial by Nath and colleagues,[302] a large number of patients ($N = 460$) were screened to create the final group of 15 patients undergoing intervention. Although this may demonstrate efficacy using rigid selection criteria, it may not represent what occurs in normal clinical practice.

Even though some may construe these findings as evidence that RF denervation is a fundamentally flawed treatment, a more plausible interpretation is that they indicate a strong need to optimize RF denervation techniques and better identify candidates likely to obtain positive outcomes. Recent studies that have used appropriate technique and needle position have clearly demonstrated sustained improvements in pain and function.[277] Several investigators have determined that placing the electrode parallel rather than perpendicular to the target nerve substantially increases the size of the lesion, thereby reducing the likelihood that the treatment will miss or only partially coagulate the target nerve.[303,304] After a literature review and cadaveric study, Lau and coauthors[305] concluded that the ideal electrode position is along the lateral neck of the superior articular process rather than at the groove between the angle of the superior articular and transverse processes, as was used in most studies.[201,202] Other investigators found the maximal lesion size to be reached within 60 seconds of lesion time,[35,304,306] independent of whether the system was temperature or voltage controlled.[307] Studies conducted in human myocardium determined that irrigation fluid has either no effect or a slightly beneficial effect on lesion size.[308] Consequently, the use of LA to prevent procedure-related pain or steroid to reduce the incidence of neuritis[309] should theoretically have no adverse effects on the efficacy of RF denervation. In an ex vivo chicken model, Provenzano and colleagues found that injection of fluid before RF denervation actually increased lesion size.[310] Ongoing studies by the same group are investigating the impact of the composition of various injectants on lesion size.

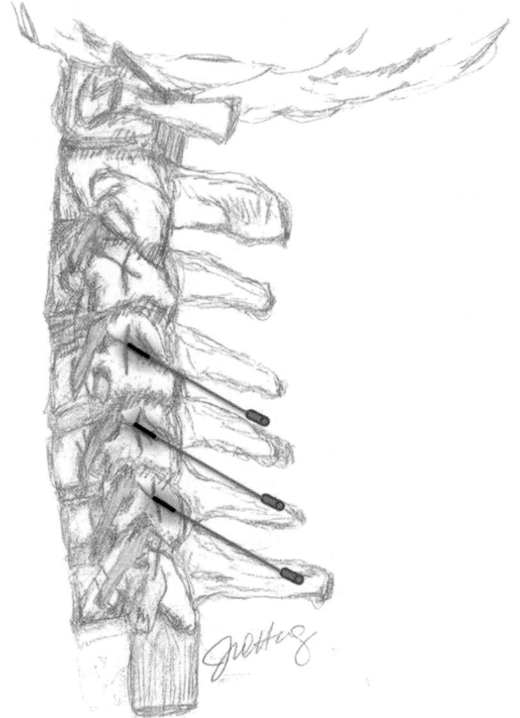

Figure 61.15 Cervical medial branch radiofrequency denervation: radiofrequency denervation of the C4, C5, and C6 medial branches. (Illustration Courtesy of Julie HY Huang, MD, MBA.)

Only two randomized, double-blind trials have evaluated percutaneous RF denervation for cervical facet pain (Fig. 61.15). Lord and colleagues randomized 24 patients with whiplash injury following an MVA and a positive response to diagnostic, placebo-controlled cervical MBB to receive either cervical medial branch denervation or a sham procedure.[154] Patients with pain stemming solely from the C2-3 z-joint were excluded. To establish a diagnosis of cervical facet pain, a series of three blocks were performed. The first block was done with either lidocaine or bupivacaine, the second block with either normal saline or the other LA, and the third block with the remaining agent. A block was deemed positive only if the patient had complete, concordant relief each time that an LA was used but no relief when normal saline was administered. Except for needle temperature, all therapeutic aspects of the procedures were the same in both groups. The mean time for return to 50% of baseline pain was 263 days in the RF group versus 8 days in the placebo group ($P = 0.04$). At 27 weeks, seven patients in the RF group and one patient in the control group remained pain free. Five of the patients in the RF group had numbness in the territory of the treated nerves, but none considered it troublesome.

In a more recent study, Stovner and coworkers randomized 12 patients in whom cervicogenic headache was diagnosed on the basis of clinical symptoms to receive either cervical facet RF denervation or a sham procedure.[123] Although the authors performed medial branch and greater occipital nerve blocks, the results were not used to select patients. The study was halted early secondary to failure to enroll subjects. At their 3-month follow-up, four of six patients in the RF denervation group obtained a meaningful clinical response versus two of six patients in the sham group. At 6 months no differences were noted between groups. Two years after the procedure, patients in the sham group felt that they had more significant improvement than did those in the RF group.

The results of sham denervation in this study are comparable to those in a previous uncontrolled study that evaluated RF for cervicogenic headache in which patients reported a 34% reduction in symptoms.[311] In an open-label prospective study comparing cervical z-joint RF results between litigant and nonlitigant patients with whiplash injuries, Sapir and Gorup found no significant differences between groups in 1-year outcomes.[312] Potential reasons for limited RF success rates for chronic neck pain and cervicogenic headache include technical difficulty denervating the frequently affected C2-3 facet joint, concomitant sources of head pain, and lack of specificity for diagnostic injections. In an observational study conducted in 56 patients with post-traumatic neck pain, provocative diskography and MBB were positive at the same level in 41% of patients.[313]

Although only two placebo-controlled trials assessed cervical facet denervation, several uncontrolled studies deserve mention. McDonald and colleagues prospectively studied patients in whom cervical facet pain was diagnosed based on controlled diagnostic blocks and found that 18 of 28 patients obtained significant pain relief lasting at least 90 days.[314] In patients with a positive response, the median duration of relief was 421.5 days. A later study by Barnsely measured the duration of pain relief following cervical facet denervation in patients with a positive response to controlled cervical MBB.[52] In the 45 patients studied, 36 (80%) experienced significant relief for a mean duration of 36 weeks. In both studies, patients who experienced a good initial response to denervation obtained comparable relief following repeated procedures.

In an uncontrolled prospective study involving 40 patient with refractory thoracic pain, Stolker and associates obtained good results following thoracic medial branch denervation.[315] Thoracic facet pain was diagnosed by clinical criteria and a positive response to diagnostic MBB. After 2 months, 47.5% of patients were pain free, 35% reported more than 50% pain relief, and 17.5% experienced minimal or no relief. At an average follow-up of 31 months (18 to 54 months), 44% of patients remained pain free, 39% continued to have more than 50% pain relief, and 17% had poor outcomes. Although these results are encouraging, the diagnosis of thoracic facet joint pain was made by using clinical predictors, which are inherently nonspecific, and by using single LA MBBs, which are known to carry a high false-positive rate.[143] In addition, the long-term relief seen in many of the patients is beyond that typically observed in the cervical and lumbar spine.

The use of sensory stimulation to corroborate proximity to the targeted medial branch is another flaw of many RF studies. Generally, a threshold of 0.5 V or less is deemed to be sufficient to effect a lesion that encompasses the target nerve. Although sensory stimulation may indicate close proximity to the target nerve at this voltage, it is our experience that many patients perceive concordant stimulation at 0.5 V or less, even when the electrode is purposefully placed in muscle, as during a sham procedure. In a prospective study involving 61 patients, Cohen and colleagues found no correlation between the mean sensory threshold and lumbar RF denervation outcomes.[316] Even though one might construe this to mean that sensory stimulation is not necessary, it should be emphasized that sensory thresholds in these patients were recorded only after repeated electrode adjustments. Consequently, a high sensory threshold (e.g., 0.8 V) might not afford the same likelihood of success when electrode manipulation could result in a lower threshold and consequently closer proximity to the target nerve.

An attractive alternative or addition to sensory stimulation in the lumbar and cervical spine regions is to attempt to elicit multifidus muscle contraction since the same medial branch that innervates the lumbar facet joint also supplies this large paraspinal muscle. Both studies in which the medial branch was identified by motor stimulation demonstrated positive outcomes.[142,203]

FACTORS ASSOCIATED WITH OUTCOME

In a large, multicenter outcome study, Cohen and coworkers attempted to identify factors associated with successful RF treatment in 192 patients who underwent denervation at three teaching hospitals after a single positive MBB.[155] Among the 15 variables analyzed for their association with treatment outcome, only paraspinal tenderness was found to predict successful treatment. Factors associated with failed treatment included increased pain with hyperextension and axial rotation (i.e., facet loading), duration of pain, and previous back surgery. The latter two variables have been associated with treatment failure not only for RF denervation but also for a host of other LBP interventions, as well as for epidural steroid injections and open surgery.[317-319] A study performed on the cervical spine by the same group of investigators found similar results. The only variable associated with a positive outcome was paraspinal tenderness. Factors associated with a negative outcome included opioid use, radiation to the occiput, and pain worsened by extension-rotation maneuvers.[124] When pain returns following RF denervation, which typically occurs between 6 months and 1 year, neurotomy can be repeated with similar efficacy, and small studies of RF denervation in the lumbar and cervical regions have demonstrated greater than 85% success rates.[320,321]

EFFICACY VERSUS EFFECTIVENESS OF RADIOFREQUENCY DENERVATION

The efficacy of RF of the medial branch has been established in well-selected patients as noted in the earlier section on RF denervation. The studies that have established efficacy, however, have screened large numbers of patients and excluded most people, usually because of strict criteria for multiple MBBs.[142,301] As described previously, Nath and colleagues enrolled approximately 10% of screened study candidates to demonstrate efficacy in the 40 patients randomized to RF or sham.[302] Excluding such a high percentage of patients through rigid MBB response criteria (including exclusion of patients for longer than anticipated pain relief) will probably lead to a high success rate, but it does not represent what happens in clinical practice. In retrospective studies, failure to derive benefit from facet interventions (defined as 50% improvement at 6 months) is estimated to occur in 45% and 39% to 47% of patients after cervical and lumbar medial branch interventions, respectively.[124,155] These studies were retrospective and intended to study predictors of failure, not the incidence of failure, so the failure rate data must be interpreted cautiously. Prospectively collected data on the effectiveness of facet interventions are incredibly limited, but such studies are ongoing.

Recently, there has been significant interest buoyed by the National Institutes of Health in comparative effectiveness research in which studies assess effectiveness, benefit, and harm relative to other treatment options.[322] Unlike efficacy studies, which generally assess outcomes in comparison to placebo under ideal circumstances (i.e., stringent inclusion and exclusion criteria), effectiveness studies aim to measure treatment outcomes under "real-life" circumstances—often in comparison to the current standard treatment. Given the challenges in appropriately diagnosing facet pain, studying the comparative effectiveness of different interventions can be extremely challenging. Despite these challenges, there are ongoing studies evaluating comparative effectiveness for the treatment of presumed facet pain.

SURGERY

Surgery is occasionally performed to treat facet arthropathy despite a lack of evidence supporting fusion for degenerative spinal disorders.[323,324] Not surprisingly, the results of studies evaluating the use of lumbar z-joint blocks to predict outcomes of lumbar arthrodesis are discouraging (Table 61.8). In the three studies that compared surgical outcomes between facet block responders and nonresponders, all three failed to show a difference between groups.[325-327] Bough and associates conducted a retrospective review of 127 facet joints surgically removed from 84 patients in an attempt to correlate histologic evidence of facet degeneration with a provocative response to preoperative facet arthrography.[156] Although the authors found the positive predictive value of concordant pain reproduction to be 85%, the negative predictive value was only 43%, which led them to conclude that provocative facet arthrography was of little value as a presurgical screening tool. In a prospective case series, Lovely and Rastogi found that 83% of 23 patients who responded to bracing and three successive facet blocks achieved 90% or greater pain relief after fusion surgery at the latest follow-up.[328] However, the large volumes used per block, the failure to exclude placebo responders, and the lack of any comparison group undermine the conclusions that can be drawn. One reason that patients with lumbar z-joint pain might respond to arthrodesis is that some surgeons, either purposefully or inadvertently, perform medial branch rhizotomies during pedicle screw placement. More recently, some surgeons have proposed total posterior arthroplasty (TOPS) to treat the pain associated with lumbar stenosis, which frequently includes facet changes. The TOPS system has articulating components that are meant to allow motion while providing stability in patients appropriate for one- or two-level decompression. In a prospective pilot study involving 29 patients, TOPS was found to improve disability (measured by the ODI) and pain.[329] No other data on this treatment are currently available, and this procedure is intended for spinal stenosis patients and is therefore probably not

Table 61.8 Studies Evaluating the Ability of Lumbar Facet Blocks to Predict Operative Results

Author, Year	Patients and Methods	Results	Comments
Esses et al.,[325] 1989	Prospective study evaluating the value of external fixation to predict fusion outcome in 35 pts. 14 pts underwent preoperative facet blocks.	Among the 9 pts who reported temporary relief from facet blocks, 5 experienced relief from external fixation. In the 5 pts who had no relief with facet blocks, 4 experienced relief after fixation.	Study not designed to assess the value of facet blocks in predicting the outcome of spinal fixation.
Bough et al.,[156] 1990	Retrospective study comparing the results of surgical pathology and preoperative provocative facet arthrography in 84 pts who underwent spinal fusion.	The specificity of pain provocation for facet disease was 75%, sensitivity 59%, positive predictive value 85%, and negative predictive value 43%. The authors concluded that symptom provocation during facet arthrography was of little value as a surgical screening tool.	Histopathology results reviewed for 127 lumbar z-joints. Clinical outcomes not discussed.
Jackson,[326] 1992	Retrospective review involving 36 pts who underwent posterolateral lumbar fusion after facet injections.	Both groups improved after fusion. The 26 pts who responded favorably to facet injections did no better clinically than the 10 pts who did not.	Mean follow-up, 6.1 yr. Response to injection not a consideration for fusion.
Esses and Moro,[327] 1993	Retrospective review involving the results of spinal fusion (*n* = 82) and nonoperative treatment (*n* = 44) in 126 pts who underwent facet blocks.	15% of pts had complete relief, 41% partial relief, and 44% no relief after lumbar z-joint blocks. Response to facet blocks was not predictive of surgical or nonsurgical success.	296 pts underwent facet blocks during the index period, but only 126 had follow-up (mean, 4.6 yr).
Lovely and Rastogi,[328] 1997	Prospective case series involving 91 pts who responded to bracing and underwent 197 facet blocks. 28 pts who obtained >70% pain relief on 3 separate occasions underwent spinal fusion.	Fusion was technically successful 77% of the time. 83% of pts reported ≥90% relief, and 13% reported partial relief.	Mean follow-up, 32 mo. No comparison group who either failed or did not receive preoperative lumbar z-joint blocks. Used 3- to 5-mL injectate per facet level.

pts, patients; z-joint, zygapophyseal (facet) joint.

generalizable to the larger facet arthropathy population. On a similar note, percutaneous fusion and open facet arthroplasty have recently been touted for treatment of facet joint pain, but there are no prospective outcome data for either procedure. In summary, there is no convincing evidence to support any surgical intervention for lumbar z-joint pain aside from that resulting from a traumatic dislocation.

COMPLICATIONS

Serious complications and side effects are extremely uncommon after facet interventions. The metabolic and endocrine sequelae of intrafacetal depot steroids have not been studied, but by extrapolating from epidural steroid injections one would expect suppression of the hypothalamic-pituitary-adrenal axis for up to 4 weeks, depending on the depot steroid used and impaired insulin sensitivity manifested as elevated glucose levels for less than a week.[330,331] Though rare, a host of infections have been associated with intra-articular injections, including septic arthritis, epidural abscess, and meningitis, but none have been reported following RF denervation.[332-334] Case reports of spinal anesthesia and post–dural puncture headache have also been published.[335,336]

A recently published study described the complications associated with more than 7400 patient encounters and more than 43,000 individual facet injections in the cervical, thoracic, and lumbar spine.[337] There were no serious complications. Intravascular injection was detected in 11.4% of the patients overall, with the highest prevalence in the cervical region (20%). Local oozing was noted in 76.3% of patients, also more frequently in the cervical region. In less than 1% of cases, patients experienced vasovagal reactions, bruising, and nerve root irritation. Catastrophic injuries have been reported, including a posterior circulation stroke during a C1-2 intra-articular steroid injection that was thought to be due to microvascular injury from accidental injection into the vertebral artery.[338]

Numbness, dysesthesias, or both have been reported after RF denervation but tend to be transient and self-limited.* Burns are rare with RF procedures and may result from electrical faults, breaks in the insulation of electrodes, and generator malfunction.[285,294,295] The most common complication following facet joint RF is neuritis, with a reported incidence of less than 5%.[347] In one study, administration of corticosteroid or pentoxifylline was found to reduce the incidence of postprocedural pain following RF denervation.[309] There is also a theoretical risk for thermal injury

*35,281,287,288,297-299,303-307,316-319,329-335,339-346

to the ventral rami if an electrode slips ventrally over the lumbar transverse process.

CONCLUSION

Pain originating from the facet joints has long been recognized as a potential source of back and neck pain. Anatomic studies suggest that with aging, the lumbar facet joints become weaker and their orientation changes from coronal to sagittal positioning, thereby predisposing individuals to injury from rotational stress. The three most caudal lumbar facet joints, L3-4, L4-5, and L5-S1, are exposed to the greatest strain during lateral bending and forward flexion and are thus more prone to repetitive strain, inflammation, joint hypertrophy, and osteophyte formation. In patients with chronic neck pain, the C2-3 and C5-6 facet joints are most commonly affected. OA of the facet joints is frequently found in association with DDD. The exact prevalence of facet disease is unclear but may be as high as 10% to 15% in patients with axial LBP, 49% to 60% in patients with chronic neck pain, and 42% to 48% in patients with axial midback pain.

No discrete historical and physical findings are pathognomonic for lumbar, thoracic, or cervical facet arthropathy. Paraspinous muscle tenderness appears to be the only physical examination finding associated with a positive response to RF of the medial branch; however, its specificity is not known. Referral patterns for pain arising from the facet joints at different levels and from different structures (e.g., facet joints and disks) overlap considerably. In addition to axial LBP, pathology arising from the lower facet joints is associated with referred pain to the buttock, thigh, groin, and sometimes the lower part of the leg, whereas pain referred from the upper lumbar facet joints extends into the flank, hip, groin, and lateral aspect of the thigh. Cervical facet disease tends to refer pain to the neck, head, shoulders, and midback region. Reports on the correlation between CT and MRI evidence of facet arthropathy and the response to diagnostic lumbar facet blocks are conflicting. Since the facet joint is innervated by medial branches arising from the posterior rami of the spinal nerve at the same level and a level above the joint, LA blocks of these nerves have been advocated for diagnostic and prognostic purposes. Intra-articular facet injections with LA have also been proposed as an alternative method for diagnosing facet joint pain, although they may be technically more challenging and the existing data suggest that MBB may be a better predictive tool for RF denervation outcomes. Similar to other blocks, the potential for false-positive and false-negative results needs to be considered and steps implemented to reduce their incidence.

In addition to providing short-term and occasionally intermediate-term pain relief, diagnostic blocks are considered predictive of the potential usefulness of subsequent neurolytic procedures such as RF denervation. In carefully selected patients who fail conservative treatments, such as physical and pharmacological therapies, intra-articular steroid injections and RF denervation are treatment options. Studies evaluating the long-term outcomes of RF denervation have demonstrated efficacy in well-selected patients; however, there are limited data on the effectiveness of this procedure in clinical practice. The results of surgical therapies for facet arthropathy are discouraging.

ACKNOWLEDGMENT

The opinions or assertions contained herein are the private views of the authors and are not to be construed as official or as reflecting the views of the Department of the Army or the Department of Defense. Dr. Brummett receives support from National Institutes of Health Grant RO1 AR060392, an American Society of Regional Anesthesia and Pain Medicine Chronic Pain Research Grant, the Michigan Genomics Initiative, and the Department of Anesthesiology at the University of Michigan. Dr. Cohen receives partial salary support from the Congressman John P. Murtha Neuroscience and Pain Institute, Johnstown, Pa, Pennsylvania, and the U.S. Army.

KEY POINTS

- The facet joints are a potential cause of axial neck and back pain.
- The most commonly affected lumbar facet joints are L3-4, L4-5, and L5-S1.
- The most commonly affected cervical facet joints are C2-3, C4-5, and C5-6.
- No pathognomonic historical, physical examination, or radiologic findings are sensitive or specific for facet pain.
- In patients who fail conservative therapies, minimally invasive facet interventions can be considered.
- Radiofrequency denervation of the medial branches in the affected area can provide pain relief for 6 to 12 months.
- Medial branch blocks are potentially prognostic of radiofrequency denervation outcomes.
- Intra-articular facet joint injections with local anesthetic and steroid may provide diagnostic value and short-term pain benefit in patients with acute inflammation.
- Surgery is not recommended for axial spine pain thought to be due to facet joint disease.

SUGGESTED READINGS

Ackerman WE, Munir MA, Zhang JM, et al. Are diagnostic lumbar facet injections influenced by pain of muscular origin? *Pain Pract.* 2004;4:286-291.

Cohen SP, Hurley RW, Christo PJ, et al. Clinical predictors of success and failure for lumbar facet radiofrequency denervation. *Clin J Pain.* 2007;23:45-52.

Cohen SP, Stojanovic MP, Crooks M, et al. Lumbar zygapophysial (facet) joint radiofrequency denervation success as a function of pain relief during diagnostic medial branch blocks: a multicenter analysis. *Spine J.* 2008;8:498-504.

Cohen SP, Strassels SA, Kurihara C, et al. Randomized study assessing the accuracy of cervical facet joint nerve (medial branch) blocks using different injectate volumes. *Anesthesiology.* 2010;112:144-152.

Dolan AL, Ryan PJ, Arden NK, et al. The value of SPECT scans in identifying back pain likely to benefit from facet joint injection. *Br J Rheumatol.* 1996;35:1269-1273.

Dreyfuss P, Schwarzer AC, Lau P, et al. Specificity of lumbar medial branch and L5 dorsal ramus blocks: a computed tomography study. *Spine.* 1997;22:895-902.

Fukui S, Ohseto K, Shiotani M, et al. Referred pain distribution of the cervical zygapophyseal joints and cervical dorsal rami. *Pain.* 1996;68:79-83.

Ianuzzi A, Little JS, Chiu JB, et al. Human lumbar facet joint capsule strains, I: during physiological motions. *Spine J.* 2004;4:141-152.

Igarashi A, Kikuchi S, Konno S. Correlation between inflammatory cytokines released from the lumbar facet joint tissue and symptoms in degenerative lumbar spinal disorders. *J Orthop Sci.* 2007;12:154-160.

Kaplan M, Dreyfuss P, Halbrook B, et al. The ability of lumbar medial branch blocks to anesthetize the zygapophysial joint: a physiologic challenge. *Spine.* 1998;23:1847-1852.

Lee CJ, Kim YC, Shin JH, et al. Intravascular injection in lumbar medial branch block: a prospective evaluation of 1433 injections. *Anesth Analg.* 2008;106:1274-1278.

Lee CK. Accelerated degeneration of the segment adjacent to a lumbar fusion. *Spine.* 1988;13:375-377.

Lord SM, Barnsley L, Bogduk N. The utility of comparative local anesthetic blocks versus placebo-controlled blocks for the diagnosis of cervical zygapophysial joint pain. *Clin J Pain.* 1995;11:208-213.

Lord SM, Barnsley L, Wallis BJ, et al. Percutaneous radio-frequency neurotomy for chronic cervical zygapophyseal-joint pain. *N Engl J Med.* 1996;335:1721-1726.

Nath S, Nath CA, Pettersson K. Percutaneous lumbar zygapophysial (facet) joint neurotomy using radiofrequency current, in the management of chronic low back pain: a randomized double-blind trial. *Spine.* 2008;33:1291-1297.

Provenzano DA, Lassila HC, Somers D. The effect of fluid injection on lesion size during radiofrequency treatment. *Reg Anesth Pain Med.* 2010;35:338-342.

Revel M, Poiraudeau S, Auleley GR, et al. Capacity of the clinical picture to characterize low back pain relieved by facet joint anesthesia: proposed criteria to identify patients with painful facet joints. *Spine.* 1998;23:1972-1976.

Tekin I, Mirzai H, Ok G, et al. A comparison of conventional and pulsed radiofrequency denervation in the treatment of chronic facet joint pain. *Clin J Pain.* 2007;23:524-529.

The references for this chapter can be found at www.expertconsult.com.

62 Radiofrequency Treatment

Maarten van Eerd | Maarten van Kleef | Jan Van Zundert

The use of electric current for pain management has a long history. As early as the second half of the 19th century, brain lesions were made in animals with the application of direct current, and empirical rules for quantifying lesion size based on current and time were developed.[1,2] One of the first uses in humans was for the management of trigeminal neuralgia in 1931, when a direct current was delivered through a needle with a 10-mm uninsulated tip placed in the gasserian ganglion.[3] This technique produced lesions with unpredictable size.[4] The use of high-frequency electric current was later found to produce lesions with predictable size.[5] Because frequencies of 300 to 500 kHz were also used in radio transmitters, the current was called radiofrequency (RF) current. Later, temperature monitoring was suggested to be the most important parameter to obtain a standardized lesion size.[6]

In pain management, RF was first used for percutaneous lateral cordotomy to relieve unilateral pain in cancer patients.[5] A few years later, RF treatment of trigeminal neuralgia was described.[7] The first use of RF current for spinal pain was reported by Shealy,[8] who performed RF lesioning of the medial branch for lumbar zygapophyseal joint pain. Another application for spinal pain was introduced by Uematsu,[9] who described RF lesioning of the dorsal root ganglion (DRG).

At the end of the 1970s, percutaneous cordotomy and RF treatment of the gasserian ganglion were the only widely accepted RF procedures. A turning point came in 1980, when small-diameter electrodes, known as the Sluijter Mehta Kit (SMK) system, were introduced for the treatment of spinal pain.[10] The system consists of a 22-gauge disposable cannula with a fine thermocouple probe inside for measurement of temperature. The smaller electrode size resulted in diminished discomfort during the procedure. Because there was less risk for mechanical injury to major nerve trunks, targets in the anterior spinal compartment were no longer off limits, and procedures such as RF lesions adjacent to the DRG (RF-DRG) and lesions of the communicating ramus[11,12] and sympathetic chain became part of the treatment armamentarium.

Over the years the concept that the clinical effect of RF current was caused by the formation of heat had not been challenged. A selective effect of heat on thin nerve fibers was thought to interfere with the conduction of nociceptive stimuli.[13]

There were several reasons why the role of heat was finally questioned. First, the classic concept presupposes a strict configuration: the RF lesion must be made in between the nociceptive focus and the central nervous system (CNS). Yet RF lesions were also successful when not performed between the nociceptive focus and the CNS. For example, in the treatment of acute radicular pain from a herniated disk, the electrode is placed distal to the nociceptive focus.[14] Second, RF-DRG induces only transient sensory loss, which is possibly heat related, whereas the pain relief may be of much longer duration.[15] Finally, the role of heat was also questioned by the publication that no differences in outcome were noted when two different tip temperatures (i.e., 40° C and 67° C) were applied.[16] It is against this background that pulsed radiofrequency (PRF) treatment was developed.[17] PRF delivers strong, fluctuating electric fields while the temperature effects are kept to a minimum. PRF was conceived as a novel, potentially safer mode of administration of RF energy.[18-20] It can be specifically useful for treatments in which RF lesioning is not indicated, such as peripheral neuropathies, arthrogenic pain, painful trigger points, and application to the DRG in patients with neuropathy or radicular pain.

RADIOFREQUENCY GENERATOR SYSTEM

A modern RF lesion generator has the following functions:

- Continuous online measurement of impedance
- Nerve stimulation
- RF delivery mode
- Pulsed current delivery mode
- Monitoring of voltage, current, and wattage during the RF procedure
- Temperature monitoring

Electrical impedance is measured to confirm continuity of the electrical circuit. After placement of the needle under fluoroscopic control, nerve stimulation is performed to confirm proper position of the electrode. Stimulation is carried out at 50 Hz to ensure proximity of the electrode to sensory fibers; 2-Hz stimulation is performed to detect muscle contractions, which indicate that the position of the needle is too close to motor fibers. If an electrode is actually resting on a nerve, the minimum stimulation level required to produce a discharge is 0.25 V.[21] At a distance of 1 cm from the nerve, 2 V would be required; thus the stimulation threshold is an indicator of the distance of the electrode from the nerve. Temperature is measured with a thermocouple electrode. A thermocouple electrode consists of a junction of two dissimilar metal elements and produces a voltage that is proportional to temperature.

THEORETICAL ASPECTS OF RADIOFREQUENCY TREATMENT

CONTINUOUS RADIOFREQUENCY TREATMENT

The generator establishes a voltage gradient between the (active) electrode and the (dispersive) ground plate. RF current flowing through the tissue results in an alternating electric field. This electric field creates an electric force on ions (electrolytes) in the tissue that causes the ions to move back and forth at a high rate. Frictional dissipation of the ionic movement within the fluid medium results in tissue heating. RF heat is therefore generated in the tissue and the electrode is heated by the tissue. The size of the lesion depends on the temperature of the tip of the electrode, and tip temperature depends on the amount of power delivered. There are also other factors that influence lesion size, for instance, heat and the type of tissue. Heat is removed from the lesion area by conductive heat loss and by blood circulation (heat "washout"). The larger the heat washout, the smaller the lesion will be for a given tip temperature. Tissue factors influence heat washout. For example, bone is an effective heat insulator, and for this reason, RF lesions close to bone will have less washout. Similarly, segmental blood vessels, which lie in close relationship to the DRG, may cause more heat washout and thereby reduce the size of the lesion.[22]

PULSED RADIOFREQUENCY TREATMENT

The treatment effect of PRF is based on the dual effect of exposure of the tissue to RF fields (Fig. 62.1). Besides the ionic friction that causes the production of heat, there is an independent, electric field effect. The mechanism of this electric current effect is thought to be an alteration in synaptic transmission in a neuromodulatory type of effect.[18,19,23] Trans-synaptic induction of gene expression in the dorsal horn has been found in both the short[24] and long term.[25]

PRACTICAL CONSIDERATIONS

It may be wise to avoid ultralow sensory thresholds (<0.05 V) because such values may reflect intraneural electrode placement.[22] In a small proportion of procedures the mean tip

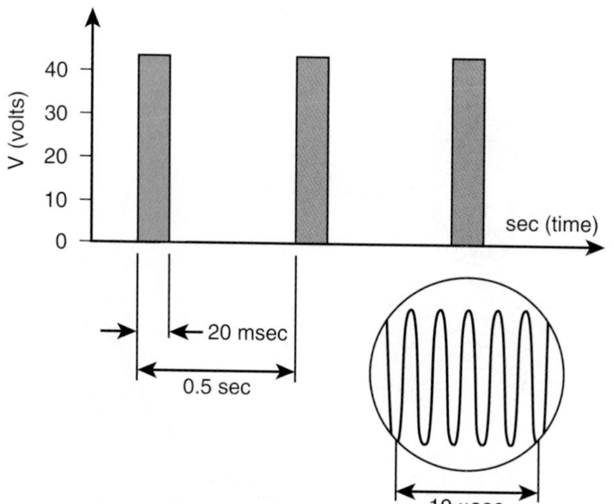

Figure 62.1 Schematic drawing of the duty cycle during pulsed radiofrequency treatment. There are two active cycles per second of 20 msec each. During the active phase, radiofrequency current is delivered at the normal frequency of 500,000 Hz. (Based on Sluijter ME. *Radiofrequency: Part I.* Meggen, Switzerland: Flivopress; 2001, with permission of the publisher.)

temperature exceeds 42° C at some point during the PRF procedure. In this case, power output should be decreased as a precaution. This can be done by lowering the voltage or by decreasing either the duration of the active cycle (typically 20 to 30 msec) or the frequency of the cycle (typically 2 Hz).

It is undesirable to adjust the voltage during a PRF procedure to reach the mean tip temperature since the mean tip temperature does not affect the outcome of the procedure.[26] Because there is a large variation in heat washout, large and unpredictable variations in voltage will occur.

INDICATIONS FOR AND CONTRAINDICATIONS TO RADIOFREQUENCY TREATMENT

RADIOFREQUENCY TREATMENT PROCEDURES ON THE HEAD

RADIOFREQUENCY TREATMENT OF THE GASSERIAN GANGLION

Trigeminal Neuralgia

Patients with trigeminal neuralgia have brief episodes of sharp, shooting pain in one or more of the trigeminal divisions that are typically provoked by touch. This so-called trigger area need not be in the division where the patient experiences pain. Many patients with pain in the first division, for example, have the trigger zone in the second division. In the classic case the patient is free of pain between episodes. However, residual pain has been reported in 42% of cases.[27] These patients were described as having a combination of trigeminal neuralgia and atypical facial pain. Some of these patients even had a continuous type of pain before the onset of trigeminal neuralgia. Trigeminal neuralgia predominantly occurs in older age groups (50+ years), although it may occasionally be seen in very young patients. It is thought to be caused by vascular compression of the trigeminal root. In patients with multiple sclerosis it occurs frequently and may indeed be the first symptom of the disease. In a study evaluating the clinical characteristics of patients with trigeminal neuralgia, 22 had multiple sclerosis. Six of them had atypical trigeminal neuralgia and 16 had signs of brainstem involvement.[28] It is not clear whether the pain is caused by plaques in the CNS in these patients, but clinically there was no distinction between patients with and without brainstem involvement. Trigeminal neuralgia may also be caused by a primary brain tumor (acoustic neuroma), which should always be excluded before symptomatic treatment is considered (red flag).

Treatment

In younger patients, posterior fossa craniotomy with microvascular decompression is the treatment of choice.[29] This treatment has a high rate of success and avoids the sensory loss that is one of the consequences of thermocoagulation of the ganglion. This procedure has a low complication rate. When complications do occur, they are mostly serious neurologic deficits.[30] In patients with multiple sclerosis the procedure should be combined with partial sectioning of the trigeminal nerve.[31] This could be an indication for a more central mechanism in these patients. Pain relief is substantially longer after microvascular decompression than after thermocoagulation of the ganglion. If the pain recurs, recurrent vascular compression is seldom found during reoperation.[32] In such cases, partial sectioning of the nerve could be performed. However, other forms of treatment such as thermocoagulation are generally recommended because the incidence of complications is distinctly higher after reoperation.[32,33] The outcome of thermocoagulation is less favorable, though, in operated patients.[34] The choice between microvascular decompression, a major operation with potentially longer effect, and RF treatment of the gasserian ganglion is a clinical decision in which age, physical condition, and personal preference of the patient have to be taken into account.

Evidence

There is extensive experience with RF treatment of trigeminal neuralgia. A review of 25 years' experience in 1600 patients undergoing percutaneous RF trigeminal rhizotomy for idiopathic neuralgia indicated acute pain relief in 97.6% and continued complete pain relief at 5 years' follow-up in 57.7%.[35] Comparisons with other techniques are based mainly on retrospective evaluations.[36-42]

The effectiveness of PRF for trigeminal neuralgia is still under debate.[43] One prospective randomized study demonstrated that PRF is not an effective method of treating pain in patients with idiopathic trigeminal neuralgia.[44]

Procedure

The technique for placing a needle (preferably an SMK-C10) in the gasserian ganglion is as follows:

The oval foramen is visualized first by using a tunnel view technique. To do this the direction of the x-rays should be reversed from the normal configuration because the image intensifier is too bulky to avoid contact with the patient's chest (Fig. 62.2). The position of the C-arm should be adjusted until the oval foramen is identified just medial to the mandibular processes and just lateral to the maxilla.

The shape of the foramen varies with the angle of the x-rays in the horizontal plane. A more vertical direction will transform the foramen into a round, almost circular shape. A more horizontal direction will make the foramen flat, like a split. The C-arm should be adjusted so that the foramen really has its oval shape. If the skin entry point is now marked over the target point, it will be seen that variation from patient to patient, in relation to the corner of the mouth, is considerable. The entry point may be just superior to the mandible, but it also may be much more superior, close to the maxilla.

The division of the trigeminal nerve that is the target for treatment also determines the choice of entry point. For the first division, the end position must be made medial and more superior (Fig. 62.3).

Adverse Events and Complications

The procedure is associated with very low morbidity and virtually no mortality. Reports vary considerably regarding recurrence of pain. This may be due to variations in technique. If a dense sensory loss is produced, there is a low incidence of recurrence.[7,45] However, loss of facial sensation and the accompanying paresthesia account for 80% of the side effects of the procedure. If RF treatment with a less intense lesion is performed, it might be associated with a lower incidence of paresthesia but potentially earlier recurrence. Other complications involve masseter weakness and paralysis (4.1%), anesthesia dolorosa (1%), keratitis (0.6%), and transient paralysis of cranial nerves III and IV (0.8%).[35]

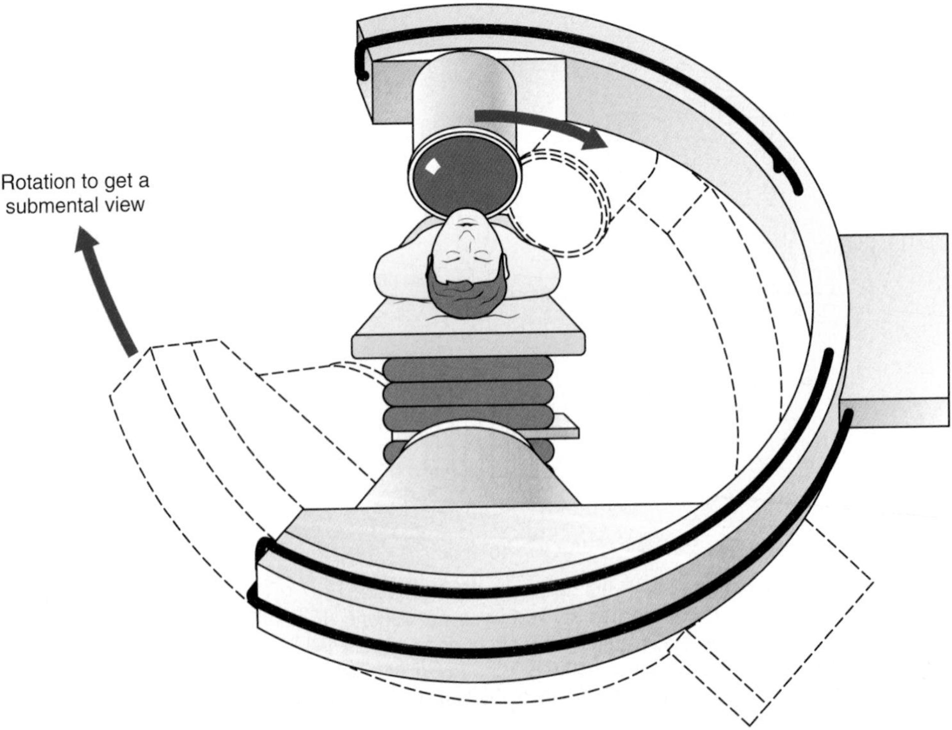

Figure 62.2 Schematic drawing of the fluoroscopy position for performing a radiofrequency procedure on the gasserian ganglion.

A much less frequent complication is permanent palsy of the abducens nerve.[46]

RADIOFREQUENCY TREATMENT OF THE PTERYGOPALATINE (SPHENOPALATINE) GANGLION

The pterygopalatine ganglion is a parasympathetic ganglion located in the pterygopalatine fossa just beneath the maxillary nerve. It is in or close to the foramen that connects the pterygopalatine fossa to the nasal cavity. Preganglionic fibers reach the ganglion from the facial nerve through the greater superficial petrosal nerve and the nerve of the pterygoid canal. There are also connections through the deep petrosal nerve that joins with the greater superficial petrosal nerve to form the vidian nerve (Fig. 62.4). Many afferent fibers originating from the nasal mucosa, the soft palate, and the pharynx cross the ganglion on their way to the maxillary nerve and eventually to the gasserian ganglion.

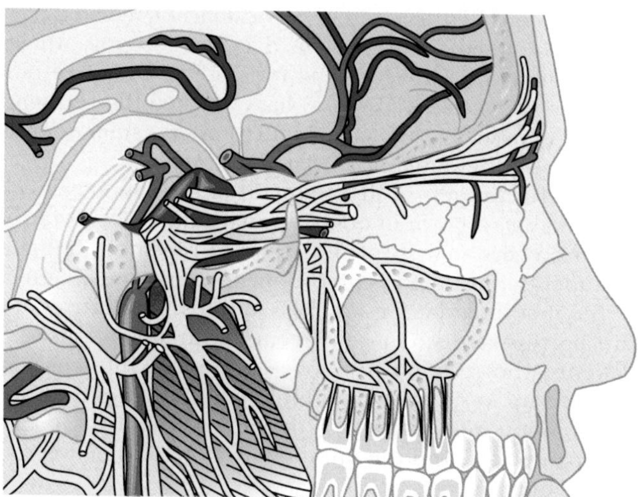

Figure 62.3 Anatomy of the gasserian ganglion and various trigeminal divisions. (From Sluijter ME. *Radiofrequency: Part I*. Meggen, Switzerland: Flivopress; 2001, with permission of the publisher.)

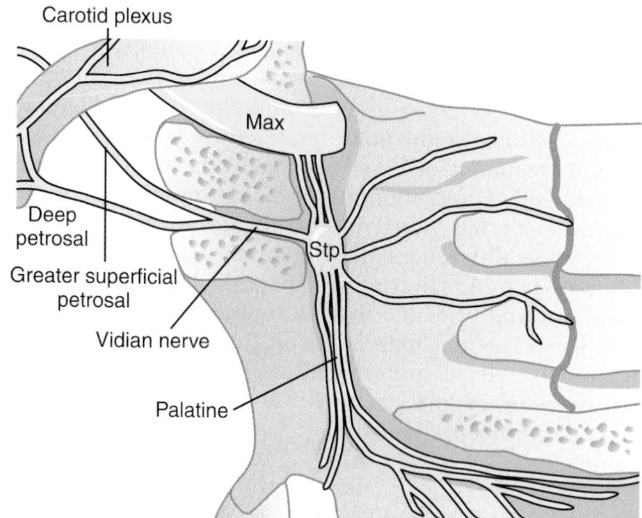

Figure 62.4 Connections of the sphenopalatine ganglion. (From Sluijter ME. *Radiofrequency: Part I*. Meggen, Switzerland: Flivopress; 2001, with permission of the publisher.)

Treatment and Evidence

The rationale for RF treatment of cluster headache is based on the parasympathetic symptoms that occur during an attack.[47] Treatment of atypical facial pain in the second division of the trigeminal nerve has also been described.[48] A case report on PRF treatment of the pterygopalatine ganglion for post-traumatic headache described 17 months of pain relief.[49] Analysis of PRF treatment of the pterygopalatine ganglion in 30 patients suffering from chronic head and facial pain showed complete relief of pain in 21% and mild to moderate relief in 65%. No side effects or complications were mentioned.[50] Evidence for the use of PRF is weak, but given the safe character of this treatment, the authors recommend the use of PRF for these conditions.

Procedure

The patient is placed in supine position with the head immobilized. The pterygopalatine fossa is identified on the lateral fluoroscopic image, and a line overlying the fossa is drawn on the skin. The intersection of this line with the inferior edge of the zygomatic arch is the entry point. After anesthetizing the skin, a 10-cm SMK cannula with a 5-mm active tip is inserted at this point and then carefully advanced under lateral fluoroscopic control in a superior and anterior direction to enter the pterygopalatine fossa (Fig. 62.5). As soon as the fossa is entered, the cannula contacts with the maxillary nerve, and the patient reports a paraesthesia, 1 to 2 mL of 2% lidocaine is injected. The cannula is advanced further until the tip reaches the pterygopalatine fossa. The pterygopalatine ganglion is located in the anterior superior corner of the fossa. It is important for the tip to actually pass the rim of the fossa to prevent damage to the maxillary nerve during the lesion.

The C-arm of the image intensifier is then placed in the anteroposterior (AP) position. The tip of the cannula

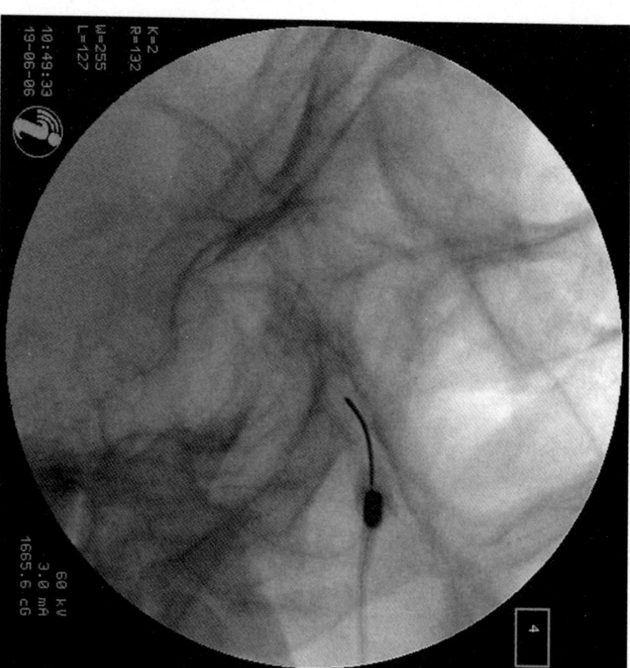

Figure 62.5 Needle placement in the pterygopalatine fossa.

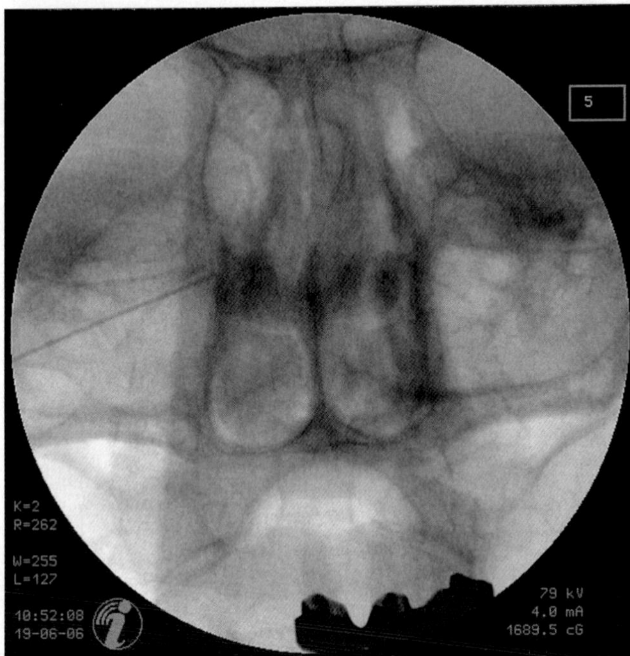

Figure 62.6 Anteroposterior view of needle placement in the pterygopalatine fossa.

should now be projected over the lateral wall of the nasopharynx (Fig. 62.6).

The stylet is removed and replaced with a thermocouple RF probe. The position of the electrode is verified by electrical stimulation at 50 Hz, and this usually results in paresthesia inside the nose at 0.2 to 1.0 V. Paresthesia occurring at the outside of the cheek or upper lip indicates stimulation of the maxillary nerve and thus that the tip of the needle is too far lateral. If the patient reports paresthesia in the palate, the cannula is advanced a few millimeters. Treatment consists of three consecutive lesions performed at 70° C to 80° C for 60 seconds.[47] In between these lesions the cannula is slowly advanced (1 to 3 mm).

Adverse Events and Complications

Total destruction of the pterygopalatine ganglion causes dryness of the eye, an "open nose" because the mucosa has less inclination to swell, and numbness of the soft palate. Following a heat RF lesion, dryness of the eye is unusual. Numbness of the soft palate does occur, but the condition is usually temporary, with gradual recovery occurring over a period of 4 to 6 weeks. Sometimes loss of taste can be permanent.

RADIOFREQUENCY TREATMENT PROCEDURES ON THE CERVICAL SPINE

CERVICAL FACET (ZYGAPOPHYSEAL) JOINT PAIN

The most common symptom associated with pain arising from the cervical facet joints is unilateral pain that does not radiate past the shoulder. Pain emanating from the cervical facet joints can be referred to the occiput, the interscapular region, or the shoulder girdle regions, depending on which cervical facet joint is involved.[51-54] Pain from the higher cervical facet joints may be the origin of cervicogenic headache.[55] Physical examination of the cervical spine usually shows paravertebral tenderness and limitation of rotation and retroflexion.[56] Computed tomography and magnetic resonance imaging may reveal morphologic abnormalities of the facet joints. However, degenerative changes of the cervical spine are present in asymptomatic patients, thus supporting the lack of correlation between radiologic findings and pain.[57,58]

Indications for RF treatment of the medial branches that innervate the cervical facet joints are degenerative and post-traumatic neck pain (i.e., whiplash-associated disorders).[59-62] The anatomy of the cervical spine is illustrated in Figure 62.7.[62,63] RF treatment of the cervical medial branches is aimed at reducing nociceptive signals from the spinal facet joints and shows some promise for the treatment of cervicogenic headache.[64] RF facet joint treatment is usually performed at two or three segmental levels.

Evidence

Percutaneous RF treatment of cervical facet–mediated pain has been studied intensively. The data from original articles were summarized in systematic reviews.[65-68] Only one randomized controlled trial (RCT) has evaluated RF treatment of the ramus medialis (medial branch) of the ramus dorsalis in patients with whiplash-associated disorders.[59]

The effectiveness of RF treatment of degenerative neck pathology was shown in observational studies.[69-71] A retrospective chart analysis of the effect of repeated RF facet treatments illustrated that the mean duration of effect of the first intervention was 12.5 months. The procedure can be repeated when pain recurs, with similar success. Patients who respond positively to the first intervention received up to six additional interventions. After each RF intervention more than 90% of the patients had satisfactory pain relief, and the duration of effect was between 8 and 12 months.[72]

Van Suijlekom and coworkers evaluated the effect of RF lesioning of the medial branch of the dorsal ramus at the C3-6 levels for the treatment of cervicogenic headache.[64] In this study the postural lateral approach was used. They demonstrated that RF cervical facet treatment leads to a significant reduction in headache severity, number of days with headache, and analgesic intake in patients with cervicogenic headache diagnosed according to the criteria of Sjaastad and colleagues.[55] In a randomized, double-blind, sham-controlled study on RF treatment of facet joints C2-3 for the treatment of cervicogenic headache, 12 patients were included and monitored for 24 months. A slight improvement was noted in the RF group at 3 months, whereas no differences were seen during the remaining follow-up period.[73] In contrast, Haspeslagh and associates[74] could not find evidence that RF treatment of the cervical facet joints is better than injection in the greater occipital nerve. However, definite conclusions on the clinical efficacy of the procedure can be drawn only from an RCT with a greater number of patients.

Procedure

Several approaches can be used to reach the medial branch of the dorsal ramus at the upper and middle cervical area. We use the posterolateral technique, which was first described with a three-quarter projection of the C-arm.[75] Since this technique is difficult to perform because it is

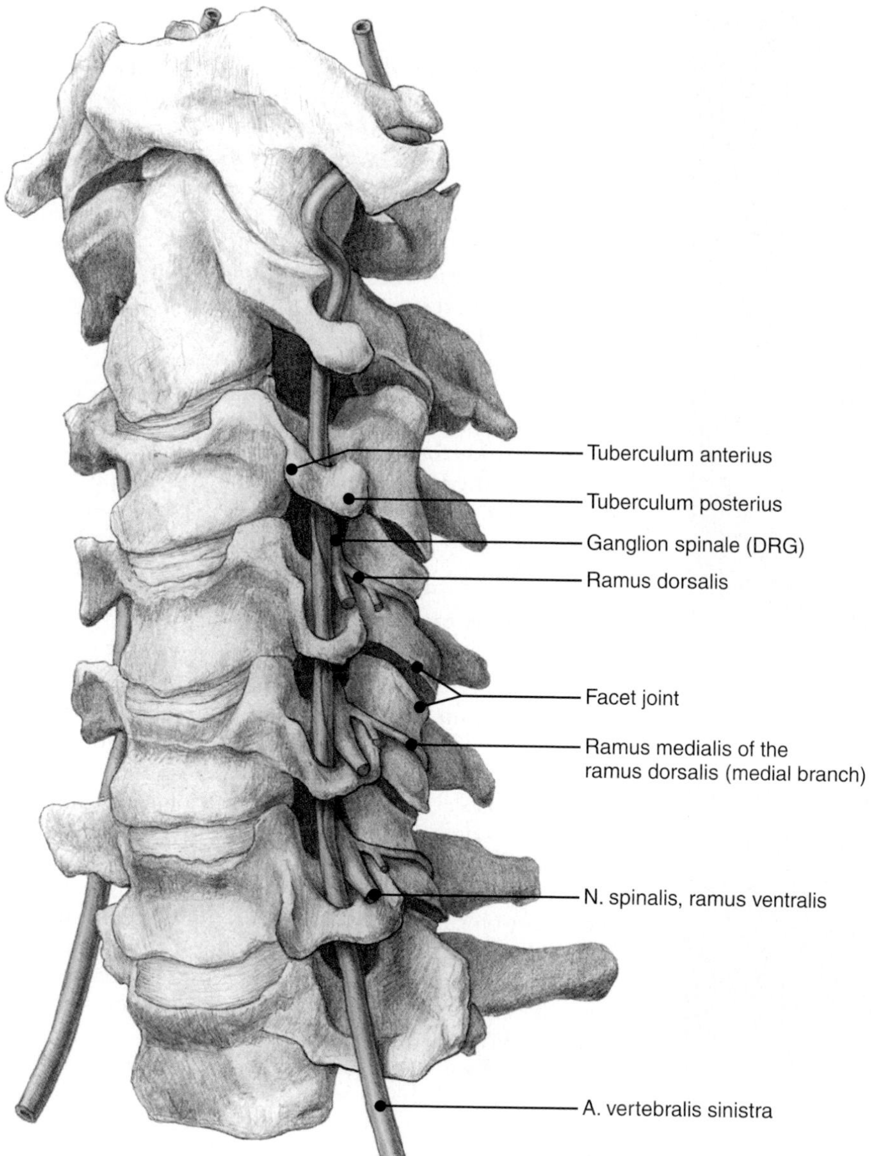

Figure 62.7 Anatomy of the cervical spine. DRG, dorsal root ganglion. (Illustration courtesy of Rogier Trompert Medical Art. Available at www.Medicalart.nl.)

not a tunnel view technique, we developed a new approach with a lateral projection. For this technique the patient is positioned supine on the operating table.

For treating the upper cervical levels, the domelike structure between C1 and C2 should be aligned without any double contours. Usually, the facet joint space of C3-4 is clearly visible, also without double contours. Adjustments of the C-arm are often necessary for the C4, C5, and C6 levels, with alignment of the facet joint spaces and the facetal column needed every time. In this position the anterior and posterior tubercles of the neuroforamen can be seen projected over the vertebral body. The medial branch runs just above the posterior tubercle, midway between the facet joints. Needle entry points should be at the dorsal side of the facetal column in a virtual vertical line exactly between the facet joint spaces. Under fluoroscopic guidance the needle electrode is carefully placed in a slightly anterior horizontal direction until contact is made with the facetal column (Fig. 62.8). The tip of the needle should be at or just above the posterior tubercle, midway or slightly rostral between the facet joint spaces. To confirm that the tip of the needle is close to the segmental nerve but not in the neuroforamen, the C-arm is placed in an approximately 30-degree oblique position in such a way that the projection of the contralateral pedicles is 50 degrees anterior to the vertebral body (Fig. 62.9). This position is sometimes preferred for

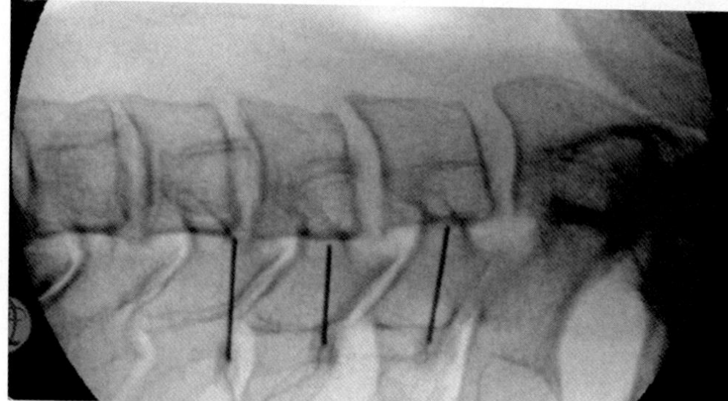

Figure 62.8 Fluoroscopic image of the position of the needle for a cervical medial branch procedure via a lateral approach.

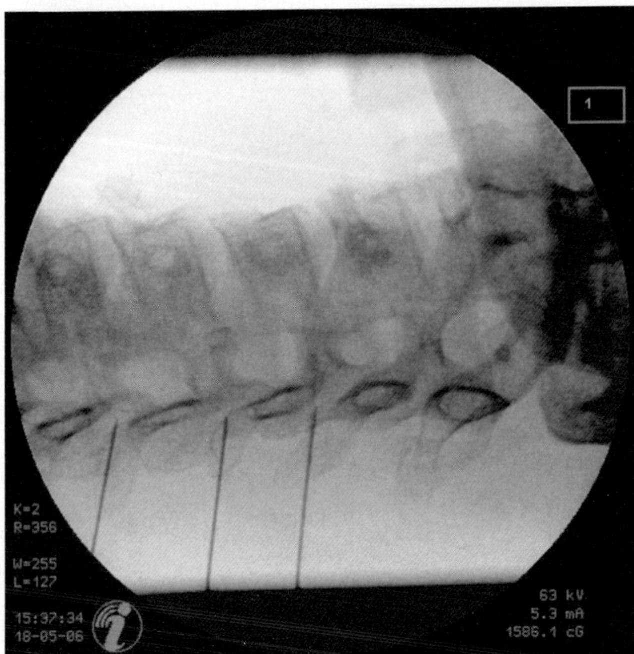

Figure 62.9 Fluoroscopic image of the position of the needle for a cervical medial branch procedure.

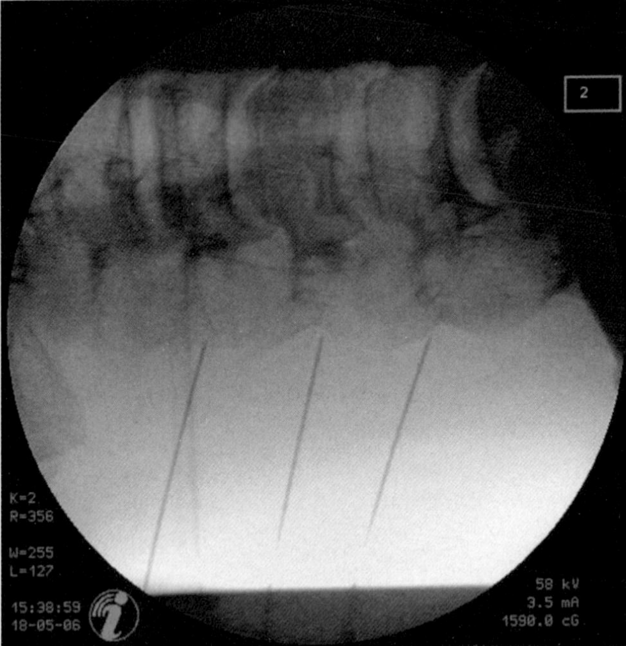

Figure 62.10 Anteroposterior view of the cervical spine–needle position for a procedure on the medial branch.

treatment of the C6 and C7 levels because of overprojection of the shoulders on the lateral view.

Positioning the C-arm in the AP direction should confirm the position of the tip of the needle adjacent to the concavity ("waist") of the articular pillars of the cervical spine at the corresponding level (Fig. 62.10). When optimal anatomic localization of the needles is achieved, an electrical stimulation is performed to confirm correct needle position. An electrical stimulation rate of 50 Hz should elicit a response (tingling sensation) in the neck at less than 0.5 V. Stimulation at 2 Hz is performed to confirm accurate needle position. Contractions of the paraspinal muscles will be noticed. Muscle contractions in the arm indicate placement of the needle too close to the exiting nerve. In this case the needle should be repositioned more posteriorly. Once proper positioning of the needle is confirmed, the medial branch of the dorsal ramus is anesthetized with 1 to 2 mL of local anesthetic solution (1% or 2% lidocaine). An 80° C RF thermal lesion is made for 60 seconds at each level.

Another method is a posterior approach to the facet joint. This was first introduced by Lord and associates in 1995.[76] For this technique the patient is positioned prone on the operating table with the head flexed (about 5 to 10 degrees) and the face resting on a padded ring. The electrode is introduced twice for each nerve: once along a parasagittal path to reach the nerve as it crosses the lateral aspect of the articular pillar and again at a 30-degree angle to the sagittal plane to reach the nerve over the lateral aspect of the articular pillar.

Adverse Events and Complications

Complications are rare. Nevertheless, one should be aware that the vertebral artery may be punctured if the needle is pushed too far anterior into the foramen intervertebral. The position of the tip of the needle should be verified with AP fluoroscopy to prevent intrathecal injection of the local anesthetic. In an observational study the incidence of inadvertent intravascular penetration for medial branch blocks at a cervical level was reported to be 3.9%, comparable to the incidence at a lumbar level (3.7%).[77] Some patients experienced short-term vasovagal reactions. Intravascular uptake of local anesthetic and contrast solution was thought to be responsible for the false-negative diagnostic blocks. No systemic effects were reported.[77] Monitoring of the saturation level and availability of resuscitation equipment are essential.

Infections have been described, but the incidence is unknown and probably very low.[78,79]

Other potential complications of facet joint interventions are related to needle placement and drug administration; they include dural puncture, spinal cord trauma, spinal anesthesia, chemical meningitis, neural trauma, pneumothorax, radiation exposure, facet capsule rupture, and hematoma formation.[68] After RF treatment, burning pain is regularly reported postoperatively, but this pain disappears in 1 to 3 weeks.[74,80] There are no incidence data on side effects and complications following cervical RF treatment of the ramus medialis (medial branch) of the ramus dorsalis. At the lumbar level the incidence of complications was lower than 1%.[62]

CERVICAL RADICULAR PAIN

Cervicobrachialgia is a common pain syndrome. Bland estimated that 9% of all men and 12% of all women experience this pain at some time in their lives.[81] Later, in 1994, Radhakrishnan and associates published a population-based survey.[82] This epidemiologic survey found the annual incidence of cervical radiculopathy to be 83.2 per 100,000 population between 13 and 91 years of age.

The pain in cervicobrachialgia is described as a continuous, dull aching pain in the neck (most commonly localized in the mid and lower cervical area) that radiates beyond the shoulder into the arm with referral to a particular spinal segment. Segmental pain in the upper extremity can be related to disk pathology, such as cervical disk protrusion with irritation of the spinal nerve. Spinal nerve irritation can also be caused by narrowing of the intervertebral foramen by spondylosis. The most common levels involved are C6, C7, and to a lesser extent, C5. Involvement of the C4 and C8 levels is uncommon. The involved spinal level can be estimated by the dermatome in which the pain is radiating[83] and can be confirmed by diagnostic nerve blocks.[78,84,85] Diagnosis of cervical radicular pain and radiculopathy requires complete history taking and clinical diagnosis using standardized methods of physical examination, medical imaging, electrophysiologic investigation, and selective nerve root blocks.

Evidence

In 1991, Vervest and Stolker published a retrospective study of 53 patients with prolonged cervical pain radiating to the occipital region, head, shoulder, or arm that did not respond to conservative treatment.[80] If the patient had local tenderness at the facet joints, a percutaneous cervical facet joint treatment was performed. If this treatment was not successful and there was cervical pain with referral to the occipital region or arm, indicative of segmental nerve irritation, diagnostic segmental nerve blocks were performed. A positive diagnostic block was followed by RF-DRG. The results were good to excellent in more than 80% of treatments. Even after a follow-up of 1.5 years, more than 80% still had satisfactory pain relief.

In an open prospective study of 20 consecutive patients with chronic intractable pain in the cervical region and referral to the head, shoulder, or arm, RF-DRG provided pain relief in 75% at 3 months and in 50% at 6 months.[15] These results indicate acceptable initial pain relief but a tendency for recurrence of the pain at 3 to 9 months. A prospective double-blind, randomized, sham-controlled trial of RF lesions adjacent to the cervical DRG for the management of chronic cervical radicular pain showed a positive outcome during the first 8 weeks after the procedure.[85] In a double-blind, randomized study with 3 months' follow-up, Slappendel and colleagues[16] found that RF treatment adjacent to the cervical DRG at 40° C is as effective as treatment at 67° C.

Despite these encouraging results, Geurts and associates[65] in a systematic review concluded that there is limited evidence that RF-DRG is more effective than placebo for chronic cervicobrachialgia. In their systematic review Niemisto and coworkers[66] came to the same conclusion.

In 2003, Van Zundert and colleagues published a clinical audit of 18 patients with cervicogenic headache or cervicobrachialgia who failed conservative treatment and underwent PRF treatment adjacent to the cervical DRG.[86] Seventy-two percent of the patients had a minimum reduction in pain of at least 50% at 8 weeks. At 1 year, 33% of the patients continued to rate the treatment outcome as good or very good. No neurologic side effects or complications were observed. These results were later confirmed in an RCT in which PRF appeared to be more effective than placebo 3 months after treatment.[87] In addition, 6 months after treatment there was a positive trend for PRF treatment, but in this study the outcome fell short of statistical significance. The need for pain medication was significantly reduced in the PRF group after 6 months. No complications were observed during the study period.[87]

There is limited evidence that PRF treatment of the DRG (PRF-DRG) on a cervical level is as effective as RF-DRG. However, PRF-DRG is safer and has fewer side effects. Therefore, the authors suggest that cervical radicular pain be treated with PRF-DRG and not with RF-DRG.

Procedure

To perform a diagnostic segmental nerve block, a viewing technique is used in which the C-arm is positioned so that the x-rays are parallel to the axis of the intervertebral foramen. This axis points 25 to 35 degrees anteriorly and 10 degrees caudally. With the C-arm in this position, entry is determined by projecting a metal ruler over the caudal part of the foramen. A 50-mm, 22-gauge neurography needle is carefully introduced parallel to the beam of the x-rays. The direction of the x-rays is then changed to the AP position and the cannula is introduced further until the tip is projecting just lateral to the facetal column. After the segmental nerve has been identified with 0.4 mL of iohexol contrast medium, 0.5 mL of 2% lidocaine is slowly infiltrated around the nerve. The resultant radiopaque mixture is closely observed during injection so that accidental overflow into the epidural space can be avoided.[85]

For the RF procedure, the same viewing technique is used. The entry point is found by projecting the metal ruler over the caudal and posterior parts of the foramen. The cannula (SMK-C5 with a 2-mm exposed tip) is introduced parallel to the beam of the x-rays, and if necessary, the approach is corrected while still in the superficial layers until the cannula is projected on the screen as a single dot (Fig. 62.11). In practice this dot should lie directly over the

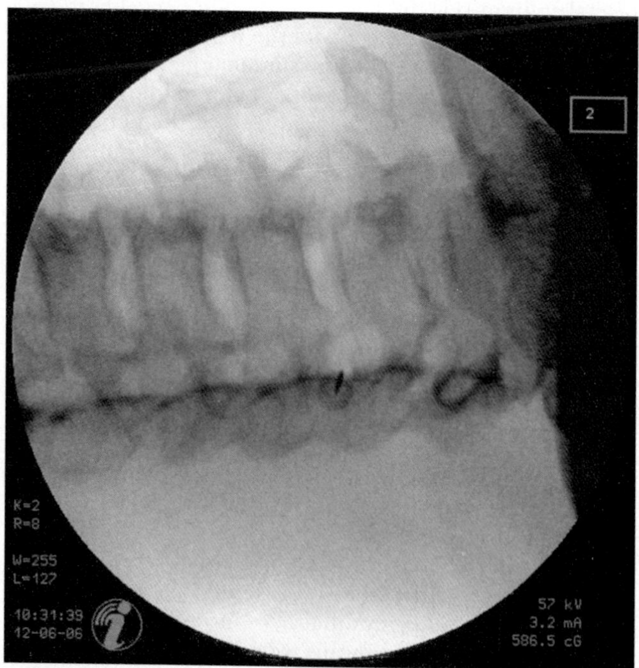

Figure 62.11 Radiofrequency lesion adjacent to the dorsal root ganglion in a 20-degree oblique, 10-degree craniocaudal projection. The needle is positioned in the posterior aspect of the fossa at the junction of the middle and caudal third part. It is projected as a dot in tunnel vision.

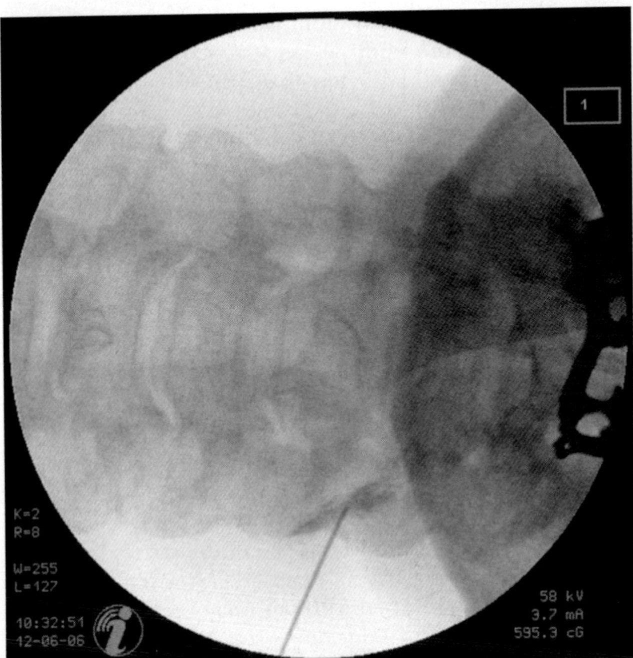

Figure 62.12 Radiofrequency treatment of the dorsal root ganglion, anteroposterior view. The tip of the needle is projected over the facetal column.

dorsal part of the intervertebral foramen at the transition between the middle and most caudal third. This dorsal position is chosen to avoid possible damage to the motor fibers of the segmental nerve and to the vertebral artery that runs anterior to the ventral part of the foramen. The direction of the x-rays is then changed to AP and the cannula is further introduced until the tip is projected over the middle of the facetal column (Fig. 62.12).

The stylet is now replaced with the RF probe. After checking the impedance, electrical stimulation is started at a rate of 50 Hz. The patient should feel a tingling sensation between 0.4 and 0.65 V. The frequency is then changed to 2 Hz and the patient is observed for muscle contractions. These contractions should not occur below a voltage of 1.5 times the sensory threshold. One-half milliliter of iohexol is injected to exclude accidental intradural positioning of the electrode, followed by 2 mL of 2% lidocaine. RF current is then passed through the electrode to increase the temperature of the tip to 67° C. This temperature is maintained for 60 seconds.

Adverse Events and Complications

A side effect that is often seen (40% to 60%) is a mild burning sensation (some deep neck soreness) in the treated dermatome, but it subsides spontaneously after 1 to 3 weeks.[75] Some sensory changes such as slight hypoesthesia may occur but invariably disappear within 3 or 4 months.[15,16,85]

Known complications of blockade of a cervical segmental nerve are epidural, intrathecal, or intravascular injection of local anesthetic. During this procedure, injectant can be placed in the adjacent venous plexus, in the vertebral artery, or even in the carotid artery. Because of the proximity of the higher cervical levels to the brain, there is a risk for local anesthetic CNS toxicity (seizure), although only a low volume of local anesthetic is used.[88]

RADIOFREQUENCY PROCEDURES ON THE THORACIC SPINE

Thoracic pain accounts for approximately 5% of all referrals to a pain clinic.[89,90] Thoracic pain may have many causes, from cardiac to lung pathology, in addition to pain referred to the chest from other affected organs (upper abdominal organs such as the gallbladder and pancreas). Pain in the lower thoracic region must be differentiated from renal pathology.[91] Thoracic pain may have an underlying pathology such as disk herniation, aneurysms, tumors,[92] postoperative sternal wound infection,[93] trauma,[94] old fractures, herpetic infection,[95] and stress fractures in athletes.[96,97] Chronic postsurgical pain has been described after many different operations, most notably thoracotomy, mastectomy, and coronary artery bypass grafting.[98-100] However, in most cases, thoracic pain is judged to be of spinal origin and emanating from nociceptive nerve endings in the periosteum, ligaments, disks, or joints.[101]

Thoracic pain can be divided into thoracic mechanical joint pain and thoracic segmental pain. The thoracic spine is a relatively immobile section. The range of motion in both flexion and extension is on the order of 10 degrees, and lateral flexion is almost impossible. Rotation is the only meaningful movement of the thoracic spine.

Thoracic mechanical pain is characterized by pain in both thoracic facet joints, as well as the thoracic disks.[102,103]

Pain emanating from thoracic facet joints is usually related to degenerative processes, vertebral collapse, and continual mechanical strain.[101] The problem can be in the facet joint but may be manifested elsewhere in the spine.[53] There are no specific pathognomonic criteria whereby thoracic facet joint pain can be diagnosed from a patient's history and physical examination. A diagnosis of thoracic facet joint pain can be based on the similarity of the symptoms to lumbar and cervical facet syndromes. Extensive examination should be performed to rule out any pathology as a primary cause of the symptoms and signs.

When thoracic spinal pain becomes chronic and resistant to conservative treatment modalities such as physical therapy, pharmacologic therapy, and transcutaneous electrical nerve stimulation, minimally invasive treatment modalities, including RF lesioning of the facet joints, can be considered.

The thoracic facet joints are more vertically oriented than the lumbar facet joints and lie almost parallel to the coronal plane (Fig. 62.13). They are oriented perpendicular to the sagittal plane and face directly anterior. The thoracic facet joints are innervated by medial branches of the posterior primary rami of the segmental nerves. Each thoracic facet joint is bisegmentally innervated by the medial branch of the same level and the medial branch of the level above. The thoracic medial branches pass through the intertransverse space and touch the superolateral corner of the transverse process. They then run medially and inferiorly across the posterior surfaces of the transverse processes before entering the posterior compartment of the back and innervating the multifidus muscles.[104] In this location they send ascending articular branches to the facet joint. An exception to this pattern occurs at the midthoracic levels (T5-8). Although the curved course remains essentially the same, inflection occurs at a point superior to the superolateral corner of the

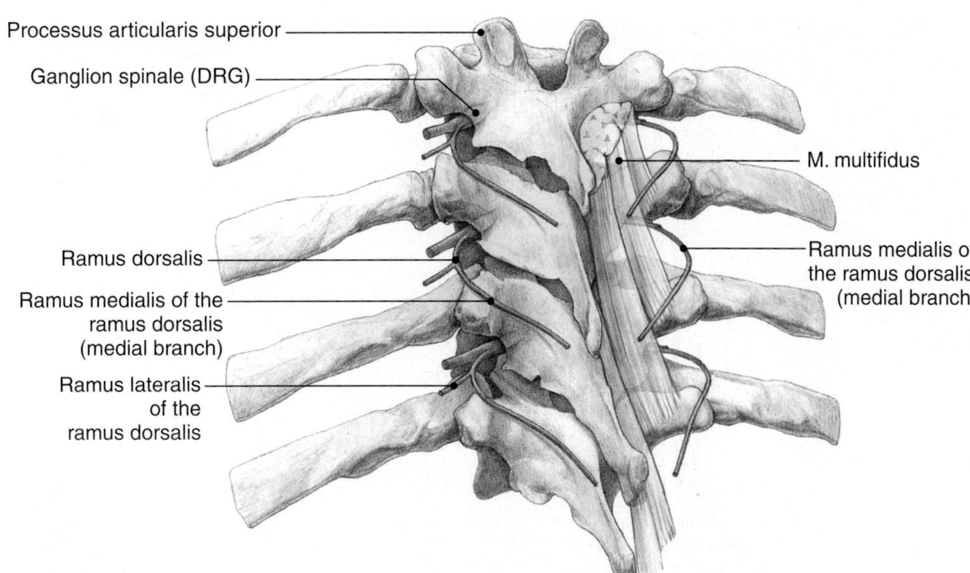

Figure 62.13 Anatomy of the thoracic spine. DRG, dorsal root ganglion. (Illustration courtesy of Rogier Trompert Medical Art. Available at www.Medicalart.nl.)

transverse process. This course is different from that seen with the lumbar medial branches, which are fixed at the junction of the superior articular process and the transverse process. The T11 and T12 medial branches have the same course as the lumbar medial branches.[105]

Evidence

Stolker and coworkers evaluated 40 patients with thoracic facet syndrome who underwent percutaneous facet joint treatment: 24 left sided, 21 right sided, and 6 bilateral. Seven study patients underwent two sessions, and two patients had three facet joint denervation sessions; 82% of the patients experienced 50% to 75% relief of their pain at 2 months. Four patients were lost to long-term follow-up (18 to 54 months, mean of 31 months), 44% of the study patients were free of pain, and 39% had a 50% or greater reduction in their pain.[103] In line with these criteria being nonspecific for thoracic facet syndrome, all patients in this study had positive diagnostic blocks performed before RF ablation. Stolker and coworkers attributed their results to the consistent course of the medial branch of the dorsal rami of the thoracic spinal nerves as they leave the intertransverse space; however, the anatomic target point (junction between the superior articular process and the transverse process) that they used in their study is at variance with the anatomic course of thoracic medial branch described by Chua and Bogduk.[104] They reported that the medial branch crosses the superolateral corners of the transverse processes and then passes medially and inferiorly along the posterior surfaces of the transverse processes before ramifying into the multifidus muscle that it supplies.[104] Bogduk and Long stated that a double-blind, controlled clinical trial of Stolker and colleagues' approach to thoracic facet nerve denervation or modification of their procedure was needed to be concordant with the surgical anatomy of the thoracic medial branches.[105]

In another study by Tzaan and Tasker in 2000 in which 17 patients with thoracic facet syndrome were evaluated, 15 had satisfactory pain relief at follow-up, with 2 patients having their procedure repeated.[106]

Procedure

The patient is placed in the prone position. Obtaining a fluoroscopic view is quite difficult for a variety of reasons. In this region one has to contend with overprojection of the ribs, a prominent transverse process that is directed slightly cranial and markedly posterior, and the size and orientation of the pedicles, which can make them difficult to visualize. In addition, the orientation of the thoracic facet joints impedes the operator's ability to differentiate between the superior and inferior articular processes.

In contrast to a diagnostic thoracic intra-articular block, which has been well described,[107] expert opinion varies on RF lesioning of medial branches in the thoracic vertebrae. Nonetheless, we describe how to perform an RF lesion of the medial branches at the thoracic level. Although we embrace this technique, some authors have suggested that the tip of the needle is actually "too far anterior" to the medial branch to result in denervation. Using the junction between the superior articular process and the superior border of the transverse process as a target point for thoracic medial branch neurotomy, Stolker and colleagues reported that the medial branch of the dorsal ramus was never within reach of the electrodes.[108] The C-arm is positioned in the axial plane, and an external radiopaque object such as a clamp is used to identify the proper level. A straight AP view of the vertebra at the anticipated target level is obtained. The end plates of the vertebra should be parallel without any visible double contours. The C-arm is then rotated slightly obliquely. This should facilitate access to the target point, which is the junction of the superior articular process and the transverse process. A proposed entry point is marked on the skin and local anesthetic (1% lidocaine) is injected with a 23-gauge needle. The RF needle is then inserted parallel to the angle of the C-arm beam until contact is made with bone at the junction of the superior articular process and the transverse process (Fig. 62.14*A*).

Subsequently, the needle is redirected slightly more cranially and laterally until it just loses osseous contact. Needle position is then checked on the lateral view. The tip of the needle should be just posterior to a line connecting the posterior aspects of the neuroforamina (see Fig. 62.14*B*).

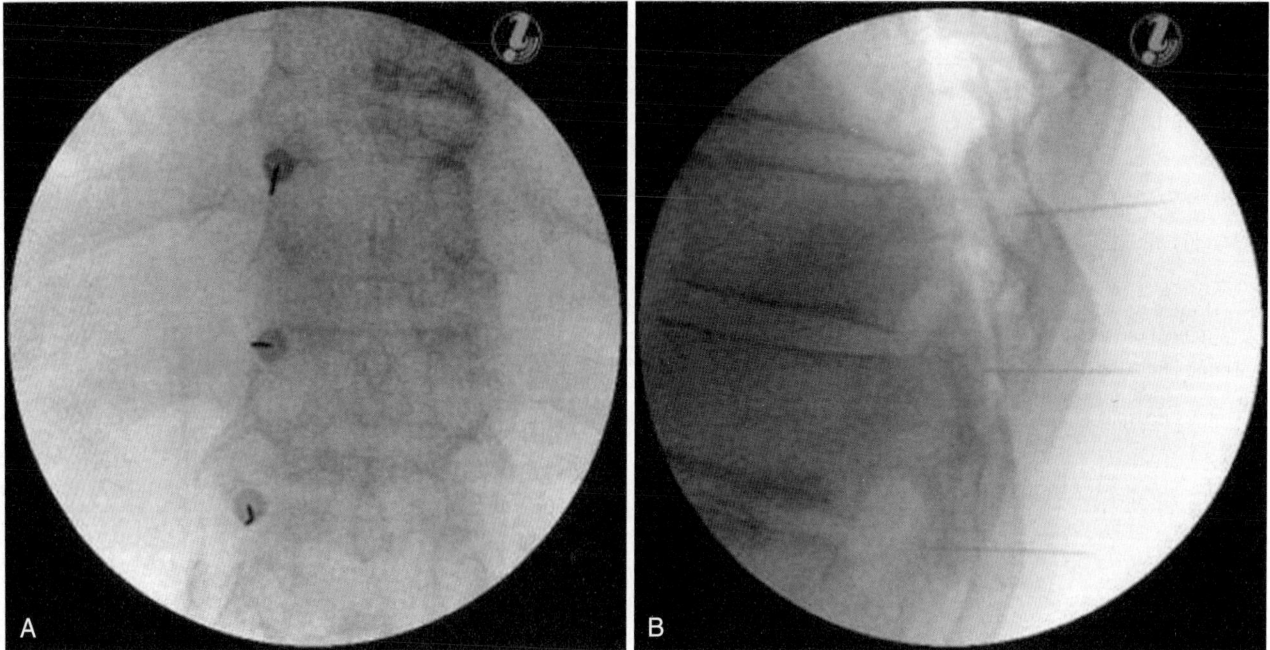

Figure 62.14 Thoracic facet joint on anteroposterior (**A**) and lateral (**B**) views.

Stimulation at 50 Hz is now performed. A paravertebral tingling sensation should be perceived with a current of less than 0.5 V. Next, stimulation at 2 Hz should provoke paravertebral muscle contractions at 1 V or less. Stimulation should be negative for anterior nerve root stimulation, which would be perceived as muscle contraction or pain in the anterior chest wall or abdominal region, depending on the level undergoing RF treatment. When proper needle position has been confirmed with fluoroscopic imaging and electrical stimulation, 0.5 mL of 1% or 2% lidocaine is administered at each level. After the local anesthetic has taken effect RF, lesioning is conducted for 60 seconds at 20 V. We typically perform RF treatment of three levels because of the multisegmental innervation of the facet joints.

Adverse Events and Complications

As with any RF procedure there is always the possibility of postprocedure exacerbation of pain. A complication unique to the thoracic region is pneumothorax. Proper technique and the use of fluoroscopic guidance for placement of the needle will minimize the risk for this complication. The patient must be warned of the possibility of the development of pneumothorax and should return to the hospital if shortness of breath or pain with inspiration develops.

THORACIC RADICULAR PAIN

Thoracic segmental pain syndromes have many causes, including disease or lesions of ribs, disorders of the thoracic skeletal spine (fractures, arthritis, metabolic disorders, and tumors), or neuropathies originating from the spinal roots, spinal nerves, or intercostal nerves.[101]

Some thoracic segmental pain syndromes are iatrogenic, such as post-thoracotomy and postmastectomy syndromes, as well as incisional pain after upper gastrointestinal surgery.[99,100,109]

Percutaneous thoracic sympathectomy is considered the most efficacious for sympathetically mediated pain, Raynaud's syndrome, hyperhidrosis, and vasculopathy.[103] Percutaneous RF treatment adjacent to the thoracic DRG has been described for segmental nerve pain related to intercostal pain, rib tip syndrome, 12th rib syndrome, vertebral collapse, and segmental peripheral neuralgia.

In the higher thoracic segments it is difficult to reach the DRGs because of overlying anatomic structures. Among the obstacles are the wide facet column, articulations of the transverse processes with the ribs, and most importantly, the lungs. The pulmonary structures prevent adopting a very lateral approach, which would have been ideal to allow one to get under the posterior osseous barriers. In successive lower thoracic segments, the anatomy gradually resembles that of the lumbar spine. This change creates an opportunity for a lower thoracic DRG to be reached as though it were a lumbar DRG.

Evidence

RF treatment adjacent to the thoracic DRG was evaluated in 45 patients who underwent 53 PRF-DRG procedures, 37 patients at one level, 1 bilaterally at one level, and 7 at two levels unilaterally. Clinical diagnoses included intercostal neuralgia, post-thoracotomy pain syndrome, postmastectomy pain syndrome, 12th rib syndrome, rib resection, osteoporosis, vertebral metastasis, and traumatic collapsed vertebra. At first follow-up 2 months after the procedure, 66.7% were pain free, 24% obtained greater than 50% pain relief, and 9% obtained no pain relief. Four patients were lost to long-term follow-up or died of their malignant disease. After a follow-up period of 13 to 46 months (median, 24 months), 49% were pain free, 37% had good pain relief, and 14.6% had no pain relief.[108]

The authors of this study advocated prognostic blockade as being essential to (1) confirm the diagnosis of segmental pain, (2) determine the appropriate level of treatment, and (3) assess the potential benefit of percutaneous RF-DRG.

In a similar study, van Kleef and Spaans[110] evaluated the effects of single-level RF-DRG for thoracic segmental pain.

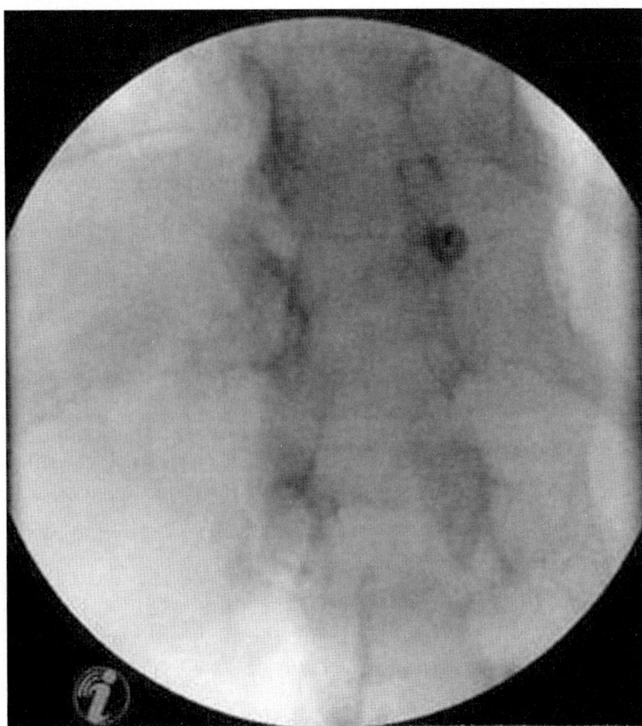

Figure 62.15 Entry point for thoracic pulsed radiofrequency treatment of the dorsal root ganglion.

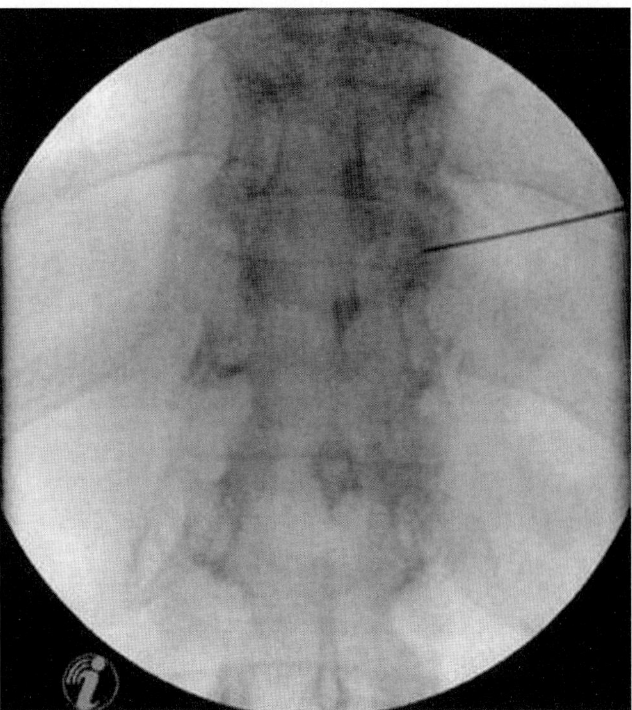

Figure 62.16 Thoracic pulsed radiofrequency treatment of the dorsal root ganglion, anteroposterior view. Note that the needle is located in the middle of the facetal column.

In this study, 43 patients with a minimum of a 6-month history of unilateral thoracic segmental pain unresponsive to conservative therapy were evaluated. Twenty-seven of the patients had pain in the distribution of only one or two segments (group 1), whereas 16 patients had pain at more than two segmental levels (group 2). Short-term analysis 8 weeks after the procedure showed that 52% of the patients in group 1 were pain free or had good pain relief whereas only 18% in group 2 were pain free or had good pain relief. Long-term follow-up (36 to 168 weeks, mean of 99 weeks) illustrated that 37% of the patients in group 1 were pain free or had good pain relief whereas only 18% of those in group 2 had such a positive outcome at long-term follow-up (40 to 60 weeks, mean of 128 weeks).

Procedure

Two or more diagnostic blocks at different levels must be performed to identify the segment involved because of frequent overlapping of thoracic segmental pain from one segment to another. An intercostal block can be used as a test block of a thoracic segmental nerve.[111] The level that provides the best temporary reduction in pain is then selected for RF-DRG treatment. As described, in the upper thoracic spine the classic approach (posterolateral approach) is not possible because the foramina face more anteriorly and accurate positioning of the needle is hindered by the angle of the ribs. Therefore, an alternative technique is used to reach the DRG of T7 and above. The patient is placed in the prone position and a dorsal approach is used. The target point is the craniodorsal part of the intervertebral foramen and is thus the same as the target point in the classic dorsolateral approach. The entry point is the midpoint of the pedicle on the AP view (Figs. 62.15 and 62.16).

This entry point is checked on a lateral view, where it should be aimed at the superior dorsal quadrant of the foramina where the DRG is supposed to be lying. Under local anesthesia a small hole is drilled with a 16-gauge Kirschner wire through the lamina of the vertebra under fluoroscopic guidance in the AP view. A potential danger is piercing of the facet joint. The RF cannula is inserted through the hole into the proper position, which is checked on the lateral view and should be in the craniodorsal part of the intervertebral foramen (Fig. 62.17).

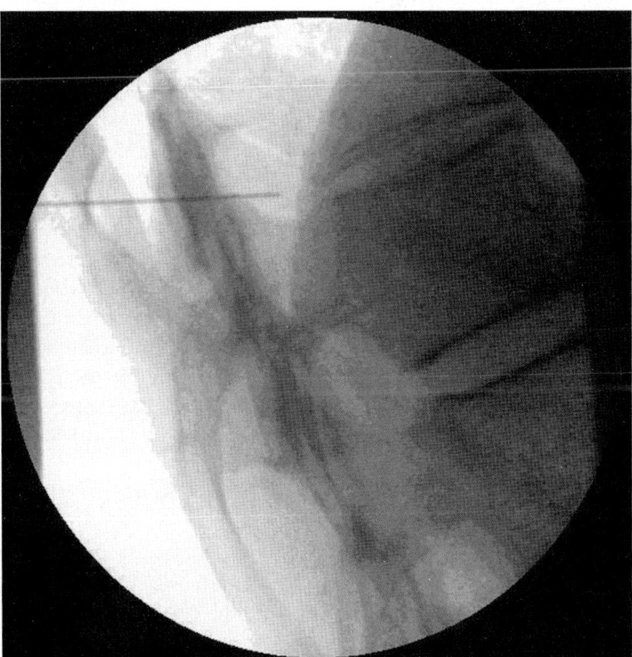

Figure 62.17 Thoracic pulsed radiofrequency treatment of the dorsal root ganglion, lateral view.

The stylet of the cannula is replaced with an RF probe, and stimulation at 50 Hz is carried out. The patient should feel tingling sensations in the selected dermatome when a 0.4- to 1.0-V stimulus is used. Stimulation at 2 Hz should not produce contractions of the intercostal muscles at a stimulation threshold below 1.5 times the sensory threshold. After satisfactory placement is achieved, 0.4 mL of iohexol contrast medium is injected to exclude intradural or intravascular spread. When correct position has been confirmed, 1 to 2 mL of 1% or 2% lidocaine is injected, and a 60-second 67° C lesion is made.

At the lower thoracic levels, the same approach can be used as at the lumbar level. The needle position, stimulation, and lesion parameters are identical. This technique is described later under RF-DRG treatment in the lumbar region.

A 10-cm SMK 22-gauge cannula with a 5-mm active tip and an RF probe can be used. This needle can be manually curved to perform the parasagittal approach. For the dorsal approach, a 16-gauge Kirschner wire can be used to make a bur hole in the lamina.

Adverse Events and Complications

One of the most important complications is the possibility of damage to the nerve root or spinal cord during placement of the needle. Another common complication is neuritis. Again, there is a slight possibility of pneumothorax and hemothorax. These particular complications should be described in detail to any prospective candidate for RF lesioning at the thoracic level. Other possible complications include infection, increased pain, bleeding, and bruising. It cannot be overemphasized that the occurrence of pneumothorax should be excluded clinically. If any doubt remains, radiographs are mandatory.

Conclusion

The data on RF facet and RF-DRG at the thoracic levels published in the years 1994 to 1996 were all collected retrospectively. For this reason the level of evidence for the different procedures is low. In the case of thoracic segmental radicular pain, for which treatment of the DRG might be considered, we prefer PRF-DRG as the first step; this is in line with policy on the cervical level. There is no formal evidence for RF or PRF, but PRF is safer on this level. When PRF-DRG on the thoracic level has a temporary effect, RF-DRG can be considered.

RADIOFREQUENCY TREATMENT PROCEDURES ON THE LUMBAR SPINE

The annual incidence of low back pain was found to be 18.6% in an adult population.[112] The prognosis for this low back pain is not as good as we once believed. Spitzer and colleagues[113] stated that 92% of these patients recover 6 months after onset of the low back pain. However, recent reviews indicate that approximately 62% of patients with low back pain still experience pain after 12 months.[114,115] At this time there are few interventions with long-term effect on chronic low back pain. However, there are some evidence-based interventions with minimal clinical short-term effect, such as behavioral therapy, back schools, manipulation, and cyclooxygenase inhibitors.[116] The minority of patients with low back pain have specific causes of their pain, such as a herniated disk, spondylolisthesis, diskitis, or fractures. Most have undiagnosed low back pain. In such patients the back pain may emanate from potential painful structures, including the lumbar facet joints, the intervertebral disks, or the sacroiliac (SI) joints. The anatomy of the lumbar spine is illustrated in Figure 62.18.

LUMBAR ZYGAPOPHYSEAL (FACET JOINT) PAIN

The prevalence of facet joint pain in an adult population with low back pain was found to be 15% to 32%.[117] Patients with lumbar facet joint pain may exhibit paramedian pain (one or both sides), absence of exacerbation by coughing ($P \leq 0.07$), absence of exacerbation by forward flexion and rising from forward flexion ($P \leq 0.002$), absence of worsening by hyperextension, and pain immediately on standing and walking ($P \leq 0.001$).[118,119] The diagnosis is confirmed by at least a 50% reduction in pain after a diagnostic local anesthetic nerve block of the medial branch of the dorsal ramus.

Evidence

Technically, two prerequisites for success of RF facet treatment are identifying the painful facet joints with a diagnostic block and precisely localizing the nerve of the targeted facet joints.[120,121] Techniques for RF facet treatment vary nevertheless.

RF treatment is frequently performed for various forms of spinal pain, although scientific evidence for this intervention remains controversial. The first controlled study was published by Gallagher and coworkers in 1994.[122] The authors selected 41 patients with chronic low back pain who responded with some relief to diagnostic intra-articular injections and randomized them to receive either "sham" or true RF treatment of the medial branches. The two study groups were then subdivided into patients who obtained good relief from the test blocks and those who did not. In a well-designed placebo-controlled study, van Kleef and associates demonstrated good results after RF treatment that lasted up to 12 months.[123] Leclaire[121] and colleagues did not find a therapeutic effect of RF treatment in a placebo-controlled trial, but this study has been criticized because the criterion for a positive "diagnostic" block was relief of pain for 24 hours or longer after lidocaine infiltration, which is inconsistent with the drug's pharmacokinetics. In addition, 94% of the screened patients with back pain were selected for participation, which is much greater than the presumed prevalence of lumbar facetogenic pain (17% to 30%) in this cohort. For this reason this study is judged to have major methodologic flaws. van Wijk and coworkers also found no difference between the treatment and control groups with regard to VAS pain score, medication use, and function.[124] However, the RF group in this study did report a 50% or greater reduction in complaints significantly more often (62% vs. 39%) than in those who received a sham procedure. The evaluation method, though, was subject to discussion. Finally, in the most recent RCT undertaken in 40 patients who obtained significant pain relief following three diagnostic blocks, a significantly greater improvement in pain symptoms, global perception of improvement, and quality of life was observed after 6 months in subjects allocated to RF treatment.[125]

In two randomized studies comparing PRF and conventional RF treatment of facetogenic pain, both showed conventional RF to be superior.[126,127] From these seven controlled and a multitude of uncontrolled studies, one can

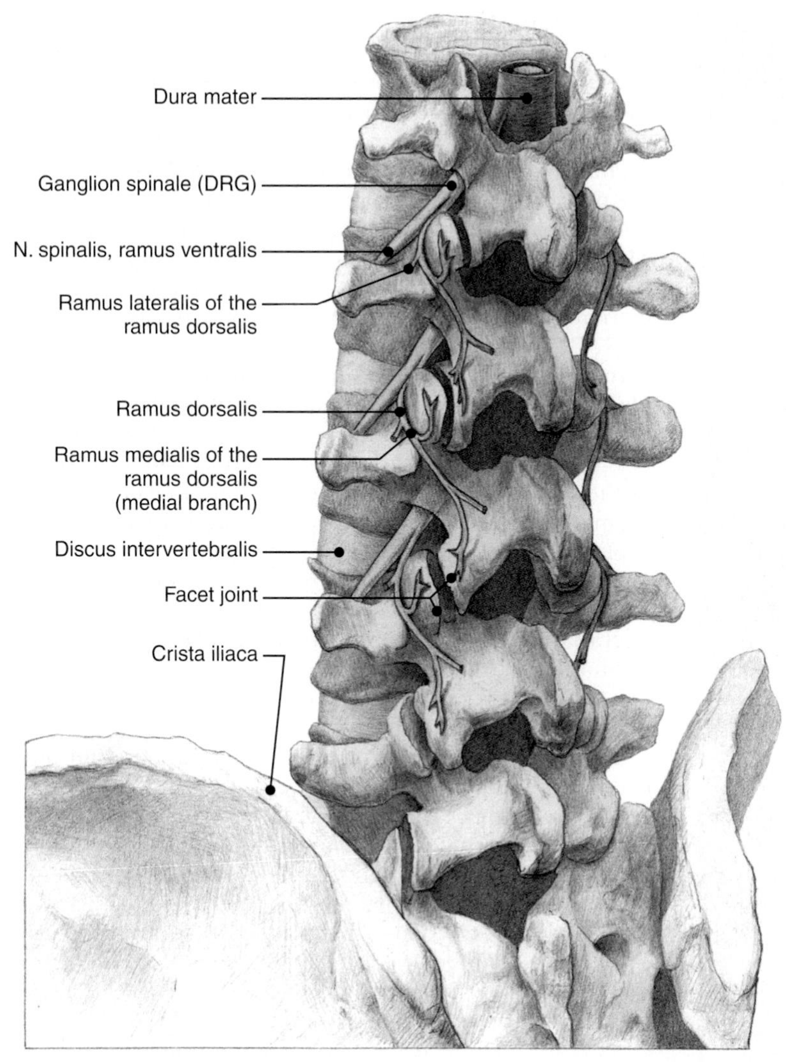

Figure 62.18 Anatomy of the lumbar spine. DRG, dorsal root ganglion. (Illustration courtesy of Rogier Trompert Medical Art. Available at www.Medicalart.nl.)

conclude that RF treatment of the facet joints can provide intermediate-term benefit in carefully selected patients.

Another prospective study, though not an RCT, is of additional importance when estimating the efficacy of RF facet treatment. Dreyfuss and associates[128] found that 60% of patients ($n = 9$) obtained at least a 90% reduction in pain at 12 months and 87% obtained at least 60% pain relief with RF facet treatment. Relief was associated with treatment of the multifidus muscle.[128] This study differs in three important aspects from all previous studies of RF facet treatment. First, the authors used a different protocol for the diagnostic blocks. Although Lord and coworkers[60] initially advocated the use of double-blind, placebo-controlled blocks to reach a precise diagnosis of "cervical" facet pain, Dreyfuss and colleagues used a modified comparative block protocol and omitted saline injections. For the first diagnostic nerve block, 0.5 mL of 2% lidocaine was injected. Patients reporting at least 80% pain relief for longer than 1 hour returned for confirmatory blocks with 0.5% bupivacaine. Patients exhibiting at least 80% pain relief for longer than 2 hours were then offered RF treatment. Second, this study used a different operative technique for RF facet treatment. Differences in comparison to other studies included the type of electrode (16-gauge Ray electrode), preoperative access to the target nerve, and coagulation of the targeted nerve 8 to 10 mm along its length, which entailed multiple lesioning. The meaning of multifidus stimulation and denervation is unclear and is still a subject of discussion.[129,130]

Procedure

The patient assumes a prone position on the fluoroscopic table. A pillow is placed under the abdomen to diminish the physiologic lumbar lordosis. First, targeted levels are identified and a straight AP projection is obtained. The C-arm is then rotated cranially or caudally until no double contours are visible on the caudal end plate of the middle vertebra. The middle vertebra of the levels to be treated is used as the reference point before the searching for the optimal position of the C-arm. Subsequently, the C-arm is rotated to an approximately 15-degree oblique view until the spinous processes are projecting over the midline but well inside the contralateral facet joints. The entry point should then be marked over the target point, which is the junction of the superior articular process and transverse process. To perform a diagnostic block, the target point should be approximately 1 mm under this junction to avoid unwanted spread of local anesthetic to segmental nerves and false-positive results. After injection of local anesthetic (1% lidocaine) into the skin, the needle is inserted at the entry point and slowly advanced via a tunnel vision technique until the tip makes contact with

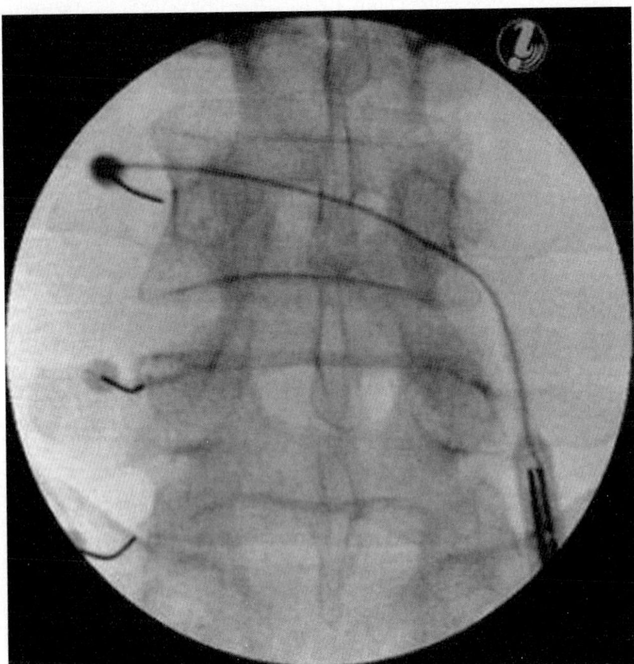

Figure 62.19 Needle position for a medial branch lumbar procedure.

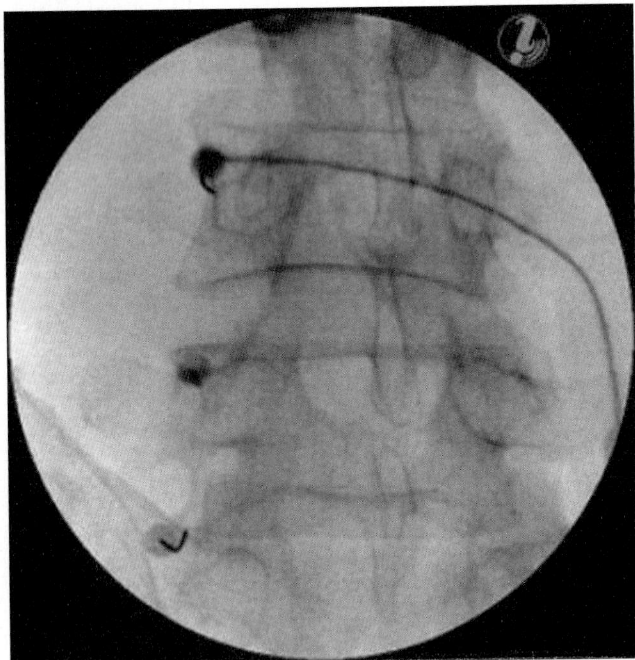

Figure 62.20 Rotated C-arm for a lumbar facet procedure.

bone. For a diagnostic block the position of the needle is checked on the lateral view and should be at the level of the inferior part of the intervertebral foramen, in line with the facet joint column. When accurate positioning is confirmed and after negative aspiration, 1 mL of local anesthetic (1% lidocaine) is injected at each level. To perform RF lesioning of the medial branch, after making bone contact with the tip of the needle, the needle is redirected slightly more cephalad until bone contact is lost, and the cannula is advanced 1 to 2 mm farther anteriorly over the superior margin of the transverse process (Figs. 62.19 and 62.20).

The C-arm is rotated into the lateral view to check the position of the needle tip, which should be in line with the facet joint column and at the level of the inferior part of the intervertebral foramen about 1 mm dorsal to the level of a line connecting the posterior aspects of the intervertebral foramina. It should be a little deeper and more cranial than the position of the needle for a diagnostic block. When this position is confirmed, stimulation at 50 Hz is conducted. The patient should feel new pressure or tingling in the back at less than 0.5 V. If sensations are felt in the ipsilateral extremity, the tip of the needle is too close to the segmental nerve. It is imperative that the needle be withdrawn slightly and stimulation checked again at 50 Hz. Subsequently, stimulation at 2 Hz is performed. The patient should experience localized contractions of the multifidus muscle and not of muscles of the leg. These local contractions can be palpated by the operator. Similarly, any contractions that occur in the leg may be detected by the operator or the assistant if a hand is placed over the muscles innervated by the exiting nerve root. If the patient perceives pain or contractions in the extremity or if muscular contractions are detected by the operator, the needle must be repositioned. After accurate positioning of the tip of the needle, 1 mL of local anesthetic (1% lidocaine) is injected at each level. RF lesioning at 67° C is performed for 60 seconds.

The fluoroscopic view for the L5-S1 facet joint and thus the medial branch of L5 is different from that for the other lumbar levels because of the difference in anatomy. The L5 medial branch lies at the junction between the superior sacral articular process and the upper border of the sacrum. Because there is no pedicle at this level to use as a radiologic landmark, the C-arm is positioned so that the junction is seen as a round curved transition. The C-arm is rotated slightly obliquely (about 15 degrees). The identified target point is the curve of the transition and is the same as the entry point. The needle is inserted via a tunnel view.

The depth of the needle is checked on a lateral radiograph to ensure that the tip projects over the posterior border of the facet column. Thereafter, the rest of the procedure is the same as described before. A 22-gauge, 10-cm SMK needle with a 5-mm active tip can be used to perform RF lesioning.

After the procedure the patient is allowed to go home, but driving a car or handling dangerous machinery is proscribed for 24 hours. In some cases there will be transient numbness of the ipsilateral extremity because of overflow of local anesthetic into the intervertebral foramen.

Side Effects and Complications

A retrospective analysis of the incidence of complications associated with fluoroscopically guided percutaneous RF treatment of the lumbar facet joints yielded a 1% overall incidence of minor complications per lesion site. With a total of 616 RF facet treatments, three cases of localized pain lasting longer than 2 weeks (0.5%) and three cases of neuritic pain lasting less than 2 weeks (0.5%) were noted. No cases of infection, new motor deficits, or new sensory deficits were identified.[131]

LUMBAR RADICULAR PAIN

Percutaneous RF-DRG was developed in the 1980s as an alternative to surgical rhizotomy for chronic refractory pain.[132] Although surgical rhizotomy initially led to impressive short-term pain relief in patients with various pain syndromes,[133] in the long term a dramatic loss of efficacy occurred, accompanied by severe adverse effects if substantial denervation had been carried out.[134]

The rationale for use of RF-DRG for lumbosacral radicular pain is based on the concept that nociceptive input at the level of the primary sensory neuron might be reduced by coagulation of a small part of the DRG without causing a sensory deficit.[135] It has been stressed that RF-DRG should be restricted to "high-input" nociceptive spinal pain syndromes. In the presence of deafferentation symptoms, RF-DRG might lead to aggravation of the pain complaints.[11] Moreover, mechanical entrapment of the nerve with combined back pain and radiculopathy must be excluded as a contributing factor before proceeding with RF-DRG. To minimize the risk for deafferentation pain, an RF-DRG heat lesion should not be used if neurologic deficits are present (i.e., reflexes, sensibility, and motor function). Thus, if diagnostic sleeve root injections were beneficial and surgical interventions are not indicated, RF-DRG can be considered.

Procedure for Radiofrequency Treatment of the Dorsal Root Ganglion

RF-DRG is aimed at creating a minimal lesion near the DRG for treating nerve root pain without causing neurologic deficits.[136] For this purpose, at the lumbar levels a 10-cm electrode (22 gauge, 5-mm active tip) is placed in the dorsal cranial quadrant of the intervertebral foramen (lateral view) and introduced with its tip between a third and about halfway across the midfacetal column on the AP projection (Fig. 62.21).

Sensory and motor stimulation is applied at 50 and 2 Hz. The position of the electrode is adjusted if necessary to reach a sensory stimulation threshold of between 0.5 and 1.0 V. The motor stimulation threshold is required to be at least 1.5 times the sensory stimulation threshold. A final check of the electrode's position is made by injecting radiopaque contrast dye to visualize the nerve root and ganglion. Subsequently, a local anesthetic is injected through the cannula to achieve dense anesthesia. RF treatment is usually performed at 65° C to 67° C for 90 seconds. At the sacral level the position of the DRG is first visualized with radiopaque contrast dye injected through a 22-gauge needle placed in the dorsal sacral foramen of the corresponding nerve root. Subsequently, a small hole is drilled with a Kirschner wire and a pneumatic drill through the overlying sacral bone to obtain access to the dorsal ganglion. The remainder of the procedure is identical to that at the lumbar level.

Evidence for Radiofrequency Treatment of the Dorsal Root Ganglion

In patients with radiating lower limb pain, one prospective[137] and several retrospective studies[10,132,138-140] reported beneficial effects of lumbosacral RF-DRG in 32% to 76% of cases. In a previous retrospective study, 279 patients underwent RF-DRG because of chronic spinal pain radiating to the leg, and an initial success rate of approximately 60% was reported.[140] In successful patients, the mean duration of reduction in pain was 3.7 years. One sham lesion–controlled RCT to assess the efficacy of RF-DRG for lumbosacral radicular pain has been performed. In this study, lumbosacral RF-DRG failed to show advantage over sham treatment with local anesthetics.[141] Since there is no clear evidence of the efficacy of RF-DRG treatment and it might be contraindicated in patients with a neuropathic component, we therefore prefer PRF-DRG.

Pulsed Radiofrequency Treatment of the Dorsal Root Ganglion

PRF-DRG uses intermittent high-frequency current, thus avoiding a rise in temperature above the critical level of 42° C, which is described as the temperature that causes neuronal damage.[142,143] Therefore, PRF-DRG is considered to be safer than conventional RF-DRG. Since the introduction of PRF-DRG in 1998, no neurologic complications have been reported, only minor postprocedural discomfort.[144]

Procedure. The approach is identical to that described for RF-DRG; however, the threshold for sensory stimulation should be less than 0.5 V to maximally reach the DRG. If this is obtained, a pulsed current (routinely a 20-msec current and 480 msec without current) is applied for 120 seconds with an output of 45 V. During this procedure the temperature at the tip of the electrode should not surpass 42° C.

RADIOFREQUENCY TREATMENT OF THE SACROILIAC JOINT

SI joint pain may result from sacroiliitis (Bechterew's disease), infections, spondyloarthropathy, pyogenic or crystal arthropathy, fracture of the sacrum and pelvis, and diastasis.[145] Primary pain emanating from the SI joint in the absence of demonstrable pathology is thought to be of mechanical origin and is termed "sacroiliac syndrome." Fifteen percent to 25% of low back pain originates from the SI joints.[146,147]

Patients with SI joint pain may have one-sided or two-sided low back pain below the level of L5. Generally, it is localized to the gluteal region (94%).[148] The typical radiation pattern of SI joint pain is illustrated in Figure 62.22. Clinical suspicion for this syndrome may increase when three of five provocative tests for SI joint pain during physical examination are positive.[149] The lateral branches of the L4-S3 dorsal rami are cited as the major innervation of the posterior SI joint.[146] Other investigators claim that L3 and S4 contribute to the posterior nerve supply.[150,151] Innervation of the anterior joint is similarly ambiguous. Currently, the diagnosis can be confirmed by means of at least one diagnostic nerve block of L4 and L5 and lateral branch blocks of S1-3. Dreyfuss demonstrated the superiority of multisite, multidepth sacral lateral blocks over single-site, single-depth blocks.[152]

Evidence

Numerous uncontrolled studies and one controlled study have been published on RF treatment of the SI joint.[146] However, these studies are characterized by wide disparities in technique, selection criteria, and standards of success. The one RCT consisted of 28 patients and sham treatment in the control group and showed significant improvement in pain and function in the treatment group. In this study cooled RF treatment was used.[153] Although these results seem promising, the efficacy of RF treatment of the SI joint for SI syndrome remains to be reproduced by larger RCTs.

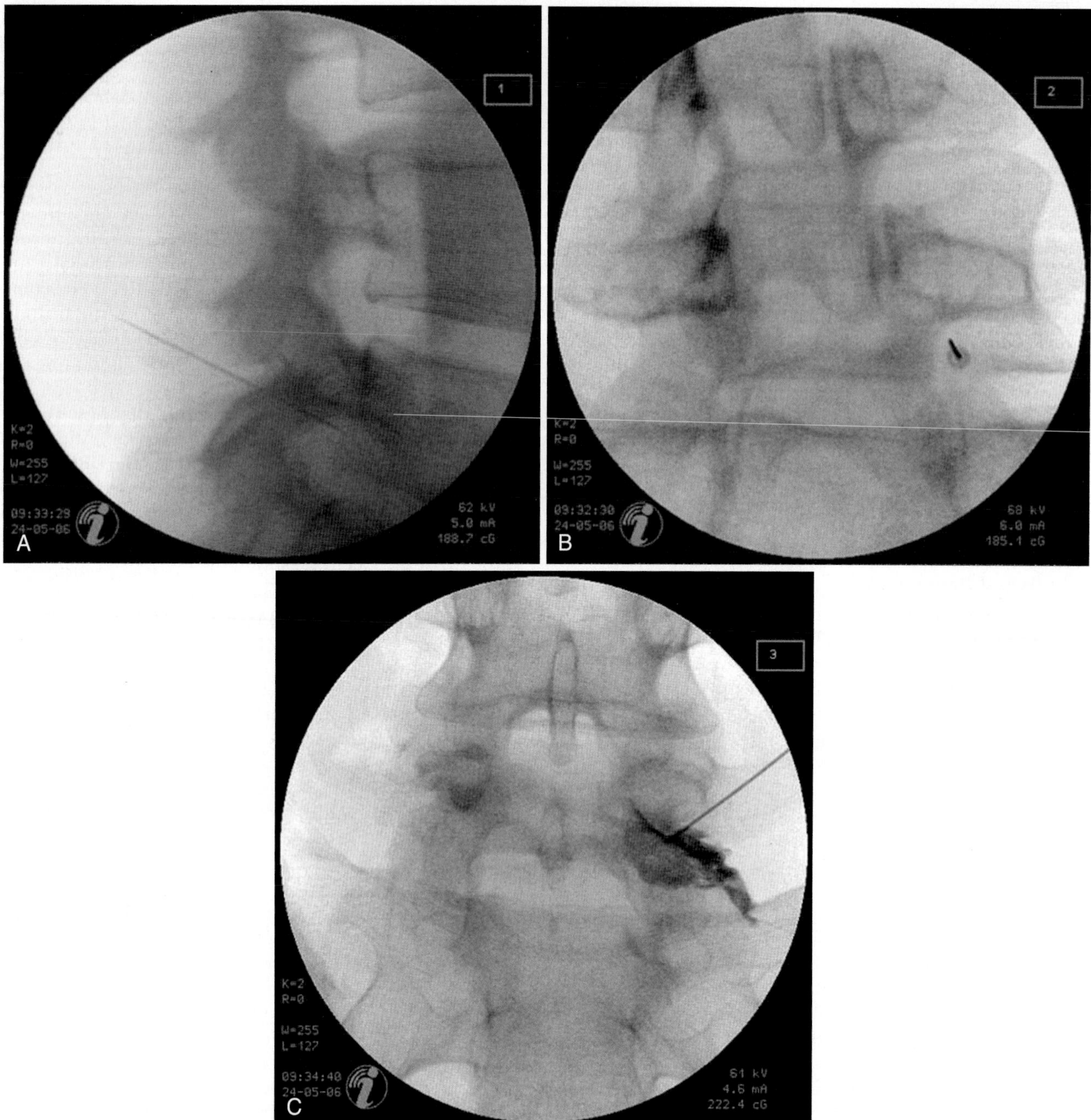

Figure 62.21 **A,** Lateral view of the needle in the superior part of the intervertebral foramen of L5. **B,** Slightly oblique view of the position of the needle for lumbar radiofrequency treatment adjacent to the dorsal root ganglion of L5. **C,** Anteroposterior view of pulsed radiofrequency treatment adjacent to the dorsal root ganglion. Note the spread of contrast medium.

Cooled Radiofrequency Treatment

The theoretical advantage of cooled RF electrodes is that they create larger lesions than conventional RF electrodes do.[154] Larger lesions may overcome anatomic variation in the targeted nerves and are more likely to interrupt the afferent lateral branches. Such lesions are created by circulation of cooling water during the delivery of RF current. The circulating water removes heat from tissue adjacent to the electrode, thereby allowing power delivery to be increased without causing high impedance and tissue charring around the electrode.[154-156]

As stated earlier, there are reports in favor of cooled RF over "classic" RF techniques for the treatment of SI joint pain, but larger, multicenter studies with long-term follow-up and comprehensive outcome measures are needed to confirm these findings. Furthermore, the additional cost of the disposable components needed for a cooled RF procedure should be taken into consideration.[157]

Procedure

Because of variable and extensive innervations of the dorsal SI joint, targeting the nerves innervating the joint with RF methods is sometimes difficult with single-lesion techniques.[132] We use the following technique. In patients with a positive diagnostic block, RF treatment is performed

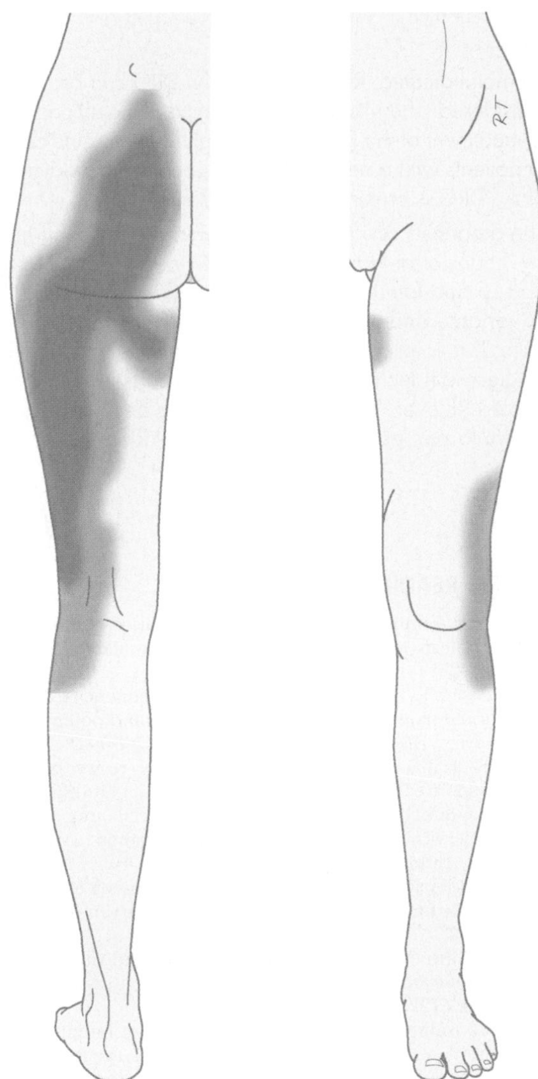

Figure 62.22 Typical pain referral pattern of sacroiliac joint pain. (Illustration courtesy of Rogier Trompert Medical Art. Available at www.Medicalart.nl.)

under fluoroscopic guidance. With the C-arm intensifier positioned to confer either a slightly oblique view (L4 dorsal ramus), AP view (L5 dorsal ramus and lateral branches), or cephalocaudad view (lateral branches), 22-gauge SMK-C10 cannulas with 5-mm active tips are inserted until bone contact is made at the location of the target nerve. Correct placement is confirmed by electrostimulation at 50 Hz, with concordant pain being noted at or below 0.6 V at all levels from L4 to S2.

With right-sided lateral branch blocks at the S1-2 levels, the optimum stimulation pattern is found anywhere between the 1:00- and 5:30-o'clock position directly outside the posterior foramen on the surface of the sacrum. For left-sided blocks, optimum stimulation was usually found between 7:00 and 11:00 o'clock. In some patients a concordant stimulation pattern cannot be obtained at less than 0.8 V for the S3 lateral branch. In such cases, two empirically made lesions are recommended, at 2:30 and 4:30 o'clock for right-sided S3 lateral branch blocks and at 7:30 and 9:30 o'clock for left-sided lateral branch blocks. Before

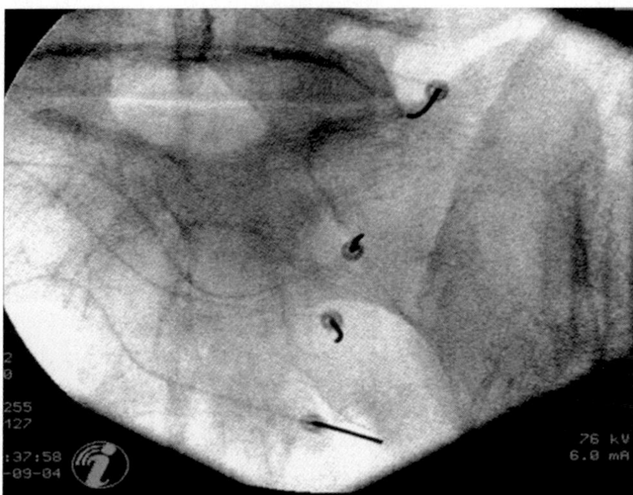

Figure 62.23 Position of the needle for radiofrequency treatment of the sacroiliac joint.

lesioning, the absence of contractions in leg muscles was verified at three times the stimulation threshold. When fluoroscopic images and stimulation parameters indicate correct electrode placement, 0.3 mL of 2% lidocaine is injected through each cannula for local anesthesia. The RF probe is then reinserted, and a 90-second 80° C lesion is made.[136] Needle placement for the RF SI procedure is illustrated in Figure 62.23.

CONCLUSION

RF treatment of chronic pain syndromes has seen a remarkable evolution over the past decade; RF current can now be applied in continuous and pulsed fashion. The former application method generates heat lesions, whereas the latter induces changes in nerve cells. Besides studies on efficacy and safety, computer modeling and in vitro and animal experiments have begun to shed light on the potential mode of action of PRF. Evidence from good-quality studies demonstrates that continuous RF and PRF can be applied to effectively treat some chronic pain syndromes. When performed in well-selected patients, who often suffer pain refractory to conventional treatment, the degree of pain relief can be higher than with conventional treatment. Moreover, in contrast to drug studies, the follow-up period is much longer and thus provides proof of long-term efficacy. RF treatment can produce minor, immediate side effects that typically resolve spontaneously within a short time. Major neurologic complications are rare but have been reported with conventional heat lesioning, though not with PRF. Because of the low neurodestructive potential, PRF is our choice for treatment of the DRG. A randomized-controlled trial comparing PRF with sham intervention adjacent to the cervical DRG for cervical radicular pain showed a higher success rate in the PRF group at 3 months.[87] These encouraging results point to the urgent need for further studies on this promising nondestructive mode of treatment. In future studies attempts should be made to assess a homogeneous patient population with specified pathology.

KEY POINTS

- Radiofrequency (RF) treatment consists of the application of a high-frequency current by a needle to specific anatomic structures. RF current heats the tissue surrounding the tip of the needle. In interventional pain procedures, these small heat lesions cause selective denervation.
- A new development is pulsed RF (PRF). Application of PRF reduces heat and probably works by creating electrical fields. Indications are neuropathic pain syndromes. Other indications are subject to research.
- An accepted indication for RF treatment of the head region is trigeminal neuralgia (RF of the gasserian ganglion). Neurologic evaluation is mandatory to exclude red flags for treatment. The first step in treatment is medication. RF treatment of the pterygopalatine ganglion can be used for cluster headache and some atypical facial syndromes.
- Indications for RF treatment of the medial branches of the cervical facet joints include degenerative and post-traumatic neck pain. RF treatment of the (higher) cervical facet joints for cervicogenic headache awaits further research. RF facet joint treatment is usually performed at two or three segmental levels since there is overlap in innervation of the facet joints.
- Segmental pain in the upper extremity can be caused by spinal nerve irritation. The involved spinal level can be estimated by the dermatome in which the pain is radiating and can be confirmed by diagnostic nerve blocks. PRF treatment of the dorsal root ganglion (DRG) is safer and has fewer side effects than RF treatment does.
- Thoracic pain may have an underlying pathology. When thoracic spinal pain becomes chronic and resistant to conservative treatment, minimally invasive treatment modalities, including RF lesioning of the facet joints, can be considered. We perform RF treatment on three levels because of the multisegmental innervation of the facet joints. Obtaining a fluoroscopic view is difficult because of overprojection of the ribs and the prominent transverse process.
- Percutaneous RF treatment adjacent to the thoracic DRG has been described for segmental nerve pain. A prognostic blockade is essential before RF treatment. PRF treatment of the DRG is preferred in cases of thoracic segmental radicular pain for which treatment of the DRG might be considered. An important potential complication is the possibility of damage to the nerve root or spinal cord during placement of the needle.
- The diagnosis of lumbar facet joint pain has to be confirmed by a diagnostic local anesthetic nerve block of the medial branch innervating the lumbar facet joints. Conventional RF, in contrast to PRF, can provide intermediate-term benefit in carefully selected patients.
- Mechanical entrapment of the segmental nerve in patients with combined back pain and radiculopathy must be excluded as a contributing factor before proceeding with RF treatment of the DRG. If diagnostic sleeve root injections were beneficial and surgical interventions

KEY POINTS—cont'd

are not indicated, RF treatment of the DRG can be considered. There is no clear evidence of the efficacy of RF treatment of the DRG, and it might be contraindicated in patients with a neuropathic component; PRF treatment of the DRG is preferred in these instances.
- The diagnosis of sacroiliac joint pain can be confirmed by means of at least one diagnostic nerve block of L4 and L5 and lateral branch blocks of S1-3. Because of variable and extensive innervations of the dorsal sacroiliac joint, RF methods are sometimes difficult with single-lesion techniques. There are reports in favor of cooled RF over "classic" RF techniques because they create larger lesions than conventional RF does.

SUGGESTED READINGS

Cahana A, Van Zundert J, Macrea L, et al. Pulsed radiofrequency: current clinical and biological literature available. *Pain Med.* 2006;7:411-423.

Chua NH, Vissers KC, Sluijter ME. Pulsed radiofrequency treatment in interventional pain management: mechanisms and potential indications—a review. *Acta Neurochir (Wien).* 2011;153:763-771.

Cohen SP. Sacroiliac joint pain: a comprehensive review of anatomy, diagnosis, and treatment. *Anesth Analg.* 2005;101:1440-1453.

Cohen SP, Bajwa ZH, Kraemer JJ, et al. Factors predicting success and failure for cervical facet radiofrequency denervation: a multi-center analysis. *Reg Anesth Pain Med.* 2007;32:495-503.

Cohen SP, Hurley RW, Christo PJ, et al. Clinical predictors of success and failure for lumbar facet radiofrequency denervation. *Clin J Pain.* 2007;23:45-52.

Dreyfuss P, Halbrook B, Pauza K, et al. Efficacy and validity of radiofrequency neurotomy for chronic lumbar zygapophysial joint pain. *Spine.* 2000;25:1270-1277.

Dreyfuss P, Henning T, Malladi N, et al. The ability of multi-site, multi-depth sacral lateral branch blocks to anesthetize the sacroiliac joint complex. *Pain Med.* 2009;10:679-688.

Kanpolat Y, Savas A, Bekar A, et al. Percutaneous controlled radiofrequency trigeminal rhizotomy for the treatment of idiopathic trigeminal neuralgia: 25-year experience with 1,600 patients. *Neurosurgery.* 2001;48:524-532: discussion 532-534.

Lord SM, Barnsley L, Wallis BJ, et al. Percutaneous radio-frequency neurotomy for chronic cervical zygapophyseal-joint pain. *N Engl J Med.* 1996;335:1721-1726.

Nath S, Nath CA, Pettersson K. Percutaneous lumbar zygapophysial (facet) joint neurotomy using radiofrequency current, in the management of chronic low back pain: a randomized double-blind trial. *Spine.* 2008;33:1291-1297: discussion 1298.

Sanders M, Zuurmond WW. Efficacy of sphenopalatine ganglion blockade in 66 patients suffering from cluster headache: a 12- to 70-month follow-up evaluation. *J Neurosurg.* 1997;87:876-880.

Stolker RJ, Vervest AC, Groen GJ. The treatment of chronic thoracic segmental pain by radiofrequency percutaneous partial rhizotomy. *J Neurosurg.* 1994;80:986-992.

Van Boxem K, van Bilsen J, de Meij N, et al. Pulsed radiofrequency treatment adjacent to the lumbar dorsal root ganglion for the management of lumbosacral radicular syndrome: a clinical audit. *Pain Med.* 2011;12:1322-1330.

van Boxem K, van Eerd M, Brinkhuizen T, et al. Radiofrequency and pulsed radiofrequency treatment of chronic pain syndromes: the available evidence. *Pain Pract.* 2008;8:385-393.

van Eerd M, Patijn J, Lataster A, et al. 5. Cervical facet pain. *Pain Pract.* 2010;10:113-123.

van Kleef M, Liem L, Lousberg R, et al. Radiofrequency lesion adjacent to the dorsal root ganglion for cervicobrachial pain: a prospective double blind randomized study. *Neurosurgery.* 1996;38:1127-1131, discussion 1131-1132.

van Kleef M, Spaans F, Dingemans W, et al. Effects and side effects of a percutaneous thermal lesion of the dorsal root ganglion in patients with cervical pain syndrome. *Pain*. 1993;52:49-53.

Van Zundert J, de Louw AJ, Joosten EA, et al. Pulsed and continuous radiofrequency current adjacent to the cervical dorsal root ganglion of the rat induces late cellular activity in the dorsal horn. *Anesthesiology*. 2005;102:125-131.

Van Zundert J, Patijn J, Kessels A, et al. Pulsed radiofrequency adjacent to the cervical dorsal root ganglion in chronic cervical radicular pain: a double blind sham controlled randomized clinical trial. *Pain*. 2007;127:173-182.

Zakrzewska JM, Thomas DG. Patient's assessment of outcome after three surgical procedures for the management of trigeminal neuralgia. *Acta Neurochir (Wien)*. 1993;122:225-230.

The references for this chapter can be found at www.expertconsult.com.

63

Sacroiliac Joint Syndrome: Sacroiliac Joint Injections and Block/Radiofrequency of the Lateral Branches

Ashley Agerson | Honorio T. Benzon | Khalid Malik

SACROILIAC JOINT SYNDROME

The pathologic conditions that affect the sacroiliac (SI) joint are myriad, including inflammatory, degenerative, traumatic, metabolic, infectious, neoplastic, and iatrogenic conditions, as well as sacroiliac joint syndrome. *Sacroiliac joint dysfunction,* or *SI joint syndrome,* is pain originating in the sacroiliac joint (SIJ) without a demonstrable anatomic lesion and presumed to be due to a biochemical abnormality.[1] Predisposing factors include conditions that cause unusual stress on the joint such as spinal deformity, previous spinal surgery, and leg length discrepancy. Pathology and pain from surrounding structures, such as intervertebral disks and lumbar facet joints, can result in SI joint pain caused by postural changes with resulting increased stress on the SI joint. Pregnancy also predisposes to SI joint pain, which is thought to result from ligament laxity mediated by the hormone *relaxin.* Patients may report a history of minor trauma, such as lifting a heavy object while in a twisted position, or mis-stepping off a curb.[2] The incidence of SI joint dysfunction in patients with back pain ranges from 15% to 30%.

Symptoms of SI joint dysfunction include pain in the superior medial quadrant of the buttock, the lateral buttock, and inferior to the posterosuperior iliac spine, with radiation to the greater trochanter, upper lateral thigh, and groin (Fig. 63.1).[1,3-6] Less commonly, the pain may radiate to the posterior thigh and leg below the knee. Two distinguishing features of the pain from SI joint dysfunction are the presence of groin pain and the absence of pain above the level of L5.[1,6] In contrast to the pain distribution of SI joint dysfunction, the typical pattern of pain from facet joint syndrome includes the low back with radiation to the posterior thigh down to the knee, whereas the pain from a herniated disk usually extends to the leg and foot. Bending, sitting, and riding typically aggravate pain in sacroiliac joint dysfunction, and walking or standing relieves it.

Physical examination of the patient with SI joint syndrome usually reveals tenderness over the posterior aspect of the joint and the sacral sulcus. There are no neurologic symptoms such as numbness or weakness. There are several provocative maneuvers designed to stress the SI joint and elicit concordant pain, including the FABER (flexion, abduction, and external rotation)-Patrick's test, Gaenslen's test, Yeoman's (extension) test,[7,8] sacroiliac or posterior shear test, and Gillet's test.[3,8,9]

FABER-PATRICK'S TEST (LEFT SACROILIAC JOINT DYSFUNCTION) (FIG. 63.2)

- Patient is supine.
- Left leg, near the ankle, is placed in front of the right thigh above the knee.
- The physician places one hand over the right iliac crest while the other hand pushes over the medial aspect of the left knee.
- Positive test: Pain over sacroiliac joint region (also back, buttock, groin).
- Comment: Test stresses sacroiliac and hip joint.

GAENSLEN'S TEST (LEFT SACROILIAC JOINT DYSFUNCTION) (FIG. 63.3)

- Patient is supine.
- Left lower thigh and leg hang over the examination table.
- The examiner flexes right hip and right knee (i.e., hip joint is maximally flexed). The examiner presses downward over the left thigh (hip joint is hyperextended).
- Positive test: Pain in the left sacroiliac joint.
- Comments: Test stresses both sacroiliac joints simultaneously by counter-rotation at the extreme range of motion of the joint. Test also stresses the hip joint and stretches the femoral nerve (examiner should ensure the absence of hip pathology or conditions affecting the femoral nerve to diagnose sacroiliac joint syndrome).

YEOMAN'S TEST (ALSO CALLED EXTENSION TEST (FIG. 63.4)

- Patient is prone.
- Examiner places one hand above the anterior aspect of the knee and elevates it slightly; the other hand presses downward over the crest of the ilium.
- Positive test: Pain over the posterior sacroiliac joint.

• Comments: The hip is extended and the ipsilateral ilium is rotated. Test stresses the sacroiliac joint; it also extends the lumbar spine and stresses the femoral nerve. More specific and reliable compared to the other tests.

GILLET'S TEST (FIG. 63.5)

• Patient is standing.
• One of the examiner's thumbs is placed on the second sacral spinous process; the other thumb is placed on the posterior superior iliac spine (PSIS).
• Normal sacroiliac joint: When the patient maximally flexes the hip, the PSIS moves inferior to the S2 spinous process.
• Dysfunctional or fixed sacroiliac joint: PSIS remains at the level of the S2 spinous process or moves superior to the sacrum.

SACROILIAC SHEAR TEST (FIG. 63.6)

• Patient is prone.
• Palm of the examiner's hand is placed over the posterior iliac wing. Shear thrust is directed inferiorly, producing a shearing force across the sacroiliac joint.
• Positive test: Pain in dysfunctional sacroiliac joint.

Pain secondary to SI joint syndrome is difficult to isolate, making these tests neither highly sensitive nor specific. The FABER-Patrick's test also stresses the hip joint, Gaenslen's test stresses the hip joint and stretches the femoral nerve, and Gillet's test can be difficult to perform. Although the Yeoman's test stretches the femoral nerve and extends the lumbar spine, it appears to be a more specific and reliable maneuver.[8] Some experts require the presence of three positive screening tests to confirm SI joint dysfunction.

The tests do not by themselves suggest the presence of SI joint dysfunction. Indeed, up to 2% of asymptomatic patients were found to have positive findings in one or more of these tests.[9] Rather, the diagnosis of SI joint dysfunction is made based on the combination of history, symptoms, and physical examination findings. The maneuvers are of added value in confirming the diagnosis when the symptoms suggest SI joint syndrome and other causes of pain have been eliminated. The presence of tenderness over the sacral sulcus, pain over the SI joint, buttock pain, and the patient pointing to the posterior superior iliac spine as the main source of pain showed better sensitivity than the other tests evaluated.[1]

Radiographic evaluation of the joint rarely aids diagnosis. Diagnostic local anesthetic block of the joint is considered

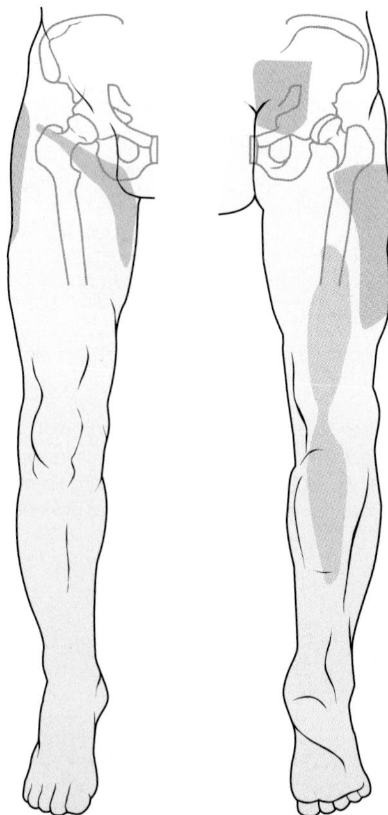

Figure 63.1 Pattern of pain from sacroiliac joint syndrome. (From Benzon HT. Pain originating from the buttock: sacroiliac joint dysfunction and piriformis syndrome. In: Benzon HT, Raja S, Molloy RE, et al, eds. *Essentials of Pain Medicine and Regional Anesthesia.* New York: Elsevier Churchill Livingstone; 2005:356-365, with permission.)

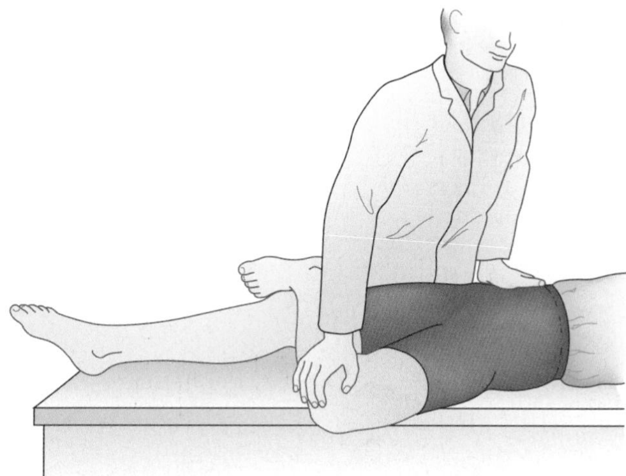

Figure 63.2 FABER-Patrick's test. (From Benzon HT. Pain originating from buttock: sacroiliac joint syndrome and piriformis syndrome. In: Benzon HT, Raja SN, Molloy RE, et al, eds. *Essentials of Pain Medicine and Regional Anesthesia.* 2nd ed. Philadelphia: Elsevier; 2005.)

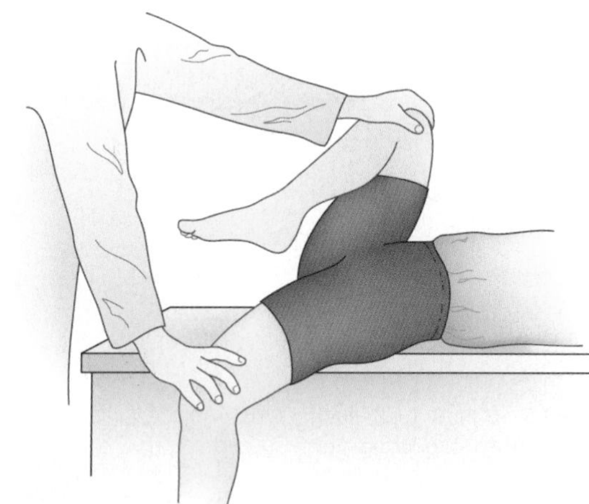

Figure 63.3 Gaenslen's test. (From Benzon HT. Pain originating from buttock: sacroiliac joint syndrome and piriformis syndrome. In: Benzon HT, Raja SN, Molloy RE, et al, eds. *Essentials of Pain Medicine and Regional Anesthesia.* 2nd ed. Philadelphia: Elsevier; 2005.)

to be the standard criterion for SI joint pain, although provocation of pain on injection of the SI joint is not a suitable criterion of SI joint dysfunction.[6]

ANATOMY

The sacroiliac (SI) joint is considered a diarthrodial joint because it contains synovial fluid, the articulating bones have ligamentous connections, the outer fibrous joint capsule has an inner synovial lining, and the cartilaginous surfaces allow motion to occur.[2] The sacral side of the joint is thicker and made up of hyaline cartilage, whereas the iliac side is made up of thin fibrocartilage. The adult joint has irregular and coarse surfaces that increase with age, reflecting the stress to which the joint is exposed.[10] The irregular contour of the joint contributes to its stability; the function of the joint is to transmit or dissipate the loading of the trunk to the lower extremities.

The ligaments of the SI joint include the anterior sacroiliac ligament, interosseous ligament, and posterior sacroiliac ligament (Fig. 63.7). The anterior sacroiliac ligament traverses the ilium to the sacrum, and the posterior sacroiliac ligament traverses the posterior iliac ridge to the sacrum. The interosseous ligament is responsible for the stability of the joint. The sacrotuberous ligament, which is superficial to the posterior SI ligament, has multiple muscle attachments including the gluteus maximus, piriformis, and long head of the biceps femoris. These multiple muscle attachments provide stability during activities such as sitting, walking, and standing, which stress the sacroiliac joint.[2] The sacroiliac joint is innervated at its anterior and posterior aspects. Its variable and extensive innervation accounts for the multiple presentations and variable referred pain patterns of sacroiliac joint pain.[7] Posteriorly, the joint is innervated by the lateral branches of the posterior primary ramus of the L4 to S4 dorsal rami.[11,12] The predominant innervation is from the dorsal ramus of S1,[13] and there are isolated dorsal innervations from S1-4.[14] The anterior innervation is from the ventral rami of the L5 to S2 and via branches from the sacral plexus.[11] The blood supply of the joint is from the anastomosis between the median sacral artery and lateral sacral branches from the internal iliac artery.

TECHNIQUE OF SACROILIAC JOINT INJECTION

For diagnostic injections, patients are asked to stop their pain medication on the day of the procedure. Sedation is usually not required but light sedation (1 to 2 mg intravenous midazolam) may be given in a nervous patient.

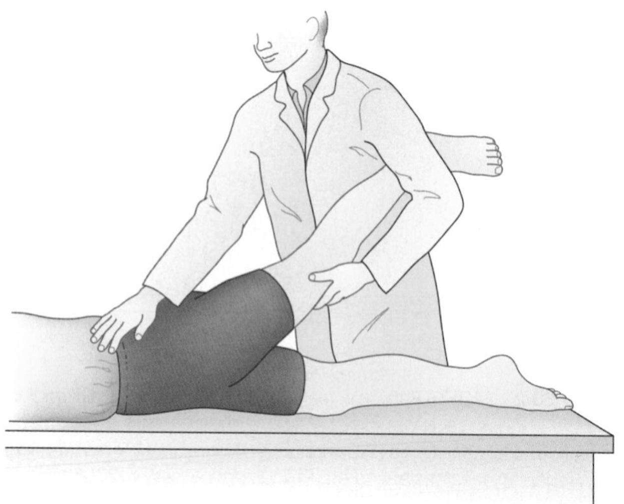

Figure 63.4 Yeoman's test (also called the extension test). (From Benzon HT. Pain originating from buttock: sacroiliac joint syndrome and piriformis syndrome. In: Benzon HT, Raja SN, Molloy RE, et al, eds. *Essentials of Pain Medicine and Regional Anesthesia.* 2nd ed. Philadelphia: Elsevier; 2005.)

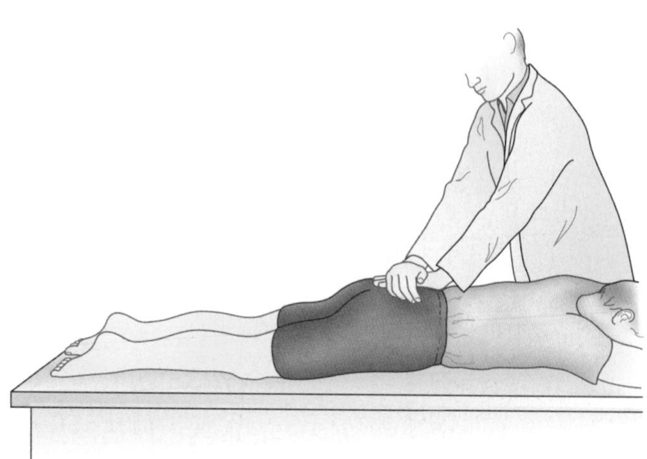

Figure 63.6 Sacroiliac shear test. (From Benzon HT. Pain originating from buttock: sacroiliac joint syndrome and piriformis syndrome. In: Benzon HT, Raja SN, Molloy RE, et al, eds. *Essentials of Pain Medicine and Regional Anesthesia.* 2nd ed. Philadelphia: Elsevier; 2005.)

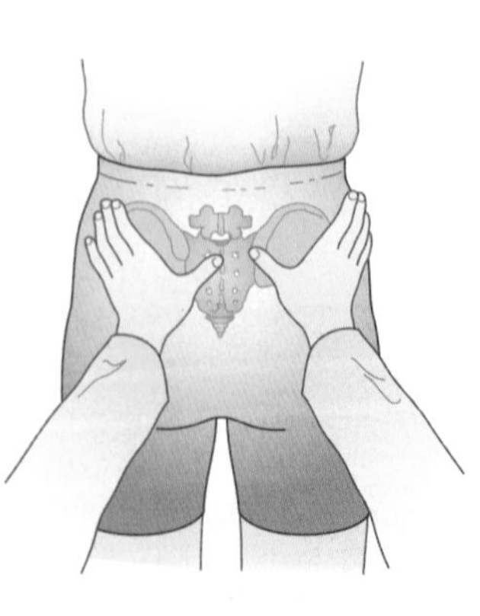

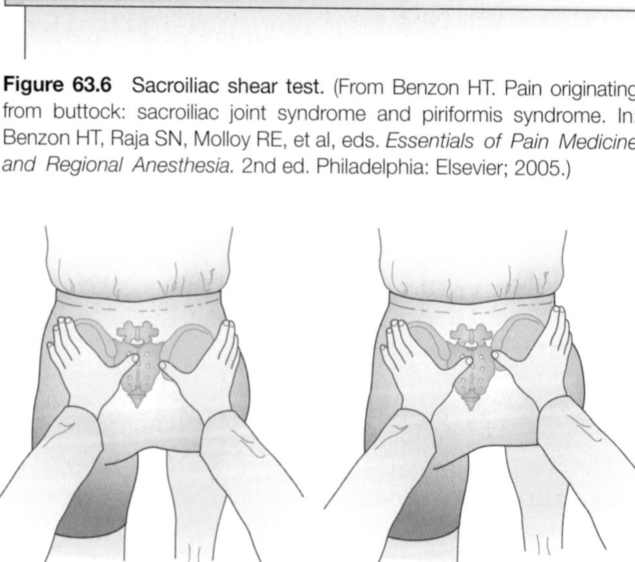

Figure 63.5 Gillet's test. (From Benzon HT. Pain originating from buttock: sacroiliac joint syndrome and piriformis syndrome. In: Benzon HT, Raja SN, Molloy RE, et al, eds. *Essentials of Pain Medicine and Regional Anesthesia.* 2nd ed. Philadelphia: Elsevier; 2005.)

Contraindications to the injection include infection in the area and bleeding diathesis. Allergy to contrast media may require pretreatment with H_1 and H_2 antagonists, whereas allergy to local anesthetics may require identification of the appropriate local anesthetic to be used for the procedure. The use of imaging is recommended during SI joint injection to ensure intra-articular needle placement, as blind injections rarely result in correct needle positioning.[15]

FLUOROSCOPY-GUIDED SACROILIAC JOINT INJECTION

The patient is positioned prone on the table, with the head turned to one side. A pillow is placed under the abdomen to flex the spine. Under a straight anteroposterior (AP) view, the SI joint presents several lines that course caudocranially in a semiparallel fashion. The lateral line represents the ventral or anterior margin of the joint, and the medial line represents the dorsal or posterior margin of the joint.[16,17] The C-arm is initially rotated approximately 30 degrees caudal to the axial plane to better visualize the area underneath the posterior superior iliac spine and iliac crest. The C-arm is then angled obliquely to the contralateral side until the inferior joint space is clearly demarcated, usually between 5 and 20 degrees. The target point lies along the inferoposterior aspect of the joint, in the area 1 to 2 cm cephalad from its most caudal end.[16]

The area is prepped and draped in the usual sterile fashion. The skin is anesthetized with 1 to 2 mL 1% lidocaine via a 25-gauge needle. A 22-gauge spinal needle is advanced coaxially toward the inferior pole of the sacroiliac joint with intermittent images obtained at regular intervals (every 2- to 4-mm advancement of the needle) to confirm trajectory. When the posterior surface of the sacroiliac joint is contacted, the needle is advanced to just penetrate the joint capsule. A change in resistance is commonly felt as the needle passes through the capsular tissue, and the needle tip is often deflected slightly as it traces the surface of the ilium. Some patients have significant osteoarthritic changes that preclude needle entry into the joint, making periarticular infiltration necessary. Once the needle is within the joint, a small amount of contrast is injected to demonstrate intra-articular spread (Fig. 63.8). The response of the patient to the injection of contrast media is noted as either "no pain," "unfamiliar pain," or "similar pain" in comparison with the pain complaint.[6] After appropriate contrast spread, a solution of steroid and local anesthetic (40 to 60 mg of methylprednisolone or triamcinolone with 1 to 2 mL of 0.5% bupivacaine or ropivacaine) is injected. Because the capacity of the sacroiliac joint is small and distension may exacerbate pain, a maximum volume of 2 to 2.5 mL has been recommended for SI joint injections.[16,18] Spillage of injectate outside the SI joint is acceptable because some of the pain receptors are located outside the joint. Nociceptive fibers and receptors containing calcitonin gene-related peptide (CGRP) and substance P immunoreactive free nerve endings have been noted in the interosseous and anterior

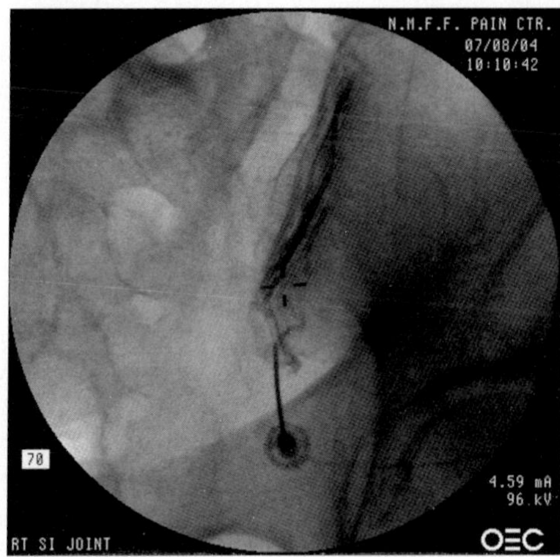

Figure 63.8 Sacroiliac joint injection. Note the spread of the dye along the joint.

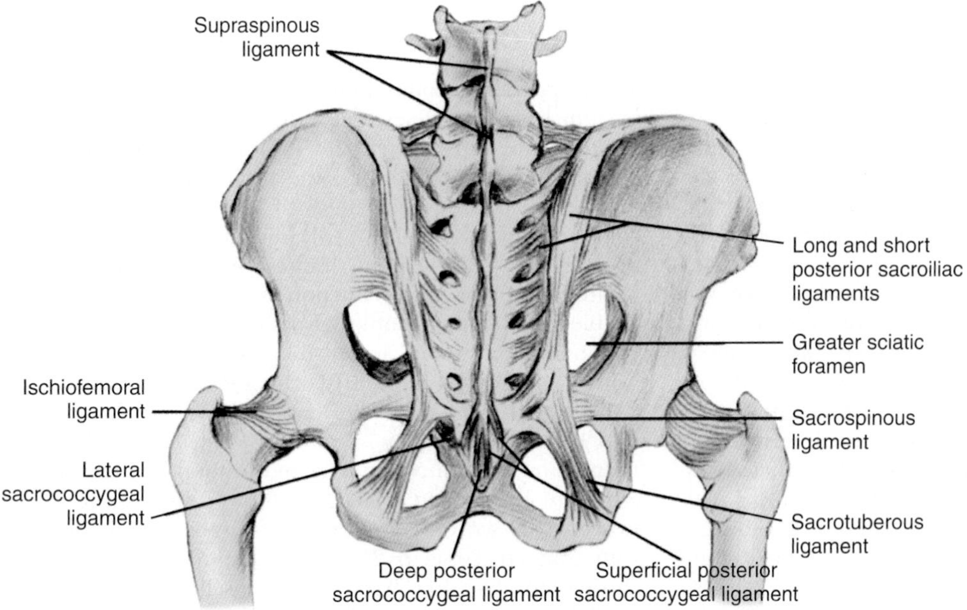

Figure 63.7 Ligaments of the sacroiliac joint. (From Cohen SP. Sacroiliac joint pain: a comprehensive review of anatomy, diagnosis, and treatment. *Anesth Analg.* 2005;101:1440-1453.)

ligaments of the SI joint by Szadek and colleagues.[19] In view of their findings, the authors recommended extra- as well as intra-articular approaches to diagnostic SI joint injection.

Other approaches include placement of the needle at the inferior end where the posterior and anterior joints overlap, if a markedly lucent zone is noted in that area.[16] The midportion of the joint also can be cannulated. With 20 to 30 degrees of contralateral obliquity, the medial and lateral planes of the joint overlap. The needle entry is at the most lucent zone of the joint space; a 20- to 30-degree medial-to-lateral and 10- to 20-degree inferior direction of the needle approach has been recommended to gain entry into the midportion of the joint.[20] Finally, the superior aspect of the joint can be accessed with a cephalocaudad approach.

Directly after the procedure the patient should be observed for 15 to 30 minutes to determine analgesic response and to monitor for complications. The local anesthetic has an immediate effect, but the anti-inflammatory effect of the steroid develops over 3 to 5 days. A greater than 75% reduction of pain over the SI joint is considered to be a positive response.[6] Provocative maneuvers can be repeated to assess improvement. Transient weakness in the ipsilateral leg is due to spillage of local anesthetic onto the sacral nerve roots or the sciatic nerve. Other complications include bleeding, infection, exacerbation of pain, fever, transient difficulty voiding, and allergic reaction to components of the prep solution or injectate.[17]

ULTRASOUND-GUIDED SACROILIAC JOINT INJECTION

The feasibility of ultrasound-guided SI joint injections was initially shown by Pekkafahli and associates[21] and was further described by Harmon and O'Sullivan.[22] The patient is positioned prone with a pillow underneath the abdomen. A curvilinear low-frequency transducer (4 to 6 MHz) is placed perpendicular to the skin over the distal sacrum in the midline in a cross-sectional view (short axis) to identify the sacral hiatus. The probe is moved laterally until the lateral edge of the sacrum comes in view, then moved cephalad to find the medial aspect of the iliac bone. At this site the SIJ appears as a hypoechoic wedge-shaped structure (Fig. 63.9). The target area for injection is at the level of the second sacral foramen, which is approximately 2 to 3 cm above the caudal pole of the SI joint. Lidocaine 1% is injected subcutaneously at the medial edge of the probe. A 22-gauge needle is inserted and advanced in-plane with a lateral and anterior trajectory into the joint. After the needle is deep to the iliac bone it is no longer visible on ultrasound. A pop is felt once the synovial joint is penetrated. Visible spread of injectate outside of the joint indicates periarticular rather than intra-articular placement.

The accuracy of this technique has been assessed. Pekkafahli and coworkers noted marked improvement with operator experience, from a 60% success rate in their first 30 injections to a 94% success rate in their second 30 injections.[21] Klauser and colleagues evaluated ultrasound-guided SI joint injection in cadavers at two levels of the joint by comparing approaches at the level of the first sacral foramen versus those at the second sacral foramen.[23] Computed tomography (CT) examination showed 90% of the needles at the lower level to be within the SIJ versus 70% in the upper level. The same procedure resulted in an intra-articular placement rate of 100% in both locations (eight in the lower and two in the upper site) when performed in live patients.

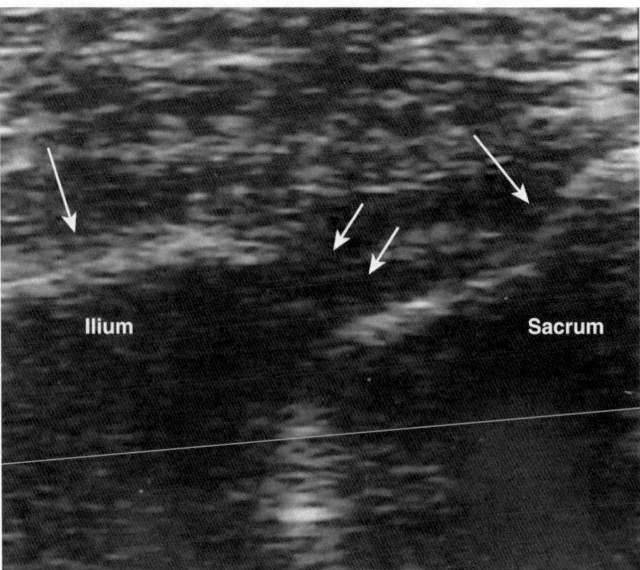

Figure 63.9 Ultrasound visualization of the sacroiliac joint. (From Pekkafahli MZ, Kiralp MZ, Basekim CC, et al. Sacroiliac joint injections performed with sonographic guidance. *J Ultrasound Med.* 2003;22: 553-559.)

COMPUTED TOMOGRAPHY–GUIDED SACROILIAC JOINT INJECTION

Injection of the SI joint has been described under computed tomography (CT) guidance.[24-26] The patient is positioned prone and the SI joint scanned. The best access point to the joint is determined and the gluteal injection point selected. The needle is inserted into the joint and steroid or local anesthetic is injected. Success rates from CT-guided injections range from 75%[26] to 92%,[24] with the duration of relief lasting 14 days[26] to 10 months.[24] The increased radiation exposure and lack of availability of CT in pain clinics restrict a wider application of this approach.

EFFICACY OF SACROILIAC JOINT INJECTIONS

The efficacy of sacroiliac joint injections has been examined in studies, meta-analyses, and reviews with discordant results. Multiple uncontrolled studies indicate that corticosteroid SIJ injections are helpful. Liliang and colleagues reported a prospective observational study of 39 patients with SIJ pain confirmed by two diagnostic SIJ injections.[27] Triamcinolone injection into the SI joint resulted in 67% of the patients having significant pain reduction for an average of 37 weeks (Table 63.1). Other studies also showed positive results in patients without spondyloarthropathies.[28-31] Bollow and associates studied CT-guided SIJ corticosteroid injections in 66 patients with back pain and known spondyloarthropathies; 92% had significant relief (average visual analog scale [VAS] reduction of 5 points) for a mean duration of 10 months.[24] Similarly, Braun and colleagues showed significant reduction in VAS score 5 months after CT-guided SIJ injection with triamcinolone in 25 of 30 patients with spondyloarthropathies and low back pain.[32] Fischer and coworkers performed corticosteroid SI joint injections in 56 children

Table 63.1 Efficacy of Sacroiliac Joint Injections

Author	Study Design	Treatment	Results	Comments
Patients with Spondyloarthropathy				
Bollow et al.[24]	Prospective case series (n = 66), patients with spondyloarthropathy	Intra-articular SIJ injection with 40 mg depot corticosteroid (CT-guided)	92% had significant decrease in pain score (from 8.8 to 3.3) at 1.7 week; duration of relief 10 months	Follow-up period up to 18 months
Braun et al.[32]	Prospective case series (n = 30), patients with spondyloarthropathy	Intra-articular SIJ injection with 40 mg triamcinolone (CT guided)	83% had improvement in pain at 5.2 months (VAS from 8.5 to 3), duration of relief 8.9 months	Follow-up period up to 18 months
Fischer et al.[33]	Prospective case series (n = 56), children with juvenile spondyloarthropathy without response to NSAIDs	Intra-articular SIJ injection with 40 mg triamcinolone (CT-guided)	88% had significant decrease in pain (VAS from 6.9 to 1.8), duration of relief 12 months	Follow-up period of 20 months
Maugars et al.[34]	Randomized, controlled, double-blind trial (n = 10), patients with spondyloarthropathy	Intra-articular SIJ injection with cortivazol versus placebo (fluoroscopically guided)	At 1 month, pain score decreased 5.3 points in treatment group, 1.8 points in placebo group; relief lasted 6 months in 67% of patients	
Patients without Spondyloarthropathy				
Lilliang et al.[27]	Prospective case series (n = 39), patients without spondyloarthropathy	Intra-articular SIJ injection with 40 mg triamcinolone (fluoroscopically guided)	67% had 50% relief for over 6 weeks, average duration of relief was 37 weeks	SIJ pain diagnosed by positive response to dual SIJ injections; history of lumbosacral fusion predicted short duration of relief
Luukkainen et al.[35]	Controlled, double-blind trial (n = 20), patients with seronegative spondyloarthropathy	Periarticular SIJ injection with 60 mg methylprednisolone + lidocaine versus saline + lidocaine	Improvement in pain score and physical exam in steroid group at 2 months	
Luukkainen et al.[36]	Controlled, double-blind trial (n = 24) patients without spondyloarthropathy	Periarticular SIJ injection with methylprednisolone + lidocaine versus saline + lidocaine	Improvement in pain score and physical exam in steroid group at 1-month follow-up	

SIJ, sacroiliac joint; CT, computed tomography; VAS, visual analog scale; NSAIDs, nonsteroidal anti-inflammatory drugs.

with spondyloarthropathy whose pain was unresponsive to nonsteroidal anti-inflammatory drugs (NSAIDs);[33] 87.5% of the patients who received injections had an improvement in pain scores that lasted 12 ± 6 months.

There have been three randomized, controlled trials that investigated corticosteroid SI joint injections; all demonstrated some benefit.[34-36] Maugars and colleagues compared steroid and local anesthetic injection with saline in 13 joints (10 patients) with spondyloarthropathy.[34] They noted improved pain control at 1 month compared to placebo (5/6 versus 1/7) and continued analgesia at 3 and 6 months. Luukkainen and associates compared periarticular injections of local anesthetic and corticosteroid with local anesthetic and saline in 20 patients with seronegative spondyloarthropathy and demonstrated significantly reduced VAS scores in the steroid group, but not the saline group, at 2 months.[35] The same investigators compared steroid and local anesthetic versus saline and local anesthetic in 24 patients with clinical sacroiliac joint dysfunction but without radiographic findings.[36] Again, they noted that the pain scores decreased significantly more in the steroid group than the local anesthetic group. These studies are limited by their small sample size, which reduced the ability to find significant differences in medication usage and functional status. In addition, all have a relatively short period of follow-up.

BLOCKADE OF THE L4 AND L5 DORSAL RAMUS AND LATERAL BRANCHES OF S1-S3

As noted, the posterior margin of the SIJ is innervated by the L5 dorsal ramus and the lateral branches of S1, S2, and

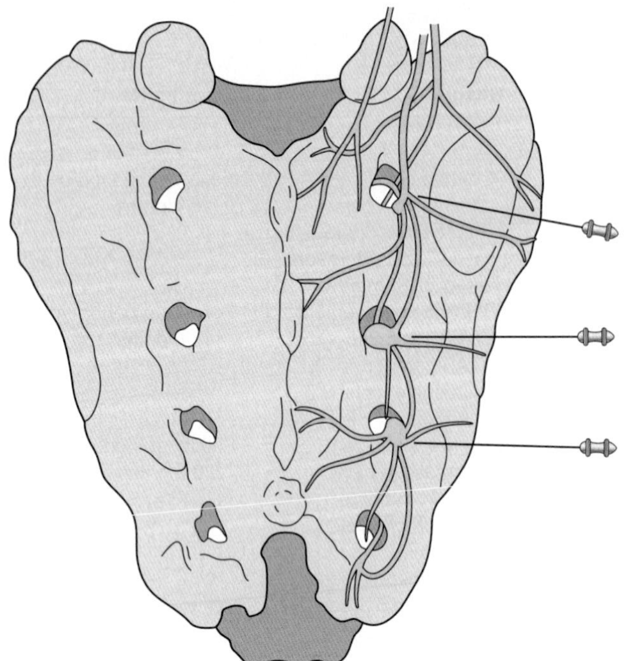

Figure 63.10 Schematic drawing showing the S1-S3 lateral branches innervating the SI joint and overlying ligaments. The needles depict the approximate location for the diagnostic lateral branch blocks (LBB). (From Cohen SP, Abdi S. Lateral branch blocks as a treatment for sacroiliac joint pain: a pilot study. *Reg Anesth Pain Med.* 2003;28:113-119.)

S3, with possible contributions from the L4 dorsal ramus. Blockade of these structures can be a diagnostic tool and is employed by some practitioners to predict response to radiofrequency (RF) ablation of the same nerves.[37] The patient is positioned prone and the fluoroscopic C-arm is either positioned AP or angled slightly cephalocaudal to optimize the appearance of the sacral foramina. After skin infiltration, 22-gauge spinal needles are advanced coaxially to a point 5 mm lateral to each foramen between the 2 and 5 o'clock positions on the right side and the 7 and 10 o'clock positions on the left side. This corresponds to the path of the lateral branch as it travels laterally and enters the ligaments of the joint (Fig. 63.10). The L5 dorsal ramus is blocked at the junction of the ala and the articular process of the sacrum. If L4 blockade is desired, the C-arm is rotated obliquely to block the L4 dorsal ramus at the junction of the transverse process of L5 and the superior articulating process. Once the position of the needle tips is confirmed, 0.5 ml of 0.5% bupivacaine is injected.[37] The patient is instructed to keep a pain diary to monitor pain relief.

RADIOFREQUENCY DENERVATION OF THE SACROILIAC JOINT

Transient pain relief from intra-articular steroid injections may require more permanent denervation of the nerve supply of the SI joint. Although chemical neurolysis with phenol can be performed, such intervention is rarely used because of possible spillage of the agent with unintended neurolysis of other structures. RF ablation of the nerves results in a more restricted neurolysis; RF ablation may target the small, terminal sensory fibers at the posterior aspect of the joint itself (strip lesioning) or the nerve supply to the joint.

STRIP LESIONING OF THE SACROILIAC JOINT

RF ablation of the terminal fibers supplying the posterior SIJ can result in analgesia in patients who previously responded to diagnostic intra-articular injections. The technique of thermal RF denervation of the SI joint utilizes two probes to create a bipolar strip lesion. The joint is visualized with the fluoroscopic C-arm as described for SIJ injection, then the first RF needle (5- to 10-mm active tip) is inserted at the inferior margin of the joint. A second RF needle is placed more cephalad, at a distance of less than 1 cm from the first probe. After anesthetizing the tissue with lidocaine, the RF probe is inserted and heated to 80° C for 90 seconds. Successive probes are placed less than 1 cm cephalad from the previous probe, and multiple lesions are created in a repetitive "leap-frog" manner as high in the joint as possible, creating a strip lesion in the posterior joint.[38] The posterior superior iliac spine obscures access to the superior portion of the joint, making only the lower third, or at most half, of the joint accessible to the lesioning. Some clinicians lesion the whole posterior border of the joint under heavy sedation.

Using this technique, Ferrante and colleagues reported a series of 50 SIJ denervations performed in 33 patients; 12 (36%) reported at least a 50% decrease in their visual analog pain scores for at least 6 months.[38] Although it was a retrospective study, it showed the efficacy of the technique.

Pino and colleagues[39] studied the ideal distance of the two probes to create a continuous strip lesion. They compared the lesions created by two needles placed at 2, 4, 6, 8, and 10 mm from each other; egg white was used as the protein medium for easy visualization and measurement of the lesions. The temperatures of the probes were raised from 40° to 90° C and held at 90° C for 190 seconds. They noted that contiguous strip lesions were produced when the cannulas were spaced 6 mm or less apart—unipolar lesions resulted when the lesions were spaced more than 6 mm apart (Fig. 63.11). Ninety percent of the final lesion area was reached by 120 seconds with the final lesions reached by 150 seconds. They concluded that the probes should be placed between 4 and 6 mm apart to maximize the surface area of the thermal lesion and that the treatment duration should be between 120 and 150 seconds at 90° C.

The size of the monopolar lesion can be increased by injecting fluid before the RF lesion is applied.[40] Using ex vivo chicken samples, Provenzano noted that preinjection of fluid other than water increased the lesion size. Hydroxyethyl starch caused the largest lesion, followed by 0.9% NaCl and lidocaine. Increasing the volume from 0.5 mL to 3 mL did not significantly change the size of the lesion. The same findings were noted with bipolar lesioning.[41] Three percent NaCl appears to be ideal in that it increased the size of the lesion between the electrodes while diminishing the spread of tissue destruction beyond the electrodes.

RADIOFREQUENCY LESIONING OF THE LATERAL BRANCHES

This technique has been performed with traditional thermal RF,[37,42,43] as well as water-cooled RF (Table 63.2).[44-46] The patient is positioned prone and the C-arm is aligned for an anteroposterior image. To target the L5 dorsal rami, an RF cannula is placed at the lateral margin of the superior articular process where it meets the sacral ala, as described previously

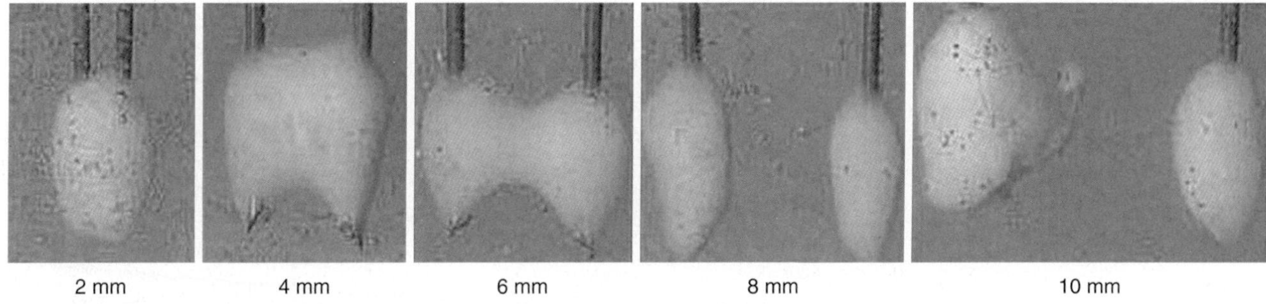

Figure 63.11 Bipolar lesions produced with the two cannulas at different distances. Note that a continuous lesion is produced when the cannulas are 6 mm or less. (Reprinted with permission from Pino CA Hoeft MA, Hofsess C, Rathmell JP. Morphologic analysis of bipolar radiofrequency lesions: implications for treatment of the sacroiliac joint. *Reg Anesth Pain Med.* 2005;30:335-338.)

Table 63.2 Efficacy of Radiofrequency Lesioning of the Lateral Branches

Author	Study Design	Treatments	Results	Comments
Gevargez et al.[25]	Prospective, observational study, n = 38	RF neurotomy in the dorsal interosseous ligament and of L5 dorsal ramus (CT guided)	At 3 months, 13 of 38 patients had no pain, 12 of 38 had substantially reduced pain	All patients had a positive response to diagnostic CT-guided SIJ injection
Cohen and Abdi[37]	Retrospective chart review (n = 9), patients with SI joint pain with short-term relief after intra-articular injection	RF neurotomy of L4, L5 dorsal rami, and S1-S3 lateral branches	8 of 9 patients reported 50% or greater pain relief at 9-month follow-up; 1 of 9 had 40% improvement	All patients had a positive response to diagnostic blocks of L4-5 dorsal rami and S1-3 lateral branches
Yin et al.[42]	Retrospective chart review (n = 14), patients with relief from dual triamcinolone and bupivacaine SIJ injection	RF neurotomy of L5 dorsal ramus and S1-3 lateral branches	9 of 14 with 60% or greater patient-perceived improvement with >50% decrease in pain scores at 6 months	
Karaman et al[46]	Prospective observational study, n = 15	Cooled RF of the L5 dorsal ramus and S1-3 lateral branches	At 6 months, 80% had >50% pain relief, 87% had a 10-point decrease in ODI	Included patients had a positive response to diagnostic SIJ injection
Patel et al.[48]	Prospective, randomized, controlled, blinded study, n = 51	Cooled RF of the L5 dorsal ramus and S1-3 lateral branches versus sham procedure	At 3 months, NRS −2.4 in treatment group and −0.8 in sham, ODI −11 in treatment group, 2 in sham; effect persisted at 9 months	Patients with axial back pain and a positive response to dual lateral branch blocks; crossover allowed at 3 months
Cohen et al[49]	Prospective, randomized, controlled study, n = 28	Conventional RF of L4-5 dorsal rami and cooled RF of S1-3 lateral branches versus sham procedure	Pain scores improved at 1 month (2.4 in treatment group, 6.3 in sham group); benefit persisted at 6 months	SIJ pain confirmed by intra-articular injection; crossover allowed at 1 month

SIJ, sacroiliac joint; ODI, Oswestry disability index; VAS, visual analog scale; NRS, numeric rating scale; RF, radiofrequency.

for the diagnostic block. Because the lesion created by conventional RF is smaller and is positioned along the active tip of the probe, the needle trajectory must preferably be parallel to the path of the nerve to maximize the chances of the neural destruction when using conventional RF. On the lateral fluoroscopic image, the needle tip should be no further anterior than the anterior third of the superior articulating process (SAP).[16] When using cooled RF, the lesion is larger and the tip should be no more anterior than the midpoint of the SAP to avoid lesioning the segmental nerve root.[45] It should be noted that some practitioners favor the use of conventional RF for the dorsal rami of L4 and L5 because the more compact lesion size seems less likely to damage the spinal nerve. This was investigated by Kapural and associates, who retrospectively reviewed 100 cases of RF ablation of the SIJ.[47] Of these patients, 82 had cooled RF of the L5 dorsal

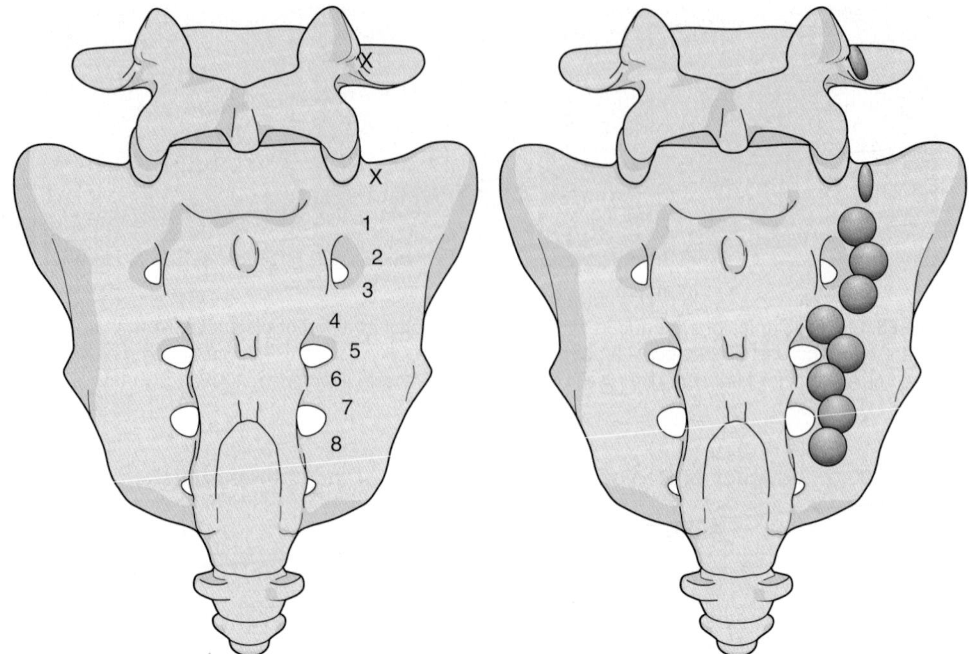

Figure 63.12 Placement of the needles in water-cooled radiofrequency ablation. (Reprinted with permission from Cohen SP, Hurley RW, Buckenmaier CC, et al. Randomized placebo-controlled study evaluating lateral branch radiofrequency denervation for sacroiliac joint pain. *Anesthesiology.* 2008;109:279-288.)

ramus, whereas others had conventional RF. The rate of acute complications was not higher in the water-cooled RF group.

For the S1-S3 lateral branches, the water-cooled RF needles are placed lateral to the sacral foramina. Three lesions are created at S1 and S2; the needles are ideally placed at 2:30, 4, and 5:30 o'clock positions on the right, and at 6:30, 8, and 9:30 o'clock positions on the left. At S3, two lesions are made at 2:30 and 4 o'clock positions on the right, and at 9:30 and 8 o'clock positions on the left (Fig. 63.12).[46] On lateral fluoroscopic images, the needle tip should not be anterior to the posterior sacrum to avoid intraforaminal positioning. Prior to lesioning at all levels, sensory nerve stimulation is applied at 50 Hz with the goal of concordant pain being reproduced below 0.6 volts. Motor stimulation is applied at 2 Hz at 2 volts, or three times the sensory threshold, to verify the absence of muscle contraction in a radicular distribution. Once the stimulation pattern is acceptable, the sites are anesthetized with 0.5 mL 1% lidocaine and lesioning begins at 80° C for 90 seconds (conventional RF) or 60° C for 150 seconds (water-cooled RF). It is customary to inject 0.5 mL of a mixture of local anesthetic (e.g., bupivacaine) and steroid (e.g., 8 mg/mL triamcinolone) after the lesioning for postoperative analgesia and to prevent neuritis.

EFFICACY OF THERMAL RF OF THE LATERAL BRANCHES

Two retrospective studies showed the efficacy of thermal RF lesioning of the lateral branches of the posterior primary ramus of the L4 to S3 dorsal rami in the treatment of SI joint syndrome. In Cohen and Abdi's study, 18 patients with SI joint pain had nerve blocks of the L4-5 primary dorsal rami and S1-3 lateral branches.[37] Thirteen of the 18 patients obtained approximately 50% relief, 2 of the 13 had relief that lasted several months, 9 of the 13 patients underwent RF lesioning (80° C for 90 seconds), and 8 of the 9 patients who had the RF denervation experienced greater than 50% relief that persisted for at least 9 months. In Yin and colleagues' study, 9 of 14 (64%) patients experienced a successful outcome (defined as > 60% patient-perceived improvement with concurrent > 50% decrease in pain score for 6 months); 5 patients (36%) had complete relief at 6 months after thermal RF of the lateral branches of S1-3.[42] Prior to the RF lesion, the patients had reproducible and consistent relief of their pain after two SI joint local anesthetic injections. Yin and associates also performed cadaver studies to follow the course of lateral branches. They noted that the lateral branches were located at the 2 to 6 o'clock positions at the right side and at the 6 to 10 o'clock positions on the left side.

The unpredictable course of the lateral branches at the S1-S3 foramina led to the recommendation of bipolar RF strip lesions at these levels.[43] In this technique, bipolar strip lesions are created approximately 5 mm lateral to the edge of the lateral half of the dorsal sacral foramina of S1, S2, and S3 by placing two 20-gauge, 10-mm exposed curved-tip RF cannulas 4 to 6 mm apart. Several sequential bipolar lesions are created by the "leapfrog" technique of moving the two cannulas along the joint edge. Initial results showed eight of nine patients had significant reductions in the severity and frequency of their back pain, as well as their analgesia requirements.[43] Bipolar strip lesioning is an alternative to making several unipolar lesions with thermal RF needles, as the burn area with thermal RF is small. It is not necessary with the water-cooled RF because the lesions created are bigger.

Complete pain relief after lesioning of the lateral branches at the posterior aspect of the SI joint has been questioned because innervation of the ventral aspect of the joint is not destroyed. However, Yin and associates as well as others noted the predominant dorsal innervation of the SI joint.[13,14,42]

A combined RF lesioning of the SI joint and the dorsal branch of L5 under CT guidance has been described.[25] The authors also lesioned the ventral and dorsal aspects of the joint. However, only an area of the joint and one nerve were lesioned. They reported that 34% of their patients had complete relief at 3 months and 32% had substantial pain reduction.

EFFICACY OF WATER-COOLED RADIOFREQUENCY

In an observational study, Karaman and colleagues investigated water-cooled RF of the L5 dorsal ramus and S1-S3 lateral branches in 15 patients.[46] The presence of SIJ pain was diagnosed by dual intra-articular blocks. They showed a significant reduction in pain scores and disability scores at 1, 3, and 6 months.

Randomized, blinded, placebo-controlled studies investigated the effect of denervation. Patel and associates reported 51 patients with SIJ pain diagnosed by positive responses to two sets of local anesthetic blocks of the L5 dorsal ramus and the S1-S3 lateral branches.[48] Either water-cooled RF or a sham procedure was performed and the patients were followed for 9 months. At 3 months, the patients were unblinded and patients who had the sham procedure were allowed to cross over. At 3 months, there was a statistically significant improvement in pain scores (an average 2.4-point decrease on the numeric rating scale in the procedure group versus a 0.8-point decrease in the sham group) as well as in the disability index (a mean 11-point decrease in Oswestry disability index in the procedure group versus a 2-point increase in the sham group). Patient-reported scores remained improved at the 9-month follow-up.

Cohen and coworkers reported a randomized, blinded, placebo-controlled pilot study that compared the efficacy of conventional RF of the L4 and L5 dorsal rami and water-cooled RF of the lateral branches of S1 to S3 to placebo.[49] Twenty-eight patients with SIJ pain confirmed by intra-articular local anesthetic injection were randomized and followed for 12 months. Baseline pain scores averaged 6.1 in the treatment group and 6.5 in the placebo group. At 1, 3, and 6 months, the pain scores in the intervention group were 2.4, 2.4, and 2.6, respectively. This was significantly better than the average pain score in the sham group, which was 6.3 at 1 month, after which patients were allowed to cross over. At 12 months only 14% of patients in the RF group continued to experience improvement.

In a follow-up retrospective study, Cohen and colleagues investigated the factors associated with success of RF ablation of the lateral branches.[44] Success was defined as a 50% reduction in pain lasting more than 6 months and a positive global perceived effect. Secondary outcomes included disability markers, medication reduction, and active duty status. Fifty-two percent of patients who underwent SIJ denervation had successful results. Pre-procedural pain intensity, pain radiating below the knee, and age over 55 were independent predictors of failure, and there was a trend toward failure in patients who were taking opioids. Water-cooled RF was associated with a higher success rate than conventional RF.

CONCLUSION

Sacroiliac joint syndrome is a common cause of buttock pain. The clinician should know the symptoms as well as the physical examination findings that help to make the diagnosis. RF lesioning of the lateral branches that innervate the SI joint, especially the water-cooled technique, may result in long-term relief.

KEY POINTS

- The pain of sacroiliac (SI) joint syndrome is felt in the SI joint area and usually radiates to the groin, lateral thigh, posterior thigh, and leg.
- The common tests that confirm the presence of SI joint syndrome include the FABER-Patrick's, Gaenslen's, Yeoman's, shear, and Gillet's tests.
- The diagnosis of SI joint syndrome is based on the patient's history, symptoms, positive confirmatory tests, elimination of the other causes of buttock pain, and a positive response to an SI joint injection.
- Relief from SI joint injection with local anesthetic and steroid can be temporary. More prolonged relief can be obtained by thermal RF lesioning of the SI joint or the lateral branches of the primary ramus of the L5-S3 nerves. Continuous RF lesions can be obtained by performing bipolar strip lesions. The use of water-cooled radiofrequency lesioning, with its larger lesions, obviates the need for bipolar strip lesions.

SUGGESTED READINGS

Benzon HT. Pain originating from the buttock: sacroiliac dysfunction and piriformis syndrome. In: Benzon H, Raja S, Molloy R, eds. *Essentials of Pain Medicine and Regional Anesthesia.* New York: Elsevier; 2005:356-365.

Bogduk N. *Practice Guidelines: Spinal Diagnostic and Treatment Procedures.* San Francisco: International Spine Intervention Society; 2004:66-86.

Cohen SP, Abdi S. Lateral branch blocks as a treatment for sacroiliac joint pain: a pilot study. *Reg Anesth Pain Med.* 2003;28:113-119.

Cohen SP, Hurley RW, Buckenmaier CC III, et al. Randomized placebo-controlled study evaluating lateral branch radiofrequency denervation for sacroiliac joint pain. *Anesthesiology.* 2008;109:279-288.

Dreyfuss P, Michaelsen M, Pauza K, et al. The value of medical history and physical examination in diagnosing sacroiliac joint pain. *Spine.* 1996;21:2594-2602.

Ferrante FM, King LF, Roche EA, et al. Radiofrequency sacroiliac joint denervation for sacroiliac syndrome. *Reg Anesth Pain Med.* 2001;26:137-142.

Grob KR, Neuhuber WL, Kissling RO. [Innervation of the sacroiliac joint of the human]. *Z Rheumatol.* 1995;54:117-122.

Harmon D, O'Sullivan M. Ultrasound-guided sacroiliac joint injection technique. *Pain Physician.* 2008;11:543-547.

Liliang PC, Lu K, Weng HC, et al. The therapeutic efficacy of sacroiliac joint blocks with triamcinolone acetonide in the treatment of sacroiliac joint dysfunction without spondyloarthropathy. *Spine.* 2009;34:896-900.

Luukkainen R, Nissila M, Asikainen E, et al. Periarticular corticosteroid treatment of the sacroiliac joint in patients with seronegative spondylarthropathy. *Clin Exp Rheumatol.* 1999;17:88-90.

Luukkainen RK, Wennerstrand PV, Kautiainen HH, et al. Efficacy of periarticular corticosteroid treatment of the sacroiliac joint in non-spondylarthropathic patients with chronic low back pain in the region of the sacroiliac joint. *Clin Exp Rheumatol.* 2002;20:52-54.

Maugars Y, Mathis C, Berthelot JM, et al. Assessment of the efficacy of sacroiliac corticosteroid injections in spondylarthropathies: a double-blind study. *Br J Rheumatol.* 1996;35:767-770.

Patel N, Gross A, Brown L, Gekht G. A randomized, placebo-controlled study to assess the efficacy of lateral branch neurotomy for chronic sacroiliac joint pain. *Pain Med.* 2012;13:383-398.

Schwarzer AC, Aprill CN, Bogduk N. The sacroiliac joint in chronic low back pain. *Spine.* 1995;20:31-37.

Szadek KM, Hoogland PV, Zuurmond WW, et al. Nociceptive nerve fibers in the sacroiliac joint in humans. *Reg Anesth Pain Med.* 2008;33:36-43.

The references for this chapter can be found at www.expertconsult.com.

64 Myofascial Injections: Trigger Point, Piriformis, Iliopsoas, and Scalene Injections

W. Evan Rivers | Honorio T. Benzon | Farooq Khan | Juan Francisco Asenjo

OVERVIEW OF MYOFASCIAL INJECTIONS

Myofascial pain is a common source of pain in the neck, low back region, and other areas of the body. The term "myofascial pain" encompasses muscle strain, myofascial trigger points, and specific muscle pain syndromes, including piriformis syndrome, iliopsoas-related pain, and pain related to compression of the brachial plexus by the scalene muscles (neurogenic thoracic outlet syndrome).

RELEVANT ANATOMY

Skeletal muscle consists of muscle fibers under somatic nervous control. Each nerve root innervates a muscle or group of muscles known as a myotome. The muscle belly of skeletal muscles is connected by tendons to the bone. Trigger points occur in the body of the muscle, most often located in the center of the muscle.

TRIGGER POINT INJECTIONS

Trigger points are nodules found in taut bands in skeletal muscle that often produce characteristic patterns of referred pain provoked by palpation.[1] A trigger point may occur in isolation, concomitantly as part of a regional myofascial pain syndrome, or as an effect of other pain syndromes through either segmental effects or biomechanical changes. Trigger points are diagnosed by the history and physical examination. A patient will complain of a localized pain or regional pain in or around skeletal muscle or replicated by palpation of a skeletal muscle.[1] The muscles commonly involved are the trapezius, splenii, cervical and lumbar paraspinal, and quadratus lumborum. On examination, localized taut bands of muscle are noted and palpation produces characteristic nondermatomal referral patterns. Trigger points may be active or latent. Active trigger points produce spontaneous pain and are painful on palpation, whereas latent trigger points produce pain only when palpated.[1] Trigger points may result from trauma, overload or overuse injury, or a prolonged period during which the muscle is in a shortened position. The pathophysiology of trigger points is not fully understood, although multiple lines of relevant research support their existence. Peripheral sensitization and central sensitization both appear to contribute to the pain from trigger points.[2-5] There is also evidence of an alteration in blood flow at trigger points.[6]

Imaging studies have only recently demonstrated anatomic changes associated with trigger points. Ultrasound (US) examination in combination with Doppler blood flow has been reported to allow visualization of trigger points, and US imaging can help direct muscle injection techniques (see later). Recently developed techniques using magnetic resonance and US elastography purport to reveal changes in intramuscular signal consistent with trigger points, but this technology has not yet been validated.[7,8]

Treatment of trigger points commonly includes physical therapy (manual release techniques, stretching and strengthening, conditioning, therapeutic modalities), trigger point injections (TPIs), dry needling and acupuncture, and transcutaneous electrical nerve stimulation.[9] A broad range of treatment modalities have been reported, but weak research methodology continues to limit interpretation of the results. Regarding medications, tizanidine, but not cyclobenzaprine, was noted to be efficacious for acute skeletal muscle spasms.[9] Diazepam, amitriptyline, and lidocaine patch were found to be effective, but literature support for the use of anticonvulsants in treating myofascial pain syndrome is limited. Although clonazepam appears to be effective, its use is limited by the side effects of depression, liver dysfunction, and difficulty weaning the patient from this drug. Nonsteroidal anti-inflammatory drugs (NSAIDs), specifically ibuprofen, appear to be effective when given with other agents, but not as monotherapy.[9]

TPIs are intramuscular injections of local anesthetic with or without corticosteroid. Some practitioners perform dry needling (needle penetration without infiltration of medication), and there is evidence that dry needling can be as effective as TPI but may cause more muscle soreness.[9] The response to TPI or dry needling is more effective when a muscle twitch reaction is elicited with needle penetration of the trigger point.[10] Some authors have suggested that botulinum toxin or tropisetron (a serotonin 5-HT_3 receptor antagonist) can be used for TPI, but the superiority of alternatives over more conventional injectants has not been consistently demonstrated.[9,11-13]

CONTRAINDICATIONS

The following conditions are contraindications to TPI: (1) infection, systemic or localized; (2) coagulopathy; (3) distorted or complicated anatomy; and (4) patient refusal.

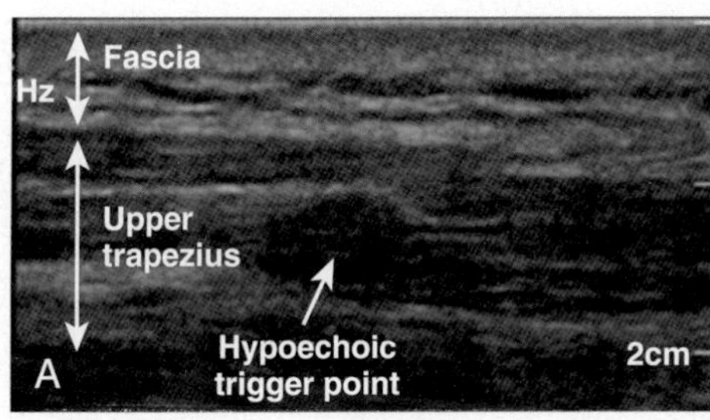

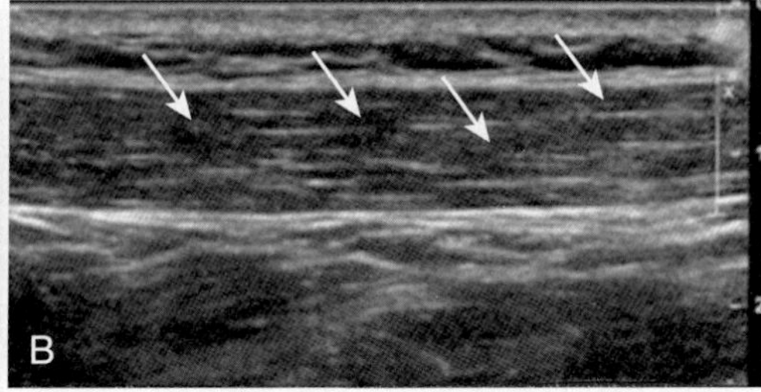

Figure 64.1 Gray-scale imaging of trigger points in the upper trapezius muscle. **A,** An isolated trigger point appears as a well-defined focal hypoechoic nodule. **B,** A series of four hypoechoic trigger points in the upper trapezius. (From Sikdar S, Shah JP, Gebreab T, et al. Novel applications of ultrasound technology to visualize and characterize myofascial trigger points and surrounding soft tissue. *Arch Phys Med Rehabil.* 2009;90:1829-1838, with permission.)

TECHNIQUE AND FOLLOW-UP

After informed consent, the muscle is palpated and the trigger points are identified and marked. The area is prepared in sterile fashion and a 25-gauge, 1.5-inch needle is inserted into the trigger point. A local twitch may be elicited at this time or the patient verbally identifies the painful area. After negative aspiration, 0.25% bupivacaine, 0.2% ropivacaine, or 1% lidocaine is injected with or without steroid, either dexamethasone (4 mg in a 30-mL bottle of local anesthetic) or a low dose of particulate steroid (e.g., 20 to 40 mg of methylprednisolone or triamcinolone diluted in the local anesthetic solution).

Possible complications include bleeding, hematoma, nerve block, and infection. The patient should be monitored closely for bleeding, development of neurologic symptoms (numbness or weakness, urinary or bowel incontinence), or signs of infection. Depending on the location of the injection, the patient should be instructed on the signs and symptoms of pneumothorax (from neck, shoulder, thoracic, and anterior chest wall injections) or local nerve blockade (for example, inadvertent median nerve block with injection of the flexor carpi ulnaris).

The success of the procedure is dependent on the diagnosis and localization of the trigger point. Patients with chronic widespread pain or psychological disorders are less likely to respond to TPI only. Patients who have focal muscle pain with the characteristics of myofascial pain can achieve significant relief for days to months with a well-performed TPI. Success of TPI is often dependent on subsequent stretching and strengthening and neuromuscular education of the muscle.[1] The most effective treatment of myofascial pain syndrome is often a multidisciplinary approach tailored to the individual needs of the patient that incorporates TPI with physical therapy and medication as noted earlier. Practitioners are counseled to provide appropriate follow-up after TPI and encourage patients to address other factors that perpetuate chronic pain (coping, employment, decreased social activity).[11,14]

ULTRASOUND-GUIDED TECHNIQUES

US guidance provides several theoretical advantages over blind needle insertion. As stated, it allows visualization of the trigger point (Fig. 64.1). The practitioner is ensured that the needle is penetrating muscle tissue, which may be of use in patients with considerable adipose tissue, and can avoid local anatomic structures that are sensitive to needle penetration or local anesthetic infiltration (i.e., neurovascular structures or viscera).[15] US imaging also allows visualization of the muscle twitch response with needle penetration, especially in muscles that are deep or small.[16] An additional use of US is to confirm local anesthetic infiltration between fascial planes.[17] It also aids in blocking the spinal accessory nerve for diagnosis of trapezius muscle–related myofascial pain.[18]

RESULTS OF TREATMENT

Research on treatment outcomes of myofascial pain has been limited by poor study methodology and reporting, inconsistent outcome selection, small sample sizes, heterogeneous patient populations, and the absence of standardized diagnostic criteria (with the exception of validated diagnostic criteria for myofascial pain of the muscles of the jaw).[19] Overall, evidence from systematic reviews supports the finding that TPI (regardless of the injectant) and dry needling of trigger points provide a benefit alone and in addition to stretching and strengthening.[9,20] Deep dry needling appears to be more effective than superficial dry needling.[21-23]

Several well-designed studies have evaluated the use of botulinum toxin for the treatment of myofascial pain, but with conflicting conclusions: although some found positive results, the preponderance did not find statistically significant effects of botulinum toxin over saline or local anesthetic. In fact, a qualitative review of published trials on botulinum toxin for myofascial TPI noted its lack of efficacy.[13] Tropisetron, a 5-HT_3 receptor antagonist, may offer longer analgesic effect than occurs with local anesthetic.[12]

Combining medication management with physical therapy and injection therapy can often offer the best opportunity for treatment. Treatment with amitriptyline, benzodiazepines, and ibuprofen (in combination with other agents) appears to be effective, and preliminary data support topical rubefacient patches, diclofenac patches, and lidocaine patches.[9] Duloxetine has recently been given an indication for musculoskeletal pain; it will probably be commonly used for the treatment of myofascial pain. The prescription of benzodiazepines must be brief and goal directed, with due diligence to minimize misuse, addiction, and diversion.

Factors associated with a lower therapeutic effect of TPI include poor coping, employment issues, decreased social activity, duration of the pain syndrome, high levels of pain, constant pain (as opposed to intermittent pain), and unresponsiveness of the pain to analgesic medication.[14]

PIRIFORMIS INJECTIONS

Piriformis syndrome consists of pain in the buttock with or without radiation in the distribution of the ipsilateral sciatic nerve. It may contribute up to 8% of buttock pain. The syndrome can be a consequence of an abnormal relationship between the sciatic nerve and the piriformis muscle that results in irritation of the sciatic nerve. A hypertrophic muscle, infection, or invasion of the muscle by tumor can cause pressure or irritation on the nerve.[24,25] In 78% to 84% of the population, the sciatic nerve passes in front of the muscle. In 12% to 21% of individuals, the divided nerve passes through or posterior to the piriformis and is exposed to muscle contractions, which trigger sciatic symptoms.[24] Piriformis syndrome is a diagnosis of exclusion since there are no standardized diagnostic criteria for it. The syndrome should be considered in patients who have buttock pain, tenderness to palpation over the piriformis muscle, and a positive response to provocative maneuvers, including the following:

1. Pace's sign: pain and weakness with seated abduction of the hip against resistance
2. Lasègue's sign (also known as the straight-leg raise test): pain with unresisted flexion, adduction, and internal rotation of the flexed hip
3. Freiberg's sign: pain with forced (i.e., against resistance) internal rotation of the extended hip[24]

Because of its small size in comparison to the gluteus muscles, its proximity to neurovascular structures, and its deep location, the piriformis muscle is usually injected under radiographic or US guidance. Piriformis injections under computed tomography (CT) or electromyographic guidance have also been described.[26-29] Contraindications are the same as those noted in the section on TPI.

FLUOROSCOPIC TECHNIQUE

The patient is placed prone on a fluoroscopy table, and the inferior margin of the sacroiliac joint is imaged and marked. The needle insertion site is 1 to 2 cm caudal and 1 to 2 cm lateral to the inferior margin of the sacroiliac joint. After sterile preparation and infiltration of local anesthetic, a 7- to 10-cm insulated needle is inserted and advanced with the nerve stimulator turned on (1 mA, 2 Hz, 0.1 msec) until an evoked motor response of the sciatic nerve is achieved (dorsiflexion, plantar flexion, eversion, inversion) at 0.4 to 0.6 mA. The needle is then withdrawn slightly until the sciatic stimulation disappears; this is to avoid intraneural injection. Steroid (40 mg of either methylprednisolone or triamcinolone) plus 5 mL of saline is injected around the sciatic nerve—this is helpful, especially in patients with signs of sciatic nerve irritation. The needle is then pulled back 1 cm into the belly of the piriformis muscle, and 1 to 2 mL of contrast agent is injected. The contrast agent should outline the piriformis muscle belly with no sign of spillage (Fig. 64.2). After the characteristic spread of dye is achieved—outline of the piriformis muscle with clean margins—the local anesthetic solution with steroid is administered. Typically, good pain relief can be attained with an injection of 5 mL of 0.25% or 0.5% bupivacaine plus 40 mg of methylprednisolone (or triamcinolone). For botulinum toxin injection, 100 mouse units in a 2-mL volume is injected.[27]

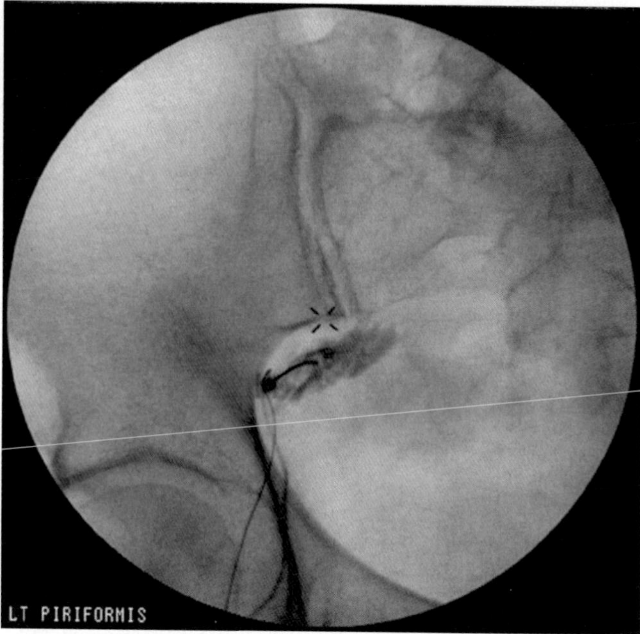

Figure 64.2 Fluoroscopically assisted piriformis muscle injection.

ULTRASOUND-GUIDED TECHNIQUE

The US-guided technique not only permits a direct view of the piriformis muscle but can also be used to examine its relationship to the sciatic nerve and rule out any anatomic variation. The patient is placed in the prone position with the US machine on the side opposite the operator. A curved, low-frequency US probe (2 to 6 MHz) is used to scan a wider and deeper area. The US machine should have Doppler to help identify the inferior gluteal artery medial to the sciatic nerve and anterior to the piriformis. A 20- to 22-gauge, 10- to 12-cm-long needle is recommended.

One technique involves positioning the transducer in short axis (transverse) over the sacroiliac joint, where medially the sacrum will be visible and laterally the ilium/gluteus maximus muscle complex will be observed.[29] While keeping the sacroiliac joint in the center of the screen, the transducer is moved caudally until the lateral view of the ilium is lost, which indicates that the transducer is over the greater sciatic notch. In this position the operator will see the hyperechoic lateral portion of the sacrum medially. In the center of the image the following are visualized: skin and fat in the near field and then the gluteus maximus muscle. Deeper to the gluteus maximus and originating from the anterior and lateral sacral edge is the piriformis muscle with its typical longitudinal fibers (Fig. 64.3). By moving the transducer slightly lower and mildly rotating the left gluteal area clockwise (counterclockwise on the right side), the sciatic nerve becomes visible deeper in the medial aspect of the piriformis. The ischium initially appears as a curved hyperechoic line (posterior acetabulum); more caudally it becomes a flat line deeper to the piriformis. Another way to find the piriformis is to place the transducer over the line between the greater trochanter and ischial tuberosity. Once the sciatic nerve is identified, it is followed cephalad until the piriformis and gluteus maximus muscles are seen over the sciatic nerve.

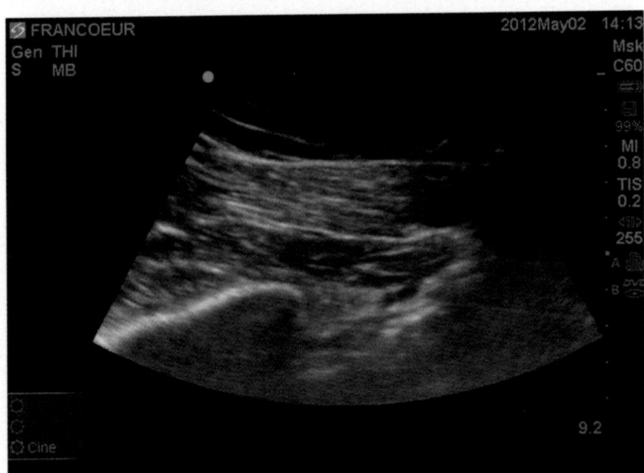

Figure 64.3 Ultrasound-assisted piriformis muscle injection.

To confirm the view of the piriformis muscle, flex the patient's knee 90 degrees and rotate the hip internally and externally. During this maneuver the piriformis will slide over the ischium while the position of the gluteus maximus remains stable. While observing the sciatic notch it is useful to identify the ischial spine since other muscles that are in similar position as the piriformis insert in the area (i.e., the gemelli and obturator muscles) and should be differentiated from it.

The piriformis runs almost horizontal between the sacrum and the femur. A lateral-to-medial, in-plane approach is ideal to maximize visualization of the needle; the needle enters the skin 3 to 4 cm lateral to the lateral edge of the transducer. The needle should cross the skin and fat in a lateral-to-medial, posterior-to-anterior direction and enter the gluteus maximus and then the piriformis in its medial half. Hydrodissection with normal saline (or a nonelectrolyte solution such as 5% dextrose if stimulation is planned) may help confirm the position of the tip of the needle. The steroid (methylprednisolone or triamcinolone) plus local anesthetic (bupivacaine or lidocaine) is then injected. After injecting the piriformis muscle, to decrease sciatic nerve irritation, the needle can be advanced and positioned between the piriformis and the sciatic nerve to create a layer of local anesthetic with steroid. Five to 8 mL of the mixture is usually adequate.

POSTPROCEDURE FOLLOW-UP

The patient should be monitored closely for the following: (1) bleeding and bruising, (2) local infection, and (3) neurologic symptoms (leg numbness and weakness, urinary or bowel incontinence). It is not uncommon for weakness or numbness to develop in the distribution of the sciatic nerve for the expected duration of the local anesthetic.

RESULTS OF TREATMENT

Injection of the piriformis may improve pain-related outcomes for several months. However, the published studies are limited by poor study methodology and reporting, inconsistent outcome selection, small sample sizes, heterogeneous patient populations, and the absence of standardized diagnostic criteria.

A retrospective study noted that 76% of patients treated with physical therapy and local anesthetic/steroid injection had greater than 50% improvement at an average 10.5-month follow-up.[30] The combination of a sciatic nerve conduction study with the flexion, abduction, internal rotation (FAIR) test may predict those who will respond to physical therapy.[30] A prospective study noted better outcomes with local anesthetic/steroid injection than with medication and physical therapy alone that were sustained for 1 year.[31] Several uncontrolled studies have evaluated the use of botulinum toxin, often in combination with physical therapy, and reported high rates of success that lasted for months (Table 64.1).[27,32-39] A controlled study demonstrated superiority of botulinum toxin over placebo injection for 10 weeks.[35] Other controlled studies have reported that the efficacy of botulinum toxin is superior to that of local anesthetic/steroid or normal saline injections for the treatment of piriformis syndrome when combined with physical therapy.[26,40] One study found good results using clonidine.[41]

ILIOPSOAS INJECTIONS

Pain emanating from the iliopsoas muscle is relatively uncommon but can be a cause of low back, hip, or inguinal pain. Patients typically have unilateral low back or anterior hip pain, although the pain can frequently be referred to the thigh or inguinal area. Patients can vary widely, from young and active athletes, particularly in hockey, soccer, and dance, to older and more sedentary individuals who spend the majority of their time sitting, such as office workers and drivers. Myofascial pain arising from the iliopsoas muscle itself is distinct from that caused by iliopsoas bursitis or tendonitis (*coxa saltans* or "snapping hip syndrome"), although these causes are frequently included in the differential diagnosis. In addition, other causes such as lumbar spinal stenosis, iliotibial band syndrome, osteoarthritis or joint infection, inguinal hernia, and nerve entrapment syndromes should be considered.[42]

On physical examination an antalgic gait as a result of a shortened stride on the affected side may be noted as the patient enters the examination room. The patient may also have pain or weakness when squatting to sit or when transitioning from a seated position to a standing one. The psoas muscle can be palpated deep in the abdomen, medial to the anterior superior iliac spine, when the ipsilateral hip is flexed. Pain on palpation while flexing the hip against resistance is an excellent tool for diagnosing psoas major myopathy but may be uncomfortable for the patient. Provocative tests are not specific for the iliopsoas muscle but can be used to aid in the diagnosis via active and passive extension of a painful muscle.[43]

- Thomas's test—The patient is supine and unable to completely extend the affected hip with the contralateral hip fully flexed; this is due to tightened hip flexors.
- Yeoman's test—The patient is prone and experiences pain with passive extension of the affected hip, typically a sacroiliac joint test but can cause anterior hip pain with passive iliopsoas extension.

Table 64.1 Results of Studies on Botulinum Toxin Injections for Piriformis, Iliopsoas, and Scalene Muscle Injections

Study	Muscle Injected	Type of Study	Groups Compared	Results
Porta[27]	Piriformis	Randomized, controlled	Botox A (100 units) vs. steroid	Pain scores significantly lower in the Botox group 60 days after injection
Lang[32]	Piriformis	Open label	Botox B, (5000 units)	Significant reduction in buttock and hip pain up to 16 wk
Fishman et al.[33]	Piriformis	Prospective, dose ranging	Botox B (5000, 7500, 10,000, 12,500 units)*	12,500 units superior to 10,000 units 12 wk after injection
Yoon et al.[34]	Piriformis	Prospective, open label	Botox A (150 units) vs. lidocaine/ dexamethasone (5 mg)	Improvement in SF-36 subscales (pain, physical and social functioning, vitality, general health) at 4 wk
Childers et al.[35]	Piriformis	Double blind, crossover	Botox A, (100 units) vs vehicle	Results better with Botox injection
Porta[27]	Iliopsoas	Randomized, controlled	Botox A (150 units) vs. steroid	Pain scores significantly lower in the Botox group 60 days after injection
De Andrés et al.[36]	Iliopsoas	Randomized, controlled	Botox A (50 units) vs. 0.25% bupivacaine or NaCl (injected into the contralateral side)	No improvement with either treatment; no difference between groups; trend toward decrease in pain scores with Botox
Jordan et al.[37]	Scalene	Prospective, open label	Botox (12-15 units per muscle)	64% of patients had >50% pain reduction for at least 1 mo
Jordan et al.[38]	Scalene	Retrospective	Botox A (12-15 units per anterior/ middle scalene); fluoroscopy/ EMG guidance compared with ultrasound/EMG guidance	Results comparable: 91% good results with ultrasound and 81% with fluoroscopy
Christo et al.[39]	Scalene	Prospective	Botox (20 units) into the scalene muscle	Significant relief of pain for 3 mo

Note: For botulinum toxin injection of myofascial trigger points, the preponderance of studies showed a lack of efficacy.[13]
*The Botox injection was combined with physical therapy.
EMG, electromyographic; SF-36, 36-Item Short-Form Medical Survey.

- Gaenslen's test—The patient is supine and feels pain with extension of the affected hip (leg hanging off the examination table) while the contralateral hip is flexed (knee held to the chest), typically a sacroiliac joint test but can cause anterior hip pain with passive iliopsoas extension.
- FABER test—The patient is supine and experiences pain with *f*lexion, *ab*duction, and *e*xternal *r*otation of the affected hip.
- Snapping hip test—"Snapping" or "clicking" is heard when the hip is rotated from flexion and abduction to extension and adduction—this rules out *coxa saltans.*

RELEVANT ANATOMY

The psoas major muscle is located in the retroperitoneal space and consists of a deep layer that originates from the transverse processes of L1-5 and a superficial layer that originates from the lateral portions of T12-L4. The lumbar plexus is located between these two layers of muscle. The psoas major also has fibrous attachments to all the lumbar disks except L5-S1. According to their position, the attachments are categorized as either "anterior" or "posterior." The attachments located on the vertebral bodies and intervertebral disks are referred to as anterior fascicles, whereas those located on the transverse processes are known as the posterior fascicles.[44]

The psoas joins the iliacus muscle, which arises from the ilium, to form the iliopsoas muscle within the iliac fascia. This muscle then runs anterolaterally through the iliopubic (iliopectineal) eminence and the muscular lacuna beneath the inguinal ligament, next forms a tendon that sits anterior to the hip joint, and finally inserts onto the lesser trochanter of the femur.[45] The psoas muscles are usually asymmetrical in size, with the right side larger than the left. Innervation of the psoas muscle is achieved via the lumbar plexus from the ventral rami of L1-3, whereas the iliacus muscle is innervated by the femoral nerve from the ventral rami of L1-4.

Occasionally, a psoas minor muscle is present and arises from T12-L1. It follows the medial border of the psoas major and inserts into the iliopectineal eminence of the innominate bone and the iliac fascia at the pelvic brim. The psoas minor is absent in 40% of adults and can therefore be mistaken for lymphadenopathy on imaging studies. This muscle is considered a weak flexor of the spine and is innervated by the ventral rami of L1.[46]

Although it is widely accepted that the iliopsoas muscle aids in flexion and external rotation of the hip, there is controversy surrounding the muscle's other functions.[47] Other electromyographic studies have demonstrated varying degrees of activation of the iliopsoas muscle during hip rotation, adduction, and abduction, as well as during lumbar spine stabilization, flexion, and lateral flexion. As a result of these investigations, the iliopsoas muscle is thought to be "dynamically active" in that it adjusts its function according to spinal position and loading.[48]

To reduce friction between the bone and muscle, a large synovial-lined bursa with only a trace amount of fluid is located at the level of the iliopubic eminence. The bursa itself is relatively undetectable on many imaging modalities, and magnetic resonance imaging (MRI) must generally be used to adequately visualize it. Additionally, the bursa communicates with the hip joint in a small percentage of adults, although the incidence rises dramatically in the setting of trauma or inflammation.[42]

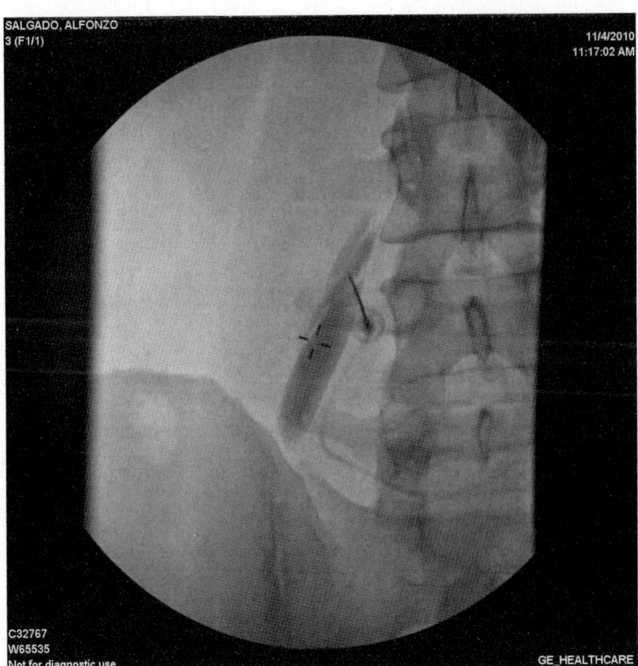

Figure 64.4 Fluoroscopically assisted iliopsoas muscle injection.

IMAGING

Iliopsoas syndrome can be confirmed via the history and physical examination alone, without the aid of special imaging. However, diagnostic imaging may be required because of the uncommon nature of the syndrome, and the diagnosis is frequently based on incidental findings. Multiple imaging modalities, including US, CT, and MRI, can be useful in providing rapid and accurate information. CT can be used to outline the extent of affected tissue and may provide a diagnosis, such as infection or tumor. MRI can be used selectively in cases in which spinal canal or vertebral involvement is suspected.[46]

US has evolved to become a very useful modality for both diagnosis and treatment of iliopsoas-associated disorders. Specifically, US can be used to quickly assess for the presence of fluid in the muscle (e.g., abscess, hematoma) and also to identify abnormal motion of the tendon. Other advantages to using US include the ability to easily scan the hip for assessment of symmetry and to direct injections into the muscle, tendon, or bursa.[49]

TECHNIQUE

BASIC CONSIDERATIONS

The same concerns that apply to any myofascial injection apply to iliopsoas injections as well. Care must also be taken to ensure that the muscle is free of tumor, abscess, or hematoma before proceeding with an injection.

FLUOROSCOPIC TECHNIQUE

Proper monitoring is applied; the patient lies prone with pillows placed beneath the abdomen to correct the lumbar lordosis. The L4 transverse process is visualized on anteroposterior fluoroscopy. After local anesthetic infiltration, a 3-inch, 22-gauge (spinal) needle is advanced until it touches the transverse process. For psoas muscle injection, the tip of the needle touches the superior aspect of the middle or the lateral third of the transverse process and is advanced 1 cm beyond the transverse process. One to 2 mL of contrast agent is injected and the muscle striation pattern is noted (Fig. 64.4). A lateral view is obtained and 6 to 8 mL of local anesthetic (0.5% bupivacaine) and steroid (40 mg methylprednisolone or triamcinolone) is injected. To inject the adjoining quadratus lumborum muscle, the needle touches the lateral tip of the transverse process and is advanced 1 cm. The same procedure as for the psoas muscle is then performed.

ULTRASOUND-GUIDED TECHNIQUE

Single-shot procedures, as well as catheter placement, can be accomplished safely with US guidance. Two US-guided techniques are described as follows.

Lateral Approach

The lateral approach is a technique modified from the one proposed by Kirchmair and colleagues.[50] This technique is recommended in patients with a body mass index lower than 35 since the US view is impaired by a thick abdominal wall. The patient is placed in the lateral decubitus position with a mild anterior tilt. A low-frequency (2 to 6 MHz) curved probe is recommended. The transducer is initially placed lateral to the spine in a cross-sectional view, just above the iliac crest, to identify the transverse process and spinous process. The scan is moved laterally around the waist, while keeping the transverse process in view, to identify the following structures as the probe is kept perpendicular to the skin over the posterior axillary line: skin, fat, lateral part of the erector spinae muscle, quadratus lumborum, part of the external and internal oblique muscles, and the transverse process of L4. At this level it is unlikely that the kidney will be seen unless the patient takes a very deep breath. The transducer is then moved laterally to obtain a full lateral view of the spine and paravertebral structures. The hyperechoic lateral portion of the vertebral body is seen as a thick line curving deeply in the anterior part; lateral to it is the cross-sectional cut of the psoas muscle between the lateral portion of the vertebral body and anterior to the transverse process (Fig. 64.5). Gentle, slow scanning of the psoas muscle while looking at the medial-posterior area will show the nerve root entering the muscle along with a segmental artery. In-plane needle access is recommended, with the entry point in the skin located about 4 cm medial to the medial/posterior end of the transducer. A 12- to 15-cm-long, 20-gauge needle is used for single-shot injections, whereas a long epidural needle is required for insertion of a catheter into the muscle. The needle is advanced toward the junction between the posterior and middle third of the muscle (in the anteroposterior plane) (see Fig. 64.5). If a catheter is placed, it should be advanced 2 to 3 cm beyond the tip of the needle under direct vision, with the bevel of the needle facing cephalad along the fibers of the muscle. The same volumes and drugs as for the fluoroscopy-guided approach are recommended.

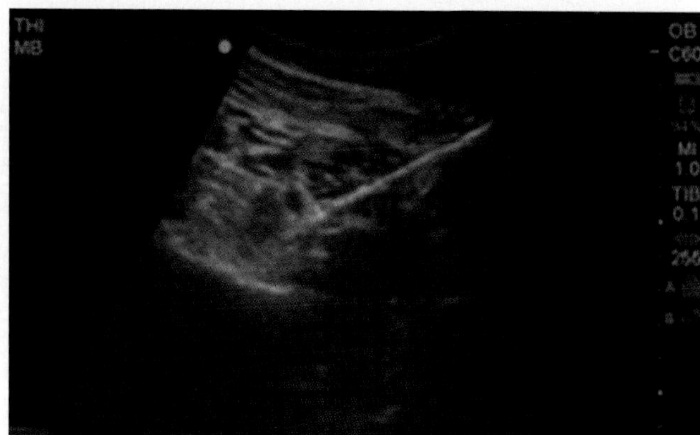

Figure 64.5 Ultrasound-assisted iliopsoas muscle injection.

Posterior Approach

The patient is prone with a pillow under the abdomen to obtain a flat, more superficial spine position. In this approach the same curved transducer probe is initially positioned longitudinally over the spinous process at the level of L3-4. The spinous processes are identified and the transducer is moved laterally to show the laminae, masses of the facet joints, and finally the transverse processes of L2-4, which look like a trident on the US monitor.[51] Careful observation while the patient pushes the ipsilateral knee against the table will show the fibers of the psoas muscle in between the transverse processes. The needle is aimed so that it crosses in between the transverse processes of L3 and L4 about 1.5 cm deeper than the distance measured from the probe to the posterior surface of the transverse process. When injecting in this location, no liquid should be seen superficial to the transverse processes. The catheter, if required, can be advanced as for the lateral US-guided approach.

The patient should be monitored for signs of intravascular injection (the aorta or vena cava when the needle is too anterior), unilateral lower extremity weakness from lumbar plexus blockade, or bilateral lower extremity weakness as a result of epidural or subarachnoid injection (the needle is too medial or larger volumes are injected).

RESULTS OF TREATMENTS

Very limited information is available on the outcome of treatment of iliopsoas syndrome. One controlled study reported the superiority of botulinum toxin injection (150 units in a 3-mL volume) over steroid and local anesthetic.[26] Another controlled study using a side-to-side comparison in the same individuals was unable to demonstrate the superiority of botulinum toxin injection over local anesthetic or saline injection (see Table 64.1).[36] Stretching in combination with dry needling was reported to be very effective in a case series.[43] Standard physical therapy interventions such as stretching, strengthening, and improving neuromuscular control with the assistance of appropriate physical modalities (such as heat and therapeutic US) are also effective in the treatment of iliopsoas syndrome and associated musculotendinous disorders.[52]

SCALENE MUSCLE INJECTIONS FOR NEUROGENIC THORACIC OUTLET SYNDROME

The incidence of thoracic outlet syndrome (TOS) varies from 3 to 80 cases per 1000 people, and it exists in three different forms: neurogenic, venous, and arterial. The most common type, neurogenic, accounts for 95% of all cases and results from compression of the brachial plexus between the anterior and middle scalene muscles and the first rib. Isolated or repeated trauma from whiplash-induced injuries to repetitive motion stress as a result of work or sports activities is a factor in up to two thirds of neurogenic TOS cases. Other causes include muscle anomalies (presence of the scalene minimus muscle, sickle-shaped middle scalene) and bone abnormalities (cervical rib, elongated transverse process). A small percentage of TOS cases are acquired through tumor metastases, osteomyelitis, or other uncommon sources.[53]

Patients often have unilateral paresthesias, usually in the ulnar nerve distribution, or weakness of the upper extremity and variable other symptoms such as headache and cold intolerance. The diagnosis is difficult to make because of a lack of specific diagnostic criteria, relative insensitivity of imaging modalities and other diagnostic testing, and a long list of differential diagnoses.[54]

Scalene muscle injections are indicated for neurogenic TOS as diagnostic, therapeutic, or prognostic blocks before surgery. Local anesthetic injections into the anterior scalene muscle alone or into both the anterior and middle scalene muscles can relieve TOS. The injection relaxes the muscle or muscles elevating the first rib and mimics the effects of first rib resection or scalenectomy. Relief with this technique correlates well with successful physical therapy and surgical treatment.[55] Successful treatment of TOS with scalene muscle injection has been shown to be independent of any brachial plexus blockade.[56]

RELEVANT ANATOMY

The scalene musculature consists of three muscles located on the lateral aspect of the neck; they have variable origin and insertion sites along the neck, as well as frequently fused fascicles between the individual muscles. A fourth muscle is occasionally present, the scalene minimus. The anterior scalene arises from the anterior tubercles of the transverse processes of the C3-6 vertebral bodies and inserts onto the scalene tubercle of the first rib proximally and anterior to the subclavian artery. The middle scalene stems from the posterior tubercles of C2-7 and inserts onto the first rib posterolateral to the anterior scalene and posterior to the subclavian artery. The anterior and middle scalene muscles contain the brachial plexus between them. The posterior scalene originates from the posterior tubercles of C4-6 and inserts posterolateral to both the anterior and middle scalenes on the posterior border of the second rib. All the scalene muscles have multiple variations in their points of origin and insertion.[57]

The scalene muscles are cervical spine flexors. Cervical spine flexion results when the scalene muscles contract bilaterally, and lateral spine flexion results when the muscles contract unilaterally. Additionally, the scalenes serve as accessory muscles of respiration when the cervical spine is stabilized, with the anterior and middle scalenes helping to elevate the first rib and the posterior scalene elevating the second rib during deep inspiration. This group of muscles also rotates the spine ipsilaterally and reaches maximal stretch with contralateral rotation.[58,59]

The scalene muscles are included in the posterior triangle of the neck, which is bordered by the trapezius posteriorly, the sternocleidomastoid anteriorly, and the clavicle inferiorly. Its apex is formed by the junction of the sternocleidomastoid and trapezius at the level of the occipital bone. Also within these demarcations are the brachial plexus (from roots to divisions), cervical sympathetic ganglia, spinal accessory nerve, phrenic nerve, subclavian artery, transverse cervical artery, and lymph nodes.

IMAGING

Imaging modalities, including MRI, usually fail to reveal any abnormalities causing TOS. However, there are reasons to obtain imaging before performing any procedure in the posterior triangle of the neck. Such reasons include confirmation of muscle anomalies (presence of the scalene minimus muscle) and bone abnormalities (cervical rib, elongated transverse process), evaluation of the surrounding soft tissue for evidence of other injuries (e.g., rotator cuff tear), and identification of the presence of tumor, osteomyelitis, or other uncommon causes.

TECHNIQUE

Contraindications to and concerns with scalene muscle injections are the same as those noted for trigger point and piriformis injections. The injections can be done blindly, which is not recommended, with fluoroscopy to visualize the spread of contrast material within the muscle, under CT guidance, or with US. The US-guided technique is preferred for safety reasons since the thyroid, esophagus, carotid, jugular vein, and brachial plexus are visualized, and hence this technique will be the one described.

ULTRASOUND-GUIDED TECHNIQUE

The patient is supine and the area is prepared in sterile fashion. US is used to visualize the anterior and middle scalene muscles through one of two approaches. The probe is placed at the level of the cricoid cartilage/C6 vertebra and moved laterally from the trachea, carotid artery, and internal jugular vein (compressible) to identify the two scalene muscles with the brachial plexus (hypoechoic nerve roots) between them. Alternatively, the US probe can be placed in the inferior (just above the clavicle) and lateral (lateral to the sternocleidomastoid) aspect of the neck. After identification of the subclavian artery and brachial plexus, the plexus is traced cephalad to the level of C7, in between the anterior and middle scalene muscles. After skin infiltration, a 1.5-cm, 21- or 22-gauge needle is advanced out of plane into the belly of the muscle away from the brachial plexus. The out-of-plane approach is preferable to avoid injection of local anesthetic into the brachial plexus (Fig. 64.6). Alternatively, an in-plane approach from the medial side for the anterior scalene muscle and from the lateral side for the middle scalene muscle can be performed. Two milliliters of 0.25% bupivacaine is injected per muscle. Although some authors inject both the anterior and middle scalene muscles, others inject only the anterior scalene muscle.[56]

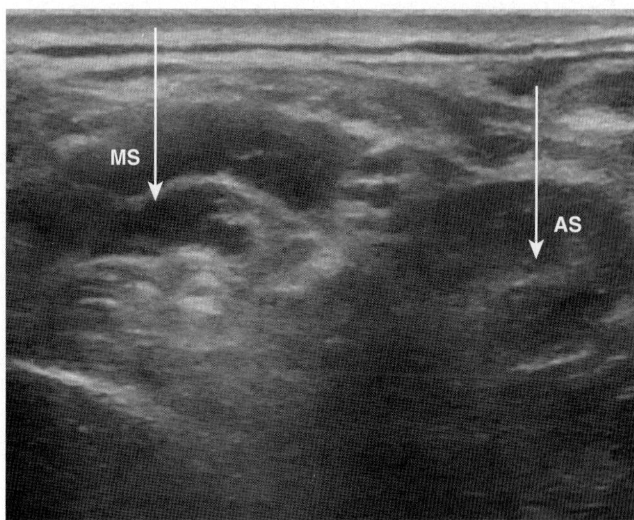

Figure 64.6 Ultrasound-assisted scalene muscle injection. AS, anterior scalene; MS, middle scalene.

Relief of symptoms can occur within 15 to 30 minutes and may last for days or weeks. The brachial plexus may be blocked, with resultant numbness of the upper extremity, since it is not uncommon for the roots of the brachial plexus to pass through the middle scalene muscle. The injected local anesthetic may spill through the fascia of the scalene muscles. If this happens, the patient should be discharged with an arm sling. Note that relief is not dependent on blockade of the brachial plexus. Either series of injections can be performed 2 to 3 weeks apart if the relief is prolonged. Even though the usual duration of relief is days to a week, it may last up to 4 weeks when a series of injections are performed.[53] If relief lasts only for hours or a few days, either injection of botulinum toxin or resection of the anterior or middle scalene (or both) can be performed. Published doses of botulinum toxin are 12 to 15 units of botulinum toxin A per muscle (see Table 64.1).[37-39] Regarding the results of surgery, a retrospective 2-year functional outcome study showed good and fair results in 49% and 35% of patients, respectively.[60]

SUMMARY

- Myofascial injections include trigger point injections and injections of the piriformis, iliopsoas, and scalene muscles.
- Trigger point is the hallmark of myofascial pain syndromes; injections of local anesthetics in conjunction with physical therapy and appropriate medication or medications may result in long-term benefit.
- Piriformis syndrome may mimic L5-S1 radiculitis, although the pain starts in the buttock. There are signs and symptoms that help aid in diagnosis of the syndrome. Injections of local anesthetic and steroid may ameliorate the pain. If relief from a series of local anesthetic/steroid injections is transient, botulinum toxin can be injected.

- Signs and symptoms of iliopsoas muscle pain are usually nonspecific. Diagnostic/prognostic local anesthetic injections may be performed, followed by botulinum toxin injection.
- The diagnosis of neurogenic thoracic outlet syndrome can be made from the patient's symptoms, physical examination, electromyographic findings, and imaging (also to rule out other pathology). Local anesthetic injections into the anterior and middle scalene muscles are preferably performed under ultrasound guidance. Either a series of local anesthetic injections or botulinum toxin injection may be performed; first rib resection and scalenectomy may result in long-term benefit.
- The use of ultrasound has revolutionized injections into the piriformis, iliopsoas, and scalene muscles. Its use with trigger point injections is increasing.
- The injections should be part of a multidisciplinary treatment program that includes physical therapy.

SUGGESTED READINGS

Annaswamy TM, De Luigi AJ, O'Neill BJ, et al. Emerging concepts in the treatment of myofascial pain: a review of medications, modalities, and needle-based interventions. *PM R.* 2011;3:940-961.

Benzon HT, Katz JA, Benzon HA, et al. Piriformis syndrome: anatomic considerations, a new injection technique, and a review of the literature. *Anesthesiology.* 2003;98:1442-1448.

Benzon HT, Rodes ME, Chekka K, et al. Scalene muscle injections for neurogenic thoracic outlet syndrome: case series. *Pain Pract.* 2011;12:66-70.

Fishman SM, Caneris OA, Bandman TB, et al. Injection of the piriformis muscle by fluoroscopic and electromyographic guidance. *Reg Anesth Pain Med.* 1998;23:554-559.

Ingber RS. Iliopsoas myofascial dysfunction: a treatable cause of "failed" low back syndrome. *Arch Phys Med Rehabil.* 1989;70:382-386.

Laulan J, Fouquet B, Rodaix C, et al. Thoracic outlet syndrome: definition, aetiological factors, diagnosis, management and occupational impact. *J Occup Rehabil.* 2011;21:366-373.

Shah JP, Danoff JV, Desai MJ, et al. Biochemicals associated with pain and inflammation are elevated in sites near to and remote from active myofascial trigger points. *Arch Phys Med Rehabil.* 2008;89:16-23.

Siddhartha S, Shah JP, Gebreab T, et al. Novel applications of ultrasound technology to visualize and characterize myofascial trigger points and surrounding soft tissue. *Arch Phys Med Rehabil.* 2009;90:1829-1838.

Simons DG, Travell JG, Simons LS. The Upper Half of the Body. *Myofascial Pain and Dysfunction: The Trigger Point Manual.* Vol. 1. 2nd ed. Baltimore: Lippincott, Williams & Wilkins; 1998.

Smith J, Hurdle MF, Locketz AJ, et al. Ultrasound-guided piriformis injection: technique description and verification. *Arch Phys Med Rehabil.* 2006;87:1664-1667.

The references for this chapter can be found at www.expertconsult.com.

Lumbar Discogenic Pain and Diskography

65

Michael M. Bottros | Steven P. Cohen

OVERVIEW OF LOW BACK PAIN

Back pain has plagued humanity since time immemorial. In most cases, the development of low back pain (LBP) is self-limited and does not require operative intervention. Fifty percent of cases of LBP resolve without medical attention within 1 week; 90% resolve within 4 months.[1] However, the remaining cases exact an enormous burden on society in terms of personal suffering and economic impact. In recent years, the prevalence of disability from back pain has exploded in industrialized societies. In the United States, it was estimated that the direct health care expenditure for back pain was $90.7 billion in 1998.[2] A recent systematic review of the global prevalence of LBP revealed that the mean "overall prevalence," which was defined as all prevalence regardless of the prevalence period, was as high as 31.0%.[3] The statistics are even more unsettling when viewed from a personal and economic perspective. In patients with LBP who have not worked in 6 months, the lifetime return-to-work rate is 50%. In those who have been off work for 1 year, only 25% will return to work. For patients whose injury has left them unable to work for 2 years, the return-to-work rate is less than 5%.[4-6] This dramatic surge in the incidence and cost of chronic LBP has led to a concurrent rise in the use of diagnostic modalities and therapeutic interventions aimed at ameliorating this growing problem. Among the various types of LBP, internal disk disruption (IDD) is widely acknowledged to be the most common source of axial symptoms.

Diskography was first described in 1948 as a diagnostic tool for herniated nucleus pulposus (HNP).[7] Since that time, simpler, safer, and more accurate imaging modalities have largely supplanted diskography as an investigative technique for nerve root compression. Yet in some circles provocative lumbar diskography continues to be a popular, albeit controversial, means of diagnosing axial LBP secondary to IDD. This is because unlike magnetic resonance imaging (MRI) or computed tomography (CT), diskography is not just an imaging modality but a provocative test purported to correlate symptoms with pathology. Although some studies have shown a high degree of correlation between the results of diskography and histologic findings[8,9] and between diskography and surgical outcomes,[10,11] others have failed to demonstrate such a relationship.[12,13]

PROVOCATIVE TESTS IN CONTEXT

Much of the criticism surrounding diskography stems from generalized disapproval about the diagnostic value of provocative procedures for other spinal disorders. In a study by Marks, no consistent segmental or sclerotomal referral patterns were found during 385 provocative lumbar facet blocks in 138 patients with chronic spinal pain.[14] Bough and coworkers assessed the histologic findings of 127 facet joints surgically removed based on the results of preoperative provocative lumbar facet arthrography.[15] The authors found the specificity of degenerative facet joint changes to be 75% but the sensitivity to be only 59%. They concluded that reproduction of symptoms during facet arthrography was of little value as a presurgical screening procedure. Schwarzer and associates conducted a prospective study of 90 patients (203 joints) to determine the relationship between pain provocation and the analgesic response to lumbar zygapophyseal joint blocks.[16] Using a single analgesic block as the diagnostic criterion, reproduction of similar or exact pain was found to predict subsequent response to analgesic facet blocks. However, when the more stringent criterion of concordant analgesic response to confirmatory blocks with lidocaine and bupivacaine was used, no significant association was found.

In 1994, Fortin and colleagues conducted two studies designed to evaluate sacroiliac (SI) joint pain referral maps generated by the distention of joints in asymptomatic volunteers. In the first study, the authors designed a pain referral map by distending the SI joint capsule in 10 asymptomatic subjects by injecting radiopaque contrast material and lidocaine.[17] Similar to a set of previous studies done on the cervical facet joints,[18,19] the authors found that the pain generated during the initial joint injection corresponded with the hypoesthesia experienced after lidocaine was administered. In the second study, independent observers chose 16 patients with chronic LBP whose pain diagrams most closely resembled the pain referral maps generated in the first study and injected their joints with bupivacaine.[20] Ten of the 16 patients obtained 50% or greater pain relief after the instillation of bupivacaine. Of note, the pain referral maps generated in the first Fortin study were significantly different from the SI joint referral zones described by other authors based solely on analgesic blocks.[21] Finally, Schwarzer and associates conducted an SI joint prevalence study in 43 patients with LBP principally below L5-S1.[22] Using the analgesic response to local anesthetic blocks as the sole criterion for diagnosis, 30% of patients were considered to have SI joint pain. Using pain relief combined with a ventral capsular tear on postarthrography CT imaging, 21% of the patients met the diagnostic criteria for SI joint pain. Using the three criteria of concordant pain provocation, abnormal findings on imaging, and analgesic response to injection of local anesthetic, just 16% were considered to have SI joint pain. Among the 27 patients with similar or exact pain reproduction during provocative testing, only 41% experienced "gratifying" pain relief following local anesthetic injection, thus suggesting that pain provocation may be associated with a significant false-positive rate. The lack of strong validity for provocative facet and SI joint injections as diagnostic tools is consistent with the findings of Slipman and coworkers, who demonstrated distinct differences between dynatomal and dermatomal maps during provocative cervical nerve root blocks.[23] In summary, there seems to be little evidence to support the use of provocative injections to diagnose other sources of LBP.

LUMBAR INTERVERTEBRAL DISK ANATOMY

The intervertebral disk complex is composed of the nucleus pulposus (NP), the annulus fibrosus (AF), and the vertebral end plates. Lying above and below the disk are the vertebral bodies or the sacrum below L5-S1. The disk is attached to the adjacent vertebral bodies via the vertebral end plates centrally and to the ligamentous attachments of the AF peripherally. Together, these components allow the principal movements exhibited by the lumbar spine, which include flexion, extension, axial rotation, and lateral flexion. Horizontal translation does not generally occur as an isolated movement but is involved in axial rotation. Posteriorly, the intervertebral disk is supported by the other two components of the three-part structure, the paired zygapophyseal joints. Working in concert, these structures function to support and stabilize the spine and prevent injury by limiting motion to specific planes of movement.[24]

The NP consists primarily of water (70% to 90%) in a matrix composed of proteoglycan, a substance with high water-binding capacity, and type II collagen. The dry weight of the intervertebral disk consists of approximately 65% proteoglycan, with the remainder of the nucleus being composed largely of type II collagen. The high water content of the disk creates a broad, relatively noncompressible weight-bearing surface that serves to cushion the spine from the stress of the truncal load.[24]

The AF is composed of primarily type I collagen arranged in highly organized, concentric lamellae. These lamellae form 10 to 20 sheets surrounding the NP and are thicker toward the center of the disk. The AF is thick and strong anteriorly and laterally but tends to be weaker posteriorly. This anatomic incongruity accounts for the disproportionate percentage of disk herniations occurring posteriorly. Posteriorly, the AF is concave in the lumbar spine. Like the NP, the AF has a high water content, in the range of 60% to 70% by weight. The annulus helps stabilize the vertebral bodies and limit excess motion.[24]

The vertebral end plate is composed of hyaline cartilage close to the vertebral body and fibrocartilage near the NP. The fibrocartilage surrounds the NP and is formed as an extension of the annular fibers. The end plates completely envelop the NP centrally but taper off peripherally, where the outermost AF lamellae directly attach to the vertebral bodies. The composition of the end plates resembles that of the annulus at its attachments to the vertebral bodies and that of the NP centrally.

A healthy adult disk is basically avascular, with its nutrition supplied through the vertebral end plates and the AF via passive diffusion. Whereas the periphery of the annulus is completely permeable, the bone-disk interface is only partially permeable to substrates.[25] The annulus contains blood vessels just in its most superficial lamellae. The nucleus itself contains no direct blood supply. The oxygen and nutrients that diffuse through the end plates come from branches of the lumbar arteries supplying the vertebral bodies.

The anabolic functions of a healthy disk are maintained by chondrocytes and fibroblasts, whereas its catabolic functions depend on the matrix metalloproteinase (MMP) enzymes collagenase (which degrades collagen) and stromelysin (which degrades proteoglycans). The metabolism of cells in the nucleus is exquisitely sensitive to changes in pH, and it is maximally active in the range of 6.9 to 7.2. Even in the presence of high oxygen concentrations, disk metabolism is mainly anaerobic.[26,27] Any number of factors can lead to a breakdown in the delicate metabolic function of the disk, including changes in pH, inflammatory mediators, and nutritional deficiencies.[24]

Functionally, innervation of the lumbar intervertebral disks stems from two extensive nerve plexuses that accompany the posterior and anterior longitudinal ligaments.[24] These are known as the posterior and anterior plexuses. The anterior plexus consists of contributions from the anterior branches of the gray rami communicantes, small medioventral branches of the sympathetic trunk, and perivascular nerve plexuses. The posterior plexus is a diffuse network of interconnecting fibers receiving somatic and autonomic input from multiple spinal levels.[28] Its visible components are derived mainly from the sinuvertebral nerves, which are formed from somatic roots arising from the ventral rami, and from autonomic contributions from the gray rami communicantes (which receive input from the sympathetic trunk), but the majority of its nerve fibers are actually microscopic. The posterior and anterior plexuses are connected via a less prominent conglomeration of nerves known as the lateral plexus, which is formed by branches of the gray rami communicantes.[24,28] Together, these plexuses provide transmission of sensory information from the entire circumference of the intervertebral disk.

In newborns, innervation of the lumbar intervertebral disk is dense, most likely because of the extensive blood supply.[29] This rich vascularization disappears around 4 years of age and is accompanied by a concomitant diminution in nerve density.[30-32] However, in later years when degenerative processes set in, there is a recrudescence of blood vessels and nerve endings. Nerve fibers are typically sparse in the lumbar intervertebral disks, with only the outer third being innervated, but in patients with degenerative disk disease (DDD), the innervation becomes both denser and deeper and frequently penetrates into the inner AF and occasionally into the NP.[33-37]

There is some evidence supporting the role that lumbar sympathetic afferent nerves play in the perception of LBP, including provocation of LBP by stimulation of the sympathetic trunk and relief of LBP following lumbar sympathetic block.[38,39] The contribution of these sympathetic afferents appears to be transmitted mainly via the L2 nerve root, as evidenced by the work of Foerster,[40] who demonstrated that L2 is the dermatome corresponding to LBP, and by the work of Nakamura and colleagues,[41] who showed that LBP disappears or significantly decreases after selective blockade of the L2 nerve root. The observation that the lumbar intervertebral disks and their adjacent ligaments are innervated by branches of the sympathetic nervous system does not necessarily mean that sensory input from these structures returns to the spinal cord via the sympathetic trunk. Rather, it has been suggested that somatic afferent fibers from the disks and surrounding pain-generating structures course with the rami communicantes and return to the central nervous system via ventral rami. Several different types of nonvascular nerve endings have been described, including simple, cluster, and partially and fully encapsulated.[32] Although the exact role of each type of nerve ending is unknown, it is speculated that under nonpathologic conditions, they function primarily as mechanoreceptors[35] (Fig. 65.1).

PATHOGENESIS OF DISCOGENIC LOW BACK PAIN

NERVE INGROWTH

Whether the lumbar intervertebral disks receive sensory innervation continues to be the subject of controversy. In the early and mid-20th century, anatomic studies failed to demonstrate nerve endings within the lumbar intervertebral disks, and it was therefore believed that the disks could not be a principal source of pain generation.[42-44] Subsequent studies have since disproved this concept. In normal human disks, sensory nerves extend into the outer third of the annulus. In degenerated and herniated disks, the innervation is deeper and more extensive, with some nerve fibers penetrating into the NP.[33-37] It is now generally acknowledged that intervertebral disks do receive sensory innervation and indeed can be a significant cause of LBP.[28,32,45-47]

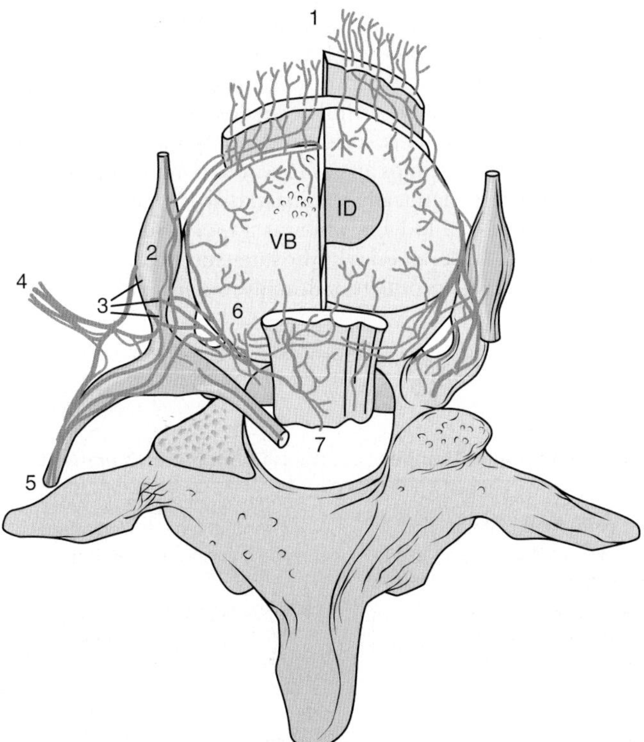

Figure 65.1 Schematic drawing of the nerve plexuses surrounding the vertebral body (VB) and intervertebral disk (ID); 1 and 7 represent the anterior and posterior plexuses, respectively. The deep, extensive penetration of the nerves indicates that degeneration has occurred. 2, Sympathetic trunk; 3, rami communicantes; 4, ventral ramus of the spinal nerve; 5, dorsal ramus; 6, sinuvertebral nerves. (Drawing courtesy of Specialist Jennifer Sempsroft, U.S. Army.)

In 1997, two groups[34,35] described ingrowth of nociceptive nerve endings into degenerate intervertebral disks. Nerve fibers were identified by using a combination of histologic nerve stains. These nerves have the morphology of nociceptive nerves and express GAP43, a marker of nerve growth, and substance P, a nociceptive (and vasoregulatory) neurotransmitter.[48] The mechanisms leading to this nerve ingrowth have been grouped into three categories.

The first of these categories is angiogenesis. During angiogenesis, endothelial cells of vessels growing into the intervertebral disk synthesize the neurogenic stimulator nerve growth factor, one of a family of neurotrophins.[49] Importantly, nerves that are structurally nociceptive in nature are seen only in intervertebral disks that are classified clinically as "pain-level disks." Hence, when these disks are stimulated (e.g., by diskography or direct probing), the patient's symptoms of back pain or sciatica, or both, are reproduced. Intervertebral disks that show similar degrees of degeneration but do not provoke concordant pain with stimulation do not exhibit nerve ingrowth.[48] The second mechanism proposed to lead to nerve ingrowth is altered intervertebral disk matrix biology. Johnson and colleagues[50] showed that aggrecan from normal intervertebral disks inhibits neurite growth but that aggrecan from degenerate intervertebral disks has less of an inhibitory effect. This suggests that with degeneration, nerve ingrowth may occur as a consequence of changed aggrecan biology. Finally, the third possible reason for ingrowth is altered cell function. Even though aggrecan normally inhibits neurite outgrowth, this could be reversed by cells derived from degenerated intervertebral disks.[51]

GENETIC PREDISPOSITION

Over the last 25 years, several genetic associations have been implicated in the predisposition to intervertebral disk degeneration, but few have been replicated consistently. Only collagen IX[52] and vitamin D receptor[53] polymorphisms have been reliably associated with degeneration in reasonably sized populations. Other possible genes currently being investigated include those for collagen I α1,[54] interleukin-6 (IL-6),[55] aggrecan,[56] MMP-3,[57] thrombospondin, cyclooxygenase, tissue inhibitor of metalloproteinases 1 (TIMP-1),[58] cartilage intermediate layer protein,[59] and IL-1. Further studies are needed to examine the functional interaction of these genes within the framework of the molecular pathology associated with the degeneration of intervertebral disks.

MECHANICAL CHANGES

In a normal disk, mechanical interplay between the AF and NP distributes weight bearing uniformly across the entire disk surface.[60,61] When a disk becomes physically stressed, such as by flexion of the spine, the nucleus acts as a noncompressible mass, with its gelatinous contents bulging in the axial, sagittal, and coronal planes. A competent annulus resists this outward bulging, thereby resulting in equal distribution of force.[24] In these circumstances the annulus is not unduly stressed since its broad surface area translates into the nucleus bearing the greatest share of the load.

Over time, age-related changes or an acute injury can lead to a breakdown in normal load bearing. Histologic studies conducted on cadaver lumbar spine specimens have revealed that as early as the second decade of life, a reduction in blood flow leads to diminished nutritional supply to the end plate. This in turn results in tissue breakdown within the disk that commences in the NP and shortly thereafter in the vertebral end plates.[31] This progressive, macroscopic degeneration, in conjunction with either low-level repetitive stress or an acute traumatic event, can lead to two possible sources of injury: microfracture of the vertebral end plate or an annular tear from torsional overload.[62] When this occurs, the ability of the NP to evenly dissipate a compressive load becomes compromised. Unlike normal disks, a compressive load in degenerated disks is not uniformly distributed. Instead, the preponderance of the weight-bearing burden is borne by the richly innervated AF.[60,61] Although this can be maintained for short periods, if the end-plate fracture does not heal, repetitive stress on the annulus can eventually lead to tearing of the fibers. These tears further decrease the load-bearing capacity of the disk since torn lamellae can no longer function as a support apparatus. This initiates a vicious circle that causes even more stress on the remaining lamellae and eventually leads to further tearing of the annular fibers, which can ultimately result in the complete loss of annular integrity.[63] The net result of this sequence of events is that the disk is now predisposed to nuclear herniation. The loss of disk height that inevitably ensues may then deteriorate into continued narrowing of the disk, accompanied by the pathologic changes commonly seen in severe DDD, such as Modic changes, sclerosis of the end plates, and bridging osteophytes[64,65] (Table 65.1). In severe cases, this is manifested as autofusion and anklylosis of adjacent segments.[66]

CHEMICAL CHANGES

Several changes can occur in degenerated disks whose end result is a decrease in the threshold for nociception. First, a break in an end plate can lead to the introduction of inflammatory cytokines into the nucleus, which results in reduced oxygen diffusion, a rise in lactate levels, and a decrease in pH. This conglomeration of factors can result in a slowdown in metabolic and reparative processes and thus lead to increased degradative metalloproteinase activity and diminished chondrocyte activity, which can accelerate disk degradation.[27,67] In certain contexts, proinflammatory cytokines can be a direct source of pain, but in the context of a functional annulus, no pain should be experienced since the inflammatory mediators cannot reach the nociceptors present in the outer part of the disk. However, when an annular tear develops, granulation tissue forms and nerve endings are able to extend through the annulus, with penetration sometimes as far centrally as the NP.[68] Thus, in the presence of a compromised AF, chemical mediators are able to reach sensitized nerve endings, the by-product of which is LBP.[69]

Sensitization and irritation of nerve endings in the end plate may also result in pain.[63] This model of chemical nociception is supported by a number of studies showing disk immunoreactivity to a variety of substances in diseased and herniated intervertebral disks, including vasoactive intestinal polypeptide,[70] substance P, and calcitonin gene–related peptide,[37,71] as well as elevated levels of nitric oxide,[67] prostaglandin E_2,[67,72] IL-2,[67] IL-6,[72] IL-8,[72] phospholipase A_2,[73-77] leukotriene B_4,[78] thromboxane B_2,[78] and tumor necrosis factor-α.[79,80]

Taken in concert, these factors provide a biochemical and mechanical rationale for performing diskography. The generation of pain at low intradiscal pressure is best explained by a preponderance of inflammatory mediators around the sensitized disk; in medical terminology, this is referred to as "chemically sensitized" disks. When disk degeneration is less severe or the disruption less acute, the disk may react to stimulation only at higher pressure, at which point the nerve fibers of the degraded annulus are stretched to the point of pain induction. This scenario describes a "mechanically sensitized" disk. Perhaps an easier way to conceptualize these models is that a chemically sensitized disk is analogous to the phenomenon of allodynia whereas a mechanically sensitive disk is akin to hyperalgesia. In the later stages of disk disease, the annulus may become functionally incompetent, in which

Table 65.1 Modic Changes on Magnetic Resonance Imaging in Patients with Degenerative Disk Disease

Category of Change in Signal Intensity*	T1-Weighted MRI	T2-Weighted MRI	Histopathologic Changes	Significance and Comments
Type I	Decreased signal intensity	Unchanged or increased signal intensity	Disruption and fissuring of the end plate and vascularized fibrous tissue within the adjacent marrow	Changes signify edema. Type I changes tend to convert to type II changes over time
Type II	Unchanged or increased signal intensity	Isointense or slightly hyperintense signal	End-plate disruption with yellow marrow replacement in the adjacent vertebral body	Signifies fatty degeneration. This is the most common type and tends to remain stable over time
Type III	Decreased signal intensity	Decreased signal intensity	Extensive bony sclerosis indicative of dense woven bone within the vertebral body rather than marrow	No marrow to produce MRI signal

*Refers to changes in signal intensity in the vertebral body marrow adjacent to the end plates of degenerative intervertebral disks.
MRI, magnetic resonance imaging.
Adapted from Modic MT, Masaryk TJ, Ross JS, et al. Imaging of degenerative disk disease. *Radiology*. 1988;168:177-186.

case injection of contrast material may fail to generate intermediate to high pressure. This can result in an uninterpretable or even false-negative pain response if manometry is not used. On CT, severely degenerated disks are likely to show a diffuse pattern of spread of contrast material with extensive leakage into the epidural space, but it is possible to miss small leaks on plain fluoroscopy. Normal disks resist pain provocation because they lack both the chemical hypersensitivity and the apparatus for mechanical overloading that are present in diseased disks. In clinical practice, these examples represent an ideal diagnostic paradigm that fails to account for the multitude of genetic, social, cultural, and psychological factors that affect pain perception. To optimize diagnosis and treatment outcomes, these factors must be considered when performing any pain-provoking procedure.

LUMBAR DISK PAIN REFERRAL PATTERNS

The premise on which diskography is based is that controlled pressurization of a painful disk will reproduce a patient's symptoms. The limitations of this paradigm have been discussed previously. In addition to the flaws inherent in any provocative test, inaccuracies may also result from oversedation with anxiolytics or opioids (or both), excessive administration of local anesthetic, anxiety, procedure-related pain, the ephemeral nature of disk pressurization, and an inability to distinguish concordant from noncordant pain in the brief moments when disk pressure exceeds the nociceptive threshold. Nevertheless, several investigators have attempted to categorize the pain patterns with positive diskograms. In a prospective study conducted in 187 patients with LBP scheduled for diagnostic CT-diskography, Ohnmeiss and coworkers found that L3-4 diskograms were likely to be positive if patients described their pain as involving the lumbar region with radiation into the anterior but not the posterior aspect of the thigh and often into the anterior aspect of the leg.[81] For L4-5 disks, the most common pain referral pattern was lumbar pain involving more equivalent proportions of the anterior and posterior thigh pain. In L5-S1 discogenic pain, the pain description generally encompassed the lumbar and posterior thigh regions, with fewer patients reporting anterior thigh or leg pain. Pain in the absence of disk pathology tended to be limited to the low back region and buttocks (Fig. 65.2).

In the late 1980s, Vanharanta and colleagues performed a series of studies to evaluate the effects of various disk abnormalities on pain referral patterns. In the first of these studies, evaluation of CT-diskograms in 91 patients showed a positive relationship between the occurrence of pain and the presence of an annular rupture.[82] The second study found that narrow disks were more likely to be associated with "exact pain reproduction" than were disks of normal height.[83] In the same study it was also suggested that the degree of pain concordance is influenced by the spinal level. Specifically, severely degenerated L3-4 disks were less likely to result in concordant pain than were comparable disks at the L4-5 and L5-S1 spinal levels. The third paper, a prospective, multicenter study evaluating the results of 300 surgical candidates with a variety of clinical diagnoses, found no significant relationship between concordant pain provocation in four diagnostic groups: disk herniation (82%), DDD (81%), lumbar syndrome (56%),

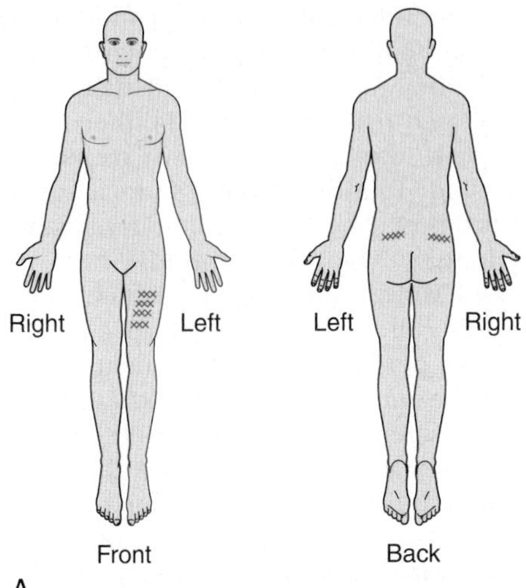

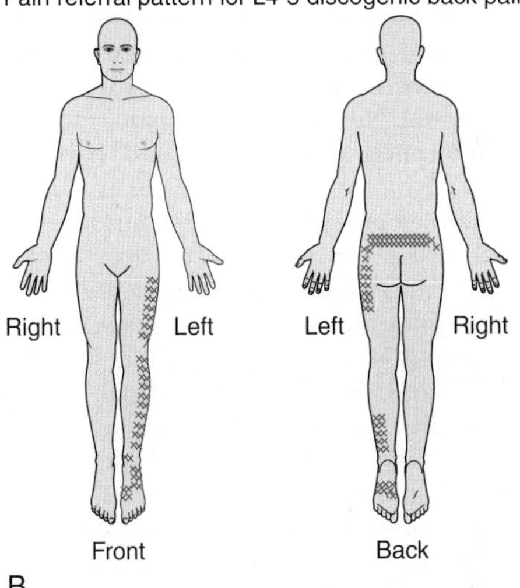

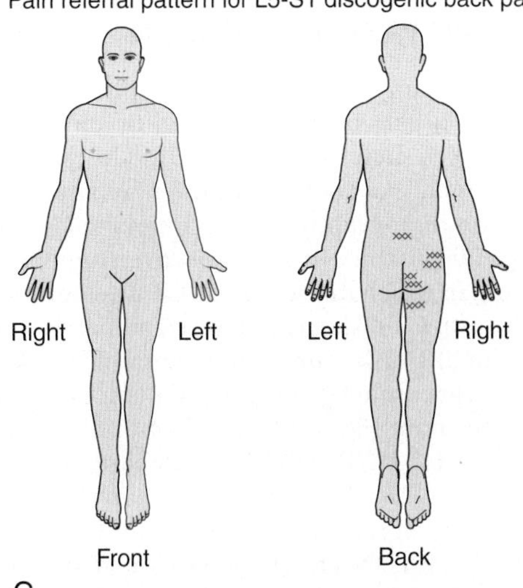

Figure 65.2 **A,** Pain referral pattern for L3-4 discogenic back pain. **B,** Pain referral pattern for L4-5 discogenic back pain. **C,** Pain referral pattern for L5-S1 discogenic back pain. (Adapted from Ohnmeiss DD, Vanharanta H, Ekholm J. Relation between pain location and disk pathology: a study of pain drawings and CT/discography. *Clin J Pain*. 1999;15:210-217.)

and radiculopathy (59%).[84] Disks that were deteriorated tended to be painful regardless of a patient's diagnostic classification. In the fourth study, based partly on the same patient population, the authors found that the percentage of degenerated disks that elicited either "no pain" or "noncordant pain" was higher in elderly patients.[85] A later retrospective study found that outer annular ruptures were the only predictors of concordant pain in a reanalysis of 833 diskograms done in 306 patients with LBP.[86]

Maezawa and Muro came to a different conclusion from Vanharanta and colleagues. In a retrospective analysis of 1477 diskograms performed in 523 patients with axial or radicular LBP, the authors found that elicitation of pain was only weakly associated with IDD whereas the presence of a herniated disk was strongly associated with pain provocation.[87] Saifuddin and coworkers performed a retrospective review of 260 lumbar diskogram reports with the aim of correlating morphologic disk abnormalities with pain referral patterns.[88] The authors demonstrated a highly significant association between annular tears and concordant back and radiating pain of any type. An association between isolated posterior tears and radiating pain was also found, but no relationship between anterior annular tears and any pain radiation was noted. No differences in pain referral patterns were identified when full-thickness and partial-thickness posterior tears were compared. There was an increased incidence of leg pain versus groin, hip, or buttock pain during L4-5 and L5-S1 disk provocation, but this trend did not reach statistical significance. Finally, a retrospective study by Slipman and colleagues did not find any correlation between the side of a patient's concordantly painful annular tear on CT-diskography and the side with the pain complaints.[89] To summarize, the presence of degenerative changes of any type is more likely to be associated with pain than are nondegenerated disks or disks with only minimal degradation. Pain provocation may also be more likely to occur in the presence of annular tears and nuclear herniations, with more evidence supporting the former assertion.

FALSE-POSITIVE PAIN PROVOCATION

In the past 30 years the use of diskography to detect disk pathology has largely been supplanted by more advanced radiologic studies such as MRI and CT. The evidence that these newer modalities are not only safer but also more accurate than plain diskography in detecting herniated nuclear material is indisputable. In a prospective study by Jackson and associates in which myelography, CT-myelography, plain diskography, and CT-diskography were compared with surgical findings in 231 disks, the authors found CT-diskography to be the most accurate test (87%) and plain diskography to be the least accurate (58%).[90] CT-diskography ranked highest in sensitivity for HNP at 92%, as compared with 78% for CT-myelography, 72% for CT, 70% for myelography, and 81% for plain diskography.[90] For specificity, CT-diskography was also the most accurate (81%), followed by CT (76%) and CT-myelography (76%), myelography (70%), and plain diskography (31%).

Since diskography is more invasive and unequivocally less sensitive in detecting most disk pathology than newer imaging techniques are, the primary justification for its continued use lies in its ability to correlate pathology with symptoms. This rationale seems reasonable given that close to two thirds of asymptomatic adults have abnormal findings on MRI of their lumbar spine, with the prevalence of these findings increasing with age.[91] LBP is an epidemic of unprecedented proportion in industrial societies, and the estimated lifetime prevalence ranges from 60% to higher than 80%.[92,93] Without a corroborative test to validate these abnormal MRI findings, it is likely that many of these patients would be conferred with incorrect diagnoses and subsequently undergo unnecessary surgical procedures. There is little doubt that unnecessary stabilization operations are performed far too frequently in the United States, but there is disagreement about whether diskography prevents or facilitates these unnecessary surgeries.[94] Proponents of diskography believe that correlating pathology with symptoms prevents unnecessary surgical intervention, whereas opponents question both the significance of diskographic pathology and the validity of provoked symptoms. These criticisms are bolstered by the relative lack of specificity of diskography, the inherent difficulty in validating provoked symptomatology, the large number of studies showing false-positive pain provocation in patients without low back symptoms, and disparities with regard to histologic findings on surgical specimens.

In phase 1 of a two-part experiment, Yasuma and coworkers studied 181 lower thoracic and lumbar disks from 30 adult cadavers diskographically and histologically.[95] Their findings revealed 32 true-positive, 15 false-positive, 122 true-negative, and 12 false-negative diskograms. Diskograms were designated false-positive when the injected contrast material was noted to extend beyond the peripheral vertebral margin but histologic sectioning of the disk was negative for protrusion. False negatives were defined as a negative diskogram despite histologically confirmed disk protrusion. In the 32 true-positive disks, both the diskograms and histologic sections showed 10 anterior protrusions, 17 posterior protrusions, and 5 posterior herniations. Among the 15 false-positive diskograms, 9 were misdiagnosed as a protrusion and 6 as a herniation. In part 2 of this study, the authors conducted a retrospective review of 77 diskography patients subsequently found to have a herniated disk during surgical exploration.[95] The diskograms were falsely interpreted as negative in 32% of the 59 patients with a protruding disk and in 56% of the 18 patients with a prolapse. In a previous study the authors found that false-positive diskograms were more likely to occur when fissures or cysts were present in a degenerated annulus but did not establish continuity with the nuclear cavity.[96]

The first study to question the validity of diskography was published in 1968 by Holt, who found false-positive results in 37% of 30 asymptomatic prisoners.[97] More than 20 years later, Walsh and colleagues performed CT-diskography on 10 asymptomatic male volunteers and 7 "control" patients with chronic LBP.[98] Sixty-five percent of the 20 disks injected in the patients with back pain showed radiologic abnormalities, with all 7 patients having at least 1 degenerated disk. In the patients without back pain, CT-diskograms were interpreted as abnormal in 17% of the 35 disks injected and in half of the 10 subjects. However none of these 5 patients experienced concordant pain associated with pain-related behavior during the injections. Thus, the false-positive rate in this study was 0%.

In 1996, Block and coworkers conducted a landmark prospective study in 90 patients with low back and leg pain who underwent CT-diskography at the three lowest lumbar levels.[99] The Minnesota Multiphasic Personality Inventory was administered to each subject before diskography and scored independently. In the 72 patients with at least one nondisrupted disk, 34 reported discordant pain provocation at a normal level, with the remaining 38 patients reporting a "concordant negative response." In the 34 patients who reported pain during pressurization of normal disks, the mean hypochondriasis, hysteria, and depression scores were significantly higher than in patients in whom stimulation of normal disks did not elicit pain.

In 1999 and 2000, Carragee and coauthors published a series of studies attempting to identify patients at high risk for false-positive diskograms. In the first study, eight patients with no history of back problems or structural spinal abnormalities who had recently undergone iliac crest bone grafting for reasons unrelated to lumbar spine, hip, or pelvic pathology were studied by provocative diskography of their three most caudal disks.[100] Four of the eight study subjects experienced severe LBP similar to the postoperative pain at their bone graft site during injection of at least one disk. All symptomatic disks had an abnormal morphologic appearance.

In the second study, the authors performed lumbar diskography on 10 patients with neck and upper extremity pain but no lower back symptoms, 6 patients with somatization disorder, and 10 control patients devoid of pain symptoms.[101] The three most caudad lumbar disks were injected in all patients, with five patients having the L2-3 disk studied as well. Eighty-three percent of patients in the somatization group, 40% of the chronic cervical pain patients, and 10% of the control patients experienced moderate or severe pain during injection of contrast material into at least one disk. Pain was provoked in 11% of disks with intermediate-grade disruption and in 37% of disks with annular tears. In contrast, injection did not result in pain in any of the 31 radiographically normal disks. In the last study, three-level diskography was performed on 47 patients who had undergone single-level diskectomy for sciatica.[102] Twenty subjects with no recurrent symptoms were designated the "study" group, and 27 patients with persistent back or leg symptoms (or both) formed the "control" group. In the asymptomatic participants, positive injections occurred in 8 of 20 (40%) operative disks. In the "control" patients with symptoms, positive injections occurred in 17 of the 27 operative disks (63%), with the pain being concordant in 15. No significant differences were found in the diskography results between symptomatic and asymptomatic participants with normal psychometric scores. In contrast, patients with abnormal prediskography psychological test scores were more likely to rate their pain as unbearable during injection of both operative and nonoperative disks than were patients in both groups with no psychopathology. All positive disks were radiographically abnormal.

There are several flaws in the studies assessing "false-positive" diskograms in asymptomatic subjects, with the main one being inherent in the study design: in subjects without preexisting LBP, one cannot provoke true concordant pain, which has become a hallmark of modern-day diskography. The second major shortcoming is that although the Carragee studies used manometry to limit intradiscal pressure, pressure readings were not a determining factor in the designation of a positive disk. The guiding principle behind diskography is to identify disks that provoke pain during stimulation, but application of excessive pressure to any bodily structure that contains nerves, including components of the spine besides disks,[17,18] will provoke pain in normal subjects.

In an effort to determine the effect that objective pressure readings have on the incidence of positive disk injections in asymptomatic volunteers, Derby and colleagues performed 43 diskograms on 13 subjects with either no history or infrequent episodes of LBP.[103] In the patients with occasional back pain, 35% of the 20 injected disks were painful versus 52% in volunteers with no history of LBP. Most disks required that high pressure be reached before pain was elicited, and even then, the pain was mild. There was no relationship between painful disk injections and abnormalities on MRI or diskography. Controlling for the intensity of response and the pressures at which pain was elicited, the authors concluded that the incidence of false-positive diskograms was less than 10%. Some potential causes of false-positive diskograms include inadvertent annular injection (Fig. 65.3), contrast-induced irritation of nervous tissue, end-plate deflection resulting from suboptimal needle placement, and stimulation of pressure receptors when excessively high pressure is generated.[104,105]

Wolfer and coauthors[106] published a systematic review in which data from five previous studies were reanalyzed by using guidelines from the International Association for the Study of Pain (IASP) and the International Spine Intervention Society (ISIS) for a positive lumbar diskogram (Table 65.2). The authors found an overall false-positive rate of 9.3% per patient and 6.0% per disk. False-positive rates dropped to 3.0% per patient and 2.1% per disk in patients without back pain or confounding factors. Chronic pain patients were found to have false-positive rates of 5.6% per patient and 3.9% per disk. Finally, the highest false-positive rates per patient and disk occurred in postdiskectomy patients (15% and 9.1%, respectively) and those with somatization disorder (50% and 22.2%, respectively).

One flaw in these criteria is that they do not consider a patient's baseline pain rating, which can lead to flagrant inconsistencies. For example, a person with significant back pain disability who rates his baseline pain as 3/10 and in whom disk stimulation provokes 5/10 pain would be considered to have a negative diskogram by ISIS guidelines because the maximum pain score did not exceed the minimum cutoff threshold for designating a disk as positive. Yet a person with less functional impairment and 9/10 baseline pain in whom disk stimulation provokes 7/10 pain could theoretically be classified as having a positive diskogram.

Despite these limitations, given the high propensity for false-positive findings in patients with previous back surgery, psychopathology, or somatization symptoms, positive diskograms should be viewed with caution in these individuals. To optimize specificity, we suggest using two adjacent control disks, a recommendation previously endorsed by Endres and Bogduk in an attempt to improve accuracy in patients at high risk for false-positive diskography.[107] Although it may seem intuitive that this would enhance specificity or improve outcomes, these issues have yet to be addressed.

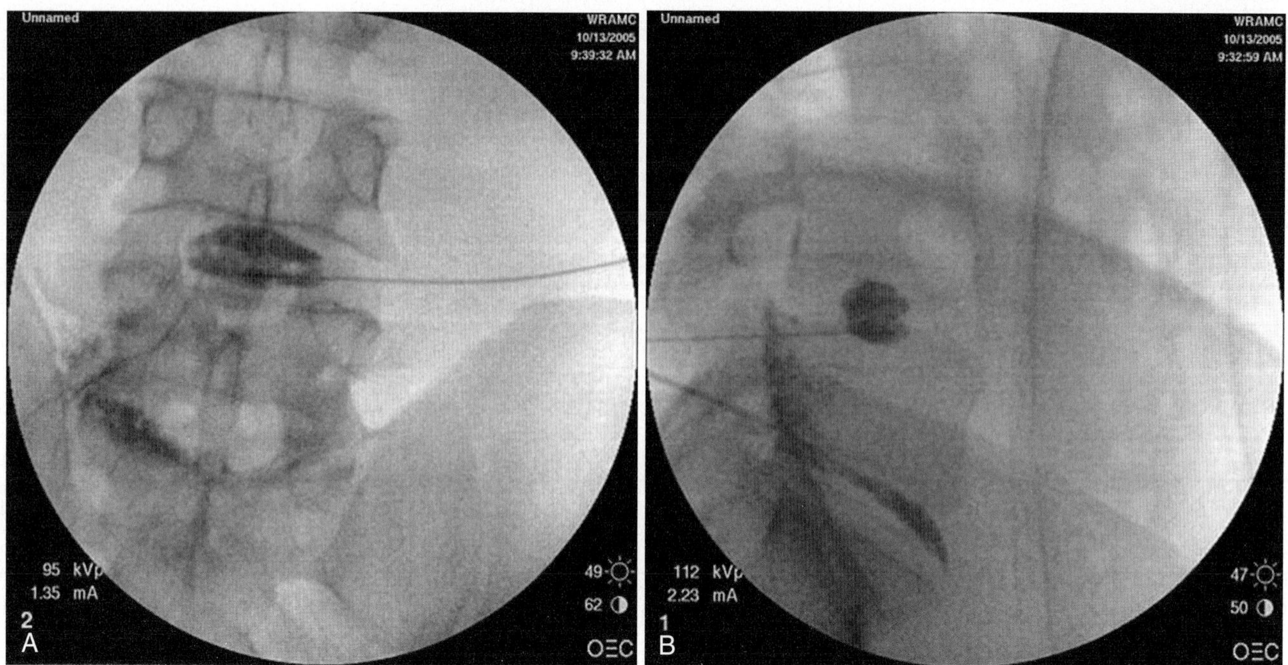

Figure 65.3 Anteroposterior (**A**) and lateral (**B**) fluoroscopic annulograms at L5-S1. **A,** Anteroposterior diskogram showing annular injection at L5-S1. **B,** Lateral diskogram showing annular injection at L5-S1.

Table 65.2 Positive Diskogram Criteria

	NRS Pain Score	Pressure (psi)	Pain Behavior	Grade 3 Annular Tear	Control Disk NRS
Walsh/Carragee	≥6/10	≤100	≥2/5	—	—
Derby	≥6/10	≤50	—	Y	<6/10
ISIS/IASP (a)	≥7/10	<50	—	Y	—
ISIS/IASP (b)	≥7/10	<50	—	Y	<6/10
ISIS/IASP (c)	≥7/10	<50	—	Y	0/10
Low pressure, <22 psi (Carragee)	≥6/10	<22	≥2/5	—	—
Low pressure, ≤15 psi (Derby)	≥6/10	≥15 psi	—	Y	<6/10

IASP, International Association for the Study of Pain; ISIS, International Spine Intervention Society; NRS, numerical rating scale.
Adapted from Wolfer LR, Derby R, Lee JE, et al. Systematic review of lumbar provocation discography in asymptomatic subjects with a meta-analysis of false-positive rates. *Pain Physician*. 2008;11:513-538.

The subject of "false-negative" diskograms has garnered far less attention but can result in inaccurate diagnoses, unnecessary interventions, and withholding of beneficial treatment from otherwise good candidates. There are several reasons that a person with discogenic pain may fail to experience pain with disk stimulation, including failure to detect an inadequate rise in intradiscal pressure because of the lack of pressure monitoring, injecting too slowly, excessive sedation, overzealous use of local anesthetic, and extensive extravasation of contrast material in severely degenerated disks. False-negative diskograms may be more likely to occur in elderly patients.[84] In a review by Cohen and associates,[108] the authors estimated that between 15% and 25% of degenerated disks fail to elicit concordant pain provocation during stimulation. The proportion of these occurrences that represent false-negative responses versus accurate reflection of a non–pain generator is a question that remains to be answered. The results of clinical studies evaluating false-positive lumbar diskography are presented in Table 65.3.

PREVALENCE OF DISCOGENIC LOW BACK PAIN

Axial back pain is one of the most common, yet challenging, problems faced by pain physicians. Numerous structures besides degenerated disks can cause axial LBP, with two of the more common ones being the lumbar facet joints and muscles. The SI and facet joints are implicated as the primary cause of chronic axial pain in 15% to 30% and 10% to 15% of cases, respectively.[110,111] In a porcine study by Indahl and coworkers, the authors determined that there is significant overlap between the neuromuscular connections of the intervertebral disks, zygapophyseal joints, and paraspinal muscles such that the relative contributions of each of these

Table 65.3 Clinical Studies Evaluating False-Positive Lumbar Diskography

Study, Year	Subjects	Criteria	Results
Massie, 1967[109]	52 male subjects, 156 disks	NR	FP rate not reported but stated "injection only occasionally produced symptoms"
Holt, 1968[97]	30 male volunteer inmates, 70 disks (20 failed injections)	Pain provocation	60% FP rate per subject, 37% per disk
Walsh, 1990[98]	10 male volunteers, 30 disks	3/5 pain provocation + 2/5 pain-related behavior	0% FP rate per subject and disk
Carragee, 1999[100]	8 males who had recently undergone iliac crest bone grafting for problems unrelated to low back pain, 24 disks	3/5 "concordant" pain provocation (to previous iliac crest pain) + 2/5 pain-related behavior	50% FP rate per subject, 38% per disk
Carragee, 2000[101]	6 subjects with somatization disorder, 10 with failed neck surgery, and 10 control patients with no pain after successful cervical spine surgery; 78 disks	3/5 "concordant" pain provocation (to previous iliac crest pain) + 2/5 pain-related behavior	FP rate per subject: 83% for somatization, 40% for failed neck surgery, and 10% for "control" group. FP rate per disk: 33% for somatization, 23% for failed neck surgery, and 3% for control group
Carragee, 2000[102]	47 subjects who underwent single-level diskectomy (20 subjects were "symptom free," whereas 27 continued to have back and/or leg pain); 138 disks	3/5 pain provocation + 2/5 pain-related behavior	FP rate per subject: 40% for asymptomatic subjects and 56% for patients with failed back surgery. FP rate per disk: 15% in the asymptomatic group
Derby, 2005[103]	13 volunteers, 43 disks	Criteria not noted. Used 0-10 pain rating and 0-4 pain behavior scales along with manometry	Using 6/10 as criterion for a positive disk, 0% FP rate. Using 4/10 pain at ≤50 psi, FP rate of 23% per subject and 9% per disk

FP, false-positive; NR, not reported.
Adapted from Cohen SP, Malik KM. Discography. In *Essentials of Pain Medicine*. 3rd ed. Philadelphia: Elsevier; 2011, 462-470.

structures to LBP may be difficult to estimate.[112] One may thus conclude that in many patients with chronic LBP, the cause of the pain is multifactorial.

The prevalence of discogenic LBP varies widely in the medical literature. In one of the most cited studies, Schwarzer and colleagues found the incidence of discogenic pain to be 39% in a prospective cross-sectional study using either zygapophyseal joint blocks or diskography in 92 consecutive patients with chronic LBP.[113] The authors based their diagnoses on exact pain reproduction during provocative disk stimulation, coupled with abnormal findings on CT-diskography and the presence of an adjacent, negative control disk. Collins and associates conducted a prospective study comparing the use of MRI and diskography in the evaluation of 29 patients with unremitting axial LBP without focal neurologic deficits.[114] The authors found exact reproduction of the symptoms to be present in 13 disks in 12 patients, for a prevalence rate of 41%. In all 13 symptomatic disks, both MRI and diskography showed degenerative changes. In another study comparing the results of MRI and diskography, Horton and Daftari performed 63 diskograms in 25 patients with nonradicular LBP.[115] Diskography yielded moderate to severe pain at 26 levels, with 19 patients reporting similar or exact pain reproduction, for a prevalence rate of 76%. Only 1 of the 26 disks was morphologically normal. Long and colleagues conducted a very large epidemiologic study in 2374 patients with LBP seen by spine surgeons at seven academic medical centers.[116] Final diagnoses were rendered after imaging studies were reviewed and treatment prescribed, with tests and therapies being performed at the discretion of the surgeon. Nonherniated degenerated disk was the final diagnosis in 6.1% of patients. Finally, in a retrospective analysis of clinical data from 127 patients with axial LBP who failed facet interventions, Cohen and coauthors reported a prevalence of 65%.[117] Based on the conflicting evidence that does exist, discogenic LBP appears to be the major source of pain in more than a third of patients with chronic axial LBP. Whereas younger and middle-aged people with axial LBP are more likely to have disks as the principal source of their symptoms, the facet joints become more important as pain generators in the elderly.

CORRELATION WITH RADIOLOGIC STUDIES

There is compelling evidence that diskography, even without CT scanning, may overestimate the prevalence of clinically significant IDD, but it is equally clear that diskography may fail to detect the disk pathology seen with other radiologic studies. In a study by Gibson and associates in which MRI and diskography were compared in making the diagnosis of DDD, agreement between the two techniques was found in 44 of the 50 disks studied.[118] In the six disks in which a discrepancy occurred, evidence of IDD was missed on five diskograms and one MRI study. In the five cases in which diskography failed to detect disk pathology, two were due to incorrect placement of the diskography needle in the annulus. Although disk stimulation symptoms were recorded in the study, the results of diskography were based only on radiographic findings.

Yoshida and coworkers sought to investigate the relationship between plain diskography and T2-weighted and gadolinium-enhanced T1-weighted MRI in 23 patients with chronic LBP.[119] A posterior annular tear was detected in 16 of the 17 positive disks with T2-weighted MRI and in 10 of 14 positive disks with gadolinium-enhanced T1-weighted MRI. The T2-weighted study also detected 11 annular tears in 39 negative disks versus 8 annular tears in 32 negative disks with T1-weighted gadolinium-enhanced MRI. The sensitivity, specificity, positive predictive value, and negative predictive value of the T2-weighted study in detecting symptomatic disks were 94%, 71%, 59%, and 97%, respectively, which compared favorably with the T1-weighted images. The authors concluded that the high sensitivity and negative predictive value of T2-weighted MRI make it a useful screening tool to avoid unnecessary diskography in patients with chronic LBP.

Simmons and coauthors compared CT-diskography with MRI in 164 patients with chronic LBP, with or without radicular symptoms.[120] Correlation between the two techniques was seen in 55% of cases. In the 371 disks in which MRI and diskography were concordant, 172 were normal and 199 were abnormal. In the disks classified as abnormal based on MRI, 37% were asymptomatic during injection. In 13% ($n = 60$) of the disks, findings on MRI were abnormal but diskograms were normal. In 7% of the disks ($n = 34$), MRI showed normal and diskography showed abnormal findings. In 21 of these 34 disks, injection of contrast material into the disk elicited exact pain reproduction.

In a comparative study evaluating MRI and diskography in patients with axial LBP, Collins and colleagues found that imaging characteristics for the two diagnostic procedures correlated in 65 of 73 disks (89%).[114] In the other eight cases, four disk levels showed evidence of early degeneration on diskography but appeared normal on MRI, whereas four disks showed decreased signal intensity on T2-weighted MRI but were diskographically normal. In the 12 patients with concordant pain on diskography, spinal fusion was performed. At their 9-month follow-up, 9 of the 12 patients reported clinical improvement.

Aprill and Bogduk[121] performed CT-diskography on 41 patients with chronic LBP who demonstrated a high-intensity zone (HIZ) on T2-weighted MRI. In all patients, CT-diskography revealed either a grade 3 or 4 annular disruption in the affected disk. The sensitivity and specificity of an HIZ for detecting similar pain reproduction during disk provocation were 63% and 97%, respectively. For detection of exact pain reproduction, the sensitivity was 82% and the specificity 89%. In the identification of a grade 4 annular disruption, the sensitivity of an HIZ was only 54%, but the specificity was 89% and the positive predictive value 90%.

Other studies have shown a much stronger correlation between MRI and diskography. Linson and Crowe found the two investigative modalites to be in agreement on 91 of 97 disks studied in 50 patients.[122] In the six disks in which a discrepancy was present, five were read as normal by MRI but abnormal by diskography. In an earlier study by Schneiderman and coworkers, MRI and diskography positively correlated in 100 of 101 levels.[123]

However, not all studies have demonstrated a high degree of correlation. Zucherman and associates[124] reported positive diskography in the face of normal MRI findings in a case series involving 18 patients. Horton and Daftari[115] conducted an observational study involving 25 consecutive patients and 63 disks studied by diskography and MRI. Abnormal diskographic morphology was noted in 42 of 59 cases, but only 23 disks were associated with significant pain. In dark disks, disk stimulation provoked pain in 7 of 11, but 0 of 5 "white" bulging disks were positive. Because of these discrepancies, the authors concluded that both MRI and diskography should be used for surgical planning. Finally, in a retrospective study of 53 consecutive patients who underwent both provocative diskography and MRI, Sandhu and colleagues[125] found poor correlation between the vertebral end plate signal changes observed on MRI and the results of provocation diskography.

Overall, diskography appears to be comparable or slightly more sensitive for the detection of IDD than MRI or CT does, especially with regard to radial annular fissures. Approximately 25% of moderately degenerative disks identified on MRI will fail to have concordant pain on diskography. The main problem with correlative studies is that when an incongruity exists, it is impossible to determine whether the discrepancy is due to a lack of sensitivity (false negatives) or specificity (false positives) in one of the diagnostic procedures (Table 65.4).

EFFECT ON OUTCOMES AFTER SPINAL FUSION

The value of spine surgery in treating DDD and axial LBP is a subject that has engendered passionate controversy in the medical and lay literature. Even though the operative results of spinal arthrodesis vary greatly, depending on the success criteria and follow-up period, it is widely acknowledged to be less beneficial than surgery for radicular pain, with success rates ranging from less than 50% to higher than 80%.[94,139,140] Moreover, these reported outcomes must be considered in light of the fact that no fusion studies have ever been conducted under strictly controlled conditions. A recent Cochrane database review concluded that there was no scientific evidence supporting any form of surgical decompression or fusion for the treatment of DDD.[141] Among the four randomized studies comparing lumbar fusion with conservative care,[142-145] only one demonstrated significant benefit at 2-year follow-up.[129] This study has been criticized because the patients allocated to nonsurgical treatment had essentially already failed most of these treatments and the improvements in pain (33%) and function (25%) were modest. The presence of concomitant pain sources in most patients with discogenic pain and the mixed clinical outcomes even when arthrodesis is technically successful[94,141,146] are factors that must be considered when evaluating clinical studies examining the correlation between the results of diskography and surgical outcomes.

Several investigators have attempted to correlate the results of diskography with surgical findings and outcomes. Colhoun and colleagues evaluated the surgical outcomes of 162 patients who underwent preoperative diskography for axial LBP.[10] In the 137 patients with concordant pain on diskography, 89% had a favorable outcome at a mean follow-up period of 3.6 years. In the 25 patients whose disks showed morphologic abnormalities but elicited no provocation of symptoms, only 52% reported significant benefit. Diskography in this study was not accompanied by manomentry, and the surgical treatments evaluated were mostly spinal fusions.

Text Continued on pg. 898

Table 65.4 Studies Comparing Lumbar Diskography with CT or MRI in Patients with Degenerative Disk Disease

Author, Year	Number of Subjects	Nature of Study	Results	Comments
Gibson, 1986[118]	22 patients, 50 disks	Compared MRI and diskography in patients with mechanical LBP	Agreement between studies in 44 of 50 disks	Diskography results based on radiographic findings only as patients were sedated. In the 6 disks that did not correlate, MRI was superior to diskography
Schneiderman, 1987[123]	36 patients with LBP with or without leg pain, 101 diskograms	Compared MRI and diskography	MRI accurate in assessing disk morphology in 100 of 101 levels. Of 52 disks with normal MRI findings, only 1 had a positive diskogram. Of 49 disks with decreased MRI signal, only 2 diskograms normal	Used only T2-weighted MRI. CT-diskography used on 39 levels
Zucherman, 1988[124]	18 patients with LBP with or without radicular symptoms	Nonconsecutive clinical case series. In most cases diskography was followed by CT	All patients had normal MRI and abnormal diskography findings	Normal MRI and abnormal diskography findings were the basis for inclusion
Yu, 1989[126]	8 cadavers, 36 disks	Compared MRI and diskography against cryomicrotomy anatomic sectioning for detecting annular tears	Diskography identified 15 radial fissures, 10 of which were seen on MRI. Two of the 15 annular fissures were missed on cryomicrotomy	Included a newborn and 2-year-old. Considered only radial tears of the annulus. Could not correlate findings with symptoms
Bernard, 1990[127]	250 patients (725 disks) with chronic LBP who underwent CT-diskography	Retrospective study comparing the accuracy of MRI, intrathecally enhanced or nonenhanced CT, or plain radiography with CT-diskography. MRI was done before diskography in 67 patients (190 disks)	Normal T2-weighted MRI findings correctly predicted 64 normal disks by CT-diskography and incorrectly predicted 12 normal disks that were abnormal by CT-diskography. In 105 disks, abnormal T2 MRI correctly predicted abnormal disks by CT-diskography. 9 disks that were normal by CT-diskography had decreased signal intensity on T2-weighted MRI. Correlation between MRI and CT-diskography was 89%	CT-diskography provided additional information affecting patient management in 93% of cases. In 94% of the 180 operations, CT-diskography correctly predicted the type of disk herniation
Collins, 1990[114]	29 patients, 73 diskograms	Compared MRI and diskography in patients with axial LBP	57 disks were abnormal on diskography, with 13 producing concordant pain in 12 patients. Diskography findings correlated with those of MRI in 90% of cases. 4 disks showed degeneration on diskography with normal MRI, and 4 had abnormal MRI with normal diskography	The 12 patients with positive diskograms underwent spinal fusion, with 9 reporting clinical improvement at 9-mo follow-up
Linson, 1990[122]	50 patients, 97 disks	Compared MRI and diskography in patients with chronic LBP	91% correlation for disk degeneration between MRI and diskography	5 of the 6 disks with negative correlation were read as normal by MRI and abnormal by diskography. No mention of control disks during diskography
Simmons, 1991[120]	164 patients, 371 disks	Compared CT-diskography and MRI in patients with chronic LBP with or without radiculopathy	55% correlation based on patients, 80% based on disks	MRI normal and diskography abnormal in 34 disks. Diskography normal and MRI abnormal in 60 disks. 37% of disks abnormal on MRI were asymptomatic on diskography. Did not include outcomes in 76 patients who underwent surgery

Continued on following page

Table 65.4 Studies Comparing Lumbar Diskography with CT or MRI in Patients with Degenerative Disk Disease (Continued)

Author, Year	Number of Subjects	Nature of Study	Results	Comments
Birney, 1992[128]	90 patients, 264 disks	Examined correlation between MRI and diskography for DDD and HNP. Compared surgical findings with diskography in 57 patients	Agreement between MRI and diskography in 86% of disks. MRI more accurate for HNP; diskography slightly superior to MRI for DDD (MRI missed 1 disk, diskography 100% sensitive)	Considered patients with LBP and radicular pain. Surgical findings correlated with diagnostic studies at 63 of 76 levels
Osti, 1992[129]	33 patients, 114 disks	Compared MRI and diskography in patients with LBP	All 54 disks identified as abnormal on MRI showed abnormal diskogram patterns. 6 of the 60 disks identified as normal on MRI were abnormal on diskography. Of the 39 disks that provoked concordant pain on diskography, 27 were abnormal on MRI. 33 of the 39 asymptomatic disks by diskography had normal MRI signal, with 24 having normal diskographic patterns	6 of 46 disks classified as degenerate on MRI were asymptomatic on diskography. Concluded that diskography is more accurate than MRI in detecting annular pathology. Patient population not well defined
Aprill, 1992[121]	41 patients (105 disks) had chronic LBP with or without radicular symptoms	Compared HIZs on T2-weighted MRI with CT-diskography	In all patients who exhibited an HIZ on MRI, CT-diskography revealed either grade 3 or 4 annular disruption. Grade 3 or 4 disruption was also present in 34 patients without an HIZ	Concordant pain provocation with diskography was present in 38 of 40 disks with HIZs and 22 of 78 disks without an HIZ. CT-diskography performed in only 41 of 500 patients in whom MRI was performed
Horton, 1992[115]	25 patients with nonradicular LBP involving 63 diskograms	Comparative study between MRI and diskography for discogenic LBP	19 patients had positive diskograms. Of the different MRI patterns, only "dark/torn," "dark/bulged," or "speckled/flat" were more likely to be associated with positive rather than negative diskograms	MRI findings classified by pattern, not by presence or absence of pathology
Brightbill, 1994[8]	7 patients with LBP	Clinical case series involving patients with discrepancy between diskography and MRI who underwent surgery and were found to have internal disk disruption	All 7 subjects had normal MRI findings and positive diskography	Did not consider surgical outcomes
Loneragan, 1994[130]	18 patients with chronic LBP thought to be discogenic (43 disks)	Compared MRI and CT-diskography for the diagnosis of DDD and HNP	MRI missed 3 of 10 disks with early degenerative changes and 1 of 3 herniations	In no cases did MRI offer more information than CT-diskography
Schellhas, 1996[131]	63 patients, 100 disks with HIZs on T2 MRI in patients with LBP and/or radicular pain	Retrospective analysis of the significance of HIZs in predicting positive diskography	All 100 disks with HIZs were abnormal on diskography, with 87 showing concordant pain. In 17 asymptomatic control patients, MRI revealed only 1 disk with an HIZ	37 patients had back surgery previously. Also included patients with radiculopathy
Braithwaite, 1998[132]	58 patients with chronic, nonradicular LBP	Retrospective study comparing vertebral end plate changes on MRI with pain provocation during diskography in 152 disks	Among 91 disks with degeneration on MRI, 78 elicited pain vs. only 12 of 61 disks without degeneration on MRI. Among 26 disks with vertebral end-plate changes on MRI, 24 were painful during diskography vs. 69 of 129 disks without end-plate changes	MRI revealed disk degeneration at 128 of 290 levels, and end-plate changes were identified at 31 levels. All patients were being investigated for discogenic LBP as a precursor to spinal fusion. 138 disks evaluated with MRI were not injected

Saifuddin, 1998[133]	58 patients (152 disks) with chronic, nonradicular LBP	Retrospective study determining the sensitivity of T2-weighted MRI in detecting painful posterior annular tears	86 annular tears on diskography, 54 of which were posterior and 26 anterior and posterior. Sensitivity, specificity, and positive and negative predictive values of MRI in diagnosing concordantly painful posterior annular tears were 27%, 95%, 89%, and 47%, respectively	Study evaluated the same patients as the Braithwaite study
Milette, 1999[134]	45 patients, 132 disks	Evaluated MRI and diskography results in patients with chronic LBP	On MRI, 71% of disks showed a normal contour and 64% showed normal signal intensity. Only 40% of diskograms were radiographically normal. Diskography demonstrated stage 2 and 3 disk disruptions in 26% of disks with a normal contour on MRI and in 13% of disks with both a normal contour and signal	Used only T2-weighted MRI. Study was designed to assess differences between disk protrusions, bulges, and loss of signal intensity on MRI, not to compare imaging studies
Sandhu, 2000[125]	53 patients with LBP, 133 diskograms	Retrospective analysis comparing diskography with vertebral end-plate signal changes on MRI	No significant correlation between diskography and end-plate signal changes	41% of disks with positive end-plate changes had positive diskograms, compared to 27% of those without. Among positive diskograms, only 23% exhibited end-plate changes on T2-weighted MRI
Yoshida, 2002[119]	23 patients, 56 disks	Examined correlation between MRI and pain response on diskography	Sensitivity, specificity, positive predictive value, and negative predictive value of T2-weighted MRI were 94%, 71%, 59%, and 97%, respectively	Did not specifically compare diskography and MRI. T2-weighted MRI superior to gadolinium-enhanced images
Kakitsubata, 2003[135]	24 disks from 5 cadavers	Compared MRI and MR-diskography with anatomic correlation for detecting annular tears	Sensitivity of MR-diskography was 100%, 57%, and 21% for radial, transverse, and concentric tears in the annulus, respectively, vs. 67%, 71%, and 21% for conventional MRI	Could not correlate findings with symptoms
Lim, 2005[136]	66 patients with chronic LBP and no neural compression	Retrospective study comparing T1- and T2-weighted MRI findings with CT-diskography results (97 disks)	Concordant pain was more common with grade 4 or 5 degeneration on MRI, in disks with HIZs, and when the disk was fissured and ruptured on CT-diskography or the contrast agent spread into or beyond the outer annulus	Concordant pain was not associated with decreased disk height, end-plate abnormalities, or facet joint arthritis
Yuan, 2006[137]	265 patients, 298 disks	Comparison of MRI and CT-diskography in patients with LBP and leg pain	96.4% of patients were accurately diagnosed via CT-diskography. MRI found to be of limited benefit in diseased disks with passive diskographic findings	MRI found to be inferior to CT-diskography, especially for contiguous disks
Kim, 2009[138]	23 patients, 24 disks	Evaluated APCD vs. MRI and CT-diskography findings in patients with LBP	Positive correlation between APCD and MRI/CT-diskography in grades 2 and 4 disk degeneration, but not in grades 3 and 5	Pain-provoking pressure was not statistically correlated with MRI grading

"Diskography" refers to diskograms performed without CT scanning.

APCD, automated pressure-controlled diskography; CT, computed tomography; DDD, degenerative disk disease; HIZ, high-intensity zone on MRI; HNP, herniated nucleus pulposus; LBP, low back pain; MRI, magnetic resonance imaging.

Adapted and updated from Cohen SP, Larkin TM, Barn SA, et al. Lumbar discography: a comprehensive review of outcome studies, diagnostic accuray, and principles. *Reg Anesth Pain Med.* 2005;30:163-183.

Esses and coworkers conducted a prospective study examining the role of external spinal fixation in predicting the success of spinal fusion in patients with chronic LBP.[147] Thirty-two of the 35 subjects underwent provocative diskography before placement of a fixator. Neither diskographic findings nor reproduction of the patients' pain predicted the results of external fixation or fusion. Even in patients with normal-appearing disks or without pain reproduction during disk injection, most improved with both procedures.

Derby and coauthors published a retrospective analysis investigating the predictive value of categorizing positive diskography findings on surgical outcomes in 96 surgical candidates with chronic LBP.[148] Patients with anterolisthesis, focal protrusion, or disk extrusion were excluded; those with previous surgery were not excluded. In patients with chemically sensitized disks (i.e., concordant pain at ≤ 15 psi above opening pressure, $n = 36$), success rates were higher (89%) for interbody/combined fusion. In patients who underwent posterior intertransverse fusion, only 20% had a favorable outcome.

Madan and associates conducted a retrospective analysis aimed at determining the predictive value of provocative diskography on surgical outcomes in 73 patients with chronic LBP.[12] The first 41 patients in this series underwent circumferential arthrodesis without preoperative diskography, with the last 32 patients undergoing surgery only if their pain was reproduced during disk provocation. In the diskography group, 75.6% of the patients had satisfactory outcomes at a minimum 2-year follow-up versus 81.2% in the group that did not undergo preoperative diskography. Manometry readings were not considered a criterion in the interpretation of diskography results, and treatment outcomes were based on a modified Oswestry scoring system.

Carragee and colleagues conducted a prospective observational study of 32 patients with nonradicular LBP to investigate whether provocative diskography with strict criteria can be used as a reference standard to identify a single painful disk.[149] Generic surgical limitations were controlled for by comparing clinical outcomes in those with a single positive diskogram and in a matched cohort of 34 patients with unstable single-level lumbar spondylolisthesis. The proportion of patients who met the "minimal acceptable positive outcome" (pain score of ≤2, minimal disability, no opioids, and return to work) was 91% in the spondylolisthesis group versus 43% in the presumed discogenic pain group. Although the authors concluded that diskography was not accurate in identifying isolated painful disk lesions, a more likely interpretation is that fusion done for IDD benefits only a small percentage of patients. Another major limitation of this study is that the authors compared two different conditions.

Willems and coauthors published a prospective observational study that aimed to determine whether the presence of "adjacent segment disease," as identified by provocative diskography, had an impact on the clinical outcome of lumbar fusion in patients with chronic LBP.[150] In 197 patients with an equivocal indication for lumbar fusion, the decision to either perform lumbar fusion or manage the patient conservatively was decided by a trial of temporary external fixation. During the diagnostic workup, all patients underwent provocative diskography that included disks adjacent to the intended fusion levels. In the 82 patients who underwent lumbar fusion, there was no difference in outcome between those with degenerative disks adjacent to the fusion and those with normal adjacent disks.

Finally, Ohtori and colleagues studied 42 patients with axial LBP in a randomized trial comparing the predictive value of provocative diskography with that of analgesic diskography, a controlled infusion of local anesthetic into the disk for the purpose of identifying symptomatic disks.[151] Despite being underpowered, the 15 patients who underwent fusion based on anesthetic diskography had superior outcomes to the 15 who underwent fusion based on provocative diskography.

In summary, the lack of strong evidence for the use of fusion to treat DDD[94,141] and the methodologic flaws in the existing studies make the interpretation of data exceedingly difficult. For the existing data, the results are conflicting regarding whether preoperative diskography improves fusion outcomes in patients with discogenic LBP. The results of studies evaluating diskography as a predictive tool for surgery are presented in Table 65.5.

CORRELATION WITH INTRADISCAL ELECTROTHERMAL THERAPY AND DISK REPLACEMENT SURGICAL OUTCOMES

The advent of new treatments for discogenic LBP such as intradiscal electrothermal therapy (IDET) and total disk replacement surgery has generated significant interest in the medical community. As a minimally invasive treatment of discogenic pain, the reported outcomes with IDET vary widely and range from minimal benefit[158] to an almost 80% success rate.[159] Of the two published placebo-controlled studies, one reported modest improvement in both pain and disability scores,[160] whereas the other failed to show a statistically significant difference from sham IDET.[161] Overall, the majority of studies report improvement rates in the 50% range in carefully chosen candidates.[162,163] Since all published studies have used preprocedure diskography as a screening test for IDET candidates, it is not possible to determine the effect that diskography has on outcomes.

There have been numerous attempts dating back to the 1950s to design implants aimed at functional reconstruction of a spinal segment. The concept of disk arthroplasty was first put into clinical use in 1966 by Fernstrom, who described using a stainless steel ball as a vertebral spacer to restore lost disk height and preserve motion.[164] Disk replacement surgery has been used in Europe as a treatment of DDD since the 1980s but has been approved in the United States only since 2004 for single-level DDD. The reported success rates in these studies vary from around 50% to greater than 80% improvement at medium-term follow-up (Table 65.6).

The studies evaluating disk replacement surgery are almost equally divided between those that have routinely used preoperative diskography as a screening test and those that have not.[165-196] Unfortunately, methodologic flaws in these uncontrolled studies, wide variability in outcome criteria, and the absence of any direct comparisons between patients who underwent preoperative diskography and those who did not preclude any meaningful conclusions from being drawn. Taken in this limited context, the use of diskography as a screening tool before disk replacement surgery does not seem to improve outcomes over choosing patients based solely on MRI and clinical findings.

Text Continued on pg. 903

Table 65.5 Clinical Studies Evaluating the Effect of Preoperative Diskography on Outcomes of Lumbar Spinal Arthrodesis

Study, Year	Number of Patients	Type of Study	Results	Comments
Kostuik, 1979[152]	350 patients with painful scoliosis who underwent spinal instrumentation	Retrospective study	Preoperative diskography improved the success rate from 65%-70% to 85%	Used L5-S1 diskography to determine whether anterior or posterior instrumentation should be used
Blumenthal,[153] 1988	34 patients with IDD at 1 level confirmed. All patients had normal CT scans, myelograms, and electromyograms	Not indicated	Clinical success rate of 74%. The successful fusion rate was 73% by plain radiographs, with an average time to union of 12 mo. The fusion rate was higher in nonsmokers	Success defined by the patient returning to work or resuming normal activities and requiring no medications or only an anti-inflammatory drug
Colhoun, 1988[10]	162 patients with axial LBP	Prospective observational study	Of 137 patients in whom diskography revealed DDD and provoked concordant pain, 89% had a favorable outcome. Only 52% of patients in whom diskography showed DDD but provoked no pain had a favorable outcome	Mean follow-up of 3.6 yr
Esses, 1989[147]	35 patients with chronic LBP and FBSS who underwent ESF before arthrodesis	Prospective study evaluating the effect of ESF before spinal fusion. 32 patients also underwent preoperative diskography	Among the 15 patients with concordant pain on diskography, 13 experienced significant or complete pain relief with ESF. 6 of these 10 patients had significant relief after arthrodesis	Study not designed to evaluate predictive value of diskography on surgical success. Not all patients underwent preoperative diskography
Gill, 1992[154]	53 patients with predominantly axial LBP and IDD at L5-S1	Retrospective study involving L5-S1 fusion	50% of patients with a type I diskogram and normal MRI scans improved vs. 75% of patients with a type II or III diskogram and abnormal MRI	Abnormal diskogram was the basis for surgery. Average follow-up of 20 months
Knox, 1993[155]	22 patients who underwent anterior spinal fusion for diskogram-concordant LBP	Retrospective study	Poor results in all 5 patients with 2-level fusions. In single-level fusions, 35% of patients had good results, 18% fair, and 47% poor outcomes	Strong correlation between subjective (clinical improvement) and objective (fusion success) results
Wetzel, 1994[13]	48 patients with axial LBP who underwent lumbar arthrodesis following provocative diskography	Retrospective study	At first follow-up (mean, 5.3 wk), 66% had a satisfactory outcome. At final follow-up (mean, 35 mo), 46% had a satisfactory outcome	CT-diskography used in all but 1 patient. Not all patients had a control disk (26 patients underwent single-level diskography)
Parker, 1996[156]	23 patients with mechanical LBP and positive diskography	Prospective case series involving spinal fusion and/or instrumentation	39% of patients reported good outcomes, 13% had fair outcomes, and 48% had poor results	Abnormal diskogram was the basis for surgery. Mean follow-up of 47 mo
Vamvanij, 1998[157]	56 patients with discogenic LBP confirmed by CT-diskography who underwent 1 of 4 fusion techniques	Not indicated	Overall rate of patient satisfaction, 46%	Success rate for patients who underwent anterior lumbar fusion with cage and facet fusion, 63%. Success rates for the other 3 groups ranged from 36% to 46%
Derby, 1999[148]	96 patients who underwent diskography for LBP	Retrospective study	In patients with chemically sensitized disks (≥6/10 concordant pain at <15 psi above opening pressure, n = 36), success rates were 89% for interbody/combined fusion, 20% for posterior intertransverse fusion, and 12% for no surgical treatment	Mean follow-up for surgical patients of 28 mo. No difference between outcomes for interbody/combined fusion and posterior intertransverse fusion for surgical sample as a whole

Continued on following page

Table 65.5 Clinical Studies Evaluating the Effect of Preoperative Diskography on Outcomes of Lumbar Spinal Arthrodesis (Continued)

Study, Year	Number of Patients	Type of Study	Results	Comments
Madan, 2002[12]	41 patients who underwent spinal arthrodesis without preoperative diskography and 32 patients who underwent surgery based on positive diskography	Not indicated	81% of patients who had surgery based on MRI and clinical findings had a satisfactory outcome vs. 76% who underwent arthrodesis based on a positive diskogram	Mean follow-up of 2.4 yr in the diskography group and 2.8 yr in the MRI/clinical group
Carragee, 2006[149]	32 patients with nonradicular LBP and a single positive low-pressure diskogram who underwent spinal fusion	Prospective observational	43% of diskography patients obtained a "satisfactory" outcome for discogenic pain vs. 91% of a matched "control" group with single-level unstable spondylolisthesis who did not undergo diskography	Compared outcomes for 2 different conditions. Follow-up period of 2 yr. Positive outcome criteria included pain score ≤2, minimal disability, no opioids, and return to work
Willems, 2007[150]	82 patients with an equivocal indication for fusion who underwent surgery based on positive ESF	Prospective observational	No difference in outcomes between patients with a positive diskogram at an adjacent segment and those with a negative diskogram	Mean follow-up of 80 mo. Outcome measures included VAS score and patient satisfaction
Ohtori, 2009[151]	42 patients with axial LBP were randomized to provocative diskography vs. anesthetic diskography	Randomized comparative	The 15 patients who underwent fusion based on anesthetic diskography had outcomes superior to the 15 who underwent fusion based on provocative diskography	Follow-up period of 3 yr. Outcomes based on VAS score, Japanese Orthopedic Association Score, ODI, and patient satisfaction

A type I diskogram is designated as IDD without extravasation of contrast material associated with concordant pain reproduction. Types II and III denote the presence of annular disruption with spread of contrast material to the periphery and epidural space, respectively.

CT, computed tomography; DDD, degenerative disk disease; ESF, external spinal fixation; FBSS, failed back surgery syndrome; IDD, internal disk disruption; LBP, low back pain; MRI, magnetic resoance imaging; ODI, Oswestry Disability Index; VAS, visual analog scale.

Adapted and updated from Cohen SP, Larkin TM, Barn SA, et al. Lumbar discography: a comprehensive review of outcome studies, diagnostic accuray, and principles. *Reg Anesth Pain Med.* 2005;30:163-183.

Table 65.6 Summary of Outcome Data for Lumbar Disk Replacement Surgery Based on Preoperative Diskography Screening

Study, Year	Preoperative Diskography?	Number of Disk Replacement Patients	Type of Surgery	Outcomes
Enker, 1993[165]	Yes	6	TDR	4 of 6 patients had satisfactory results (1 excellent, 2 good, 1 fair)
Zeegers, 1999[166]	In 36 of 50 patients	50	TDR	32 of 46 patients monitored for 2 yr had a positive clinical result. Did not provide separate data for patients undergoing diskography
Bertagnoli, 2002[167]	No	108	TDR	Results "excellent" in 91%, "good" in 7%, "fair" in 2%, and poor in no (0%) patients at 3-mo to 2-yr follow-up
Hochshuler, 2002[168]	Yes	56	TDR	52.7% improvement in mean VAS scores at 6-wk follow-up. In the 22 patients monitored for ≥1 yr, improvements in VAS and ODI scores were maintained
Mayer, 2002[169]	No	34	TDR	Mean VAS score decreased from 6.3 preoperatively to 3.4 at 1-yr follow-up (not all patients monitored for 1 yr). 61% of patients "completely" satisfied and 22% "satisfied"
Delmarter, 2003[170]	Not routinely	35	TDR	Mean VAS score decreased from 7.4 to 4.4 and ODI from 31 to 15 at 6-mo follow-up. No significant differences between the patients who underwent TDR and the 18 randomized to fusion
Blumenthal, 2003[171]	Yes	57	TDR	63% of patients improved at 2-yr follow-up (based on >20-point improvement in the VAS score)
Shim, 2003[172]	In patients with DDD at more than 1 level	46	PDR	Mean VAS score 8.5 preoperatively and 3.1 at 1-yr follow-up. 11% had excellent and 67% had good results
Van Ooij, 2003[173]	Yes	27	TDR	Good outcome obtained in 12 of 26 patients, with variable follow-up period (range, 1 mo-10 yr)
Tropiano, 2003[174]	No	53	TDR	87% of patients "entirely satisfied." Mean ODI of 56 preoperatively and 14 at last follow-up (mean, 1.4 yr)
McAfee, 2003[175]	Yes	41	TDR	Mean VAS score of 73.5 preoperatively and 30.4 at 1-3 yr of follow-up
Kim, 2003[176]	Not mentioned except for a negative diskogram being a contraindication	11 patients with juxtafusional DDD	TDR	Of the 5 patients monitored for >6 mo, mean ODI decreased from 64% to 24%
Jin, 2003[177]	No	45	PDR	Mean ODI decreased from 52.2% to 16.5% in the 30 patients seen at 6-mo follow-up. 87% of patients were clinically improved
Zigler, 2003[178]	Not routinely	28	TDR	Decrease in VAS score from approximately 7.8 to 5.6 after 6 mo
Guyer, 2004[179]	Yes	100	TDR	Mean ODI score decreased from 71 to 30 at 2-yr follow-up vs. from 70 to 28 in 44 patients who underwent anterior interbody fusion
Lemaire, 2005[180]	Yes	107	TDR	62% of patients had excellent results (≥70% resumption of activity), 28% had good results 60%-70%, and 10% had poor outcomes at a mean follow-up of 11.3 yr
Blumenthal, 2005[181]	Yes	205	TDR	Mean reduction in VAS pain score of 42.4% and mean reduction in ODI of 48.5% at 24-mo follow-up. 71.3% were satisfied. Study was designed to compared disk replacement with lumbar fusion
Cakir, 2005[182]	Yes	29	TDR	VAS pain score decreased from a mean of 67 to 22 in 25 patients with physiologic segmental lordosis and from 71 to 23 in those with nonphysiologic lordosis. Minimum follow-up of 12 mo. Study was not designed to measure outcomes. Main finding was that although total lumbar lordosis did not change significantly, segmental lordosis usually increased
Tropiano, 2005[183]	No	55	TDR	60% of patients had excellent (>70% improvement) outcomes, 15% had good (60-70%) outcomes, and 25% had a poor result. Mean follow-up, 8.7 yr
Le Huec, 2005[184]	Yes	64	TDR	Minimum follow-up of 2 yr. LBP VAS score decreased from 76 to 32; ODI decreased from 43.8 to 23.1
Bertagnoli, 2005[185]	Yes, "when indicated"	104	TDR	Single-level DDD. Minimum follow-up of 2 yr. 58.3% were "completely satisfied" and 38.8% were "satisified." ODI decreased from 54 to 29. There was a 3-fold increase in return to work full-time and a 5-fold decrease in not returning to work

Continued on following page

Table 65.6 Summary of Outcome Data for Lumbar Disk Replacement Surgery Based on Preoperative Diskography Screening (Continued)

Study, Year	Preoperative Diskography?	Number of Disk Replacement Patients	Type of Surgery	Outcomes
Bertagnoli, 2005[186]	No	25	TDR	Multilevel DDD. Minimum follow-up of 2 yr. 75% were "completely satisfied" and 17% were "satisified." ODI decreased from 65 to 21.6. There was a 5-fold increase in return to work full-time and a 4-fold decrease in not returning to work
Regan, 2005[187]	No	100	TDR	Preoperative VAS score of 73.2 vs. 39.2 at 6 mo postoperatively. Preoperative ODI decreased from 53.4 to 37.6. Follow-up of 6 mo
Chung, 2006[188]	Yes	36	TDR	Minimum follow-up of 2 yr. LBP VAS score decreased from 75 preoperatively to 30 at follow-up. Leg pain VAS score decreased from 47 to 12. ODI decreased from 69.2 to 21
Siepe, 2006[189]	No	92	TDR	Mean follow-up of 34.2 mo. 68.1% of total patients returned to work. 65.2% of patients were "completely satisfied"; 17.4% were "satisfied"
Gioia, 2007[190]	In 28 of 36 patients	36	TDR	Mean follow-up of 6.9 yr. Preoperative VAS score of 80 vs. 14 at follow-up. ODI decreased from 44 to 9
Ross, 2007[191]	Yes	160	TDR	Mean follow-up of 79 mo. Patient satisfaction scores were "much better" in 41%, "better" in 28%, "same as before" in 11%, and "worse than before" in 20% of patients
Siepe, 2007[192]	No	99	TDR	Mean follow-up of 25.8 mo. VAS score decreased from 70 to 30. ODI decreased from 42 to 21. 66.3% of patients returned to work
Zigler, 2007[193]	Yes	286	TDR	At 2-yr follow-up, VAS score decreased from 76 to 37 and ODI decreased from 63.4 to 34.5 in the ProDisc group
Sasso, 2008[194]	Not required, although the senior authors used this exclusively to diagnose DDD	67	TDR	Comparison of FlexiCore TDR with standard circumferential fusion. At 2 yr, mean ODI decreased from 62 to 6 in the FlexiCore vs. 58 to 12 in the standard group. Mean VAS score decreased from 86 to 16 in the FlexiCore vs. 82 to 20 in the standard group
Guyer, 2009[195]	Yes	233	TDR	Minimum follow-up of 5 yr. Mean VAS score decreased from 72 to 30. 68% of patients in the Charite group had an improvement in ODI of ≥15 points
Pimenta, 2011[196]	Yes	36	TDR	Study was designed to evaluate a new extreme lateral approach to TDR. Mean VAS score improved by 69.6% and mean ODI improved by 61.4% in all patients. Minimum follow-up of 2 yr

Note: The table does not include studies lacking information about patient selection criteria.
DDD, degenerative disk disease; LBP, low back pain; ODI, Oswestry Disability Index; PDR, partial disk replacement (prosthetic disk nucleus); TDR, total disk replacement; VAS, visual analog scale.
Adapted and updated from Cohen SP, Larkin TM, Barn SA, et al. Lumbar discography: a comprehensive review of outcome studies, diagnostic accuray, and principles. *Reg Anesth Pain Med*. 2005;30:163-183.

ANALGESIC DISKOGRAPHY

In the past 10 years there has been kindled interest in the role of analgesic diskography as a more robust means of detecting which disks may be contributing to a patient's LBP. The rationale behind analgesic diskography is that using pain relief provided by the intradiscal placement of local anesthetic as the reference standard for a positive test rather than pain provocation could reduce the false-positive rate. This is consistent with the diagnostic tests used to identify painful facet and SI joints.

DePalma and coauthors published a retrospective analysis examining whether painful annular fissures during provocative diskography were the source of LBP.[197] After injecting 0.8 mL of 4% lidocaine into the disks of a cohort of 28 patients, 50% or greater pain relief occurred in 80% of positive disks based on provocative diskography.

There has been some debate regarding which painful disks are more prone to a positive response with analgesic diskography. In 2007, Bartynski and Rothfus evaluated intradiscal lidocaine administration after provocative lumbar diskography by comparing disks that retained contrast material (n = 82) with those in which contrast material was extravasated (n = 100).[198] In disks with a nonfunctional annulus that extravasated contrast material, 74% demonstrated complete or nearly complete pain reduction versus only 20% of disks with a functional annulus. Possible explanations for this finding include greater distribution throughout the annulus via fissures in the disks that demonstrated extravasation and "false-positive" pain relief in the leaky disks secondary to inadvertent epidural spread of contrast material.

Alamin and coworkers compared clinical outcomes after analgesic and provocative diskography in a prospective clinical trial of 41 patients with LBP.[199] After a positive provocation diskogram, a catheter was placed in the proposed painful disk or disks and local anesthetic was administered. A positive analgesic result was defined as 50% or greater pain reduction following painful movements. Seventeen percent of patients with two-level findings on provocation diskography had only one positive level with analgesic diskography, and 27% with pain during disk stimulation had a negative analgesic test. Fifty-one percent had corroborating results between provocative and analgesic tests. In 49% of patients the results of analgesic diskography changed the plan of treatment that would have been developed with the results of provocation. Those with a changed treatment plan had improved Oswestry Disability Index and visual analog scale scores over a 6- to 24-month follow-up.

Alamin and colleagues later performed a follow-up cohort study investigating the difference between provocative diskography and functional analgesic diskography in 52 patients with LBP.[200] Forty-six percent of the patients experienced discordant results between the two tests, with 26% having positive provocation diskography and a negative analgesic test, 16% of individuals having single-level findings on analgesic testing versus two or more positive levels with provocation testing, and 4% of individuals having new positive findings on analgesic testing after negative provocation diskography.

As discussed earlier, Ohtori and coauthors published a randomized study comparing fusion outcomes in 42 patients who underwent either provocative or analgesic diskography.[151] At the 3-year follow-up in the 30 patients who proceeded to surgery on the basis of positive diskography, those who underwent analgesic diskography had lower pain scores and less disability. Not all studies have shown superior outcomes with analgesic diskography. Derby and associates investigated 70 consecutive patients with LBP who underwent either provocative (n = 23) diskography or provocation in conjunction with analgesic (n = 47) diskography.[201] The authors found that adding local anesthetic to provocative diskography did not affect the number of positive results (73.9% in the provocation-only group vs. 70% in the combination group). The average subjective pain relief 15 minutes after the procedures also did not differ significantly between the two groups.

The main problems with analgesic diskography revolve around inconsistencies in its use and the potential for accelerated disk degeneration as a result of the larger needles required for insertion of the catheter or catheters. Because of the lack of vascularity within the disk, the duration of analgesia following intradiscal injection of local anesthetic may be prolonged and variable. In a randomized controlled study, Simmons and coauthors reported that only 9% of patients experienced significant pain relief 10 to 14 days after injection.[202] However, Kotilainen and colleagues reported that two thirds of patients obtained pain relief 2 weeks following intradiscal bupivacaine administration.[203] In individuals with suspected multilevel disease who do obtain prolonged benefit after the first disk injection, evaluation of subsequent disks at the same visit would not be possible. Although the conceptual appeal and early reports of analgesic diskography are encouraging, further studies are needed to determine the true clinical utility of the test.

DISKOGRAPHY VERSUS BONY VIBRATION TEST

The main argument for diskography is that it is the only test available that correlates symptoms with pathology.[204,205] In an attempt to find a less invasive replacement for diskography, Yrjämä and Vanharanta devised the bony vibration test (BVT) whereby a blunt, vibrating object such as the shaft of an electric toothbrush is compressed against the skin overlying successive spinous processes to provoke pain. In the pilot study conducted in 57 patients with LBP, the authors found the sensitivity and specificity of BVT to be 0.71 and 0.63, respectively, in comparison to provocative diskography.[206] When patients with failed back surgery syndrome and painful disk herniations were excluded (n = 40), the sensitivity increased to 0.96 and the specificity to 0.72. The difference in accuracy resulted from the finding that the prolapsed lumbar disks that provoked pain during diskography were almost always painless during vibration testing. In two follow-up studies comparing BVT findings with MRI and CT-diskography, the authors found similarly high sensitivity and specifity when patients with previously operated backs and complete annular tears were excluded.[207,208]

In an attempt to combine vibration provocation with noninvasive imaging capability, Yrjämä and colleagues added ultrasonic disk imaging to vibratory stimulation in the evaluation of 38 patients with chronic LBP.[209] In the 26 patients in whom pain was provoked during diskography, BVT was painful in 17; in the 12 with negative diskography, BVT was painless in 7. However, in the 14 patients in whom annular fissures were present, the combination of ultrasound and vibration testing yielded only one "false-positive" and one "false-negative" result in comparison to diskography. To date, the findings of Yrjämä and colleagues have yet to be replicated by other authors, and no studies correlating vibration provocation with surgical outcomes are available.

COST-EFFECTIVENESS

Several third-party payers have recently opted to decline reimbursement for diskography despite evidence that this test is one of the most cost-effective screening tools available. Anterior or anterior-posterior lumbar fusion with rehabilitation costs an average of $61,000, and diskography costs an average of $3400; the rate of positive diskography is 42%. Assuming that all patients with negative diskography do not undergo spinal fusion whereas those with a positive diskogram do proceed to fusion, the use of diskography with its existing flaws has the potential to save approximately $32,000 per patient. This is, of course, overly simplistic because many patients will require ongoing nonsurgical treatment. Nonetheless, this simple calculation emphasizes the need for an effective screening test to eliminate unwarranted surgical intervention in those with discogenic pain.

Cost-effectiveness is an artificial construct in that variations in one parameter can dramatically affect the conclusions that one can draw. For example, should the cost of diskography increase or spinal fusion decrease or either short-term (e.g., diskitis) or long-term (e.g., disk herniation) complications develop after disk stimulation, the cost savings per patient will decrease accordingly. Experienced spine surgeons are also less likely to refer "poor surgical candidates" for screening than inexperienced surgeons are, so the higher positive diskography rate will result in less cost savings per patient.

STANDARDIZATION OF DISKOGRAPHY

Several important variables should be assessed during diskographic examination, including the volume of contrast agent injected, the degree and pattern of pain provocation, morphologic changes in the disk, and the pressure at which pain is elicited. One criticism of diskography is that except for the volume injected and radiologic findings, all other parameters depend on the pain response of the patient. Pain is always subjective, and what one person considers painful may be innocuous to another. In an attempt to standardize diskography, several investigators have sought to objectify the criteria for positive diskography. In their prospective studies in asymptomatic patients, both Walsh and coworkers[98] and Carragee and colleagues[100-102] used a 0 to 5 pain-related behavior scale that was subsequently correlated with pain intensity and disk morphology. In the Walsh study, disparities between reported pain and pain-related behavior occurred in 6 of 51 disks, with all cases involving patients reporting significant pain (≥3/5) in the absence of corresponding pain behavior (≤2/5 actions). In the three combined Carragee studies, the agreement between pain behavior and numerical pain score was higher than 90%. In both investigations the authors videotaped the pain response for further review.

Stojanovic and associates performed a prospective analysis of diskography-associated changes in heart rate in 26 patients with 75 diskograms.[210] The authors found that positive diskograms were associated with greater changes in heart rate than were diskograms that elicited no pain or noncordant pain, with all positive disks exhibiting pathologic radiographic changes. When greater than a 5-beat/min increase from baseline was used as the cutoff value, the sensitivity of the heart rate response was 85% and its specificity 100%. The rationale for the use of heart rate changes and pain behavior to validate the reported pain response is based on numerous studies showing both variables to be valid indicators of pain perception.[211]

The problem with the use of secondary variables to corroborate interpretation of diskography is that even though they may be useful in identifying the small subset of patients in whom secondary gain issues and extensive psychological overlay contribute to self-reported pain scores, their effects on treatment outcomes remain unknown.

Although numerous investigators have used manometry during disk stimulation, the use of discrete cutoff values as a reference standard for what constitutes a positive test has been surprisingly scarce. In 1999, Derby and colleagues introduced a three-tiered system whereby concordant pain of 6/10 or greater in severity at less than 15 psi above opening pressure was designated to be a "chemically sensitized disk," concordant pain of 6/10 or greater in intensity at between 15 and 50 psi above opening pressure was considered a "mechanically sensitive disk," and concordant pain between 51 and 90 psi was termed indeterminate or normal[148] (Table 65.7). In a retrospective analysis, intermediate-term (mean of 16 months) outcomes were assessed in 96 patients who were treated either conservatively or by spinal fusion. No differences in outcomes were found between patients who underwent interbody/combined fusions and those who received intertransverse fusions across the entire sample. However, subgroup analysis found that patients with chemically sensitized disks who underwent interbody/combined fusions experienced better outcomes than did those who underwent intertransverse fusions. One serious flaw in this diagnostic scheme is that it does not control for baseline differences in pain between patients. Thus, a diskogram that provokes 5/10 in a patient with incapacitating 4/10 baseline pain would be considered negative, whereas a diskogram that provokes 6/10 pain in a patient with 10/10 baseline pain would be positive. A second problem is that significant numerical differences may exist between manometric systems, so a scale developed for one system may not be valid when used in a different system. Factors that may affect the accuracy of diskography are listed in Table 65.8.

PERFORMING DISKOGRAPHY

PATIENT PREPARATION

A detailed history and physical examination should always be performed before the procedure. It is the responsibility of the diskographer to review all pertinent information, including preprocedural laboratory tests, electromyograms, plain films, and MRI scans. It may be helpful to record a description of the pain symptoms or create a pain diagram for reference during the procedure. Although the diskographer reports the final diagnostic conclusions, it is the patient who ultimately communicates the provoked symptoms and their degree of concordance with the typical pain. Patients who have a difficult time describing their typical pain syndrome may have an equally difficult time describing the provoked symptoms. Indications for diskography

Table 65.7 Interpretation of Disk Stimulation Data

Disk Classification	Intradiscal Pressure at Pain Provocation	Pain Severity	Pain Type	Interpretation
Chemical	Immediate onset of pain occurring as <1 mL of contrast is visualized reaching the outer annulus or pain provocation at <15 psi above opening pressure	≥6/10	Concordant	Positive
Mechanical	Pain noted between 15 and 50 psi above opening pressure	≥6/10	Concordant	Positive (but other pain generators may be present; further investigation is warranted)
Indeterminate	Pain noted between 51 and 90 psi	≥6/10	Concordant	Generally negative, but further investigation may be indicated
Normal	>90 psi	No pain or pressure	Not applicable	Negative

Modified from Derby R, Howard MW, Grant JM, et al. The ability of pressure-controlled discography to predict surgical and nonsurgical outcomes. *Spine*. 1999;24:364-372.

Table 65.8 Factors That May Affect the Accuracy of Diskography

Factor	Effect on Interpretation	Preventive Measure
Needle placement in the annulus	False-positive result	Use of multiplanar fluoroscopic views and contrast injection
Needle placement too close to the vertebral end plate	False-positive result	Use of anteroposterior fluoroscopic views
Increasing the pressure too rapidly or slowly	False-positive or false-negative result	Use of standardized contrast delivery device
Overpressurization	False-positive result	Use of manometry, cutoff value for designating the diskogram as positive
Diffuse contrast extravasation/ underpressurization	False-negative result	Use of lateral fluoroscopy in real time and manometry
Pain sensitization	False-positive result	Inject the "control" disk first and the suspected disk or disks last. Make sure that the patient has realistic expectations and understands the nature of the procedure. Treat anxiety and pain from needle placement appropriately
Oversedation or undersedation	False-negative or false-positive result	Judicious use of sedation
Overuse or underuse of local anesthetic	False-negative or false-positive result	Judicious use of local anesthetic, especially near the foramina and disks. Use smaller needles
Psychological (e.g., somatization disorder, depression), physiologic (e.g., fibromyalgia, multiple comorbid pain conditions), or anatomic (e.g., previous back surgery) factors	False-positive result	Treatment of poorly controlled conditions (e.g., antidepressants and therapy for psychiatric conditions) beforehand. Use two adjacent control disks to reduce the false-positive rate. Consider the use of facial expressions and heart rate monitoring in addition to pain report as the criteria for designating a diskogram as positive

have previously been outlined in numerous guidelines and reviews[107,127,205,212-221] and include the following:

1. Evaluation of patients with unremitting spinal pain, with or without extremity pain, of greater than 3 months' duration that has been unresponsive to appropriate conservative therapy.
2. Patients with severe, persistent, severe symptoms in whom other diagnostic tests have failed to reveal clear confirmation of a suspected disk or disks as the source of the pain.
3. Evaluation of persistent pain in a postsurgical patient whose symptoms may be arising from intervertebral disk degeneration, recurrent herniation, or pseudoarthrosis of a spinal fusion.
4. To determine the number of levels to be fused in spinal surgery or the primary symptomatic disk level.
5. To determine whether levels adjacent to a planned spinal arthrodesis are either normal or painful.
6. To diagnose lateral disk herniations.
7. If the patient prima facie satisfies the criteria for intradiscal treatment. In these cases, CT-diskography may be undertaken to assess disk morphology and determine the optimal placement (if any) of the device (e.g., IDET electrode).
8. For assessment of candidates for minimally invasive surgical decompression to confirm contained disk herniations or to investigate the distribution of dye before chemonucleolysis or other percutaneous decompression procedures.

At our institutions, before the start of the procedure we review the MRI studies to identify levels with decreased signal intensity on T2-weighted images, increased signal consistent with an HIZ, decreased disk height, or other evidence of degeneration with the idea that we will probably inject all abnormal levels. This notion is supported by studies showing that even though MRI is sensitive in identifying disk pathology, it is less accurate in detecting the pattern of disk morphology.[118,123]

Previous ISIS guidelines recommended that two control levels be obtained for optimal interpretation of disk stimulation.[107] However, given the inherent risks associated with diskography, most authors have not adhered to these stringent guidelines.[127,205,222] At our institutions we consider one adjacent, unequivocal negative disk adequate for control purposes. For the most commonly symptomatic L5-S1 disk, only one adjacent control disk is possible.

Preparation of the patient for disk stimulation begins with the initial visit before diskography. It is during this time that the patient is briefed on what to expect during the procedure. Patients must realize that diskography is performed for diagnostic information rather than therapeutic benefit. Some patients may be surprised to learn that the short-term goal of diskography is pain provocation rather than analgesia. They should be familiar with use of the pain scale that will be used during the procedure and be prepared to note whether the pain induced by diskography is concordant with or dissimilar to their typical pain.

Absolute contraindications to the procedure include patient refusal, inability to adequately report their response to the procedure, untreated localized infection, untreated coagulopathy, and pregnancy. Relative contraindications include allergy to the contrast medium, local anesthetic, or antibiotics; systemic infection; and anatomic derangements that preclude safe, successful conduct of the procedure.

PROCEDURAL PREPARATION

The operative suite should be equipped with oxygen, emergency medications, and all appropriate monitors. It is our practice that all individuals in the procedure room wear caps and masks and that the operators wear sterile gowns and gloves, as is routinely practiced with open surgical procedures. Whereas ISIS recommends draping the entire patient, as well as the image intensifier and remote console,[223] other diskographers create only a small sterile field.

Diskographers vary in their use of sedation. Many different methods of sedation have been described, from none at all to benzodiazepines alone and in various combinations with opioids.[127,224] If used, sedation should be aimed toward relieving anxiety and promoting tolerance to the procedure without compromising the patient's ability to assess symptoms. Excessive use of sedation increases the risk for false-positive results, neurologic injury, and other complications.

Because of the possibility of inadvertent intrathecal administration, only nonionic contrast material should be injected. Nonionic dye also minimizes the risk for allergic reactions, which may be delayed until the contrast material is systemically absorbed from the disk. In patients with known previous contrast reactions, premedication is necessary. Some diskographers use no contrast or contrast only to confirm placement of the needle in the NP and inject saline to elevate intradiscal pressure. Another option is to use gadolinium as the contrast agent.[225]

NEEDLE PLACEMENT

Diskography is an invasive procedure that should be performed only by experienced clinicians. ISIS recommends that anyone performing this procedure should have extensive experience with less technically challenging interventional procedures such as facet blocks. There are numerous different ways to perform this procedure,[127,205,222,223,226-228] but this section describes only one (Figs. 65.4 and 65.5).

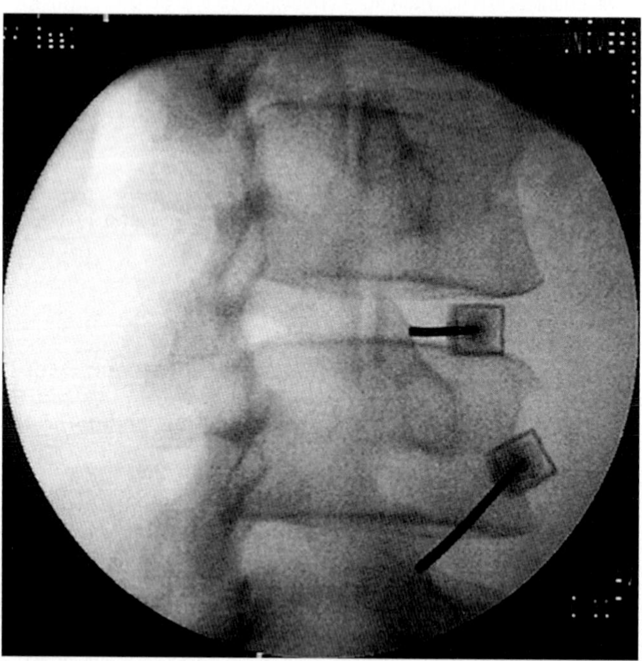

Figure 65.4 Oblique fluoroscopic view for diskography needle placement via an extrapedicular approach.

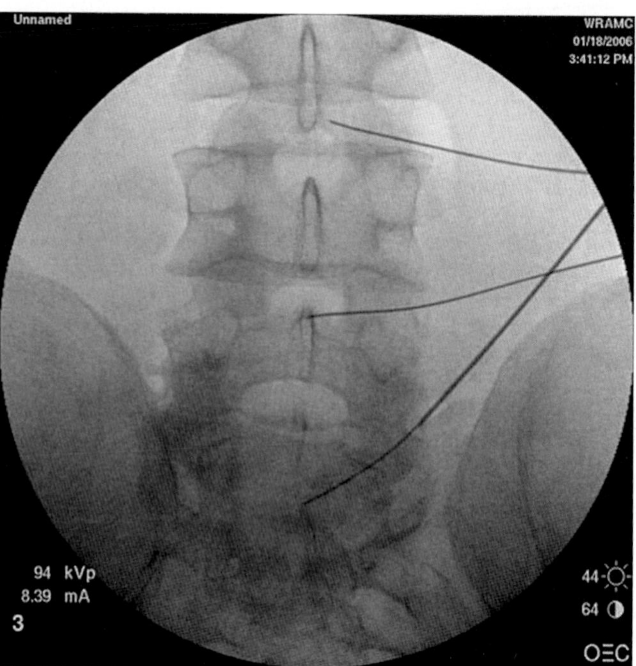

Figure 65.5 Needle placement in the anteroposterior view for a three-level diskogram.

Image guidance for needle placement is ideally achieved with C-arm or biplanar fluoroscopy. Interspinous and interlaminar approaches have been advocated following fusion with a paraspinal bone graft but are otherwise rarely used because of the necessity for penetration of the dura. Patients can be placed in the left lateral decubitus or prone position. In the prone position, the side of approach is usually determined by the preference of the diskographer unless unilateral pathology or an anatomic obstacle is suspected. Though recommended by some authors,[223,227] we have shown that an approach from the side ipsilateral to a patient's symptomatology does not affect the rate of false-positive diskograms.[117]

Assuming prone positioning, craniocaudal angulation is adjusted so that the imaging beam parallels the disk space at selected levels. This can be done by lining up the image so that the x-ray beam passes parallel to the subchondral border of the inferior vertebral end plate of the disk. The C-arm is then rotated laterally until the superior articulating process of the lower vertebra is positioned just posterior to the geometric center of the disk. After superficial injection of local anesthetic, an 18-gauge introducer needle is advanced lateral to the superior articular process, preferentially at the midpoint of the superior-inferior margin of the disk (see Fig. 65.4). At this point the fluoroscope is changed from an oblique to a lateral view. A 22- or 25-gauge (150 mm) diskography needle is advanced through the introducer needle into the annulus. The annular fibers provide a firmer feel than do the nucleus and surrounding soft tissue. The needle is then advanced through the annulus until it is situated halfway between the anterior and posterior borders of the disk. The tip of the needle should remain close to the midpoint of the superior-inferior margins of the disk because injection into the end plates can result in a false-positive response. When the needle is satisfactorily positioned on lateral imaging, the fluoroscope is rotated to an anteroposterior view, where the final needle position in the middle third of the disk should be confirmed. If the needle has not passed far enough on the anteroposterior view, the skin entry point was too medial; if the needle has passed clear to the opposite side of the disk, the entry point may have been too lateral. In a normal disk or mildly degenerated one, central needle placement is necessary to avoid injection into the richly innervated AF, which may result in a false-positive diskogram.

At L5-S1, the iliac crests often prohibit use of a needle trajectory aimed directly at the center of the disk. Entry into this level is subject to higher failure rates, which may be substantially reduced by using a curved needle technique.[226] Identification of the target at this level begins with a sharp, caudal angulation of the beam that passes parallel to the subchondral plate of the inferior end plate of the disk. At this point the C-arm is rotated laterally until either the superior articulating process of the S1 vertebra is positioned just posterior to the geometric center of the disk or the iliac crests begin to encroach on the target point. Usually, a small triangular window can be appreciated that is bordered laterally by the iliac crest, medially by the superior articular process, and superiorly by the subchondral border of the superior end plate. Once the entry point is identified, an introducer is advanced toward the lateral margin of the superior articulating process of S1 and walked off just beyond its edge. The C-arm is then positioned in the lateral view. Especially at L5-S1, it is important to adjust the angulation of the camera so that the superior and inferior end plates appear sharp and are discernable. A diskography needle is then bent slightly about 1 cm from its tip and advanced through the introducer until it meets the outer edge of the annulus. A bend may facilitate steering the needle around bony obstacles and, with proper rotation, may promote more central placement. As the needle is advanced toward the edge of the disk, it is not uncommon to have the patient experience paresthesias. If this occurs, either the needle is withdrawn and an approach is made at a different angle or the position of the introducer is moved superiorly or inferiorly. As for the upper disks, the final needle position for L5-S1 should ideally be in the middle third of the disk, but it is not unusual at this level for it to end up in a more peripheral location.

DISK STIMULATION AND INTERPRETATION

After all needles have been positioned properly, the patient is prepared for the injection. If patients are still experiencing persistent effects of sedation, it is prudent to wait until they are more awake and answering directed questions. Patients should be questioned again regarding their pain level while care is taken to ensure that they can distinguish residual procedural pain from their typical pain. They should be able to respond appropriately to questions pertaining to the quality, intensity, location, and concordance of the provoked pain, which will provide critical diagnostic information.

Responses may be more reliable if the patient is not informed that an injection is occurring. The patient should also be blinded to the level of injection. The sequence of disk injection depends on the diskographer's expectation for provocation of pain at each level. Once severe pain is produced, the patient may be less able to tolerate or judge subsequent injections. Therefore, the level considered likely to cause the most intense pain should be injected last.

One modification that is occasionally used is for the diskographer to be blinded to the MRI findings. Although this may remove physician bias from the equation, it can interfere with proper disk selection and the optimal sequencing of injection. After injecting all levels, it is sometimes necessary to confirm the initial reactions by injecting levels a second time.

Verbal and nonverbal reactions, including facial expressions, should be closely monitored and recorded on a diskogram worksheet (Box 65.1). Besides pain response, other data that should be recorded include the total volume of contrast agent, injection end point (reason why the injection was stopped), and nucleogram appearance. Normal disks take less than 1 mL of contrast agent before firm resistance is reached (high-pressure end point). Degenerated disks generally accept larger volumes of contrast and demonstrate moderate or low resistance to injection (low-pressure end point). When the disk communicates with the epidural space because of complete annular disruption, higher (or unlimited) volumes can be injected with little to no resistance (volume end point). When severe symptoms are provoked, the injection should be stopped even if minimal contrast agent has been injected[224] (pain end point).

Injection pressure can be measured with specialized commercially available devices, which is recommended by ISIS.[223] Proponents of manometry state that a pressure-recording

Box 65.1 Data Collection for Diskography

- Technical success of the procedure (are the needles positioned properly?)
- The pressure observed when contrast agent is first visible in the disk (opening pressure)
- The pressure at which pain is first noted
- The amount of contrast agent injected (maximum volume)
- The maximum pressure noted (peak pressure)
- Injection end point (reason why the injection was stopped):
  - High-pressure end point (firm)
  - Low-pressure end point
  - Volume end point
  - Pain end point
- The pattern of contrast distribution (e.g., diffuse, fissuring, posterior or anterior, right or left, extravasation into the epidural space)
- The pain response. Where does it hurt? Is it identical, similar, or different in location and character from your typical pain? On a 0 to 10 rating scale, how do you rate the intensity? This pain score must be taken in the context of the preinjection pain score
- The presence of control disks. If none is obtained, the procedure is nondiagnostic

device allows objective designation of painful disks as either chemically or mechanically sensitive.[148,223] Others have not endorsed the use of these devices[127,219,227] and claim that an experienced diskographer can determine relative pressure with only a syringe. To date, no studies have evaluated the effect that manometry has on surgical outcomes or diskographic results. However, it is our opinion that the proper use of manometry can both enhance the accuracy of diskography and reduce the likelihood of inadvertent disk injury. Any bodily structure containing mechanoreceptors, whether diseased or normal, can be a source of pain when subjected to excessive pressure. This effect can be even more pronounced when the pressure is elevated too rapidly, thereby resulting in false-positive diskograms. Conversely, if pressure cannot be generated in a severely degenerated disk because of annular incompetence, a diskogram may be mistakenly interpreted as negative. An additional benefit of pressure measurement is that it alerts the diskographer to overpressurization of disks, which can result in permanent injury.

If manometry is used, one should first determine the opening pressure of the disk, which in practical terms is the pressure at which contrast material is first visualized entering the disk (usually <15 psi). Once opening pressure is determined, the disk is slowly filled with contrast in aliquots of 0.25 to 1 mL. As alluded to earlier, raising the pressure too rapidly may result in a false-positive result. The end point is usually a high-pressure end point at around 100 psi or the point at which pain is experienced. In patients with severely degenerative disks, it may not be possible to achieve pressures above 50 psi. If either 100 psi or 50 psi above opening pressure is reached without pain being noted, the disk is considered negative and can serve as a control. Generating pressures higher than 100 psi greatly increases the risk for iatrogenic injury. If pain is noted at low pressures (<15 psi above opening pressure), the disk is considered chemically sensitive. If pain is noted between 15 and 50 psi above opening pressure, the disk is considered mechanically sensitive, and the diskogram may or may not be positive. If pain is noted at greater than 50 psi above opening pressure, "the response cannot be considered clinically significant."[106] Pain at higher pressures may be due to mechanical irritation, end-plate deflection, or stimulation of mechanoreceptors (see Table 65.7). Although numerous diskographic classification systems have been advocated, including some devoid of pressure measurements,[148,223,224] no single set of criteria is universally accepted as standard (Table 65.9).

Some authors have advocated videotaping to document patient reactions during disk injections.[98,99,127] Videotaped findings are later correlated with fluoroscopy or compared with simultaneous changes in physiologic parameters such as heart rate and blood pressure. If relevant, the videotape can be made available to the referring surgeon.

IMAGE INTERPRETATION

For morphologic interpretation of fluoroscopic images, even though plain diskography is clearly inferior to CT-diskography, useful information may nevertheless be garnered from the overall appearance of spread of contrast material. A small central "cotton ball" appearance usually indicates a normal painless disk. Normal disks may also have a central bilobular appearance, like a "hamburger in a bun." A thin line of contrast that extends to the posterior edge of the disk is consistent with an annular tear, and it is not unusual for patients to complain of pain when the contrast agent moves posteriorly. Small lines of anterior extravasation are sometimes seen but are less likely to elicit pain. More diffuse posterior spread of contrast can indicate a large annular tear. Spread of contrast into the epidural space is consistent with a complete tear of the annulus and loss of integrity of the outer annular wall. Diffuse spread in all directions, with or without spread into the epidural space, is indicative of a severely degenerated disk (Figs. 65.6 to 65.8).

Fluoroscopy can show morphologic differences between normal and degenerated disks but poorly characterizes the locations of annular tears and their relationship to nerve roots. Disk architecture is much better assessed by CT because of its cross-sectional acquisition of thin slices parallel to the disk spaces. Thus, many annular tears seen on CT images are invisible with fluoroscopy. For this reason, we perform procedures requiring a functional annulus, such as percutaneous disk decompression, only after CT-diskography.[214] Contiguous helical CT images enable longitudinal reformations in the identical coronal and sagittal planes obtained with MRI. Coronal and sagittal CT reformations demonstrate the distribution of contrast in relation to both the internal and external annulus, as well as focal contour abnormalities relative to the central spinal canal, lateral recesses, neural foramina, and nerve roots (Figs. 65.9 to 65.11).

The most commonly used terminology of disk disease was adapted for MRI. This terminology is difficult to apply to CT-diskography because it addresses only contour abnormalities, such as disk bulges, extrusions, and sequestrations. Internal disk abnormalities that cannot be detected on MRI become obvious on CT because they are filled with contrast material. On CT-diskographic images, morphologic analysis of disk architecture, including the NP and AF, can be applied to disks with normal MRI contours, as well as to

Table 65.9 Scoring and Interpretation of Diskograms

Concordant Levels	Points	L2-3	L3-4	L4-5	L5-S1	Sum of Rows
		Segments Studied				
Concordant pain	30					
Pain >5/10	5					
Pain >7/10	5					
Pressure <50 psi	10					
Pressure <15 psi	10					
SUBTOTAL						
Divide the subtotal by the number of concordant disks. Enter the result in this row.						

Control Levels	Points	L2-3	L3-4	L4-5	L5-S1	Sum of Rows
		Segments Studied				
No pain	30					
Pain at <50 psi	-10					
Pain at <15 psi	-10					
TOTAL of sums of rows below the double line						

Interpretation: >70 points is positive, 40-60 points is indeterminate, and <40 points is negative.

1. For each disk studied (see columns), enter the appropriate score for each of the variables indicated (rows).

For disks with concordant pain:
- Enter 30 if the concordant pain is produced.
- Enter 5 if the pain produced is greater than 5/10.
- Enter another 5 if the pain produced is also greater than 7/10.
- Enter 10 if the pressure at which pain occurred is anything less than 50 psi.
- Enter another 10 if the pressure is also less than 15 psi.

For disks at conrol levels (i.e., not concordant pain):
- Enter +30 if the disk was painless.
- Enter −10 if pain occurred at a pressure less than 50 psi.
- Enter another −10 if pain occurred at a pressure also less than 15 psi.

2. For the concordant disks, add up the scores in each row and record the sum of each row in the column labeled Sum of Rows.
3. Add up the sums of the rows for all concordant disks, that is, all scores above the double line. Divide this total by the number of concordant disks, and record the quotient in the cell indicated, immediately below the double line, in the column labeled Sum of Rows.
4. For the nonconcordant disks, add up the scores in the rows while taking heed of any negative numbers, and record the sum of each row in the column labeled Sum of Rows.
5. Add up the total of the sums column below the double line while taking care to heed negative numbers.
6. Interpret the results.

Adapted from Standards Committee of the International Spine Intervention Society. Lumbar disc stimulation. In: Bogduk N, ed. *Practice Guidelines: Spinal Diagnostic and Treatment Procedures*. San Francisco: International Spine Intervention Society; 2004:20-46.

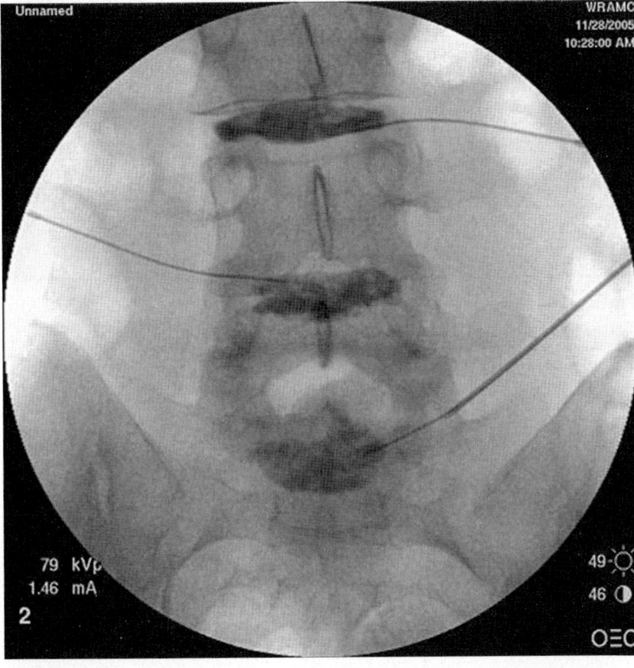

Figure 65.6 Anteroposterior view of a diskogram showing early degenerative changes in the L3-4 and L4-5 intervertebral disks.

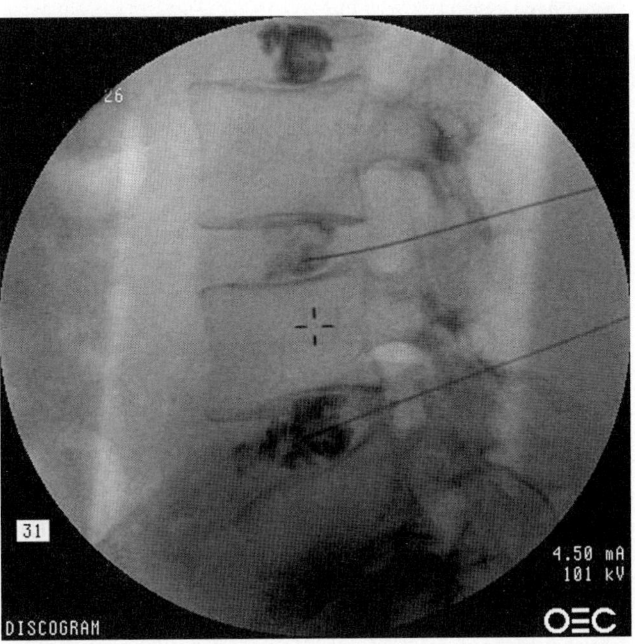

Figure 65.7 Lateral view of normal L3-4 and L4-5 diskograms. The L5-S1 diskogram reveals a partial tear in the anterior annulus that was clinically insignificant.

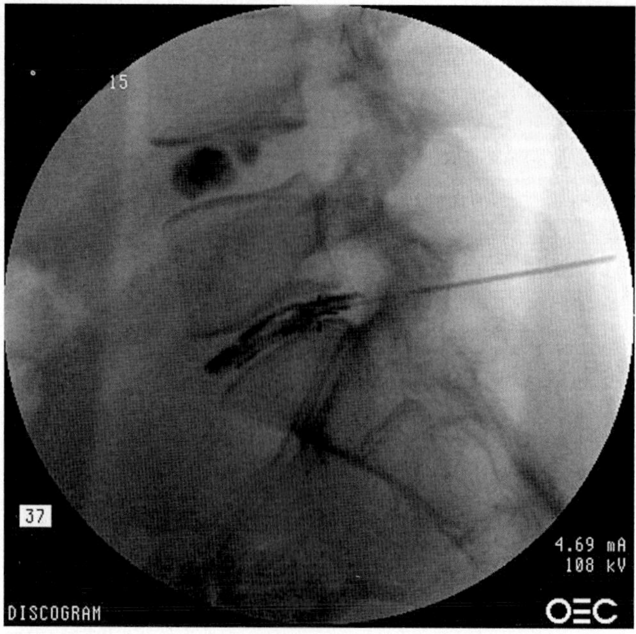

Figure 65.8 Lateral view of a two-level diskogram revealing a normal L4-5 disk and a diffusely degenerated L5-S1 disk with a complete posterior annular tear. (Adapted from Bernard TN. Lumbar discography followed by computed tomography. Refining the diagnosis of low-back pain. *Spine*. 1990;15:690-707; and Sachs BL, Vanharanta H, Spivey MA, et al. Dallas discogram description: a new classification of CT/discography in low-back disorders. *Spine*. 1987;12:287-294.)

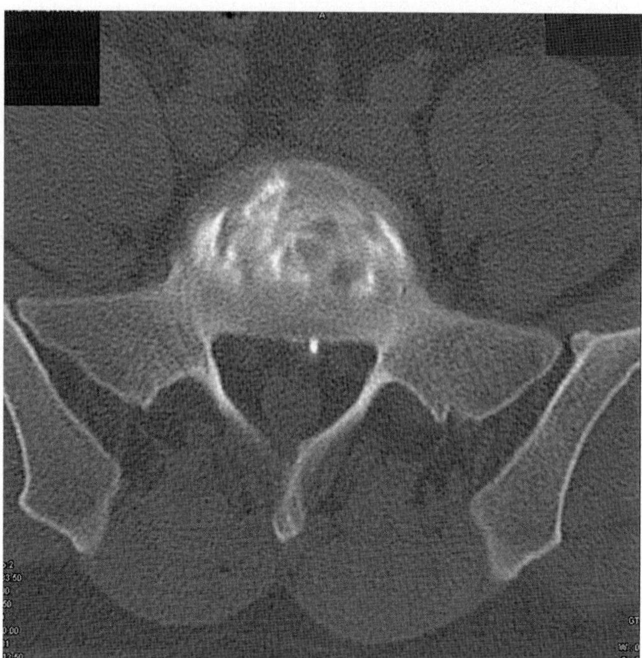

Figure 65.10 Axial computed tomographic diskogram of a diffusely degenerated L5-S1 disk.

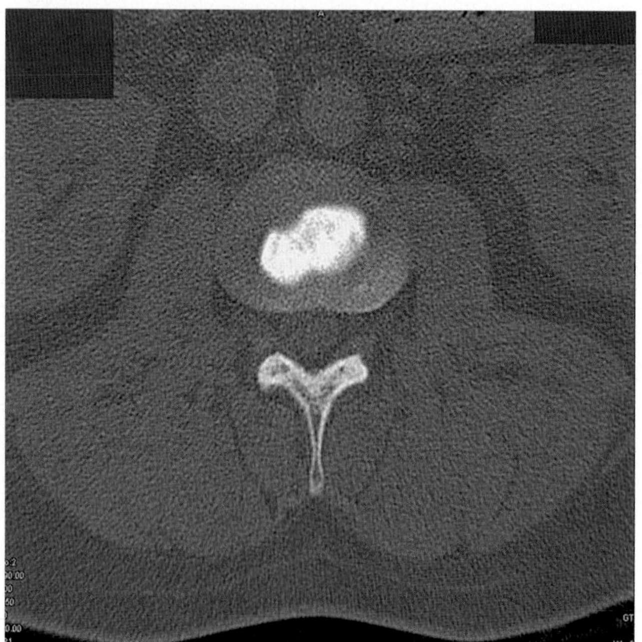

Figure 65.9 Axial view of a normal computed tomographic diskogram. Note the "cotton ball" appearance of the contrast material within the confines of the nucleus pulposus.

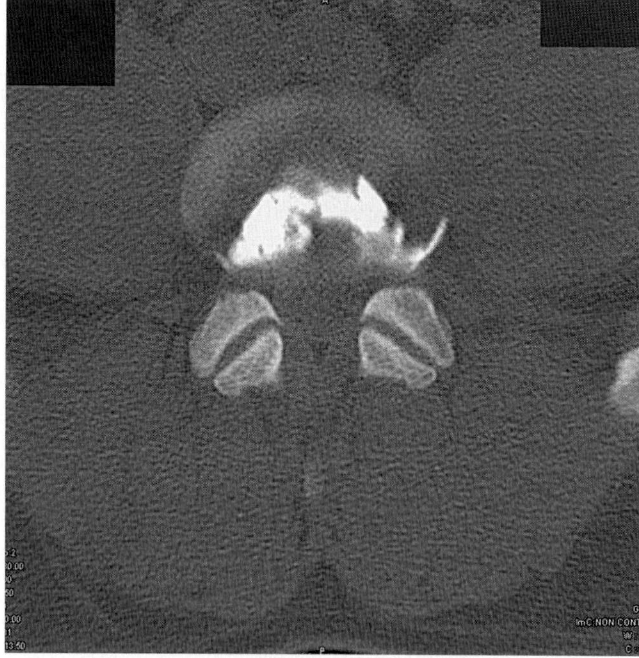

Figure 65.11 Axial view of a computed tomographic diskogram demonstrating bilateral posterolateral annular tears.

herniated disks. The Dallas diskogram scale was originally developed to describe and grade annular tears and has subsequently undergone several modifications[127,224] (Fig. 65.12). The modified Dallas classification for disk morphology takes into account annular tears, as well as extra-annular contrast leakage and diffuse degenerative changes. In this modified scheme, disk morphology is graded from 0 to 7[127] (Fig. 65.13; Box 65.2).

The final interpretation of lumbar diskography should take into consideration not only disk stimulation data and morphology but also less tangible factors such as a patient's psychological profile, expectations, behavior, and physiologic parameters during pain provocation, as well as potential confounding factors such as secondary gain and return-to-work issues. In a well-chosen diskography candidate, pain is

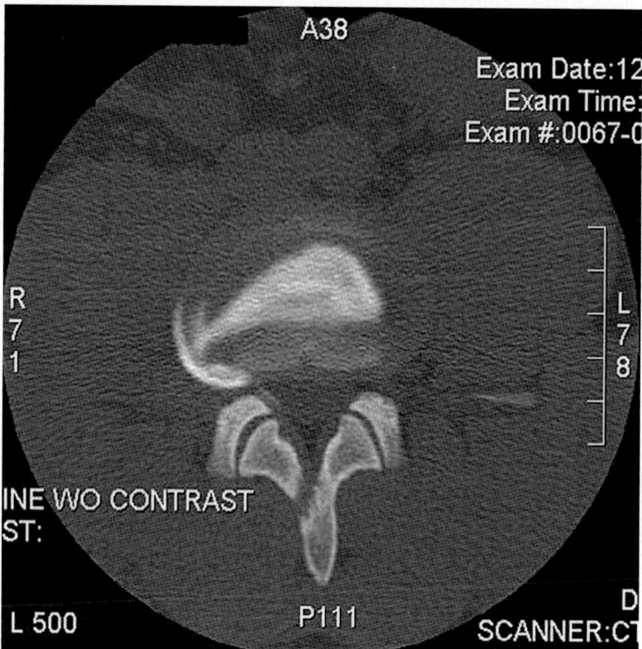

Figure 65.12 Computed tomographic diskogram demonstrating a large right posterolateral annular tear. On this axial image, the spread of contrast material appears to be contained within the annulus.

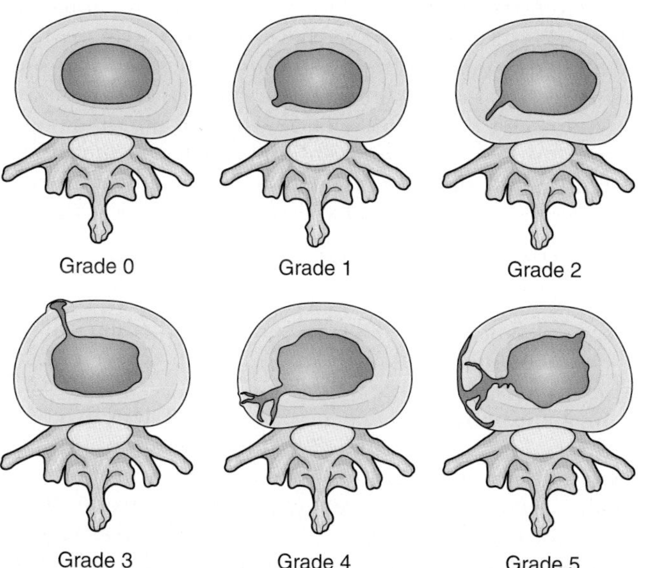

Figure 65.13 Modified Dallas diskogram scheme for the classification of annular tears by computed tomographic diskography. (Drawings by Jee Hyun Kim. From Cohen SP, Larkin TM, Barna SA, et al, Lumbar discography: a comprehensive review of outcome studies, diagnostic accuracy, and principles. *Reg Anesth Pain Med.* 2005;30:163-183.)

infrequently reproduced in a disk that is morphologically, manometrically, and volumetrically normal. In the rare instances when this does occur, the diskographer must consider the patient's clinical picture, including historical and physical examination findings, the presence of spinal and psychological pathology, additional radiologic and diagnostic tests, and the technical success of the diskogram, before deciding on a treatment course.

Box 65.2 Computed Tomography Classification of Diskography

Type 1: The diskogram is normal manometrically, volumetrically, and radiologically and produces no pain. CT-diskography shows contrast material to be centrally located in both the axial and sagittal projections.

Type 2: Identical to type 1 except that it is positive for pain reproduction.

Type 3: The annular tears lead to a radial fissure. This group can be further subdivided into the following:

- **Type 3a:** The radial fissure is posterior.
- **Type 3b:** The fissure radiates posterolaterally.
- **Type 3c**: The fissure extends laterally to a line drawn from the center of the disk tangential to the lateral border of the superior articulating process.

Type 4: When the radial fissure reaches the periphery of the annulus fibrosus, nuclear material protrudes and causes the outer annulus to bulge.

Type 5: When the outer annular fibers rupture, nuclear material may extrude beneath the posterior longitudinal ligament and directly contact either the dura or a nerve root.

Type 6: When the extruded fragment is no longer in continuity with the interspace, it is said to be sequestrated. Manometrically, volumetrically, and radiologically, these diskograms are always abnormal. Concordant pain may be reproduced only if enough pressure is generated against the free fragment to cause stimulation of pain-sensitive structures.

Type 7: The end stage of the degenerative process is internal disk disruption, in which multiple annular tears occur. The diskograms are abnormal manometrically and volumetrically, and familiar pain may or may not be reproduced. Radiologically, the contrast material usually fills the entire interspace in a chaotic fashion. CT-diskography shows extravasation of contrast material throughout multiple annular tears.

Adapted from Bernard TN. Lumbar discography followed by computed tomography. Refining the diagnosis of low-back pain. *Spine.* 1990;15:690-707; and Sachs BL, Vanharanta H, Spivey MA, et al. Dallas discogram description. A new classification of CT/discography in low-back disorders. *Spine.* 1987;12:287-294.

POSTPROCEDURAL CARE

At the conclusion of disk stimulation, disks may be injected with local anesthetic. In a small case series by Kotilainen and colleagues, the authors found that 83% and 67% of patients who received 0.5% bupivacaine intradiscally obtained good pain relief 1 day and 2 weeks after the procedure, respectively.[203] In clinical practice, the amount injected into the disk is largely determined by the disk itself since trying to force fluid into a fully pressurized disk may do more harm than good. Typically, in a degenerative disk with an annular tear, 0.5 mL of local anesthetic should safely help reduce postprocedural pain. It may also be helpful to reanesthetize the track of the needle, but care must be taken to avoid unintentionally anesthetizing a nerve root. Although these measures are often sufficient to alleviate postprocedural pain, it is our practice to routinely administer nonsteroidal anti-inflammatory drugs at the termination of the procedure. Occasionally, a patient may require extra analgesic medication to treat postdiskography pain. Although one retrospective study concluded that intradiscal steroids confer adequate pain relief,[229] two placebo-controlled trials failed to demonstrate any benefit.[202,230]

COMPLICATIONS

DISKITIS

Diskitis is the most feared complication of diskography because infection can be extremely difficult to treat as a result of the poor blood supply that intervertebral disks receive. Procedure-related pain is commonplace following diskography, yet any patient who experiences a new neurologic finding or complains of increased pain 1 week after the procedure warrants re-evaluation. At minimum the postdiskography workup should include a focused history, physical examination, and laboratory screening tests. The erythrocyte sedimentation rate (ESR) and C-reactive protein are the most sensitive indicators of diskitis, but elevation does not usually occur until 3 weeks after the procedure.[231,232] If the ESR is higher than 50, a bone scan or MRI is needed to rule out diskitis. The most common etiologic agent in postprocedure diskitis is *Staphylococcus aureus*.[232]

In a retrospective study conducted in 432 patients, Fraser and colleagues found that the incidence of diskitis was reduced from 2.7% to 0.7% when a through-and-through double-needle technique was used.[233] However, a confounding factor when interpreting these results is that no stylet was used during the single-needle technique. A review by Guyer and Ohnmeiss found an overall incidence of diskitis of less than 0.15% by patient and less than 0.08% by disk, with most of the studies included not administering prophylactic antibiotics.[234] Osti and associates advocated mixing 1 mg/mL of cefazolin with the injected contrast agent as a safe and effective means of preventing diskitis following a two-part study.[235] In the first phase of the study, intradiscal cefazolin was found to be equivalent to parenteral antibiotics administered 30 minutes before the procedure in preventing diskitis in sheep inoculated with intradiscal *Staphylococcus epidermidis*. In the second phase of the study, radiographic or clinical evidence of diskitis developed in 0% of 127 patients following diskography conducted by mixing 1 mg/mL of cefazolin with the contrast material. A recent in vitro study by Klessig and colleagues supports the prophylactic use of intradiscal antibiotics in lieu of systemic therapy for patients undergoing provocative diskography.[236]

The administration of prophylactic antibiotics is by no means universal. Willems and colleagues performed a literature review of postdiskography diskitis cases with and without the use of prophylactic antibiotics.[237] Inclusion criteria were use of the double-needle technique and stringent reporting of complications and dropouts. Including their own report on 200 patients who underwent 435 diskograms, 11 studies were analyzed, only 1 of which administered prophylactic antibiotics. Among the 4981 patients included in the analysis who did not receive prophylactic antimicrobial therapy, the incidence of diskitis was 0.25% (0.09% of 12,770 diskograms). The authors concluded that there was not enough evidence to support prophylactic antibiotics as a means of preventing diskitis.

A more recent systematic review by Sharma and coworkers concluded that although preclinical animal models support the use of prophylactic antibiotics before iatrogenic disk innoculation, neither intravenous nor intradiscal antibiotics have been conclusively shown to reduce the incidence of infection following diskography.[238] Another review conducted by Kapoor and associates for cervical diskography similarly found that the overall evidence for the use of prophylactic antibiotics to prevent diskitis was not definitive.[239]

In view of the inherent difficulties in treating diskitis and the fact that no serious complications have ever been reported from the use of low-dose intradiscal antibiotics, the authors believe that the prophylactic use of intradiscal cefazolin or clindamycin is justified in patients (e.g., diabetes, human immunodeficiency virus infection, steroid use) or circumstances that may increase the risk for infection (Box 65.3). Collectively, we have performed more than 8000 diskograms with intradiscal antibiotics and had only a single case of diskitis in a patient with diabetes. If diskitis should occur, the mainstay of treatment is antibiotics and pain control; surgical intervention is not usually necessary. Potential complications of diskitis include epidural abscess, intervertebral fusion, and paralysis.[240]

Box 65.3 Antibiotic Prophylaxis Guidelines

Intravenous

Cefazolin, 1 g in 50 mL normal saline 30 to 60 minutes before the procedure or

Clindamycin (for patients with cephalosporin or penicillin allergy), 900 mg in 50 mL normal saline 30 to 60 minutes before the procedure or

Ciprofloxacin (for patients with cephalosporin or penicillin allergy), 400 mg in 50 mL normal saline 30 to 60 minutes before the procedure

Intradiscal

Cefazolin, 1 mg (10 mg/mL) either before the start of contrast injection or mixed with the contrast agent or

Clindamycin, 0.6 mg (6 mg/mL) either before the start of contrast injection or mixed with the contrast agent

DISKOGRAPHY AND THE PROGRESSION OF DISK DEGENERATION

A key question surrounding diskography is whether artificial elevation of intervertebral disk pressure can worsen existing LBP or injure the intervertebral disk.

In an experimental biochemical model tested in 113 cadavers, Iencean determined that the amount of pressure required to rupture the annulus was inversely proportional to the degree of degeneration and ranged from 108 to 188 psi.[241] However, vigilance should be exercised at all times during disk stimulation because there are many reports of diskography-induced lumbar disk herniation occurring at lower pressures.[242]

Carragee and associates attempted to answer this question by conducting a controlled, prospective study to examine whether provocative lumbar diskography is associated with long-term low back symptoms in 26 subjects without low back complaints.[243] In the 10 patients who were pain free after unrelated neck surgery, none reported persistent LBP 1 year following diskography. In 10 patients with chronic neck or arm pain after cervical spine surgery, 2 reported persistent pain 1 year after diskography. In the six patients with somatization disorder, two thirds (four of six) reported ongoing pain after diskography. In two control groups composed of somatization patients who did not undergo diskography and LBP patients with positive diskograms but no other nondiscogenic spine abnormalities, no significant change in low back symptomatology was noted during the 1-year follow-up. After a 4-year follow-up study, the authors concluded that painful disk injections and annular disruptions are poor and weak predictors of future low back problems in patients without preexisting low back complaints, respectively.[244] Conversely, the authors found psychological distress and preexisting pain complaints not involving the low back region to be stronger predictors of the subsequent development of LBP.

In three studies evaluating the clinical and anatomic sequelae of diskography, Johnson,[245] Flanagan and Chung,[246] and Saifuddin and coworkers[247] all found no evidence that diskography causes damage to intervertebral disks based on repeated diskograms, clinical and radiographic findings, and MRI findings, respectively. Although the study by Saiffudin and colleagues used the reference standard (i.e., MRI) for detecting disk pathology, only a small number of patients (n = 7) were involved, and repeated imaging was done at a mean follow-up period of just 72 days, which may not be sufficient to detect long-term sequelae.

In an effort to better elucidate this issue, Carragee and associates[248] performed a prospective, matched-control cohort study to evaluate disk degeneration over a 7- to 10-year period in patients who underwent diskography. The rationale behind this endeavor was that annular puncture has been used for many years as an animal model of disk degeneration,[249,250] but little is known about its long-term effects in humans. Seventy-five patients without serious LBP underwent a protocol MRI and L3-4, L4-5, and L5-S1 diskography as part of previous studies designed to identify "false-positive" responders. A matched group enrolled at the same time underwent the same protocol MRI examination. Seven to 10 years after the baseline assessment, subjects underwent a repeated MRI examination. In all measured parameters, disks that had undergone diskographic evaluation demonstrated greater progression of the degenerative findings (35% vs. 14%) and more new disk herniations (35% vs. 15%) than did control (noninjected) disks. Moreover, new disk herniations were disproportionately found on the side of annular puncture. Quantitative measures of disk height and disk signal also showed significantly greater progression in the diskography group. This was the first study of its kind showing that diskography using a small-gauge needle (25 and 22 gauge) with limited pressurization could result in accelerated disk degeneration.

OTHER COMPLICATIONS

In a study analyzing 146 lumbar diskograms in 52 patients, Tallroth and colleagues found that 2% of patients experienced nausea, 4% convulsions, and 6% severe back pain during the procedures.[251] Ten percent of patients reported severe headache and 81% worsening LBP 1 day after the procedure. The headaches were attributed to neuraxial leakage of contrast material. In a retrospective study assessing complications in 4400 cervical diskograms performed in 1357 patients, Zeidman and coauthors reported a complication rate of 0.6%, or 0.16% of disk injections.[252] Adverse events included seven cases of diskitis and one abscess. Prophylactic antibiotics were administered only to patients deemed to be at high risk for infection. Pilet and colleagues reported a patient with worsening pain following diskography in whom herniation through the vertebral end plate (Schmorl's node) was found to have developed.[253] Other possible complications of diskography include meningitis, spinal headache, subdural or epidural abscess, intrathecal and retroperitoneal hemorrhage, arachnoiditis, nerve root injury, paravertebral muscle pain and contusions, postprocedural pain exacerbation, vasovagal reactions, allergic reactions, and damage to the disk, including but not limited to herniation.[205,254-259]

CONCLUSION

Considering the long history of diskography in diagnosing disk pathology and the advent of more advanced imaging techniques, wherein lies the future of disk stimulation? Diskography has already come under scrutiny by third-party payers, with many refusing to reimburse for the procedure. Nonetheless, diskography appears to be a cost-effective screening test in view of the high cost of spinal fusion. Because of the high lifetime prevalence of LBP, which approaches 80% by some estimates, and the fact that various stages of disk degeneration can be detected in a majority of people—even without low back symptoms—it is clear that some sort of test is needed to determine whether a causative relationship exists between the two phenomena. Even though diskography, with or without CT, remains the only imaging tool that ostensibly allows a clinician to relate pathology with symptoms, the value of this test remains unclear.

When assessing diskographic pathology, proponents of diskography argue that it is necessary to correlate provoked pain with anatomic abnormalities. In regard to symptomatic disk herniations, the enhanced accuracy and safety of MRI have rendered plain diskography obsolete for this purpose. For IDD, CT-diskography is a more sensitive diagnostic tool than plain MRI, although T2-weighted MRI may detect some pathology missed with plain diskography. Based on cadaveric studies, diskography seems to be more accurate in identifying radial than transverse or concentric tears in the AF. Disk stimulation studies have consistently found that degenerated disks of all types are more likely than normal disks to provoke pain and that annular disruption seems to be a prominent source of pain generation. However, the significance of these findings is limited by the high prevalence of abnormal features, the fact that in clinical contexts diskography is almost exclusively performed on disks already noted to be abnormal on CT or MRI, and the observation that a substantial percentage of patients with LBP may be at increased risk for "false-positive" diskograms.

As a diagnostic procedure that carries substantial risk, including possible acceleration of disk degeneration in some patients, the critical question that will determine whether diskography remains a viable preoperative screening tool or becomes merely another footnote in history is whether it improves patient outcomes, and presently, evidence for this is lacking. In studies directly comparing fusion outcomes between patients who underwent routine preoperative diskography screening and those who did not, the results are conflicting. For intradiscal procedures targeting discogenic pain, the controversy surrounding its efficacy and the fact that all published studies have consistently used preprocedure diskography prevent any conclusions from being drawn. With disk replacement surgery, although the studies are almost evenly divided between those that used preoperative diskography and those that did not, the lack of direct comparison between groups, the presence of methodologic flaws, and differences in outcome measures, length of follow-up, and surgical technique render any comparisons futile. Given the lack of evidence supporting any interventional treatment of discogenic LBP, even if prospective, randomized studies were to be conducted on the benefits of diskography, they would be unlikely to definitively resolve this controversy.

There clearly exists a wide discrepancy in the use of lumbar diskography to treat discogenic LBP. Routine use of diskography as a screening tool before minimally invasive surgical procedures is inconsistent, and the procedure is used sporadically before spinal arthrodesis and disk replacement surgery. After weighing the risks and benefits of diskography, the authors believe that the procedure should be strongly considered before any invasive surgical procedure used to treat discogenic LBP except when the evidence implicating a particular disk or disks as the pain generator is strong or definitive. Consequently, diskography may be more beneficial when screening patients for an inexperienced surgeon than it is for selecting patients for an experienced surgeon, in whom the positive diskography rate may be much higher. Inherent in this recommendation is that the procedure be conducted according to evidence-based standards, which remain the subject of ongoing debate. These standards might include the routine use of manometry, obtaining two adjacent control disks in patients at high risk for "false-positive" pain provocation, performing psychological screening similar to that used routinely before spinal cord stimulation, and requiring at least one objective measure to confirm a positive diskogram, such as a significant increase in heart rate or elicitation of certain facial expressions. This recommendation is also contingent on the results of disk stimulation being considered in the context of other diagnostic screening tests and with the understanding that patients with preexisting psychopathology and somatization symptoms may be prone to false-positive pain provocation. Although anesthetic diskography was developed as a tool to reduce the high false-positive rates in selected individuals, whether the purported increased specificity outweighs the increased risk for iatrogenic disk injury, increased cost, and potential for false-negative results has yet to be determined. One point on which there does seem to be consensus is that clinical studies are needed to better elucidate the role that diskography will assume in the diagnosis of disk pathology in the future and to determine what effect, if any, it has on the surgical treatment of discogenic LBP.

SUGGESTED READINGS

Brox JI, Reikeras O, Nygaard O, et al. Lumbar instrumented fusion compared with cognitive intervention and exercises in patients with chronic back pain after previous surgery for disc herniation: a prospective randomized controlled study. *Pain.* 2006;122:145-155.

Carragee EJ, Don AS, Hurwitz EL, et al. 2009 ISSLS prize winner: does discography cause accelerated progression of degeneration changes in the lumbar disc: a ten-year matched cohort study. *Spine.* 2009;34:2338-2345.

Colhoun E, McCall IW, Williams L, et al. Provocation discography as a guide to planning operations on the spine. *J Bone Joint Surg Br.* 1988;70:267-271.

Derby R, Howard MW, Grant JM, et al. The ability of pressure-controlled discography to predict surgical and nonsurgical outcomes. *Spine.* 1999;24:364-371.

Fairbank J, Frost H, Wilson-MacDonald J, et al, for the Spine Stabilisation Trial Group. Randomised controlled trial to compare surgical stabilisation of the lumbar spine with an intensive rehabilitation programme for patients with chronic low back pain: the MRC spine stabilisation trial. *BMJ.* 2005;330:1233.

Freemont AJ, Peacock TE, Goupille P, et al. Nerve ingrowth into diseased intervertebral disc in chronic back pain. *Lancet.* 1997;350:178-181.

Madan S, Gundanna M, Harley JM, et al. Does provocative discography screening of discogenic back pain improve surgical outcomes? *J Spinal Disord Tech.* 2002;15:245-251.

Nakamura S, Takahashi K, Takahashi Y, et al. The afferent pathways of discogenic low-back pain. *J Bone Joint Surg Br.* 1996;78:606-612.

Ohtori S, Kinoshita T, Yamashita M, et al. Results of surgery for discogenic low back pain: a randomized study using discography versus discoblock for diagnosis. *Spine.* 2009;34:1345-1348.

Schwarzer AC, Aprill CN, Derby R, et al. The prevalence and clinical features of internal disc disruption in patients with chronic low back pain. *Spine.* 1995;17:1878-1883.

Sharma SK, Jones JO, Zeballos PP, et al. The prevention of discitis during discography. *Spine J.* 2009;9:936-943.

Valdes AM, Hassett G, Hart DJ, et al. Radiographic progression of lumbar spine disc degeneration is influenced by variation at inflammatory genes: a candidate SNP association study in the Chingford cohort. *Spine.* 2005;30:2445-2451.

Vanharanta H, Sachs BL, Spivey MA, et al. The relationship of pain provocation to lumbar disc deterioration as seen by CT/discography. *Spine.* 1987;12:295-298.

Wolfer LR, Derby R, Lee JE, et al. Systematic review of lumbar provocation discography in asymptomatic subjects with a meta-analysis of false-positive rates. *Pain Physician.* 2008;11:513-538.

The references for this chapter can be found at www.expertconsult.com.

66

Intradiscal Procedures for the Treatment of Discogenic Lower Back and Leg Pain

Leonardo Kapural

SUMMARY

Although establishing the diagnosis of lumbar disk herniation with associated leg pain is usually intuitive, diagnosis and treatment of lumbar discogenic pain remain difficult. It may account for one third of patients with lower back pain. The mechanism of this pain is still unclear, clinical presentation can vary, and imaging may be misleading. Provocative diskography remains the only diagnostic test that can relate changes observed on imaging tests and the patient's pain, despite questioned validity of provocative diskography as an appropriate diagnostic test.

Percutaneous treatments for diskogenic lower back pain emerged in the early 2000s, and these therapeutic approaches seem to be more efficacious and less invasive alternatives to currently available surgical options. They are cost-effective, when compared to surgical approaches, and may cause fewer side effects. However, the true therapeutic value of these therapies has yet to be established. Proper patient selection may significantly improve successes of those minimally invasive treatments, so that fewer patients elect to undergo open spinal surgery.

Percutaneous disk decompression procedures when used as minimally invasive approaches to treat back and leg pain caused by contained disk herniation clinically had generally favorable clinical outcomes and complication rates were low. However, studies with higher level of evidence are lacking.

INTRODUCTION

Frequently cited causes of lower back pain include myofascial, discogenic, facetogenic origins, conditions originating from the sacroiliac joint, compression fractures, and lumbar stenosis.[1,2] Low back pain is one of the most common causes of lost work time and is becoming a major economic burden.[1] Discogenic pain remains one of the main causes of lower back pain.[3]

This chapter highlights some interesting, novel, and minimally invasive therapeutic interventions, and those procedures should be used as a part of comprehensive, multidisciplinary treatment in order to produce the best results in a patient's functional capacity and improvements in pain scores.

Intervertebral disk as a pain generator is difficult to evaluate using conventional and conservative methods. Patients frequently describe unrelenting low back discomfort and groin or occasionally leg pain that worsens with axial loading that improves with recumbency. Patients complain of increased pain in their lower back with Valsalva maneuver, prolonged sitting, or driving a car. The signs and symptoms provide a clue to the causative factors so that further steps can be taken to determine an accurate diagnosis.[1-4] Imaging (e.g., magnetic resonance imaging [MRI]) correlates poorly with clinical findings, leaving open the question of pain causality.[1-4] One approach to substantiate clinical findings and correlate the patient's pain to the imaging study is to conduct a provocative or analgesic diagnostic diskography. Currently, this approach is the only diagnostic method to correlate anatomic abnormalities with clinically observed lower back pain. Despite wide clinical use, the diagnostic value of this test has been repeatedly questioned, mainly because of potentially high false-positive rates.[5-7]

After a provisional diagnosis of discogenic pain has been established, an effective treatment is desired. Several commonly used minimally invasive intradiscal therapies involve careful denervation of the annulus fibrosus (Fig. 66.1). So-called annuloplasty procedures have been clinically used, despite a lack of objective histologic findings of nociceptive fiber denervation or any changes in collagen fiber structure expected after intradiscal heat is used.[8-12] The minimally invasive approach, low cost, and relative simplicity of these procedures, as well as a short recovery time, are major advantages of annuloplasty procedures when compared to surgical approaches such as lumbar fusion or disk replacement. Intradiscal electrothermal therapy (IDET; Smith and Nephews, London, United Kingdom), DiscTRODE (Valleylab, Boulder, Colorado), and Intradiscal Biacuplasty (Baylis Medical, Inc., Montreal, Canada) (see Fig. 66.1) have been historically used to treat discogenic pain.

The process of intervertebral disk degeneration includes induced dehydration of the intervertebral disk and a loss of nuclear material. Delamination and fissuring of the lamellar layers are physical changes, and the production of certain cytokines and other mediators is one of the biochemical and cellular changes occurring within the disk. Inside the intervertebral disk, the production of inflammatory cytokines including tumor necrosis factor-α (TNF-α), nitric oxide, and matrix metalloproteinases (MMPs) can be greatly altered.[13,14] Nociceptors, normally limited to the outer third of the annulus, could be the substrate for discogenic pain when they are expanded over the larger annular area and penetrate further into the degenerated disk along the vasculature and fissures.[15-18] Those C- and Aδ fibers are

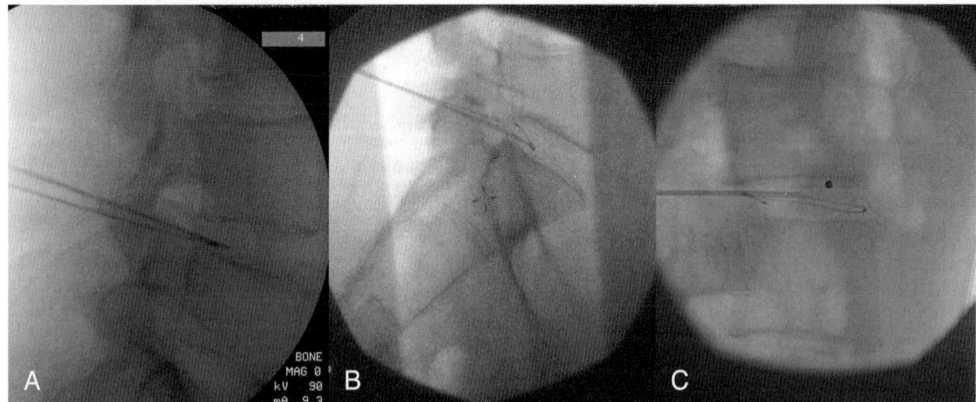

Figure 66.1 Lateral fluoroscopic view of the final electrode positions during three different intervertebral disk heating (annuloplasty) procedures used for the treatment of discogenic pain. **A,** Bipolar intradiscal biacuplasty probes within the intervertebral disk. Lateral fluoroscopic view of two biacuplasty probes within the intervertebral disk and away from vertebral end plates. **B,** DiscTRODE electrode (ValleyLab, Boulder, Colorado) positioned across the posterior annulus. A second straight probe is a temperature probe. **C,** IDET coil is shown within the intervertebral disk. Lateral fluoroscopic view of the L4-5 disk and properly positioned IDET coil.

likely responsible for transmitting pain responses,[14,17] and their elimination may, in theory, disrupt transmission of the pain signal.

Minimally invasive thermal procedures deliver heat inside the disk annulus via a resistive heating coil in, for example, IDET, bipolar biacuplasty (Kimberly Clark, Atlanta, Georgia), or unipolar, flexible (DiscTRODE; Valleylab, Boulder, Colorado) radiofrequency (RF) electrode to denervate nociceptive fibers and coagulate collagenous tissues.

During the application of RF, similar to any other tissue, alternating flow of electrical current causes ions in the tissue to alternate fast movements. This molecular vibration results in frictional heating and ablation.[19,20] Ionic heating produces thermal injury of the cells when tissue temperature reaches > 42° C.[21] The extent of cellular damage depends on multiple factors including the temperature, position, thickness of electrodes, and duration of heating.[22] An increase in tissue temperature is a function of current density, which is greatest at the proximity of the electrode and decreases with increasing distance from the electrode. However, by increasing the power output, current density around the electrode is increased and lesion size is limited by the given current density.

Cooling the RF electrode internally can increase lesion size and is currently used during intradiscal biacuplasty procedures.[23-28] Cooled RF probes have cooling sink lumens that extend to the tip of the electrode. The cooling fluid (water) circulates from the tip of the electrode to a synchronized water pump. As coolant removes heat from the tissue adjacent to the electrode, larger lesion volumes are produced by increasing power deposition and the duration of the current interval.[23] An even larger lesion volume can be produced by using two internally cooled RF electrodes in a bipolar arrangement at significantly lower temperatures.

INTRADISCAL ELECTROTHERMAL THERAPY (IDET)

IDET technology, although limited in its use clinically, is still considered a valuable intradiscal procedure and will be briefly discussed (see Fig. 66.1*C*). It provides focal heat via an elongated resistive coil of very small diameter to the limited area of the posterior annulus. Possible mechanisms of pain relief were already discussed. The limited use results from the high temperatures attained just around the electrode itself and quick dissipation of the heat at 2- to 4-mm radius away from the coil. Positioning of the resistive coil within the posterior annulus of the disk can be prolonged, and multiple attempts may be required, or it may be necessary to pass another coil from the opposite side of the posterolateral disk to achieve optimal electrode placement within the interface between the annulus and the nucleus (see Fig. 66.1*C*). This may further damage the intervertebral disk, and sometimes placing the tip of the coil within the posterior annular fissure may extend too close to the neural canal. Indications for IDET include persistent discogenic low back pain despite prolonged and comprehensive conservative treatments including physical therapy and a directed home exercise program, similar to other annuloplasty procedures.[29-31] Provocative or analgesic diskography should replicate or eliminate concordant pain at low disk pressurization (< 50 PSI). The clinical outcome studies on intradiscal electrothermal therapy (IDET) are listed with other annuloplasty studies in Table 66.1.[29-43]

Multilevel disk degeneration seen on magnetic resonance imaging (MRI) appears to be an important negative predictor for the success of annuloplasty, especially when compared to a group of patients with one or two degenerated disks as shown on the MRI. There are few patients with a single disk disease compared to those with multilevel degeneration present on the MRI.[41] Two other groups of patients who have much lower chance of successful functional capacity improvement after annuloplasty are overweight patients[44] and patients receiving workers' compensation benefits.[40,45]

Another approach to annuloplasty utilizes a flexible radiofrequency electrode and is called DiscTRODE or percutaneous intradiscal radiofrequency thermocoagulation (PIRFT).[46,47] Two studies, utilizing proper patient selection, showed minimal or no benefit from PIRFT. Kvarstein and coworkers reported minimal or no improvements in functional capacity,[46] as did Kapural and associates.[47] It appears that the design of the PIRFT electrode provided minimal heat dissipation, which, in turn, could not adequately denervate the posterior annulus.[47]

Table 66.1 Selected Published Articles on Three Annuloplasty Procedures*

Study	Year	Type of Annuloplasty	Indications	Number of Patients	Type of Study	Outcomes	Complications	Conclusions
Kapural et al. (41)	2004	IDET	Single-or two-level DDD and p.disco., > 50% disk height versus multilevel DDD	34	Prospective Matched study	1,2-DDD > 50% improvement in VAS and PDI	None	IDET effective, but only in one-or two-level DDD
Assietti et al. (42)	2010	IDET	Single-level DDD and p.disco., > 60% disk height	50	Prospective	VAS 68% decrease; ODI from 59.0+/−7.6% to 20.1+/−11% at 24 m	None	Effective/safe
Kapural et al., Kapural (49, 50)	2008	Biacuplasty	Single- or two-level DDD and p.disco., > 50% disk height	15	Prospective pilot	7 of 13 > 50% VAS ODI to 17.5 and SF-36-PF from 51 to 67 @12 m	None	Effective/safe
Kvarstein et al. (46)	2009	DiscTRODE	Chronic LBP, p.disco	23	Prospective randomized, double blind	No improvement study or sham at 12 m	None	Ineffective
Pauza et al. (35)	2004	IDET	DDD and p.disco., > 80% disk height	64	Randomized sham-controlled prospective	56% > 2 VAS change; 50% patients > 50% relief at 6 m	None	Effective/safe
Jawahar et al. (43)	2008	IDET	DDD and positive discogram, > 80% disk height, WC patients	53	Prospective	VAS reduction 63%, ODI 70%	None	Useful in carefully selected WC patients
Karaman et al. (51)	2011	Biacuplasty	Axial pain > 6 m; one or two levels DDD	14	Prospective observational	78% of patients > 10 points Oswestry improvement	None	Effective/safe
Kapural et al. (52)	2012	Biacuplasty	Single- or two-level DDD and p.disco., > 50% disk height	64	Randomized, sham-controlled prospective	1 level DDD: VAS −2.78, SF-36-PF +18 2 level DDD:VAS −1.3, SF36-PF+10.5 (Table 66.2)	None	Effective/safe

*Patient selection varied, possibly resulting in the differences in clinical outcomes.
LBP, low back pain; DDD, degenerative disk disease; ODI, Oswestry Disability Index; p. disco, positive discogram; VAS, visual analog scale.

INTRADISCAL BIACUPLASTY (IDB)

Intradiscal biacuplasty (IDB) is the latest, and seems to be the most promising, of the minimally invasive posterior annulus heating techniques (see Fig. 66.1*B*). This technology employs bipolar cooled RF electrodes named *transdiscal electrodes* (Kimberly Clark, Atlanta, Georgia). Initial data are encouraging.[48-52] Internally cooling the electrodes provides more substantial and even heating over the wider area of the posterior annulus (Fig. 66.2).[26-28]

The procedure itself is fluoroscopy guided with the patient lying in the prone position. Electrodes are percutaneously inserted bilaterally in the posterior annulus of the intervertebral disk (see Fig. 66.1*A* and Fig. 66.2). The generator delivers RF energy led by a temperature thermocouple near the tip of the electrode. The temperature increases gradually to 50° C, with an overall heat time of 15 minutes. During this time, the patient should be awake and conversant to decrease the probability of neurologic injury.

Initially, clinical biacuplasty data from two case series of 14 and 15 patients were completed. Both studies demonstrated significant pain relief following the disk biacuplasty procedure at 3, 6, and 12 months.[50-52] The Turkish case series suggested > 50% improvement in pain scores at 6 months with good patient satisfaction. The U.S. pilot study involving 15 patients described reduction in the median visual analog scale (VAS) pain score from 7 to 3 cm at 6 and 12 months' follow-up, respectively; an improvement in the Oswestry index from 23.3 to 16.5 points; and a significant increase in the SF-36 bodily pain scores.[50,52]

The authors completed a sham, prospective randomized study on IDB (Table 66.2).[52] The aim of the study was to compare the efficacy of intradiscal biacuplasty with placebo using 1:1 randomization. Sixty-four patients were enrolled using the same selection criteria as in the pilot study (see the previous discussion and Table 66.2). Patients in the IDB group exhibited statistically significant improvements in physical function, decreased pain, and disability at 6 months' follow-up as compared to patients who received the sham treatment (see Table 66.2).

Those who had one-level degenerative disk disease (DDD) had better outcomes than those with two disks involved; therefore, IDB is not as successful in alleviating pain for many patients with multilevel DDD and should be recommended only to properly selected patients.[52]

Intradiscal biacuplasty may offer several advantages over the earlier techniques. There is negligible disruption to the native tissue architecture, and thus the biomechanics of the spine are likely unchanged and the relative ease of electrode placement abolishes the need to thread a long heating catheter (e.g., IDET).

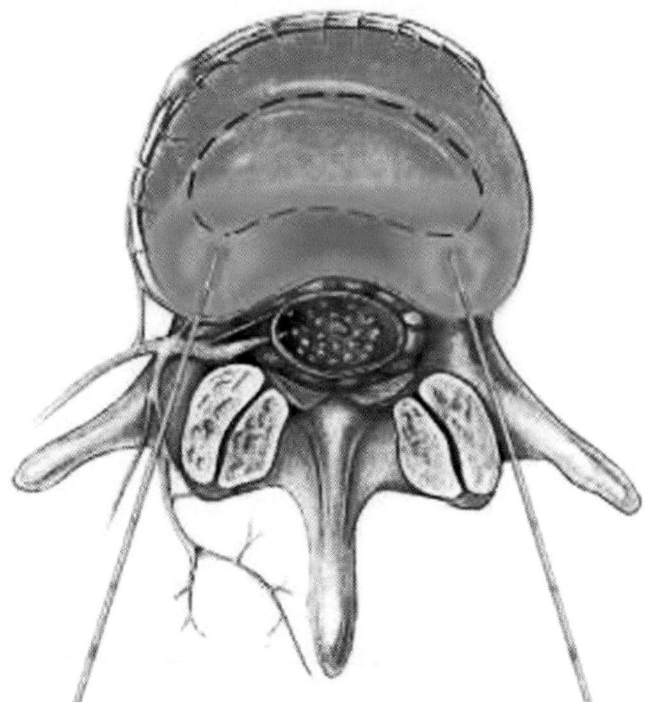

Figure 66.2 Lumbar intervertebral disk schematic with two cooled electrodes for biacuplasty and their positioning within the posterior annulus of the lumbar disk. Providing a distance of less than 3 cm between the electrodes, a proper heat distribution is achieved across the posterior annulus without causing injury to posterior neural elements.

Table 66.2 Physical Function, Pain, and Disability Scores in Patients Who Received IDB Treatment in 1 and 2 Disk Levels

	One Level (n = 16)		Two Levels (n = 11)		
Outcome Measure	**Mean**	**SD**	**Mean**	**SD**	***P* Value**
SF-36 Physical Functioning (0-100)					
Baseline	48.75	17.08	44.55	24.95	0.607
6 months	66.88	18.34	55.00	25.50	0.171
6-month change	18.13	15.37	10.45	18.23	0.248
NRS for Pain (0-10)					
Baseline	7.47	1.45	6.64	1.76	0.191
6 months	4.69	2.38	5.32	1.81	0.465
6-month change	−2.78	2.59	−1.32	1.95	0.126
Oswestry Disability Scale (0-100)					
Baseline	38.88	8.48	42.55	16.64	0.457
6 months	28.88	13.04	38.85	18.90	0.116
6-month change	−10.00	8.91	−3.70	10.99	0.113

IDB, intradiscal biacuplasty; SF, short form; NRS, numeric rating scale; SD = standard deviation.

From Kapural L, Vrooman B, Sarwar S, et al. A randomized, placebo-controlled trial of intradiscal biacuplasty for treatment of discogenic lower back pain. Abstract of 11th Annual Pain Medicine Meeting (ASRA); 2012; Miami.

COMPLICATIONS OF ANNULOPLASTY PROCEDURES

The incidence of various complications related to annuloplasty could be as high as 10%,[53,54] but serious complications are rare. If the radiofrequency electrode or resistive coil is positioned in close proximity to the neural elements, the high temperatures that are delivered may cause nerve injury manifested as radicular pain, or transient palsy. Transient radiculopathy and even motor deficit with footdrop were previously reported following the IDET procedure.[54]

Catheter breakage,[54] vertebral osteonecrosis,[55] and cauda equina[56] syndrome were also reported after the IDET procedure. The classic risk factors such as the duration of back pain, obesity, smoking, history of leg pain, and diabetes may not be associated with the higher incidence of complications.[53,57] Discitis is a rare complication of any intradiscal procedure.[57-62] The appropriate timing of the intravenous antibiotic seems to be effective in preventing discitis after provocative diskography and any minimally invasive intradiscal procedure.[57-62] The incidence of disk herniation following annuloplasty could be as high as 0.3%, which was assumed to be due to a thermally mediated loss of tensile strength of the collagen fibers.[63] There were reports on disk herniation after the IDET procedure.[53,54,57]

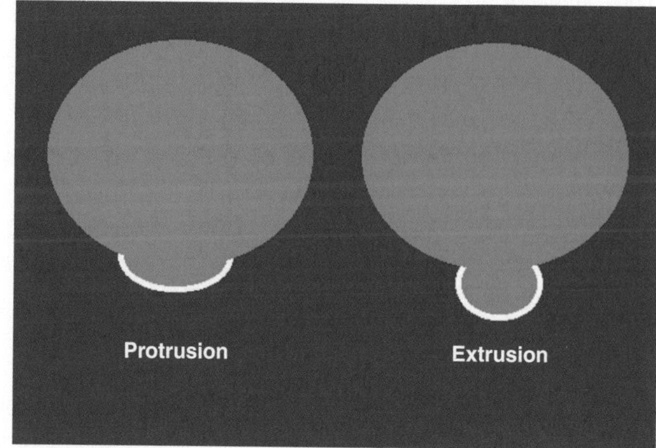

Figure 66.3 Two basic types of intervertebral disk herniation. Protrusion is defined by the fact that the greatest distance, in any plane, between the edges of disk material beyond the disk space is less than the distance between the edges of the disk base in the same plane *(left)*. Extrusion is present if any one distance between the edges of the disk material beyond the disk space is greater than the base.

DISK HERNIATION AND PAIN RELIEF FROM PERCUTANEOUS DISK DECOMPRESSION

A herniated disk can cause radicular pain that manifests over an appropriate dermatomal area. Abnormal weight-bearing loads with internal disk disruption (IDD) could cause changes in shape or disruption of the annular fibers. Contained disk herniation or even extrusion of the disk may compress the nerve root.[64]

Inflammatory mediators present in the intravertebral disk—such as phospholipase A_2, prostaglandin E_2, interleukin-1α, interleukin-1β, interleukin-6, tumor necrosis factor-α, and nitric oxide (NO)—may be additional pain culprits.[65] Nuclear material, in addition to or without mechanical pressure, may produce painful chemical radiculitis.

Contained disk herniation may exert pressure on a nerve root, and possibly the dorsal root ganglion, providing a basis for intradiscal percutaneous disk decompression. Removal of a small amount of the nuclear material from the affected disk or applying heat through radiofrequency within the nucleus can cause a decrease of intradiscal pressure and, possibly, retraction of the herniation away from the nerve. A significant drop in intradiscal pressure may not be produced if the elasticity of the disk is not preserved and the disk contains a high-grade (Dallas 5) fissure. This may be less likely if disk extrusion is present (Fig. 66.3).

The appropriate candidate for percutaneous, minimally invasive intradiscal disk decompression is the patient who experiences radicular pain that correlates with the imaging findings, has contained disk herniation, and experiences predominantly leg pain. Patients with spinal stenosis, extruded disk herniation, progressive neurologic motor deficits, and cauda equina syndrome are not candidates for this minimally invasive approach.

THE DEKOMPRESSOR DEVICE

During percutaneous decompression of the disk in patients with contained disk herniation, the Dekompressor device extracts variable amounts of nuclear disk material via an auger that ends inside the nucleus and collects extracted material into the specially designed chamber. Depending on the volume extracted, a decrease in intradiscal pressure follows. The annular wall must be intact (without completed annular disruption) in order for the herniated portion to retract. Provocative diskography is needed before this procedure to detect complete annular disruption.[66-68]

The technique of needle placement of the Dekompressor is similar to nucleoplasty, or standard diskography. First, the introducer is placed in the nucleus of the disk, and the probe is advanced via an introducer contrast that is injected to delineate the size of the treated disk nucleus. A collection chamber is attached to the probe, which can be removed to be inspected together with the probe for the amount of collected nuclear tissue. Assessment of the tissue volume removed should include measurement of the tissue volume in the collection chamber and that along the probe. The Dekompressor probe is removed when a sufficient amount of material has been taken out from the disk.

Although it has been used clinically for the treatment of contained, symptomatic disk herniation since the early 2000s, the Dekompressor device still has not been tested in a controlled, randomized study. There are a few observational studies that provided positive outcomes. Lierz and coworkers (Table 66.3)[66] studied 64 patients and reported an average decrease in pain scores from 7.3 to 2.1 at 12 months. Similar data were provided by Amoretti and associates,[67] who reported that 50 patients had a > 70% decrease in pain in 72% of cases, and Alo and colleagues,[68] who reported an 80% success rate (see Table 66.3).

COBLATION: NUCLEOPLASTY

Nucleoplasty (ArthroCare Corporation, Austin, Texas) uses coblation technology to ablate and coagulate nucleus pulposus to decompress the disk and minimize contained disk herniation.[69] Therapeutic decompression is more likely in a nondegenerated intervertebral disk.[70-74] Similar to the Dekompressor, the disk is accessed by an introducer using fluoroscopy. Once the introducer is in place, the SpineWand coblation electrode is then placed through the introducer. Channels are created across the nucleus during forward

Table 66.3 Selected Outcome Studies on Nucleoplasty

Study	Year	Type of Intervention	Indications of Procedure	Number of Patients	Type of Study	Outcomes	Complications	Conclusions
Mirzai et al. (72)	2007	Nucleoplasty	Lumbar herniated disk, and radicular pain for at least 3 mo	52	Prospective	VAS from 7.5 to 3.1; ODI 42.2 to 24.8 @ 6 m	None	Effective/safe
Singh et al. (70)	2002	Nucleoplasty	Contained herniation; Radicular > 3 m; disk height > 50%; pos.discogram	80	Prospective Observational	75% decrease in numeric pain score @12 m	None	Effective/safe
Lierz et al. (66)	2009	Dekompressor	Contained herniation	64	Prospective Observational	VAS down 5.2; decreased medication use 80% @ 12 m	None	Effective/safe
Calisaneller et al. 2007 (73)	2007	Nucleoplasty	Contained herniation	29	Prospective	VAS from 6.95 to 4.53	None	Effective/safe
Amoretti et al. (67)	2004	Dekompressor	Contained herniation	10	Retrospective	VAS > 70% decrease; 80% no analgesics	None	Effective/safe
Zhao et al. (75)	2005	PLDD	Contained herniation	173	Prospective	Properly selected group 82% excellent and good outcomes	None	Effective/safe
Gronemeyer et al. (76)	2003	PLDD	Herniated disk	200	Observational	73% "good outcomes"	1 diskitis	Effective
Casper et al. (77)	1996	PLDD	Herniated disk	100	Prospective	87% "surgical success"	None	Effective/safe

PLDD, percutaneous laser disk decompression; Dekompressor (visual analog scale [VAS]).

movement of the cannula and then withdrawn to the starting position five to six times all within the nucleus.[69]

Again, this relatively simple procedure is intended only for radicular pain without large disk protrusions or disk extrusions. The best candidate for nucleoplasty is someone who has a contained disk protrusion of < 6 mm with preserved annular integrity.[69-75] To date, no randomized, prospective studies have been conducted to prove the efficacy of nucleoplasty. Multiple observational and prospective studies have shown an improvement in functional capacity in treated subjects (see Table 66.3).[70-74]

OTHER INTRADISCAL METHODS FOR TREATMENT OF CONTAINED DISK HERNIATION

Two other commonly used percutaneous disk decompression methods have been applied sparingly in recent years. One is the Nucleotome (Clarus Medical, Minneapolis, Minnesota), which uses an automated shaver with continuous irrigation to remove nuclear disk material. Although it can remove large amounts of disk material, it also employs a bulky probe, which can potentially produce significant annular damage. The same concerns are shared by most practitioners who had an experience with the percutaneous laser disk decompression (PLDD) device (see Table 66.3).[75-77]

COMPLICATIONS OF PERCUTANEOUS DECOMPRESSIVE PROCEDURES

A higher prevalence of leg pain and increased weakness in patients who received nucleoplasty, compared to a conservative group, has been documented. The most common postoperative complaint was soreness at the site of the needle insertion.[78] Discitis is a serious complication described after PLDD (see Table 66.3).[76] Another complication with the Dekompressor was probe breakage within the disk nucleus.[79]

KEY POINTS

- Discogenic pain continues to be a major diagnostic and therapeutic problem.
- Few minimally invasive treatments can claim therapeutic effectiveness for discogenic pain, and these are mainly radiofrequency annuloplasties performed in selected subpopulations of patients.
- There have been developments in basic science research and a few ongoing clinical studies in the area of intradiscal biologics, but clinical data are lacking.
- DiscTRODE annuloplasty and conventional nuclear radiofrequency are ineffective when used to treat discogenic back pain.

KEY POINTS—cont'd

- Biacuplasty produces positive therapeutic effects in properly selected patients.
- Future areas of clinical research in discogenic pain may include cytokine inhibitors, ablative agents, and growth factors.
- It is less clear if any of the percutaneous disk decompression procedures will show long-term pain relief when tested in a randomized, sham-controlled study format.

SUGGESTED READINGS

Amoretti N, Huchot F, Flory P, et al. Percutaneous nucleotomy: preliminary communication on a decompression probe (Dekompressor) in percutaneous discectomy. Ten case reports. *Clin Imaging.* 2005;29: 98-101.

Andersson GBJ. Epidemiological features of chronic low-back pain. *Lancet.* 1999;354:581-585.

Appleby D, Andersson G, Totta M. Meta-analysis of the efficacy and safety of intradiscal electrothermal therapy (IDET). *Pain Med.* 2006;7: 308-316.

Casper GD, Hartman VL, Mullins LL. Results of a clinical trial of the holmium: YAG laser in disc decompression utilizing a side-firing fiber: a two-year follow-up. *Lasers Surg Med.* 1996;19:90-96.

Derby R, Howard MW, Grant JM, et al. The ability of pressure-controlled discography to predict surgical and nonsurgical outcomes. *Spine.* 1999;24:364-371.

Grönemeyer DH, Buschkamp H, Braun M, et al. Image-guided percutaneous laser disk decompression for herniated lumbar disks: a 4-year follow-up in 200 patients. *J Clin Laser Med Surg.* 2003;21:131-138.

Kapural L, Deer T. Radiofrequency and other heat applications for the treatment of discogenic pain. In: Kapural L, Kim P, eds. *Diagnosis, Management and Treatment of Discogenic Pain: Interventional and Neuromodulatory Techniques for Pain Management Series.* Vol. 3. Philadelphia: Elsevier; 2011:80-87.

Kapural L, De la Garza M, Ng A, et al. Novel transdiscal biacuplasty for the treatment of lumbar discogenic pain: a 6 months follow-up. *Pain Med.* 2008;9:60-67.

Kapural L, Houra K, Radic A. Complications associated with discography and intradiscal treatment techniques. In: Neal JM, Rathmell JP, eds. *Complications in Regional Anesthesia and Pain Medicine.* 2nd ed. Philadelphia: Lippincott Williams & Wilkins; 2012:317-326.

Kapural L, Mekhail N, Sloan S, et al. Histological and temperature distribution studies in the lumbar degenerated and non-degenerated human cadaver discs using novel transdiscal radiofrequency electrodes. *Pain Med.* 2008;9:68-75.

Kapural L, Vrooman B, Sarwar S, et al. *A randomized, placebo-controlled trial of intradiscal biacuplasty for treatment of discogenic lower back pain.* Abstract of 11th Annual Pain Medicine Meeting (ASRA); Miami; 2012.

Mirzai H, Tekin I, Yaman O, Bursali A. The results of nucleoplasty in patients with lumbar herniated disc: a prospective clinical study of 52 consecutive patients. *Spine J.* 2007;7:88-92.

Pauza KJ, Howell S, Dreyfuss P, et al. A randomized, placebo-controlled trial of intradiscal electrothermal therapy for the treatment of discogenic low back pain. *Spine J.* 2004;4:27-35.

Singh V, Piryani C, Liao K, Nieschulz S. Percutaneous disc decompression using coblation (Nucleoplasty™). *Pain Physician.* 2002;5:250-259.

The references for this chapter can be found at www.expertconsult.com.

67 Minimally Invasive Procedures for Vertebral Compression Fractures

Ronil V. Chandra | Thabele M. Leslie-Mazwi | James D. Rabinov | Albert J. Yoo | Joshua A. Hirsch

One in two women and one in five men older than 50 years will experience an osteoporotic fracture, which can result in substantial pain, morbidity, and health care utilization. A new osteoporotic vertebral fracture occurs every 22 seconds; 1.4 million occur worldwide every year.[1] The majority are asymptomatic or result in tolerable symptoms, with only a third of patients with a new fracture seeking medical attention.[2] In the vast majority, the acute back pain symptoms subside over a period of 6 to 8 weeks as the fracture heals.[3]

Vertebroplasty and kyphoplasty are minimally invasive, image-guided procedures that involve the injection of cement into a fractured vertebral body (Figs. 67.1 and 67.2). The majority of these vertebral augmentation procedures are performed in a small subset of patients with symptomatic osteoporotic compression fractures that fail conservative medical therapy. Failure of medical therapy is variably defined but can be considered if the pain persists at a level that severely compromises mobility or activities of daily living despite analgesic therapy or if unacceptable side effects such as confusion, sedation, or constipation occur as a result of the doses of medication required to reduce the pain to tolerable levels. Notably, the first report of augmentation (published in 1987) was for neoplastic disease.[4] As survival rates in cancer patients continue to improve, symptomatic neoplastic vertebral fractures and neoplastic vertebral tumors have increased in prevalence. A selected subgroup of these patients, in particular, those with symptomatic fractures from multiple myeloma and metastasis that fail to respond to conservative therapy, also benefit from vertebral augmentation.[5] The primary goal of augmentation is pain relief and enhanced functional status with the secondary goal of vertebral body stabilization in cases of fracture. Key points, indications for, and contraindications to vertebral augmentation are summarized at the end of the chapter.

CONSERVATIVE MEDICAL THERAPY FOR VERTEBRAL COMPRESSION FRACTURES

The goals of conservative therapy are pain reduction (with analgesics, bed rest, or both), improvement in functional status (with orthotic devices and physical therapy), and prevention of future fractures (with vitamin D and calcium supplementation and bisphosphonate therapy).

Although conservative management of those with mild pain and no limitation of function is appropriate, conservative treatment of those with more severe pain or limitation of function is not benign. In this cohort, conservative therapy often involves a period of bed rest, which may lead to undesirable side effects such as loss of bone mass and muscle strength, decubitus ulceration, and venous thromboembolic disease, all of which can prolong the recovery period and result in loss of independence. Bone loss occurs at a rate of approximately 2% per week,[6] muscle strength is reduced by 10% to 15%,[7] and infectious complications can lead to septicemia and osteomyelitis. Moreover, the presence of fracture or malignancy combined with bed rest elevates the risk for venous thromboembolic disease in this cohort. Overall, the complications of prolonged bed rest, combined with opioid analgesic use and its associated side effects, can result in a vicious cycle of physical deconditioning, poor nutrition, and subsequent increased risk for vertebral insufficiency.

TECHNICAL ASPECTS OF VERTEBRAL AUGMENTATION

Evaluation of patients for vertebral augmentation should identify those likely to benefit from vertebral augmentation, as well as screen for contraindications. The decision to proceed with treatment must be based on a good history, physical examination, appropriate laboratory evaluation, and imaging, as summarized in Boxes 67.1 and 67.2.

SEDATION

Analgesia is typically necessary for vertebroplasty and kyphoplasty. In the majority of cases, it is achieved with a combination of local analgesics (e.g., lidocaine with bicarbonate or bupivacaine) and moderate sedation (intravenous midazolam and fentanyl). In some cases, general anesthesia is needed to provide adequate comfort and safety, particularly in patients at high risk for airway or respiratory complications with prone positioning or those with significant preprocedure narcotic analgesic requirements. However, having the patient awake is desirable because it allows feedback (e.g., increasing pain, neurologic dysfunction) that can alert the operator to potential complications. In all cases, continuous monitoring is performed with a minimum of electrocardiography, blood pressure measurements, and pulse oximetry. Sedation and monitoring are performed by anesthesiologists, nurse anesthetists, or certified nursing

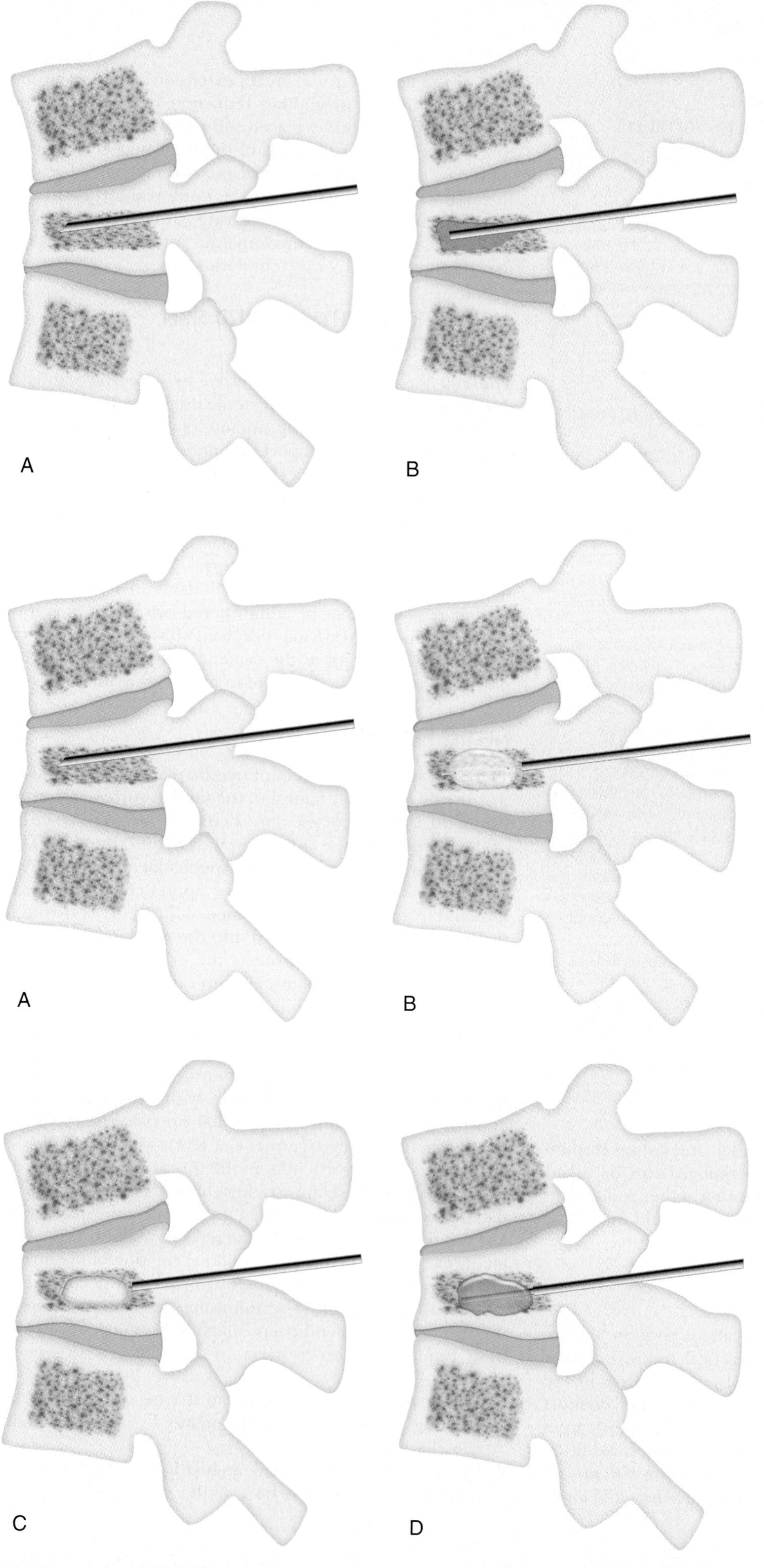

Figure 67.1 Vertebroplasty involves insertion of a needle into the vertebral body (**A**) with subsequent delivery of cement (**B**) into the vertebral body.

Figure 67.2 Kyphoplasty. Once access to the vertebral body is achieved (**A**), the inner stylet is removed and a balloon tamp is inflated within the vertebral body (**B**) to create a cavity within the bone (**C**) into which cement is delivered (**D**).

Box 67.1 Indications for and Contraindications to Vertebral Augmentation

Indications

1. Treatment of symptomatic osteoporotic vertebral body fractures that are refractory to conservative medical therapy
2. Treatment of symptomatic vertebral bodies weakened or fractured because of neoplasia that are refractory to medical therapy

Absolute Contraindications

1. Active systemic infection, in particular, spinal infection
2. Uncorrectable bleeding diathesis
3. Insufficient cardiopulmonary health to safely tolerate sedation or general anesthesia
4. Myelopathy resulting from fracture retropulsion or epidural tumoral extension
5. Known allergy to bone cement

Relative Contraindications (Should Be Treated Only by Experienced Practitioners)

1. *Marked loss of vertebral body height* (greater than 75% loss of height), which makes the procedure more difficult since there may be little space for placement of a cannula.
2. *Vertebroplasty above T5*, which is challenging because of the small size of the vertebral bodies and pedicles. The shoulders often limit fluoroscopic imaging at these levels.
3. *Severe osteopenia resulting in poor visualization of osseous structures on fluoroscopy*, which increases the risk for improper needle placement and cement leakage. This can be overcome with guidance by computed tomography.
4. *Disruption of the posterior cortex*, which increases the risk for posterior cement leakage and therefore the risk for spinal cord or nerve root compression. This is frequently seen with burst fractures and neoplasm. The integrity of the posterior cortex is best evaluated with computed tomography.
5. *Substantial canal narrowing* (without neurologic dysfunction), which increases the risk that even a small amount of cement leakage will produce neurologic compromise.
6. *Retropulsion of fracture fragments*, which increases the risk for further canal compromise with vertebral augmentation, particularly if the posterior vertebral body wall is unstable.
7. *Epidural extension of tumor*, which in the setting of pathologic fractures results in significantly higher rates of spinal canal leakage than osteoporotic fractures do.

personnel. In patients with substantial preexisting respiratory or cardiac disease, an anesthesiologist can be asked to evaluate the patient and determine whether monitored anesthesia care is warranted. The patient should not eat or drink for at least 4 to 6 hours before the procedure.

PATIENT POSITIONING

Prone or oblique prone is the ideal patient position for thoracic and lumbar procedures. In practical terms, we allow patients an amount of freedom to place themselves in the prone oblique position should it promote greater comfort throughout the procedure. This can introduce 10 to 15 degrees of obliquity, depending on the patient's position. In addition to the clear advantage of easy access, this position with proper cushion support under the upper part of the chest and lower part of the abdomen maximizes extension of the fractured segments, thereby promoting reduction of kyphosis.[9] The patient's arms should be placed sufficiently toward the head to keep them out of the path of the fluoroscope. Analgesia should be considered before placement on the table because this part of the procedure may be quite painful. Particular care must be taken when transferring patients who are aged or have osteoporosis or myelomatous infiltration since this may result in new rib or vertebral fractures.

ANTIBIOTIC PROPHYLAXIS AND SKIN PREPARATION

The risk for infection is minimized by following standard operating room guidelines for sterile preparation of the skin, draping, operator scrubbing, and use of sterile gowns, masks, and gloves. Few data support or oppose antibiotic administration, but there are reports of spine infections after these procedures,[10,11] and the presence of polymethyl methacrylate (PMMA) makes these infections difficult to treat successfully. We routinely use antibiotic prophylaxis. Prophylaxis for these procedures comes in one of two forms. An intravenous antibiotic such as cefazolin (1 g) or clindamycin (600 mg with penicillin allergy) may be administered before skin incision. Alternatively, the PMMA may be mixed with an antibiotic, such as tobramycin (1.2 g), as the cement is being prepared; this practice has diminished in favor of intravenous antibiotics.

NEEDLE PLACEMENT

The most important aspect of needle placement is to keep the needle trajectory lateral to the medial cortex and superior to the inferior cortex of the pedicle. This prevents entry of the needle into the spinal canal or neural foramen. The needle may be placed via a transpedicular or parapedicular approach. In the transpedicular approach, the needle is directed from the posterior surface of the pedicle, through the length of the pedicle, and into the vertebral body. The long intraosseous path protects the postganglionic nerve roots and other soft tissues. However, the pedicle configuration can limit one's ability to achieve a final needle tip position near the midline. In the parapedicular approach, the needle is directed along the lateral surface of the pedicle, with the pedicle being penetrated along its path or the vertebral body at its junction with the pedicle. This approach may permit more medial tip placement, which can be useful during treatment of levels with anatomically small pedicles, in particular, in the thoracic spine.

For either of these approaches there are multiple potential image guidance strategies, including anteroposterior (AP) and end-on ("down the barrel") views, with the latter technique involving ipsilateral oblique rotation of the image intensifier to place the fluoroscopy beam and needle track parallel to each other. The following description assumes the use of two perpendicular image intensifiers simultaneously (biplanar fluoroscopy):

1. Rotate the image intensifier to a true AP position by aligning the spinous process midway between the pedicles (Fig. 67.3).
2. Change the craniocaudad angulation by bringing the pedicles to the midportion of the vertebral body. Use

Box 67.2 Preprocedure Workup

Identify patients who will probably benefit from vertebral augmentation.
Screen for absolute contraindications.
Document failure of conventional medical therapy.
Symptoms:
- Fractures possibly occurring with little or no trauma
- Deep pain with a sudden onset
- Midline location
- Exacerbation by axial mechanical loading (worsened with standing or weight bearing and often at least partially relieved by recumbency)
- Exacerbation with motion (especially flexion)
- Referred lateral radiation in a dermatomal pattern possibly present

Signs:
- Point tenderness at the spinous process of the fractured vertebra. Local signs may be surprisingly absent. However, up to 30% of patients may have subjective off-midline pain or tenderness over nontarget vertebrae and still gain significant benefit.[8]
- Localization to a specific level if possible is important in targeting treatment in patients who have multiple compression fractures, some of which may be healed and do not require treatment. In difficult cases, examination can be performed with fluoroscopic assistance to localize the pain to a specific anatomic level.

Assess lower extremity neurologic function.

Laboratory evaluation:
- Screen for infection, coagulopathy, and metabolic abnormality.
- Additional tests such as urinalysis, electrocardiography, and/or chest radiography are left to the discretion of the practitioner.

Imaging:
- Its role is to confirm the clinical diagnosis, identify and assess the acuity of the acute painful fracture, identify potential difficulties, and plan the procedure.
- MRI with STIR or T2-weighted sequences with fat saturation should be obtained in all patients if not contraindicated. These sequences identify marrow edema, which distinguishes acute from chronic fractures. MRI also distinguishes between benign osteoporotic and pathologic fractures and assesses the degree of fracture retropulsion, epidural tumor extension, spinal canal compromise, and compression of the spinal cord or nerve roots. Fracture clefts appear as a linear band of T1 hypointensity and T2 hypointensity or hyperintensity within the vertebral body.
- In patients who cannot undergo MRI, nuclear scintigraphic bone scanning or single-photon emission computed tomography in combination with CT are the tests of choice. Acute fractures will take up the injected ^{99m}Tc-MDP tracer in much higher concentrations; CT evaluates bone integrity and the spinal contents. In patients with pathologic fractures, CT also helps define the extent of sclerosis and posterior wall osteolysis, which in turn predict increased technical challenges associated with the procedure.

CT, computed tomography; MDP, methylene diphosphate (medronate); MRI, magnetic resonance imaging; STIR, short tau inversion recovery.

the lateral fluoroscopic view to aid in determination of the correct craniocaudad adjustment required.

a. For the end-on view, rotate image intensifier approximately 20 degrees ipsilateral to the target pedicle so that the medial cortex of the pedicle is at the middle third of the vertebral body. The vertebra adopts the "Scotty dog" configuration. Place the needle so that it is "end on" to the image intensifier and appears as a dot.

3. Plan the trocar trajectory. For the AP and partial ipsilateral oblique views, the trocar entry site should be at the 3-o'clock position of the right pedicle or the 9-o'clock position of the left pedicle for the transpedicular approach. In the end-on view, it is centered within the circle formed by the cortex of the pedicle. For parapedicular approaches an entry site just lateral to the 3- or 9-o'clock position of the pedicular cortex is best.
4. Anesthetize the skin and periosteum by subcutaneous injection of lidocaine or bupivacaine via a 22-gauge needle along the planned trajectory. Use this smaller-gauge needle to assess and adjust the planned trajectory.
5. Make a small vertical skin incision (allows easier craniocaudal needle angulation), and insert the 11- or 13-gauge diamond-tipped needle stylet (sheathed in a cannula).
6. Advance the needle to the bone surface while making small corrections in craniocaudad angulation on the true lateral view (care is needed to angle the image intensifier so that a true lateral view is obtained). For the parapedicular approach, the position at which bone is encountered (i.e., at the junction of the pedicle and vertebral body) is more anterior on the lateral view.
7. Once in the bone, advance the needle either with a drilling motion and controlled forward pressure or by carefully tapping the needle handle with an orthopedic mallet.
8. Maintain a true AP view of the image intensifier for advancement of the needle unless using the end-on view, in which case the needle is kept as a dot during initial placement through the pedicle. The needle must remain lateral to the medial cortex of the pedicle until it has traversed the entire pedicle on the lateral view.
9. Once the needle has traversed the pedicle, one can replace the diamond-tipped needle with a straight bevel-tipped needle or curved needle for better maneuverability (Fig. 67.4). Advance the needle further via the lateral view to the anterior third to quarter of the vertebral body.

ADDITIONAL STEPS FOR KYPHOPLASTY

For vertebroplasty, the PMMA is delivered through the cannula after placement of the needle as just described. Kyphoplasty involves the additional steps of balloon tamp insertion and inflation to create a cavity within the bone (Fig. 67.5). For kyphoplasty, pull the cannula back to the posterior aspect of the vertebral body to allow the insertion of the balloon tamp. After the needle stylet is removed, insert the balloon tamp through the cannula and slowly inflate with iodinated contrast medium. The balloon is attached to a locking syringe with a digital manometer

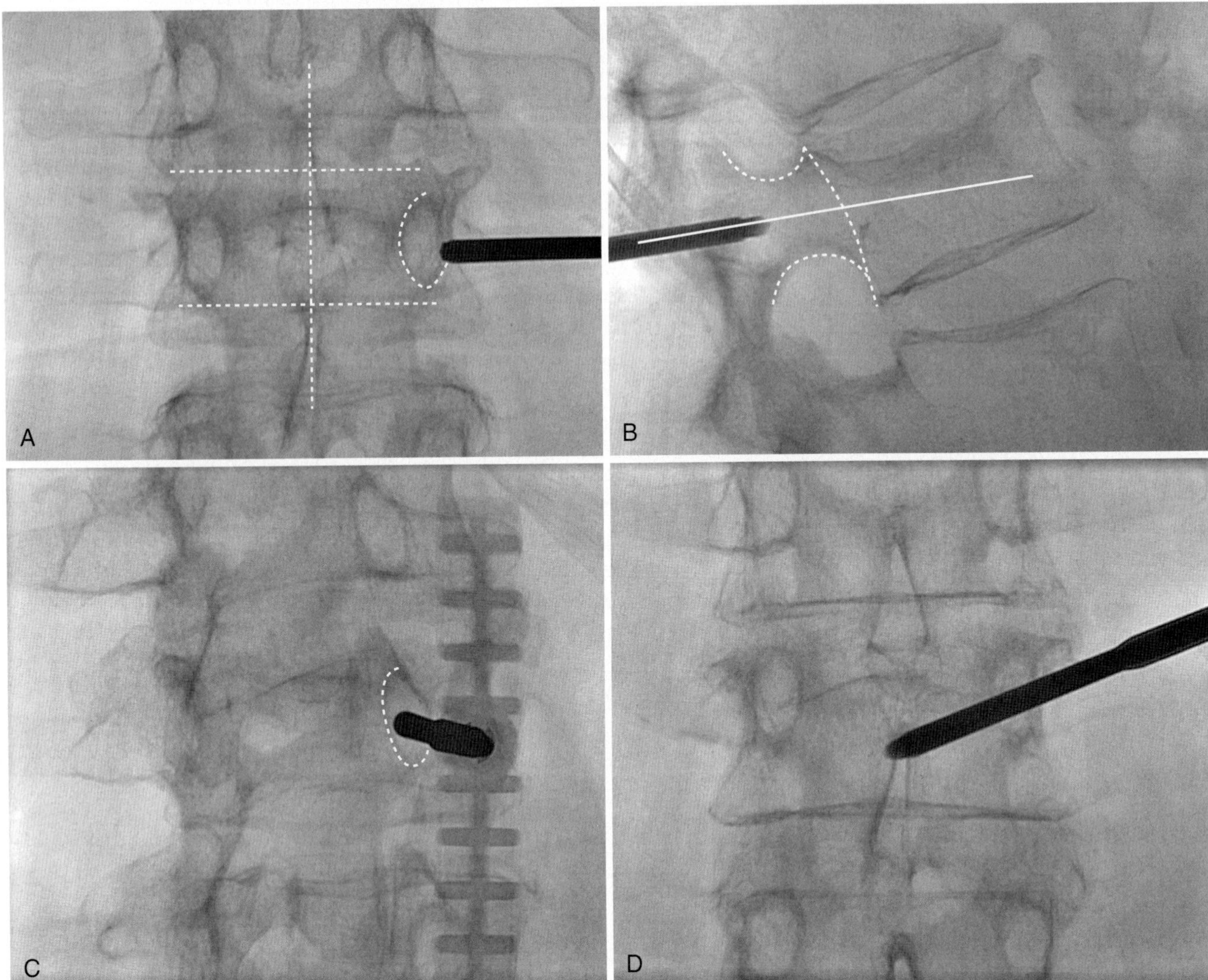

Figure 67.3 Initial positioning of the needle for a transpedicular approach. **A,** Anteroposterior (AP) fluoroscopic image. The image intensifier is first rotated to a true AP position to align the spinous process midway between the pedicles (vertical dotted line). The craniocaudad angulation is changed to bring the pedicles to the midportion of the vertebral body (horizontal dotted lines). **B,** Lateral fluoroscopic image. The image intensifier is rotated to a true lateral position by overlapping the cortices of both pedicles and ensuring that the posterior margin of the vertebral body is aligned (dotted lines). Note that the entire needle trajectory within the vertebral body should be considered during initial transpedicular access for optimal final needle position (solid line). **C,** Near "end-on" projection during needle placement with preservation of the medial and inferior cortices of the pedicle. Note that a "T-grip" needle handle can obscure bony landmarks and slight rotation of the image intensifier may be required. **D,** Midline needle position obtained via a unilateral transpedicular approach, which can be achieved with larger target pedicles, typically in the lumbar vertebrae.

(Fig. 67.6). Monitor the inflation with both the pressure transducer and intermittent fluoroscopy. Continue inflation until one of two conditions is met: the system reaches significant pressure or maximum balloon volume or further inflation results in patient discomfort. Balloon placement can be either unipedicular or bipedicular. Deflate and then remove the balloon.

CEMENT PLACEMENT

The consistency of the cement, when ready for injection, is similar to that of toothpaste. Wong and Mathis recommend a drip test, in which the cement should ball up at the end of the needle and not drip downward, which will result in a cement consistency that is slightly more viscous than toothpaste.[12] Working time varies from 10 to 20 minutes, depending on temperature and the specific PMMA formulation being used. A variety of delivery systems are available for the cement. These systems vary from a few 1-mL syringes with a spatula and a mixing bowl to self-contained delivery devices. A screw-syringe injector with long, flexible delivery tubing has the advantage of minimizing exposure of the operator to radiation.[13]

VERTEBROPLASTY

- After removing the needle stylet, fill the cannula with saline to prevent pressurized injection of air and air embolism. Connect the delivery system to the cannula and inject the cement slowly.

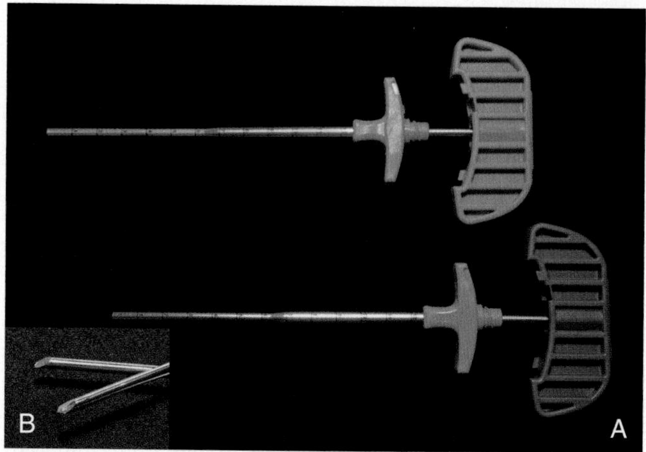

Figure 67.4 Photographs of typical vertebroplasty needles. **A,** Typical coaxial vertebroplasty needle—the inner stylet locks into the outer cannula. Note the large handles to facilitate insertion and removal from the bone. Manufacturers may use different colored or marked handles to indicate the type of needle tip (magnified in **B**). A needle with a beveled tip can be used to facilitate directing the needle along the desired trajectory.

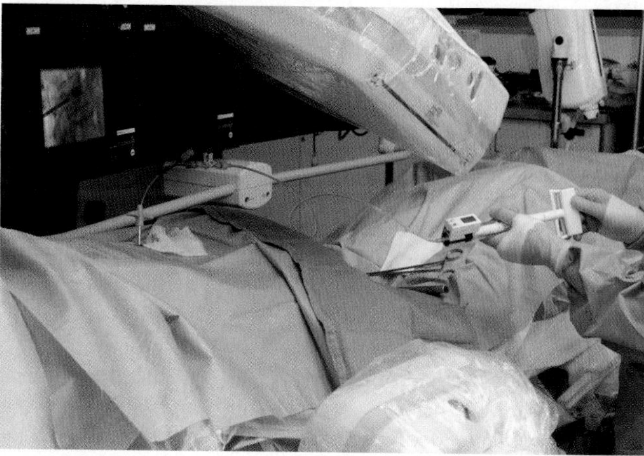

Figure 67.6 Balloon kyphoplasty. The balloon is attached to a digital manometer, which allows assessment of balloon pressure. Note the long flexible tubing, which permits the operator's hands to remain out of the primary radiation beam during fluoroscopic assessment of balloon inflation.

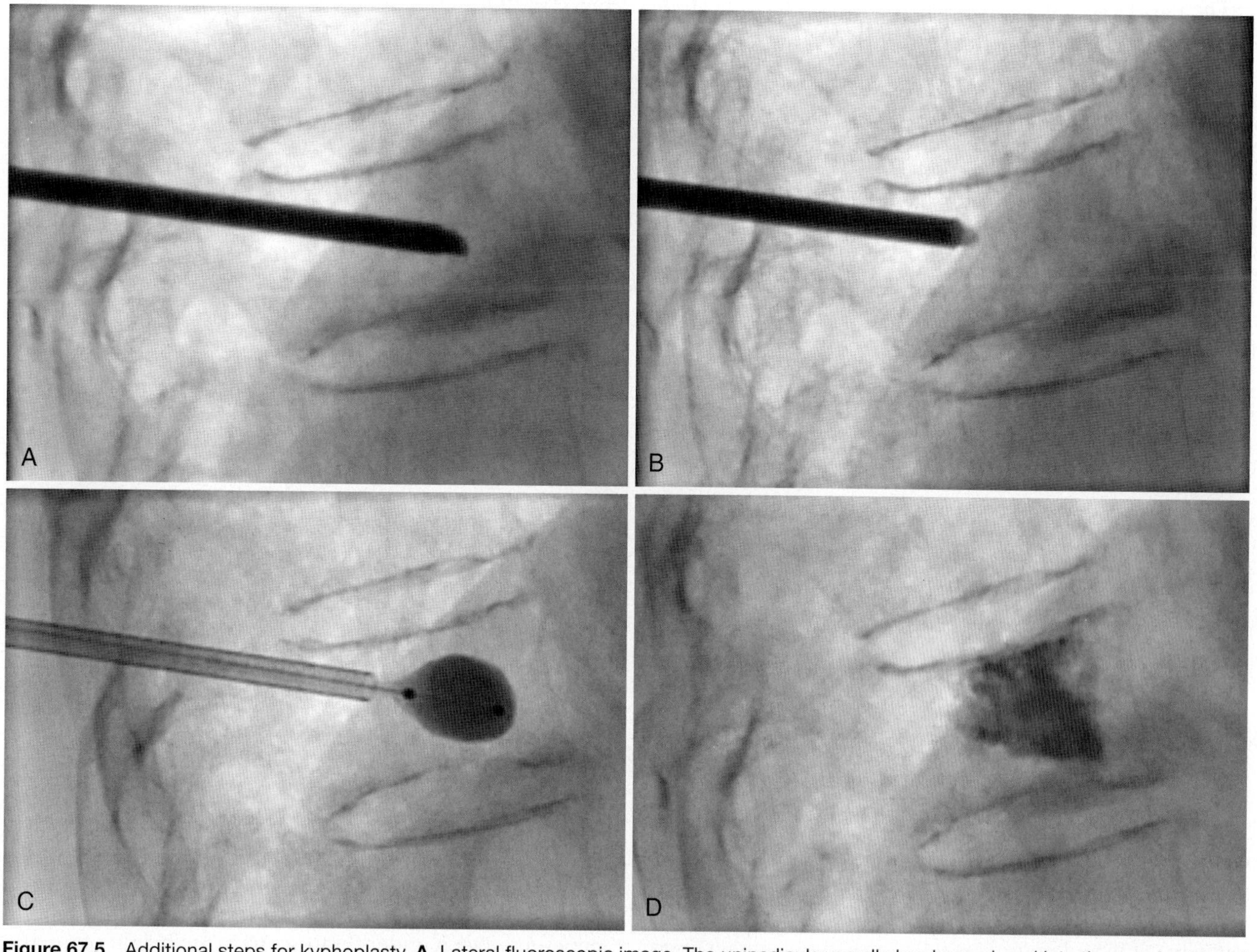

Figure 67.5 Additional steps for kyphoplasty. **A,** Lateral fluoroscopic image. The unipedicular needle has been placed into the anterior third of the T10 vertebral body. **B,** The needle is withdrawn to the posterior third of the vertebral body and the inner stylet removed. **C,** The balloon tamp is introduced into the needle track and inflated to create a cavity within the bone. **D,** Cement opacifies both the cavity and extends into adjacent trabecular bone.

- Monitor carefully with fluoroscopic imaging to ensure that the cement remains within the vertebra. Posterior or posterolateral leakage could result in irritation of or damage to the spinal cord or nerve roots and should be avoided. New pain with a different character should prompt an immediate pause in the procedure and additional views.
- End points for cement injection include passage of cement beyond the marrow space or cement reaching the posterior quarter of the vertebral body on the lateral projection. In the case of cement leakage, one may wait 1 to 2 minutes to allow the cement to harden and then reinject to see whether the cement is redirected within the vertebral body.[14] Ideally, the cement will extend across the midline to the opposite pedicle by the end of the injection. The optimal volume of cement remains a matter of controversy.
- The final portion of cement may be delivered by inserting the needle stylet. Alternatively, the cement may be allowed to harden and the needle removed with a gentle rocking motion to ensure that the cement within the cannula separates at the tip of the cannula.

KYPHOPLASTY

- The cavity created by the balloon tamp allows injection of cement that is more viscous than that typically used for vertebroplasty. The cavity and more viscous cement theoretically minimize the risk for extravasation of cement. Sufficient time is allowed for the cement to reach a doughy consistency, with loss of the "sheen" of the initially mixed cement.
- Many practitioners use manual bone filler devices to inject cement, although one can use injector systems. The delivery system is connected to the cannula and the cement is injected slowly under fluoroscopic guidance. The cavity is filled with cement from anterior to posterior until it matches or slightly exceeds the volume of the inflated balloon tamp.

CONTROVERSIES AND SPECIAL TOPICS

BIPEDICULAR VERSUS UNIPEDICULAR APPROACH

Vertebroplasty and kyphoplasty can be performed with placement of bilateral needles or a single needle.[15] In either case the goal is to place cement across the midline within the vertebral body—we use placement of PMMA to the opposite pedicle as our general landmark. Therefore, use of a single needle with a relatively medial position of the needle tip is sufficient in many cases. If a unilateral approach is attempted during kyphoplasty and balloon expansion does not cross midline, a second system may then be placed on the other side, depending on the distribution of cement fill. In many cases, cement fill will continue across the midline, thereby obviating the need for a second needle. Moreover, hemivertebral fill (cement traverses <10% of the contralateral unfilled vertebra) has been shown to be as efficacious in reducing pain and improving function without an increased risk for fracture.[16]

Importantly, there is no statistically significant difference in the pain relief achieved with unipedicular and bipedicular vertebroplasty[17] or kyphoplasty.[18] There are advantages to each approach. Advantages of a unipedicular approach include a decrease in procedure time and elimination of the risk associated with placement of a second needle. A unipedicular approach is also associated with lower rates of cement leakage.[19] The major advantage of a bipedicular approach is that access is typically transpedicular with a less aggressive lateral to medial approach that may result in less paravertebral vessel and nerve injury and a potential biomechanical advantage for bilateral delivery of cement.

VOLUME OF CEMENT INJECTED

The optimal volume of cement is a matter of controversy, with some practitioners advocating injection of maximal amounts of cement to completely fill the vertebral body and others advocating lower cement volumes with an emphasis on safety. The theoretical goal of more complete filling is to achieve restoration of biomechanical strength within the vertebral body to prevent refracture without creating excessive stiffness that may be transmitted to the adjacent levels. Based on an in vitro biomechanical study, Mathis and Wong recommended filling 50% to 70% of the residual volume of the vertebral body with cement.[20] However, much smaller amounts of cement (as little as 0.5 mL) appear to result in similar clinical outcomes as do larger-volume injections in terms of the primary goal of pain relief, with no association between the volume of cement injected and the clinical outcomes of pain and medication use.[20] The decreased risk for extravasation of cement with smaller-volume injections and meticulous attention to the end-of-injection criteria outlined earlier favor an approach using a smaller volume of cement.

VERTEBRA PLANA

When the vertebral body loses 70% of its original height, safe needle placement becomes a challenge. According to Stallmeyer and associates, at least 8 mm of residual height is required for cannula placement.[21] Vertebra plana often adopts a bow-tie configuration in which the center is compressed the most. This usually requires a lateral needle position with placement of bilateral needles.[22] Only a small amount of cement is needed to achieve pain relief.[23] If there is a cystic cleft within the fracture (Kummel's disease), the needle may be placed near the midline within the cleft in the hope of expanding the height of the vertebra during needle placement and cement injection.

FRACTURES WITH AN INTRAOSSEOUS VACUUM PHENOMENON (KUMMEL'S DISEASE)

The intraosseous vacuum phenomenon is thought to be related to osteonecrosis. A fluid-filled cleft seen on magnetic resonance imaging (MRI) is an equivalent finding. Pain in this setting is believed to arise from motion between the unhealed fracture fragments. In some cases this motion can even be seen under fluoroscopy as the height of the vertebral body changes with respiration. Prone positioning during the procedure promotes restoration of height because of the traction placed across the vertebral body. The needle should be placed into or as close to the cleft as possible so that cement will fill the cleft. Vertebral augmentation yields significant rates of pain relief in the setting of an intraosseous vacuum phenomenon,[24,25] and in our experience it can provide considerable restoration of height. It is important to keep the patient prone for 15 to 20 minutes after injection of the cement to allow the cement to harden within the cleft before moving the patient off the fluoroscopy table.

MALIGNANT FRACTURES WITH POSTERIOR WALL OSTEOLYSIS OR EPIDURAL TUMOR EXTENSION

Although vertebral augmentation may be performed in the setting of posterior wall osteolysis or epidural tumor extension, there should be heightened awareness of the potential neurologic complications related to epidural extension of cement or posterior displacement of tumor. In a study of 51 patients with a vertebral lesion and epidural extension treated by vertebroplasty, 30% had preprocedure symptoms of partial or complete cord compression/cauda equina syndrome.[26] These patients were terminally ill and did not undergo surgical decompression because their paraplegia was deemed irreversible (present for more than 1 month or associated with spinal cord atrophy) or their general condition was a contraindication to surgery. Although no further clinical deterioration was observed in this subgroup after vertebroplasty, in 1 of the 36 patients without neurologic symptoms, cauda equina syndrome developed 2 days after vertebroplasty and required surgical decompression.[26] Cement leakage (as detected on postprocedure computed tomography [CT]) occurred in 62%, with half of these leaks extending into the epidural space. Importantly, extension of cement beyond the confines of the vertebral body but within the epidural tumor was still classified as a leak.[27] Nonetheless, the aforementioned was the only symptomatic cement leak. No systemic complications occurred. Analgesic efficacy, based on 50% or greater improvement in pain as compared with baseline, was impressive—94% (48 of 51 patients) at day 1, 86% (31 patients) at 1 month, 83% (19 patients) at 6 months, and 92% (11 patients) after 1 year (data are from surviving patients).[26] Safeguards to prevent complications in this cohort include performing the procedure with the patient awake (new pain may be the first sign of dangerous cement leakage) and more modest cement injection than used for routine cases. Limiting the cement to the anterior two thirds of the vertebral body may be a good rule of thumb, as well as injection of thicker cement, which may in turn reduce the risk for epidural cement leakage.[28]

SAFETY OF MULTILEVEL TREATMENT

A patient scheduled for vertebral augmentation may have multiple fractures that require treatment. Ideally, all the levels would be treated at one time. However, treating an excessive number of levels in a single session raises many concerns, including PMMA toxicity, difficulty for the elderly to lie prone and cooperate for the extended amount of time that this would require, discomfort after the procedure related to placement of multiple needles, and fat emboli being extruded from marrow during the cement injection. There have been two reported deaths in patients who underwent vertebral augmentation at eight or more levels.[29] Even though there is no established guideline, a good rule of thumb is to treat a maximum of three levels per session.[30,31]

OUTCOMES ASSOCIATED WITH VERTEBRAL AUGMENTATION

The mechanism by which vertebroplasty and kyphoplasty relieve pain is uncertain.[32] Hypotheses include mechanical stabilization of mobile fracture fragments, thermal or chemical neurolysis, or inherent tumoricidal or cytotoxic effects on malignant fractures. A cadaveric study has also demonstrated new bone formation after PMMA injection.[33]

Two highly publicized placebo-controlled randomized clinical trials on vertebroplasty have been published in the *New England Journal of Medicine*. Both trials used a sham procedure in the placebo arm that involved injection of local anesthetic down to the periosteum of the pedicle[34] or injection of local anesthetic combined with passage of a 13-gauge needle to rest on the lamina.[35] Both studies found that there was no significant reduction in pain or pain-related disability in patients undergoing vertebroplasty versus the sham procedure.

The INvestigational Vertebroplasty Efficacy and Safety Trial (INVEST) included 131 patients, with 68 randomized to vertebroplasty and 63 to the sham procedure.[34] Even though at 1 month there was a trend toward a higher rate of clinically meaningful improvement in pain (30% decrease from baseline), no statistical difference in regard to pain scores, back pain–related disability, or quality of life was noted.[34] Buchbinder and colleagues studied 78 patients, with 38 randomized to vertebroplasty and 40 to the sham procedure.[35] After the procedure, both groups had similar improvements in pain, physical functioning, and quality of life. There were no significant differences between the groups at 1 week, 1 month, 3 months, and 6 months of follow-up.[35]

These reports are in contrast to previous retrospective case series that had documented impressive rates of pain relief with these procedures.[36] The *New England Journal of Medicine* trials were criticized for potential inclusion of patients with chronic fractures of up to 12 months in duration. The average duration of back pain was 18 weeks in INVEST, with a third of all randomized patients having pain for longer than 6 months. The trial of Buchbinder and coworkers had four patients randomized after 6 months. In the INVEST trial, marrow edema seen on MRI or increased uptake on bone scanning was required only for fractures of an uncertain age (rate of use was not reported). In the trial of Buchbinder and colleagues, MRI demonstrating marrow edema or a fracture line (or both) was required; however, determination of bone marrow edema was not described. Further criticisms include inconsistent use of physical examination, difficulties in recruitment, and absence of a control group without intervention.

Since then, the vertebroplasty versus conservative treatment in acute osteoporotic vertebral compression fractures (VERTOS II) investigators[37] performed a nonblinded trial in which 202 patients with severe back pain for 6 weeks or less, focal tenderness at the fracture level, and MRI demonstration of bone edema were randomized equally into the vertebroplasty or conservative arms. All patients were prescribed analgesics that were individually titrated, bisphosphonates, and calcium and vitamin D supplements. Vertebroplasty was performed at a mean of 5.6 weeks after the onset of symptoms. There were statistically significant reductions in mean visual analog scale (VAS) scores in favor of vertebroplasty at 1 month ($P < 0.0001$), with the benefit persisting at 1 year ($P < 0.0001$).[37] There were significant reductions in the use of drugs in the vertebroplasty group at 1 day ($P < 0.0001$), 1 week ($P = 0.001$), and 1 month ($P = 0.033$).[37] Moreover, significant pain relief (reduction in VAS score of 3 or more points) was achieved earlier and in more patients after vertebroplasty (29.7 days; 95% confidence interval [CI], 11.45 to 47.97) than after conservative treatment (115.6 days; 95% CI, 85.87 to 145.40).[37] Notably, the same investigators have already planned VERTOS IV—a prospective, multicenter, randomized controlled trial using the same strict inclusion criteria as in VERTOS II that is designed to compare pain relief after vertebroplasty and a sham intervention in patients with acute osteoporotic vertebral compression fractures.[38]

The FREE trial was another large trial supporting the efficacy of vertebral augmentation. A total of 300 patients were randomized to undergo kyphoplasty ($n = 149$) or conservative therapy ($n = 151$).[39] Fractures were to have a minimum of 15% loss of height and MRI evidence of edema. Although both osteoporotic and malignant fractures were included, 96% of the fractures were related to primary osteoporosis. At randomization, fractures were a mean of 6 weeks old, kyphoplasty was performed at a mean of 7 days after randomization, and patients with fractures older than 3 months were excluded. The primary outcome measure was the mean 36-Item Short-Form Health Survey (SF-36) physical component summary (PCS) scale, a validated global quality-of-life measure weighted on physical ability.[39] Statistically significant improvements in SF-36 PCS scores in favor of kyphoplasty were noted at 1 month ($P < 0.0001$) and 12 months ($P = 0.0004$). There were greater reductions in Roland-Morris Disability Questionnaire (RDQ) scores in favor of kyphoplasty at 1 month ($P < 0.0001$) and 12 months ($P = 0.0012$).[39] Patients in the kyphoplasty group also had greater reductions in back pain scores, lower rates of narcotic analgesic use, and fewer days of restricted activity than did those managed with conservative therapy.[39] By 12 months, the differences between the conservative therapy arm and kyphoplasty group were diminished, most likely because of fracture healing.[39]

Further randomized controlled trial evidence comes from the Cancer Patient Fracture Evaluation (CAFE) study, which reported a benefit of kyphoplasty over conservative therapy for malignant painful vertebral compression fractures.[5] The CAFE study investigators recruited 134 patients with malignant fractures at 22 sites in Europe, the United States, Canada, and Australia. Approximately 50% of the patients had breast, lung, or prostate cancer metastasis, and 40% had multiple myeloma–related fractures. Patients with osteoblastic tumors, primary bone tumors such as osteosarcoma, or plasmacytoma at the index compression fracture were excluded. Patients were randomly assigned to kyphoplasty ($n=70$) or conservative therapy ($n=64$). The median estimated symptomatic fracture age was 3.5 months (interquartile range, 1.2 to 6.8); 87 of 129 patients had edema on MRI. The primary end point was back-specific functional status as measured by the RDQ at 1 month. There was a statistically significant reduction in RDQ scores in favor of kyphoplasty at 1 month ($P < 0.0001$).[5] The mean RDQ score in the kyphoplasty group was reduced from 17.6 at baseline to 9.1 at 1 month, as opposed to a mean change in score from 18.2 to 18.0 in the control group, and the kyphoplasty treatment effect on the RDQ score was −8.4 points at 1 month (95% CI, −7.6 to −9.2; $P < 0.0001$). Patients in the kyphoplasty group also had greater reductions in back pain—both groups had baseline mean back pain score of 7.3; the mean score at 7 days was 3.5 versus 7.0 in the conservative arm ($P < 0.0001$), which remained significant at 1 month ($P < 0.0001$). In addition, there were significant reductions in analgesic use and days of bed rest and improvement in quality of life (as measured by the SF-36 PCS) and Karnofsky performance status in the kyphoplasty group versus the conservative arm. These improvements in pain, overall functional status, and quality of life continued for the 12 months of the study period.[5]

With regard to longer-term outcomes, there are few data. Two-year outcome data from the FREE trial revealed that although there were no longer statistically significant differences in SF-36 PCS or RDQ scores at 24 months, patients in the kyphoplasty arm maintained a statistically significant reduction in back pain scores relative to conservative therapy at 24 months ($P = 0.009$).[40] A similar benefit was also reported at 36 months following kyphoplasty in a smaller prospective nonrandomized study of 60 patients.[41]

For height restoration, the results are less dramatic. Studies have shown that the magnitude of partial height restoration after vertebroplasty ranges from 2.5 to 8.4 mm and is overall similar to that reported after kyphoplasty.[42] However, many of these studies did not report the incidence of fracture clefts. Overall, restoration of height appears to be related to dynamic mobility of fracture fragments from the presence of a fracture cleft.[43] Dynamic mobility refers to a change in vertebral body height during changes in position, typically an increase in vertebral body height with supine or prone positioning versus the erect position; this typically occurs with fractures at the thoracolumbar junction (T11-L1), where the relatively fixed thoracic spine joins the more mobile lumbar spine. A study of 65 vertebral compression fractures referred for vertebroplasty revealed dynamic mobility in a third of treated levels.[44] All fractures that were mobile had a fracture cleft, and all fractures that were fixed did not have a fracture cleft. Fractures that were mobile had an average absolute increase in anterior vertebral height of 8.4 mm (range, 2.0 to 17.4 mm) and a decreased kyphosis angle of 7.2 degrees (40%) after vertebroplasty. There was no restoration of height or correction of kyphosis in fixed fractures.[44] In general, restoration of vertebral body height and correction of kyphosis may be desirable to improve postural endurance, reduce abdominal crowding, and improve overall pulmonary capacity. However, it remains unclear whether these results have any clinical significance.[42]

COMPLICATIONS ASSOCIATED WITH VERTEBRAL AUGMENTATION

With adherence to careful technique and optimal visualization, the risk for morbidity or mortality from vertebral augmentation is low (Box 67.3). For treatment of benign osteoporotic fractures, complication rates are approximately 1%.[31] Not surprisingly, they are higher for inexperienced practitioners or those attempting the procedure without

Box 67.3 Potential Complications

- Infection (osteomyelitis, epidural abscess)
- Paraspinal hematoma
- Fracture (of a rib, pedicle, or vertebral body)
- Failure to improve pain or worsening of pain
- Pneumothorax (for thoracic levels)
- Cement leakage
    - Nerve or spinal cord damage resulting in paralysis or bowel/bladder dysfunction
- Pulmonary embolism (secondary to cement or fat emboli)
- Hypotension or depressed myocardial function (secondary to free methylmethacrylate monomer or fat emboli)
- Death from cardiovascular collapse or anaphylaxis to the cement

adequate image guidance or cement opacification.[31] In the VERTOS II trial, the only complications referable to vertebroplasty that occurred in the 101 patients treated were a urinary tract infection in 1 patient and asymptomatic cement deposition into a segmental pulmonary artery in another.[37] Similarly, in the FREE trial, complications referable to kyphoplasty in the 149 patients treated were one soft tissue hematoma and one urinary tract infection.[39] Of note, almost all kyphoplasty procedures in the FREE trial were performed under general anesthesia, and in neither cohort were rates of urinary catheterization reported. In our experience, both vertebroplasty and kyphoplasty can be performed with local anesthesia and conscious sedation in most cases, and urinary catheterization is not required.

The risks are greater in patients with malignancy-related fractures, with an overall complication rate of 5% to 10% being reported.[45] In the CAFE trial, of the 70 patients treated with kyphoplasty for malignancy-related fractures, the only complications referable to kyphoplasty were one superficial wound infection and one patient with leakage of cement to the adjacent disk who had an adjacent fracture the day after the procedure.[5] There were no serious adverse events that were deemed device related. Importantly, kyphoplasty was not performed on those who had vertebral fracture morphology deemed unsuitable as determined by the treating physician. Thus, patients with vertebra plana, comminuted fractures, fractures with posterior wall involvement, or those with epidural involvement, which would incur higher risk, were excluded.

Extraosseous passage of cement is an important source of complications during vertebral augmentation. With vertebroplasty for osteoporotic fractures, small amounts of cement leakage are very common—in VERTOS II, 72% of treated vertebral bodies demonstrated cement leaks on postprocedure CT, with the majority being discal or into segmental veins; none extended into the spinal canal.[37] All patients remained asymptomatic. There was one patient (1%) with an asymptomatic cement segmental pulmonary embolus.[37]

In performing kyphoplasty, a cavity is created and will fill first, which theoretically results in a lower rate of cement leakage.[46-49] In the FREE trial, extravasation of cement occurred in 27% of treated vertebrae; however, this was assessed with intraoperative fluoroscopy and postoperative radiographs.[39] Most were end-plate or discal leakages; there was one foraminal leakage, none extended into the spinal canal, and no cement embolisms occurred. All patients remained asymptomatic.[39] In a small retrospective series with postprocedure CT, the rate of local leakage of bone cement was 87.5% (21/24) with percutaneous vertebroplasty and 49.2% (29/59) with kyphoplasty.[50]

Cement leaks are also common with pathologic fractures.[45,51,52] A recent retrospective study of CT-guided vertebroplasty for 331 malignant vertebral lesions revealed local cement leaks in 59 (194 of 331 vertebrae).[53] Although osteolysis of the posterior wall was evident in 49% (162 of 331 vertebrae), only 5% (15 of 331) of leaks extended into the spinal canal through the posterior cortex. Pulmonary cement emboli were detected on 1 of 53 (2%) chest radiographs and 10 of 88 (11%) chest CT scans.[53] A large single-center study of 106 patients with multiple myeloma treated by vertebroplasty revealed CT-detected extravasation of cement in 23% of the treated vertebrae, mainly into perivertebral (85%) and epidural (9%) veins. In five patients (5%), cement emboli were detected in the lungs. All leaks were asymptomatic.[54]

Although most extraosseous cement produces no symptoms or long-term morbidity, even small amounts of PMMA adjacent to a nerve root, including cement within the foraminal veins, can produce radicular pain.[45] When radiculopathy is produced by cement leakage, the pain can be treated with a nerve root block or systemic steroids. The need for surgical decompression is rare,[30] but it may be necessary when there is sufficient foraminal cement to cause frank root compression or when sufficient cement has been placed in the spinal canal to cause cord compression or cauda equina syndrome.[26]

POSTPROCEDURE AND FOLLOW-UP CARE AFTER VERTEBRAL AUGMENTATION

Immediately following the procedure, manual compression is applied over the needle access sites for 5 minutes to promote clotting and prevent hematoma formation, which might increase postprocedure pain. Transfer to the stretcher using logroll precautions may be performed immediately after the procedure, except in the setting of a vertebral cleft, where we keep the patient prone on the fluoroscopy table for 15 to 20 minutes. The patient is kept supine and flat in bed for 2 hours, followed by a further hour with the head of the bed inclined 30 degrees after the procedure. To alleviate immediate postprocedure pain, the patient may be given 15 to 30 mg of intravenous ketorolac, unless renal insufficiency is present. Most patients can be discharged later the same day, although more fragile patients may be observed overnight in the hospital. Assessment of the patient shortly after the procedure commonly reveals improvement in the back pain. Frequently, the patient will be able to differentiate any new procedure-related pain, which is typically treated with nonsteroidal anti-inflammatory drugs and should resolve over a period of 24 to 72 hours. In the setting of clinical deterioration suggestive of cement leakage, cross-sectional imaging should be performed.

Postprocedure follow-up of the patient is important. The patient's progress should be reviewed in the near term (e.g., 3 weeks) to assess pain and mobility levels and the need for analgesia. It is important to counsel the patient to report any sudden increase in back pain or new back pain because it may indicate a new fracture, and imaging should be performed. Importantly, up to a third of patients will suffer a repeated fracture within 1 to 3 years, with the greatest risk in those with steroid-induced osteoporosis.[55,56] Thus, prevention of future fractures is particularly important. Although the vast majority of recurrent fractures occur at new levels, a small percentage of patients suffer recurrent fracture at a previously treated level and may gain pain relief from repeated vertebral augmentation.[57] This being said, caution should be taken when interpreting marrow edema at a previously treated level because according to one study, normal MRI findings following vertebroplasty include persistent or progressive marrow edema at the treated level in up to a third of patients and for up to 6 months after the procedure.[58]

KEY POINTS

- Vertebral compression fractures are a common cause of pain and loss of independence in the middle-aged and elderly.
- Vertebroplasty and kyphoplasty are minimally invasive, image-guided vertebral augmentation procedures that involve the injection of cement into a fractured vertebral body that fails conventional medical therapy. The primary goal of augmentation is pain relief and enhanced functional status with the secondary goals of vertebral body stabilization in cases of fracture.
- Although two recent high-profile trials in the *New England Journal of Medicine* found no benefit with vertebroplasty, more recent randomized controlled trials of vertebral augmentation versus conservative therapy for both osteoporotic and malignant fractures have demonstrated significant improvements in back pain, reduction in disability, and improvement in quality of life in favor of vertebral augmentation.
- Complications are rare and generally result from unrecognized extraosseous leakage of the injected polymethyl methacrylate. Complications include radiculopathy, paralysis, and pulmonary embolism. These risks can be minimized and vertebral augmentation performed safely by experienced operators with the use of high-quality imaging, preferably with biplane fluoroscopy.

SUGGESTED READINGS

Berenson J, Pflugmacher R, Jarzem P, et al. Balloon kyphoplasty versus non-surgical fracture management for treatment of painful vertebral body compression fractures in patients with cancer: a multicentre, randomised controlled trial. *Lancet Oncol.* 2011;12:225-235.

Buchbinder R, Osborne RH, Ebeling PR, et al. A randomized trial of vertebroplasty for painful osteoporotic vertebral fractures. *N Engl J Med.* 2009;361:557-568.

Kallmes DF, Comstock BA, Heagerty PJ, et al. A randomized trial of vertebroplasty for osteoporotic spinal fractures. *N Engl J Med.* 2009;361:569-579.

Klazen CA, Lohle PN, de Vries J, et al. Vertebroplasty versus conservative treatment in acute osteoporotic vertebral compression fractures (VERTOS II): an open-label randomised trial. *Lancet.* 2010;376:1085-1092.

Wardlaw D, Cummings SR, Van Meirhaeghe J, et al. Efficacy and safety of balloon kyphoplasty compared with non-surgical care for vertebral compression fracture (free): a randomised controlled trial. *Lancet.* 2009;373:1016-1024.

The references for this chapter can be found at www.expertconsult.com.

68

Biopsychosocial Prescreening for Spinal Cord and Peripheral Nerve Stimulation Devices

Robert J. Gatchel | Robbie Haggard

Pain is a complex and serious medical condition, affecting more than 75 million Americans.[1,2] Moreover, Gatchel[3] and Gremillion[4] have reported that the most frequently cited reason patients in the United States seek medical care is due to pain. Besides the human suffering, there are enormous economic costs as well associated with chronic pain, in terms of medical care and lost productivity.[5-7] According to recent statistics from the National Academy of Sciences, the societal costs of chronic pain and related disability in the United States alone is $560 billion to $635 billion each year. Gaskin and Richard[8] have also reported similar costs and note that these annual costs for pain were greater than the annual costs for heart disease, cancer, and diabetes. Unfortunately, many chronic pain conditions are not being successfully treated. Indeed, the important and influential Institute of Medicine (IOM) report, *Relieving Pain in America*,[9] has highlighted the urgent need for the development of more cost-effective approaches to pain management because the ever-increasing costs associated with current treatment approaches cannot be sustained. Moreover, ongoing pain has been underdiagnosed and undertreated in nearly all health care settings. Therefore, there is still an urgent need for the development of treatment- and cost-effective methods for managing chronic pain, especially when it becomes intractable.

As Gatchel noted,[3,10] since the early 2000s there has been an expanding role of spinal cord and peripheral nerve stimulation as a potential treatment option for intractable chronic pain. Stimulated by Melzack and Wall's gate-control theory of pain,[11] which proposes that the activation of low-threshold afferent nerve fibers decreases the response of dorsal horn neurons to unmyelinated nociceptors (thereby "closing the gate" to pain transmission from the spinal cord), a number of clinical applications of this theory have been developed. For example, Shealy and colleagues[12] were the first to apply this theory when they stimulated the dorsal columns for the treatment of chronic, intractable pain. Since that time, implantable dorsal column stimulation (i.e., spinal cord stimulation [SCS]) was developed to treat a wide variety of pain syndromes. As Cameron and Elliot[13] noted, since the time that the SCS procedure was first prompted by the gate-control theory, its potential efficacy has been linked to a number of other mechanisms, such as the activation of spinal pain inhibitory circuits, as well as regional blood flow to various regions at the cerebral level. Subsequently, several groups started to use implantable peripheral nerve stimulators.[14,15] Peripheral nerve stimulation (PNS) applies an electrical current to the peripheral nerves to relieve the chronic pain symptoms. PNS techniques are used for treating pain in a nerve region that is not accessible by SCS. Nerve regions that are more easily accessed by PNS include the trigeminal nerve, occipital nerve, and subcutaneous peripheral nerves. Conditions for which PNS might be indicated include trigeminal neuropathic pain, occipital neuralgia, supraorbital neuralgia, and inguinal neuralgia. Headache disorders, including migraines and cluster headaches, might also benefit from cranial forms of PNS currently under investigation.

Thousands of stimulators were implanted in the decade following the first attempts. However, successful results with SCS and PNS have been difficult to define empirically, although some consensus in the literature has identified greater than 50% relief of index pain 12 months following implantation as a potential benchmark.[16] Although success rates vary widely from 40% to 80%, conditions commonly treated by SCS include failed back surgery syndrome, peripheral vascular disease, neuropathic pain, multiple sclerosis (MS), and reflex sympathetic dystrophies.[17-22] Moreover, the initial short-term expense of these implantable therapies has proven to be potentially offset in the long term by the benefits and resultant reduction in treatment expenses. For example, Kumar, Malik, and Demeria[20] evaluated costs for patients who received SCS and compared them to the costs for treatment by conventional pain therapies (CPT) in a control group. Although the cost for SCS was significantly higher than for CPT in the first 2.5 years, after that time point the cost of treating patients with SCS not only became less than the cost for CPT, but it also remained less expensive during the rest of the 5-year follow-up period.[19] Demonstrated success rates are no greater than 50%, although these initial high costs for implantable therapies make it necessary in the current evidence-based medicine environment to find means of better identifying those 50% of patients who are more likely not to benefit from the procedure.

It should also be noted that various side effects (e.g., neural impairment and scarring) have been observed. There were reports of high complications and failure rates.[23-27] In an attempt to determine both the positive and negative outcome indicators for surgical procedures, Spengler and Freeman[28] initially performed a retrospective analysis of 30 patients who had unsuccessful outcomes from various surgical procedures for low back pain, sciatica, or both. Among their findings, the most commonly reported cause of the poor results was a poor initial candidate-selection process, despite initial indications for the surgical procedures. A more focused investigation identified instances of drug abuse, alcoholism, marital discord, and personality factors that were likely to have played a role in the patients' postsurgical success or failure. Spengler and colleagues[28] therefore recommended presurgical psychological evaluation in order to reduce the likelihood of unsuccessful procedures. Following closely on the heels of the report by Spengler and colleagues,[28] Long and colleagues[24] performed a retrospective analysis of their own patients, who received surgically implanted dorsal column stimulators between 1970 and 1973. At that time, the only method for identifying candidates for this procedure was a persisting self-report of pain after failing all other treatments. Long and colleagues[24] found that too few patients achieved satisfactory pain relief with SCS and that approximately half of those patients originally selected for the procedure would have been rejected using updated inclusion criteria. Psychosocial factors were the most frequent reasons for failures, including substance use disorders.

Thus, it was soon recognized that not all patients were good candidates for such implantable devices. Indeed, starting with spinal surgery, clinical researchers became more involved in prescreening patients for these invasive interventions.[29] Before discussing an example of more current attempts, a discussion of the biopsychosocial approach to assessment is warranted.

THE BIOPSYCHOSOCIAL APPROACH TO ASSESSMENT

The biopsychosocial approach is recognized as the most comprehensive and heuristic approach to the evaluation of medical disorders.[3,7,29-31] The biopsychosocial model focuses on the complex interaction among biologic, psychological, and medicolegal variables that patients encounter when coping with a persistent, distressing medical condition. This interaction may perpetuate, and even worsen, the clinical presentation. This complex interaction accounts for the likelihood that a patient's life will be adversely affected in a variety of ways by his or her medical condition, thus requiring a comprehensive assessment and treatment approach designed to address all aspects of required care (i.e., biologic and psychosocial). This approach is in contrast to the former biomedical reductionist approach, which mistakenly assumed that most medical conditions, such as chronic pain, can be separated into distinct, independent physical and psychosocial components. Each patient experiences a medical condition uniquely. The complexity of a condition can be especially evident when it persists over time as a range of psychological, social, and economic factors emerge. These factors interact with the physical pathology to modulate a patient's discomfort and disability associated with the condition. Therefore, any successful assessment of patients needs to comprehensively evaluate these various factors.

A review by Gatchel and coworkers[32] highlighted how individuals significantly differ in the frequency of reporting physical symptoms, in their tendency to visit physicians when experiencing identical symptoms, and in their responses to the same treatment. Moreover, the nature of a patient's response to treatment has little to do with his or her objective physical condition. A comprehensive assessment of a patient proceeds from a global biopsychosocial diagnosis of the disorder in question, to a more detailed evaluation for the most important interactive factors needed for the diagnosis.[3,7] For example, for a patient reporting low back pain, a comprehensive physical examination would initially be conducted to assess the bio-component of the equation. This examination would consist of the assessment of range of motion, tenderness, gait, posture, sciatic stretch tests, and the neurologic components of myotomal/dermatomal deficits or reflex change. The examination is valuable when it defines objective signs that may lead to further diagnostic or treatment recommendations. It is less valuable when it is nonspecific or demonstrates pain inhibition. Waddell and colleagues[33] were the first to describe behaviors of back pain patients on physical examination that they termed *nonorganic* or *behavioral* signs. They suggested that a patient might not have a simple, straightforward physical diagnostic problem. Thus, a comprehensive biopsychosocial assessment of each patient is needed before the development of a treatment plan. The same such comprehensive assessment is needed before prescribing use of implantable devices for chronic pain.

THE BIOPSYCHOSOCIAL PRESCREENING PROCESS

SUMMARY OF CLINICAL RATIONALE AND PROCESS OF PRESCREENING

The process of test selection for prescreening can be difficult for the clinician not experienced with this process. The instruments described herein are a comprehensive battery, based on the work of Block and colleagues.[29,34,35] These can be used as a foundational starting point for the clinician who has been asked to screen and evaluate patient candidates for SCS or PNS (Block's work will be reviewed at greater length in the next section of this chapter). A general survey of pain symptoms is a necessary starting point for any pretreatment evaluation in a pain program. A general intake assessment should include a survey of pain symptoms, along with other self-report items such as demographic information, date of onset and pertinent details of the pain condition, prior treatments or surgeries, employment status, education level, disability payment status, workers' compensation or personal injury litigation involvement, health care utilization, additional contact numbers, and other comorbid chronic health problems. A brief summary of these assessment tools is provided here:

- First developed in 1976, the *visual analog scale* (VAS), also referred to as the *pain drawing analog* (PAD),[36] is a scale designed to rate the patient's degree of pain on a scale from 0 (no pain) to 10 (worst possible pain). It is made up of a 10-centimeter horizontal line divided at two-point intervals, and patients mark an "X" on the line to represent current levels of pain. The psychometric properties and utility with chronic pain populations of the VAS/PDA are further described in the literature.[37,38]

- A further development of the VAS/PDA is the *million visual analog scale* (MVAS).[39] The MVAS consists of 15 self-report items specific to perceived pain and disability. Patients respond on a similar 10-centimeter line, representing a range of possible answers from 0 to 10, in which the total score is the sum of all responses. Various cutoff points have been described based on psychometric testing of the MVAS. Scores of 0 to 39 indicate "mildly disabling" pain, scores of 40 to 84 indicate "moderately disabling pain," and scores of 85 and above indicate "severely disabling pain." The MVAS is especially helpful for discrepancies, such as when self-reported pain is higher than expected based on physical findings. This is often suggestive of a potential psychosocial component in the patient's experience of pain.[40]
- The *Oswestry Disability Questionnaire*[41] is another self-report scale designed to assess the degree of functional impairment. Consisting of 10 items regarding limitations of activities of daily living due to pain, the Oswestry has demonstrated test-retest reliability of .99 with a 24-hour interval between administrations, as well as acceptable levels validity.[42,43] Each item is scored on a 0- to 5-point scale, with a potential range of scores from 0 to 50, with higher scores significant for higher levels of pain-related limitations.
- Adams and colleagues[44] developed the *Pain Medication Questionnaire* to determine the risk of medication misuse among chronic pain patients. Identified behavioral correlates and attitudes suggestive of medication misuse were used to develop the 26 self-report items that make up the PMQ. Higher scores indicate a likely greater incidence of substance abuse potential, emotional distress, impaired coping skills, reduced physical functioning, as well as higher rates of unemployment.[44]
- The *Beck Depression Inventory* (BDI-II) is a 21-item self-report inventory designed to assess the intensity of depressive symptomatology.[45] Each item is scored from 0 to 3, with a potential range of scores from 0 to 63. A total score of 0 to 9 is considered normal, 10 to 15 is mild depression, 16 to 19 represents mild to moderate depression, 20 to 29 reflects moderate to severe depression, and 30+ indicates severe depression. Being able to identify symptoms of depression is important in chronic pain populations, as is being able to delineate between cognitive and somatic specific symptoms, which is an option allowed by the BDI-2. To obtain more than the subjective self-reported symptoms of depression available with the BDI-2, an experienced clinician will also want to perform a more objective assessment of depression to validate or clarify his or her findings. One such tool that is widely available, but does require some training and experience, is the Hamilton Rating Scale for Depression (HAM-D),[46] which is administered by the clinician in a brief interview format and could potentially be incorporated into the overall clinical interview.

In addition to examining the current emotional status of the patient candidate prior to SCS or PNS implantation, long-standing personality traits are important to consider before a patient begins a life-changing process that implantable therapies entail. Although these inventories are lengthy and time consuming, they have been used extensively in chronic pain populations. Third-party payers may limit the type or extent of testing that is performed with presurgical candidates, but the two inventories reviewed here provide valuable insight into the characteristic way these patients relate to the people and situations around them. If time and the situation allow, they should be considered as part of the comprehensive prescreening evaluation. The *Millon Behavioral Medicine Diagnostic* (MBMD)[47] is a 165-item, self-report inventory that examines psychosocial factors that may impact treatment outcomes with medical patients. The MBMD includes 29 clinical scales, three response pattern scales, one validity indicator, and six negative health habits indicators. It is intended for adult clinical and rehabilitation patients (ages 18 to 85) who are undergoing medical care or surgical evaluation, making this a valuable resource for the prescreening process.

A more widely recognized personality assessment, which has been used extensively in chronic pain research, is the *Minnesota Multiphasic Personality Inventory-2* (MMPI-2).[48] Although the MMPI-2-RF is gaining popularity in clinical settings, most research relating to pain is based on the MMPI-2, so this chapter will focus solely on that particular inventory. The MMPI-2 is a 567-item, self-report measure of personality functioning and psychiatric symptoms. It is the most commonly used personality assessment for patients with chronic pain, who often demonstrate a higher prevalence of emotional distress, specifically depressive symptoms and potential personality disorders, relative to the general population.[49] There are 10 empirically derived clinical scales, various supplementary scales, and validity scales provided to assess the test-taking attitudes of the patient. The MMPI-2 has a great deal of utility when used as part of the prescreening process with chronic pain patients. Findings from the MMPI-2 can help in the identification of psychopathology, personality and behavioral characteristics, treatment planning, and prediction of treatment outcomes.[49]

Current quality of life is also an important factor for patients being considered for an implantable therapy device, as this can interrupt current lifestyle during training and adjustment and can also improve quality of life for many of those receiving this option. The *Medical Outcomes Survey 36-Item Short Form Health Survey* (SF-36)[50] is a 36-item questionnaire that assesses health-related quality of life, both physical and mental, from the patient's perspective. The SF-36, and variants of this measure, is widely used for assessment and follow-up monitoring of health care treatment outcomes. The SF-36 consists of eight subscales and two standardized summary scales, the Mental Component Scale (MCS) and the Physical Component Scale (PCS). The MCS and PCS provide an overall gauge of the patient's sense of physical and mental well-being.

The coping skills that patients already rely on are necessary for the clinician performing the prescreening to identify, as these will likely be the set of coping skills employed during the training and postimplant phase of treatment. If there is a notable lack of healthy coping skills, this is something that might be managed prior to, and following, surgery with biobehavioral therapy. The *Coping Strategy Questionnaire* (CSQ)[51] is a 42-item self-report inventory that assesses how often pain patients use six cognitive coping strategies and two behavioral coping strategies. These strategies include diverting attention or distraction, reinterpreting pain sensations, ignoring pain, praying and hoping, coping self-statements, increasing behavioral activities, and catastrophizing. Additionally, the CSQ measures the subjective ability to control and decrease pain. Patients rate on a 6-point scale activities they engage in when experiencing pain, where 0 = never do that, 3 = sometimes do that, and 6 = always do that.

Although all of the aforementioned assessment tools are useful for performing a comprehensive prescreening evaluation, again it is up to the clinician to obtain the proper training to perform these assessments, along with a thorough clinical interview. These data can then be used to prepare a detailed report of the findings for both the patient and the physician performing the implantation procedure. In addition to performing these tasks, it should also be within the clinician's repertoire to know how to ask about what treatments the patient has found helpful in the past, what prescriptions and over-the-counter medications the patient is taking, what the patient's activities of daily living entail now and prior to the pain condition, and what the patient's realistic expectations are for life postprocedure.

THE PRESCREENING PROCESS DEVELOPED BY BLOCK AND COLLEAGUES

As noted earlier, there have been attempts to prescreen patients who were being considered for surgery.[35,52-54] Epker and Block[53] reviewed the methods for predicting positive outcomes for spine surgery in general and highlighted the positive and negative psychosocial risk factors that appeared to impact recovery from spine surgery. They delineated specific risk factors that had been shown to predict a poor surgical outcome and suggested the evaluation and quantification of these factors before performing spine surgery in order to predict positive outcomes. Three major categories of psychosocial factors were described: (1) personality/emotional, (2) cognitive/behavioral, and (3) environmental/historical. Scale elevations on the MMPI-2 associated with pain sensitivity (scales 1 and 3), depression (scale 2), anger (scale 4), and anxiety (scale 7) were the most noteworthy factors negatively influencing outcomes. Other significant factors included maladaptive coping strategies, workers' compensation status, litigation related to pain, and drug and alcohol abuse. Epker and Block[53] also discussed "quasi-medical" risk factors that could predict poor results: the duration of pain and number of previous surgeries for pain are negatively correlated with positive outcomes, and smoking and obesity can also have a negative effect on recovery from surgery. Finally, they noted that the presence of nonorganic Waddell signs (see Waddell and coworkers[33]) can help identify candidates who will have poor outcomes.

Subsequently, the most comprehensive screening approach for spine surgery was presented by Block and colleagues.[29] They developed a "scorecard" to clarify the spine surgery candidate's biopsychosocial risk factors, using an array of factors. The scorecard lists and quantifies each of psychosocial risk factors, along with additional medical risk factors. Based on the extant research demonstrating predictive ability, each risk factor is assigned an *a priori* weight of high risk (2) or medium risk (1), and the risk factors in each group (medical and psychosocial risks) are then totaled to arrive at a surgical prognosis. They based this approach on a study conducted by Block and colleagues.[35] In that study, 204 patients were referred for psychosocial screening and were evaluated no more than 1 month prior to surgery. A semistructured interview and two psychosocial questionnaires, the MMPI-2 and the Coping Strategy Questionnaire (CSQ),[55] were used to evaluate the psychosocial and medical risk factors. Based on the results of screening, patients were placed into one of three predictive categories ("good," "fair," or "poor"). Analyses of results showed the screening achieved an 82% accuracy rate, with 82.3% of patients in the "good" group experiencing a good outcome and 83.0% of patients in the "poor" prognostic group resulting in poor outcome. Logistic regression analyses were also conducted to determine which variables were the most significant predictors of outcome. These analyses yielded psychosocial test data as the most significant cluster of variables to correctly classify patients, with a correct classification rate of 78.4%. The addition of psychosocial interview data brought the model up to an 83.3% correct classification rate. Finally, the addition of the medical risk factors contributed slightly, bringing the total model to 84.3% correctly classified. This study was the first empirical investigation to show that a large number of psychosocial and medical risk factors can be identified, quantified, and used to accurately predict surgical outcomes.

The original screening scorecard, developed by Block and associates,[35] was subsequently replaced with a new prognostic algorithm by the same group.[29] This algorithm added several new features that enhanced its predictive utility. The changes involved the following:

- The algorithm placed psychosocial risk factors above all others because they have proven to have the most predictive power.
- A category termed *adverse clinical features* was also included to account for factors such as inconsistency, compliance issues, and medication seeking (which were often found in the patients' medical charts and observed during the clinical interview).
- A set of general treatment recommendations was added. The psychologists' recommendations fell into five categories: (1) proceed with surgery; (2) surgery, but with postoperative psychosocial treatment sessions; (3) preoperative treatment psychosocial sessions prior to surgery; (4) only noninvasive therapy recommended; or (5) no treatment of any kind is recommended.

REVIEW OF CLINICAL STUDIES

In the past, only a few studies have systematically evaluated the predictive value of biopsychosocial risk factors and treatment outcomes for implantable devices.[55-57] Moreover, they have varied in their methodologies. Our clinical research group therefore decided to use a more structured, standard approach. Using the presurgical screening algorithm developed by Block and colleagues, we were the first to evaluate its validity and application in categorizing patients' potential suitability as candidates for a subset of implantable modalities (specifically, spinal cord stimulators and intrathecal opioid pump systems).[58,59] The rationale for using an algorithm developed for spinal surgery for patients being considered for potential implantable devices was noted as follows:

Of course, one might argue that, because neuromodulation is quite different from spine surgical intervention, this algorithm would not be applicable to the former. However, for any type of presurgical screening that involves stress and uncertainty, such as the current one, the global psychological resilience of the patient (including the psychological strengths and weaknesses in dealing/coping with stress) is the key entity that is evaluated. That is to say, the global capacity of the patient to respond adaptively, whatever the specific challenges of any particular surgery, is the key ingredient. With this in mind, it was expected that Block's algorithm would be clinically applicable to neuromodulation procedures. We attempted to delineate differences found among prognostic groups with regard to psychosocial, functional and medical risk factors. (p. 238)[59]

The algorithm used in the investigation by Schocket and colleagues[59] included both psychosocial and medical risk factors, as delineated in Box 68.1. On the basis of this algorithm, patients were classified into one of five groups: *Green* (proceed with surgery); *Yellow I* (proceed with surgery, but administer postoperative psychosocial intervention); *Yellow II* (administer preoperative psychosocial intervention before surgery); *Red I* (only noninvasive intervention is recommended); and *Red II* (no treatment of any kind is recommended). Although this investigation did not provide the opportunity for long-term follow-up of all patients, data were collected from patients who were able to complete a 6-month follow-up evaluation. The results of this evaluation revealed a trend among the groups in terms of additional medications being taken. As expected, the Green group showed 40% of patients to be taking no new medications at the 6-month follow-up. This percentage decreased as prognosis worsened (Yellow I, 27.3%; Yellow II, 25%; and Red I and II, 0%). Although these were only statistical trends, due to limited power because of a relatively small sample size, the results do suggest a clinically significant change. Obviously, additional clinical research of this type is needed.

SUMMARY AND CONCLUSIONS

In this chapter, we initially highlighted the fact that chronic pain is a very prevalent and costly medical condition in the United States. When it becomes intractable in nature, more invasive methods often must be employed. One category of methods consists of implantable devices, such as SCS and PNS. This category of methods was then reviewed, as well as the pain syndromes they have been used for. It soon became apparent, though, that not all patients experienced positive outcomes after implantation. This prompted the need for more careful prescreening methods to help determine which patients would be good versus bad candidates for such an implantable-device intervention. A comprehensive biopsychosocial evaluation was presented as the best method to use for prescreening purposes. The various instruments that have been/could be used in the evaluation were reviewed.

In terms of the evaluation, as recently reviewed by Gatchel,[10] many complex biopsychosocial interactions can significantly affect how individuals respond to implantable devices, such as spinal cord and peripheral nerve stimulation. Indeed, again, appropriate biopsychosocial screening before such interventions are essential to maximize the benefits of the devices. As discussed in this chapter, we are beginning to make promising advances in this area by developing standardized prescreening protocols. For example, Block and colleagues[29,35] have developed an impressive screening algorithm for patients being considered for spine surgery. As an extension of this screening algorithm, Gatchel and colleagues[58,59] were the first to develop a modified prescreening protocol (based on that developed by Block and colleagues) for patients being considered for surgically installed implantable devices, specifically spinal cord stimulators and intrathecal pump devices. The results of this novel approach have been found to be quite promising, but it was pointed out that additional clinical research is still greatly needed to both refine the screening technique and examine long-term outcomes of its efficacy. There is also still a great need for evaluating the short- and long-term cost-effectiveness of these implantable devices, relative to

Box 68.1 The Psychosocial and Medical Risk Factors Used by Schocket and Colleagues

Psychosocial Risk Factors

- Job dissatisfaction
- Workers' compensation status
- Pending litigation
- Spousal solicitousness or lack of support
- Abuse or abandonment history
- Substance abuse
- History of psychosocial disturbance
- Pain sensitivity
- Chronic or reactive depression
- Pathologic depression profile
- Anger
- Anxiety

Medical Risk Factors

- Duration of pain
- Type of surgery
- Presence of nonorganic signs
- Abnormal pain drawing
- Previous surgeries
- Prior medical problems
- Smoking status
- Obesity

From Schocket KG, Gatchel RJ, Stowell AW, et al. Presurgical behavioral medicine evaluation: categorizing patients for potential treatment efficacy for spinal cord stimulation and intrathecal drug therapy. *Neuromodulation.* 2008;11:237-248.

less invasive forms of treatment. The final conclusion is that despite the promising results reviewed in this chapter, there is still a dearth of well-controlled evidence-based clinical research studies addressing this potentially useful approach for relieving unremitting chronic pain using palliative approaches. This research has been called for a great many times, starting with Gatchel in the early 2000s,[6] but to no avail.

KEY POINTS

- Drug abuse, alcoholism, marital discord, and personality factors have been noted to play a role in the success or failure of surgical procedures for either low back pain or sciatica.
- The biopsychosocial approach to preoperative assessment focuses on the complex interaction among biologic, psychological, and medicolegal variables that patients encounter when coping with a persistent, distressing medical condition.
- Individuals significantly differ in the frequency of reporting physical symptoms, in their tendency to visit physicians when experiencing identical symptoms, and in their responses to the same treatment.
- A general assessment should include a survey of pain symptoms, along with other self-report items such as demographic information, date of onset and pertinent details of the pain condition, prior treatments or surgeries, employment status, education level, disability payment status, workers' compensation or personal injury litigation involvement, health care utilization, additional contact numbers, and other comorbid chronic health problems.
- In addition to assessing the current emotional status of the patient prior to SCS or PNS implantation, long-standing personality traits are important to consider.
- Several assessment tools include the Oswestry Disability Questionnaire, Beck Depression Inventory, Pain Medication Questionnaire, MMPI, SF-36, and Coping Strategy Questionnaire.

KEY POINTS—cont'd

- The major categories of psychosocial factors that negatively influence outcomes include the following: (1) personality/emotional, (2) cognitive/behavioral, and (3) environmental/historical aspects. Scale elevations on the MMPI-2 associated with pain sensitivity (scales 1 and 3), depression (scale 2), anger (scale 4), and anxiety (scale 7) were the most noteworthy factors negatively influencing outcomes.
- Based on prognostic algorithms, a patient's suitability as a candidate can be classified into the following categories: Green (proceed with surgery), Yellow I (proceed with surgery, but administer postoperative psychosocial intervention), Yellow II (administer preoperative psychosocial intervention before surgery), Red I (only noninvasive intervention is recommended), and Red II (no treatment of any kind is recommended).

SUGGESTED READINGS

Adams LL, Gatchel RJ, Robinson RC, et al. Development of a self-report screening instrument for assessing potential opioid medication misuse in chronic pain patients. *J Pain Symptom Manage.* 2004;27:440-459.

Block AR, Ohnmeiss DO, Guyer RD, et al. The use of presurgical psychological screening to predict the outcome of spine surgery. *Spine J.* 2001;1:274-282.

Epker J, Block AR. Presurgical psychological screening in back pain patients: a review. *Clin J Pain.* 2001;17:200-205.

Gatchel RJ. A biopsychosocial overview of pre-treatment screening of patients with pain. *Clin J Pain.* 2001;17:192-199.

Heckler D, Gatchel RJ, Lou L, et al. Presurgical behavioral medicine evaluation (PBME) for implantable devices for pain management: a one-year prospective study. *Pain Pract.* 2007;7:110-122.

Prager J, Jacobs M. Evaluation of patients for implantable pain modalities: medical and behavioral assessment. *Clin J Pain.* 2001;17:206-214.

Schocket KG, Gatchel RJ, Stowell AW, et al. Presurgical behavioral medicine evaluation: categorizing patients for potential treatment efficacy for spinal cord stimulation and intrathecal drug therapy. *Neuromodulation.* 2008;11:237-248.

Waddell G, McCulloch JA, Kummel E, Venner RM. Nonorganic physical signs in low-back pain. *Spine.* 1980;5:117-125.

The references for this chapter can be found at www.expertconsult.com.

Spinal Cord and Peripheral Nerve Stimulation

69

Robert W. Hurley | Allen W. Burton

SPINAL CORD STIMULATION

Spinal cord stimulation (SCS), sometimes called dorsal column stimulation, describes the use of pulsed electrical energy near the spinal cord to control pain.[1] This technique was first applied in the intrathecal space and later in the epidural space as described by Shealy and associates in 1967.[2] In the present day, neurostimulation commonly involves the implantation of leads in the epidural space to transmit this pulsed energy to the spinal cord or the desired nerve roots. This technique has notable analgesic properties for neuropathic pain states, anginal pain, and peripheral ischemic pain. The same technology can be applied in deep brain stimulation, cortical brain stimulation, and peripheral nerve stimulation.[3-5] These latter techniques are typically in the realm of the neurosurgeon, although more and more pain physicians are using peripheral nerve stimulation techniques. This chapter concentrates on the modality of spinal cord (dorsal column) stimulation.

MECHANISM OF ACTION

Neurostimulation began shortly after Melzack and Wall proposed the gate control theory in 1965.[6] This theory posed that painful peripheral stimuli carried by unmyelinated C fibers and lightly myelinated Aδ fibers terminated at the substantia gelatinosa of the dorsal horn (the gate). Large myelinated Aβ fibers responsible for touch and vibratory sensation also had collateral input to "the gate" in the dorsal horn. It was hypothesized that their input could "close the gate" to the cephalad transmission of painful stimuli. As an application of the gate control theory, in 1967 Shealy implanted the first spinal cord stimulator device for the treatment of chronic pain.[2] This technique was noted to control pain and has undergone numerous technical and clinical refinements in the ensuing years.

Although the gate theory was initially proposed as the mechanism of action, the underlying neurophysiologic mechanisms are not clearly understood. Research has given us insight into effects occurring at the local and supraspinal levels and through dorsal horn interneuron and neurochemical mechanisms.[7-9] Linderoth and colleagues[8] have noted that the mechanism of analgesia when SCS is applied in neuropathic pain states may be very different from those involved in analgesia as a result of limb ischemia or angina. Experimental evidence points to SCS having a beneficial effect at the dorsal horn by favorably altering the local neurochemistry, thereby suppressing the hyperexcitability of the wide dynamic range (WDR) neurons. Specifically, there is some evidence for increased levels of gamma-aminobutyric acid (GABA) release, serotonin, and perhaps suppression of levels of some excitatory amino acids including glutamate and aspartate. In the case of ischemic pain, analgesia seems to be obtained through restoration of a favorable oxygen supply and demand balance, perhaps through alteration of sympathetic tone. Guan and colleagues[9] made three substantial findings in an in vivo model of SCS and neuropathic pain: (1) stimulation of either the dorsal horn or dorsal nerve roots at intensity and frequency to selectively activate Aβ fibers reduced WDR neurons spontaneous firing in animals with neuropathic injuries; (2) this same stimulation reduced WDR responses to mechanical stimulation of normal and injured animals; and (3) stimulation of the dorsal columns, but not the dorsal root, reduced activity-dependent neuronal excitability (wind-up). Other experimental evidence has suggested that antidromic stimulation from dorsal column stimulation of cutaneous fibers plays a role in the analgesic effect of SCS[10] and possibly the result of antidromic inhibition of orthodromic transmission.[11]

PATIENT SELECTION

Patient selection is the most challenging and important step in the decision to offer neurostimulation. Although it can be viewed as a burden or barrier by both the patient and the physician, the additional time dedicated to the selection of patients who are most likely to positively respond to the therapy in the short and long term is time well invested. The challenge pain physicians face is being able to predict who will respond well with durability. There are relatively few data to guide pain physicians in this realm; most of the studies examining who is a good candidate for SCS therapy are small prospective or retrospective studies. In a study examining 36 patients with complex regional pain syndrome (CRPS) treated with SCS, the authors found that mechanical allodynia of the affected limb was negatively correlated with SCS therapy success, and patient age, duration, or intensity of pain had no relationship to SCS outcome.[12] In patients with CRPS, response to a sympathetic nerve block may positively correlate with SCS therapy outcome.[13] Many patients with chronic pain have some symptoms of depression; psychological screening can be extremely helpful for avoiding failed implants in patients with major psychological disorders. An interesting study by Olson and colleagues revealed a high correlation between many items on a complex psychological testing battery and favorable response to trial stimulation.[14] In a systematic review, it was noted

Box 69.1 Overview of the Stages of Spinal Cord Stimulator Placement

Stage 1: Pain physician visit. This stage is performed to evaluate the pain condition and thereby determine whether the patient's pain syndrome is amenable to spinal cord stimulation therapy.
Stage 2: Psychological evaluation. This stage is performed to understand the patient's needs and expectations of therapy.
Stage 3: Trial stimulation. This stage is performed to evaluate the effectiveness of pain reduction (3 to 8 days).
*Stage 4: Diagnostic imaging.** An MRI will be ordered to determine whether the patient has obstructions within the high lumbar and thoracic spinal space for thoracic placement or cervical space that would lead to concerns about safe lead placement.
Stage 5: Permanent implantation. This may be performed by a neurosurgeon or a pain physician depending on the patient's comorbidities, pain distribution, or patient preference.

*This stage may be performed prior to stage 3 (trial implant) if there are clinical signs or symptoms of stenosis or other anatomic impediments to percutaneous cylindrical lead placement.

that symptoms of depression, somatization, anxiety and poor coping skills were predictors of poor SCS outcome.[15] It appears that overall mood is an important predictor of outcomes. Paradoxically, the psychological construct of catastrophizing, which has been negatively associated with other pain therapies, was not detrimental to the positive SCS outcome in patients with CRPS.[16] Sex and age of patients as well as laterality of pain have also been examined for predictive value and none have been found to impact the results of the SCS therapy.[17] Relatively few randomized controlled studies have been performed that evaluate long-term predictors of success or failure from SCS therapy for specific pain disease processes.[18-22]

The evaluation of a patient for spinal cord stimulation is a staged process (Box 69.1). Appropriate patients for a trial of neurostimulation must meet the following criteria: (1) the diagnosis is amenable to this therapy (e.g., neuropathic pain syndromes), (2) the patient has failed conservative therapy, and (3) significant psychological issues have been ruled out.[23]

IMAGING

Magnetic resonance imaging (MRI) or computed tomography (CT) to determine patency and sufficiency of the high lumbar and low to mid thoracic epidural space should be used to evaluate patients progressing forward to the implantation phase of the thoracic SCS. Ruling out moderate to severe stenosis increases the safety of the procedure. This evaluation may also guide the pain physician's decision to refer the patient to a surgeon for implantation—for instance, if a surgical decompression is needed prior to implantation of the lead system. Cases of mild (nonoperative) spinal stenosis at the target levels could lead the physician to choose a smaller cylindrical lead rather than the paddle-type leads.

CONSERVATIVE THERAPY

Despite the increase in the number of agents available to treat neuropathic pain, a substantial number of patients still suffer from poorly controlled neuropathic pain. Puig estimates as many as 50% of patients with neuropathic pain have ineffective pain relief even with appropriate pharmacological management.[24] Recommended selection criteria from these authors include (1) confirmed diagnosis of neuropathic pain; (2) chronicity of greater than 6 months; (3) failed trials of polypharmacy including anticonvulsants, antidepressants, and other drugs (such as opioids) because of lack of efficacy or side effects; (4) a lemniscal pathway (spinal connection to painful site) that has been preserved so that stimulation-induced paresthesias can be felt; and (5) the absence of contraindications including nociceptive pain syndromes, psychological disturbance, infection at site, systemic bacterial infections, and a lifestyle that is incompatible with longevity of therapy (patient employed in field requiring excessive repetitive flexion and extension, MRI technician, etc.).

TRIAL

A careful trial period is essential to avoid a failed implant. Trials of different lengths have been advocated; the risk of a longer trial is mainly infection, whereas the primary risk of too short a trial is a false-positive result. We use a 5- to 8-day trial and encourage patients to be as active as possible in their usual environment, with the exception of limiting bending and twisting movements. In rare circumstances, the author (RWH) uses a permanent trial implantation (discussed later) whereby the percutaneous leads are placed and secured in the same fashion and the entire permanent system is placed with the exception of the implantable pulse generator (IPG); a tunneled lead extension is externalized and connected to the trialing system. Patient selection and physician discretion are exceptionally important in these cases, as there is a natural bias to going forward with the remainder of the implant because of the commitment that has already been made by implantation of the permanent leads. In "perm-trial" cases, the trial period is often much longer than the percutaneous trial, as in this author's (RWH) experience of up to 3 weeks.

Despite advances in our understanding of diagnoses that respond to neurostimulation, improved psychological screening, and the availability of improved multilead systems, clinical failures of implanted neurostimulator devices remain all too common. Pain physicians must critically evaluate their own outcomes and adhere to the strict selection criterion outlined here. Simpson published a neurosurgeon's perspective on the use of SCS in treating chronic pain.[25] To paraphrase Simpson,

> *The mindset of the public and many physicians favors drugs over physical treatments such as surgery and neurostimulation, and many physicians exhibit a "protective" reluctance to refer for these procedures, but are prepared to persist with polypharmacy despite the real risks of mental impairment, nausea, constipation, weight gain, and addiction. The worst thing a neurostimulator can do is fail to work.*

Many pain specialists are beginning to side with Simpson on this issue, preferring a trial of SCS before committing a patient to chronic opioid therapy. Although this is true, the corollary is also the case and would suggest caution against the overly liberal application of the technology.

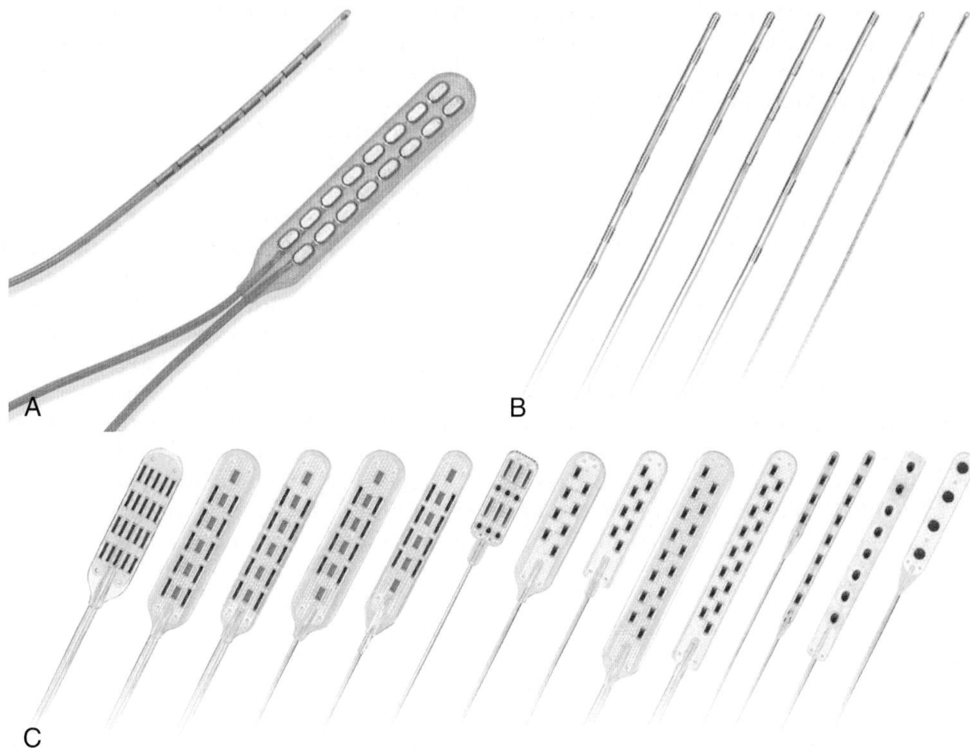

Figure 69.1 Neurostimulator Leads. A, Left to right—cylindrical type to paddle type. **B**, Cylindrical type. **C**, Paddle type. (*A*, Image courtesy of Boston Scientific Corporation. *B*, Image courtesy of St. Jude Medical [ANS]. *C*, Image courtesy of St. Jude Medical [ANS].)

In examining one's own outcomes with SCS therapy, several factors must be considered:

1. Examination of your trial to permanent ratio data. These data will tell you what percentage of the patients you trial go on to have a permanent implantation. All things being equal (with the assumption that all permanent implantations were the correct decision) this ratio will give a hint to your ability to select appropriate patients for this therapy. A ratio below 50% would suggest you are not being selective in your application of the therapy, and a ratio of 95% would suggest you are being too selective and more than likely not offering the therapy to those who could benefit.
2. Examination of your permanent implantation data:
   a. Number of patients who continued to use the SCS in the long term
   b. Number of patients who had the permanent system removed
   c. Number of surgical site infections (within 1 year of implant) and proximate cause
   d. Number of clinically significant migrations
      i. How many were resolved with re-programming
      ii. How many were resolved with re-operation
   e. Number of other adverse events (not already listed)
3. Long-term pain relief success of therapy. This applies to follow-up with your SCS patients at regular intervals to reassess their success or lack thereof. A common interval recommended is every 6 months to every year (at the maximum).
4. Assessment of other quality-of-life indicators:
   a. Improvement in activities of daily living (household chores, fitness activities)
   b. Improvement in psychological factors (mood, pain coping, anxiety)
   c. Improvement in patients' sleep, personal relationships
5. Assessment of medication intake. What reductions in pain medication have occurred? (Have you, as the physician, addressed this issue and attempted to wean medications?)

TECHNICAL CONSIDERATIONS

SCS is a technically challenging interventional/surgical pain medicine technique. It involves the placement of an electrode array (leads) in the epidural space, a trial period, anchoring the lead(s), positioning and implantation of the pulse generator or radiofrequency (RF) receiver, and the tunneling and connection of the wires. This is one of the more complex procedural skills in pain medicine and is an excellent example of why pain medicine is a subspecialty of the practice and should not be performed by a nonphysician or non-pain medicine trained physician.

A spinal cord stimulator system is made up of three parts: (1) electrodes or leads (Fig. 69.1), (2) IPGs or the battery (Fig. 69.2), and (3) the charging and programming systems (see Fig. 69.2). Electrodes are of two types: cylindrical (formerly known as percutaneous) and paddle (formerly known as surgical) (see Fig. 69.1). These electrodes are connected to an IPG or (historically, but no longer available) an RF unit. Currently, three companies—Medtronic, Inc., St. Jude Medical, Inc., and Boston Scientific Corp. (formerly Advanced Bionics, Inc.)—make neurostimulation equipment (Appendix A). Historically the paddle-type lead could only be implanted via a laminotomy or more extensive laminectomy. In 2011, one neuromodulation company introduced a system by which a surgical paddle lead (single 8-contact column) could be implanted in a percutaneous fashion using a wide flat introducer that is placed via the Seldinger technique (Fig. 69.3). This has allowed advanced pain physicians who are not spine surgeons to take advantage of these lead systems.[22]

A spinal cord stimulator trial may be accomplished in two ways: percutaneous or permanent lead trial. In both trial methods, under fluoroscopy and sterile conditions (Table 69.1), a lead is introduced into the epidural space with a standard epidural needle or curved epidural needle. To facilitate threading of the lead cephalad in the dorsal midline region, it is imperative to have the needle at a shallow angle (often less than 45 degrees). It is essential to avoid perpendicular or near perpendicular needle placement into the epidural space (unless using a curved needle) because of the consequent 75- to 90-degree bend then required to introduce the stimulator lead. The lead is directed under fluoroscopic imaging into the posterior or dorsal paramedian epidural space up to the desired anatomic location—generally the low thoracic cord region (commonly T8 to T10) to obtain paresthetic coverage of the lower extremities or the midcervical level to obtain coverage of the upper extremities (i.e., the lead is moved cephalad and caudad in the epidural space until the pattern of resulting electrical stimulation overlies the painful region; Fig. 69.4). Trial stimulation is undertaken to attempt to cover the painful area with an electrically induced paresthesia. After the painful area is captured with either one or more leads, the two techniques of trialing differ.

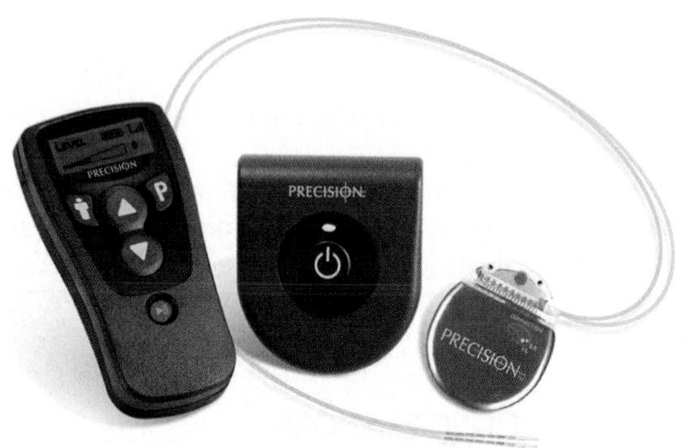

Figure 69.2 IPG and charging system. (Image courtesy of Boston Scientific Corporation.)

In the percutaneous trial, the needle is withdrawn, the lead is adhered in place (with a suture, surgical skin glue, or surgical adhesive), a chlorhexidine impregnated patch (RWH) and a sterile dressing is applied. The lead passes from the epidural space, through the skin to the external pulse generator throughout the trial period. When the patient returns after a trial of several days, the dressing is removed, and the lead is removed and discarded regardless of the success of the trial. When the patient returns for an implant, a new lead is placed in the final location of the trial lead contacts and connected to an IPG.

In the permanent lead trial, after successful positioning of the trial lead(s), local anesthetic is infiltrated around the needle(s) and an incision is made, cutting down to the supraspinous fascia to anchor the leads securely using nonabsorbable suture. The anchoring device should be placed as closely as possible to the fascia entry site, ideally with the "nose" of the anchor protruding into the fascia to lessen the bending angle of the lead. The anchor is secured using nonabsorbable suture, such as 2.0 silk. At this point, two approaches can be used. The first method requires opening up the midline back incision. In this technique, the proximal end of a temporary extension wire is connected to the permanent lead, and the distal end is tunneled away from the back incision and out through the skin. The second method does not require reopening the midline back incision; instead a pocket for the IPG is created. With this technique, the IPG pocket is created and the permanent lead is tunneled to this pocket; an extension lead is then connected to the permanent lead and the distal end is tunneled away from the IPG pocket. The IPG pocket is then sutured closed. With either technique, this exiting connector is secured to the skin using a suture (or surgical skin glue), antibiotic ointment, and a sterile dressing. If the trial is successful, at the time of implant the back incision (or IPG site incision) is opened and the percutaneous lead extension is cut, pulled out through the

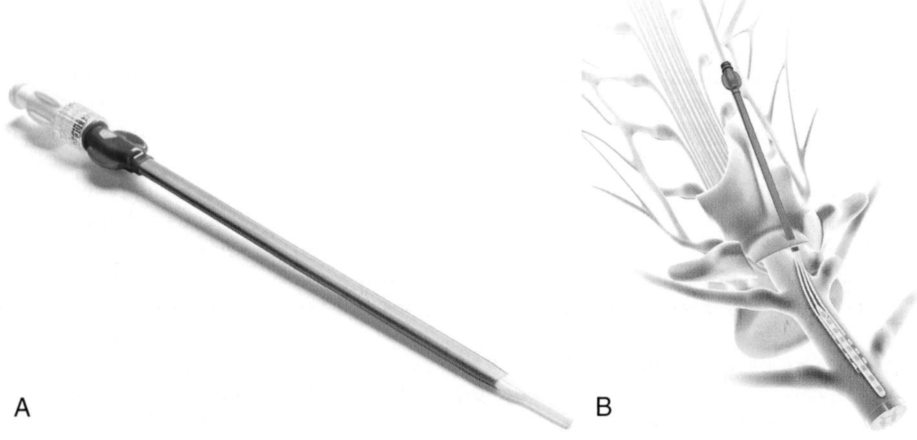

Figure 69.3 Epidural introducer for delivery of multiple leads through a single needle insertion or for the introduction of a paddle-type lead through a percutaneous approach. **A**, The Epidural introducer (Epiducer). **B**, Epidural introducer with single paddle-type lead *(center)* and two cylindrical leads. (Image courtesy of St. Jude Medical [ANS].)

skin site, and discarded. The permanent lead(s) that was used for the trial is attached to a new sterile extension(s) (not needed if at the IPG site) and tunneled (or directly connected) to the IPG.

The permanent lead trial method has the advantages of saving the cost of new electrodes at implant and ensuring that the implanted lead position matches the trial lead position. Advantages of the "percutaneous lead" approach include avoiding the costs of two trips to the operating room (even for an unsuccessful trial, this is necessary to remove the anchored trial lead); avoiding an incision and postoperative pain during the trial, which may confuse trial interpretation by the patient; and avoiding the risk of infection associated with the percutaneous temporary extension. The percutaneous extension must be anchored and meticulously dressed or the risk of infection may be higher than with the straight percutaneous technique.[26] The majority of clinicians favor the percutaneous trial method. Most consider 50% or more pain relief to be indicative of a successful trial, although the ultimate decision also should include other factors such as activity level and medication intake. Some combination of pain relief, increased activity level, and decreased medication intake is indicative of a favorable trial.

A trial with paddle-type electrodes (with the exception of the previously mentioned percutaneous paddle introduction technique) requires the implanted lead approach with the significant addition of a laminotomy to slip the flat plate electrode into the epidural space. Some physicians trial the patient with the percutaneous approach and if successful send the patient to a neurosurgeon for a paddle-type implant.

The IPG is generally implanted in the flank, occasionally in the posterior superior gluteal area or rarely the lower abdominal area or pectoral region. It should be in a location the patient can access with the dominant hand for adjustment of the settings with the patient-held remote control unit. The decision to use a rechargeable implantable IPG is based on several considerations. If the patient's pain pattern requires the use of many anode or cathode settings with high power requirements during the trial, consider a rechargeable, higher-capacity unit. The IPG battery life largely depends on the power settings used, but the newer IPG units generally last several years at average

Table 69.1 Sterile Setup for Spinal Cord Stimulator Trial and Permanent Implant

	Surgeon	Patient	Instruments
Percutaneous Trial Lead	Hair coverage, eye protection	Pre-procedure chlorhexidine shower	Sterile covering for fluoroscopic machine
	Surgical scrub	Sterile skin preparation with alcohol-based chlorhexidine scrub	Lead kit from company
	Sterile gown, gloves	Towels and full surgical drape	
		Bio-patch (chlorhexidine) application	
Permanent or Perm Trial Lead	Hair coverage, eye protection	Pre-procedure chlorhexidine shower	Sterile covering for fluoroscopic machine
	Surgical scrub	Pre-operative antibiotics for coverage of skin flora (cefazolin or clindamycin)	Lead kit from company
	Sterile gown and gloves	Sterile towels	Implantable pulse generator (IPG) from company (if IPG implantation is intended)
		Iodine-impregnated adhesive dressing (unless iodine allergic)	
		Full surgical drape	

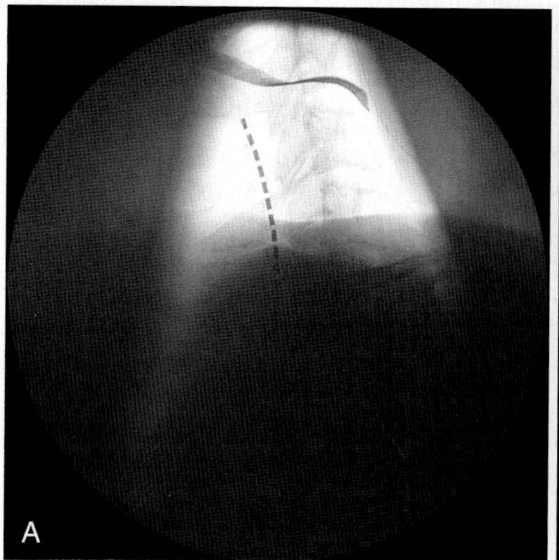

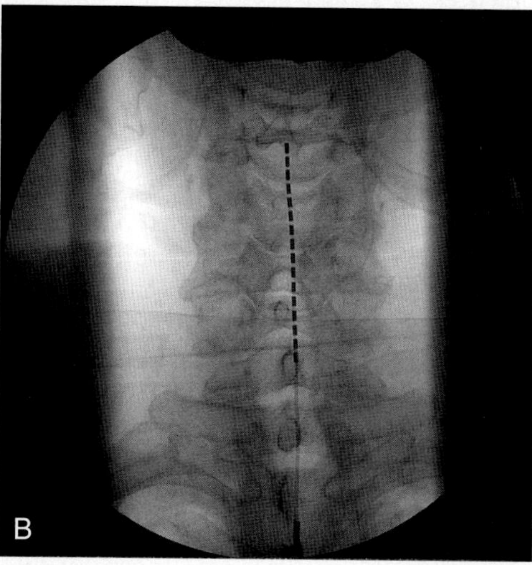

Figure 69.4 Fluoroscopic image of a 16-contact stimulator lead placed in the cervical spine to simultaneously treat upper and lower extremity pain. **A**, Lateral view. **B**, Anteroposterior view. (Courtesy R.W. Hurley, MD, PhD.)

power settings. All three manufacturers offer rechargeable IPG systems with two significant advantages over the previous IPG devices: (1) the patient may use higher voltage settings without worry of prompt battery depletion, allowing more flexibility in programming, and (2) the promise of a much longer interval until replacement is required, perhaps 10 years or more. The unit is recharged via an external recharger every 7 to 14 days as needed.

COMPLICATIONS

Complications associated with spinal cord stimulation range from simple, easily correctable problems—such as lack of appropriate paresthesia coverage—to devastating paralysis, nerve injury, and death. Prior to implantation of the trial lead, an educational session should occur with the patient and family members. This meeting should include a discussion of possible risks and complications. In the postoperative period, the caregiver should be involved in identifying problems and alerting the health care team.

North and colleagues reported their experience in 320 consecutive patients treated with SCS between 1972 and 1990.[27] A 5% rate of subcutaneous infection was observed, which is consistent with other published trials. The most frequent complication was lead migration or breakage, and that remains the predominant weakness of neurostimulation. The revision rate for patients with modern multichannel devices was 16%. Failure of the electrode lead was observed in 13% of patients and steadily declined over the course of the study as the lead systems were modernized. When analyzed by implant type (single-channel percutaneous, single-channel laminectomy, and multichannel), the lead migration rate for multichannel devices was approximately 7%. Analysis of hardware reliability for 298 permanent implants showed that technical failures (particularly electrode migration and malposition) and clinical failures had become significantly less common as implants had evolved into programmable, multichannel devices and anchoring technique and equipment have improved.

Occasionally, a short-lived series of SCS complications can occur at sites. In 2008, an outbreak of staphylococcus aureus infections related to interventional procedures including SCS resulted in temporary closure of a private pain practice.[28] Other outbreaks of infection have been noted during quality assessments of current practices. One such assessment of the experience at the Johns Hopkins Pain Clinic in 2010 revealed that, during a 6-month period in 2010, five patients with SCS trial lead implantations became infected as compared to one trial lead in the previous 3.5 years.[29] The median time to infection diagnosis was 4.5 days. The infections associated with the five trial lead infections in 2010 ranged from superficial cellulitis to radiographically confirmed epidural abscess. Unfortunately, no independent risk factors (implanting pain fellow, SCS company, use of pre-operative antibiotics, lead location, or patient comorbidities) were identified as the causative agent.

In a 5-year experience prior to 2006 at the Cleveland Clinic, Rosenow and colleagues reported a 43% revision or removal rate among 289 patients implanted with SCS systems.[30] Thirty-three percent of all leads required revision, with the most common reasons being lead breakage, poor pain coverage, migration, and infection in descending order of frequency. Ten percent of patients had a lead migration requiring revision. Paddle-type leads broke twice as often as percutaneous leads. Twenty-two percent of all patients required more than one revision procedure; 49% requiring at least one lead revision underwent multiple revisions. Anatomically, cervical leads were the most likely to require revision. Their overall infection rate was 3.6%. This experience was somewhat exceptional and the data are no longer current, so they are included only for historical guidance. A more recent retrospective review from the same institution shows the progress made in SCS therapy complication rates.[31] In this review, the only documented complication associated with SCS trials was lead migration in 5 of 707 patients (0.7%). There were no permanent neurologic deficits or deaths as a result of SCS permanent implantation. The most common complications were hardware related (38% of all complications) and included lead migration (22.6%), lead connection failure (9.5%), and lead breakage (6%). Revisions or replacements were required in these cases. Related complications included pain at the generator site (12%) and clinical infection (4.5%; 2.5% with positive culture). The rates of infection varied among the different diagnoses with the highest in failed back surgery syndrome (6.3%). Patients with diabetes had an infection rate of 9%, over the 4% rate in nondiabetics. Infections were managed successfully with explantation and antibiotic therapy without permanent sequela.

May and coworkers and Barolat and associates reported lead revision rates caused by lead migration of 4.5% and 13.6% and breakage of 0% and 13.6%, respectively.[26,32] Infections occurred in 7% and 2.5% of cases, respectively. No serious complications were observed in either study. These studies are representative of the complication rate of neurostimulation therapy. Kumar and colleagues in Saskatchewan have quantified the costs of SCS complications and published suggestions to improve outcomes.[33] Their series included 160 patients treated over 10 years with SCS implantation. They noted 42 patients with 51 complications classified as hardware related (39) or biologic (12) with the range of costs of treatment from $130 (hematoma aspiration) to $22,406 (system reimplantation) (in 2005 Canadian dollars). Their most common hardware failures were lead displacement (11% of patients), followed by fractured electrode (5.6% of patients). Their most common biologic complication was wound infection at 4.4% overall, with subcutaneous hematoma next at 3% overall. These authors presented an analysis of engineering work done at Medtronic, Inc. with regard to lead migration and fracture. This manufacturer recommends the use of a silicon anchor (not hard plastic) with the tip of the anchor pushed through the deep fascia to reduce the pressure point or fatigue point on the lead with repeated bending. Further, the manufacturer recommends a strain relief loop between the anchor and the IPG, with the flank being the preferred site of IPG implant because of less stress on the leads during bending. Another poorly understood phenomenon described by Kumar is late tolerance to stimulation in 16 of 160 patients (10%).

Infections range from simple infections at the surface of the wound to epidural abscess. The patient should be instructed on wound care and recognition of signs and symptoms indicative of infection. Many superficial infections can be treated with oral antibiotics or simple surgical incision and drainage followed by wound irrigation. For an excellent review on infectious complications of SCS, the reader is referred to Follett and colleagues' review of 114 cases with recommendations for avoidance.[34] They found that the most common sites of infection were the IPG (54%), the connector tract (17%), and the back incision (8%). Staphylococcus species were the most common pathogen, cultured in 18% of cases, with system explant required in 82% of cases. One death related to infection and one case of epidural abscess leading to paralysis caused by SCS have been reported.[35,36] Standard practice includes prophylactic preoperative antibiotics (30 minutes pre-incision).

If infection reaches the tissues involving the devices, in most cases the implant should be removed. In such cases, one should have a high index of suspicion for an epidural abscess. Abscess of the epidural space can lead to paralysis and death if not identified quickly and treated aggressively. The likelihood of epidural abscess from a percutaneous SCS trial is exceptionally low,[31] although exceptions do exist.[29]

PROGRAMMING

There are four basic parameters in neurostimulation that may be adjusted to create stimulation paresthesias in the painful areas, thereby mitigating the patient's pain. They are amplitude, pulse width, rate, and electrode selection.

Amplitude is the intensity or strength of the stimulation measured in volts. Typically, voltage may be set from 0 to 10 volts, with lower settings used over peripheral nerves and with paddle-type electrodes. Pulse width is a measure in microseconds (μs) of the duration of a pulse. Pulse width is usually set between 100 and 400 μs. A larger pulse width typically gives the patient broader coverage. Rate is measured in hertz (Hz) or cycles per second, between 20 and 120 Hz. At lower rates the patient feels more of a thumping, whereas at higher Hz the feeling is more of a buzzing. Electrode selection is a complex topic that has been the subject of research by Barolat and colleagues, who provided mapping data of coverage patterns based on lead location in 106 patients.[37] The primary target is the cathode (−), with electrons flowing from the cathode(s) (−) to the anode(s) (+). The newest stimulator systems allow for partial anode and cathode arrangements at different contacts, which have been termed "current steering." This expands the ability to cover most painful areas with a well-placed lead or leads and makes the number of possible configurations available for programming almost infinite. Thus, a programming strategy is important, and each company has developed computer-assisted programming to narrow down the possible choices. Most patients' stimulators are programmed with electrode selection changes until the patient obtains anatomic coverage, then the pulse width and rate are adjusted for maximal comfort. The patient is left with full control to (1) turn the stimulator on and off, (2) choose between numerous programs in the device (which have different effects), and (3) adjust the intensity of stimulation up and down for comfort.

The lowest acceptable settings on all parameters are generally used to conserve battery life unless using the newer rechargeable systems. Other programming modes that save battery life include a cycling mode during which the stimulator cycles full on and off at patient-determined intervals (minutes, seconds, or hours). The patient's programming may change over time, and reprogramming needs are common. The neurostimulator manufacturing companies help clinicians with patient reprogramming. Many busy pain practices designate a nurse practitioner or physician's assistant to handle patient reprogramming needs.

Box 69.2 Evidence Classification Scheme for a Therapeutic Intervention

Class I: An adequately powered prospective randomized controlled clinical trial with masked outcome assessment in a representative population or an adequately powered systematic review of prospective randomized controlled clinical trials with masked outcome assessment in representative populations. The following are required:

a. Randomization concealment
b. Primary outcome(s) is/are clearly defined
c. Exclusion/inclusion criteria are clearly defined
d. Adequate accounting for dropouts and crossovers with numbers sufficiently low to have minimal potential for bias
e. Relevant baseline characteristics are presented and substantially equivalent among treatment groups or there is appropriate statistical adjustment for differences

Class II: Prospective matched-group cohort study in a representative population with masked outcome assessment that meets a through e above or a randomized controlled trial in a representative population that lacks one criteria in a through e

Class III: All other controlled trials (including well-defined natural history controls or patients serving as own controls) in a representative population, where outcome assessment is independent of patient treatment

Class IV: Evidence from uncontrolled studies, case series, case reports, or expert opinion

Rating of Recommendations

Level A rating (established as effective, ineffective, or harmful) requires at least one convincing class I study or at least two consistent, convincing class II studies

Level B rating (probably effective, ineffective, or harmful) requires at least one convincing class II study or overwhelming class III evidence

Level C (possibly effective, ineffective, or harmful) rating requires at least two convincing class III studies

From Brainin M, Barnes M, Baron JC, et al. Guidance for the preparation of neurological management guidelines by EFNS [European Federation of Neurological Societies] scientific task forces: revised recommendations 2004. *Eur J Neurol* 2004;11:577-581.

OUTCOMES

The most common use for SCS in the United States is failed back surgery syndrome (FBSS), whereas in Europe, peripheral ischemia is the predominant indication. With respect to clinical outcomes, it makes sense to subdivide the outcomes based on diagnosis (Boxes 69.2 and 69.3). There have been prospective randomized controlled trials (RCTs) examining SCS therapy in FBSS, CRPS, angina, and peripheral vascular disease (PVD) meeting Class II evidence requirements. However, in a review of the available SCS literature, most evidence falls within the Class III (limited) category, as a result

Box 69.3 Spinal Cord Stimulation by Disease

Failed back surgery syndrome. Level A (favorable pain relief, functional capacity, health-related quality of life, and return to work all favorably affected)
Complex regional pain syndrome. Level B (favorable global perceived effect, pain reduction, and a variety of other quality of life/disability measures)
Peripheral ischemia. Level A (favorable limb salvage rates and quality of life measures)
Angina pectoris. Level A (fewer anginal attacks, lower nitrate requirements, improved exercise capacity and equivalent cardiovascular outcomes to revision coronary bypass surgery, and lower complication rate—no meta-analysis done)

of the invasiveness of the modality and difficulties inherent in blinding treatment with SCS, because much of the available literature used older technologies. Recognition must also be given to the time frame within which a study was performed because of rapidly evolving SCS technology. Basic science knowledge, implantation techniques, lead placement locations, contact array designs, and programming capabilities have changed dramatically from the time of the first implants. These improvements have led to decreased morbidity and a much greater probability of obtaining adequate paresthesia coverage with subsequent improved outcomes.[27] For these reasons the literature on SCS outcomes is limited to year 2000 to the present day. Coffey and Lozano,[38] among others,[39] called for future study designs to include unambiguous entry criteria, randomization, parallel control groups receiving sham treatment, and blinding of patients, investigators, and programmers. They also suggested a minimum follow-up time of 1 year for chronic pain conditions, with a Kaplan-Meier–type analysis of ongoing pain relief.[38,40]

SPINAL CORD STIMULATION OUTCOMES: FAILED BACK SURGERY SYNDROME

Cruccu and the European Federation of Neurological Societies (EFNS) reviewed this topic extensively and found significant supportive literature for SCS in the patient with FBSS.[41] Other reviews have similar results and specifically pointed out sufficient evidence for sustained long-term pain relief with medication reduction, improvement in quality of life, increased ability to return to work, increased patient satisfaction, minimal side effects, and cost-effectiveness compared with alternative therapies.[42] Further advantages noted include the trial period for SCS, which limits treatment failures, and the reversibility of the technique.

There has been one prospective randomized study looking specifically at reoperation versus SCS in patients with FBSS as well as others that are under way.[19,43] North and associates[19] selected 51 patients as candidates for repeat laminectomy. All the patients had undergone previous surgery and were excluded from randomization if they presented with severe spinal canal stenosis, extremely large disk fragments, a major neurologic deficit such as footdrop, or radiographic evidence of gross instability. In addition, patients were excluded for untreated dependency on narcotic analgesics or benzodiazepines, major psychiatric comorbidity, the presence of any significant or disabling chronic pain problem, or a chief complaint of low back pain exceeding lower extremity pain. Crossover between groups was permitted. The 6-month follow-up report included 27 patients. At this point they became eligible for crossover. Of the 15 patients who had undergone reoperation, 67% (10 patients) crossed over to SCS. Of the 12 who had undergone SCS, 17% (2 patients) opted for crossover to reoperation. For 90% of the patients, long-term (3-year follow-up) evaluation has shown that spinal cord stimulation continues to be more effective than reoperation, with significantly better outcomes for SCS. Overall, 47% of patients in the SCS group achieved 50% or greater pain relief compared with 12% in the reoperation group ($p < 0.01$). Additionally, patients randomized to reoperation used significantly more opioids than those randomized to spinal cord stimulation. Other measures assessing activities of daily living and work status did not differ significantly.[32]

More recently, Kumar and colleagues published a study examining the real-world comparison of SCS therapy versus conventional medical management (CMM) in patients with FBSS.[20] One hundred FBSS patients with predominant leg pain of neuropathic radicular origin received spinal cord stimulation plus conventional medical management or conventional medical management alone for at least 6 months. In the intention-to-treat analysis at 6 months, 24 SCS patients (48%) and 4 CMM patients (9%) ($p < 0.001$) achieved the primary outcome of 50% pain reduction. Compared with the CMM group, the SCS group experienced improved leg and back pain relief, quality of life, and functional capacity, as well as greater treatment satisfaction. Between 6 and 12 months, 5 SCS patients crossed to CMM, and 32 CMM patients crossed to SCS. In a 2-year follow-up study of these same patients, Kumar and colleagues noted that the 42 patients continuing SCS (of 52 randomized to SCS) reported significantly improved leg pain relief, quality of life, and functional capacity. At 24 months, 46 of 52 patients randomized to SCS and 41 of 48 randomized to CMM remained in the study, and the primary outcome was achieved by 17 (37%) randomized to SCS versus 1 (2%) to CMM and by 34 of 72 patients who received SCS (including crossovers) as final treatment versus 1 (7%) of 15 for CMM. In subsequent analysis of secondary measures, it was noted that SCS improved health related quality of life measures up to the last time point examined at 24 months following implantation.[44]

In an effort to identify those patients who are likely to benefit from SCS therapy, Turner and colleagues undertook a prospective cohort trial that examined the success of SCS therapy in patients receiving workers'compensation insurance.[18] They examined patients who received at least a trial of SCS ($n = 51$) versus those who (1) were evaluated at a multidisciplinary pain clinic and did not receive SCS ($n = 39$) or (2) received neither SCS nor a pain clinic evaluation ($n = 68$). Patients then completed measures of pain, function, medication use, and work status at baseline and 6, 12, and 24 months later. The most important finding of this study was that very few (< 10%) patients in any group achieved success at any follow-up on the composite primary outcome (reduced daily opioid use, reduced leg pain, and improved overall function). At 6 months, the SCS group showed modestly greater improvement in leg pain and function, but with higher rates of daily opioid use. These differences were not present at 12 months. Patients who received a permanent spinal cord stimulator did not differ from patients who received some pain clinic treatment on the primary outcome at any follow-up, and 19% had them removed within 18 months. The authors concluded that there is no evidence for greater effectiveness of SCS versus alternative treatments in the workers' compensation FBSS population after 6 months. Unfortunately, this study suffered from numerous design flaws, author biases, and patient inclusion flaws as criticized in subsequent publications.[39,45] The most substantial finding in this study may be that patients in these clinics did not improve no matter what therapy they received, which is not consistent with the remainder of the literature in patients with FBSS treated in other clinics.

SPINAL CORD STIMULATION OUTCOMES: COMPLEX REGIONAL PAIN SYNDROME

Research of high quality regarding SCS and CRPS is limited, but existing data are positive in terms of pain reduction, quality of life, analgesic use, and function. Kemler and colleagues published a prospective randomized comparative trial to compare SCS versus conservative therapy for CRPS.[21] Patients with a 6-month history of CRPS of the upper extremities were randomized to undergo trial SCS (and implant if successful) plus physiotherapy versus physiotherapy alone. In this study, 36 patients were assigned to receive a standardized physical therapy program together with SCS, whereas 18 patients were assigned to receive therapy alone. In 24 of the 36 patients randomized to spinal cord stimulation along with physical therapy, the trial was successful, and permanent implantation was performed. At a 6-month follow-up assessment, the patients in the spinal cord stimulation group had a significantly greater reduction in pain, and a significantly higher percentage rated themselves as "much improved" for the global perceived effect. However, there were no clinically significant improvements in functional status. The authors concluded that in the short term, spinal cord stimulation reduces pain and improves the quality of life for patients with CRPS involving the upper extremities. A subsequent publication including a 2-year follow-up of the same patients showed durability of these positive findings in SCS.[46] The 5-year follow-up data had such significant patient dropout rates to render the positive and negative findings essentially meaningless.[47]

Taylor performed a meta-analysis on the use of SCS to treat CRPS and concluded that level A (the highest level) evidence is available supporting the use of SCS to treat CRPS.[48] Stanton-Hicks recently expanded upon the usefulness on SCS in the treatment of CRPS in the context of an overall treatment strategy, which included analgesics, physiotherapy, psychological therapies, and other interventions in a time-contingent manner because of the progressive debility of untreated or undertreated CRPS, stressing a step up in the aggressiveness of therapy every 12 to 16 weeks in the face of lack of response.[49] This treatment algorithm is from a 2002 consensus panel and review of the literature (Fig. 69.5).[50]

SPINAL CORD STIMULATION OUTCOMES: PERIPHERAL ISCHEMIA AND ANGINA

Cook and associates reported in 1976 that SCS effectively relieved pain associated with peripheral ischemia.[51] This result has been repeated and noted to have particular efficacy in conditions associated with vasospasm such as Raynaud's disease.[52] Many studies have shown impressive efficacy of SCS to treat intractable angina.[53] Reported success rates are consistently high and these indications, already widely used in other countries, are certain to expand within the United States. SCS increases distal extremity skin temperature. The beneficial effects of SCS on the ischemic limb are attributed to an improvement in the microcirculatory status of the limb, as the nutritional health of the skin and nerves is dependent on this microcirculatory blood flow. Microvascular perfusion is measured by multiple methods; the most sensitive is the transcutaneous partial pressure of oxygen ($TcPO_2$) measurement.[54] $TcPO_2$ is increased by sympathetic blockade or SCS therapy.[55] However, the relationship between pain relief and limb survival has not been demonstrated.

Ubbink and Vermeulen performed a meta-analysis on SCS for peripheral ischemia or critical leg ischemia (CLI).[56] The authors used Cochrane Review criteria for inclusion of an article into their analysis. They found nine reports describing six clinical trials, five of which were randomized. The overall sample size was 444 patients and a variety of end points were evaluated, but consistently the primary end point was limb salvage at 12 months. The limb amputation rate was 11% lower in the SCS group versus the conservative treatment group. Overall, SCS-treated patients showed higher quality-of-life indices and less analgesic consumption. Only two of these six trials used $TcPO_2$ measurements, which should lead to optimal outcomes. One of the latter trials suggested a $TcPO_2$ of less than 10 is likely to require amputation regardless of treatment, and a $TcPO_2$ of greater than 30 is likely to improve regardless of treatment. Further, that group advocates an increase in $TcPO_2$ of at least 10 mm Hg during the SCS trial.[54] By using these selection criteria, limb salvage rates approach 83% versus conservative care rates, which run between 20% and 64%. Thus, existent high-level grade A recommendation exists for the use of SCS in CLI. Further RCTs should show higher success rates (versus conservative therapy) based on the refined $TcPO_2$ selection criteria.

A European RCT of SCS in the treatment of nonreconstructable chronic critical leg ischemia (NR-CCLI) did not conclusively show prevention of major amputation of limbs in patients.[57] A subsequent European trial replicated this study but included measures of microvascular perfusion including $TcPO_2$.[58] The researchers again found no global improvement in limb salvage but found in a subgroup of patients with poor baseline (pre-SCS) microcirculation ($TcPO_2 < 10$ mm Hg), 78% of those who responded with increased $TcPO_2$ (delta > 20 mm Hg) with SCS therapy had improved wound healing and limb salvage.[58]

SCS has been used in the treatment of refractory angina pectoris states since first reported by Murphy and Giles in Australia.[59] It is estimated that millions of patients suffer refractory angina in spite of the endoluminal revascularization

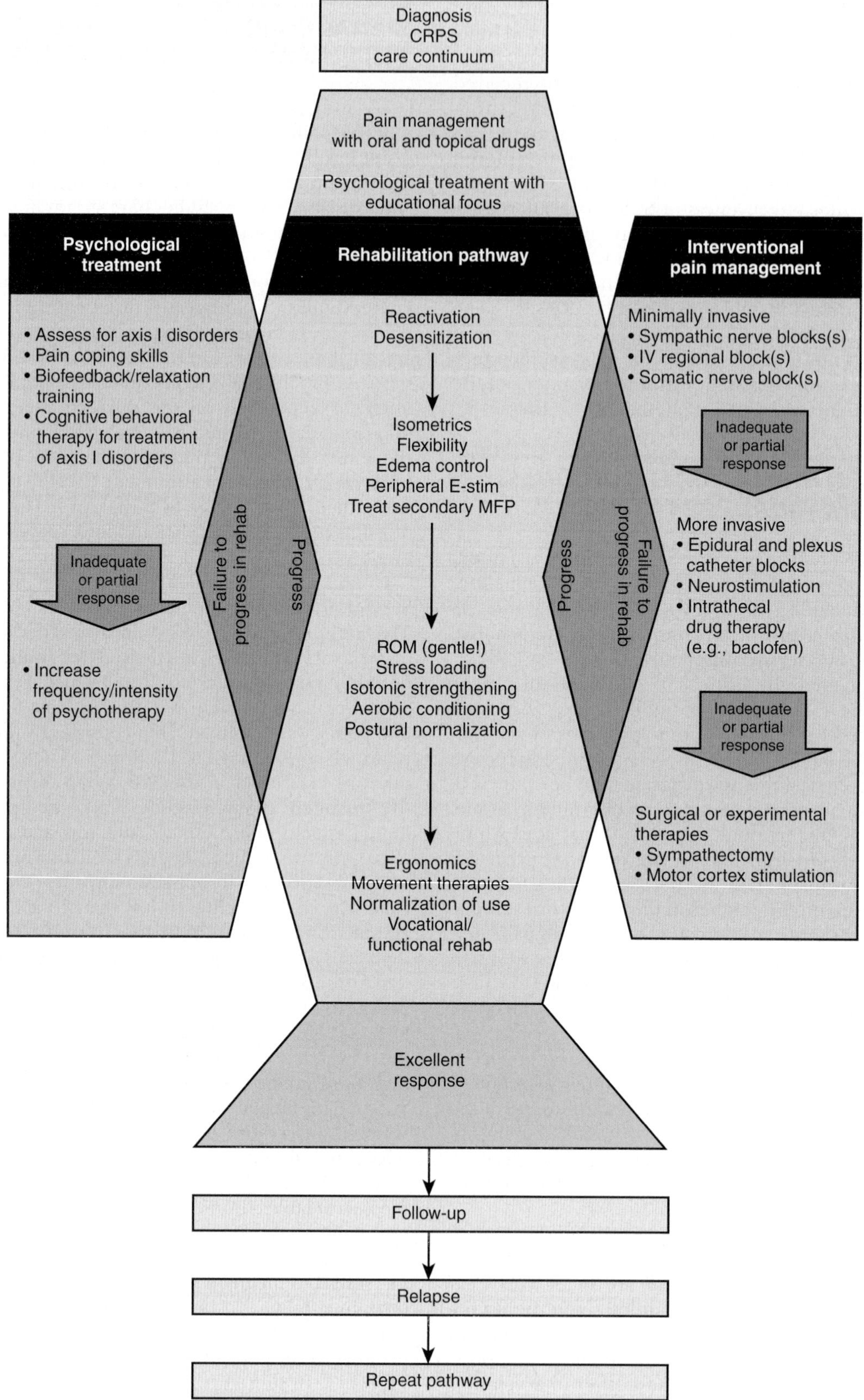

Figure 69.5 Treatment algorithm for complex regional pain syndrome (CRPS). IV, intravenous; MFP, myofascial pain; ROM, range of motion. (From Stanton-Hicks M, Burton AW, Bruehl SP, et al. An updated interdisciplinary clinical pathway for CRPS: report of an expert panel. *Pain Pract.* 2002;2:1-16.)

strategies currently used in clinical cardiology. Buchser and coworkers reviewed the topic, and in spite of numerous favorable studies, little support for this technique has been forthcoming in the cardiology realm.[60] The lead or leads are placed at the T1-2 level just to the left of midline with manipulation of the lead until the chest is covered with paresthesia in the usual anginal region. SCS has been shown to have similar efficacy to coronary bypass surgery in treating refractory angina, but with lower morbidity and mortality rates acutely.[61] The mechanism of action of SCS in the angina pectoris patient, as with the CLI patient, is a relief of the ischemia with a favorable shift of the oxygen supply and demand relationships.

Although SCS is thought to be effective in treating refractory angina (at least in Europe), blinded RCTs have been absent from the literature because of the perceived need for SCS-related chest paresthesia that has made placebo-controlled trials exceptionally difficult to perform. Lanza and associates circumvented this problem in an interesting model in which they examined subliminal (non-paresthetic) SCS on anginal pain in a small blinded RCT.[22] In this trial they compared subliminal SCS with paresthetic SCS and with sham SCS. After 1 month, no SCS patients (sham SCS, SCS implanted but not turned on) were randomized to either group (paresthetic SCS or subliminal SCS). After 1 month, changes in angina episodes ($p = 0.016$), nitroglycerin use ($p = 0.015$), angina class ($p = 0.02$), quality-of-life score ($p = 0.05$), and items 2 ($p = 0.008$) and 3 ($p = 0.009$) of the Seattle angina questionnaire differed significantly among groups. The group with paresthetic SCS showed significant improvement in outcomes compared to the group with no SCS, whereas there were no significant differences between the subliminal SCS group and the no SCS group. At 3 months, a significant difference between the paresthetic SCS group and the subliminal SCS group was observed in angina attacks ($p = 0.002$), but not in other variables. Thus, in this study, paresthetic, but not subliminal, SCS was superior to sham SCS in improving clinical status in refractory angina patients.[22]

COST-EFFECTIVENESS (IN U.S. DOLLARS)

The cost-effectiveness of SCS therapy has been a secondary outcome measure in the RCTs examining SCS therapy in CRPS and FBSS patients as well as economic models. North and colleagues examined the cost utility of the 2005 trial in which lumbar spine reoperation was compared to SCS therapy.[19] Three years after the initial trial, 13 of 21 patients (62%) crossed from reoperation to SCS versus 5 of 19 patients (26%) who crossed from SCS ($p < 0.025$) to reoperation. The mean cost per success was $117,901 for patients who crossed over to SCS. There were no crossovers to reoperation that achieved pain relief despite the mean per-patient expenditure of $260,584. Regardless of the success, the mean per-patient cost was $31,530 for SCS versus $38,160 for reoperation without crossover (intention to treat), and $48,357 for SCS versus $105,928 for reoperation with crossover (treated as intended). SCS was more effective and less expensive in the incremental cost-effectiveness ratios and incremental cost-utility ratios. Therefore, the authors concluded SCS was less expensive and more effective than reoperation in selected failed back-surgery syndrome patients and should be the initial therapy of choice. SCS is most cost-effective when patients forego repeat operation. Should SCS fail, reoperation is unlikely to succeed and should be discouraged.[62] This contrasts with the results from the analysis of the cohort study of workers' compensation patients with SCS treatment for FBSS.[18] Hollingworth and colleagues found that the mean medical cost per SCS patient over 24 months was $52,091.[63] This was $17,291 higher than in the group treated conservatively in a pain clinic and $28,128 higher than in the group treated by the group members' primary care physicians. Adjusting for baseline covariates, the mean total of medical and productivity loss costs per patient of the SCS group were $20,074 higher than those of the pain clinic group and $29,358 higher than those of the primary care group. The authors concluded that in the workers' compensation patient population, SCS was unlikely to be the most cost-effective intervention.[63] In an economic modeling study, Taylor used a decision analytic model to examine the cost-effectiveness of SCS versus conventional medical management and versus reoperation in patients with FBSS.[64] In this study the costs were from the National Health Service of Great Britain and the British pound has been converted into U.S. dollars. The incremental cost-effectiveness of SCS compared with medical management was ~$8000 per quality-adjusted life-year, with an 89% probability that SCS is cost-effective at a willingness-to-pay threshold of ~$31,300. Compared with reoperation, the incremental cost-effectiveness of SCS was ~$10,000 per quality-adjusted life-year, with an 82% probability of cost-effectiveness at the ~$31,300 threshold.

In 2002 Kumar and colleagues evaluated the cost-effectiveness of SCS (in the treatment of chronic back pain).[65] They prospectively followed 104 patients with FBSS. Of the 104 patients, 60 were implanted with a spinal cord stimulator using a standard selection criterion. Both groups were monitored over 5 years. The annual cost for the stimulation group was $29,000 versus $38,000 for the control group. The authors found that 15% returned to work in the stimulation group versus 0% in the control group. The higher costs in the nonstimulator group were in the categories of medications, emergency center visits, x-rays, and ongoing physician visits.

Kemler and Furnee performed a similar study but looked at "chronic reflex sympathetic dystrophy (RSD)" using outcomes and costs of care before and after the start of treatment.[66] This essentially is an economic analysis of the outcomes paper. Fifty-four patients with chronic RSD were randomized to receive either SCS together with physical therapy (SCS + PT; $n = 36$) or physical therapy alone (PT; $n = 18$). Twenty-four SCS and PT patients responded positively to trial stimulation and underwent SCS implantation. During 12 months of follow-up, costs (routine SCS, out of pocket) and effects (pain relief by visual analog scale [VAS], health-related quality of life [HRQL] improvement by EuroQol [EQ]-5D) were assessed in both groups. Analyses were carried out up to 1 year and up to the expected time of death. SCS was both more effective and less costly than the standard treatment protocol. As a result of the high initial costs of SCS, in the first year, the treatment per patient was $4000 more than control therapy. However, in the lifetime analysis, SCS per patient was $60,000 cheaper than control therapy. In addition, at 12 months, SCS resulted in pain relief (SCS + PT [−2.7] versus PT [0.4] [$p < 0.001$]) and improved HRQL (SCS + PT [0.22] versus PT [0.03] [$p = 0.004$]). The authors found SCS to be both more

Box 69.4 Principles of Neurostimulation

- The mechanism of action for spinal cord stimulation (SCS) is not completely understood but influences multiple components and levels within the central nervous system (CNS) with both interneuron and neurochemical mechanisms.
- SCS therapy is effective for many neuropathic pain conditions. The entire painful area may experience stimulation-evoked paresthesia.
- Stimulation should be applied with low intensity, just suprathreshold for the activation of the low-threshold, large-diameter fibers, and should be of nonpainful intensity. To be effective, SCS must be applied continuously (or in cycles) for at least 20 minutes before the onset of analgesia. This analgesia develops slowly and typically lasts several hours after cessation of the stimulation.
- SCS has demonstrated clinical benefit and cost-effectiveness in limb ischemia, failed back surgery syndrome (FBSS), and complex regional pain syndrome (CRPS). Clinical effectiveness also has been shown in angina pectoris and occipital neuralgia, with favorable preliminary reports in visceral pain states.
- Multicontact, multiprogram systems improve outcomes and reduce the incidence of surgical revisions. The role of the paddle versus percutaneous leads is uncertain with islands of support for each.
- Anchoring technique is one of the most important skills to obtain. Two of the three SCS companies now have anchoring systems that lock the lead to the anchor, reducing the risk of lead migration within the anchor.
- Serious complications are exceedingly rare but can be devastating. Meticulous care must be taken during implantation to minimize procedural complications. The most frequent complications are lead breakage or migration (approximately 13% for permanent percutaneous leads and higher for paddle leads) and wound infections (approximately 3% or less).
- The frequent need for revision procedures as outlined in this chapter is important in many ways. Although the revision procedures entail relatively minimal risk, there are numerous costs and risks for the patient and health system. The patient's analgesia is interrupted, entailing the expense and time of lost work or productivity, increased medication use, SCS hardware expenses, operative expenses, and other direct costs. Correction of this high hardware failure rate must be addressed in future technology systems in the face of increased scrutiny over shrinking health care resources if this expensive therapy is to remain a viable choice.
- One of the greatest threats to the viability of this therapy is the cost of the therapy and the poor selection of appropriate patients. Poor selection results in a low trial to permanent ratio that imposes huge costs to the health care system with no benefit to the patient. A trial to permanent ratio should be on the order of 75%. Trial to permanent ratios below 50% should be empirically examined.

effective and less expensive compared with the standard treatment protocol for chronic RSD.

PERIPHERAL, CORTICAL, AND DEEP BRAIN STIMULATION

Although this chapter concentrates on the SCS technique, it must be noted that neurostimulation can be used successfully at other locations in the peripheral and central nervous systems to provide analgesia.

Peripheral nerve stimulation was introduced by Wall and Sweet as well as others in the mid-1960s.[67] This technique has shown efficacy for peripheral nerve injury pain syndromes as well as CRPS, with the use of a carefully implanted paddle lead using a fascial graft to help anchor the lead without traumatizing the nerve.[68] There are numerous potential applications for peripheral nerve stimulation including occipital, supratrochlear, supraorbital, ilioinguinal, genitofemoral nerves, and sacral nerve roots; however, the level of evidence for this technique has not exceeded class III.[69] Good blinded RCTs in this domain are essential to continue this work.

Motor cortex and deep brain stimulation have been explored to treat highly refractory neuropathic pain syndromes including central pain, deafferentation syndromes, trigeminal neuralgia, and others.[70] Deep brain stimulation (DBS) has become a widely used technique for movement disorders and much less so for painful indications, although there have been many case reports on treating highly refractory central pain syndromes.[71] Unfortunately, a multicenter study, promoted by the Food and Drug Administration (FDA), showed negative results of DBS therapy in the treatment of neuropathic pain.[72] These findings hinder the use of DBS in clinical practice in the United States, leaving only class III level evidence for DBS for phantom limb pain, trigeminal neuralgia, and other peripheral nerve pain syndromes. Motor cortex stimulation for the treatment of pain is supported by several blinded RCTs (Class I evidence) including the most recent trial in 2009.[73] This trial involved 16 patients who had neuropathic pain related to peripheral lesions. Patients were followed up for 12 months and evaluated by VAS, brief pain inventory (BPI), McGill Pain Questionnaire (MPQ), and Sickness Impact Profile scores. VAS and Sickness Impact Profile scores had significantly improved by 1 year postimplantation.[73]

CONCLUSION

Spinal cord stimulation is an invasive, interventional surgical procedure that is useful in refractory chronic pain syndromes. Meyerson and Linderoth have proposed principles of neurostimulation that are cornerstones of SCS theory and practice (Box 69.4).[74,75] The evidence for spinal cord stimulation in properly selected populations with neuropathic pain states is good to moderate. The evidence for SCS therapy in the FBSS patient population (who are not covered by workers' compensation) supports a level A recommendation. The evidence for CRPS supports a level B recommendation, and the evidence for critical limb ischemia and angina is Class I and supports a level A recommendation. However, this therapy should be reserved for patients who have failed more conservative therapies and who are extremely well selected and educated regarding the goals and expectations of therapy. With appropriate selection and careful attention to technical issues, the clinical results are overwhelmingly positive. It is now time to focus on providing evidence of quality of life and overall function improvement with this therapy.

KEY POINTS

- Shealy implanted the first spinal cord stimulator device for the treatment of chronic pain in 1967.
- Stimulation of either the dorsal horn or dorsal nerve roots at intensity and frequency to selectively activate Aβ fibers reduced the spontaneous firing of wide dynamic range (WDR) neurons in animals with neuropathic injuries. This same stimulation reduced WDR responses to mechanical stimulation of normal and injured animals. Stimulation of the dorsal columns, but not the dorsal root, reduces activity-dependent neuronal excitability (wind-up).
- Patient selection is the most challenging and important step in the decision to offer neurostimulation.
- Appropriate patients for a trial of neurostimulation must meet the following criteria: (1) the diagnosis is amenable to this therapy (e.g., neuropathic pain syndromes), (2) the patient has failed conservative therapy, and (3) significant psychological issues have been ruled out.
- Schedule a 5- to 8- day trial and encourage patients to be as active as possible in their usual environment, with the exception of limiting bending and twisting movements.
- A spinal cord stimulator system is made up of three parts: (1) electrodes or leads, (2) implantable pulse generators (IPGs) or the battery, and (3) the charging and programming systems.
- Most consider 50% or more pain relief to indicate a successful trial, although the ultimate decision should include other factors such as activity level and medication intake. Some combination of pain relief, increased activity level, and decreased medication intake indicates a favorable trial.
- SCS is a cost-effective treatment modality for patients with radicular and back/neck pain following spine surgery (FBSS).

KEY POINTS—cont'd

- SCS is a cost-effective treatment modality for patients with neuropathic pain of an extremity (e.g., complex regional pain syndrome [CRPS]).
- SCS (or neuromodulation) is effective in the treatment of pain associated with angina, peripheral vascular disease, and occipital neuralgia.

SUGGESTED READINGS

Guan Y, Wacnik PW, Yang F, et al. Spinal cord stimulation-induced analgesia: electrical stimulation of dorsal column and dorsal roots attenuates dorsal horn neuronal excitability in neuropathic rats. *Anesthesiology*. 2010;113:1392-1405.

Kemler MA, Barendse GA, van Kleef M, et al. Spinal cord stimulation in patients with chronic reflex sympathetic dystrophy. *N Engl J Med.* 2000;343:618-624.

Kemler MA, Furnee CA. Economic evaluation of spinal cord stimulation for chronic reflex sympathetic dystrophy. *Neurology*. 2002;59:1203-1209.

Kumar K, Taylor RS, Jacques L, et al. Spinal cord stimulation versus conventional medical management for neuropathic pain: a multicentre randomised controlled trial in patients with failed back surgery syndrome. *Pain.* 2007;132:179-188.

Lame IE, Peters ML, Patijn J, et al. Can the outcome of spinal cord stimulation in chronic complex regional pain syndrome type I patients be predicted by catastrophizing thoughts? *Anesth Analg.* 2009;109:592-599.

Lanza GA, Grimaldi R, Greco S, et al. Spinal cord stimulation for the treatment of refractory angina pectoris: a multicenter randomized single-blind study (the SCS-ITA trial). *Pain.* 2011;152:45-52.

Melzack R, Wall PD. Pain mechanisms: a new theory. *Science.* 1965;150: 971-979.

North RB, Kidd DH, Farrokhi F, et al. Spinal cord stimulation versus repeated lumbosacral spine surgery for chronic pain: a randomized controlled trial. *Neurosurgery*. 2005;56:98-107.

Turner JA, Hollingworth W, Comstock BA, et al. Spinal cord stimulation for failed back surgery syndrome: outcomes in a workers' compensation setting. *Pain.* 2010;148:14-25.

Ubbink DT, Vermeulen H. Spinal cord stimulation for critical leg ischemia: a review of effectiveness and optimal patient selection. *J Pain Symptom Manage.* 2006;31:S30-S35.

The references for this chapter can be found at www.expertconsult.com.

A Appendix

NEUROSTIMULATOR COMPANIES

- Medtronic, Inc., 710 Medtronic Parkway, Minneapolis, MN 55432-5604; 763-514-5604; www.medtronic.com.
- St. Jude Medical, Inc., 6501 Windcrest Drive, Ste. 100, Plano, TX 75024; 800-727-7846. www.sjm.com.
- Boston Scientific, Corp. 25129 Rye Canyon Loop, Valencia, CA 91355; 800-678-2575; www.bostonscientific.com/home.bsci.

70

Intrathecal Drug Delivery: Patient Selection, Trialing, and Implantation

Timothy Furnish | Mark S. Wallace

Intrathecal drug delivery for the treatment of pain is an outgrowth of pioneering research into spinal cord mechanisms and receptors that modulate nociceptive signal transmission to and within the central nervous system. Starting in the 1970s, researchers identified the peptide substance P in small dorsal root ganglion cells[1] and observed that opiates with a spinal action would produce selective analgesia.[2] These findings as well as the observation that substance P release evoked from C fibers is blocked by morphine[3] marked the beginning of the current trend toward focusing on the selective regulation of spinal afferent processing. Since then, there has been much research in this area, leading to widespread use of intrathecal therapy to treat chronic intractable pain. Although this therapy has proven to be extremely beneficial to many patients, it is also associated with high costs, high maintenance, and risks requiring careful patient selection. This chapter focuses on the patient selection, technologies used for chronic intrathecal drug delivery, system implantation, and troubleshooting.

INTRASPINAL DRUG DELIVERY TECHNIQUES

There are essentially three methods of intraspinal drug delivery: (1) externalized systems, (2) partially externalized systems, and (3) totally implanted systems. The selection of the technique will depend on the goal of therapy, ranging from short-term intrathecal trialing to long-term therapy to treat chronic pain. Each technique has associated risks and costs, which are taken into account when selecting the technique.

EXTERNALIZED SYSTEMS

An externalized intrathecal catheter is the most widely used technique for trialing intrathecal drugs. Such a system is designed for short-term (hours to days) use but has been successfully used for longer-term delivery in the terminally ill (weeks to months). The use of an externalized catheter raises the concern for a local infection at the catheter exit site or that the catheter may serve as a conduit for either epidural or intrathecal spread of infection. Using strict aseptic technique for catheter insertion can minimize the risk of insertion site infection, and the placement of a chlorhexidine impregnated catheter patch at the insertion site further reduces this risk (Fig. 70.1). There is no evidence that systemic antibiotics prevent these infections. In the terminally ill patient, the risk-benefit ratio may favor the use of an externalized catheter for intrathecal drug delivery. Some practitioners tunnel these catheters under the skin for some distance to provide stability and reduce the likelihood of inadvertent catheter withdrawal. Currently, the U.S. Food and Drug Administration (FDA) has not approved any externalized intrathecal catheters, and it is common to use epidural or lumbar drain catheters for this purpose.

PARTIALLY EXTERNALIZED SYSTEMS

Partially externalized systems are those in which the intrathecal catheter is tunneled and connected to a subcutaneous port. A needle then accesses the port percutaneously and medication is delivered with tubing connected to an external pump. Compared to an externalized system, this permits greater patient freedom of movement and reduces the risk of inadvertent catheter removal. Partially externalized systems are intended for single bolus injections. There continues to be a risk of colonization and infection of the port pocket with prolonged or repeated needle access. These systems have limited application for long-term, continuous intrathecal drug delivery.

IMPLANTED INTRATHECAL INFUSION PUMPS

Totally implanted systems are those with both the catheter and pump system completely internalized by surgical implantation. They have the advantages of a lower risk of infection, potential for long-term use, and much greater freedom of movement for the patient. The totally implanted systems are more expensive and require a more invasive surgical procedure than the externalized or partially externalized systems. Although it is generally recommended that implanted pumps be reserved for patients with a life expectancy of greater than 6 months, this therapy may improve quality of life in patients with life expectancy as low as 2 to 3 months. However, patients with a life expectancy of less than 6 months should be carefully selected.

There are two main types of intrathecal infusion systems, fixed-rate and variable-rate programmable pumps. All implanted pumps have two percutaneous access ports. One port is for refilling the drug reservoir, and there is a separate intrathecal catheter access port for bolus injection through, or aspiration from, the catheter. The

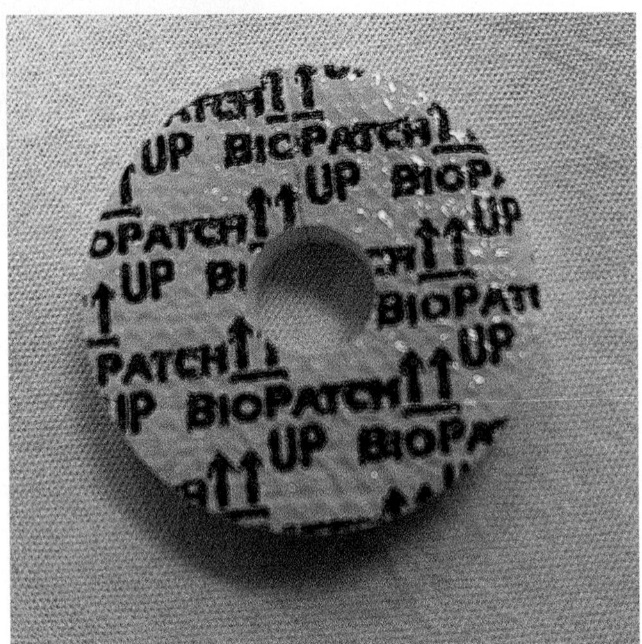

Figure 70.1 Chlorhexidine impregnated patch, BioPatch, Johnson & Johnson.

infusion systems are generally implanted in the lower abdominal subcutaneous fat and connected to a catheter, which is tunneled subcutaneously around the abdominal wall into the intrathecal space.[4,5] However, the pumps may also be implanted subcutaneously in the lower back in rare, selected patients (see the discussion that follows). The septum puncture life of the percutaneous refill port is very high: 500 punctures for the most commonly used, Medronic Synchromed II, pump. It would be unlikely to reach this number of punctures during the life of the pump (7 years for the Synchromed II).[6]

The first intrathecal pump, manufactured by Shiley Infusaid, became commercially available in 1982.[7] The Infusaid and other early pumps were nonprogrammable fixed-rate infusion systems. These pumps were simple devices without batteries, in which pressurized gas pushes the drug from a reservoir through a valve and into the catheter. The chief advantage of these pumps is simplicity of design and lack of batteries. Unfortunately, they are unable to vary the dose delivered without changing the concentration of drug in the reservoir. Currently the Codman 3000 (Fig. 70.2) is the only fixed-rate infusion pump on the market in the United States and is no longer used with significant frequency. The pump is available in three sizes (16, 30, and 50 mL reservoir), and each size is available in three flow rates. The low and medium flow rates are 0.5 and 1 mL/day, respectively, for all sizes. The high flow rates are 1.3, 1.7, and 3.4 mL/day, respectively, for the 16, 30, and 50 mL pumps. The flow rate is controlled by a flow restrictor. Flow rates may vary for different drugs, drug combinations, and especially with high drug concentrations, based on differences in viscosity.[8] In addition, changes in body temperature and atmospheric pressure will change flow rate by affecting the gas pressure within the system.

Programmable pumps, on the other hand, allow the clinician to vary infusion rates to increase or decrease the dose without changing the concentration of the drug or drugs in the pump. The original programmable pump was the Medtronic

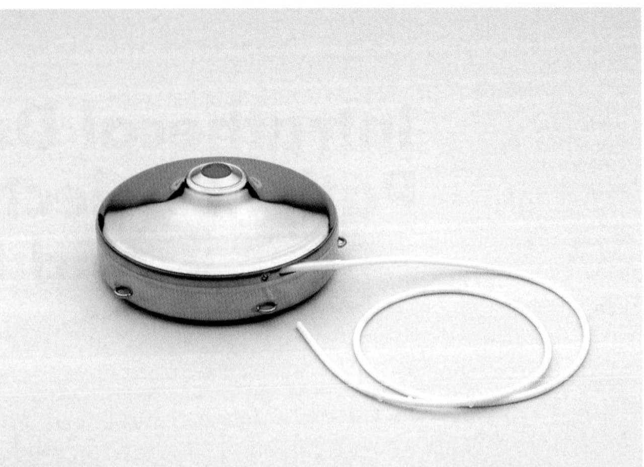

Figure 70.2 Codman 3000 fixed-rate infusion pump, Codman & Shurtleff, Inc.

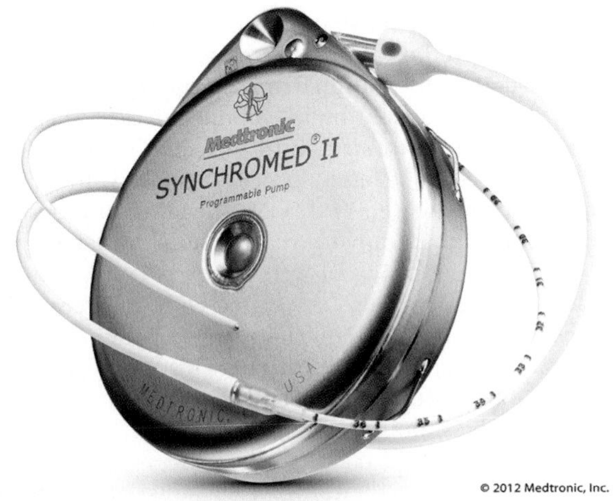

Figure 70.3 Syncromed II intrathecal pump, Medtronic, Inc.

Synchromed, first introduced in 1991.[9] More recent programmable pumps such as the Medtronic Synchromed II (Fig. 70.3) allow patient-controlled intrathecal bolus dosing via a remote control device. The Synchromed II uses a peristaltic roller system (Fig. 70.4) to move the drug from the reservoir to the implanted intrathecal catheter. The Synchromed II is available in a 20-mL and a 40-mL reservoir size and is FDA approved for baclofen, morphine, and ziconotide.

In 2012, the FDA gave marketing approval for the Flowonix Prometra implantable pump (Fig. 70.5). This device uses a pressurized gas chamber as the driving force. Unlike the older fixed-rate infusion pumps, a programmable flow-metering valve allows for a variable drug delivery rate.[10] The Prometra pump's low energy requirement is its main advantage. Since the batteries are used to control the electronics only, not to pump the drug, the battery has a 10-year life span before the need to surgically replace the pump. The Prometra is available in a 20-mL reservoir and is FDA approved for morphine. The issues with variable flow resulting from viscosity, temperature, and residual reservoir volume have been addressed by the advanced flow-metering valve.

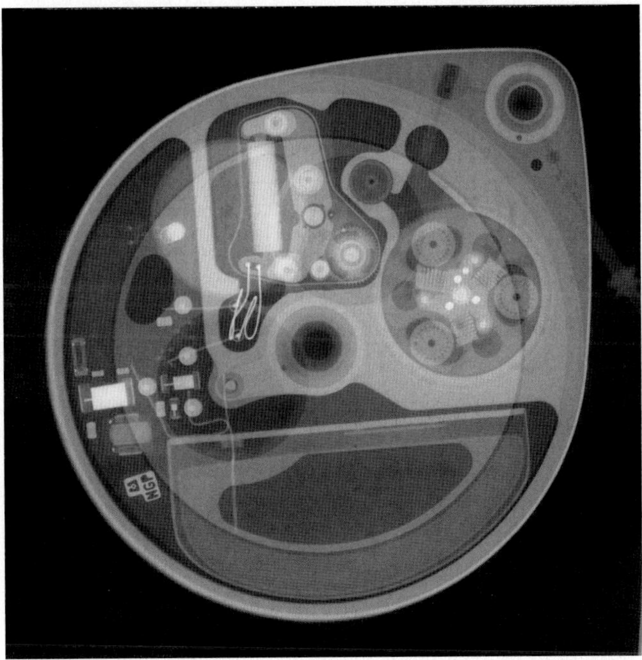

Figure 70.4 Synchromed II internal structures, Medtronic, Inc.

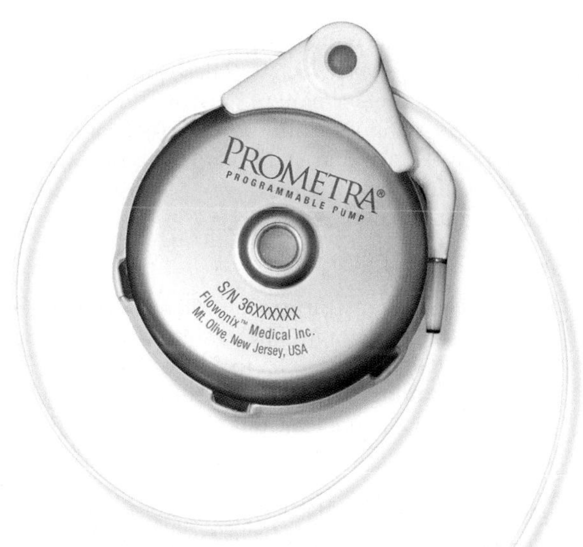

Figure 70.5 Prometra intrathecal pump, Flowonix, Inc.

The MedStream Programmable Infusion System is another implantable device currently FDA approved only for the delivery of intrathecal baclofen (Fig. 70.6). This implantable drug delivery system offers improved catheter technology and pump durability. Its intrathecal catheter has been designed to resist kinking and tearing (similar to the newest Medtronic catheters). The MedStream uses compressed gas as the driving force and a ceramic drive flow valve system to maintain the infusion rate. The pump has either a 20-mL or a 40-mL reservoir and measures 76 mm by 21.6 mm (20 mL) or 28.2 mm (40 mL).[11,12]

The Medallion is an implantable drug delivery system currently in clinical trials. The Medallion system offers safety improvements with the use of a negative pressure reservoir.

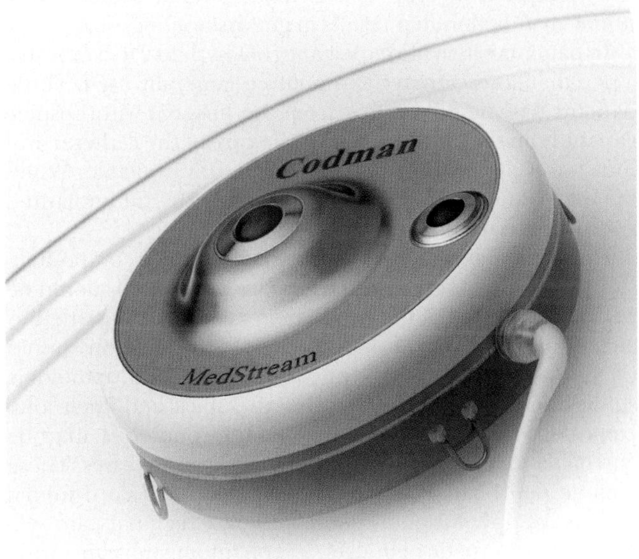

Figure 70.6 MedStream Programmable Infusion Pump, Codman & Shurtleff, Inc.

The negative pressure draws medication from the syringe during pump refills rather than requiring positive pressure from the syringe plunger. This reduces the risk of inadvertent injection into the pump pocket rather than the pump reservoir. The Medallion will be available in either a 20- or a 40-mL reservoir.[12]

PATIENT SELECTION

PAIN TYPE

Intrathecal drug delivery systems (IDDSs) are reserved for treating severe and refractory pain in two types of patients: those with cancer pain and those with noncancer pain who have failed more conservative therapies.[13] The cost and invasive nature of IDDSs necessitate a careful evaluation to determine whether each individual patient is appropriate and likely to achieve benefit. A thorough assessment includes an evaluation of pain-generating pathology, medical comorbidities, psychosocial issues, patient compliance history, economic and health care coverage, and anatomic and technical considerations.[14]

In advanced stages of cancer, the prevalence of pain exceeds 60%. One third of those patients report moderate to severe pain.[15] Comprehensive medical management (CMM) can significantly reduce pain and manage the adverse effects of opioids and other analgesics.[16] Despite aggressive therapy, however, some patients continue to endure severe pain. Others are unable to tolerate systemic opioids due to toxicity. A 2002 multicenter randomized trial compared CMM alone versus CMM plus an IDDS. They found that cancer patients receiving CMM plus an IDDS had reduced pain, fewer drug toxicities, and prolonged survival compared to controls.[17] Patients with significant toxicity or with refractory pain that has been inadequately controlled by the systemic administration of opioids and other analgesics are potential candidates for an IDDS.[18] Intrathecal therapy may be especially valuable in patients with neuropathic pain from tumor invasion of neural plexuses, unstable pathologic fractures, painful impending spinal cord compression, and visceral tumors with or without autonomic dysfunction that results in gut dysmotility.

In patients with a life expectancy of less than 2 to 3 months, a percutaneous catheter and pump is generally used. These patients may be discharged from the hospital with hospice care or home-health services for the care of the catheter and infusion if appropriate services are locally available. When life expectancy is greater than 3 to 6 months, an implanted system is generally recommended.[19,20]

For the patient with chronic noncancer pain, a comprehensive evaluation to establish the etiology of the pain should be performed as part of the decision process regarding whether an intrathecal pump is appropriate. The evaluation should include a detailed history, physical examination, radiologic studies, and assessment of prior therapies and their outcomes.[21] Many diagnoses and painful conditions may be amenable to intrathecal drug delivery in certain cases. These include neuropathic syndromes such as spinal cord injury, diabetic peripheral neuropathy, complex regional pain syndrome, postherpetic neuralgia, and phantom limb pain. Additionally, mixed nociceptive and neuropathic conditions such as postlaminectomy pain syndrome or chronic pancreatitis as well as nociceptive pain conditions such as chronic vertebral compression fractures and severe spinal degeneration may be appropriate for an IDDS in some circumstances.[14,21,22]

Implanted drug delivery therapy should be reserved for those patients who are refractory from more conservative treatment. A stepwise approach starting with the least invasive and costly therapies is recommended.[13,14] This may begin with exercise programs, relaxation techniques, and over-the-counter analgesics. Subsequent steps include adjuvant analgesics, muscle relaxants, physical therapy, and psychological therapies. More invasive therapies include neuraxial somatic and sympathetic blocks and spinal cord stimulation. More aggressive medication therapy can then be introduced with oral opioids. The top tier of this stepwise treatment pyramid is reserved for the most invasive therapies, including intrathecal drug delivery and neurodestructive procedures.[21,23] There are few controlled trials of intrathecal therapy for chronic *noncancer* pain, but observational studies suggest such therapy can provide pain relief in certain patients who have failed to achieve relief with more conservative treatments.[24,25] Determining the efficacy of long-term intrathecal drug therapy remains one of the greatest challenges in chronic noncancer pain management. One of the reasons for the lack of randomized controlled trials is that the high cost and invasiveness of such treatment pose ethical challenges in designing a double-blind, placebo-controlled study. Therefore, one can only rely on the retrospective reviews of patients receiving this therapy and attempt to make conclusions on the efficacy of this treatment. Many studies have attempted to determine the efficacy of long-term intrathecal morphine therapy based on classification of the pain. However, a review of these articles reveals large discrepancies in pain classification between studies. Because pain is often multifactorial (e.g., failed back syndrome versus HIV neuropathy versus complex regional pain syndrome), it is difficult to determine what pain syndromes are the most responsive to this therapy.

PATIENT COMORBIDITIES

The aging chronic pain patient may experience some of the same age-related comorbidities as any individual. Many of these comorbid conditions can complicate the implantation and use of an intrathecal pump. These medical issues and their potential interaction with intrathecal therapy must be considered during the patient selection process.

Diabetes Mellitus

Diabetes mellitus affects over 8% of the U.S. population and nearly 27% of those over the age of 65.[26] Patients with diabetes experience poor wound healing and suffer from an increased incidence of surgical site infections.[27] Implantable devices pose a special risk of surgical wound infections. With implantable intrathecal pumps, wound infections have been found to be the most common device-related complication.[28] Patients with diabetes, especially if blood glucose control is poor, should be counseled on the increased risk, and implanters should maintain extra vigilance for signs of site infections.

Anticoagulant Therapy

Anticoagulant therapy has become increasingly common as more indications for anticoagulation such as coronary artery stent placement have arisen. Additionally, newer anticoagulant therapies have improved management and dosing of anticoagulants. Patients on anticoagulant therapy are at increased risk of epidural hematoma formation after placement or removal of epidural or spinal catheters.[29,30] The American Society of Regional Anesthesia publishes guidelines regarding the performance of neuraxial injection and catheter placement with concomitant administration of anticoagulants (Fig. 70.7).[30] These guidelines do not specifically address the permanent implantation of intrathecal drug delivery systems. Scattered case reports of anticoagulant therapy restarted after implantation of intrathecal pumps offered no clear evidence for or against the safe use of intrathecal pumps in these patients.[14]

Infections

Any active infection puts the patient at high risk of seeding the pump with bacteria. The resulting pump pocket infection is virtually impossible to clear completely and will require explanting the entire pump and catheter system. Any active or chronic bacterial or fungal infectious

Drug/Dose	Hold Prior to Needle/Catheter Placement	Restart after Neuraxial Placement
Heparin SQ	1 hour	1 hour
Enoxaparin 40 mg SQ/day	12 hours	2 hours
Enoxaparin > 40 mg SQ/day	24 hours	2 hours
Warfarin	5 days & check INR < 1.3	Same day
NSAIDS/Aspirin	Not necessary	—
Clopidogrel (Plavix)	7 days	Same day
Ticlopidine (Ticlid)	14 days	Same day

Figure 70.7 Summary of American Society of Regional Anesthesia (ASRA) Neuraxial Analgesia Anticoagulation Guidelines. (From Horlocker T, Wedel D, Rowlingson J, et al. Regional anesthesia in the Society of Regional Anesthesia and Pain Medicine evidence-based guidelines (3rd ed.). *Reg Anesth Pain Med.* 2010;35:64-101.

process, particularly with noncancer pain patients, should be regarded as an absolute contraindication to implantation.

Pulmonary Disease

More than 18 million Americans have obstructive sleep apnea (OSA).[31] In addition to the risks of carbon dioxide retention and both systemic and pulmonary hypertension, the OSA patient has increased sensitivity to the respiratory depressant effects of opioids.[32] There are no studies of intrathecal opioid use in OSA patients. However, case reports suggest that chronic use of oral opioids in those with OSA may increase apnea duration and hypoxia severity.[32] Chronic obstructive pulmonary disease (COPD) also results in carbon dioxide retention and increased risk of respiratory depression with administration of opioids. A retrospective case-controlled study of postoperative COPD patients administered opioids found an increased risk of respiratory events (odds ratio [OR] 5.09; 95% confidence interval [CI]) compared to patients without chronic lung disease.[32] Most of these events occurred within 24 hours of surgery. The long-term risk of intrathecal opioid administration in patients with severe pulmonary disease is unknown. However, known risks of perioperative opioid administration in this population warrant careful monitoring during trialing as well as after implantation and initiation of therapy.

PSYCHOLOGICAL SCREENING

The Centers for Medicare and Medicaid Services require a psychological assessment prior to the implantation of spinal cord stimulator systems. No such requirement exists for IDDS. Although not required, it is widely accepted that a pre-procedure psychological assessment is warranted and is at least as important for appropriate patient selection for an IDDS as spinal cord stimulation.[13,14,20] Ideally, a psychological evaluation would aid in predicting positive response to an implantable therapy. In reality, there is limited evidence regarding the efficacy of psychological screening to predict long-term success. Much of the literature in this area concerns implantable spinal cord stimulators, and it is from this body of literature that guidelines regarding the use of psychological evaluation for IDDS have been extrapolated.[13,14,20]

The presence of suicidal or homicidal ideation, uncontrolled depression, active psychosis, severe cognitive deficits, and active drug abuse are absolute contraindications to implantation. In a study by Celestin and colleagues, certain psychological factors and traits were associated with poor analgesic outcome after implantation. These include somatization, depression, anxiety, and poor coping skills.[33] However, a study by Doleys and Brown found that those with mild abnormality on the Minnesota Multiphasic Personality Inventory (MMPI) personality profiles had better long-term analgesic efficacy than those with more normal scores.[34] Consensus guidelines have recommended the use of some form of psychological assessment in the selection process for IDDS candidates but caution against using the results to categorically rule out implantation in patients with psychological issues.[14]

The psychological evaluation should be used to identify factors that may affect the outcome of a trial or long-term therapy, either positively or negatively. In addition to identifying severe psychopathology, the screening examination can evaluate for cognitive deficits, coping mechanisms, social supports, patient expectations, and comprehension of treatment goals that may affect therapy. This screening may also identify the need for psychological treatment that can improve the outcome of therapy. The psychologist should not be asked to give "clearance" but rather act as an additional source of information as to whether IDDS therapy is appropriate, the patient has rational expectations, and this therapy is likely to succeed for an individual patient.

TRIALING

Some type of therapy trial prior to permanent system implantation has been commonly performed and is often required by insurance (Medicare). Trial options include a single bolus intrathecal injection, multiple bolus injections, or a continuous infusion via percutaneous intrathecal or epidural catheter. Unfortunately, there are no commonly accepted guidelines regarding how to perform a trial. Further, the data are limited, suggesting that trialing can accurately predict efficacy after implantation.[14] An expert consensus statement regarding guidelines for selection of patients for noncancer pain recently recommended against the requirement of a pre-implant trial because of the trial's unsubstantiated predictive value.[14]

The selection of a trialing method for noncancer pain will be made largely based on physician preference along with payer requirements. The majority of trials are performed in a hospital inpatient setting via epidural or intrathecal infusion. The advantage of epidural infusion is simplicity of catheter placement and a much lower risk of postdural puncture headache (PDPH). The development of a PDPH during trial may impair the patient's ability to determine the efficacy of the trial. An intrathecal trial more closely mimics the permanent implant conditions. Both of these options are more costly than single or multiple intrathecal injections. Although injections, whether single or multiple, provide simplicity with a low incidence of PDPH, they fail to mimic the chronic infusion conditions of a permanent implant.[14]

Trials for cancer pain are performed in a similar fashion. However, the lack of prognostic evidence for trials calls into question their value in patients with rapidly progressive disease near the end of life. According to one consensus guide to intrathecal therapy for cancer pain, the risks associated with the trial and delay of therapy may not outweigh the alleged prognostic benefits.[20] However, other experts have recommended the use of a trial in the event of cancer pain in order to give the patient and physician the opportunity to evaluate potential responses as well as possible side effects.[18]

Trials of baclofen therapy for spasticity are considerably more straightforward than those for cancer and noncancer pain. There are clear, objective outcome measures of spasticity that can be assessed to determine response. The commonly used criterion for a successful trial is a 2-point reduction on the Modified Ashworth Scale for grading spasticity (Fig. 70.8).[35,45] Patients may also demonstrate improvements in joint range of motion.

The baclofen trial consists of a bolus intrathecal injection of 25 to 50 mcg of baclofen and is performed in an outpatient setting. The onset of effect occurs in 1 to 3 hours and may last 6 to 8 hours.[36] The patient is then evaluated with serial examinations to determine response. If the patient fails to respond, the trial may be repeated on a subsequent day at a higher dose.

Ashworth Number	Description
0	No increase in muscle tone
1	Slight increase in tone manifested by a catch or minimal increased resistance at the end of ROM
1+	Slight increase in tone manifested by a catch followed by minimal resistance throughout the remainder of ROM
2	More marked increase in tone throughout ROM
3	Considerably increased tone, passive movement difficult
4	Affected part(s) rigid in flexion or extension

Figure 70.8 Modified Ashworth Scale for spasticity. ROM, range of motion. (From Bohannon RW, Smith MB. Interrater reliability of a modified Ashworth scale of muscle spasticity. *Phys Ther.* 1987;67:206-207.)

Most patients that reach the level of intrathecal therapy to treat chronic pain are on some amount of systemic opioids. It is controversial whether to detoxify patients off of the opioids prior to trialing. There are many advantages to detoxifying the patient prior to a trial. First, the drug holiday will provide the opportunity to observe the patient without the systemic opioids and allows a better assessment of addiction. There is often a gray area between addiction and treating chronic pain, as there is frequently some overlap between treating valid chronic pain complaints and the presence of addiction that needs to be assessed prior to implant. Second, the drug holiday will reduce tolerance, allowing for a better assessment of response to intrathecal therapy during the trial. Third, weaning patients off of the opioid prior to implant will likely result in lower doses of intrathecal opioids in the long term. Patients that are titrated up on intrathecal opioids as they are being weaned from systemic opioids often experience withdrawal symptoms resulting in overly aggressive increases in the intrathecal dose. One disadvantage to weaning the systemic opioid prior to trialing includes the pain and suffering that the patient may experience during the drug holiday. There is currently no clear consensus on whether to wean or maintain the systemic opioid prior to trialing. The decision should be based on a discussion between the physician and patient. An addictionology consult may be considered for patients who are unable to wean from the opioids because of severe withdrawal symptoms.

IMPLANTATION

LOCATION OF PUMP PLACEMENT

There are several considerations when choosing where to locate the pump. Patient comfort is of primary importance. The pump must be located away from bony prominences, including the iliac crest and ribs, to avoid rubbing. The amount of subcutaneous fat is also important. In the average-sized patient there may be too little space and tissue in the flank, whereas in the morbidly obese patient there may be too much subcutaneous fat in the abdomen. Have the patient sit up to mark the site to ensure that the pump will not lie below the belt line. Discuss the patient's sleeping habits to determine if the patient is a side sleeper. If so, then place the pump in the contralateral abdomen. In the majority of cases, the most appropriate location for pump placement is in either the left or right lower quadrant of the abdomen.[37] Unlike spinal cord stimulator pulse generators, the size of intrathecal pumps makes placement in the flank or upper gluteal region uncomfortable for average-sized patients. Placement of the pump pocket in the abdomen necessitates positioning the patient in lateral decubitus for the surgical procedure. Proper attention to positioning is necessary to ensure that both the pump site and catheter insertion site are accessible without breaking scrub and repositioning.

Patients who have had multiple abdominal surgeries may pose a challenge in locating the pump pocket. If an abdominal site is impossible, a smaller 20-mL pump may be placed in the superior gluteal region. In larger patients, there may also be room to place the pump in the flank midway between the 12th rib and the iliac crest. A consultation with a plastic surgeon may be helpful in patients with limited implant site options.

When re-implanting a pump after previous pump site infection, it is best to use a new location such as the contralateral abdomen to minimize re-infection risk. Placement of a pump into scar tissue is not recommended, as the blood supply can be erratic, limiting the flow of antibiotics to the area during implantation. This is evident with pump re-implantations for battery failure in which the capsule surrounding the pump has minimal bleeding when opened. In these cases, meticulous care must be taken with sterile technique to minimize the risk of infection with the re-implant.

ANESTHESIA FOR PUMP IMPLANTATION

Intrathecal pump implantation can be performed under local anesthesia with sedation, spinal anesthesia, or general anesthesia. The anesthesia method of choice is to place the catheter under local anesthesia followed by either a spinal anesthetic or local anesthetic infiltration for catheter anchoring, tunneling, and pump placement. This method allows for communication with the patient during catheter placement to minimize the risk of nervous system injury. It is also acceptable to use general anesthesia, but the risks must be disclosed to the patient. The choice of anesthesia will depend on surgeon and patient preference. Nonsurgically trained pain physicians may be more comfortable with an awake patient under local anesthesia who can communicate with the implanter during needle and catheter placement and allow for the assessment of neurologic status.[37] Orthopedic and neurosurgeons may be more accustomed to a patient under general anesthesia. In addition, general anesthesia may be more comfortable and better tolerated by some patients. If implanting under spinal anesthesia, the implanter will first place the Tuohy needle into the intrathecal space under local anesthesia. The implanter can then thread the intrathecal catheter through the Tuohy, communicating with the patient to make sure there is no pain or paresthesias. Once the catheter is confirmed to be in the intrathecal space radiographically and by free flow of cerebrospinal fluid (CSF), injection of 20 to 30 mg of preservative-free lidocaine will achieve adequate spinal anesthesia for both the posterior midline incision and abdominal pump pocket incision.

PATIENT POSITIONING

Most commonly the pump will be located in the abdomen, which necessitates either a lateral decubitus position or repositioning of the patient from prone to supine midway through the surgery. Most implanters use the lateral decubitus position to avoid the time delay and potential infection risk of repositioning. Careful positioning with pressure points padded and an axillary roll in place is necessary for patient comfort and to avoid intraoperative nerve compression injuries. The use of sticky rolls to support the upper abdomen or posterior thorax may assist in positioning the patient in a true lateral decubitus. Taking the time to ensure the patient is well supported and the sagittal axis is perpendicular to the operating room table will ensure a true anterior-posterior (AP) view with fluoroscopy. Position the patient's arms to avoid interfering with fluoroscopic visualization. As stated before, it is critical to mark the pump implantation site with the patient in the sitting position because tissue will shift when in the lateral position. Marking the patient while in the lateral position risks having the pump end up in an uncomfortable location.

SURGICAL TECHNIQUE

STERILE TECHNIQUE

Good sterile technique and pre-operative antibiotics are the two most important controllable factors in preventing wound infections. In a study of primary implantations and revisions of intrathecal baclofen pumps in pediatric and adult patients, an infection rate of 4% to 5% was found.[38] In more than half of the infections, the primary organism was *Staphylococcus aureus*. In a multicenter prospective study of intrathecal pump implantations for both pain and spasticity, Follett found that the most common complication was infection, with an incidence of 7%.[39] Most surgical site infections in clean surgeries are due to skin microorganisms.[40] Careful cleansing of both the surgeon's hands and the patient's skin at the operative site with either a chlorhexidine-alcohol or povidone-iodine scrub reduces skin bacterial counts. Scrubs of 2 to 3 minutes are superior to shorter scrub times. Several studies have suggested that chlorhexidine-alcohol scrubs may be superior to povidone-iodine scrubs.[40] Body hair should be removed only if excessive, and removal should be performed with clippers instead of shaving. Shaving results in microtrauma of the skin, resulting in the inability of the antiseptics to reach the cracks and crevices that may be hiding bacteria.[41] Use of chlorhexidine skin preparation of the surgical site followed by the use of povidone-iodine-impregnated adhesive skin drapes is recommended, as this produces another barrier between the skin flora and wound. If using these drapes, allow extra time for the skin prep to dry so that the adhesive will stick firmly to the skin. Adherence to the patient's skin is necessary for the antiseptic effect. Surgeons and assistants should double glove to reduce the infection risk associated with glove puncture. Prophylactic systemic antibiotics against the most likely pathogens (skin flora) should be administered within 60 minutes of skin incision. If patient allergy to cephalosporins and penicillin precludes their use, one recommended alternative is clindamycin. There is no evidence supporting the postoperative administration of oral antibiotics to prevent wound infections.[40]

Additional practices that may reduce the risk of infection include (1) soaking the pump in a mixture of saline and povidone-iodine solution, (2) packing the wounds with povidone-iodine-soaked sponges for a few minutes, (3) painting the edge of the wound with povidone-iodine and redraping the edge of the wound prior to placing the pump into the wound, and (4) regloving after surgical dissection is complete and before handling the pump. These practices may reduce the risk of skin flora colonization of the pump and pocket.

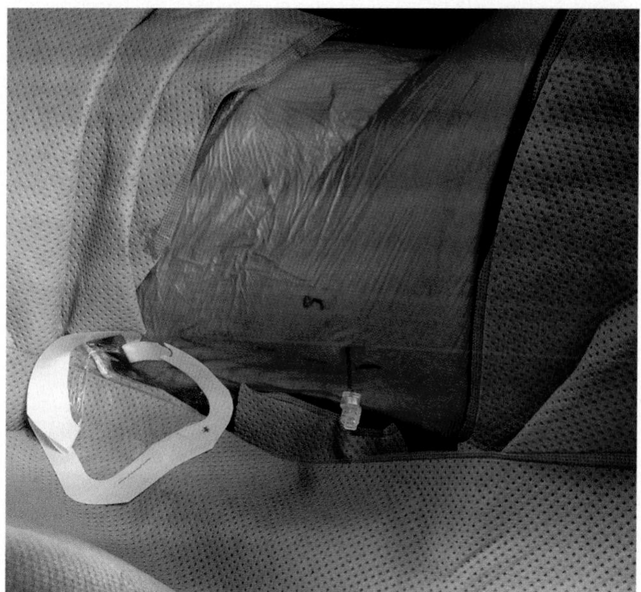

Figure 70.9 Paramedian needle insertion, same side as the abdominal pump pocket.

CATHETER PLACEMENT AND ANCHORING

Prior to needle insertion, the spinous processes of the levels of insertion should be marked on the skin. This will identify the midline incision to be used for dissection and anchoring. Insert the introducer needle using a shallow-angle, paramedian oblique technique (Fig. 70.9). An angle of approximately 30 degrees off of the spine is ideal. For an average-sized patient, the skin entry point will be 1 to 2 cm lateral to the midline on the side of the intended pump pocket, and 1 to 1.5 vertebral levels caudad to the targeted interlaminar entry site. The typical entry site will range from the L2 to L4 interlaminar spaces unless anatomic considerations or previous surgery dictates otherwise.

With the stylet in place, the introducer needle should be advanced to the superior edge of the caudad lamina for the target space. After touching the lamina to gauge depth, the needle is then walked off the edge to the midline of the interlaminar space and, using the loss of resistance technique, the epidural space should be identified (Fig. 70.10). It is best to enter the epidural space just lateral to the midline. Further advancement into the intrathecal space will then be more midline. Once the epidural space is identified, the bevel of the needle is rotated 90 degrees toward the midline so that the needle bevel will be parallel to the longitudinal fibers of the dura. This will spread rather than cut the fibers to reduce the chance of postdural puncture headache. The fluoroscopic view should then be rotated to the lateral view to monitor the needle depth as it is advanced into the intrathecal space. With gentle aspiration, the needle is advanced until there is a return of CSF. If there is no return of CSF in spite of adequate depth on lateral fluoroscopic view, rotate the needle

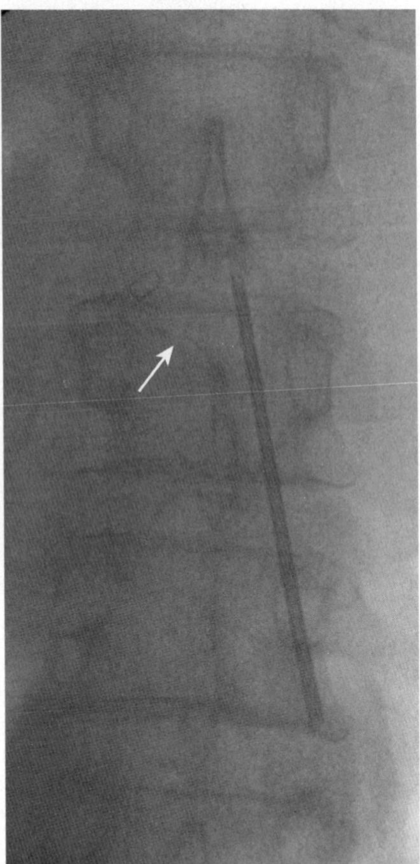

Figure 70.10 Needle advanced into the epidural space after walking off the superior edge of the L3 lamina. White arrow indicates edge of lamina.

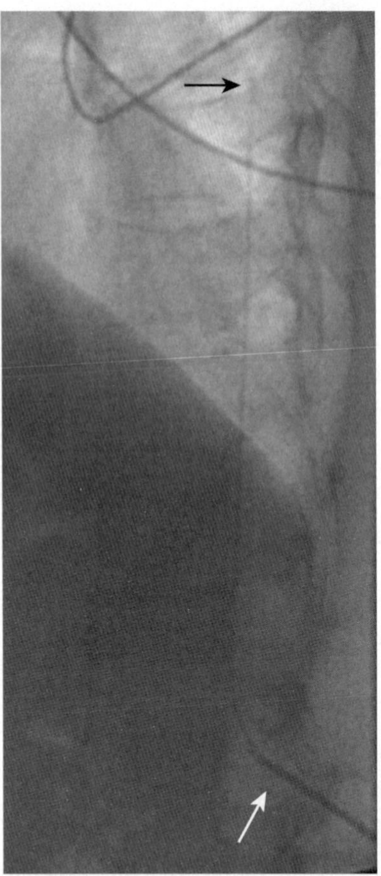

Figure 70.11 Lateral image with needle *(white arrow)* in the intrathecal space and the catheter tip visible five vertebral levels above the entry site *(black arrow).*

back 90 degrees to the original position, which may result in CSF return. If there is no CSF return, rotate 90 degrees and gently advance the needle. Periodically rotate the needle if no CSF returns. Keeping the patient awake and communicating provides an increased margin of safety. Replace the needle stylet to stop CSF flow until ready to place the catheter. Turn the bevel tip cephalad. Ensure that the catheter guidewire is fully advanced into the catheter and is in place during insertion and positioning of the catheter. Advance the catheter through the introducer to the desired level under fluoroscopic guidance (Fig. 70.11). Once the catheter tip is beyond the distal portion of the needle, extreme caution should be used should the catheter need to be withdrawn, as catheter sheering or damage may occur. If there is the slightest resistance when attempting to withdraw the catheter through the needle, it is recommended that the needle and catheter be removed together and the process restarted with needle placement.

Leaving the needle in place to protect the catheter, make an incision in the midline over the spinous processes medial to the needle entry site down to the supraspinous ligament. The incision must be large enough to create a pocket for anchor placement, approximately 5 cm. Undermine the edges of the incision laterally to expose the fascial plane for anchor placement and fully expose the traversing introducer needle (Fig. 70.12).

With the catheter guide wire still in place, carefully remove the needle. To prevent inadvertent withdrawal of the catheter, hold the catheter steady just proximal to where it enters into

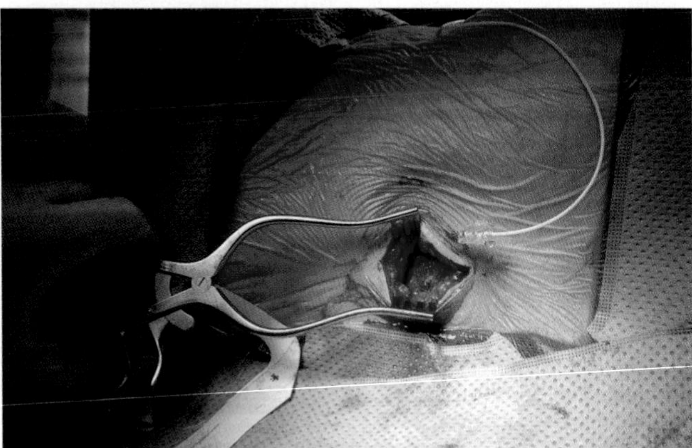

Figure 70.12 Posterior incision medial to needle insertion down to the supraspinous ligament. Pocket undermined laterally to expose the needle within the pocket.

the needle. Once the needle is removed, hold the catheter firmly at the entry site into the fascia at the level of the supraspinous ligament, and withdraw the guide wire. Recheck the catheter position under fluoroscopy to ensure proper placement (Fig. 70.13). Injection of a small amount of contrast may be necessary to make the catheter visible under fluoroscopy. While still holding the catheter at the fascia, bring the external portion of catheter through the skin into the posterior pocket (Fig. 70.14). Clamp the end of the catheter with a rubber

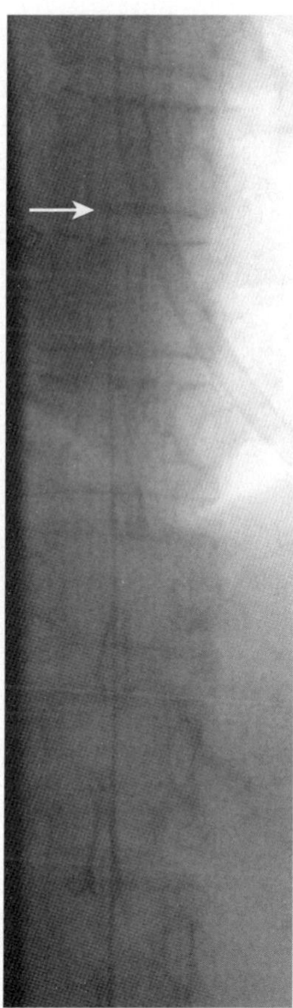

Figure 70.13 Confirm catheter tip *(white arrow)* location on fluoroscopic image prior to anchoring.

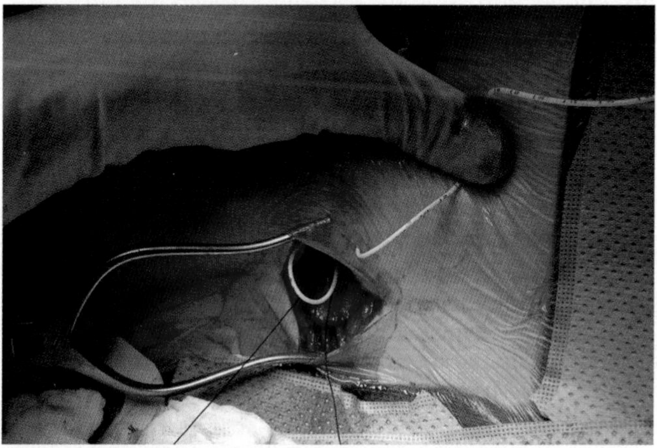

Figure 70.14 After carefully removing the needle and guidewire, bring the external section of the catheter into the pocket.

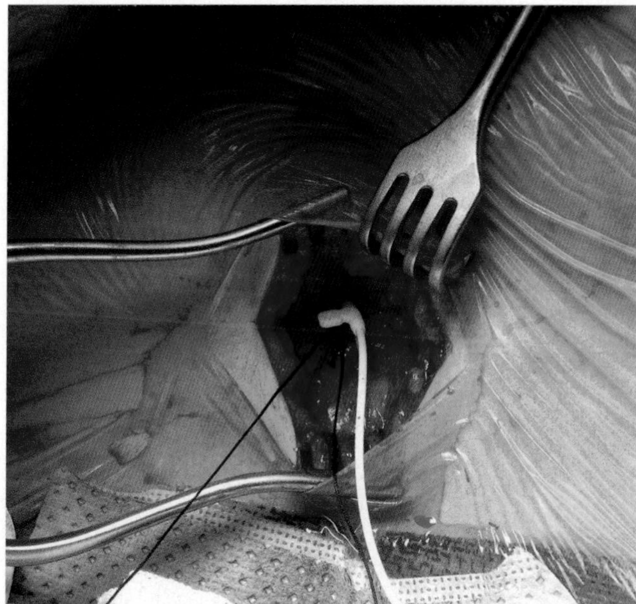

Figure 70.15 After placing a suture through the supraspinous ligament, slide the butterfly anchor over the catheter down to the fascia. Then tie the two wings of the butterfly anchor together with the suture.

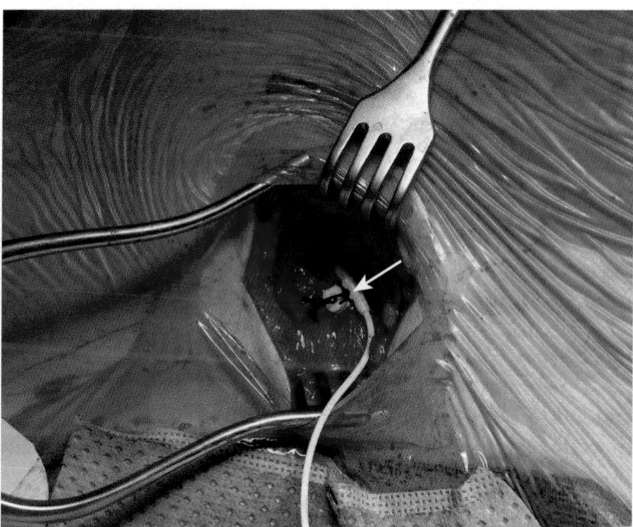

Figure 70.16 A second suture placed through the supraspinous ligament and tied around the neck of the butterfly wings *(white arrow).*

shod clamp to prevent CSF loss while anchoring and tunneling. Using nonabsorbable suture, tie a purse string suture through the fascia around the catheter to prevent CSF leak tracking back along the catheter.[9] Place an 0 silk suture into the supraspinous ligament next to the catheter as it penetrates the fascia and tie the suture. Next, place the butterfly (V-wing) anchor onto the catheter and advance it to the fascial entry site (Fig. 70.15). Use the 0 silk suture placed in the ligament to close the anchor wings together. A second 0 silk suture is then tied around the neck of the anchor, making sure the suture fits in the groove on the anchor (Fig. 70.16). This will ensure a tight fit to hold the catheter. Make sure the anchor is attached firmly to the supraspinous ligament and not to subcutaneous fat and that the distal tip of the anchor is as close as possible to the catheter entry point into the fascia. Catheter migration out of the intrathecal space may occur if the anchor is not firmly attached to fascia. Extra catheter between the anchor and fascial entry point may also increase the risk of catheter migration. Catheter migration distal to the anchor can further be avoided by bringing a layer of tissue together over the anchor and suturing with absorbable suture (discussed later).

PUMP POCKET

Once the catheter is securely anchored, the implanter can then turn attention to creating a subcutaneous pocket for

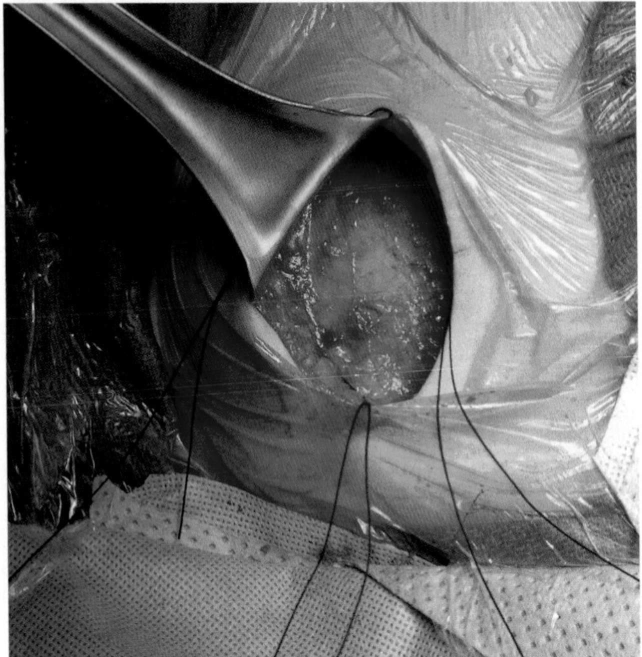

Figure 70.17 Sutures placed in three corners to tie down the pump through the attached suture rings.

the pump. Anesthesia for this and subsequent portions of the surgery can be achieved by injecting spinal lidocaine through the catheter. Alternatively, local anesthetic infiltration into the site can be used. At the abdominal site previously marked, make an incision down through the scarpas fascia to subcutaneous fat. Obtain hemostasis with electrocautery as necessary and extend the incision to a depth of at least 1.5 cm but no more than 2.5 cm. Using careful scissor dissection, undermine along a horizontal plane to create a pocket that just fits the pump. An oversized pocket increases the risk of seroma and shifting or flipping of the pump. The pocket should be undermined predominantly cephalad or caudad to the incision so that the final incision does not lie directly over the refill port of the pump. Accessing the refill port is much easier if the incision scar is not directly over the port. After ensuring proper fit of the pump, place 0 silk sutures into at least three corners of the pocket for anchoring the pump (Fig. 70.17). These sutures should be firmly anchored to the fascia if possible. However, in obese patients this may not be possible, so using a large needle, take big bites of fat and gently tie the knot. The scaring that subsequently results around the sutures will eventually anchor the pump.

TUNNELING

Once the pocket is prepared, the catheter must be tunneled from the posterior incision to the pump pocket (Fig. 70.18). The supplied tunneling device may be bent in a gentle curve to facilitate passage subcutaneously from posterior to anterior trunk. Start at the posterior pocket with pressure and a gentle twisting motion to begin passing the tunneling device toward the pump pocket. Place one hand on the skin surface over the tunneling device tip. The tip should be palpable without piercing the skin throughout the course to ensure it is neither too deep nor too superficial. Once the

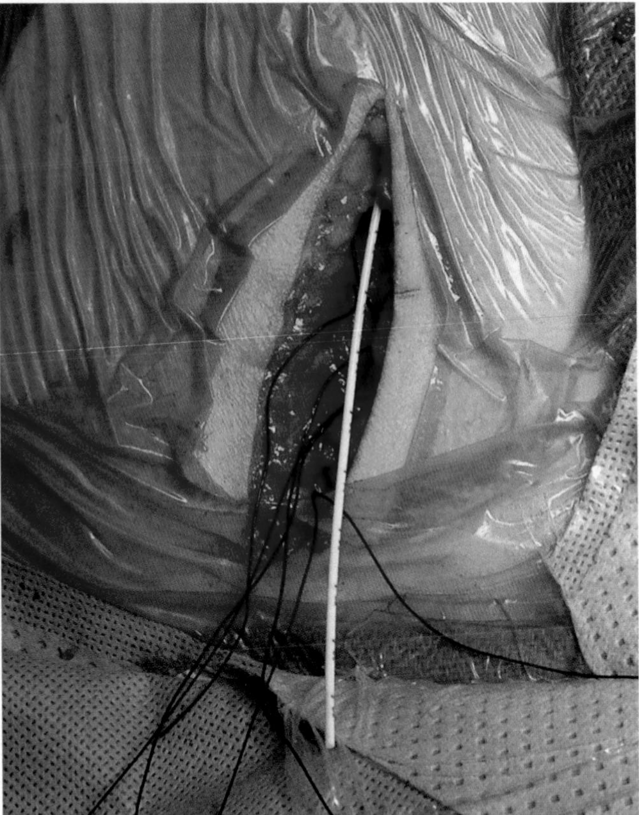

Figure 70.18 The catheter is tunneled into the pump pocket using the provided tunneling device.

introducer has entered the pump pocket, remove the handle and begin passing the catheter through the introducer toward the pocket. Remove the introducer from the pump pocket side. Excess catheter length will be coiled beneath the pump.[6] Once the catheter has been tunneled, irrigate each pocket with copious amounts of normal saline with or without bacitracin.

Unclamp the catheter tip and ensure patency by observing CSF flow from the catheter. Attach the catheter to the provided catheter connector. The connector is then attached to the pump. Ensure that it is firmly connected. Access the side port using the appropriate side port access needle and gently aspirate to make sure there is a flow of CSF. Insert the pump into its pocket and use the previously placed 0 silk sutures to tie it down in three of the corner suture loops. Make sure the catheter is not entangled in these sutures to prevent kinking. Tying the pump down will prevent it from flipping over in the pocket. Place coils of excess catheter behind the pump and ensure that the pump refill port is facing up (Fig. 70.19).[6]

CLOSURE

Before closure of the posterior pocket, pass one 2-0 Vicryl suture through the dorsolumbar fascia alongside the anchor, then cross the suture over the anchor and through the fascia on the opposite side (Fig. 70.20). Pull the two sides together to tightly cover the anchor site and tie down (Fig. 70.21). This tight pocket over the anchor will help prevent catheter migration out of the intrathecal space. For deep incisions, the deep fascia may need to be closed

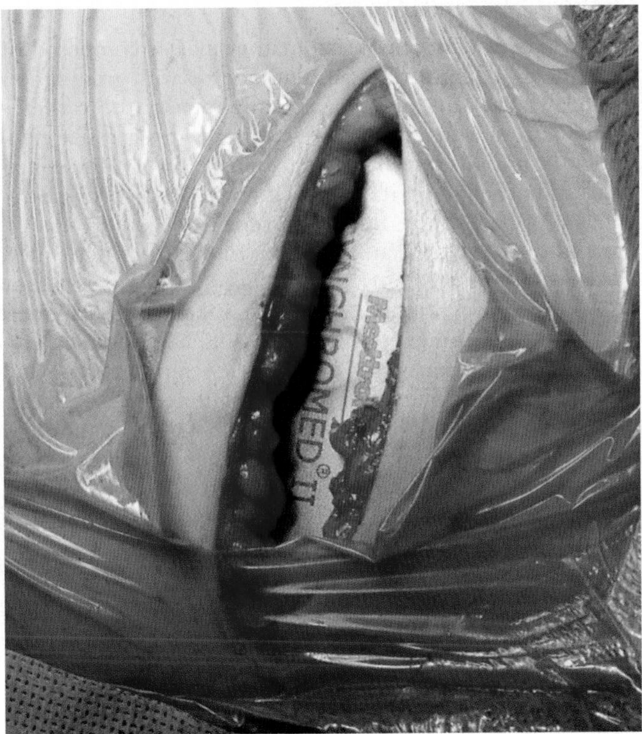

Figure 70.19 Pump tightly in place within the pocket with the access port facing out.

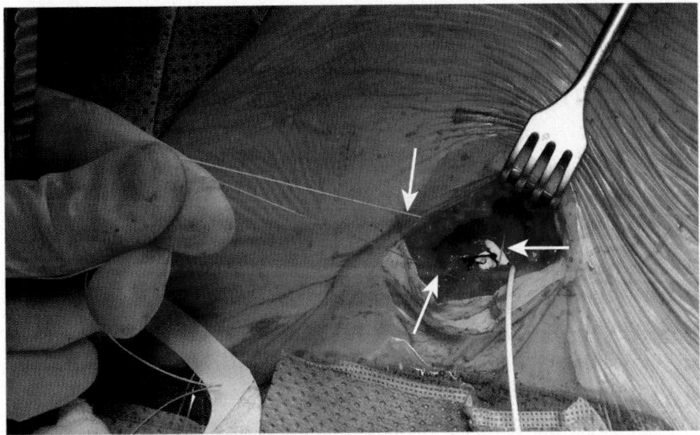

Figure 70.20 One suture placed through the dorsolumbar fascia on one side of the anchor then crossed over to the other side *(arrows)* to close a flap of tissue over the top of the anchor. This will help prevent migration of the catheter out of the intrathecal space.

using interrupted inverted absorbable sutures. For shallower incisions, only the subcutaneous fascia will need to be closed, using interrupted inverted sutures with the spacing close enough that a fingertip placed between sutures is unable to pass below the fascia into the subcutaneous fat. For the pump site, only the subcutaneous fascia will require closure, using interrupted inverted absorbable sutures similar to the back incision closure technique. Skin closure of both incisions may be performed with a running subcuticular closure of 3-0 Monocryl with Steri-strips or with staples. For dressings, place Telfa directly over the incision, followed by 4×4 gauze, then a clear occlusive dressing.

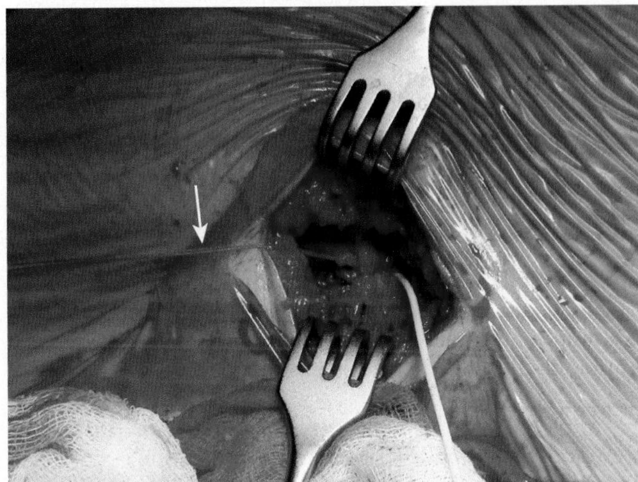

Figure 70.21 Suture pulled tight *(white arrow)* to close a flap over the top of the anchor.

COMPLICATIONS

PERIOPERATIVE COMPLICATIONS

The implantation of an IDDS exposes the patient to risks similar to those of other surgical or invasive procedures such as bleeding, infection, wound dehiscence, and neurologic injury. In addition there is a risk of CSF leakage, migration of the intrathecal catheter, and pump site complications such as seroma formation.

BLEEDING

Intraoperative bleeding is most likely to be problematic in patients with a history of bleeding diathesis or hepatic disease, or those on anticoagulant therapy. Patients with suspected coagulation disorders should be evaluated carefully prior to implantation. The American Society of Regional Anesthesia and Pain Medicine guidelines regarding anticoagulants for neuraxial analgesia should be followed to reduce the risk of potentially catastrophic spinal or epidural hematoma formation.[30]

INFECTION

The incidence of infection following intrathecal pump implantation has been reported to be between 2.5% and 9%.[28] The majority of infections occur at the pump pocket site and present within 15 to 45 days after implantation. Pediatric patients implanted for treatment of spasticity have been found to have slightly higher rates of postimplantation infections.[42] In addition to local infection at the pump site, there is a risk of infection spreading to the CSF with resulting meningitis. This risk necessitates good infection control practices to prevent surgical site infections as well as careful evaluation of any suspected infection (discussed previously). In the majority of cases, a pump pocket infection will require explanting both the device and the catheter.

The clinical presentation of a local pump pocket infection may include increased pain, fever, erythema, tenderness, swelling, purulent drainage, and warmth at the pump site. In the case of CSF infection and meningitis, the patient may present with nuchal rigidity, headache, nausea, vomiting, and fever. In either case the patient may have an elevated white blood count (WBC), C-reactive protein, or erythrocyte sedimentation rate. The formation of a seroma within the pump pocket may mimic a local infection with swelling and erythema. Percutaneous drainage and culture of fluid may assist in making the diagnosis. The most common pathogens implicated are *Staphalococcus*.[28]

If an infection is suspected, the pump and catheter should be removed immediately. Antibiotics should not be administered until the pump is removed and wound cultures are obtained. Antibiotics administered before cultures are obtained can make it difficult to identify the bacteria, thus committing the patient to a longer course of broad coverage antibiotic therapy.

CEREBROSPINAL FLUID LEAKS

Cerebrospinal fluid leaks may occur around the catheter via the dural puncture site or as a result of disconnection, fracture, or puncture of the catheter. The leakage of CSF may result in a postdural puncture headache. Generally, CSF leaks that are not due to catheter fracture or disconnection are self-limiting and may be treated conservatively. However, if the leak and symptoms persist, an epidural blood patch may be performed under fluoroscopic guidance in order to avoid damage to the catheter.[4,42]

Severe CSF leaks may result in CSF fluid collections in the posterior catheter site pocket. These can be difficult to treat, and if an epidural blood patch does not resolve the leak, injection of 1 mL of fibrin glue at the dural entry site under fluoroscopy can be considered. If this does not resolve the leak, explantation of the system may be necessary.

Persistent or recurrent fluid collection in the pump pocket after percutaneous drainage should raise the suspicion of a catheter disconnect from the pump with a CSF leak into the pump pocket. Percutaneous side port access with injection of contrast under fluoroscopy can diagnose this complication.

CATHETER COMPLICATIONS

Catheter-related problems are the most common complications following implantation of an intrathecal drug delivery system. Although the reported occurrence varies, Follet and Naumann found a rate of 18.6% in a prospective study of catheter-related complications.[43] These problems include fracture, puncture, disconnection, migration, or dislodgement from the intrathecal space. Among these, catheter migration is the most common and usually is the result of improper anchoring of the catheter to the fascia.[43] Catheter failures may present as inadequate analgesia, CSF leaks, or withdrawal symptoms. Evaluation of catheter complications starts with accessing the side port. If CSF can be aspirated freely, then a fluoroscopic evaluation with injection of contrast may help identify leaks and the location of the catheter within the intrathecal space. If CSF cannot be aspirated, one must fill the pump with saline and clear the catheter of the drug before injecting contrast in order to avoid bolus injection of drug intrathecally. Contrast studies may not detect small leaks, kinks, or breakage. A computed tomography (CT) myelogram following injection of contrast through the side port may be required to identify the location of a leak or the formation of a granuloma at the catheter tip.

GRANULOMA FORMATION

Granulomas are aseptic inflammatory masses composed of macrophages, neutrophils, and monocytes with granulation tissue.[19,42] The formation of a granuloma at the catheter tip may cause a loss of analgesic efficacy, progressive neurologic symptoms resulting from a mass effect on the spinal cord, and permanent neurologic injury. In a study of granulomas reported to the manufacturer of one pump system, the authors calculated an incidence of 0.49% of implanted systems.[44] Because many granulomas go undetected or unreported, the actual incidence is likely much higher. The most commonly reported symptoms are decreased efficacy of analgesia and pain. Neurologic symptoms reported include weakness, numbness, and incontinence.[44] Risk factors for granuloma formation include a high dose and high concentration infusion of opioids (all except fentanyl). The most commonly implicated drug has been morphine, but other opioids and, rarely, baclofen have been associated with granuloma formation. Imaging by magnetic resonance imaging (MRI) with contrast or CT myelogram can aid in the evaluation of a suspected granuloma. However, in the authors' experience, CT myelogram is superior, as catheter identification can be difficult with MRI, and we have seen two cases where MRI with contrast failed to demonstrate a granuloma whereas subsequent CT myelogram diagnosed the granuloma. The treatment employed will depend on the presence and severity of any neurologic symptoms. Options include replacement of the intrathecal infusate with saline, removal of the catheter, or surgical exploration and mass resection.[19]

CONCLUSION

Since the 1980s, intrathecal drug delivery of opioids and nonopioid analgesics has become a promising option when more conservative therapies have failed. There are an increasing number of choices with regard to implanted intrathecal pump systems for the management of spasticity as well as cancer and chronic noncancer pain. The challenges involved in the successful use of intrathecal therapy start with patient selection. Understanding the issues in selecting an appropriate candidate with cancer pain, chronic noncancer pain, or spasticity will go a long way toward ensuring adequate therapy once the system is implanted. The main risks associated with implantation of an intrathecal system are infection and catheter migration. Careful attention to good sterile technique during the surgical implantation as well as catheter anchoring can minimize these risks.

KEY POINTS

- Intrathecal analgesia therapy has proven to be extremely beneficial to many patients; it is also associated with high costs, high maintenance, and risks requiring careful patient selection.
- The cost and invasive nature of an intrathecal drug delivery system (IDDS) necessitate a careful evaluation to determine whether each individual patient is appropriate and likely to achieve benefit.

KEY POINTS—cont'd

- A 2002 multicenter randomized trial compared comprehensive medical management (CMM) alone versus CMM plus an IDDS. The researchers found that cancer patients receiving CMM plus an IDDS had reduced pain, fewer drug toxicities, and prolonged survival compared to controls.
- The psychologist should not be asked to give "clearance" but rather act as an additional source of information as to whether IDDS therapy is appropriate, the patient has rational expectations, and the treatment is likely to succeed for an individual patient.
- Granulomas are aseptic inflammatory masses composed of macrophages, neutrophils, and monocytes with granulation tissue. The formation of a granuloma at the catheter tip may cause loss of analgesic efficacy, progressive neurologic symptoms due to a mass effect on the spinal cord, and permanent neurologic injury.

SUGGESTED READINGS

Celestin J, Edwards R, Jamison R. Pretreatment psychosocial variables as predicators of outcomes following lumbar surgery and spinal cord stimulation. *Pain Med.* 2009;10:639-653.

Horlocker T, Wedel D, Rowlingson J, et al. Regional anesthesia in the Society of Regional Anesthesia and Pain Medicine evidence-based guidelines. 3rd ed. *Reg Anesth Pain Med.* 2010;35:64-101.

Lawson E, Wallace M. Current developments in intraspinal agents for cancer and noncancer pain. *Curr Pain Headache Rep.* 2010;14:8-16.

Schuster J, Rechtine G, Norvell D. The influence of perioperative risk factors and therapeutic interventions on infection rates after spine surgery: a systematic review. *Spine.* 2010;35:S125-S137.

van den Beuken-van Everdingen M, de Rijke J, Kessels A, et al. Prevalence of pain in patients with cancer: a systematic review of the past 40 years. *Ann Oncol.* 2007;18:1437-1449.

Yaksh TL, Rudy TA. Analgesia mediated by a direct spinal action of narcotics. *Science.* 1976;192:1357-1358.

The references for this chapter can be found at www.expertconsult.com.

71 Joint Injections

David A. Provenzano | Kailash Chandwani

Intra-articular (IA) joint and bursa injections are used to treat pain in the joint and surrounding structures. Musculoskeletal system disorders, including osteoarthritis, are some of the most common medical conditions for which patients seek care. Musculoskeletal diseases are associated with high levels of disability and significant economic costs.[1,2] Osteoarthritis, a noninflammatory rheumatologic condition, is the most prevalent form of arthritis. It is projected that more than 59 million individuals in the United States (18% of the population) will suffer from osteoarthritis by 2020.[3]

In the 1950s, Hollander introduced the IA corticosteroid injection for the treatment of rheumatoid arthritis (RA).[4-6] In 1958, the first clinical trial for IA joint injections for osteoarthritis was performed.[7] Currently, joint injections continue to be used extensively in a multimodal treatment platform for musculoskeletal conditions. In the updated American College of Rheumatology (ACR) guidelines for the medical management of osteoarthritis, IA injections were recommended as alternative and augmentative treatment approaches to oral medications and physical therapy.[8]

This chapter provides an updated review of IA joint injections. Four major areas are covered: (1) pharmacology of common injectable agents, (2) indications for treatment, (3) image-guided injection techniques, and (4) IA injection-associated adverse effects and complications. The three major joints addressed are the shoulder, hip, and knee. Assessments of the accuracy and therapeutic efficacy of each technique are provided.

PHARMACOLOGY OF AGENTS UTILIZED FOR JOINT INJECTIONS

Intra-articular needle placement is routinely used to deliver therapeutic agents to reduce pain and improve function. The three agents routinely employed for IA injections are local anesthetics, corticosteroids, and viscosupplements.

LOCAL ANESTHETICS

INDICATIONS AND MECHANISM OF ACTION

Local anesthetics (LAs) are often utilized in combination with corticosteroids for IA and extra-articular injections. The rationale for utilizing LAs includes providing pain relief for the needle insertion itself and diagnostic purposes as well as diluting and distributing the steroid preparation within the joint.

Local anesthetics act by reversibly binding to sodium channels on neuronal cell membranes, thereby blocking nerve conduction.[9] Local anesthetics also have transient anti-inflammatory effects and inhibit several leukocyte functions.[10]

LOCAL ANESTHETIC AGENT SELECTION (STRUCTURE AND FUNCTION)

Local anesthetics commonly employed for joint injections include the short-acting LA, lidocaine, and the long-acting LAs, bupivacaine and ropivacaine.

ADVERSE EFFECTS AND COMPLICATIONS ASSOCIATED WITH LOCAL ANESTHETIC INJECTION

Local anesthetics are associated with both local and systemic side effects. Local effects of LAs include myotoxicity and chondrotoxicity. Myotoxicity can occur from LA administration in or around muscle tissue, although it is usually not clinically relevant and muscle regeneration occurs.[11] Bupivacaine is more myotoxic than lidocaine and ropivacaine. Local anesthetics produce myonecrosis through the lytic degeneration of the sarcoplasmic reticulum and mitochondria. The addition of corticosteroids to LA injection amplifies the muscle damage and prolongs the recovery phase.[12] Myonecrosis rarely presents any clinically discernible manifestations in the course of routine use of local anesthetics for IA joint injections.

Local anesthetics are also chondrotoxic.[13-17] Most reported cases of chondrolysis occurred after use of continuous IA local anesthetic infusions to manage postoperative pain rather than single IA injections.[17] In vitro studies have demonstrated that LAs cause mitochondrial dysfunction and apoptosis in human chondrocytes.[14] Chondrotoxic effects are influenced by the LA type and concentration. Grishko and colleagues[14] demonstrated that 2% lidocaine caused massive necrosis of cultured chondrocytes after 24 hours of exposure, whereas 1% lidocaine caused a detectable but insignificant decrease in cell viability. For longer-acting LAs, in vitro studies indicate that 0.5% ropivacaine is significantly less chondrotoxic to cultured human articular cartilage than 0.5% bupivacaine.[15] Similar to myotoxicity, combining LA with corticosteroids amplifies chondrotoxicity.[18] Further studies are needed to determine the clinical significance and exact mechanisms of LA toxicity to cartilage cells.

When combining LA with corticosteroids, flocculation—aggregation of the particles of steroid—may occur.[19] Indeed, dilution with either saline or LA may influence the size of corticosteroid particles.[20] Betamethasone sodium phosphate/betamethasone acetate (Celestone Soluspan) should not be mixed with LAs that contain the excipients methylparaben, propylparaben, or phenol because of an increased risk of flocculation.[19] Flocculation leads to larger particles that may clog smaller bore needles, preventing injection. The effect of flocculation of the injected steroid on its therapeutic effect is unclear; theoretically, the change in the size of the microaggregates of the steroid could significantly alter the bioavailability of the steroid over time as well the distribution within the joint after injection, altering the therapeutic effect.

Systemic effects of LAs include allergic reactions and central nervous system and cardiac toxicity.[9] When appropriate steps are taken to avoid intravascular injection, including frequent aspiration and using small volumes for musculoskeletal injections, the incidence of these occurrences are low. Allergic reactions are more common with amino-ester LAs secondary to the production of metabolites related to *para*-aminobenzoic acid. Allergic reactions may also be due to the preservatives contained within the carrier solution (e.g., methylparaben). Cross-sensitivity does not exist between LA structural classes. The American Society of Regional Anesthesia published a practice advisory on local anesthetic toxicity and provided a checklist for managing local anesthetic toxicity (Fig. 71.1).

CORTICOSTEROIDS

INDICATIONS AND MECHANISM OF ACTION

Corticosteroids are often used for pain associated with symptomatic arthritis and soft tissue conditions (e.g., tendinitis, bursitis, and tenosynovitis). Numerous guidelines with specific focus on osteoarthritis of the knee recommend IA corticosteroid injection for short-term pain relief.[8,21,22] Intra-articular steroid injections should be part of a multimodal treatment plan that includes aerobic and muscle-strengthening programs. Contraindications to IA injection are shown in Box 71.1.

The exact mechanism of action of corticosteroids in reducing arthritic joint pain has not been completely defined. Corticosteroids placed in the joint exert both local and systemic effects.[19,23] In individuals with RA, changes in the non-injected knee thermographic index, a quantitative measure of radiated energy from a defined area of the joint surface, have been demonstrated after IA prednisolone and triamcinolone hexacetonide (TH) injection into the symptomatic knee.[23,24] Intra-articular placement of methylprednisolone acetate (MPA), 40 or 80 mg, resulted in detectable serum levels with peak levels occurring between 2 and 12 hours after injection. Additionally, endogenous serum cortisol levels were suppressed for up to 1 week after injection.[25] The systemic effects are further confirmed by reduction of systemic inflammatory marker levels, including erythrocyte sedimentation rate (ESR) and C-reactive protein (CRP).[19]

Corticosteroids have significant anti-inflammatory and immune effects and are active at the cellular level by combining with receptors to alter the rate of messenger RNA synthesis and specific protein production. Specifically, corticosteroids result in increased synthesis of annexin-1 (lipocortin-1). Annexin-1 has phospholipase A_2-inhibitory activity that reduces production of multiple inflammatory mediators, including eicosanoids, lysosomal enzymes, interleukin-1, leukotrienes, and prostaglandins.[26-28] The clinical response to IA steroids is accompanied by histologic improvement and decreased expression of genes that are involved in articular cartilage destruction.[29] Additionally, corticosteroids reduce microvascular permeability and synovial perfusion, and they increase synovial fluid viscosity.[30]

Corticosteroids seem to exert greater therapeutic effects with IA injection versus either systemic or intramuscular (IM) administration. Injection of corticosteroid into multiple joints in RA patients greatly improved ACR criteria, patient disease activity, number of tender points, and reduced systemic side effects, when compared to equivalent IM dosing.[31]

CORTICOSTEROID SELECTION (STRUCTURE AND FUNCTION)

The first steroid used for IA injection was hydrocortisone.[5,6] Although over the past 50 years pharmacologic developments have resulted in the advancement of steroid preparations, substantial variation still exists for agent selection. However, there remains a paucity of randomized controlled trials comparing the efficacy of different corticosteroids for osteoarthritis. Thus, evidence-based recommendations to guide steroid selection cannot be made. In 1994, a survey of ACR members indicated that agent selection was usually determined empirically and was strongly influenced by the geographic region of training. The three most commonly utilized agents were MPA, TH, and triamcinolone acetonide (TA).[32]

Table 71.1 lists commonly utilized corticosteroids that have been certified by the United States Food and Drug Administration (FDA) for IA injection. The only other corticosteroid approved for IA injection is dexamethasone. Dexamethasone, a highly water soluble, nonparticulate steroid preparation, exerts primarily systemic effects even after IA injection and is not routinely utilized for IA injections.[19,20]

The selection of a depot corticosteroid can be based on cost and multiple pharmacologic properties including solubility as well as crystal and molecular structure. Chemical structures important to depot steroids include the presence of an ester group and the addition of a fluorine group. Ester groups decrease corticosteroid solubility.[33] Inserted fluorine groups increase corticosteroid absorption and increase steroid potency.[19]

Corticosteroid solubility may influence duration of action, although published studies are conflicting. Triamcinolone hexacetonide is the most insoluble injectable corticosteroid. Some IA injection studies have demonstrated prolonged duration of activity with TH compared to other corticosteroids with higher solubility. Derendorf and associates[34] demonstrated that TH was associated with lower levels of systemic absorption and higher synovial levels than similar IA administration of TA. Comparison of TH and MPA for knee osteoarthritis did not support steroid solubility as the only factor influencing drug duration of action and therapeutic efficacy.[35] After 3 weeks, TH was more effective but at 8 weeks only MPA resulted in continued improvement in pain and disability scores. Another study comparing TH and MPA for RA treatment demonstrated a longer therapeutic effect with TH.[36] Thus, available data are conflicting.

The adverse-effect profile of a corticosteroid should also be considered. Methylprednisolone acetate may be utilized for both joint and soft tissue injections, whereas TH is not recommended for soft tissue injections because of the higher risk of calcification, necrosis, and atrophy of soft tissues.[9,33,37]

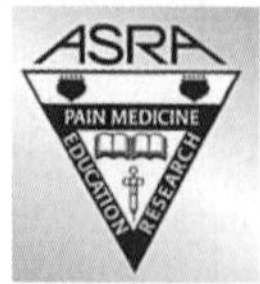

AMERICAN SOCIETY OF
REGIONAL ANESTHESIA AND PAIN MEDICINE

Checklist for Treatmentof
Local Anesthetic Systemic Toxicity

The Pharmacologic Treatment of Local Anesthetic Systemic Toxicity (LAST) Is Different from Other Cardiac Arrest Scenarios

- ☐ **Get Help**
- ☐ **Initial Focus**
  - ☐ **Airway management:** ventilate with 100% oxygen
  - ☐ **Seizure suppression:** benzodiazepines are preferred; **AVOID propofol** in patients having signs of cardiovascular instability
  - ☐ **Alert** the nearest facility having **cardiopulmonary bypass** capability
- ☐ **Management of Cardiac Arrhythmias**
  - ☐ **Basic and Advanced Cardiac Life Support (ACLS)** will require adjustment of medications and perhaps prolonged effort
  - ☐ **AVOID vasopressin, calcium channel blockers, beta blockers, or local anesthetic**
  - ☐ **REDUCE individual epinephrine doses to <1 mcg/kg**
- ☐ **Lipid Emulsion (20%) Therapy** (values in parentheses are for 70 kg patient)
  - ☐ **Bolus 1.5 mL/kg** (lean body mass) intravenously over 1 minute (~100 mL)
  - ☐ **Continuous infusion 0.25 mL/kg/min** (~18 mL/min; adjust by roller clamp)
  - ☐ Repeat bolus once or twice for persistent cardiovascular collapse
  - ☐ Double the infusion rate to 0.5 mL/kg/min if blood pressure remains low
  - ☐ **Continue infusion** for at least 10 minutes after attaining circulatory stability
  - ☐ Recommended upper limit: Approximately 10 mL/kg lipid emulsion over the first 30 minutes
- ☐ **Post LAST events at** www.lipidrescue.org and report use of lipid to www.lipidregistry.org

BE PREPARED

- We strongly advise that those using local anesthetics (LAs) in doses sufficient to produce local anesthetic systemic toxicity (LAST) establish a plan for managing this complication. Making a *Local Anesthetic Toxicity Kit* and posting instructions for its use are encouraged.

RISK REDUCTION (*BE SENSIBLE*)

- Use the least dose of LA necessary to achieve the desired extent and duration of block.
- Local anesthetic blood levels are influenced by site of injection and dose. Factors that can increase the likelihood of LAST include: advanced age, heart failure, ischemic heart disease, conduction abnormalities, metabolic (e.g., mitochondrial) disease, liver disease, low plasma protein concentration, metabolic or respiratory acidosis, medications that inhibit sodium channels. Patients with severe cardiac dysfunction, particularly very low ejection fraction, are more sensitive to LAST and also more prone to "stacked" injections (with resulting elevated LA tissue concentrations) due to slowed circulation time.
- Consider using a pharmacologic marker and/or test dose, e.g. epinephrine 5 mcg/mL of LA. Know the expected response, onset, duration, and limitations of "test dose" in identifying intravascular injection.
- Aspirate the syringe prior to *each* injection while observing for blood.
- Inject incrementally, while observing for signs and querying for symptoms of toxicity between each injection.

DETECTION (*BE VIGILANT*)

- Use standard American Society of Anesthesiologists (ASA) monitors.
- Monitor the patient during and after completing injection as clinical toxicity can be delayed up to 30 minutes.
- Communicate frequently with the patient to query for symptoms of toxicity.
- Consider LAST in any patient with altered mental status, neurological symptoms or cardiovascular instability after a regional anesthetic.
- Central nervous system signs (may be subtle or absent)
  - *Excitation* (agitation, confusion, muscle twitching, seizure)
  - *Depression* (drowsiness, obtundation, coma or apnea)
  - *Non-specific* (metallic taste, circumoral numbness, diplopia, tinnitus, dizziness)
- Cardiovascular signs (often the only manifestation of severe LAST)
  - *Initially may be hyperdynamic* (hypertension, tachycardia, ventricular arrhythmias), then
  - *Progressive hypotension*
  - *Conduction block,* bradycardia or asystole
  - *Ventricular arrhythmia* (ventricular tachycardia, torsades de pointes, ventricular fibrillation)
- Sedative hypnotic drugs reduce seizure risk but even light sedation may abolish the patient's ability to recognize or report symptoms of rising LA concentrations.

TREATMENT

- Timing of lipid infusion in LAST is controversial. The most conservative approach, waiting until after ACLS has proven unsuccessful, is unreasonable because early treatment can prevent cardiovascular collapse. Infusing lipid at the earliest sign of LAST can result in unnecessary treatment since only a fraction of patients will progress to severe toxicity. The most reasonable approach is to implement lipid therapy on the basis of clinical severity and rate of progression of LAST.
- There is laboratory evidence that epinephrine can impair resuscitation from LAST and reduce the efficacy of lipid rescue. Therefore it is recommended to avoid high doses of epinephrine and use smaller doses, e.g., <1 mcg/kg, for treating hypotension.
- Propofol *should not be used* when there are signs of cardiovascular instability. Propofol is a cardiovascular depressant with lipid content too low to provide benefit. Its use is discouraged when there is a risk of progression to cardiovascular collapse.
- Prolonged monitoring (>12 hours) is recommended after any signs of systemic LA toxicity, since cardiovascular depression due to local anesthetics can persist or recur after treatment.

Figure 71.1 American Society of Regional Anesthesia (ASRA) checklist for treatment of local anesthetic toxicity. (Reprinted with permission from Neal JM, Mulroy MF, Weinberg GL. American Society of Regional Anesthesia and Pain Medicine checklist for managing local anesthetic toxicity: 2012 version. *Reg Anesth Pain Med.* 2012;37:16-18.)

Continued

The ASRA Practice Advisory on Local Anesthetic Toxicity is published in the society's official publication *Regional Anesthesia and Pain Medicine*, and can be downloaded from the journal website at www.rapm.org.

Neal JM, Bernards CM, Butterworth JF, Di Gregorio G, Drasner K, Hejtmanck MR, Mulroy MF, Rosenquist RW, Weinberg GL. ASRA practice advisory on local anesthetic systemic toxicity. *Reg Anesth Pain Med* 2010;35:152-161.

Figure 71.1, cont'd.

Box 71.1 Absolute and Relative Contraindications for Intra-articular Joint Injections with Corticosteroids or Viscosupplementation

Absolute Contraindications

Overlying skin infection
Fracture site
Severely compromised immune status
Suspected bacteremia
Suspected infectious arthritis
Hypersensitivity to previous viscosupplementation

Relative Contraindications

Coagulopathy
Hypersensitivity to avian products (proteins, feather, and egg products)*
Joint prosthesis
Poorly controlled diabetes mellitus
Previous lack of efficacy

*Consider using nonavian viscosupplementation products.

CORTICOSTEROID DOSING AND POSTINJECTION PROTOCOLS

Corticosteroid dosing ranges for various joints are listed in Table 71.1. Evidence-based recommendations for dosing and the maximum injection frequency do not exist. Standard recommendations for weight-bearing joints include a maximum of three to four injections per year, typically with 3 to 4 months between injections.[30,33] Long-term corticosteroid safety was studied by Raynauld and colleagues [38] in a randomized, double-blind, placebo-controlled trial that compared IA knee injections of TA or saline every 3 months for up to 2 years. No detrimental effects or joint space destruction was observed on radiographs. Balch and coworkers[39] found no radiographic evidence of corticosteroid-induced joint destruction after long-term repeated IA injections (from 4 to 15 years) on knee joints affected by RA and osteoarthritis.

Following IA corticosteroid injection, patients are often advised to avoid overusing the joint for 2 to 3 days postinjection.[40] Studies investigating potential benefits of rest following corticosteroid injections have reported conflicting results.[19] Chakravarty and colleagues[41] demonstrated additional improvement in individuals who rested for 24 hours after IA injection whereas Chatham and associates[42] found no benefit in individuals who rested for 48 hours.

If an individual is going to undergo a total hip or knee joint replacement in the near future, caution should be exercised in performing IA injections close to the surgical date.[43] Retrospective comparative studies demonstrated increased risk for deep infection in individuals who received IA corticosteroid injections shortly before the surgical replacement procedure.[44,45] However, Joshy and colleagues[46] did not observe increased deep infection rates for individuals who underwent IA injections shortly prior to total knee replacement.

ADVERSE EFFECTS AND COMPLICATIONS ASSOCIATED WITH CORTICOSTEROID INJECTION

The adverse effects and complications of corticosteroid injections can be divided into local and systemic effects. Local adverse effects include tissue (skin or fat) atrophy, Nicolau's syndrome, tendon rupture, cartilage damage, postinjection flare, hemarthrosis, joint destruction, avascular necrosis, and septic arthritis.[9,33,47,48] Local tissue atrophy is one of the most common local adverse effects occurring in 1% to 8% of cases and is often associated with superficial injection, inaccurate placement, and less soluble agents (e.g., triamcinolone compounds). Skin atrophy typically develops between 1 and 4 months after injection.[30,47] Methylprednisolone acetate is less frequently associated with soft tissue atrophy. Another common adverse effect is postinjection flare in pain, with a prevalence of 2% to 25%. Postinjection flare typically presents within a few hours of injection and resolves within 1 to 3 days.[33]

Concern also exists for corticosteroid-specific effects on cartilage, tendon, and bone. Current data on corticosteroid effects on cartilage are conflicting. Animal studies have been inconsistent, with some demonstrating cartilage destruction and others revealing a cartilage-protective effect during acute inflammatory events.[49-55] Clinical studies suggest that cartilage loss may occur more frequently with repeated injections in large numbers.[9] Avascular necrosis has also been reported after joint injections, with the hip being the most commonly affected joint. This complication typically occurs after multiple joint injections within a short period of time and is seen more often in individuals who are concurrently taking oral steroids.[47] Tendon disruption has also occurred following corticosteroid injection and care should be taken to avoid direct injection within tendons.[47,56]

Hemarthrosis and septic arthritis are two infrequent complications that carry significant morbidity. No specific guidelines exist for performance of IA steroid injections in individuals on anticoagulants, and surveys have demonstrated substantial practice variation.[57] A small study demonstrated a low risk of hemorrhage in individuals taking warfarin sodium who received IA injections.[58] Septic arthritis has a reported incidence ranging from 1 in 3000 to 1 in 50,000.[19,59,60] To limit this adverse event it is important to understand contraindications to injection (see Box 71.1) and utilize a stringent aseptic technique. When performing a joint injection, if synovial fluid appears abnormal, the aspirated fluid should be sent for a complete white blood cell (WBC) count including differential, crystal analysis, Gram stain, and culture. Steroid should not be placed until the synovial fluid analysis (Table 71.2) has been reviewed and interpreted. Septic arthritis is a medical emergency and can result in cartilage destruction, septicemia, and death within a few days if untreated. When septic arthritis is suspected, orthopedic surgery and infectious disease specialists should

Table 71.1 Common Corticosteroid Preparations for Intra-articular and Periarticular Injections.

Preparation	How Supplied	Equivalent Dosage (mg)*	Anti-Inflammatory Potency†	Solubility (%wt/vol)	Fluorinated	Dose Based on Joint Size
Betamethasone sodium phosphate/ betamethasone acetate (BSP/BA)	3 mg BSP/3 mg BA per 1 mL	0.75	25	Not mentioned‡	Yes	Large: 1-2 mL Medium: 0.5-1 mL Small: 0.25-0.5 mL
Methylprednisolone acetate (MPA)	20, 40, 80 mg/mL	4	5	0.001	No	Large: 20-80 mg Medium: 10-40 mg Small: 4-10 mg
Triamcinolone acetonide (TA)	10, 40 mg/mL	4	5	0.004	Yes	Large: 5-15 mg Small: 2.5-5 mg
Triamcinolone hexacetonide (TH)	5, 20 mg/mL	4	5	0.0002	Yes	Large: 10-20 mg Small: 2-6 mg

*Equivalent to 5 mg prednisone. For TA and TH the specific dosing for medium-sized joints was not mentioned.
†Relative potencies based on equivalent milligram doses with hydrocortisone being the relative baseline with a potency of 1.
‡The betamethasone preparation consists of the highly soluble ester BSP, which is devoid of particles, and the less soluble BA.
(Data from references 19, 28, 30, 33, and 40.)

Table 71.2 Synovial Fluid Analysis

Diagnosis	Color	Clarity	WBC Count per mm³	% Neutrophils	Gram Stain
Normal	Clear	Transparent	<200	<25	Negative
Noninflammatory	Straw	Translucent	200-2000	<25	Negative
Inflammatory (crystalline)	Yellow	Cloudy	2000-100,000	>50	Negative
Septic arthritis	Yellow	Cloudy	>25,000-50,000	>75	Variable
Pseudosepsis	NA	NA	5000-80,000*	NA	Negative

NA, not available
*Unlike septic arthritis, aspirate from joints with suspected pseudosepsis may contain an elevated eosinophil count suggestive of an immune-mediated inflammatory reaction.[82]
(Data from references 170-172.)

be consulted immediately. Arthrocentesis and synovial fluid analysis (see Table 71.2) are mandatory for diagnosis and to guide treatment. Blood tests including a WBC, erythrocyte sedimentation rate, and CRP are neither sensitive nor specific in diagnosing or excluding septic arthritis.[61] Broad-spectrum antibiotics are initially started after obtaining the synovial fluid, and antibiotic selection is further guided by culture and sensitivity results. Septic arthritis has also been reported following viscosupplementation injections.[62]

Systemic adverse effects of IA corticosteroids include endocrine, metabolic, and vascular effects.[63] The most common and predictable endocrine effect is rapid suppression of endogenous cortisol production. Maximal suppression of serum cortisol levels occur by 24 to 48 hours after IA injection; adrenocorticotropic hormone (ACTH) levels typically return to normal between 1 and 4 weeks, indicating recovery of normal endogenous steroid production.[25,63,64] Metabolic effects include elevation of blood glucose levels in diabetic patients.[65] In diabetics with appropriate glucose control, acute hyperglycemia may persist for 2 to 3 days with peak glucose levels reaching 300 mg/dL.[63,66] Facial flushing is an unpleasant adverse effect seen in 15% to 40% of patients.[9] The effect occurs, on average, 19 hours after injection and is self-limiting, lasting approximately 36 hours. Triamcinolone administration is associated with a higher rate of facial flushing.[63]

VISCOSUPPLEMENTATION

INDICATIONS AND MECHANISM OF ACTION

Viscosupplementation refers to IA administration of synthetic hyaluronic acid (HA). Intra-articular HA administration (IAHA) is recommended by numerous specialty guidelines, including the ACR, Osteoarthritis Research Society International (OARSI), and European League Against Rheumatism (EULAR), as a treatment option for the management of knee osteoarthritis.[8,67,68] Intra-articular HA administration is approved by the FDA only for knee osteoarthritis. Off-label application of IAHA has been reported for the shoulder, hip, and ankle. Selection criteria include unresponsiveness to standard noninvasive treatment programs with clinical and radiologic signs of knee osteoarthritis.[8,69] Osteoarthritis severity may be an important predictor in determining the magnitude of clinical response to IAHA injection. In general, IAHA seems most beneficial in individuals with early osteoarthritis and radiographic evidence of joint space preservation.[70-72] Contraindications to IAHA injection are shown in Box 71.1.

Table 71.3 Commonly Used Hyaluronic Acid Preparations for IA Viscosupplementation.

Product Structure	Product Name	Origin	Molecular Weight (kDa)	Injection Interval	Dosing Volume	Recommended Dosing Regimen*
Cross linked	Synvisc	Sodium hyaluronate	6000	1 week	2 ml	3
	Synvisc-One	Sodium hyaluronate	6000	N/A	6 ml	Once
Non–cross linked	Supartz	Sodium hyaluronate (naturally derived)	620-1170	1 week	2.5 ml	3 or 5*
	Hyalgan	Sodium hyaluronate (naturally derived)	500-730	1 week	2 ml	3 or 5*
	Orthovisc	Bacterial fermentation (nonavian)	1000-2900	1 week	2 ml	3-4*
	Euflexxa	Bacterial fermentation (nonavian)	2400-3600	1 week	2 ml	3

*Treatment schedule: Please refer to manufacturers' specific recommendations.
kDa, kilodalton. N/A, not applicable.

Although the exact mechanism of action is unknown, the treatment goal is to restore the viscoelastic properties of synovial fluid.[73] Observed treatment benefits are not entirely explained by IA residence time, which is considerably shorter than the duration of clinical benefit. Several in vitro and preclinical studies have proposed additional mechanisms of action for IAHA, including inhibition of inflammation and cartilage degradation, reduction of pain mediators, and induction of in vivo HA synthesis.[74,75]

VISCOSUPPLEMENTATION AGENT SELECTION (STRUCTURE AND FUNCTION)

Viscosupplementation formulations differ in their origin, method of production, molecular weight, treatment schedule, and physicochemical properties.[75] Six hyaluronic acid preparations are approved for knee osteoarthritis in the United States (Table 71.3). Formulations are classified as cross-linked or non-cross-linked and are further defined by chemical modifications and production method (avian- versus non-avian-derived products). Non-avian products are produced by bacterial fermentation. All available avian preparations are derived from rooster combs and are purified natural products. The sole exception is hylan G-F 20, which is chemically modified (cross-linked HA) to increase the molecular weight to more closely replicate the properties of native synovial fluid and to lengthen IA residence half-life.[73,76] No conclusive evidence exists that differences in viscosupplement physical properties translate into superior clinical efficacy.[77]

DOSING AND POSTINJECTION PROTOCOLS

The recommended dosing regimens for particular viscosupplementation products are based on the physical properties and the manufacturers' prescribing recommendations. Currently, there is insufficient evidence to guide the appropriate injection frequency and dosing intervals. Common recommendations are either for a single injection or a total of three to five weekly injections based on the selected product (see Table 71.3), but these are solely based on the manufacturer's recommendations that arose from the premarketing registry trials for each product.[78] Evidence-based recommendations do not exist for interval timing for repeating treatment. Insurance providers typically require a minimum of 6 months between repeated treatment courses. Pre-injection synovial fluid aspiration and avoidance of excessive weight bearing activities for 48 to 72 hours postinjection may yield better outcomes.[70,72,79]

ADVERSE EFFECTS AND COMPLICATIONS ASSOCIATED WITH VISCOSUPPLEMENTATION INJECTION

In general, viscosupplementation is well tolerated with more local reactions but fewer systemic side effects compared to other medical interventions for the management of knee osteoarthritis.[80] Frequently reported local adverse effects include injection site pain, short-term erythema, and joint effusion development. These effects are typically mild and resolve within 24 to 48 hours.

Other infrequent local adverse effects include pseudosepsis and pseudogout.[81] Pseudosepsis, a severe acute inflammatory reaction (SAIR), is considered an extreme local adverse reaction. It is characterized by a large effusion, severe pain, and cellular infiltration occurring within 24 to 72 hours after the injection. Pseudosepsis often requires clinical intervention such as arthrocentesis, IA corticosteroids, and systemic analgesics.[82] Pseudosepsis may be misdiagnosed as septic arthritis.[82] The proposed mechanisms of pseudosepsis include an immune reaction to cross-linked products. Inappropriate injectate placement has also been suggested as a causative factor in pseudosepsis.[70,83] When pseudosepsis is suspected, it is imperative that other clinical conditions such as septic arthritis are ruled out.

Pseudogout is a type of crystal-induced arthropathy characterized by calcium pyrophosphate crystal deposition. Individuals with pseudogout present with acute pain, joint swelling, and decreased function. The pathophysiology leading to pseudogout after IAHA is not clearly understood. Pseudogout occurs more frequently in patients with preexisting chondrocalcinosis; therefore, IAHA should be used with a caution in these individuals.[84,85] Pseudogout may also be mislabeled as pseudosepsis. Synovial fluid analysis is helpful in making the correct diagnosis (see Table 71.2).

JOINT INJECTION TECHNIQUES

Three injection techniques (palpation, ultrasound guided, and fluoroscopy guided) may be used for the placement of drugs into the IA space. Palpation-guided IA injections are associated with inappropriate needle placement rates as high as 50% to 60%.[86,87] Fluoroscopy- and ultrasound-guided methods have evolved to increase injection accuracy. Although both techniques allow for needle visualization, ultrasound guidance has advantages. Benefits of ultrasound-guided injection include dynamic real-time multiplanar imaging of relevant anatomic structures, direct visualization of injected therapeutic agents, and absence of ionizing radiation.

Improved injection accuracy with visually guided techniques ensures correct IA compound placement and may significantly influence clinical outcomes. In a randomized control trial evaluating clinical outcomes in individuals who received either anatomic palpation-guided or ultrasound-guided IA joint injections, the benefit of accurate IA placement was demonstrated.[87] A total of 148 joint injections were studied with 95% of injections occurring in large joints (knee, hip, shoulder, elbow, wrist, and ankle). The remaining 5% of the injections occurred in small joints (interphalangeal or metacarpophalangeal joints). Intra-articular knee injections represented the largest category at 42%. Sonographic needle guidance was found to be statistically superior in multiple areas. In comparison to palpation-guided injections, ultrasound-guided injections resulted in a 43% reduction in procedural pain, 58.5% reduction in absolute pain scores at 2 weeks, 26% increase in responder rate, and 62% reduction in the nonresponder rate. Sonographic needle placement also improved detection of joint effusion by 200% and increased aspirated fluid volume by 337%. The authors concluded that sonographic guidance for IA injections is associated with significant short-term clinical advantages.

In this section we will describe the injection techniques for the three major joints: shoulder, hip, and knee. Emphasis will be placed on the visual-guided techniques. The efficacy for IA and viscosupplementation will also be discussed. Strict aseptic technique should be utilized for all injections.

SHOULDER

ANATOMY

The shoulder is a complex anatomic structure allowing multidirectional movement. The shoulder girdle refers to several articulations associated with important muscle groups that provide a wide range of shoulder movement. Three important shoulder joints are the glenohumeral, acromioclavicular, and sternoclavicular. The glenohumeral joint is a ball and socket joint that allows abduction, adduction, flexion, extension, rotation, and circumduction. The acromioclavicular joint is situated superficially between the lateral end of clavicle and acromion process of scapula. The rotator cuff muscles include the supraspinatus, infraspinatus, teres minor, and subscapularis. The subacromial bursa is positioned within the subacromial space between the overlying deltoid muscle and the underlying supraspinatus tendon, and it provides rotator cuff lubrication.

Injection techniques for the shoulder include palpation (anatomic landmarks) and visually guided (ultrasound and fluoroscopy) approaches. We will focus the discussion on visually guided techniques for the three major anatomic locations for shoulder injections: (1) subacromial/subdeltoid bursa, (2) glenohumeral joint, and (3) acromioclavicular (AC) joint. Shoulder injection using only anatomic landmarks may be inaccurate,[88-92] which may adversely affect short-term clinical outcomes.[88,93]

SUBACROMIAL/SUBDELTOID BURSA INJECTIONS

INDICATIONS AND MUSCULOSKELETAL PATHOPHYSIOLOGY

Subacromial injections are used to diagnose and treat various shoulder conditions including rotator cuff pathology, subacromial bursitis, and subacromial impingement.[94,95] Impingement refers to the narrowing of space available for the rotator cuff resulting in compression of rotator cuff tendons against the undersurface of the coracoacromial arch.[96] Rotator cuff impingement may result in the development of bursitis, subacromial inflammation, secondary tendinitis, and degenerative tears.[97]

Clinical outcomes following subacromial injections have been linked to the accuracy of injection, the severity of imaging findings, and the duration of symptoms.[88,93,98] Specifically, a magnetic resonance imaging (MRI) finding of isolated bursitis without rotator cuff tear, younger age, and shorter duration of symptoms (less than 1 year) are associated with better postinjection clinical outcomes.[98]

PALPATION-GUIDED ANATOMIC INJECTION TECHNIQUE

Commonly utilized portals for palpation-guided subacromial injections include the posterior-lateral and anterior-lateral approach.[89,97,99,100] In the posterior approach, the needle is inserted 1 to 2 cm inferior to the posterior-lateral aspect of the acromion process. The needle is directed anteriorly and cephalad. In the anterior approach, the needle is inserted approximately 1 cm inferior to the anterior/inferior aspect of the acromion process. The needle is directed posteriorly and cephalad. The posterolateral approach is preferred because of the existence of a larger subacromial space.[100]

FLUOROSCOPY-GUIDED INJECTION TECHNIQUE

Limited information exists detailing subacromial joint injections performed under fluoroscopic guidance. The utilization of fluoroscopy with radiographic contrast IA injection has been employed as a confirmatory adjunct to palpation-guided injections, to ensure appropriate needle[98] and injectate placement.[88,99,101]

ULTRASOUND-GUIDED INJECTION TECHNIQUE

The patient sits in the upright position with the shoulder extended, elbow flexed, and palm of the hand placed over the ipsilateral back pocket (modified Crass position).[95,102] Initially the IA portion of the biceps tendon is identified over the anterior shoulder with a high frequency linear-array ultrasound probe. The probe is oriented in the coronal plane and is moved superiorly and posteriorly until it is aligned with the supraspinatus tendon longitudinal axis. The supraspinatus tendon in this position has a typical beak-shaped appearance.[102] The subacromial-subdeltoid bursa is visualized as a thin hypoechoic band outlined by highly

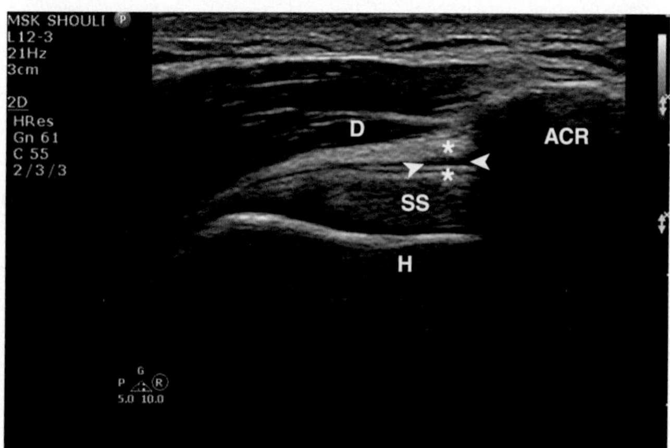

Figure 71.2 Ultrasound view of the subacromial-subdeltoid bursa along the long axis of the supraspinatus tendon. Asterisks (*) indicate peribursal fat; arrowheads identify the subacromial bursa. ACR, acromion process; D, deltoid; H, humerus; SS, supraspinatus tendon. (Please see text for a detailed description of patient and ultrasound probe positioning.)

reflective lines corresponding to peribursal fat between the deltoid muscle and supraspinatus tendon (Fig. 71.2).[95,103] Other structures visualized include the acromion process at the medial end and the greater tuberosity at the lateral end of the scan plane. The lateral end of the transducer is marked for the skin entry. A procedure needle is advanced with an in-plane technique into the subacromial-subdeltoid bursa. After confirming needle position within the bursa, the desired medication is injected slowly while noting the expansion of the bursa.[104] Injection without bursa distention suggests intramuscular or intratendinous needle insertion and requires needle tip repositioning.

GLENOHUMERAL JOINT INJECTIONS

INDICATIONS AND MUSCULOSKELETAL PATHOLOGY

Glenohumeral joint injections are used as a nonoperative management technique for glenohumeral arthrosis or adhesive capsulitis (frozen shoulder).[94]

FLUOROSCOPY-GUIDED INJECTION TECHNIQUE

The patient is placed in the lateral decubitus position with the head resting on the nontargeted arm with the targeted shoulder in the nondependent position. A bolster is placed in front of the patient and then the patient rotates onto the bolster with the targeted arm internally rotated until the glenohumeral joint space is aligned under the fluoroscopic anterior-posterior view (Fig. 71.3).[105] The skin entry site is marked over the inferiomedial quadrant of the humeral head.[106] A 22-gauge needle is advanced with a coaxial fluoroscopy-guided technique to the humeral head. After negative aspiration, radiographic contrast is injected to confirm IA needle placement. Although the posterior approach is commonly used, additional fluoroscopic techniques have been described utilizing the anterior[107] and rotator cuff interval approaches.[108]

ULTRASOUND-GUIDED INJECTION TECHNIQUE

The patient is placed in either the semiprone position resting on the contralateral shoulder or in an upright sitting

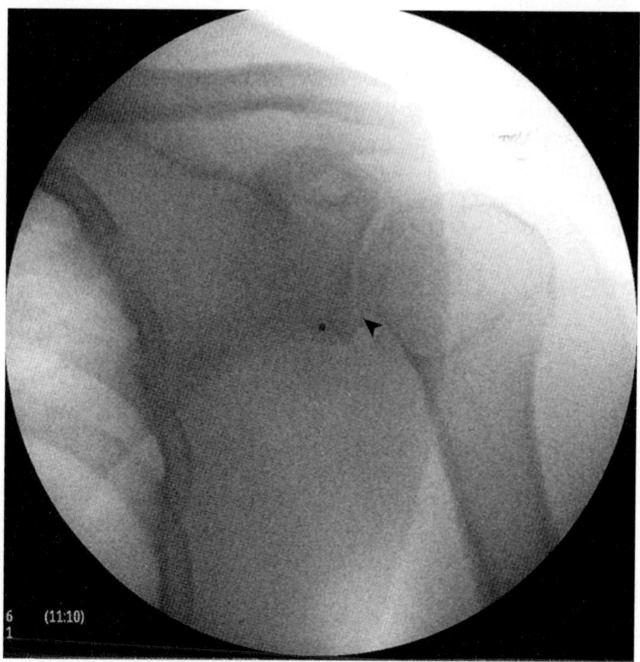

Figure 71.3 Glenohumeral joint visualization by fluoroscopy. The posterior aspect of the glenohumeral joint space is viewed tangentially under fluoroscopic guidance. The inferomedial quadrant of the humeral head is marked (arrowhead) as the needle entry site. (Please see text for a detailed description of patient positioning.)

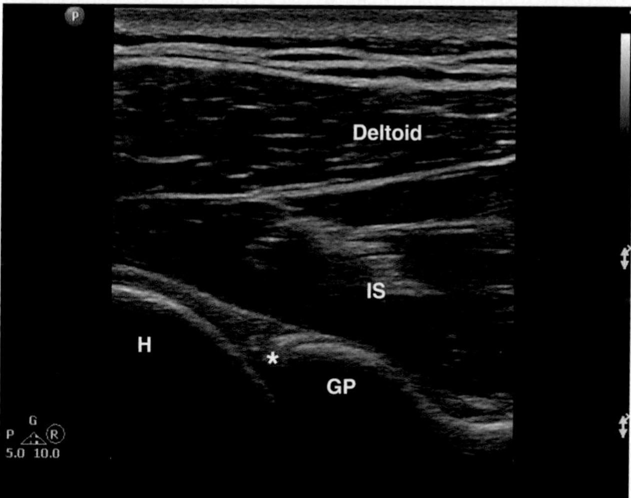

Figure 71.4 Glenohumeral joint visualization by ultrasound. The posterior aspect of the glenohumeral joint space is viewed using ultrasound guidance. Asterisk (*) indicates the glenoid labrum. GP, glenoid process; H, humerus head; IS, infraspinatus muscle. (Please see text for a detailed description of patient and ultrasound probe positioning.)

position with the ipsilateral arm placed on the contralateral shoulder to open up the glenohumeral joint space.[91] A high-frequency linear-array probe facilitates visualization of superficial structures including the infraspinatus muscle, glenoid cavity, glenohumeral joint, and associated labrum. The probe is positioned over the infraspinatus fossa inferior and parallel to the scapular spine. The field of view is adjusted to encompass the posterior glenoid rim and the glenohumeral junction (Fig. 71.4). The posterior glenoid labrum appears as a triangular structure. The lateral end of the transducer is marked for the skin entry. A 22-gauge needle is advanced with an in-plane approach into the joint deep to the infraspinatus tendon, between the posterior glenoid labrum and the hypoechoic humeral articular cartilage.[109] Resistance at the time of injection suggests a needle tip position within articular cartilage or labrum and necessitates needle repositioning. Alternative techniques include the anterior[110] and rotator cuff interval approaches.[111]

ACROMIOCLAVICULAR JOINT INJECTION

INDICATIONS AND MUSCULOSKELETAL PATHOLOGY

AC joint injections are employed for diagnostic and therapeutic purposes for AC joint arthritis.[94,112]

FLUOROSCOPY-GUIDED INJECTION TECHNIQUE

Few reports exist describing fluoroscopically guided AC joint injections. With the patient in the supine position, a 25-gauge needle is advanced into the AC joint using either an anterior or superior approach. Less than 0.5 mL of radiographic contrast is utilized to confirm IA placement.[113,114]

ULTRASOUND-GUIDED INJECTION TECHNIQUE

Both in-plane[115] and out-of-plane[95,104,116] ultrasound-guided techniques have been described. However, the out-of-plane technique is preferred due to this joint's small size and superficial location.[95] The patient is positioned in the sitting position, and a high-frequency linear-array probe is placed in an anatomic coronal plane over the superficially located AC joint (Fig. 71.5). The acromion process, clavicle, joint capsule, and wedge-shaped fibrocartilaginous disk are visualized. A 25-gauge needle is advanced using an out-of-plane technique. Because of the shallow AC joint depth, needle insertion must be carefully controlled to avoid misplacement into the subacromial space.[95,112]

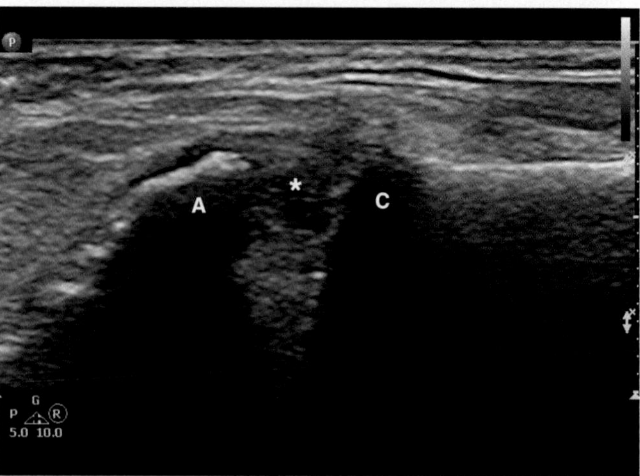

Figure 71.5 Ultrasound view of the acromioclavicular joint. Asterisk (*) indicates the acromioclavicular joint. C, clavicle; A, acromion. (Please see text for a detailed description of patient and ultrasound probe positioning.)

GENERAL EFFICACY OF SHOULDER INJECTIONS

GENERAL EFFICACY OF SUBACROMIAL/SUBDELTOID BURSA INJECTIONS

Evidence for the efficacy of subacromial/subdeltoid bursa injections is conflicting. This incongruity may correlate with the lack of selection of specific shoulder diagnoses in some study populations or inaccurate injectate placement.[93,98,117] A randomized controlled trial of palpation-guided subacromial injections demonstrated greater short-term pain reduction and functional outcome improvement at 1 and 6 weeks with the combined subacromial injection and exercise protocol versus exercise alone.[118] However, the study did not demonstrate continued differences in clinical outcomes at 12 weeks. Predictors of success following subacromial injections have been investigated. MRI findings consistent with low-grade impingement and bursitis without evidence of a rotator cuff tear are positive predictors of injection response.[98]

GENERAL EFFICACY OF GLENOHUMERAL JOINT INJECTIONS

The majority of available evidence for therapeutic glenohumeral joint injection relates to adhesive capsulitis.[117] A systematic review evaluated the efficacy of repeated IA corticosteroid injections in treating adhesive capsulitis.[119] Nine randomized controlled trials were included in this review. This review concluded that multiple injections improve pain and range of motion in the short term (6 to 16 weeks). Another systematic review investigated the efficacy of IA glenohumeral joint corticosteroid injection compared to other treatments including oral corticosteroid, subacromial injection, joint manipulation, joint distension, and physical therapy. This review concluded that IA corticosteroid injection improves pain and range of motion in the short term, with no significant long-term differences in comparison to other treatments.[120] Limitations to the studies included in these reviews were use of diverse outcome measures, injection techniques (palpation versus image guidance), injection site (concurrent subacromial and AC joint injection in some studies), drug types and preparations, and physical therapy regimens. Future studies with improved design are required to definitively assess IA glenohumeral injection efficacy for shoulder joint disorders.

GENERAL EFFICACY OF ACROMIOCLAVICULAR JOINT INJECTIONS

To date, no randomized controlled trials have been published evaluating the effectiveness of AC joint injections. Retrospective case series and prospective cohort studies reported short-term improvement.[121,122] In studies examining pain relief beyond 3 months, decreasing levels of efficacy were documented with only 14% to 19% of patients reporting sustained pain relief.[123,124] In one study, a predictor of short-term procedural success was capsular hypertrophy (more than 3 mm) on MRI.[114]

COMPARISONS OF ACCURACY AND EFFICACY FOR SPECIFIC SHOULDER JOINT INJECTION TECHNIQUES

ACCURACY AND EFFICACY OF SUBACROMIAL/ SUBDELTOID BURSA INJECTION TECHNIQUES

When directly comparing visually guided techniques to palpation-guided techniques, Naredo and associates[93] demonstrated improved technique accuracy and outcomes (shoulder functional assessment) with ultrasound-guided injection versus palpation-guided injection. Palpation-guided injection resulted in a 30% accuracy rate when validated with ultrasound confirmation of injectate placement. Although fluoroscopic confirmation of injectate placement has been described in other clinical studies, no direct comparative data have been presented with regard to fluoroscopy- versus palpation-guided injection techniques.[88,98,99,101] In a systematic review, image-guided (fluoroscopy or ultrasound) injection had an average accuracy rate of 100% compared to an average accuracy rate of 72% for palpation-guided injections.[125] When examining individual studies for palpation-guided anatomic injection techniques, clinical and cadaveric studies have reported variable accuracy rates in the range of 29% to 91%.[88-90, 99,101,126] Improved injection accuracy resulting from ultrasound guidance[93] or fluoroscopic confirmation[88] positively affects short-term clinical outcomes

Studies directly comparing the efficacy and safety of various image-guided techniques have not been conducted. However, Mathews and coworkers[127] questioned the reliability of fluoroscopy-guided injections in a cadaveric study. Approximately 7% of injections considered to be accurately placed under fluoroscopic guidance were found to be placed inaccurately on subsequent cadaveric dissection. Because of the complex soft tissue anatomic structures of the shoulder joint, fluoroscopic guidance may not guarantee accurate needle placement in the subacromial space. Better visualization of soft tissues using ultrasound guidance potentially favors this method for subacromial joint injections and diagnostic shoulder imaging.[93,97,102] Diagnostic evaluation of rotator cuff tears with high-resolution ultrasound has been shown to be comparable in utility to MRI.[102,128]

COMPARISON OF ACCURACY AND EFFICACY FOR GLENOHUMERAL INJECTION TECHNIQUES

When directly comparing ultrasound-guided techniques to palpation-guided techniques, Cunnington and colleagues[129] demonstrated that junior trainees with basic ultrasound skills achieved higher IA injection accuracy rates using ultrasound-guided (63%) compared to palpation-guided (40%) approaches. No studies exist that directly compare fluoroscopy- versus palpation-guided glenohumeral injection techniques. In one review, image guidance (fluoroscopy, ultrasound, and MRI) had an average accuracy rate of 95% compared to an average accuracy rate of 79% with palpation guidance.[125] When examining individual studies for palpation-guided anatomic injection techniques, clinical and cadaveric studies have reported variable glenohumeral injection accuracy rates in the range of 27% to 100%.[88,126,130-132]

Improved glenohumeral injection accuracy resulting from ultrasound guidance[129,133] or fluoroscopic confirmation[88,129] significantly enhances short-term clinical outcome. In a study involving multijoint interventions, Sibbitt and colleagues[87] demonstrated that ultrasound guidance significantly improves clinical outcome. When directly comparing ultrasound guidance with fluoroscopic guidance, Rutten and coworkers[91] demonstrated that ultrasound guidance improved procedural outcomes. Ultrasound guidance resulted in a first pass accuracy rate of 94% compared to 72% obtained with fluoroscopic guidance, and it also comparatively reduced procedural time and patient discomfort levels.

COMPARISON OF ACCURACY AND EFFICACY FOR ACROMIOCLAVICULAR JOINT INJECTION TECHNIQUES

Because of the small size and variable morphology of the AC joint, needle placement into the joint is often difficult and inaccurate.[90,123] In a direct comparison cadaveric study, ultrasound-guided AC injections using in-plane technique demonstrated a 100% accuracy rate compared with the 40% accuracy rate for palpation-guided injections.[115] No direct comparative data have been generated between fluoroscopy- versus palpation-guided injection techniques. For anatomically guided palpation techniques, clinical and cadaveric studies have reported variable accuracy rates in the range of 40% to 66% when confirmation of needle or injectate placement was validated with fluoroscopy or cadaveric dissection.[90,123,134] Sabeti-Aschraf and associates[116] observed similar clinical outcomes following palpation-guided and ultrasound-guided AC injections when performed by experienced physicians.

HIP

ANATOMY

The hip joint is a ball-and-socket type of synovial joint situated deeply within the pelvis. Hip joint stability is attributed to the articulation of the convex femoral head (ball) into the concave acetabulum (socket), with additional reinforcement arising from the articular capsule and surrounding muscles and ligaments. The fibrous articular capsule extends from the acetabular rim across the joint to the base of the femoral neck. This capsular anatomy allows for accurate IA injectate placement into the capsule at the femoral head/neck junction without going directly into the joint space. The femoral neurovascular bundle lies medially to the hip joint in the femoral triangle.

INDICATIONS AND MUSCULOSKELETAL PATHOLOGY

Intra-articular injections are used to diagnose and treat the symptoms of inflammatory and noninflammatory arthritis of the hip joint. Osteoarthritis is a significant cause of hip pain and disability. Intra-articular hip injections are used as a nonoperative treatment for hip osteoarthritis. Intra-articular hip injections are also utilized for diagnostic purposes to assist in determining and distinguishing IA hip pathology from extra-articular sources of pain.[135] Clinical predictors of a successful response include the presence of joint effusion[136] and lack of an atrophic radiologic pattern.[137] The radiographic severity of hip arthritis does not predict pain relief outcome for therapeutic IA hip injection.

PALPATION-GUIDED ANATOMIC INJECTION TECHNIQUE

Multiple hip joint injection techniques are described in literature including palpation- (anatomic landmarks) and visually (fluoroscopy and ultrasound) guided techniques. Palpation-guided injections include both anterior and lateral approaches. Intra-articular hip injections using anatomic landmarks are often inaccurate due to the joint's deep location.[138,139] Here we focus on descriptions of visually guided techniques, which are associated with improved injection accuracy.[140-142]

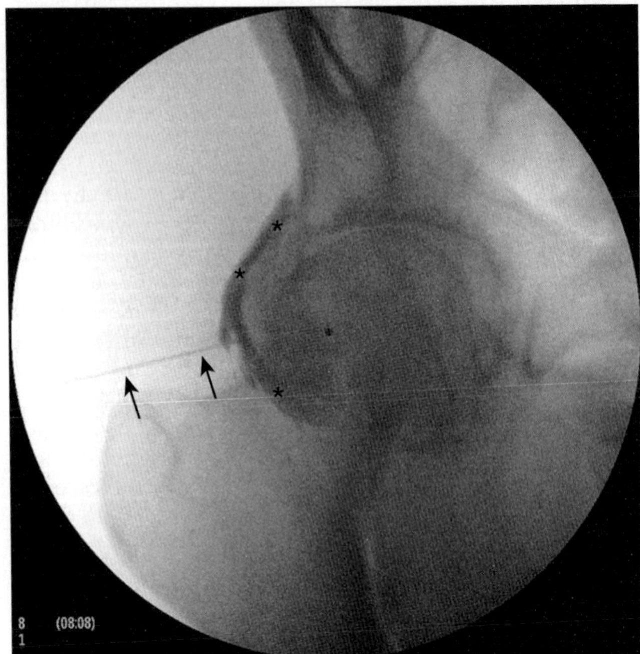

Figure 71.6 **Fluoroscopy-guided lateral-approach hip joint injection.** An anteroposterior fluoroscopy-guided view used to position the needle for a lateral-approach hip joint injection. The needle tip is positioned at the lateral femoral head/neck junction. Injection of radiographic contrast medium confirms accurate intracapsular needle placement. The arrows point to the needle. Asterisk (*) outlines the intracapsular radiographic contrast agent spread. (Please see text for a detailed description of patient positioning.)

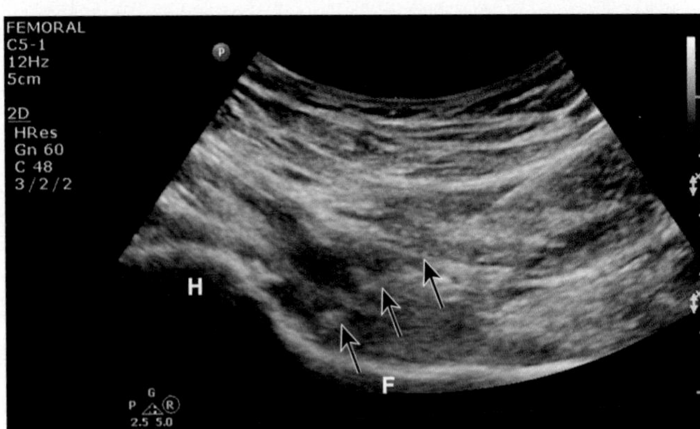

Figure 71.7 **Ultrasound-guided intra-articular hip injection.** The arrows indicate the needle tip accurately placed within the synovial recess at the femoral head/neck junction. F, femoral shaft; H, femoral head. (Please see text for a detailed description of patient and ultrasound probe positioning.)

FLUOROSCOPY-GUIDED INTRA-ARTICULAR HIP INJECTION TECHNIQUES

Anterior Approach

The patient is placed in the supine position on the fluoroscopy table. First, the femoral artery is identified with palpation along the inguinal crease.[143] With fluoroscopy under an anterior-posterior view, the lateral aspect of the femoral head/neck junction is identified.[113] A needle is then directed coaxially under fluoroscopic guidance to the lateral femoral head/neck junction while avoiding the previously marked femoral artery. After reaching the lateral aspect of the femoral head/neck junction, the needle is slightly withdrawn. Following negative aspiration, radiographic contrast agent is injected to confirm intracapsular needle placement. Corticosteroids, often with local anesthetics, are then injected (see Table 71.1).

Lateral Approach

The patient is placed in the lateral decubitus position on the fluoroscopy table with the targeted hip in the nondependent position. The skin entry point is identified immediately proximal to greater trochanter. The center of the hip joint often corresponds to midplane between the anterior and posterior aspects of the thigh.[144] In the anterior-posterior view, the needle is advanced to the lateral aspect of the femoral head/neck junction (Fig. 71.6). Care is taken to avoid an anterior or posterior needle trajectory to the femoral head/neck junction. On the fluoroscopy image, if the needle has passed the femoral head/neck junction without contacting bone the needle needs to be repositioned to ensure intracapsular injection. Corticosteroids, often with local anesthetics, are then administered (see Table 71.1). Proposed advantages of the lateral approach include a skin entry distant from the femoral neurovascular bundle and visualization of the needle throughout placement.[143]

ULTRASOUND-GUIDED INTRA-ARTICULAR HIP INJECTION TECHNIQUES

The patient is placed in the supine position on the procedure table. Typically, a low frequency curvilinear probe is employed to allow for adequate penetration and a larger field of view.[145] The femoral neurovascular bundle is identified in the short axis view. Then, the probe is moved laterally and oriented to align it parallel to the long axis of the femoral neck. In the anterior-oblique-sagittal (anterior-longitudinal) view, the femoral neck, femoral head, acetabular rim, and anterior synovial recess should be visualized.[142,145,146] The anterior synovial recess, at the femoral head/neck junction, is the target location. In this view, the femoral neurovascular bundle is located 20 to 30 mm medial to the desired needle trajectory.[146] Power or color Doppler is utilized to identify any overlying vascular structures such as the ascending branch of lateral femoral circumflex artery.[147] The ultrasound view is adjusted to provide a needle trajectory that is clear of any vascular structures. A 22-gauge needle is advanced with an in-plane approach into the anterior synovial recess (Fig. 71.7). After confirming needle position within the synovial recess, the medication is injected slowly while noting expansion of anterior hip capsule.

EFFICACY OF INTRA-ARTICULAR HIP INJECTIONS

Limited data exist that evaluate the efficacy of IA hip injections for osteoarthritis. Efficacy data for IA knee injections cannot be extrapolated to the IA hip injections because of differences in anatomic and functional characteristics. Three prospective randomized controlled studies suggest short-term efficacy for pain relief and functional outcome with visually guided (ultrasound or fluoroscopy) administration of corticosteroids.[136,148,149]

ACCURACY AND EFFICACY FOR INJECTION TECHNIQUE COMPARISONS

Although multiple studies have recommended image guidance to improve accuracy, no studies to date have directly compared image-guided versus palpation-guided techniques.[137,138,140-142] Conventional palpation-guided IA injections may result in inaccurate needle placement. The femoral neurovascular bundle is the primary anatomic structure at risk of injury.[138] Accuracy rates of 60% to 80% for IA injectate placement have been documented with palpation-guided techniques.[138-140,150]

Ultrasound-guided IA hip injections have demonstrated accuracy rates of 97% to 100%, which are comparable to the accuracy rates associated with computed tomography (CT)- or fluoroscopy-guided injections.[142,150] Given the paucity of clinical outcome studies, no conclusive relationship can be established between improved accuracy rates and clinical and functional outcomes. One study demonstrated that ultrasound guidance significantly improved performance and clinical outcomes for small and large joint IA injections.[87] Further evaluation is warranted regarding the safety and efficacy of IA hip injections, with direct comparison necessary between fluoroscopy- and ultrasound-guided techniques.

KNEE

ANATOMY

The knee joint is a synovial joint composed of three bones: the patella, femur, and tibia. The four major ligaments providing stability to the knee are the anterior cruciate, posterior cruciate, medial collateral, and lateral collateral.[151,152]

The medial and lateral menisci are fibrocartilaginous structures that provide stability, lubrication, and nutrition to the joint space. Meniscal tears occur three times more frequently in the medial meniscus. Knee flexion and extension are the main motion planes. The knee is divided into three major compartments: medial, lateral, and patellofemoral. Knee arthritis typically occurs in two or more compartments.[152,153]

INDICATIONS AND MUSCULOSKELETAL PATHOLOGY

Intra-articular knee injections with either corticosteroids or viscosupplements are part of nonoperative management of knee osteoarthritis. In 1997, viscosupplementation was approved in the United States to treat knee osteoarthritis. For knee osteoarthritis, clinical predictors of a positive response to IA corticosteroids have not been conclusively identified.[154] Multiple attempts have been made to identify clinical predictors of response to IA corticosteroids. Jones and Doherty[154] were not able to identify clinical predictors. Gaffney and colleagues[155] reported greater improvements in pain relief when there was clinical evidence of an effusion and aspiration of synovial fluid at the time of injection. Based on these data, it is difficult to determine whether an effusion predicts clinical response or if synovial fluid is just a surrogate marker for appropriate needle placement.

PALPATION-GUIDED ANATOMIC KNEE INJECTION TECHNIQUES

Commonly utilized knee portals for IA injections include superior anteromedial, superior anterolateral, inferior anteromedial, inferior anterolateral, and lateral and medial midpatellar approaches. Multiple studies have examined different injection techniques in specific populations. In individuals without knee effusions, confirmation of appropriate needle placement can be difficult when using a palpation-guided technique. Jackson and colleagues[156] demonstrated that the lateral midpatellar approach resulted in a higher accuracy rate (93%) in comparison with both the anteromedial (75% accuracy) and anterolateral (71% accuracy) approaches. The anteromedial and anterolateral injections were performed inferior to the patella with the affected leg over the side of the examination table and the knee flexed to approximately 90 degrees.

A cadaver study compared four different IA injection sites (anteromedial, anterolateral, lateral midpatellar, and medial midpatellar).[157] The midpatellar approaches were performed with the knee extended on an examination table. The anteromedial and anterolateral injections were performed inferior to the patella with the leg over the side of the examination table and the knee flexed to approximately 90 degrees. The accuracy rate was highest for the anterolateral approach (85%) and lowest in the medial midpatellar approach (56%).

Wind and Smolinski[158] examined injection portals superior to the patella (superolateral and superomedial) for low-volume (2 to 3 mL) injections, consistent with viscosupplementation treatment. Injections were performed with the knee extended. In this study, the lateral joint line injection was unreliable and resulted in IA placement less than 50% of the time.

FLUOROSCOPY-GUIDED KNEE INJECTION TECHNIQUES

Techniques have been described for both fluoroscopic needle advancement and fluoroscopic confirmation of appropriate injectate location following palpation-guided IA injection.[113,159] The fluoroscopy-guided injection technique can be performed above (Fig. 71.8), below, or at the level of the patella. When the injection is performed at the patellofemoral joint with either a medial or lateral approach, the patella is manually displaced away from the needle and the needle is advanced into the joint.[113] In individuals with severe patellofemoral joint arthritis, access into the joint may be difficult with this technique.

Anterior approaches have also been described.[160,161] Moser and associates[161] assessed the infrapatellar anterolateral and anterior paramedian needle insertion approaches for technical success and patient tolerance levels during knee arthrography. For the anterior paramedian approach, the knee is flexed to 60 degrees and the needle is introduced just lateral to the inferior patellar ligament and directed cephalad and medial toward the femoral notch. For the anterolateral approach, the knee is flexed to 90 degrees and the joint space is located. The needle is placed at the joint line and directed posteriorly and slightly medial toward the lateral femoral articular condyle.

For the fluoroscopy-guided techniques, radiographic contrast agent may be injected to confirm appropriate needle placement. If radiographic contrast cannot be utilized, IA placement has also been verified by mini-air arthrography.[159] For the superior patellar approach, mini-air arthrography is able to confirm IA placement when

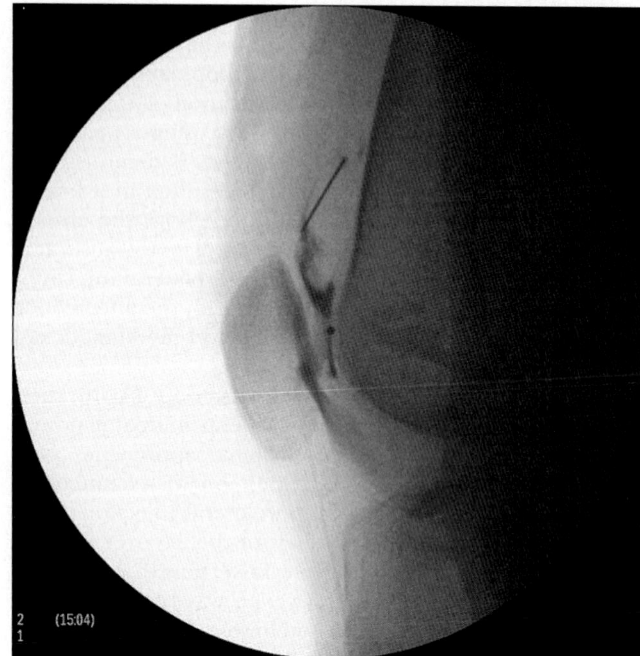

Figure 71.8 Fluoroscopy-guided lateral approach for suprapatellar intra-articular knee injection. Accurate needle tip placement in the suprapatellar synovial recess is confirmed by appropriate localization of injected radiographic contrast medium. (Please see text for a detailed description of patient positioning.)

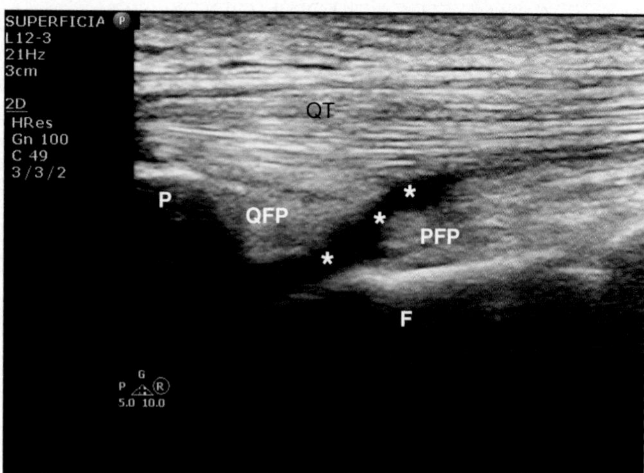

Figure 71.9 Long-axis view of the suprapatellar synovial recess. P indicates patella; F, femur; PFP, prefemoral fat pad; QFP, quadriceps fat pad; QT, quadriceps tendon. Asterisk (*) indicates the outline of the suprapatellar synovial recess communicating with the intra-articular joint space. (Please see text for a detailed description of patient and ultrasound probe positioning.)

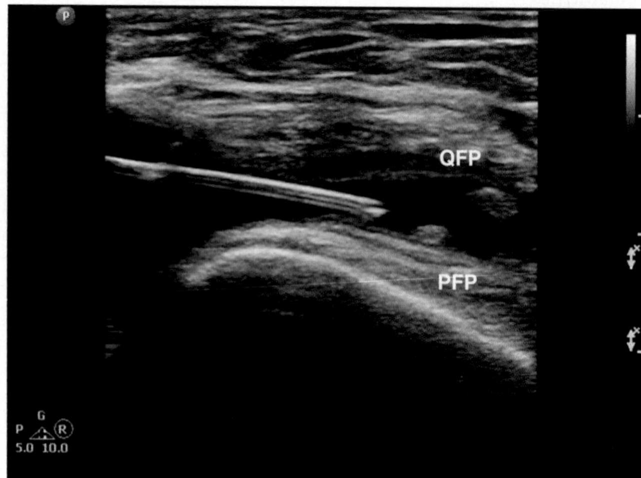

Figure 71.10 Short-axis (transverse) view of the suprapatellar synovial recess. The needle was accurately placed in the suprapatellar synovial recess between the prefemoral fat pad (PFP) and quadriceps fat pad (QFP). (Please see text for a detailed description of patient and ultrasound probe positioning.)

a sharply defined shadow of air is found in the suprapatellar pouch after 0.5 to 5 mL of air is injected.[159,162] Extra-articular placement is suggested when the air is found diffusely in the surrounding tissues. Although air arthrography has been suggested as a safe procedure, the Doppler function for ultrasound or a negative aspiration for fluoroscopy-guided injections should be utilized prior to injecting air to prevent an intravascular injection and the possible development of an air embolism.

ULTRASOUND-GUIDED INJECTION TECHNIQUES

Ultrasound-guided approaches include the midpatellar lateral,[162] the midpatellar medial,[163] and the suprapatellar synovial recess[164] approaches. With both the medial and lateral midpatellar approaches, the patella prevents direct visualization of the needle and injectate in the IA space. Therefore, the preferred technique is the suprapatellar synovial recess approach. This approach also minimizes the risk to soft tissue structures and the articular cartilage.[164] One disadvantage of this approach is that the suprapatellar synovial recess can be difficult to visualize in individuals without knee effusions.

For the suprapatellar approach, the patient is in the sitting or supine position with the knee flexed approximately 20 to 30 degrees.[165] The knee can be supported with a pillow. A high-frequency linear-array probe is utilized. First the knee is scanned with the transducer parallel to the longitudinal axis of the quadriceps tendon (Fig. 71.9). Then the skin and subcutaneous tissues, quadriceps tendon, patella, quadriceps fat pad, prefemoral fat pad, femur, and suprapatellar synovial recess are identified. The suprapatellar synovial recess is located between the prefemoral and quadriceps fat pads, and it communicates directly with the knee joint. It is important that transducer pressure is minimized to prevent compression of the synovial recess. In some individuals, a significant effusion will be visualized in the synovial recess. Next the transducer is rotated 90 degrees to the axial (transverse) plane for the short axis view (Fig. 71.10), and the same structures are identified. The needle is advanced in the short axis view with an in-plane technique from lateral to medial into the suprapatellar synovial recess. Synovial fluid may be aspirated. Then the injectate is placed into the joint under direct ultrasound visualization. The Doppler function can also be utilized to enhance visualization of the injected fluid.

The suprapatellar synovial recess injection may also be performed with the ultrasound transducer along the longitudinal axis.[164] With this technique, the superior margin of the patella is the inferior landmark of the suprapatellar synovial recess. The transducer is moved laterally to avoid insertion into the quadriceps tendon. The cephalad end of the transducer is positioned more laterally than the caudal end. The needle is advanced in-plane in the long axis. This approach may be advantageous when it is difficult to view the suprapatellar synovial recess in the short axis (transverse) plane.

GENERAL EFFICACY OF INTRA-ARTICULAR KNEE INJECTIONS

One review evaluated the efficacy of IA-injected corticosteroids for treating knee osteoarthritis.[166] Twenty-eight trials were included in the analysis. Corticosteroids were compared to placebo, viscosupplementation (hyaluronan and hylan derivatives), and joint lavage. For pain relief at 1 week, injected corticosteroids were found to be superior to placebo with a number needed to treat (NNT) of three. Increased pain reduction by injection versus placebo lasted up to 3 weeks. From 4 to 24 weeks there was a lack of evidence to support prolonged therapeutic efficacy. Functional outcomes were difficult to evaluate secondary to a lack of data. Corticosteroid injection and viscosupplementation benefits were similar between 1 and 4 weeks postinjection. From weeks 5 to 13, viscosupplementation was assessed as superior, with improvements maintained in functional and pain outcomes.

A systematic review of viscosupplementation for the treatment of osteoarthritis evaluated 76 trials.[80] In comparison to placebo, viscosupplementation was found to be superior. From 5 to 13 weeks postinjection, viscosupplementation improved pain relief from baseline by 28% to 54%, and enhanced function by 9% to 32%. Although slower in onset, viscosupplementation appears to have a more prolonged therapeutic effect than IA corticosteroids.[167] Comparisons between different formulations of viscosupplementation could not be made secondary to differences in study designs and outcome measures.[80]

COMPARISONS OF ACCURACY AND EFFICACY FOR INTRA-ARTICULAR KNEE INJECTION TECHNIQUES

In direct comparison of visually guided techniques to palpation-guided techniques for IA knee injections, numerous studies have demonstrated greater accuracy with visually guided methods.[87,163-165,168] For the suprapatellar approach, ultrasound-guided IA injection resulted in greater accuracy rates (96% to 100%) than palpation-guided injections (55% to 84% accuracy).[164,165] For the medial patellar portal, injection accuracy increased from 77% for blind injections to 96% for ultrasound-guided injections.[163] Improvement in accuracy from ultrasound needle guidance positively and significantly influences clinical outcomes and cost effectiveness.[87,168] Improvement in outcomes using ultrasound guidance for arthrocentesis of the effusive knee included a 48% reduction in procedural pain and a 183% increase in aspirated synovial fluid volumes.[169] Short-term pain outcomes were also improved at 2 weeks postinjection. Although fluoroscopic guidance assists with needle placement, data have not yet been presented that demonstrate improvements in clinical or functional outcomes.

CONCLUSION

Joint injections are an important part of multimodal treatment for painful musculoskeletal conditions. Ultrasound- and fluoroscopy-guided IA injections assist in improving the accuracy of needle placement. Ultrasound is particularly helpful for interventional musculoskeletal procedures, offering advantages for specific procedures due to its ability to visualize periarticular soft tissues and provide real-time needle tracking without using ionizing radiation. The improvement in the accuracy of needle placement with ultrasound guidance for some joints is associated with significant clinical outcome benefits when compared with palpation-guided techniques. Future comparative studies are needed to develop guidelines for selecting the most appropriate IA corticosteroid and viscosupplementation agents and selecting the best methods to deliver these agents. Particular attention must be paid to the efficacy and adverse effects associated with treatment of each particular joint and underlying musculoskeletal condition. Furthermore, optimal protocols for the timing of injection, postprocedure activity, and specific dosing regimens need to be defined. For some joint injections, larger-scale studies are needed to directly compare the safety and efficacy of ultrasound-guided IA techniques with traditional landmark-based and fluoroscopy-guided techniques.

KEY POINTS

- Musculoskeletal diseases, including symptomatic arthritis and soft tissue conditions, are associated with high levels of disability and significant economic costs. Osteoarthritis is the most prevalent form of arthritis.
- When joint injections are used, they should be incorporated into a multimodal treatment plan.
- Agents utilized for joint injections include corticosteroids, local anesthetics, and viscosupplements.
- Multiple corticosteroid and viscosupplementation formulations exist with differing pharmacologic properties.
- Viscosupplementation seems to have a more prolonged analgesic effect than intra-articular corticosteroids.
- It is important to understand the adverse effects and complications associated with each injectate class. Appropriate management strategies should be employed when these events occur.
- Joint injections may be performed with palpation, ultrasound-guided, or fluoroscopically guided injection techniques.
- Visually guided techniques (ultrasound and fluoroscopy) have been shown to improve the accuracy of needle placement.
- Ultrasound offers advantages for specific procedures because of its ability to visualize periarticular soft tissues and to provide real-time needle tracking without ionizing radiation.
- Appropriate intra-articular placement with ultrasound has been shown to positively influence clinical and economic outcomes.

SUGGESTED READINGS

Bannuru RR, Natov NS, Obadan IE, et al. Therapeutic trajectory of hyaluronic acid versus corticosteroids in the treatment of knee osteoarthritis: a systematic review and meta-analysis. *Arthritis Rheum.* 2009;61:1704-1711.

Bellamy N, Campbell J, Robinson V, et al. Viscosupplementation for the treatment of osteoarthritis of the knee. *Cochrane Database Syst Rev.* 2006:CD005321.

Bellamy N, Campbell J, Robinson V, et al. Intraarticular corticosteroid for treatment of osteoarthritis of the knee. *Cochrane Database Syst Rev.* 2006:CD005328.

Bum Park Y, Ah Choi W, Kim YK, et al. Accuracy of blind versus ultrasound-guided suprapatellar bursal injection. *J Clin Ultrasound.* 2011;40:20-25.

Cole BJ, Schumacher HR Jr. Injectable corticosteroids in modern practice. *J Am Acad Orthop Surg.* 2005;13:37-46.

Habib GS. Systemic effects of intra-articular corticosteroids. *Clin Rheumatol.* 2009;28:749-756.

Habib GS, Saliba W, Nashashibi M. Local effects of intra-articular corticosteroids. *Clin Rheumatol.* 2010;29:347-356.

MacMahon PJ, Eustace SJ, Kavanagh EC. Injectable corticosteroid and local anesthetic preparations: a review for radiologists. *Radiology.* 2009;252:647-661.

Peng PW, Cheng P. Ultrasound-guided interventional procedures in pain medicine: a review of anatomy, sonoanatomy, and procedures, part III: shoulder. *Reg Anesth Pain Med.* 2011;36:592-605.

Peterson C, Hodler J. Evidence-based radiology (part 2): is there sufficient research to support the use of therapeutic injections into the peripheral joints? *Skeletal Radiol.* 2010;39:11-18.

Rutten MJ, Collins JM, Maresch BJ, et al. Glenohumeral joint injection: a comparative study of ultrasound and fluoroscopically guided techniques before MR arthrography. *Eur Radiol.* 2009;19:722-730.

Sibbitt WL Jr, Peisajovich A, Michael AA, et al. Does sonographic needle guidance affect the clinical outcome of intraarticular injections? *J Rheumatol.* 2009;36:1892-1902.

Zhang W, Moskowitz RW, Nuki G. OARSI recommendations for the management of hip and knee osteoarthritis, part II: OARSI evidence-based, expert consensus guidelines. *Osteoarthritis Cartilage.* 2008;16:137-162.

The references for this chapter can be found at www.expertconsult.com.

72

Radiation Safety and Use of Radiographic Contrast Agents in Pain Medicine

James P. Rathmell

OVERVIEW OF RADIATION SAFETY

Pain practitioners have come to rely on fluoroscopy and, to a lesser but growing extent, on computed tomography (CT) to facilitate image-guided pain treatment techniques. Fluoroscopy and computed tomography employ ionizing radiation to produce the x-rays needed for imaging. Understanding the physics and biology underlying the biologic effects of ionizing radiation will help pain practitioners to minimize radiation exposure to their patients, other involved personnel, and themselves during image-guided injection. The basic elements of the fluoroscopy unit are illustrated in Figure 72.1. X-rays emanate from an x-ray tube, typically positioned beneath the table and the patient to minimize radiation exposure. The x-rays pass through the table and the patient to strike the input phosphor of the image intensifier, where they are converted to visible light and, in turn, detected by an output phosphor that transfers the signal to a digital camera for visual display on a monitor or transfer to film. The size and shape of the x-ray beam can be adjusted after exiting the x-ray tube and before entering the patient, from side to side by an adjustable linear collimator or in a circular, concentric fashion by an iris collimator. The C-arm allows variation in the axis of the x-ray beam in numerous planes relative to the patient.

The use of CT has become more commonplace, particularly among radiologists. With the advent of fluoroscopy units that can rotate around the patient and acquire images at numerous angles and then reconstruct the images in multiple planes, the distinction between CT-fluoroscopy and traditional CT has become blurred. These CT-fluoroscopy units yield data that can be reformatted in multiple planes and produce final images rivaling the quality of conventional CT. However, acquiring images in multiple planes with either CT-fluoroscopy of conventional CT requires significantly greater radiation exposure than conventional fluoroscopy.[1] In most instances, the superior anatomic information provided does not warrant the routine use of these advanced imaging modalities (see the further discussion of radiation dose later in this chapter). Patients undergoing high-risk procedures where small variations in anatomy can alter the risk/benefit ratio of a given technique may benefit from CT-fluoroscopy or conventional CT guidance.

BASIC RADIATION PHYSICS

Radiation is energy radiated or transmitted as rays, waves, or in the form of particles. X-rays are one portion of the spectrum of electromagnetic radiation. As x-rays pass through matter, they impart enough energy to dislodge electrons (ionizing radiation), yielding free radicals that can lead to harmful biologic effects. In radiography, it is the x-rays that penetrate the body without effect that emerge to strike an image intensifier where they are converted to visible light and can be displayed on a monitor or transferred to film, producing an image based on x-ray penetrability of various tissues.

Several factors and definitions are central to any basic understanding of radiation safety. The biologic effects of ionizing radiation are proportional to the time of exposure, whereas radiation exposure is inversely proportional to the *square* of the distance from the radiation source. Radiation exposure is expressed as roentgen (R) or coulomb per kilogram, whereas the energy absorbed from radiation is expressed as radiation absorbed dose (rad) or as gray (Gy). Because different types of radiation can have different biologic effects, units of exposure are converted from rad to radiation equivalent in man (rem) or Sievert (Sv). The units used to express radiation exposure are listed in Table 72.1.[2] For x-rays, 1 R ~ 1 rad ~ 1 rem.

The electrical input to the tube that generates the x-rays can be varied to produce x-rays that differ in number and energy. Increased current applied to the x-ray tube (expressed as milliamps or mA) produces more x-rays, and the more x-rays that strike the image intensifier, the darker the image. Lengthening the exposure time will also increase the number of x-rays reaching the image intensifier, thus variations in current and exposure time are expressed as mAs (mA × seconds). Increased voltage (expressed as kilovoltage peak or kVp) applied to the x-ray tube results in x-ray emission at higher energy levels (i.e., with greater ability to penetrate). In general, high kVp (75 to 125 kVp) and low mA (50 to 1,200 mA) are employed for fluoroscopy with short exposure times. This combination optimizes image quality while minimizing radiation exposure. High kVp/low mA combinations expose the patient to significantly less radiation than low kVp/high mA combinations. Modern fluoroscopy units typically employ automatic brightness control (ABC), which automatically adjusts kVp and mA to yield optimal brightness and contrast.

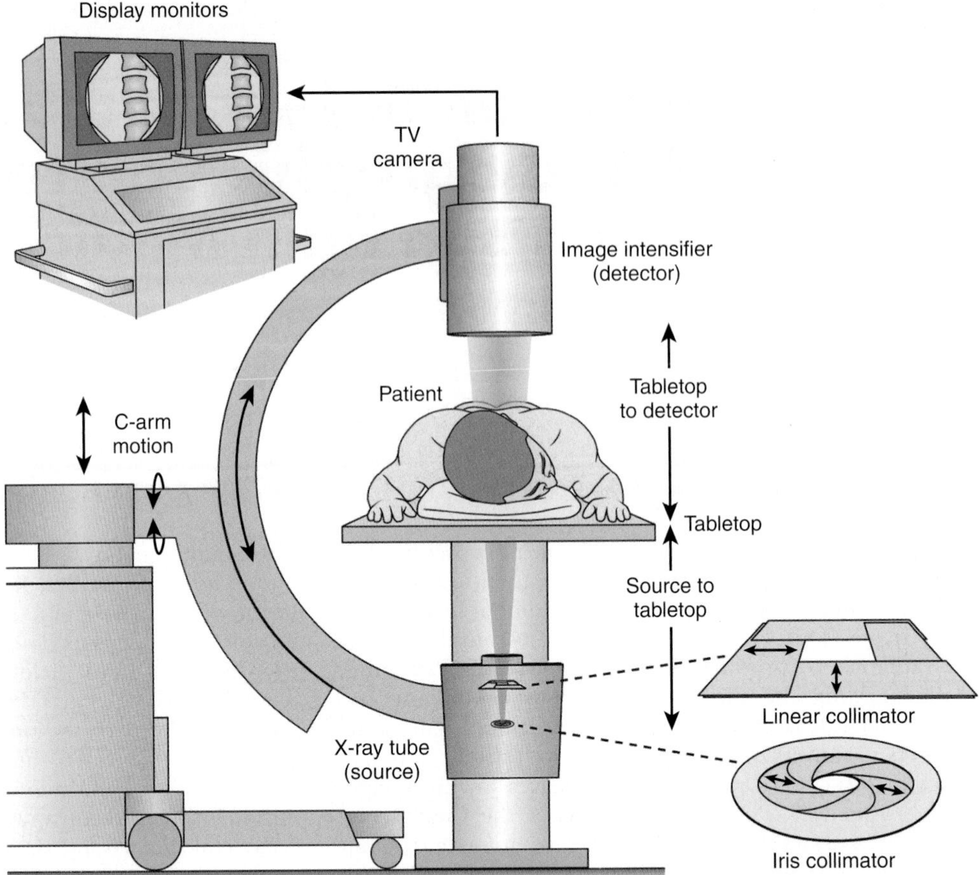

Figure 72.1 Diagram of the components of a typical fluoroscopy unit. (Reproduced with permission from Rathmell JP. *Atlas of Image-Guided Intervention in Regional Anesthesia and Pain Medicine.* 2nd ed. Philadelphia: Lippincott Williams & Wilkins; 2012, Figure 2-1.)

Table 72.1 Units Used to Express Radiation Exposure and Dose

Term	Traditional Units	SI Units	Conversion
Exposure	Roentgen (R)	Coulomb/kg (C/kg)	1 R = 2.5 × 10^{-4} C/kg
Radiation absorbed dose	rad	Gray (Gy)	100 rad = 1 Gy
Radiation equivalent in man	rem	Sievert (Sv)	100 rem = 1 Sv

The x-rays generated during fluoroscopy are a form of ionizing radiation and have the potential to produce significant biologic effects. Small doses of ionizing radiation can produce molecular changes that take years to manifest in the form of cancerous transformation. Exposure to low doses of ionizing radiation is likely inconsequential because normal cellular mechanisms repair the damage. The International Committee on Radiation Safety Protection (ICRP) has produced estimates of the maximum permissible dose (MPD) of annual radiation to various organs (Table 72.2). Exposure below these levels is unlikely to lead to any significant effects, but the ICRP recommends that workers should not receive more than 10% of the MPD.

Use of fluoroscopy for interventional procedures grew rapidly during the late 1980s, leading to increased concerns about radiation exposure.[3] In 1994, the U.S. Food and Drug Administration (FDA) issued a public health advisory about serious radiation-related skin injuries

Table 72.2 Annual Maximum Permissible Radiation Doses

Area/Organ	Annual Maximum Permissible Dose
Thyroid	0.5 mSv (50 rem)
Extremities	0.5 mSv (50 rem)
Lens of the eye	0.15 mSv (15 rem)
Gonads	0.5 mSv (50 rem)
Whole body	0.05 mSv (5 rem)
Pregnant women	0.005 mSv to fetus (0.5 rem)

Data from the National Council on Radiation Protection and Measurements (NCRP). Report No. 116. *Limitation of exposure to ionizing radiation*. Bethesda, MD: NCRP Publications; 1993.

resulting from some fluoroscopic procedures.[4] Today's equipment and techniques have reduced the risks of radiation exposure dramatically. Radiation exposure during a typical epidural steroid injection carried out with fluoroscopy and assuming the practitioner is at least 1 meter from the x-ray tube has been reported to be as low as 0.03 mR. In contrast, the typical entrance skin exposure during fluoroscopy ranges from 1 to 10 R per minute. A typical single chest radiograph leads to a skin entrance exposure of 15 mR. Thus, 1 minute of continuous fluoroscopy at 2 R per minute is equivalent to the exposure during 130 chest radiographs. Minimum target organ radiation doses that lead to pathologic effects are shown in Table 72.3. Radiation dermatitis still occurs in fluoroscopists with unknown long-term consequences. Estimates of the relative radiation dose to the patient during use of fluoroscopy in comparison to other common diagnostic radiologic procedures are shown in Table 72.4.

Table 72.3 Minimum Target Organ Radiation Doses to Produce Organ Pathologic Effects

Organ	Dose (rad)	Dose (Gy)	Results
Eye lens	200	2	Cataract formation
Skin	500	5	Erythema
	700	7	Permanent alopecia
Whole body	200-700	2-7	Hematopoietic failure (4-6 weeks)
	700-5000	7-50	Gastrointestinal failure (3-4 days)
	5000-10,000	50-100	Cerebral edema (1-2 days)

MINIMIZING PATIENT RADIATION EXPOSURE

MINIMIZE DOSE AND TIME

Practitioners using ionizing radiation should adhere to the ALARA principle ("as low as reasonably achievable"),

Table 72.4 Comparative Radiation Doses for Common Diagnostic X-ray and Fluoroscopic Procedures

Procedure	Dose
X-ray—Chest	0.1 mSv (10 mrem)
X-ray—Mammography	0.42 mSv (42 mrem)
X-ray—Skull	0.1 mSv (10 mrem)
X-ray—Cervical spine	0.2 mSv (20 mrem)
X-ray—Lumbar spine	6 mSv (600 mrem)
X-ray—Upper GI	6 mSv (600 mrem)
X-ray—Abdomen (kidney/bladder)	7 mSv (700 mrem)
X-ray—Barium enema	8 mSv (800 mrem)
X-ray—Pelvis	0.6 mSv (60 mrem)
X-ray—Hip	0.7 mSv (70 mrem)
X-ray—Dental bitewing/image	0.005 mSv (0.5 mrem)
X-ray—Extremity (hand/foot)	0.005 mSv (0.5 mrem)
*Fluoroscopy, intermittent (e.g., for lumbar transforaminal or facet injection)	0.007-0.03 mSv (0.7-3 mrem)
*Fluoroscopy, high dose	(three- to sixfold the radiation exposure of standard dose)
*Fluoroscopy, continuous, pulsed mode	0.2-1 mSv/minute of exposure (20-100 mrem/minute of exposure)
*Fluoroscopy, continuous	2-10 mSv/minute of exposure (200-1000 mrem/minute of exposure)
*Fluoroscopy, continuous, high dose	10-20 mSv/minute of exposure (1000-2000 mrem/minute of exposure)
*Fluoroscopy, continuous, digital subtraction	20-40 mSv/minute of exposure (2000-4000 mrem/minute of exposure)
Computed tomography—Head	2 mSv (200 mrem)
Computed tomography—Chest	7 mSv (700 mrem)
Computed tomography—Abdomen/pelvis	10 mSv (1000 mrem)
Computed tomography—Extremity	0.1 mSv (10 mrem)
Computed tomography—Angiography (heart)	20 mSv (2000 mrem)
Computed tomography—Angiography (head)	5 mSv (500 mrem)
Computed tomography—Spine	10 mSv (1000 mrem)
Computed tomography—Whole body	10 mSv (1000 mrem)
Computed tomography—Cardiac	20 mSv (2000 mrem)

*Fluoroscopy exposure values are approximate and vary widely based on the region of the body examined and the body habitus of each patient. The values presented are extrapolated from data provided by Philips Medical Systems for the Pulsera 9-inch mobile C-arm and the following references: Wagner AL. Selective lumbar nerve root blocks with ct fluoroscopic guidance: technique, results, procedure time, and radiation dose. *AJNR Am J Neuroradiol*. 2004;25:1592-1594; and Mahesh M. The AAPM/RSNA Physics Tutorial for Residents. Fluoroscopy: patient radiation exposure issues. *RadioGraphics*. 2001;21:1033-1045.

Data adapted from American Nuclear Society. Radiation dose chart. Available at www.new.ans.org/pi/resources/dosechart. Accessed January 9, 2011.

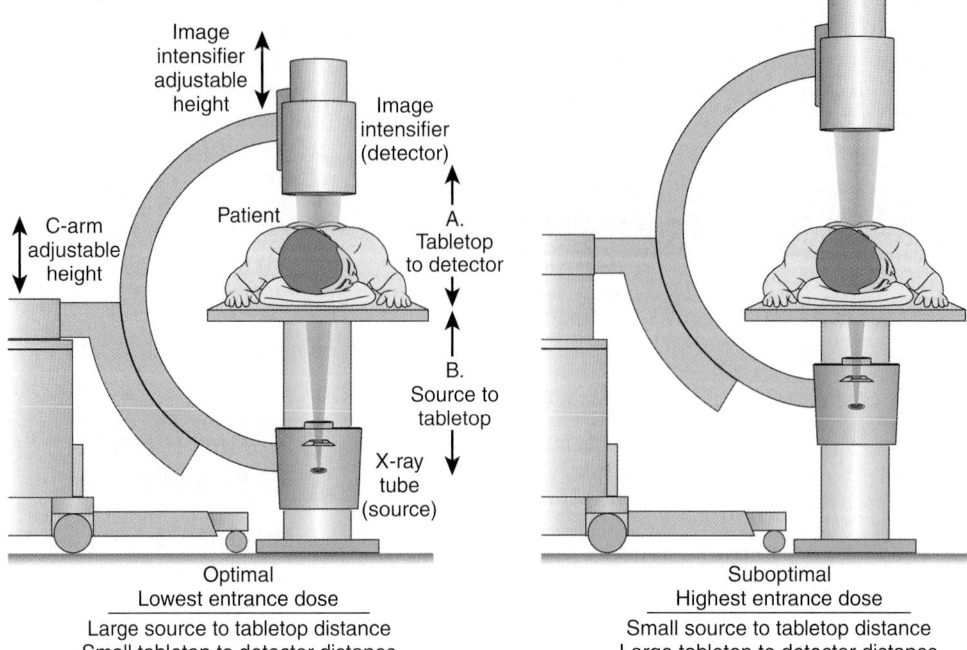

Figure 72.2 Effect of pulsed fluoroscopy on radiation dose (patient entrance skin dose). For example, by switching from continuous fluoroscopy (typically 30 pulses per second) to 15 pulses per second, for a dose savings of nearly 22%. (Adapted with permission from Mahesh M. The AAPM/RSNA Physics Tutorial for Residents. Fluoroscopy: Patient Radiation Exposure Issues. *RadioGraphics.* 2001;21:1033-1045.)

combining optimal technique and shielding to minimize patient and personnel exposure.[5,6] Because no dose of ionizing radiation is without biologic effects and can be considered absolutely safe, radiographs should be used only when necessary, and the dose and exposure time should be limited. Dose is a factor of both the number of x-rays (proportional to mA × seconds of exposure) and the energy of the x-rays (proportional to kVp).[7] Modern fluoroscopy units employ ABC, which automatically controls mA and kVp settings to optimize brightness and contrast while minimizing dose. However, if you choose to use fluoroscopy in the manual mode (e.g., to increase penetration in an obese patient), the kVp should be increased while minimizing mA. For an equivalent increase in exposure, the mA must be doubled, whereas the kVp must be raised only 15%. When using ABC mode, the only element under practitioner control is the exposure time, and this should be held to the minimum required to complete the procedure. Short pulses of exposure rather than continuous exposure should be employed whenever feasible. Continuous fluoroscopy in the form of movies (cineradiography) and digital subtraction exposes patients to markedly higher doses than brief spot images (see Table 72.4). Many modern units include an option termed *pulsed* mode for use in place of a continuous technique. This mode substitutes brief, periodic spot images separated by an interval without exposure (e.g., a new image is displayed one to two times per second). Use of this mode in place of continuous fluoroscopy can reduce overall exposure dramatically and is suitable for procedures in the pain clinic where continuous fluoroscopy is needed (e.g., while threading an epidural catheter or spinal cord stimulation lead; see Fig. 72.2).

OPTIMIZE THE POSITION OF THE X-RAY TUBE

Radiation exposure to the patient is best minimized by ensuring optimal distance between the patient and the x-ray tube (Fig. 72.3). When the x-ray tube is positioned close to the patient, a small area of skin will be exposed to radiation, but because of the close proximity of the x-rays, the dose that this smaller area will be exposed to is much higher. When the tube is positioned further from the patient, a larger area is exposed to a smaller dose of radiation. The x-ray tube should be positioned as far from the patient as possible, without including unnecessary structures in the field of view.

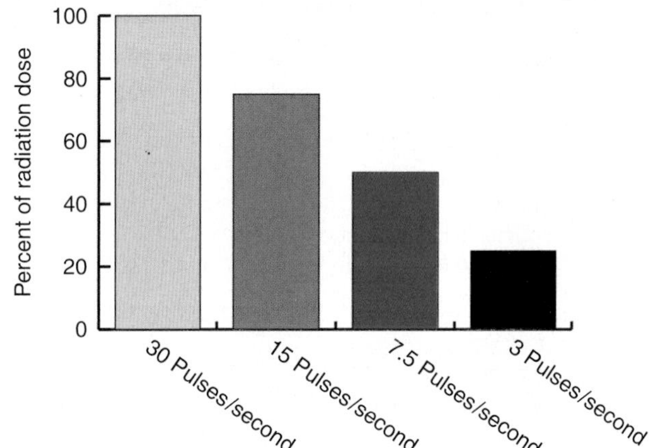

Figure 72.3 Optimal spacing between the x-ray source and the patient to minimize radiation exposure. (Reproduced with permission from Rathmell JP. *Atlas of Image-Guided Intervention in Regional Anesthesia and Pain Medicine.* 2nd ed. Philadelphia: Lippincott Williams & Wilkins; 2012, Figure 2-3.)

EMPLOY SHIELDING WHENEVER POSSIBLE

The use of lead shielding can prevent exposure of regions adjacent to the area that is to be imaged from being exposed to any ionizing radiation. Small lead shields can be placed on the table underneath the patient, directly in front of

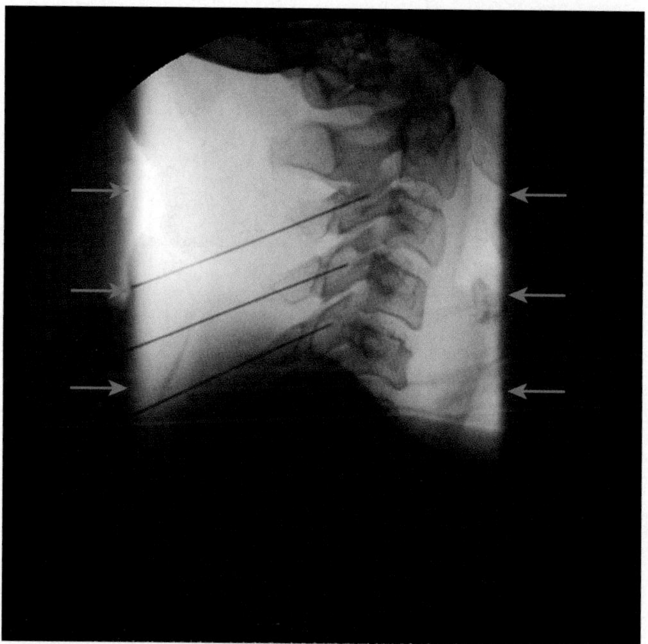

Figure 72.4 Use of adjustable (linear) collimator to decrease radiation exposure to the patient, while improving image resolution by decreasing the range of tissue density included in the image field. (Reproduced with permission from Rathmell JP. *Atlas of Image-Guided Intervention in Regional Anesthesia and Pain Medicine.* 2nd ed. Philadelphia: Lippincott Williams & Wilkins; 2012, Figure 2-4.)

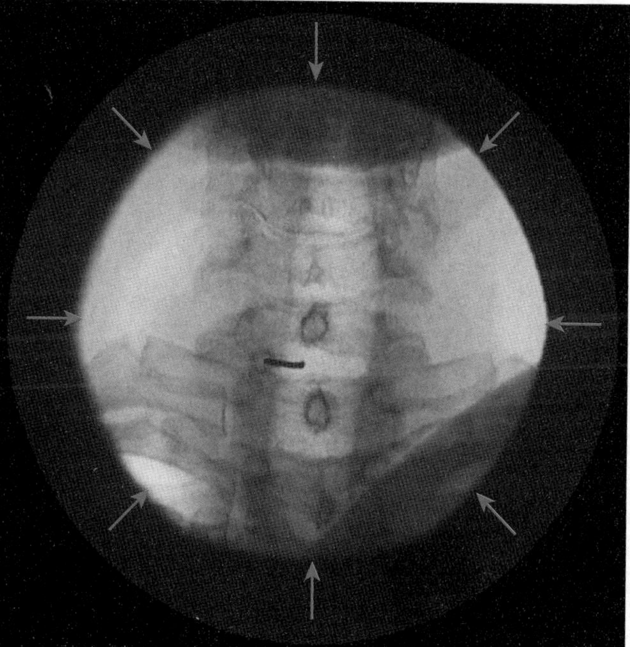

Figure 72.5 Use of adjustable (iris) collimator to limit the field to the area of interest reduces radiation exposure to the patient and improves image resolution by decreasing the range of tissue density included in the image field. (Reproduced with permission from Rathmell JP. *Atlas of Image-Guided Intervention in Regional Anesthesia and Pain Medicine.* 2nd ed. Philadelphia: Lippincott Williams & Wilkins; 2012, Figure 2-5.)

the x-ray beam *before* it penetrates the patient to protect the gonads or the fetus in the rare instance where fluoroscopy is necessary in a pregnant patient. Although lead shields should be readily available in the fluoroscopy suite, they are seldom practical for use during image-guided injection of the lumbosacral spine because the shield would lie directly in the path of the structures to be imaged.

EMPLOY COLLIMATION

Fluoroscopy units have built-in mechanisms that allow the emitted x-ray beam to be reduced in size and changed in shape (or *collimated*) so the area of the patient exposed is minimized. All units have both linear and circular collimation. Linear collimation employs shutters that can be moved in from either side of the exposure field and are helpful in imaging long, thin structures such as the spine (Fig. 72.4). Circular or *iris* collimation can be helpful when a small, circular area is to be imaged (Fig. 72.5). Collimation is also helpful in optimizing image quality because the ABC mode attempts to optimize the image quality by taking into account the exposure needed across the entire field of exposure; it is often difficult to visualize radiodense and radiolucent areas in the same image. Useful employment of collimation can exclude areas of greatly varying radiodensity to improve image quality by reducing the range of densities included in the field. Two good examples are imaging of the thoracic spine, where the large density differences between the spine and the adjacent air-filled lungs can make it difficult to see the bony elements of the spine with any resolution. Linear collimation to limit the field to the spine itself will dramatically improve the image quality. Likewise, imaging in the cervical spine is fraught with the same difficulties when the air on either side of the neck is included in the x-ray field (see Fig. 72.4). Either linear collimation or circular collimation (see Fig. 72.5) can be used to limit the field to the area of interest, improving image quality and reducing radiation exposure. Modern fluoro units may also allow for *magnification* of the image by electronically magnifying the area of interest. Magnification allows better visualization of a smaller area but leads to increased radiation exposure as the system increases output to compensate for losses in gain. To minimize the dose to the patient, the largest field of view, in conjunction with the tightest collimation, should be employed.

MINIMIZING PRACTITIONER EXPOSURE

EMPLOY PROPER SHIELDING

Only the personnel needed to conduct the procedure should be in the fluoroscopy suite. All personnel should be shielded with lead aprons *before* use of fluoroscopy begins. The practitioner using the fluoroscopy unit should alert everyone in the room that he or she is about to begin and ensure that personnel are shielded. Routine use of thyroid shields can minimize the long-term risk of thyroid cancer. Although protective lead gloves can reduce the exposure of the hands to radiation, they can produce a false sense of security. When leaded gloves are employed and the practitioner's hands are in the field of exposure, units with ABC will increase their output to compensate for the radiodense leaded gloves and negate their protective effects. Using techniques that eliminate the practitioner's hands from direct exposure within the x-ray field should be used at all times. Protective eyeglasses are available that dramatically reduce eye exposure during fluoroscopy; leaded eyewear is recommended for practitioners who accumulate monthly readings on collar badges above 400 mrem (4 Sv). Levels of exposure in this range are typically encountered only in areas where continuous cineangiography is conducted frequently (e.g., the cardiac catheterization laboratory).

PRACTITIONER POSITION

The practitioners must understand the geometry of the radiation path as it passes from the x-ray tube to the image intensifier and adopt positions that minimize their exposure during fluoroscopy (Fig. 72.6). The dose drops proportionally to the square of the distance from the x-ray source. Thus, standing as far from the x-ray tube as practical is the first means to minimize exposure. Using an intravenous extension tube and taking a step back from the table during periods where contrast is injected under continuous or live fluoroscopy will reduce exposure. When the x-ray tube is rotated to obtain a lateral image, the practitioner should step completely away from the table beneath the x-ray tube and out of the path of the x-ray beam or move to the side of the table of the image intensifier. Inverting the C-arm so the x-ray tube is above the table and the image intensifier is below the table is a means some practitioners use to increase the C-arm's range of lateral movement beyond the typical 45 to 55 degrees allowed by the unit. This practice dramatically increases exposure to both patient and practitioner by bringing them in close proximity to the x-ray source.

OPTIMIZING IMAGE QUALITY

Modern fluoroscopy units use ABC, which automatically adjusts mA and kVp to optimize image brightness and contrast while minimizing radiation exposure. These controls can be adjusted separately. Increased kVp produces x-rays of higher energy that penetrate without attenuation, thus the resulting image is brighter with less contrast between different tissues, thereby reducing image detail. The clarity of small structures, or image detail, can be improved by lowering kVP, reducing the distance between the patient and the image intensifier, and by using collimation to limit the field of exposure to only those structures of interest. Fluoroscopic images also have less sharpness at the periphery of the image because of a fall off in brightness and spatial resolution, a phenomenon called *vignetting*. Placing the structure of interest in the center of the image will yield maximum image detail. Finally, *pincushion distortion* occurs toward the periphery of the image because the x-rays emanate from a spherical surface and are detected on a flat surface. This results in an effect much like a fisheye camera lens with a splaying outward of objects toward the periphery of the image. This can lead to particular difficulties when attempting to advance a needle using a coaxial technique if the needle is toward the periphery of the image. Within the past several years, several manufacturers have developed electronic flat plate detectors to replace conventional image intensifiers. Flat plate detectors employ a gridlike

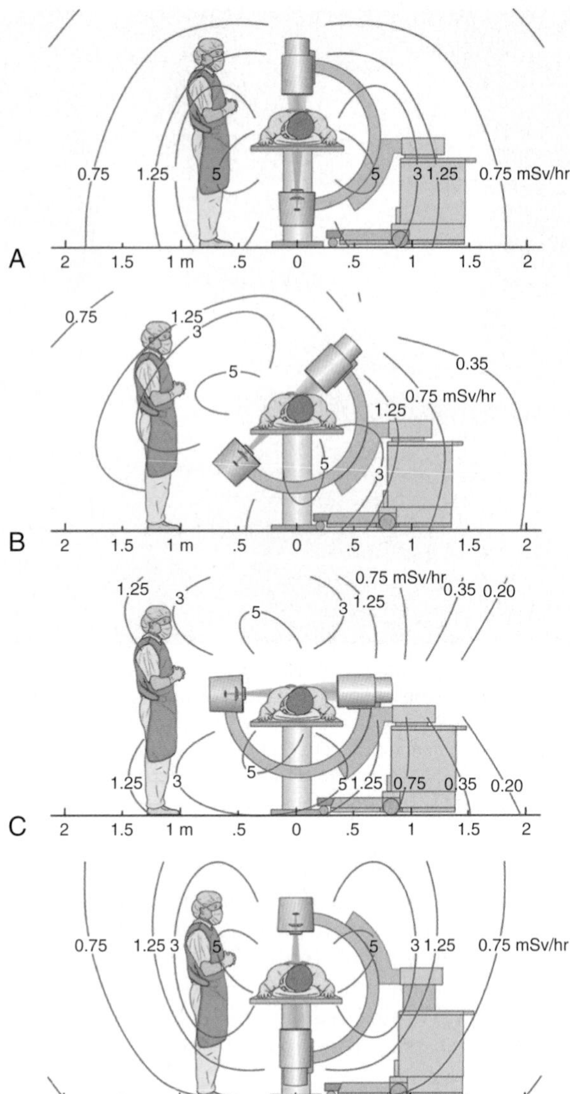

Figure 72.6 Radiation exposure dosage during fluoroscopy. **A,** During routine use in the anterior-posterior plane, the x-ray tube (source) should be positioned below the patient and the detector above the patient to minimize radiation exposure to both the patient and the practitioner. **B,** The oblique projection results in markedly increased exposure to the practitioner. **C,** During use in the lateral projection, the practitioner should step completely behind the x-ray tube (source) to minimize radiation exposure. When it is necessary to work close to the patient during lateral fluoroscopy, the practitioner should step away from the x-ray tube and move to the side of the table opposite the x-ray tube to minimize exposure. **D,** Radiation exposure to both patient and practitioner is dramatically increased when the x-ray tube (source) is inverted above the patient. Some practitioners invert the C-arm to allow for more extreme lateral angle (e.g., rotation beyond 35 to 45 degrees oblique to the side opposite the C-arm is not possible without inverting the C-arm on some units). Radiation exposure can be reduced by rotating the patient on the table and keeping the x-ray source below the table. (Reproduced with permission from Rathmell JP. *Atlas of Image-Guided Intervention in Regional Anesthesia and Pain Medicine.* 2nd Edition. Philadelphia: Lippincott Williams & Wilkins; 2012, Figure 2-6.)

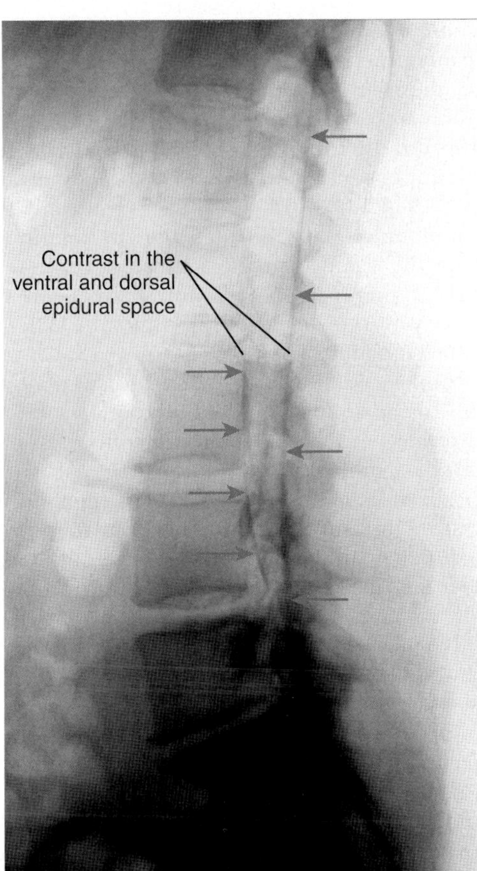

Figure 72.7 Epidural contrast injection. This typical lateral lumbar epidurogram demonstrates the "double-line" or "railroad track" appearance of radiographic contrast in the anterior and posterior epidural space *(arrows).* (Reproduced with permission from Rathmell JP, Torian D, Song T. Lumbar epidurography. *Reg Anesth Pain Med.* 2000;25:541.)

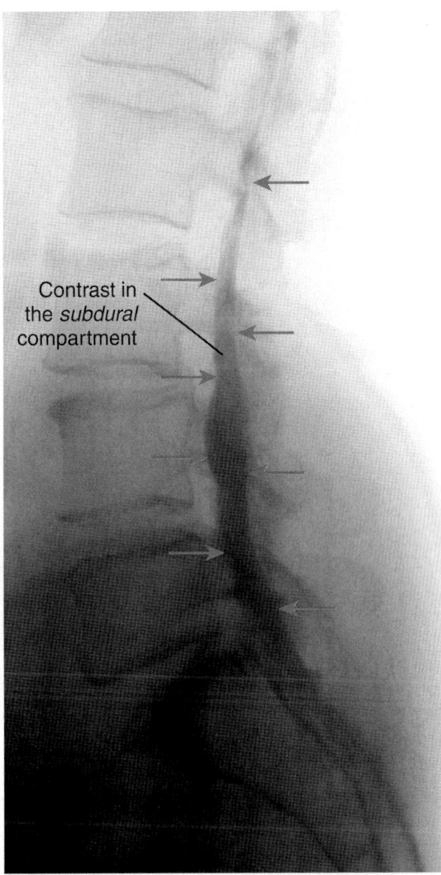

Figure 72.8 Subdural contrast injection. Injection of contrast in the subdural (epi-arachnoid) space is recognized by the regular posterior border and irregular anterior border of loculated contrast collection on this lateral radiograph of the lumbar spine. The contrast is contained posteriorly by the dural membrane, but it extends only partially anteriorly, as the thin arachnoid membrane contains it. Compare with Figure 72.9, subarachnoid administration, where the contrast extends all the way from the posterior to the anterior limits of the thecal space. Although the contrast does not extend to the anterior portion of the thecal sac, it is not limited to the epidural space. (Reproduced with permission from Ajar A, Rathmell JP, Mukerji S. The subdural compartment. *Reg Anesth Pain Med.* 2002;27:73.)

electronic detector that eliminates both vignetting and pincushion distortion, providing optimum image quality from the center to the peripheral portions of each image. Flat plate digital detectors are rapidly replacing traditional image intensifiers. Digital flat plate detectors are capable of dramatically reducing radiation while improving image quality and eliminating the distortion of the image at the periphery of the detector that occurs with traditional image intensifiers.

OVERVIEW OF RADIOGRAPHIC CONTRAST MEDIUM

Iodine is the only element that has proven satisfactory as an intravascular radiographic contrast medium (RCM).[8,9] Iodine produces the radiopacity whereas the other portions of the molecule act as the carriers for the iodine, improving solubility and reducing the toxicity of the final compound. Organic carriers of iodine are likely to remain in widespread use for the foreseeable future.[10] During image-guided injection, injection of RCM can prove invaluable in determining the final location and distribution of the injectate (Figs. 72.7 to 72.9). Use of RCM can improve the safety of many techniques by allowing for detection of intravascular (Figs. 72.10 and 72.11), subdural (see Fig. 72.8), or intrathecal (see Fig. 72.9) needle location before local anesthetic or steroid is placed.

PHARMACOLOGY OF RADIOGRAPHIC CONTRAST MEDIA

Currently, there are four chemical varieties of iodinated RCM in widespread use: ionic monomers, nonionic monomers, ionic dimers, and nonionic dimers.[11] On intravascular injection, all four are redistributed rapidly via capillary permeability to the extravascular space, they do not enter the interior of blood or tissue cells, and they are rapidly excreted, more than 90% eliminated via glomerular filtration within 12 hours of administration. None of the four varieties have marked pharmacologic actions. All RCM agents come in a range of concentrations that vary in their radiopacity and viscosity. Because iodine is the element that is responsible for the radiopacity, the iodine concentration

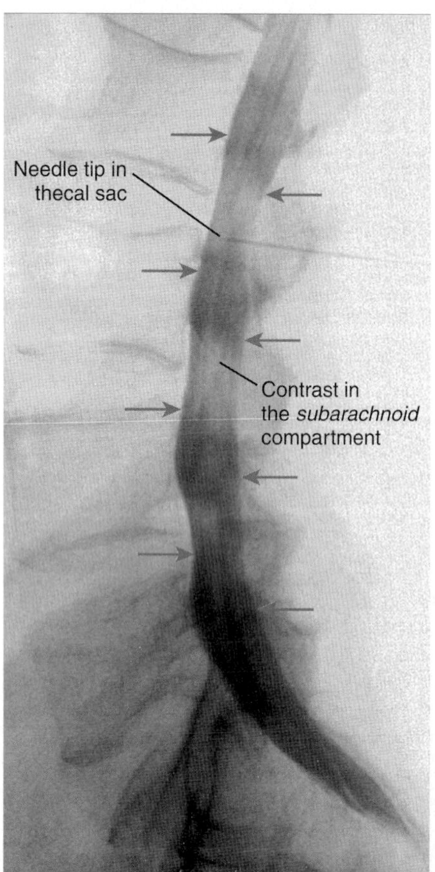

Figure 72.9 Subarachnoid (intrathecal) contrast injection. This typical myelogram demonstrates contrast within the thecal sac *(arrows)* on this lateral radiograph of the lumbar spine. The spinal cord and spinal nerves are visible as hypodense regions within the contrast collection. (Reproduced with permission from Rathmell JP, Torian D, Song T. Lumbar epidurography. *Reg Anesth Pain Med.* 2000;25:543.)

in milligrams per milliliter represents the radiopacity. The nonionic monomers are now used almost exclusively in pain medicine; the nonionic dimers offer increased radiopacity at low osmolar concentrations but are not in widespread clinical use and offer questionable clinical advantages.

Several important chemical properties determine the characteristics of RCM in clinical use. Osmolality depends on the number of particles of solute in solution and is highest for the ionic contrast agents. Adverse reactions, particularly discomfort on injection, have been reduced dramatically with the advent of low-osmolar RCM. Contrast media with osmolality below 500 mOsm per kg of water are virtually painless. Radiopacity depends on the iodine concentration of the solution and, therefore, on the number of iodine atoms per molecule and the concentration of the iodine-carrying molecule in solution. Digital subtraction electronically enhances the image, reducing the amount of contrast medium needed by twofold to threefold. With the use of digital subtraction, RCM with as little as 150 to 200 mg per mL of iodine can be used even for intra-arterial use. Ionic molecules dissociate into cation and anion in solution. Non-ionicity, or a molecule that does not dissociate in solution, is essential for myelography or use along the neuraxis, where inadvertant placement within the cerebrospinal fluid (CSF) is possible during injection. The chemical properties of common RCM used in clinical practice are compared in Table 72.5.

The most frequently used ionic monomers are diatrizoate (Urografin), iothalamate (Conray), and metrizoate (Isopaque). All ionic monomers are the salts of meglumine or sodium as the cation and a radiopaque tri-iodinated fully substituted benzene ring as the anion. The ionic monomers are still used for intravenous pyelography and similar applications; however, they have been completely replaced by the low-osmolar, nonionic RCM for many applications, including intrathecal administration. The most common nonionic

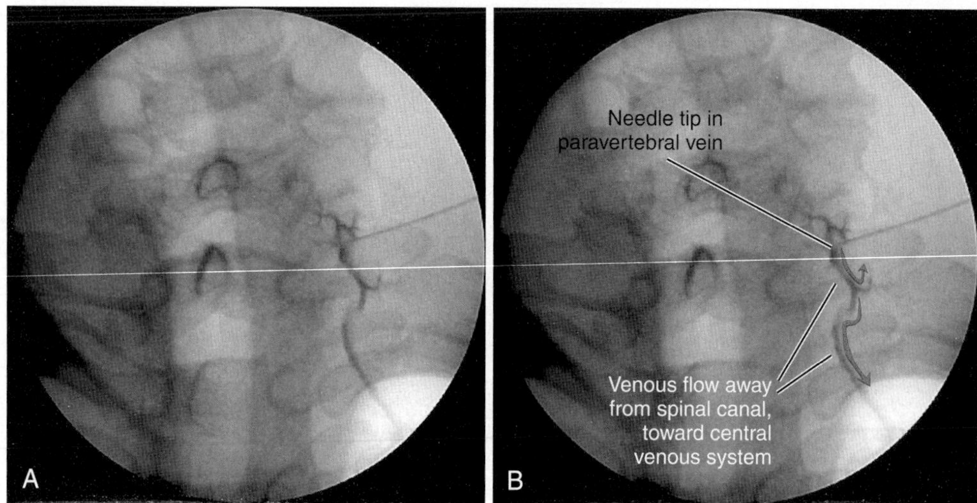

Figure 72.10 Intravenous contrast injection. **A,** Intravenous contrast injection is typically not seen on still images because the contrast material is rapidly diluted in the bloodstream. During real-time or live fluoroscopy, intravenous contrast injection appears as in this anterior-posterior radiograph of the cervical spine taken during cervical transforaminal injection. The contrast can be seen flowing away from the spinal canal and toward the central venous circulation with the venous blood. **B,** Labeled image showing direction of contrast flow. (Reproduced with permission from Rathmell JP. *Atlas of Image-Guided Intervention in Regional Anesthesia and Pain Medicine.* 2nd ed. Philadelphia: Lippincott Williams & Wilkins; 2012, Figure 3-4.)

monomers in clinical use include iodixanol (Visipaque), iohexol (Omnipaque), iopamidol (Isovue), and ioversol (Optiray); only iohexol and iopamidol are labeled for intrathecal use. The nonionic monomers appeared in the 1970s and now represent the most common RCM in clinical use. They are more stable in solution and less toxic than the ionic monomers.

ADVERSE REACTIONS TO RADIOGRAPHIC CONTRAST MEDIA

Modern contrast agents have reduced, but not eliminated, the risk of adverse reactions.[10] To minimize the risk, RCM should be used in the smallest concentrations and in the smallest total dose that will allow adequate visualization. Adverse reactions associated with RCM can be divided into idiosyncratic anaphylactoid reactions, nonidiosyncratic reactions, and combined reactions.[12] The risk of adverse reactions is significantly greater with use of high-osmolar, ionic agents when compared with low-osmolar, nonionic agents. This discussion is limited to the risks associated with low-osmolar, nonionic agents because they are used almost exclusively in pain medicine applications.

IDIOSYNCRATIC ANAPHYLACTOID REACTIONS

Idiosyncratic reactions are the most feared and most serious complications associated with RCM. At present, we cannot predict or prevent this type of reaction reliably, and they

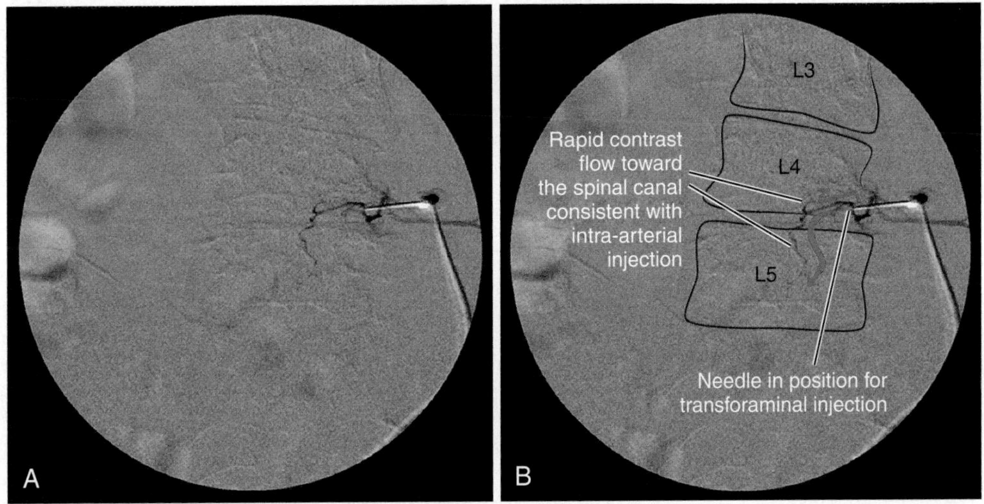

Figure 72.11 Intra-arterial contrast injection (digital subtraction). **A,** Intra-arterial contrast injection is typically not seen on still images because the contrast material is rapidly diluted in the bloodstream. During real-time or live fluoroscopy, intravenous contrast injection appears as in this anterior-posterior digital subtraction radiograph of the lumbar spine taken during lumbar transforaminal injection. The contrast can be seen flowing toward the end organ (in this image, toward the lumbar spinal cord) with the arterial blood. Use of digital subtraction cineradiography allows for detection of intravascular injection with small doses of radiographic contrast material. **B,** Labeled image showing direction of contrast flow. (Reproduced with permission from Rathmell JP. *Atlas of Image-Guided Intervention in Regional Anesthesia and Pain Medicine.* 2nd ed. Philadelphia: Lippincott Williams & Wilkins; 2012, Figure 3-5.)

Table 72.5 Comparison of Common Radiographic Contrast Agents Used in Clinical Practice*

Chemical Composition	Trade Name	Iodine (mg/mL)	Osmolality (mOsm/kg H_2O)	Viscosity (cps @ 37°C)	RCM Agent Type
Sodium/meglumine diatrizoate 30%	Urografin 150	146	710	1.4	Ionic, high-osmolar
Sodium/meglumine diatrizoate 67%	Urografin 325	325	1650	3.3	Ionic, high-osmolar
Iohexol 180 mg/mL	Omnipaque 180	180	360	2.0	Nonionic, low-osmolar
Iohexol 300 mg/mL	Omnipaque 300	300	640	6.1	Nonionic, low-osmolar
Iopamidol 41%	Isovue 200	200	413	2.0	Nonionic, low-osmolar
Iopamidol 61%	Isovue 300	300	616	4.	Nonionic, low-osmolar

*The ionic, high-osmolar agent diatrizoate and the nonionic, low-osmolar, agents iohexol and iopamidol. Iohexol and iopamidol are commonly used in image-guided pain treatment. These agents provide a nonionic low-osmolar RCM that balance a low risk of adverse reaction, demonstrated safety for intrathecal use, and sufficient radiopacity for identifying intravascular and intrathecal placement.
RCM, radiographic contrast media.

Table 72.6 Incidence of Severe Adverse Drug Reactions

Clinical History	Severe ADR (%)*
No history of allergy or previous ADR to RCM	0.03
Renal disease	0.04
Diabetes mellitus	0.05
Heart disease	0.10
History of allergy	0.10
Atopy	0.11
History of previous ADR to RCM	0.18
Asthma	0.23

*ADR following intravenous injection of low-osmolar, nonionic RCM.
ADR, adverse drug reaction; RCM, radiographic contrast media.
Adapted with permission from Katayama H, Yamaguchi K, Kozuka T et al. Adverse reactions to ionic and non-ionic contrast media: a report from the Japanese Committee on the Safety of Contrast Media. *Radiology*. 1990;175:621-628.

Table 72.7 Type and Relative Incidence of Adverse Drug Reactions

Patient Characteristics in Trial	
Total number of patients	163,363
Total ADRs	3.13%
Total severe ADRs	0.04%
Death	(1)
Symptoms	**% of ADR***
Nausea	1.04
Heat	0.92
Vomiting	0.45
Urticaria	0.47
Flushing	0.16
Venous pain	0.05
Coughing	0.15
Dyspnea	0.04

*ADR following intravenous injection of low-osmolar, nonionic radiographic contrast media.
ADR, adverse drug reaction.
Adapted with permission from Katayama H, Yamaguchi K, Kozuka T et al. Adverse reactions to ionic and non-ionic contrast media: a report from the Japanese Committee on the Safety of Contrast Media. *Radiology*. 1990;175:621-628.

occur without warning. These reactions usually begin within 5 minutes of injection and may be mild and self-limited or proceed rapidly to life-threatening cardiovascular collapse and death. The risk of anaphylactoid reaction is increased in patients with previous reaction to RCM (sixfold), in asthmatics (eightfold), in allergic and atopic patients (fourfold), and in those with advanced heart disease (threefold) (Table 72.6). Regarding patients with seafood allergy, their risk of a reaction to RCM appears to be similar to patients with other food allergies or asthma, and experts concluded that allergy to shellfish does not increase reaction to contrast any more than other allergies.[13]

NONIDIOSYNCRATIC ANAPHYLACTOID REACTIONS

Nonidiosyncratic reactions can be divided into chemotoxic reactions (chemical reactions to the iodine-carrying molecule) and osmotoxic reactions (those caused by high osmolality of the contrast medium). These nonidiosyncratic reactions are dose dependent; therefore, this type of reaction should be exceedingly rare in patients receiving the small volumes of RCM required to facilitate needle localization during image-guided pain treatment.

Chemotoxic reactions are rare and may result in direct organ toxicity and include cardiac (direct and prolonged decrease in cardiac contractility), neurologic (seizures), and renal toxicity (oliguria, impaired creatinine clearance, and reduced glomerular filtration rate that may progress to acute renal failure).[14]

Osmotoxic reactions were much more common with the high-osmolar contrast media, where the osmolality of the RCM can reach several times that of physiologic osmolality of 300 mOsm per kg H_2O (see Table 72.5).[15] Osmotoxic reactions have been dramatically reduced with the advent of low-osmolar, nonionic agents such as iohexol and should be exceedingly rare after administration of the small volumes used in pain medicine applications. Hyperosmolar reactions include erythrocyte damage (hemolysis), endothelial damage (capillary leak and edema), vasodilation (flushing, warmth, hypotension, cardiovascular collapse), hypervolemia, and direct cardiac depression (reduced cardiac contractility). The relative incidence of various adverse reactions to RCM is listed in Table 72.7.

RECOGNITION AND TREATMENT OF REACTIONS TO RADIOGRAPHIC CONTRAST MEDIA

Reactions can be generally grouped as mild, moderate, or severe. The incidence of these reactions following the small volumes of RCM used in pain medicine has not been reported, but the incidence following intravenous administration of larger volumes of contrast is given here. Mild reactions occur in 5% to 15% of those receiving intravenous contrast and include flushing anxiety, nausea, arm pain, pruritus, vomiting, headache, and mild urticaria. These are generally mild and self-limiting, and require no specific treatment. Occasionally, an oral antihistamine (diphenhydramine 25 mg) can be useful in managing pruritus and anxiety. More serious reactions occur in 0.5% to 2% of those receiving intravenous contrast and include more pronounced severity of mild symptoms, as well as moderate degrees of hypotension and bronchospasm. Suggested treatments for moderate reactions are given in Table 72.8.

Severe reactions are life threatening, occur in less than 0.04% of those receiving intravenous RCM, and include convulsions, unconsciousness, laryngeal edema, severe bronchospasm, pulmonary edema, severe cardiac arrhythmias, and cardiovascular collapse.[16] Treatment of these life-threatening reactions is urgent, necessitating the immediate

Table 72.8 Suggested Treatment for Reactions to Radiographic Contrast Media of Moderate Severity

Adverse Reaction	Suggested Treatment
Urticaria	Diphenhydramine 25-50 mg PO, IM, or IV
Anxiety	Diazepam 5-10 mg PO or midazolam 1-2 mg IV
Bronchospasm	Mild: Inhaled albuterol Severe: Hydrocortisone 100 mg IV Epinephrine 0.05-0.1 mg SQ, IM, IV
Anaphylaxis	Epinephrine 0.01 mg/kg SQ, IM, IV (maximum adult dose 0.5 mg)

PO, by mouth; IM, intramuscularly; IV, intravenously; SQ, subcutaneously.

availability of full resuscitation equipment and trained personnel, along with a practiced routine for responding to these rare events. The airway must be secured, and oxygen, mechanical ventilation, external cardiac massage, and electrical cardiac defibrillation must be administered as required. Epinephrine is the drug of choice for the treatment of anaphylaxis; the usual adult starting dose is 0.01 mg/kg (maximum of 0.5 mg) subcutaneously, intravenously, or intramuscularly. Death may ensue following this type of severe adverse reaction; the incidence is not known with accuracy but likely lies between 1/14,000 to 1/170,000 intravenous administrations of RCM.

PREVENTION OF REACTIONS TO RADIOGRAPHIC CONTRAST MEDIA

Recognition of the factors that predispose patients to adverse reactions when receiving RCM is the first step in prevention (see Table 72.6). The risk of reaction is increased in those with previous reaction to RCM (sixfold), in asthmatics (eightfold), in allergic and atopic patients (fourfold), and in patients with advanced heart disease (threefold). If there is any chance that the injectate will end up in the subarachnoid space, then a low-osmolar, nonionic contrast agent must be used. Infrequent deaths have been reported following the inadvertent intrathecal administration of ionic RCM. Most pain medicine practitioners have adopted the universal use of a low-osmolar, nonionic RCM in a moderate concentration (e.g., iohexol 180 mg/mL or iopamidol 41%) for all applications.

There is no known premedication regimen that can reliably eliminate the risk of severe reactions to RCM.[17] The most common strategies suggested combine pretreatment with corticosteroids (e.g., oral prednisone 50-mg doses 12 and 2 hours before RCM administration) and antihistamines (e.g., oral diphenhydramine 50-mg doses 1 to 2 hours before RCM administration). Some authors recommend the addition of H2-antagonists (e.g., oral ranitidine). This approach has proven to reduce the incidence of subsequent adverse reactions in those with a history of previous reaction

Box 72.1 Patients Considered at Greater than Usual Risk of Severe Adverse Reactions to Radiographic Contrast Media

Those with a history of previous adverse reactions to RCM (excluding mild flushing and nausea)
Asthmatics
Allergic and atopic patients
Cardiac patients with congestive heart failure, unstable arrhythmia, or recent myocardial infarction
Patients with diabetic nephropathy or renal failure of any etiology
Feeble, elderly patients
Those with severe, general debility or dehydration
Extremely anxious patients
Patients with specific hematologic or metabolic disorders (e.g., sickle cell anemia, polycythemia, multiple myeloma, pheochromocytoma)

RCM, radiographic contrast media.
Adapted with permission from Grainger RG. Intravascular radiologic iodinated contrast media. In: Grainger RG, Allison DJ, Adam A et al., eds. *Grainger & Allison's Diagnostic Radiology.* 4th ed. New York: Churchill Livingstone; 2001.

to high-osmolar contrast agents; however, it is less clear whether prophylactic treatment is needed prior to the use of a low-osmolar, nonionic contrast agent such as iohexol. Patients believed to be at greater than usual risk are listed in Box 72.1. It has been our practice to avoid radiographic contrast altogether in those at elevated risk for adverse reaction. Most procedures in pain medicine can be carried out safely without use of radiographic contrast. In some instances (e.g., epidural placement), the location can be established using loss of resistance alone, and final needle position can be verified using anterior-posterior and lateral radiography without contrast. However, some injections should not be attempted without radiographic contrast injection (e.g., transforaminal injection); in this case, injection of contrast under live or real-time fluoroscopy (with or without digital subtraction) is the only means to detect intra-arterial needle location (see Figs. 72.10 and 72.11) and to prevent catastrophic injection of particulate steroid directly into critical vessels supplying the spinal cord. Performing interlaminar epidural steroid injection without contrast may well be a safe and effective alternative to transforaminal injection in the patient with a greater than usual risk for adverse reaction to RCM.

USE OF GADOLINIUM AS AN ALTERNATIVE TO IODINATED RADIOGRAPHIC CONTRAST MEDIA

Gadolinium chelates, such as gadopentetate dimeglumine (Magnevist), are commonly used intravenous contrast agents used to enhance vascular structures during diagnostic magnetic resonance imaging. Gadolinium chelates also have an intrinsic ability to attenuate x-rays and have been used successfully in place of iodinated contrast media for angiography and spinal injections used in image-guided

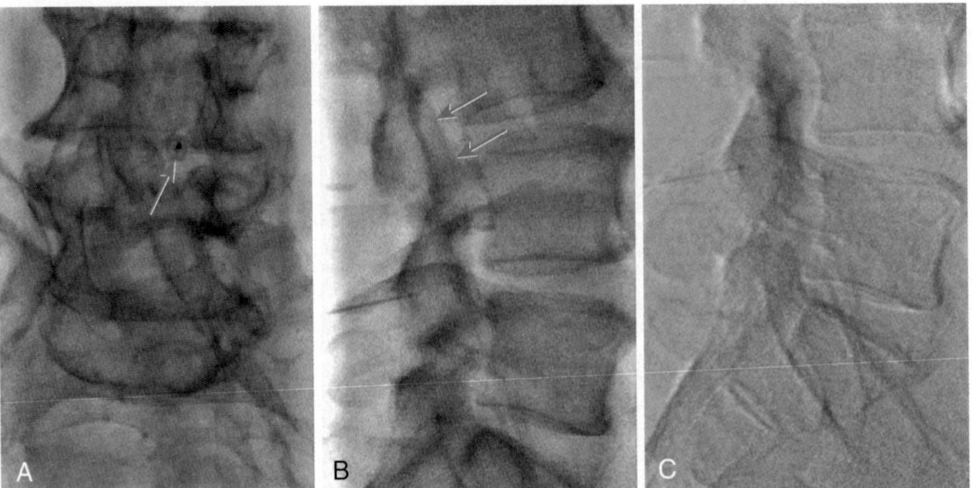

Figure 72.12 Utility of digital subtraction fluoroscopy for visualization of the gadolinium-based contrast epidurogram. A nonselective epidural steroid injection performed in a 62-year-old male at L4-L5 employing an interlaminar approach. **A**, Right anterior oblique (RAO) projection of the lumbar spine shows a needle *(arrow)* inserted into the interlaminar space at L4-L5. **B**, Conventional fluoroscopy permits visualization of an epidurogram in the lateral projection *(arrows)*. **C**, Digital subtraction fluoroscopy in the lateral projection more clearly demonstrates the distribution of the gadolinium chelate in the epidural space. (Adapted with permission from Shetty SK, Nelson EN, Lawrimore TM, Palmer WE. Use of gadolinium chelate to confirm epidural needle placement in patients with an iodinated contrast reaction. *Skeletal Radiol.* 2007;36:301-307, Figure 2.)

pain treatment. They have also been used as an alternative to iodinated contrast agents in patients with known contrast allergy. The radiopacity of gadolinium is less than that of iodinated contrast agents, resulting in a less conspicuous appearance on fluoroscopic images (Fig. 72.12, A, B). Nonetheless, 1 to 3 mL of undiluted gadopentetate dimeglumine (Magnevist) has been used successfully and reliably for identification of the epidural space; the visualization can be further enhanced through the use of digital subtraction in combination with gadolinium (Fig. 72.12, C). Limited experience with intrathecal administration of gadolinium chelates suggests that it is safe when administered directly within the CSF.[18] Use of gadolinium-based contrast agents has been linked to the subsequent development of nephrogenic systemic fibrosis in patients with renal disease.[19] The risk depends on the degree of renal dysfunction, dose of contrast agent, and severity of concomitant illness and varies from negligible in healthy patients to up to 2% to 5% in select high-risk patients. The use of gadolinium-based contrast is contraindicated in patients with GFR < 30 mL/min/1.72 m^2, and caution is recommended in patients with moderately reduced kidney function (30 to 60 mL/min).[20] Given the small dose of gadolinium used in most pain treatment applications, the risk of renal toxicity should be negligible, making gadolinium a viable and readily available alternative in those at risk of reaction to iodinated agents.

ACKNOWLEDGMENTS

Much of the material in this chapter was originally prepared and published by the author in Rathmell JP, *Atlas of Image-Guided Intervention in Regional Anesthesia and Pain Medicine,* 2nd edition, Philadelphia, Lippincott Williams & Wilkins, 2012. I am grateful to Lippincott Williams & Wilkins, the original publisher, and Brian Brown, executive editor with Lippincott, for providing permission for the material to appear here in a modified format.

KEY POINTS

- The biologic effects of ionizing radiation are proportional to the time of exposure, whereas radiation exposure is inversely proportional to the *square* of the distance from the radiation source.
- Modern fluoroscopy units typically employ automatic brightness control (ABC), which automatically adjusts kVp and mA to yield optimal brightness and contrast.
- The International Committee on Radiation Safety Protection (ICRP) has produced estimates of the maximum permissible dose (MPD) of annual radiation to various organs. Exposure below these levels is unlikely to lead to any significant effects, but the ICRP recommends that workers should not receive more than 10% of the MPD.
- A minute of continuous fluoroscopy at 2 R per minute is equivalent to the exposure during 130 chest radiographs.
- Practitioners using ionizing radiation should adhere to the ALARA principle ("as low as reasonably achievable"), combining optimal technique and shielding to minimize patient and personnel exposure.
- The x-ray tube should be positioned as far from the patient as possible, without including unnecessary structures in the field of view.
- To minimize the dose to the patient, the largest field of view, in conjunction with the tightest collimation, should be employed.
- Although protective lead gloves can reduce the exposure of the hands to radiation, they can produce a false sense of security.
- Leaded eyewear is recommended for practitioners who accumulate monthly readings on collar badges above 400 mrem (4 Sv).

KEY POINTS—cont'd

- Iodine is the only element that has proven satisfactory as an intravascular radiographic contrast medium (RCM). Iodine produces the radiopacity, whereas the other portions of the molecule act as the carriers for the iodine, improving solubility and reducing the toxicity of the final compound.
- Digital subtraction electronically enhances the image, reducing the amount of contrast medium needed by twofold to threefold.
- Of the common nonionic monomers in clinical use, only iohexol and iopamidol are labeled for intrathecal use.
- The most common premedication regimen to reduce the risk of severe reactions to contrast media combines pretreatment with corticosteroids and antihistamines; some recommend the addition of H2-antagonists.
- Gadolinium chelates have been used as an alternative to iodinated contrast agents in patients with known contrast allergy. Its use has been linked to the subsequent development of nephrogenic systemic fibrosis in patients with renal disease.

SUGGESTED READINGS

Ellis JH, Cohan RH. Prevention of contrast-induced nephropathy: an overview. *Radiol Clin North Am.* 2009;47:801-811.

Fishman SM, Smith H, Meleger, et al. Radiation safety in pain medicine. *Reg Anesth Pain Med.* 2002;27:296-305.

Greenberger PA, Patterson R. The prevention of immediate generalized reactions to radiocontrast media in high-risk patients. *Clin Immunol.* 1991;87:867-872.

Norris TG. Radiation safety in fluoroscopy. *Radiol Technol.* 2002;73:511-533.

Simons FE. Anaphylaxis. *J Allergy Clin Immunol.* 2010;125(2 suppl 2):S161-S181.

The references for this chapter can be found at www.expertconsult.com.

PART 8

PAIN MANAGEMENT IN SPECIAL SITUATIONS AND SPECIAL TOPICS

ROBERT W. HURLEY | CHRISTOPHER L. WU, EDITORS

PART OUTLINE

73

The Management of Pain from Sickle Cell Disease

Carlton Dampier

Sickle cell disease (SCD) refers to a related group of genetic hemoglobin disorders. Sickle hemoglobin has a single mutation resulting in the replacement of glutamine with valine at the sixth amino acid position in the beta-globin subunit. Molecules of this abnormal hemoglobin polymerize upon deoxygenation into long polymers that physically deform the erythrocyte into the characteristic sickle shape and ultimately obstruct blood flow.[1] This polymerization largely ceases when sickle hemoglobin is combined with adult hemoglobin, so-called sickle trait, or with high levels of fetal hemoglobin, resulting in a relatively benign condition. In contrast, this polymer formation is promoted to varying degrees by the co-occurrence of sickle hemoglobin with other abnormal hemoglobins, such as hemoglobin C, D, E, or O^{arab}, or mutations that reduce the production of normal hemoglobin (thalassemias), resulting in sickling disorders of varying degrees of severity.[2]

The sickle mutation is believed to have arisen independently many thousands of years ago in several areas of Africa and the Middle East or Indian subcontinent.[3] Its prevalence was maintained and expanded in these areas by reproductive advantage as sickle trait provided some degree of protection from severe malaria.[4] Thus, most of the 100,000 to 150,000 individuals with SCD in the United States trace their ethnic origins to Africa, the Middle East, or the Mediterranean where malaria was endemic; the slave trade to the Caribbean and South America also led to the spread of the sickle mutation to many individuals of Hispanic ethnicity.

The pathophysiology of vaso-occlusive pain in SCD is quite complex (Fig. 73.1) and involves mechanisms beyond sickle polymer formation,[5] especially the adhesion of sickled erythrocytes, and perhaps other cellular elements including leucocytes and platelets,[6] to abnormal vascular endothelium.[7] As part of the vicious cycle of sickling, the subsequent ischemic tissue injury from initial vaso-occlusion results in the accumulation of endogenous factors released from cells that reside within or infiltrate into the injured area (including mast cells, basophils, platelets, macrophages, neutrophils, endothelial cells, keratinocytes, and fibroblasts). Collectively, these factors, referred to as the "inflammatory soup," represent a wide array of signaling molecules, including neurotransmitters, peptides, eicosanoids and related lipids, neurotrophins, cytokines, and chemokines, as well as extracellular proteases and protons, which damage local nociceptive nerves leading to increased spontaneous firing that is perceived as acute pain.[8]

Although considerable further research is needed to confirm this process, the intense and repetitive nature of vaso-occlusive events and resulting chronic tissue/bone damage likely drive the experience of chronic pain in adults with SCD (Fig. 73.2) through a process termed *central sensitization,* which represents an activity- or use-dependent form of functional synaptic plasticity that can occur after intense repetitive noxious stimuli. Central sensitization with its augmented pain response occurs by complex processes involving changes in neurotransmitters, receptors, ion channels, and signaling pathways in spinal cord and cortical neurons that change the response elicited by normal sensory inputs, including those that usually evoke innocuous sensations, resulting in the sensation of persistent pain.[9] Further changes in the pain experienced in chronic pain disorders occur as a result of anatomic and functional connectivity changes in various brain regions[10] and can reverse with treatment.[11]

EPIDEMIOLOGY OF VASO-OCCLUSIVE PAIN

SCD is a relatively unique pain disorder, as pain can begin early in the first year of life as levels of fetal hemoglobin decline in susceptible individuals.[12] Most children reported to have pain in the first year of life have pain locations (hands/feet) and signs/symptoms (swelling or tenderness) consistent with dactylitis, often referred to as "hand-foot syndrome," which becomes progressively less prevalent in older children and rare after 5 to 7 years of age.[13] Almost all children with SCD experience increasingly frequent pain throughout childhood and into adolescence and young adulthood;[14] however, the majority of these painful episodes are managed at home rather than in acute care settings.[15,16] Most episodes are relatively brief, typically 2 to 3 days, with pain of moderate intensity located in a small number of body sites, usually the lower legs, back, and chest wall.[17] However, a small number of children transition, often in their early adolescent years, from a pattern of sporadic episodes of brief acute pain to frequent, recurrent, acute pain or chronic pain, and these individuals represent the majority of pediatric patients hospitalized for acute pain.[18,19] Pain is a more complex experience in adults with SCD, with features of both acute recurrent and chronic pain,[20,21] and is more often managed in an acute care setting compared to pain in children.[22] Family characteristics and mental health issues are often comorbidities contributing to frequent health care utilization in SCD adults with chronic pain.[23,24]

OTHER PAIN ETIOLOGIES IN SCD

Vaso-occlusive pain in SCD remains a clinical diagnosis as laboratory and imaging studies largely show nonspecific increases in inflammatory markers and increased hemolysis.[25] Other pain syndromes distinct from vaso-occlusive episodes are not uncommon and always need to be considered when evaluating an individual with SCD and pain (Table 73.1). Children and, occasionally, young adults can experience acute left-upper-quadrant visceral pain from rapid enlargement of the splenic capsule consistent with acute splenic sequestration, an often life-threatening trapping of sickled erythrocytes and platelets in the spleen.[26] Almost all children with SCD will experience episodic right-upper-quadrant colicky abdominal pain and jaundice from cholelithiasis or bile duct obstruction and ultimately require cholecystectomy,[27] as chronic hemolysis results in bilirubin accumulation in the gallbladder and the subsequent production of pigment stones. Avascular necrosis in the vertebral column, shoulder, or hips can be a source of acute pain as well as chronic pain in adolescent and young adult patients, who often respond to physical therapy for initial symptom management of hip pain; some patients, however, have progressive collapse, particularly in the head of the femur, that will ultimately require joint replacement for relief of chronic pain or to improve physical functioning.[28] Although uncommon in the pediatric age group, leg ulcers, typically over the medial malleolus of either or both ankles, can be a source of considerable pain and disability and are difficult to manage.[29] Headaches, as an isolated pain syndrome or as part of a vaso-occlusive event, can occur but are not well characterized.[30] Some have features characteristic of migraine headaches, others may be more typical of tension-type headaches, and a small number of individuals satisfy current diagnostic criteria for chronic daily headache. Use of the triptan class of medications to treat migraine-like headaches in SCD individuals is contraindicated because of cardiovascular concerns.

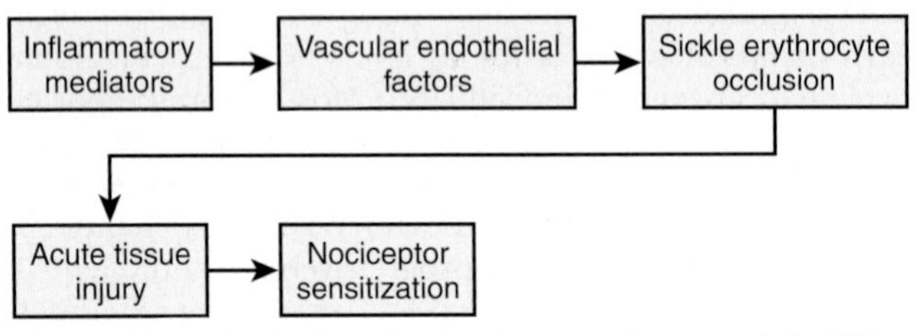

Figure 73.1 Mechanisms for development of acute pain in SCD.

SCD PAIN MANAGEMENT

EDUCATION IS THE FOUNDATION

A lifespan approach is most applicable for these sickling disorders, as pain will likely be experienced throughout childhood and adult life. A focus on the family is essential for children,[31] whereas adolescents must be encouraged and supported to accept progressively more responsibility for their own pain management so that they can function appropriately in the adult health care system. Thus, initial disease and pain management education involves parents and other caregivers for young children and broadens to include the school system in older children; finally, organized transition programs starting in early adolescence focus on self-management skill education.[32] Self-management skill development should include learning psychological approaches to pain management,[33] similar to other pediatric chronic pain disorders for which one meta-analysis indicated the superiority of cognitive-behavioral interventions (multicomponent, relaxation, and biofeedback approaches) for pain management.[34]

HOME MANAGEMENT: "IT TAKES A VILLAGE"

A number of studies in children[15] and adults[20] suggest the preference to manage vaso-occlusive pain at home. The home setting is likely to be more comfortable for children

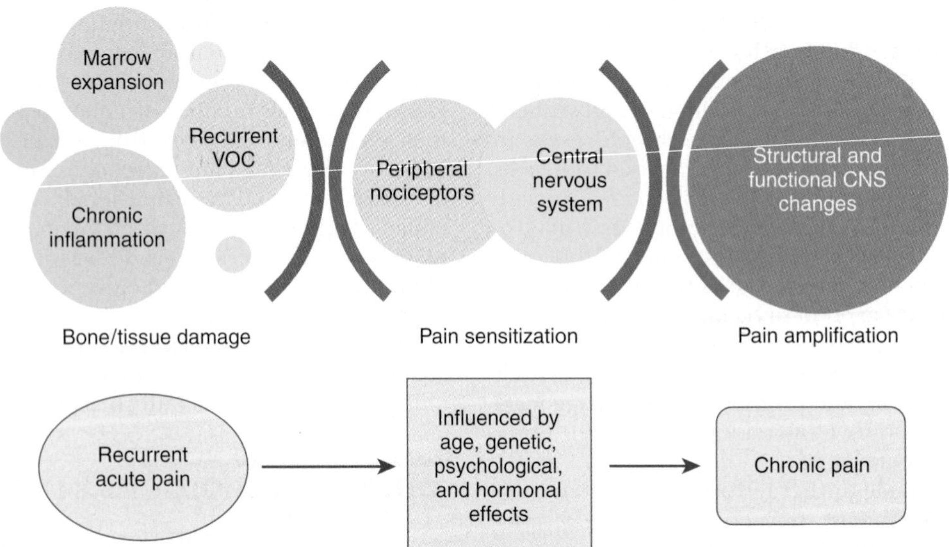

Figure 73.2 Mechanisms for development of chronic pain in SCD. CNS, central nervous system; VOC, vaso-occlusive crisis.

and less disruptive to the families' normal activities and routines. Surprising to most health care providers, many SCD individuals avoid care in acute care settings, as they frequently encounter negative attitudes toward patients with SCD and a pervasive fear among health care providers of catering to opioid addiction, which often compromises analgesic therapy.[35] Successful home management requires a parent or other caregiver skilled in pain assessment and administration of appropriate analgesic medications. Extended family also is critical for psychological and physical support, as most pain episodes may last for several days and usually require around-the-clock medication for adequate management.[15] Support by trusted medical health professionals with experience in SCD and pain management also facilitates home management and appropriate emergency department utilization. Clergy and local complementary and alternative medicine practitioners and mental health professionals also can facilitate the use of both medical and psychological interventions to assist with the management of pain symptoms. Several studies of caregivers of children with SCD have found that a large percentage of families use prayer, spiritual healing, massage, and relaxation in addition to medication to manage their child's pain at home.[36,37] In both studies, complementary medicine approaches were used more frequently with higher levels of pain or medication use.

Low-potency analgesics, such as acetaminophen and ibuprofen, are recommended as initial therapy at the onset of typical vaso-occlusive pain and are often adequate for mild to moderate pain, particularly in younger children. These analgesics are often chosen out of concern for the adverse consequences of opioid analgesics and have the advantage of less sedation and subsequent disruption of age-appropriate activities. A substantial number of oral hydrocodone and oxycodone analgesics of varying potency, often in combination with acetaminophen, are available in liquid and tablet formulations for management of more intense pain in children with SCD. There has been some shift away from the use of codeine containing analgesics because of pharmacogenetic issues of excessive toxicity or inadequate efficacy.[38] Although labeled dose amounts and frequency of potent oral opioid analgesics are usually prescribed, the enhanced hepatic and renal clearance of morphine in this population[39,40] and the potential impact of prevalent pharmacogenetic genotypes impacting morphine metabolism[41] suggests that the dose and frequency of these opioids may need to be further individualized.

There have been few comparative studies of adjunctive nonopioid analgesic medications in this population. A study using pharmacy claims data suggested that pharmacologic treatments for sickle pain consisted mainly of nonsteroidal anti-inflammatory drugs (NSAIDs) and weak opioids.[42] Significantly more severe SCD patients, those with more than three yearly inpatient or emergency department (ED) visits for pain management, were prescribed more potent opioids, antidepressants, or anticonvulsants. Prescription of both stronger opioids and antidepressants or anticonvulsants was significantly associated with lower frequencies of acute sickle pain visits. Further clinical trial data are needed in SCD individuals to support these observations and to establish comparative efficacy and safety data for various analgesic and anticonvulsant or antidepressant combinations, particularly as many of these classes of medications are not currently labeled for use in pediatric age groups.

MANAGEMENT OF SCD PAIN IN THE ACUTE CARE SETTING

Authoritative guidelines have been published for the management of severe SCD pain in the acute care setting,[43,44] but they are somewhat outdated. However, a number of pediatric hospitals have published more contemporary single site pain management practices,[45,46] and an update of the National Institutes of Health's Sickle Cell Treatment Guidelines will be available in 2013. Nurse-initiated ED analgesic protocols for adults with SCD also have been developed[47] and their implementation has been shown to improve pain relief over the period of ED treatment.[48]

Table 73.1 Pain Syndromes in SCD Not Directly Involving Vaso-Occlusion

Pain Syndrome	Typical Locations	Pain Characteristics
Acute splenic sequestration	Spleen	Acute visceral pain related to stretch of splenic capsule from splenic enlargement
Splenic infarction	Spleen	Acute visceral pain from splenic infarction involving splenic tissue extending to splenic capsule
Acute bone infarction	Ribs, sternum, or long bones	Acute pain from necrosis of bone marrow
Avascular necrosis	Hips, shoulders, or vertebrae	Acute and chronic pain from progressive collapse of bone cortex related to persistent vascular compromise
Osteomyelitis	Any bone	Acute and chronic pain from bacterial infection of bone cortex or marrow, often related to chronic ischemia
Acute cholelithiasis	Gallbladder	Acute visceral pain from irritation or common bile duct obstruction by pigment gallstones
Leg ulcers	Medial or lateral ankles	Acute and chronic pain from ischemic damage to skin and underlying soft tissue
Headache	Head	Acute or chronic headache pain with or without migrainous aura or characteristics

Intravenous doses of potent opioids, usually morphine or hydromorphone, are the typical initial treatment for vaso-occlusive pain in both adults and children, as all are assumed to have failed a course of oral analgesics at home prior to arrival in the ED. In some pediatric centers, intravenous nalbuphine is also used, as it is often associated with fewer complaints of nausea and pruritis,[49] but it is seldom used for SCD adults because it may precipitate opioid withdrawal symptoms in opioid tolerant individuals. The use of oral and subcutaneous routes of opioid administration is increasing in adults with limited intravenous access.[48] Administration of opioids by patient-controlled analgesia (PCA) devices is not a common practice in the ED, but where available it allows more frequent dosing, which can be problematic in a busy ED.[46] The concurrent use of a parenteral NSAID, usually ketorolac, is a widespread clinical practice in the ED setting as an additional analgesic, and it may have additional benefit as an anti-inflammatory agent given the increased evidence for the role of inflammation in SCD pathophysiology.[50] Parenteral NSAID doses administered to SCD adults are often reduced for renal insufficiency, which is not uncommon.[51]

SCD PAIN MANAGEMENT IN THE INPATIENT SETTING

A snapshot of current analgesic practice, across a large number of pediatric and adult hospitals that participated in an observational study after hospitalization for sickle pain management, documented the widespread use of opioid-based PCA.[52] Opioid doses varied over a wide range but appeared to be somewhat higher for individuals receiving PCA compared to scheduled opioid dosing, as well as for those receiving hydromorphone compared to morphine. The relationship between opioid dosing and prior daily opioid usage was not described in this cohort, but adult chronic pain patients with chronic opioid use have been shown to report higher postoperative pain scores after surgery and have a slower rate of pain resolution;[53] a similar pattern is likely in SCD. A small clinical trial of opioid PCA dosing suggested that adult SCD individuals have a more rapid improvement in pain when using PCA largely delivered by continuous infusion rather than demand dosing, likely because individuals with severe pain had difficulty obtaining adequate pain relief with frequent demand doses.[54] Parenteral NSAIDs, usually ketorolac, are commonly used as an additional analgesic. Evidence of efficacy of other adjuvant analgesics for acute sickle pain, as have been proposed for post-operative pain,[55] have not been subjected to controlled trials. Refractory sickle pain that persists beyond 3 to 5 days can present a difficult management problem, particularly in adolescents and young adults. The use of concurrent low-dose ketamine infusions has been described for this situation,[56] as has the use of epidural anesthesia,[57] but further research and clinical experience are needed.

Nausea, pruritus, and constipation are common opioid-related adverse effects[54] and require symptomatic management during the course of hospitalization, with constipation often being quite problematic.[58] The use of concurrent administration of low doses of an opioid antagonist (naloxone) has been shown in several small pediatric cohorts[59,60] to ameliorate many central nervous system (CNS) opioid-related symptoms without altering analgesia, and it may be of particular importance in SCD where respiratory depression may increase the risk for symptomatic hypoxia and SCD pulmonary complications, such as acute chest syndrome. Common opioid -related adverse effects of nausea and constipation can be ameliorated by peripherally acting nonabsorbable opioid antagonists, such as methylnaltrexone,[61] but they have not been studied in SCD and are not yet approved for children. Similar to its use for other critically ill patients,[62] transdermal or oral clonidine, an α2-adrenergic agonist, is often used in SCD adolescents and adults with prolonged hospitalizations and opioid exposure to reduce symptoms of opioid withdrawal after discharge, which otherwise might result in a subsequent readmission.

MANAGEMENT OF PERIOPERATIVE PAIN IN SCD

Pre-operative management of individuals with SCD relies on adequate, usually overnight, intravenous hydration and red blood cell transfusion if the hemoglobin is less than 10 grams/dl.[63] In some low-risk surgeries, transfusion may not be necessary, and in some high-risk surgeries, individuals with higher hemoglobin levels may require exchange transfusion.[64] Intra-operative management focuses on the prevention of sickling by maintaining adequate hydration, oxygenation, and ambient temperature. Effective pain control is a primary goal in the perioperative management of patients with SCD and may require additional analgesics compared to that used to treat other patients. For example, postoperative pain scores after laparoscopic cholecystectomy, one of the most common surgeries in SCD, were higher in SCD patients than in controls, and morphine consumption was more than double that compared to control children, as was the duration of PCA use.[65] SCD children also had a longer duration of postoperative hospital stay (3.4 ± 1.6 days versus 1.5 ± 0.5 days). These differences likely reflect alterations in pain perception from frequent vaso-occlusive episodes,[66,67] enhanced clearance of opioids,[39,40] and psychosocial variables.[24,68]

MANAGEMENT OF CHRONIC PAIN IN SCD: LARGELY UNCHARTED TERRITORY

The management of chronic daily pain, which is likely prevalent in adolescents and young adults, is largely uncharted territory with few case series or clinical trials to guide therapy selection. Currently, pain management in SCD has largely relied on the use of long-acting opioid preparations,[14] sometimes using very large daily doses and putting these individuals at risk for opioid tolerance and opioid-induced hyperalgesia. Studies focusing on the U.S. population suggest that daily opioid usage is more frequent in individuals with comorbid psychological and psychiatric disorders,[69] and clinical experience suggests similar findings in the SCD population.[70] Adolescents and young adults with SCD started on daily opioids should also receive concurrent psychosocial and psychiatric support given the negative role that emotional, social, and psychiatric issues play in an individual's pain experience.[71] SCD chronic pain management strategies may benefit from extrapolations from other chronic pain syndromes where antidepressants and anticonvulsants have proven track records of efficacy,[72] but further research and clinical experience are again needed before definitive treatment recommendations can be made.

SUMMARY

SCD is unique as a lifelong pain disorder with features of acute recurrent pain in childhood that often transforms in adolescents or young adults into a chronic pain syndrome complicated by exacerbations of acute pain. Health providers and patients often have difficulty changing treatment goals and strategies during this transformation, which can be further complicated by transitioning from pediatric to adult health care systems. As with other chronic pain syndromes, mental health problems are frequent comorbidities; poverty and health disparities unique to urban minority populations are additional challenges. Pain management optimally requires a multidisciplinary team of hematologists, psychologists, physical therapists, alternative medicine practitioners, and pain specialists. Further clinical collaborations are also important for expanding the evidence base for acute and chronic pain management in this population, which currently is distressingly limited. A further understanding of the pathophysiology of pain in this complex pain syndrome, likely driven by peripheral and central sensitization from repeated ischemic insults and chronic inflammation, could lead to the identification of new therapeutic targets and agents to ameliorate the pain and suffering currently experienced by individuals with SCD.

KEY POINTS

- The pathophysiology of sickle vaso-occlusion in sickle cell disease (SCD) involves intracellular polymer formation and related biochemical changes, a host of cellular interactions, and multiple inflammatory pathways, making the development of targeted therapeutics challenging.
- Pain from sickle vaso-occlusion likely represents acute nociceptor stimulation by inflammatory mediators from hypoxia and reperfusion injury, as well central sensitization from repeat episodes of severe pain.
- SCD is a relatively unique pain disorder, as pain can begin early in the first year of life and almost all children with SCD experience increasingly frequent pain throughout childhood and into adolescence and young adulthood.
- Pain is a more complex experience in adults with SCD, with features of both acute recurrent and chronic pain.
- Mental health issues are often comorbidities contributing to frequent health care utilization in SCD adults with chronic pain.
- Other pain syndromes distinct from vaso-occlusive episodes are not uncommon in children and adults with SCD, and they always need to be considered when evaluating an individual with SCD and pain.

KEY POINTS—cont'd

- Low-potency analgesics, such as acetaminophen and ibuprofen, are recommended as initial therapy at the onset of typical vaso-occlusive pain, and they are often adequate for mild to moderate pain, particularly in younger children, whereas oral hydrocodone and oxycodone analgesics, often in combination with acetaminophen, are available in liquid and tablet formulations for the management of more intense pain in children with SCD.
- Cognitive-behavioral approaches—specifically deep breathing and progressive muscle relaxation, guided imagery, and calming self-talk—are effective psychological therapies for SCD pain in children and adolescents.
- Support by trusted medical health professionals with experience in SCD and pain management facilitates home management and appropriate emergency department utilization.
- Intravenous doses of potent opioids, usually morphine or hydromorphone, are the typical initial treatment for vaso-occlusive pain in both adults and children, as most have failed a course of oral analgesics at home prior to arrival in the emergency department (ED).
- The concurrent use of a parenteral nonsteroidal anti-inflammatory drug (NSAID), usually ketorolac, is a widespread clinical practice in the ED setting as an additional analgesic, and it may have additional benefit as an anti-inflammatory agent.
- The efficacy of adjuvant analgesics for acute sickle pain has not been subjected to controlled trials, and refractory sickle pain that persists beyond 3 to 5 days is a difficult management problem with few new therapeutic options.
- Chronic daily pain, which is likely prevalent in SCD adolescents and young adults, is currently managed with long-acting opioid preparations.
- Adolescents and young adults with SCD started on daily opioids should also receive concurrent psychosocial and psychiatric support and may benefit from antidepressants and anticonvulsants, but further research and clinical experience are needed.

SUGGESTED READINGS

Anie KA, Green J. Psychological therapies for sickle cell disease and pain. *Cochrane Database Syst Rev.* 2012;2:CD001916.

Brandow AM, Stucky CL, Hillery CA, et al. Patients with sickle cell disease have increased sensitivity to cold and heat. *Am J Hematol.* 2013;88:37-43.

Carroll PC, Haywood C, Hoot MR, et al. A preliminary study of psychiatric, familial, and medical characteristics of high-utilizing sickle cell disease patients. *Clin J Pain.* 2013;29:317-323.

Conran N, Franco-Penteado CF, Costa FF. Newer aspects of the pathophysiology of sickle cell disease vaso-occlusion. *Hemoglobin.* 2009;33:1-16.

Dampier C, Ely B, Brodecki D, et al. Characteristics of pain managed at home in children and adolescents with sickle cell disease by using diary self-reports. *J Pain.* 2002;3:461-470.

Dampier CD, Smith WR, Kim HY, et al. Opioid patient controlled analgesia use during the initial experience with the IMPROVE PCA trial: a phase III analgesic trial for hospitalized sickle cell patients with painful episodes. *Am J Hematol.* 2011;86:E70-E73.

Darbari DS, Neely M, van den Anker J, et al. Increased clearance of morphine in sickle cell disease: implications for pain management. *J Pain.* 2011;12:531-538.

Jerrell JM, Tripathi A, Stallworth JR. Pain management in children and adolescents with sickle cell disease. *Am J Hematol.* 2011;86:82-84.

Miller ST, Kim HY, Weiner D, et al. Inpatient management of sickle cell pain: a "snapshot" of current practice. *Am J Hematol.* 2012;87:333-336.

Platt OS, Thorington BD, Brambilla DJ, et al. Pain in sickle cell disease: rates and risk factors. *N Engl J Med.* 1991;325:11-16.

Smith WR, Penberthy LT, Bovbjerg VE, et al. Daily assessment of pain in adults with sickle cell disease. *Ann Intern Med.* 2008;148:94-101.

Smith WR, Scherer M. Sickle-cell pain: advances in epidemiology and etiology. *Hematology.* 2010;2010:409-415.

Sogutlu A, Levenson JL, McClish DK, et al. Somatic symptom burden in adults with sickle cell disease predicts pain, depression, anxiety, health care utilization, and quality of life: the PiSCES project. *Psychosomatics.* 2011;52:272-279.

Taylor LE, Stotts NA, Humphreys J, et al. A review of the literature on the multiple dimensions of chronic pain in adults with sickle cell disease. *J Pain Sympt Manage.* 2010;40:416-435.

Williams TN, Weatherall DJ. World distribution, population genetics, and health burden of the hemoglobinopathies. *Cold Spring Harb Perspect Med.* 2012;2:a011692.

Zempsky WT. Treatment of sickle cell pain: fostering trust and justice. *JAMA.* 2009;302:2479-2480.

The references for this chapter can be found at www.expertconsult.com.

Burn Pain

74

Jason C. Brookman | Kanupriya Kumar | Christopher L. Wu

Management of pain from burns is extremely challenging for the clinician due in part to the complex physiology and potential chronic nature of burn pain. Although there may be variability in the etiology and extent of burn pain, the treatment options of pain management are similar. While traditional analgesic agents such as opioids are a mainstay for the treatment of different types of burn pain, adjuvant agents and nonpharmacologic techniques also play important roles in the management of burn pain. A multidisciplinary approach involving not only pain management but also psychological support and physical rehabilitation may be the ideal method for treating patients with burns.

Attempts have been made in the past to present a reasonable approach for managing the complex pain associated with burn injuries.[1] However, because evidence continues to evolve in our understanding of the mechanisms of pain therapeutics in burns, evidence-based treatment regimens and algorithms for burn pain management remain limited. Despite this evolution in our knowledge, practice standards for burn pain management have remained and continue to remain inadequate, inconsistent, and mostly unchanged in many centers since the 1990s, with opioid- and benzodiazepine-based regimens as the mainstay of therapy in the acute setting.

EPIDEMIOLOGY

Burn injuries occur in approximately 1.25 million people in the United States alone each year, with up to 71,000 people requiring hospitalization.[2] The majority of burns are a result of flame-related (55%) or scald burns (40%).[3] The age of the person correlates with the type of injury, with scald burns occurring more frequently in children and flame-related burns more common in adults.[3] Burns disproportionately affect people in developing countries with an estimated 90% of the global burns occurring in low- and middle-income countries.[4] Globally, there are also gender differences in burn injuries with a greater proportion of women injured in fires from cooking/heating fuels in the developing world and a predominance of men injured in fires from industrial accidents in developed nations.[4]

A national review of burn data (approximately 140,000 cases) in the United States revealed that 58% were Caucasian, 17% were African American, 13% were Hispanic, 2% were Asian, and 0.6% were native American (the remainder had missing data).[5] Approximately 16% of cases had a burn surface area (BSA) of greater than 20%.[5] The elderly (age > 70 years) accounted for 8% of reported burns.[5] Of the 60% of cases with a defined etiology for the burn injury, fire/flame accounted for 44%, followed by scald (36%), contact with a hot object (8%), electrical (4%), and chemical (3%).[5]

PATHOPHYSIOLOGY

Depending on the location and extent of the insult, burn injury (which may originate from different sources such as heat, cold, electricity, or chemicals/radiation) is a potentially traumatic event that may result in a systematic inflammatory response affecting all organ systems.[3] At the molecular level, there is a massive activation of toxic inflammatory mediators, including histamine, prostaglandins, thromboxane, bradykinin, serotonin, catecholamines, platelet aggregation factor, angiotensin II, vasopressin, oxygen radicals (superoxide, hydrogen peroxide, hydroxyl ion), and corticotropin-releasing factor. At the cellular level there is protein denaturation and coagluation with surrounding tissue hypoperfusion and capillary vasoconstriction. These may lead to disruption of structures deep to the skin (e.g., dermal tissue, muscle). When combined, these local responses to burn trauma become systemic and manifest as myocardial dysfunction, increased systemic vascular resistance, increased pulmonary vascular resistance, increased pulmonary capillary wedge pressure, organ ischemia, peripheral capillary leak causing interstitial and pulmonary edema secondary to hypoproteinemia, temperature dysregulation from loss of body heat, and increased evaporative water loss. If severe enough, they may then result in potentially fatal systemic complications such as infection, respiratory distress, shock, or multiple organ failure.[3]

PHASES OF BURN RECOVERY

Recovery from burn injuries can be broadly divided into four phases (Table 74.1[6]). The first phase is the initial evaluation and resuscitation that occurs over 1 to 3 days postinjury. This is when the patient often requires large volume fluid resuscitation. The second phase is when the burn wounds are excised and temporarily closed with auto- or allografting of skin to accelerate the natural healing process. This generally occurs over weeks to months, depending on the size of the burn injury. The third phase occurs with definitive wound closure and reconstruction. Finally, the last stage of recovery is rehabilitation and reconstruction, which eventually leads to discharge and reintegration into society.[7]

TYPES OF PAIN IN BURN PATIENTS

Acute postburn injury pain is often severe and extremely challenging to treat, usually necessitating powerful doses of opioids for analgesia. Burn depth, total body surface area

Table 74.1 Features of Burn Depths, Association of Pain, and Approximate Healing Times

Burn Depth		Appearance	Blistering	Sensation	Healing Time
Epidermal		Red	None	Painful	7 days
Partial Thickness	Superficial	Pink with wet appearance Brisk cap-refill	(+)	Painful	14 days
	Deep	Pale/fixed red staining Poor cap-refill	(+/–)	Painful or painless	21 days; (+/–) burn excision and skin grafting
Full Thickness		Leathery white or brown	None	None in burned area (+/–) Pain at edges	Usually requires burn excision and skin grafting

*Adapted from Gandhi M, Thomson C, Lord D, Enoch S. Management of pain in children with burns. *Int J Pediatrics*. 2010. Epub. Accessed October 20, 2010.

affected, mechanism of injury, and various patient factors play a significant role in acute burn pain. Differences in the mechanism of burn injury may also alter the severity and complexity of pain experienced. For example, pain from a partial-thickness (second-degree) burn results from loss of dermis and epidermis exposing raw nerve fibers. In contrast, nerves are also burned with the upper skin layers in full-thickness (third-degree) burns and result in lower levels of acute pain.[8] Pain from burns may be both nociceptive and neuropathic in origin.[9] Pain in burn patients can be divided into four different categories, which may intensify as tissues heal:

1. *Rest pain.* Constant, dull background pain.
2. *Breakthrough pain.* Intermittent, short duration, rapid onset/offset, sometimes excruciating pain.
3. *Procedural pain.* Short duration, greatest intensity, occurring with certain activities (i.e., wound cleaning, debridement, dressing changes, joint range of motion exercises).
4. *Psychogenic pain.* Anticipatory pain in the absence of mechanical stimulation.

PAIN MANAGEMENT OPTIONS

Modern day clinical burn injury care necessitates a multifaceted approach to effective postburn pain management, using both pharmacologic and nonpharmacologic methods. There are many pharmacologic agents (Table 74.2) available to manage the various types of pain related to burn injuries. Because these have been presented in greater detail elsewhere in this text, we will only provide a cursory review of the various agents in context appropriate for burn pain management.

PHARMACOLOGIC ANALGESIA

OPIOIDS

Opioids including morphine, hydromorphone, and fentanyl have been the cornerstone of effective burn pain management for decades. They are widely available, can be administered by a variety of routes (e.g., oral [PO], intravenous [IV], transdermal) are inexpensive, and have a relatively ubiquitous familiarity among health care providers. In experimental studies utilizing burn injury, opioids (μ-receptor agonists) have been shown to produce antinociceptive effects, although there may be reduced efficacy of morphine antinociception in chronic burn injury.[10,11] Opioid doses required by patients in the acute phase of burn injury to control pain may be many times greater than maximum recommended doses. An early negative consequence of (and possibly result from) this rapid and massive dose escalation is the development of acute opioid tolerance. A later consequence of this opioid escalation may be opioid-induced hyperalgesia. Longer-acting opioids, such as methadone, may mitigate or even reverse this acute tolerance and hyperalgesia, as might using other nonopioid analgesics, including ketamine, dextromethorphan, and clonidine. Although opioids are an important modality for the treatment of burn pain, clinicians should be aware of the side effects (including respiratory depression and hyperalgesia) associated with their use in any patient. For burn patients, the immunosuppressant effects of opioids could theoretically lead to an increase risk of infectious complications, although opioids should not be withheld in patients with burn-related pain.[12]

Methadone is a unique opioid because of its receptor binding properties. It is both a mu-opioid and *N*-methyl-D-aspartate (NMDA)-receptor antagonist, and it also has serotonin and norepinephrine reuptake inhibitor properties. Administration can occur via oral, parenteral, and rectal routes. However, because of variable and unpredictable potency, dosing efficacy is dependent on chronicity. The long-acting analgesia provided by methadone makes this an ideal opioid for maintenance in burn pain management.[1] Further, the NMDA antagonist properties may be responsible for reducing or reversing opioid tolerance and hyperalgesia from other shorter-acting opioids, as well as modulating neuropathic pain. Methadone may be a viable option for some burn patients who are opioid tolerant and have developed chronic neuropathic pain unrelieved by conventional pharmacotherapies.[13]

Fentanyl is a synthetic lipophilic opioid analog with high potency. These properties facilitate rapid onset of action and quick redistribution from the central circulation. Lipophilicity allows for transmucosal absorption via nasal or buccal routes with rapid onset and peak effect similar to that achieved by IV administration. Although fentanyl is generally administered intravenously, it can be given orally or intranasally. These properties make this opioid a useful

Table 74.2 Pharmacologic Management of Burn Pain

Agents	Examples	Mechanism of Action	Administration
Opioids	Fentanyl, morphine, Hydromorphone	*mu*-R agonism	IV, PO, IM, TD
Methadone		*mu*-R agonism, NMDA-R antagonism, serotonin- and NE-reuptake inhibition	IV, PO
NMDA antagonists	Ketamine Dextromethorphan	Noncompetitive NMDA-R antagonism	IV, PO (dextromethorphan)
NSAIDs	Ketorolac Ibuprofen APAP	Cyclooxygenase (COX-1 and -2) inhibition	IV, PO, PR; intrathecal/local (experimental)
Gabapentinoids	Gabapentin Pregabalin	Ca^{2+} channel blockade ($\alpha_2\delta$-1 subunit-containing channels)	PO
Local anesthetics	Lidocaine Bupivacaine Ropivacaine	Na^+ channel blockade	IV (lidocaine), epidural/intrathecal, perineural, TD
α_2 adrenergic agonists	Clonidine Dexmedetomidine	Central and peripheral α_2-adrenergic blockade/sympatholysis	IV (dexmedetomidine), PO

R, receptor; NMDA, *N*-methyl-D-aspartate; NE, norepinephrine; APAP, *N*-acetyl-p-aminophenol/acetaminophen; NSAIDs, nonsteroidal anti-inflammatory drugs; IV, intravenous; PO, per os; IM, intramuscular; TD, transdermal; PR, per rectum.

adjunct for procedural burn care activities, such as dressing changes and hydrotherapy.[14] The use of oral transmucosal fentanyl citrate and patient-controlled intranasal fentanyl for procedural wound care in burn patients has been reported.[14,15]

N-METHYL-D-ASPARTATE (NMDA)-RECEPTOR ANTAGONISTS

NMDA antagonists such as ketamine and dextromethorphan may be valuable agents for the treatment of burn pain, as the NMDA receptor plays a central role in neuropathic pain processing and tolerance. In an experimental human study, ketamine significantly reduced the area of secondary hyperalgesia resulting from local first-degree burn injury.[16] Similarly, dextromethorphan reduced the magnitude of secondary hyperalgesia from experimentally produced burn injuries.[17]

Ketamine is a noncompetitive NMDA-receptor antagonist with antihyperalgesia and anti-allodynia properties. It reduces NMDA-R–mediated central transmission and processing of pain, thereby inhibiting central wind-up. Thus, there are many benefits to initiating ketamine early in the course of burn wound care. When administered with opioids, ketamine has synergistic effects with superior pain relief and reduced opioid consumption compared to placebo. When administered with opioids, ketamine appears to have a synergistic analgesic effect on experimentally induced wind-up–like pain in humans.[18,19] At analgesic doses, it has significantly less risk of respiratory depression and negligible psychomimetic or dissociative effects.[20] Analgesic maintenance dosing ranges from about 1 to 3 mcg/kg/min (or 0.05 to 0.15 mg/kg/hr or 4 to 10 mg/hr). Furthermore, there appears to be no risk of developing tolerance to the drug, even with extended-duration infusion at analgesic doses.[21,22] A survey of 188 European burn centers noted that ketamine was preferred for analgesia in 12% and for sedation in 13% of all substances used.[23] A systematic review of studies investigating intravenous ketamine as an analgesic agent for burn pain suggested that ketamine demonstrated analgesic efficacy for burn injuries with attenuation of secondary hyperalgesia and that no subjects withdrew from the studies as a result of ketamine-related side effects.[24] Delivery of ketamine via patient-controlled analgesia for burn dressing changes has been reported.[25] Ketamine has been used for long-term sedation and analgesia in burn patients.[21,25] Finally, ketamine may be an effective analgesic agent for painful procedures in the pediatric burn patient.[26]

Dextromethorphan (DXM) is a noncompetitive NMDA-receptor antagonist that acts by reducing excitatory transmission of primary afferent pathways and is effective in managing challenging neuropathic/wind-up pain in patients who, for a variety of reasons, may be unable to receive ketamine. It has a reduced affinity for the NMDA-receptor compared to ketamine, and it also has a significant first-pass effect in the liver via CYP2D6 microsomal enzymes. Clinically, DXM has synergistic effects when administered with opioids and has superior analgesic and opioid-reducing effects when compared to placebo. Most studies describe doses in the 60 mg twice a day to 90 mg three times a day range. It is effective in 70% to 90% of patients but has been shown to have better efficacy at lower doses when coadministered with a CYP2D6-inhibitor such as quinidine. There are virtually no psychomimetic effects at the doses used clinically.[27] Clinically, however, ketamine appears to be used more frequently than dextromethorphan.

NONSTEROIDAL ANTI-INFLAMMATORY AGENTS (NSAIDS)

Analgesia from nonsteroidal anti-inflammatory drugs (NSAIDs) occurs by reducing inflammation and inflammatory mediators via cyclooxygenase-specific inhibition (COX-1 and COX-2). In the burn trauma population, NSAIDs may be useful adjuncts to help reduce the neurogenic inflammatory pain and fever associated with burns. In the acute setting, however, their use should be time and dose limited as they may present increased risks of bleeding from platelet dysfunction, gastric ulcers and gastrointestinal bleeding from COX-1 inhibition in the setting of acute stress, and renal dysfunction in the setting of reduced renal perfusion, especially in patients with larger total body surface area (TBSA) burns.[28] COX-2–specific inhibitors (i.e., celecoxib) may offer a better overall safety profile compared to nonspecific COX inhibitors like ibuprofen and ketorolac, but data in the burn patient population are lacking and the subject needs to be better studied. NSAIDs may be especially useful for the treatment of burn pain, as experimental studies suggest that intrathecal or local administration of NSAIDs may decrease postburn hyperalgesia and reduce hypersensitivity in skin sensitized by ultraviolet burn.[29,30] Intravenous ketorolac administered to volunteers increased the pressure pain tolerance threshold and attenuated secondary hyperalgesia from an experimental skin burn injury.[31] In addition, experimental animal studies suggest that NSAIDs may enhance tissue perfusion and reduce edema formation after burns.[32] Few studies have specifically examined NSAIDs or acetaminophen alone in the treatment of burn pain as the majority of these agents have been used as part of a multimodal approach to pain management in burn patients. A prospective, multicenter, randomized, double-blind trial evaluating intravenous ibuprofen for treatment of fever and pain in burn patients found that use of intravenous ibuprofen was associated with a significant reduction in fever and that use of the maximum daily recommended dose (800 mg every 6 hours) over 5 days was well tolerated.[28] Finally, acetaminophen (also called paracetamol, or APAP) may be useful in the management of background postburn pain in children at doses in the 10- to 15-mg/kg/4 hr range. It is available for administration via oral, rectal, and intravenous routes. In one observational study 50% of children received only acetaminophen to control background pain.[33]

GABAPENTINOIDS

The gabapentinoids gabapentin and pregabalin are lipophilic structural analogs of γ-amino butyric acid (GABA) that selectively block Ca^{2+} channels containing the $\alpha_2\delta$-1 subunit. In injured dorsal root ganglion neurons, gabapentin has been shown to selectively silence spontaneous discharges but failed to block propagation of normal impulses.[34] In peripheral nerve injury, as occurs in burn trauma, gabapentin activates and enhances the efficacy and release of descending noradrenergic neuronal activity from the locus coeruleus. By using central neuronal plasticity, it induces more spinal noradrenaline release after nerve injury,[35] suppresses transmission of pain signals to the brain, and may facilitate a more natural sleeplike state in the acute setting owing to the upregulation of activity in the locus coeruleus.[36] Gabapentinoids may be effective for the treatment of burn pain, as experimental studies demonstrate that oral gabapentin (in humans) may decrease primary mechanical allodynia in acute inflammation following a thermal injury and that intrathecal gabapentin (in rats) may produce a dose-dependent reversal of thermal hyperalgesia evoked by mild thermal injury.[37,38]

Despite the potential benefits of gabapentinoids in the treatment of burn pain especially considering the presence of neuropathic pain in burn patients, few studies have actually been undertaken to examine the analgesic efficacy of this modality. One of the few double-blind, randomized placebo-controlled trials examining the analgesic efficacy of pregabalin found that administration of pregabalin (up to 300 mg twice a day over a period of 28 days) significantly reduced several aspects of the neuropathic pain and pain associated with procedures.[39] A relatively small retrospective review of pregabalin noted that 69% of patients in a burn outpatient clinic experienced some reduction in pain score after treatment with pregabalin.[40] Observational data also suggest that gabapentin may be useful in reducing neuropathic burn-related pain, as administration of gabapentin rapidly reduced the severity of the neuropathic burn pain and decreased opioid consumption.[41,42] Another potentially useful role for gabapentin is for the treatment of postburn pruritus in patients where pruritus is not relieved with antihistamines.[43]

Na^+-CHANNEL BLOCKERS: LOCAL ANESTHETICS

Sodium channel blockers such as local anesthetics have been shown to reduce primary and secondary hyperalgesia from experimental heat trauma in humans.[44] Human experimental studies indicate that intravenous lidocaine may attenuate long-term inflammation-induced tissue responses to thermal injury,[45] and it has been shown to attenuate cytokine-induced cell injury in endothelial and vascular smooth muscle cells.[46] Local anesthetics for analgesia can be administered via nerve blocks or intravenously in some cases.

Intravenous lidocaine has been used as an analgesic agent for postoperative pain control and for the treatment of neuropathic pain. There is only one randomized controlled trial[47] and a few observational reports[48,49] describing the use of intravenous lidocaine for the treatment of burn pain. The sole randomized controlled trial examined intravenous lidocaine (versus placebo) in 45 severely burned patients undergoing wound care procedures on two consecutive days. Subjects were randomized to either the intravenous lidocaine or control on the first dressing day and crossed over to the alternate treatment on the second dressing day. Although pain scores were significantly lower for lidocaine, there were no significant differences with regard to opioid consumption or satisfaction.[50] A systematic Cochrane review was unable to recommend routine use of intravenous lidocaine in burn pain management at this time.[50]

Neuraxial and peripheral regional nerve blockade have been used as analgesic techniques in the treatment of postoperative pain; however, these techniques have not been widely used for the treatment of burn pain. A variety of single-injection regional analgesic techniques have been described in burn patients, typically for reducing pain at skin graft donor site.[51,52] One case report described using double continuous peripheral nerve block catheters in a child who had suffered a burn injury.[53,54] Despite the potential benefits that peripheral and neuraxial catheter blocks can offer, clinicians should be aware of the potential infectious complications associated with continuous regional analgesic techniques, especially if indwelling catheters are used for any duration.

α_2-ADRENERGIC AGONISTS

Clonidine and dexmedetomidine are both highly selective central and peripheral α_2-adrenergic agonists that decrease noradrenaline release at presynaptic receptor sites causing sympatholysis, thereby reducing autonomic outflow. Both drugs significantly reduce pain intensity and have a morphine-sparing effect.[55] Other potential benefits include anti-inflammatory effects, improved macrophage function, antiapoptotic activity, reduced delirium, and reduced mortality by approximately ~70% for dexmedetomidine when compared to using benzodiazepines for sedation in critically ill patients.[56] Analgesic dosing for these agents depends on the route of administration. For clonidine, dosing regimens may include 2 to 5 mcg/kg PO, 0.1 to 0.3 mg/24 hr TTD, or 30 mcg to 300 mcg IV for procedural sedation in chronic opioid/chronic pain patients. Dexmedetomidine is given exclusively IV as an infusion at 0.2 to 1 mcg/kg/hr but may be bolused intermittently in small doses of 4 to 8 mcg IV push with minimal side effects. In terms of nociception, α_2-adrenergic agonists may have a role in the prevention or treatment of burn pain. Experimental data suggest that α_2-adrenoceptor-mediated mechanisms may be involved in nociceptor sensitization to heat stimuli in normal skin and produce antinociceptive effects in a thermal hyperalgesia model.[57] Clinically, α_2-adrenergic agonists may be used for analgesia and sedation in burn patients. A report of oral clonidine in a burn patient who had severe pain noted that administration of clonidine resulted in improved analgesia and sedation.[58] The addition of low-dose intravenous clonidine in a child with severe burns requiring large doses of morphine causing severe opioid-related side effects resulted in a significant decrease in morphine consumption with attendant improvement in ventilatory, gastrointestinal and psychological functions.[59] When administered to burn patients, dexmedetomidine is typically used for sedation for procedures or in critically ill mechanically ventilated patients.[60]

NONPHARMACOLOGIC ANALGESIA

Although management of burn pain is typically achieved primarily by pharmacologic agents, nonpharmacologic techniques (Table 74.3) may be particularly helpful in the treatment of burn pain, especially considering the long-term nature of rehabilitation and possible development of chronic pain and stress-related disorders. A variety of nonpharmacologic modalities (e.g., cognitive therapies, relaxation techniques) have been examined, although there are significant methodological limitations in many available studies.

VIRTUAL REALITY

Virtual reality utilizes computer-simulated environments that primarily incorporate sight to simulate physical presence in an alternate environment. The application of virtual reality may be most useful during painful procedures, and it is typically used in conjunction with pharmacologic analgesic agents (rather than as a sole modality for analgesia). By distracting a patient's attention from the real world (and possibly decreasing processing of incoming nociceptive signals), virtual reality may potentially reduce pain from procedures by approximately 35% to 50% with a corresponding decrease in pain-related brain activity as documented by functional magnetic resonance imaging (fMRI).[61] A systematic review of virtual reality for burn pain revealed that use of virtual reality (mostly for wound dressing changes) as an adjunct to systemic analgesics was associated with a significant reduction in procedural pain.[62] Although virtual reality can be used for patients in any age group, this technique may be especially useful for pediatric patients.[63] Depending on the type of virtual reality system used, there may be a significant time commitment from staff for implementation of such a system.[64]

Table 74.3 Nonpharmacologic Management of Burn Pain

Method	Purported Mechanism of Action
Virtual reality	Mostly visual distraction/decrease in processing of incoming nociceptive signals
Music therapy	Auditory distraction/attenuation of stress response to pain
Relaxation techniques	Behavioral management of anxiety, especially immediately pre-procedure/dressing changes

MUSIC THERAPY

Although in some sense music therapy can be considered a form of virtual reality, in some ways it should be examined separately, as virtual reality generally implies a visual rather than an auditory input in most virtual reality studies in burn patients. There is some evidence suggesting that the use of music may be of benefit in decreasing pain, especially during dressing changes or debridement procedures.[65,66] Music may attenuate some measures of the cognitive and physiologic component of the stress response with a lower heart rate and anxiety in subjects who listened to music versus those who did not.[67] However, not all data have demonstrated a decrease in burn pain with music therapy,[68] and reporting guidelines for music-based interventions have been proposed.[69] Nevertheless, music therapy may be a valuable nonpharmacologic intervention for the treatment of procedural pain after burn injury.

RELAXATION TECHNIQUES

Relaxation techniques (e.g., breathing relaxation techniques) may be a useful adjunct to pharmacologic agents for the treatment of burn, as these techniques in essence do not increase patient risk, are easily mastered and implemented, and generally do not require expensive equipment.[70] A systematic review of simple relaxation techniques for burn pain was unable to definitively determine the efficacy of simple relaxation techniques for the treatment of burn pain, although concentration on breathing, in combination with jaw relaxation, was suggested to be the most promising technique. Future research should address some of the methodological limitations of currently available studies in this area.[71]

SUMMARY

Pain following burn injuries requires an aggressive multimodal and multidisciplinary approach to analgesia. Typically, burn pain consists of both nociceptive and neuropathic components and the use of pharmacologic agents to address each component as part of a multimodal approach is optimal. Unfortunately, there are few large-scale randomized controlled trials to guide our analgesic management for burn patients, and we currently are guided by our pathophysiologic understanding of the nociceptive processing of burn pain. Nevertheless, we recognize that both pharmacologic and nonpharmacologic modalities are needed for the successful treatment of pain in burn patients.

KEY POINTS

- Burn injuries occur in approximately 1.25 million people in the United States alone each year, with up to 71,000 people requiring hospitalization.
- Modern-day clinical burn injury care requires an aggressive multimodal and multidisciplinary approach to effective postburn pain management, using both pharmacologic and nonpharmacologic methods.
- Acute postburn injury pain is often severe and extremely challenging to treat, usually necessitating intense doses of opioids for analgesia.
- Pain from burns may be both nociceptive and neuropathic in origin.
- Pain in burn patients can be divided into four different categories: rest pain, breakthrough pain, procedural pain, and psychogenic pain.
- In experimental burn injury, opioids (μ-receptor agonists) have been shown to produce antinociceptive effects.
- Consequences of rapid and massive opioid dose escalation may include acute opioid tolerance and opioid-induced hyperalgesia.
- Longer-acting opioids, such as methadone, may be a viable option for some burn patients who are opioid tolerant and have developed neuropathic pain.
- Fentanyl is a useful adjunct for procedural burn care activities, such as dressing changes and hydrotherapy due to rapid onset of action and quick redistribution.
- NMDA antagonists such as ketamine and dextromethorphan may be valuable agents for the treatment of burn pain, as the NMDA receptor plays a central role in neuropathic pain processing and tolerance.
- NSAIDs may be useful adjuncts to help reduce the neurogenic inflammatory pain and fever associated with burns.
- Gabapentinoids are potentially effective for the treatment of burn pain, as they decrease primary mechanical allodynia in acute inflammation following a thermal injury.

KEY POINTS—cont'd

- Peripheral regional nerve blockade may be useful for reducing pain at the skin graft donor site, but it should be used with care due to potential issues of infection.
- Dexmedetomidine may reduce mortality by approximately ~70% when compared to benzodiazepines for sedation in critically ill patients.
- Nonpharmacologic techniques, including cognitive therapies, relaxation techniques, music therapy, and virtual reality, may be particularly helpful in the treatment of burn pain.

SELECTED READINGS

Cuignet O, Pirson J, Boughrouph J, Duville D. The efficacy of continuous fascia iliaca compartment block for pain management in burn patients undergoing skin grafting procedures. *Anesth Analg.* 2004;98:1077-1081.

Cuignet O, Pirson J, Soudon O, Zizi M. Effects of gabapentin on morphine consumption and pain in severely burned patients. *Burns.* 2007;33:81-86.

de Klaver MJM, Buckingham MG, Rich GF. Lidocaine attenuates cytokine-induced cell injury in endothelial and vascular smooth muscle cells. *Anesth Analg.* 2003;97:465-470.

Faucher L, Furukawa K. Practice guidelines for the management of pain. *J Burn Care Res.* 2006;27:659-668.

Gray P, Kirby J, Smith MT, et al. Pregabalin in severe burn injury pain: a double-blind, randomised placebo-controlled trial. *Pain.* 2011;152:1279-1288.

Hoffman HG, Chambers GT, Meyer WJ, et al. Virtual reality as an adjunctive non-pharmacologic analgesic for acute burn pain during medical procedures. *Ann Behav Med.* 2011;41:183-191.

Lin H, Faraklas I, Sampson C, et al. Use of dexmedetomidine for sedation in critically ill mechanically ventilated pediatric burn patients. *J Burn Care Res.* 2011;32:98-103.

McGuinness SK, Wasiak J, Cleland H, et al. A systematic review of ketamine as an analgesic agent in adult burn injuries. *Pain Med.* 2011;12:1551-1558.

Meyer 3rd WJ, Nichols RJ, Cortiella J, et al. Acetaminophen in the management of background pain in children post-burn. *J Pain Symptom Manage.* 1997;13:50-55.

Pacreu S, Fernandez Candil J, et al. The perioperative combination of methadone and ketamine reduces post-operative opioid usage compared with methadone alone. *Acta Anaesthesiol Scand.* 2012 Nov;56:1250-1256.

Promes JT, Safcsak K, Pavliv L, et al. A prospective, multicenter, randomized, double-blind trial of IV ibuprofen for treatment of fever and pain in burn patients. *J Burn Care Res.* 2011;32:79-90.

Shah H, Smythe J, Hanafiah Z, et al. Factors in the choice of oral transmucosal fentanyl citrate dose for adult burns dressings. *Burns.* 2009;35:798-801.

Siu A, Drachtman R. Dextromethorphan: a review of N-methyl-D-aspartate receptor antagonist in the management of pain. *CNS Drug Rev.* 2007;13:96-106.

Trupkovic T, Kinn M, Kleinschmidt S. Analgesia and sedation in the intensive care of burn patients: results of a European survey. *J Intensive Care Med.* 2011;26:397-407.

Zachariah JR, Rao AL, Prabha R, et al. Post burn pruritus: a review of current treatment options. *Burns.* 2012;38:621-629.

The references for this chapter can be found at www.expertconsult.com.

75

Pain Management in the Emergency Department

James R. Miner | Knox H. Todd

Emergency physicians provide acute care for an extraordinarily broad range of illnesses and injuries, the majority of which involves some degree of pain. Emergency providers also cause pain in the course of therapeutic and diagnostic procedures. This chapter considers the prevalence of pain in the emergency department (ED), barriers to its adequate treatment, and a variety of treatment modalities. Space limitations prohibit a discussion of the wide variety of specific painful conditions that present to the ED. These can be found in other chapters of the text.

PREVALENCE AND ASSESSMENT OF PAIN IN THE EMERGENCY DEPARTMENT

The prevalence of pain among emergency department (ED) patients is as high as 78%, and among those with pain, underlying chronic pain conditions are present in 40%.[1-5] A national survey suggests that 24 million adults with chronic pain visit the ED annually and that 12 million visits are due to exacerbations of chronic pain syndromes.[6] Although arriving at a diagnosis and choosing the appropriate therapy to treat underlying conditions are principal goals for physicians, those who present to the ED with pain also desire recognition of their pain and rapid, effective pain treatment.

Patients face many barriers in their efforts to obtain superior medical care, especially in regard to pain. The ED serves as a fail-safe mechanism for our fragmented health care system, and pain is but one of the many conditions in which we not only face the problem of acute clinical presentations but also care for those with chronic pain who are seeking access to specialized pain care.

Notwithstanding the issue of providing compassionate care, pain that is not acknowledged and managed appropriately causes anxiety, depression, sleep disturbances, increased oxygen demands with the potential for end-organ ischemia, and decreased movement with an increased risk of venous thrombosis.[7,8] Failure to recognize and treat pain may also result in dissatisfaction with medical care, hostility toward the physician, unscheduled returns to the ED, delayed complete return to full function, and an increased risk of litigation.[9]

Pain is inherently subjective and inevitably complex. Our patients experience pain and suffering as individuals; we assess it only indirectly. The ED's task is to use a commonly understood vocabulary and classification system in assessing pain so that our findings can be communicated consistently. Only by quantifying the pain experience in meaningful ways can we move beyond myth and opinion toward a scientific approach to our many questions regarding the pain experience. This challenge is at the root of our difficulties in treating pain; thus issues surrounding pain assessment have primacy in our approach to understanding. Only when we use comparable methods in assessing pain can we begin to accumulate the scientific evidence that should drive our practice.

The most common response of physicians confronted by patient pain reports is skepticism. The validity of patient self-reports is often questioned, and attempts to "objectify" the pain experience are sought. This search is bound to disappoint the querulous clinician, as neither blood tests, tissue pathology, diagnostic imaging, physical assessments, nor patient behavior reliably reflects the internal pain experience.

A number of practical pain assessment tools are available. The subjective nature of pain makes such instruments necessary, and revised standards of The Joint Commission (TJC) have fostered their widespread use. Pain intensity should be assessed for all patients presenting to the ED with either an 11-point numeric rating scale (NRS) or a graphic rating scale (GRS). The NRS is sensitive to the short-term changes in pain intensity associated with emergency care.[10] The GRS or picture scales are particularly useful for populations with limited literacy, including children.[11,12] In one study of patients who have advanced cancer and pain, 81% were able to complete a picture scale, whereas only 75% could complete the visual analog scale.[13] In another study, the authors noted that male patients were uncomfortable with scales depicting severe pain using tears.[14] Picture scales with such depictions might profitably be avoided because they may be biased in the direction of less severe pain in male patients. No matter the specific pain scale used, assessments should be repeated after therapeutic interventions and at the time of ED discharge.

THE PROBLEM OF EMERGENCY DEPARTMENT OLIGOANALGESIA

Although adequate analgesia in the ED is an important goal of treatment, the underuse of analgesics, termed "oligoanalgesia" by Wilson and Pendleton in 1989, occurs in a significant proportion of ED patients.[15-19] A variety of factors are felt to give provenance to pain undertreatment[20] (Box 75.1).

Recognized risk factors for ED oligoanalgesia include extremes of age[21-23] and minority ethnicity.[24-26] It has been suggested that patients' expectations for pain treatment and perceptions of pain intensity do not differ by ethnic groups

Box 75.1 Factors Underlying Emergency Department Oligoanalgesia

1. Lack of educational emphasis on pain management
2. Inadequate emergency department (ED) quality improvement systems
3. Lack of ED pain research, particularly among older adult and pediatric populations
4. Emergency providers' concerns regarding opioid addiction and abuse
5. Fear of opioid adverse effects
6. Racial and ethnic bias

when patients are matched for socioeconomic factors.[27-29] Differences have been noted, however, in the way that patients of different cultural backgrounds express their pain.[29] Differences in the interactions of physicians and patients of a different ethnic group have been described and may affect physician assessment.[30,31] When affect, actual patient-physician interaction, and cultural expressions of ethnicity are removed from a case presentation, such as with written clinical vignettes, patients with similar pain are similarly treated by physicians.[32] Cultural discordance between the patient and the physician may hinder the ability of patients to confer an understanding of their pain to their physician.

Although there is a general reluctance to accept patient report as the most reliable indicator of pain and disparities between patients' and physician's pain intensity ratings may lead to inadequately treated pain, patients themselves may be reluctant to report pain presence and intensity. This may be a result of low expectations of obtaining pain relief, fear of analgesic side effects, and a notion that pain is to be expected as part of the underlying disease or from medical treatments. Some patients have a fear of addiction when prescribed opioids or fear the stigma associated with opioid use.

Although patients may decline opioid analgesics due to concerns about addiction, the emergency department may also be targeted by patients seeking controlled substance for misuse or diversion. Unfortunately, prescription opioid abuse is a continuing concern in the U.S. population. The National Survey on Drug Use and Health estimates that among those aged 26 or older, 3.2 % reported using pain relievers nonmedically within the past 12 months. It is encouraging that the misuse of pain relievers by youth and young adults appears to be in decline. Among youths aged 12 to 17, nonmedical pain reliever use fell from 3.2% to 2.3% between 2002 and 2011, and among young adults aged 18 to 25, rates have fallen to 3.6% from a high of 5.0% in 2006.[33]

Although pain is far more common than substance abuse, emergency physicians frequently encounter both among patients. Professional discussions of pain in the ED often center on concerns of being duped by patients who fabricate symptoms to obtain opioids, so-called drug-seeking behavior. Complicating this issue, such behaviors may represent an appropriate response by those with untreated chronic pain for whom treatment resources are lacking. In managing pain complaints, emergency physicians are responsible for beneficence and nonmaleficence. They must treat pain and ameliorate suffering while minimizing the extent to which their decisions enable substance abuse by patients and increase the supply of prescription opioids available for abuse by the general public. The increasing functionality of online prescription monitoring programs is a promising development that can aid emergency physicians in differentiating appropriate and problematic requests for opioid analgesics.[34]

PAIN TREATMENT AND PROCEDURAL SEDATION

Effective pain management involves both pharmacologic and nonpharmacologic modalities. Simply asking about pain and validating the pain reports has a potent effect on patients' satisfaction with ED pain management. In one study, patient satisfaction with pain management was predicted more strongly by the perception that ED staff asked about pain than by the actual administration of an analgesic.[35] Other modalities such as reassuring the patient that pain will be addressed, immobilizing and elevating injured extremities, and providing quiet, darkened rooms for patients with migraine headaches are essential aspects of quality pain management.

Pharmacologic therapies should begin as soon as is practical after presentation to the ED. Analgesic protocols allowing early pain treatment can decrease the time to effective treatment and improve patient outcomes.[36-38] Analgesics may be administered by a variety of routes; however, the majority of medications are administered by the oral or parenteral routes. Oral therapies are most commonly used because they are convenient and inexpensive for patients who can tolerate oral intake. When pain is severe, analgesics must be given immediately and titrated to effect. The intravenous rather than intramuscular (IM) route is indicated in this context. IM injections are painful, they do not allow for titration, absorption is unpredictable, and they result in slow onset of drug action. Unless intravenous access is elusive, there is little to recommend the IM route.

In general, it is inappropriate to delay analgesic use until a diagnosis has been made. In the case of acute abdominal pain, a large number of studies find no deleterious effect of intravenous opioid therapy on our ability to make appropriate diagnoses.[39]

SPECIFIC TREATMENT MODALITIES

A wide variety of analgesics are used in emergency medicine practice. In a 20-site survey of ED analgesic practice, a total of 735 doses of 24 different analgesics were administered to 506 patients receiving analgesics while in the ED. The majority of analgesics administered were opioids (59%), morphine being the most commonly used analgesic (20%), followed by ibuprofen (17%). Analgesics recorded as being administered in the report are listed in Table 75.1.[5]

NONOPIOIDS

Commonly available analgesics include opioid and nonopioid agents. When opioids are required for pain treatment, nonopioids should be included to potentiate the opioid analgesic effect and decrease the severity of side effects. Nonopioids include salicylates, nonsteroidal anti-inflammatory drugs (NSAIDs), and acetaminophen. Unfortunately,

Table 75.1 Analgesics Administered in the Emergency Department (735 Doses Given to 506 Patients)

Medication	N (%)
Morphine	148 (20.1)
Ibuprofen	127 (17.3)
Hydrocodone/acetaminophen	93 (12.7)
Oxycodone/acetaminophen	83 (11.3)
Ketorolac	60 (8.2)
Acetaminophen	53 (7.2)
Hydromorphone	36 (4.9)
Antacid	26 (3.5)
Meperidine	24 (3.3)
Fentanyl	23 (3.1)
Metoclopramide	13 (1.8)
Codeine/acetaminophen	12 (1.6)
Oxycodone	10 (1.4)
Naproxen	9 (1.2)
Other	18 (2.4)
Total	735 (100)

From Todd KH, Ducharme J, Choiniere M, et al. Pain in the emergency department: results of the Pain and Emergency Medicine Initiative (PEMI) multicenter study. *J Pain.* 2007;8: 460-466.

nonopioid agents exhibit an analgesic ceiling effect and cannot be titrated to effect. This limits their usefulness in the setting of severe or fluctuating pain; however, they should be used as an adjunct to opioid therapies unless contraindicated, for the reasons noted earlier.

Acetaminophen is indicated for mild to moderate pain and is often combined with opioid agents. Acetaminophen, unlike NSAIDs, has no antiplatelet activity or anti-inflammatory effect. Although a great deal of attention has been paid to acetaminophen hepatotoxicity, especially in the setting of chronic malnutrition, alcoholism, or liver disease, such effects are uncommon, particularly as compared to NSAID-related gastrointestinal toxicity.

NSAIDs, including salicylates, inhibit prostaglandin synthesis by interfering with cyclooxygenase (COX) enzymes. They cause platelet dysfunction and can precipitate renal failure in patients with renal insufficiency or volume depletion. They increase the risk of gastrointestinal bleeding when taken chronically.

OPIOIDS

Opioid combination analgesics are commonly used for moderate to severe pain. Although the opioid component in these agents does not exhibit ceiling analgesic effects, the nonopioid component dose must be limited; thus, one cannot titrate these analgesics. The convenience of combination therapy must be balanced against this limitation. Hydrocodone and oxycodone combination agents are associated with less nausea and vomiting and are preferable to codeine combination agents. Also a significant proportion of the population is made up of poor metabolizers of codeine, which must be metabolized to morphine in order to manifest analgesic effects, further limiting its effectiveness.

The tramadol-acetaminophen combination agent is indicated for acute pain; however, experience with this agent in the ED setting is limited. Its mechanism of action is unclear: the tramadol component binds only weakly to opioid receptors and inhibits the reuptake of both norepinephrine and serotonin.

Opioids are the mainstay of ED therapy for moderate to severe pain, and morphine is the standard of comparison for all agents of this class. If contraindicated because of allergy or other sensitivity, hydromorphone or fentanyl may be substituted. These opioids can be rapidly titrated intravenously to control severe pain, allowing institution of an oral regimen. Fentanyl has the advantage of being relatively short acting and is preferred in the setting of multiple trauma, head injury, and potential hemodynamic instability. Intravenous morphine is the standard of treatment for severe pain in the ED. Morphine 0.1 mg/kg bolus has been found to be safe but not usually adequate to effect pain relief.[40] Repeat boluses of 0.05 mg/kg every 5 minutes until pain relief represents a safe incremental strategy.[41,42]

Meperidine is a problematic opioid for a number of reasons. Many EDs have completely eliminated the use of meperidine because of its metabolism to normeperidine, a toxic metabolite causing central excitation and seizures, as well as its contraindication in patients taking monoamine oxidase inhibitors.[43] It is, however, frequently used. In a review of ED patients treated in the United States for isolated benign headache, meperidine was found to be the most common prescribed treatment, despite national recommendations for the use of nonopioid therapies supported by strong evidence.[44] This likely has more to do with the persistence of medical tradition than with pharmacology. Subtherapeutic doses of intramuscularly administered meperidine have been used to treat a wide variety of acute pain complaints by generations of physicians. The availability of other opioid agents of equal efficacy with fewer contraindications and fewer adverse effects argues against its continued use.

Agonist-antagonist opioids, such as nalbuphine and butorphanol, have mixed effects on opioid receptor subtypes, exhibiting ceiling effects on both analgesia and respiratory depression. Because clinically important respiratory depression is distinctly rare in the setting of acute pain treatment, it is difficult to justify their routine use. One possible exception is for patients with advanced pulmonary disease. In particular, one cannot titrate these drugs to maximal effect because of analgesic ceiling effects. Additionally, these drugs are contraindicated and will induce withdrawal symptoms in patients who are physically dependent on opioids, either because of opioid therapy for chronic pain, methadone maintenance therapy, or active opioid addiction.

PATIENT-CONTROLLED ANALGESIA

The use of patient-controlled analgesia (PCA) has been described in emergency medicine in adults and children.[45,46] Although no specific advantage has been found over the titration of opioids, PCAs were found to be at least as effective. In the setting of high demands on nursing resources, PCAs could serve to ensure pain treatment.

ALTERNATIVE DELIVERY ROUTES

Multiple alternative delivery routes for the administration of pain medications have been described. The use of nebulized fentanyl has been described and holds great promise as a route of opioid delivery that can be initiated before an intravenous (IV) needle has been placed.[47-49] Intranasal fentanyl has also been described and shown to be effective in the ED and the prehospital setting.[50,51] The promise of nebulized and intranasal pain medications, especially in children who have severe pain but have not had an IV needle placed yet, could be very useful in the ED.

PROCEDURAL SEDATION AND ANALGESIA

Minimal, moderate, and deep sedation have all been described in the ED. Patients often present to the ED in need of painful or complex procedures that require compliance that must be done emergently, and procedural sedation and analgesia (PSA) has adopted a specialized format for procedures in the ED. Unlike most patients who are undergoing sedation in other settings, patients in the ED have unpredictable nothing by mouth (NPO) status, often have concurrent severe systemic disease, and usually are in severe pain before the procedure begins. In addition, unpredictable concurrent events and time or bed constraints in the ED complicate these procedures.

The indications for ED PSA range from pain control for short painful procedures to the need for patient compliance with a complex emergent procedure. Goals for level of sedation during ED PSA range from minimal through moderate and deep sedation, depending on the needs for the procedure. Although it is acknowledged that deep sedation can inadvertently result in patients achieving a level of sedation consistent with anesthesia, this is not typically the goal of ED PSA. Minimal sedation, a drug-induced state during which patients respond appropriately to their developmental age to verbal commands, is generally performed for procedures that require compliance but are not typically painful with the use of local anesthesia. Minimal sedation has been described for lumbar puncture, evidentiary examinations, simple fracture reductions (in combination with local anesthesia), and abscess incision and drainage.

During minimal sedation, cardiovascular and ventilatory functions are usually maintained, although patients should be monitored for inadvertent oversedation to deeper levels with oxygen saturation monitors and close nursing supervision. Agents typical of minimal sedation include fentanyl, midazolam, combinations of the two, and low-dose ketamine.

Moderate sedation is performed on patients who would benefit from either a deeper level of sedation to augment the procedure or from amnesia of the event. Moderate sedation is a drug-induced depression of consciousness during which patients respond appropriately to their developmental age to verbal commands, either alone or with light tactile stimulation. Patients usually have an intact airway and maintain ventilatory function without support. As with minimal sedation, inadvertent oversedation to deeper levels can occur with moderate sedation; appropriate monitoring, including that for oxygen saturation as well as for cardiac and blood pressure, should be done throughout the sedation, and direct observation of the patient's airway should be maintained throughout the procedure. Agents used for moderate sedation in the ED include propofol, etomidate, ketamine, and the combination of fentanyl and midazolam.

Deep sedation is performed on patients who would benefit from a deeper level of sedation in order to complete the procedure for which they were being sedated. Generally, amnesia of the procedure is similar between moderate and deep sedation, and it is not necessary to sedate patients to a deep level only to obtain amnesia of the procedure.[52] Deep sedation generally is achieved in the ED with the same agents as moderate sedation; the difference is in the intended level of sedation. Monitoring for deep sedation is the same as for moderate with oxygen saturation, cardiac and blood pressure monitoring, and direct observation of the airway. End-tidal carbon dioxide has also been described in ED PSA, but its use over direct observation of the patient's airway has not been established.[53,54] Deeply sedated patients can develop respiratory depression but generally maintain a patent airway and adequate ventilation. Patients sedated to this level can progress to a level of sedation consistent with anesthesia,[41,55-58] and there is some evidence that this may occur more frequently in patients intended to undergo deep sedation than in those who are to undergo moderate sedation.[59] For this reason, it is usually safer to use moderate than deep sedation in the ED unless the procedure for which the patient was being sedated requires a deeper level of sedation (such as hip reduction).[60]

Patients who progress to an unintended level of sedation consistent with anesthesia are not arousable, even to pain. The ability to independently maintain ventilatory function is usually impaired, and patients often require assistance in maintaining a patent airway. Because patients can quickly progress to this level using the agents typical of moderate and deep sedation, physicians performing moderate and deep sedation must be prepared to provide ventilatory support until the patient has regained consciousness. To decrease the likelihood of aspiration, patients who are undergoing moderate or deep sedation in the ED should be kept NPO. It is difficult to find a consensus on the amount of time a patient should be kept NPO prior to PSA.[61,62] Many departments use 3 to 6 hours as a minimum.[63] The risk of aspiration must be balanced with the urgency of the procedure, and it is often necessary to perform sedation on patients who have recently eaten when they have an emergent requirement for sedation. In general, the least deep level of sedation possible to complete the procedure should be used in patients who have not been NPO.[64] ED PSA has been described in patients who are medically stable (American Society of Anesthesiologists Physical classes 1 and 2) and in those who are not (classes 3 and 4). PSA for critically ill children has been described using ketamine[65] and in adults using propofol or etomidate.[42] The degree of respiratory depression noted in these patients was similar to that for patients with physical status scores of 1 or 2, but an increased rate of hypotension was seen in physical status 3 and 4 patients who received propofol. It may be that ketamine and etomidate are better suited for the emergent sedation of critically ill patients, but data are not yet sufficient to make a definite recommendation.

Sedated patients are generally monitored by pulse oximetry, which is a sensitive measure of oxygenation. If a patient receives supplemental oxygen before starting PSA, this monitor may not be as sensitive to changes in the patient's ventilatory status.[54,66,67] Preoxygenation is generally recommended for ED PSA; however, there is no evidence that it decreases the incidence of transient hypoxia that has been noted as a complication of PSA. End-tidal carbon dioxide has been recommended as an additional modality for the monitoring of sedated patients.[63,68] Monitoring expired carbon dioxide during PSA allows for a graphic display of the patient's ventilatory status that can be a detector of respiratory depression before it becomes clinically apparent. In the event of hypoventilation, the end-tidal CO_2 value increases as the respiratory rate decreases. In the event of increasing airway obstruction, the baseline end-tidal CO_2 value decreases along with a blunting of the waveform as a result of increased mixing of the nasal expiratory sample with ambient air caused by the turbulence from the obstruction.

Ketamine has been described in adults[69,70] but predominantly in children for use in ED PSA.[71] It is a dissociative anesthetic that provides 15 to 20 minutes of sedation when given intramuscularly, with a return to baseline mental status in 30 to 60 minutes. It can be given in doses of 1 to 4 mg/kg IM and should be combined with atropine 0.01 mg/kg to prevent hypersalivation. The addition of 0.1 mg/kg of midazolam to ketamine has been described to prevent emergence phenomena, but this has been shown to have unclear use.[72] The 1-mg/kg dose achieves light sedation sufficient for such procedures as lumbar puncture, dressing changes, and simple laceration repair. The doses ranging from 2 to 4 mg/kg result in increasingly deep levels of sedation but have all been shown to generally achieve moderate or deep sedation with a decreasing responsiveness to pain as the dose is increased. Patients sedated with ketamine usually maintain a patent airway and ventilate normally. Laryngospasm has been described with its administration at a fairly rare rate.[73] Patients undergoing PSA with ketamine should be monitored for respiratory depression and possible laryngospasm.[71] Emergence phenomena, described as an unpleasant perceptual experience by patients as they regain consciousness from sedation with ketamine, have been described in adults and children.[72,74,75] The use of ketamine IV has also been described for ED PSA.[69,76] It is generally given at 1 mg/kg IV and has an onset of 1 to 2 minutes, followed by moderate sedation lasting 8 to 12 minutes. The side effects have been described as similar to IM ketamine, and similar precautions should be taken. The combination of ketamine with propofol has also been described, with the theoretical advantage of decreased respiratory depression from propofol alone and decreased vomiting and emergence phenomena over ketamine alone. Several case studies and small trials have shown this combination to be generally safe and efficacious, but data are not sufficient to determine if there are situations in which the combination is superior to propofol for ketamine alone.[77-80]

The combination of fentanyl and midazolam has been described for minimal, moderate, and deep sedation in the ED.[54,59,74,81,82] These medications result in the longest sedation of the agents described here and have been noted to have a high rate of respiratory depression that increases with the dose. For this reason, this combination of agents, whereas adequate for minimal sedation, is less useful for moderate and deep sedation, and its use for these levels of sedation is not recommended. Dosing for minimal sedation has been described as 0.1 mg/kg IV midazolam followed by 0.5 µg/kg IV fentanyl, with repeated fentanyl boluses every 3 minutes until the patient is adequately sedated. The sedation typically lasts 30 to 60 minutes, with a return to baseline mental status of 45 to 120 minutes. This method of PSA has increasing respiratory depression with increasing levels of sedation, and close respiratory monitoring is required. A sedation regimen similar in duration but without analgesic properties is pentobarbital. It is usually used to sedate children for radiologic procedures.[83,84] The medication is usually started at 2.5 mg/kg IV, followed by 1.25 mg/kg IV every 5 minutes until sedation is achieved. This is usually used for minimal or moderate sedation, and pulse oximetry is required. The rate of respiratory depression is lower than for other protocols but the sedation is inadequate for painful procedures.[85]

Methohexital has also been described for moderate and deep PSA.[41,86,87] It is a very short-acting agent with dense amnestic capabilities. It can be given at 1 mg/kg IV with 0.5-mg/kg repeat boluses every 2 minutes as needed. It has an onset of 30 seconds. The sedation generally lasts 2 to 4 minutes with a return to baseline mental status of 10 to 15 minutes. It has been associated with respiratory depression and a quick progression to deeper levels of sedation than intended, and it can result in oversedation even when carefully titrated. This agent therefore requires close respiratory monitoring throughout the sedation, as with other agents. When compared directly with propofol, it was found to be similarly effective and safe when only a single bolus was given and less safe than propofol when multiple doses were required.[41] It therefore should be used principally for very brief procedures that are expected to last less than 2 to 4 minutes, such as simple fracture and dislocation reductions.

Propofol is well described for ED PSA.[41,42,54-58,88-92] It is generally administered as a 1-mg/kg bolus with repeat boluses of 0.5 mg/kg every 3 minutes until the patient is adequately sedated for the procedure. The sedation persists 2 to 5 minutes after a single bolus and longer for patients receiving multiple boluses, with a return to baseline mental status in 10 to 15 minutes. This medication has been associated with rates of clinically apparent respiratory depression from 4% to 7.7% in ED PSA, so close respiratory monitoring is required as with the other agents. It has also been associated with hypotension in critically ill patients and should be used with caution in this group.[42]

Another agent used in ED PSA is etomidate.[42,93-98] It is usually given as a single bolus of 0.1 to 0.3 mg/kg, with an onset of sedation in 30 to 60 seconds and sedation lasting 7 to 10 minutes. It is not associated with hypotension and is therefore optimal in patients who are at risk for this condition. It is, however, associated with myoclonic jerking in up to 25% of patients receiving the medication, which can sometimes complicate the procedure for which the patient has been sedated.[43] This makes it slightly suboptimal relative to propofol in healthy patients. Etomidate has been associated with adrenal suppression. This has been noted in studies of single boluses of 0.3 mg/kg, but no significant changes in cortisol levels were found, and the significance of this outcome remains unclear.[99]

KEY POINTS

- Failure to recognize and treat pain may cause unnecessary increases in anxiety and delayed return to function among emergency department patients.
- Barriers to superior emergency department pain management include knowledge deficits among providers and inadequate quality improvement efforts.
- The true prevalence of opioid addiction among emergency department patients is unknown and likely overestimated by emergency physicians and nurses.
- Few specialty-specific treatment guidelines exist to promote best practices for emergency department pain management.
- Emergency providers tend to disbelieve pain reports that do not conform to expectations.

SUGGESTED READINGS

McHale PM, LoVecchio F. Narcotic analgesia in the acute abdomen: a review of prospective trials. *Eur J Emerg Med.* 2001;8:131-136.

Pletcher MJ, Kertesz SG, Kohn MA, Gonzales R. Trends in opioid prescribing by race/ethnicity for patients seeking care in US emergency departments. *JAMA.* 2008;299:70-78.

Todd KH. Pain and prescription monitoring programs in the emergency department. *Ann Emerg Med.* 2010;56:24-26.

Todd KH, Cowan P, Kelly N, Homel P. Chronic or recurrent pain in the emergency department: a national telephone survey of patient experience. *West J Emerg Med.* 2010;11:409-416.

Todd KH, Ducharme J, Choiniere M, et al. Pain in the emergency department: results of the Pain and Emergency Medicine Initiative (PEMI) multicenter study. *J Pain.* 2007;8:460-466.

The references for this chapter can be found at www.expertconsult.com.

76

Pain Management in the Critically Ill Patient

Michael A. Erdek | Andrew H. Gordon

Pain in the critically ill is poorly understood. Only recently has attention and investigation turned toward the issues of pain assessment and treatment in this patient population, and existing literature is scant. The prevalence of poorly treated pain in the critically ill is considerable and greater than commonly believed among health care physicians. This chapter examines some salient issues as well as the modern, pertinent literature detailing barriers to assessing and treating pain in a critical care setting, as well as some strategies for dealing with this challenging clinical dilemma.

PREVALENCE OF PAIN IN THE INTENSIVE CARE UNIT

Patients admitted to the intensive care unit (ICU), although often unable to communicate as a result of the severity of their disease process or the presence of impediments such as artificial airways or endotracheal tubes (ETTs), experience pain and discomfort that often goes unrecognized and untreated. Between 63% and 77% of patients report experiencing pain while in the ICU.[1]

An observational study in 128 Italian ICUs of 661 postoperative patients found that 36.3% of patients did not receive any analgesia in the first 48 hours of their ICU stay.[2] "Pain control" was the reason for the opioid administration in only 54.5% of instances in which an opioid was given. Fentanyl was the most commonly administered opioid. Although fentanyl's rapidity of onset makes it perhaps desirable in an ICU setting, its use by prolonged infusion may be counterproductive in that its lipophilicity contributes to a prolonged offset of action when weaning or discontinuing this medication.

One study attempted to characterize the experience of a group of critically ill patients at high risk for hospital death.[3] Between 55% and 75% of 100 cancer patients reported the experience of pain, discomfort, anxiety, sleep disturbance, or unsatisfied hunger or thirst.

One prospective cohort study of 400 medical ICU patients found that those patients for whom analgesics were prescribed had a higher concomitant incidence of hemodynamic monitoring, greater use of neuromuscular blocking agents, more mechanical ventilation days, and longer ICU and hospital lengths of stay.[4] Consistent with these findings, patients who received analgesics also had higher trauma injury severity scores (TISS) and predicted mortality.

BARRIERS TO PAIN ASSESSMENT IN THE INTENSIVE CARE UNIT

Given the potential compromise of patients' physiologic stability and communication skills secondary to underlying disease processes, the ICU presents a unique environment for the assessment and treatment of pain. This presents unique challenges to clinicians that may not commonly be seen in other arenas of pain control. As mentioned, the presence of impediments to communication such as the presence of an endotracheal tube (ETT) or the severity of underlying critical illness may prevent typical ICU patients from communicating with the nursing or physician staff their level of discomfort (Box 76.1). Indeed, critical care patients have a much higher risk of enduring untreated pain because they often cannot communicate secondary to altered mental status, mechanical ventilation, and sedation.[5] A clinician's observation and subjective rating of ICU patient pain often underestimates that patient's pain, and whenever possible, ICU patients should rate their own pain.[6]

A critically ill patient may be obtunded secondary to the underlying disease process or physiologically compromised by a process such as sepsis or shock. The question has been raised as to how much real pain the patient is experiencing, and this question is difficult to answer. Many patients may not remember these experiences, and even if these experiences can be recalled, there are limitations of assessing pain retrospectively.[7] A chief challenge in assessing pain in the ICU comes when assessing patients in whom communication may be compromised. Increased vigilance by physicians and nursing staff, as well as the development and use of alternative means of pain assessment, are necessary when patients cannot verbalize pain.

One study examined the assessment and treatment of pain in two surgical ICUs in a university hospital setting.[8] After the investigators found poor results in both of these areas, the following action plans of improvement were sequentially implemented: (1) education of the physician and nursing staff regarding the importance of pain and to measure pain with a modified visual analog scale (VAS) that is similar to a numeric rating scale (Fig. 76.1), (2) assurance that these modified VAS scales were readily available at patients' bedsides, (3) documentation of patients' pain scores on daily ICU rounds, and (4) creation of an expectation in these ICUs that a pain score greater than 3 is a cause for intervention. Although 42% of nursing interval assessments were not measured on a standard 10-point scale at baseline, after the 5-week period of

Box 76.1 Barriers to Pain Assessment and Treatment in the Intensive Care Unit

- Severe critical illness causing mental status compromise
- Endotracheal intubation or positive pressure mask ventilation
- Sleep deprivation
- Failure to recognize pain issues in the face of hemodynamic/septic/other issues

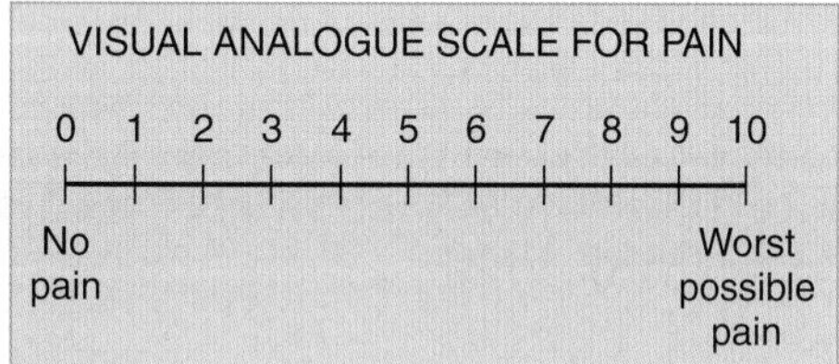

Figure 76.1 Modified visual analog scale for pain.

implementation of these strategies, pain assessments according to this scale increased to more than 70%. The study also found that patients whose pain scores were less than 3/10 increased from 59% before these interventions were begun to greater than 90% after they were completed.

Additional methods of evaluating pain in patients unable to communicate verbally have been developed from similar techniques in the pediatric arena. This would include the various behavioral pain assessment scales, in which pain scores are recorded by assessing a variety of patients' nonverbal behaviors and sometimes including changes in vital signs. An investigation described earlier found that placing VAS cards at the patients' bedsides permits some patients to point at a spot on the scale that corresponds to their pain score.[8]

Moreover, pain in critically ill and postoperative pediatric patients is essential for their comfort and benefit, and the use of pain protocols in these regards improves patient comfort.[9] More compliance and implantation of such protocols is very much needed in the pediatric critical care population. Another study attempted to compare three different pain assessment tools—the Critical-Care Pain Observation Tool (CPOT), the adult Nonverbal Pain Scale (NVPS), and the Faces, Legs, Activity, Cry, and Consolability scale (FLACC)—in nonverbal critically ill patients in a cardiac postanesthesia care unit. These scales were compared immediately before, 1 minute, and 20 minutes after two discomforting events: suctioning and repositioning. Both the CPOT and NVPS were found to be more reliable than the FLACC, which is predominantly used in a pediatric setting.[5] After standardized implementation, the CPOT resulted in more a consistent assessment of pain in critically ill patients and fewer analgesic and sedative agents being administered.[10]

One group[11] attempted to validate a behavioral pain scale (Fig. 76.2)[12] for use in the ICU environment, noting that no pain scale for patients incapacitated by critical illness had yet been validated. Noting a significant difference between physiologic variables such as heart rate and mean arterial pressure, the observers were able to validate a behavioral pain scale at rest and during painful procedures. The behaviors evaluated in determining a score for pain were facial expression, upper limb movements, and compliance with mechanical ventilation. This scale was also felt to be feasible from a time standpoint, with an average assessment time of 4 minutes.

BARRIERS TO PAIN TREATMENT IN THE INTENSIVE CARE UNIT

The difficulty of treating pain in those hospitalized in the ICU has been clearly documented, and there is a defined lack of high-level evidence for clinical decision making in these regards. Frequent need for rapid drug titration can contribute significantly to interpatient variability in response, which is likely more magnified in those who are critically ill. Moreover, there can be significant difficulty in distinguishing adverse drug events from other comorbid medical conditions in ICU patients.[13]

Highlighting this clinical dilemma of treating pain in ICU patients, the SUPPORT investigators examined more than 4000 ICU patients over 2 years. In the data-gathering phase I portion, family members reported moderate to severe pain at least half the time for 50% of conscious patients who died in the hospital.[14] Similar results were found in another study, in which a sample of 24 surgical patients from two different hospitals was interviewed after transfer from the ICU. Sixty-three percent of the patients rated their pain as being moderate to severe in intensity while in the ICU.[15]

Another study analyzed the adequacy of pain control for 17 trauma patients during the initial aspect of their ICU admission.[16] In contrast to 47% of patients rating their pain as severe, 95% of house staff and 81% of nurses reported the patients had received adequate pain control. This is underscored by the fact that 53% of house staff did not ask patients if pain control was satisfactory. The impact of insufficient analgesia was evidenced by the fact that 68% of patients reported that pain affected their ability to cough and 55% had trouble deep breathing. Presumed barriers to adequate pain control were felt to include a disparity in the perception of pain between patients and caregivers, patients refusing to request pain medicine despite the presence of moderate to severe pain, and physician and nurse concerns about patients' adverse physiologic response to further or increased doses of analgesics. It was noted that 19% of patients reported a fear of addiction to opioids. Misconceptions regarding opioid pharmacology on the part of caregivers have been reported.[16] In one report, some members of a nursing staff felt that the use of anxiolytics negated the need for larger doses of opioids.

A critically ill patient's ability to communicate pain may be impaired by the severity of the injury or the presence of factors that impede communication, such as the presence of endotracheal or positive pressure ventilation. One study attempted to put forth guidelines regarding sedation and analgesia in the critically ill patient nearing death[17] (Box 76.2). In doing so, the panel recognized the difficulty of pain assessment in this setting as a result of several factors including communication problems particular to the ICU environment, the severity of critical illness and potential presence of multisystem organ failure, the possibility of a decreased level of consciousness resulting from illness and drugs, and difficulty in the interpretation and reporting of

Item	Description	Score
Facial expression	Relaxed	1
	Partially tightened (e.g., brow lowering)	2
	Fully tightened (e.g., eyelid closing)	3
	Grimacing	4
Upper limb movements	No movement	1
	Partially bent	2
	Fully bent with finger flexion	3
	Permanently retracted	4
Compliance with mechanical ventilation	Tolerating movement	1
	Coughing but tolerating ventilation for most of the time	2
	Fighting ventilator	3
	Unable to control ventilation	4

Figure 76.2 Behavioral pain scale.

Box 76.2 Guidelines for Relief of Pain and Suffering in the Intensive Care Unit

Relief of Pain and Suffering

To relieve pain and suffering at the end of life, both pharmacologic and nonpharmacologic means should be used. Nonpharmacologic interventions include ensuring the presence of family, friends, and pastoral care (if desired) and changing the technological intensive care unit (ICU) environment to a more private and peaceful one.

Initial Dosage

Most ICU patients require narcotics and sedatives to ease the pain and suffering associated with their critical illness. The amount of drugs needed varies on an individual basis. As in active disease treatment, palliative care *must* be individualized.

Titration of Analgesics and Sedatives

Once analgesics and sedatives are initiated, they are increased in response to (1) the patient's request; (2) signs of respiratory distress; (3) physiologic signs—unexplained tachycardia, hypertension, diaphoresis; (4) facial grimacing, tearing, vocalizations with movements, turns or other nursing care; and (5) restlessness.

Does a Maximum Dose Exist?

No maximum dose of narcotics or sedatives exists. The goal of palliative care is to provide relief of pain and suffering, and whatever amount of drugs accomplishes this goal is the amount needed for that individual patient.

Should Analgesics and Sedatives Be Administered in Response to Signs and Symptoms of Pain and Suffering or Before They Begin?

Support for both approaches exists among intensivists. The treatment of signs and symptoms of pain and suffering is good palliative care. When appropriate doses of narcotics and sedatives are used and the intent of the physician is clear and well documented, pre-emptive dosing in anticipation of pain and suffering is not euthanasia or assisted suicide but good palliative care.

clinical signs. In the treatment of terminal disease, there are several possibilities for titrating sedation and analgesia: patient request, signs of respiratory distress, and physiologic signs such as tachycardia, hypotension, diaphoresis, facial grimacing, tearing, vocalization, or patient restlessness.

One investigation used a questionnaire to collect data on patients' stressful experiences associated with being in an ICU and with mechanical ventilation.[18] Of those who remembered the ETT, 68% were significantly bothered by not being able to speak (68%), pain associated with the ETT (56%), and anxiety regarding the ETT (59%). It is not surprising that this study found that those who did not remember the ETT or ICU were on average more severely ill and subject to a longer duration of mechanical ventilation than the group who remembered these experiences. It is quite possible, given the severity of their disease process, that the former group may have been more likely to be chemically paralyzed or heavily sedated.

BENEFITS OF ASSESSING AND TREATING PAIN IN THE INTENSIVE CARE UNIT

ICU patients who are intubated may be at higher risk for pulmonary complications after surgery. Postoperative pain in these patients results in a pattern of shallow breathing with fewer sigh breaths. Complications of retention of secretion, atelectasis, hypoxemia, and pulmonary infections may be seen among this group.[19] Epidural analgesia, intrapleural analgesia, intravenous patient-controlled analgesia (PCA), and intercostal nerve blockade (the duration of which is based on the duration of the local anesthetic used) are options in this situation. Clinical situations in which placement of thoracic epidural analgesia may be of significant benefit to the patient in the ICU include patients with post-thoracotomy pain; these catheters may be left in place to provide coverage of chest tube site pain until the chest tubes are discontinued. The placement of epidural catheters for pain control may aid trauma patients with rib fractures and also may help to facilitate weaning from mechanical ventilation.[20]

PCA in the ICU is useful in an awake and alert patient by allowing the patient to receive on-demand dosing of analgesic agents, either via the epidural or intravenous route. Ballantyne and colleagues published a meta-analysis of randomized, controlled trials to examine postoperative analgesic therapies and their effects on pulmonary outcomes.[21] Epidural opioids tended to decrease the incidence of atelectasis (respiratory rate [RR] = 0.53, 95% cardiac index [CI] = 0.33 to 0.85) and showed a less impressive tendency to decrease the incidence of pulmonary infections (RR = 0.53, 95% CI = 0.18 to 1.53) and overall pulmonary complications (RR = 0.51, 95% CI = 0.20 to 1.33) when compared with systemically administered opioids. Epidural local anesthetics, compared to systemically administered opioids, were found to decrease the incidence of pulmonary infections (RR = 0.36, 95% CI = 0.21 to 0.65) and overall pulmonary complications (RR = 0.58, 95% CI = 0.42 to 0.80). No clinically or statistically significant differences were found in other measures of pulmonary outcome, including forced expiratory volume in 1 second (FEV_1), forced vital capacity (FVC), and peak expiratory flow rate (PEFR). This meta-analysis sheds light on the value of postoperative epidural analgesia in reducing postoperative pulmonary morbidity and questions the correlation of these spirometry values as predictors of postoperative pulmonary morbidity.

The benefit of controlling perioperative pain to attenuate the perioperative stress response has been debated. This response brings about an increase in sympathetic tone, increased secretion of catecholamines and catabolic hormones such as glucagon and cortisol, and decreased secretion of anabolic hormones such as insulin. It also increases antidiuretic hormone (ADH) and aldosterone secretion, electrolyte abnormalities, and protein catabolism. One theory suggests that opioids diminish the hyperglycemic and epinephrine responses because of efferent nerve blockade to the adrenal medulla yet have no effect on the cortisol response as a result of incomplete afferent nerve block.[22]

One group attempted to study the quality of the dying process in the ICU by retrospectively interviewing family members of 38 ICU decedents.[23] This investigation found that family members perceived that the patients experienced substantial physical symptoms during the last week of life, but they felt that their loved ones' pain was under satisfactory control less than half the time. A review of the hospital records showed a near universal absence of data regarding pain assessment as well as records of how sedatives and analgesics were titrated to pain and symptom relief. Of the many items measured, the perception of how well the patient's pain was under control correlated strongly with the quality-of-dying ratings as measured in the study. The authors concluded that end-of-life care efforts in the ICU include management of pain as well as support of dignity, respect, peace, and maximizing patient's pain control.

Implementing a structured and scheduled approach to pain management in the ICU may also be of significant value, both to the patient and to the medical institution providing care. ICU patients whose pain regimens were titrated based on standardized sedation, analgesia, and delirium scores attained better analgesia, received fewer opiates, and, despite comparable sedation, endured a shorter duration of mechanical ventilation.[24] Also, based on a wellness model and the World Health Organization's multimodal analgesic ladder, pain outcomes after cardiac surgery were improved. Where "as needed" analgesics were previously implemented, scheduled dosing around the clock and prior to procedural pain provided effective pain relief in 95% of 120 patients over a 3-month period, for every ICU staff shift for the first 6 days after cardiac surgery postoperatively. Side effect profiles improved, and median length of stay after surgery decreased. Moreover, implementation of a structured ICU pain protocol at the University of Iowa medical ICU reduced the number of ventilator days required from 10.3 to 8.9, the cost per patient by $10,500, and a savings of nearly $2 million for the hospital over a 26-month period.[25]

METHODS OF PAIN CONTROL IN THE INTENSIVE CARE UNIT

This topic is limited to a discussion of methods of pain control (Box 76.3) as pertinent to the ICU setting, given that these issues are discussed in detail in other chapters in this text.

Analgesia may be administered by blocking afferent impulses carried along neural pathways, affecting integration in the central nervous system (which may display plasticity and central sensitization in response to pain), and blocking efferent impulses modulated by the neuroendocrine or sympathetic nervous system.[22]

Opioids mediate analgesia by binding with both central and peripheral opioid receptors, with the μ and κ receptors most important for analgesia. An "ideal" opioid would have rapid onset, ease of titration, lack of accumulation of the drug or its metabolites, and low cost.[26] Morphine has ideal characteristics but may precipitate histamine release and theoretically might cause hypotension in the ICU patient with diminished volume status. In addition, active metabolites such as morphine-3- and morphine-6-glucuronide may accumulate in the presence of renal insufficiency. Meperidine is a poor drug for use in the ICU. It is metabolized to normeperidine, the accumulation of which may lead to delirium and seizures in patients with renal compromise. Opioids are discussed in more detail in Chapter 37.

The Society of Critical Care Medicine put forth practice parameters with regard to the use of opioids in the intensive care unit.[27] The authors suggested that morphine is the initial agent of choice and is best started at a loading dose of 0.05 mg/kg administered over 5 to 15 minutes. It was suggested that most adults require 4 to 6 mg/hr after an adequate loading dose. This report also suggested that fentanyl (1 to 2 mcg/kg/hr after one or more loading doses of 1 to 2 mcg/kg) or hydromorphone (initiated at 0.5 mg and titrated by 0.5-mg increments to a general range of 1 to 2 mg every 1 to 2 hours) are acceptable alternatives to morphine. It is important to remember that opioid-tolerant patients often require higher doses of opioid analgesia than their opioid-naïve counterparts.

The use of opioids may lead to hypotension in patients with intravascular volume compromise or those reliant on

Box 76.3 Methods of Pain Control in the Intensive Care Unit

- Opioids
- Nonsteroidal anti-inflammatory drugs (NSAIDs)
- Neuraxial (epidural and intrathecal) local anesthetics and opioids
- Peripheral nerve blocks (including sympathetic nerve blocks)
- Pre-emptive strategies before major surgery
- Nonpharmacologic approaches (i.e., hypnosis)

sympathetic tone for end-organ perfusion, which may be a significant issue in the ICU population. The route of administration is important. Subcutaneous and intramuscular injections, never optimal for pain relief in any setting, are not advisable given the uncertain perfusion and absorption seen in many ICU patients.[28] Transdermal fentanyl presents similar issues and is suboptimal for acute pain management given the 12- to 24-hour delay in both onset and offset of analgesia.[29] Patients who are able to cooperate may benefit from the institution of intravenous patient-controlled analgesia (IVPCA). IVPCA possesses an inherent safety mechanism in that the patient stops using the demand feature when pain is controlled and when side effects such as sedation are more prominent. This property of IVPCA helps minimize the chance of opioid overdose and resultant respiratory depression while optimizing the timely delivery of analgesic agent to the patient.[30]

A group of authors examined the effect of thoracic epidural bupivacaine-morphine versus IVPCA morphine after thoracoabdominal esophagectomy.[31] Pain scores at rest and with mobilization were better in the epidural group on postoperative day 1, as were the opioid-mediated side effects such as sedation. It was noted, however, that one third of those in the epidural group had their infusion discontinued earlier than planned because of technical failures such as insufficient analgesia or catheter displacement. Group assignment had no effect on ICU stay, duration of hospitalization, or mortality. Given the ability of epidural analgesia to decrease sympathetic tone, it is not surprising that this study found that the epidural group received larger amounts of colloid and crystalloid intravenously in the first 24 hours.

Intrathecal dosing of opioids may be done perioperatively, before a patient's transfer to the ICU. Questions have been raised regarding the need for monitoring these patients for delayed respiratory depression, as well as the subsequent timing of analgesics. This issue was examined by a prospective, randomized, double-blind study in postoperative lumbar spinal fusion patients.[32] Patients were randomized to receive intraoperative injection of 0.2 mg (group 1), 0.3 mg (group 2), or 0.4 mg (group 3) of morphine into the subarachnoid space under direct visualization. Pain levels were similar in groups 2 and 3 at zero hours and at 12 hours after surgery, but they were significantly higher in group 1. The patients' respiratory rates were significantly lower in group 3 than in groups 1 and 2. The Pa_{CO_2} was also higher in group 3. No difference, however, was found in pruritus or nausea among the three groups. Some intensivists have suggested that this would argue for 0.3 mg as an optimal perioperative intrathecal morphine dose. Nonsteroidal anti-inflammatory agents (NSAIDs) should not be discounted as useful adjuncts in some ICU patients. Ketorolac, an intravenous NSAID, has been shown to have opioid-sparing effects and therefore may limit opioid-mediated side effects. This and other nonselective inhibitors of cyclooxygenase (COX) may have adverse effects on gastric mucosal perfusion, platelet aggregation, and renal perfusion in patients with suboptimal intravascular volume status. Therefore, it is recommended that ketorolac be limited to only 5 days' use and administered with caution in older adults.[33] Newer, highly selective COX-2 inhibitors are not in common use in the ICU setting and may be inappropriate in older adults given the documented increase in adverse cardiac events in this population.[34]

The ICU burn patient population is particularly important to take note of, as pain is often one of their most serious and persistent complaints. As an adjunct approach to their pain management, hypnosis was demonstrated in burn patients to reduce pain intensity and anxiety, improve efficiency of administering opioids, improve wound outcome, decrease costs, and overall improve patient care of burn ICU patients without pharmacologically induced side effects.[35]

Interventional pain procedures also may have a role in the ICU. Thoracic epidural infusion of local anesthetic, with or without the addition of an opioid, may be useful for patients with traumatic rib fractures, who often encounter difficulty weaning from mechanical ventilation secondary to significant chest wall pain.[20] The use of intercostal nerve blocks is debatable given that the relief only lasts as long as the duration of action of the local anesthetic used.

Another potential role for an interventional pain procedure in the ICU is poor distal perfusion in an extremity. Sympathetic blocks may prove useful in such situations.[36] This may be achieved by the direct performance of either a sympathetic ganglion block, such as a stellate ganglion block, or lumbar sympathetic block to improve perfusion in an affected upper or lower extremity, respectively. An indwelling axillary or femoral nerve sheath catheter might also be a means of providing local anesthetic on a continual basis, either with or without superimposed patient-demand dosing.[37]

One study examined a pre-emptive strategy for reducing opioid consumption in elderly patients undergoing cardiac surgery by pretreating surgical candidates with 150 mg of pregabalin prior to surgery and then with 75 mg of pregabalin twice daily for 5 days after surgery in a randomized, double-blind placebo-controlled trial. The group of patients administered pregabalin demonstrated a marked reduction of postoperative opioid consumption, to almost 50%, from the time of extubation to the fifth postoperative day, as compared to those on placebo. Patients treated with pregabalin also experienced reduced incidence of postoperative confusion on the first postoperative day, suggesting an opioid-sparing benefit in this instance. However, time to extubation was 138 minutes shorter in the placebo group. Interestingly, patients on the short-term pregabalin regimen experienced less pain 3 months postoperatively than the placebo group. Therefore, pregabalin appears to have potential short- and long-term benefits for critically ill patients undergoing cardiac surgery, and its use should be further investigated in these regards.[38]

EPIDURAL INFUSIONS IN THE INTENSIVE CARE UNIT

Epidural infusions may consist of a combination of a local anesthetic and an opioid. This allows the synergy of two mechanisms of action: local anesthetics work by blocking sodium channels on the nerve membrane, and opioids work through opioid receptors in the substantia gelatinosa of the dorsal horn of the spinal cord. This combination also minimizes the potential toxicity or side effects from each agent. The potential for seizures or cardiac toxicity from the local anesthetic or sedation or respiratory depression from the opioid may be attenuated because less of each agent is used when they are used in combination.[39]

Many local anesthetic–opioid combinations include fentanyl. Fentanyl is relatively lipophilic and tends to affect the neuraxis at or near the level of the spinal cord, where it is infused.[40] It will also achieve plasma levels relatively quickly because of its lipophilicity. Morphine, conversely, has relatively hydrophilic properties. It tends to ascend cephalad in the neuraxis, potentially contributing to delayed respiratory depression.

The clinical situation in the ICU may dictate the choice of opioid in the infusion. Thoracic epidural analgesia (TEA) may be beneficial for pain control in post-thoracotomy patients to cover incisional pain as well as pain from chest tube sites, which can be particularly problematic with regard to pain control.[41] Given the restricted use of intravenous fluids associated in many thoracic surgical cases, the patient may arrive in the ICU with a picture of uncontrolled pain in the face of relatively low blood pressure. A dose of local anesthetic given via the epidural catheter may precipitate hypotension as a result of interruption of sympathetic tone and may lead to compromise of end-organ perfusion. Given the desirability of maintaining the epidural catheter for ongoing pain control, one solution to this problem is to provide a continuous epidural infusion of morphine.[42] Excellent neuraxial anesthesia can be given without the hypotension that might ensue from a local anesthetic. There is a possibility of progressing to a local anesthetic–opioid combination as the patient progresses to euvolemia.

Attention has been given to the use of epidural analgesia in the ICU in the presence of post-traumatic rib fractures. Epidural analgesia has been compared with IVPCA and found to improve patients' pain scores.[20] This study reviewed the charts of 64 patients with three or more rib fractures after a motor vehicle accident and had initiation of intravenous (IV) PCA morphine or TEA with bupivacaine and fentanyl within 24 hours of admission. Despite the fact that the patients who received epidural analgesia were older and sustained more rib fractures, their pain scores on a 5-point scale were significantly lower for up to 80 hours from baseline. Another study examined epidural approaches in patients with chronic obstructive pulmonary disease undergoing open surgery for abdominal aortic aneurysm, and it was determined that both epidural anesthesia and postoperative epidural analgesia improved postoperative respiratory function and reduced postoperative pain in comparison with general anesthesia and systemic analgesia.[43]

One review also suggested that TEA may be a cornerstone of a multifaceted strategy for improving (pain) outcomes in lung transplantation. TEA was demonstrated to decrease the duration of mechanical ventilation, as well as ICU length of stay and number of respiratory complications. This is based on a low level of evidence of published studies, however, so further prospective trials are warranted.[44]

A study retrospectively reviewed more than 64,000 patients from the National Trauma Data Bank with one or more rib fractures.[45] The authors found that mortality and pulmonary morbidity increased with the number of rib fractures. It was found that only 2% of all patients with fractured ribs received epidural analgesia. This use was increased in patients who suffered six or more rib fractures. The use of epidural analgesia was associated with a significant decrease in hospital mortality compared to alternative forms of analgesia, leading the authors to conclude that this modality of pain control appears to be underused.

SEDATION IN THE INTENSIVE CARE UNIT

The main indications for sedation in an ICU setting include patient tolerance for ventilation, tolerance for medical and nursing interventions, and actual patient symptoms, with more systematic assessments of patient pain and sedation level needed to properly administer the ideal level of pharmacologic sedation.[46] Before treating anxiety in the critically ill patient, it is also crucial to identify other underlying disorders that can contribute to this problem. These include hypoxemia, hypoglycemia, hypotension, metabolic disturbances, and drug and alcohol withdrawal. Agitation may lead to harmful sequelae such as breathing against the ventilator, increase in oxygen consumption, and removal of monitoring devices and catheters.[26] No one gold standard exists to quantify sedation, and the Ramsay, Riker, Motor Activity Assessment, and Vancouver scales all have been used for this process[47-50] (Tables 76.1 to 76.4).

Common sedatives used in the care of the critically ill patient include benzodiazepines such as midazolam and lorazepam, hypnotic agents such as propofol, and centrally acting α_2 agents such as dexmedetomidine. Titrating a given sedative to a defined end point has been recommended with subsequent systematic tapering of the dose or, alternatively, daily interruption of sedation with retitration to minimize prolonged sedation.[26]

A report in the *Journal of the American Medical Association (JAMA)* offered a broad view regarding the use of dexmedetomidine in comparison with both midazolam and propofol in mechanically ventilated ICU patients. Two randomized controlled trials demonstrated that dexmedetomidine was noninferior to propofol and midazolam in maintaining target levels of sedation in ICU patients who required prolonged mechanical ventilation. Moreover, dexmedetomidine also appears to reduce the duration of mechanical ventilation as compared to midazolam, and it reduces time to extubation in comparison with both midazolam and propofol. Dexmedetomidine also reduced delirium and improved patient communication with nursing staff as compared to propofol. However, dexmedetomidine use had no effect on length of ICU or hospital stay and also induced higher rates of hypotension and bradycardia as compared with midazolam. Overall, the *JAMA* study

Table 76.1 Ramsay Scale

Score	Item
1	Anxious and agitated or restless or both
2	Cooperative, oriented, and tranquil
3	Responding to commands only
4	Brisk response to light glabelar tap
5	Sluggish response to light glabelar tap
6	No response to light glabelar tap

From Ramsay MA, Savege TM, Simpson BR, et al. Controlled sedation with alphaxalone-alphadolone. *BMJ.* 1974;2:656-659.

Table 76.2 Riker Sedation-Agitation Scale

Score	Category	Description
7	Dangerous agitation	Pulling at endotracheal tube, trying to remove catheters, climbing over bed rail, striking at staff, thrashing side to side
6	Very agitated	Does not calm despite frequent verbal reminding of limits, requires physical restraints, biting endotracheal tube
5	Agitated	Anxious or mildly agitated, attempting to sit up, calms down on verbal instructions
4	Calm, cooperative	Calm, easily arousable, follows commands
3	Sedated	Difficult to arouse, awakens to verbal stimuli or gentle shaking but drifts off again, follows simple commands
2	Very sedated	Arouses to physical stimuli but does not communicate or follow commands, may move spontaneously
1	Unarousable	Minimal or no response to noxious stimuli, does not communicate or follow commands

From Riker RR, Picard JT, Fraser GL. Prospective evaluation of the Sedation-Agitation Scale for adult critically ill patients. *Crit Care Med.* 1999;27:1325-1329.

Table 76.3 Motor Activity Assessment Scale

Score	Description	Definition
0	Unresponsive	Does not move with noxious stimulus
1	Responsive only to noxious stimulus	Opens eyes *or* raises eyebrows *or* turns head toward stimulus *or* moves limbs with noxious stimulus
2	Responsive to touch or name	Opens eyes *or* raises eyebrows *or* turns head toward stimulus *or* moves limbs when touched or name is loudly spoken
3	Calm and cooperative	No external stimulus is required to elicit movement *and* patient is adjusting sheets or clothes purposefully and follows commands
4	Restless and cooperative	No external stimulus is required to elicit movement *and* patient is picking at sheets or tubes *or* uncovering self and follows commands
5	Agitated	No external stimulus is required to elicit movement *and* attempts to sit up *or* moves limbs out of bed *and* does not consistently follow commands (e.g., will lie down when asked but soon reverts back to attempts to sit up or move limbs out of bed)
6	Dangerously agitated, uncooperative	No external stimulus is required to elicit movement *and* patient is pulling at tubes or catheters *or* thrashing side to side *or* striking at staff *or* trying to climb out of bed *and* does not calm down when asked

From Devlin JW, Boleski G, Mlynarek M, et al. Motor activity assessment scale: a valid and reliable sedation scale for use with mechanically ventilated patients in an adult surgical intensive care unit. *Crit Care Med.* 1999;27:1271-1275.

concluded that dexmedetomidine is a viable long-term sedative in the ICU setting that can reduce duration of mechanical ventilation and improve comfort.[51]

The effect of the specific agent on weaning from mechanical ventilation was examined.[52] A remifentanil-based regimen (started at 0.1 to 0.15 mcg/kg/minute and titrated in 0.025-mcg/kg/minute increments every 5 to 10 minutes to optimum levels based on clinical judgment), when compared with a midazolam-based regimen (administered by infusion or by boluses and titrated to optimum levels based on clinical judgment), resulted in a decreased duration of mechanical ventilation by more than 2 days. It also reduced, by 1 day, the time from the start of the weaning process to the time of extubation. The authors did not comment on the relative cost of the two agents and whether an overall cost savings was appreciated in the remifentanil-based group.

Implementation of a guided, structured protocol for sedation of mechanically ventilated patients at the Brigham and Women's Hospital medical intensive care unit was reviewed by retrospective analysis. Adopting a formalized protocol for sedation management in these regards resulted in more goal-directed administration of sedatives, frequency of sedation assessment documentation, and increased percentage of assessments of mechanically ventilated patients at or near the sedation goal. Although compliance with such a protocol improved, this did not result in improved clinical outcomes, highlighting the continued challenges associated with successfully implementing sedation and pain protocols in an intensive care setting.[53]

KEY POINTS

1. Pain in the critically ill patient is often difficult to assess due to existent communication barriers.
2. Use of several behavioral scales may be helpful in attempting to quantify pain and discomfort in the critically ill.
3. Despite appropriate focus on what may be life-threatening physiologic abnormalities in the critically ill patient, pain control is not to be ignored as an essential component of care for this population.

CONCLUSION

Assessment and treatment of pain in the critically ill population are challenging tasks given the frequent lability in patients' physiologic status and the compromise in their ability to communicate. Intensivists have an array of therapeutic

Table 76.4 The Vancouver Interaction and Calmness Scale

Interaction Score/30	Strongly Agree	Mildly Agree	Agree	Mildly Disagree	Disagree	Strongly Disagree
Patient interacts	6	5	4	3	2	1
Patient communicates	6	5	4	3	2	1
Information communicated by patient is reliable	6	5	4	3	2	1
Patient cooperates	6	5	4	3	2	1
Patient needs encouragement to respond to questions	1	2	3	4	5	6
Calmness Score/30	**Strongly Agree**	**Mildly Agree**	**Agree**	**Mildly Disagree**	**Disagree**	**Strongly Disagree**
Patient appears calm	6	5	4	3	2	1
Patient appears restless	1	2	3	4	5	6
Patient appears distressed	1	2	3	4	5	6
Patient is moving around uneasily in bed	1	2	3	4	5	6
Patient is pulling at lines/tubes	1	2	3	4	5	6

From de Lemos J, Tweeddale M, Chittock D, et al. Measuring quality of sedation in adult mechanically ventilated critically ill patients: the Vancouver Interaction and Calmness Scale. *J Clin Epidemiol.* 2000;53:908-919.

options available including NSAIDs, opioids (both by infusion and by IVPCA), and central and peripheral nerve blockades (i.e., sympathetic nerve blocks and continuous epidural analgesia). Although undertreatment of pain in ICU patients is well documented, data suggest that organizational changes, implementation of standardized pain regimens and sedation/analgesia protocols, and appropriate use of pharmacologic therapy may improve pain control in the critically ill patient. Sedation is equally important as analgesia in pain control, and newly studied agents such as dexmedetomidine, with shorter ventilation times and better comfort, offer more promise in overall pain control.

SUGGESTED READINGS

A controlled trial to improve care for seriously ill hospitalized patients. The study to understand prognoses and preferences for outcomes and risks of treatments (SUPPORT): the SUPPORT principal investigators. *JAMA.* 1995;274:1591-1598.

Ahlers SJ, van Gulik L, van der Veen AM, et al. Comparison of different pain scoring systems in critically ill patients in a general ICU. *Crit Care.* 2008;12:R15.

Ballantyne JC, Carr DB, deFerranti S, et al. The comparative effects of postoperative analgesic therapies on pulmonary outcome: cumulative meta-analyses of randomized, controlled trials. *Anesth Analg.* 1998;86:598-612.

Erdek MA, Pronovost PJ. Improving assessment and treatment of pain in the critically ill. *Int J Qual Health Care.* 2004;16:59-64.

Erstad BL, Puntillo K, Gilbert HC, et al. Pain management principles in the critically ill. *Chest.* 2009;135:1075-1086.

Freire AX, Afessa B, Cawley P, et al. Characteristics associated with analgesia ordering in the intensive care unit and relationships with outcome. *Crit Care Med.* 2002;30:2468-2472.

Horlocker TT, Hebl JR, Kinney MA, Cabanela ME. Opioid-free analgesia following total knee arthroplasty: a multimodal approach using continuous lumbar plexus (psoas compartment) block, acetaminophen, and ketorolac. *Reg Anesth Pain Med.* 2002;27:10510-10518.

Jacobi J, Fraser GL, Coursin DB, et al. Clinical practice guidelines for the sustained use of sedatives and analgesics in the critically ill adult. *Crit Care Med.* 2002;30:119-141.

Jakob SM, Ruokonen E, Grounds RM, et al. Dexmedetomidine for Long-Term Sedation Investigators. Dexmedetomidine vs midazolam or propofol for sedation during prolonged mechanical ventilation: two randomized controlled trials. *JAMA.* 2012;307:1151-1160.

Panaretou V, Toufektzian L, Siafaka I, et al. Postoperative pulmonary function after open abdominal aortic aneurysm repair in patients with chronic obstructive pulmonary disease: epidural versus intravenous analgesia. *Ann Vasc Surg.* 2012;26:149-155.

Pasero C, Puntillo K, Li D, et al. Structured approaches to pain management in the ICU. *Chest.* 2009;135:1665-1672.

Shapiro BA, Warren J, Egol AB, et al. Practice parameters for intravenous analgesia and sedation for adult patients in the intensive care unit: an executive summary. Society of Critical Care Medicine. *Crit Care Med.* 1995;23:1596-1600.

Skrobik Y, Ahern S, Leblanc M, et al. Protocolized intensive care unit management of analgesia, sedation, and delirium improves analgesia and subsyndromal delirium rates. *Anesth Analg.* 2010;111:451-463.

The references for this chapter can be found at www.expertconsult.com.

77

Pain Management at the End of Life

Perry G. Fine | Stephen J. Bekanich

The end stages of chronic, progressive, life-limiting diseases bring a host of difficult symptoms and causes of suffering. There are disease-mediated symptoms, such as pain, dyspnea, fatigue, and loss of mobility, and there are the accompanying emotional states, such as depression, anxiety, and a sense of uselessness.[1] These symptoms and states intertwine and interact in a complex manner, and each one deserves attention.

Of the many symptoms experienced by those at the end of life (EOL), pain is one of the most common and most feared.[2,3] Pain is often undertreated, even when prevalence rates and syndromes are well understood and the means of relief are within all physicians' capabilities to provide, directly or through consultation. With careful assessment and a comprehensive plan of care that addresses the various aspects of the patient's needs, pain can be controlled in the majority of cases. Awareness and provision of basic and specialized interventions can ensure comfort for all patients through the final stages of a terminal illness. This is equally important in order to prevent prolonged and pathologic grief in surviving loved ones.

All the members of a palliative care team play important roles in comprehensive pain management. The roles of both physicians and nurses begin with assessment and continue throughout the development of a plan of care and its implementation. Rehabilitation specialists, clinical pharmacists, psychologists, social workers, and spiritual counselors also provide important elements in helping patients optimize their quality of life, stay comfortable, heal relationships, complete unfinished business, and find peace as they approach death. To provide optimal pain control, all health care professionals must understand the causes and prevalence of pain at the end of life, the treatments used to provide relief, and the barriers that prevent good management. To champion this position there are now multiple guidelines regarding pain assessment and management during this time. One example is from the American College of Physicians, which also, for the first time in the medical literature, defines the EOL period as "a phase of life when someone is living with an illness that will worsen and eventually cause death. It is not limited to the short period of time when the patient is moribund."[4] This challenges providers to think about EOL pain in a much more upstream fashion as many of these patients will be in this phase of their lives for years.

To illustrate some common scenarios, we present three different fictional, but typical, case studies.

CASE 77.1 Pain Assessment and Care Planning in a Cognitively Intact Patient

Judith is a frail 81-year-old who lives on her own with assistance from a home care nurse and from a daughter, who lives nearby. She was admitted to the hospital with acute respiratory failure resulting from bronchitis. She has advanced chronic obstructive pulmonary disease (COPD), with general fatigue, a poor appetite, and a sleep disorder. She also reports severe, debilitating pain in the midthoracic region from postherpetic neuralgia (PHN). She also struggles with congestive heart failure (CHF), coronary artery disease, and attendant angina pectoris that is usually relieved with nitrates. Judith says that she has been feeling "pretty low" lately and finds herself becoming irritated at small events. She characterizes her pain as "bad as it can be" (Fig. 77.1). After a 2- to 3-day intensive care unit (ICU) stay, she will be ready for discharge. However, her pain from PHN is still not controlled, and her life expectancy is most likely limited because of her ongoing comorbidities. She does not have a written advance directive. The hospital staff discusses the next step.

PREVALENCE OF PAIN AT THE END OF LIFE

Assessing pain in patients approaching the end of life requires a multifactorial evaluation. It is important to acknowledge and address the prevalence, high incidence, and serious adverse consequences of pain in the end-stage conditions that affect patients with advanced medical illness, such as controlled and uncontrolled cancer, heart disease, human immunodeficiency virus (HIV) disease, neurodegenerative diseases (e.g., amyotrophic lateral sclerosis [ALS] and multiple sclerosis), and end-stage renal and respiratory diseases (Box 77.1 and Fig. 77.2).[5,6] These conditions may also be accompanied by other pain-producing disorders that may require separate treatments, as in the case mentioned.

The prevalence of pain in the terminally ill varies by diagnosis and demographics. Approximately one third of the people who are actively receiving treatment for cancer and two thirds of those with advanced malignant disease experience pain.[7-10] Almost 75% of patients with advanced cancer who are admitted to the hospital report pain on admission.[11] In a study of cancer patients who were very near the

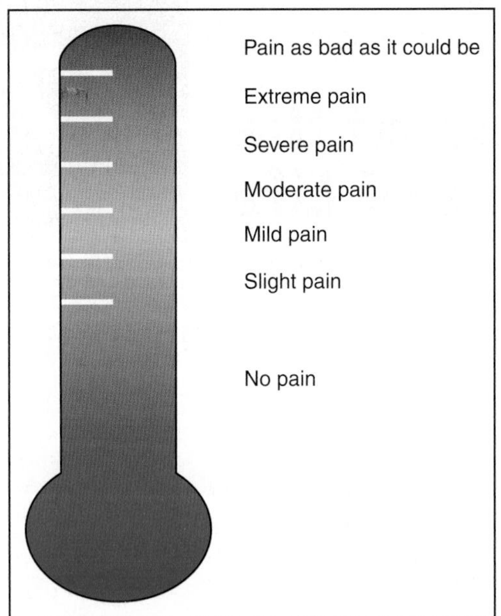

Figure 77.1 Pain thermometer. (Used with permission of Keela Herr, PhD, RN, College of Nursing, The University of Iowa, 2007.)

Box 77.1 Common Causes of Persistent Pain in Advanced Medical Illness

- Low back pain from facet joint arthritis and spondylosis
- Osteoarthritis
- Osteoporosis
- Previous bone fractures
- Rheumatoid arthritis
- Polymyalgia rheumatica
- Paget's disease
- Peripheral neuropathies
- Neuropathic pain associated with stroke
- Shingles; postherpetic neuralgia
- Diabetes
- Trigeminal neuralgia
- Nutritional neuropathies
- Peripheral vascular disease
- Coronary artery disease

end of life, pain occurred in 54% and 34% at 4 weeks and 1 week prior to death, respectively.[12] Uncontrolled cancer pain also predicts hospital admissions.[13] In an outpatient cancer center, an evaluation of more than 5000 patient encounters where the pain intensity scores were high (7 to 10 on a scale of 0 to 10) demonstrated that 29% of these patients were hospitalized within 30 days of those visits. In another study of more than 13,000 cancer patients in U.S. nursing homes, an average of 30% of the patients reported daily pain. In those patients, pain varied according to age, sex, race, marital status, physical function, depression, and cognitive status.[14]

In other studies of patients admitted to palliative care units, pain often is the dominant symptom, along with fatigue and dyspnea.[2] Until recently it was widely believed that patients dying from nonmalignant disease did not have high levels of pain. However, it is now known that patients dying from cardiac failure, COPD, end-stage renal disease, and other end-stage diseases suffer similar levels of pain to those found in patients with malignant disease.[15,16] In fact, comparing advanced cancer patients to those with symptomatic congestive heart failure (CHF), it is now clear that the symptom burden is as great, or greater, in the latter.[17] In a multicenter Veterans Administration (VA) study of the symptoms CHF patients experience, it was noted that over 55% of the them had pain, the majority of which rated their pain as moderate to severe. This was more common than the sensation of dyspnea.[18] People at particular risk for undertreatment include older adults, minorities, and women.[19,20]

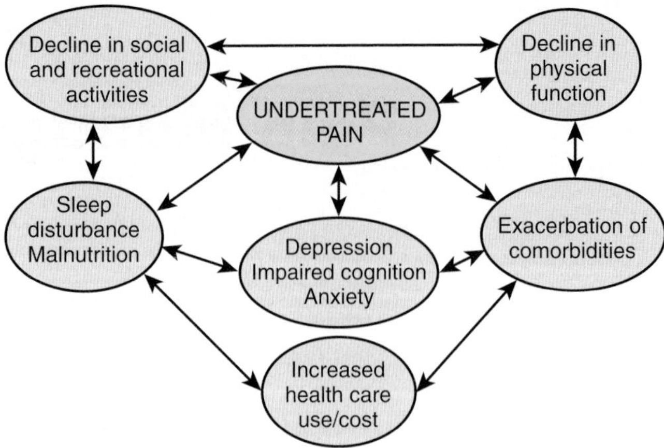

Figure 77.2 Consequences of undertreatment of pain. (Data from Davis MP, Srivastava M. Demographics, assessment, and management of pain in the elderly. *Drugs Aging.* 2003;20:23-57.)

An attempt has been made to characterize the pain experience of those with HIV disease because of the frequency for this disorder to be seen in palliative care settings. More than 56% of patients with HIV disease report pain, with the most common manifestations being headache, abdominal pain, chest pain, and neuropathies.[5,6,21,22] Lower $CD4^+$ cell counts and HIV-1 ribonucleic acid (RNA) levels are associated with higher rates of neuropathy.[22,23] There have been many reports of undertreatment of patients with HIV disease, including those patients with a history of addictive disease.[24]

ASSESSING PAIN AT THE END OF LIFE

Assessment of pain, including a thorough history and comprehensive physical examination, guides the choice of diagnostic studies and the development of the pharmacologic and nonpharmacologic treatment plan. The primary source of information in a pain assessment should be a patient's self-report. Many different pain rating scales are available, ranging from complex multidimensional tools to very simple numeric and picture scales, which can help patients identify pain and then document the efficacy of treatment. Widely used examples of this include the FACES Pain Scale, the McGill Pain Questionnaire, and the Brief Pain Inventory. When using pain scales, be sure to follow the directions for administration carefully.

A pain scale that suits a given patient's ability to self-report should be part of each patient's medical record. Health professionals should teach patients and their families to use these scales themselves to help in longitudinal pain assessment and continuity of care. Patients with terminal illnesses should be encouraged to describe their experiences of pain in their own words. However, many patients near the end of life are unable to provide detailed descriptions of their pain character, intensity, or location. Particularly for patients with cognitive impairment, self-assessments may be difficult to interpret. Nevertheless, even in these patients, self-assessments remain the cornerstone of pain management. For these patients, the use of the "pain thermometer" has been validated as a self-report instrument for pain intensity in patients with mild to moderate cognitive impairment.[25]

CASE 77.1 Pain Assessment and Care Planning in a Cognitively Intact Patient (continued)

Judith describes her PHN as a "burning, needling pain" near her spine, spreading out across her back on the right, beneath her axilla, and around to her breast. Her pain subsides sometimes, but rarely goes away altogether. Knowing the character and location of her neuropathic pain allows her caregivers to pinpoint adjuvant pain relief. In contrast, Judith's angina pain is "a deep, heavy ache" in her chest. She notes that it is intermittent and stressful, because she never knows quite when to expect it. By asking her to keep track of when her angina occurs, her caregivers are able to predict more precisely when it may be triggered and advise her accordingly, perhaps reducing both severity and frequency.

A comprehensive evaluation of pain should include an assessment of the pain intensity, character, frequency, onset, duration, and location as well as a detailed history of pain, a physical and neurologic examination, and psychosocial assessment. Diagnostic evaluation that includes tests to determine the cause of pain are important to corroborate clinical impressions of the cause of pain and mechanisms, but diagnostic workup should neither delay empiric treatment nor add excessive burden to the patient, especially when death is imminent. It also is important to take into account common pain- and advanced illness–related comorbidities, such as sleep disturbances and depression, which can affect pain levels, suffering, and functioning.[26,27]

Terminally ill patients sometimes complain of pain as a way of expressing other forms of suffering, distress, grieving, anxiety, or depression. When this is the case, psychosocial or spiritual evaluation and intervention will be more effective than analgesics. It is well established that attention and emotion influence pain processing and perception, and conversely inadequately managed pain can lead to anxiety and depression.[8-10] Therefore, comprehensive assessment is required to determine the optimal plan of care, as specific to pain etiology as possible. Particularly for health care providers unfamiliar with the care of patients near the end of life, involvement of other disciplines (e.g., nursing, social work, chaplaincy) can be very valuable in uncovering other sources of emotional or spiritual suffering that may be confusing the pain assessment.

DIFFERENTIATING PAIN MECHANISMS AND CHOOSING APPROPRIATE THERAPIES AT THE END OF LIFE

Patients in the terminal stage of an illness often experience multiple mechanisms of pain simultaneously (e.g., both nociceptive and neuropathic). Nevertheless, it is important to differentiate among different types of pain because the type of treatment and its success are largely dictated by the pain mechanism and its original source.[28,29] In some conditions, especially metastatic cancer, pain is often caused by a complex mix of nociceptive and neuropathic factors. Though neuropathic pain afflicts 7% to 8% of the general population,[30] its effective recognition and management might be wanting given the lack of exposure in medical education on this topic. An evaluation of 104 U.S. medical schools found only 48 of them include neuropathic pain as a required topic and on average only 0.5 hour is spent teaching about it.[31] Evidence-based guidelines are available[30,32] and should be utilized while keeping in mind that an important strategy for treating EOL patients is using one medication that might treat more than one type of pain or multiple symptoms. For example, an opioid might be helpful for neuropathic pain as well as angina. A tricyclic antidepressant can be employed for both postherpetic neuralgia and a sleep disorder. This strategy is supported in the medically frail population.[33]

EFFECTS OF UNRELIEVED PAIN ON THE PATIENT AND CAREGIVER

There is growing evidence that inadequate pain relief might hasten death, not only via the well-recognized morbid effects of increasing physiologic stress, reducing mobility, increasing proclivities toward pneumonia and thromboembolism, and increasing the work of breathing and myocardial oxygen requirements, but also through immune suppression.[34] Pain may lead to a spiritual despair and significant decrease in emotional well-being because the individual's quality of life is impaired.[5,6] It is the professional and ethical responsibility of clinicians to focus on and attend to adequate pain relief for their patients and to properly educate patients and their caregivers about analgesic therapies.[35]

Palliative care and hospice programs are charged with caring for not just the patient but the family/caregivers as well. Caregiving is a risk factor for mortality.[36] This carries not only physical consequences but emotional, economic, and social ones.[37] When pain and other distressing symptoms are properly attended and advance directives are completed to guide the caregiver, quality scores for EOL care increase, costs and resource utilization decrease, and caregiver stress is diminished.[38-40]

CASE 77.1 Pain Assessment and Care Planning in a Cognitively Intact Patient (continued)

Returning to Judith, who has COPD, coronary artery disease, and PHN, it is clear that discussions about care preferences (i.e., advance directives) are optimal before a medical crisis and while there is cognitive capacity for decision making. However, under the current circumstances, a care planning meeting with the attending clinician, consultant clinicians (e.g., palliative care/hospice team), and designated responsible family member is of paramount importance. The team must adequately control her pain before discharge with a follow-up plan in place, or they must transfer her to a skilled facility, such as an inpatient palliative care/hospice unit, where pain management expertise and focused attention are immediately available. Alternatively, with a prognosis of 6 months or less, if Judith prefers to go home immediately, a hospice program with the ability to manage her pain condition should be consulted. Regardless of setting, nonpharmacologic approaches to pain control along with titration of "first-line" agents for neuropathic pain (anticonvulsants, topical local anesthetic, and opioids) should proceed with close monitoring to balance therapeutic and adverse effects.

CASE 77.2 Pain Assessment and Care Planning in a Severely Cognitively Impaired Patient

Grace is a 74-year-old in the late stages of Alzheimer's disease with severe osteoarthritis in her knees and spine. She lives with her married daughter and two grandchildren. Her daughter and a son living nearby provide her essential care, and until recently she has remained active and ambulatory. She is beginning to experience severe pain from her arthritis, manifest by grimacing, crying, and moaning. The current caregivers are not always sure what she is expressing, but they understand that she is in some distress and are eager to help alleviate it. They meet with their family physician to talk about options. Because Grace is in the far-advanced stage of Alzheimer's disease, the physician refers her to hospice for comprehensive care and support of her family. During her initial evaluation, the family stresses that their primary goal is to make sure that Mom is comfortable. The hospice nurse evaluates Grace and determines that she responds well to a variety of nonpharmacologic interventions. Her family members express a willingness to use a variety of hands-on and nonpharmacologic techniques to help Grace live her last days relatively free of pain and suffering. Meanwhile, she is started on a regimen of around-the-clock acetaminophen (1000 mg three times daily) with the option for more potent pharmacologic therapies left open.

NONPHARMACOLOGIC APPROACHES TO PAIN MANAGEMENT IN PALLIATIVE CARE

An important aspect of any management strategy is the use of nonpharmacologic treatments.[26,41] Various nonpharmacologic approaches to pain are effective in alleviating pain for patients with advanced illness. These include physical interventions, such as positioning and active or passive mobilization (therapeutic exercise); techniques, such as transcutaneous electrical nerve stimulation (TENS), massage, and heat or cold; and complementary and alternative medicine techniques, music, and relaxation or imagery exercises. Table 77.1 offers a list of some of the most common nonpharmacologic interventions.

The type of intervention, or combination of interventions, depends on the source and severity of pain as well as the physical condition and receptivity of the patient. In an investigation of the prevalence of complementary and alternative medicine use in an end-of-life population, Tilden and colleagues,[42] through a series of phone interviews with family caregivers of recently deceased patients, found that 53.7% of the deceased used some kind of complementary therapy, were more likely to be younger with college degrees and higher household incomes, and were more likely to have used one or more life-sustaining treatments. Symptom relief was the most frequent reason given for complementary and alternative medicine use. A study by Weiner and Ernst[43] that reviewed common complementary and alternative treatment modalities for the treatment of persistent musculoskeletal pain found that the use of these modalities is increasing in older adults. The study authors concluded that rigorous clinical trials examining efficacy are still needed before definitive recommendations regarding the application of these modalities can be made.

Aside from their objective efficacy, a medical sociologic study by Garnett[44] on the use of complementary therapies by palliative care nurses sees these therapies as an "emotional inoculation" that builds resiliency and an important bond between patient and caregiver. Nonpharmacologic interventions often comfort the patient while involving and empowering family and other caregivers. The necessity of feeling effective for caregivers should not be overlooked—it can have a direct effect on the experience of the patient as well as the emotional survival of the family caregiver in particular. A study by Keefe and colleagues[45] on the self-efficacy of family caregivers of cancer patients found that caregivers who rated their self-efficacy as high reported much lower levels of caregiver strain as well as lower negative mood and higher positive mood. Caregiver self-efficacy in managing the patient's pain was related to the patient's physical well-being. When the caregiver reported high self-efficacy, the patient reported having more energy, feeling less ill, and spending less time in bed.

Table 77.1 Nonpharmacologic Approaches to Pain Management in Palliative Care

Intervention	Details
Rehabilitation/physical therapy	• Physical, occupational, and speech therapy can be beneficial in managing pain. • Mobility may be improved by strengthening, stretching, and using assistive devices. • Home settings vary in their use for a debilitated person, as does the degree of hands-on physical assistance that friends and family can provide. • The decision to use these modalities is made on a case-by-case basis.
Massage	• Family members can be taught simple, safe techniques of massage. • Hospice programs can often provide trained, certified massage therapists who are familiar with the clinical issues faced by cancer and noncancer patients with far-advanced disease.
Transcutaneous/percutaneous	• Evidence exists to support the use of percutaneous electrical nerve stimulation for persistent low electrical nerve stimulation back pain.
Acupuncture	Popular complementary therapy for patients with cancer and other end-stage pain: • Many patients with cancer use acupuncture when symptoms persist with conventional treatments, or as a complement to their ongoing treatments. • Several researchers have found acupuncture to be an effective antidepressant. • Studies show that acupuncture has a significant positive effect on chronic obstructive pulmonary disease (COPD), dyspnea associated with end-stage cancer, and asthma.
Cognitive interventions	Some common cognitive interventions: • Psychological tools and strategies for the purposes of self-regulating emotions • Distraction from noxious sensations and thoughts • Methods for reducing negative attitudes • Involving patients in cognitive self-care may improve mood and increase coping behaviors
Music therapy	Music effectively reduces anxiety and improves mood for: • Medical and surgical patients • Patients in intensive care units • Patients undergoing procedures • Children as well as adults • Low-cost intervention • Often reduces chronic pain • Music improves the quality of life, enhancing a sense of comfort and relaxation • Music to caregivers may be a cost-effective and enjoyable strategy for improving empathy, compassion, and relationship-centered care without interfering with technical aspects of care

REHABILITATION AND PHYSICAL THERAPY

Functional rehabilitation and physical therapy techniques in appropriately selected patients can add to quality of life even in the face of limited life expectancy. In the case presented, Grace typifies patients who respond well to nonpharmacologic pain interventions. A study by Montagnini and colleagues,[46] assessing the use of physical therapy in a hospital-based palliative care setting, found that a significant proportion demonstrated improvement in function after 2 weeks. The study authors found that patients with a diagnosis of dementia were most likely to show improvement in functional status and concluded that physical therapy assessment and use were uncommon in the studied group, but when implemented, 56% of the patients benefited.

MASSAGE

Research suggests that patients with cancer, particularly in the palliative care setting, are increasingly using aromatherapy and massage. There is good evidence that these therapies may reduce anxiety for short periods. A study by Soden and colleagues[47] was designed to compare the effects of 4-week courses of aromatherapy with massage and massage alone on physical and psychological symptoms in patients with advanced cancer. The study authors were unable to demonstrate any significant long-term benefits of aromatherapy or massage in terms of improving pain control, anxiety, or quality of life, but sleep scores improved significantly in both groups, and there were statistically significant reductions in depression scores in the massage group, suggesting that patients with high levels of psychological distress respond best to these therapies. When massage has been evaluated for impact in treating osteoarthritis of the knee, it has been found to lower pain scores and improve functionality.[48] In this 8-week study with 125 participants receiving either usual care or weekly massage regimens, it was reported that there is an increasing effect with greater total time of massage until a plateau was reached at 60 minutes per week.

ACUPUNCTURE AND TRANSCUTANEOUS NERVE STIMULATION (TENS)

These modalities may be effective in selected patients based on meta-analyses of the literature and findings of National

Institutes of Health (NIH) consensus panels.[49] When looked at for osteoarthritis of the knee, TENS has been found to require further study based on a Cochrane review.[50] Patients with the following characteristics appear to benefit most from acupuncture: a diagnosis of osteoarthritis, living in a multiperson household, being female, and failing other therapies.[51] For percutaneous procedures, appropriate cautions, skilled certified practitioners, and fastidious aseptic techniques are required to protect patients and staff from untoward adverse outcomes. Similarly, for therapies involving electrical stimulation, awareness of implanted devices (pumps, stimulators, implantable cardioverter defibrillators, or pacemakers) and precautions to prevent malfunction must be taken.

COGNITIVE INTERVENTIONS

Simple psychological interventions can have a significant impact on pain. As an example, Paqueta and colleagues[52] explored the idea that everyday emotion regulation through self-supporting maintenance or change in positive and negative emotions can help reduce pain intensity in the hospitalized older adult. Emotion regulation was found to be prospectively related to pain intensity for both overall emotion and anxiety-specific regulation. The study authors suggested that promoting emotion regulation as a self-management strategy could contribute to cost-effective pain management in general or targeted older adult populations.[52]

MUSIC THERAPY

There is growing interest in the therapeutic use of music. The difficulties inherent in the medical treatment of this population make the use of music, as a noninvasive therapeutic modality, attractive.[53] Five studies with a total of 175 participants in a Cochrane review suggested a benefit for patients near the EOL, though the results were subject to a high risk of bias.[54] Music is often used to enhance well-being, reduce stress, and distract patients from unpleasant symptoms. Although there are wide variations in individual preferences, music appears to exert direct physiologic effects through the autonomic nervous system.[55]

CHOOSING THE BEST APPROACH

Although pain at the EOL is often thought to come from cancer or HIV, discomfort from osteoarthritis needs much more attention. An observational study of more than 4700 older adult decedents found the prevalence of pain in the last month of life to be 60% in those with arthritis and 26% in those without ($P < 0.001$).[56] A combination of treatments is usually most effective when using nonpharmacologic approaches to pain management. When cognition is compromised, constant vigilance for the presence of pain by monitoring behavior and nonverbal cues that deviate from a patient's baseline is advised. If the presence of pain is unclear, it might be warranted to attempt analgesic intervention.[57] Similar to pharmacotherapy, multimodal approaches offer the potential benefit of additive and synergistic effects. Because nonpharmacologic therapies need to be tailored to individual likes, dislikes, and effectiveness, knowledge of the various modalities, management of expectations, open-mindedness, and a "trial-and-error" approach should be embraced.

CASE 77.2 Pain Assessment and Care Planning in a Severely Cognitively Impaired Patient (continued)

The hospice nurse was able to offer Grace's family a variety of hands-on and alternative modalities that could be used in addition to pharmacologic interventions to successfully comfort the patient. The nurse found that simple stretches and strengthening and mobilization exercises were effective for reducing the stiffness that was associated with Grace's musculoskeletal disease. This helped to relax the patient and prevent the usual anxiety that is associated with getting her out of bed in the morning and daily personal care, such as bathing and toileting. A simple TENS unit appeared to ease the patient's knee pain. The nurse was also able to guide the family in some interventions that reduced Grace's anxiety and increased the family's sense of involvement and effectiveness. They found that songs from her youth brought Grace a great deal of pleasure, and her son, a fan of the music, enjoyed spending listening time with her. Physical contact often calmed Grace, and the nurse trained Grace's granddaughter in simple massage techniques. These interventions seemed to be effective and helped the family to feel that they were contributing to Grace's care and well-being.

CASE 77.3 Complex Symptom Management in the Home Setting

Ben is a 79-year-old with metastatic colon cancer who has just returned to his home in an assisted-living facility postoperatively after a bowel resection. He sees a geriatric nurse practitioner, in collaboration with a family physician, for ongoing primary care. It has become clear that there are widespread metastases, and his oncologist agrees that the current goal of care is comfort only. Ben is still ambulatory and in the early stages of his terminal illness. No further chemotherapy or radiation therapies are indicated, but the patient reports progressive abdominal pain, and symptoms suggestive of intermittent bowel obstruction have developed. Ben refuses further hospitalization and surgery, and prefers noninterventional therapies, if at all possible. A consulting pharmacist and medical director from the local hospice are asked to come in and help the nurse practitioner choose the best pharmacotherapy for pain and bowel-related signs and symptoms, including types of drugs, route of drug administration, and the best way to minimize possible side effects. The explicit goals of care are a comfortable, dignified death, crisis prevention, and self-determined life closure (no prolongation of dying by medical intervention).

PAIN MANAGEMENT AND PALLIATIVE CARE FOR CANCER PATIENTS

Cancer, arguably more than any other disease process, has been the model from which the evidence base has sprung for aggressive attention to pain control and palliation of the whole person and for their families.[4] It is also a driving force for quality improvement measures. Pain is the most frequent complaint for cancer patients presenting to the emergency department.[58] Compared to cancer patients who die in a hospital, those who die at home have higher quality of life scores and their bereaved family members are at less risk for developing psychiatric illness.[59] Because of data such as these, the cancer community has developed evidence-based recommendations on pain management.[60] It is also now recommended that all cancer patients have access to palliative care services so that patient-centered care is seamlessly integrated into standard oncology practice.[61]

DRUGS FOR PAIN RELIEF IN PALLIATIVE CARE

Pharmacologic therapies for pain include nonopioids, opioids, adjuvant analgesics, disease-modifying therapies, and (in some cases) interventional techniques. Intractable pain and symptoms that are not responsive to basic therapeutic techniques, although not common, must be treated appropriately and aggressively.[1] In some highly selective cases, palliative sedation may be warranted.[62] A sound understanding of pharmacotherapy for pain treatment allows the palliative care/hospice team to create a comprehensive plan of care as well as recognize and assess medication-related adverse effects, understand drug-drug and drug-disease interactions, and educate patients and caregivers regarding appropriate medication usage. Recognition of the limits of usual therapies and the ability to muster expert assistance are important skills. This will ensure a comfortable process of dying for the well-being of the patient and for the sake of those in attendance.

Genetic factors, pathologic processes, concurrent medication, and aging all influence drug response and disposition. However, there are also a variety of nonmedical factors that influence responses to drug treatment in patients with far-advanced disease, including the social, environmental, and psychological milieus as well as the general vulnerability of this population. Understanding the clinical pharmacology of the drugs in question is essential for professional caregivers.[28] Commonly, there is a need to use drugs for non–U.S. Food and Drug Administration (FDA)–approved indications or routes of administration, simply because randomized controlled clinical trials have not been performed, because (usually) of financial constraints. Rational polypharmacy (combining drugs with different mechanisms of action to produce additive or synergistic effects and minimize adverse effects) is often necessary, but there is a high potential for drug interactions, so close monitoring is required.

The principles of effective symptom control are always paramount: diagnose the underlying cause of each symptom and tailor the treatment to individual circumstances and clinical context. Keep in mind that normal pharmacokinetics and pharmacodynamics may be considerably altered by end-stage disease states. For example, in patients with chronic liver disease or hepatic metastases, drugs may bypass hepatic metabolism altogether, increasing bioavailability. Similarly, renal clearance is almost always diminished during the dying process, leading to the accumulation of drug metabolites, some of which (e.g., those of morphine) may be toxic.[6,63]

COMMUNICATING WITH PATIENTS, FAMILIES, AND OTHER HEALTH CARE PROFESSIONALS

Communicating clearly about pharmacologic pain control with patients, families, and other members of the palliative care/hospice team is essential to providing effective pain management. It is important to be specific about the types of drugs that are available, how they are likely to affect the patient, how they are to be administered, and how they may interact with existing medications. Despite the importance of pain management at the end of life, there are often substantial roadblocks to overcome in getting patients the treatment that they need. Professional health care workers may have unsubstantiated but strong beliefs about analgesic use, especially opioid use, that lead to underprescribing.[14,64]

Several surveys show that physicians, nurses, and pharmacists express concerns about addiction, tolerance, and side effects of morphine and related compounds.[65] These fears are pervasive among patients and family members as well. Studies have suggested that these fears lead to undermedication and increased pain intensity.[66] Concerns about being a "good" patient or belief in the inevitability of cancer pain lead patients to hesitate in reporting pain. In these studies, less educated and older patients were most likely to express these beliefs.

Often a physician or other providers may be reluctant to offer the patient direct and objective information on his or her health, especially toward the end of life, seeking to "soften the blow" by keeping the details vague. Most patients, however, prefer complete information about their condition.[67,68] However, patients may wish to defer decision making to the physician or family members.[69,70] Physicians have a professional duty to determine patients' medical wishes. As a purely practical matter, by default or situational necessity, this responsibility may fall to the nurse or nurse practitioner. It is important to know that there are helpful tools, such as simple card sorting, that can be used to facilitate this exchange; for example, the five-card Control Preference Scale uses cards to portray different roles in treatment decision making with a statement and a picture.[71]

DISPELLING COMMON MYTHS ABOUT PAIN MANAGEMENT

Understanding the barriers that are faced when treating pain can lead professionals to better educate and counsel patients and their families.[45] Patients should be asked whether they are concerned about addiction and tolerance (often described as becoming "used to" or "immune" to the drug).[72] At the end of life, patients may need to rely on family members or other support persons to dispense medications. Studies suggest that patients' pain experiences and family members' perceptions about them do not correlate well, leading to inadequate provision of analgesia.[73,74] The interdisciplinary palliative care/hospice team is essential in the communication effort, with nurses, social workers, chaplains, physicians, volunteers, and others providing support in exploring the meaning of pain and barriers to pain relief. Education, counseling, reframing, and spiritual support are imperative.

Providers can also be concerned about precipitating death with the use of medications such as opioids or benzodiazepines that are used aggressively during the EOL phase or when someone is actively dying (aberrant respirations, hypotension, diminished cognition, low urine output). It has been established that patients have legal and ethical rights to symptom management during this time.[75] Furthermore, and importantly, there is no evidence to suggest that administration of these medications will hasten death. Indeed the opposite has been observed with patients living longer periods of time when symptom-driven medications are delivered compared to those without the medications.[76,77] The reason for this is unsettled but physiologic-based theories have been published.[78] The provider has a duty to address the ethical, legal, and physiologic rationale for medications with patients and caregivers in this situation.

OVERVIEW OF NONOPIOID AND OPIOID THERAPY IN ADVANCED DISEASE

This section provides a brief overview of commonly used pharmaceutic agents available in the United States for the treatment of persistent pain associated with advanced disease. Pain-relieving drugs can be categorized as nonopioid analgesics, opioid analgesics, and adjuvant analgesics. Detailed knowledge of these classes of agents is necessary to provide quality palliative care, and although a comprehensive review is beyond the scope of this chapter, links to more detailed lists of all drugs used for pain control throughout the world can be found in Table 77.2. Of note, newer formulations or delivery systems are coming on to the market regularly. They may have a place in the EOL medication repertoire in the future. For now it is important to recognize that currently none of the new or renovated analgesic agents have been shown to be superior to the medications described in this chapter in the EOL population.

There are several possible methods of approaching pharmacologic pain management for patients with advanced diseases. Patients may require several different medications to deal with a variety of pain syndromes and disease- or treatment-related discomfort. For expedient and thorough treatment, it is often wise to adopt a stepwise approach to the use of pain medications. The World Health Organization (WHO) has developed a simple three-step model for managing cancer pain that can be applied to many different situations. It has been modified over time to adapt to the evolving fields of pain and palliative medicine (Fig. 77.3).[1] This revised approach recommends that mild pain (1 to 3 on a numeric analog scale) should be treated with nonopioid pain relievers, such as aspirin, acetaminophen, and nonsteroidal anti-inflammatory drugs (NSAIDs), with or without adjuvant therapy. Higher pain intensities indicate the use of nonopioid analgesics along with opiate derivatives, such as hydrocodone, oxycodone, or tramadol. If pain is not relieved, then titration of opioids, such as morphine, hydromorphone, and fentanyl, in combination with nonopioid analgesics and adjuvants, is indicated. Refractory pain syndromes often require more invasive techniques, such as spinal opioids, nerve block, or neurostimulation.[1,29,79]

Table 77.2 Drugs for Pain Control at the End of Life

Web Address	Content
www.palliativedrugs.com	Palliative care formulary online
www.pallmed.net	Generic site, with drug-compatibility database
http://nccam.nih.gov	Information on complementary medicines
www.fda.gov/orphan	Information on orphan drugs

From Doyle D, Hanks G, Cherny NI, Calman K, eds. *Oxford Textbook of Palliative Medicine.* 3rd ed. Oxford, UK: Oxford University Press; 2003.

NONOPIOID ANALGESICS

ACETAMINOPHEN

Acetaminophen has been determined to be one of the safest analgesics for long-term use in the management of mild pain or as a supplement in the management of more intense pain syndromes. It is especially useful in the management of nonspecific musculoskeletal pain or pain associated with osteoarthritis, but it should be considered an adjunct to any chronic pain regimen. It is often forgotten or overlooked when severe pain is being treated in terminally ill patients, but it can be quite effective as a "coanalgesic." It is important to take into account acetaminophen's limited anti-inflammatory effect and its hepatic effects. Reduced doses or avoidance of acetaminophen is recommended for patients with renal insufficiency or liver failure, particularly individuals with significant alcohol use.[41,80] In 2011, one of the manufacturers of acetaminophen announced that the historic 4 grams per day limit placed on it was voluntarily reduced to a lower maximum dose of 3 grams per day for all patients. How this new limit should impact hepatic dysfunction, if at all, is to be determined.

NSAIDs

NSAIDs reduce the biosynthesis of prostaglandins by inhibiting cyclooxygenase (COX) and the cascade of inflammatory events that cause, amplify, or maintain nociception. NSAIDs also appear to directly affect the peripheral and central nervous systems. COX has been identified in spinal

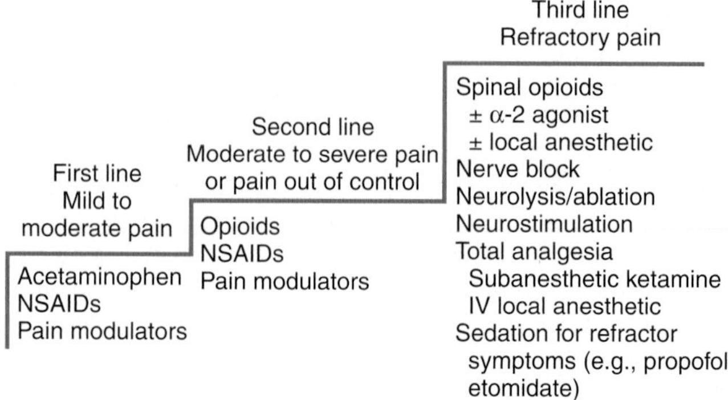

Figure 77.3 Modification of WHO 3-Step Ladder. NSAIDs, nonsteroidal anti-inflammatory drugs. (From Fine PG. The evolving and important role of anesthesiology in palliative care. *Anesth Analg.* 2005;100:183-188.)

cord neurons and may play a role in the development of neuropathic pain, but these agents do not appear to be useful in the treatment of neuropathic pain.[28] The "classic" NSAIDs (e.g., aspirin or ibuprofen) are relatively nonselective in their inhibitory effects on the enzymes that convert arachidonic acid to prostaglandins, so gastrointestinal ulceration, renal dysfunction, and impaired platelet aggregation are common.[5] The COX-2 selective NSAIDs rofecoxib and valdecoxib have been taken off the market, and because of potential problems and concerns with gastrointestinal bleeding and thrombosis, celecoxib should be used with caution in high-risk palliative care patients for protracted periods.[81]

NSAIDs are useful in treating many pain conditions mediated by inflammation, including those caused by cancer.[82-84] These agents cause minimal nausea, constipation, sedation, or effects on mental function, although there is evidence that their use can impair short-term memory in older patients.[85] These agents may be very useful for moderate to severe pain control, either alone or as an adjunct to opioid analgesic therapy. Adding NSAIDs to an opioid regimen may allow a reduced opioid dose when sedation, obtundation, confusion, dizziness, or other central nervous system effects of opioid analgesic therapy alone become problematic.[83] Extended-release formulations are likely to increase compliance and adherence.[28] As with acetaminophen, decreased renal function and liver failure are relative contraindications for NSAID use. Platelet dysfunction or other potential bleeding disorders also contraindicate use of the nonselective NSAIDs because of their inhibitory effects on platelet aggregation, a clear advantage of the coxib class of NSAIDs. If NSAIDs are effective but there is need for prolonged use or there is a history of gastrointestinal complications, proton pump inhibitors can be given to lower the risk of gastrointestinal bleeding.[86] For more information on NSAIDs, see Chapter 41.

OPIOID ANALGESICS

Opioid analgesics are the most useful agents for the treatment of pain associated with advanced disease, including neuropathic pain.[87,88] There are few, if any, indications for the mixed agonist-antagonist agents, especially in older patients at end of life.[89,90] The pure antagonists are used to treat acute overdose and, in selected cases, to prevent opioid-induced bowel dysfunction.[91,92] The opioids used most commonly in palliative care are morphine, hydromorphone, fentanyl, oxycodone, and methadone.

The only absolute contraindication to the use of an opioid is a history of a hypersensitivity reaction (e.g., rash, wheezing, and edema). Allergic reactions are almost exclusively limited to the morphine derivatives, and the prevalence of true allergic reactions to synthetic opioids is much lower. There is significant inter- and intra-individual variation in clinical responses to the various opioids, so dose titration is the best approach to initial management. Idiosyncratic responses may require trials of different agents in order to determine the most effective drug and route of delivery for any given patient. Table 77.3 lists more specific suggestions regarding optimal selection of opioids in end-of-life care, and Table 77.4 lists the commonly used opioids.

Opioid analgesics may accumulate toxic metabolites over time, especially when drug clearance and elimination decrease as disease progresses and organ function deteriorates.[93] Use of meperidine is specifically discouraged for repeated dosing over time because of its neurotoxic metabolite, normeperidine.[90] In the United States, propoxyphene has been taken off the market because of the active metabolite norpropoxyphene, its weak analgesic efficacy, and the significant acetaminophen dose found in some formulations.[89] The mixed agonist-antagonist agents—typified by butorphanol, nalbuphine, and pentazocine—are not recommended for the treatment of pain in patients with advanced disease. They have limited efficacy, and their use may cause an acute abstinence syndrome in patients using pure agonist opioids.[94] For further information on opioids and chronic opioid therapy, see Chapters 37 and 38.

MORPHINE, THE PROTOTYPE OPIOID RECEPTOR

Morphine, the prototype agonist, is considered the gold standard of opioid analgesics and is used as a measure for dose equivalence.[89] Although some patients cannot tolerate morphine because of pruritus, headache, dysphoria, or other adverse effects, common initial dosing effects, such as sedation and nausea, often resolve within a few days.[95] It is best to anticipate these adverse effects, especially constipation, nausea, and sedation, and prevent or treat appropriately (see the following discussion). Morphine-3-glucuronide, a metabolite of morphine, may contribute to myoclonus, seizures, and hyperalgesia, particularly when patients cannot clear the metabolite as a result of renal impairment.[93,96] Side effects and metabolite effects can be differentiated over time. Side effects generally occur soon after the drug is absorbed, whereas metabolite effects are generally delayed by several days. Morphine's bitter taste may be prohibitive, especially if "immediate-release" tablets are left in the mouth to dissolve. In this case, several options are available. One available type of long-acting morphine comes in a capsule that can be opened, releasing small pellets that can be mixed in applesauce or other soft food.[97] Oral morphine solution can be swallowed, or small volumes (0.5 to 1 mL) of a concentrated solution (e.g., 20 mg/mL) can be placed in the mouth of patients whose voluntary swallowing capabilities are significantly limited.[98]

FENTANYL

Fentanyl is a lipophilic opioid that can be administered several ways including parenterally, spinally, transdermally, and transmucosally. Because of its potency, dosing is usually conducted in micrograms. It should be noted that on July 15, 2005, the FDA issued a public health advisory to alert health care professionals, patients, and their caregivers of reports of death and other serious side effects from overdoses of fentanyl in patients using transdermal fentanyl for pain control.[99] Careful fentanyl dosing is particularly important in older patients; a study of transdermal fentanyl in postoperative patients found that absorption was significantly delayed in men 64 to 82 years of age compared with men 25 to 38 years of age.[100]

In consideration of the these cautions, transdermal fentanyl, often called the fentanyl patch, is particularly useful when patients cannot swallow, do not remember to take medications, or experience adverse effects from other opioids.[101] Opioid-naïve patients should begin with titrated immediate-release opioids to establish the needed 24-hour dose of

Table 77.3 Choosing an Opioid: A Matrix of Factors Leading to a "First Best Choice"

General Pharmacomedical Considerations	Pharmacoclinical Considerations	Pharmacogenetic Considerations	Pharmacoeconomic Considerations
Allergies/sensitivities (e.g., morphine and its derivatives)	• Prior experience (subjective responses and preferences) • Adherence (compliance) issues • Social circumstances (cognitive capacity, reliable caregiver, etc.)	Cytochrome P-450 enzyme system genotypes (e.g., "slow metabolizers" at CYP2D6 ineffectively convert the prodrug codeine to the active drug morphine)	Insurance coverage and formulary restrictions
Drug-disease interactions (e.g., renal insufficiency; pulmonary disease)	Administration or absorption preferences and limitations (e.g., oral versus transdermal formulation; once-a-day dosing versus multiple dosings per day; G-tube "sprinkle" formulations)	Future possibilities of genotyping to match patient-specific opioid phenotypes to physiochemically different opioids	Indirect costs (e.g., caregiver time, use of clinical services, treatment of side effects such as constipation, etc.)
Drug-drug interactions (e.g., CNS depressants; MAOIs; SSRIs; shared metabolic pathways [i.e., inducers and inhibitors of CYP2D6 and CYP3A4])	Monitor efficacy (e.g., activity, sleep, mood, pain intensity scores)		
Monitor changes in clinical condition (e.g., resolution or progression of disease; new disease; change in medications)	Monitor adverse effects (e.g., sedation, nausea, bowel function, ataxia, cognitive effects, "tolerance"/hyperalgesia)		

CNS, central nervous system; CYP, cytochrome P-450 isoenzyme; G-tube, gastrostomy tube; MAOIs, monoamine oxidase inhibitors; SSRIs, selective serotonin reuptake inhibitors.

Originally published in Fine PG. Opioid-induced hyperalgesia and opioid rotation. *J Pain Palliat Care Pharmacother.* 2004;18:75-79. Reprinted with permission from Haworth Press, Inc.

opioid before determining that the lowest available dose, currently a 12.5-mcg/hour patch, can be tolerated. A responsible caregiver should monitor patients for the first 24 to 48 hours of therapy until steady-state blood levels are reached. Transdermal fentanyl may not be appropriate for patients with fever, diaphoresis, cachexia, morbid obesity, and ascites, all of which may have a significant effect on the absorption, blood levels, and clinical effects of the drug.[102,103]

Some patients experience reduced analgesic effects within 48 hours of applying a new patch. If so, determine whether a higher dose can be tolerated with increased duration of effect or whether a more frequent (every 48 hours) patch change is the better alternative. Under most circumstances, breakthrough pain medications should be available to patients using continuous-release opioids, such as the fentanyl patch. Several novel transdermal fentanyl delivery systems are under development, including ones that allow bolus dosing. There are insufficient data or experience to make recommendations about their relative safety or efficacy at this time.

Oral transmucosal fentanyl citrate is composed of fentanyl on an oral applicator to provide rapid absorption of the drug. This formulation of fentanyl is particularly useful for breakthrough pain, as demonstrated in the first clinical report of its use for this indication in a terminally ill patient.[104]

OXYCODONE

Oxycodone is a synthetic opioid available in a long-acting formulation (OxyContin), as well as immediate-release tablets (alone or with acetaminophen) and liquid. It is approximately as lipid-soluble as morphine but has better oral absorption.[105] Side effects appear to be similar to those experienced with morphine, but one study comparing the two formulations in patients with advanced cancer found that oxycodone was less likely to cause nausea and vomiting.[106]

METHADONE

Methadone has several characteristics that make it useful in the management of severe, chronic pain.[107-109] Methadone has a half-life of 24 to 36 hours with a much longer terminal half-life, allowing for prolonged dosing intervals. However, the analgesic half-life of methadone is often much shorter. Methadone is an *N*-methyl-D-aspartate (NMDA) receptor antagonist, which may be of particular benefit in neuropathic pain.[110] Methadone is much less costly than comparable doses of proprietary continuous-release formulations, making it potentially more available for patients without sufficient financial resources for more expensive drugs.

Despite these advantages, much is unknown about the appropriate dosing ratio between methadone and morphine,

Table 77.4 Pure μ-Agonists Used in End-of-Life Care for Pain Control in the United States

Drug	Equianalgesic (Mg) Doses*†	Half-Life (Hr)	Peak Effect (Hr)	Duration (Hr)	Toxicity	Comments
Morphine	10 IM/IV/subcutaneous 20-30 PO‡	2-3 2-3	0.5-1 1-2	3-4 3-6	Constipation, nausea, sedation most common; respiratory depression is rare when titrated to effect	Standard for comparison for opioids; multiple routes available
Controlled-release morphine	20-30 PO‡	2-3	NA	8-12	Typical opioid effects	Brand name and generics available
Sustained-release morphine	20-30 PO‡	2-3	4-6	12-24	Typical opioid effects	Once-a-day approved in the United States
Hydromorphone	1.5 IM/IV/subcutaneous 7.5 PO	2-3 2-3	0.5-1 1-2	3-4 3-6	Typical opioid effects	Potency and high solubility may be beneficial for patients requiring high opioid doses and for subcutaneous administration.
Oxycodone	20-30 PO	2-3	1-2	3-6	Typical opioid effects	Available as a single entity or combined with NSAIDs or acetaminophen
Controlled-release oxycodone	20-30 PO	NA	3-4	8-12	Typical opioid effects	
Oxymorphone	1 IM/IV/subcutaneous 10 PR 10-15 PO	NA NA	0.5-1 1.5-3	3-6 4-6	Typical opioid effects	Oral immediate releases and extended-release formulations available
Levorphanol	2 IM/IV/subcutaneous 4 PO	12-15 12-15	0.5-1 1-2	3-6 3-6	Typical opioid effects	With long half-life, accumulation possible after beginning or increasing dose
Methadone	Variable	12-150	1-2	6-8	Typical opioid effects	Highly variable half-life and potential for accumulation require greater vigilance for development of opioid toxicity; can prolong the QTc interval
Hydrocodone	30 PO	2-4	1-2	3-6	Typical opioid effects	Only available combined with acetaminophen or NSAIDs
Fentanyl	50-100 mcg IV/subcutaneous	7-12	< 10 min	1-2	Typical opioid effects	Can be administered as a continuous IV or subcutaneous infusion
Fentanyl transdermal system	NA	NA	12-24	48-72 per patch	Typical opioid effects	Refer to package for equianalgesic dosing guidelines for oral and parenteral medication. Not recommended for opioid-naïve patients; not recommended for acute pain
Oral transmucosal fentanyl citrate	NA	7-12	15-30 min	1-2	Typical opioid effects	Not recommended for opioid-naïve patients. Recommended starting dose for breakthrough pain, 200-400 mcg, even with high "baseline" opioid doses

*Dose provides analgesia equivalent to 10 mg of morphine given by IM route. These ratios are useful guides when switching drugs or routes of administration. In clinical practice, the potency of the IM route is considered to be identical to the IV and subcutaneous routes.

†When switching from one opioid to another, incomplete cross-tolerance requires a reduction in the dose of the new drug by 25% to 50% to prevent excessive opioid effects. Provision of "rescue" medication during the conversion period (a few days) prevents breakthrough pain that may result from relative underdosing. When switching to methadone from another drug, the reduction in the equianalgesic dose should be greater, usually 75% to 90%.

‡Extensive survey data suggest that the relative potency ratio of IM to PO morphine, which has been shown to be 1:6 in an acute dosing study, is 1:2 to 1:3 with chronic dosing.

FDA, U.S. Food and Drug Administration; IM, intramuscular; IV, intravenous; NA, not applicable or no data available; NSAIDs, nonsteroidal anti-inflammatory drugs; PO, per mouth; PR, per rectum.

Originally published in Fine PG, Portenoy RK. *A Clinical Guide to Opioid Analgesia.* Minneapolis: McGraw-Hill Healthcare Information; 2004.

as well as the safest and most effective time course for conversion from another opioid to methadone.[111] Current data suggest that the dose ratio increases as the previous dose of oral opioid equivalents increases, and although the long half-life is an advantage, it also increases the potential for drug accumulation prior to achieving steady-state blood levels.[109] There may be a risk of oversedation and respiratory depression after 2 to 5 days of treatment with methadone. Close monitoring of these potentially adverse or even life-threatening effects is required.[28,63] Data suggest that methadone can lead to life-threatening QT interval prolongation.[111] As a result, patients not in hospice programs, and even selected hospice patients, should have interval QT screening before and during methadone treatment.[112]

Patients currently receiving methadone as part of a maintenance program for addictive disease often develop cross-tolerance to opioids and require higher doses than opioid-naïve patients.[113] Prescribing methadone for addictive disease requires a special license in the United States, so prescriptions for methadone to manage pain in palliative care should specify "for pain."

HYDROMORPHONE

Hydromorphone is a synthetic opioid that can be a useful alternative to morphine in patients at end of life. It is available in oral tablets, liquids, suppositories, and parenteral formulations, but the only long-acting U.S. formulation was recalled by the FDA because of interactions with alcohol that could lead to excessively rapid drug release.[114] As a synthetic opioid, hydromorphone can be useful if there is inadequate pain control or when patients experience true allergic responses to morphine or intolerable side effects occur. The metabolite hydromorphone-3-glucuronide may lead to the same opioid neurotoxicity seen with morphine metabolites: myoclonus, hyperalgesia, and seizures.[115] This is particularly likely in patients with renal dysfunction.[116,117]

ROUTES FOR ADMINISTERING OPIOIDS

The oral route is generally preferred when patients are capable and enteral absorption is not problematic. In the palliative care setting, alternative routes of administration must be available for patients who can no longer swallow or when other dynamics preclude the oral route.[5] These include transdermal, transmucosal, rectal, vaginal, topical, epidural, and intrathecal. In a study of cancer patients at 4 weeks, 1 week, and 24 hours before death, more than half of the patients required more than one route of opioid administration. As patients approached death and oral use diminished, the use of intermittent subcutaneous injections and intravenous or subcutaneous infusions increased.[12] Therefore, in caring for patients near the end of life, it is essential to identify alternatives to oral administration that can be used if necessary.

Enteral feeding tubes can be used to access the gut when patients can no longer swallow. The rectum, stoma, or vagina can be used to deliver medication, although fecal contents, mucosal dryness, thrombocytopenia, or painful lesions may preclude the use of these routes. For morphine, commercially prepared suppositories, compounded suppositories, or micro-enemas can be used to deliver the drug directly to the rectum or stoma.[118] Sustained-release morphine tablets have been used rectally, with resultant delayed time to peak plasma level and approximately 90% of the bioavailability achieved by oral administration.[119]

Because the vagina has no sphincter, a tampon covered with a condom or an inflated urinary catheter balloon may be used to prevent early discharge of the drug.[118] Although useful, the rectal or vaginal routes may be unacceptable to many patients and their caregivers, especially when the patient is obtunded or unable to assist.[6]

Parenteral administration in palliative care is usually limited to subcutaneous and intravenous delivery because repeated intramuscular opioid delivery is excessively noxious. The intravenous route provides rapid drug delivery but requires vascular access that may not be easily obtained or maintained in a home or long-term care setting. In the absence of intravenous access, it must be remembered that subcutaneous boluses, although effective, have a slower onset and lower peak effect when compared with intravenous boluses.[5] Subcutaneous infusions as much as 10 mL/hour are usually absorbed, although most patients tolerate 2 to 3 mL/hour with the least difficulty.[120,121]

Intraspinal routes, including epidural or intrathecal delivery, may allow administration of drugs, such as opioids, local anesthetics, and α-adrenergic agonists. A randomized controlled trial demonstrated benefit for cancer patients experiencing pain.[79] However, the equipment used to deliver these medications is complex, requiring specialized knowledge for health care professionals and potentially greater caregiver burden. Risk of infection and other complications along with up-front and maintenance costs are significant concerns when contemplating high-technology procedures. Selection should be based on greater than 6 months' life expectancy for implanted programmable pumps, and adequate organizational infrastructure to manage these devices should be in place.

ADJUVANT THERAPIES

The term *adjuvant analgesics* is often used synonymously with *coanalgesics, pain-modifying drugs,* and similar descriptives. A wide variety of nonopioid medications from several pharmacologic classes have been demonstrated to reduce pain caused by various pathologic conditions (e.g., tricyclic antidepressants) or modify the ongoing disease process in a way that specifically reduces pain (e.g., bisphosphonates).[122] Under most circumstances these drugs are indicated for the treatment of severe neuropathic pain or bone pain, and opioid analgesics are used concurrently to provide adequate pain relief. Typical adjuvants include tricyclic antidepressants, serotonin-norepinephrine reuptake inhibitor (SNRI) antidepressants, anticonvulsants, corticosteroids, and other disease-modifying drugs, such as bisphosphonates for metastatic bone pain. See Table 77.5 for a listing of current adjuvant therapies for neuropathic pain. For more information on adjuvant analgesics, see Chapters 39 and 40.

ANTIDEPRESSANTS

The analgesic effect of tricyclic antidepressants appears to be related to inhibition of norepinephrine and serotonin reuptake, making these neurotransmitters more available within

Table 77.5 Adjuvant Therapies for Neuropathic Pain

Category/Agents	Comments
Corticosteroids	
Dexamethasone Prednisone Prednisolone	• Shown to reduce spontaneous discharge in injured nerves • Dexamethasone has the least mineralocorticoid effect (long duration of action for once-daily dosing) • May be dosed orally, intravenously, subcutaneously, or epidurally • May produce psychosis, proximal muscle wasting
Anticonvulsants	
Carbamazepine Gabapentin Valproate Phenytoin Clonazepam Tiagabine Levetiracetam Lamotrigine Topiramate Zonisamide Oxcarbazepine Pregabalin	• Older agents are used extensively, but potential for adverse events requires careful monitoring; clinical experience is extensive for carbamazepine, but propensity for bone marrow suppression (i.e., leukopenia) limits its use in patients with cancer • Lamotrigine has demonstrated efficacy in HIV sensory neuropathy, painful diabetic neuropathy, and post-stroke pain, but requires slow titration; also associated with Stevens-Johnson syndrome and severe rash • The role of newer agents (e.g., levetiracetam, oxcarbazepine, tiagabine, etc.) has not been established • Gabapentin approved for PHN • Pregabalin approved for painful diabetic neuropathy
Tricyclic Antidepressants	
Amitriptyline Nortriptyline Desipramine Imipramine Clomipramine	• Use is associated with significant tolerability issues • Nortriptyline has fewer anticholinergic/anti-α-adrenergic effects, and therefore has better tolerability, especially in older adults • Should be administered at night to reduce daytime sedation and support good sleep hygiene
Local Anesthetics	
Mexiletine Lidocaine IV	• Oral lidocaine analogues are effective in some patients, but long-term use may lead to clinically significant adverse events • Infusional lidocaine is gaining greater acceptance; may be particularly effective for visceral or central pain • A lidocaine challenge can assess whether a patient's pain is responsive (i.e., 1-3 mg/kg IV or subcutaneous over 30-60 min.); if challenge is effective or partially effective, continuous infusion consists of 1-2 mg/kg/hr • Perioral numbness suggests toxicity. Infusion should be halted and restarted at a slower rate on resolution
Anticancer Therapies	
Radiation therapy	• Local, half-body, or whole-body radiation therapy can enhance efficacy of analgesia by directly affecting tumor and other causes of pain • Curative excision or palliative debulking of tumor may relieve pain directly, decrease symptoms of obstruction or compression, and improve prognosis

HIV, human immunodeficiency virus; PHN, postherpetic neuralgia.
Adapted and reprinted with permission from Fine PG, Miaskowski C, Paice JA. Meeting the challenges in cancer pain. *J Support Oncol.* 2004;2(suppl 4):5-22.

central nervous system pain inhibitory pathways. There are many significant, controlled clinical trials for several pain conditions, and guidelines list tricyclic antidepressants as one of the first-line therapies for neuropathic pain.[30,123,124] The significant side effects, especially in older patients, require careful titration and monitoring in palliative care populations, but their sleep-enhancing and mood-elevating effects may be beneficial enough to outweigh their disadvantages.[125] The newer mixed SNRIs—selective serotonin reuptake inhibitors (SSRIs), such as venlafaxine and duloxetine—may offer some of the advantages of tricyclic antidepressants without the anticholinergic side effects.[126] See Chapter 39 for a more complete discussion of antidepressants.

ANTICONVULSANTS

The older anticonvulsants, such as carbamazepine and clonazepam, putatively relieve pain by blocking sodium channels.[125] These compounds are very useful in the treatment of certain types of neuropathic pain, especially pain with episodic, lancinating qualities such as trigeminal neuralgia. Gabapentin seems to have several different mechanisms of action, although calcium ion channel blockade is thought to be its main pain-inhibiting mechanism.[127]

The analgesic doses of gabapentin reported to be effective in a typical and common neuropathic pain condition, painful diabetic neuropathy, ranged from 900 mg/day to

3600 mg/day in divided doses.[128] Additional evidence supports the use of gabapentin in neuropathic pain syndromes seen in palliative care, such as thalamic pain, pain due to spinal cord injury, cancer pain, and restless legs syndrome and HIV-associated sensory neuropathies.[27,129] Withdrawal from gabapentin, if indicated due to ineffectiveness or adverse effects, should be gradual to prevent possible seizures.[130] In the authors' experience, other anticonvulsants that have been used effectively to treat neuropathies causing pain in patients at end of life include lamotrigine, pregabalin, levetiracetam, tiagabine, and oxcarbazepine, but no clinical trials in this specific population are available.[26,28,131]

CORTICOSTEROIDS

Corticosteroids are particularly useful for neuropathic, visceral, and bone pain syndromes in patients with far advanced disease, including plexopathies and pain associated with stretching of the liver capsule as a result of metastases.[132,133] Dexamethasone produces the least amount of mineralocorticoid effect, making it the least toxic choice. Dexamethasone is available in oral, intravenous, subcutaneous, and epidural formulations. The standard dose is 16 to 24 mg/day and can be administered once daily due to the long half-life of this drug, but divided doses are usually used to mitigate high-dose toxic effects, such as psychosis and severe blood sugar abnormalities in diabetic patients. Doses as high as 100 mg may be given with severe pain crises, similar to the doses used in acute neurologic emergencies. Intravenous bolus doses should be administered over several minutes to reduce untoward reactions, such as burning sensations.

LOCAL ANESTHETICS

Local anesthetics are useful for relieving neuropathic pain. They can be given orally, topically, intravenously, subcutaneously, or spinally.[134] Mexiletine has been reported to be useful when anticonvulsants and other adjuvant therapies have failed. Doses start at 150 mg/day and increase to levels as high as 900 mg/day in divided doses.[135,136] Pretreatment electrocardiogram evaluation is recommended to evaluate for conduction blocks that can be exacerbated by oral local anesthetics. Local anesthetic gels and patches have been used to prevent the pain that is associated with needlestick and other minor procedures. Both gel and patch (lidocaine 5% patch) versions of lidocaine have been shown to reduce the pain of PHN.[137] Intravenous lidocaine at 1 to 5 mg/kg (maximum, 500 mg) administered over 1 hour, followed by a continuous infusion of 1 to 2 mg/kg/hour, has been reported to reduce patients' intractable neuropathic pain in inpatient palliative care and home hospice settings.[26] Epidural or intrathecal lidocaine or bupivacaine delivered with an opioid can reduce neuropathic pain.[138]

BISPHOSPHONATES

Bisphosphonates inhibit osteoclast-mediated bone resorption and alleviate pain related to metastatic bone disease and multiple myeloma, reduce the incidence of pathologic fractures, and are used to treat tumor-related hypercalcemia.[139] In patients with breast cancer and multiple myeloma, zoledronic acid has demonstrated improved safety and efficacy compared with pamidronate.[140,141] Similarly, there appears to be more sustained pain relief with zoledronic acid compared with other bisphosphonates in patients with metastatic prostate cancer.[142] Clinical trials in patients with lung and renal cell carcinoma have also shown therapeutic benefit from regular infusions of zoledronic acid.[143]

CHEMOTHERAPY AND RADIATION THERAPY

Palliative chemotherapy is the use of antitumor therapy to relieve the symptoms that are associated with malignancy. Patient goals, performance status, sensitivity of the tumor, and potential toxicities must be considered.[5] Examples of symptoms that may improve with chemotherapy include relief of chest wall pain from reduced tumor ulceration through the use of hormonal therapy in breast cancer. Some newer agents, such as docetaxel, reduce pain and improve quality of life in hormone-refractory prostate cancer, and topotecan and epidermal growth factor receptor inhibitors accomplish similar results for patients with lung cancers.[144-146]

Radiation therapy is also a highly useful adjunct to control pain from bone metastasis and pressure-inducing and ulcerative malignancies. Single-fraction and hypofractionated regimens are proving to be effective in very sick patients and those with limited life expectancy in whom the opportunity costs of multiple treatment sessions are untenable.[147,148] These therapies are often underused in hospice or palliative care, and they should be considered for any patient with a life expectancy of more than a few weeks.[149]

OTHER OPTIONS

Medications typically seen in the setting of the operating room or the intensive care unit can have a role in severe or refractory pain that range from neuropathic pain from chemotherapeutics to opioid-induced hyperalgesia. Examples are ketamine and dexmedetomidine. Ketamine is a potent NMDA-receptor channel blocker available for administration intravenously, subcutaneously, orally in solution, sublingually, and via nasal passages. It has been evaluated for both pain and mood disorders.[150] In these relatively small trials or case series as well as the authors' experience, it can be extremely useful in select situations. Dexmedetomidine is an alpha-2 adrenergic agonist. The mechanism of action is similar to that of clonidine but it is significantly more alpha specific. The benefit of this drug is that it can produce sedation and analgesia but does not cause respiratory depression. Reports have emerged in using this for refractory pains.[151]

Palliative sedation is a procedure in which medications are used to lower the level of consciousness to limit the awareness of suffering that a patient finds intolerable and intractable. Though it has met resistance in the past, it has been through the scrutiny of both ethicists and judges and has been determined to be an acceptable practice for properly selected patients. A prospective study has demonstrated that patients undergoing palliative sedation experience no life-shortening effect.[152] The procedure should not be done without experience or guidance. The National Hospice and Palliative Care Organization released a position paper on the topic.[153]

Emerging nonpharmacologic therapies should also be watched with interest. One involves use of the MC5-A Calmare device, also known as Scrambler therapy. This novel machine provides electrocutaneous nerve stimulation for neuromodulation. This attempts to provide cutaneous nerves with "nonpain" information, thus blocking the effect of pain information. The small studies show promise. One of them found that chronic neuropathic pain was more effectively controlled with Scrambler therapy than guideline-based management.[154,155]

BEGINNING THERAPY, ADDING OR CHANGING DRUGS, AND BREAKTHROUGH PAIN

Application of practical and mechanism-based approaches, coupled with context-appropriate follow-up, will optimize drug and other palliative therapies. The "best first choice" and subsequent timing of opioid rotation will depend on patient-specific medical, psychological, and social considerations and a sound knowledge of opioid pharmacotherapy. If adverse effects exceed the analgesic benefit of the drug, conversion to an equianalgesic dose of a different opioid is recommended. Because cross-tolerance is incomplete, it is important to reduce the calculated dose by one third to one half and titrate upward based on the patient's pain intensity scores.[5]

Titration and combining drugs that may provide additive or synergistic effects should proceed along rational lines, based on the pharmacokinetics and monitored pharmacodynamics of the drugs. Frail patients and those with pain crises may require observation in a monitored setting in order to provide safe and effective relief within an acceptable time frame.

Transitory flares of pain, or breakthrough pain, can be expected both at rest and during movement. If breakthrough pain lasts longer than a few minutes, rescue doses of the patient's current analgesics may provide relief.[156] In patients without parenteral access, oral transmucosal fentanyl may be useful for rapid episodic pain relief or during a brief but painful dressing change. Frail older adults or severely debilitated patients should start with the 200-mcg dose and efficacy should be monitored, advancing to higher-dose units as needed.[157] Clinicians must be aware that unlike other breakthrough pain drugs, the around-the-clock dose of opioid does not predict the effective dose of oral transmucosal fentanyl. Some pain relief can usually be expected in about 5 to 10 minutes after administration. Patients should use oral transmucosal fentanyl citrate over a period of 15 minutes because more active sucking will result in more swallowing and less transmucosal absorption.

Because misunderstandings lead to undertreatment, all clinicians involved in the care of patients with advanced illness and pain must be able to differentiate and clearly explain to patients and their families the clinical conditions of tolerance, physical dependence, and the rarity of addiction related to opioid use at end of life. It also is critically important to be aware that there is no established relationship between titration of opioid analgesics to affect pain relief and timing of death in palliative care or hospice settings.[158,159]

MINIMIZING AND MANAGING ADVERSE EFFECTS

Drugs for pain can cause a variety of adverse effects for patients in palliative care. The normal side effects associated with pain-relief medications are often exacerbated by changes in metabolism caused by end-stage disease, polypharmacy associated with advanced age, and other factors. Following are some of the more common adverse effects and an overview of possible approaches to preventing or alleviating them.

CONSTIPATION

Patients in palliative care frequently experience constipation, in part because of opioid therapy.[66] Always begin a prophylactic bowel regimen when commencing opioid analgesic therapy. Avoid bulking agents such as psyllium because these tend to increase desiccation time in the large bowel, and debilitated patients can rarely take in sufficient fluid to facilitate the action of bulking agents. Instead, starting with cost-effective and palatable products, such as senna tea and fruit or senna plus docusate sodium (Colace) for patients with a history of "sluggish" bowel function, is advised. If this is ineffective at creating regular laxation, then prescription therapies are indicated (e.g., bisacodyl, senna derivatives, propylene glycol).[63] Tables listing recommended regimens are readily available in clinical guidelines and texts. When traditional regimens have failed to bring about the desired effect, using a peripherally acting mu opioid receptor antagonist such as methylnaltrexone can be useful. This new drug class is a targeted therapy for opioid-induced constipation, and because it does not enter the central nervous system there are no symptoms of opioid withdrawal or increased pain. These have been studied in patients with advanced illness.[160,161]

SEDATION

Excessive sedation may occur with the initial doses of opioids. If sedation persists after 24 to 48 hours and other correctable causes have been identified and treated, psychostimulants may be beneficial. These include dextroamphetamine 2.5 to 5 mg by mouth every morning and midday or methylphenidate 5 to 10 mg by mouth every morning and 2.5 to 5 mg midday (although higher doses are frequently used, and use later in the day may be required for wakefulness throughout the evening hours, if desired).[5] Adjust both the dose and timing to prevent nocturnal insomnia, and monitor for undesirable psychotomimetic effects (such as agitation, hallucinations, and irritability). Once-daily dosing of modafinil, a newer agent approved to manage narcolepsy, has been reported to relieve opioid-induced sedation.[162]

RESPIRATORY DEPRESSION

Respiratory depression is rarely a clinically significant problem for opioid-tolerant patients who are in pain.[63] When respiratory depression occurs in a patient with advanced disease, the cause is usually multifactorial.[163,164] When depressed consciousness occurs along with a respiratory rate less than 8/minute or hypoxemia (O_2 saturation less than 90%) associated with opioid use, slow, cautious titration of naloxone can be instituted (0.4 mg [one ampule, 400 mcg, diluted in 10 mL injectable saline = 0.4 mcg/mL]) every 3 to 5 minutes while providing respiratory support and supplemental oxygen). This should be done according to the patient's goals or in conjunction with their surrogate decision maker. Excessive administration may cause abrupt opioid reversal with pain and autonomic crisis.

NAUSEA AND VOMITING

Nausea is common and vomiting is an occasional adverse effect associated with opioids as a result of activation of the chemoreceptor trigger zone in the medulla, vestibular sensitivity, and delayed gastric emptying, but habituation occurs in most cases within several days.[5] Assess for other treatable causes. In severe cases or when nausea and vomiting are not self-limited, pharmacotherapy is indicated. Usually, low doses of an H_1 blocker (e.g., diphenhydramine) are all that is required while the patient habituates to this unpleasant side effect. If there is no relief within a few days, metoclopramide or a different opioid is recommended; also consider transdermal rather than enteral therapy.[28,63]

MYOCLONUS

Myoclonic jerking can occur with high-dose opioid therapy. If myoclonus develops, switch to an alternate opioid, especially if using morphine. Evidence suggests that this symptom is associated with metabolite accumulation, particularly in the face of renal dysfunction.[5] A lower relative dose of the substituted drug may be possible because of incomplete cross-tolerance. Clonazepam 0.5 to 1 mg by mouth every 6 to 8 hours, to be increased as needed and tolerated, may be useful in treating myoclonus in patients who are still alert, able to communicate, and take oral preparations.[165] Lorazepam can be given sublingually if the patient is unable to swallow. Otherwise, parenteral administration of diazepam is indicated if symptoms are distressing. Grand mal seizures associated with high-dose parenteral opioid infusions have been reported and may be caused by preservatives in the solution.[166] Preservative-free solutions should be used when administering high-dose infusions.

PRURITUS

Pruritus can occur with most opioids, although it appears to be most common with morphine. Fentanyl and oxymorphone may be less likely to cause histamine release. Most antipruritus therapies cause sedation, so the patient must see this as an acceptable trade-off. Antihistamines (such as diphenhydramine) are the most common first-line approach to this opioid-induced symptom. Ondansetron and paroxetine have been reported to be effective in relieving opioid-induced pruritus, but no randomized controlled studies exist.[167,168]

CASE 77.3 Complex Symptom Management in the Home Setting (continued)

After examination and consultation, it was determined that Ben could continue to reside in the assisted-living facility, attended to by home-based hospice staff. Treatment proceeded with subcutaneous administration of octreotide and hydromorphone to relieve bowel symptoms and provide analgesia on an as-needed basis. In this way the unpleasantness of nasogastric suctioning, nausea, and vomiting was avoided, and he was able to die in a manner consistent with his preferences.

CONCLUSION

Effective pain management in advanced medical illness and at the end of life is a critical component of quality medical care to ensure dignified, safe, and comfortable dying. To quote Sir William Osler, the "father of modern medicine," "The study of morbid anatomy combined with careful clinical observations has taught us to recognize our limitations and to accept the fact that a disease itself may be incurable and that the best we can do is to relieve symptoms and make the patient comfortable."

Principles to help improve this important domain of clinical care can be summarized with the following key points regarding pharmacotherapy for the relief of pain in far-advanced illness.

KEY POINTS

- Ensure that communications about goals of care and treatment plans among professional caregiving staff and the patient and family members are clear and understood in order to optimize outcomes and minimize potential conflicts.
- Determine the etiology of pain and the social and prognostic circumstances that will affect the pain experience and pain therapy.
- Focus on discernible clinical end points:
  - Pain reduction
  - Functional capacities
  - Mood
  - Sleep
  - Relationships
  - Pleasure in living
- Match the mechanism of pain with the class of drug whenever possible; initiate therapy and adjust dose according to therapeutic response, side effects, and known pharmacokinetics of the drug.
  - Anticipate and monitor for adverse effects.
  - Prevent side effects.
  - Actively treat side effects.

KEY POINTS—cont'd

- Acetaminophen should be the first consideration in the treatment of mild to moderate pain of musculoskeletal origin.
- Use adjunctive drug therapies, especially for neuropathic pain.
- Opioid analgesic drugs are often necessary to relieve moderate to severe pain, and long-acting or sustained-release analgesic preparations should be used for continuous pain.
- Breakthrough pain should be identified and treated by the use of fast-onset, short-acting preparations.
- Last, and perhaps most important, know your limits. When a patient is not responding to therapy, be prepared to consult with someone who has more training, expertise, and experience.

SUGGESTED READINGS

Attal N, Crucco G, Baron R, et al. EFNS Guidelines on the pharmacological treatment of neuropathic pain: 2010 revision. *Eur J Neurol.* 2010;17:1113-1123.

Bakker J, Jansen TC, Lima A, et al. Why opioids and sedatives may prolong life rather than hasten death after mechanical ventilator withdrawal in critically ill patients. *Am J Hosp Palliat Care.* 2008;25:152-155.

Davis MP, Walsh D. Methadone for relief of cancer pain: a review of pharmacokinetics, pharmacodynamics, drug interactions and protocols of administration. *Support Care Cancer.* 2001;9:73-83.

Dy SM, Asch SM, Naeim A, et al. Evidence-based standards for cancer pain management. *J Clin Oncol.* 2008;26:3879-3885.

Fine PG. The ethical imperative to relieve pain at life's end. *J Pain Symptom Manage.* 2002;23:273-277.

Hartsell WF, Scott CB, Bruner DW, et al. Randomized trial of short- versus long-course radiotherapy for palliation of painful bone metastases. *J Natl Cancer Inst.* 2005;97:798-804.

Herr K, Bjoro K, Decker S. Tools for assessment of pain in nonverbal older adults with dementia: a state-of-the-science review. *J Pain Symptom Manage.* 2006;31:170-192.

Kirk TW, Mahon MM. Nation Hospice and Palliative Care Organization position statement and commentary on the use of palliative sedation in imminently dying terminally ill patients. *J Pain Symptom Manage.* 2010;39:914-923.

Meisel A, Snyder L, Quill T. Seven legal barriers to end-of-life care: myths, realities, and grains of truth. *JAMA.* 2000;284:2495-2501.

Pergolizzi J, Boger RH, Budd K, et al. Opioids and the management of chronic severe pain in the elderly: consensus statement of an international expert panel with focus on the six clinically most often used World Health Organization step III opioids. *Pain Pract.* 2008;8:287-313.

Qaseem A, Snow V, Shekelle P, et al. Evidence-based interventions to improve the palliative care of pain, dypnea, and depression at the end of life: a clinical practice guideline from the American College of Physicians. *Ann Intern Med.* 2008;148:141-146.

Ripamonti C. Pharmacology of opioid analgesia: clinical principles. In: Bruera E, Portenoy RK, eds. *Cancer Pain: Assessment and Management.* Cambridge, UK: Cambridge University Press; 2003:124-149.

Thomas J, Karver S, Cooney GA, et al. Methylnaltrexone for opioid-induced constipation in advanced illness. *N Engl J Med.* 2008;358:2332-2343.

Tilden VP, Drach LL, Tolle SW. Complementary and alternative therapy use at end-of-life in community settings. *J Altern Complement Med.* 2004;10:811-817.

Zhang B, Wright AA, Huskamp HA, et al. Health care costs in the last week of life. *Arch Intern Med.* 2009;169:480-488.

The references for this chapter can be found at www.expertconsult.com.

78 Pain Management in the Home: Using Cancer Patients as a Model

Nessa Coyle | Myra Glajchen

Pain management in the home is a family experience, as every aspect of care provided to the patient affects the family system as a whole. Successful pain management at home depends on a patient and family who understand and are invested in the pain management regimen and express confidence in implementing the plan as prescribed. This includes understanding the difference between around-the-clock and prn dosing; knowing when to use "rescue" doses; being able to identify and report changes in the pain site, character, and severity; as well as having the ability to recognize and report adverse side effects from the analgesic prescribed and to manage the technical aspects of the pain treatment plan.

Pain associated with cancer must be viewed within a cluster of symptoms that need to be monitored and managed by the family. Pain changes, its assessment and management, are made more complex by the presence of other symptoms, the likelihood that increased pain may be associated with disease progression, and the component of suffering frequently experienced by family caregivers. Various family dynamics also can change the pain experience.

Because of the complexity of cancer pain management, the patient and family can rarely manage pain in the home setting on their own. Rather, they need guidance and support from the oncology team. Effective communication among the primary physician, advanced practice nurse, home care, nurse and family, as well as ready access to the point person among these professionals, is essential for the success of the home care plan. A system of ongoing monitoring and support for the patient and family needs to be in place to ensure the effectiveness of pain relief measures and early identification of caregiver burden and unmet needs. Careful discharge planning followed by regular assessment and reassessment can facilitate effective pain management and support for the patient at home as well as minimize pain "emergencies."

Chronic pain associated with cancer is an extremely stressful situation for both patient and family. Surveys indicate that pain is experienced by 30% to 60% of cancer patients during active therapy and in more than two thirds of those with advanced disease.[1-7] In addition, symptom clusters and multiple symptoms tend to be the norm, not the exception, in advanced cancer patients with pain.[8-10] These patients spend minimal time in the hospital and most of the time in their homes. The experience of chronic pain, therefore, is mainly a home experience, one that involves not only pain but also multiple other symptoms, and one that involves not only the patient but also the patient's family and friends.[11-13] Unrelieved pain is incapacitating and undermines quality of life; it interferes with physical functioning and social interaction and is strongly associated with heightened psychological distress.[14-18] Uncontrolled severe pain, or episodes of excruciating pain in this setting, can lead to a desire for hastened death.[18]

FAMILY CAREGIVERS ON THE FRONT LINES

The literature is replete with discussions about the prevalence of pain, its undertreatment, and barriers to adequate pain management.[19-24] Less attention had been given to factors affecting pain management in the home, although a growing literature explores issues particular to this topic. These issues include knowledge and attitudes about cancer pain and its management among patient and family members,[22,25,26] stress in family caregivers and community nurses,[26-31] management of the technical aspects of pain in the home,[31,32] and communication.[33] Recognition of the "responsibility without adequate training or power" phenomenon that nurses commonly experience in the home care setting has been an impetus for the development of training programs for home care nurses in pain management. Many families experience the same phenomenon. Family caregivers are expected to play a primary role in cancer pain relief across all stages of the disease and yet are frequently given little or no training on how to do so.[29-31,34-37] Structured pain education programs have been shown to result in positive outcomes for patients and their family caregivers.[38-40]

Understanding the factors that influence adequacy of pain management in the home has become increasingly important in the face of the current trend toward shorter inpatient hospital stays, earlier hospital discharges, and the expectation that extremely sick patients will be managed at home.[41-43] This trend is likely to continue in light of health care reform and new systems of care such as the medical home. Family members, with community nursing support, are on the front line of home pain management.

BARRIERS TO PAIN MANAGEMENT IN THE HOME

Generally speaking, the home environment offers substantial benefits to the individual with cancer and pain, but home care also can result in intense burdens for family caregivers resulting in compromised care.[35,44] Home care is best viewed as a family experience with the recognition that every aspect of care provided to the patient will affect family caregivers.[44]

At the same time, barriers have been described that hinder pain management in the home, including patient and family fears of addiction, failure to report pain, and limited access to care.[27,35,36,38,39] The intense demands on family caregiving at home, especially in the provision of 24-hour physical caregiving, is well described.[41-43,45] Less attention has been placed on the emotional burden to the family of assuming responsibility for the patient's well-being in the home.[46,47] In addition, little has been written about the care of cancer patients with pain who are discharged home to a high-risk, drug-abuse environment. Encompassing a relatively small group of individuals, their needs can be great. However, with careful planning and close monitoring, safe pain management at home can be achieved for most people with cancer.[48]

An early small descriptive study (trial of 10), which investigated the experience of managing pain at home from the perspectives of the patient, the primary family caregiver, and the home-care nurse, encapsulated many of the important areas that affect pain management in the home.[26] Areas of decision making and conflict mainly centered around the use of medications. Patients were preoccupied with decisions about which pain medication to take and how much. Negative side effects and meaning in regard to these medications contributed to conflicts in patients' minds about whether they were doing the "right thing" in taking the pain medication.[49]

Nearly all the patients assumed that their pain would increase with impending death. Patients' decisions about how to live with the pain included considerations about the impact of their actions and words on family members and health care professionals. Sometimes these factors led the patient to deny the pain. Similarly, the decisions and conflicts that arose most frequently for family caregivers were related to pain medication, making decisions about which pill to give, and when to give the medication. Exacerbating these decisions were concerns related to overdosing, adverse side effects, and addiction. Sometimes the family member admitted to withholding information from the patient or the nurse in an attempt to benefit the patient in some way. For example, depending on the decision-making process of the family member, more or less medication might be given. Other studies conducted on knowledge and beliefs about pain management in cancer patients and their families found that although patients and families share similar beliefs about pain, family members tend to have a higher degree of emotional distress associated with observing pain in their loved ones.[50]

PAIN MEDICATION ADMINISTRATION AND ADHERENCE IN THE HOME

For family caregivers of cancer patients, effective medication management involves a complex set of activities, which include filling the prescription, safely storing the pain medication, organizing and dispensing medication as needed or on a fixed dosing schedule, monitoring effectiveness and adverse events, and communicating about those symptoms with the oncology team.[51]

Nonadherence, defined as the inability of patients to take medications as prescribed, is a major concern in pain management. Nonadherence is usually multifactorial and may lead to undertreatment or even potentially dangerous medication errors. Caregivers' lack of experience with opioids, fears of addiction, and fears about managing pain medications in the home setting can lead to under-reporting of pain and undermedication. This was the case in a study involving 89 days of oncology inpatients and their primary caregivers. In this study, patient-caregiver ratings of pain were noncongruent, with patients reporting higher pain and poorer performance status levels.[52] The authors concluded that patients were reluctant to report their pain to family members for fear of causing them distress. As a consequence, 45% of family caregivers underestimated their loved ones' pain, whereas 55% overestimated it. In another study involving caregivers of patients with advanced cancer, caregiver distress led to hypervigilance by caregivers, exaggeration of the patient's pain experience by caregivers, and over-reporting of the patient's pain experience. These studies suggest that caregivers' burden and distress can influence symptom management in patients.[53]

THE ROLE OF CAREGIVERS IN THE ASSESSMENT OF PAIN

Effective pain management is dependent on an accurate assessment. When the patient is being cared for at home, the physician frequently relies on second- or third-hand information supplied by the patient, family, or home care nurse on the severity of the pain, adequacy of relief, presence of side effects, and associated toxicity. Correct interpretation of the patient's and caregiver's report of pain is essential. According to Elliot and colleagues,[54] and suggested by the preceding studies, three dimensions constitute a patient's pain experience: cognitive factors (including attitudes, beliefs, and knowledge), sensory or physical input, and affective or emotional experience. Elliot and coworkers found that although patients and families reported parallel perceptions of the patient's cancer pain, family members consistently assessed the patient's level of pain somewhat higher than the patient. This suggested to them the effect of observing rather than experiencing the pain. In addition, Ward and colleagues reported that patients with increased concerns were less likely to use analgesics adequately.[27] These studies, as well as others, document that family caregivers are often as affected by pain as the patient, and sometimes more so.

There are important implications here for evaluating the efficacy of a pain management strategy, if the assessment is largely dependent on a family member's report.[27,31,35,45] The report of poorly controlled pain may indicate the family member's distress as well as that of the patient. Areas of family distress include fatigue, lack of knowledge about pain management, concern about addiction, concern about harming the patient, and an overwhelming feeling of responsibility.[25,26,34] Family concerns as well as patient distress must be addressed if pain is to be adequately managed. There is a close relationship between the two.

In a comprehensive review of 129 quantitative research studies on family caregivers and palliative care in the home setting, family caregivers reported providing extensive help to dying relatives in the areas of medication and symptom management.[55] Other studies have reported an inverse relationship between the health and function of the cancer patient and the amount of caregiver burden with caregiver strain, depression, and anxiety reaching its peak as the patient enters the terminal phase.[56]

In another comprehensive review of more than 100 qualitative studies on family caregiving at home at the end of life,[57] the general consensus across studies was that caregivers reported a lack of preparation, knowledge, and skills in symptom, pain, and medication management, especially with the technical aspects of medication administration. Recommendations included teaching family caregivers about the practical aspects of care at the end of life and making sure caregivers were routinely provided with general information about the nature and course of the patient's disease. Yet caregiving is not uniform and the needs of caregivers of cancer patients are neither identical nor static. Caregiver burden and comfort with home pain management regimens must be assessed and reassessed over time.

A national survey of 1677 family caregivers, including caregivers of cancer patients, documented the complexity of medical management in the home setting. More than 90% of caregivers ordered, picked up, and paid for the patient's medication. Caregivers dispensed pills, prepared pillboxes, or gave medication in the form of injections, inhalers, eye and eardrops, and infusion pumps. Although caregivers found medication-related tasks to be inconvenient, repetitive, and time consuming, fewer than half had received counseling or training in the area of medication management.[58]

The difficulties that patients and family caregivers commonly encounter when trying to put a pain management regimen into place at home are summarized in Box 78.1. They illustrate that patients and family caregivers need ongoing support and help with problem solving in order to optimize their pain management regimen.[59] Most caregivers rely on nurses for information related to medications.[60]

Box 78.1 Difficulties Patients and Family Caregivers Encounter When Trying to Put a Pain Management Regimen into Place at Home

1. Obtaining the prescribed medication(s)
2. Accessing information
3. Tailoring prescribed regimens to meet individual needs
4. Managing side effects
5. Cognitively processing information
6. Managing new or unusual pain
7. Managing multiple symptoms simultaneously

NONDRUG INTERVENTIONS USED BY PATIENTS FOR PAIN MANAGEMENT IN THE HOME

In addition to the numerous and sometimes overwhelming responsibilities related to the pharmacologic management of pain in the home, patients and family caregivers use many nondrug strategies for pain relief. Although some of these techniques are taught in the hospital setting, they are seldom reinforced by the medical team once the patient is discharged home. Nondrug interventions include both physical and cognitive approaches. Physical approaches include interventions such as heat, cold, and massage. Cognitive strategies include a variety of relaxation techniques, imagery, meditation, and prayer.[28,61-64] These nondrug strategies, especially those that are a "fit" with the patient's values and belief system, can be enormously helpful in not only enhancing pain relief but also in helping the individual to regain a sense of control.[65]

PLANNING FOR HOME PAIN MANAGEMENT: TRANSITION FROM HOSPITAL TO HOME

Hospitalization and discharge episodes are notorious for interrupting the pain regimens of cancer patients as a new treatment team is involved or as new medications are added or withdrawn in light of new medical conditions or side effects. Common to all groups, however, is the need for basic education on cancer pain management with the individualized home pain management regimen clearly written out in a language that the patient and family can understand; a pain management plan that is financially feasible for the patient; verification that prescribed analgesics are available in the community; confirmation that the patient and family are secure with the discharge and follow-up plans; and assurance that the patient is not discharged (if at all possible) within 24 hours of a change in opioid drug or route of administration (Box 78.2).[48]

CLASSIFICATION OF PATIENTS INTO GROUPS HELPS INDIVIDUALIZE AND ORGANIZE CARE

To facilitate discharge planning for patients with cancer-related pain and ease the transition from hospital to home, it is useful to classify patients into different groups, depending on specific needs and risk factors (Table 78.1).[66] This is important because discharge-planning needs and home care needs are specific to each group.

Group 1 comprises patients who have stable pain, and are, for example, using an oral, transmucosal, rectal, or transdermal route of opioid administration. These patients may or may not be pursuing a course of curative or life-prolonging therapy. The patient is usually followed on an outpatient basis with ongoing prescriptions written by the primary physician or nurse practitioner. The patient is instructed to contact the primary physician or nurse practitioner for any change in the quality, severity, or site of the pain and the occurrence of adverse side effects. Prior to the patient's discharge home, it is important that the community pharmacy be contacted to make sure that it has the necessary opioid in stock or is willing to obtain it.[48,67,68] It is good practice for the physician or pain management nurse to initiate contact with the patient within the first week of discharge to confirm that pain is adequately controlled and that the patient and family feel confident with the pain management approach. This initial telephone contact also confirms that pain management is a priority and the patient's pain will continue to be monitored closely with resources readily available even though care is now on an ambulatory basis. The cost of medication on an outpatient basis can be a significant barrier for patients without a prescription plan.[69-72] The ability of a patient to both pay for and obtain the outpatient analgesic prescription must be established prior to discharge home. Often the patient does not volunteer this information unless specifically asked for it. The social worker can be very helpful in this area. Several pharmaceutical companies have specific patient "hardship" programs. A social worker can again be very helpful in evaluating a patient's eligibility for these programs and accessing these resources.

If a patient's pain escalates once at home, it is crucial to explore with the patient or family caregiver whether the pain medication is being taken as prescribed. It is not unusual that a pain management regimen is not adhered to once an individual goes home, for the variety of reasons described earlier.[73] The reasons for nonadherence need to be discussed in an open and frank manner. Tailoring a pain management regimen that fits in with the patient's and family caregiver's values, goals, and capabilities is essential if symptoms are to be controlled at home.

Group 2 consists of patients who require a parenteral route of drug administration to control their pain. Although the majority of patients do well on the oral or transdermal route of opioid administration, some will require ongoing administration through a parenteral route.[74-76] The most common indications for a parenteral infusion in the cancer population are bowel obstruction or malabsorption, severe stomatitis, intractable nausea and vomiting, and dysphagia.[74-76] A parenteral opioid infusion also is considered for patients with rapidly escalating and unstable pain or those with frequent and severe episodes of breakthrough pain. In these situations, the use of patient-controlled analgesia in combination with the continuous parenteral infusion helps ensure more effective pain relief.[74] Finally, an opioid parenteral infusion may be considered if the oral route produces severe gastrointestinal side effects. Similar to the patients in group 1, these patients may or may not be pursuing a

Box 78.2 Paying Attention to Detail Can Make a Huge Difference to Patient Comfort

These factors will facilitate continued pain control during the transition period from hospital to home.

Do *not* discharge a patient in the following conditions:

1. Within 24 hours of a change in route of opioid administration.
2. Within 24 hours of a change in opioid drug.
3. Without written instructions regarding the patient's analgesic regimen.
4. Without a 24-hour resource telephone number for pain management issues.
5. Without a bowel regimen.

If a patient is being discharged on other than the parenteral route of drug administration, *make sure* of the following:

1. That the prescribed drugs are available in the patient's community pharmacy.
2. That the patient has an outpatient prescription plan and, if not, will be able to pay for the pain medication out of pocket.
3. That the patient is given sufficient medication at the time of discharge to continue on the pain management regimen until able to fill the prescription at a community pharmacy.

If a patient is being discharged on a parenteral infusion, do the following:

1. *Avoid* sending the patient home on the weekend if possible.
2. *Give* the patient a 48-hour supply of oral or injectable opioids to take home in case there is a mechanical problem with the pump.

Table 78.1 Grouping of Patients to Help Individualize and Organize Care

Group	Status	Nature of pain	Medications	Setting
1	May or may not pursue curative or life-prolonging treatment	Stable	Oral	Outpatient
2	May or may not pursue curative or life-prolonging treatment	Escalating, unstable	Parenteral (intravenous, subcutaneous)	Outpatient
3	End stage of life	Focus on quality of life	Oral, parenteral as needed	Home-based hospice programs
4	Patients for whom drug diversion is an issue	—	Oral, parenteral	Home or environment where drug diversion may occur
5	Elderly, debilitated (unable to take care of themselves)	—	Oral, parenteral	Extended care facility
6	Cancer survivors	Pain secondary to cancer or its treatment (e.g., neuropathic pain)	Oral, parenteral	Outpatient
7	Older adults, cognitively impaired	—	Oral, parenteral	Extended care facility

course of curative or life-prolonging therapy. They are not imminently dying and do not meet hospice criteria for long-term follow-up. Discharge planning is more complex than for those in group 1 and requires a team approach, with good communication between the hospital and the community. In some institutions, a specific discharge planner, usually a nurse, plays an important role in organizing the home care plan once the needs have been identified by the team. The discharge planner facilitates referral to home care agencies (e.g., a home infusion company) and is able to identify insurance constraints or availability of drug constraints so that alternative avenues may be sought to provide the patient and family with the care that they need.

It is rarely feasible to maintain peripheral intravenous access for continuous infusion in the home. Continuous infusions are usually only considered in patients who have an indwelling central venous port or other long-term central venous device. Placement of one of these devices is occasionally necessary prior to the patient's discharge home in order to accommodate a large volume of fluid—for example, in the case of a fentanyl infusion. In most cases, however, a continuous subcutaneous infusion can accomplish the goals of therapy without the need for intravenous access.

The degree of support that is needed to maintain a parenteral infusion at home varies widely, depending on the patient and family characteristics. Specific educational issues need to be addressed with all patients and caregivers. These include knowledge of drug effects and side effects; the use of rescue doses; operation of the infusion device, specifically turning the pump on and off and changing the battery; and knowledge of how to change the cassette or infusion bag. A minority of patients/families never achieve a comfort level in changing the infusion cassette or bag. In those instances, the infusion home care nurse will usually make the necessary changes. It is mandatory that all patients and their families who are receiving a parenteral infusion at home have a 24-hour resource person available to them to troubleshoot the system (Box 78.3). The most common error encountered in a continuous infusion at home using a computerized pump is incorrect programming—for example, failure to reprogram the pump when the concentration of the opioid in the cassette or bag is changed.[74] This leads to an inadvertent overdosing or underdosing of the patient. Such errors can be largely circumvented through the use of a flowchart kept in the patient's home. Errors will be picked up rapidly if the patient is being adequately monitored. The first sign of an incorrectly programmed pump might be increasing pain or the occurrence of side effects such as increasing sedation or nausea and vomiting.

Box 78.3 Parenteral Opioid Infusion at Home: Troubleshooting the System

Complaints of Increased Pain

1. Evaluate in context of the disease and psychological state.
2. Check needle site, pump setting, cassette/bag content, and concentration.
3. Evaluate the use and amount of "rescue doses."

Complaints of Increased Side Effects (e.g., sedation)

1. Evaluate in context of the disease and psychological state.
2. Check cassette/bag for drug and concentration.
3. Check pump setting and correlate it with cassette/bag content.
4. Evaluate use and amount of "rescue doses."
5. Evaluate other drugs being used.

The cost of a parenteral opioid home infusion may be high.[77] It includes rental of the pump, involvement of a home infusion agency including pharmacy overheads, delivery of the premixed medication to the home, and availability of home infusion nurses on a 24-hour basis. However, the cost of poorly controlled pain is even higher in both human terms and from the need to rehospitalize the patient for uncontrolled pain.[78] Medicare, Medicaid, and most private insurances cover the cost of home infusion pain management, as long as there is a clearly documented indication for such an approach. For Medicare and Medicaid patients, if an opioid other than morphine is being used, a letter is usually needed to explain why the alternative opioid has been chosen. The specific insurance requirements regarding drug specificity must be clarified prior to the patient's discharge.

Group 3 includes patients who are imminently dying and want to go home. Patients in this group may or may not require a parenteral route of drug administration to control their pain. Systems are in place, however, to manage even the most complex patients at home if the family is strongly committed to this end. Various models are in place to facilitate good pain control. Regardless of which model is selected as the optimal mechanism for the delivery of home pain management at the end of life, the common theme for all models is one of an interdisciplinary team approach to care, with the patient and family at the center of such care.

Family caregivers play a major role in home-based palliative care and hospice programs. Generally speaking, higher symptom burden for patients is associated with higher caregiver burden, but most cancer patients opt for care at home during this end stage of life. Anxiety related to ineffective symptom control and fear of administering medication are frequently reported by caregivers across many palliative home care studies, suggesting that education, skill building, and ongoing support for caregivers are essential components of home cancer care and pain management.[79,80]

Hospice care, the most widely available model of home care for the dying, focuses on optimizing quality of life in those not seeking, and unlikely to benefit from, life-sustaining treatment.[70,81] Hospice programs are run by both profit and not-for-profit organizations and have become part of the standard of care offered to patients nearing the end of life. Eligibility requirements for enrollment in a hospice program include a life expectancy of 6 months or less. A major advantage for patients and families followed in a hospice home care program is regular home visits by the hospice nurse and 24-hour emergency support from skilled hospice nurses with backup from the hospice medical staff. In addition, the cost of all medication related to the terminal illness is included in the hospice benefit without additional charge to the patient. Because of the variety of hospice models, levels of sophistication, and depth of services offered, the needs of the patient and the services offered through the program should be evaluated before referral. For example, although most hospice programs have changed their policy toward the use of technology in end-of-life care, in contrast to an earlier "no high-tech" approach, severe restrictions on the financial reimbursement for programs may limit their ability to deliver care to patients requiring the parenteral route of opioid infusion to manage their pain. The physician who refers the dying patient to hospice care can remain as actively involved in the patient's ongoing pain management as he or she chooses to be. In some instances, the referring physician remains the patient's primary physician and works with the hospice team in titrating the opioids to ensure comfort. In other instances, the referring physician asks the hospice physician to assume that role.

Group 4 consists of patients with chronic cancer-related pain who are going home to an environment where it is suspected that drug diversion may occur. The patients themselves may or may not have a history of illicit drug use. In general, patients with a history of drug abuse are at risk for having their pain undertreated.[82,83] Three subgroups of patients can be identified: (1) patients who are actively using street drugs, (2) patients who are in methadone maintenance programs, and (3) patients who have not used illicit drugs for many years.[82]

Patients in the first subgroup strain the resources of even the most sophisticated home management pain team and require strict monitoring during opioid therapy. It must be recognized that these patients, like any other patients, may experience severe pain associated with their cancer but will probably require larger doses of opioids to control the pain because of the development of tolerance. One physician or advanced practice nurse should be identified as the point person to adjust analgesics and write all prescriptions, and one nurse should be identified as the person to organize and coordinate the patient's plan of care.[84] If the patient is on an oral drug regimen, it may be necessary to give only a 1-week supply of the opioid at a time. Giving a larger amount at one time invariably results in the patient "running out of the drug" regardless of the amount given. Psychiatric symptoms and comorbidities such as anxiety, depression, and bipolar disorders are frequently seen in this population and need to be addressed.[82-84] A team approach is essential in the care of these patients. If the patient is in a methadone maintenance program, it is important that the program is contacted for assistance in planning the patient's overall care.

For some patients being discharged home into a drug-abuse or chaotic environment, the use of an oral route of opioid administration is not feasible because of constant drug loss. Occasionally these patients are placed on a parenteral route of opioid administration to ensure adequate pain control and safety, maintain tighter control on the amount of drug used, and minimize the risk of drug diversion. In these situations, no extra opioid cassettes or infusion bags are left in the home and neither the patient nor family is taught how to change the infusion cassette. The home infusion nurse performs bag or cassette changes. In addition, in some situations, cassettes and not bags are used for the infusion, as there is less risk of "siphoning off" the medication. Personal experience using this approach with several patients has been extraordinarily successful. The patient's pain has been controlled and unaccounted for drug usage kept to a minimum. Patients also appear to appreciate the considerable amount of attention they receive. It is, however, time intensive and requires close coordination and communication among the prescribing physician or advanced practice nurse, the home infusion pharmacist, and the home infusion nurse.

Group 5 includes patients with cancer and pain who are unable to be cared for at home and are to be discharged to an extended-care facility. These facilities are rarely able to accommodate a patient whose pain requires a parenteral route of opioid administration. These patients are frequently elderly, debilitated, and receiving polypharmacy for chronic medical conditions. They are at high risk for inadequate pain assessment and consequent undermedication for pain.[85] In addition, the elderly and debilitated patient's therapeutic margin may be narrow, and the patient may be at increased risk for developing troublesome side effects including sedation and confusion.[86] Close monitoring is required, with careful dose titration and adjustment based on ongoing assessment. This requires training, skill, and an institutional system in place that screens for the presence of pain and adequacy of relief on a regularly scheduled basis. Until recently, the staff in long-term care facilities had little training in pain management and end-of-life care. This training is still limited, although the Joint Commission on Accreditation of Healthcare Organizations standards has made such training mandatory.[87]

In the current situation, it is essential that verbal communication be established between the physician/advanced practice nurse or pain management nurse from the discharging institution and the physician and nursing supervisor from the extended-care facility. This communication should take place prior to the patient's discharge to the facility. The two teams can then work together to ensure adequate pain relief for the patient. Some long-term care facilities have established contracts with community hospice programs and have developed palliative care approaches to the care of their residents. As this is still not the norm, the selection of a long-term care facility for someone with cancer and pain must be done with great care.

Group 6 is made up of cancer survivors with chronic pain related to their cancer treatment. With advances in cancer therapy, increasing numbers of patients are being cured of their cancer or living with cancer as a chronic disease. A proportion of this population will develop a pain syndrome and neuropathies as a consequence of the cancer itself or its treatment. Sometimes these conditions resolve over time but irreversible damage to tissue and nerves may have occurred and the pain syndrome becomes chronic.[88]

Neuropathic pain syndromes associated with neurotoxic chemotherapies, surgery such as a mastectomy or thoracotomy, lymph node dissections, and radiation therapy have long been recognized as chronic pain syndromes in cancer survivors. Pain associated with osteoporosis and vertebral fractures, a direct effect of treatment in breast and prostate cancer, or long-term steroid use in brain tumor patients, has more recently been recognized as a significant problem for cancer survivors. Alerting cancer survivors to the possibility that pain can persist following cancer treatment increases the likelihood that such ongoing pain will be reported and addressed.[23] Overall, pain in cancer survivors is probably under-reported and undertreated. Concerns about addiction may be raised for clinicians as well as the patients or their families.

Box 78.4 Home Care Challenges When Managing Pain in Older Adults or the Medically Frail

1. Multiple concurrent medical problems
2. Multiple symptoms
3. Multiple medications and forgetting which to use for which symptom
4. Cognitive impairment including poor memory (confused by instructions, forget what they have been told)
5. Sensory loss including vision and hearing (cannot hear instructions or read them)
6. Under-report pain (fear of hospitalization, taking medications, and being a "complainer")
7. Fearful of using opioids (side effects, addiction)
8. Feelings of being overwhelmed, powerless, demoralized, and hopeless when given information they cannot understand
9. Depression
10. Partner may be an older adult and infirm too
11. Money worries

Group 7 consists of older adults with pain. Pain assessment and management at home presents unique challenges in this group. Older patients frequently under-report their pain. They may have concurrent medical illnesses as well as a variety of painful musculoskeletal disorders unrelated to cancer or its treatment. In addition, older individuals have a higher incidence of cognitive impairment, hearing and visual deficits, and medication side effects than those in younger age groups. This complicates pain management.

Because older adults may have hearing and visual deficits and take longer to process information than younger patients, enough time must be built into the system to allow for effective communication. Speech should be clear and unhurried, words and questions should be rephrased to be sure that they are understood, and the patient should be allowed plenty of time to ask and respond to questions. These same principles apply for the medically frail or terminally ill and are outlined in Box 78.4.

ADDITIONAL ASPECTS OF THE TRANSITION FROM HOSPITAL TO HOME

In preparing patients with chronic pain and their family members to go home, the focus should be on security, clarification of the pain management plan, and communication.[48] A family meeting is often a useful method of consolidating this information.

The central role of the family is acknowledged in the management of pain in the home. It is emphasized that the family will be given ongoing support and backup for day-to-day pain management decisions—for example, the when and how of rescue dose use and the management of opioid side effects should they occur. Of note, the needs of the family when the patient is initially discharged home and their needs later on may be different. When the patient is first discharged home, the family is still learning the basic principles and skills required for pain management. Once these skills have been learned and a routine established, the need is for continuing support and validation.

CLARIFICATION AND WRITTEN INSTRUCTIONS

It is essential that the patient and family are given specific, detailed, written instructions, in layman's language, of the pain management approach to be used, both pharmacologic and nonpharmacologic. The principle underpinning the pain management approach, that analgesics should be used to prevent pain rather than having to be "earned" through experiencing severe pain, is underscored. This principle encompasses addressing the concerns surrounding the prevalence of addiction when opioids are used to manage pain and the clinical significance of tolerance (e.g., that the opioids may no longer be effective if they are used early on in a disease process). In addition, safety issues surrounding opioids in the home need to be reviewed. These include that the opioids be kept in a safe place out of the reach of children; that unused opioids be flushed down the toilet or returned to the prescribing institution for disposal; that if parenteral opioids are used, a syringe and needle disposal kit be obtained; and that needles and syringes, however well wrapped, should not be disposed of in household garbage containers.[48]

COMMUNICATION: THE CORNERSTONE OF GOOD PAIN MANAGEMENT IN THE HOME

The patient and family must have no ambiguity as to whom to call on a 24-hour basis if pain is not well controlled or if the patient experiences troublesome side effects. Tools of communication are reinforced, which include keeping a daily diary to record pain level (using a numeric estimate [e.g., a 0-10 scale] or a categorical scale [e.g., none, slight, moderate, severe]), medication taken, other pain-relieving strategies used, extent and duration of pain relief, activity level, and interference with quality of life. Keeping a pain diary has been found to heighten patient and caregiver awareness of the pattern of pain, guide pain management behaviors, enhance a sense of control, and facilitate communication.[89]

To ensure that the pain management plan instituted in the hospital can be maintained at home, a series of steps can be taken. First, if home care nursing has been instituted, the home care nurse should be contacted to discuss the pain management plan. Second, the community pharmacy should be contacted to ensure that it has the prescribed opioids in stock, or if not, is willing to obtain the medication. In addition, it should be established specifically when the drugs will be available in the home pharmacy so that the patient is not left uncovered. In the event that the local pharmacy neither has nor can obtain the prescribed opioid, an alternative source for the patient must be located prior to discharge from the hospital. Third, the physician or nurse practitioner who will be responsible for writing the opioid prescriptions and titrating the drug must be clearly identified. Fourth, the family should be instructed to establish a routine where the amount of medication remaining is checked on a scheduled basis so that the medication does

Box 78.5 Factors That Place Cancer Patients at High Risk for Poorly Controlled Pain in the Home

Includes patients who have the following conditions:

1. Complex pain syndromes.
2. Advanced disease and rapidly escalating opioid requirements and the need for a parenteral or "unfamiliar" route of drug administration
3. Advanced disease and desire to die at home but with poor community or social supports
4. High levels of physiologic, psychological, and social fatigue or an overwhelmed family
5. Memory or cognitive impairment
6. Discharge to an extended-care facility that does not have a pain management program in place
7. No outpatient prescription plan and financially burdened
8. A history of drug abuse or discharge to a high-risk home environment

not "run out" (the Friday night and holiday syndrome). Some families find it helpful to keep a 1-week supply of the medication to the side, and when they need to go into that supply, it reminds them to call their prescribing clinician for a new prescription. These simple steps can help ease the transition from hospital to home for the patient with chronic pain and the family.[48] Factors that place cancer patients at risk for poorly controlled pain in the home are reflected in Box 78.5.

PROVIDING CONTINUITY OF CARE AND SUPPORT FOR COMPLEX PAIN MANAGEMENT AT HOME

Continuity of care for cancer patients with pain is particularly important. Frequently, patients receive their care in a variety of medical settings.[90-92] Numerous physicians, nurses, and health care professionals are involved. Pain management may or may not have been considered a priority. Effective management approaches may be changed because of unfamiliarity with a specific technology (such as a continuous subcutaneous infusion) or with the community resources (such as a "high-tech" agency's ability to initiate or maintain an infusion in the home) or concern over the amount of opioid a patient is receiving. The hospice movement has addressed the need for continuity of care of the dying patient.[81] A similar need of the cancer patient with chronic pain who is not imminently dying, and the importance of bridging the gap between hospital and community, has been recognized.[91] A palliative care approach, using hospital-based continuity of care or supportive care programs, which bring the expertise of a cancer center to the community, is seen as a valuable component to patient care and addresses the needs of the cancer patient with chronic pain earlier on in the disease process. This model of care is also important for dying patients who either do not have access to a hospice program or who, for a variety of reasons, choose not to be followed by the hospice system of care.

COMMUNICATION TOOLS FOR MONITORING PATIENTS WITH PAIN AT HOME

The use of the telephone is an important aspect of monitoring and managing pain on an outpatient basis.[93,94] In addition, it makes expert resources available to communities where this might not otherwise be the case. Continuity of care also can be fostered through 24-hour telephone availability of a pain management expert (usually an advanced practice nurse) to the patients, their families, and community professionals. Telemonitoring has been widely used in a variety of chronic diseases. For the cancer patient with chronic pain, a telemonitoring system may be a useful tool to reinforce patient and family teaching around medication use and nonpharmacologic approaches to pain control. The system is reasonably inexpensive and can be used through a television or computer screen. As computers have become more commonplace in the home, the use of websites, e-mail, and computer programs to reinforce patient and family teaching and to document changes in the management approach is becoming more commonplace.

SUMMARY

Although the basic principles of pain management are the same whether the patient is being cared for in an acute care setting, at home, or in a long-term care facility, there is a major shift in responsibility for day-to-day pain management when the patient is to be cared for at home. What was primarily the responsibility of the nurse/physician team in the inpatient setting becomes the responsibility of the patient and family. Pain management in the home becomes a family experience, as every aspect of care provided to the patient affects the family system as a whole.

Successful pain management at home depends on an informed and confident patient and family with collaboration and effective communication among the physician or advanced practice nurse, home care nurse, and patient and family. Most important, a system of ongoing monitoring and support for the patient and family must be in place to ensure the effectiveness of pain relief measures and early identification of undue stress on the part of the family. Careful discharge planning helps facilitate appropriate pain management and support for the patient at home and for the family caregivers.

KEY POINTS

- There is a major shift in responsibility for day-to-day pain management when a patient is to be cared for at home.
- What was primarily the responsibility of the nurse/physician team becomes the responsibility of the patient and family.
- Pain management in the home is a family experience.

KEY POINTS—cont'd

- When the patient is seriously ill, frail, or an older adult, assessment and management of pain become more complex. Multiple symptoms and polypharmacy become the norm.
- A family is expected to keep track of and administer multiple medications frequently with minimal training, which may lead to an overwhelmed family, nonadherence to a pain management plan, and poorly controlled pain.
- Comprehensive patient and family assessment helps identify factors that make the patient at risk for having poorly controlled pain in the home setting.
- Tailoring a pain management regimen that fits the patient's and family caregiver's values, goals, and capabilities is important if pain control is to be maintained in the home.
- Family and patient education in pain and symptom management as well as ongoing support from competent pain practitioners are essential.
- Clear, straightforward communication, both verbal and in writing, is a critical component of this education and support.
- Continuity of care can be fostered through the 24-hour telephone availability of a pain management expert to the patients, their families, and community professionals.

SUGGESTED READINGS

Bennett MI, Bagnall AM, Closs SJ. How effective are patient-based educational interventions in the management of cancer pain? Systematic review and meta-analysis. *Pain.* 2009;143:192-199.

Coyle N. Facilitating cancer pain control in the home: opioid related issues. *Curr Pain Headache Rep.* 2001;5:217-226.

Coyle N, Khojainova N, Francavilla JM, Gonzales GR. Audio-visual communication and its use in palliative care. *J Pain Symptom Manage.* 2002;23:171-175.

Coyle N, Layman-Goldstein M. Pain management and pharmacologic and nonpharmacological interventions. In: Matzo M, Witt Sherman D, eds. *Palliative Care Nursing: Quality Care to the End of Life.* New York: Springer Publishing Company; 2010:357-410.

Fletcher BS, Miaskowski C, Given B, Schumacher K. The cancer family caregiving experience: an updated and expanded conceptual model. *Eur J Oncol Nurs.* 2012;16:387-398.

Gilbertson-White S, Aouizerat BE, Jahan T, Miaskowski C. A review of the literature on multiple symptoms, their predictors, and associated outcomes in patients with advanced cancer. *Palliat Support Care.* 2011;9:81-102.

Grant M, Ferrell B. Nursing role implications for family caregiving. *Semin Oncol Nurs.* 2012;28:279-282.

Higginson IJ, Gao W. Caregiver assessment of patients with advanced cancer: concordance with patients, effect of burden and positivity. *Health Qual Life Outcomes.* 2008;6:42.

Kirkova J, Walsh D, Aktas A, Davis MP. Cancer symptom clusters: old concept but new data. *Am J Hosp Palliat Care.* 2010;27:282-288.

Mehta A, Cohen SR, Ezer H, et al. Striving to respond to palliative care patients' pain at home: a puzzle for family caregivers. *Oncol Nurs Forum.* 2011;38:E37-E45.

Moryl N, Coyle N, Essandoh S, Glare P. Chronic pain management in cancer survivors. *J Natl Compr Canc Netw.* 2010;8:1104-1110.

Nguyen LM, Rhondali W, De la Cruz M, et al. Frequency and predictors of patient deviation from prescribed opioids and barriers to opioid pain management in patients with advanced cancer*J Pain Symptom Manage.* Aug 30, 2012:[Epub ahead of print].

Oldham L, Kristjanson L. Development of a pain management program for family careers of advanced cancer patients. *Int J Palliat Nurs.* 2004;10:91-99.

Portenoy RK. Treatment of cancer pain. *Lancet.* 2011;377:2236-2247.

Reinhard SC, Levine C, Samis S. Home alone: family caregivers providing complex chronic care. New York: United Hospital Fund; 2012. Available from www.uhfnyc.org/publications/880853.

Schumacher KL, Koresawa S, West C, et al. Putting cancer pain management regimens into practice at home. *J Pain Symptom Manage.* 2002;23:369-382.

Sun V, Borneman T, Piper B, et al. Barriers to pain assessment and management in cancer survivorship. *J Cancer Surviv.* 2008;2:65-71.

The references for this chapter can be found at www.expertconsult.com.

79

The Health Implications of Disparities in Cancer and Pain Care: Unequal Burdens and Unheard Voices

Carmen R. Green

Several federal agencies have acknowledged and set goals toward eliminating racial and ethnic disparities in health (and health care) and promoting health equity.[1-3] The literature discussing health and health care inequities based on social determinants (e.g., age, race, gender, class) has mostly failed to address the quality of pain care or the impact that pain has on overall health and well-being.[4-9] However, the health and health care disparity literature has often focused on diseases frequently associated with pain, such as cardiovascular disease, cancer, diabetes, osteoarthritis, and obesity.[4,10,11] Unfortunately, pain has been viewed as a symptom and not a disease, even when it persists and has long-term physical (e.g., disability) and emotional (e.g., depression) health implications. In fact, a report of the Institute of Medicine (IOM), *Unequal Treatment: Confronting Racial and Ethnic Disparities in Health Care*, devoted only a few pages to analgesic care for acute and cancer pain, although pain has important and unique health considerations and socioeconomic implications.[12,13] The lack of attention to pain in general and to disparate pain care in particular is also missing from other well-publicized public health agendas designed to improve the nation's colloquial health-related quality of life.[14] Fortunately, the IOM's recent report *Relieving Pain in America: A Blue Print for Transforming Prevention, Care, Education, and Research* acknowledges pain's unique implications, as well as disparate care, while including important policy recommendations.[15]

Race, gender, and age-related health disparities impair public health and are national problems.[6,16-18] An emerging literature has begun to highlight differences in pain perception, as well as disparities in pain care, in racial and ethnic minorities for all types of pain and across all settings.[19,20] Consistent with the social justice literature, in which pain relief is acknowledged to be a fundamental human rights issue, this chapter provides a platform to discuss the impact of pain, pain assessment, and management as a unique and significant public health problem.[21-26]

IMPACT OF PAIN ON OVERALL HEALTH AND WELL-BEING

Pain is defined by the International Association for the Study of Pain (IASP) as an unpleasant sensory and emotional experience associated with actual or potential tissue damage.[27] Pain can further be defined by its cause or duration in terms of acute pain (i.e., pain that is short-lived, usually lasting less than 3 months), cancer-related pain (i.e., pain caused by cancer or its treatment), chronic benign or nonmalignant pain (i.e., pain persisting for longer than 6 months that is not due to cancer), or some combination (e.g., cancer-related chronic pain).[10,27] Aging and increased survival from cancer, diabetes, and trauma have yielded an increase in pain complaints.[28] Regardless of the etiology, pain diminishes overall physical, social, and emotional health.[29,30]

The IOM estimates that more than 100 million Americans live with chronic pain.[15] The increasing prevalence of pain has significant socioeconomic and health ramifications for the individual and progressively impairs collective health in the United States.[13,31-33] The third largest global health problem, pain causes significant psychological, physical, and social perturbations that result in needless suffering and subsequent disability.[12,24,32,34-37] Yet pain is a neglected topic in medicine that leads to concomitant depression, anxiety, post-traumatic stress disorder (PTSD), sleep disturbance, fatigue, and decreased overall physical functioning.[28,33,38,39] Living with pain may also cause an individual to withdraw from societal roles, thereby leading to impaired family, community, and career relationships, and diminish health and quality of life.[29,34,40-43] With these facts in mind, the World Health Organization (WHO) joined the IASP and the European Federation of IASP Chapters to host the first Global Day Against Pain in 2004 to document the tremendous disease burden associated with acute, chronic, and cancer-related pain.[44] The literature suggests that racial and ethnic minorities are disproportionately affected by pain.

THE COST OF PAIN

Currently, pain complaints are the most frequent cause of disability in the United States and lead to more than 700 million lost workdays. The second leading cause of all U.S. physician visits, pain complaints account for more than $500 billion in annual health care expenditures.[45-47] Americans also spend an additional $40 billion per year on chronic pain.[48-50] Older adults use more health care resources (e.g., prescription pain medications, procedures) than younger adults do.[51-54] The prevalence of chronic pain will increase as the U.S. population ages, especially among baby boomers (i.e., those born between 1946 and 1964). Nearly 50% of older Americans live with pain, and racial and ethnic minorities are at increased risk for suboptimal care regardless of age and type of pain.[55-59] By 2030 there will be an estimated 71.5 million people older than 65 years and 137 million individuals of racial and ethnic minorities in the United States.[60,61] More specifically, by 2030 the number of hip and knee replacements is expected to grow by 154% (572,000 procedures) and by 673% (3.48 million procedures), respectively.[62] Without improvements in the quality and availability of care, pain will have devastating socioeconomic and health ramifications for an increasingly aging society. Unfortunately, the medical advantages yielding increased longevity for most white Americans have not been uniformly applied to all Americans.[63-66] For example, racial and ethnic minorities experience many chronic illnesses (e.g., diabetes, cancer) associated with aging and pain and report pain at an earlier age than whites do.[51-54]

Both positive and negative life experiences have an impact on health and pain.[67-70] Chronic pain often coexists with other medical conditions associated with aging (e.g., sleep problems, arthritis, Parkinson's disease, and depression), thereby further impairing health.[71-74] The pain literature focusing on the intersection between race, gender, and aging has primarily dealt with younger adults and white women; the findings from these studies are not readily generalizable to large and growing population groups such as older racial and ethnic minority women.[5,18,75-78] A key concept common to health disparities and the life course perspective is "multiple exposures over the life-course have combined effects on health" (e.g., poverty's negative cumulative effect).[79] It follows that impoverished individuals and racial and ethnic minorities may be particularly vulnerable to diminished health when faced with pain.[80,81] Thus, age, race, gender, and class are important factors in understanding health, pain, and disability.[10,82] Furthermore, the significant gap in the literature will escalate as more Americans (especially women and racial and ethnic minorities) age.

Chronic pain in older adults often accompanies musculoskeletal conditions (e.g., arthritis) and physical disability, and functional limitations arise as a result of muscle disuse, weakness, and atrophy.[52] Older adults often cope with pain by restricting their activities, which leads to depression, dependence, and social isolation.[83-88] Sleep disturbance, anxiety, and increased PTSD symptoms are also associated with chronic pain.[89-92] Women have more pain across the life course than men do, yet chronic pain studies comparing health outcomes and potential racial, ethnic, gender-related, and class disparities across the life span are lacking.[71-74]

HEALTH DISPARITIES AND PAIN

Despite scientific advances and the ability to alleviate suffering, pain and health disparities remain critical public health issues.[28,93] However, the science of health disparities with respect to pain is in its infancy. In 1998 the National Institutes of Health (NIH) held a symposium on pain in women, yet potential variations attributable to race, ethnicity, and aging were not addressed.[94] According to 2000 U.S. census data, 12.4% of the U.S. population was 65 years or older (29% of whom consisted of racial and ethnic minorities and 59% were women).[52,95] By 2030, 20% of the U.S. population will be 65 years or older (50% of the total projected to be members of racial and ethnic minorities and >60% of the total to be women).[95,96] The 2008 NIH exploratory workshop on pain in the elderly acknowledged the importance of social determinants, but data on race, ethnicity, and gender differences were not provided.[3] New knowledge aimed at clarifying the health domains affected and potential racial and ethnic differences at the individual and group level is essential for health care planning. Consistent with the health disparity literature, older adults, racial and ethnic minorities, women, and impoverished individuals (especially low-income racial and ethnic minority women) may be particularly vulnerable to chronic pain's negative sequelae, but few prospective and longitudinal studies have examined pain's impact on vulnerable and underserved populations.[97]

In a retrospective study of 7000 black and white Americans with chronic pain seen at a tertiary care pain center, important differences were found in health based on race and ethnicity.[89,98] Overall, African Americans reported significantly more comorbid conditions, higher pain scores, increased pain severity, more suffering, and less pain control than did white Americans across the age continuum. Black Americans also reported increased physical disability in activities of daily living as a result of pain (e.g., sexual activity, self-care, occupation, family life) and more problems with falling and staying asleep. The mental health of black Americans living with chronic pain was also more negatively affected than that of whites living with chronic pain. Although both black and white Americans met the criteria for clinical depression, black Americans (regardless of age and gender) were significantly more depressed and reported more symptoms consistent with PTSD and anxiety across the age continuum regardless of gender. It is unclear whether these findings reflect undertreatment, over-reporting of differences in pain sensitivity, or some combination of both. Racial and ethnic minorities are frequently more reluctant than white Americans to seek treatment of mental health disorders, and such disorders are often poorly addressed, misdiagnosed, and inadequately treated when they do seek care.[81,99] Nonetheless, it is well documented that most individuals with depression go without treatment. Thus, it follows that pain and its negative sequelae are more likely to decrease the overall health and well-being of racial and ethnic minorities than that of white Americans.

THE PAIN RESPONSE

An individual's response to pain is influenced by complex interactions between biologic, physiologic, emotional, social, and cultural factors.[14,100-105] Differences in pain learning, culturally imposed factors, pain care attitudes and beliefs, comorbid conditions, coping styles, and social roles (i.e., career, community, and family responsibilities) may work cooperatively and competitively to influence the pain experience.[106-109] These differences may predispose some toward multiple actions that maximize rather than minimize threats to bodily integrity and thereby amplify or exacerbate chronic pain.[110,111] People with similar disease activity report differences in pain intensity and its impact.[10,14,100-102]

Experimental models have shown wide variability in response to a painful stimulus.[20,103,104,106,112-120] Race, ethnicity, gender, disease, age, culture, socioeconomic status (SES), past experiences, response bias, and the experimental setting influence pain measurement, coping, health, and the pain response.[31,121-130] However, the clinical relevance of experimentally induced pain and how sociodemographic factors influence clinical pain syndromes remain unknown.

Folkman and colleagues described coping as "a person's cognitive and behavioral efforts to manage the internal and external demands of the person-environment transaction appraised as taxing or exceeding their resources."[131] Maladaptive coping styles (e.g., catastrophizing, repression) and poor adjustment (e.g., poor information seeking, passivity) influence the response to pain.[107,108,132,133] Passive coping and catastrophizing are detrimental to successfully coping with a pain problem.[102,132,134,135] Social support also has a significant role in coping with many chronic conditions and plays an important role in pain management.[136] Well-validated models support the role of pain-related fear and postulate behavioral responses (e.g., confrontation, avoidance) that ultimately determine outcome. Most models propose that people in pain become enmeshed in a downward spiral of increased fear, avoidance, anxiety, depression, disability, and pain.[130,137,138] When there is no pain-related fear and rapid confrontation, an adaptive response yielding recovery and better functioning occurs.[139-141] Unfortunately, most coping illness models were tested on primarily homogeneous white and younger adult populations and did not consider social roles. Thus, these models are not generalizable to growing populations, which is a critical limitation in an aging and diversifying society.[137]

Differences in coping have been identified. Several studies have revealed that blacks with chronic pain report more suffering from the pain than do whites regardless of age or gender.[89,98] Blacks tend to use religious coping (e.g., church participation), wishful thinking, and social support systems when dealing with stress more than whites do.[142,143] They often describe stoicism and believe that pain is inevitable but fear reporting their pain because family and friends may not understand. Associations between John Henryism (i.e., actively coping with stressors by working increasingly harder against potentially insurmountable obstacles) and higher blood pressure, hypertension, and bodily pain were described in a general population of older blacks.[130,137,138] In view of the high prevalence of hypertension in racial and ethnic minorities, further investigations are necessary to see whether John Henryism is actually detrimental or helpful to racial and ethnic minorities with chronic pain. Green and associates showed that blacks with chronic pain tend to believe more so than whites that race and ethnicity affect the health care and pain care that they receive.[144] Black patients also tend to believe that good patients avoid talking about pain and that pain medications cannot really control pain.[144]

SES also influences pain.[145] Living in a resource-poor neighborhood was found to affect older blacks more than older whites, thus confirming that neighborhood resources contribute to the negative consequences of chronic pain.[128] A study comparing younger black and white Americans reported that increasing neighborhood resources is associated with decreased negative chronic pain outcomes.[146] In other studies, racial and ethnic minorities, low-income individuals, and older adults were found to face structural barriers to obtaining prescription analgesics in their local pharmacies even when their pain was assessed and treated.[59,147] Comorbid diseases commonly associated with pain (e.g., cancer) also influence health and well-being more frequently in blacks than in whites.[78] Differences in coping styles, health status, health service access and use, social roles, sociodemographic characteristics, and stressors may also predispose some individuals to an adaptive or ineffective response to pain.[20,114,148-151] Thus, race, ethnicity, SES, neighborhood resources, and comorbid conditions are important considerations when examining the impact of pain on health and health care.[128]

ACCESS TO PAIN CARE

System-related variables (e.g., health services access and use, health insurance), as well as stressors (e.g., social roles, comorbid conditions) and resources (e.g., wealth, poverty), influence health and health care.[8,59,152,153] Health insurance coverage does not ensure quality health or pain care.[154] Regardless of age, black Americans with chronic pain had diminished health when compared with whites with chronic pain.[98] Racial and ethnic minorities with health insurance also reported increased difficulty accessing and paying for quality health and pain care than did similar white Americans.[144] Black Americans also believed that race, ethnicity, culture, and gender influenced access to both health care and pain care more than white Americans did.[144] These disparate attitudes have significant implications in potentially vulnerable, marginalized, and underserved populations already at risk for decreased access to primary care and specialty pain care, as well as suboptimal pain assessment and management.[155]

The absence of health insurance, a primary care physician, or a usual source of medical care diminishes access to quality pain care and contributes to the use of emergency services for preventable problems.[44,144] Racial and ethnic minorities and low-income individuals are less likely to have a regular primary care physician and have less access to specialty care.[156,157] The literature has revealed that blacks and low-income people with chronic pain believe more frequently than whites do that they should have been referred to a pain center sooner, report decreased access to health care overall, and believe that race and ethnicity influenced pain care.[144] Since racial and ethnic minority status and income are often interrelated, rising co-payment for health care services and economic downturns tend to have a greater impact on racial and ethnic minorities, who also have increased disease burden for many comorbid conditions associated with pain (e.g., diabetes, cancer), disproportionately more so than whites even when access to quality pain care is available.[16,64,158] Nonetheless, these individuals report less access to pain management specialists, receive less pain medication, and are at risk for having their pain poorly assessed and undertreated.[19,93,159]

PAIN ASSESSMENT

The first building block to ensure quality pain care is optimizing pain assessment. Disability, depression, and pain intensity issues often complicate pain assessment and treatment.[19,56,160] Overall, the failure to optimize pain assessment and treatment contributes to poor health.[19] Despite the economic, psychological, familial, and social impact of pain, as well as an extensive literature documenting the benefits of optimizing pain management and guidelines designed to improve pain management, this information is not universally taken into account.[115-120] One major challenge in optimizing pain care is that pain is subjective with no objective measures, and thus implementing quality pain care can be problematic across the continuum of care. Another important limitation is that most guidelines rarely address the role of social determinants despite evidence that age, race, ethnicity, gender, and SES influence communication and pain care.[161]

Patient-physician communication is fraught with difficulties.[144,162-168] The literature describes racial and ethnic differences in the ability to discuss pain complaints and negotiate pain treatment plans with physicians. Women and racial and ethnic minorities are at risk for receiving poorer quality pain care than men are.[56,57] Patient expectations for the patient-physician relationship do not differ by race and ethnicity, but their experiences, perceptions, and satisfaction differ significantly.[169] Physicians were more verbally dominant, engaged in less patient-centered communication, used less rapport building, rated conditions as less severe (even when there were no differences), and provided less information in encounters with racial and ethnic minorities than they did with whites.[166,170-175] Racial and ethnic differences in patient-physician interactions help explain the disparities in patient satisfaction, but not in use of health services.[175,176] When tested in an experimental design, cancer patients receiving coaching discussed their pain concerns more, thereby reducing disparities.[174,177] Thus, empowered patient-physician communication that encourages patients to ask questions and express concerns, as well as racial concordance, has been shown to reduce disparities.[178-181]

PATIENT VARIABILITY

Intra-race variability in pain complaints has been observed. Younger blacks reported higher pain intensity and depression than older blacks did.[89] When comparing health status and pain treatment perceptions in older adults, blacks were significantly younger; reported more bodily pain, poorer health, and more problems with social functioning; and had greater role limitations because of emotional problems than white Americans did.[89,92] After controlling for age, marital status, education, and pain duration in younger women with chronic pain, black women were found to have greater pain intensity, depression, disability, and PTSD symptoms than did white women.[182] Another study identified three clusters of patients with chronic pain within age, race, and gender groups: (1) chronic pain syndrome, (2) good pain control, and (3) disability with a mild pain syndrome.[130] Blacks and younger adults were more likely to have chronic pain syndrome.[138] Blacks with "chronic pain syndrome" or disability with mild pain syndrome reported higher disability than did their counterparts.[130] Older patients and women in the good pain control group reported lower levels of pain and depression, whereas those with "disability with mild pain syndrome" had lower pain and depression.[182] Thus, the response to chronic pain varies according to race, gender, and age.[130]

Race and ethnicity influence pain management–seeking behavior, but the mechanisms remain unclear. What is clear is that the pain complaints of racial and ethnic minorities, older adults, impoverished people, and women are often not treated the same as the pain complaints of white men, who receive better-quality care.[103,183,184] Patient behavior, how patients communicate (e.g., language barriers), physician-patient communication, and stereotyping can complicate assessment.[185-191] Communication differences increase the likelihood of pain complaints being discounted. In addition, most measures used to assess pain lacked cultural and linguistic sensitivity and were not validated in racially and ethnically diverse populations, thus contributing to the persistence of disturbing racial and ethnic disparities in health and pain care.[192-196]

CLINICIAN VARIABILITY IN PAIN MANAGEMENT DECISION MAKING

Although pain complaints are very common, they are often poorly managed. Patients report that their pain complaints are frequently unheard and undertreated by physicians.[115,167-169] In addition, clinicians report that they are not knowledgeable or satisfied with the pain care that they provide.[55-57,160] Given these considerations, it is surprising that pain education remains a neglected topic in most medical, nursing, dental, and pharmacy school curricula, a shortcoming that further contributes to poor pain care.[123,197-201] A study of practicing Michigan physicians revealed that nearly 30% reported that they had not received any medical school, residency, or continuing medical education specifically directed at managing pain.[57] Thus, physicians and other health care providers are ill equipped to assess and treat pain. Consequently, it is not surprising that most clinicians express low satisfaction, confidence, and goals when treating pain while also prescribing better treatment (e.g., referral to specialist) for men than for women, even when women had similar or more pain than men did.[55-57,89,202] In addition, health care system factors, trust, legal factors, and health care provider decision making influence pain assessment regardless of guidelines designed to ensure adequate pain care.

The worker's compensation literature also provides evidence of disparate pain care.[153,203] Blacks were twice as likely to be disabled 6 months following an occupational back injury, and blacks without legal representation received less treatment and lower disability ratings than did whites without legal representation.[204,205] Overall, Tait and Chibnall found that race and SES disparities are present in the worker's compensation system, with black men receiving less compensation than white men for similar injuries.[203]

The quality of physician-prescribed pain care also varies with respect to race, ethnicity, and gender for similar pain problems.[19,93,185,206-209] In a retrospective study of emergency care, a twofold difference in receiving analgesics based on ethnicity was noted in emergency room patients with isolated long-bone fractures, and 55% of Hispanics received no pain medications for similar injuries as whites.[206]

The cancer pain literature shows health care and cancer care disparities, with blacks suffering more severe cancer-related pain, inaccurate pain assessment, and inadequate pain treatment in comparison to whites.[19,82,210] The cancer survivor literature reveals similar results, with women having higher rates of pain and blacks suffering greater interference. Multiple factors influence the disparities in cancer care: (1) environmental variables (e.g., segregation, exposure to toxins), (2) patient sociodemographic factors and differences in pain sensitivity (e.g., health behavior, beliefs, attitudes, and coping strategies), (3) health care provider factors (e.g., pain knowledge and education, cultural competence, language barriers, stereotypes, and bias), and (4) health care system variables (e.g., health insurance, access to care). It follows that these factors may play a significant role in disparities in pain care.

Racial and ethnic minority cancer patients were prescribed less potent analgesics and were significantly undertreated with respect to the WHO recommendations for managing cancer pain. Those treated at university centers or centers primarily caring for racial and ethnic minorities were more likely to receive inadequate analgesia than were whites treated elsewhere and in the community.[30,211-213] Other studies have shown that physicians underestimate pain severity in Hispanic and black patients.[214,215] For instance, Bernabei and coworkers showed that black nursing home residents were less likely to have their pain assessed; if their pain was assessed, they still received less pain medication than white residents did.[159] Although 40% of blacks with cancer pain reported daily pain, 25% received no analgesics whatsoever. Green and colleagues recently revealed shortcomings in assessing and treating breakthrough pain (pain flares interrupting well-controlled baseline pain) in advanced cancer, with women and racial and ethnic minorities reporting increased pain and worse health.[216,217]

Green and associates showed that chronic pain was poorly assessed and treated, with blacks and women being adversely affected.[56,89] Suboptimal pain care in all clinical settings combined with clinician variability in pain management decision making complicates pain therapy in racial and ethnic minorities and women.[89] A Michigan study revealed that 20% of cancer survivors experienced cancer-related chronic pain, with women and blacks disproportionately affected.[218] Green and Ndao-Brumblay also showed that blacks used less complementary and alternative medicine techniques (including acupuncture) and significantly less manipulation, biofeedback, or relaxation training than did whites for chronic pain.[219] Thus, poor pain assessment, inadequate pain treatment, and decreased ability to obtain pain medications (even when prescribed) complicate appropriate and quality pain management of racial and ethnic minority persons, thereby impairing their overall health and well-being. In general, these studies illustrate that racial and ethnic minorities and low-income people experience more disease burden, receive less pain relief, and are less likely than whites to be adequately assessed for all types of pain and in all settings.

Racial and ethnic minorities face additional barriers to adequate pain management. In two pharmacy studies, those located in minority neighborhoods were less likely to carry opioid analgesics than were those in nonminority neighborhoods.[147] After accounting for zip code median income and stratifying by income, Green and coworkers found structural barriers for racial and ethnic minorities, low-income whites, and older adults, who experienced increased difficulty getting their opioid analgesic prescriptions filled in their local pharmacies across Michigan.[59] Surprisingly, low-income whites had better access to opioid analgesics than did high-income racial and ethnic minorities. Thus, clinician perceptions and goals may lead to the undertreatment of pain (especially in racial and ethnic minorities).

CRITICAL QUESTIONS AND NEW DIRECTIONS

The potential implications of poorly treated pain are devastating for the individual, and the cost to society is staggering. Pain profoundly affects morbidity, mortality, quality of life,[3] and health care expenditures. Therefore, ensuring optimal pain management is critically important from a public health perspective.[220,221] Both patient and physician variability in attitudes and beliefs contributes to suboptimal pain care (with racial and ethnic minorities, low-income people, older adults, and women receiving lower-quality pain care).[82,93,168,222] Pain's impact and prevalence will increase as Americans live longer and have a profound effect on morbidity and health care expenditures. Assessment remains the cornerstone of quality pain care.[54,122,223-228] Despite chronic pain's individual and socioeconomic impact, documented benefits in optimizing pain care, therapeutic advances currently available to treat chronic pain, and guidelines for managing pain, physicians and other health care providers are ill equipped to assess and treat chronic pain.* There are also important questions regarding estimates of the amount of pain (severity) and its correlates (physical, emotional, and social burden) in different groups, the extent of poorly assessed and treated pain, planning for the amount of health care required, improving pain care delivery, and differences and variability in quality and the way that health services are provided based on social determinants.

There is evidence that all types of pain have unique health implications in racial and ethnic minorities that are often unrecognized or overlooked.[19,89,98,115] No longitudinal and prospective studies have examined the long-term effects of pain on overall health and well-being in an ethnically diverse population. In addition to race and ethnicity, other social determinants may make certain racial and ethnic minorities more vulnerable to pain. Thus, racial and ethnic minority individuals who are elderly, impoverished, or women are extremely vulnerable to the distressing effects of pain.[84,89,98,130,233-237] Culturally and linguistically appropriate interventions must be developed to ensure quality pain assessment and management so that racial and ethnic disparities in pain care can be eliminated. The role of clinician and patient-provider variability in pain management decision making, as well as health insurance, health care system, and regulatory factors, must be examined. By improving pain care for the most underserved and

*56,57,89,116,119,121,123,144,229-232

vulnerable populations in our society, it will be improved for all.[154,238,239] In a climate of increasing patient safety concerns, inadequate pain assessment and treatment must be viewed as a quality-of-care issue.[240-242] Pain relief is fundamentally a human rights issue, whereas inadequate pain care is fundamentally a medical error.[243,244] Beyond being a quality issue, inequitable pain care based on sociodemographic characteristics is fundamentally a social justice issue. There is a critical need for increased awareness, advocacy, and health care and pain care policy to rectify these ills. Also needed are physician, health care provider, and health system leadership and interventions that ensure (1) access to quality and equitable patient-centered primary care and multidisciplinary pain care that is culturally and linguistically sensitive; (2) the ability to optimize pain assessment and the comorbid conditions often associated with pain by increasing pain education for both patients and clinicians; (3) comprehensive and multidisciplinary approaches, evidence-based guidelines, and research and policy initiatives; and (4) establishment of mechanisms to ensure access to the resources needed to prevent and manage pain at the neighborhood level.

KEY POINTS

- More than 100 million Americans live with chronic pain, and racial and ethnic minorities and women are disproportionately affected.
- Both positive and negative life experiences have an impact on pain and contribute to differences in the pain experience in racial and ethnic minorities, women, older adults, and impoverished persons.
- By 2030, 20% of the U.S. population will be 65 years or older (50% of the total projected to be members of racial and ethnic minorities and >60% of the total to be women).
- Racial and ethnic minorities have decreased access to pain care, are at risk for suboptimal pain assessment and management, and have adverse health outcomes.
- Race and ethnicity, socioeconomic status, gender, and age also influence the quality of pain care, use of health services, clinician decision making, and health outcomes.
- Both patient intra- and inter-race variability and clinician variability contribute to disparities in health and pain care.

SUGGESTED READINGS

Anderson KO, Green CR, Payne R. Racial and ethnic disparities in pain: causes and consequences of unequal care. *J Pain.* 2009;10:1187-1204.

Anderson KO, Richman SP, Hurley J, et al. Cancer pain management among underserved minority outpatients: perceived needs and barriers to optimal control. *Cancer.* 2002;94:2295-2304.

Bonham VL. Race, ethnicity, and pain treatment: striving to understand the causes and solutions to the disparities in pain treatment. *J Law Med Ethics.* 2001;29:52-68.

Chibnall JT, Tait RC. Disparities in occupational low back injuries: predicting pain-related disability from satisfaction with case management in African Americans and Caucasians. *Pain Med.* 2005;6:39-48.

Cousins MJ, Brennan F, Carr DB. Pain relief: a universal human right. *Pain.* 2004;112:1-4.

Edwards RR, Moric M, Husfeldt B, et al. Ethnic similarities and differences in the chronic pain experience: a comparison of African American, Hispanic, and white patients. *Pain Med.* 2005;6:88-98.

Green CR. Being present: the role of narrative medicine in reducing the unequal burden of pain. *Pain.* 2011;152:965-966.

Green CR, Anderson KO, Baker TA, et al. The unequal burden of pain: confronting racial and ethnic disparities in pain. *Pain Med.* 2003;4:277-294.

Green CR, Baker TA, Smith EM, et al. The effect of race in older adults presenting for chronic pain management: a comparative study of black and white Americans. *J Pain.* 2003;4:82-90.

Green CR, Hart-Johnson T. The adequacy of chronic pain management prior to presenting at a tertiary care pain center: the role of patient socio-demographic characteristics. *J Pain.* 2010;11:746-754.

Green CR, Hart-Johnson T. The association between race and neighborhood socioeconomic status in younger black and white adults with chronic pain. *J Pain.* 2012;13:176-186.

Green CR, Hart-Johnson T, Loeffler DR. Cancer-related chronic pain: examining quality of life in diverse cancer survivors. *Cancer.* 2011;117:1994-2003.

Green CR, Montague L, Hart-Johnson T. Consistent and breakthrough pain in diverse advanced cancer patients: a longitudinal examination. *J Pain Symptom Manage.* 2009;37:831-847.

Green CR, Nado-Brumblay SK, Nagrant AM, et al. Race, age, and gender influences among clusters of African American and white patients with chronic pain. *J Pain.* 2004;5:171-182.

Green CR, Nado-Brumblay SK, West B, et al. Differences in prescription opioid analgesic availability: comparing minority and white pharmacies across Michigan. *J Pain.* 2005;6:689-699.

Green CR, Wheeler JR, LaPorte F. Clinical decision making in pain management: contributions of physicians and patient characteristics to variations in practice. *J Pain.* 2003;4:29-39.

Kalauokalani D, Franks P, Oliver JW, et al. Can patient coaching reduce racial/ethnic disparities in cancer pain control? Secondary analysis of a randomized controlled trial. *Pain Med.* 2007;8:17-24.

Smedley BD, Stith AY, Nelson AR. *Unequal Treatment: Confronting Racial and Ethnic Disparities in Health Care.* Washington, DC: National Academies Press; 2002.

Todd K, Samaroo N, Hoffman J. Ethnicity as a risk factor in inadequate emergency department analgesia. *JAMA.* 1993;269:1537-1539.

The references for this chapter can be found at www.expertconsult.com.

PART 9

RESEARCH, ETHICS, AND REIMBURSEMENT IN PAIN

DENNIS C. TURK, EDITOR

PART OUTLINE

80 Clinical Trial Design Methodology for Pain Outcome Studies

Thomas R. Vetter | Roger Chou

It is traditionally held that the first comparative clinical trial was performed in 1747 by Dr. James Lind (1716-1794) of the British Royal Navy to identify a treatment for scurvy. Lind evenly assigned 12 scurvy-afflicted sailors aboard the HMS *Salisbury* to receive cider, vitriol (a weak acid), vinegar, seawater, oranges and lemons, or nutmeg paste.[1] After 6 days, only the two sailors who had received oranges and lemons (and thus adequate amounts of vitamin C) had sufficiently recovered to return to duty. Two centuries later, the advent of the pharmaceutical industry and the evolution of methodological concepts led to the first controlled clinical trial in which patients were randomly assigned to different treatments. Performed in 1947-1948, it observed the effects of streptomycin on pulmonary tuberculosis to be significantly better than those of a placebo.[2,3]

EVIDENCE-BASED MEDICINE

In contrast, common acceptance of the merit of individual medical or surgical practice—the proverbial "in my experience" (N of one), "in case after case, I have seen" (N of two), and "in my series" (N of three)—evidence-based medicine (EBM) acknowledges that simple intuition, unsystematic clinical experience, and a pathophysiologic rationale are inadequate bases for clinical decision making.[4] EBM stresses the critical examination of evidence from clinical research. EBM likewise offers a formal set of steps to complement medical training and "common sense" for clinicians to effectively interpret the results of clinical research ("how to read a paper") and apply them in their practice (Box 80.1). Last, EBM places a lower value on expert authority than the traditional medical paradigm.[5-8]

Many systems for grading the level or quality of evidence and the strength of recommendations have been created. Unfortunately, guideline developers around the world are inconsistent in how they rate quality of evidence and grade strength of recommendations—resulting in confusion among guideline users.[9] Although the Grading of Recommendations Assessment, Development and Evaluation (GRADE) Working Group is not without limitations,[10] it defines and clearly delineates all of the major domains that affect the reliability of research evidence, including the quantity, quality, consistency, and types of studies of the published evidence, resulting in one of three grades of evidence (high, moderate, or low). GRADE also assigns a rating for strength of evidence of strong or weak, based on the estimate of net benefit relative to harms and other factors, including the quality of evidence, importance of patient preferences and values, as well as costs and burdens. Each recommendation is thus assigned one of six possible grades, based on the strength of the recommendation and the quality of evidence (Table 80.1). Many groups—including the Cochrane Collaboration, the American College of Physicians (ACP), the American College of Chest Physicians (ACCP), the U.S. Agency for Healthcare Research and Quality (AHRQ), the UK National Institute for Health and Clinical Excellence (NICE), and the World Health Organization (WHO)—have adopted GRADE.

Since the term was coined about 30 years ago,[12] evidence-based medicine (EBM) has progressed from a novel concept to a buzzword to a mantra.[13] Along these lines, it has been observed: "Clinical decisions should, as far as possible, be evidence based. So runs the current clinical dogma. We are urged to lump all the relevant randomised controlled trials into one giant meta-analysis and come out with a combined odds ratio for all decisions."[14] EBM is thus often misconstrued as being only about randomized clinical trials, when it has actually evolved, along with the efforts of GRADE, specifically to take into account evidence from observational studies.

THE SPECTRUM OF OUTCOMES RESEARCH

The appraisal of a new or existing treatment modality—including for pain management—involves three steps (Fig. 80.1).[15-19] First, the efficacy, or whether a treatment achieves its intended clinical benefits ("Can it work?"), is demonstrated under "optimal" circumstances in highly controlled settings with carefully selected patients, typically in a randomized controlled trial. Subsequently, the effectiveness, or whether these benefits are also seen under more ordinary or "naturalistic" circumstances, is assessed ("Does it work?"), often by way of an analytic cohort study, though randomized controlled trials can also be designed to evaluate effectiveness. The efficiency or cost-effectiveness (the health status improvement realized for a given amount of resources expended) is sometimes determined via a health care economic evaluation ("Is it worth it?"). An economic evaluation can also provide crucial insight into the value of providing a health care intervention to a specific population.[20]

Importantly, in order for an intervention to be cost-effective, it must first be shown to be effective. For example, routine imaging for low back pain in the absence of red flags is associated with no benefit in pain or function compared to usual care without routine imaging.[21] Therefore, even though lumbar x-rays are relatively inexpensive, routine imaging with them cannot be cost-effective. On the other hand, interventions associated with relatively high upfront costs can still be cost-effective if the clinical benefits are substantial or the upfront costs are offset by decreased downstream costs. For example, some studies suggest that spinal cord stimulators for failed back surgery syndrome may be a cost-effective treatment compared to medical management,[22] though others suggest that the high upfront costs may not be offset by lower costs of subsequent care.[21]

EXPERIMENTAL VERSUS OBSERVATIONAL STUDY DESIGNS

Many clinician scientists (not to mention journal editors and reviewers) have viewed the randomized controlled trial as the de facto gold standard of clinical trial design for evaluating the efficacy and safety of a treatment or intervention.[23] However, although a well-conducted randomized trial is generally more valid than other study designs for providing valid (true) results, there are a number of other study designs, which may on a situational basis be more appropriate to apply in conducting human research.[24] For example, for evaluating harms, it may be unethical to randomize patients, or for rare or long-term harms, adequately powered randomized trials may not be feasible.[25]

Box 80.1 The Five Steps of Evidence-Based Medicine and Related Clinical Practice[8]

1. Asking focused questions: Translation of uncertainty to an answerable question.
2. Finding the evidence: Systematic retrieval of best evidence available.
3. Critical appraisal: Testing evidence for validity, clinical relevance, and applicability.
4. Making a decision: Application of results in practice.
5. Evaluating performance: Auditing evidence-based decisions.

The array of quantitative study designs are classified as experimental or observational, with observational studies being further divided into descriptive and analytic categories (Fig. 80.2).[23,26-30] Observational studies can complement findings from often smaller-scale randomized controlled trials by assessing treatment effectiveness in patients in more realistic day-to-day clinical practice.[31] However, it is important to note that a randomized trial is not necessarily an efficacy study, nor is an observational study necessarily an effectiveness study. Rather, the methods used to ensure that a study evaluates more representative populations, interventions, and comparisons; evaluates patient-centered outcomes; and is conducted in settings typically encountered in clinical practice are what determine whether a study is an efficacy or effectiveness study.[32]

RANDOMIZED CONTROLLED TRIAL

In contrast to observational studies, in which the allocation of interventions is outside of the control of the researchers, clinical trials are a type of experimental study in which the interventions are allocated by the researchers. A controlled

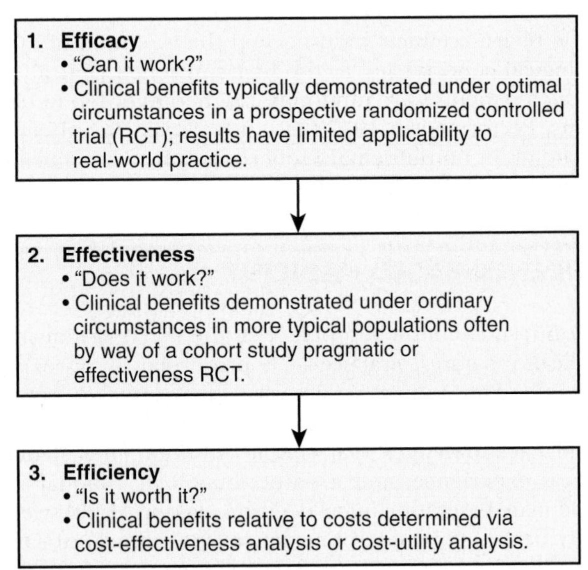

Figure 80.1 The three sequential steps involved in the appraisal of a new or existing health care intervention.[15,19]

Table 80.1 System for Grading Evidence Incorporating the Quality of Published Evidence and Strength of Recommendations (GRADE system)[9,11]

Strength of recommendations ↓	**Quality of evidence →**	A = High quality: consistent evidence from RCTs without important limitations or exceptionally strong evidence from observational studies	B = Moderate quality: RCTs with limitations or very strong evidence from observational studies	C = Evidence for at least one critical outcome from observational studies, case series, RCTs with serious flaws, or indirect evidence
1 = Strong: Desirable effects clearly outweigh undesirable effects		1A	1B	1C
2 = Weak: Desirable effects closely balanced with undesirable effects		2A	2B	2C

RCTs, randomized controlled trials.

clinical trial involves the comparison of two or more interventions in order to assess their relative benefits and harms.

The manner in which treatments are assigned in controlled clinical trials is critical. When treatment determinations are based in part on known patient characteristics, the allocation of treatments is typically based in part on the assessed likelihood to benefit, overall health status, socioeconomic considerations, or other factors that influence clinical outcomes. Therefore, an inherent shortcoming of such nonrandomized controlled clinical trials is that it is not possible to determine whether differences in outcomes between interventions are due to the interventions themselves or to other confounding variables.

A randomized controlled trial (RCT) on the other hand, is a type of controlled clinical trial predicated on participants being assigned to the possible exposures or interventions purely by the play of chance ("flip of a coin").[23] When successfully implemented, random allocation produces two or more treatment groups that are free of selection and confounding bias—by both known and unknown factors.[33] When those involved in an RCT are blinded (masked) as to the intervention each participant receives, treatment and assessment bias are also reduced.[34] Thus, when properly designed and performed, an RCT has internal validity: it accurately and reliably measures what it is intended to measure—that is, the relative benefits and harms of two or more interventions. When sample sizes are determined based on an appropriate power analysis, an RCT can efficiently detect small to moderate group outcome differences with the minimum sample size, which exposes the least number of study subjects to the risks of treatment and nontreatment.[35]

A randomized trial of transcutaneous electrical nerve stimulation (TENS) for low back pain illustrates an example of how an RCT can be designed to overcome potential sources of bias and address critical clinical questions.[36] By randomizing patients to TENS versus sham TENS, rather than usual care or no treatment, the trial was better able to control for potential effects that knowledge of receiving an active treatment might have. In addition, the trial randomized patients to exercise or no exercise. Because exercise and TENS are often used together in clinical practice, it is important to understand whether there are any additive benefits. Finally, blinding can be a challenge because TENS is associated with sensations that patients can perceive. Therefore, the researchers designed the study to exclude patients with prior experience with TENS (who would be familiar with the sensations), used sham units identical to functioning units, and performed follow-up, lead placements, and adjustments in an identical fashion. Subsequent analysis showed that blinding was in fact successful. Unlike previous studies of TENS, this RCT found no difference between TENS and sham TENS in pain scores.[37]

CLUSTER RANDOMIZED CONTROLLED TRIAL

A cluster randomized trial (CRT) is a trial in which individuals are randomized in groups—the group as a whole is randomized and not the individual. Physicians, group practices, health plans, or even geographic regions (counties or states) can be defined as clusters. In a CRT, all individuals within a given cluster are assigned to the same study arm.[38] The methodology of cluster randomized trials has been widely discussed.[39-41] In evaluating a therapy, unlike a standard RCT, a CRT typically focuses on effectiveness by evaluating outcomes under conditions of actual use. A CRT is often done when individual randomization is not feasible. For example, if a clinician is implementing a new low back pain evaluation and treatment study protocol, it would be difficult to randomize some patients in a clinic to one protocol and other patients to another protocol, because there is too much shared knowledge of the different protocols and overlap in clinic personnel. The CRT can also offer considerable cost and time efficiencies when implemented by a health insurance plan that has extensive existing information about its members and their treatments and outcomes, along with an existing research infrastructure.[38] However, compared with individually randomized trials, cluster randomized trials are more complex to design, require more participants to

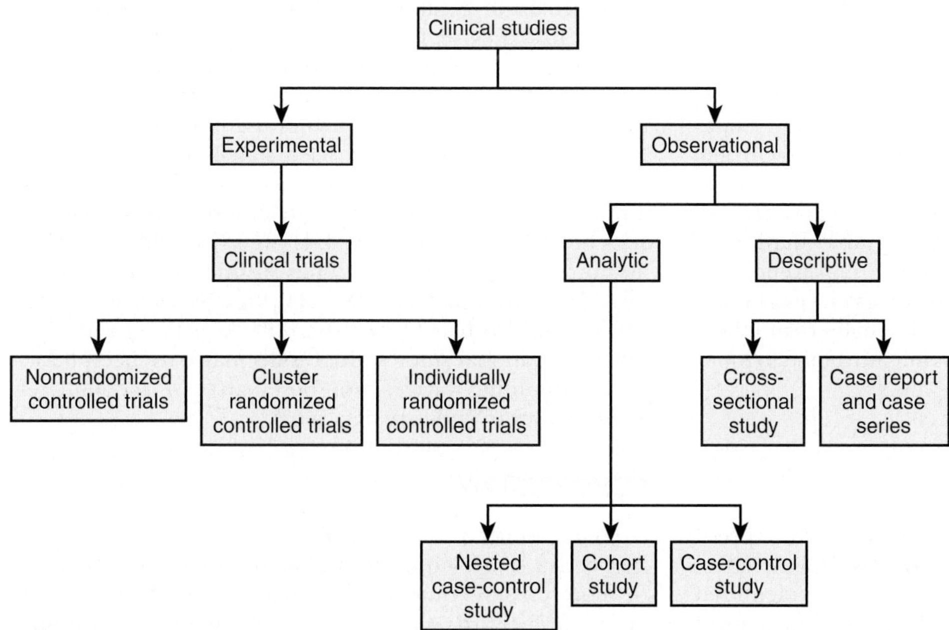

Figure 80.2 Classification of clinical study designs.

obtain equivalent statistical power, and require more complex analysis (e.g., adjustment for the intracluster correlation coefficient of the cluster randomization).[42-44] A CRT is also typically not blinded. Thus, not surprisingly, the use of this trial design has been fraught with challenges, undermining the validity of some published findings.[43,45]

For example, a cluster randomized clinical trial investigated the effect of an evidence-based psychosocial educational program (PSEP) on low back pain (LBP) beliefs for 3792 soldiers completing military training.[46] The military training environment requires living in close quarters with other members of the military unit (company), thus making individual randomization unfeasible. A cluster randomization strategy was thus used for assigning entire companies of soldiers to receive or not receive the PSEP. This meant that for a given company, every soldier who consented to the study received either the PSEP or no education (the control group). The primary outcome measure was the back beliefs questionnaire (BBQ), which assesses the inevitable consequences of and ability to cope with LBP. Compared to baseline, at 12 weeks follow-up, soldiers who received the PSEP had an improvement in their BBQ scores ($P < 0.0001$). Unfortunately, the cluster correlation coefficient was not reported. In addition, it was not possible to blind soldiers to the educational intervention received, though analyses suggested that differences in attrition across groups had little effect on the conclusions.

CROSS-SECTIONAL STUDY

A cross-sectional study determines the prevalence (i.e., the existing presence) of a disease at a given point or period in time. If its sample is randomly chosen, such a frequency survey provides a valid snapshot of the characteristics of the source population. It thus can provide an estimate of the magnitude of a problem and thus the significance and rationale for further investigation. A cross-sectional study cannot assess possible causality between a predictor variable (e.g., gender and socioeconomic status) and an outcome variable (e.g., pain intensity). Although a cross-sectional study also cannot assess the comparative outcomes (benefits and risks) of an intervention, the findings of a cross-sectional study can generate hypotheses for further studies.[26-30,47,48]

For instance, a cross-sectional study was conducted in a nationally representative sample of 27,035 United States (U.S.) adults to estimate the point prevalence of chronic pain and to describe sociodemographic and other characteristics of chronic pain.[49] The results of this cross-sectional, Internet-based survey revealed a considerable burden of chronic pain among U.S. adults. Although experienced by 31% of overall respondents, chronic pain was more common with lower socioeconomic status and in females than males. Primary chronic pain was most commonly attributed to lower back pain, followed by osteoarthritis pain.[49]

CASE-CONTROL STUDY

A case-control study is aimed at determining the relationship between a single outcome (disease) and one or more previous possible contributing factors (exposures). Case-control studies look or work backward, starting with the identified outcome or disease (exposures ← disease). Case-control studies are retrospective, relying on existing data or recall of exposures, and therefore are generally less time consuming and less costly to perform than studies using a prospective design. This study design is particularly suited to outcomes that are rare or have a protracted onset. Cases are subjects with the outcome of interest, whereas controls are subjects without the outcome of interest. It is crucial that the controls be drawn from the same source population (study base) as the cases, such that the controls are comparable to the cases in all important respects except for the outcome of interest.[50] Controls thus must also be chosen independent of their exposure status. Primary validity threats with a case-control study include selection bias (noncomparable controls without the disease) and recall bias (differential recollection about exposure among cases with the disease). Overmatching can also occur if the cases and controls are matched on a variable that is also associated with the exposure of interest. If one thus matches on a factor that is both affected by exposure and a cause of disease, this will obscure a disease association.[51] There is no denominator in a case-control study, so an event rate, relative risk, or risk ratio cannot be calculated. Instead an odds ratio (the ratio of the odds of exposure in the cases and the odds of exposure in the controls) is conventionally generated as the measure of association between the exposure and the disease in a case-control study. When the outcomes occur at an infrequent rate, the odds ratio should approximate the relative risk.[26-30,52]

The potential adverse effect of various nonsteroidal anti-inflammatory drugs (NSAIDs) on patient outcome, in particular acute myocardial infraction (AMI), has been a major clinical concern, with a number of published observational studies.[53,54] For example, a case-control study was performed to assess the relative risk of AMI among users of celecoxib and rofecoxib in Medicare beneficiaries 65 years of age or older.[55] Each of the 10,895 identified cases of AMI was matched to four controls on the basis of age, gender, and the month of index date. Current use of rofecoxib was associated with an elevated relative risk of AMI when compared with celecoxib, with an odds ratio (OR) of 1.24 (95% confidence interval [CI]: 1.05 to 1.46, $P = 0.011$). Dosages of rofecoxib of greater than 25 mg were associated with a higher risk (OR of 1.70; 95% CI, 1.07 to 2.71; $P = 0.026$) than dosages of 25 mg or less (OR of 1.21; 95% CI, 1.01 to 1.44; $P = 0.036$). Interestingly, the risk of AMI with rofecoxib was elevated in the first 90 days of use but not thereafter.[55] Of note, because this study used state-level administrative claims data on all beneficiaries over a 3-year period and applied a broad set of inclusion criteria, recall bias and selection bias were minimized. However, as addressed by its authors, there may have been misclassification of end point of AMI in the Medicare data set, though such misclassification tends to bias toward the null. As with all retrospective observational studies, the results may have been biased by confounding factors not observable or incompletely assessed in the Medicare data set.[55]

COHORT STUDY

A cohort study is aimed at determining the relationship between a single contributing factor (exposure) and one or more possible outcomes (diseases). Cohort studies look or work forward, starting with the identified exposure

(exposure → diseases). Cohort studies are by definition longitudinal. However, the collection of data can be prospective, retrospective, or ambispective—if the study groups were identified and the needed historical data have been collected from a previous starting point. The key design element is that all participants in a cohort study are outcome or disease free prior to the exposure (intervention) and at the outset of data collection. Outcome data are then sequentially collected. Prospective and retrospective cohort studies may be less prone to recall bias compared to case-control studies, but they are subject to differential attrition bias, whereby participants in one group exit the study at a disproportionate rate. Cohort studies are also vulnerable to confounding by indication, a form of selection bias in which a variable is a risk factor for a disease among the nonexposed persons and is associated with the exposure of interest in the population from which the cases are derived, without being an intermediate step in the causal pathway between the exposure and the disease (e.g., a marked increase in gastrointestinal bleeding in patients prescribed an NSAID plus a proton-pump inhibitor versus only an NSAID).[56,57] Prospective cohort studies are also typically more time-consuming and costly than other observational studies, especially for rare outcomes (diseases) and those with a protracted onset. The cohort study allows for direct estimation of an incidence (new event) rate, relative risk, and relative risk ratio.[26-30,58] Of note, a randomized controlled trial is essentially a type of prospective cohort study in which premeditated assignment to exposure (intervention) randomly occurs.[23]

An illustrative observational cohort study was undertaken to determine whether self-reported chronic headache predicts stroke.[59] During the longitudinal follow-up of 35,056 randomly selected Finnish men and women, aged 25 to 64 years at baseline, a total 2167 incident (new) stroke events were recorded. After adjusting for age, smoking, serum cholesterol level, systolic blood pressure, diabetes, and body mass index, among men, the headache-associated hazard ratios (95% confidence intervals) for stroke were 3.92 (2.01-7.66) and 1.76 (1.26-2.47) at 1-year and 5-year follow-up. No significant association was observed between headache and the risk of stroke among women.[59] However, the observed gender-associated difference in stroke risk may have been due to a higher prevalence and a more heterogeneous etiology of headache in women (with their more common migraine and muscular tension headache) compared with men (with their more common vascular or of other intracranial origin). This likely reduced the sensitivity of detecting an association between headache and the risk of stroke among women.[59]

NESTED CASE-CONTROL STUDY

A nested case-control study is a case-control study in which the cases and controls are selected from members of an existing longitudinal cohort.[60] The members of the base cohort are followed for a certain period of time until the specific outcome or end point occurs.[28,61] The nested case-control design differs from the non-nested case-control design in that patients are selected from a well-defined cohort, for which data on all members can be obtained.[62] This design makes it easier to satisfy the fundamental assumption of the case-control study: that cases and controls represent random samples from the same study base.[62] If all data are collected prospectively before the outcome occurs, a nested case-control study is also unlikely to be impacted by recall bias.[27]

As noted earlier, the association between patient NSAID use and cardiac complications has been the focus of a number of published observational studies.[53,54] In another example, data from a large health maintenance organization were used to assemble a cohort of all patients age 18 to 84 years treated with an NSAID over a 3-year period, within which a nested case-control study was performed.[63] Each of 8143 identified cases of serious coronary heart disease (acute myocardial infarction and sudden cardiac death) was matched with four controls from the study base based on age, sex, and health plan region. The adjusted odds ratio for rofecoxib (all doses) versus celecoxib was 1.59 (95% CI: 1.10 to 2.32, $P = 0.015$), and for naproxen versus remote NSAID use, the adjusted odds ratio was 1.14 (95% CI: 1.00 to 1.30, $P = 0.05$).[63]

HEALTH CARE ECONOMIC EVALUATION

Health care economic evaluation has matured considerably since the 1980s. However, despite its widespread promotion to this audience, many physicians and researchers remain reluctant to apply economic evaluation methods in their clinical decision making and clinical trials—including for chronic pain treatment modalities.[64,65] Much of this reluctance has been attributed to physicians and their innate propensity to think more in terms of clinical effectiveness and advocacy at the individual patient level rather than about cost-effectiveness at the population or policy level.[15,66]

Furthermore, as witnessed by the intense United States health care reform debate, there is a strong unwillingness among Americans and hence their elected officials to consider whether an intervention may be cost-effective—often because of fears of government-mandated rationing of care and geriatric discrimination. A provision of the American Recovery and Reinvestment Act (ARRA) of 2009 created and funded the Patient-Centered Outcomes Research Institute (PCORI) to undertake rigorous comparative effectiveness research. The Patient Protection and Affordable Care Act (PPACA) of 2010 in turn specifically prohibited PCORI from undertaking any comparative cost-effective analyses using cost per quality-adjusted life year (QALY) as a common metric.[67-69] Nevertheless, given the aging U.S. population, the associated increasing health care utilization but decreasing active workforce, and the unsustainably growing percentage of the United States gross domestic product (GDP) devoted to health care, there is a clear and imminent need for valid health care economic evaluation data to establish health care funding priorities—including for chronic pain treatment modalities.[15,70]

Efforts to provide optimal care, while controlling unnecessary or wasteful health care expenditures, should focus on delivering "high-value, cost-conscious health care."[71] Whether an intervention provides such high value depends on assessing whether its health benefits justify its costs. There are three key concepts for understanding how to assess the value of health care interventions. First, assessing the benefits, harms, and costs of an intervention is essential to understand whether it provides good value. Second, assessing the cost of an intervention should include not only the cost of the intervention itself but also any downstream costs that occur because the intervention was performed. Third, the incremental cost-effectiveness ratio estimates the additional cost required to obtain additional health benefits and provides a key measure of the value of a health care intervention. In the United States, most decision makers conclude that interventions that cost less than $50,000 to $60,000 per quality-adjusted life year (QALY) gained is highly cost-effective.[71] The point at which an intervention is not cost-effective varies, though many decision makers would consider up to US$100,000 per QALY gained as reasonably cost-effective.

Full health care economic evaluation techniques conventionally include cost-minimization analysis, cost-benefit analysis, cost-effectiveness analysis, and cost-utility analysis.[65,72-75] A cost-utility analysis is a cost-effectiveness analysis that measures outcomes using quality-adjusted life years or another similar measure. Such full economic evaluations require that two or more therapeutic interventions be compared in relation to both costs and effects.[72,76] The six fundamental steps in undertaking a full economic evaluation include (1) identifying the perspective of the study, (2) identifying the alternatives that will be compared, (3) identifying the relevant costs and effects, (4) determining how to collect the cost and effect data, (5) determining how to perform calculation for cost and effects data, and (6) determining the manner in which to depict the results, draw comparisons, and make conclusions.[72,76,77]

With proper planning, a health care economic evaluation can be validly performed and reported alongside a clinical randomized controlled trial.[15,78-82] However, given the logistical challenges of such a conjoint study,[83] researchers often combine previously published cost and clinical outcome data to create a decision-analysis model.[15,84] The validity of such studies depends on how well the model reflects the key clinical issues and on the reliability of the parameters used to estimate costs, outcomes, and utilities. Sensitivity analyses are therefore critical for understanding how conclusions might change depending on variability or uncertainty in key parameters.

Given its high prevalence and high associated direct and indirect medical costs, the cost-effective management of migraine headache has received considerable attention.[85] For example, applying decision-analysis modeling demonstrated greater cost-effectiveness of rizatriptan and sumatriptan compared to a combination of ergotamine tartrate plus caffeine in the abortive treatment of an acute migraine attack. The net annual cost savings associated with use of rizatriptan and sumatriptan was US$622.98 per patient, with an incremental QALY of 0.001, meaning that the two triptans dominated ergotamine bolus caffeine (lower costs plus greater utility). The findings were not sensitive to changes in key variables such as efficacy, utility, drug costs, hospitalization cost, and patient preference over alternative therapies.[86] In a comparison of five treatments for acute migraine prophylaxis (amitriptyline 75 mg/day, topiramate 100 and 200 mg/day, timolol 20 mg/day, divalproex sodium 1000 mg/day, or propranolol 160 mg/day), a Markov decision-analysis model, with Monte Carlo simulation, indicated that among these preventive medications, probabilistic sensitivity analysis suggested that when the societal willingness to pay is less than US$18,000 per QALY gained, amitriptyline is the most likely cost-effective option.[87]

STANDARDS FOR REPORTING STUDY DESIGN AND FINDINGS

In 1858, Pasteur introduced the methods section of the scientific report, creating what is now known as the IMRAD format (introduction, materials and methods, results, and discussion).[88,89] Not surprisingly, in the interim heady 150 years, as investigators have applied these various basic study designs, there has been wide variability in their application as well as the content and organization of their published reports. In response, standards for reporting of study design and findings have been promulgated—several of which are applicable to acute and chronic pain management (Table 80.2).

Table 80.2 The Various Publication Guidelines

Acronym	Full Title of Guideline	Notes
EQUATOR	Enhancing the Quality of and Transparency of Health Research	www.equator-network.org
CONSORT*	Consolidated Standards of Reporting Trials[92]	www.consort-statement.org
STROBE	STrengthening the Reporting of OBservational studies in Epidemiology[93]	www.strobe-statement.org
QUOROM	Quality of Reporting of Meta-analyses[94]	QUOROM has been replaced by PRISMA
PRISMA	Preferred Reporting Items for Systematic Reviews and Meta-Analyses[95]	www.prisma-statement.org
SQUIRE	Standards for Quality Improvement Reporting Excellence[96]	http://squire-statement.org
MOOSE	Meta-analysis of Observational Studies in Epidemiology[97]	
COREQ	Consolidated Criteria for Reporting Qualitative Research[98]	
STARD	Standards for Accurate Reporting of Diagnostic Tests[99]	www.stard-statement.org
TREND	Transparent Reporting of Evaluations with Nonrandomized Designs[100]	www.cdc.gov/trendstatement

*The main CONSORT Statement is based on the "standard" two-group parallel design. However, there are several types of randomized trials, some of which have different designs (e.g., cluster, noninferiority and equivalence, or pragmatic trials), interventions (e.g., herbal medicinal, nonpharmacologic, or acupuncture), and data (e.g., harms), for which specific CONSORT extensions exist.

The EQUATOR (enhancing the quality of and transparency of health research) network has been created to monitor and propagate the proper use of these guidelines[90] and thus "to improve the quality of scientific publications by promoting transparent and accurate reporting of health research."[91] Furthermore, an increasing number of major (high-impact) clinical and health care journals require or recommend adherence to the applicable set of such guidelines for submitted manuscripts.

STANDARDIZATION OF PAIN-RELATED OUTCOME MEASURES

Regardless of the study design used, pain-related research should assess and report outcomes that are valid, reproducible, and clinically meaningful to patients. Unfortunately, even though measures such as joint range of motion, dynamometer measures of muscle strength, or imaging evidence of successful spinal fusion are often seen as objective, pain is an inherently subjective outcome and correlates only modestly with such measures. Fortunately, research shows that pain can be measured in a valid and reproducible fashion, using measures such as numeric rating or visual analog scales. However, although pain may reflect a patient's subjective experience, it is insufficient by itself, as self-reported pain often does not correlate well with actual ability to function. Therefore, it is important for studies of pain to go beyond self-reports of pain and to also routinely examine outcomes that measure patients' behavior and function in their daily lives.

Since its inception in 2002, the Initiative on Methods, Measurement, and Pain Assessment in Clinical Trials (IMMPACT) has enlisted a broad array of experts in its efforts to improve the design, execution, and interpretation of clinical trials of treatments for pain.[101] IMMPACT has developed a series of consensus reviews and recommendations regarding trials for chronic pain in adults, trials for acute pain in adults, and trials for pediatric acute and chronic pain.[102-109] IMMPACT recommends that trials routinely measure outcomes in multiple core domains—including pain, physical functioning, emotional functioning, global improvement, satisfaction with treatment, and adverse events—and includes a list of suggested measurement tools for each of these domains.

DISTINGUISHING BETWEEN STATISTICAL AND CLINICAL SIGNIFICANCE

A key concept when interpreting the results of clinical research is that statistically significant results are not always clinically meaningful.[110] For example, with a large enough sample size, a study may report a difference in pain scores between the treatment and no treatment groups of an average of 3 points on a 0 to 100 scale, with a *P* value of 0.01. Although such a difference is statistically significant, the clinical significance is very small or trivial. Another challenge in interpreting results of studies that report mean or differences in outcomes related to pain or function is that such data do not indicate whether they reflect a situation in which some patients experienced a very good outcome and others experienced no benefit, or a situation in which patients generally experienced a small, similar average result.[111]

The minimal clinically important difference (MCID) is defined as the smallest change in an outcome that a patient would perceive as clinically meaningful.[112] The IMMPACT group proposed defining the MCID as a 30% or greater improvement in self-reported pain and function. The IMMPACT group also recommended that studies report the proportion of patients in each group who meet the MCID threshold. Based on the absolute difference between groups in the proportion of patients who experienced the MCID, the number needed to treat to achieve one clinically meaningful outcome can be calculated (100/[the percentage of individuals with the MCID in group A minus the percentage of individuals with the MCID in group B]).[113] Therefore, in a study in which 40% of patients in group A experience the MCID for pain relief compared with 20% in group B, the number needed to treat would be 100/20 or 5. By contrast, a study in which 40% of patients in group A experience the MCID compared with 37% in group B, the number needed to treat would be 100/3 or 33.

The effect size is a way of assessing results across studies that report similar outcomes (e.g., pain relief) using different measures (e.g., 0 to 4 verbal rating scale, 0 to 10 numerical rating scale, and 0 to 100 visual analogue scale). The effect size (also called the Z score) is a unit-less measure that standardizes results across studies by dividing the difference in the mean scores between groups by the standard deviation. Each point in the effect size is equivalent to a difference in one standard deviation. Although clinical interpretation of effect sizes can vary depending on the outcome being measured, the population assessed, the sample sizes of the studies, and other factors, a general rule of thumb is that an effect size of 0.2 to 0.5 indicates a small effect, >0.5 to 0.8 a moderate effect, and >0.8 a large effect.[114]

ASSESSING AND ADDRESSING BIAS AND CONFOUNDING IN CLINICAL RESEARCH

Bias refers to any systematic process, effect, or error in the design or conduct of a study that favors one outcome over others.[115] Therefore, studies at greater risk of bias are more likely to be misleading. Important types of bias include (1) *selection bias* resulting in differences between groups other than the intervention of interest; (2) *performance bias* due to effects of knowledge of patient assignment to different therapies; (3) *attrition bias* due to differences between those persons who do versus those who do not complete a study; (4) *detection bias* resulting in differential interpretation of outcomes based on knowledge of assigned interventions; (5) *reporting bias* from the selective presentation results, typically those that are more favorable or statistically significant; and (6) *publication bias* resulting from the preferential publication of studies reporting positive findings.

Methods to reduce the risk of bias in randomized trials include (1) use of adequate randomization and allocation concealment to prevent selection bias; (2) assessment of similarity of groups at baseline to detect important imbalances and failure of randomization to control for known confounders; (3) blinding of patients, caregivers, and research staff to avoid performance and detection bias; (4) low loss to follow-up and use of intention-to-treat analysis to avoid attrition bias; and (5) full reporting of prespecified primary and secondary outcomes to avoid reporting bias. Given a randomized trial with a large enough sample and successful implementation of randomization, the problem of selection bias is largely eliminated because all confounders—including those that are unmeasured or unknown—are equally distributed among groups. Successful blinding of patients and research staff should largely eliminate performance and detection bias.[116]

As noted earlier, observational studies by their nature are susceptible to selection bias and confounding by indication, and they cannot blind patients and treating clinicians to the interventions received. Confounding refers to a situation in which the association between an intervention (I) and an outcome (O) is distorted by another factor (C).[117] This occurs when I is associated with C, and C is also an independent risk factor for O. For example, patients with back pain may have poorer outcomes when prescribed opioids compared with persons not prescribed opioids. However, if back pain is also associated with psychological comorbidities, and psychological comorbidities are independently associated with poorer outcomes, a study that does not address this confounder would provide misleading results about the effects of opioid use on back pain. To address this during the assembly of the cohort, a study could match patients on key confounders such as psychological comorbidities or restrict enrollment to patients without psychological comorbidities. After a cohort has been assembled, a study could evaluate baseline differences among groups in psychological comorbidities to assess the likely impact of this confounder, and it could perform statistical adjustment through regression or other methods (e.g., propensity score matching) to control for its effects or stratification to evaluate how effects vary in defined subgroups.

When considering multiple studies at the level of a body of evidence, it is also important to consider the possibility of publication and related biases due to the selective publication of studies.[118] Steps to address publication bias include efforts to locate unpublished studies, and performance of graphical or statistical tests to determine whether publication bias may be present and its potential magnitude.

Different types of evidence studies vary in their susceptibility to bias. Therefore, when evaluating the validity of a study, it is important to consider any design-specific methodological shortcomings, as well as its place on the study design hierarchy. For example, a well-conducted randomized controlled trial will generally be less susceptible to bias than a well-conducted cohort study.

External validity (generalizability or applicability) is separate from risk of bias but also critical for interpreting research evidence. Studies may be at low risk of bias and therefore valid (i.e., give true results), but only apply to very specific situations. It is therefore always important to consider whether the study evaluates effectiveness—or the extent to which a treatment works on average patients in everyday settings—as compared to efficacy—the extent to which a treatment works in highly selected patients in tightly controlled settings.[32]

KEY POINTS

- Evidence-based medicine offers a formal set of steps for clinicians to follow in order to effectively interpret the results of clinical research ("how to read a paper") and to apply them in their practice.
- The Grading of Recommendations Assessment, Development and Evaluation (GRADE) system is widely used to grade the quality of published evidence and strength of recommendations.
- A randomized controlled trial is a type of controlled clinical trial predicated on participants being assigned to the possible exposures or interventions purely by the play of chance.
- A cluster randomized trial is a trial in which individuals are randomized in groups—the group as a whole is randomized, and not the individual.
- A case-control study determines the relationship between a single outcome (disease) and one or more previous possible contributing factors (exposures).
- A cohort study determines the relationship between a single contributing factor (exposure) and one or more possible outcomes (diseases).
- A nested case-control study is a case-control study in which the cases and controls are selected from members of an existing longitudinal cohort.
- Efforts to provide optimal care, while controlling unnecessary or wasteful health care expenditures, focus on delivering high-value, cost-conscious health care, which can be determined using health care economic evaluation techniques.
- A key concept when interpreting the results of clinical research is that statistically significant results are not always clinically meaningful (minimal clinically important difference [MCID]).
- *Bias* refers to any systematic process, effect, or error in the design or conduct of a study that favors one outcome over others, whereas *confounding* refers to a situation in which the association between an intervention and an outcome is distorted by another factor.

SUGGESTED READINGS

Arnett DK, Claas SA. Chapter 35: Introduction to Epidemiology. In: David R, Gordon HW, eds. *Clinical and Translational Science.* San Diego: Academic Press; 2009:527-541.

Chou R, Aronson N, Atkins D, et al. AHRQ Series Paper 4: assessing harms when comparing medical interventions: AHRQ and the Effective Health-Care Program. *J Clin Epidemiol.* 2010;63:502-512.

Gordis L. *Epidemiology.* Philadelphia: Elsevier/Saunders; 2009.

Greenhalgh T. *How to Read a Paper: the Basics of Evidence-Based Medicine.* Chichester: J. Wiley; 2010.

Grimes DA, Schulz KF. An overview of clinical research: The lay of the land. *Lancet.* 2002;359:57-61.

Guyatt GH, Oxman AD, Vist GE, et al. GRADE: an emerging consensus on rating quality of evidence and strength of recommendations. *BMJ.* (Clinical research ed.) 2008;336:924-926.

Hartung DM, Touchette D. Overview of clinical research design. *Am J Health Syst Pharm.* 2009;66:398-408.

Mann CJ. Observational research methods. Research design II: cohort, cross sectional, and case-control studies. *Emerg Med J.* 2003;20:54-60.

Ostelo RW, Deyo RA, Stratford P, et al. Interpreting change scores for pain and functional status in low back pain: towards international consensus regarding minimal important change. *Spine.* 2008;33:90-94.

Owens DK, Qaseem A, Chou R, Shekelle P. High-value, cost-conscious health care: concepts for clinicians to evaluate the benefits, harms, and costs of medical interventions. *Ann Intern Med.* 2011;154:174-180.

Petrou S, Gray A. Economic evaluation alongside randomised controlled trials: design, conduct, analysis, and reporting. *BMJ.* (Clinical research ed.) 2011;342:d1548.

Psaty BM, Siscovick DS. Minimizing bias due to confounding by indication in comparative effectiveness research. *JAMA.* 2010;304:897-898.

Schulz KF, Grimes DA. Case-control studies: research in reverse. *Lancet.* 2002;359:431-434.

Silverman SL. From randomized controlled trials to observational studies. *Am J Med.* 2009;122:114-120.

Vetter TR. The application of economic evaluation methods in the chronic pain medicine literature. *Anesth Analg.* 2007;105:114-118.

The references for this chapter can be found at www.expertconsult.com.

81 Ethics of Research in Patients with Pain

Meredith G. van der Velden | David B. Waisel

Ethics and Science need to shake hands.

DR. RICHARD CLARKE CABOT, 1936

Medical experimentation has a long history. Biblical references suggest that as early as the sixth century BCE, King Nebuchadnezzar tested nourishment as an outcome of variation in diet in his subjects.[1] Although scattered reports of other rudimentary experimentation have been documented, most historical accounts indicate that Dr. James Lind inaugurated modern-day clinical research through the first controlled clinical trial in the mid-1700s. Lind, a physician stationed on a British naval vessel, compared the administration of citrus fruit with other therapies for the treatment of patients with scurvy.[2] Using hypothesis generation and testing, he found a cure for the once mysterious disease of scurvy. Dr. Lind set the stage for a rich history in human subject research that has since evolved in sophistication, influence, and magnitude.

Although the scope of clinical research has changed in sophistication and complexity over the centuries, what has not changed are the basic tenets—to understand the causes, evolution, and effects of human disease and to improve our ability to prevent, diagnose, and treat it.[3] However, this privilege of investigation requires professional responsibility to protect the subjects. This assertion underlies the field of research ethics and is the focus of this chapter.

The underlying principles of research ethics are the same as the generally accepted medical ethics. Professional morality is often considered to be based on four overarching principles that form the framework for the ethics that guide us in our practice—respect for autonomy, nonmaleficence, beneficence, and justice.[4] These principles are germane to research ethics.

Respect for autonomy. Respect for autonomy addresses the respect for decision making by autonomous persons. It prioritizes a person's right to hold views, make choices, and take actions based on personal values and beliefs.[4] It is the core of the informed consent and informed refusal discussions that are central to research ethics. The principle of respect for autonomy becomes particularly relevant in vulnerable patients with potentially diminished autonomy, such as those with chronic pain, who may clutch at any opportunity for relief.[5]

Nonmaleficence. Nonmaleficence is the moral norm of *primum non nocere*: "above all do no harm."[4] Pertinent to this principle are considerations of the acceptable risk incurred by doing research and balancing these risks with the prospect of benefit.

Beneficence. Beneficence describes actions that promote the welfare of a person, patient, or subject. It tangles with respect for autonomy when patient preferences are at odds with physician judgment.[4] In research ethics, beneficence encompasses the scientific and social value and integrity of the research, as well as any potential benefits to the subject when balanced with the risks.[4]

Justice. Justice describes fair, equitable, and appropriate treatment in light of what is due persons.[4] It demands stalwart vigilance to avoid the exploitation of socioeconomically and medically disadvantaged individuals, and it requires systems to ensure that all have a fair opportunity to receive the benefits. Flagrant exploitation in the past has led us to the current guidelines and controversies. From this infrastructure we will build an understanding of research ethics as an application of these principles in general and as it is relevant to research involving pain medicine.

RESEARCH ETHICS

HISTORY OF RESEARCH ETHICS

Advances in research ethics have primarily been instigated by the exploitation of human subjects.[2] Even though some evidence suggests that ethical issues in human experimentation had been recognized and addressed as early as the late 1800s,[6] the 1947 Nuremberg Code is commonly cited as the first document to govern the conduct of human research. This code arose from the war trials of Nazi physicians accused of conducting "murderous and torturous human experiments" on prisoners in concentration camps in the name of medical science.[7] The Nuremburg Code was the first to formally outline standards for the ethical conduct of research on humans.[8] It declared that voluntary consent is "absolutely essential," subjects should be protected from "unnecessary physical and mental suffering and injury," subjects may withdraw at any time from the experiment, researchers should stop the experiment if continuation is likely to be harmful to the subject, and the experiment has a legitimate likelihood of bearing fruit.[9]

The period following World War II was marked by a time of increased medical research activity and the development of new methods. To further define the requirements for human experimentation, the World Medical Association published the "Declaration of Helsinki."[3] First adopted in 1964 at the meeting of the World Medical Association in Helsinki, Finland, the document has undergone multiple, often contentious revisions, most recently in 2008, to address evolving issues in human experimentation.[10] The document builds on and reinforces many of the principles in the Nuremberg Code but excludes 2 of the 12 items in an effort to address perceived deficiencies in the Nuremberg Code. The requirement for voluntary consent of subjects was replaced by a statement that allows guardians to consent for research in subjects who are "legally incompetent, physically or mentally incapable of giving consent or is a legally incompetent minor."[3] In doing so, the Declaration of Helsinki became the first document to address experimentation in children and others with limited decisional capacity. The other substantive changes included indications for cessation of research by the investigator, notification of subjects that they may withdraw at any time, and the distinction between therapeutic and nontherapeutic research.[3,11]

The Declaration of Helsinki did not halt all questionable research activities in the United States.[8] In 1966, Dr. Henry K. Beecher, a former anesthetist in chief at the Massachusetts General Hospital, published a landmark paper in the *New England Journal of Medicine* in which he exposed multiple instances of contemporaneous research that were in direct violation of what was declared at Helsinki. Beecher documented studies that withheld known effective treatment, administered known harmful therapy, and exploited incompetent patients and children. In the face of soaring research funding, Beecher placed a necessary and influential pause on the process to re-examine the ethics of the field and remind investigators, the field of medicine, and society about our moral responsibilities to research subjects. He also suggested that journal editors were responsible to reject manuscripts of unethical research in the hope that "failure to obtain publication would discourage unethical experimentation."[12]

In 1972, the Tuskegee Study of Untreated Syphilis became the impetus for the next page in the history of research ethics. The U.S. Public Health Service conducted the Tuskegee study from 1932 through 1972. The study withheld effective therapy for syphilis from hundreds of African American men to observe the progression of syphilis, presumably for the sake of medical research.[13] In response to the horror generated by the discovery and exposure of this study, the U.S. Congress enacted the National Research Act in 1974. This act created the National Commission for the Protection of Clinical Subjects of Biomedical and Behavioral Research to oversee human experimentation in the United States. In 1979, the commission drafted the Belmont Report.[5] The Belmont Report describes the basic ethical principles underlying the conduct of research—respect for persons, beneficence, and justice—and it applies them to research conduct by addressing the specific issues of informed consent, risk-benefit assessment, and selection of research subjects.[5] In addition to establishing the commission, the National Research Act led to the Common Rule in 1991, a set of federal regulations necessitating oversight of government-funded research in the United States. Elements of the policy center on the presence and procedures of institutional review boards (IRBs) and general requirements for informed consent. Subsequent revisions of the regulations addressed vulnerable research subjects, including children.[8,14,15]

Even though there is widespread support for the basic ethical principles addressed in these documents, their practical use is continuously debated and refined. Some researchers think that the regulations are necessary to operationalize these principles, whereas others see them as an excessive obstacle to research.[16] The dilemma between promoting scientific advancement and protecting subjects is real and complex; staying on the narrow road that protects both interests requires thoughtful calibration and imaginative solutions.

ETHICS OF RESEARCH ON HUMAN SUBJECTS

Applying ethical principles in performing research requires dedication to adherence. Emanuel and colleagues proposed seven requirements for ethical research that comprehensively define and guide evaluations of clinical studies on humans. These requirements provide an inclusive and detailed framework that should ensure performance of ethical research (Box 81.1).[17]

The requirement for social or scientific value requires that to justify potential risks and use of resources, the research should add knowledge to the field, regardless of whether it leads directly to changes in patient care.[17] This requires avoiding unnecessary or needlessly repetitive research.[18] Researchers are obligated to publish their research to benefit society.[17,19] In pain research, value may include "immediate value," which may immediately improve health, or "potential value," which comes from the knowledge of better understanding the science of pain.[20]

Scientific validity requires the research to have adequate methodologic rigor to potentially produce meaningful results regardless of the value of the proposed research. The scientific value of an idea alone does not ensure its validity.[17]

Clinical equipoise is a requirement for interventional research validity and, accordingly, becomes a requirement for ethical research. It describes a state of uncertainty about the superiority of the prospective intervention over existing interventions and must be present for an interventional study to be considered ethical.[21,22] Although clinical equipoise is the accepted basis for many clinical trials, its practical utility has not been without controversy.[23] Because this stipulation has the potential to present a significant obstacle to initiating clinical trial research, distinctions have been made between individual versus community equipoise by delineating whether the uncertainty must lie with the individual investigator or within the expert medical community.[21,23]

Box 81.1 The Seven Requirements for Ethical Clinical Research

Social or scientific value
Scientific validity
Fair subject selection
Favorable risk-benefit ratio
Independent review
Informed consent
Respect for potential and enrolled subjects

From Emanuel EJ, Wendler D, Grady C. What makes clinical research ethical? *JAMA*. 2000;283:2701-2711.

The requirement for scientific validity is also based on the idea that risks cannot be incurred nor resources used without a functional study design.[17] In pain research, adequate study design may dictate the inclusion of a placebo arm, as often required by the Food and Drug Administration (FDA),[24] a somewhat controversial topic addressed below.

Independent review of research by outside parties is conducted in an attempt to mitigate potential conflicts of interest and address inadequately designed research. In concept, it entails review of all research activity, including project proposal and design, data collection, ongoing monitoring of the research, and final analysis of the results. In practice, it is performed by funding agencies, IRBs, and safety-monitoring boards.[17] Independent review bodies should specifically consider these seven requirements when analyzing the research being reviewed. Independent review is notably concerned about taking advantage of vulnerable patients such as those in chronic pain. Review processes are also pivotal in addressing conflicts of interest.[25]

The requirement for respect for potential and enrolled subjects seeks to ensure privacy and confidentiality, allow subjects to freely withdrawal from research, inform subjects of the results of the study, and maintain the welfare of subjects.[17] Though seemingly simple operationally, the complexity of this requirement lies in including all the principles and many of the requirements mentioned. In short, it demands placing the research subject as the primary center while still conducting useful research.[19]

With reference to pain research, it is worth highlighting the idea of opportunity for withdrawal. People with pain may have unique barriers to accepting their freedom to withdraw from a study because of concerns about obtaining appropriate and effective alternative treatments once they have withdrawn.[20]

Fair subject selection specifies that subject selection and opportunities for participation be based on the goals of the research rather than unrelated factors such as privilege or vulnerability and that those bearing potential risks by participating be able to experience the benefits.[17] An example of research that would violate fair subject selection is testing a new medication primarily on a socioeconomically disadvantaged population for a disease that equally or primarily affects a more advantaged group. This may occur because academic centers are often centered in socioeconomically disadvantaged areas. An example of a different concern is not offering research participation to women when the disease and intervention being studied equally pertain to women.[17,19] In this case, exclusion of women, perhaps for practical research reasons, may result in subsequent therapeutic recommendations that may not be applicable to the excluded group.

The converse of the requirement for equal opportunity inclusion is exploiting vulnerable populations for research that will not benefit that population or will not result in generalizable knowledge.[17] Nazi experimentations were one such example. Another relevant study is the Willowbrook Hepatitis Study. At the Willowbrook State School for disabled children in Staten Island, New York, numerous disabled children were deliberately infected with infectious hepatitis to study the disease, as well as to test the effects of potential therapies, thus raising concern for exploitation.[8,26]

For research to be justified, there must be a favorable risk-benefit ratio. Because much of the goal of research is to test untested interventions, the risks and benefits associated with such interventions will in part be unknown or uncertain.[17] To justify research, however, potential risks must be minimized, potential benefits must be enhanced, and the risks and benefits must be commensurate.[3,5,17]

When considering the potential benefit side of the balance, discussions should pertain to the benefits received by the subject or the subject's population and, except in unusual circumstances, not those gained by society at large. Potential benefits do not include providing proper medical care.[17] The Tuskegee Study of Untreated Syphilis highlights this point in that the men in this study were thought to be receiving a "benefit" that more properly should have been considered standard health care.[27] Finally, benefits such as money or gifts could conceivably be increased to the point, particularly in certain subjects, that even the most risk-laden endeavors will be outweighed by the non–health-related benefit.[17,19] In pain research, potential benefits are manifested as the potential to benefit future patients or more immediately benefit the patient or the patient's population with either access to medications or access to study results that may help the patient choose between medications.[20]

Conceptually, the requirement for assessment and minimization of risk in research is derived from the principle of nonmaleficence. Most would agree that limiting the harm imposed by research activities is appropriate and necessary for the protection of all subjects. U.S. federal regulations governing research on human subjects require that risk to subjects be minimized "(i) by using procedures which are consistent with sound research design and which do not unnecessarily expose subjects to risk, and (ii) whenever appropriate, by using procedures already being performed on the subjects for diagnostic or treatment purposes."[28] The regulations also place large responsibility for the oversight of this standard in the hands of review bodies, such as IRBs.[28]

Even though minimizing risk has accepted value, dissension arises in defining risks for any individual subject and study. Delineating risk includes consideration of both the probability and magnitude of the harm.[5,29] It is meant to include physiologic, psychological, social, economic, and legal risks and to represent aggregate risk for participation, not for any single individual potentially harmful encounter. In light of this, it is difficult to quantify risk, and attempts have been made to create categorical distinctions to guide researchers and review bodies in assessment of the appropriateness of the research activity.[29]

"Minimal risk" is a categorical distinction of risk that is delineated in the federal regulations. The purpose of the category of minimal risk is to set a threshold that triggers closer examination of the risks and benefits of the research.[29] It is defined as follows: "the probability and magnitude of harm or discomfort anticipated in the research are not greater in and of themselves than those ordinarily encountered in daily life or during the performance of routine physical or psychological examinations or tests."[28] As with defining risk itself, the ambiguity inherent in making such a distinction has sparked criticism of the concept.[8] Difficulty in defining minimal risk complicates weighing whether the risks and benefits of a study meet the minimal risk standard. Operationally, the presence of minimal risk can be a reason for altered or "expedited" review processes for research approval.[28]

In pain research, examples of risks include potential medication side effects, persistence of pain symptoms if randomized to the placebo arm without breakthrough dosing available, risks associated with sham procedures, and pain associated with travel and paperwork.[20] It may also include the intentional use of noxious stimuli to test potential pain relief mechanisms.[30]

Those involved in research and oversight should systematically analyze and define the risks and benefits as much as possible to allow the risk-benefit relationship to be elucidated.[5] In the end, potential benefits need to be commensurate with potential risks.[17]

Informed consent is a process that has at its core the principle of respect for autonomy. The purpose of the informed consent process is to ensure that the subject understands the purpose, methods, risks, benefits, and alternatives to the research to the extent that the subject can make a voluntary informed decision about participation.[17] The quality of the informed consent is married to good study design[20] and involves the remaining six requirements.

The initial step in the process of informed consent is the interactive and iterative process of conveying information and discussing all aspects of the research. This interaction also requires the ethereal but essential assessment of sufficient comprehension. Finally, the potential participant may agree to participation.[31]

Consent must be free of coercion. Coercion can take the form of obvious pressure or inducement to participate or may be more subtle in the form of perceived pressure that the potential participant may feel in light of an existing clinical relationship with the investigator on whom the participant depends for medical care.[19] Another form of coercion is offering better medical care not otherwise available. Consider the pressure to participate on a patient in unremitting chronic pain who is desperate for any shot at relief.[32] One way to mitigate this problem is to limit inclusion to patients who have access to excellent pain treatment services before enrollment.[20]

Relevant to this latter point is the seminal concept of therapeutic misconception. The term, coined by Applebaum and colleagues in 1982, refers to the misperception of study participants that their involvement in the study is focused on their individual therapeutic medical care rather than on scientific purposes.[33] It poses a direct threat to informed consent in clinical trials[34] and is particularly relevant to patients in chronic pain, who have vulnerabilities that would particularly predispose them to therapeutic misconception.[24]

ADDITIONAL CONSIDERATIONS FOR RESEARCH ON PAIN

A few ethical concerns are particularly germane to research on pain medicine. Tait delineated three characteristics that render pain research challenging: pain is highly subjective, it is composed of sensory, affective, and cognitive elements, and its correlation with actual injury is uncertain and variable.[24] These characteristics, among others, contribute to the potential classification of these research subjects as vulnerable. This is particularly pertinent to patients with chronic pain, whose complexity complicates the design and ethics of research.[24,35] Notably, included in this is the common comorbidity of psychiatric disturbance in the chronic pain population, conditions that may affect cognition in a way that threatens the informed consent process.[24] However, similar to other vulnerable populations, patients in pain should be entitled to the same opportunities for research on behalf of their condition, and efforts should be made to manage these tensions.

PLACEBOS

Placebos are often necessary for sound research design and are often required by the FDA for studies evaluating efficacy.[24,36] In line with the prevailing principles that have already been discussed, the ethical use of placebo-controlled studies assumes that the following conditions have been met: no effective treatment is available that can be used for comparison, the risks potentially incurred by use of a placebo are acceptable, study validity requires its use, and informed consent includes disclosure of the potential use of placebo.[24,36-38] Some studies may benefit from a placebo arm that involves an intervention, such as inserting an epidural catheter and infusing a sham drug so that clinicians do not realize what the patient is receiving. Determining whether the benefits of a placebo arm are necessary for study validity depends on the incremental improvement in the validity of the study and the potential harm of the intervention. Although minimal risk with the intervention requires that the intervention be done if it improves study validity, more significant risks must hurdle greater standards, such as a study result that would directly benefit the patient subsequently.[38]

Particular attention has been paid to the use of placebo-controlled trials in pain research. The highly subjective nature of pain and the related tendency toward powerful placebo responses in patients who experience pain make the use of placebo particularly compelling in research involving interventions directed at the pain experience.[24,37] Although further discussion of the merits of placebo use in research design is beyond the scope of this chapter, several threats to ethical integrity are relevant to the use of placebo in analgesia research on patients with chronic pain, namely, therapeutic misconception, coercion related to a reliant relationship with the physician, and risk for irrecoverable exacerbation of symptoms when withholding therapies.[24] These risks are not absolute barriers to the use of placebo; however, they do suggest the need for more oversight at the level of the investigator and regulatory parties.

INDUSTRY AND CONFLICTS OF INTEREST

Conflicts of interest in performing and publishing research may rise from external or internal pressure. It is important to think of conflict of interest not as a statement of fact (i.e., the researcher is doing something wrong because of external benefits), but as a potential situation. It is, of course, impossible to know the intent of a researcher. Nonetheless, we can certainly recognize situations that may potentially lead to conflict.

External pressure, such as continued funding from industry, is a well-recognized concern, and procedures are in place to publicly identify such conflicts in an attempt to prevent them. However, public identification is not a panacea. In one study, only 80% of physicians reported industry funding related to their research. Fewer reported funding from the same company but unrelated to the specific product.[39]

Perhaps more insidious than the conflicts that may arise from industry's financial pressure is the unrecognized desire for academic promotion and enhanced reputation. In our view, one of the most dangerous conditions is the ownership that physicians feel for their ideas, which may lead to the well-meaning conviction that their idea is the right answer. This can lead to bias, overlooking of contrary data, and even "correcting" of data because they have the solution. Investigators must be mindful of this phenomenon.

The subjectivity of pain assessment puts an investigator at risk for potential conflicts of interest throughout a study—inclusion/exclusion criteria, risk-benefit ratios, overestimating responses to treatment, and underestimating symptoms. In light of the increasingly complex relationships between pain physicians and industry, the American Academy of Pain Medicine has published recommendations related to conflicts of interest in research, with a particular focus on disclosures and review.[25]

Pain management has recently had two scandals that show the potential harm related to research and conflicts of interest. In 2009, the lead researcher who was responsible for publishing influential data that encouraged multimodal pain therapy was found to have significant irregularities in data that required retraction of multiple articles. Pain management physicians were left without data to support their current clinical practices.[40]

Researchers must also be sure that agreements with industry permit publication of data regardless of the outcomes. Although it is widely accepted that industry-provided materials and representatives overstate the benefits and understate the risks associated with a drug, it is perhaps less appreciated that drug companies may do the same on a larger scale. This is most clearly seen with the anti-inflammatory drug rofecoxib (Vioxx), in which Merck intentionally distorted and obfuscated information on an increased rate of myocardial infarction.[41,42]

These two events violated the requirement of research ethics to perform fruitful studies, which includes accurate reporting so that clinicians may act on the results.

GUIDELINES AND STANDARDS

The International Association for the Study of Pain, the American Pain Society, and the American Academy of Pain Medicine endorse the ethics outlined in the seminal documents addressed earlier and have developed standards and guidelines addressing such. In addition to the general principles and requirements, the statements notably give mention to the vulnerability of the pain population and provide guidance on the use of placebo, including sham interventions, and set expectations for the use of noxious stimuli in pain research.[43-45]

KEY POINTS

- The fundamental principles of research ethics are respect for autonomy, nonmaleficence, beneficence, and justice.
- The principle of respect for autonomy demands promoting knowledgeable and voluntary decision making by potential and active research subjects.
- The principle of nonmaleficence requires researchers to vigilantly ensure that they "do no harm" in selecting and performing research activities.
- The principle of beneficence obligates researchers to "do good" in selecting and performing research activities.
- The principle of justice demands fairness and equity throughout pain medicine research, particularly in the selection of human subjects and research areas.
- Our history of exploitation of human subjects has shaped our current approach to clinical research ethics.
- Historical documents central to the modern ethical and legal approach to protection of research subjects are the Nuremburg Code, the Declaration of Helsinki, and the Belmont Report.
- Requirements for ethical research include social or scientific value, scientific validity, independent review, respect for subjects, fair subject selection, favorable risk-benefit ratio, and informed consent.
- Special considerations for pain medicine research include subject vulnerability, use of placebo, conflicts of interest with industry, and use of noxious stimuli.
- The International Association for the Study of Pain, the American Pain Society, and the American Academy of Pain Medicine are leaders in promoting ethical research and in addressing the ever-changing dilemmas in pain medicine research.

SUGGESTED READINGS

Beecher HK. Ethics and clinical research. *N Engl J Med.* 1966;274:1354-1360.

Casarett DJ, Karlawish J. Beyond informed consent: the ethical design of pain research. *Pain Med.* 2001;2:138-146.

Emanuel EJ, Wendler D, Grady C. What makes clinical research ethical? *JAMA.* 2000;283:2701-2711.

Protection of human subjects; Belmont Report: notice of report for public comment. *Fed Regist.* 1979;44:23191-23197.

Tait RC. Vulnerability in clinical research with patients in pain: a risk analysis. *J Law Med Ethics.* 2009;37:59-72.

The Nuremberg Code. *JAMA.* 1996;276:1691.

World Medical Association Declaration of Helsinki: ethical principles for medical research involving human subjects. *JAMA.* 2000;284:3043-3045.

The references for this chapter can be found at www.expertconsult.com.

82

Postoperative Pain Management: Trends and Future Directions and Areas in Need of Investigation

Jason C. Brookman | Honorio T. Benzon | Asha Manohar | Christopher L. Wu

Significant progress in the management of postoperative pain has been made since the 1990s. Increased awareness of the undertreatment of postoperative pain, improved analgesic techniques, and new analgesic agents have contributed in part to improvements in its management. Despite the advances made in the management of postoperative pain, many challenges remain in improving the quality of pain control for patients.

CURRENT STATUS OF POSTOPERATIVE PAIN MANAGEMENT

Although a comprehensive overview of the current state of postoperative pain management is beyond the scope of this chapter, many facets are described elsewhere in this book. One of the persistent issues in the management of postoperative pain is that a relatively high percentage of patients still experience moderate to severe levels of pain, despite increased awareness by health care providers of the issue (e.g., pain as the "fifth vital sign"). Data suggest that postoperative pain continues to be undermanaged. For instance, one survey found that 80% of United States (U.S.) adult patients experienced acute pain postoperatively after outpatient surgery with approximately 85% of these patients experiencing moderate to severe pain.[1] A similar assessment in Europe noted that 41% of adult surgical patients experienced moderate to severe pain on the day of surgery.[2] The parents of pediatric patients undergoing tonsillectomy and adenoidectomy felt that 86% of their children experienced significant overall pain.[3] The reasons for the continued relative undertreatment of postoperative pain is uncertain but may be related to multiple factors including heightened awareness leading to an improved identification of undertreatment of pain, the continued lack of pain assessment or documentation, underutilization of more effective analgesic techniques such as regional analgesic techniques, and the lack of adherence to available pain management guidelines.[4-7]

Our current understanding of the perioperative pathophysiology basically is that a wide range of pathophysiologic responses are initiated when nociceptors are activated after tissue injury that ultimately results in a local inflammatory, behavioral, and physiologic responses.[8] Sympathoneural and neuroendocrine activation and postoperative pain resulting from tissue injury may eventually produce potentially detrimental responses,[8] which may be especially harmful in high-risk patients or those undergoing high-risk procedures and lead to increases in morbidity or even mortality.

Because the use of regional techniques utilizing a local anesthetic-based analgesic solution may attenuate these pathophysiologic responses to a greater extent than that seen with systemic analgesics, it is possible that use of these techniques may be associated with an improvement in some patient outcomes as well as patient satisfaction. For instance, several meta-analyses suggest that the use of regional analgesic techniques is associated with a decreased risk of postoperative pulmonary complications in patients undergoing abdominal-thoracic procedures.[9,10] In addition, several systematic reviews in patients undergoing high-risk cardiothoracic-vascular procedures suggest that a decrease in pulmonary complications, cardiac dysrhythmias, and overall cardiac complications may be seen with perioperative thoracic epidural analgesia with a local anesthetic-based analgesic regimen.[11,12] In patients undergoing abdominal surgery, the perioperative use of thoracic epidural analgesia with a local anesthetic-based regimen is associated with faster resolution of postoperative ileus.[9,13,14] Finally, numerous randomized controlled trials indicate that utilizing continuous peripheral regional catheters may facilitate postoperative rehabilitation and decrease costs associated with surgery.[15,16]

Different analgesic agents may have different effects when compared to one another with respect to patient-centered outcomes such as analgesia or patient satisfaction. When compared to conventional "as needed" opioid analgesia, the use of intravenous patient-controlled analgesia with opioids for postoperative pain control results in superior analgesia and greater patient satisfaction.[17] Regional analgesic techniques utilizing a local anesthetic-based regimen provide superior postoperative analgesia versus systemic opioids.[18,19] Despite the analgesic benefits of regional analgesic techniques, it is not clear whether this improved analgesia can be translated to improvements in some other patient-centered outcomes such as quality of life and quality of recovery.[9,20]

To improve postoperative analgesia, utilization of multimodal analgesia, typically a combination of an opioid and nonopioid analgesic with or without a regional anesthetic

signs. For children with cognitive impairment, the revised Face, Legs, Activity, Cry, and Consolability (r-FLACC) tool and the Nursing Assessment of Pain Intensity (NAPI) may have higher utility than the Non-Communicating Children's Pain Checklist-Postop Version (NCCPC-PV).[61]

The IMMPACT group recommended the following self-report measures for acute pain intensity: (1) poker chip tool for patients 3 to 4 years of age, (2) Faces Pain Scale Revised for patients 4 to 12 years of age, and (3) visual analog scale for patients 8 years of age or older.[43] For observational pain scales, the IMMPACT group recommended the FLACC, CHEOPS, Parents Postoperative Pain Measure (PPPM), and the COMFORT Scale for patients 1 year and older and the Toddler-Preschooler Postoperative Pain Scale for patients 1 to 5 years. For the cognitively impaired children, the Non-Communicating Children's Pain Checklist–Postop Version (NCCPC-PV)[62] may be useful. The COMFORTneo Scale appears to be a promising tool for the assessment of pain in neonates.[63]

For emotional assessment in pediatric patients, the IMMPACT group recommended the Adolescent Pediatric Pain Tool for use in children 8 years of age or older and the Facial Affective Scale as the single-item scale of the affective component of pain.[43] For observational measures of the assessment of behavioral distress during procedures, the Procedure Behavior Checklist (PBCL) and Procedure Behavioral Rating Scale Revised (PBRS-R) was recommended. Both measurement tools can be used for patients 1 year of age or older. The VAS Anxiety Scale in children aged 7 to 16 years compares favorably with other measures of preoperative anxiety in children.[64]

FUTURE AREAS FOR INVESTIGATION

Although there are in essence endless possibilities for research in the area of postoperative pain management, we have highlighted areas in the prior section where the greatest need appears to be in upcoming decades. The trends that we have described appear to be sustainable (e.g., increase in the percentage of the elderly or obese, increase in the U.S. federal deficit) for the foreseeable future; however, we also discuss other areas of potential interest for investigation.

POSTOPERATIVE DELIRIUM AND POSTOPERATIVE COGNITIVE DYSFUNCTION

Increasing age is one of the primary risk factors for the development of postoperative delirium.[28] The prevention (if possible) of postoperative delirium is a significant health care concern, as the presence of this complication is a predictor of mortality and increased length of hospitalization.[28] With the growing percentage of elderly in the population, we would expect that the incidence of this complication will only increase.

Several avenues for investigation in this area would be needed. In terms of the correlation of the postoperative pain and postoperative delirium, this general correlation would have to be evaluated and the severity of postoperative pain per se should be confirmed as an independent risk factor for the incidence or severity of postoperative delirium or postoperative cognitive dysfunction. Once this has been confirmed, the utilization of different analgesic regimens or perioperative interventions should be investigated to examine their effect on influencing the incidence or severity of postoperative delirium. For instance, it is clear that regional analgesic technique (either epidural or peripheral nerve catheter) utilizing a local anesthetic-based regimen provides superior analgesia compared to systemic opioids including those delivered via intravenous patient-controlled analgesia.[18,19] The superior analgesia along with the minimization of opioid use would lead one to believe that utilization of this regimen in elderly postoperative patients would result in a lower incidence or severity of postoperative delirium. However, a somewhat related systematic review[65] examining the incidence of postoperative cognitive difference after general versus neuraxial anesthesia noted no difference between the techniques, although the authors elucidated several methodological issues (e.g., perioperative use of benzodiazepines) in the available published literature.

A more recent systematic review examined prospective and retrospective clinical trials and case studies on delirium and drug therapy in all adult patients.[32] The authors indicated that the quality of available evidence was limited and called for additional well-designed randomized, double-blind, placebo-controlled trials investigating the drug management of delirium, including dose-ranging studies and optimal duration of therapy.[32] In addition to avoidance of medications known to increase the risk of postoperative delirium and providing superior pain control, prophylactic interventions with antipsychotic and cholinesterase inhibitors in high-risk patients may be investigated in an attempt to minimize drug-induced delirium potential.[32] Ultimately, successful attempts to decrease the incidence or severity of postoperative delirium and cognitive dysfunction will most likely require a multimodal approach including optimal drug/analgesic therapy, physical rehabilitation, and other nontraditional approaches. (e.g., cognitive stimulation).

ECONOMIC CONSIDERATIONS

It is clear that there will be more emphasis on cost control in the delivery of health care, and the arena of postoperative pain management will most likely not be exempt from scrutiny. Although health care workers who manage postoperative pain most likely would tend to believe in the added value of a discrete postoperative pain management service, there are few meaningful cost data on these services.[66] It is likely that postoperative patients who are managed by an acute pain service will have superior pain control and decreased analgesic-related side effects,[66] but whether this translates into improved satisfaction, quality, or duration of recovery is uncertain at this time.

There has been an increasing interest by policymakers on cost-effectiveness despite potential resistance from current stakeholders (e.g., health care providers, insurance companies, drug manufacturers, patients, and legislators).[67] Cost-effectiveness data have been used in other countries to guide health care decisions. For instance, Britain's National Institute for Health and Clinical Excellence's (NICE) decision-making process utilizes cost-effectiveness thresholds based in part on the number of quality-adjusted life-years (QALYs) gained with a particular intervention such as a drug, device, or procedure.[68] It is important to note that the goal of NICE is not to ration health care per se and the decisions made incorporate not only cost-effectiveness data but also social values.[68] There are many fears regarding cost-effectiveness, including a possible shift of medical decision making by organizations from individual physicians, lack of transparency of the decision-making process, and suspicion of the methods utilized in a cost-effectiveness analysis.[69] Although there are concerns regarding the implementation of cost-effectiveness data and research, cost-effectiveness analysis is not a cost-containment tool but a method to improve value when implemented properly.[69]

With increased funding for cost-effectiveness research available (approximately $1 billion to support research on the comparative effectiveness of drugs and medical devices in 2009),[70] are there any areas for postoperative pain research that would be particularly amenable for this type of analysis? Although comparative/cost-effectiveness analysis is more common in other areas of medicine, it has been infrequently used in pain management or anesthesiology, and analgesic drugs and techniques/devices lend themselves to this type of analysis. For instance, the use of a regional analgesic technique is associated with potential benefits (e.g., superior analgesia, decreased morbidity)[11,18-20] and complications (e.g., failure of technique, neurologic injury, infectious complication).[70,71] Clinicians generally will present these benefits and risks during the informed consent process to allow patients to decide whether to choose or decline this technique; however, it is often difficult to combine both benefits and risks into a meaningful single analysis. Inserting the currently available data into this type of analysis may demonstrate a preferred method of treatment (i.e., to choose or decline the technique or drug),[72] although patient preferences would need to be incorporated into any meaningful analysis.[73] Nevertheless, both efficacy (high internal validity, low generalizability) and effectiveness (low internal validity, high generalizability) studies will be needed in the future.

Although there has been a relative paucity of research on the effect of postoperative pain on economic outcomes, there are several examples in the literature. For instance, a multivariate regression analysis was used in a prospective observational/surveillance study to determine how acute pain contributes to recovery and discharge. Pain was the most common cause of delayed discharge from postanesthesia care units, affecting 24% of patients in this study. Pain was a significant independent predictor of total recovery duration, and patients who did require analgesics were discharged 54 minutes later than patients who did not require analgesic therapy.[74] The use of regional analgesic techniques instead of general anesthesia with volatile anesthetics is associated with a reduction of postoperative nausea and vomiting, pain, and the need for postoperative intravenous opioids. Ultimately, recovery room length of stay is reduced (if not eliminated). Reductions in recovery room use, including via recovery room bypass, has been shown to lead to a decrease in hospital cost due in part to including reduced postoperative nursing interventions, reduced unanticipated admissions, and faster discharge times.[75]

OBSTRUCTIVE SLEEP APNEA

Surgical patients with obstructive sleep apnea pose significant challenges for the management of postoperative pain. This issue is complicated by the fact that a large percentage of patients with obstructive sleep apnea are not diagnosed at the time of surgery.[37] The standard tool to diagnose obstructive sleep apnea is polysomnography (i.e., sleep study); however, the accuracy of making the diagnosis of obstructive sleep apnea based on preoperative history only is under investigation. The postoperative management of monitoring these patients is also somewhat nebulous.

Although it would seem intuitive to avoid opioids and sedatives postoperatively as has been recommended in published guidelines,[38] it should be recognized that there are few data to guide clinicians in managing these patients. Guidelines recommended using regional analgesic techniques with only a local anesthetic-based regimen when possible, yet there are no high-quality data to support a decreased incidence of complications with use of this technique. It should be recognized that using adjuvant agents (e.g., nonsteroidal anti-inflammatory agents, acetaminophen) to produce an opioid sparing effect may not necessarily translate into a decrease in severe adverse events such as respiratory depression.[76,77] Clearly, well-designed and -executed randomized controlled trials are needed to compare perioperative regional analgesic techniques utilizing a local anesthetic regimen to systemic opioids; however, these trials will need to be adequately powered and designed to assess the adverse events of interest (i.e., respiratory complications).

PREVENTION OF CHRONIC PAIN AFTER SURGERY

Persistent postsurgical pain (PPP) is a persistent pain state that occurs more than 2 months postoperatively that cannot be explained by other causes such as disease or inflammation.[78] The incidence of PPR ranges from 5% to 50%, and the mechanisms causing it are multifactorial.[79,80] Potential mechanisms include inflammatory (release of inflammatory prostaglandins and cytokines) and neuropathic (sustained ectopic activity of injured nerve and changes in spinal inhibition and facilitation) causes.[81] The factors involved in PPP are either patient or surgery related.[79,82] Preoperative causes include psychological factors, presence of pain, genetic factors, gender, and age.[78,83,84] Intraoperative factors include the type of anesthesia, surgical approach, and nerve injury. Most studies on PPP have been retrospective.

The FDA, through its critical path initiative, embarked on a project to help facilitate the development of novel analgesics for the prevention of PPP. The Analgesic Clinical Trial Innovations, Opportunities, and Network (ACTION) initiative was designed as a public-private partnership to bring together experts from academic, government, and private organizations to share data, nest practices, and innovative ideas.[85] Under the ACTION initiative, the Food and Drug Administration (FDA) anticipates that projects will be developed among the stakeholders, resulting in expedited development of drugs that are effective in preventing and treating PPP. Preclinical applications involving long-term neurobiologic and behavioral changes have been proposed.[81] An ideal clinical study design has been proposed (Box 82.2), and the criteria for clinically meaningful improvements and the factors to consider in determining the clinical importance of the results of clinical trials on

Box 82.2 Elements of an "Ideal" Study Design of Persistent Postsurgical Pain

Preoperatively

- Presence of preexisting pain (locally and remote)
- Measurement of the functional consequences of preexisting pain
- Neurophysiologic assessment
- Psychological assessment
- Analysis of "pain genes"

Intra-operatively

- Descriptive characteristics about the incision
- Descriptive characteristics about handling of nerves and muscles
- Information about the disease being treated
- Early postoperatively
- Pain intensity and character
- Pain treatment modality used
- Neurophysiologic assessment
- Late preoperatively
- Psychological consequences
- Neurophysiologic assessment

From Kehlet H, Rathmell JP. Persistent postsurgical pain: the path forward through better design of clinical studies. *Anesthesiology.* 2010;112:514-515.

preventive analgesia have been proposed.[86] Preclinical and clinical trials that are better designed and more clinically applicable results will lead to better management of persistent pain after surgery.

SAFE KIDS INITIATIVE

Research conducted by the FDA's National Center for Toxicological Research (NCTR) showed that exposure to some sedatives and anesthetics may cause harmful changes in the central nervous systems of laboratory animals. These include loss of nerve cells and later abnormal behavior when the anesthetics were administered during rapid brain growth in rodents.[87-92] A study in newborn monkeys, a higher-level animal, showed harmful effects of ketamine.[93] These studies attributed the cognitive behavioral dysfunctions to the transient suppression of neurogenesis or widespread neuroapoptosis in the early postnatal period. In a series of in vitro and in vivo experiments, Briner and associates demonstrated that during the early stage of postnatal brain development in rats, synapse development is altered by exposure to the volatile anesthetics isoflurane, sevoflurane, or desflurane.[94] This elegant study added synaptic remodeling to the list of possible mechanisms by which anesthetics may cause long-lasting changes in the developing brain (of rodents).[95] The developing brain is most vulnerable during the period of rapid synaptogenesis.[95,96]

There are limited human clinical data on this issue. One study showed learning disabilities after several anesthetics given before the child was 4 years of age.[97] Another study showed a lower than expected normative academic achievement test value and more than expected scores below the fifth percentile in academic achievement.[98] It should be noted that the duration of surgery and anesthesia correlated negatively with achievement scores.[98] To make anesthetic drugs as safe as possible for infants and children, the FDA launched the SAFEKIDS Initiative in March 2009. It is a partnership between the FDA and nongovernment organizations with the International Anesthesia Research Society managing the initiative and fundraising efforts (www.iars.org/.../SAFEKIDS%20FAQ%20FINAL%20101609.pdf, accessed December 8, 2012).

SUMMARY

There have been significant improvements and awareness of the prevalence and importance of postoperative pain and its potential deleterious effects on patient outcomes. Surveys suggest that postoperative pain is still undermanaged. The use of more effective analgesic techniques such as regional analgesic techniques and multimodal analgesia may help to improve postoperative analgesia. Outcome domains and measurement tools have been recommended in clinical trials on chronic pain and pediatric acute pain. Several measurement tools have been identified to assess the functional and emotional domains of pain as well as patient satisfaction.

The future areas of potential research in the area of postoperative pain management may be reflected in the macrotrends that are already in place. Additional research is needed to examine the effect of postoperative analgesia on obstructive sleep apnea (obesity), postoperative delirium (elderly), and economic outcomes. It is hoped that drugs to prevent persistent pain after surgery will be developed from the FDA's Analgesic Clinical Trials Innovations, Actions, and Networks (ACTION) initiative. The FDA's SAFEKIDS initiative will optimistically make anesthetic drugs safe for infants and children.

KEY POINTS

- Postoperative pain is still undertreated. The reasons may be related to multiple factors including heightened awareness leading to an improved identification of undertreatment of pain, the continued lack of pain assessment or documentation, underutilization of more effective analgesic techniques such as regional analgesic techniques, and the lack of adherence to available pain management guidelines.
- The use of regional techniques utilizing a local anesthetic-based analgesic solution may attenuate these pathophysiologic responses to a greater extent than that seen with systemic analgesics. The use of these techniques may be associated with an improvement in some patient outcomes as well as patient satisfaction.
- Utilization of multimodal analgesia, typically a combination of an opioid and nonopioid analgesic with or without a regional anesthetic block, has been encouraged to concurrently reduce opioid-related side effects. Studies on the use of multimodal techniques appear to improve pain management, but the results are not consistent.

KEY POINTS—cont'd

- An increasing number of elderly individuals are having surgery, and there is a higher incidence of postoperative delirium with increased age.
- There continues to be an increase in the incidence of obese adults. Perioperative patients who are obese are potentially at higher risk for postoperative complications.
- The increasing federal debt results in an unsustainable increase in health care spending. There is political pressure to control health care spending, partly through the implementation of clinical programs that allow for high-quality and cost-effective standards in the delivery of clinical care.
- Outcome domains and measurement tools have been recommended by the IMMPACT group. Appropriate measurement tools have been identified for pain, side effects, functional conditioning, emotional functioning, and patient satisfaction.
- The FDA, through its ACTION initiative, promotes public-private partnership to develop drugs and interventions to prevent and treat persistent pain after surgery.
- The FDA's SAFEKIDS initiative, in partnership with the International Anesthesia Research Society, is a multiyear research endeavor to make anesthetic drugs safer for infants and children.

SUGGESTED READINGS

Apfelbaum JL, Chen C, Mehta SS, Gan TJ. Postoperative pain experience: results from a national survey suggest postoperative pain continues to be undermanaged. *Anesth Analg.* 2003;97:534-540.

Block RI, Thomas JJ, Bayman EO, et al. Are anesthesia and surgery during infancy associated with altered academic performance during childhood? *Anesthesiology.* 2012;117:494-503.

Crosby G, Culley DJ, Patel PM. At the sharp end of spines: anesthetic effects on synaptic remodeling in the developing brain. *Anesthesiology.* 2010;112:521-523.

Kehlet H, Jensen TS, Woolf CJ. Persistent postsurgical pain: risk factors and prevention. *Lancet.* 2006;367:1618-1625.

Kehlet H, Rathmell JP. Persistent postsurgical pain: the path forward through better design of clinical studies. *Anesthesiology.* 2010;112:514-515.

McGrath PJ, Walco GA, Turk DC, et al. Core outcome domains and measures for pediatric acute pain and chronic/recurrent pain clinical trials: PedIMMPACT recommendations. *J Pain.* 2008;9:771-783.

Myles PS, Hunt JO, Fletcher H, et al. Relation between quality of recovery in hospital and quality of life at 3 months after cardiac surgery. *Anesthesiology.* 2001;95:862-867.

Neal JM, Bernards CM, Hadzic A, et al. ASRA Practice Advisory on Neurologic Complications in Regional Anesthesia and Pain Medicine. *Reg Anesth Pain Med.* 2008;33:404-415.

Practice Guidelines for the Perioperative Management of Patients with Obstructive Sleep Apnea: a report by the American Society of Anesthesiologists Task Force on Perioperative Management of Patients with Obstructive Sleep Apnea. *Anesthesiology.* 2006;104:1081-1093.

Wilder RT, Flick RP, Sprung J, et al. Early exposure to anesthesia and learning disabilities in a population-based birth cohort. *Anesthesiology.* 2009;110:796-804.

Wu CL, Raja SN. Treatment of acute postoperative pain. *Lancet.* 2011;377:2215-2225.

The references for this chapter can be found at www.expertconsult.com.

83 Future Directions and Trends in Pain Medicine

Robert W. Hurley | Honorio T. Benzon | Dennis C. Turk

This chapter is divided in two main sections. The first section addresses the future of pain medicine, and the second tackles the newest trends in pain treatment. The overarching principle guiding the authors of this chapter is the delivery of the highest quality of pain care in a manner that is most consistent with empiric medical evidence. Although the comprehensive treatment of pain has long been a goal of the profession, the practice of pain medicine has become laden with divisions, sub-sub-specialization that has resulted in a field with an unclear core mission. It is also challenged by the definitions imposed by nonpain clinicians. The future of the field of pain medicine relies on greater rigor in at least three domains: (1) defining the medical specialty of pain medicine, (2) educating future pain medicine clinicians, and (3) advancing the basic, clinical, and translational sciences related to the etiology and treatment of pain.

As in this textbook, the practice of pain medicine is often divided into acute, recurrent, and chronic pain medicine (or management). The historical application of this terminology has equated brief episodes of pain (e.g., post-surgical pain) with being an "acute" pain, recurrent, episodic acute pain (e.g., migraine, sickle cell disease), and most other pain conditions with "chronic" pain (associated with persistent cancer and noncancer-related painful disorders). This subtyping by duration is no longer helpful when it is applied to the current, complex, and highly specialized health care environment. For instance, the outpatient pain clinician manages the pain of patients who have recent injuries, thereby fitting the definition of acute pain, not just persistent pain. The hospital "acute" pain service often takes care of patients with persistent pain conditions. As acute, recurrent acute, and chronic (persistent) pain patients are seen in the inpatient and outpatient settings and the employed treatment modalities differ among the populations, the more appropriate distinction may be between the treatment of hospitalized patients with pain and that for nonhospitalized patients with pain.

RECENT HISTORY OF OUTPATIENT PAIN MEDICINE

In the late 1960s, an anesthesiologist, John J. Bonica, founded the first multidisciplinary clinic for the treatment of patients with chronic pain. The practice approached pain from biologic models involving neurologists, internists, orthopedists, and neurosurgeons. After much frustration in treating patients debilitated by their persistent pain, Dr. Bonica, at the urging of the behavioral scientist Wilbert E. Fordyce, adopted the biopsychosocial model of the treatment of pain. The behavioral psychology approach of not rewarding pain behaviors (and, in some instances, ignoring the verbal pain complaints and related behaviors such as moaning and facial grimaces) but focusing on rehabilitation and increased function of the patient was integrated into a multidisciplinary pain clinic. Throughout the 1970s, this clinic and others that incorporated the principles used in the original pain clinic were very successful in treating patients with persistent pain. In the early 1980s, the neurosurgeon John Loeser took over Bonica's pain clinic and credited the interactions between the providers as the reason why patients did so well.

It would be a logical extension to believe that this model would be adopted by pain treatment facilities throughout the United States because of the revolutionary success the multidisciplinary pain clinic had in treating this challenging patient population. The reality was, unfortunately, far from that assumption. Currently, in the United States, there are relatively few truly multidisciplinary pain clinics that involve management of pain in patients in the inpatient and outpatient settings. The architecture and economics of medicine have been redirected in a way that undermines this successful treatment model. The changes that occurred include the increasing cost of health insurance, the shifting of health insurance costs from employers to employees, and the decreasing coverage of a number of health and mental health care services. These changes have negatively impacted the practice of multidisciplinary pain medicine. The health care economic bottom line meant that physicians had to practice reimbursable medicine for pain treatment clinics to remain viable. The paradox is that there is more evidence supporting the clinical effectiveness and cost-effectiveness of multidisciplinary rehabilitation than any traditional medical or surgical treatment for patients with problems of persistent pain.

This economic shift promoted the unidisciplinary model of pain care in the 1990s, in which physicians focused on the treatment algorithm most closely associated with their medical training and specialty. Anesthesiologists focused on interventional analgesic procedures, and opioid and nonopioid adjuvant medications to treat pain reports, taking the biologic approach to pain care. Physiatrists (physical medicine and rehabilitation) focused on musculoskeletal exams, electrodiagnostic tests, and medical management of pain with opioids. Psychiatrists focused on the medical management of pain, the treatment of addiction disorders resulting from the treatment of pain with opioids and benzodiazepines, and the treatment of psychiatric comorbidities. Psychologists continued to follow behaviorist or cognitive-behaviorist approaches in concert with group therapy to teach pain patients coping skills to live with their chronic daily pain in those institutions where financial support existed, but often as adjuncts to biologically based treatments rather than as components of an integrated approach that had been shown to be effective.

In the late 1990s and 2000s, the continued contraction of medical and health care services covered by government and private insurance and a shift in emphasis even further from the integrated, rehabilitation approach to procedures performed have changed the pain medicine landscape again. Across the United States, anesthesiologists further specialized in interventional pain medicine procedures (transforaminal epidural steroid injections, facet joint interventions, radiofrequency procedures, spinal cord stimulation, and intrathecal pump therapy) with a more modest medical management clinic where opioid and nonopioid medications were recommended to others to prescribe. Physiatrists began performing interventional pain therapies copying the anesthesiologist's interventional model. Psychiatrists, neurologists, and neurosurgeons reduced or eliminated their pain management practices. Pain psychologists became fewer and fewer, and those who remained focused on pain research and small clinical practices. This less integrated, silo approach that focused on interventional therapies has provided good (though not ideal) care to some patients because of the advancement in some of the pain procedures employed, such as spinal cord stimulation. However, this fundamental conflict has left few options for the significant set of patients with pain that is not amenable to these therapies.

WHERE TO GO FROM HERE?

In going forward, it is essential to reduce the confused terminology and purpose:

1. Pain is a distinct disease entity when it is no longer associated with an ongoing injury or the immediate repercussions of the injury.
2. The treatment of pain with medications, procedural or surgical therapies, and psychological and physical rehabilitation are all components of the integrated practice of pain medicine.
3. The goal of pain treatment is not simply to relieve pain but to return the patient to satisfactory physical and psychological function.
4. Clinicians with appropriate medical, psychological, or rehabilitative (e.g., physical therapy, social work) training, certification, and credentialing practice within the field of pain medicine. The use of the descriptor "pain management" for the field has led to an overly broad definition of who is able to safely provide these complex pain services and should therefore be retired as a descriptor of the practice.

PAIN MEDICINE EDUCATION OF PHYSICIANS

Comprehensive and multidisciplinary education of future pain medicine physicians is paramount to the optimal care of patients. Unfortunately, the training of physicians in pain treatment traditionally had a narrow focus on pharmacological or interventional management, with little more than passing reference to the psychological and physical rehabilitative components of pain treatment. This deficit was recognized on a national level, and in 2007 the Accreditation Council for Graduate Medical Education (ACGME) redefined the pain medicine fellowships by setting new standards for achieving the goal of comprehensive pain training. The four medical specialty boards (Anesthesiology, PM&R, Neurology, Psychiatry) administering pain medicine board examinations agreed to a single ACGME-approved pain medicine training fellowship curricula and a single pain medicine subspecialty board examination. In a post-2007 pain medicine fellowship, trainees are required to have training in pain medicine from the medical, rehabilitative, and psychological perspectives. This change in education and certification has been a step in the right direction and has been responsible for the closure of "pain" fellowships that had a predominant or exclusive focus on interventional training. Unfortunately, this unidisciplinary approach to training continues in some of those closed programs as non-ACGME-approved "Interventional Spine" fellowships. This shift has been a disservice to those who train in these programs for numerous reasons including the inability to take the pain medicine board exams as well as to the patients who believe they are receiving care from a comprehensively trained pain physician. Even with these exceptions, the changes made by the ACGME in 2007 have been a good step toward the patient-centered model of multidisciplinary pain medicine developed by John Bonica. However, it is only a single piece of the puzzle.

Additional changes include a future match program for pain medicine fellowship positions that has been approved by the Association of Pain Program Directors. The match should provide a better opportunity for applicants to get their desired training program. For pain medicine clinicians, patient simulation will be included in future maintenance of certification accreditation (MOCA) requirements. Although simulation training is now offered in regular anesthesiology recertification testing and has been proven to be successful,[1] it is new in pain medicine. The American Society of Anesthesiologists Committee on Simulation has already approved simulation centers and aims to establish testing centers in different regions in the country. The curriculum and case scenarios for simulation in pain medicine have been aptly described by Brenner and colleagues.[2]

FUTURE OF PAIN MEDICINE

The appropriate changes in pain medicine education have not been accompanied by reform of the reimbursement methodologies. Our insurance system is still heavily biased toward remunerating for procedures and not for clinician decision making. It is also biased toward reports of pain relief and not toward the increased functionality of pain patients. The face of pain medicine will likely change to more of a patient-centered model of reimbursement. We have seen the beginnings of this shift, in which Medicare has begun to associate payment to physicians and hospitals with quality metrics (e.g., refusing to pay for readmission resulting from iatrogenic infections). The future of pain medicine will progress to paying for therapeutic approaches that have successfully returned patients to function and a resumption of their activities of daily living. Based on the positive historical experience of the Bonica-style pain programs, the multidisciplinary model with inpatient and outpatient treatment might be the best goal. The challenge of revisiting this model is the costs associated with these programs in light of low levels of reimbursement for these services. The questions that remain include, can the cost-efficiencies of modern medicine be applied to the old model of comprehensive pain medicine, and will the insurance companies recognize its long-term cost savings and pay for the services in order to make the old model fiscally viable? With respect to chronic low back pain, the answer may be yes.[3]

The manner of education and the modalities used in pain medicine will continue to change, as previously addressed, and the manner in which research or lack thereof influences our practice will become foremost concerns. Physician experience and medical teaching are becoming less and less acceptable rationales for the treatments pain physicians employ. The challenge is that a substantial number of treatments have few rigorous data to support their use. And unfortunately, even when evidence exists, it is often ignored. One of the most common procedures in pain medicine, the epidural steroid injection for back and extremity pain, has been shown to have no benefit for axial low back pain, minimal benefit for back pain associated with spinal stenosis, and moderate short-term benefit for extremity pain related to disk herniation.[4] Yet a subset of physicians continue to perform steroid injections for low back pain and promise long-term benefit for radicular symptoms in spite of studies that showed its short-term efficacy.[5] The medicinal treatment of radicular symptoms is managed as though they are the same as neuropathic pain of disparate etiology including diabetic and postherpetic neuralgia, yet evidence of the efficacy of the most commonly used medications is minimal.[6] These are only two examples of misguided therapies. The challenge will be to produce evidence of effectiveness and safety for medications and procedures that are etiology specific, cost-effective, and widely applicable.

PHARMACOLOGICAL MANAGEMENT OF CHRONIC PAIN

This section deals with topics that were not discussed or emphasized in the previous chapters on pharmacological management. The management of cancer pain will probably remain as it has been (i.e., opioid as the mainstay of treatment in combination with other medications including the anticonvulsants). It is in the area of chronic noncancer pain (e.g., osteoarthritis, diabetic painful neuropathy) where drugs that are effective with minimal side effects are being constantly sought. Guidelines from groups of well-respected experts have been proposed in the management of neuropathic pain. These include the European Federation of Neurological Sciences (EFNS), the International Association for the Study of Pain (IASP) Neuropathic Pain Special Interest Group (NeuPSIG), and the Canadian Pain Society.[7-9] The guidelines recommended the anticonvulsants, serotonin and norepinephrine reuptake inhibitors (SNRIs), and antidepressants as the first-line treatments for neuropathic pain. More recent data, coupled with the SNRIs reduced side effects, made the EFNS and the IASP NeuPSIG recommend these as the first-line drugs. These guidelines continue to evolve based on the results of randomized controlled studies.

Pregabalin, with its linear pharmacokinetics, quicker analgesic onset than gabapentin,[10] and efficacy with lower doses,[11] will continue to be used. Although pregabalin and gabapentin are well known, lacosamide has been shown to be effective in diabetic painful neuropathy (DPN).[12] Its clinical use in DPN is awaiting approval from the United States Food and Drug Administration (FDA).

The SNRIs are definite improvements over the tricyclic antidepressants, particularly in their side effect profiles. Milnacipran lacks anticholinergic, antihistaminic, and alpha-adrenergic receptor blocking activity; is weakly protein bound; and has no effect on the P450 system, resulting in fewer drug interactions.[13,14] Randomized controlled studies in fibromyalgia showed positive results with improvements in fatigue, physical conditioning, and discomfort.[14,15]

A combination of drugs with different mechanisms of action maybe more effective than any drug alone. Randomized controlled studies showed beneficial effects when drugs with different mechanisms of action are combined. The combination of gabapentin and morphine in patients with postherpetic neuralgia (PHN) and DPN resulted in less pain, lower doses, and fewer side effects from the drugs.[16] The same salutary effects were noted with the combination of gabapentin and nortriptyline,[17] gabapentin and lidocaine plaster for PHN/DPN,[18] and gabapentin and oxycodone in DPN.[19] For neuropathic cancer pain, a combination of opioid and gabapentin was noted to be more effective than opioid monotherapy.[20] However, not all drug combinations showed positive results. No beneficial effects were noted when pregabalin and oxycodone were combined in the treatment of PHN or DPN[21] or with morphine and nortriptyline for lumbosacral radiculitis.[22] Whether the lack of additive effects with the combinations was due to the dosages used (the doses of pregabalin in the study by Zin and colleagues were up to 600 mg/day, whereas the oxycodone dose was 10 mg/day) or to inappropriate drugs being used (radiculitis may not respond to antidepressants) is not known. More studies are needed to determine which drug combinations work best in which chronic pain syndrome. Moreover, in addition to concerns about the side effects of individual medications, with drug combinations there is the added concern about potential drug-drug interactions among some of the medications most frequently combined (such as opioids that also have serotonergic effects, e.g., tramadol and tapentadol, and selective serotonin reuptake inhibitors [SSRIs] and SNRIs where serotonin syndromes may be created by the combination).

For neuropathic pain, clinicians are using nonsteroidal anti-inflammatory drugs (NSAIDs).[23] Although animal models showed the efficacy of NSAIDs for neuropathic pain treatment,[24] clinical studies showed some efficacy,[25,26] no efficacy,[27] or inconclusive results.[28] The unequivocal results call for randomized studies on the role of NSAIDs in neuropathic pain. However, there are significant concerns about NSAIDs because of their gastrointestinal and renal toxicities, and there are concerns about the cardiac effects of the newer cyclooxygenase-2 inhibitor (COX2) drugs.[29]

It is important to note that regardless of the medication used to control pain, the actual benefits, while statistically significant, are modest, with fewer than 35% of patients obtaining at least a 50% reduction in pain. Moreover, the effects of even the most recently developed medications have shown that they do little to improve physical functioning.

INTRAVENOUS INFUSIONS AND TOPICAL ANALGESICS

Intravenous infusions, especially ketamine, are being used more frequently and studies have shown their efficacy. Unfortunately, these publications were either case series or retrospective studies or consisted of patients with different pain syndromes.[30,31] It is in the treatment of complex regional pain syndromes that controlled studies showed the efficacy of ketamine infusions.[32,33] Randomized controlled studies are welcome. These studies should involve specific pain syndromes (e.g., spinal cord injuries) and the doses and duration of infusions sought, especially as there may be hepatotoxicity from the infusion;[34] the mechanism of hepatic injury should also be investigated.

The high-dose capsaicin patch is an improvement over the low-dose patch and needs to be applied only every 3 months. The patch has been shown to be effective in the treatment of PHN, DPN, and human immunodeficiency virus (HIV) neuropathy.[35,36] However, it is expensive and its application is painful even when a local anesthetic cream is pre-applied. Topical clonidine gel was noted to be effective in DPN patients with functional (and possibly sensitized) nociceptors in the affected skin.[37] The use of topical doxepin or topical doxepin and capsaicin was noted to be superior to placebo in treating neuropathic pain.[38] A randomized study showed topical ketamine, amitriptyline, or a combination to be effective for patients with neuropathic pain.[39] Open-label studies on topical amitriptyline and ketamine for neuropathic pain showed encouraging results.[40,41] The same results were noted with topical ketamine for PHN.[42] More controlled studies are required, especially in view of the advantages of drugs applied topically or as patches in patients who cannot tolerate oral medications.

PRESCRIPTION PATTERNS OF PAIN MEDICINE PHYSICIANS

It is gratifying to note that the prescription patterns of pain physicians reflect evidence-based treatments. Most ask for opioid agreements, electrocardiograms (ECGs) are ordered when methadone is prescribed, the maximum dose of acetaminophen is decreased in moderate alcohol drinkers, opioids are prescribed for cancer pain, and the majority follow the guidelines recommended by the EFNS and the IASP's NeuPSIG (i.e., anticonvulsants and SNRIs followed by drug combinations).[43] However, several gaps in knowledge were also identified, including the prescription of codeine for patients who have difficulty metabolizing codeine to its active morphine metabolite (i.e., Caucasians, Asians, and pediatric populations).[44-46] Although only a small percentage responded that they prescribe carisoprodol, this drug is metabolized to meprobamate, which causes dependence and has been shown to be no more effective than placebo.[47] It would be interesting to know the prescription patterns of primary care physicians who take care of most pain problems.

Although opioids are the most commonly prescribed medication for pain, prescriptions for chronic, noncancer pain patients are more controversial. This class of medication may have significant and unintended effects on immune and hormonal function and there is some evidence of the paradoxical effect of opioid-induced hyperalgesia. There are also growing concerns about the misuse and abuse of these drugs. Moreover, opioids appear to have little effect on improving physical functioning. Finally, there is no long-term evidence of the analgesic benefits of opioids.[48]

INTERVENTIONAL PAIN PROCEDURES

DISK HERNIATION, SPINAL STENOSIS, AND INFLAMMATORY MARKERS

Disk herniation results in the release of phospholipase A2 (PLA2), resulting in the production of prostaglandins. Increased levels of inflammatory cytokines interleukin (IL)-6 and IL-8 were noted in disk materials taken from patients with known disk disease.[49] Cytokines such as IL-1 and IL-6 and tumor necrosis factor alpha (TNF-α) have been strongly linked to radicular pain.[50,51] IL-1 beta, IL-6, and TNF-α have been noted to increase the discharge rates and mechanosensitivity of the dorsal root ganglion and peripheral receptive fields in rats.[52] Disks express TNF-α, which causes morphologic and functional changes when applied to spinal nerve roots.[53] Levels of IL-6 in the cerebrospinal fluid (CSF) of patients with radicular pain from spinal stenosis correlated with the degree of spinal stenosis.[54]

These studies led investigators to inject TNF-α inhibitors into the epidural space of patients with a herniated disk or spinal stenosis. Studies of epidural etanercept or tocilizumab, a TNF-α inhibitor and an anti-IL6 receptor antibody, respectively, showed some efficacy. The epidural injection of etanercept has been shown to have salutary effects, in terms of pain and numbness, in patients with a herniated disk[55] or spinal stenosis.[56] The epidural injection of tocilizumab decreased low back pain and numbness in patients with spinal stenosis.[57] The follow-ups in these studies were for 1 month[56] or 6 months.[55] These beneficial results should be contrasted with the findings that intravenous infliximab had similar efficacy as placebo in relieving lumbar radicular pain from a herniated disk.[58] More studies are needed in this area, especially to evaluate the risks involved; patients on TNF-α inhibitors are prone to infection.

EPIDURAL STEROID INJECTIONS

CNS INJURIES AFTER TRANSFORAMINAL EPIDURAL STEROID INJECTIONS

Epidural steroid injections (ESIs) are given to patients to relieve low back and radicular pain. It has been postulated that inflammatory changes in the nerve root cause the pain, and nerve root edema has been demonstrated on computed tomography (CT) scans of patients with herniated disks.[59] The rationale for ESIs includes their anti-inflammatory effect[59] and a specific anti-nociceptive effect.[60] The results of studies on epidural steroids were not uniform. Overall, the studies showed short-term relief.[5]

There have been reports of central nervous system (CNS) injuries, including spinal (paraplegia) and brain (brainstem hemorrhage and cerebellar infarct) events. These unfortunate events are probably secondary to arterial injury (trauma or spasm) or embolism of the particulate steroid.[61] The ascending and deep cervical arteries have been shown to send medullary branches to the anterior spinal artery; these two arteries anastomose with the vertebral artery and are very close to the superior articular process, a landmark in transforaminal epidural steroid injections.[62] Intravascular injection of the contrast into the radicular artery accompanying the nerve root has been demonstrated.[63] Injection of the particulate steroid into the anterior spinal artery (through the medullary branches or the radicular artery) or into the vertebral artery (through the ascending and deep cervical arteries) is possible.

Particulate steroids cause more problems than nonparticulate steroids. The CNS injuries reported with nonparticulate injectates were temporary,[64,65] compared to permanent injuries with the particulate injectates.[61] Animal studies support the catastrophic lesions/events associated with particulate steroids in comparison to nonparticulate injectates. Animals injected with the particulate steroid became unconscious and required ventilator support[66] or showed cerebral hemorrhage.[67] In contrast, the animals injected with dexamethasone, a nonparticulate steroid, had no evidence of injury and had full recovery.

The reported cases of CNS injuries led a Working Group of Experts and the FDA Safe Use Initiative to formulate recommendations on the prevention of these injuries. The recommendations will probably include knowledge of the anatomy, use of live fluoroscopy or digital subtraction technology (DST), ability to correctly interpret the images, use of nonparticulate steroids in cervical transforaminal injections, and others. Obviously, particulate steroids are acceptable in interlaminar injections. These recommendations will come out in late 2013 or early 2014.

COMPOUNDING STEROIDS

Some physicians use compounded depot steroids for epidural injections to avoid the vehicles and preservatives in the depot steroid and for reasons of price. Avoidance of the preservatives is unnecessary, as the studies on the neurolytic lesions caused by these preservatives used concentrations that were 8- to 10-fold higher than the concentrations of these preservatives in the depot steroids.[68-70] A case report of flaccid paralysis occurred after an unintentional subarachnoid injection of 40 mL of 0.9% NaCl that contained 1.5% benzyl alcohol.[71] In addition to the lower concentrations of the preservatives in the commercially available steroids, the steroid is diluted with 1 to 3 mL of saline or local anesthetic, further decreasing the concentrations of the preservatives.

An outbreak of fungal meningitis occurred after an epidural injection of compounded methylprednisolone.[72,73] The episode was traced to contaminated steroid produced by the New England Compounding Company, exposing the lax regulations that oversee compounding companies.[74-76] Clinicians will continue to use compounded medications because of the lack of availability of other medications (e.g., oral ketamine, intrathecal pump drugs) or because of their lower cost. Pain medicine interventional physicians can assure themselves of a safe product by purchasing compounded drugs from companies accredited by the Pharmacy Compounding Accreditation Board. A list of accredited companies is available on the agency's website (www.pcab.org). There are now bills pending in Congress mandating supervision of compounding companies by the FDA instead of the state where they are located.

OTHER INTERVENTIONAL PROCEDURES

Minimally invasive lumbar decompression (MILD) procedures for symptomatic central lumbar canal stenosis have been described, wherein the hypertrophied ligamentum flavum is thinned percutaneously. An initial review of the safety of MILD showed no incidents of dural puncture, nerve injury, hematoma, or blood transfusion.[77] A 1-year follow-up of results showed a decrease in pain scores and improvements in the Oswestry Disability Index,[78] Zurich Claudication Questionnaire, and SF-12 Health Survey.[79] There were no major device-related or procedure-related complications. These great results were questioned by a single-center experience of complications including nondecompression of supposedly decompressed levels, persistent neurogenic complications, cerebrospinal fluid (CSF) leak, and transected nerve roots.[80] Obviously, more prospective studies are required to determine the long-term efficacy and complications associated with this procedure.

For intrathecal pain management, an interdisciplinary panel of experts published recommendations that included the proper methods of trialing for long-term intrathecal drug delivery; an update of the algorithms for the rational use of intrathecal medications for the treatment of neuropathic and nociceptive pain; guidance on the how to minimize the risk of respiratory depression, infection, granuloma, device-related complications, endocrinopathies, and human error; and instruction on the prevention, diagnosis, and management of intrathecal granulomas.[81-84] No new pharmacological developments are anticipated in the near future.

PSYCHOLOGICAL TREATMENT OF PATIENTS EXPERIENCING PAIN

Research performed since the 1990s confirms that psychology-based pain treatments (e.g., cognitive-behavior therapy, relaxation, positive reinforcement of activity, exposure to activities avoided, realistic goal setting) are more effective than no treatment, standard care, and treatment conditions that control for the effects of time, therapist attention, and treatment outcome expectancies (such as pain education or relaxation training only). However, despite the fact that different treatments are often based on different theoretic perspectives, most psychological treatments result in similar outcomes,[85] and not one of them completely eliminates pain for the majority of patients.[86] However, this is not unique to psychological treatment. Of all treatment modalities, the pharmacological and nonpharmacological, the best evidence for pain reduction averages approximately 30% to 40% in approximately half of treated patients, and this does not always occur with concurrent improvement in physical and emotional function.[87] Thus, none of the most commonly prescribed treatment regimens, by themselves, are sufficient to eliminate pain and to have a major impact on physical and emotional functioning in the majority of patients with persistent pain. This is hardly surprising given the complexity of pain and the myriad of psychological, contextual, historical, and genetic along with neurophysiologic factors involved. In the absence of a cure, there is a need to maximize symptom relief so that patients are able to lead the highest quality of life possible.

Although psychological factors have been demonstrated consistently to play an important role in one's perception and response to acute and postsurgical pain, the greatest emphasis of psychological treatments has been to help patients manage, cope with, and adapt to the presence of persistent pain and its associated symptoms. Consequently, rarely are psychological treatments applied in the absence of medical and pharmacological treatments for patients with chronic pain.

We anticipate several trends and directions for the application of psychological treatments and psychological principles in the management of patients with persistent pain in the future, specifically (1) combination treatments, (2) matching of treatment components to specific patient characteristics, (3) development and use of maintenance-enhancing strategies based on psychological principles and technological advances, and (4) availability of psychologists and reimbursement. We outline these approaches in the following sections.

COMBINATION TREATMENTS: PHARMACOLOGICAL AND NONPHARMACOLOGICAL TREATMENTS

Turk[88] suggested that the combination of pharmacological and nonpharmacological interventions (somatic, behavioral) might be particularly advantageous given the nature and impact of pain syndromes and the fact that cure is rarely possible and therefore patients will need to learn to cope with at least some level of pain. Several studies have reported on the additive benefits of pharmacological and psychological treatments[89-91] where combinations had a greater effect than *either* the pharmacological or the psychological treatments alone.

Interdisciplinary pain rehabilitation programs, by definition, are combination treatments in that they often combine psychological and physical treatment approaches, medications, and at times other interventions.[92] Meta-analyses and systematic reviews have provided support for both the clinical effectiveness and cost-effectiveness of such interdisciplinary treatment programs.[93,94] However, to date few studies have been designed to dismantle these comprehensive treatments in order to determine the necessary and sufficient treatment components or identify the characteristics of patients most likely to benefit from intensive rehabilitation programs.

One systematic review recommended cognitive interventions combined with exercise for chronic low back pain,[95] and two evidence-based clinical practice guidelines recommended the combination of medication, exercise, and cognitive-behavioral therapy (CBT) for fibromyalgia patients.[96,97] If research confirms the initial positive results, various combination treatments may become common practice.

RESPONDERS AND TREATMENT MATCHING

Pain patients are typically bundled into classifications based on pain location (e.g., head, neck, back) or known pathology (e.g., neuropathic) and treated as if they were a homogeneous group. Patients with persistent pain, however, even when they have the same diagnosis, are heterogeneous and differ from one another on many important variables (e.g., demographic, symptom presentation, psychosocial style, and adaptation).[98] Indeed, patients' responses to a standardized interdisciplinary treatment vary based on each individual's psychosocial and behavioral characteristics.[99,100]

It is important to consider that treatment responses depend on a range of individual differences, and no one approach is likely to benefit all patients. Matching patients to particular treatments based on relevant predictive characteristics would probably be ideal, if we had knowledge of the appropriate matching variable. Research can be conducted to identify treatment responders (e.g., 30% improvement in pain severity, 20% improvement on a functional outcome) and then use regression analyses to identify the characteristics (predictors) of treatment response. For example, Thieme and colleagues[101] identified different pretreatment characteristics that were associated with different response rates to cognitive-behavior therapy, relative to a treatment based on operant conditioning. A prospective study can then be conducted to determine whether treatments customized to address specific patient characteristics do, indeed, produce the desired effects. Research in this area can provide an empirical basis for prescribing treatments to those most likely to benefit, and it can serve as an impetus for the development of treatments that will match the characteristics of patients who may not have responded. This strategy would improve patient outcomes and would be more cost-effective than the current approach of treating all patients with the same treatment—the treatment selected based on the preferences and training of the providers rather than the results of clinical trials. There is a great need for research that goes beyond asking whether a particular treatment is effective to addressing what treatment is effective for which patients, and under what circumstances.

To maximize efficiency, improve outcomes, control costs, and reduce patient burden, the research needs to identify treatment responders and the components of the treatment that make the greatest contribution to successful outcomes. In the future, clinicians need to focus more on patient-centered approaches so that they can tailor treatment approaches to patient characteristics. We anticipate that this will be a focus of great interest.

ADHERENCE AND MAINTENANCE OF EFFECTS

A general caution about all symptomatic treatments is that of maintenance. Treatments that are tested in clinical trials are rehabilitative, not curative, and rely for their continued success on patient self-management. It is reasonable to assume that patients will continue to manage some pain and disability and that they will experience inevitable flare-ups. Maintenance of therapeutic efforts by patients is critical for long-term success. However, significant problems can arise related to adherence to self-management programs and maintenance of initial positive benefits over long periods of time—years, if not decades. Studies that have examined maintenance of lifestyle changes (e.g., weight loss, smoking reduction, reduction of substance abuse) have demonstrated significant relapse rates. It is naïve to assume that benefits from brief treatments for patients with pain will be maintained unless the benefits are sufficiently reinforcing; otherwise, relapse will be a significant problem. Thus, strategies are needed to facilitate adherence to long-term change. Psychological principles have been used as the bases for maintenance enhancement strategies and may guide and be incorporated into treatments over time.

TECHNOLOGICALLY ENHANCED VIRTUAL TREATMENTS

It is inconvenient for some patients with significant physical impairments to travel to treatment programs that extend over time and that may be at great distances from their homes. Importantly, as noted previously, none of the currently available pharmacological, medical, or psychological treatments are able to provide cures for the majority of people who experience persistent pain, although many can offer patients a reduction in symptoms and improvements in physical and emotional functioning.[87] Consequently, many individuals with chronic pain are going to have to learn how to function with at least some pain persisting for extended periods.

Psychological treatments tend to focus on teaching skills that foster self-management. However, limitation of resources, inconvenience, and lack of maintenance have been shown to be recalcitrant problems and present significant challenges.

One approach to addressing these long-term maintenance issues is to make use of sophisticated and rapidly evolving technologies. Web-based technologies, smartphone applications, use of e-mail communication, and other service delivery platforms offer opportunities that can address both treatment barriers and issues of maintenance and generalization (also noted by Naylor and colleagues[102]), often with the added benefits of convenience and privacy. Findings from a number of preliminary studies support the potential of these approaches with adults[103] and adolescents.[104]

In a meta-analysis, Macea and colleagues[105] identified 11 studies, involving 2953 patients, that evaluated the effects of Web-based interventions for chronic pain. The pooled effect sizes for pain reduction (standardized mean difference between intervention and waiting-list group means) were modest but significant, favoring the Web-based interventions. Other positive outcomes reported in different studies included reductions in pain behaviors, decreased depression and anxiety, greater capacity for work, reductions in medication, and a reduction in physician visits. These studies demonstrate not only the potential value of taking advantage of advanced technologies but also the acceptance of such interventions and modalities. For reasons of both access and effectiveness, we anticipate that technological innovations will be used more frequently as modes for delivering psychological treatments and as tactical maneuvers, incorporating psychological principles, to facilitate and enhance maintenance.

AVAILABILITY OF PSYCHOLOGISTS AND REIMBURSEMENT

The availability of appropriately trained therapists to provide psychological treatments for patients with pain is often limited to large urban areas and academic centers. Thus, in the future telehealth may become essential for patients who seek the services of psychologists. There are and will likely continue to be concerns about the availability of psychological services, whether remotely or at the point of care. This chronic problem occurs despite substantial evidence demonstrating both the clinical utility and cost-effectiveness of behavioral health strategies.[106,107] How best to address the evidence-based paradox—more evidence to support the benefits of behavioral health interventions as part of interdisciplinary programs than most alternative treatments for chronic pain, coupled with a denial of payment—remains unresolved.

In addition to the use of advanced technologies to take advantage of psychological interventions, there are a number of important psychological principles that all health care providers can use—for example, paying attention to provider-patient communication, with particular attention placed on providing realistic expectations for treatment, identifying and addressing patient concerns and fears, emphasizing self-management in the absence of complete symptom elimination, stressing the importance of adhering to the treatment plan, and offering positive reinforcement to patient efforts, not just outcomes. Psychologists may serve as consultants to other health care providers even when they do not deliver services directly to patients. This consultant role may be an important one in the future.

SUMMARY AND CONCLUDING COMMENTS

There are exciting new developments in pain medicine, including the areas of education and training (e.g., the match program for pain medicine fellowships), accreditation (MOCA), pharmacological advances (guidelines from respected groups of experts), and interventional management approaches (patient safety, the MILD procedure, recommendations from the interdisciplinary expert panel on intrathecal drug management). The American Society of Regional Anesthesia (ASRA) is in the process of formulating guidelines on interventional pain procedures for patients on anticoagulants. When appropriate, a combination of psychological and nonpsychological (pharmacological, interventional, rehabilitative) treatments is more effective than either treatment alone. Rapidly evolving technologies may address the long-term maintenance of patients' improvement. We cannot predict the specific areas where future developments will occur. However, some developments are on the horizon (Box 83.1). Pain medicine has become an exciting specialty. In view of the talented trainees, researchers, and young faculty entering the field of pain medicine, the future is promising.

Box 83.1 Possible Future Developments in Education and Pharmacological, Interventional, Rehabilitative, and Psychological Management in Pain Medicine

Education

- Greater integration of psychological and rehabilitative modalities into education of pain medicine fellows
- Match program in pain medicine fellowships
- Maintenance of certification accreditation (MOCA) using simulation
- Eventual development of pain medicine into its own independent multidisciplinary specialty

Pharmacological and Interventional Management

- Update of the different guidelines on the treatment of neuropathic pain
- Controlled studies on intravenous infusions and topical treatments
- Studies on treatment combinations for different chronic pain syndromes
- Education of primary care physicians on evidence-based pharmacological management of the different chronic pain syndromes
- FDA Safe Use Initiative and Working Group recommendations on the safety of transforaminal epidural steroid injections
- Improved regulation of compounding companies
- ASRA recommendations on interventional pain procedures in patients on anticoagulants

Psychological Rehabilitation Management

- Combination with pharmacological and interventional modalities
- Identify predictors of favorable response to treatments
- Match treatment or components of treatment with patient characteristics
- Long-term maintenance of positive response to treatment

There is a growing awareness that single treatments are inadequate for patients with persistent pain. Combinations of medications and, perhaps even more important, of pharmacological and nonpharmacological modalities may provide the greatest outcome for the greatest number of patients with recalcitrant conditions. The pendulum appears to be swinging back to the patient-centered approach characteristic of multidisciplinary treatments from monotherapies. There is growing evidence of both the clinical benefit and cost-effectiveness of these programs for those who do not achieve sufficient relief from biomedical treatments alone. Cost-effectiveness is an important issue to address in research and to communicate to payers. Outcomes other than subjective ratings of pain reduction are becoming essential, and clinicians are going to have to provide evidence that the treatments they offer also reduce health care consumption, return people to improved function (including, when appropriate, to gainful employment), and close disability cases.

Comprehensive programs that adopt the biopsychosocial perspective and that are multidisciplinary may be the best alternative. Practitioners who treat patients with persistent pain are going to have to consider the psychosocial and environmental factors as well as the medical ones. By the time patients come to the attention of pain specialists, they have had long learning histories and unique phenotypes. Moreover, they do not live in isolation but in a psychosocial context with many external influences that have an impact on their reports of pain, their adaptation to their plight, and how they respond to treatment. It is not a body part that needs to be treated, but that body part as part of a whole person with a history, who lives in a societal context. Failure to adopt this broader, biopsychosocial perspective may explain the inadequacies of treatment for those with intractable chronic pain in contrast to inpatients with brief episodes of pain (e.g., postsurgical).

KEY POINTS

- Pain can become a distinct disease entity when it is no longer associated with an ongoing injury or the immediate repercussions of the injury.
- The treatment of pain with medications and procedural or surgical therapies is probably inadequate, at least for patients with persistent pain, and thus the practice of pain medicine needs to be multidisciplinary and must include clinicians such as physical therapists and psychologists as well as representatives from a number of other medical specialties.
- Physicians with appropriate medical training, board certification, and credentialing do practice pain medicine, but as part of a multidisciplinary environment. The use of the descriptor "pain management" lacks precision and opens an inappropriate discussion on who may provide these health care services, and the term should therefore be retired.
- Integrated, rather than fragmented, treatment of pain patients ideally focuses on the multidimensional nature of pain within a biopsychosocial context.
- Favorable changes in the education of trainees and maintenance of accreditation include the adoption of a match program and the addition of simulation.
- Although the norepinephrine reuptake inhibitors and anticonvulsants are advancements over the traditional nonsteroidal anti-inflammatory drugs and opioids by themselves, they are often inadequate for the treatment of patients with persistent pain and need to be used in combination with other pharmacological and nonpharmacological interventions.
- There are gaps in the knowledge of pain medicine physicians regarding the safe and effective treatment of patients with persistent pain.
- The Food and Drug Administration Safe Use Initiative and a Working Group of Experts, together with some of the national pain organizations, will have recommendations on improving the safety of transforaminal epidural steroid injections.
- There will be improved regulations on the safety of compounding depot steroid and other drugs for pain management.

KEY POINTS—cont'd

- A combination of psychological and other (pharmacological, rehabilitation) interventions is a clinically effective and cost-effective treatment approach for patients who do not achieve adequate improvement from any monotherapy.
- Strategies to maintain therapeutic improvements are necessary and may include rapidly evolving technologies such as Web-based tools, smartphone applications, and e-mail communication.

SUGGESTED READINGS

Attal N, Cruccu G, Haanpaa M, et al. EFNS guidelines on pharmacological treatment of neuropathic pain: 2010 revision. *Eur J Neurol.* 2010;17:1113-1123.

Benzon HT, Chew TL, McCarthy R, et al. Comparison of the particle sizes of the different steroids and the effect of dilution: a review of the relative neurotoxicities of the steroids. *Anesthesiology.* 2007;106:331-338.

Dworkin RH, O'Connor AB, Aydette J, et al. Recommendations for the pharmacological management of neuropathic pain: an overview and literature update. *Mayo Clin Proc.* 2010;85:S3-S14.

Guzman J, Esmail R, Karjalainen K, et al. Multidisciplinary rehabilitation for chronic low back pain: systematic review. *BMJ.* 2001;322:1511-1516.

Hocking G, Cousins MJ. Ketamine in chronic pain management: an evidence-based review. *Anesth Analg.* 2003;97:1730-1739.

Hoffman BM, Papas RK, Chatkoff DK, Kerns RD. Meta-analysis of psychological interventions for chronic low back pain. *Health Psychol.* 2007;26:1-9.

Huntoon MA. Anatomy of the cervical intervertebral foramina: vulnerable arteries and ischemic neurologic injuries after transforaminal epidural injections. *Pain.* 2005;117:104-111.

Kainer MA, Reagan DR, Nguyen DB, et al. Fungal infections associated with contaminated methylprednisolone in Tennessee. *N Engl J Med.* 2012;367:2194-2203.

Macea DD, Gajos K, Daglia Calil YA, et al. The efficacy of Web-based cognitive behavioral interventions for chronic pain: a systematic review and meta-analysis. *J Pain.* 2010;11:917-929.

Noppers IM, Niesters M, Aarts LP, et al. Drug-induced liver injury following a repeated course of ketamine treatment for chronic pain in CRPS type 1 patients: a report of 3 cases. *Pain.* 2011;152:2173-2178.

Outterson K. Regulating compounding pharmacies after NECC. *N Engl J Med.* 2012;367:1969-1972.

Pinto RZ, Maher CG, Ferreira ML, et al. Drugs for relief of pain in patients with sciatica: systematic review and meta-analysis. *BMJ.* 2012;344:e497.

Pinto RZ, Maher CG, Ferreira ML, et al. Epidural corticosteroid injections in the management of sciatica. *Ann Intern Med.* 2012;157:865-877.

Turk DC. The potential of matching treatments to characteristics of chronic pain patients: lumping vs. splitting. *Clin J Pain.* 2005;21:44-55.

Turk DC, Wilson HD, Cahana A. Treatment of chronic non-cancer pain. *Lancet.* 2011;377:2226-2235.

Vo T, Rice ASC, Dworkin RH. Non-steroidal anti-inflammatory drugs for neuropathic pain: how do we explain continued widespread use? *Pain.* 2009;143:169-171.

The references for this chapter can be found at www.expertconsult.com.

Index

Page numbers followed by f indicate figures; t, tables; b, boxes.

C

D

H

M

O

Q

R

U

V

W

X

Y

Z